FOUNDATIONS FOR OSTEOPATHIC MEDICINE

SECOND EDITION

FOUNDATIONS FOR OSTEOPATHIC MEDICINE

Published under the auspices of the American Osteopathic Association

SECOND EDITION

Executive Editor

ROBERT C. WARD, D.O., F.A.A.O.

Professor
Department of Osteopathic Manipulative Medicine and Family Medicine
College of Osteopathic Medicine
Michigan State University
East Lansing, Michigan

Section Editors

RAYMOND J. HRUBY, D.O., M.S., F.A.A.O.
Professor and Chairman
Department of Osteopathic Manipulative Medicine
College of Osteopathic Medicine of the Pacific
Western University of Health Sciences
Pomona, California

JOHN A. JEROME, Ph.D., B.C.F.E.
Associate Professor of Clinical Medicine
Department of Osteopathic Medicine
Michigan State University
East Lansing, Michigan
Clinical Director
Pain Clinic
Pain Management Specialists, PLLC
Lansing, Michigan

JOHN M. JONES, III, D.O., AOBFP
Professor
Department of Osteopathic Manipulative Medicine
College of Osteopathic Medicine of the Pacific
Western University of Health Sciences
Pomona, California

ROBERT E. KAPPLER, D.O., F.A.A.O.
Professor and Chair
Department of Osteopathic Manipulative Medicine
Chicago College of Osteopathic Medicine
Midwestern University
Downer's Grove, Illinois

MICHAEL L. KUCHERA, D.O., F.A.A.O.
Professor of Osteopathic Manipulative Medicine
Director of Osteopathic Manipulative Medicine Research
Philadelphia College of Osteopathic Medicine
Philadelphia, Pennsylvania

WILLIAM A. KUCHERA, D.O., F.A.A.O.
Professor Emeritus of Osteopathic Manipulative Medicine
Kirksville College of Osteopathic Medicine
Kirksville, Missouri

MICHAEL M. PATTERSON, Ph.D.
Professor and Assistant Chair
Department of Osteopathic Principles and Practice
College of Osteopathic Medicine
Nova Southeastern University
Ft. Lauderdale, Florida

BERNARD R. RUBIN, D.O., M.P.H.
Professor of Medicine
Chief, Division of Rheumatology
Department of Medicine
University of North Texas Health Science Center
Fort Worth, Texas

MICHAEL A. SEFFINGER,
D.O., C.S.P.O.M.M., F.A.A.F.P.
Assistant Professor
Department of Osteopathic Manipulative Medicine
College of Osteopathic Medicine of the Pacific
Western University of Health Sciences
Pomona, California

SARAH A. SPRAFKA, Ph.D.
Director, Predoctoral Education
College of Osteopathic Medicine
University of New England
Biddeford, Maine

RICHARD VAN BUSKIRK, D.O., Ph.D.
Private Practice
Sarasota, Florida

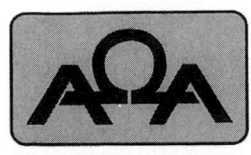

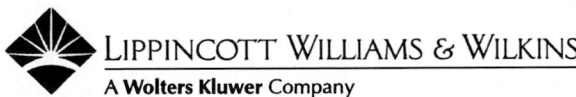
LIPPINCOTT WILLIAMS & WILKINS
A Wolters Kluwer Company
Philadelphia • Baltimore • New York • London
Buenos Aires • Hong Kong • Sydney • Tokyo

Acquisitions Editor: Timothy Y. Hiscock
Developmental Editor: Michelle LaPlante
Production Editor: Robin E. Cook
Manufacturing Manager: Tim Reynolds
Cover Designer: Mark Lerner
Compositor: TechBooks
Printer: Courier Westford

Library of Congress Cataloging-in-Publication Data

Foundations for osteopathic medicine / edited by Robert C. Ward . . . [et al.].— 2nd ed.
        p. ; cm.
    Includes bibliographical references and index.
    ISBN 13: 978-0-7817-3497-4
    ISBN 10: 0-7817-3497-5
    1. Osteopathic medicine.   2. Osteopathic medicine—Philosophy.
I. Ward, Robert C., DO.
    [DNLM: 1. Osteopathic Medicine—methods. WB 940 F771 2002]
    RZ342 .F68   2002
    615.5'33—dc21   2002016285

Care has been taken to confirm the accuracy of the information presented and to describe generally accepted practices. However, the authors, editors, and publisher are not responsible for errors or omissions or for any consequences from application of the information in this book and make no warranty, expressed or implied, with respect to the currency, completeness, or accuracy of the contents of the publication. Application of this information in a particular situation remains the professional responsibility of the practitioner.

The authors, editors, and publisher have exerted every effort to ensure that drug selection and dosage set forth in this text are in accordance with current recommendations and practice at the time of publication. However, in view of ongoing research, changes in government regulations, and the constant flow of information relating to drug therapy and drug reactions, the reader is urged to check the package insert for each drug for any change in indications and dosage and for added warnings and precautions. This is particularly important when the recommended agent is a new or infrequently employed drug.

Some drugs and medical devices presented in this publication have Food and Drug Administration (FDA) clearance for limited use in restricted research settings. It is the responsibility of the health care provider to ascertain the FDA status of each drug or device planned for use in their clinical practice.

10 9 8 7 6

This second edition of **Foundations for Osteopathic Medicine** *is dedicated to three icons of osteopathic medicine. Each, in his own very special way, made remarkable contributions to the growth and evolutions of the osteopathic profession, and all it stands for.*

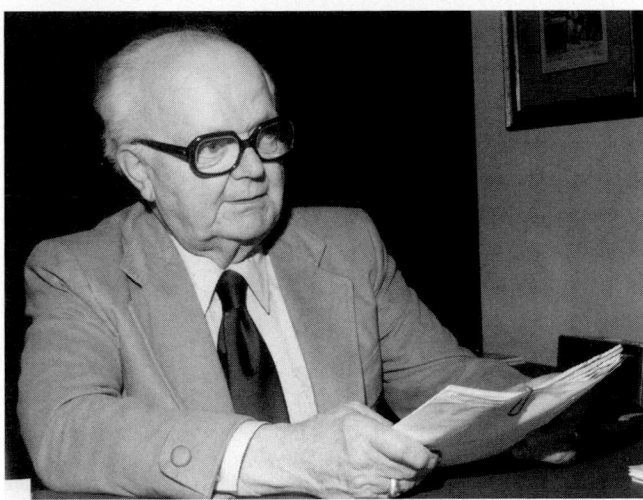

George Northup

George Northup, D.O., F.A.A.O. (1915–1996), was the son of Thomas Northup, D.O., the first secretary treasurer of the American Academy of Osteopathy. Among his many accomplishments, Dr. Northup was the 1958–1959 president of the American Osteopathic Association (AOA). Born in Syracuse, New York, he lived for a short time in Kirksville, Missouri, while his father was a student. In 1939, he graduated from the Philadelphia College of Osteopathic Medicine and established practices in Morristown and Livingston, New Jersey. From the beginning, he dedicated his career to "... [gaining] ... acceptance of the profession by the rest of organized medicine and the public" (1). Particularly skilled at politics, Dr. Northup worked diligently for greater osteopathic recognition as a full-service health profession. Always dedicated to excellence, he was appointed editor-in-chief for AOA publications in 1961, serving 26 years until his retirement in 1987. Among his greatest successes were his many insightful editorials dealing with a wide array of osteopathically oriented and general health policy issues. Among his many publications is his classic book, *Osteopathic Medicine: An American Reformation* (2).

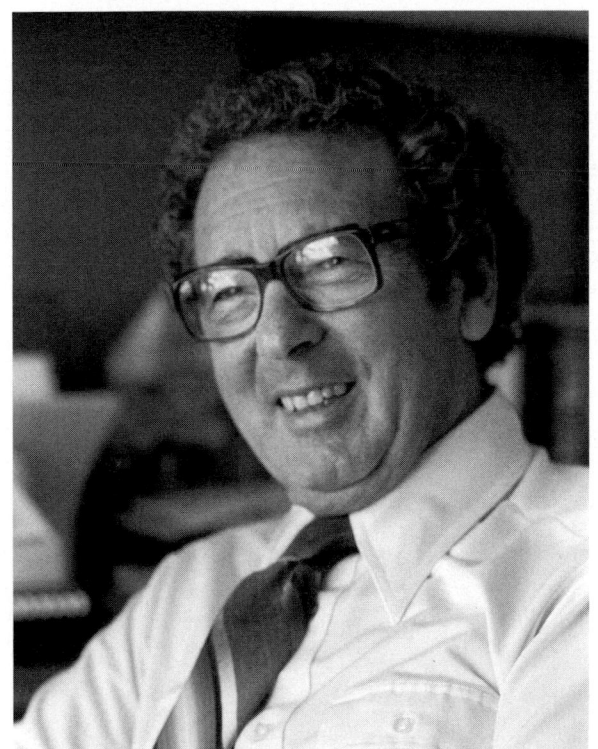

Irving M. Korr

Irvin M. Korr, Ph.D., (1910–), led a distinguished career as both a respected researcher and educator at the Kirksville College of Osteopathic Medicine (KCOM). Beginning his career as a cellular physiologist, he received his PhD from Princeton University in 1935. From 1936 to 1942, he was an instructor in physiology at the New York University School of Medicine in New York City. During World War II he worked for the U.S. War Department researching aspects of aviation medicine, wound ballistics, and climate physiology. After the war, Korr was recruited to Kirksville College of Osteopathic Medicine by J. Stedman Denslow, D.O., himself a distinguished faculty member actively pursuing osteopathically related research. Shortly after arriving at Kirksville, Dr. Korr realized that his real interests lay in exploring the relationship of the autonomic nervous system to somatic dysfunction. Some refer to Korr's tenure at Kirksville as a golden age for osteopathic research. After a 30-year career, he retired from KCOM having written or cowritten many papers that continue to be widely quoted and used in most osteopathic curricula. After leaving Kirksville, he spent a number of years teaching osteopathic philosophy and principles of healthy lifestyles at both Michigan State University College of Osteopathic Medicine, and the University of North Texas College of Osteopathic Medicine.

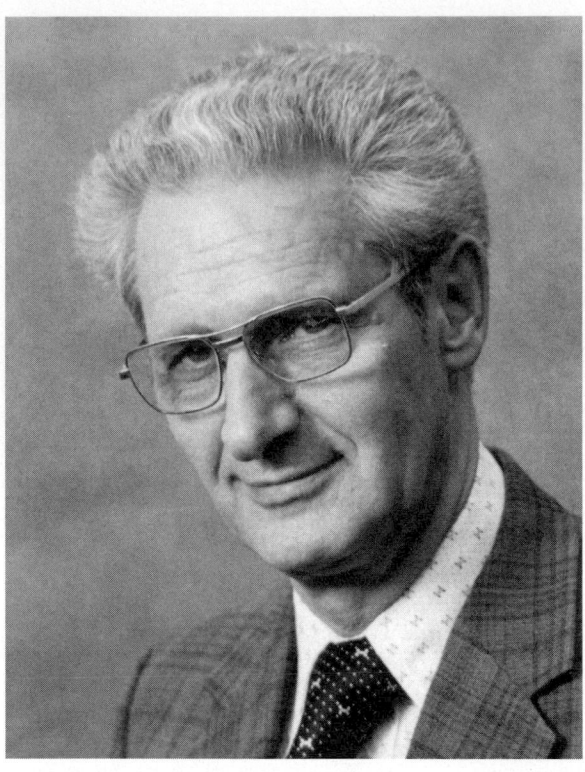

Paul E. Kimberly

Paul F. Kimberly, D.O., F.A.A.O., Professor and Chairman Emeritus, Kirksville College of Osteopathic Medicine (1915–) a quiet and unassuming osteopathic giant, was born into an osteopathic family. He graduated from the Des Moines Still College of Osteopathic Medicine in 1940. Through a mixture of preclinical and postdoctoral teaching, writing, and pragmatically useful approaches to osteopathic patient care, Dr. Kimberly's contributions are legendary for over three generations of osteopathic physicians. He is renowned for his detailed and clinically useful grasp of functional anatomy and credits much of his career to his first mentor, H. Virgil Halliday, D.O., Professor of Anatomy at the Des Moines School. Halladay, himself a consummate functional anatomist, was a student of A.T. Still. Recognizing Kimberly's special combination of anatomical knowledge and communication skills, Halladay hired the rising young star as a teaching assistant. Eventually, the opportunity led Kimberly to directly involve himself in the development of many aspects of contemporary osteopathic skills teaching programs. Among his contributions are the following:

A collaboration with O. Edwin Owen, D.O., that collated and published the first edition of *Chapman's Reflexes*. Publication rights now lie with the American Academy of Osteopathy.

Collaboration with Fred L Mitchell, Sr, of Chattanooga, Tennessee, in the development of the original muscle energy concepts.

Organization and development of the first detailed anatomy courses highlighting W.G. Sutherland's cranial osteopathy concepts. Several decades later, he published a manual on cranial osteopathic methods that is widely in use today.

Development and participation in the first clinical teaching teams sponsored by the American Academy of Osteopathy.

His central role in helping the Educational Council on Osteopathic Principles (ECOP) develop and clarify its long-range agenda, much of which is represented in this text.

His major role in introducing and developing international cooperation among allopathic and American osteopathic physician groups in collaboration with the International Federation of Musculoskeletal and Manual Medicine (FIMM).

His major participation in developing and standardizing postdoctoral continuing education programs at the Michigan State University College of Osteopathic Medicine, which were begun at the request of the North American Academy of Musculoskeletal and Manual Medicine (NAMM) and FIMM.

(1) Fitzgerald M. Hail to our ex-chief, *The DO,* 1997:32
(2) Northup G. *Osteopathic Medicine: An American Reformation,* Chicago: American Osteopathic Association, 1966.

CONTENTS

Contributing Authors xi
Mission Statement xv
Preface xvii
Preface to the First Edition xix
Foreword xxi
Acknowledgments xxiii

SECTION I: OSTEOPATHIC PHILOSOPHY AND HISTORY 1

1. Osteopathic Philosophy 3
Michael A. Seffinger, Hollis H. King, Robert C. Ward, John M. Jones, III, Felix J. Rogers, and Michael M. Patterson

2. Major Events in Osteopathic History 19
Barbara E. Peterson

SECTION II: OSTEOPATHIC CONSIDERATIONS IN THE BASIC SCIENCES 31

Introduction 32
Michael M. Patterson

3. Rules of Anatomy 37
Lex C. Towns

4. Anatomy 44
Allen W. Jacobs and William M. Falls

5. Biomechanics: An Osteopathic Perspective 63
Michael R. Wells

6. Autonomic Nervous System 90
Frank H. Willard

7. Neurophysiologic Mechanisms of Integration and Disintegration 120
Michael M. Patterson and Robert D. Wurster

8. Nociception, the Neuroendocrine Immune System, and Osteopathic Medicine 137
Frank H. Willard

9. Tissue Respiration and Circulation 157
Harvey V. Sparks, Jr.

10. Microbiologic Considerations and Infectious Diseases 165
Lauritz A. Jensen and James B. Jensen

11. Endocrine System and Body Unity: Osteopathic Principles at a Chemical Level 179
Ronald Portanova

12. Pharmacologic and Osteopathic Basic Principles 189
Robert J. Theobald, Jr.

SECTION III: OSTEOPATHIC CONSIDERATIONS IN THE BEHAVIORAL SCIENCES 195

Introduction 196
John A. Jerome

13. Health Promotion and Maintenance 197
Gerald G. Osborn

14. Introduction to Psychoneuroimmunology 208
David A. Baron

15. Pain Management 212
John A. Jerome

16. Life Phases and Health 227
Jed Magen

17. Stress Management in Primary Care 233
John A. Jerome

18. Osteopathic Psychiatry 245
Ronald H. Bradley, Gerald G. Osborn, John A. Jerome, and Mary C. Williams

SECTION IV: OSTEOPATHIC CONSIDERATIONS IN CLINICAL PROBLEM SOLVING 255

19. Clinical Problem Solving 257
Sarah A. Sprafka

SECTION V: OSTEOPATHIC CONSIDERATIONS IN FAMILY PRACTICE AND PRIMARY CARE 281

Introduction 282
Richard L. Van Buskirk and Robert E. Kappler

20. Osteopathic Family Practice: An Application of the Primary Care Model 289
Richard L. Van Buskirk and Kenneth E. Nelson

21. General Internal Medicine 298
Donald R. Noll, John M. Willis, and Terri Turner

22. General Pediatrics 305
Shawn Centers, Mary Anne Morelli, Colleen Vallad-Hix, and Michael A. Seffinger

23. Geriatrics 327
Thomas A. Cavalieri

SECTION VI: OSTEOPATHIC CONSIDERATIONS IN THE CLINICAL SPECIALTIES 339

Introduction 340
Michael A. Seffinger

24. An Osteopathic Perspective on Cardiology 345
Felix J. Rogers

25. Osteopathic Management of Ear, Nose, and Throat Disease 370
Harriet H. Shaw and Michael B. Shaw

26. Osteopathic Medicine in the Practice of Emergency Medicine 383
Peter Adler-Michaelson, Bernadette Brandon, and Raul Garcia

27. General Surgery 399
Constance Cashen and Sydney P. Ross

28. Gynecology 409
Melicien Tettambel

29. Neuromusculoskeletal Medicine and Osteopathic Manipulative Medicine 420
Raymond J. Hruby

30. Neurology 435
Mitchell L. Elkiss and Louis E. Rentz

31. Obstetrics 450
Melicien Tettambel

32. Oncology 462
Michael I. Opipari, Augustine L. Perrotta, and David R. Essig-Beatty

33. Orthopedics 477
Richard A. Scott, Michael L. Kuchera, and Jeff J. Patterson

34. Pulmonology 500
Gilbert E. D'Alonzo, Jr. and Samuel L. Krachman

35. Osteopathic Physical Medicine and Rehabilitation 516
J. Michael Wieting and James A. Lipton

36. Rheumatology 526
J. Michael Finley

37. An Osteopathic Approach to Sports Medicine 534
P. Gunnar Brolinson, Kurt Heinking, and Albert J. Kozar

SECTION VII: OSTEOPATHIC CONSIDERATIONS IN PALPATORY DIAGNOSIS AND MANIPULATIVE TREATMENT 551

Introduction 552
John M. Jones, III and Robert E. Kappler

Part A: Overview: Evaluation and Management 557

38. Palpatory Skills and Exercises for Developing the Sense of Touch 557
Robert E. Kappler

39. Examination and Diagnosis: An Introduction 566
Michael L. Kuchera

40. Diagnosis and Plan for Manual Treatment: A Prescription 574
Robert E. Kappler and William A. Kuchera

41. Considerations of Posture and Group Curves 580
Michael L. Kuchera and Robert E. Kappler

42. Radiographic Aspects of the Postural Study 591
Michael L. Kuchera and William A. Kuchera

43. Postural Considerations in Coronal, Horizontal, and Sagittal Planes 603
Michael L. Kuchera

44. Musculoskeletal Examination for Somatic Dysfunction 633
William A. Kuchera and Robert E. Kappler

Part B: Regional Examination and Treatment 660

45. Head: Diagnosis and Treatment 660
Robert E. Kappler and Kenneth A. Ramey

46. Cervical Spine 684
Robert E. Kappler

47. Upper Extremities 690
Robert E. Kappler and Kenneth A. Ramey

48. Thoracic Region 705
Raymond J. Hruby

49. The Rib Cage 718
Raymond J. Hruby

50. Lumbar Region 727
William A. Kuchera

51. The Abdominal Region 751
Raymond J. Hruby

52. Pelvis and Sacrum 762
Kurt P. Heinking and Robert E. Kappler

53. Lower Extremities 784
Michael L. Kuchera

Part C: Palpatory Diagnosis and Manipulative
Treatment 819

54. Soft Tissue Techniques 819
Walter C. Ehrenfeuchter, David Heilig, and
Alexander S. Nicholas

55. Articulatory Techniques 834
David A. Patriquin and John M. Jones, III

56. Thrust (High-Velocity/Low-Amplitude)
Techniques 852
Robert E. Kappler and John M. Jones, III

57. Muscle Energy Techniques 881
Walter C. Ehrenfeuchter and Mark Sandhouse

58. Fascial-Ligamentous Release: Indirect
Approach 908
Anthony G. Chila

59. Balanced Ligamentous Tension Techniques 916
Jane E. Carreiro

60. Integrated Neuromusculoskeletal Release and
Myofascial Release 931
Robert C. Ward

61. Functional Technique: An Indirect Method 969
William L. Johnston

62. Osteopathy in the Cranial Field 985
Hollis H. King and Edna M. Lay

63. Strain and Counterstrain Techniques 1002
John C. Glover and Paul R. Rennie

64. Facilitated Positional Release 1017
Stanley Schiowitz, Eileen L. DiGiovanna, and
Dennis J. Dowling

65. Progressive Inhibition of Neuromuscular
Structures Technique 1026
Dennis J. Dowling

66. Myofascial Trigger Points as Somatic
Dysfunction 1034
Michael L. Kuchera and John M. McPartland

67. Chapman Reflexes 1051
David A. Patriquin

68. Lymphatic System: Lymphatic Manipulative
Techniques 1056
Elaine Wallace, John M. McPartland, John M. Jones,
III, William A. Kuchera, and Boyd R. Buser

69. Visceral Manipulation 1078
Kenneth Lossing

70. Treatment of Somatic Dysfunction with an
Osteopathic Manipulative Method of
Dr. Andrew Taylor Still 1094
Richard L. Van Buskirk

71. Treatment of the Acutely Ill Hospitalized
Patient 1115
Hugh Ettlinger

72. Efficacy and Complications 1143
Michael L. Kuchera, Eileen L. DiGiovanna, and
Philip E. Greenman

73. Somatic Dysfunction 1153
H. James Jones

SECTION VIII: BASIC AND CLINICAL RESEARCH FOR OSTEOPATHIC THEORY AND PRACTICE 1163

Introduction 1164
Albert F. Kelso and Bernard R. Rubin

74. Foundations for Osteopathic Medical
Research 1167
Michael M. Patterson

75. The Research Status of Somatic
Dysfunction 1188
Deborah M. Heath and Norman Gevitz

76. Outcomes Research and Design 1194
Richard J. Snow, John C. Licciardone
and Russell G. Gamber

77. Biobehavioral Interactions with Disease
and Health 1203
Brian H. Foresman, Gilbert E. D'Alonzo, Jr.,
and John A. Jerome

78. Clinical Research and Clinical Trials 1215
Bernard R. Rubin

79. Osteopathic Research: Challenges of the
Future 1219
Michael M. Patterson

Glossary of Osteopathic Terminology 1229
Appendix I 1255
Appendix II 1258
Subject Index 1263

CONTRIBUTORS

Peter Adler-Michaelson, D.O., Ph.D. Assistant Professor of Osteopathic Medicine, Philadelphia College of Osteopathic Medicine, Philadelphia, Pennsylvania

David A. Baron, M.S.Ed., D.O. Professor and Chair, Department of Psychiatry, Temple University School of Medicine, Philadelphia, Pennsylvania

Ronald H. Bradley, D.O., Ph.D. Clinical Professor of Internal Medicine, Michigan State University, East Lansing, Michigan, and Vice Chairman, Department of Psychiatry, Ingham Regional Medical Center, Lansing, Michigan

Bernadette Brandon, D.O. Emergency Medicine Residency Director, St. Barnabas Hospital, Bronx, New York

P. Gunnar Brolinson, D.O. Private Practice, Toledo, Ohio

Boyd R. Buser, D.O. Associate Dean, Clinical Affairs, University of New England, Biddeford, Maine

Jane E. Carreiro, D.O. Associate Professor and Chair, Department of Osteopathic Manipulative Medicine, University of New England College of Osteopathic Medicine, Biddeford, Maine

Constance Cashen, D.O., F.A.C.O.S. Clinical Associate Professor of General Surgery, St. Vincent Mercy Medical Center, Toledo Surgical Associates, Toledo, Ohio

Thomas A. Cavalieri, D.O. Professor of Clinical Medicine, Chairman, Department of Medicine, School of Osteopathic Medicine, University of Medicine and Dentistry, Stratford, New Jersey

Shawn Centers, D.O. Clinical Attending and Assistant Professor of Pediatrics, Department of Osteopathic Manipulative Medicine, Osteopathic Center for Children of Western University of Health Sciences, San Diego, California

Anthony G. Chila, D.O. Professor of Family Medicine, Ohio University College of Osteopathic Medicine, Athens, Ohio

Gilbert E. D'Alonzo, Jr., D.O., F.A.C.O.I. Professor of Medicine, Division of Pulmonary and Critical Care, Temple University School of Medicine, Deputy Chief Division of Pulmonary and Critical Care, Temple University Hospital, Philadelphia, Pennsylvania

Eileen L. DiGiovanna, D.O. Professor of Osteopathic Manipulative Medicine, New York College of Osteopathic Medicine, Old Westbury, New York, and Attending Physician, Department of Family Practice, Good Samaritan Hospital, West Islip, New York

Dennis J. Dowling, D.O. Professor and Chairman Department of Osteopathic Manipulative Medicine, New York College of Osteopathic Medicine, Old Westbury, New York, and Director of Manipulation, Attending Physician, Department of Physical Medicine and Rehabilitation, Nassau University Medical Center, East Meadow, New York

Walter C. Ehrenfeuchter, D.O., F.A.A.O. Clinical Professor of Osteopathic Manipulative Medicine, Philadelphia College of Osteopathic Manipulative Medicine, Bala Cynwyd, Pennsylvania

Mitchell L. Elkiss, D.O. Assistant Clinical Professor of Internal Medicine, Michigan State University, East Lansing, Michigan, and Associates in Neurology, P.C., Farmington Hills, Michigan

David R. Essig-Beatty, D.O. Associate Professor of Osteopathic Principles and Practice, West Virginia School of Osteopathic Medicine, Lewisburg, West Virginia

Hugh Ettlinger, D.O. Associate Professor of Osteopathic Manipulative Medicine, New York College of Osteopathic Medicine, Old Westbury, New York, and St. Barnabas Hospital, Bronx, New York

William M. Falls, Ph.D. Associate Dean of Student Services, College of Osteopathic Medicine, Professor, Department of Radiology, Division of Anatomy and Structural Biology, East Lansing, Michigan

J. Michael Finley, D.O. Department of Internal Medicine, Western University College of Osteopathic Medicine, Pomona, California

Brian H. Foresman, D.O., M.S. Associate Professor of Clinical Medicine, Indiana University School of Medicine, Indianapolis, Indiana

Russell G. Gamber, D.O. Department of Osteopathic Manipulative Medicine, University of North Texas Health Science Center, Fort Worth, Texas

Raul Garcia, D.O.   Senior Emergency Medicine Resident, New York College of Osteopathic Medicine, St. Barnabas Hospital, Bronx, New York

Norman Gevitz, Ph.D.   Professor and Chair, Department of Social Medicine, Ohio University College of Osteopathic Medicine, Athens, Ohio

John C. Glover, D.O.   Physicians Health Care Center, Oklahoma State University College of Osteopathic Medicine, Tulsa, Oklahoma

Philip E. Greenman, D.O.   Professor Emeritus of Osteopathic Manipulative Medicine, College of Osteopathic Medicine, Michigan State University, East Lansing, Michigan

Deborah M. Heath, D.O., M.D.(H)   Private Practice, Arizona Center for Health and Medicine, Scottsdale, Arizona

David Heilig, D.O. (Deceased)   Emeritus Professor, Department of Osteopathic Manipulative Medicine, Philadelphia College of Osteopathic Medicine, Philadelphia, Pennsylvania

Kurt Heinking, D.O.   Assistant Chair, Department of Osteopathic Manipulative Medicine, Chicago College of Osteopathic Medicine, Midwestern University, Downer's Grove, Illinois, and Staff Member, Department of Family Medicine, Hinsdale Hospital, Hinsdale, Illinois

Raymond J. Hruby, D.O., M.S., F.A.A.O.   Professor and Chair, Department of Osteopathic Manipulative Medicine, Western University of Health Sciences, College of Osteopathic Medicine of the Pacific, Pomona, California

Allen W. Jacobs, D.O., Ph.D. (Deceased)   Dean, College of Osteopathic Medicine, Professor and Team Physician, Department of Osteopathic Manipulative Medicine, Michigan State University, East Lansing, Michigan

Lauritz A. Jensen, D.A.   Director of Pre-Clinical Education, Nova Southeastern University College of Osteopathic Medicine, Ft. Lauderdale, Florida

James B. Jensen, D.O.   Microbiology Department, Brigham Young University, Provo, Utah

John A. Jerome, Ph.D.   Associate Professor of Clinical Medicine, Michigan State University College of Osteopathic Medicine, East Lansing, Michigan, and Clinical Director, Pain Clinic, Pain Management Specialists, PLLC, Lansing, Michigan

William L. Johnston, D.O., F.A.A.O.   Professor Emeritus, Department of Family and Community Medicine, Michigan State University, College of Osteopathic Medicine, East Lansing, Michigan

John M. Jones, III, D.O.   Professor, Department of Osteopathic Manipulative Medicine, College of Osteopathic Medicine of the Pacific, Western University of Health Sciences, Pomona, California

H. James Jones, D.O.   Assistant Professor of Neurology/Osteopathic Manipulative Medicine, Western University of Health Sciences, College of Osteopathic Medicine of the Pacific, Pomona, California

Robert E. Kappler, D.O., F.A.A.O.   Professor and Chair, Department of Osteopathic Manipulative Medicine, Chicago College of Osteopathic Medicine, Midwestern University, Downer's Grove, Illinois

Albert F. Kelso, Ph.D., D.Sci. (Hon.)   Professor Emeritus, Center for Osteopathic Education and Research, University Health Sciences, Chicago College of Osteopathy, Chicago, Illinois

Hollis H. King, D.O., Ph.D.   Associate Professor of Osteopathic Manipulative Medicine, College of Osteopathic Medicine, Pacific Western University of the Health Sciences, San Diego, California

Albert J. Kozar, D.O.   Sports Care, Toledo, Ohio

Samuel L. Krachman, D.O.   Director, Sleep Disorders Center, Tuberculosis Program, Department of Pulmonary Medicine, Temple University, Philadelphia, Pennsylvania

Michael L. Kuchera, D.O.   Professor of Osteopathic Manipulative Medicine, Director of Osteopathic Manipulative Medicine Research, Philadelphia College of Osteopathic Medicine, Philadelphia, Pennsylvania

William A. Kuchera, D.O., F.A.A.O.   Professor Emeritus, Department of Osteopathic Manipulative Medicine, Kirksville College of Osteopathic Medicine, Kirksville, Missouri

Edna M. Lay, D.O.   Private Practice, Bozeman, Montana

John C. Licciardone, D.O., M.S., M.B.A.   Professor of Family Medicine, Director of Grants and Funding, Department of Family Medicine, Texas College of Osteopathic Medicine, University of North Texas Health Science Center, Fort Worth, Texas

James A. Lipton, D.O., F.A.A.O., F.A.A.P.M.R.   Adjunct Clinical Professor, Osteopathic Manipulative Medicine, New York College of Osteopathic Medicine, Adjunct Clinical Associate Professor, Family Medicine, Midwestern University, Downer's Grove, Illinois

Kenneth Lossing, D.O.   Private Practice, San Rafael, California

Jed Magen, D.O.   Director, Residency Education, Department of Psychiatry, Michigan State University College of Osteopathic Medicine, East Lansing, Michigan

John M. McPartland, M.S. (Hons), D.O. Faculty of Health and Environmental Sciences, UNITEC, Auckland, New Zealand

Mary Anne Morelli, D.O. Private Practice, Osteopathic Center for Children, San Diego, California

Kenneth E. Nelson, D.O., F.A.A.O., F.A.C.O.F.P. Associate Professor, Osteopathic Manipulative Medicine, Department of Osteopathic Manipulative Medicine, Chicago College of Osteopathic Medicine, Midwestern University, Downer's Grove, Illinois

Alexander S. Nicholas, D.O. Pennsylvania College of Osteopathic Medicine, Philadelphia, Pennsylvania

Donald R. Noll, D.O. Associate Professor, Kirksville College of Osteopathic Medicine, Kirksville, Missouri

Michael I. Opipari, D.O. BiCounty Community Hospital, Warren, Michigan

Gerald G. Osborn, D.O. Kirksville College of Osteopathic Medicine, Kirksville, Missouri

David A. Patriquin, D.O. Professor Emeritus, Department of Family Medicine, Ohio University College of Osteopathic Medicine, Athens, Ohio

Michael M. Patterson, Ph.D. Professor and Assistant Chair, Department of Osteopathic Principles and Practice, College of Osteopathic Medicine, Nova Southeastern University, Ft. Lauderdale, Florida

Jeff J. Patterson, D.O. Professor of Family Medicine, Department of Family Medicine, University of Wisconsin, Northeast Family Medical Center, Madison, Wisconsin

Augustine L. Perrotta, D.O. Clinical Professor of Medicine, Michigan State University College of Osteopathic Medicine, East Lansing, Michigan, and Chairman, Department of Medicine, Chief, Section of Hematology/Oncology, BiCounty Community Hospital, Warren, Michigan

Barbara E. Peterson, D.Litt. Evanston, Illinois

Ronald P. Portanova, Ph.D. Chair, Department of Biomedical Sciences, Ohio University College of Osteopathic Medicine, Athens, Ohio

Kenneth A. Ramey, D.O. Oviedo, Florida

Paul R. Rennie, D.O. Clinical Assistant Professor, Department of Osteopathic Manipulative Medicine, Michigan State University College of Osteopathic Medicine, and President, RennieMatrix, Inc., Williamston, Michigan

Louis E. Rentz, D.O. Michigan Institute for Neurological Disorders, Farmington Hills, Michigan

Felix J. Rogers, D.O. Downriver Cardiology Consultants, Trenton, Michigan

Sydney P. Ross, D.O. Kirksville College of Osteopathic Medicine, Kirksville, Missouri

Bernard R. Rubin, D.O. Professor of Medicine, Chief, Division of Rheumatology, University of North Texas Health Science Center, Fort Worth, Texas

Mark Sandhouse, D.O. Assistant Professor, Department of Osteopathic Principle and Practice, Nova Southeastern University College of Osteopathic Medicine, Fort Lauderdale, Florida

Stanley Schiowitz, D.O. New York College of Osteopathic Medicine, Old Westbury, New York

Richard A. Scott, D.O. Associate Clinical Professor, Department of Osteopathic Medicine and Orthopedic Surgery, Michigan State University College of Osteopathic Medicine, East Lansing, Michigan, and Department of Orthopedic Surgery, BiCounty Community Hospital, Warren, Michigan

Michael A. Seffinger, D.O. Assistant Professor, Department of Osteopathic Manipulative Medicine, College of Osteopathic Medicine of the Pacific, Western University of Health Sciences, Pomona, California

Harriet H. Shaw, D.O. Clinical Professor Department of Family Medicine, College of Osteopathic Medicine, Oklahoma State University Center for Health Sciences, Tulsa, Oklahoma

Michael B. Shaw, D.O. Clinical Professor of Family Medicine, College of Osteopathic Medicine, Oklahoma State University Center for Health Sciences, Tulsa, Oklahoma

Richard J. Snow, D.O., M.P.H. Doctor's Hospital Family Practice, Grove City, Ohio

Harvey V. Sparks, Jr., M.D., Ph.D. Department of Physiology, Michigan State University, East Lansing, Michigan

Sarah A. Sprafka, Ph.D. Director of Predoctoral Education, College of Osteopathic Medicine, University of New England, Biddeford, Maine

Melicien Tettambel, D.O. Chair, Division of Female and Child Health and Professor of Osteopathic Manipulative Medicine, Department of Obstetrics and Gynecology, Kirksville College of Osteopathic Medicine, Kirksville, Missouri

Robert J. Theobald, Jr., Ph.D. Professor and Chairman, Department of Pharmacology, Kirksville College of Osteopathic Medicine, Kirksville, Missouri

Lex C. Towns, Ph.D. Professor and Chair, Department of Anatomy, Kirksville College of Osteopathic Medicine, Kirksville, Missouri

Terri Turner, D.O. Sebastopol, California

Colleen Vallad-Hix, D.O. Apnea Clinic, Michigan State University, Lansing, Michigan

Richard L. Van Buskirk, D.O., Ph.D. Sarasota, Florida

Elaine M. Wallace, D.O. Professor and Chair, Department of Osteopathic Practices and Principles, Nova Southeastern University Health Conference Division, College of Osteopathic Medicine, Ft. Lauderdale, Florida

Robert C. Ward, D.O. Professor, Department of Osteopathic Manipulative Medicine, Michigan State University, East Lansing, Michigan

Michael R. Wells, Ph.D. Associate Professor and Chairman, Department of Biomechanics and Bioengineering, New York College of Osteopathic Medicine, New York Institute of Technology, Old Westbury, New York

J. Michael Wieting, M.A., D.O. Associate Professor, Department of Physical Medicine and Rehabilitation, Michigan State University College of Osteopathic Medicine, East Lansing, Michigan

Frank H. Willard, Ph.D. College of Osteopathic Medicine, University of New England, Biddeford, Maine

Mary C. Williams, D.O. Roanoke, Virginia

John M. Willis, D.O. Assistant Professor, Internal Medicine, Chief, Division of General Internal Medicine, University of North Texas Health Science Center, Texas College of Osteopathic Medicine, Ft. Worth, Texas

Robert D. Wurster, D.O. Professor, Department of Physiology, Loyola University Medical Center, Maywood, Illinois

MISSION STATEMENT

Welcome
Medicine
tion is c
preface
perspecti

Seve
areas, bu
shortene
overlappi
family m
now in o
restructu
and their
Only two
Chapter
add a ne
current n
importan

Alon
lowing ar
Chap
Chap
tious Dis
Chap
Chap
Chap
gency Me
Chap
pathic Ma
Chap
itation
Chap
Chap
Structures
Chap
Chap
Osteopath
Still
Chap
Chap
Chap
Chap
Health
Chap
Here

Part VII. Osteopathic Considerations in Palpatory Diagnosis and Manipulative Treatment

As with the first edition, this comprises almost half the book. The associate editors and previous authors have done masterful work expanding, clarifying, and illustrating their material. We hope you agree. Five new chapters strengthen the material even more:

Chapter 65: Progressive Inhibition of Neuromuscular Structures (PINS)

Chapter 69: Visceral Manipulation

Chapter 70: Treatment of Somatic Dysfunction with an Osteopathic Manipulative Method of Dr. Andrew Taylor Still

Chapter 71: Treatment of the Acutely Ill Hospital Patient

Chapter 73: Somatic Dysfunction

Part VIII. Basic and Clinical Research for Osteopathic Theory and Practice

Under new leadership, this important section has been changed considerably to reflect the important and evolving roles of both basic and clinical research methodologies as they relate to the osteopathic philosophy and its principles.

Glossary of Osteopathic Terminology

The Glossary, first published in 1981, is an ongoing project under continuing revision by the Educational Council on Osteopathic Principles. This edition is the most current.

PREFACE TO THE FIRST EDITION

Osteopathic medical students and physicians alike have expressed the need for a major text dealing with the broad aspects of osteopathic medicine. For this and many other reasons, the American Osteopathic Association concluded that a wide variety of venues would benefit from a straightforward and practical explanation of osteopathic philosophy and its principles as practiced in a modern context. *Foundations for Osteopathic Medicine* reflects the current understanding and knowledge of osteopathic philosophy and principles as reflected by more than 70 osteopathically oriented authors and even greater number of peer reviewers from a variety of basic science, behavioral, and clinical disciplines.

This text provides an up-to-date multidisciplinary overview of osteopathic philosophy and principles with examples of clinical perspectives gleaned from a variety of disciplines. The book has been organized in ten sections, many of which are introduced with an editorial overview from the section editor. A brief overview of the ten sections follows.

I. Osteopathic Philosophy

This consensus statement comes from the Editors of Foundations for Osteopathic Medicine after an extensive peer-review process. The reader will note that many other philosophy references are scattered throughout the text, including the Mission Statement.

II. History

No text of this sort gives proper perspective to its essential ideas and practices without discussing its ancestry and evolution. In the United States, accelerating reorganization of health care services of all types emphasizes the importance of this profession's historical memory. Sometimes forgotten are the many individual and collective struggles for full medical licensure in all 50 states; general ostracism, then acceptance into military and public sector positions; moves from within sectors of the profession to restrict osteopathic physician licensure for their own short-term gain; and, most recently, the substantial growth of osteopathic education and training programs in universities, colleges, and schools, while at the same time there is a merging/closure and downsizing of hospitals in response to economic pressures.

III. Basic Sciences

From its earliest beginnings, osteopathic medicine emphasized the scientific basis for applications of its fundamental ideas. In the 19th century, there was little to go on other than clinical instincts and intuition. On the other hand, formal scientific investigation was exploding in many areas. Now, a century later, research and evidence-based clinical practices are becoming rules rather than exceptions. With this in mind, the section editors recognized the need for presentation of current osteopathic perspectives among the basic science disciplines. To this end, authors from a variety of basic science disciplines have skillfully crafted creative, pertinent, and current perspectives representing their fields of inquiry. A number of clinically applicable discussions relating the particular disciplines to neuromusculoskeletal structure and function perspectives are of particular interest.

IV. Behavioral Sciences

This offering is a first effort from within osteopathic medicine to highlight some of the important and complex behavioral, psychosocial, and cultural issues in a context that uses osteopathic philosophy and its principles as a frame of reference. Patients and physicians alike behave and are affected by their genetic endowments, cultural values, belief systems, gender, age, family background, education, and working environments. Health, impairment, and disease/illness outcomes are often determined by individual, family, and social group responses and choices deriving from these background elements. Authors highlight some of these important issues, such as life stages, stress, and depression.

V. Clinical Problem Solving

Like the Behavioral Science Section, this too is an osteopathic textbook first. Written by one of the pioneers in the field, the offering lays out both general and specific problem-solving strategies that enhance comprehensive clinical evaluations in a context that highlights osteopathic philosophy and principles. Emphasis is placed on integrative thinking processes in the clinical setting.

VI. Family Practice and Primary Care

Family practice and primary care form the backbone of osteopathic medicine. When these chapters were written, approximately 60% of graduates nationwide were entering the fields of family practice, general pediatrics, and general internal medicine. If general obstetrics and gynecology is added, the figures are higher. The authors have given general overviews of their disciplines, with an emphasis on osteopathic philosophy and principles.

VII. Clinical Specialties

In our complex, high technology, medically oriented society, applications of osteopathic medicine principles may, at times, be difficult to articulate. One outcome has been the inaccurate notion that osteopathic philosophy and its principles reflect alternative or complementary medicine rather than mainstream practices. Among many complex reasons for this view is the reality that some specialties and subspecialties seem less holistic than others, often inappropriately so.

VIII. Palpatory Diagnosis and Manipulative Treatment

Approximately half of this text presents a perspective on aspects of osteopathic palpatory diagnosis and manipulative treatment processes. Survey chapters cover the major curriculum content areas taught in American colleges of osteopathic medicine. Contributions have been peer reviewed by members of the Educational Council on Osteopathic Principles, an osteopathic manipulative skills teaching arm of the American Association of Colleges of Osteopathic Medicine.

IX. Health Restoration

Osteopathic palpatory diagnosis, manipulative treatment, and rehabilitative procedures are essential components of an osteopathic medical treatment program. These survey chapters address some of the pertinent issues.

X. Applications of Basic and Clinical Research for Osteopathic Theory and Practice

This section discusses appropriate research methods and opportunities confronting osteopathic medical practice. Particular emphasis is placed on appropriate research planning, data acquisition and documentation, basic science perspectives, clinical trials, epidemiologic considerations, and outcomes research in relation to somatic dysfunction.

In addition, the Glossary of Osteopathic Terminology, prepared by the Educational Council on Osteopathic Principles of the American Association of Colleges of Osteopathic Medicine, endorsed by the American Osteopathic Association, is included. The text concludes with a comprehensive Index.

The time for this text has been long in coming. One idea for such a textbook was informally discussed during the 1970s as part of a longitudinal osteopathic principles curriculum effort by the Educational Council on Osteopathic Principles. Other such forums had discussed additional alternatives over the years. However, the concept and plan for this text was developed within the Bureau of Research of the AOA. The Bureau officially termed the development activity the "Osteopathic Principles Textbook Project." Our goal has been to introduce both future and present osteopathic physicians to the rationale behind applications of osteopathic principles and the appropriate use of palpatory diagnosis and manipulative treatment in a wide range of disciplines. After years of soul-searching and peer review, our efforts are in your hands. We have given our best. We hope you agree.

FOREWORD

"The theory of a free press is that truth will emerge from discussion, not that it will be presented perfectly and instantly in any one account."
—Walter Lippmann[1]

As Editor-in-Chief of the American Osteopathic Association, it is my pleasure to present the second edition of *Foundations for Osteopathic Medicine*. In the spirit of Walter Lippmann, this text reflects many illustrations of ongoing and evolving discussions within the osteopathic profession. For those seeking greater insight and perspective, this authoritative text explores the osteopathic philosophy and its evolving relationships with the behavioral, basic and clinical sciences. It is our hope that readers will find it a useful addition for classrooms, offices, hospitals, and osteopathic principles' learning laboratories.

As in the first edition, 79 chapters and the Glossary of Osteopathic Terminology blend osteopathic principles and practices with contemporary multidisciplinary health care. Over half of the book is dedicated to palpatory diagnosis and osteopathic manipulative treatment. In addition, many aspects of osteopathically oriented problem solving as it applies to primary care and specialty practices are also highlighted. Through extensive cross-referencing, osteopathic considerations are repeatedly emphasized in order to give the reader better insights.

Robert C. Ward, D.O., his 11 associate editors, almost 100 authors, and numerous peer reviewers have worked extremely hard producing a more valuable, meaningful, and relevant textbook for our profession. Seventy-seven have been extensively revised, and several others added.

In the foreword to the first edition, Howard Levine, D.O. asked readers to use the textbook to "think osteopathically." Through the vision and commitments of both Dr. Levine and Dr. Ward, this textbook has come to life. With further editions, it is expected that additional changes will occur.

This text is significant not for only students, but also for osteopathic physicians already in practice. More than five years ago, having already been in practice for many years, I read portions of the first edition that focused on the etiology and clinical applications relating to somatic dysfunction. In these materials, I found plausible scientific information that helped me better understand this particular concept in greater depth. The result was that it allowed me to apply osteopathic principles and practices to pulmonary and critical care medicine in ways I had never envisioned before. Visceral disease and its effect on the musculoskeletal system took on new meaning. The relationship between somatic dysfunction and visceral physiology and its pathophysiology had always been appreciated, but after reviewing these materials carefully, these special osteopathically oriented relationships became more understandable. As an osteopathic physician, I became much stronger. More importantly, my inquisitive and scientifically oriented mind undertook numerous new journeys, the first steps in pursuing newly directed research.

As a pulmonologist, the second edition of *Foundations* has taken my personal understanding to a higher level than ever expected. An example of how one pair of authors' evolving osteopathic insights are changing is found by comparing the first and second edition respiratory systems chapters, coauthored by Samuel Krachman and myself. Not only are there numerous content changes, but our method of presentation and osteopathic perspectives have changed dramatically.

It is my hope that my personal experience with this project provides some insight for future readers of this text. As Dr. Levine recommends, use this text as a template for learning "to think osteopathically," while using all available scientific and clinical information that make the science and art of practicing of osteopathic medicine so special and distinctive.

GILBERT E. D'ALONZO, D.O., F.A.C.O.I.
Editor-in-Chief, AOA Publications
American Osteopathic Association

---

[1] Walter Lippmann, Pulitzer Prize winner, syndicated columnist, and editor of the New York World.

ACKNOWLEDGMENTS

Development of this second edition of *Foundations for Osteopathic Medicine* has been a remarkable, often stress-inducing, but worthwhile experience for all concerned. Initial planning began at the October 2000 AOA meeting in New Orleans. Only two face-to-face meetings were needed to implement and evaluate project goals and objectives. The first occurred over two days in Philadelphia in March 2001 at the corporate offices of Lippincott Williams & Wilkins. The second took place over a two-hour breakfast meeting at the AOA convention in San Diego, California in October 2001. As expected, there were a number of conceptual and detail type problems putting the project together. Most noteworthy, however, is the fact that virtually all the work occurred in cyberspace. Among the benefits were fast turnaround times and reasonably quick fixes for major problems. One comes away with a sense that a diverse group of associate editors, authors and staff have worked unbelievably hard meeting project expectations deadlines. Dedication to our profession, once again, has been the byword. In literal terms, the project moved from concept to production in less than 12 months! What more can be said, except an enormous thank you to everyone involved.

On a sad note, one of our anatomy coauthors, Allen Jacobs, D.O., Ph.D., Dean of the Michigan State University College of Osteopathic Medicine, died suddenly and unexpectedly in December 2001. His dedication to osteopathic medicine, and its students in particular, was legendary.

Special thanks goes to the following:

Section Editors:
Raymond J. Hruby
John A. Jerome
John M. Jones, III
Robert E. Kappler
Michael L. Kuchera
William A. Kuchera
Michael M. Patterson
Bernard R. Rubin
Michael A. Seffinger
Sarah A. Sprafka
Richard L. Van Buskirk

Project Managers:
For the Osteopathic Principles Textbook Project
    Jane A. Walsh

For Lippincott Williams & Wilkins
    Timothy Y. Hiscock, Acquisitions Editor
    Michelle M. LaPlante, Senior Developmental Editor
    Robin E. Cook, Senior Production Editor

For the American Osteopathic Association
    John Crosby, J.D., Executive Director, American Osteopathic Association
    Gilbert A. D'Alonzo, D.O., F.A.C.O.I., Editor-in-Chief, Publications, American Osteopathic Association
    Philip A. Saigh, Jr., Director of the Department of Communications, American Osteopathic Association
    Michael Fitzgerald, Director of the Division of Publications, American Osteopathic Association

Peer Reviewers
Constance Cashen, D.O., F.A.C.O.S.
Anthony G. Chila, D.O., F.A.A.O.
Eileen L. DiGiovanna, D.O., F.A.A.O.
Lori Dillard, D.O.
Chester DeGroat, Ph.D.
Dennis Dowling, D.O., F.A.A.O.
John Duhn, MS III: MSU-COM
Walter Ehrenfeuchter, D.O., F.A.A.O.
Mitchell Elkiss, D.O., F.A.C.N.
Thomas Gilson, D.O.
Philip Greenman, D.O., F.A.A.O.
Andra Grosser, MS II:COMP, OMM Teaching Fellow
Raymond J. Hruby, D.O., F.A.A.O.
Sheru Hurlong, MS II:COMP, OMM Teaching Fellow
John A. Jerome, Ph.D.
William L. Johnston, D.O., F.A.A.O.
Robert E. Kappler, D.O., F.A.A.O.
Albert F. Kelso, Ph.D.
Hollis King, D.O., Ph.D., F.A.A.O.
Steven Kopka, M.A.
Michael L. Kuchera, D.O., F.A.A.O.
William A. Kuchera, D.O., F.A.A.O.
Edna M. Lay, D.O., F.A.A.O.
Wesley Lockhart, D.O.
Jayne H.-W. Martin, D.O.
Chindeum Olsekeka, MS II:COMP, OMM Teaching Fellow
Gerald G. Osborn, D.O., F.A.C.N.
David A. Patriquin, D.O., F.A.A.O.
Michael M. Patterson, Ph.D.

Christopher Pohlod, MS III:MSU-COM, OMM Teaching Fellow
Felix J. Rogers, D.O., F.A.C.O.I.
Bernard R. Rubin, D.O., F.A.C.O.I.
Jesus Sanchez, MS II:COMP, OMM Teaching Fellow
Michael A. Seffinger, D.O.
Seth Torregiani, MS II:COMP, OMM Teaching Fellow
Richard L. VanBuskirk, D.O., F.A.A.O.
Angela Wagner, D.O.
Elaine Wallace, D.O.
Robert C. Ward, III, D.O.
Robert Wurster, Ph.D.

Major Project Contributors
Michael Fitzgerald, AOA
Philip Saigh, AOA
Ms. Jane Walsh, Project Coordinator, Department of Osteopathic Manipulative Medicine, MSU-COM
Ms. Patricia Grauer, Information officer, MSU-COM
Ms. Sharon Husch, Executive secretary, Department of Osteopathic Manipulative Medicine, MSU-COM

ROBERT C. WARD, D.O., F.A.A.O.
Executive Editor

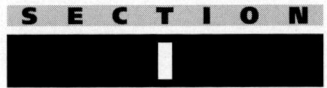

SECTION
I

OSTEOPATHIC PHILOSOPHY AND HISTORY

1

OSTEOPATHIC PHILOSOPHY

MICHAEL A. SEFFINGER
HOLLIS H. KING
ROBERT C. WARD
JOHN M. JONES, III
FELIX J. ROGERS
MICHAEL M. PATTERSON

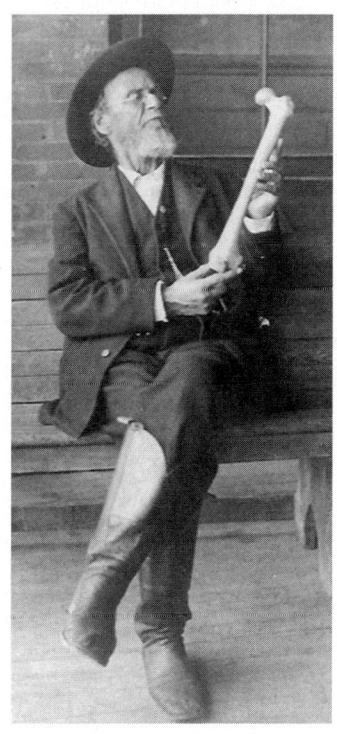

Andrew Taylor Still, M.D., D.O. (1828–1917)

KEY CONCEPTS

- Origin of osteopathic philosophy
- Classic osteopathic philosophy
- Historical development of osteopathic concepts
- Evolution of the osteopathic philosophy from A.T. Still to present
- Applications of osteopathic principles as guidelines to patient care

INTRODUCTION

The osteopathic philosophy, deceptively simple in its presentation, forms the basis for osteopathic medicine's distinctive approach to health care. The philosophy acts as a unifying set of ideas for the organization of scientific knowledge in relation to all phases of physical, mental, emotional, and spiritual health, along with distinctive patient management principles. As such, its concepts form the foundation for practicing osteopathic medicine.

Viewpoints and attitudes arising from osteopathic principles give osteopathic practitioners an important template for clinical problem solving and patient education. In the 21st century, this viewpoint is particularly useful as practitioners from a wide variety of disciplines confront increasingly complex physical, psychosocial, and spiritual problems affecting individuals, families, and populations from a wide variety of cultures and backgrounds.

HOW IT ALL BEGAN

Andrew Taylor Still (1828–1917) was an American frontier doctor who was convinced that 19th century patient care was severely inadequate. This resulted in an intense desire on his part to improve surgery, obstetrics, and the general treatment of diseases, placing them on a more rational and scientific basis.

As his perspectives and clinical understanding evolved, Still created an innovative system of diagnosis and treatment with two major emphases. The first highlights treatment of physical and mental ailments (i.e., diseases) while emphasizing the normalization of body structures and functions. Its hallmark was a detailed knowledge of anatomy that became the basis for much of his diagnostic and clinical work, most notably palpatory diagnosis and manipulative treatment. The second emphasizes the importance of health and well being in its broadest sense, including mental, emotional, and spiritual health, and the avoidance of alcohol and drugs, and other negative health habits.

ORIGINS OF OSTEOPATHIC PHILOSOPHY

Historically, Still was not the first to call attention to inadequacies of the health care of his time. Hippocrates (c. 460–c. 377 B.C.E.), Galen (c. 130–c. 200), and Sydenham (1624–1689) are others. Each, in his own way, criticized the inadequacies of existing medical practices, while focusing contemporary thinking on the patient's natural ability to heal.

In addition, Still was deeply influenced by a number of philosophers, scientists, and medical practitioners of his time. There is also evidence he was well versed in the religious philosophies and concepts of the Methodist, Spiritualist, and Universalist movements of the period (1).

Following the loss of three children to spinal meningitis in 1864, Still immersed himself in the study of the nature of health, illness, and disease (2). His goal was to discover definitive methods for curing and preventing all that ailed his patients. He implicitly believed there was "a God of truth," and that: "All His works, spiritual and material, are harmonious. His law of animal life is absolute. So wise a God had certainly placed the remedy within the material house in which the spirit of life dwells." Furthermore, he believed he could access these natural inherent remedies "... by adjusting the body in such a manner that the remedies may naturally associate themselves together, hear the cries, and relieve the afflicted" (2). In this quest, he combined contemporary philosophical concepts and principles with existing scientific theories. Always a pragmatist, Still accepted aspects of different philosophies, concepts, and practices that worked for him and his patients. He then integrated them with personal discoveries of his own from in-depth studies of anatomy, physics, chemistry, and biology (1). The result was the formulation of his new philosophy and its applications. He called it: "Osteopathy."

Still's moment of clarity came on June 22, 1874. He writes, "I was shot, not in the heart, but in the dome of reason" (2). "Like a burst of sunshine the whole truth dawned on my mind, that I was gradually approaching a science by study, research, and observation that would be a great benefit to the world" (2). He realized that all living things, especially humans, were created by a perfect God. If humans were the embodiment of perfection, then they were fundamentally made to be healthy. There should be no defect in their structures and functions.

Since he believed that "the greatest study of man is man," he dissected numerous cadavers to test his hypothesis (2). He believed that if he could understand the construction (anatomy) of the human body, he would comprehend Nature's laws and unlock the keys to health. Still found no flaws in the concepts of the body's well-designed structure, proving to him that his hypothesis was correct.

A corollary to Still's revelation was that the physician does not cure diseases. In his view, it was the job of the physician to correct structural disturbances so the body works normally, just as a mechanic adjusts his machine. In *Research and Practice* he wrote, "The God of Nature is the fountain of skill and wisdom and the mechanical work done in all natural bodies is the result of absolute knowledge. Man cannot add anything to this perfect work nor improve the functioning of the normal body. . . . Man's power to cure is good as far as he has a knowledge of the right or normal position, and so far as he has the skill to adjust the bones, muscles and ligaments and give freedom to nerves, blood, secretions and excretions, and no farther. We credit God with wisdom and skill to perform perfect work on the house of life in which man lives. It is only justice that God should receive this credit and we are ready to adjust the parts and trust the results" (3).

While Still practiced the orthodox medicine of his day from 1853 to 1879, including the use of oral medications such as purgatives, diuretics, stimulants, sedatives, and analgesics, and externally applied salves and plasters, once he began using his new philosophical system he virtually ceased using drugs. This occurred after several years where he experimented with combinations of drugs and manipulative treatment. In addition, he compared his results with those of patients who received no treatment at all (2). After several years' experience, he became convinced that his mechanical corrections consistently achieved the same or better results without using medications.

It was at that point that Still philosophically divorced himself from the orthodox practices of 19th century medicine (2). He writes, "Having been familiar myself for years with all their methods and having experimented with them I became disheartened and dropped them"(3). His unerring faith in the natural healing capabilities of the mechanically adjusted body formed the foundation for his new philosophy.

Unsure of what to call his new hands-on approach in the early years, Still at times referred to himself as a "magnetic healer" and "lightning bone-setter" (1,4). In the 1880s Still began publicly using the term "osteopathy" as the chosen name for his new profession (1,5). He writes: "Osteopathy is compounded of two words, osteon, meaning bone, (and) pathos, (or) pathine, to suffer. I reasoned that the bone, 'Osteon,' was the starting point from which I was to ascertain the cause of pathological conditions, and so I combined the 'Osteo' with the 'pathy' and had as a result, Osteopathy" (2).

As the name osteopathy implies, Still used the bony skeleton as his reference point for understanding clinical problems and their pathological processes. On the surface, he was most interested in anatomy. On the other hand, he taught that there is more to the skeleton than 206 bones attached together by ligaments and connective tissue. In his discourses, Still would describe the anatomy of the arterial supply to the femur, for example, trace it back to the heart and lungs, and relate it to all of the surrounding and interrelated nerves, soft tissues, and organs along the way. He would then demonstrate how the obstruction of arterial flow anywhere along the pathway toward the femur would result in pathophysiologic changes in the bone, producing pain or dysfunction.

He writes of his treatment concepts: "Bones can be used as levers to relieve pressure on nerves, veins and arteries" (2). This can be understood in the context that vascular and neural structures pass between bones or through orifices (foramina) within a bone. These are places where they are most vulnerable to bony compression and disruption of their functions. In addition, fascia is a type of connective tissue that attaches to bones. Fascia also envelops all muscles, nerves, and vascular structures. When strained or twisted by overuse or trauma myofascial structures not only restrict bony mobility, but also compress neurovascular structures and disturb their functions. By using the bones as manual levers, bony or myofascial entrapments of nerves or vascular structures can be removed, thus restoring normal nervous and vascular functions.

The Philosophy Involves More Than Neuromusculoskeletal Diagnosis and Treatment

Osteopathy is not only a neuromusculoskeletal-oriented diagnostic and treatment system, it is also a comprehensive and scientifically based school of medicine that embraces a philosophy. In answer to the question, "What is osteopathy?" Still stated, "It is a scientific knowledge of anatomy and physiology in the hands of a person of intelligence and skill, who can apply that knowledge to the use of man when sick or wounded by strains, shocks, falls, or mechanical derangement or injury of any kind to the body" (6).

Furthermore, osteopathy had a greater calling. In what could be considered a mission statement, Still wrote, "The object of Osteopathy is to improve upon the present systems of surgery, midwifery, and treatment of general diseases" (2). And, "To find health should be the object of the doctor. Anyone can find disease" (6).

CLASSIC OSTEOPATHIC PHILOSOPHY OF HEALTH

Health Is a Natural State of Harmony

Still believed health to be the natural state of the human being (Table 1.1). In his own words:

> Osteopathy is based on the perfection of Nature's work. When all parts of the human body are in line we have health. When they are

TABLE 1.1. CLASSIC OSTEOPATHIC PHILOSOPHY

A. T. Still's fundamental concepts of Osteopathy can be organized in terms of health, disease, and patient care.

Health
1. Health is a natural state of harmony.
2. The human body is a perfect machine created for health and activity.
3. A healthy state exists as long as there is normal flow of body fluids and nerve activity.

Disease
4. Disease is an effect of underlying, often multifactorial causes.
5. Illness is often caused by mechanical impediments to normal flow of body fluids and nerve activity.
6. Environmental, social, mental, and behavioral factors contribute to the etiology of disease and illness.

Patient Care
7. The human body provides all the chemicals necessary for the needs of its tissues and organs.
8. Removal of mechanical impediments allows optimal body fluid flow, nerve function, and restoration of health.
9. Environmental, cultural, social, mental, and behavioral factors need to be addressed as part of any management plan.
10. Any management plan should realistically meet the needs of the individual patient.

not the effect is disease. When the parts are readjusted disease gives place to health. The work of the osteopath is to adjust the body from the abnormal to the normal, then the abnormal conditions give place to the normal and health is the result of the normal condition (3).

Mechanics and Health

Still's concept of a healthy person is insightful. It places his belief of the importance of structural and mechanical integrity within the perspective of a comprehensive view of a human being within society:

> When complete, he is a self-acting, individualized, separate personage, endowed with the power to move, and mind to direct in locomotion, with a care for comfort and a thought for his continued existence in the preparation and consumption of food to keep him in size and form to suit the duties he may have to perform (6).

Still believed that life exists as a unification of vital forces and matter. Since the body is controlled by the mind to exhibit purposeful motion in attaining the needs and goals of the organism, he stated that, "Osteopathy . . . is the law of mind, matter and motion" (2). Once Still accepted that motion is an inherent quality of life itself, it was a small step to inquiring into what is moving and how it moves. Through his in-depth study of anatomy, he could see the interdependent relationships among different tissues and their component parts. He observed that each part developed as the body was moving, growing, and developing from embryo to fetus to newborn and throughout life. Thus, each tissue, organ, and structure is designed for motion. "As motion is the first and only evidence of life, by this thought we are conducted to the machinery through which life works to accomplish these results" (7).

If "life is matter in motion"(6), then what is the effect on a body part that is not moving? Still reasoned that a lack of motion is not conducive to life or health. "[The osteopath's] duties as a philosopher admonish him that life and matter can be united, and that that union cannot continue with any hindrance to free and absolute motion" (6). Further, he boldly states that the practice of osteopathy "covers all phases of disease and it is the law that keeps life in motion" (2).

Normal Nerve Activity and Flow of Body Fluids

A machine cannot run without proper lubrication, fuel, and mechanisms to remove the by-products of combustion. In teaching his students, Still identified each component of the body's intricate mechanisms as he knew them. In the process, he discussed various forces that he reasoned create motion and maintain life. He explained how lubricating and nourishing fluids flow through the arteries, veins, lymphatics, and nerves. He also noted that they turn over by-products of metabolism through the venous and lymphatic systems. "The human body is a machine run by the unseen force called life, and that it may be run harmoniously it is necessary that there be liberty of blood, nerves and arteries from their generating point to their destination" (2).

Another component of Still's machine concept was the power source. He identified the brain as the dynamo, the electric battery that keeps the body moving and working:

> The brain furnishes nerve-action and forces to suit each class of work to be done by that set of nerves which is to construct forms and to keep blood constantly in motion in the arteries and from all parts back to the heart through the veins that it may be purified, renewed, and re-enter circulation (6).

CLASSIC OSTEOPATHIC PHILOSOPHY OF DISEASE

Disease Is an Effect of an Underlying Cause or Causes

From the time of Hippocrates through the first half of the 20th century, diseases were identified primarily through simple and complex descriptions of symptoms and signs. Many afflictions were without clear etiology. In spite of our current greater levels of knowledge and understanding, this is still true in many cases.

Still taught that disease is the effect of an abnormal anatomic state with subsequent physiologic breakdown and decreased host adaptability. Germs were first discovered in the 17th century with the invention of the microscope, but the germ theory of disease was not accepted until Pasteur provided convincing scientific evidence in the mid-19th century. However, experienced clinicians like Still, as well as an emerging group of laboratory scientists, saw germs as opportunists to decreased host function, not as primary in themselves. They speculated that infections resulted from an interaction between the degree of virulence and quantity of the infecting agent and the level of host immunity.

Still also realized that there were multifactorial components to disease processes (8,9). He believed that disease was a combination of influences arising from decreased host adaptability and adverse environmental conditions. He recognized that symptoms often were a manifestation of nerves irritated by pathophysiologic processes commonly created by an accumulation of fluids (congestion and inflammation). This diminished the patient's ability to adapt to the environment (2). Additionally, Still was keenly aware of the deleterious effects of environmentally induced trauma, or abrupt changes in the atmosphere, causing physical or emotional "shock" or inertia, and therefore obstructing normal metabolic processes, body fluids, and nerve activity (3).

Mechanical Impediments to Flow of Body Fluids and Nerve Activity

Still's study of pathology found that in all forms of disease there is mechanical interruption of normal circulation of body fluids and nerve force to and from cells, tissues, and organs (3). "Sickness is an effect caused by the stoppage of some supply of fluid or quality of life" (2). He understood that it is the combination of free circulation of wholesome blood and motor, nutrient, and sensory nerve activity that creates tissues and organs, and facilitates their growth, maintenance, and repair. Through cadaver dissection studies he reasoned that strains, twists, or distortions in fascia, ligaments, or muscle fibers surrounding the small capillaries and nerve bundles could very well be the cause of ischemia

and congestion by mechanical obstruction, interruption, or impediment to normal flow of vital fluids.

Still understood that the flow of body fluids was under the control of the nerves that innervated the blood vessel walls, adjusting the diameter of the vessels and thus controlling the amount and rate of blood flow to the tissues and organs. "While the vascular and nervous systems are dependent upon each other, it must be remembered that the bloodstream is under the control of the nervous system, not only indirectly through the heart, but directly through the vasoconstrictor and vasodilator nerve fibers, which regulate the caliber and rhythm of the blood vessels" (9). Still writes: "All diseases are mere effects, the cause being a partial or complete failure of the nerves to properly conduct the fluids of life" (2). Although he emphasized that "the rule of the artery is absolute, universal, and it must be unobstructed, or disease will result"(2), he also pointed out the importance of unimpeded flow of lymphatics: "[W]e must keep the lymphatics normal all the time or see confused Nature in the form of disease. We strike at the source of life and death when we go to the lymphatics" (6). However, even if the blood and lymph are flowing normally, Still pointed out that, "the cerebro spinal fluid is the highest known element that is contained in the human body, and unless the brain furnishes this fluid in abundance a disabled condition of the body will remain. He who is able to reason will see that this great river of life must be tapped and the withering field irrigated at once, or the harvest of health be forever lost" (7).

Holistic Aspects—Environmental, Social, Mental, and Behavioral Etiologies

For the most part, Still described the origins of disease and illness as a result of "anatomic disturbances followed by physiologic discord." However, at the same time, he acknowledged the potential detrimental influences of heredity, lifestyle, environmental conditions, contagious diseases, inactivity and other personal behavior choices, and psychological and social stress on health (6,8,9).

Still also recognized that substance abuse (e.g., alcohol and opium) as well as poor sanitation, personal hygiene and dietary indiscretion, lack of exercise or fitness all contributed to illness and disease. He lectured passionately against the social forces that promulgated these deleterious behaviors and social situations, including slavery and economic inequities. Indeed, he talked from personal experience as he and his family members suffered from these challenging social circumstances during the pioneer days of the 19th century Midwest.

CLASSIC OSTEOPATHIC PHILOSOPHY AND PATIENT CARE

The Body Provides Its Own Drug Store

Like many others, Still observed that some people are more susceptible to epidemic diseases than others. It was also recognized that host resistance to disease is more apparent in certain individuals (10); so-called natural immunity, that is either inherited or acquired (11,12). Still believed that promoting free flow of arterial blood to an infected area would enable "Nature's own germicide" to eradicate the infectious agent (3). Still's philosophy places complete trust in the innate self-healing ability of the body. Removing all hindrances to health wasn't enough however, as it was incumbent upon the physician to ensure that the body's natural chemicals were able to work effectively in alleviating any pathophysiologic processes (2).

Use of Medications

I was born and raised to respect and confide in the remedial power of drugs, but after many years of practice in close conformity to the dictations of the very best medical authors and in consultation with representatives of the various schools, I failed to get from drugs the results hoped for and I was face to face with the evidence that medication was not only untrustworthy but was dangerous (3).

Initially, Still conceived of osteopathy as "a system of healing that reaches both internal and external diseases by manual operation and without drugs" (2). Although he stated, "Osteopathy is a drugless science," he clarified this statement by explaining that he believed that drugs "should not be used as remedial agents," since the medications of his era only addressed symptoms or abnormal bodily responses to an unknown cause. In osteopathy, there is no place for injurious medications, whose risks outweigh their benefits, especially if safer and equally effective alternatives exist.

Specifically, Still was against the irrational use of drugs that (a) showed no benefit, (b) had proven to be harmful, and (c) had no proven relationship to the cause of disease processes. He accepted anesthetics, poison antidotes, and a few others that had proven beneficial. "Osteopathy has no use for drugs as remedies, but a great use for chemistry when dealing with poisons and antidotes" (13). Still supports his reasons by listing the life-threatening risks of using drugs commonly employed in the late 19th century, namely, calomel, digitalis, aloe, morphine, chloral hydrate, veratrine, pulsatilla, and sedatives (2). Still persuasively argued that a detailed physical examination, with focus on the neuromusculoskeletal system, followed by a well-designed, manipulative treatment, often removes impediments to motion and function. Where he differed from others was his view that manipulative treatment should always be used before deciding that the body has failed in its own efforts.

Vaccinations

Jenner introduced the smallpox vaccine in the 17th century, with considerable success. Still acknowledged this by stating, "I believe the philosophy of fighting one infection with another infectious substance that could hold the body immune by long and continuous possession is good and was good" (6). Without disrespect to Jenner, he describes shortcomings of Jenner's methods, pointing out that there were many patients on whom the vaccine did not work or who became disabled or fatally ill. He states his belief that there is a less harmful method of vaccination and requests that Jenner's methods be improved.

His rejection of drugs and vaccinations showed up in the initial mission statement for the American School of Osteopathy (ASO) (3). However, in 1910, even while Still was president, the school changed its stance and accepted vaccinations and serums as part of osteopathic practices.

First and foremost, Still clearly believed that the osteopathic physician should strive to help the patient's body release its own medicine for a particular problem. He writes:

The brain of man was God's drug store, and had in it all liquids, drugs, lubricating oils, opiates, acids, and antacids, and every quality of drugs that the wisdom of God thought necessary for human happiness and health (13).

The Mechanical Approach to Treating the Cause of Disease

Still reasoned that the cause of most diseases was mechanical, therefore, treatment must follow the laws of mechanics. As a consequence, he used manipulative approaches designed to release bony and soft tissue barriers to nervous and circulatory functions in order to improve chances for healing (Fig. 1.1). He claimed that mobilization of these structures improved the outcomes of his patients (3). However, manipulation procedures were not only applied to relieve musculoskeletal strains and injuries, but to treat internal organ diseases as well. For example, he found characteristic paraspinal muscle rigidity and other abnormal myofascial tensions in patients with infectious diseases. He noted improvement in the health of these patients as well when the musculoskeletal and myofascial impediments to normal physiologic processes were alleviated. In a majority of cases the patient's condition was seemingly cured, leading him to believe that the mechanical aspects of dysfunction or disease were vitally important (3). Still thus proposed, that in all diseases, mobilization of all the spinal joints not in their proper positional and functional relationships was necessary to ensure proper nerve activity and blood and lymph flow throughout the body. This included everything from the occiput to the coccyx, and indicated adjustment of the pelvis, clavicles, scapulae, costal cage, and diaphragm.

Comprehensive Treatment

While heavily committed to the use of palpatory diagnosis and manipulative treatment, Dr. Still continued many other aspects of patient care. He practiced surgery and midwifery (obstetrics), although little is documented about specific activities.

His patient education strategies highlighted moderation. He included advice for removing noxious or toxic substances from the diet and environment and behavioral adjustments such as adding exercises and stopping smoking. He also admonished his patients for abusing alcohol, opium, and heroin.

Mental illness and stress-related problems were also important to Still (2,3). He wrote about the role the physician can take in providing emotional support and encouragement to patients with end-stage medical problems. He described the importance of giving hope to patients and, at the same time, providing them with a realistic approach to managing their clinical condition (3).

Individualized Treatment

Each person is treated as a unique individual, not as a disease entity. Still taught that the history and physical evaluation of each person would turn up unhealthy self-care behaviors or circumstances and parts of the body not moving normally; the

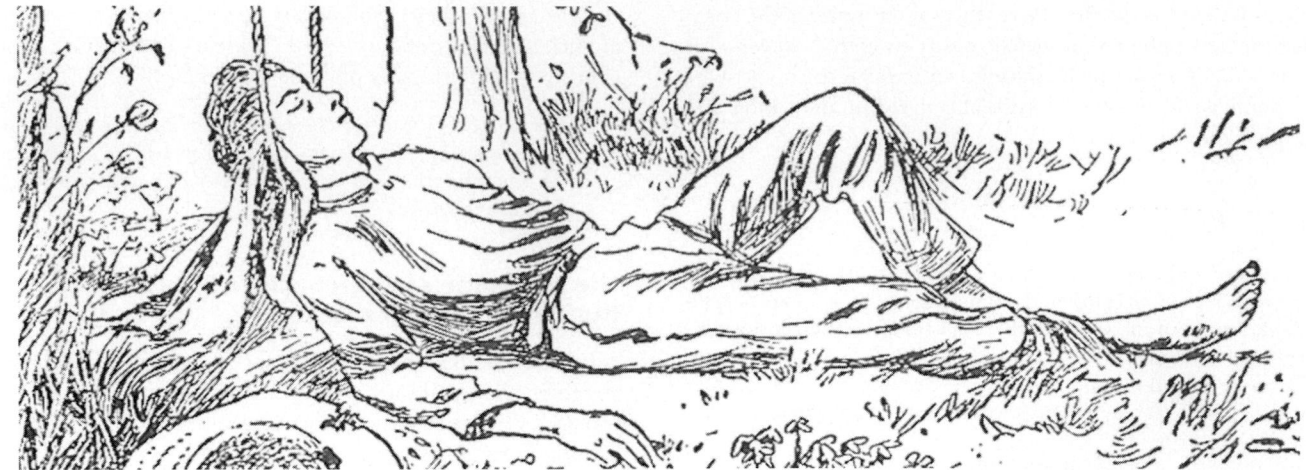

FIGURE 1.1. Like many physicians before and after him, Dr. Still applied his new philosophy first to himself and then to his patients. In a famous early anecdote, he stopped a headache by suspending his neck across a low-lying rope swing. He later applied self-adjustments of spinal joint dysfunction to abate an attack of "flux" (bloody dysentery). After he was successful at curing 17 children of the same affliction by adjusting their spinal joint dysfunctions, he realized he was onto something worthwhile. (From Still AT. *Autobiography of Andrew T. Still.* Rev ed. Kirksville, MO: Published by the author; 1908. Distributed, Indianapolis: American Academy of Osteopathy.)

combination interfering with the body's natural ability to heal itself. The treatment would need to be tailored specifically for each patient's particular needs.

HISTORICAL DEVELOPMENT OF OSTEOPATHIC CONCEPTS

Exactly how much influence previous or contemporary philosophies and practices had on Still is purely speculative, since he never discussed specific attachments for any particular philosopher or scientist. The writings of contemporary philosophers of science and biology, like Herbert Spencer (1820–1903) and Alfred Russel Wallace (1823–1913), resonated with those of Still (1). They promoted the theories of evolution and the interdependence of the environment and the organism in all biologic processes, including the origins of disease. They also promoted the concepts of the interdependence of structure and function, the importance of differentiating cause and effect, and emphasized the unity of the organism and interrelatedness of its parts. Throughout his life, however, Still maintained that his discoveries and thoughts were based on personal observation, experimentation, applications of factual knowledge, and the power of reasoning. After nearly 50 years of developing his concepts, he stated:

> I have explored by reading and inquiry much that has been written on kindred subjects, hoping to get something on this great law written by the ancient philosophers, but I come back as empty as I started (2).

A number of scholars and educators have attempted to trace both the historical development and evolution of thoughts and practices that may have influenced Still's thinking (10–12, 14–18). In general, the authors compare Still's ideas with well-known discourses passed on principally through Western cultural ideas. In 1901, Littlejohn wrote, "Osteopathy did not invent a new anatomy or physiology or construct a new pathology. It has built upon the foundation of sciences already deeply seated in the

philosophy of truth, chemistry, anatomy and physiology, a new etiology of diseases, gathering together, adding to and reinforcing natural methods of treating disease that have been accumulating since the art of healing began" (10). However, C.M.T. Hulett emphatically stated that "Osteopathy is a new system of thought, a new philosophy of life" (19). Whereas Littlejohn (14) finds the foundation of osteopathy in Greek and Roman medicine, G.D. Hulett (12) and Downing (15) trace the origins of various osteopathic concepts to the philosophy and practice of medicine found in other ancient writings, such as those of the Ptolemies, Brahmins, Chinese, and Hebrews. All agree on the further development of medicine throughout Europe as a precursor to American osteopathic medical practice. Northup compares osteopathy to the concepts of Hippocrates and the Cnidian schools (18). Korr contrasts the contributions of Asclepian and Hygeian roots (17). Whereas G.D. Hulett (12) and Korr (17) describe osteopathy as part of an *evolution* of the philosophy of medicine, Lane (11) and Northup (18) consider it a *reformation* of medical theory and practice.

Still's use of spinal manipulation had many precedents. Schiötz and Cyriax (20) and Lomax (21), among many, document the use of manual treatments for millennia. Hippocrates discussed "subluxations" or minor displacements of vertebra in his treatise "On the Articulations" and the manual adjustments used to correct them (22). In the 18th and 19th centuries many American and European practitioners acknowledged that there are relationships among displaced or "subluxed" vertebrae, and "irritated" spinal nerves in relation to both musculoskeletal and visceral disorders (23).

EVOLUTION OF OSTEOPATHIC PHILOSOPHY

In his unique way, Still integrated many of these concepts into his new system and molded it into a distinctive medical school curriculum that continues to evolve to this day. Still was adamant that he did not expect his students and colleagues to take what he advocated as dogma. He taught, "You must reason. I say reason, or you will finally fail in all enterprises. Form your own opinions, select all facts you can obtain. Compare, decide, then act. Use no man's opinion; accept his works only" (6). He urged his students to study, test, and improve upon his ideas.

An example of this evolution is a shift from Still's early, and virtually exclusive, emphasis on anatomy to a more inclusive stress on primary physiologic functions that strengthen his concepts. Initially, J. Martin Littlejohn (14), and later, Burns (24), Cole (25), Denslow (26), and Korr (27,28) promoted integrative neurophysiologic and neuroendocrine concepts.

Whereas Littlejohn interpreted Still's concepts in light of 19th century physiologic theories, Burns, Cole, Denslow, and Korr pioneered distinctive osteopathic approaches to physiologic investigations, making significant scientific contributions. Korr was particularly influential in interpreting osteopathic concepts in light of the rapidly developing science of physiology in the 20th century. He has been referred to as "the second great osteopathic philosopher" (29).

Irvin Korr, Ph.D., received his physiology degree from Princeton University. Most of his teaching and research career was spent at the Kirksville College of Osteopathic Medicine in Missouri, with later appointments at both Michigan State University College of Osteopathic Medicine and The Texas College of Osteopathic Medicine (University of North Texas). A multitalented individual, Korr was an accomplished violinist, sometimes playing chamber music with Albert Einstein, who was in residence at the time of his postgraduate training. He published extensively with several colleagues, including J.S. Denslow, A.D. Krems, Martin J. Goldstein, Price E. Thomas, Harry M. Wright, and Gustavo S.L. Appeltauer. In 1947, Korr's initial publication, with Denslow and Krems, focused on facilitation of neural impulses in motoneuron pools. Original research papers followed this on dermal autonomic activity, electrical skin resistance, and trophic function of nerves (28). As Korr gained insight into Still's concepts, he lectured widely and published a number of important treatises tying osteopathic concepts together with proven physiologic models that emphasized the important roles played by the neuromusculoskeletal system. Whereas Still emphasized a focus on bones as the starting place from which he was to discern the cause of pathology, Korr expanded this concept to include the integrative activity of the spinal cord and its relationships with the musculoskeletal and the sympathetic nervous systems (28). Similar to Still, however, Korr often referred to the neuromusculoskeletal system as the "Primary Machinery of Life." (See Korr's "An Explication of Osteopathic Principles" later in this chapter).

The Definition of Osteopathy

Osteopathic philosophy has been defined various ways over the years. To get a better sense of the evolution of the osteopathic philosophy since its inception, it is instructive to follow how it has been defined over time. In his autobiography, Still gave a "technical" definition as follows:

> Osteopathy is that science which consists of . . . knowledge of the structure and functions of the human mechanism . . . by which nature

under the scientific treatment peculiar to osteopathic practice . . . in harmonious accord with its own mechanical principles . . . may recover from displacements, disorganizations, derangements, and consequent disease and regain its normal equilibrium of form and function in health and strength. (2)

Besides Still, several other American osteopathic scholars wrote treatises on osteopathic philosophy and principles (11,12, 15,16,25,30–36). Each author had his or her own definition and explanation of osteopathic philosophy. There have been several attempts over the past century to obtain consensus, or agreement, on a unifying definition and clearly stated tenets or principles that govern the practice of osteopathic medicine.

According to Littlejohn, the first consensus definition of osteopathy, among multiple faculty members, representing several osteopathic medical schools, was published in 1900 (10). In 1922, another consensus statement was developed and published by the A.T. Still Research Institute as a revised edition of a popular classic textbook by G.D. Hulett (12). By this time in medical thought, it was widely accepted that cellular level activity was a strong determinant of health or disease states. In an attempt to update osteopathic philosophy in light of emerging concepts in cellular biology, the authors applied Still's mechanistic viewpoint to cellular physiology. The following passage not only illustrates this approach, but demonstrates the desire of the profession to state osteopathic philosophy and principles in terms of concise tenets based on contemporary scientific knowledge:

> The osteopathic view of the cell . . . is largely covered by the following statements:
>
> ■ Normal structure is essential to normal function.
> ■ Normal function is essential if normal structure is to be maintained.
> ■ Normal environment is essential to normal function and structure, though some degree of adaptation is possible for a time, even under abnormal conditions.
>
> In the human body, with its diversified functions, we may add also,
>
> ■ The blood preserves and defends the cells of the body.
> ■ The nervous system unifies the body in its activities.
> ■ Disease symptoms are due either to failure of the organism to meet adverse circumstances efficiently, or to structural abnormalities.
> ■ Rational methods of treatment are based upon an attempt to provide normal nutrition, innervation and drainage to all tissues of the body, and these depend chiefly upon the maintenance of normal structural relations (12).

The addition of medications in the practices of osteopathic physicians and surgeons over the years affected how the philosophy was stated. For example, in 1948, the faculty at the College of Osteopathic Physicians and Surgeons in Los Angeles added the following phrase to their basic osteopathic principles statement: "Like a machine, the body can function efficiently only when in proper adjustment and when its chemical needs are satisfied either by food or medical substances" (37). Further evolution occurred in 1953, when the faculty of the Kirksville College of Osteopathy and Surgery (KCOS) agreed on the following:

> Osteopathy, or Osteopathic Medicine is a philosophy, a science and an art. Its philosophy embraces the concept of the unity of body structure and function in health and disease. Its science includes the chemical, physical and biological sciences related to the maintenance

of health and the prevention, cure, and alleviation of disease. Its art is the application of the philosophy and the science in the practice of osteopathic medicine and surgery in all its branches and specialties.

Health is based on the natural capacity of the human organism to resist and combat noxious influences in the environment and to compensate for their effects; to meet, with adequate reserve, the usual stresses of daily life and the occasional severe stresses imposed by extremes of environment and activity. Disease begins when this natural capacity is reduced, or when it is exceeded or overcome by noxious influences.

Osteopathic medicine recognizes that many factors impair this capacity and the natural tendency towards recovery, and that among the most important of these factors are the local disturbances or lesions of the musculoskeletal system. Osteopathic medicine is therefore concerned with liberating and developing all the resources that constitute the capacity for resistance and recovery, thus recognizing the validity of the ancient observation that the physician deals with a patient as well as a disease (38).

They then combined several concepts and restated them as four principles:

The osteopathic concept emphasizes four general principles from which are derived an etiological concept, a philosophy and a therapeutic technic that are distinctive, but not the only features of osteopathic diagnosis and treatment.

1. The body is a unit.
2. The body possesses self-regulatory mechanisms.
3. Structure and function are reciprocally inter-related.
4. Rational therapy is based upon an understanding of body unity, self-regulatory mechanisms, and the inter-relationship of structure and function (38).

Over the ensuing 40 years, advances in the biologic sciences elucidated many mechanisms in support of the concept that optimal health calls for integration of countless functions ranging from the molecular to the behavioral level. When this integration breaks down, dysfunction and disease commonly follow. Infectious and metabolic diseases, as well as diseases of aging and genetics are frequent examples. Interdisciplinary fields of study have been developed to investigate and delineate the complex interactions of numerous coordinated body functions in health and disease. Psychoneuroimmunology, for example, provides substantial evidence linking mind, body, and spiritual activities with a wide variety of biologic observations (39–42).

Clinical applications of the advances in molecular, cellular, neurologic, and behavioral sciences, combined with the decreased emphasis on mechanical factors within osteopathic medical practice, demanded a new consensus statement. Using the 1953 Kirksville faculty statement as a beginning, the associate editors of the first edition of this text (1997) stated:

Health is the adaptive and optimal attainment of physical, mental, emotional, and spiritual well-being. It is based on our natural capacity to meet, with adequate reserves, the usual stresses of daily life and the occasional severe stresses imposed by extremes of environment and activity. It includes our ability to resist and combat noxious influences in our environment and to compensate for their effects. One's health at any given time depends on many factors including his or her polygenetic inheritance, environmental influences, and adaptive response to stressors (43).

The editors modified the four key principles of osteopathic philosophy as follows:

1. The body is a unit; the person is a unit of body, mind, and spirit.
2. The body is capable of self-regulation, self-healing, and health maintenance.
3. Structure and function are reciprocally interrelated.
4. Rational treatment is based upon an understanding of the basic principles of body unity, self-regulation, and the interrelationship of structure and function (43).

Although Korr applies 20th century physiologic concepts in his explication of osteopathic principles, he maintains Still's basic premise: "It is the patient who gets well, and not the practitioner or the treatment that makes them well" (44).

In order to represent an increasingly diverse group of osteopathic physicians, the American Osteopathic Association (AOA) adopted a general statement regarding osteopathic medicine. Since 1991, the official AOA definition of *osteopathic medicine* has been reviewed periodically. The latest rendition is available by consulting the AOA website at *www.aoa-net.org* and clicking on the "yearbook" icon. It was last reviewed and accepted as policy by the AOA House of Delegates in 1998:

Osteopathy (Osteopathic Medicine): A complete system of medical care with a philosophy that combines the needs of the patient with current practice of medicine, surgery and obstetrics; that emphasizes the interrelationship between structure and function; and that has an appreciation of the body's ability to heal itself.

The Educational Council on Osteopathic Principles

In the contemporary era, the evolution, growth, and teaching of osteopathic philosophy have been coordinated through the Educational Council on Osteopathic Principles (ECOP) of the American Association of Colleges of Osteopathic Medicine. This organization consists of the chairs of the departments of osteopathic manipulative medicine and osteopathic principles and practice from each osteopathic medical school. It is the "expert panel" in the osteopathic profession in regard to osteopathic manipulative medicine and osteopathic philosophy and principles. These osteopathic physicians are considered leading-edge thinkers in terms of osteopathic philosophy and principles.

One of ECOP's charges is to obtain consensus on the usage of terms within the profession. *The Glossary of Osteopathic Terminology* was first published in 1981 (45), and is updated annually. The 2002 edition is included at the back of this text. The Glossary elaborates upon the AOA definition of osteopathic medicine:

Osteopathic medicine is a philosophy of health care and a distinctive art, supported by expanding scientific knowledge; its philosophy embraces the concept of unity of the living organism's structure (anatomy) and function (physiology). Its art is the application of the philosophy in the practice of medicine and surgery in all its branches and specialties. Its science includes the behavioral, chemical, physical, spiritual and biological knowledge related to the establishment and maintenance of health as well as the prevention and alleviation of disease.

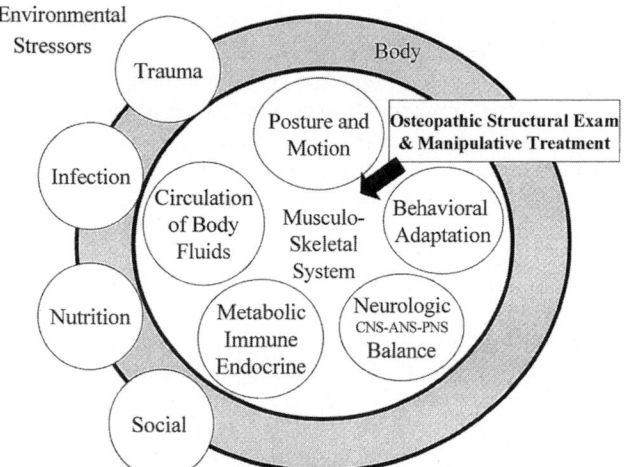

FIGURE 1.2. Osteopathic philosophy of health displayed as the coordinated activity of five basic body functions, integrated by the musculoskeletal system, adapting to environmental stressors. Evaluation and treatment of the musculoskeletal system is performed in light of its ability to affect not only the five functions, but also how it ultimately affects the person's ability to adapt to internal and external stressors.

One of the products of ECOP's work is the development of a method of organizing osteopathic concepts using systems theory and modern concepts in physiology. The primary approach taken was to adopt a health-oriented perspective while also focusing on competent diagnosis and clinical management.

Five basic integrative and coordinated body functions and coping strategies are considered in a context of healthful adaptation to life and its circumstances:

1. Posture and motion, including fundamental structural and biomechanical reliability
2. Neurologic integration, including central, peripheral, autonomic, neuroendocrine, neurocirculatory, and somatic elements
3. Macro- and microrespiratory and circulatory factors
4. Metabolic processes of all types
5. Psychosocial, cultural, behavioral, and spiritual elements

Figure 1.2 depicts the musculoskeletal system as the core or hub of a five-spoked wheel. Careful observation and educated palpation help make the musculoskeletal system a natural entry point for both diagnosis and treatment. Importantly, the musculoskeletal system often reflects numerous signs relating to internal diseases.

OSTEOPATHIC PRINCIPLES AS PRACTICE GUIDELINES

The contributions of A.T. Still and the osteopathic medical profession affect many aspects of general patient care. First, irrespective of diagnoses or practitioner, the patient is of central importance. Second, a competent differential diagnosis is essential. This includes all aspects of the person (body, mind, and spirit) (Table 1.2). Third, clinical activities integrate realistic expectations with measurable outcomes. Finally, and ideally, patient-oriented educational efforts pragmatically address both personal and family-related concerns. The patient is ultimately responsible

TABLE 1.2. OSTEOPATHIC PATIENT EDUCATION AND GUIDANCE FOR SELF-CARE

While osteopathically oriented medical care emphasizes competent comprehensive patient management, it also places importance on restoration of well being appropriate for the patient's age and health potential. This includes addressing:

- Physical, mental, and spiritual components
- Personal safety, such as wearing seat belts
- Sufficient rest and relaxation
- Proper nutrition
- Regular aerobic, stretching, and strengthening exercises
- Maintaining rewarding social relationships
- Avoidance of tobacco, and other abused substances
- Eliminating or modifying abusive personal, interpersonal, family, and work-related behavior patterns
- Avoidance of environmental radiation and toxins

for long-term self-health care. Emphasis is on health restoration and disease prevention.

An ad hoc interdisciplinary committee of osteopathic educators, philosophers, and researchers recently proposed osteopathic principles for patient care:

The Patient Is the Focus for Health Care

All osteopathic physicians, irrespective of the specialty of the practitioner, are trained to focus on the individual patient. The relationship between clinician and patient is a partnership in which both parties are actively engaged. The osteopathic physician is an advocate for the patient, supporting his or her efforts to optimize the circumstances to maintain, improve, or restore health.

The Patient Has the Primary Responsibility for His or Her Health

While the physician is the professional charged with the responsibility to assist a patient in being well, the physician can no more impart health to another person than he or she can impart charm, wisdom, wit or any other desirable trait. Although the patient–physician relationship is a partnership, and the physician has significant obligations to the patient, ultimately the patient has primary responsibility for his or her health. The patient has inherent healing powers and must nurture these through diet and exercise, as well as adherence to appropriate advice in regard to stress, sleep, body weight, and avoidance of abuse.

An Effective Treatment Program for Patient Care

An effective treatment program for patient care is founded on the above tenets and incorporates evidenced-based guidelines, optimizes the patient's natural healing capacity, addresses the primary cause of disease, and emphasizes health maintenance and disease prevention. The emphasis on the musculoskeletal system as an integral part of patient care is one of the defining characteristics of osteopathic medicine. When applied as part of a coherent philosophy of the practice of medicine, these tenets represent a distinct and necessary approach to health care . . . .

Evidence-based guidelines should be used to encourage those treatments with proven efficacy and to discourage those that are not beneficial, or even harmful. Osteopathic medicine embraces the concept of evidence-based medicine as part of a valuable reformation of clinical practice.

Andrew Taylor Still told his students to "look for health; anyone can find disease." This precept provides a useful orientation in patient care. An emphasis on health rather than disease helps to promote optimism. It may facilitate efforts to engage the patient as an active participant in recovery from illness. It may also encourage the realization that no single treatment approach is successful for every patient. Rather, optimal approaches will use diet, exercise, medications, manipulative treatment, surgery, or other modalities according to the needs and wishes of the patient and the skill and aptitude of the practitioner (46).

In end-stage conditions, treatment may be only palliative, yet, as Korr points out,

[I]t is the physician's responsibility, while giving palliative and remedial attention to the patient's immediate problem, to support each patient's internal health care system, to remove impediments to its competence, and above all, to do it no harm. It is also the responsibility of physicians to instruct patients on how to do the same for themselves and to strive to motivate them to do so, especially by their own example (44).

Osteopathically oriented problem-solving and treatment plans help guide the application of osteopathic principles in medical, behavioral, and surgical care. In 1987, ECOP developed guidelines for use by osteopathic physicians in developing an osteopathic management plan (47). The extent to which palpatory diagnosis and manipulative treatment are specifically useful interventions for a wide variety of neuromusculoskeletal problems remains to be seen through research. However, since many clinical presentations commonly interfere with a patient's ability to meet the requirements of normal daily activities, including appropriate exercise, it stands to reason that improving the efficiency of the neuromusculoskeletal system would benefit each patient. "There is a somatic component in all clinical situations. The somatic component is addressed to the extent that it influences patient well-being. Conceptually, osteopathic manipulative treatment is designed to address both structural abnormalities and self-regulatory capabilities."

SUMMARY

Based on a health-oriented medical philosophy, osteopathic medicine uses a number of concepts to implement its principles. The neuromusculoskeletal system is used as a common point of reference, because it directly relates the individual to the physical environment on a day-to-day basis. The practitioner's primary roles are to:

- Address primary cause(s) of disease using available evidence-based practices
- Enhance the patient's healing capacity
- Individualize patient management plans with an emphasis on health restoration and disease prevention
- Use palpatory diagnosis and manipulative treatment to focus on and affect somatic signs of altered structural, mechanical, and physiologic states

Osteopathic philosophy is meant to guide osteopathic physicians in the best use of scientific knowledge to optimize health and diminish disease processes. Upon founding his profession and school, Still expressed the hope that "the osteopath will take up the subject and travel a few miles farther toward the fountain of this great source of knowledge and apply the results to the relief and comfort of the afflicted who come for counsel and advice" (6). It is the intention of the authors to organize current medical knowledge and place it on a foundation of osteopathic philosophy. We do this in order to provide the osteopathic medical student with a road map that will lead to the further study of the science of osteopathy and the practice of the highest quality patient-centered health care possible.

Editor's note: For 50 years, Irwin M. Korr, scientist, philosopher, and humanist, has led and inspired several generations of osteopathic physicians and educators. His final treatise on osteopathic philosophy was written for the first edition of this text.

AN EXPLICATION OF OSTEOPATHIC PRINCIPLES

IRVIN M. KORR

At this stage of your medical training, you have become familiar with osteopathic principles and can recite them in their usual brief, maxim form. The purpose of this section is to explore more fully the meaning, biological foundations, and clinical implications of the founding principles of osteopathic medicine.

Remember that these principles began to evolve centuries ago, even before the time of Hippocrates. However, their basis in animal and, more specifically, human biology did not begin to become evident through research until late in the 19th century. The origin of these principles, therefore, was largely empirical; that is, they were the product of thoughtful and widely shared observations of ill and injured people. For example, it could hardly escape notice, even in primitive societies, that people (and animals) recovered from illness and wounds healed without intervention and, therefore, some natural indwelling healing power must be at work.

Even at the time of the founding of the osteopathic profession in 1892, the available knowledge in the sciences of physiology, biochemistry, microbiology, immunology, and pathology was meager. Indeed, immunology, biochemistry, and various other neurosciences and biomedical sciences had yet to appear as distinct disciplines. Therefore, these principles could only be expressed as aphorisms, embellished perhaps with conjectures about their biological basis. It is to the credit and honor of the osteopathic profession that it contributed cogent elaboration of the principles, developed effective methods for their implementation, built a system of practice upon those principles, and disclosed much about their basis in biological mechanisms through research.

In view of the enormous amount of biomedical knowledge recorded throughout the 20th century, it is timely to examine the principles that guide osteopathic practice in the light of that knowledge and to explore their relevance to clinical practice and to current and future health problems. What follows is an effort in that direction, without detailed reference to individual research.

THE PERSON AS A WHOLE

The Body

The principle of the unity of the body, so central to osteopathic practice, states that every part of the body depends on other parts for maintenance of its optimal function and even of its integrity. This interdependence of body components is mediated by the communication systems of the body: exchange of substances via circulating blood and other body fluids and exchange of nerve impulses and neurotransmitters through the nervous system.

The circulatory and nervous systems also mediate the regulation and coordination of cellular, tissue, and organ functions and thus the maintenance of the integrity of the body as a whole. The organized and integrated collaboration of the body components is reflected in the concept of homeostasis, the maintenance of the relative constancy of the internal environment in which all the cells live and function.

In view of this interdependence and exchange of influences, it is inevitable that dysfunction or failure of a major body component will adversely affect the competence of other organs and tissues and, therefore, one's health.

The Person

Important and valid as is the concept of body unity, it is incomplete in that it is, by implication, limited to the physical realm. Physicians minister not to bodies but to individuals, each of whom is unique by virtue of his or her genetic endowment, personal history, and the variety of environments in which that history has been lived.

The person, obviously, is more than a body, for the person has a mind, also the product of heredity and biography. Separation of body and mind, whether conceptually or in practice, is an anachronistic remnant of such dualistic thinking as that of the 17th century philosopher-scientist, René Descartes. It was his belief that body and mind are separate domains, one publicly visible and palpable, the other invisible, impalpable, and private. This dualistic concept is anachronistic because, while it is almost universally rejected as a concept, it is still acted out in much of clinical practice and in biomedical research.

Clinical and biomedical research (as well as everyday experience) has irrefutably shown that body and mind are so inseparable, so pervasive to each other, that they can be regarded—and treated—as a single entity. It is now widely recognized (whether or not it is demonstrated in practice) that what goes on (or goes wrong) in either body or mind has repercussions in the other. It is for reasons such as these that I prefer unity of the person to unity of the body, conveying totally integrated humanity and individuality.

The Person as Context

Phenomena assigned to mind (consciousness, thought, feelings, beliefs, attitudes, etc.) have their physiological and behavioral counterparts; conversely, bodily and behavioral changes have psychological concomitants, such as altered feelings and perceptions. It must be noted, however, that it is the person who is feeling, perceiving, and responding not the body or the mind. It is you who feels well, ill, happy, or sad, and not your body or mind. What goes on in body and mind is conditioned by who the person is and their entire history.

In short, the person is far more than the union of body and mind, in the same sense that water is more than the union of hydrogen and oxygen. Nothing that we know about either oxygen or hydrogen accounts for the three states of water (liquid, solid, and gas), their respective properties, the boiling and freezing points, viscosity, and so forth. Water incorporates yet transcends oxygen and hydrogen. To understand water we must study water and not only its components. In the same way, at an enormously more complex level, the person comprises yet transcends body and mind.

Moreover, once hydrogen and oxygen are joined to form water, they become subject to the laws that govern water. In the same but infinitely more complex sense, it is you who makes up your mind, changes your mind, trains and enriches your mind, and puts it to work. It is you who determines from moment to moment whether and in what way you will express, through your body, what is in or on your mind.

Thus the person is the context, the environment, in which all the body parts live and function and in which the mind finds expression. Everything about the person—genetics, history from conception to the present moment, nutrition, use and abuse of body and mind, parental and school conditioning, physical and sociocultural environments, and so on—enters into determining the quality of physical and mental function. The better the quality of the environment provided by the person for the mental and bodily components, the better they will function. For example, someone who has a peptic ulcer is not ill because of the ulcer. The ulcer exists because of an unfavorable internal environment.

In conclusion, just as the proper study of mankind is man (Alexander Pope), so is the study of human health and illness also man. As will become evident, the principle of the unity of the person leads us naturally to the next principle.

THE PLACE OF THE MUSCULOSKELETAL SYSTEM IN HUMAN LIFE

The Means of Expression of Our Humanity and Individuality

Structure determines function, structure and function are reciprocally interrelated, and similar aphorisms have traditionally represented another osteopathic principle. That principle recognizes the special place of the musculoskeletal system among the body systems and its relation to the health of the person. We examine now the basis for the osteopathic emphasis on the musculoskeletal system in total health care.

Human life is expressed in human behavior, in humans doing the things that humans do. And whatever humans do, they do with the musculoskeletal system. That system is the ultimate instrument for carrying out human action and behavior. It is the means through which we manifest our human qualities and our personal uniqueness—personality, intellect, imagination, creativity, perceptions, love, compassion, values, and philosophies. The most noble ethical, moral, or religious principle has value only insofar as it can be overtly expressed through behavior.

That expression is made possible by the coordinated contractions and relaxations of striated muscles, most of them acting upon bones and joints. The musculoskeletal system is the means through which we communicate with each other, whether it be by written, spoken, or signed language, or by gesture or facial expression. Agriculture, industry, technology, literature, the arts and sciences—our very civilization—are the products of human action, interaction, communication, and behavior, that is, by the orchestrated contractions and relaxations of the body's musculature.

Relation to the Body Economy

The musculoskeletal system is the most massive system in the community of body systems. Its muscular components are collectively the largest consumer in the body economy. This is true not only because of their mass, but because of their high energy requirements. Furthermore, those requirements may vary widely from moment to moment according to what the person is doing, with what feelings and in what environments.

The high and varying metabolic requirements of the musculoskeletal system are met by the cardiovascular, respiratory, digestive, renal, and other visceral systems. Together, they supply the required fuels and nutrients, remove the products of metabolism, and control the composition and physical properties of the internal environment. In servicing the musculoskeletal system in this manner, these organ systems are at the same time servicing each other (and, of course, the nervous system).

The nervous system is also, to a great degree, occupied with the musculoskeletal system, that is, with behavior and motor control.

Indeed, most of the fibers in the spinal nerves are those converging impulses to and from the muscles and other components of the musculoskeletal system. In addition, the nervous system, its autonomic components, and the circulatory system mediate communication and exchange of signals and substances between the soma and the viscera. In this way, visceral, metabolic, and endocrine activity is continually tuned to moment-to-moment requirements of the musculoskeletal system, that is, to what the person is doing from moment to moment.

Consequences of Visceral Dysfunction

Impairment or failure of some visceral function or of communication between the musculoskeletal system and the viscera is reflected in the musculoskeletal system. When the resulting dysfunction is severe and diffuse, motor activity and even maintenance of posture are difficult or impossible and automatically imposed.

The Musculoskeletal System as Source of Adverse Influences on Other Systems

In view of the rich afferent input of the musculoskeletal system into the central nervous system and its rich interchange of substances with other systems through the body fluids, it is inevitable that structural and functional disturbances in the musculoskeletal system will have repercussions elsewhere in the body.

Such structural and functional disturbances may be of postural, traumatic, or behavioral origin (neglect, misuse, or abuse by the person). Further, it must be appreciated that the human framework is, compared with other (quadruped) mammals, uniquely unstable and vulnerable to compressive, torsional, and shearing forces, because of the vertical configuration, higher center of gravity, and the comparatively small, bipedal base.

The human musculoskeletal system, therefore, is the frequent source of aberrant afferent input to the central nervous system and its autonomic distribution, with at least potential consequences to visceral function. Which organs, blood vessels, etc. are at risk is determined by the site of the musculoskeletal dysfunction and the part(s) of the central nervous system, (e.g., spinal segments) into which it discharges its sensory impulses.

When a dysfunction or pathology has developed in a visceral organ, that disturbance is reflected in segmentally related somatic tissues. Viscus and soma become linked in a vicious circle of afferent and efferent impulses, which sustain and exacerbate the disturbance. Appropriate treatment of the somatic component reduces its input to the vicious circle and may even interrupt that circle with therapeutic effect.

Importance of the Personal Context

Whether or not visceral or vasomotor consequences of somatic dysfunction occur, and with what consequences to the person, depends on other factors in the person's life, such as the genetic, nutritional, psychological, behavioral, sociocultural, and environmental. As research has shown, however, the presence of somatic dysfunction and the accompanying reflex and neurotrophic effects exaggerate the impact of other detrimental factors on the person's health. Effective treatment of the musculoskeletal dysfunction shields the patient by reducing the deleterious effects of the other factors. Such treatment, therefore, has preventive as well as therapeutic benefits.

Such treatment directed to the musculoskeletal system assumes even greater and often crucial significance when it is recognized that the other kinds of harmful factors, such as those enumerated above, are not readily subject to change and may even require social or governmental intervention. The musculoskeletal system, however, is readily accessible and responsive to osteopathic manipulative treatment. I view these considerations as the rationale for osteopathic manipulative treatment and its strategic role in total health care.

Finally, the osteopathic philosophy and the unity of the person concept enjoins the physician to treat the patient as a whole and not merely the affected parts. Hence, appropriate corrective attention should also be given to other significant risk factors that are subject to change by both patient and physician.

OUR PERSONAL HEALTH CARE SYSTEMS

The Natural Healing Power

Appreciation, even in ancient times, of our inherent recuperative, restorative, and rehabilitative powers is reflected in the Latin phrase, *vis medicatrix naturae* (nature's healing force). We recover from illnesses, fevers drop, blood clots and wounds heal, broken bones reunite, infections are overcome, skin eruptions clear up, and even cancers are known to occasionally undergo spontaneous remission. But miraculous as is the healing power (and appreciated as it was until we became more impressed by human-made miracles and breakthroughs), the other, more recently revealed components of the health care system with which each of us is endowed are no less marvelous.

The Component System That Defends against Threats from Without

This component includes, among others, immune mechanisms that defend us against the enormous variety and potency of foreign organisms that invade our bodies, wreaking damage and even bringing death. These same immune mechanisms guard us against those of our own cells that become foreign and malignant as the result of mutation. Included also are the mechanisms that defend against foreign and poisonous substances that we may take in with our food and drink or that enter through the skin and lungs, by disarming them, converting them to innocuous substances, and eliminating them from the body. They defend us (until overwhelmed) even against the toxic substances that we ourselves introduce into the atmosphere, soil, water, or more directly into our own bodies.

Mechanisms That Defend against Changes in the Internal Environment

We humans are exposed to, and adapt to, wide variations in physical and chemical properties of our environment (e.g., temperature, barometric pressure, oxygen, and carbon dioxide concen-

trations) and sustain ourselves with chemically diverse food and drink. But the cells of our body can function and survive only in the internal environment of interstitial fluids which maintain body functions within relatively narrow limits as regards variations in chemical composition, temperature, tissue, osmotic pressure, pH, etc.

This phenomenon, called homeostasis, is based on thousands of simultaneously dynamic equilibria occurring throughout the body. Examples include rates of energy consumption and replenishment by the cells. Homeostasis constancy and quick restoration of constancy must be accomplished regardless of the variations in the external environment, composition of food and drink, and the moment-to-moment activities of the person. It is accomplished by an enormously complex array of regulatory mechanisms that continually monitor and control respiratory, circulatory, digestive, renal, metabolic, and countless other functions and processes. Maintenance of optimal environments for cellular function is essential to health. The homeostatic mechanisms may, therefore, be viewed as the health maintenance system of the body.

Commentary

These, then are the three major components of our indwelling health care system, each comprising numerous component systems. In the order in which humans became aware of them, they are (a) the healing (remedial, curative, palliative, recuperative, rehabilitative) component; (b) the component that defends against threats from the external environment; and (c) the homeostatic, health-maintaining component. These major component systems, of course, share subcomponents and mechanisms.

When the internal health care system is permitted to operate optimally, without impediment, its product is what we call health. Its natural tendency is always toward health and the recovery of health. Indeed, the personal health care system is the very source of health, upon which all externally applied measures depend for their beneficial effects. The internal health care system, in effect, makes its own diagnoses, issues its own prescriptions, draws upon its own vast pharmacy, and in most situations, administers each dose without side effects.

Health and healing, therefore, come from within. It is the patient who gets well, and not the practitioner or the treatment that makes them well.

THE THREE PRINCIPLES AS GUIDES TO MEDICAL PRACTICE

The Unity of the Person

In caring for the whole person, the well-grounded osteopathic physician goes beyond the presenting complaint, beyond relief of symptoms, beyond identification of the disease and treatment of the impaired organ, malfunction, or pathology, important as they are to total care. The osteopathic physician also explores those factors in the person and the person's life that may have contributed to the illness and that, appropriately modified, compensated, or eliminated, would favor recovery, prevent recurrence, and improve health in general.

The physician then selects that factor or combination of factors that are readily subject to change and that would be of sufficient impact to shift the balance toward recovery and enhancement of health. The possible factors include such categories as the biological (e.g., genetic, nutritional), psychological, behavioral (use, neglect, or abuse of body and mind; interpersonal relationships; habits; etc.), sociocultural, occupational, and environmental. Some of these factors, especially some of the biological, are responsive to appropriate clinical intervention, some are responsive only to social or governmental action, and still others require changes by patients themselves. Osteopathic whole-person care, therefore, is a collaborative relationship between patient and physician.

The Place of the Musculoskeletal System in Human Biology and Behavior: The Strategic Role of Osteopathic Manipulative Treatment

It is obvious that some of the most deleterious factors are difficult or impossible for patient and physician to change or eliminate. These include (at least at present) genetic factors (although some inherited predispositions can be mitigated by lifestyle change). They include also such items as social convention, lifelong habits (e.g., dietary and behavioral), widely shared beliefs, prejudices, misconceptions and cultural doctrines, attitudes, and values. Others, such as the quality of the physical or socioeconomic environments, may require concerted community, national, and even international action.

Focus falls, therefore, upon those deleterious factors that are favorably modifiable by personal and professional action, and that, when appropriately modified or eliminated, mitigate the health-impairing effects of the less changeable factors. Improvement of body mechanics by osteopathic manipulative treatment is a major consideration when dealing with these complex interactions.

OUR PERSONAL HEALTH CARE SYSTEMS

This principle has important implications for the respective responsibilities of patient and physician and for their relationship. Since each person is the owner and hence the guardian of his or her own personal health care system, the ultimate source of health and healing, the primary responsibility for one's health is each individual's. That responsibility is met by the way the person lives, thinks, behaves, nourishes himself or herself, uses body and mind, relates to others, and the other factor usually called lifestyle. Each person must be taught and enabled to assume that responsibility.

It is the physician's responsibility, while giving palliative and remedial attention to the patient's immediate problem, to support each patient's internal health care system, to remove impediments to its competence, and above all, to do it no harm. It is also the responsibility of physicians to instruct patients on how to do the same for themselves and to strive to motivate them to do so, especially by their own example.

The relationship between patient and osteopathic physician is therefore a collaborative one, a partnership, in maintaining and enhancing the competence of the patient's personal health care system. The maintenance and enhancement of health is the most effective and comprehensive form of preventive medicine, for health is the best defense against disease. As stated by A.T. Still, "To find health should be the object of the doctor. Anyone can find disease."

Relevance to the Current and Future Health of the Nation

The preventive strategy of health maintenance and health enhancement, intrinsic to the osteopathic philosophy, is urgently needed by our society today. One of the greatest burdens on the nation's health care system and on the national economy is in the care of victims of the chronic degenerative diseases, such as heart disease, cancer, stroke, and arthritis, which require long-term care.

The incidence of these diseases has increased and will continue to increase well into the next century as the average age of our population continues to increase. The widely accepted (but usually unspoken) assumption that guides current practice (and national policy) is that the chronic degenerative diseases are an inevitable aspect of the aging process; that is, that aging is itself pathological. It is now increasingly apparent, however, that the increase of their incidence with age is because the longer one lives, the greater the toll taken by minor, seemingly inconsequential, inconspicuous, treatable impairments and modifiable contributing factors in and around the person. They are, therefore, largely the natural culmination of less-than-favorable lifestyles, and, hence, they are largely preventable.

The great national tragedy is that, while the nation's health care system is so extensively and expensively absorbed in the care of millions of older adult victims of chronic disease (at per capita cost 3.5 times that of persons under the age of 65 years), tens of millions of younger people and children are living on and embarking on life paths that will culminate in the same diseases. The health care system simply must move upstream to move people from pathogenic to salutary paths. And the osteopathic profession can show the way.

The osteopathic profession has a historic opportunity to make an enormous contribution to the enhancement of the health of our nation. It can do this by giving leadership in addressing this great tragedy by bringing its basic strategy of whole-person, health-oriented care to bear on the problem and demonstrating its effectiveness in practice.

Having reviewed and enlarged on the principles of osteopathic medicine, their meaning, biological foundations, and clinical implications, it seems appropriate to propose a definition of osteopathic medicine. The author offers the following: Osteopathic medicine is a system of medicine that is based on the continually deepening and expanding understanding of (a) human nature; (b) those components of human biology that are centrally relevant to health, namely the inherent regulatory, protective, regenerative, and recuperative biological mechanisms, whose combined effect is consistently in the direction of the maintenance, enhancement, and recovery of health; and (c) the factors in and around the person that both favorably and unfavorably affect those mechanisms.

The practice of osteopathic medicine is, essentially, the potentiation of the intrinsic health-maintaining and health-restoring resources of the individual. The methods and agents employed are those that are effective in enhancing the favorable factors and diminishing or eliminating the unfavorable factors affecting each individual. Osteopathic medical practice necessarily includes the application of palliative and remedial measures, but always on the condition that they do no harm to the patient's own health-maintaining and health-restoring resources. This stipulation governing the choice of methods and agents is based on the recognition that all therapeutic methods depend on the patient's own recuperative power for their effectiveness and are valueless without it and that health and the recovery of health come from within.

The art and science of osteopathic medicine are expressed in the identification and selection of those factors in each individual that are accessible and amenable to change and that, when changed, would most decisively potentate the person on health-supporting resources.

Osteopathic physicians give special emphasis to factors originating in the musculoskeletal system, for the following reasons:

1. The vertical human framework (a) is highly vulnerable to compressive (gravitational), torsional, and shearing forces, and (b) encases the entire central nervous system.

2. Since the massive, energy-demanding system has rich two-way communication with all other body systems, it is, because of its vulnerability, a common and frequent source of impediments to the functions of other systems.

3. These impediments exaggerate the physiological impact of other detrimental factors in the person's life, and, through the central nervous system, focus it on specific organs and tissues.

4. The musculoskeletal impediments (somatic dysfunctions) are readily accessible to the hands and responsive to the manipulative and other methods developed and refined by the osteopathic medical profession.

REFERENCES

1. Trowbridge C. *Andrew Taylor Still.* Kirksville, MO: Thomas Jefferson University Press, Northeast Missouri State University; 1991:95–140.
2. Still AT. *Autobiography of Andrew T. Still.* Rev ed. Kirksville, MO: Published by the author; 1908. Distributed, Indianapolis: American Academy of Osteopathy.
3. Still AT. *Osteopathy Research and Practice.* Seattle, WA: Eastland Press; 1992. Originally published by the author; 1910.
4. Still CE Jr. *Frontier Doctor Medical Pioneer.* Kirksville, MO: Thomas Jefferson University Press, Northeast Missouri State University; 1991.
5. Hildreth AG. *The Lengthening Shadow of Dr. Andrew Taylor Still.* Macon, MO: Privately published, 1942. Reprinted and distributed, Kirksville, Mo: Osteopathic Enterprises, Inc.
6. Still AT. *The Philosophy and Mechanical Principles of Osteopathy.* Original copyright by the author, Kirksville, Mo: 1892. Then, Kansas City, Mo: 1902. Reprinted, Kirksville, MO: Osteopathic Enterprises; 1986.
7. Still AT. *Philosophy of Osteopathy.* Kirksville, MO: 1899. Reprinted, Academy of Applied Osteopathy, Carmel, CA;1946.
8. Booth ER. Summation of causes in disease and death. *J Am Osteopath Assoc.* 1902;2(2):33–41.
9. Lyne ST. Osteopathic philosophy of the cause of disease. *J Am Osteopath Assoc.* 1904;3(12):395–403. Reprinted in *J Am Osteopath Assoc.* 2000; 100(3):181–189.
10. Littlejohn JM. Osteopathy: an independent system co-extensive with the science and art of healing. *J Am Osteopath Assoc.* 1901;vol 1. Reprinted in *J Am Osteopath Assoc.* 2000;100(1):14–26.
11. Lane MA. *Dr. A.T. Still. Founder of Osteopathy.* Chicago, IL: The Osteopathic Publishing Co; 1918.
12. Hulett GD. *A Text Book of the Principles of Osteopathy,* 5th ed. Pasadena, CA: A.T. Still Research Institute; 1922.
13. Schnucker RV, ed. *Early Osteopathy: In the Words of A.T. Still.* Kirksville, MO: Thomas Jefferson University Press, Northeast Missouri State University; 1991.
14. Littlejohn JM. The physiological basis of the therapeutic law. *J Sci Osteopath.* 1902;3(4).
15. Downing CH. *Osteopathic Principles in Disease.* Originally published, San Francisco, CA: Ricardo J. Orozco; 1935. Reprinted and published, Newark, OH: American Academy of Osteopathy; 1988.
16. Page LE. *Principles of Osteopathy.* Kansas City, MO: Academy of Applied Osteopathy; 1952.
17. Korr IM. The osteopathic role in medical evolution. *The DO.* 1973;(Nov).
18. Northup GW. *Osteopathic Medicine; An American Reformation.* Chicago, IL: American Osteopathic Association; 1979.
19. Hulett CMT. Relation of osteopathy to other systems. *J Am Osteopath Assoc.* 1901;1: 227–233.
20. Schiötz, EH and Cyriax, J. *Manipulation. Past and Present.* London, England: William Heinemann Medical Books, Ltd; 1975.
21. Lomax E. Manipulative therapy: a historical perspective from ancient times to the modern era. In: Goldstein M, ed. *The Research Status of Spinal Manipulative Therapy,* Bethesda, MD: U.S. Dept. of Health, Education and Welfare; 1975:11–17. NIH publication 76–998.
22. Adams F. *The Genuine Works of Hippocrates.* First published his translation in 1849, then again in 1886, and again in 1929. However, the published editions that are usually available today were published in Philadelphia, PA: Williams & Wilkins; 1939.
23. Harris JD, McPartland JM. Historical perspectives of manual medicine. In: Stanton DF, Mein EA, eds. *Physical Med Rehabil Clin North Am.* 1996;7(4): 679–692.
24. Burns L. *Pathogenesis of Visceral Disease Following Vertebral Lesions.* Chicago, IL: American Osteopathic Association; 1948.
25. Beal MC, ed. *The Cole Book of Papers Selected From the Writings and Lectures of Wilbur V. Cole, D.O., F.A.A.O.* Newark, OH: American Academy of Osteopathy; also see Hoag JM, Cole WV, Bradford SG, eds. *Osteopathic Medicine.* New York, NY: McGraw-Hill; 1969.
26. Beal MC, ed. *Selected Papers of John Stedman Denslow, DO.* Indianapolis, IN: American Academy of Osteopathy; 1993.
27. Korr IM. *The Neurobiologic Mechanisms of Manipulative Therapy.* New York, NY: Plenum Press; 1977.
28. Peterson B, ed. *The Collected Papers of Irvin M. Korr.* Colorado Springs, CO: The American Academy of Osteopathy (currently in Indianapolis, IN); 1979.
29. Jones JM. Osteopathic philosophy. In: Gallagher RM, Humphrey FJ. eds. *Osteopathic Medicine: A Reformation in Progress.* New York, NY: Churchill Livingstone; 2001.
30. McConnell CP, Teall CC. *The Practice of Osteopathy,* 3rd ed. Kirksville, MO: The Journal Printing Co, 1906.
31. Tasker D. *Principles of Osteopathy.* Los Angeles, CA: Baumgardt Publishing Co; 1903.
32. Burns L. *Studies in the Osteopathic Sciences; Basic Principles,* Vol I. Los Angeles, CA: Occident Printery; 1907.
33. Downing CH. *Principles and Practice of Osteopathy.* Kansas City, MO: Williams Publishing Co; 1923.
34. Barber E. *Osteopathy Complete.* Kansas City, MO: Hudson-Kimberly Publishing; 1898.
35. Booth ER. *History of Osteopathy and Twentieth Century Medical Practice.* Cincinnati, OH: Jennings and Graham, 1905.
36. Hildreth AG. *The Lengthening Shadow of Andrew Taylor Still.* Macon, MO and Paw Paw, MI: Privately published by Mrs. AG Hildreth and Mrs. AE Van Vleck; 1942.
37. College of Osteopathic Physician and Surgeons documents, 1948. University of California at Irvine, Library Archives, Special Collections.
38. Special Committee on Osteopathic Principles and Osteopathic Technic,

Kirksville College of Osteopathy and Surgery. An interpretation of the osteopathic concept. Tentative formulation of a teaching guide for faculty, hospital staff and student body. *J Osteopath.* 1953;60(10):7–10.

39. Felton DL. Neural influence on immune responses: underlying suppositions and basic principles of neural-immune signaling. *Prog Brain Res.* 2000(122), Ch. 27.

40. Pert CB. *Molecules of Emotion: The Science Behind Mind-Body Medicine.* New York, NY: Touchstone, Simon and Schuster; 1997.

41. Damasio A. *The Feeling of What Happens: Body and Emotion in the Making of Consciousness.* New York, NY: Harcourt; 1999.

42. Dossey L. *Prayer Is Good Medicine: How to Reap the Healing Benefits of Prayer.* San Francisco, CA: HarperCollins; 1996.

43. Seffinger MA. Development of osteopathic philosophy. In Ward RC, exec ed. *Foundations for Osteopathic Medicine.* Baltimore: Williams & Wilkins; 1997:3–7.

44. Korr IM. An explication of osteopathic principles. In Ward RC, exec ed. *Foundations for Osteopathic Medicine.* Baltimore: Williams & Wilkins; 1997:7–12.

45. Ward R, Sprafka S. Glossary of osteopathic terminology. *J Am Osteopathic Assoc.* 1981;80(8):552–567.

46. Rogers FJ, D'Alonzo GE, Glover J, Korr IM, et al. Proposed tenets of osteopathic medicine and principles for patient care. *J Am Osteopath Assoc.* 2002;102(2):63–65.

47. Educational Council on Osteopathic Principles. Core Curriculum Outline. Washington, DC: American Association of Colleges of Osteopathic Medicine; 1987.

MAJOR EVENTS IN OSTEOPATHIC HISTORY

BARBARA E. PETERSON

KEY CONCEPTS

- Beginnings of osteopathic medicine
- Growth of the osteopathic profession
- Educational issues
- Areas of conflict and agreement with allopathic medicine
- Osteopathic professional organizations
- Recognition by state and federal governments
- Role in specialties, hospitals, and primary care

Osteopathic medicine has from its beginning been a profession based on ideas, tenets that have lasted through all sorts of adversity and have been credited with bringing the profession to its present level of success. The previous chapter outlines in some detail the growth of these ideas. It is perhaps significant that the profession's founder never wrote clinical manuals, only books of philosophy (1–4).

It is striking that these ideas, still quoted extensively today (5), came not from universities or medical centers, but from the creative problem solving of an informally educated American frontier doctor named Andrew Taylor Still. Looking back more than a century, it seems surprising that his ideas were so controversial when first put forward. But perhaps history has caught up with this eccentric, inventive man.

The story of Andrew Taylor Still is worth knowing in detail but must be told superficially.

He was born in a log cabin in Virginia in 1828, the year Andrew Jackson was elected president. Still's family were farmers, as most people were then; his father was also a Methodist circuit rider who preached and treated people's ills. He later would teach his five sons to be doctors in the usual frontier apprentice system of the time.

Still's mother came from a family that was nearly all wiped out by a Shawnee Indian massacre (6), and it must have seemed a supreme irony when in 1851 she and her husband moved to Kansas as missionaries to the descendants of these same Indians. However, the family course first took them to Tennessee and then to Missouri, where they also were frontier missionaries.

Andrew Still had the sketchy education of a frontier child (3), but he was an inventive person, and he liked to read. Eventually he would become familiar with many of the major practical and ideological trends of his time. But learning to survive had to come first; Missouri and Kansas were true frontiers. The Stills first eked out a living by hunting for food and making some of their clothes from animal skins. The family also plowed their land claim and established a farm while the father rode a circuit among scattered settlers, ministering to minds and bodies. It was a lifestyle that gave substance to the word "survivor" (7).

Andrew Still would later say how important animal dissection had been as a preparation for study of human anatomy. He also recorded another prophetic childhood experience in his *Autobiography*:

One day, when about ten years old, I suffered from a headache. I made a swing of my father's plow-line between two trees; but my head hurt too much to make swinging comfortable, so I let the rope down to about eight or ten inches of the ground, threw the end of a blanket on it, and I lay down on the ground and used the rope for a swinging pillow. Thus I lay stretched on my back, with my neck across the rope. Soon I became easy and went to sleep, got up in a little while with the headache gone. As I knew nothing of anatomy at this time, I took no thought of how a rope could stop headache and the sick stomach which accompanied it. After that discovery I roped my neck whenever I felt one of those spells coming on (3).

To the end of his life, Still continued to "rope his neck" (see Fig. 1.1). In his old age he would lie down daily with his neck on a version of a Chinese pillow, known among country folk as a "saint's rest"—a wooden frame with a leather strap suspended across it—giving the same effect as a plow rope suspended between two trees. In his middle years he discovered other crude but effective methods for self-treatment, notably a croquet ball, upon which he lay down at the correct point when the problem was in his back rather than his neck (8).

In the 1840s the issue of slavery divided the Methodist church, and the Stills stayed with the northern (abolitionist) branch. By the early 1850s, most of the family had moved to Kansas, including Andrew and his young wife. At that time Andrew began seriously to read and practice medicine with his father. They gave the Indians "such drugs as white men used [and] cured most of the cases [they] met" (3).

In 1855 the government forced the Shawnees further west, and Kansas became a virtual war zone, as both abolitionist and pro-slavery settlers rushed in. The fate of Kansas as a free state depended on a popular vote. The Stills chose to be active abolitionists. Still recalled:

> I could not do otherwise, for no man can have delegated to him by statute a just right to any man's liberty, either on account of race or color. With these truths before me I entered all combats for the abolition of slavery at home and abroad, and soon had a host of bitter political enemies, which resulted in many thrilling and curious adventures (3).

The Stills met John Brown and fought under the command of Jim Lane, two of the abolitionist leaders active on the western frontier. There are numerous stories of "abolitionist encounters" during the pre-Civil War days (9–11). The struggle lasted, said Still, until Abraham Lincoln "wrote the golden words: 'Forever free, without regard to race or color.' I will add—or sex" (3).

The territorial political situation was volatile and confusing, with even the elections seemingly decided by gun battles. There are many accounts of "bloody Kansas" in the pre-Civil War period, including those in early osteopathic writings. But somehow a free-state legislature was elected in 1857, and Andrew Still was a proud member of that group (12).

Andrew Still's first wife, née Mary Margaret Vaughn, died in 1859, leaving three children. In late 1860 Still married a young schoolteacher, who had learned to mix prescriptions for her physician father and who was prepared by her background to accept Still's medical and spiritual speculations (9). It was a most important partnership; Mary Elvira Turner Still was to support her husband and family through the long period of doubt and disgrace that preceded successful establishment of the osteopathic profession, and again through the heady days of unexpected success. But all this was in the future.

When the Civil War officially began, Andrew Still enlisted first in a cavalry division of a force assigned to Jim Lane. Later he organized a company of Kansas militia, which was in turn consolidated with other militia battalions. He was commissioned a major and saw active combat; some experiences are recounted in his *Autobiography* (3). He also served as a military surgeon, though he had been listed as a hospital steward on the official record (13). His unit was disbanded in October 1864, and Still went home to resume normal civilian life.

It was not exactly a joyful homecoming. In February 1864 three Still children had died of cerebrospinal meningitis, despite the best efforts of the physicians called to help. All around him, Still saw people who had become addicted to alcohol or morphine, and he considered that these were "habits, customs, and traditions no better than slavery in its worst days" (3).

Mainstream Civil War medicine still depended heavily on purging, bloodletting, and an armamentarium of medicines that could only be characterized as violent. On both sides there were many more casualties from sickness than from battle injuries (14). A history of American medicine recounts:

> Even the most erudite and experienced physician had few effective medicines at his command. Some of those which were effective were unknown to the poorly educated practitioner; others he knew not how to use. The short list of effective agents in the 1870s included

the anesthetics (ether, chloroform, and nitrous oxide); opium and its alkaloids (morphine was first used extensively during the Civil War to ease the pain of the wounded); digitalis, which was used chiefly for cardiac edema [congestive heart failure]; ergot, to stimulate uterine contractions and to control postpartum hemorrhage; mercury in the form of an inunction for syphilis and in the form of calomel to purge and salivate; various cathartics of botanical origin; iron, usually in the form of Blaud's pills for anemia; quinine for malaria; amyl nitrite, which was first recommended for the relief of angina pectoris by Sir Thomas Lauder Brunton in 1867 but was still not well known in 1876; sulfur ointment for the itch (scabies); green vegetables or citrus fruit for the prevention or treatment of scurvy. These various medicines were administered either by mouth, by rectum, by inhalation, or by application to the skin. The hypodermic syringe had been introduced by the French surgeon Pravaz in 1851. He employed it to inject "chloride of iron" into vascular tumors to coagulate their contents. Although it was subsequently used for other restricted purposes, the danger of infection limited its use until the physician had learned how to prevent infections by the preparation of sterile solutions (15).

This description of the *best* of the armamentarium available was recorded about a decade after the Civil War. The urban populations certainly benefited most from these breakthroughs; frontier doctors and their patients were very much worse off. Still agonized over the situation:

> My sleep was well nigh ruined; by day and night I saw legions of men and women staggering to and fro, all over the land, crying for freedom from habits of drugs and drink.... I dreamed of the dead and dying who were and had been slaves of habit. I sought to know the cause of so much death, bondage, and distress among my race.... I who had had some experience in alleviating pain found medicine a failure. Since my early life I had been a student of nature's book. In my early days in windswept Kansas I had devoted my attention to the study of anatomy. I became a robber in the name of science. Indian graves were desecrated and the bodies of the sleeping dead exhumed in the name of science. Yes, I grew to be one of those vultures with the scalpel, and studied the dead that the living might be benefited. I had printed books, but went back to the great book of nature as my chief study (3).

He also wrote that he attended a course of lectures at a Kansas City medical school that was long defunct at the time of writing (16).

The next decade of Still's life was devoted to a search for a better way. He farmed, and he invented a butter churn and a version of a grain reaper. More children were born, the sons and daughter who would eventually become prominent in the profession their father was soon to found.

The search for a better way had many potential bypaths. The post-Civil War period was a time of great diversity in the healing professions, both in terms of how one became identified as a physician and how one approached the practice (17). In the mid-19th century there were no licensing boards and only scattered state laws governing medical practice. There were a few medical schools, but there were no standard curricula. Most physicians, especially on the frontiers, were trained as apprentices, doing some reading and serving as a physician's assistant for an unstated length of time.

A majority of physicians followed a standard pattern, heavily influenced by the "heroic medicine" of Benjamin Rush, who said that "there is but one disease in the world," and that it was treatable by "depletion," which translated as blood-letting, blistering, and purging. One influential textbook writer, John Esten Cooke, wrote that:

> All diseases, particularly fevers, arose from cold or malaria, which weakened the heart and thus produced an accumulation of blood in the vena cavae and in the adjoining large veins of the liver. Consequently, calomel and other cathartics which acted on that organ were the cure. "If calomel did not salivate and opium did not constipate, there is no telling what we could do in the practice of physic" (18).

Calomel and other mercury compounds were still listed as late as 1899 in the first Merck's manual, along with opium and morphine and many alcohol-based compounds (19). The practice of "heroic" dosing was well established and well defended. By the time of the Civil War, the system was also called "allopathy," now defined as "that system of therapeutics in which diseases are treated by producing a condition incompatible with or antagonistic to the condition to be cured or alleviated" (20).

The damage caused by the "heroic" techniques was obvious to thinkers before Still, and there were alternative systems of medicine available for consideration. Home remedies and Indian herbal preparations were a basic choice, and this lore was substantial and widely used (18). Numerous resources for botanic preparations were available as well; many of these manuals were widely circulated.

Homeopathy was a major influence in the 19th century. Articulated by Samuel Hahnemann (1755–1843), it was a system of therapy in which "diseases are treated by drugs which are capable of producing in healthy persons symptoms like those of the disease to be treated, the drug being administered in minute doses" (20,21). Eclecticism was another choice, described as "a once popular system of medicine which treats diseases by the application of single remedies to known pathologic conditions, without reference to nosology, special attention being given to developing indigenous plant remedies" (17). Magnetic healing, which "combined spiritualism and healing by seeking to restore the balance of an invisible magnetic fluid circulating throughout the body" (17), and its variants that attempted to use electrical current to restore health were employed. The water cure, movements emphasizing hygiene, anti-alcoholism or temperance, fresh air and sunlight, nutritional programs, and physical education, and popular versions of mental healing, including hypnotism, spiritualism (table rapping), and phrenology were additional alternatives. And, there were the bone-setters.

At least two of these methods attracted A.T. Still and he linked his name to each for a time. A professional card in the Still Museum in Kirksville, Missouri, identifies Still as a "lightning bonesetter." In 1874 he advertised himself in Kirksville as a "magnetic healer," possibly because he was persuaded by "the metaphor of the harmonious balance of the interaction of body parts and the unobstructed flow of body fluids" (17).

After a decade of study, in 1874, Still "flung to the breeze the banner of osteopathy" (3). He did not say precisely what that meant—perhaps a decision, perhaps a sudden coming together of creative thought—but it was followed by attempts to present his findings at Baker University, an institution his family had helped to found (22). He could not get a hearing. Further, he was ejected from the Methodist church on the basis that only Christ was allowed to heal by the laying of hands. Still's description of that experience makes it clear that his "laying on of hands" was therapeutic manipulation.

During the next year Still spent some time with his brother, who had become addicted to morphine through medical treatment. This experience, added to the uselessness of medications in saving his family and others, roused in Still a hatred for the drugs of the day. This enmity sometimes appeared to be nearly absolute, even when the armamentarium of drugs began to move from harmful toward helpful (1–4,23). However, there is evidence in his own writings that he sometimes used topical medications. For example, for snakebites, he washed the wounds with spirits of ammonia, and washed areas bitten by a dog with hydrophobia/rabies with a diluted sulfuric acid solution, and used alcohol to wash a spasmodic tetanic joint (4).

Late in 1875 Still moved from Kansas to Kirksville, Missouri, where he spent the rest of his life. For several years Still used Kirksville as a base to conduct a marginal itinerant practice (24). His practice evolved as he gained experience, so that the main treatment modality became manipulation. Although this treatment included some of the traditions of magnetic healing and bone setting, it emphasized detailed knowledge of anatomy and body mechanics so that treatment could be said to restore normal function. He held that the body is an efficient chemical laboratory that, in health, makes all the "drugs" it naturally needs. The object of treatment was to discover what caused the sickness and remove the interference so that the body could heal itself (2).

By 1887 enough patients came to Kirksville so that Still could stop his itinerant practice. Word of dramatic successful outcomes began to spread via the newspapers and word of mouth, and once that happened, the burden of practice quickly became heavy. Still began to think about teaching others his methods; unlike many alternative practitioners of his day, he never intended to keep therapeutic secrets to himself or to grow rich from his methods. There were abortive attempts first to train apprentices and then to teach a class of operators to assist in the practice of osteopathy. The attempts were unsuccessful largely because the students lacked Still's detailed knowledge of anatomy and bodily function.

The term "osteopathy" was coined by Still in about 1889. The story is told (25) that when challenged because this word was not in the dictionary, Still replied, "We are going to put it there." The word became for Still and his followers a symbol for medical reform, for a science that would refocus medicine on the restoration of normal function. Osteopathy aimed to work with and facilitate the natural machinery of the body for normal and reparative function, rather than working against it, as seemed to be the case with purgatives, emetics, bloodletting, and addictive drugs.

PROFESSIONAL EDUCATION AND GROWTH

First School

The first successful school where osteopathy was taught, the American School of Osteopathy, was chartered in May 1892 and opened that fall with a class of about 21 men and women, including members of Still's family and other local people. The faculty consisted of Still and Dr. William Smith, a physician trained in Edinburgh, Scotland, who taught anatomy in exchange for learning osteopathy. The goal, as stated in the revised (1894) charter for the school, was "to improve our present system of surgery, obstetrics, and treatment of diseases generally, and [to] place the same on a more rational and scientific basis, and to impart information to the medical profession." The charter would have permitted granting the doctor of medicine (MD) degree, but Still insisted on a distinctive recognition for graduates, DO, for diplomate in osteopathy (later doctor of osteopathy) (26).

The first course was just a few months long; most of the students voluntarily returned for a second year of additional training. By 1894 the course was 2 years long, two terms of 5 months each. In addition to their study of anatomy, students worked in the clinic under experienced operators, at first only under Still but later under graduates as well.

During the last 5 years of the 19th century the growth of both clinic and school were spectacular. Patients came from near and distant places, having heard by word of mouth or by printed accounts of near-miraculous cures. There were enough of such "miracles" that the osteopathic profession was widely promoted by grateful patients. A significant number of early DOs were either former patients or family members of patients who came to their studies with a kind of evangelical fervor. The town of Kirksville prospered and came to regard Still, who once was ridiculed, as a citizen of immense importance. He was lavishly praised, and he lived to see his statue, with the inscription "Demonstrate the Vision," erected in the town square (27,28).

Data on numbers of enrolled students illustrate the school's dramatic growth. In October 1895 there were 28 students. By the following summer there were 102. By 1900, there were over 700 students, with a faculty of 18 (26). By the turn of the century there were also more than a dozen "daughter" schools founded by graduates of the original school (29). Some of the schools were well organized under the model established by Still; others were established as diploma mills with the anticipation of generating large incomes for the persons establishing them. Still considered many of these to be for training "engine wipers" who were incapable or inexperienced in the practice of osteopathy. Many of these closed as standards were established by the American Osteopathic Association and by state licensure; by 1910, only eight remained.

Conflict with the American Medical Association

Medical education in the late 19th century was not well regulated. Many schools, allopathic, eclectic, homeopathic, and osteopathic, had virtually no entrance requirements except tuition payments, and many schools were for-profit institutions. Licensing laws had not yet reached a stage where they were effective in setting educational standards. The American Medical Association (AMA), founded in 1847, later a powerful influence on raising educational standards, was, in the 1890s, weak and in need of reorganization.

A new, reorganized AMA, observing that there were too many doctors, made its first order of business, under a revised constitu-

tion, the regulation of medical education. Its Council on Medical Education was formed in 1904, with a charge (among others) to improve the academic requirements for medical schools. This was fulfilled by rating all medical schools as class A (approved), B (probation), or C (unapproved), and making the findings available to state licensing boards (30).

Even before the AMA formed its Council on Medical Education, the young American Osteopathic Association (AOA) had adopted standards of its own for approval of osteopathic colleges (1902) and began inspections (1903) (31). This caused many small osteopathic colleges to close or merge with larger institutions.

Osteopathic schools were not included in the first AMA survey, but they were included in the influential Flexner Report, published in 1910 (32). After this report, which harshly condemned osteopathic schools along with many medical schools, more marginal schools closed, and the surviving ones converted to a not-for-profit status. Few of the schools established for teaching black physicians survived this period (33), and all but two or three of the schools for women closed (34,35). State licensing boards began to enforce stricter requirements; this probably was a more decisive influence than the Flexner Report (17,36).

Curriculum

Many medical schools formed affiliations with universities; by doing so, they gained both experienced science faculty and stable funding. This was not an option for osteopathic institutions at that time, and they faced a difficult dilemma: raise entry standards and lose major portions of tuition payments, which represented their only income, or adopt a "go slow" attitude. They chose the latter, which meant that they were perhaps two decades behind in the educational reforms that many agreed were desirable (37). AOA standards did increase the required length of osteopathic curricula, to 3 years in 1905 and to 4 years in 1915 (31).

The profession responded officially to external criticism by pointing out the differences between osteopathic and orthodox medical education. However, when there was an opportunity to raise general standards, as came about in the 1930s, the profession did so. By the mid-1930s, osteopathic colleges were requiring at least 2 years of college before matriculation; in 1954, 3 years were required; by 1960, over 70% of students had either baccalaureate or advanced degrees prior to entry (37). At present, virtually all students enter colleges of osteopathy with at least baccalaureate degrees; many have advanced degrees as well.

Curriculum content similarly grew and changed with the times. An 1899–1900 Kirksville catalogue describes the school's course of study as follows (38):

> The course of study extends over two years, and is divided into four terms of five months each.
>
> The first term is devoted to Descriptive Anatomy, including Osteology, Syndesmology and Myology; lectures on Histology illustrated by micro-stereopticon; the principles of General Inorganic Chemistry, Physics and Toxicology.
>
> The second term includes Descriptive and Regional Anatomy with demonstrations; didactic and laboratory work in Histology;

Physiology and physiological demonstrations; Physiological Chemistry and Urinalysis; Principles of Osteopathy; Clinical Demonstrations in Osteopathy.

The third term includes Demonstrations in Regional Anatomy; Physiology and physiological demonstrations; lectures on Pathology illustrated by micro-stereopticon; Symptomatology; Bacteriology; Physiological Psychology; clinical demonstrations in Osteopathy and Osteopathic diagnosis and therapeutics.

The fourth term includes Symptomatology; Surgery; didactic and laboratory work in Pathology; Psycho-Pathology and Psycho-Therapeutics; Gynecology; Obstetrics; Hygiene and Public Health; Venereal Diseases; Medical Jurisprudence; Dietetics; clinical demonstrations; Osteopathic and Operative clinics.

The major difference between this 1899–1900 curriculum and that of an allopathic medical school of the same period, in addition to the distinctive osteopathic content, was the exclusion of *materia medica* (pharmacology).

Early in osteopathic history a difference appeared between so-called lesion osteopaths and broad osteopaths: those who limited their therapeutic practice essentially to manipulation, and those who used all the tools available to medicine, including *materia medica.*

Andrew Taylor Still practiced midwifery (obstetrics) and surgery; both were taught under his guidance. Indeed, when the issue of surgery became controversial among later DOs, Still's son provided an affidavit concerning his father's practice (39). As already noted, A.T. Still remained skeptical about using or teaching any form of pharmaceutical therapy.

Still's general opposition to drugs did not prevent some early DOs from using them for treatment. Quite a few had been trained as MDs before they came to osteopathic schools; others went on to earn MD degrees after they became DOs; still others simply decided to use all the adjunctive treatments available. Most "broad" osteopaths felt that after new safer medications were developed it was consistent with being a completely trained physician to incorporate them into osteopathic practice. The most direct early confrontation came in 1897 when a DO-MD opened the short-lived Columbian School of Osteopathy in Kirksville, with the announced intention of offering DO and MD degrees upon graduation from a course in manipulation, surgery, and *materia medica.* The competitive and personal issues in this case extended beyond the academic questions, and the school closed after graduating only three classes (26). The issue was professionally divisive for many years thereafter.

Adjunctive treatments became a major subject of debate within the AOA and the Associated Colleges of Osteopathy (now the American Association of Colleges of Osteopathic Medicine) for many years. The question finally was resolved in favor of the "broad" osteopaths, not by consensus over the idea but by recognizing that state licensing laws required fuller training. In 1916, against the direct protest of Still (40), the trustees revoked a previous year's action condemning individuals and colleges that taught drug therapy, effectively opening the way for the colleges to form their own curricula. The profession's great success in using manipulative treatment during the 1918 influenza epidemic (41) probably slowed the integration of *materia medica* into the osteopathic curriculum. However, by the late 1920s it became officially permissible to institute courses in "comparative

therapeutics," of which pharmacology was one subheading (37). By the mid-1930s the integration was complete. The change was validated as drugs were greatly improved, making it possible to offer pharmaceutical treatment where benefits outweighed risks.

Curricular improvement continued as clinical teaching facilities grew and as budgets permitted the hiring of full-time faculty, particularly in the basic sciences. While instruction by physicians in active practice was an advantage for students who were developing clinical skills, the basic sciences and laboratory-based research required faculty who could give these interests their full attention. All the colleges had full-time basic science faculty by the time the first osteopathic medical school became affiliated with a major American university; such affiliations had been the route by which allopathic schools had strengthened their basic science teaching earlier in the 20th century.

One other curricular improvement deserves mention. For many years, teachers of osteopathic principles and practice developed courses in their area of expertise as traditions within their individual schools, sometimes jealously guarded and always zealously defended. In 1968, a small intercollegiate group of osteopathic principles professors met for the first time. The initial agenda was a response to the new initiative of uniform medical coding, in light of a movement to change the term "osteopathic lesion" to "somatic dysfunction." This change had to be discussed and agreed upon as part of preparation for diagnostic coding. The group continued to meet, and it became known as the Educational Council on Osteopathic Principles, and later it became affiliated with the American Association of Colleges of Osteopathic Medicine. Its agenda grew to include a uniform glossary of osteopathic terminology (a current edition is included at the back of this text), systematic development of agreement about the content of a multidisciplinary-oriented osteopathic principles curriculum, and finally this textbook, *Foundations for Osteopathic Medicine.* Its continuing role also includes development of osteopathic-oriented questions for national board/licensure and specialty board examinations.

Research

On one level, since its earliest days, osteopathic medicine has been a profession based on a research question: "Can we find a better way?" Osteopathic manipulation developed as an experimental approach to clinical conditions that did not respond to the conventional treatments of the time, and its practical success became the empirical research results that led to another level: the questions of "why" and "what if" appropriate to laboratory study. Medical research, in parallel with medical education, underwent a process of developing new traditions and controls, as well as better equipment, all of which would shape future clinical studies.

Laboratory studies began among osteopathic physicians almost as soon as there was an organized osteopathic school (42). Study of the scientific questions raised by osteopathic manipulative practice has never been easy; the difficulty can be illustrated by one obvious clinical question: "What is a manipulative placebo?" In spite of these and other difficulties, a number of significant accomplishments have been recorded (43). Section VIII of this book offers an extensive survey of osteopathic research efforts from past to present.

Growth of the Profession's Schools

Enthusiastic graduates of the first osteopathic college—for reasons evangelistic or pecuniary—quickly began to establish new schools throughout the country. Some of these were short-lived because they were unable to meet the rising standards of the AOA. Others merged with stronger institutions and survived in a new organization. Still others strengthened their positions and survived. This was the general trend for medical education in the 19th century, and the smaller schools, whether allopathic, osteopathic, or homeopathic, had similar closures, consolidations, or rebuilding.

As noted previously, by 1910 only eight of the early osteopathic schools were still in operation. Six of these have survived into the new millennium; all have had complicated histories of name changes, relocations, charter changes, mergers, and affiliations with other educational institutions. The five original schools still accredited (29) are:

Kirksville College of Osteopathic Medicine, successor to the first school (1892);

Philadelphia College of Osteopathic Medicine (1898);

Chicago College of Osteopathic Medicine at Midwestern University (1900);

University of Health Sciences, College of Osteopathic Medicine, Kansas City (1916)—there had been an osteopathic college in Kansas City as early as 1895; and

Des Moines University, College of Osteopathic Medicine and Surgery (1905)—there had been a school in Des Moines as early as 1898.

One school, the College of Osteopathic Physicians and Surgeons, Los Angeles, has survived as a medical school (University of California at Irvine). The California conflict and merger in the 1960s, described briefly under "State Licensure," resulted not only in the change of an osteopathic college to an allopathic college, but in a revival of interest in osteopathic education in the profession. The first new educational focus was in Michigan, and it began not only a new tradition in osteopathic education but became an impetus for nationwide growth that continues to this day.

In 1964, the Michigan Association of Osteopathic Physicians and Surgeons committed itself to develop a new, independently funded college of osteopathic medicine. This initiative occurred because more than 1,000 osteopathic physicians practiced in the state, representing about 5% of the state's physician total and providing care for about 20% of the state's patients. None of these DOs had received their education in the state. In 1969, 18 students enrolled in the first class at a new campus in Pontiac, Michigan. Within 2 years, it was clear that a program of such complexity could not survive financially as a freestanding institution. A number of strong supporters in the Michigan legislature, and Michigan's governor, were willing to support a bill for state funding with one major stipulation: the college had to be integrated with an existing, accredited university program. After complex negotiations, the program transferred to the cam-

pus of Michigan State University in 1971, where it became the first university-based osteopathic college.

After this affiliation proved successful, 13 more osteopathic schools (some public, some private) were developed over the next 25 years. In 2002, 19 colleges were accredited by the AOA for predoctoral osteopathic education (29). In addition to the "surviving five," they are:

Michigan State University College of Osteopathic Medicine (1964)

University of North Texas Health Science Center at Fort Worth, Texas College of Osteopathic Medicine (1966)

Oklahoma State University College of Osteopathic Medicine (1974)

West Virginia School of Osteopathic Medicine (1974)

Ohio University College of Osteopathic Medicine (1975)

University of Medicine and Dentistry of New Jersey, School of Osteopathic Medicine (1976)

University of New England, College of Osteopathic Medicine (1976)

Western University of Health Sciences, College of Osteopathic Medicine of the Pacific (1977)

New York College of Osteopathic Medicine (1977)

Nova Southeastern University College of Osteopathic Medicine (1981)

Lake Erie College of Osteopathic Medicine (1992)

Arizona College of Osteopathic Medicine (1995)

Pikeville College, School of Osteopathic Medicine (1997)

Touro University, College of Osteopathic Medicine (1997)

As of 2002, a 20th school, Edward Via Virginia College of Osteopathic Medicine, was undergoing provisional accreditation and planning to admit its first class in fall of 2003.

STATE LICENSURE

Closely related to the issue of educational standards was licensure under increasingly strict state laws.

The first legislative recognition of osteopathic practice came from Vermont in 1896 (44), where graduates of the American School of Osteopathy, Kirksville, were accorded the right to practice in that state. Missouri had a successful bill as early as 1895, but it was vetoed by the governor; what was hailed as a better bill was passed and signed into law in March 1897 (23,45).

Such laws as these, greeted with much rejoicing, made tremendous growth possible in the osteopathic profession in states where legislation provided a friendly welcome. Osteopathic history includes numerous stories about legal action against DOs for practicing without a valid license, David-and-Goliath encounters of DOs with MD-dominated legislatures, and testimony or influence offered by prominent people who were osteopathic patients. These colorful tales were the war stories of an energetic first generation of DOs, who managed to secure legislative rights to at least limited practice in a majority of states.

Registration and licensure were related, but often different, matters. Some states provided for the formation of separate osteopathic licensing boards; some permitted the addition of an osteopathic representative to an existing or composite board; and a few permitted DOs to apply through a medical board without osteopathic representation.

The roles of these boards were not immediately clear at the time of their formation. There was opposition on ideological grounds even to the idea of licensure. Some populists, not partisan to either osteopathic or allopathic physicians, said that medical licensure was in itself discriminatory. Others said that licensing would interfere with freedom of medical research. Some social Darwinists went so far as to say that if the poor died of their own foolishness in choosing bad medical practitioners, the species would improve (33).

By 1901, however, every state had some form of legislation requiring at least registration, with a diploma from an accepted school, or a state examination of some type. When the Missouri board began to function in 1903, the first certificate it issued was to A.T. Still (46).

Licensure to practice a full scope of medicine was another matter, and in most places it was related first to the content of the osteopathic curriculum and later to the results of examinations. Again using Missouri as an example, by 1897 the subjects taught had expanded to include anatomy, physiology, surgery, midwifery, histology, chemistry, urinalysis, toxicology, pathology, and symptomatology. Everything was included except *materia medica* and academic consciences were temporarily satisfied. By 1937, however, only 26 states had any provision to provide unlimited licenses to DOs.

In some states DOs were ineligible to apply because their education did not meet specific criteria. As late as 1937, osteopathic standards did not meet pre-professional college requirements in 16 states; in 8 states, a year's internship was needed. Originally, DOs who took examinations under medical or composite boards showed a much lower pass rate. Whether this was a difference in osteopathic curricula or an educational deficiency, as it was argued, in due course, the curricula were altered and the pass rates increased. The major changes were addition of more basic science courses, more faculty, and larger clinical facilities (37).

After World War II, a major effort was made to change the old limited practice laws. These efforts, along with major changes in osteopathic education, enabled the enactment of new practice laws for all 50 states (47).

A final dramatic chapter in the American licensing story of the osteopathic professional came when the California Osteopathic Association agreed in 1961 to merge with the California Medical Association, and the College of Osteopathic Physicians and Surgeons, Los Angeles, became the California College of Medicine. Consenting DOs were given MD degrees as a preparation for a referendum approved by voters in 1962, which discontinued licensure of DOs in that state (37).

A new state osteopathic group, Osteopathic Physicians and Surgeons of California, was chartered by the AOA. This group fought against the referendum but lost; they then began a long legal battle that culminated in a 1974 decision by the California Supreme Court that licensure of DOs must be resumed (48). A new college was chartered in that state, and professional continuity was restored.

By the end of the 20th century, state licensure could be attained in various ways: through the standard national osteopathic licensing examination and/or through the standard national medical licensing examination, depending on state requirements. Some states maintained separate osteopathic and allopathic licensing boards; many were composite boards. Graduate education required for new licenses still varied from state to state. In every state, however, as well as in a number of foreign countries, it was possible for DOs to be licensed for unlimited practice.

OSTEOPATHIC ORGANIZATION

The AOA began as a student organization in Kirksville, under the name American Association for the Advancement of Osteopathy, in 1897. Its present name was adopted in 1901 (49). The second national association was the Associated Colleges of Osteopathy (now the American Association of Colleges of Osteopathic Medicine), formed in 1898. Both groups sought to protect and raise standards for education and practice of DOs. The AOA became the regulatory group, no longer under student control; the Associated Colleges became a discussion and consensus group for faculty and officers of the schools.

In 1907 the first organization devoted to osteopathic research began, though the first recorded osteopathic research was done almost a decade earlier (42). The AOA played a vital role in encouraging and supporting osteopathic research. Money for research has never been plentiful; a major portion of the support for osteopathic research, especially in earlier days, has come from financial contributions by DOs themselves. More recently qualified researchers have been recipients of public grant funds, but the role of AOA-affiliated research organizations has been essential for start-up projects.

State (divisional) and local (district) osteopathic organizations were established to serve DOs in their own localities. When the AOA grew too large for general membership meetings, state societies began (in 1920) to name representatives to serve in an AOA House of Delegates. That body thereafter became the chief policy-making group for the osteopathic profession. A board of trustees, elected by the house, oversaw the implementation of those policies, a role it still fills. Students participate as voting members of delegations from the states in which their schools are located, are appointed to AOA boards, bureaus, and committees; and they have a number of organizations of their own.

A major early effort of the AOA was to produce a code of ethics; this was accomplished in 1904. A participant in those deliberations observed that the problem was not because anyone really wished to practice unethically, but rather that on some points it was difficult to agree upon what was ethical (50). To put this in perspective: the issue of advertising was a hard-fought question among all professionals at that time. The question was resolved by declaring advertising unethical except for brief professional card listings. By the 1990s advertising by professionals was ultimately considered ethical, though not of course to condone unfounded claims.

Over time many osteopathic organizations grew, from starting points as various as special tasks, geographic or school affinity, and practice interest. A current guide to all AOA-recognized osteopathic organizations is available online (51).

The AOA has always been the umbrella group that recognizes and coordinates its efforts on behalf of the profession. The AOA itself has many important functions. Through its bureaus, councils, and committees, it is the osteopathic accrediting organization for undergraduate, graduate, and continuing medical education and for health care facilities. It certifies specialists in all fields, through a network of specialty boards and its own central bureau. Research grants and related projects, as well as educational meetings, are arranged through AOA bureaus and councils.

Staff, directed by elected officers and trustees, provide professional services, including: maintenance of central records on all DOs, public and legislative education, member services, educational activities including publications and conventions, and coordinated special efforts on a variety of concerns. Position papers on various topics are approved by the House of Delegates and presented as the profession's position on questions of public health and professional interest.

In addition to activities of the AOA itself, a network of divisional and affiliate societies is recognized by the AOA. Certain major "sub-umbrella" organizations have networks of their own: the associations of osteopathic colleges, health care organizations, licensing groups, and foundations.

Specialty colleges, distinct from the certifying boards, conduct educational affairs and recognize their own members' achievements through fellowships and other awards. State (divisional) and local (district) societies typically deal with state legislative and regulatory affairs, conduct educational programs, and provide a variety of member services.

Colleges typically have student and alumni groups, student chapters of certain specialty organizations, fraternities and sororities, and a variety of special interest groups. Many of the physicians' and students' organizations have auxiliary organizations for spouses.

All organizations recognized by the AOA accept such ongoing controls as approval of any changes in basic documents and designation of how many representatives (if any) are sent to the AOA House of Delegates for voice and vote in professional policy affairs.

FEDERAL GOVERNMENT RECOGNITION

The first major attempt by the AOA to obtain federal government recognition was during World War I, when it tried to gain commissions for DOs as military physicians (41). This effort was unsuccessful, in spite of active support by such prominent advocates as the former president of the United States, Theodore Roosevelt (52).

At that time, an examination was set, and it was understood that if DOs (along with MDs) took this and passed it, they could be commissioned as medical officers. About 25 DOs took the examination and were recommended for commissions. The Surgeon General unilaterally ruled that only MDs were eligible. Bills were then introduced (1917) in both the House of Representatives and the Senate to correct this inequity. The bills were referred to the Military Affairs Committees, and hearings were held. The committee then referred the issue to the Surgeon General, who in his statement of opposition claimed that regular physicians would withhold their services if DOs were allowed to serve. The bills remained in committee without resolution until the end of

the war. Meanwhile, DOs served as regular soldiers, unable to use their medical training.

The situation remained uncorrected when World War II began. Again there were efforts to obtain commissions for DOs, this time emphasizing regulatory rather than legislative barriers (41,53). DOs were deferred rather than drafted, waiting for the possibility to serve in a medical capacity that never came. Ironically, the DOs left behind became family physicians to the thousands of the patients left by the MDs in military service, which enhanced the public's view of DOs as full-service physicians.

The pressure for federal recognition continued after World War II ended, and in 1956 a new law specifically provided for the appointment of DOs as commissioned officers in the nation's military medical corps. However, implementation of that law was blocked for another 10 years, until the Vietnam conflict created another special need for military physicians. The first DO was finally commissioned in May 1966. The next year the AMA withdrew its long-standing opposition, and DOs were included in the doctor draft. It was another 20 years, in 1983, before the first DO was promoted to be a flag officer in the U.S. military medical corps (31).

Acceptance of DOs as medical officers in the U.S. Civil Service was accomplished in 1963. Careers in this field became possible after that date.

Nearly every federal recognition for DOs came after a long and difficult fight. Among the important federal recognitions were the following (31,37):

1951: The U.S. Public Health Service first awarded renewable teaching grants to each of the six osteopathic colleges.

1957: The AOA was recognized by the U.S. Office of Education, Department of Health, Education and Welfare (DHEW), as the accrediting body for osteopathic education.

1963: The Health Professions Educational Assistance Act included a provision for matching construction grants for osteopathic colleges and loans to osteopathic students.

1966: The AOA was designated by the DHEW (now the Department of Health and Human Services [DHHS]) as the official accrediting body for hospitals under Medicare.

1967: The AOA was recognized by the National Commission on Accrediting as the accrediting agency for all facets of osteopathic education.

1983: The first osteopathic flag officer in the U.S. military was appointed.

1997: The first osteopathic surgeon-general of the army was appointed.

The AOA continues to maintain a presence in Washington, D.C., where it attempts to ensure inclusion of DOs and osteopathic institutions as active partners in all legislative and regulatory initiatives.

Specialties

Perhaps the first osteopathic activity in what now is called a medical specialty began only 3 years after Wilhelm Roentgen announced the discovery of radiographs. The second x-ray machine west of the Mississippi was installed in Kirksville in 1898. With it, Dr. William Smith formulated a method to inject a radiopaque substance in cadaveric veins and arteries to demonstrate the normal pattern of circulation. Two articles were published late that year, one in the *Journal of Osteopathy*, a Kirksville journal associated with the American School of Osteopathy, and the other in the fledgling *American X-Ray Journal*. These were reprinted for modern reference in AOA publications in 1974 (54). When formal certifying boards for osteopathic specialties were organized, radiology was first (1939) (31).

Along with these events came the long story of the development of osteopathic hospitals, internships, residencies, specialty organizations, specialty standards, examinations, and recognition for those standards. By the 1990s a full complement of specialties, training programs, and certifying boards were well established in the osteopathic profession, including a board recognizing osteopathic manipulative medicine, now referred to as neuromusculoskeletal medicine. At the same time, the profession was unknowingly developing what would come to be the most needed type of practice for the 1990s: primary care.

Throughout its history, osteopathic clinical education has taken place in primary care settings: community hospitals and clinics. The profession has supported very few academic medical centers. By the 1990s, this disadvantage became an advantage because of the profession's success in producing primary care physicians, including many willing to work in underserved communities.

Many factors have been cited as influential in the choice of practice type and venue, but the chief ones seem to be undergraduate experiences and role models (55). Students trained in academic medical centers tend to have only subspecialists as role models and their clinical contacts tend to be cases typically referred to tertiary medical centers. Meanwhile, osteopathic students have continued to have regular contact with community clinics and hospitals and have many faculty role models who are primary care physicians.

For instance, rural clinics, long a mainstay of clinical education for the Kirksville college and later for other osteopathic schools, have become a model for primary care education (56). In the last decade of the 20th century, the osteopathic profession found itself in the enviable role of advisor on how to replicate its educational processes in other places.

HOSPITALS

As with medicine in general, hospitals had their share of developmental problems in the 19th century. Inadequate facilities and staff, infection, disagreement over who should get patient fees, social stigma, and hospital ownership all entered the picture. By about 1900, however, with the growth of an educated nursing profession and a new sense of sanitation, hospitals began to be—at the very least—safe. Many small institutions were privately owned by surgeons who furnished hotel services and nursing for their own patients. New general hospitals began to appeal to patients other than the poor, and patient fees began to help with hospital development (36).

There were osteopathic hospitals early in the 20th century; at the time of Flexner's inspection, Kirksville had the largest, with 54 beds. Chicago had 20 beds; the Pacific College, 15; Boston, 10; and Philadelphia, 3. No others were listed in that report (37). Eventually the numbers and size of osteopathic hospitals grew, but few reached the size and diversity of specialties that characterized the academic medical centers associated with university medical schools. However, the osteopathic profession did set hospital standards, first for the training of interns and residents, and then for accreditation of the institutions themselves.

The growth of osteopathic hospitals was especially marked in the period during and after World War II, when MD-run hospitals did not permit DOs to join their medical staffs. When U.S. government programs were approved to help with construction of hospitals, osteopathic institutions participated along with MD-run institutions. Many community teaching hospitals were constructed during those years.

In 1954, a landmark court decision in Audrain County, Missouri, made it illegal for public hospitals to deny staff membership and admitting privileges to qualified DOs. This initiated a series of changes in areas outside California, where for many years DOs had been in charge of half the Los Angeles County Hospital. By the 1960s, most public hospitals were open to DOs; by the 1980s most private hospitals were open as well.

By the 1990s, with medical residencies open to both MDs and DOs, the need for a network of osteopathic hospitals for training purposes was much reduced. Mechanisms were adopted to recognize training that took place in allopathic institutions as acceptable for osteopathic board certification. This is now possible either by affiliation of the MD institution with an accredited osteopathic college or by direct AOA accreditation of the training institution (51). By 1999, osteopathic graduate training institutes (OPTIs), were the standard, linking resources through hospital–college consortiums.

Reorganization of the health care system itself made these changes necessary. Payment mechanisms led to the formation of large networks of health care providers, including hospitals, outpatient facilities, home care, extended and long-term care, and multiple independent contractors and physician organizations. Community hospitals, including many osteopathic institutions, were merged with larger groups or simply closed. The lines between osteopathic and allopathic hospitals blurred, as both came under the umbrella of managed care organizations.

In a case of history repeating itself, economic factors control health care delivery, and the profit motive is once again a respectable part of medical practice. This is placed against a call for serious reform of medical education and better distribution of primary care physicians. The goal is to provide excellence in patient care and in physician education, while seeking through corporate management tools the funds to survive in a competitive environment.

CONCLUSION

At the start of the 21st century, the "parallel and distinctive" osteopathic profession is respected in many quarters for a variety of reasons. First and foremost is the osteopathic emphasis on primary care. This arose not only from the earlier circumstances of training opportunities and role models but also from the profession's traditional whole-person philosophy.

Additionally, there has been a rebirth of interest in manual medicine and other osteopathic methods. In most osteopathic colleges and graduate education programs, there is increased emphasis on historic tenets and clinical skills. The profession's horizons have been expanded by a global emphasis of its own and an interest in international groups devoted to manual medicine (57–60).

Osteopathic physicians have gained a positive voice in public affairs. In the public arena, DOs are regarded as "parallel and distinctive" in regulatory and legislative affairs, and the profession is consulted on most matters of public health policy. The profession has also launched clinical initiatives in such categories as women's health, minority health care, and pediatric end-of-life care. Continued emphasis on preventive care and health maintenance is in line with traditional osteopathic values. An ambitious strategic plan launched in 2001 by the AOA formalized some of these emphases and added others, including international recognition of U.S.-trained DOs, an AOA Center for International Affairs, and a new World Osteopathic Medical Association (61).

One of the dedicatees of this volume, George W. Northup, wrote in 1988:

> Today, the practice of medicine needs as never before the guiding light of a fundamental philosophy. It needs to recognize the action and interaction of all body systems. It should apply known truths and explore new frontiers founded on the osteopathic profession's basic philosophy.... Dr Still did not say he was giving the world a philosophy that should act as a guide to the future. Rather, in his book, *The Philosophy of Osteopathy,* he stated his desire was "... to give the world a start in a philosophy that may be a guide to the future"(62).

The purpose of medical history has long been a subject for discussion. At its best and fullest, it can be said to "provide a wonderful schooling in prudence" (63). The caution follows that the historical record must be "considered in terms of its own circumstances and standards. This demands insight into the viewpoints, thoughts, emotions, reactions, likes and dislikes of people of the past." Such insight requires a more thorough study than an introductory chapter can offer.

Some care has been taken to offer to the interested student a list of references that can facilitate deepened insights. But beyond these readings, there is much more to explore and understand.

ACKNOWLEDGMENTS

Appreciation is expressed to the following, who contributed substantively to the current version of this chapter: Dr. G. D'Alonzo, Dr. E. DiGiovanna, Dr. D. Dowling, Dr. N. Gevitz, Ms. P. Grauer, Dr. M. Kuchera, Dr. G. Osborn, Dr. D. Ward, and Dr. R. Ward.

REFERENCES

Note: Concerning reference 3: There is a typographic error on page 18 of the edition currently in print, concerning the date of the Still's move to Missouri: The date should be 1837, not 1827.

Concerning references 41 and 52: A number of interesting anecdotal accounts were published in JAOA *by various authors: 18:247–248, Jan 1919; 18:277–278 and 18:299–302, Feb 1919; 18:335–338 and 18:357–368, Mar 1919; 18:396–398 and 18:415–418, Apr 1919. Also: An attempt was made by the editors of the publication* Osteopathic Physician *to quantify treatment results. See OP 34:1–2, Dec 1918 and 36:1, Jul 1919. Some suggestive details on type of treatment also were published and reprinted in* Time Capsule, *The DO 1980;(Jan):31–36. See also Booth ER:* History of Osteopathy and Twentieth Century Medical Practice, *1924 edition.*

1. Still AT. *The Philosophy and Mechanical Principles of Osteopathy.* Kansas City, MO: Hudson-Kimberly Publishing Co; 1892 and 1902.
2. Still AT. *Philosophy of osteopathy.* Published by the author, Kirksville, MO; 1899.
3. Still AT. *Autobiography of Andrew T. Still with a History of the Discovery and Development of the Science of Osteopathy.* Rev ed. Published by the author, Kirksville, MO; 1908.
4. Still AT. *Osteopathy, Research and Practice.* Published by the author, Kirksville, MO; 1910.
5. Tenets of osteopathic medicine, American Osteopathic Association. Available at: http://www.aoa-net.org/AOAGeneral/tenets.htm. Accessed April 15, 2002.
6. Brown JM, Woodworth RB. *The Captives of Abb's Valley; a Legend of Frontier Life.* New ed. Staunton, VA: Printed for the author by the McClure Co; 1942.
7. Dick E. *The Sod-House Frontier.* Lincoln, NE: Johnsen Publishing Co; 1954.
8. Personal communication: Mrs. J.S. Denslow (Dr. Still's granddaughter); 1972.
9. Trowbridge C. *Andrew Taylor Still, 1828–1917.* Kirksville, MO: Thomas Jefferson University Press, Northeast Missouri State University; 1991.
10. Thomas JL, ed. *Slavery Attacked: The Abolitionist Crusade.* Englewood Cliffs, NJ: Prentice-Hall; 1965.
11. Monaghan J. *Civil War on the Western Border, 1854–1865.* New York, NY: Bonanza Books; 1965.
12. Eldridge SW. First free-state legislature. In: *Recollections of Early Days in Kansas; Publications of the Kansas State Historical Society.* Vol II. Topeka, KS: Kansas State Printing Plant; 1920:149–158.
13. A.T. Still Pension File. Still National Osteopathic Museum, Kirksville, MO.
14. Duffy J. *From Humors to Medical Science; A History of American Medicine,* 2nd ed. Urbana, IL: University of Illinois Press; 1993.
15. Bordley J, Harvey AM. *Two Centuries of American Medicine, 1776–1976.* Philadelphia, PA: WB Saunders Co; 1976:97.
16. Laughlin GM. Asks if A.T. Still was ever a doctor. *Osteopathic Physician.* 1909;15(Jan):8.
17. Osborn GG. The beginning: nineteenth century medical sectarianism. In: Humphrey RM, Gallagher FJ, eds. *Osteopathic Medicine: A Reformation in Progress.* London, England: Churchill Livingstone; 2001: 3–26.
18. Pickard ME, Buley RC. *The Midwest Pioneer; His Ills, Cures & Doctors.* Crawfordsville, IN: R.E. Banta; 1945.
19. *Merck's 1899 Manual of the Materia Medica, Together with a Summary of Therapeutic Indications and a Classification of Medicaments; a Ready-Reference Pocket Book for the Practicing Physician.* New York, NY: Merck & Co; 1899. Reprinted in facsimile by Merck & Co; 1999.
20. *Dorland's Illustrated Medical Dictionary,* 26th ed. Philadelphia, PA: WB Saunders Co; 1981.
21. Danciger E. *The Emergence of Homeopathy; Alchemy into Medicine.* London, England: Century Hutchinson Ltd; 1987.
22. Ebright HK. *The History of Baker University.* Baldwin, KS: Published by the University; 1951.
23. Schnucker RV, ed. *Early Osteopathy in the Words of A.T. Still.* Kirksville, MO: Thomas Jefferson University Press, Northeast Missouri State University; 1991.
24. Still CE. A.T. Still: the itinerant years. In: From the Archives. *The DO.* 1975;(Mar):27–30.
25. Riley GW. Following osteopathic principles. In: Hildreth AG, ed. *The Lengthening Shadow of Dr. Andrew Taylor Still.* Published by the author, Macon, MO; 1938:411–435.
26. Walter GW. *The First School of Osteopathic Medicine; A Chronicle, 1892–1992.* Kirksville, MO: Thomas Jefferson University Press, Northeast Missouri State University; 1992.

27. Violette EM. *History of Adair County.* Kirksville, MO: Denslow History Co; 1911:253.

28. Still CE Jr. *Frontier Doctor, Medical Pioneer; The Life and Times of A.T. Still and His Family.* Kirksville, MO: Thomas Jefferson University Press, Northeast Missouri State University; 1991.

29. Historic reference of osteopathic colleges. American Osteopathic Association. Available at: http://www.aoa-net.org/Education/collegehist.htm. Accessed.

30. Johnson V, Weiskotten HG. *A History of the Council on Medical Education and Hospitals of the American Medical Association.* Chicago, IL: American Medical Association; 1960.

31. Important dates in osteopathic history. American Osteopathic Association. Available at: http:///www.aoa-net.org/Publications/yearbooktoc. htm. Accessed April 15, 2002.

32. Flexner A. *Medical Education in the United States and Canada; a Report to the Carnegie Foundation for the Advancement of Teaching.* Boston, MA: Merrymount Press; 1910.

33. Morais HM. The history of the Negro in medicine. In: *International Library of Negro Life and History.* Vol 4. The Association for the Study of Negro Life and History. New York, NY: Publishers Co; 1968.

34. Lopate C. *Women in Medicine.* Published for the Josiah Macy, Jr. Foundation. Baltimore, MD: Johns Hopkins Press; 1968.

35. Walsh MR. *Doctors Wanted: No Women Need Apply; Sexual Barriers in the Medical Profession.* New Haven, CT: Yale University Press; 1977.

36. Starr P. *The Social Transformation of American Medicine.* New York, NY: Basic Books; 1982.

37. Gevitz N. The D.O.s: *Osteopathic Medicine in America.* Baltimore, MD: Johns Hopkins University Press; 1982:75–87.

38. *Catalogue of the American School of Osteopathy, Session of 1899–1900.* Kirksville, MO; seventh annual announcement.

39. The memoirs of Dr. Charles Still; IV. A postscript. In: From the Archives. *The DO.* 1975;(Jun):25–26.

40. Booth ER. *History of Osteopathy and Twentieth-Century Medical Practice.* Cincinnati, OH: Printed for the author by the Caxton Press; 1924.

41. Gevitz N. The sword and the scalpel: the osteopathic 'war' to enter the Military Medical Corps, 1916–1966. *JAOA.* 1998(May);279–286.

42. Peterson B. How old is osteopathic research? In: Time Capsule. *The DO.* 1978;(Dec):24–26.

43. Cole WV. Historical basis for osteopathic theory and practice. In: Northup GW, ed. *Osteopathic Research: Growth and Development.* Chicago, IL: American Osteopathic Association; 1987:57.

44. A Vermont story and Contacts with the law. In: From the Archives. *The DO.* 1972;(Nov):46–50.

45. Hildreth AG. *The Lengthening Shadow of Dr Andrew Taylor Still.* Published by the author, Macon, MO; 1938.

46. The Old Doctor gets first certificate. *J Osteopathy.* 1904;11(Jan):28.

47. Years states passed unlimited practice laws. American Osteopathic Association. Available at: http://www.aoa-net.org/Recognition/laws.htm. Accessed.

48. Fryman VM. Alexander Tobin, 1921–1992. In: *The Collected Papers of Viola M. Frymann, DO.* Indianapolis, IN: American Academy of Osteopathy; 1996.

49. Students form association. American Osteopathic Association. Available at: http://www.aoa-net.org/Assocation/aoa.htm. Accessed.

50. Evans AL. The beginnings of the AOA (1928 manuscript). In: From the Archives. *The DO.* 1972;(Sep):34–38.

51. American Osteopathic Association. Available at: http://www.aoa-net. org. Accessed April 15, 2002.

52. They passed the exam, but they could not serve: the DO doughboys. In: From the Archives. *The DO.* 1975;(Aug):39–46.

53. How DOs gained commissions. In: Time Capsule. *The DO.* 1980;(Apr): 25–32.

54. 1898: Radiology in Kirksville. In: Time Capsule. *JAOA.* 1974;74(Oct): 167–172.

55. Rodos JJ, Peterson B. *Proposed Strategies for Fulfilling Primary Care Manpower Needs; a White Paper Prepared for the National Advisory Council, National Health Service Corps, U.S. Public Health Service.* Rockville, MD: National Health Service Corps; 1990.

56. Blondell RD, Smith IJ, Byrne ME, Higgins CW. Rural health, family practice, and area health education centers: a national study. *Fam Med.* 1989;3(May–Jun):183–186.

57. Svoboda J. C'mon, take your medicine—global. *The DO.* 2000(Dec): 56–58.

58. Vitucci N. Healing hands around the world. *The DO.* 2002(Mar): 36–40.

59. Vitucci N. Finding common ground. *The DO.* 2002(Mar): 42–45.

60. Kuchera ML. Global alliances: advancing research and the evidence base. *JAOA.* 2002;102:5–7.

61. AOA's annual report: 2000–01 and beyond. *The DO.* 2001;(Sep):65–70.

62. Northup GW. Mission accomplished? *JAOA.* 1988;9(Sep). Reprinted in Beal MC, ed. *1995–96 Yearbook: Osteopathic Vision.* Indianapolis, IN: American Academy of Osteopathy; 1996:124.

63. Rosen G. Purposes and values of medical history. In: Galdston I, ed. *On the Utility of Medical History.* New York, NY: International Universities Press; 1957:11–19.

OSTEOPATHIC CONSIDERATIONS IN THE BASIC SCIENCES

INTRODUCTION

MICHAEL M. PATTERSON

Osteopathic medical practice is built on the foundation of both scientific knowledge and a medical philosophy that guides the application of facts within the art of treatment. Too often, in the practice of medicine, we overlook the fact that medical knowledge must be delivered in the context of a philosophy of how life, health, and disease processes function. The interaction between physician and patient then flows from that philosophy and directly affects the patient's response.

OSTEOPATHIC PHILOSOPHY

The philosophy of osteopathic medicine was initially formulated by Andrew Taylor Still, MD, DO and has been elaborated by leaders of the profession for almost 110 years. Still's initial formulations had their roots in the earliest of medical thought and practice. To these ideas, Still added important insights and understandings gained from his own experience and knowledge. As new medical knowledge and understandings of human function have been discovered, the philosophy has been refined and its implications better elucidated. However, its basic tenets have remained as fundamental guides for osteopathic physicians, scientists, and teachers in optimizing health and diminishing disease processes in their patients, guiding the scientific process in formulating new knowledge, and passing the profession to new generations.

Within osteopathic philosophy, one of the most important aspects is that for optimal function, there must be integration of the various constituent functional levels, from the subcellular to organ systems to the psychological. When a breakdown in the integration of these functions develops, the individual can no longer maintain the best level of health, and disease symptoms are increasingly likely. This leads to another of the basic tenets of the profession, that the underlying cause of disease is disturbance of function; homeostatic mechanisms can no longer ward off invasions of bacteria or viruses or contain the degeneration of aging or use. Osteopathic philosophy suggests that one of the most important things for the osteopathic physician to understand is how body functions are integrated, how that integration can be degraded, and how it can be restored.

The amount of knowledge available to the student of human function is not beyond the wildest dreams of those in the field only a few years ago. Information of human function is increasing at an astounding rate, and all indications are that it will continue to compound even more rapidly in the years ahead. The Human Genome Project alone promises to provide insights into the basic nature of human disease that is beyond our comprehension. It is

becoming increasingly difficult for any one person to have even a basic understanding of all the fields of medical knowledge, let alone a mastery of them. Rather than decreasing the need for a philosophic basis for medical practice, the increasing knowledge base makes it even more important to have a means of organizing the vast numbers of facts and theories to make a coherent medical practice. Without such a philosophy, the practitioner is prone to being whipsawed by the medical treatment *du jour* and hence not serving the patient well.

It is the purpose of this section to present ways to look at and organize various areas of knowledge in the basic sciences for the student of osteopathic medicine, in light of an important part of osteopathic philosophy; the integration of function. It is not possible for one or often even a series of texts to present all the knowledge of the various scientific areas underlying biomedical science. Some physiology texts alone are longer than this book and the same holds true for most of the other basic sciences. This section is meant to serve as material to supplement the basic science training of the osteopathic student or to refresh and enhance the practicing osteopathic clinician's knowledge. Chapters in this section provide information and knowledge in these areas in terms of integration of function and, in some cases, ways in which the lack of integration, or disintegration, can occur. Some of the chapters present information or syntheses of areas not readily available elsewhere, but that are important to interpreting osteopathic clinical practice. Thus, the chapters do not attempt to cover all areas of basic science or even to summarize the current knowledge in these areas, but rather provide ways of conceptualizing areas within an osteopathic understanding of health and loss of health.

Anatomy

The first three chapters of the section deal with the very important area of anatomy and build on each other. The study of anatomy is of utmost importance to the osteopathic student. Without a thorough understanding of not only the structures of the body, but also how the structures provide function, the osteopathic physician will be unable to best use the basic principles of palpation and manipulation. In Chapter 3, "Rules of Anatomy," Towns uses his years of experience in teaching anatomy to draw attention to some of the important ways to view the body's structures and the principles that combine these structures with function. He points out that it is important for the osteopathic physician to be able to visualize the true relationships between structures, not only to understand their function, but also to know when they are not functioning correctly and how to use the best manipulative techniques to improve functional capacity. How fluids move into and out of an area is vital to understanding normal and abnormal function. This includes not only the arterial and venous supply, but also lymph movement and drainage. Improper fluid movement is a vital and primary cause of loss of integrated function. Knowledge of what is connected to what and how pain can be used or misunderstood is a vital part of understanding anatomy. It contributes to a physician's ability to help the patient. These topics are discussed here.

Chapter 4, by Jacobs and Falls, provides an overview of the concepts of anatomy. The authors point out that a thorough understanding not only of anatomic structures but of how they interrelate is key to understanding the basis of health. They discuss the often overlooked, all-encompassing fascial tissues as important contributors to continuity throughout the body. They also emphasize the importance of myofascial continuity throughout the body as a means to understanding the disparate effects of disturbances in an often-distant structure.

Chapter 5, by Wells, completes this trilogy with a presentation of biomechanics. This chapter brings together the basic concepts of the Chapters 3 and 4 into a functional whole. Many of the concepts presented here are necessary to interpret the findings of palpatory diagnosis and to determine the best means of treatment of biomechanical problems. Key elements include the idea of constant remodeling of tissues, including bone, functional stress, the changes of these properties with age, and the storing of energy during movement by elastic properties of tissues.

These three chapters provide the student of osteopathic medicine with an excellent introduction to the important issues in anatomy. They should supplement well the basic knowledge gained in the anatomy laboratory and during the study of palpation and manipulation.

Autonomic Nervous System

The autonomic nervous system is one of the most important, and yet one of the most poorly understood, systems of the body. Usually thought of as a rather dull and even uninteresting part of the nervous system, dealing with only visceral functions, it is actually one of the most important of the integrating systems. The sympathetic nerves actually innervate almost all body structures and have tremendous influence over the body's immune function. In Chapter 6, Willard provides a glimpse of the vast complexity of this system as it influences all body function. He examines not only the structure of the system, but outlines many of the neurochemical aspects of this great integrating system, and the complexity of the process involved. He emphasizes the importance of this system in coordinating the activities of the visceral systems to meet the demands imposed by the musculoskeletal system. An understanding of the autonomic system is vital to the osteopathic physician's understanding of total body integration, and to the often confusing and seemingly contradictory symptoms that are produced when the system malfunctions.

Neurophysiology

Chapter 7, by Patterson and Wurster, and Chapter 8, by Willard, present a picture of the workings of the neurophysiological sys-

tems as they relate to the integration of body function. While obviously not separate from the autonomic nervous system, the information in these two chapters focuses on the organization of the somatovisceral and viscerosomatic interactions of the body and the functional changes brought about by afferent input to these systems. In Chapter 7, Patterson and Wurster review the structural basis for somatovisceral and viscerosomatic interactions and present an example of these pathways. The four stages of reflex alterations, from short-term to permanent alterations in reflex function are reviewed and some of their implications for function are outlined. The authors then review the evidence for axoplasmic or nonimpulse-based actions of nerves on end organs and the implications for function of this neural activity.

In Chapter 8, Willard presents the neurochemical basis for reflex change and reviews the implications of nociceptive activity for higher neural or brain function. The results of pain inputs for psychological and immune function are given, along with a basic outline of the brain processes involved. Willard presents a model for interpreting aspects of the somatic dysfunction in terms of these changes, and provides good evidence for an organized dysfunctional pattern that evolves from abnormal responses to pain inputs.

The coordinated picture emerging from various areas of neurophysiology and neuropsychology fully supports the clinical observations of the osteopathic profession regarding the integrated nature of physiological and psychological function. The effects of pain inputs have consequences for reflex function at the spinal cord level that were seen by Denslow and Korr in their studies of the 1940s and 1950s. It is now becoming clear that these types of alterations that disrupt normal function also occur at higher centers and cause psychological, immune, and adaptive dysfunction. By understanding these sequences of change and how to minimize, reverse, or enable adaptation to them, the osteopathic physician will be much better able to help a wide spectrum of patients once thought to be intractable to health restoration.

Respiration/Circulation

The topic of respiration and circulation was one of the most important issues in the thinking of Still and early osteopathic practitioners. The flow of fluids and the proper balance of respiratory products in the tissues were vitally important in the maintenance of proper function. While the nerves controlled the flow of blood, the arteries supplied the route and means for the fluids to reach the tissues and the veins and lymphatics allowed for the return and purification of blood and extracellular fluids. Any disruption of these flows was looked on as the moment of the start of disease, or dysfunction. When discussing respiration, Still generally meant respiration at a cellular level, and the fluid circulation was the key to that process.

Chapter 9, by Sparks, begins by acknowledging this fact, that the circulation is the cell's connection to the outside world. The chapter reviews the cellular requirements for activity and how the basic cellular processes require regulated energy resources. From there, the author advances to the regulation of tissue circulation at the local and regional levels. The coronary circulation is used as an example of the interactions between local and neural circulatory regulation. Finally, he discusses blood flow regulation in the skin. Thus, the contrasts between skin and coronary blood flow regulation show the differences in regulation in vital versus nonvital organs. This discussion of blood flow regulation and circulatory demands should allow the student to begin to see the complexity of cellular respiration and circulation and how the requirements differ in various tissues, as well as how the moment-to-moment circulatory requirements and flows directly affect cellular function and, hence, health.

Microbiology

The area of microbiology is one that was in its infancy at the time the osteopathic profession was founded. Still clearly recognized the role of the microbe as a pathological process affecting human morbidity and mortality. The germ theory of disease was well delineated by the time Still founded his school, and he referred to it often. While recognizing the role of microorganisms in pathologic processes of illness, Still also recognized that in many, if not all cases, in order to have symptomatic consequences for the human being, the microorganism must have a fertile ground in which to grow. Under normal function, the pathological organism would be kept in check by the host. When the circulatory or other functions were disturbed, the often naturally occurring organism could produce illness or death. Thus, for Still, the primary cause of disease was not the microorganism, but the lack of proper function. Indeed this is a very important distinction to make. Thus, the root cause of a disease process is function, not a microorganism.

In Chapter 10, the Jensens masterfully outline the background of microbiology and the germ theory of disease. They point out just what the constraints of this theory are and how osteopathic philosophy recognized the theory within its own framework. The chapter introduces the student to the concepts of virulence and virulence factors as they affect the operation of pathogenic organisms. The role of the host is identified and discussed. The authors outline the factors that affect the success of microbes in their assault on the human, and the various countermeasures humans have evolved to thwart microbial assault. They show the reader the important role of nutrition, fever, and immune mechanisms in discouraging microbial pathology. Of particular importance is the discussion of the role and pitfalls of antibiotics in medical practice. This should be read by all osteopathic medical students, as should the discussion of hygiene and vaccinations. The distinction the Jensens make between a microbe and a pathogen at the end of Chapter 10 is very important. Many microbes coexist peacefully with every human being until the controlling mechanisms of the host human are compromised, allowing the microbe to change to a pathogen, sometimes killing the host. It is this principle that was recognized by Still and that must be reemphasized today. In most cases, the proper function of the host is sufficient unto itself to control the microbe. When the host's function is compromised, the pathogenic properties of the microbe are allowed to be manifest. The major problem is not the microbe, but in the host's function, and that is where major restorative efforts must be directed. Too often in medicine today, the only effort is to externally control the microbe and the role of the host is forgotten.

Endocrinology

The endocrine system is treated uniquely by Portanova in Chapter 11. As with all other systems discussed in this section, the author has room only to provide an overview of the endocrine system as it applies to the concept of functional integration. Portanova uses the complexity and ubiquity of endocrine function to illustrate the beauty of interactions at every level of function. He points out that, while the level of knowledge in Still's time was very rudimentary (but then, what will our grandchildren say of our understanding?), the concepts of functional integration held by Still are beautifully shown by the control loops and feedback pathways within the endocrine system. Indeed, Portanova uses several of the basic tenets of the osteopathic philosophy as tenets of endocrine function. This allows the reader to see the application of these concepts at a systems level. Indeed, the author points out that the osteopathic philosophy is so "deeply rooted in the fabric of life" that even knowledge gained in the future will be embraced by this philosophy. Perhaps this is one of the beauties of Still's philosophy and conceptualization of function. Certainly, the reader will gain a new and deeper appreciation for both the osteopathic philosophy and the endocrine system while reading this chapter.

Pharmacology

In the early days of the osteopathic profession, drug use was looked upon with great suspicion. In fact, Still forbade the use of drugs and the teaching of pharmacology in his school. In retrospect, it is easy to see why Still took this attitude. Most, if not all, common drugs of the time were detrimental to function and health, or were used in harmful ways. It was common to use mercury in sufficient amounts to cause teeth to fall out. Now, the use of Pharmacopoeia is common and viewed as a necessary adjunct for complete medical practice. There is little doubt, however, that drugs are often overprescribed, incorrectly used, and abused. In Chapter 12, Theobald presents parallels between the concepts of osteopathic medicine and the use of modern pharmacologic agents. He points out that the rational use of any pharmacologic agent necessitates understanding that each individual is unique. Chemical agents used properly can help the body regain control of systems that are functioning improperly and help redress balance of function. The author's description of the treatment of hypertension with pharmacologic agents using the principles of integration is a wonderful example of how endogenous agents can help the body restore properly integrated function. There can be little doubt that Still's attitude, were he alive today, would be somewhat different toward the proper use of some pharmacologic agents, although just as surely, not appreciating the widespread and profligate use seen in many medical practices today.

CONCLUSION

The chapters of this section show various levels of integration within and between various body systems and units. In addition, the correspondence of the osteopathic philosophy with principles used in human function is evident. These examples provide a basis for understanding ways in which structure and function are interrelated. The interrelatedness of structure with function provides an integration that is the hallmark of health. The examples used in many of the chapters show how the integration of health can become disrupted, producing the first and necessary cause of disease, but as an effect, not a cause. Osteopathic philosophy is admirably demonstrated in these chapters, with the authors showing the fit between the emerging scientific understanding of human function and osteopathic philosophy. Thus, the authors have provided a means for a deeper understanding of the application of osteopathic philosophy to the optimization of human health.

3

RULES OF ANATOMY

LEX C. TOWNS

KEY CONCEPTS

Seven "rules" of anatomy will help guide the study and use of anatomy in medical practice:

■ Understanding three-dimensional relationships is fundamental to using anatomy.
■ Knowing what things do is the companion goal of knowing their location.
■ The integrity of arteries and nerves is essential to health.
■ Healthy homeostasis requires that fluid entering be drained away, too.
■ Pain is almost always an anatomic symptom.
■ No organ or organ system exists in isolation in the body.
■ Each person has a different anatomy.

An understanding of anatomy is fundamental to the rational practice of medicine. To assess health and disease, physicians must have a detailed knowledge of the structures of the body with which they deal. The detailed anatomic knowledge of many physicians may be restricted to the particular body area or functional system that they use in a specialized practice. However, effective physicians, even those in specialized practices, need and use a working knowledge of the reciprocal, interactive nature of the body's structure and function. Osteopathic physicians need sufficient knowledge of body structure and function to understand how focal destructive causes may not only lead to localized effects but may also contribute to more subtle, widespread, or distant degenerative, morbid events. The payoff for mastering anatomy is to develop the ability to practice medicine—especially osteopathic medicine—in a more intelligent, predictable, and effective manner.

This chapter does not attempt to thoroughly review anatomy. Numerous excellent books and programs are available on human anatomy, and the effective methods of teaching anatomy vary from school to school. The purpose of this chapter is to provide the beginning student with some conceptual bases to guide the study of anatomy and thereby to help maximize the positive impact of anatomic knowledge on the eventual osteopathic medical practice. These concepts are sketched here as a series of "rules." These "rules" are not mutually exclusive or exhaustive;

indeed, faculty at each school will add or subtract as they see fit. Nevertheless these rules are intended to illustrate that attention to fundamental concepts of anatomy will assist the student in learning anatomy and, hopefully, will also convince the student that effective osteopathic medical treatment proceeds from an accurate understanding of structure.

RULE 1: RULE OF PROXIMITY

Understanding spatial relationships forms the essence of the use of anatomy in medical practice. The most usable admonition is also the most obvious: in any particular part of the body, you must know the spatial arrangement of all the organs and tissues. Knowledge of spatial relations, gained from lectures, readings, and dissections, allows one to mentally reconstruct the entire anatomy of an area when only limited cues are available. For example, when palpating the abdomen, the physician must be able to accurately place the entire abdominal contents based on a few large organs or surface landmarks that can be seen or felt manually. Another example: when casting a limb, the physician must understand the placement of important arteries, veins, and nerves to avoid the disastrous consequences that would result from compromise to these vital structures, the locations of which are inferable only from bony or muscular surface landmarks.

A necessary first step is often to learn basic facts of anatomy, such as: What is the attachment of the biceps brachii? What are the branches of the femoral artery? How is the brachial plexus formed and what are its branches? However, the more important task is to place those isolated facts into a larger morphologic context. For example, a student might initially memorize the layout of the brachial plexus; but the brachial plexus is spatially related to other crucial structures in the arm, axilla, and root of the neck. The ventral rami of spinal nerves that form the brachial plexus pass through and among the scalene muscles of the neck; the cords of the brachial plexus surround the brachial artery; and the nerves derived from the cords pass around and among the muscles of the arm. Without this subsequent understanding, the memorization is largely a wasted effort.

With the advent of powerful new imaging technologies, some might assume that the eventual task of the practicing physician would be greatly simplified, that the study of relational anatomy would become unnecessary. In fact, a new level of complexity is added by the ready availability of computerized tomography (CT), magnetic resonance imaging (MRI), and other modern imaging technologies. Recognizing and reconstructing whole anatomic structures on the basis of their sectional representation is not an inconsequential mental task. Most teaching programs of anatomy now emphasize how the three-dimensional morphology seen in dissection and represented in textbooks and atlases appears when imaged via various technologies. Physicians must now be conversant with the contemporary images of structure, and they must also become facile at translating these static or dynamic images into complete, inclusive, three-dimensional living patients. Realistically, the advent of modern imaging technology has replaced the need to infer deep anatomy from subtle surface landmarks. However, the clarity with which previously unviewable structures can now be seen is offset by the necessity to mentally reconstruct whole regions of the body three-dimensionally from slices.

Also, despite the power of these remarkable new tools, many important small structures are not visualized. Physicians must still rely on a detailed knowledge of relational anatomy in order to be able to place small nerves and vessels into the context of structures seen on CT or MRI images. For example, the esophagus is easily visualized in CT or MRI, and many pathological conditions (i.e., esophageal cancer) would be readily detected. The esophageal plexus, on the other hand, would not be visualized. This plexus of nerves, embedded in the external fascia of the esophagus, is the sole source of parasympathetic fibers to many abdominal organs and contains important sensory fibers as well. Thus, the knowledgeable physician would want to be attentive to the possibility of symptoms that would result from destruction of the esophageal plexus as a result of esophageal disease.

The rule of proximity is also powerfully applied with the reconstruction of spatial relations as osteopathic physicians use the most distinctive features of their practice: palpatory diagnosis and musculoskeletal manipulative therapy. The osteopathic physician must have a clear comprehension of the anatomic relationships of muscles, muscle attachments, and bones to each other and to vessels, nerves, lymphatics, fascia, and organs. This is prerequisite to most osteopathic diagnostic and therapeutic strategies. Together, palpation and manipulation can be thought of as anatomy in practice. This mental reconstruction of the anatomic structure of a region proceeds from only a few palpable or visible superficial landmarks.

The accurate diagnosis and treatment of many conditions and diseases proceeds from knowing where things are located. Virtually all the utilization of anatomy in a clinical setting, as well as all of the other rules described in this chapter, are based on the rule of proximity.

RULE 2: RULE OF FUNCTION

Most gross anatomy courses appropriately limit the discussion of function for many of the structures, organs, or organ systems. For example, the function of the lung is to provide gas exchange between the air and the blood; the function of the kidneys is to filter the blood and excrete urine; and the function of the gastrointestinal tract is to digest and absorb nutrients and water. Details of these functions are left to the other basic sciences, which in turn assume an understanding of gross structure. Nevertheless it remains important to grasp the intimate relationship of structure and function. The human organism is a complex, unified organism; relating structure and function is one basic and necessary strategy to understand the functioning, integrated, whole human being.

The musculoskeletal system is approximately 75% of the body mass; this vast system gives stability in health, provide clues to dysfunction and disease, and offers a mode of treatment to support the patient who is diseased or stressed. Osteopathic physicians must understand well the function of the individual components of the musculoskeletal system. This function is seen from two fundamental, complementary perspectives: What action or function does a muscle (joint, bone, ligament, etc.) produce? And, Which muscle (joint, bone, ligament, etc.) produces a specific action or function?

In a clinical evaluation, the physician may be presented with a patient who has, among other symptoms, a weakness in abducting the arm. Abducting the arm—that is, moving the upper limb from aside the body to a position overhead—requires the coordinated, sequential action of several muscles. A small muscle attached to the scapula (the supraspinatus) initiates abduction. Movement of the arm to a horizontal position is accomplished by contraction of the deltoid, the large muscle making up the rounded point of the shoulder. For the arm to be raised overhead, the scapula has to be rotated by muscles that attach the scapula to the spine (principally the trapezius).

Working from the complaint or observation, the physician must recall which muscle(s) produces the action and then assess the strength of each in its various movements. Let's assume in this scenario that the physician has demonstrated a weakness of the deltoid muscle. The physician must then use his or her knowledge of anatomy to move to the question of why the deltoid is weak. First, the physician must recall the innervation of the muscle (the axillary nerve) and assess the strength of other muscles (teres minor) innervated by that nerve. The axillary nerve also provides sensory fibers to the point of the shoulder; thus, the physician would want to examine sensation to the area. Working proximally up the brachial plexus, the physician then checks the function of muscles that, like the deltoid via the axillary nerve, receive their motor supply from branches of the posterior cord of the brachial plexus (this would be all the extensor muscles of the upper limb). More proximally still, the innervation of the deltoid muscle is principally from the fifth cervical spinal nerve. From this cervical spinal segment also arises some of the motor fibers that innervate the thoracic diaphragm. Thus, starting with a relatively simple functional loss in the deltoid muscle, the physician looks for answers to the following questions: Does teres minor contract properly? Is sensory loss evident over the point of the shoulder? Are the extensor muscles of the upper limb weak? Is there any compromise in respiratory function?

The physician may then proceed to enlarge the domain of the functional examination. What postural or functional compensation has the patient made for weakness of the deltoid? Is weakness of abduction unrelated to the deltoid and simply a function of pain in the shoulder; that is, does the patient not raise the arm because it hurts to do so? Is the pain in the joint itself or does it result from disease of some internal organ?

Understanding the rule of function in the musculoskeletal system leads inevitably to a series of questions predicated on more complex structural and functional interrelationships: How might dysfunction of the muscle (or other musculoskeletal component) affect total body efficiency and health? How might dysfunction of some visceral element degrade the structural or functional integrity of the musculoskeletal system? These questions form the core of some of the following rules.

RULE 3: RULE OF SUPPLY

Two structural entities, arteries and nerves, are important for the health and maintenance of any organ or area. Arteries supply nutrients, oxygen, and a variety of hormonal regulatory substances to the area of their distribution. Nerves provide ongoing neural control of skeletal and smooth muscle and glandular tissue and deliver trophic or regulatory factors to the muscles or organs that they innervate. The rule of supply illustrates a major source for maintenance of health or, conversely, origin of pathology when disrupted.

Few statements are more cogent than A.T. Still's insightful dictum: "The rule of the artery is supreme" (1). An adequate blood supply during varying physiologic conditions is a prerequisite for health of an organ or region. Conversely, compromise to the blood supply often leads to functional capacity being diminished, cascading, in turn, toward disease. The osteopathic physician must work to ensure continued blood supply in the healthy state and, when treating injury or disease, should attempt to enhance arterial supply to affected regions. One important condition of compromise is bleeding due to trauma or disease. The physician must have sufficient understanding of anatomy to be able to halt hemorrhage quickly and subsequently restore adequate blood flow to ischemic areas. But the physician must also be able to recognize the clinical signs of ischemia due to blockage of arterial supply and work to relieve the blockage.

To optimize strategies that continue arterial supply (and vigor) in the healthy state, and to use appropriate therapeutic interventions in disease or injury to restore adequate blood supply, a physician must have an accurate knowledge of the arterial supply to an area. Consistent with rule 1, as previously outlined, it is not sufficient simply to know the name of the artery that provides supply; rather, the passage of the arterial supply must be placed in the context of surrounding muscles, bones, organs, lymphatics, fascia, and so forth.

One of the goals of an osteopathic approach to medical treatment is, first, to recognize which piece of surrounding tissue might be compressing an artery and, having visualized the mechanical impediment to blood flow, adopt appropriate therapies to relieve the compression and thereby restore normal flow. Similarly, the osteopathic physician works to recognize in the healthy individual those areas or organs that might be at risk for reduced blood flow caused by lifestyle, activities, posture, obesity, and so on, and adopt a treatment plan to maintain health in zones at risk.

As do arteries, nerves also supply vital components to every portion of the body. Nerves supply control; they are a major component of the body's homeostatic mechanisms. Nerve cell bodies in the central nervous system (CNS) send nerve fibers to control contraction of smooth (involuntary) muscles and skeletal (voluntary) muscles and to control secretion of glands. Nerves also provide sensory input; they convey either exteroceptive input concerning physical forces that impinge on the body or interoceptive feedback about the status of the internal milieu. Nerve fibers also supply chemical materials from the CNS to the periphery and vice versa. Through the mechanism of axoplasmic transport, trophic (growth promoting) chemicals are manufactured in the neuron cell body and carried to target muscles or organs where, after release into the synaptic space, they are taken into the target tissue to promote healthy function. Passing in the opposite direction, chemicals from the muscle or organ can cross the synapse, be taken up, and be transported retrogradely to the neuron cell bodies where the chemicals can then alter basic neuronal function.

Individual peripheral nerves have specific segmental relationship to the CNS and, therefore, to the entire body. The segmental origin of nerves is pertinent to three general targets of innervation: skin, muscles, and internal organs. The dermatomal (skin) innervation pattern is relatively straightforward. Pain or sensory loss over some specific dermatomal zone leads the knowledgeable physician to inferences about the integrity of restricted areas of the CNS or nerves near their origin. Innervation of the skin of the limbs becomes a bit more complicated because the sensory nerves from specific spinal cord segments are drawn together into specific cutaneous nerves that contain sensory fibers from more than one segment. A specific peripheral nerve (e.g., the medial cutaneous nerve of the forearm) will contain fibers from two or more segments (in this case C8 and T1), although those fibers will distribute at their termination in the skin in a dermatomal pattern. Here the notion is that the examining physician must have sufficient understanding of anatomy to be able to differentiate sensory disturbances that arise in a particular peripheral nerve as opposed to an entire segmental level.

The innervation pattern of muscles is particularly pertinent to osteopathic medicine because changes in the tone, texture, or function of a muscle may be related to the segmental source of nerve supply to that muscle. The innervation of muscles of the trunk is relatively simple and follows a pattern similar to that of the dermatomes. Nerve fibers to the muscles of the limbs, on the other hand, arise from the spinal cord and are woven through complex networks (the brachial plexus and lumbosacral plexus) that combine fibers from several spinal cord segments into motor nerves that typically serve functional groups of muscles. A physician must understand innervation of limb muscles well enough to reconstruct those nerve fibers from their termination, through the plexus to their spinal cord origin. As with the sensory nerves, the goal for the physician is to be able to differentiate motor losses due to compromise of a distal, peripheral nerve versus losses associated with a lesion of one or more spinal cord segments or associated spinal nerves.

The internal viscera receive abundant autonomic nerve supply, and the sensory innervation to the internal viscera that signals functional status, distention, and pain typically accompanies the autonomic innervation to the target organ. The pattern by which this autonomic and sensory nerve supply arises from the spinal cord or brainstem and passes to target tissue is schematically simple but anatomically complex; as such, its pattern will not be summarized here. The key point to be made, however, is that because of developmental and maturational events, the segmental origin of autonomic and sensory innervation of a specific organ may be relatively distant from that particular viscus. As a result, changes in a particular visceral organ may appear as pain or changes in muscle texture some distance from the organ. On the other hand, localized musculoskeletal misalignment may produce alteration in autonomic outflow from the related segmental zone of the spinal cord and may disturb function in an internal organ some distance away from that segment. The physician must understand both the general segmental origin and anatomic pathway by which autonomic nerve fibers and the accompanying sensory nerve fibers pass to the various internal organs.

Nerves supply important functional and trophic control to all parts of the body. An important aspect of osteopathic medical practice is to recognize and treat conditions that alter nerve supply to a region or organ. The success of palpation and treatments in recognizing and relieving compression or irritation to nerves and the effectiveness of maintenance of nerve traffic by healthy lifestyles depend directly on how well the physician understands the route that nerves take from their origin to their destination.

RULE 4: RULE OF DRAINAGE

While the arterial supply is the only means by which fluid and blood cellular components are taken to an area, two pathways remove fluids and blood cells from a region. The venous network collects the deoxygenated blood from the capillary bed; the lymphatic channels drain the relatively cell-free extracellular fluid that accumulates outside the vascular system. Compromising either of these return channels leads to edema in the affected area: more fluid goes in than comes out.

To alleviate edema, the osteopathic physician may choose to use protocols to enhance venous and/or lymphatic return. The strategy selected depends, of course, on the medical condition of the patient as well as on a thorough knowledge of the anatomy of the venous and lymphatic systems. As with the arterial system, the knowledge of anatomy places venous and lymphatic channels into the context of surrounding organs, muscles, bones, fascia, and so forth, usually by appreciating those structures on the basis of subtle palpable or surface landmarks.

Peripheral venous channels tend to be somewhat variable, with considerable anastomoses. For general medical application, it is acceptable to understand the overall pattern of peripheral venous drainage and concentrate one's effort on the larger, more predictable central veins. Understanding the anastomoses of peripheral venous channels is useful in the treatment of the venous system. For example, venous anastomoses offer therapeutic strategies for the physician as alternate routes of venous drainage are established. Understanding the routes of venous anastomoses is vital to also correctly diagnose pathology, as significant venous blood flow through some anastomoses is unusual and may

indicate a pathologic condition. Most venous blood from the gastrointestinal system, for example, is drained through the portal venous system to the liver. But most of the blood from the lower half of the body wall and lower limbs drains into the inferior vena cava. Some small, usually insignificant anastomoses between these two major venous channels do exist. However, when large amounts of blood are shunted from the portal system to the caval system, these anastomotic vessels become enlarged. Internal anal hemorrhoids or esophageal varices are engorgements of these anastomotic vessels and indicate shunting of blood from the portal venous system to the vena caval system and may, therefore, indicate blockage of venous drainage to the liver—so-called portal hypertension—that results when the liver is diseased.

The rule of venous drainage is to know by which veins an area is typically drained of blood, by what routes blood drains if the typical route is blocked, and where the veins lie relative to the surrounding structures.

Lymphatic channels are typically even more variable than veins in their gross morphology; knowing general patterns and spatial relations of lymph drainage is usually sufficient. Although they are less well defined anatomically, they are important to understand. As with venous return, selecting osteopathic approaches to treatment of edema assumes a working knowledge of the location of lymph channels and how to augment lymphatic flow. Lymph collects into blind-ended endothelial tubes in the periphery. These channels merge into ever-larger channels throughout the body, are filtered at predictable intervals by lymph nodes, and finally converge on (usually) two large lymphatic ducts in the root of the neck. These two lymphatic ducts then empty into the venous system near the heart.

As the lymphatic system has no intrinsic pump, fluid is moved from peripheral to central regions by osmotic pressure, muscular contractions, external pressure, and pressure differences between the thorax and the abdomen. There are various techniques to increase lymphatic return. When using techniques of muscle contraction or applying local pressure or lymphatic pump mechanisms, one needs prerequisite knowledge of the anatomy of lymphatic flow.

In addition to returning extracellular fluid to the general circulation, the lymphatic system and the lymph nodes are often indicators of disease. The lymphoid system houses important cells of the immune system. As a result of infection, lymphocytes proliferate and are sequestered in lymph nodes, where they attack pathogens (bacteria, viruses, etc.) in the lymph. Because of this important immune function, lymph nodes draining an infected area are often swollen and palpable.

Cancer in an organ will often metastasize to adjacent lymph nodes and will also cause node enlargement. It is therefore crucial that the examining physician understand the potential significance of enlarged lymph nodes. For example, breast cancer may metastasize to the lymph nodes on the lateral thoracic wall or in the axilla that drain lymph from the breast. Or, illustrating a less obvious anatomic relationship, an enlarged node above the clavicle in the root of the neck may indicate disease of the stomach. When enlarged lymph nodes are detected, the examining physician can use knowledge of the anatomic pattern by which lymph drains to infer the source of a disease process.

RULE 5: RULE OF PAIN

Pain brings more people to the physician than any other single complaint. Because of the prevalence of pain as a symptom, it is important to understand the anatomy of pain. Pain is almost always a symptom, not the disease or disturbance itself.

Pain—whether sharp or dull, constant or intermittent, recent or long-standing—can usually be localized by the patient. Where the pain is easily attributed to an identifiable injury, the physician's use of anatomy is somewhat simplified; the pain is generally alleviated by administering analgesics and adopting therapies to support wound healing. Even in these cases, however, a working knowledge of the anatomy of the damaged area is a useful tool in the treatment of pain resulting from injury. The structural and functional integrity of the arterial supply, venous and lymphatic drainage, and nerve supply to the wounded area must be optimized to treat pain caused by a localized wound.

A common medical scenario, however, is of a patient who has a symptom of localized pain, yet no superficial tissue damage is visible. Swelling or redness may help direct the examination, but often the complaint is without an obvious external physical manifestation. Whether local signs are present or not, the physician must be able to appreciate the structures in that area and their spatial relationships. Using this mental map of the area, and guided by the history, the physician gently palpates in an effort to more clearly identify the source of the pain. Such palpatory examinations are of limited use without an understanding of anatomy and, indeed, proceeding in ignorance may risk further injury.

The task of inferring anatomy from surface palpation is somewhat simpler in the limbs. These areas are not intrinsically easier (some of the most complex spatial relationships of structure are associated with the limbs), but a proportionally greater amount of the limbs are available for direct visual inspection and palpation. Similarly, much of the superficial neck anatomy can be assessed with palpation, but deep prevertebral structures are inaccessible to palpation. The walls of the thorax, abdomen, or pelvis are readily palpated; superficial pain in these walls can often be assessed with limited necessity to recall deep anatomy. However, to address a patient's pain inside the thorax, abdomen, or pelvis, one must know the normal anatomy of the affected region. Preliminary judgments of the size, integrity, and health of the viscera are based on superficial cues.

In most medical environments, the initial visual or palpatory inference of anatomy may be rapidly checked with one or more medical imaging modalities, such as plane radiographic films, CT, MRI, or ultrasound. The information given the physician is anatomically more concrete, but in some cases requires an even more sophisticated level of anatomic knowledge. The examining physician must call on a detailed mental image of the anatomy of an area during initial examination. The physician must then reconstruct three-dimensional spatial relations from CT or MRI sections, inferring placement of structures from shades of gray in a radiograph, or visualizing unseen structures in the shadows of an ultrasound sector, which also requires a detailed knowledge of anatomy. It is difficult to localize and interpret the source of that most common symptom, pain, without an accurate understanding of the anatomy of a region.

Physicians must also be alert to referred pain (i.e., when an organ or structure is diseased or damaged but the pain is felt somewhere else). The most coherent hypothesis of referred pain postulates that individual pain transmission neurons in the spinal cord receive afferents from both somatic pain fibers from the body wall and visceral pain fibers from deep organs. Individual pain transmission cells are almost always stimulated by somatic pain; higher somatosensory centers thus come to interpret that cell's firing as localized to a somatic site. In the rare circumstance that a pain transmission cell in the spinal cord is stimulated by visceral pain afferents, the pain is nevertheless interpreted by higher centers as originating at the somatic site.

Referred pain is often difficult to localize and may move as the state of the disease progresses. Initially, pain may be vague and gnawing, and felt in the midline of the body. Later, pain may become paravertebral and then follow a segmental or dermatomal pattern. Examples of referred pain are numerous. The following are two examples: Damage to heart tissue invokes a sensation of pain in the left arm, shoulder, neck, and jaw; or gallbladder irritation causes referred pain in the right flank.

Physicians recognize referred pain by experience and further understand its significance in a patient. The osteopathic physician should be particularly attentive to pathways of sensory innervation and pain innervation. The somatic innervation to the body wall and limbs is via spinal nerves, while the pain innervation of thoracic, abdominal, and pelvic viscera is via peripheral processes of dorsal root ganglia cells that generally accompany the distribution of autonomic fibers.

Pain is the most anatomic of symptoms. The proper localization and identification of the source of pain, whether superficial or deep, direct or referred, is essential to understanding the significance of the pain and a necessary prerequisite to comprehensive treatment of the underlying condition.

RULE 6: RULE OF CONNECTEDNESS

It has not been customary in modern medicine to point out that the human is a complex, unified organism made up of many overlapping, interconnected systems. Recently, conventional medicine has attempted to reassemble its various specialties and subspecialties, each focused on a body region or functional system, into a holistic understanding of health and disease. Nevertheless, the structure of medicine retains much of its compartmentalization; it is difficult for even the most thoughtful physician, particularly those in a demanding specialty practice, to step back routinely and holistically assess a patient.

A physician's understanding of body unity and the propensity to view the patient holistically is heightened by remembering a basic unifying principle: although the body is made up of many structurally and functionally discrete elements, the elements are linked together by a number of connectors. These connectors, or the connectedness of the body, make up a significant portion of the study of medicine in general and the study of anatomy in particular.

Some of the connectors are easily listed and we have already touched on their importance. The circulatory system obviously connects distant body parts and, among other things, serves as a means of communication and connection. The nervous system, although traditionally divided into component parts (central, peripheral, autonomic, and enteric), is one continuous, functional entity. The nervous system constantly receives external and internal stimuli filters, sorts and integrates those stimuli, and then produces the coordinated contraction of muscles and/or secretion of glands in response to those stimuli. The nervous system can even impel muscular contraction and/or glandular secretion independent of external stimulation. The endocrine and immune systems, interconnected to each other and to the nervous systems, are also major connectors, serving to bring tissues distant from each other under unified, coordinated control.

One class of connectors is connective tissue in general, and fascia in particular. Connective tissue binds organ to organ, muscle to bone, and bone to bone, and literally is the fundamental connector that allows structural and functional systems to be physically grouped into a unified package. Without connective tissue, the body is a dissociated mass of dying cells. It is the connective tissue, most of it a proteinaceous extracellular matrix, that enforces form and thereby permits function. Connective tissue plays a critical role in body health and disease, but ironically it is so pervasive that it is easily overlooked in the study of anatomy, in the maintenance of health, and in the diagnosis and treatment of disease.

Fascia is one component of body connective tissue that is readily identified in gross anatomy. Fasciae are sheets of connective tissue that envelop specific structures and segregate one structure, organ, or area from another. For example, each individual muscle is wrapped in a layer of tightly investing connective fascia. Groups of muscle of similar location and function are further ensheathed in an enveloping fascia.

At a basic anatomic level, these fasciae define the individual muscles and muscle groups. For example, each of the muscles in the anterior compartment of the leg has its own investing fascia. The entire group is bounded laterally by a wall of fascia, the anterior crural septum, medially by fascia that is continuous with the periosteum of the tibia, and anteriorly by the encasing deep fascia of the leg. As is typical, the blood and nervous supply to these muscles, as well as venous and lymphatic return, are principally contained within this fascial compartment. These fasciae collectively define the anterior compartment. More important, they enhance the extensor functions of the muscles, while simultaneously providing protection, support, and separation from other muscle groups. The fasciae define the normal, healthy limit of the group; they tend to constrain destructive states and prevent the spread of bleeding, infection, tumor growth, and so forth, into adjacent compartments.

Fascial compartments also separate muscles of the trunk. For example, the muscles of the anterior abdominal wall are easily divided into planes and groups by tough, enveloping fascia. The external oblique, internal oblique, transversus abdominis, and rectus abdominis are delineable as a group and from one another not only by their attachments and orientations but also by the tight-fitting sheets of fascia that enclose them. Planes of fascia are also found in the subcutaneous space, external to the deep fascia that bounds the surfaces of the muscles. Understanding the placement of these fasciae is important in a variety of medical and surgical settings.

Many of the layers of fascia, whether subcutaneous or investing, merge together and/or have common points of attachment. The fasciae that separate and ensheathe the external and internal abdominal oblique muscles merge posteriorly. They also merge with the thick connective tissue, thoracolumbar fascia, which continues upward, encasing and separating the erector spinae, the deep muscles of the back. Anteriorly the fasciae of the abdominal muscles merge, split, and are reflected to contribute to the inguinal anatomy and abdominal aponeurosis. These fasciae are continuous with connective tissue sheets that flow over the crest of the pelvis and become the fascia lata of the thigh. The fascia of the thigh is continuous, in turn, with the crural fascia of the leg. As a consequence of the widespread continuity of fascia, distortion or damage to fascia in one area can have effects in a distant, seemingly unrelated area.

The subcutaneous fasciae are also continuous from one body region to another. The deep layer of superficial fascia of the abdomen (Scarpa's fascia) defines a space that is more or less continuous from the flank onto the abdominal wall. It continues inferiorly into the perineum, where it is the superficial perineal space (bounded by Colles' and dartos fasciae, continuations of Scarpa's fascia). Fluid or infection in the abdominal subcutaneous space can, thus, spread to the lumbar area or into the perineum.

The importance of the two-faceted aspect of fascia, that it at once not only separates and segregates but is also continuous structure-to-structure and area-to-area, should not be overlooked. This pervasive connector (along with muscle and bone) helps to regionalize the body and also connects region-to-region. Such a dualism is apparent in many physical manifestations of both health and disease.

The body, so often represented as a group of discrete regions or functional systems, is in reality an integrated whole. The integration of the body region-to-region and system-to-system is accomplished by a series of connectors. Some of these connectors, the endocrine and immune systems, are more commonly included in the context of physiology, biochemistry, or immunology. The nervous system, the vascular system, and the lymphatics are also important connectors, the structural components of which are part of anatomic disciplines. Finally, the visible connective tissues of the body, and particularly the fascia, are great physical connectors that bind organs or muscles into larger groups.

Coherent medical practice requires attention to the connected nature of the unified human organism. Typically, one disturbing force (a localized injury, lesion, or infection) causes a cascade of altered structural and functional changes in other areas or systems. Similarly, the treatment of localized disease or injury must be not only localized but must also attempt to bring the whole organism into healthy equilibrium. Planned treatments must account for not only the effect of the treatment protocol on the target site or organ system, but also the so-called side-effect alterations brought about in distant, relatively healthy systems by the treatment.

Observe the obvious examples of body unity. Take time to appreciate the connected nature of the body. For didactic reasons the body is traditionally disassembled into component parts or regions such as bones, muscles, vessels, nerves, thorax, gastrointestinal system, or upper limb. Yet it is important to be able mentally to reconstruct the intact specimen. The fundamental idea of holistic medicine is predicated on this.

RULE 7: RULE OF DIFFERENCE

The human body is not always built the way it is "supposed" to be: Sometimes it does not look like the picture in the atlas. The important rule to be stated is, again, the most obvious: The structure of each human body is different from all others. As our faces differ person-to-person, so, too, does the rest of our anatomy. There are two reasons for variation of human form: developmental and historical. Variation in structure may be based on either or both.

During development and maturation of the human form, each person's genetic information, along with extrinsic influences, determines their ultimate form. Developmental deviations of structure are so common that descriptions of normal anatomy can more usefully be translated as usual anatomy, with variations assumed. For example, the pattern of venous drainage of surface structures (the limbs and neck are all good examples) is so variable that only a general plan can be described, and even with the propensity of anatomists to name everything, only the larger elements can typically be identified. Similar normal variation is common in arterial supply. The branching of the celiac trunk to supply the stomach, liver, pancreas, spleen, and duodenum follows a general pattern, but there are numerous deviations. However, deviation of structure from the "norm" does not necessarily imply a pathologic condition.

As you continue the study of anatomy, you will also see how each individual's anatomy has been altered by injury or disease that is part of their life history. Virtually every cadaver has localized and/or widespread, visible, pathologic alteration of structure, caused by ravages of atherosclerotic disease, metastatic carcinoma, prolapsed rectum or uterus, arthritic changes, or any of the nearly endless list of diseases, injuries, or dysfunctions that characterize the physical, human condition. The structural outcome of systemic disorders, be they cardiovascular, pulmonary, gastrointestinal, musculoskeletal, or other, are often visible in the morphologic condition of those organs.

The cadavers available for teaching anatomy are usually of older individuals and, in addition to the types of systemic pathology outlined previously, these bodies also show the structural changes caused by the wear and tear of seven or eight decades. One can find arthritic joints, muscles withered by disuse, worn or infected teeth, or resorbed bones of the jaw when teeth are missing. The list of the normal alterations of anatomy that accompany aging is lengthy; these are important consequences of each person's life history. Many patients show morphologic evidence of age-related deterioration, and the physician can benefit from recollecting the texture and appearance of those changes first seen in cadaver dissection.

CONCLUSION

The rules that have been outlined here are, for the most part, self-evident. Anatomy is the study of structure and general function. It is imperative to learn where things are, what they do, how they are connected, how they influence each other, and how they change with time and life's experience.

REFERENCE

1. Still AT. *Autobiography of A. T. Still.* Published by the author, Kirksville, MO; 1897:219.

4

ANATOMY

ALLEN W. JACOBS
WILLIAM M. FALLS

KEY CONCEPTS

- How the fully developed human body's segmental nervous system is directly related to embryological growth patterns
- Differences among major types of connective tissue, the constituents of each, and their functional significance
- Differences between synovial and nonsynovial joints; joint play and its significance in the diagnosis of joint-related dysfunctions
- Structures in synovial joints and their functional basis
- Examples of nonsynovial joints and the differences between fibrous and cartilaginous types
- Anatomy of the muscle–tendon complex and its functional significance
- How the innervation from spinal segments is distributed throughout the body and how the limbs are supplied from this source
- Structural implications of myofascial continuity and its impact on the osteopathic diagnosis and treatment of musculoskeletal dysfunction

A fundamental understanding of basic human anatomy forms the foundation of osteopathic medicine. The embryologic development of the neuromusculoskeletal system provides the basis for understanding the segmental dermatomal representation of the nervous system as well as the distribution of somatic and visceral nerve supply to the entire body.

The microscopic structure of connective tissue is a key element in understanding myofascial continuity of the body. The gross structure of the musculoskeletal system is based on the microscopic structural and functional components of connective tissue and their interrelationship with skeletal muscle. The ability of the tissues of the musculoskeletal system to heal and repair following injury is directly related to their cellular content and microscopic structure. At the macroscopic level the arrangement of neurovascular bundles, which supply somatic tissue, is intimately related to connective tissue spaces and fascial planes.

The functional units of the musculoskeletal system are the synovial joint, muscle-tendon complex, and fascial elements, which support skeletal muscles and their neurovascular supply.

At the macroscopic level, the embryologic segmental organization of the body is represented in the axial skeleton. The arrangement of nerve and arterial supply, as well as venous and lymphatic drainage, is repeated segmentally throughout the axial skeleton and is modified to serve the upper and lower limbs. An understanding of this segmental organization is essential for diagnosis and treatment of neuromusculoskeletal system dysfunction and disorders.

The functional adaptation of the limbs is best understood through the concept of myofascial continuity. Posture, balance, and stability during dynamic activity are directly related to the functional capacity and adaptability of the myofascial elements of the body.

The discussion of the embryologic development, microscopic anatomy, functional units, and segmental organization of the neuromusculoskeletal system is based on an anatomic understanding that can be obtained by studying the detail presented in major anatomy textbooks (1–8). The application of this knowledge and an understanding of myofascial continuity are the foundations of osteopathic medicine, which are utilized in the diagnosis and treatment of neuromusculoskeletal dysfunctions and disorders.

NEUROMUSCULOSKELETAL EMBRYOLOGY

The embryologic development of the neuromusculoskeletal system exemplifies the segmental organization of the body. The formation of somites in the developing embryo, composed of embryonic mesoderm (mesenchyme), is specifically related to the segmentation of the neural tube. Each somite differentiates into two parts: a sclerotome and a dermomyotome (Fig. 4.1). As the mesenchyme migrates from these parts of the somites during development to form the segmental elements of the axial skeleton (e.g., vertebral column and ribs from the sclerotome; deep back muscles and intercostal muscles from the myotome), segmental nerve (spinal nerve) supply from the developing neural tube (spinal cord) is maintained (Figs. 4.2 and 4.3). Each myotome divides into an epimere innervated by the posterior primary ramus of a spinal nerve and a hypomere innervated by the

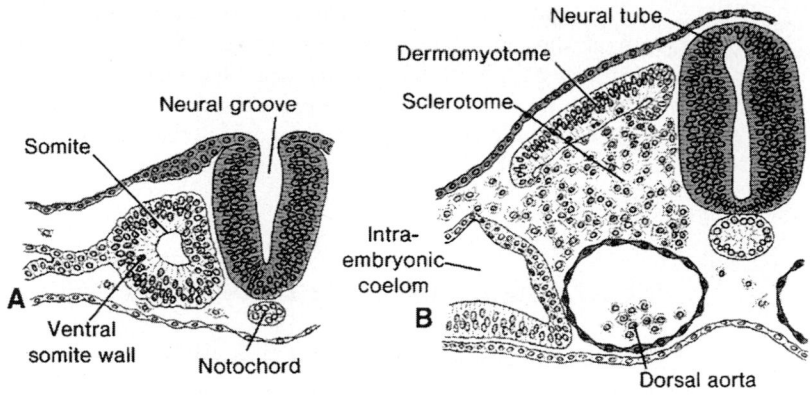

FIGURE 4.1. A and **B**: Transverse sections showing differentiation of a somite in relation to development of neural tube.

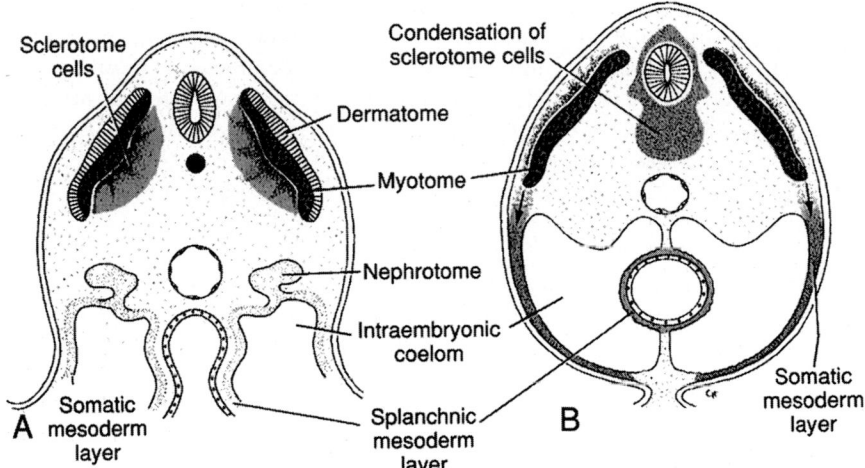

FIGURE 4.2. A and **B**: Transverse sections showing migration of cells from sclerotome and myotome during development.

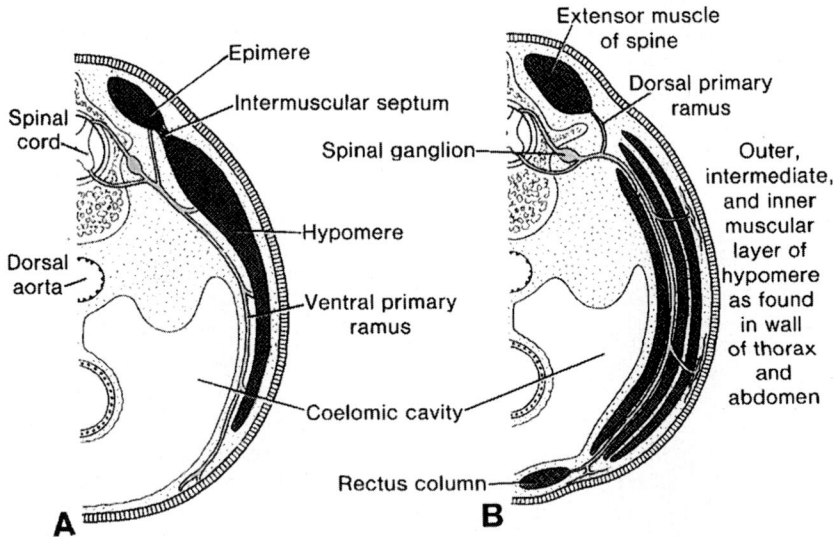

FIGURE 4.3. A and **B**: Transverse sections showing segmental nerve from developing spinal cord innervating developing musculature of thorax and abdomen.

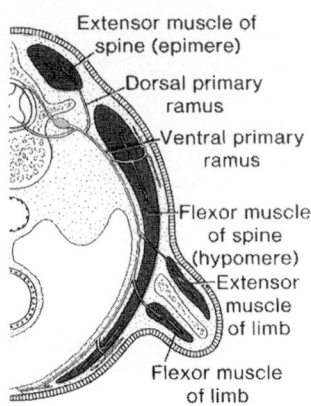

FIGURE 4.4. Transverse section showing that muscles (as well as bone and connective tissues) of developing limbs maintain segmental innervation from developing spinal cord.

anterior primary ramus of a spinal nerve (Fig. 4.3). This segmentation in the axial skeleton is sustained in the adult. The mesenchymal cells in the epimere become the deep back muscles in the adult, while the mesenchymal cells in the hypomere become the muscles of the anterolateral wall of the thorax and abdomen (Fig. 4.3).

With the development of the upper and lower limbs the mesenchyme, which forms bone, connective tissue, and muscle (derived from the hypomere) maintains segmental connections with the developing spinal cord through the anterior primary rami of spinal nerves growing into the developing limbs (Fig. 4.4). However, through differential limb growth and development (e.g., mesenchymal cells from different segments combining to form a single muscle in the adult) the initial segmental representation of the embryo is modified in the adult.

The segmentally organized nervous system provides the link between the somatic tissue and the viscera, which develop internally in a similar segmental manner. Therefore, through the segmental organization of the nervous system there is a structural relationship between the nerve supply to the somatic tissue and the autonomic visceral nerve supply of each segment of the developing embryo.

MUSCULOSKELETAL MICROSCOPIC ANATOMY

The connective tissues of the body are derived from mesenchyme. These developing tissues (connective tissue, bone, and cartilage) contain cells (fibroblasts, osteoblasts, and chondroblasts) that produce a matrix of ground substance and fibers surrounding the cells. Each type of connective tissue has a unique arrangement of cell types (fibrocytes, osteocytes, and chondrocytes) within a specific matrix of ground substance and fibers. By changing these three elements (cells, ground substance, and fibers) the variable composition and consistency of each type of connective tissue in the musculoskeletal system is produced. Connective tissue is classified on the basis of the arrangement of these three elements.

Connective Tissue

Loose connective tissue forms an open meshwork of cells (fibrocytes, fibroblasts) and fibers (collagen, elastic, reticular) with a large amount of fat cells and ground substance in between. Loose connective tissue also surrounds neurovascular bundles and fills the spaces between individual muscles and fascial planes (Fig. 4.5).

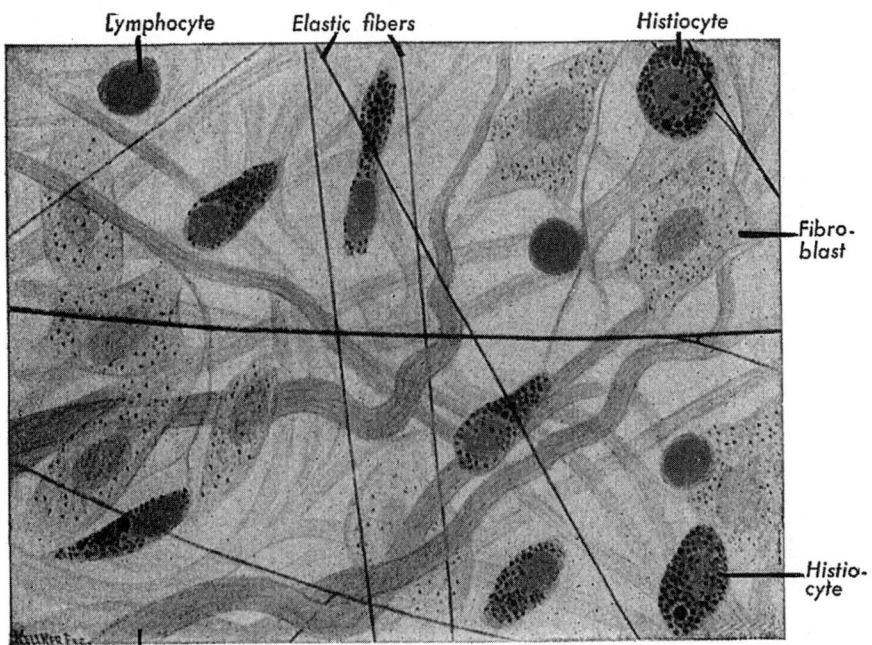

FIGURE 4.5. Cellular elements of loose connective tissue.

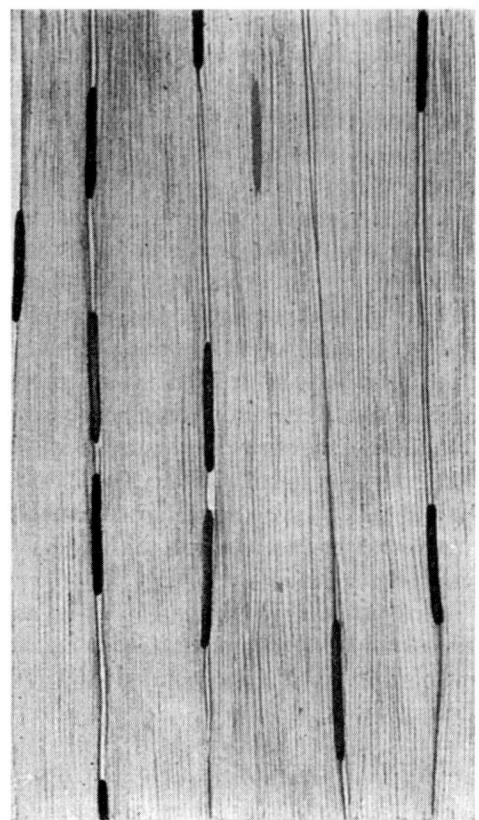

FIGURE 4.6. Cellular elements of dense, regular fibrous connective tissue. Dark fibroblast nuclei lie between bundles of regularly arranged collagen fibers.

Dense fibrous connective tissue is classified on the basis of the dense, regular arrangement of the predominant collagen fiber bundles, which run in the same direction. This tissue forms the substance of periosteum, tendons, ligaments, and deep fascia. It is commonly described as regular or irregular (e.g., periosteum and deep fascia) depending upon the arrangement of the closely packed collagen fiber bundles (e.g., tendons and ligaments) (Fig. 4.6).

Cartilage and Bone

Cartilage and bone are highly specialized connective tissues in which the ground substance of the matrix is predominant over the cellular and fibrous elements.

The chondroblast is responsible for producing the ground substance and fibers of the three types of cartilage: hyaline (articular; found in synovial joints), elastic (found in the external ear, auditory tube, larynx, and epiglottis), and fibrous (found in intervertebral discs). These three cartilage types vary in histologic makeup on the basis of their ground substance and predominant fiber type (collagen or elastin) and are avascular (Figs. 4.7–4.9).

The osteocytes of bone are maintained in a rigid matrix, which is calcified and reinforced by connective tissue fibers, which are produced by the osteoblasts. The structural unit of bone, the osteon (haversian system), is formed by concentric lamellae of bone surrounding a microscopic neurovascular bundle in the haversian canal. The osteocytes are located within microscopic spaces (lacunae) between the concentric bone matrix lamellae and extend processes into the matrix (Fig. 4.10).

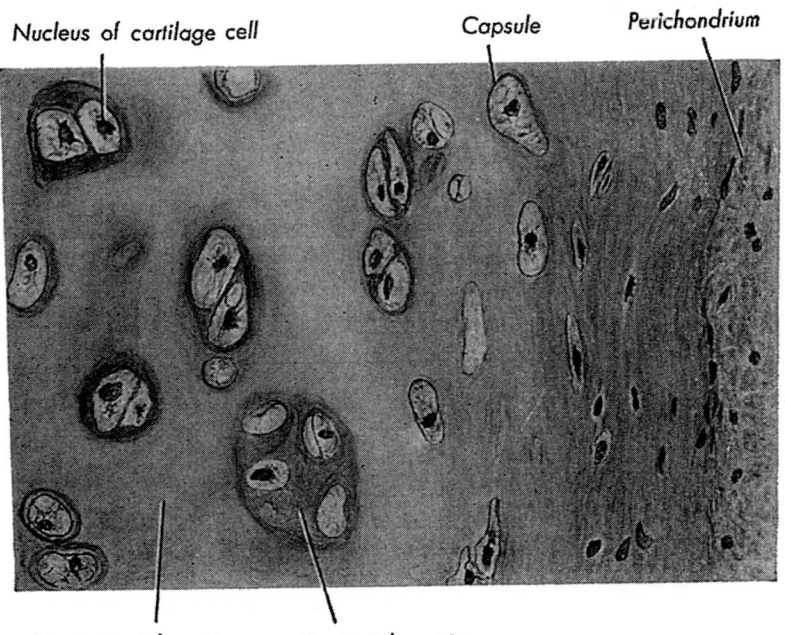

Nucleus of cartilage cell   Capsule   Perichondrium

Interterritorial matrix   Territorial matrix

FIGURE 4.7. Cellular elements of hyaline (articular) cartilage.

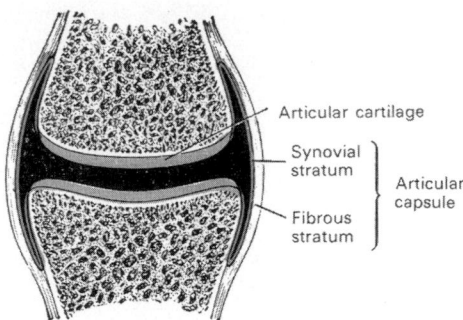

FIGURE 4.12. Typical synovial joint.

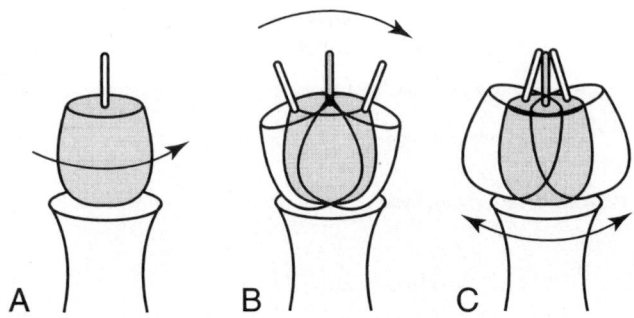

FIGURE 4.14. Motion at a synovial joint. **A:** Spin. **B:** Roll. **C:** Slide.

and distal bones, which form the synovial joint, and it is classified as dense, irregular fibrous connective tissue. At the point where the articular hyaline cartilage ends the bone tissue is covered by the periosteum. The fibrous outer layer of the joint capsule could be described as the free periosteum, which envelops the freely movable joint and connects the proximal and distal bones at the articulation. The unique inner layer is the synovial membrane, which lines the fibrous outer layer. This membrane secretes the synovial fluid, which lubricates the internal joint surfaces and the articular hyaline cartilage. The uniqueness of this membrane is that it is derived from mesenchyme. However, microscopically and functionally this tissue is similar to epithelial tissue, which is an ectodermal derivative.

Each synovial joint is stabilized by specific ligaments. Ligaments may be classified as capsular or accessory. A capsular ligament is a part of the fibrous outer layer of the joint capsule, while accessory ligaments are either located within the joint cavity (intracapsular) or outside the joint capsule, separated from the fibrous outer layer (extracapsular). All ligaments are histologically composed of dense, regular fibrous connective tissue and have microscopic, structural, and functional continuity with the periosteum of adjacent bone.

The temporomandibular, sternoclavicular, ulnomeniscotriquetral, and knee joints are highly specialized types of synovial joints. These joints have the unique feature of either a disc or meniscus (incomplete disc) within the joint cavity (Fig. 4.13). The fibrocartilaginous disc provides for additional support and stability as it separates the two hyaline cartilage articular surfaces. Peripherally discs are connected to the fibrous outer layer of the

joint capsule. A disc extends across a synovial joint, dividing it structurally and functionally into two synovial cavities. The disc, which is derived from mesoderm, represents a highly specialized form of connective tissue, which is distinct in that the fibrous element of the matrix predominates. A synovial joint with a fibrocartilaginous disc displays a structure similar to the embryologically developing synovial joint. This type of synovial joint maintains the fibrocartilaginous element, which is developmentally lost in the "typical" synovial joint.

Synovial joints are commonly classified according to the shape of the articular surfaces and/or the movements permitted. None of the articular surfaces are truly flat. Biomechanically these joint surfaces permit motion, which is described as spin, roll, or slide (Fig. 4.14). Spin represents rotation about the longitudinal axis of a bone. Roll is the result of decreasing and increasing the angle between the two bones at an articulation. Slide is the result of a translatory motion of one bone gliding/sliding on the other at the joint. Specific details regarding the classification system and individual synovial joints can be found in any anatomy textbook (1,2,4,5,7,8).

Nonsynovial joints are subdivided into fibrous and cartilaginous types. These joints, where the articulating bones are directly connected by either fibrous tissue or cartilage, have no free surface for movement, but provide for strength and stability between adjacent bones. The fibrous joints include the sutures of the skull (Fig. 4.15), teeth in the mandible and maxilla, and the distal tibiofibular joint. The fibrocartilaginous intervertebral discs between adjacent vertebral bodies and the pubic symphysis (Fig. 4.16) are examples of cartilaginous joints.

The sutures of the skull provide a classic example of the interrelationship between structure and function. Each suture (joint) between adjacent cranial bones uniquely provides support and mobility. Unlike the freely moveable synovial joints, the sutures are highly restricted to slight gliding motion. However, motion loss/restriction is the clinically significant factor in describing somatic dysfunction of the joint.

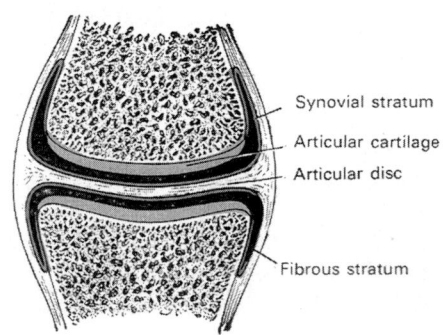

FIGURE 4.13. Synovial joint with an articular disc.

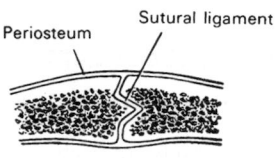

FIGURE 4.15. A suture is an example of a fibrous joint.

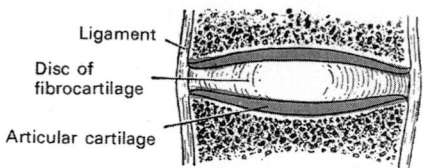

FIGURE 4.16. A symphysis is an example of a cartilaginous joint.

Cranial bone motion is also influenced by the tension of the cranial dura mater, which covers the brain and forms the internal lining of the skull. Cranial dura mater consists of two layers: periosteal and meningeal. The periosteal layer is the periosteal lining of the cranium and there is histologic continuity of this layer with the fibrous tissue (sutural ligament) at each cranial suture. The meningeal layer of cranial dura mater has continuity with the spinal dura mater (thecal sac) at the foramen magnum of the occipital bone (Fig. 4.17). The direct effect of these connective tissues on cranial bone motion has been described by Sutherland (9) as the reciprocal tension membrane.

In summary, synovial and nonsynovial joints exemplify the osteopathic concept of the interrelationship between structure and function. Synovial joints, which are freely moveable, allow for the body to have mobility and greater range of motion. The nonsynovial joints (fibrous and cartilaginous) provide strength and stability within a limited range of motion.

Joint Play

The voluntary movement of synovial joints is accommodated by joint play as described by Mennell (10). Joint play is defined as a

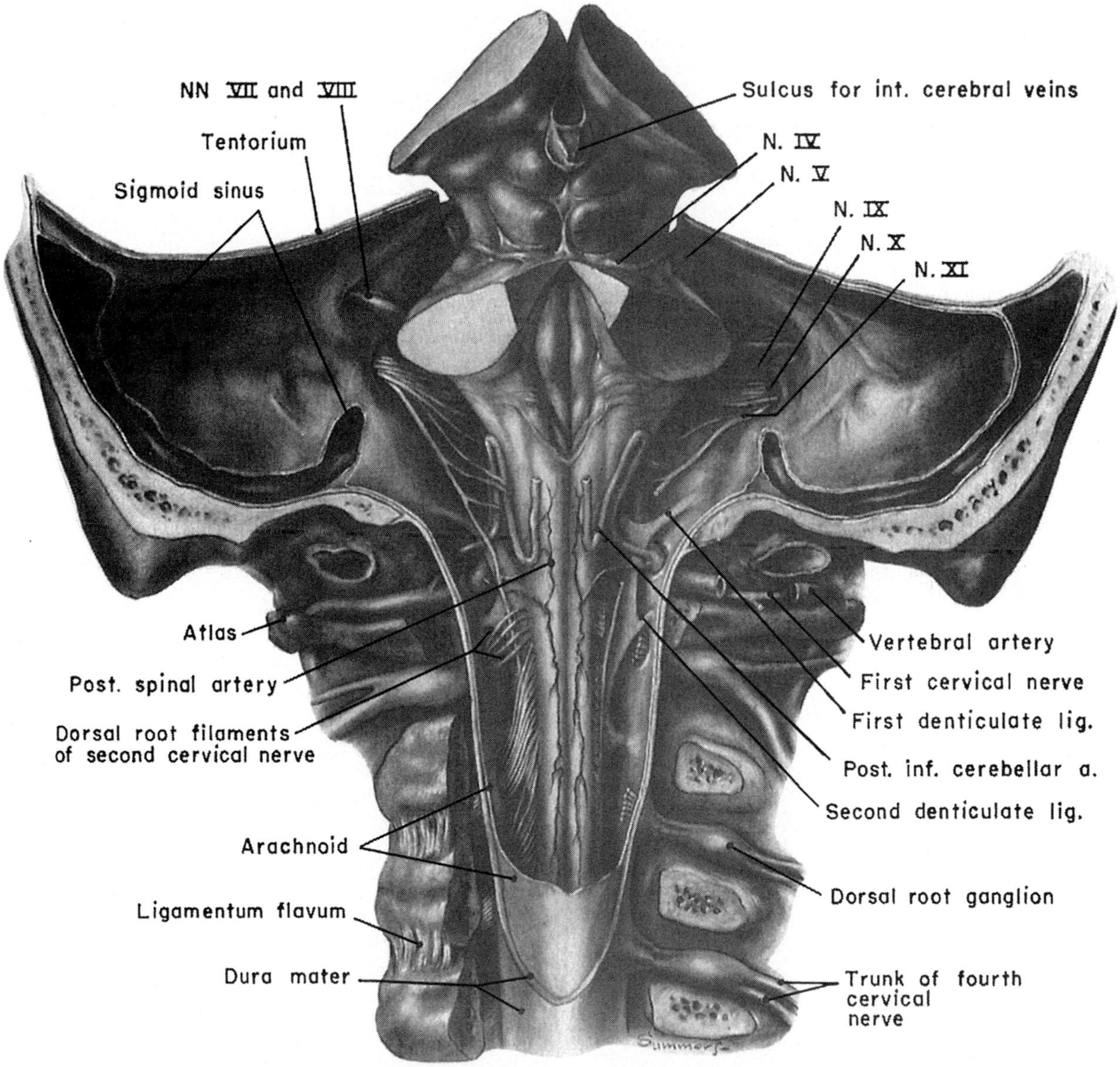

FIGURE 4.17. Area of foramen magnum. Cranial dura mater lines the internal surface of cranium, is continuous with fibrous tissue of sutures, and is continuous with spinal dura mater of foramen magnum.

small but precise amount of movement (less than one-eighth of an inch), which is independent of the action of voluntary muscle function. The normal, easy, voluntary range of active motion at a synovial joint is dependent upon the integrity of joint play. Joint play is only present in the living synovial joint. The movement of joint play can only be demonstrated by passive examination. Each synovial joint has one or more joint play movements. Joint dysfunction is defined as the loss of joint play and therefore a limitation of the voluntary range of motion at a synovial joint. Joint dysfunction is a component of somatic dysfunction (acute or chronic) which is diagnosed in the evaluation of the neuromusculoskeletal system. The restoration of joint play appears to be the basis for the success of synovial joint mobilization using direct or indirect action treatment techniques in osteopathic manipulation.

Muscle-Tendon Complex

A delicate network of fine connective tissue surrounds individual skeletal muscle fibers. At each end of the muscle this connective tissue forms a tendon composed of dense, regular fibrous connective tissue. The tendon is attached to bone through a microscopic interlacing of its connective tissue with the periosteal connective tissue covering the bone (Fig. 4.18). Each muscle has two parts: a predominant connective tissue at its ends that attaches to bones and a predominance of muscle tissue in its functional contractile belly. The change to connective tissue at its ends provides the muscle a firm attachment to bone. The musculotendinous junction represents the point at which there is a significant change in the histologic composition of skeletal muscle from predominantly muscle fibers to predominantly collagen fibers. Muscle contraction exerts force on the musculotendinous junction and then the tendon, which moves a bone at a joint.

Fascia and Neurovascular Bundle

Fascia is a derivative of mesoderm. Throughout the body there is a subcutaneous layer of loose connective tissue called the su-

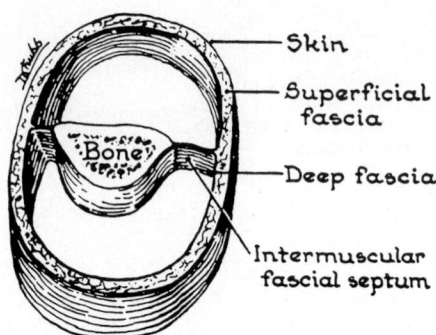

FIGURE 4.19. Diagrammatic representation of a transverse section through the arm, illustrating the organization of superficial and deep fascia. Deep fascia divides the arm into compartments by way of intermuscular septa.

perficial fascia (Figs. 4.5 and 4.19). It contains collagen fibers as well as variable amounts of fat. Superficial fascia serves to increase skin mobility, acts as a thermal insulator, and stores energy for metabolic use. The dense connective tissue envelope, which invests and separates individual muscles of the limbs and trunk, is deep fascia. It is also composed primarily of collagen fibers. Between individual muscles there is a fascial plane, which represents the separation of the connective

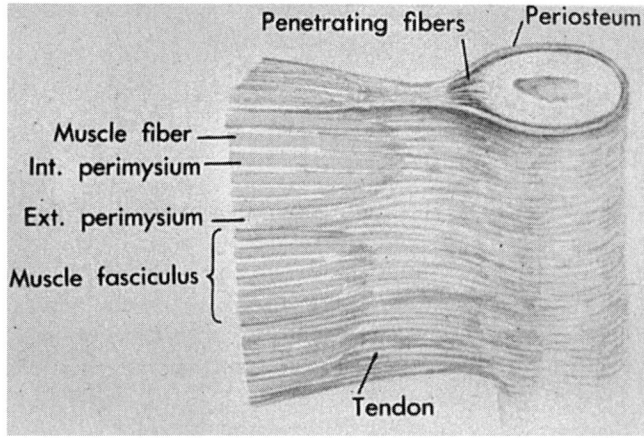

FIGURE 4.18. Diagrammatic representation of how muscle attaches to bone. (Source unknown.)

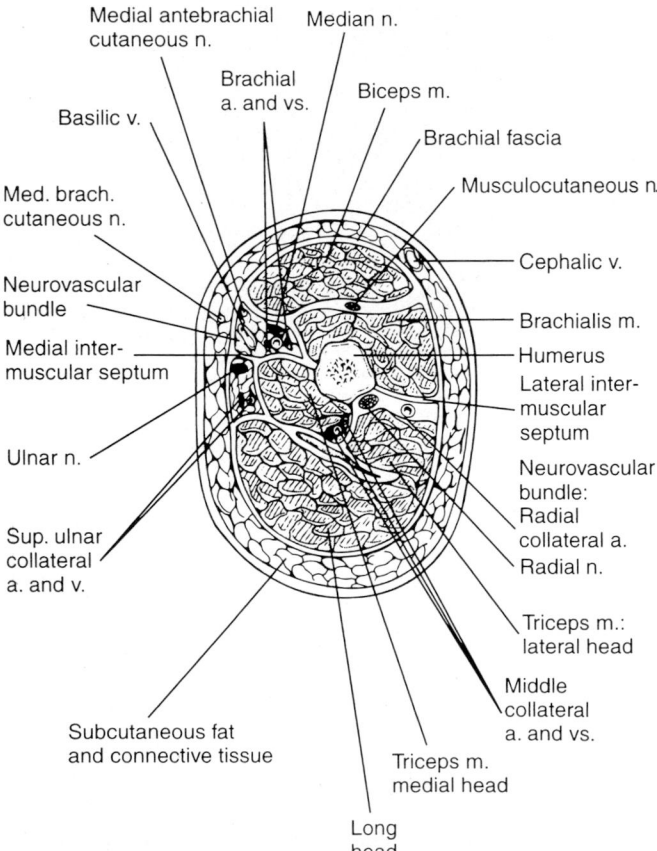

FIGURE 4.20. Transverse section through the arm. Neurovascular bundles are found between skeletal muscles in anterior and posterior compartments.

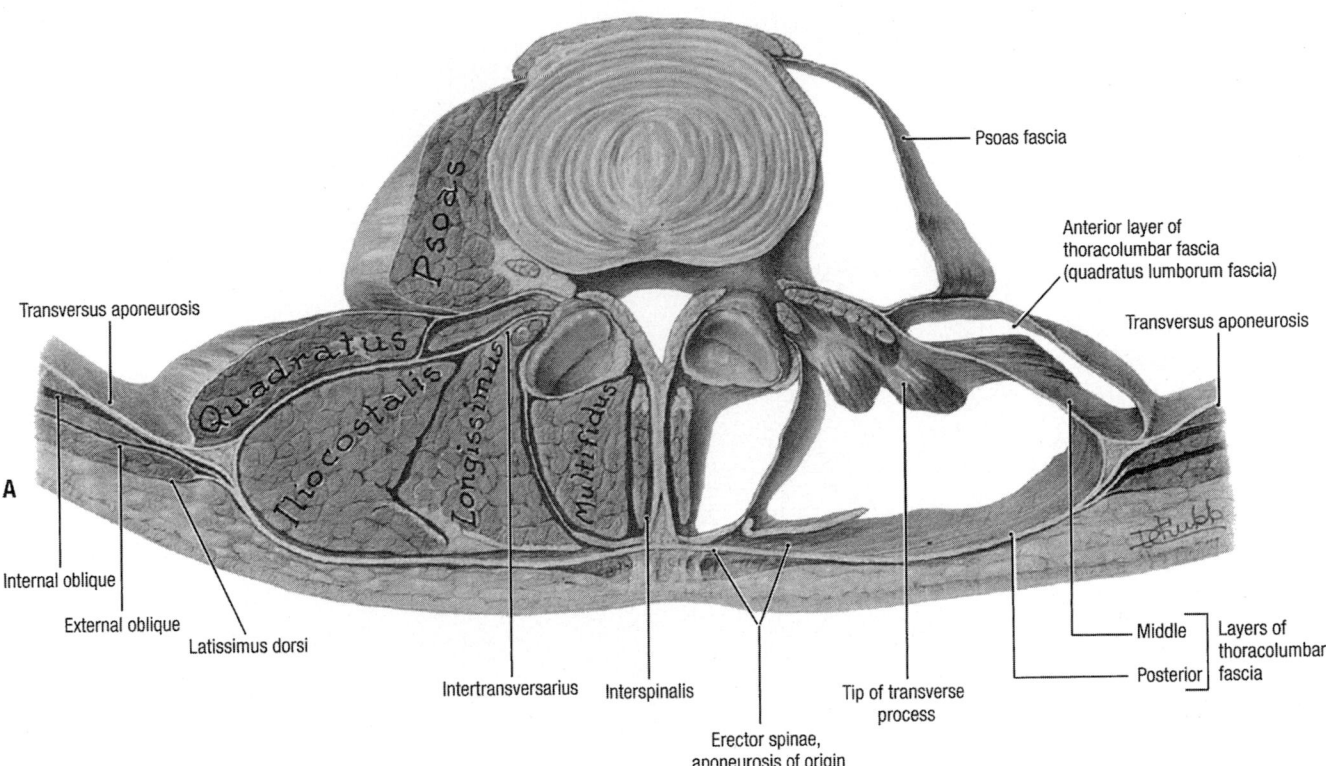

Psoas fascia

Anterior layer of thoracolumbar fascia (quadratus lumborum fascia)

Transversus aponeurosis

Middle ⎫
       ⎬ Layers of thoracolumbar fascia
Posterior ⎭

Transversus aponeurosis

Internal oblique

External oblique

Latissimus dorsi

Intertransversarius

Interspinalis

Erector spinae, aponeurosis of origin

Tip of transverse process

A

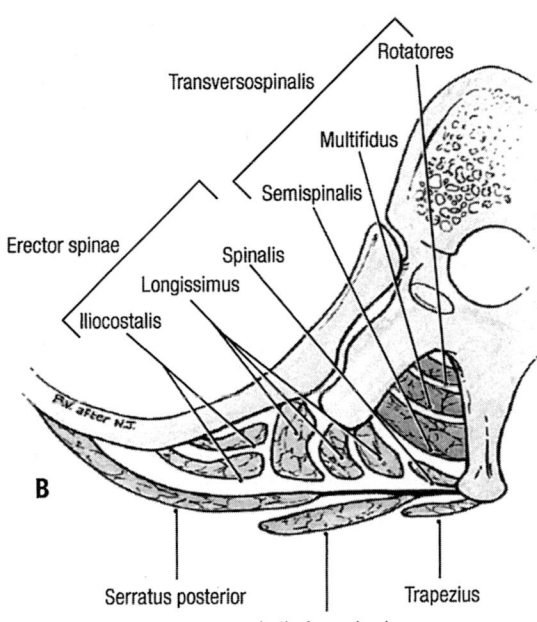

Rotatores

Transversospinalis

Multifidus

Semispinalis

Erector spinae

Spinalis

Longissimus

Iliocostalis

Serratus posterior

Latissimus dorsi

Trapezius

B

FIGURE 4.21. Transverse section through the back, illustrating the organization of deep fascia. The deep fascia serves to divide the back into compartments for muscles of similar function.

tissue investment (wrapper) of the individual muscles. In the limbs, back, and neck, deep fascia passes over and between muscle groups and connects to bone periosteum. The deep fascia passing between muscle groups in the limbs is called intermuscular septa. These intermuscular septa, together with the deep fascia in the limbs and deep fascia in the back and neck, pass over and between muscle groups serving to compartmentalize muscle groups of similar functions and innervations (Figs. 4.20–4.22). Deep fascia between individual muscles, which move ex-

tensively, is loose connective tissue and facilitates movement. As a connective tissue, fascia provides for mobility and stability of the musculoskeletal system. Myofascial continuity can be found throughout the body. This will be discussed in detail later in the chapter. Further details regarding the structure and function of fascia can be found in Chapter 3, "Rules of Anatomy" (11).

Peripheral nerves and blood and lymph vessels lie in fascia, loose connective tissue, between muscles. This fascia serves to

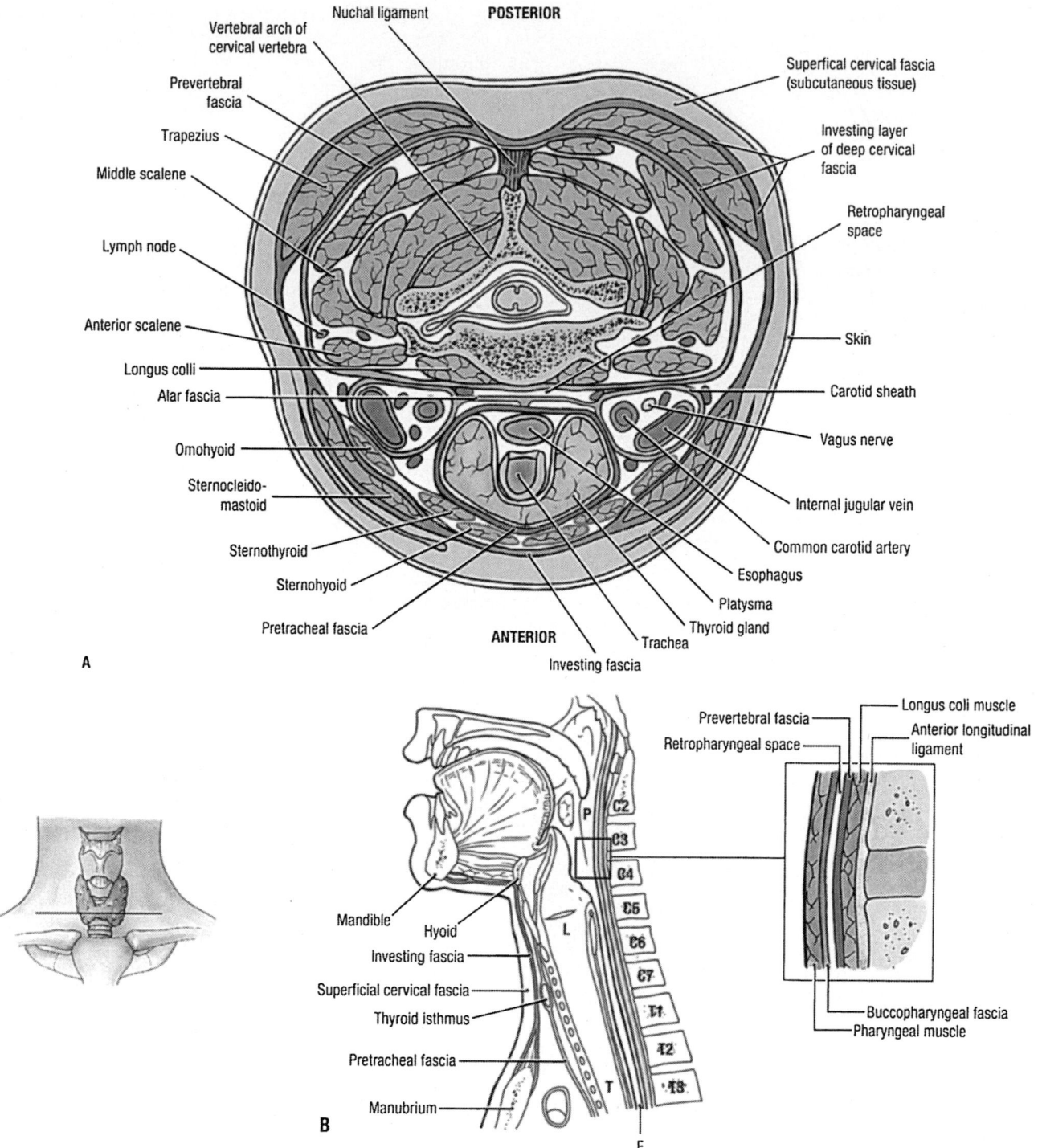

FIGURE 4.22. Transverse section through the neck, illustrating the organization of the deep fascia. The deep fascia divides the neck into muscular, visceral, and neurovascular compartments.

bind together these nerves and vessels, and collectively the components form the neurovascular bundle (Fig. 4.20).

Muscle Action

A muscle contracts because it is stimulated by a motor nerve. A single motor nerve fiber innervates more than one skeletal muscle fiber. The nerve fiber and all the muscle fibers it innervates are called the motor unit (Fig. 4.23). In general, small muscles that react quickly (e.g., extraocular muscles) have ten or fewer muscle fibers innervated by a single nerve fiber. In contrast, large muscles which do not require fine central nervous system control (e.g., deep back muscles) may have up to 1,000 muscle fibers in a motor unit. When a muscle is resting, some motor units are always discharging. It may not be the same motor units at each instance in time. This type of motor activity (muscle tone) is the

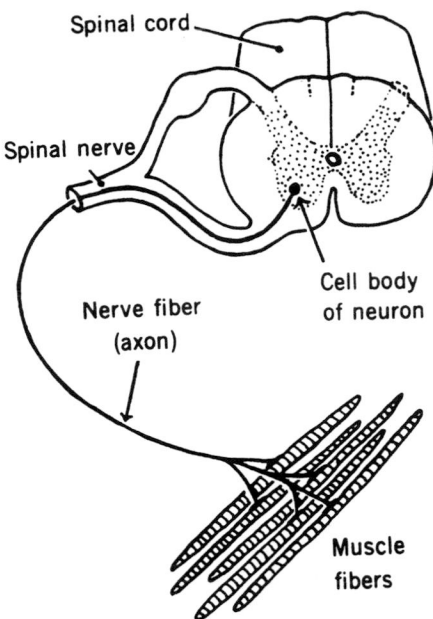

FIGURE 4.23. A motor unit.

Most movements require the combined action of several muscles. The term "prime mover" is used for those muscles that act directly to bring about the desired movement. Every muscle, which acts on a joint, is paired with another muscle that has the opposite action on the same joint. These muscles are antagonists of each other (e.g., biceps brachii, flexor; triceps, extensor). An antagonist does not significantly block the action of the prime mover. Its primary effect only occurs at the initiation of the movement after which it relaxes until the movement is finished. There are times when prime movers and antagonists contract together and are called fixators. This occurs to stabilize a joint or hold a part of the body in an appropriate position. Muscles that contract at the same time as prime movers are called synergists. These can be either muscles that aid the prime movers in the performance of the desired action or antagonist muscles that contract at the same time as a prime mover and thereby prevent unwanted movement, which would be counterproductive to the desired action. Individual muscles should not always be considered as units with a single function. Different parts of the same muscle may have different, even antagonistic, actions (e.g., deltoid muscle).

background for muscular contraction in the performance of a purposeful movement.

When most muscles contract, their fibers act through tendons on moveable bones to get the desired action (Fig. 4.18). Movements result in the activation of motor units in some muscles and the simultaneous relaxation of motor units in other muscles. Movement that comes about from muscle contraction causes the muscles to change in length. When this occurs, tension created within the muscle remains constant and the contraction is called isotonic. If movement does not occur as a result of muscle contraction and muscle length stays constant with elevated tension generated within the muscles, the contraction is called isometric (e.g., posterior compartment muscles of the leg in standing). Isotonic contractions may be concentric (shortening of the muscle) or eccentric (lengthening of the muscle).

SEGMENTAL ORGANIZATION OF THE NEUROMUSCULOSKELETAL AND VASCULAR SYSTEMS

A typical transverse section through the thoracic region demonstrates the basic organization of the axial skeleton (Figs. 4.3 and 4.24). Throughout the thoracic region, each vertebral level is organized symmetrically about a central axis composed of the vertebra, spinal cord, and aorta. The distribution of a typical spinal nerve and posterior intercostal artery are repeated at each segmental level of the thoracic spine (T1 through T12).

The typical spinal nerve is formed by the union of the anterior and posterior roots just lateral to the intervertebral foramen. Within a short distance, the spinal nerve divides to form a posterior primary ramus and an anterior primary ramus (Fig. 4.24).

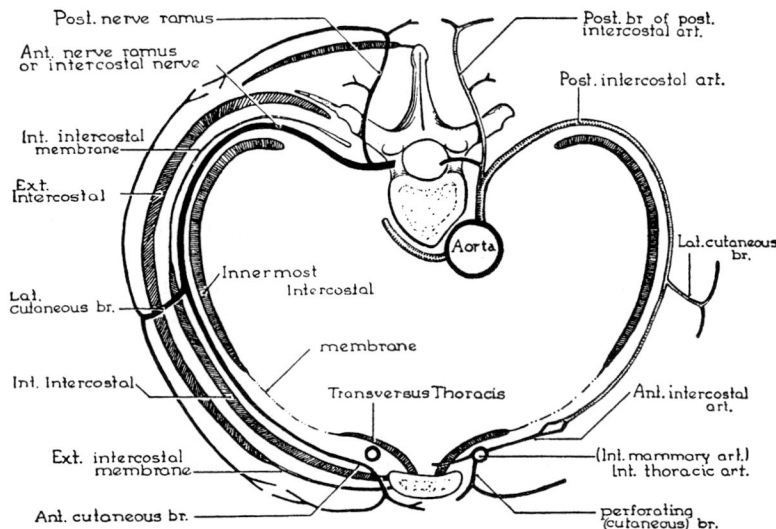

FIGURE 4.24. Transverse section illustrating contents of a segmental level through the thorax.

LIMB ANATOMY

Upper and Lower Limbs

The anatomy of the upper and lower limbs is comparable. If one is to understand this basic anatomy, as well as how the limbs function, then one must understand limb development. The limbs are divided into four major parts. The upper limb is divided into the shoulder (shoulder girdle), arm, forearm, and hand while the lower limb consists of the pelvic girdle, thigh, leg, and foot. The bones of the upper and lower limbs form the appendicular skeleton. These bones form *in situ* in the developing limb buds. They begin as mesenchyme, which condenses and differentiates into hyaline cartilage bone models. These cartilaginous models eventually ossify through endochondral ossification. Limb musculature is also derived from mesenchyme but, unlike that which form the bones, muscle mesenchyme is derived from somites adjacent to the developing neural tube and migrates into the limb bud from the hypomere, where it condenses adjacent to the developing bones (Fig. 4.4). As the limb elongates, the muscular tissue splits into flexor (anterior) and extensor (posterior) components. Initially the muscles of the limbs are segmental in character, but in time, they fuse and are composed of muscle tissue from several segments. Upper limb buds are opposite neural tube (spinal cord) segments C5-8 and T1, while lower limb buds lie opposite segments L2-5 and S1 and S2. As the limbs grow, posterior and anterior branches derived from anterior primary rami of spinal nerves penetrate into the developing muscles (Fig. 4.4). Posterior branches enter extensor musculature while anterior branches enter flexor musculature.

With development, the segmental posterior and anterior branches from each anterior primary ramus unite to form large posterior and anterior nerves. This union of the original segmental posterior and anterior branches from each anterior primary ramus is the basis for the formation of the brachial and lumbosacral plexuses (Fig. 4.26), and comes about with the fusion of segmental muscles. The large posterior and anterior nerves are represented in the adult upper limb as the radial nerve supplying extensor musculature and the median and ulnar nerves innervating flexor musculature, respectively (Fig. 4.26). In the adult lower limb, the large posterior and anterior nerves are represented as the femoral and common fibular nerves supplying extensor musculature and the tibial nerve supplying flexor musculature, respectively (Fig. 4.26). Contact between nerves and differentiating muscle cells is a prerequisite for complete functional muscle differentiation. The segmental spinal nerves also provide sensory innervation of the limb dermatomes. The original segmental dermatomal pattern is modified with growth of the limbs, but an orderly sequence is present in the adult (Fig. 4.27).

As discussed earlier, the development of the upper and lower limbs is similar. However, there are two differences. First, the lower limb develops later than the upper limb. Second, the limbs rotate in opposite directions. The upper limb rotates 90 degrees laterally so that the elbow points posteriorly; the extensor musculature lies on lateral and posterior surfaces while the flexor musculature lies on anterior and medial surfaces; and the thumb lies laterally on the anterior facing palm. The lower limb rotates 90 degrees medially so that the knee points anteriorly, the extensor muscles are on the anterior surface while the flexor muscles

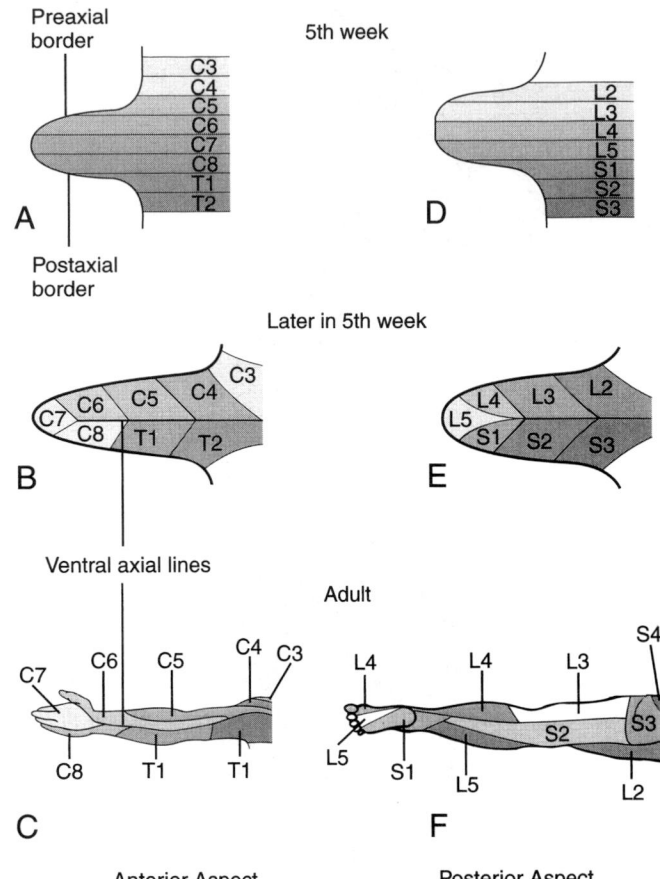

FIGURE 4.27. Developing dermatomal patterns in upper (**A–C**) and lower (**D–F**) limbs. **A–C:** Anterior view, upper limb. **D** and **F:** Posterior view, lower limb. **A, B, D** and **E:** Limb buds in embryo. **C** and **F:** Adult limbs.

are on the posterior surface, and the big toe is medial. These rotations are necessary based on the functions that the limbs perform. Deep fascia and intermuscular septa connecting with bone in the limbs separate or compartmentalize groups of muscles. The muscles in each compartment share similar functions, developmental histories, nerve and arterial supply, as well as venous and lymphatic drainage.

Functional Adaptation

Through their development, the upper and lower limbs have anatomically adapted to perform different functions. The upper limb is involved in manual activity. It moves freely, especially the hand, which is adapted for manipulating and grasping. The stability of the upper limb has been sacrificed for mobility. The digits are the most mobile parts of the upper limb. The lower limb is involved in locomotion, weight bearing, and maintaining equilibrium. Because of its weight-bearing function, some movement has been sacrificed in order to achieve stability.

MYOFASCIAL CONTINUITY

The concept of myofascial continuity is best understood by examining the attachment of a tendon to a bone. The dense fibrous

Through the attachment of the dense regular fibrous tissue of tendon and ligament to bone a microscopic fiber continuity is found, with the periosteum covering the substance of each bone. The tendon attachment provides direct continuity of a muscle at its origin and insertion to bone. The connection of tendon to bone provides functional integrity of each part of the body across each synovial joint by way of the muscle-tendon complex, which can best be described as myofascial continuity (Fig. 4.18).

The latissimus dorsi muscle exemplifies the myofascial continuity concept. Through attachment to the lumbar spine and iliac crest by way of the lumbodorsal (thoracolumbar) fascia the latissimus dorsi tendon/aponeurosis has continuity with the flat sheet of skeletal muscle, which covers the posterior and lateral trunk. The latissimus dorsi muscle then converges to a narrow flat tendon, which crosses the posterior axilla and inserts into the floor of the intertubercular groove on the anterior aspect of the humerus (Figs 4.28 and 4.29). The latissimus dorsi

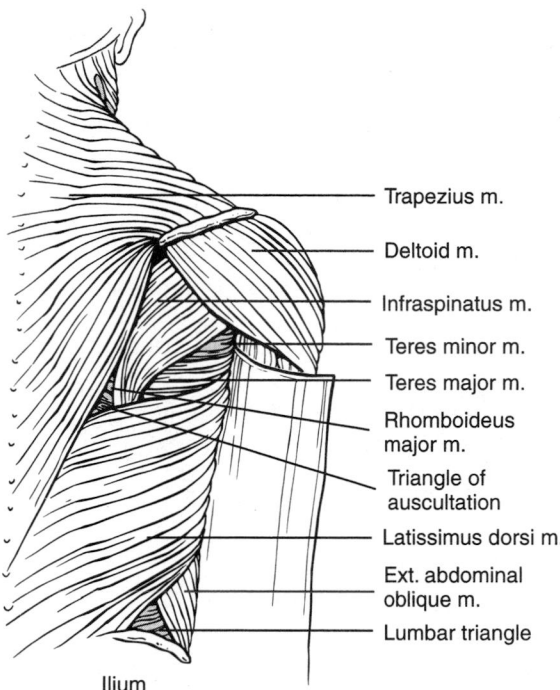

FIGURE 4.28. Superficial muscles of the upper limb located on the back. Notice extensive broad attachment of latissimus dorsi muscle as it covers the posterior and lateral trunk.

connective tissue is anchored to the compact cortical substance of bone by microscopic connective tissue penetrating fibers (Sharpey fibers). The connective tissue, which then forms the mass of the tendon, becomes feathered to interdigitate with the skeletal muscle fibers, which will form the substance of a given muscle. The same architecture is duplicated at the proximal and distal muscle attachments to bone (Fig. 4.18).

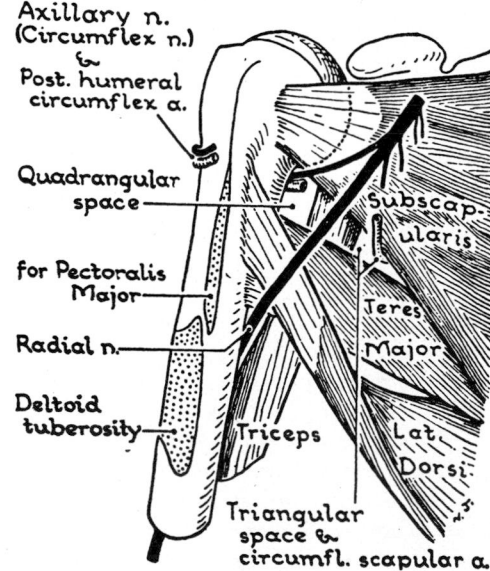

FIGURE 4.29. Posterior wall of axilla showing attachment of latissimus dorsi muscle into the intertubercular groove of humerus.

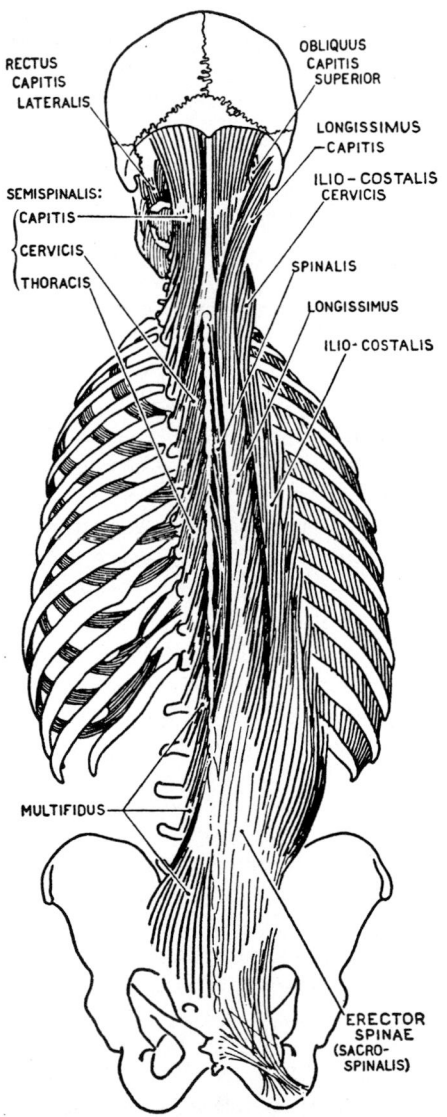

FIGURE 4.30. Deep muscles of back provide myofascial continuity from the cranium through the vertebral column to the pelvis.

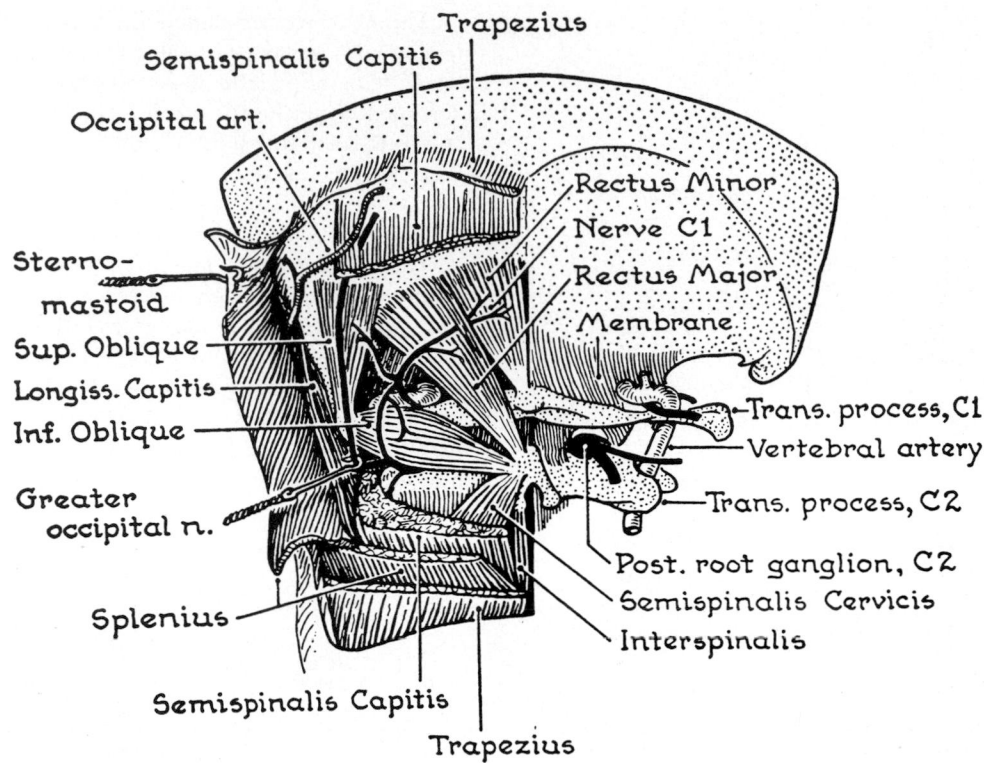

FIGURE 4.31. Suboccipital region. Suboccipital muscles (obliquus capitis superior and rectus capitis posterior minor) provide myofascial continuity between the cranium and C1/atlas.

muscle then provides functional and structural continuity between the upper limb, spine (thoracic, lumbar, and sacral), ribs, and pelvis through an attachment to the crest of the ilium and pelvis. Dysfunction of the latissimus dorsi muscle can therefore have a direct effect on the glenohumeral joint, scapulothoracic articulation, acromioclavicular joint, thoracic facet joints, costovertebral joints, lumbar facet joints, and stability of the pelvis at the sacroiliac joint.

Myofascial continuity from one region of the body to another can best be understood through consideration of the regional structure of the body which includes the cranium, cervical spine and upper limb, thoracic spine and trunk, lumbosacral spine, and the pelvis and lower limb (Fig. 4.30).

The myofascial continuity of the cranium is best understood by studying the internal and external structure of the skull as it articulates with the first cervical vertebra (C1/atlas). Suboccipital muscles (obliquus capitis superior and rectus capitis posterior minor) provide for this continuity (Fig. 4.31).

The meningeal layer of cranial dura mater is continuous with the spinal dura at the occipital foramen magnum (Fig. 4.17). The spinal dura surrounding and supporting the spinal cord is free within the vertebral canal. The inferior aspect of the spinal dura mater at the S2 vertebral level is attached to the coccyx by the coccygeal ligament (Fig. 4.32). Through the dura mater there is a direct connection between the internal aspect of the neurocranium and the inferior aspect of the vertebral column.

The bones of the face (viscerocranium) and the cranial vault (neurocranium) are covered externally by a thin layer of connective tissue periosteum. This periosteum provides a protective covering of each bone and a mechanism for attachment of specific muscles (e.g., muscles of facial expression; Fig. 4.33).

It is important to understand the concept of myofascial continuity and the fact that many muscles in the body cross more than one joint and exert their actions on those joints, as well as different areas of the body. Because of this, the physician should always examine joints and muscle groups well removed from an area of discomfort in order to discover the true source of injury or dysfunction.

DEDICATION

Allen W. Jacobs, DO, PhD, a nationally recognized leader in osteopathic medicine, dean of the Michigan State University College of Osteopathic Medicine, and co-author of this chapter, died unexpectedly on December 2, 2001. The thing that I remember most about Al was his great compassion and love for his family, the college, the osteopathic profession, and the discipline of anatomy. This chapter reflects his belief that a solid understanding of anatomic principles is the foundation of osteopathic medicine. I honor his passing by dedicating this chapter to keeping alive the belief that he so devoutly expounded.

William M. Falls, PhD

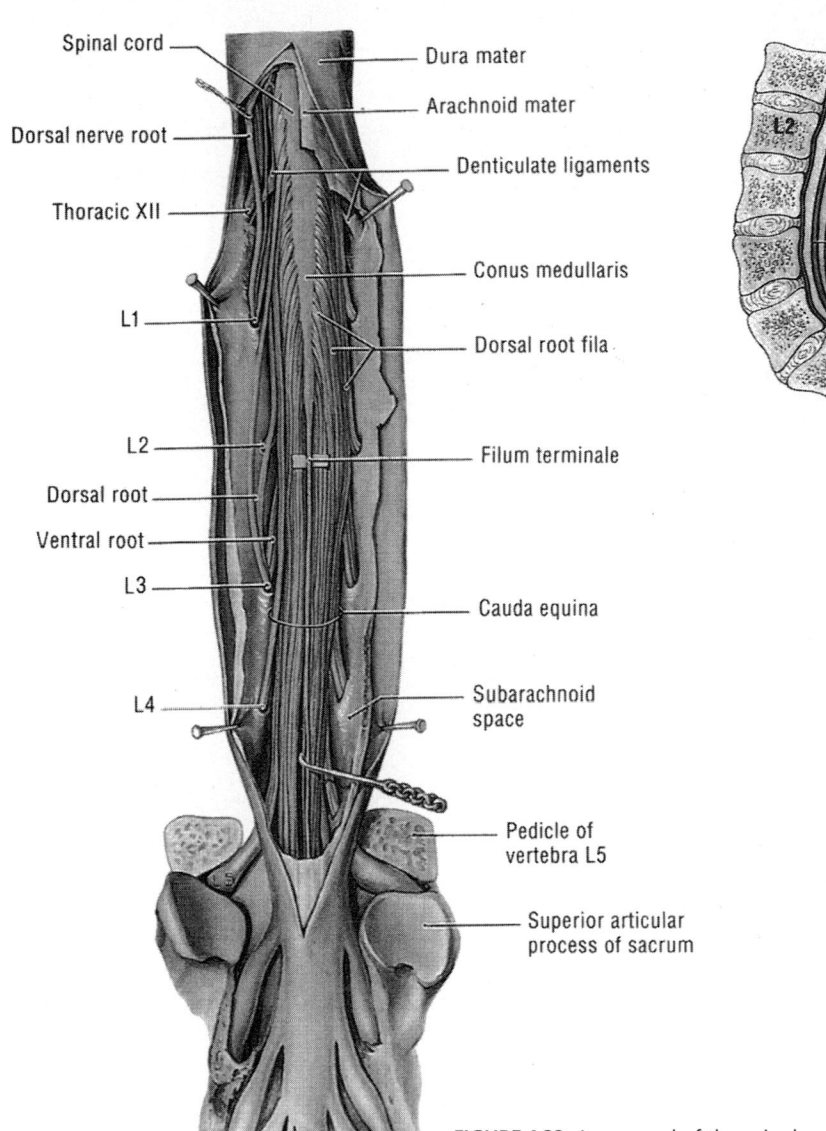

Spinal cord

Dorsal nerve root

Thoracic XII

L1

L2

Dorsal root

Ventral root

L3

L4

Dura mater

Arachnoid mater

Denticulate ligaments

Conus medullaris

Dorsal root fila

Filum terminale

Cauda equina

Subarachnoid space

Pedicle of vertebra L5

Superior articular process of sacrum

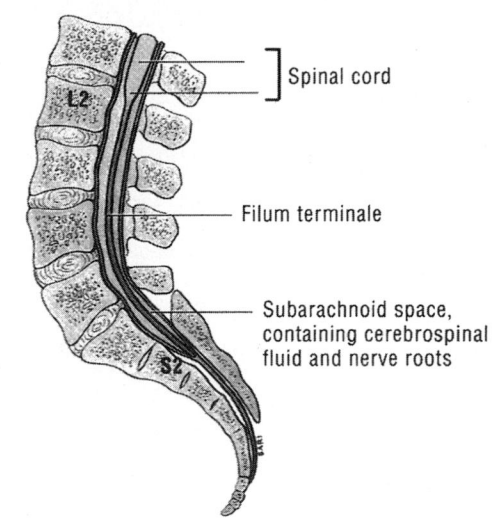

Spinal cord

Filum terminale

Subarachnoid space, containing cerebrospinal fluid and nerve roots

L2

S2

FIGURE 4.32. Lower end of the spinal cord, including cauda equina, and its coverings. Inferior end of dura mater at S2 is attached to coccyx by coccygeal ligament. Dura mater provides a direct connection from the internal surface of the cranium to the coccyx.

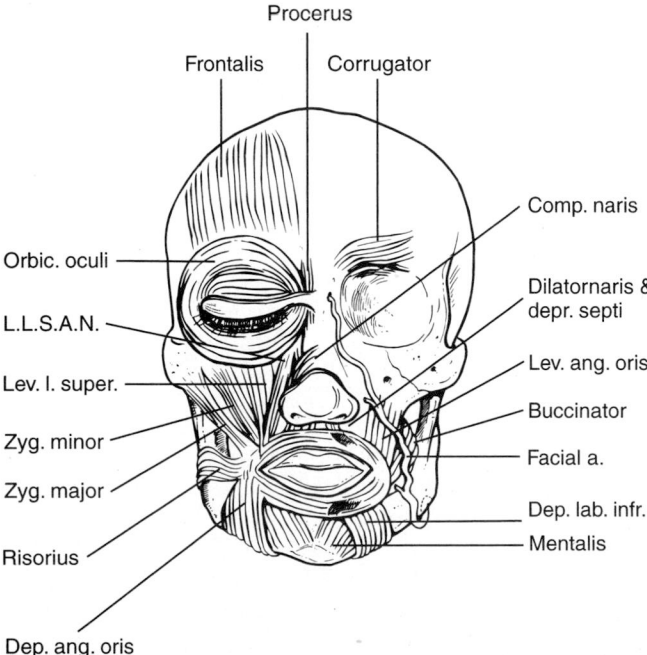

Procerus

Frontalis

Corrugator

Comp. naris

Orbic. oculi

L.L.S.A.N.

Lev. l. super.

Zyg. minor

Zyg. major

Risorius

Dep. ang. oris

Dilatornaris & depr. septi

Lev. ang. oris

Buccinator

Facial a.

Dep. lab. infr.

Mentalis

FIGURE 4.33. Muscles of facial expression. Periosteum covering bones of viscerocranium provides attachment for these muscles inserting into skin.

REFERENCES

1. Basmajian JV, Slonecker CE. *Grant's Method of Anatomy,* 11th ed. Baltimore, MD: Williams & Wilkins; 1989.
2. Clemente CD. Gray's Anatomy of the Human Body (American ed.), 3rd ed. Philadelphia, PA: Lea & Febiger; 1985.
3. Copenhaver WM, Bunge RP, Bunge MB. *Bailey's Textbook of Histology,* 16th ed. Baltimore, MD: Williams & Wilkins; 1971.
4. Hollinshead WH, Rosse C. *Textbook of Anatomy,* 4th ed. Philadelphia, PA: Harper & Row; 1985.
5. Moore KL. *Clinically Oriented Anatomy,* 3rd ed. Baltimore, MD: Williams & Wilkins; 1992.
6. Sadler TW. *Langman's Medical Embryology,* 6th ed. Baltimore, MD: Williams & Wilkins; 1990.
7. Williams PL, Warwick R, Dyson M, Bannister LH. *Gray's Anatomy* (British ed.), 37th ed. London, England: Churchill Livingstone; 1989.
8. Woodburne RT, Burkel WE. *Essentials of Human Anatomy,* 9th ed. New York, NY: Oxford University Press; 1994.
9. Magoun HI. Osteopathy. In: *The Cranial Field,* 3rd ed. Kirksville, MO: The Journal Printing Company; 1976.
10. Mennell J. *Joint Pain.* Boston, MA: Little, Brown and Company; 1964.
11. Towns LC. Rules of anatomy. In: *Foundations for Osteopathic Medicine,* 2nd ed. Philadelphia: Lippincott Williams & Wilkins; 2002.

5

BIOMECHANICS: AN OSTEOPATHIC PERSPECTIVE

MICHAEL R. WELLS

KEY CONCEPTS

- Biomechanics describes the relationship between structure and function.
- Motion and forces in three-dimensional space can be divided into components with a magnitude of action in each dimension.
- Stress, strain, and force moments are terms used to describe how forces act on objects and how objects respond to those forces.
- The biomaterial properties of tissues such as bone, cartilage, muscles, tendons, and ligaments, are based on a hierarchy of biomechanical properties from the molecular, cellular, tissue, and gross anatomic levels.
- Tissues are constantly remodeling in response to the stresses placed upon them.
- Excessive stresses or inadequate responses to them (loss of homeostasis) result in injury or disease in tissues.
- The basic biomaterial properties and remodeling capacity (adaptability) of tissues change with age, generally to render them more vulnerable to stresses and injury.
- The gross biomechanical properties of the skeleton are defined by bony structure and the attachment of muscles and tendons which produce forces across joints.
- The primary motions at the surfaces of articulations are gliding (translation), rotation, rolling, compression, and distraction.
- Basic properties of joint kinetics can be described by measuring the forces produced by muscles and the length of moment arms acting across joints.
- The elastic properties of muscles, tendons, and ligaments allow them to store energy in some phases of movements for release during others.
- Normal movement in the spinal column is a composite of smaller motions of individual vertebrae. Restrictions of movement in one area can result in a compensatory increased mobility in others.
- The orientation of intervertebral joint facets in the spine, in association with the direction of spinal muscle

contraction, produces a motion coupling of vertebral movement. These coupling relationships differ over areas of the spine.
- It is necessary to consider the biomechanical relationships of the body as a whole when attempting to define the consequences of injury or altered function of a body segment.

BIOMECHANICS DESCRIBES THE RELATIONSHIP BETWEEN STRUCTURE AND FUNCTION

The interrelationship of structure and function in the body is one of the basic principles of osteopathy. The science of biomechanics is dedicated to describing this relationship more generally in biologic systems. This can apply to the organism as a whole (as with kinesiology) or even on a subcellular level (as with microtubular transport mechanisms). The approach to the mechanics of biologic systems is similar to the mechanics of inanimate objects, and consists largely of how they respond to forces applied to them. When struck with a hammer, an object may shatter or absorb the force and be accelerated into movement. The response will depend upon a variety of factors including the material comprising the object, the object's shape, internal structure, where and how the force is applied, and so forth. The response of the human body to either externally or internally applied forces can be described similarly, as it must obey the same basic laws of physics. However, the human body and other biologic systems have extremely intricate structural arrangements of highly variable materials down to the molecular level. This can make the accurate biomechanical modeling of even simple movements very challenging. Additionally, the body also has the essential biologic ability to adapt and structurally remodel itself according to the stresses placed upon it. Some of these adaptations, as in the mechanical properties of tissues, can occur relatively rapidly. This "moving target" property can add an additional layer of difficulty for accurate description.

The capacity of the body to adapt appropriately to environmental stress will make the difference between health and disease. The goal of the osteopathic physician is to assist the body in regaining a balance with the stressors of the patient's environment, usually at multiple levels of consideration. From a biomechanical standpoint, this may involve the correction of somatic dysfunctions or to break cycles of inappropriate responses that have produced them. In doing so, the primary biomechanical considerations for the osteopathic physician must include broad characteristics encompassing both biomaterial characteristics of tissues and the primary mechanical operation of the body as a unit. As opposed to other medical disciplines, this must include a literal "feel" for the characteristics of tissues in addition to figurative "feel" for the understanding of body mechanics derived from a knowledge of anatomy. The primary goal of this chapter is to assist the reader in obtaining this latter knowledge. For this reason, an emphasis will be placed on basic biomaterial and biomechanical concepts rather than mathematical modeling of properties. As with other chapters in this volume, this chapter is intended to be a summary of biomechanical concepts that are of particular relevance to those who study osteopathic medicine. More comprehensive discussions may be readily obtained from texts on particular topics. It will be assumed that the reader has a basic working knowledge of gross anatomy and the concepts relating anatomy to function.

Motion and Forces Can Be Described as Components With a Magnitude in Each Dimension of Three-Dimensional Space

The strategy for describing the mechanics of biologic materials begins with the same terms and methods employed to describe inanimate objects. The process of interest is broken down into components that can be measured and characterized. These components and their properties are then incorporated into models (often mathematical) that can be used to describe the system and predict its reaction to defined stresses. The terminology used is common to areas of mechanical sciences, and can be categorized into terms related to:

1. Dimensions and movement in three-dimensional space
2. The nature of applied forces
3. Properties of biomaterials

Objects and Movements in Three-Dimensional Space Can Be Described as Components in Each of the Three Dimensions

An object can be described by the magnitude of its size in each of its dimensions (length, width, height; Fig. 5.1). Similarly, simple movement (translation) of an object in three-dimensional space can be described as three different components *(vectors)* of movement (up/down, back and forth, in and out relative to the page) that can occur simultaneously. Vectors will have a magnitude and direction similar to describing the dimensions of an object, except that the magnitude of movement is expressed as velocity (meters per second). Vector components are shown on

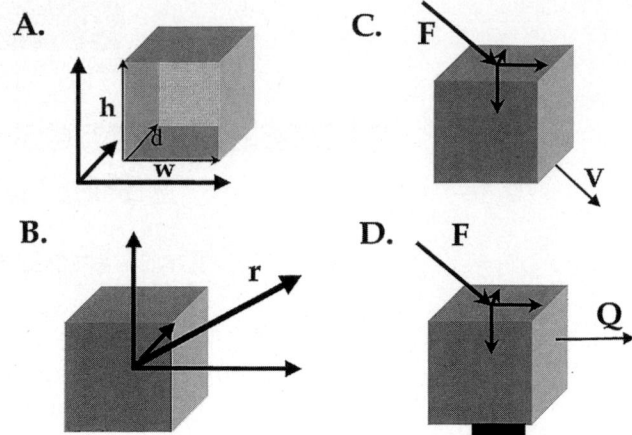

FIGURE 5.1. A: An object in three-dimensional space (axes) can be described by the length vectors (height [*h*], width [*w*], depth [*d*]). **B:** The motion of an object can be described as three separate primary vectors of velocity. The actual movement of the object is represented by the resultant vector (*r*). **C:** A force (*F*) that is applied to an object may also be represented by separate force vectors in each dimension directed into the object. The object may be moved in a direction (*v*) by the force. **D:** If one component of the accelerating force is resisted, the object will move in a new direction (*Q*), determined by the magnitude of the remaining vector components.

an axis system (Fig. 5.1) that is used to model three-dimensional space. By describing the vectors of movement in each of these three dimensions, the motion of the object can be characterized. The actual path of the object is referred to as the *resultant velocity vector.* Biomechanical analysis uses similar vector systems to describe most parameters in space, such as velocity, acceleration, and pressure.

Beyond simple models, the properties of each component of a resultant vector can become increasingly complex. For example, an object of irregular shape will require more than a simple length measurement in each dimension to describe it. Similarly, an object moving in space may also rotate about an axis. Because of this, even relatively simple movements of body segments may require sophisticated mathematical modeling to describe the movement.

Applied Forces Can Also Be Expressed as Three-Dimensional Vectors

Applied *forces,* such as a manipulative thrust, are essentially *pressure* (force per unit area) applied to an object. By definition, forces act to accelerate an object of a given mass. Accordingly, an object at rest must have a force applied to it in order to achieve movement through acceleration. An object moving at a constant velocity will require no forces to sustain movement, unless other forces (e.g., friction) are acting to resist the movement. The object's resistance to change of velocity (*inertia*) is also described as the force required to accelerate it from rest (zero velocity) or to decelerate it from movement.

The magnitude of forces and associated force vectors are used to describe external pressures applied to the body and internal forces like those generated in muscles to achieve limb movement. Force magnitudes are expressed as the mass of the object times the acceleration (F = ma). The metric unit of force is a newton (N) or 1 kilogram accelerated to a velocity of 1 meter per second each second (kg × m/s^2). Like velocity, forces are characterized as a combination of vector components of a certain magnitude in each of the three axes defining space (Fig. 5.1). The *resultant force* is the sum of the individual force vectors. The manner in which the object might be moved or mobilized by the force will depend upon which of the vector components are resisted and which are not (Fig. 5.1). Similarly, a resultant force vector arising from a manipulative thrust would be characterized by describing force components not only directly into the body, but also in lateral directions (rostral, caudal, medial, or lateral) as well as rotational components. Mobilization of body segments by the force will depend upon which components of the thrust meet with direct resistance and obviously how the body is positioned. In biomechanics, it is important to characterize the different components that a force may have in order to understand the ensuing reaction of the material or body structures.

Moments Are Forces that Act at a Distance and/or Produce Rotation of an Object

Forces that act to produce rotation of an object about an axis, or in two-dimensional models, a center point (Fig. 5.2), are called *force moments* (also *moment* or *torque*). The magnitude of a force moment is the product of the force applied and the distance of application from the center of rotation (force × distance). The latter distance is referred to as the *moment arm*. This is essentially a process of using a lever to produce rotation about an axis. Because of this relationship, it is important to note that moments of the same magnitude may be produced by increasing the force applied while proportionately reducing the moment arm or vice versa (Fig. 5.2). A common example of the properties of force

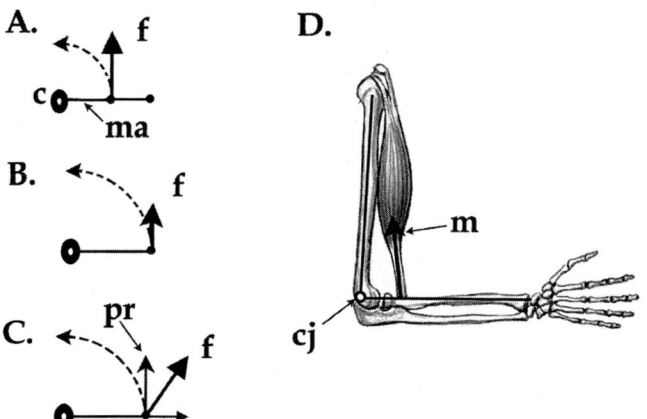

FIGURE 5.2. Force moments on an object such as a door. **A:** A force (*f*) applied at a distance (moment arm, *ma*) in the middle of the door can produce rotation (*dotted arrow*) around a center or axis (*c*) located at the hinge. The moment is the force applied times the distance (*d*) from the center (f × d). A smaller force acting on a longer moment arm at the doorknob (**B**) will produce the same moment (f × d). **C:** If the force is applied in a direction other than directly against the moment arm, only part (*pr*) of the force will be used to produce the rotation. **D:** In the body, force moments are generated by muscle contraction forces (*m*) that produce rotation of a mobile body segment about a center in the joint (*cj*).

moments can be obtained from pushing open a door (Fig. 5.2). Pushing the door open at the handle usually is relatively easy (low force), because of the long distance (moment arm) between the handle and the center of rotation at the hinge. Note, however, that opening the door at the handle requires a relatively large distance of movement (large displacement). Attempting to push the door open at a point near the hinge (short moment arm) is much more difficult (greater force), but requires less displacement to open the door. Note also that the direction or angle at which the push is applied to the door will determine how much of the force applied is actually used to push the door open (Fig. 5.2). This rotation component of the applied force is at a right angle to the surface of the door (directly into the door) at any instant. The remaining force component will be in a direction along the surface of the door. For the same opening force to be maintained, the direction of the applied force must change constantly to move in a circle with the door.

The strategy of changing the force or the length of the moment arm and the direction at which forces are applied is often employed in body mechanics and in manipulation techniques, depending upon the need for more or less force at the cost of greater or lesser displacement.

Moments are used in the biomechanical modeling of body motion because most movements are composites of rotational movements of individual body segments around joints. Force moments are generated from the contraction of muscles attached between two body segments causing the movement of the more mobile segment around a center of rotation (Fig. 5.2). The center of rotation is usually near the articulation surface in the less mobile segment. The moment arm of the contracting force is related to the distance of the muscle insertion on the mobile segment from the center of rotation. In simple biomechanical models of body movement, this center of rotation in the joint is usually shown as immobile. In actual movements, both segments may be mobile and motions within the joint may also occur to change the center of rotation.

Stresses Are Forces Applied to Objects in Various Orientations

The characteristics of forces applied to an object are described as *stresses* (Fig. 5.3). The magnitude of basic stresses is described as force applied over a defined unit of object surface area or pressure. This may be described as pounds per square inch (psi) or in the metric form, pascals (N per square m). Particular types of stresses are identified to describe their relationship to the object acted upon (Fig. 5.3). For convenience, stresses are usually described for an object that is immobilized or constrained, such that the object must resist the stress and not undergo acceleration or movement other than deformation (see "Strain Is Deformation Produced by Stress," later in the chapter). *Tension* is a force applied perpendicularly outward from the surface of an object (pull), such that the object would be elongated or stretched. *Compression* stress is a force applied perpendicularly inward (push) to the surface of an object, such that the object would be shortened or compressed. *Shear stresses* are forces applied parallel to the surface of an object. *Torsion stresses* are rotation-like forces, which on a constrained object, act to twist it about a neutral axis (that is, an axis that

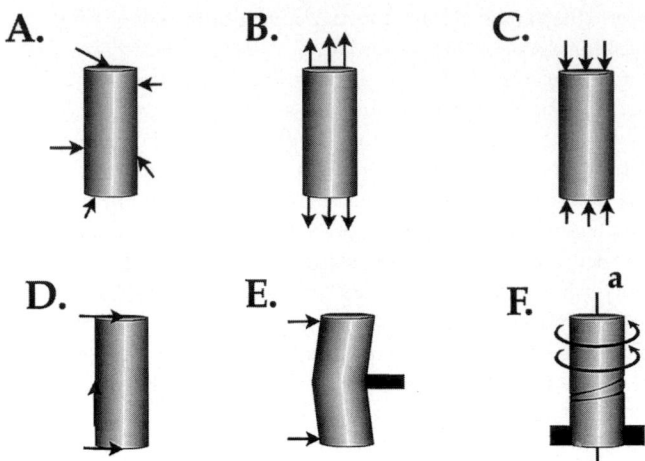

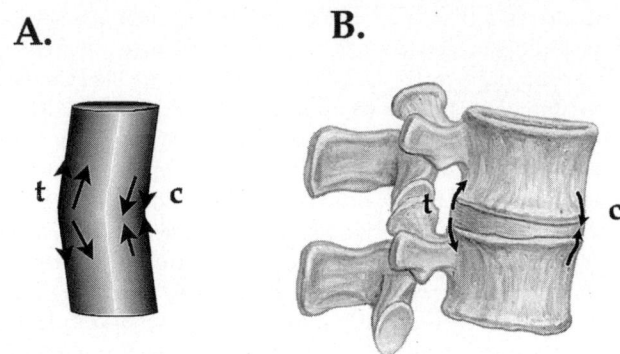

FIGURE 5.4. **A:** Bending strain produces tensile stress (*t*) on one side of an object and compressive stress (*c*) on the other. **B:** This same principle applies directly to biologic materials, such as spinal discs.

FIGURE 5.3. **A:** Stresses are forces acting from various orientations relative to the object. Stresses are named according to their action upon the object. **B:** Tensile stresses act to stretch an object. **C:** Compressive stresses compact the object. **D:** Shear stresses act parallel to the surface of an object. **E:** Bending stress acts to fold an object about an axis. **F:** Torsion stresses twist an object about an axis.

would not be translated or moved by the force). *Bending* is also technically a rotation-like force (or coupled coactive forces) that acts to fold or bend an appropriately constrained object along a neutral axis. The sum of all stresses on an object is termed *load*.

BEHAVIOR OF MATERIALS SUBJECTED TO FORCES

The Behavior of an Object or Material May Be Isotropic or Anisotropic

While stresses may originate from external forces applied to an object's surfaces, they are also transmitted from the area of contact through the entire substance comprising the object. The primary factors affecting the transmission of forces through an object are its shape and material composition including infrastructure. The characteristics of the material composition of the object will determine if the object can be accelerated or rotated by a stress of sufficient magnitude or physically broken by it. The shape of an object may dramatically affect the manner in which it responds to similar stresses exerted in different places on the object. An object, such as a sphere of homogenous composition, will respond in the same way to a particular type and magnitude of stress applied to any point on its surface. This type of object is referred to as *isotropic* in relation to stresses. Objects having a nonuniform surface shape (such as an irregular cube) or heterogeneous composition will respond to the same stress differently depending upon the point of application. These objects or materials are referred to as *anisotropic*. Most biologic structures fall into this category.

As with surface characteristics, the internal structure or composition of an object will also determine its response characteristics to stresses. The object's composition and molecular infrastructure determine how a force applied to a particular location is transmitted to the remainder of the object's mass. In objects that have an anisotropic internal composition, such as biologic mate-

rials, localized internal stresses are often the primary determinant of the toleration of the material for stresses of a particular magnitude and orientation of a stress. As discussed subsequently, bone, muscle, tendons, and ligaments have a linear cellular/molecular structure that causes the response to loads to differ dramatically depending upon the orientation of the applied stress.

Strain Is Deformation Produced by Stress

As muscles contract, they apply primary localized tensile stresses to bone to accelerate the mobile segment(s) and to stabilize the immobile segment(s). Under this condition, the applied stresses produce a change in the shape of the bone or object (*deformation*). The magnitude of deformation produced by stress is referred to as *strain*. The actual deformation of an object will depend upon the same factors defining stress distribution (internal composition and infrastructure) and is characterized as a sum of different strain vectors. These vectors are usually named for the type of stress producing them (e.g., tensile strain, compressive strain, etc.). Many different strain vectors may be produced within an object by a particular type of stress. A simple example is a bending stress that produces tensile strain on the side of the object opposite the neutral axis and compressive strain in the direction of bending (Fig. 5.4). A similar condition exists with strain on a spinal disc with bending between segments.

The Elastic Modulus Shows the Relationship Between Stress and Strain

While it can generally be assumed that increases in stress on an object will produce an increase in strain, the relationship is not direct, particularly for biologic materials. The relationship between the amount of a particular stress applied to an object and the resulting deformation or strain is shown by a stress/strain curve (Fig. 5.5). In this instance, a material is subjected to a defined stress such as tension. In this model, the strain may be quantified as the change in length of the object (as with a tendon or ligament). A similar result could be obtained by the displacement of the center of a bending load (as with a bone). Stress/strain relationships for most materials have a linear region (elastic behavior) in which increasing stress produces a corresponding amount of deformation (Fig. 5.5). Reducing the stress or unloading of the

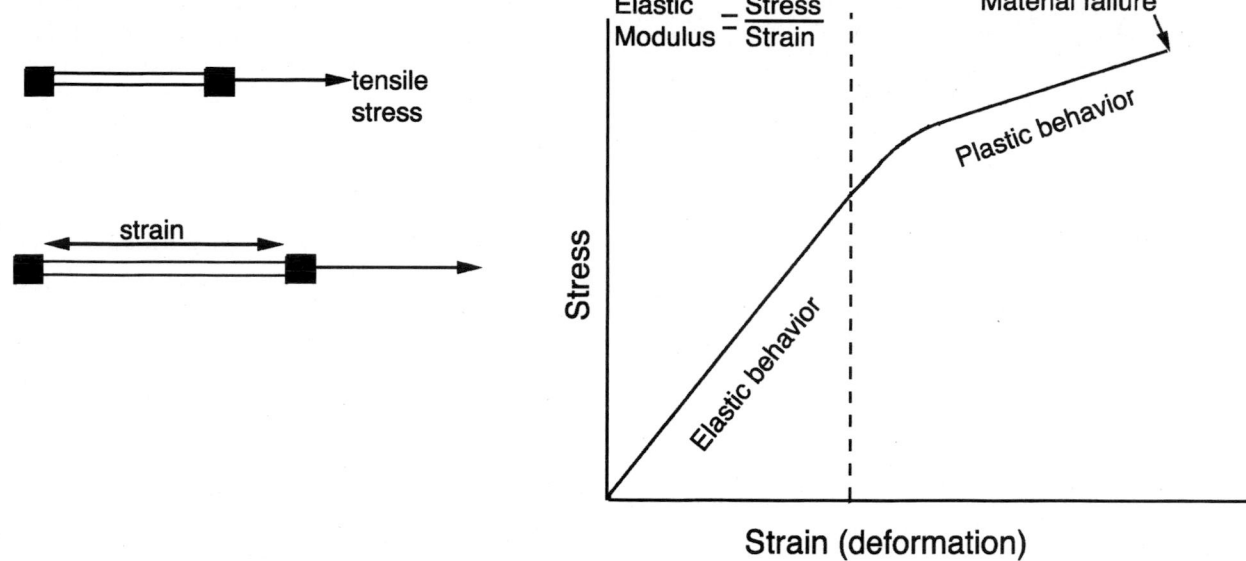

FIGURE 5.5. A stress/strain curve **(right)** of an object undergoing increasing tensile stress **(left)**. The change in length can be used as a measure of strain. The curve has an area of elastic behavior, in which a release of stress will allow the object to return to its original shape. In this area, the stress/strain relationship can be expressed as elastic modulus. With increasing stress, the material has permanent deformation or plastic behavior, followed by material failure.

object will allow it to return to its former shape without a permanent change in shape. In this elastic area of the stress/strain curve, the slope of the line (stress/strain) is termed the *elastic modulus.* The elastic modulus is also a quantitative description of *stiffness,* a term commonly associated with the amount of force necessary to bend an object.

When an applied stress is greater than that defined by the elastic area (Fig. 5.5), a permanent deformation of the material or plasticity will result. The plastic behavior area of the curve ends with the material *failure* or breaking of the object. Materials may also be described as *brittle* or *ductile* depending upon the amount of deformation they can undergo before failure. *Brittle* objects such as glass will undergo little deformation before they break (fail), and the pieces after breaking retain their shape such that pieces will fit together to produce a puzzlelike reproduction of the object with little deformation. *Ductile* materials such as a copper wire will have a permanently altered shape beyond their elastic region and after failure. Many factors other than basic structure of a material may significantly affect the stress/strain relationship. The most common of these are temperature and the rate at which a stress is applied.

Viscoelasticity Is the Combination of Elastic and Viscous Properties of Materials in Response to Stress

The rate at which a stress is applied can be a particularly important determinant in the response of materials that exhibit a combination of both elastic and viscous behavior in response to an applied stress. Viscous behavior can be described as resistance to flow, such as that observed with cold syrup. Viscosity in biologic materials arises largely, but not completely, from the resistance of their water content to flow into and out of the material with

applied stress. For example, spaces between molecules of collagen in ligaments contain a large amount of water with salts and other small relatively mobile molecules. Tensile stress (stretching) of the ligament will decrease the available space between collagen molecules, forcing the fluid between them out of the ligament. This process is similar to stretching a wet sponge (Fig. 5.6). If the structure is stretched rapidly, there is an increasing resistance to fluid movement out of (and into) these spaces, since this

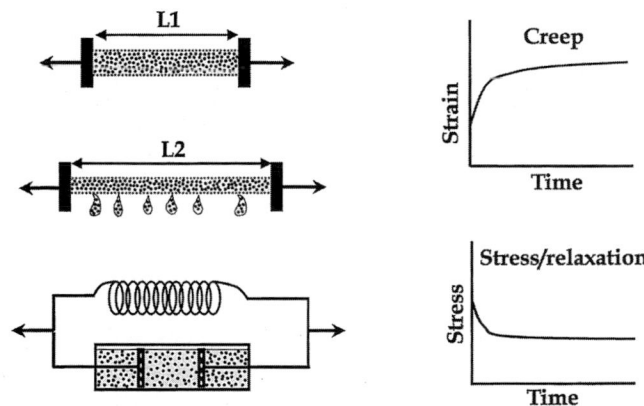

FIGURE 5.6. Left: Viscoelastic behavior occurs when a material containing a mobile fluid phase is stretched (or compressed) from a resting length (*L1*) to force fluid out of an elastic matrix similar to a sponge to a greater length (*L2*). This can be modeled schematically **(bottom)** as a spring in parallel with a fluid containing resistance compartment with porous baffles. **Right:** Time-dependent viscoelastic behavior of a material under tensile stress. Creep **(top)** is a measure of deformation (strain) over time with stress (stretch force) held constant. Stress/relaxation **(bottom)** is a measure of stress over time with strain held constant. (Portions of this figure have been adapted from Carlstedt CA, Nordin M. Biomechanics of tendons and ligaments. In: Nordin M, Frankel VH, eds. *Basic Biomechanics of the Musculoskeletal System,* 2nd ed. Philadelphia, PA: Lea & Febiger; 1989:59–74, with permission.)

requires time. The time required for fluids to move out of intermolecular spaces acts to slow the rate of deformation of an elastic material. This alters the elastic and plastic regions of the stress/strain curve. In combination with the elastic properties of the material, this behavior is described as *viscoelasticity.* This property is usually modeled as a spring acting in parallel to a resistance provided by a fluid compartment (Fig. 5.6).

Besides the flow of small molecules from intermolecular spaces, frictional resistance due to molecular movement and ionic interactions between molecules also contributes to the viscosity in a material. These molecular interactions, along with the elastic properties of the material, are important in the return of water and other small molecules back into the matrix, again much as a sponge reabsorbs fluid after being squeezed. This recovery process is important if the biomaterial properties of the tissue are to be maintained under repeated loading. Additionally, since viscoelastic behavior involves the movement of small molecules and the interaction between molecules, temperature can significantly affect this property.

Viscoelastic properties can produce significant alteration of material behavior when the rate of loading is too fast for the fluid exchange to occur. Under these conditions, a material may exhibit a higher elastic modulus (that is, appear stiffer or more brittle) under high loading rates, as compared to the same load applied over a longer period of time. If a viscoelastic material is stretched rapidly and the load is sustained after the initial loading period, there will be a rapid initial deformation of the material followed by a slower deformation as the remaining fluid in the matrix reaches a new equilibrium at a slower rate (Fig. 5.6). Two types of measurements are used to describe this property. First, if the material is subjected to an initial load, such as tensile stress (Fig. 5.6), which is then maintained, the material will stretch to an initial length and then more slowly increase in length as the more resistant fluid in the matrix effuses. The slower phase after the initial stretch is called *creep.*

Another measurement looks at the load necessary to maintain a constant deformation or, in the case of Fig. 5.6, the length of the material. As the matrix reaches equilibrium, the load necessary to maintain the length will decrease. This property is referred to as *stress/relaxation.*

Because of their high water and solute content, bone, muscle, ligament, tendon, and other biologic materials have viscoelastic properties that are important for their function. Due to the differences in the cellular structure and the matrix between cells in these materials, the actual viscoelastic properties of these tissues differ markedly.

Fatigue is the Failure of a Material as a Result of Repeated Stress

Fatigue is a multifaceted term that is used to describe material failure after repeated application of stresses that, if applied individually, would not produce failure. In nonbiologic materials such as metals, a significant part of fatigue failure can result from the accumulated breakdown of crystalline structure as the result of repeated stress, such as breaking a steel or copper wire by repeated bending. In biologic systems, the process of fatigue failure becomes more complicated, because of the ability to repair and adapt materials to repeated stress. For example, bone under repeated stress may undergo microfractures in its structure (see the following section). Depending upon the frequency of the stress and the ability of the bone to repair these microfractures, the bone may suffer a fatigue fracture or adapt to the stress by increasing its mass.

PROPERTIES OF BIOLOGIC MATERIALS: BONE

Bone Is an Anisotropic Material Comprised of Osteons

Mechanical models describing nonbiologic materials are difficult to apply to biologic systems directly, due in part to their complicated structure. The response of biologic materials to stresses is determined by structural properties layered down to the subcellular level. Still, the material properties of bone structure as a whole are clearly traceable from tissue structure (1). Bone consists of connective tissue cells organized and embedded in a highly mineralized extracellular matrix. Although lower than other tissues, this matrix also contains significant amounts of water and other small molecules, giving bone viscoelastic material properties. The basic unit of organization is the osteon or haversian system. These systems consist of concentric rings of bone cells or osteocytes around a central cavity (the haversian canal) through which the blood vessels and nerves supplying the bone travel (Fig. 5.7). The osteons are arranged in a dense, regular pattern around the shaft of long bones to form cortical or compact bone. The border between osteons is the *cement line.* The cement line is structurally weaker than the substance of the circularly oriented osteons and can often be identified microscopically as the site of failure of bone tissue under high stresses (2). Osteocyte lacunae may also be a site of structural weakness (3). Beneath the cortical layer of compact bone is a central core of more porous bone

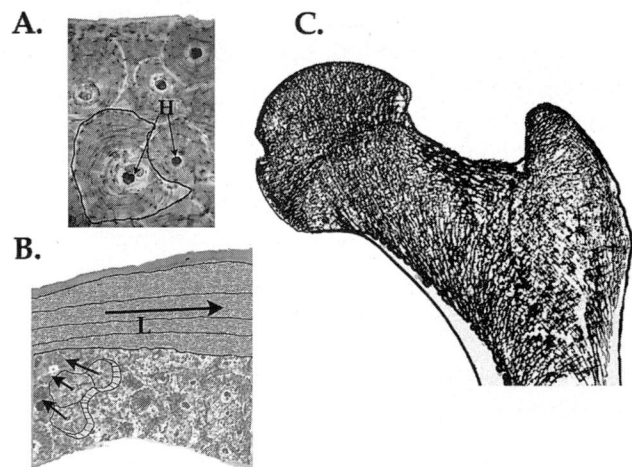

FIGURE 5.7. Histologic and structural properties of bone. **A:** Compact bone structure is organized into cylinder-shaped osteons with haversian canals *(H)* that are separated by a cement line *(outline).* **B:** In long bones, osteons are oriented longitudinally along the axis of the bone and surrounded by circumferentially oriented lamellar bone *(L).* Both surround a marrow space that contains marrow and cancellous bone. **C:** The organization cancellous bone is not random in structures such as the femur, where the trabeculae *(black)* help to distribute stresses through the internal structure of the bone.

(termed cancellous, trabecular, or spongy bone), with lacunae comprising the marrow space. While the structure of cancellous bone may initially appear as a random mesh of thin bone, it can be readily shown that areas of organization do exist and contribute to the structural stability of the bone as a whole by distributing stresses internally in the bone structure (4) (Fig. 5.7).

Bones Are Structured to Resist the Primary Functional Stresses Placed Upon Them

As might be expected, the highly organized cellular and gross structure of bone causes it to behave in an anisotropic manner to applied stresses. The outward structure and infrastructure of bones are organized to resist the major stresses to which they are subjected under normal physiologic conditions. For the structure of a long bone such the tibia, the compressive loading lengthwise will require much higher stress before failure compared to a stress of similar magnitude applied perpendicularly to the long axis. In this manner, from the subcellular to gross structure, bone represents one of the most obvious examples of the structure-to-function relationship. This anisotropic behavior also defines the manner in which bones will undergo material failure when excessive stresses are placed upon them.

Different Stress Vectors Produce Varying Types of Bone Failure (Fracture)

The material failure (fracture) of bone can be observed clinically for all major categories of stresses, with the mechanism of material failure varying with type of loading (1). Also, the viscoelastic behavior of bone gives it sensitivity to loading rate. At rapid loading rates, bone appears stiffer as the movement of fluid and molecular friction increasingly resists deformation. This causes bone to store more energy before failure. When bone does fail at high loading rates, its more brittle behavior makes it more likely to fragment, much like shattering glass (comminuted fracture) (5). Accordingly, fractures can also be categorized into different types according to the energy absorbed with the resulting failure, low energy, high energy, and very high energy. Higher energy fractures (automobile accidents, gunshot wounds) are typically accompanied by bone fragmentation and soft tissue damage, as the energy stored under rapid loading is dissipated with biomaterial failure.

Under physiologic conditions, bones will experience a combination of stress vectors at the same time and failures may result from the combination rather than a particular stress type. However, fractures do begin in the stress component direction most prone to failure according to the material properties of the bone. This allows the description of some types of fracture resulting from particular stress categories. Muscles pulling on bone typically generate tensile stress fractures. The tensile fracture of the calcaneus adjacent to the Achilles tendon insertion is a frequent example (Fig. 5.8). Compression fractures are most commonly found in the vertebral column, which is subject to high compressive load and a weakening of the bones with age. Shear forces act parallel to bone surfaces, typically at articulations, where bones are in contact. Shear fractures can occur under conditions of compression loading of a joint, coupled with a shear or lateral force across the articulation with a failure of the joint bony plateau.

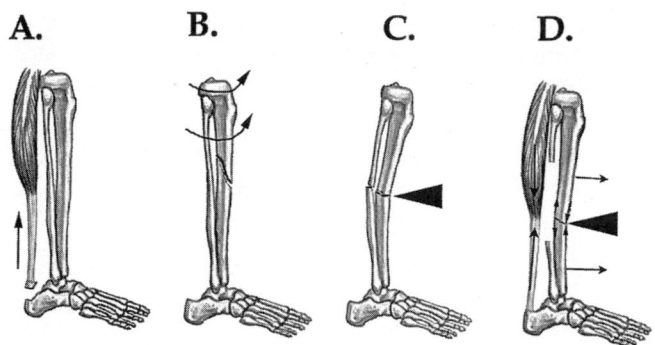

FIGURE 5.8. Examples of fracture types resulting from a material failure due to a primary stress component. **A:** Tensile fracture of the calcaneus. **B:** Spiral fracture from torsional stress of the tibia. **C:** Bending stress fracture. **D:** Example of how muscle contraction forces can act to counter bending stress. Bending stress produces tensile forces on one side of the tibia and compressive stress on the other (see Fig. 5.4). Muscle contraction can act to counter the tensile component by producing a compressive moment. (Portions of this figure have been adapted from Gollnick PD, Matoba H. The muscle fiber composition of skeletal muscle as a predictor of athletic success. An overview. *Am J Sports Med.* 1984;12:212–217, with permission.)

Bending and torsional loading produce multiple types of material stresses on bone depending upon the direction of the loading. As described earlier, bending of an object produces tensile stress on one side of an object and compression on the other (Fig. 5.4). Bone is weaker in tension than compression, so bone material failure begins upon the tensile stress side (Fig. 5.8). Immature bone, which is less calcified and more ductile, may be more sensitive to compression and fractures may occur on the compressive side first. Torsional loading (Fig. 5.8), or usually twisting around the long axis of bones, produces shear stresses around the neutral axis while compression and tension loading are diagonal to the axis. The resulting failure (spiral fracture) is initially due to shear stress followed by tensile stress failure along a diagonal axis. As should be expected, if there are weaknesses in the bone structure, such as during rehabilitation after injury, failure will occur at the weakest point or at the site of bony defect with bending loads.

The biomaterial failure of bone under stresses is greatly influenced by the attachment and contraction of muscles. Muscle activity can decrease or counter stresses produced on bone by altering the direction of the resultant stress vectors to those to which bone may be more tolerant. Fig. 5.8 shows how muscle activity may alter a bending or tensile stress to produce compression stress. As bone is very resistant to compressive stress (such as weight on the long axis of the tibia), this redistribution of stress can be important to avoiding stress fracture. Consequently, the physiologic tiring of muscle during strenuous exercise can contribute significantly to fractures because the protective mechanism is lost.

While sudden, large stresses are usually associated with bone fracture, failure of the material itself can result from repetitive loading over a period of time. This fatigue-type fracture of bone involves an accumulation of smaller failures within the bone microstructure and is dependent upon the magnitude, frequency, and rate of loading. Even low-level repetitive loads may produce fatigue microfractures in bone (6). In living bone, these microfractures will be repaired by cellular reactions to the injury. If the fatigue process outpaces the repair, failure will eventually occur as a repetitive stress fracture. A common example of this is the fatigue fracture of metatarsal bones in long distance runners (7).

Bone Remodels Its Structure in Response to Stress and Depends upon Stresses to Maintain Its Material Properties

In the presence of stresses, bone can alter size, shape, and structure to withstand stresses placed upon it. The unusual corollary to this property is that bone must be subjected to stress in order to maintain its biomaterial properties. The underlying principle of this process in bone has been expressed as Wolff law, which states that bone is increased where needed and resorbed where not needed (8). The resorption of bone under conditions of reduced usage or immobilization (9) are of particular concern clinically, since mechanical stress on bone is reduced during casting or in more limited conditions, such as weightlessness in space travel (10). Immobilization results in the resorption of periosteal and subperiosteal bone (11) and a decrease in bone strength and stiffness (12). Conversely, the hypertrophy (13,14) and increase in density of bone (15) may be observed in normal bones in response to strenuous exercise. Both hypertrophy and resorption of bone may be observed around implant screws and plates used to surgically stabilize bone defects or to attach prosthetic joints (16).

Bone properties also are altered with aging, with a progressive loss of bone density and size (17,18). This is independent of the condition of osteoporosis. The result is a decrease in bone strength and stiffness and altered stress/strain properties, including an increase in brittleness and a reduction in energy storage capacity. These properties make bones more susceptible to material failure under high stress conditions with increasing age.

ARTICULAR CARTILAGE

The Surfaces of Contact Between Bones in Synovial Joints Is Hyaline Cartilage

There are three identified primary types of cartilage in the human body: hyaline cartilage, fibrocartilage, and elastic cartilage. Hyaline cartilage covers the surface of the articulations of almost all diarthrodial joints, and will be the focus of our description of basic biomaterial properties of cartilage. Cartilage has some similarity to bone in that it consists of cells (chondrocytes) surrounded by an extensive extracellular matrix that they secrete. However, cartilage is avascular; lacking blood vessels, lymph channels, or nerves within its matrix and the matrix secreted is not calcified as in bone. The extracellular matrix of cartilage consists primarily of collagen (type II), proteoglycans, and 60% to 87% water with inorganic salts and other minor matrix proteins and lipids (19,20). The collagen and proteoglycans form the major structural elements of cartilage, and these interact extensively on a molecular level with the smaller molecules, including water. The interaction of these elements with each other within cartilage and their interaction with the water in the matrix determine the primary biomaterial properties of cartilage.

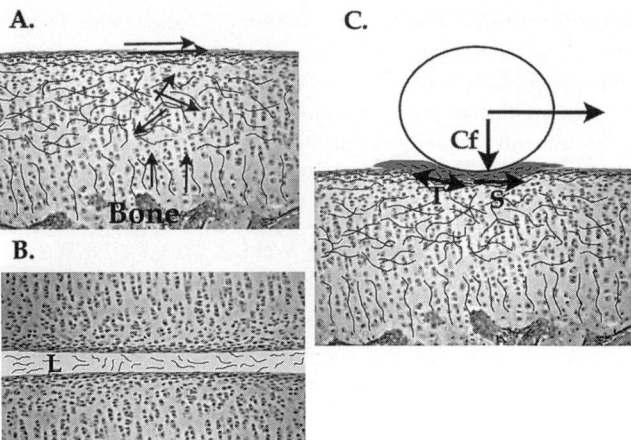

FIGURE 5.9. A: Schematic of the orientation *(arrows)* of collagen fibrils *(drawn lines)* in articular cartilage. The orientation varies from the articular surface to the bone interface. **B:** Representation of cartilage surface separated by a thin layer of lubricating fluid *(L)* that prevents direct surface contact. **C:** With a compressive force on the surface *(cf)* additional fluid is exuded and the matrix is compressed. Lateral movement produces tensile *(t)* and shear *(s)* stress on the cartilage surface and matrix components.

The major collagen and proteoglycan structural element on the cartilage of articular surfaces is not randomly organized and can be divided into histologic zones that differ in cellular organization from the surface to the underlying subchondral bone (20) (Fig. 5.9). The orientation of collagen fibril bundles within the matrix differs between the layers (Fig. 5.9) with a tangential orientation at the surface, random organization in the middle zone, and radial orientation near the subchondral bone surface. This orientation provides the basic structural framework for the cartilage and resistance to the loads placed upon it. Depending upon the particular joint function, the primary stresses may be compression, which, as the joint moves, contributes to shear and tensile stresses on the cartilage surfaces (Fig. 5.9).

Cartilage Has Significant Viscoelastic Properties That Are Essential to Its Function

The collagen and proteoglycan structural elements of cartilage have spaces between them filled with water, salts, and other small molecules, forming a matrix with viscoelastic properties as previously described. Further, the structural elements contain molecules such as hyaluronic acid and have ionically charged groups throughout their structure. This property allows them to strongly bind water and inorganic salt within the cartilaginous matrix. The cartilage matrix has properties of flexibility from a pliable, porous collagen superstructure containing small molecules that can be forced out, but with some molecular and ionic interaction based resistance to the efflux. The properties of this matrix allow a viscoelastic behavior in which the cartilage allows rapid, but declining deformation (cushioning) in response to compressive loads followed by creep or stress/relaxation (21) (Fig. 5.7). The slower deformation will continue until equilibrium is reached between the load and the forces resisting it within the matrix. The differing mechanical properties of the layers of articular cartilage interact dynamically to reach equilibrium in response to a sustained compressive force (22).

On a tissue level more closely related to normal function, the viscoelastic response of cartilage can be explained by a compressive stress that produces a rapid efflux of fluid forced out of the extracellular matrix directly beneath it and in areas immediately adjacent to it (Fig. 5.9). The resistance to this efflux of fluid is dependent upon the effective porosity or space available in the cartilage matrix for fluid to move. Other resistance to matrix deformation includes the internal friction generated by movement between long polymer molecules such as collagen and attached proteoglycans and the ionic binding of these chains to the water and other small molecules. The time required for the fluid phase to reach a full equilibrium between cartilage layers under the applied load may require hours (21). However, because of the elasticity of the collagenous structural elements and ionic interactions with the small molecules of the matrix, this fluid exchange is reversible and supplies a pumping action of nutrients into and waste products out of cartilage in addition to normal diffusion. This action is particularly important because of the avascular nature of cartilage.

Articular Cartilage Has Several Properties That Act to Prevent Wear Damage

Under physiologic conditions, cartilage surfaces of joints contact each other under a variety of loading conditions while showing little wear. This occurs in spite of the fact that joint surfaces are not perfectly smooth. The prevention of wear is due in part to a system of lubrication of synovial articular surfaces provided by synovial fluid and the properties of the cartilage itself. Fluids lubricate surfaces by preventing their direct contact (Fig. 5.9). The first level of lubrication of joint surfaces is the absorption of lubricin, a glycoprotein in synovial fluid that is absorbed onto articular surfaces. This provides a thin boundary of lubricant on the joint surface. The synovial fluid itself also provides a thin film of fluid between the joint surfaces that can be redistributed under loading conditions. Further, during loading the fluid extruded as a result of the compressive deformation of the cartilage will provide a fluid layer to separate the opposed surfaces (23).

Under normal conditions, the fluid lubricating properties of the joint will prevent the direct contact of uneven sections or asperities of joint surfaces to contact each other. If contact does occur, wear of the joint surfaces or interfacial wear (mechanical removal of material from a solid surface) may occur. This may consist of abrasion of the joint surface because of contact of uneven elements of the surface or small fragments of joint surfaces may adhere to each other and be dislodged. The efficient lubricating properties of normal joint usually preclude interfacial wear, but it may occur in damaged or degenerated joints (22).

Cartilage Wear May Result from Several Different Mechanisms, Including Intrinsic Changes with Aging

While cartilage can be damaged as a result of traumatic injury as in shearing stress applied to the meniscal cartilage of the knee, the mechanisms of abnormal wear are not as clear. Hypotheses of the mechanism of cartilage wear include the disruption of the structural molecules of the cartilage matrix through repeated stress (24,25) and the alteration of the matrix content under the same conditions. As with bone, rapid loading of a viscoelastic matrix increases the stiffness of cartilage, and the loss of the fluid component of the matrix will also increase stiffness. This loss of fluid may include soluble proteoglycans from the cartilage surface that are important in the maintenance of its properties. Under conditions of rapidly repeated high-impact loading, the fluid forced from the matrix that would normally provide a cushioning effect cannot be reabsorbed in time to cushion subsequent impacts. This may also produce plastic deformation of cartilage surfaces that does not sufficiently recover for smooth surface contact upon subsequent loading. The increased stiffness and deformation of the matrix increases the likelihood of mechanical wear in addition to rendering the subchondral bone surface more vulnerable to damage.

Cartilage wear may also be complicated by the limited capacity of cartilage to repair or regenerate. This property gives it a limited capacity to adapt to stress. In conjunction with repeated stresses and minor injuries, a cycle of damage, wear, and insufficient recovery may occur, leading to joint degeneration and/or osteoarthritis. The inability of cartilage to recover during repeated high stress loads may be one source of macroscopic structural defects observed in cartilage (26) and responsible for the high incidence of specific joint degeneration and the development of osteoarthritis in persons with certain occupations (football players and dancers).

The intrinsic composition and properties of cartilage also change with age (27). The matrix composition changes and permeability increases, decreasing cartilage stiffness and rendering it less resistant to rapid loading. Along with the accumulation of injuries from which the tissue cannot recover, these age-related changes may contribute to the increased incidence of joint degeneration with age.

LIGAMENTS AND TENDONS

Ligaments and Tendons Are Dense, Regular Connective Tissue with a High Resistance to Tensile Loading

Ligaments and tendons, along with joint capsules, surround the articulations of the skeletal system. Their functions are, in the case of ligaments and joint capsules, to structurally connect, stabilize, and guide the bones forming the articulation (28). They may also act as a sensor for joint position and strain for the joint. Tendons connect muscle to bone and transmit forces from muscle to bone to produce motion. Both tendons and ligaments are classified as dense, regular connective tissues. They have sparse cellular elements and abundant extracellular matrix in a highly organized array. The extracellular matrix is rich in collagen and water with a small amount of elastin, again producing a viscoelastic behavior under stress. The collagen molecules are linked together in lengthwise overlapping arrays to microfibrils, that are in turn combined in similar overlapping arrays to form fibrils, then fibers, and bundles of fibers to form the macroscopic tendon (Fig. 5.10). This successive parallel linkage down to the molecular

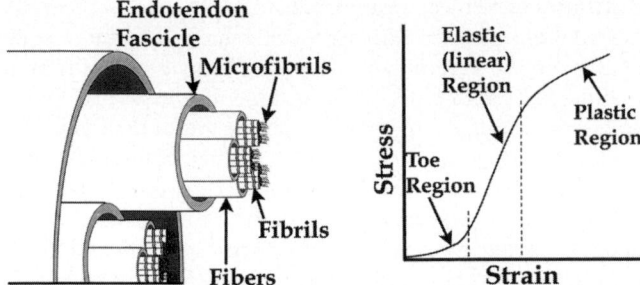

FIGURE 5.10. Left: Schematic view of the structural organization of tendon. Microfibrils are the smallest component consisting of collagen molecules. Microfibrils are organized into fibrils that are grouped into fibers. Fibers are grouped into fascicles that comprise the tendon. **Right:** Idealized version of a stress/strain curve for tendon under tensile stress. The toe region is a nonlinear behavior attributed to the "slack" between collagen molecules. The elastic region has a linear relationship between stress and strain. In the plastic region, permanent deformation occurs, eventually resulting in failure.

level makes ligaments and tendons capable of handling high tensile loads. The arrangement of fibrils in ligament tissue is less parallel than tendon and accounts for its higher resistance to tensile loading in orientations other than along the tissue axis. The collagen molecules are also linked to each other by cross-links. While there are some important biomechanical differences between ligaments and tendons, most of their properties are basically similar and will be described together here.

The Primary Biomaterial Characteristics of Ligaments and Tendons Are Described by Elastic Modulus and Viscoelastic Properties

The primary stress response characteristics of ligaments and tendons are described by their modulus of elasticity properties. Under tensile loading (stretch), ligaments and tendons exhibit a modulus of elasticity that is variable with load (Fig. 5.10). Under low loading, there is a relatively large increase in length in response to the load applied (low elastic modulus). This is attributed to lengthening as the result of macromolecular "slack" within the collagen fiber structure that offers less resistance to an imposed load. As the slack is taken up, fibers slide relative to each other and fluid is extruded from the matrix. The elastic modulus then increases (stiffness increases) gradually with increasing load and shows a linear response up to the point where failure begins. The behavior of tendons and ligaments is similar except for ligament tissue such as the ligamentum flavum of the spinal column, where a high elastic content produces a different pattern of the elastic modulus.

The extracellular matrix of tendons and ligaments between the collagen fibrils has proteoglycans, a high water content, and other small ionically charged molecules that can interact with structural elements. This matrix is comparatively more porous than cartilage or bone, and is structured to resist tensile rather than compressive stresses. The viscoelastic properties become evident at high loading rates, where the tissue will demonstrate increased stiffness and offer increased resistance to tensile stress (stretch). As with cartilage, repeated tensile loading in cycles can result in a slow increase in elastic stiffness due to plastic de-

formation (29,30). This plastic deformation is presumably due to molecular deformation in the fibrous structural elements of the tendon or ligament, and also to the inability of fluid and small charged molecules to reequilibrate within the molecular structure.

Ligaments and tendons also demonstrate the viscoelastic properties of stress or load relaxation and creep. To characterize these properties, the tissue is placed under a tensile load (stretch) within the linear region of the elastic modulus and maintained at a constant length (stress relaxation) or a constant load (creep). Ligament and tendon tissue adjusts its molecular structure and fluid distribution to the load primarily within the first 6 to 8 hours, but will continue over a period of months. The creep phenomenon is used clinically as plaster casts or braces are employed to place a constant load to correct a soft-tissue deformity, such as some spinal curvatures (31).

Material Failure of Ligaments and Tendons Is Preceded by Microfailure of the Molecular Structural Elements

Overall failure of the ligament or tendon is usually sudden and preceded by the microfailure of the attachments between collagen fibers within the tissue and loss of the ability of the tendon or ligament to recover its length. With tendon and ligament, it is also important to distinguish eventual failure due to a sustained load (creep failure) from sustained cyclic loading and unloading (fatigue failure). Both are important biomaterial properties for tendon and ligament. As with bone, a smaller degree of microfailure may occur within the range of physiologic loading, suggesting that repeated stress may lead to declining strength or fatigue over time (32). There may be a range of damage depending upon the total deformation and extent of partial failure. Inflammation resulting from such damage is associated with tendonitis (32).

Failure of both tendons and ligaments may also occur at the bone interface. The site of failure may depend upon the loading rate (33). Tendons, with their attached muscles, typically have a higher tensile strength than muscle, and rupture of muscle is more common than tendon. The instability of the joint that may result from tendon, or especially ligament, damage can contribute to and be complicated by damage to the joint capsule. This damage and associated abnormal loading patterns may contribute to osteoarthritis (31).

Ligaments and Tendons Can Adapt to Stresses

Like other tissue, ligament and tendon structurally remodel in response to the stresses placed upon them within the limits of damage (32). They become stronger and stiffer with increased stress and weaker and less stiff with a reduction in stress (34). Physical training can increase the strength of tendons and ligaments along with the ligament-bone interface (35,36). Immobilization (such as from casting) can decrease the strength and stiffness of ligaments. While reconditioning can occur, it can require a considerable length of time (34,37).

The Properties and Structure of Ligaments and Tendons Change with Age

During maturation, the number and quality of cross-links increases in the collagen of ligaments and tendons and fibril diameter increases as well (38), producing increased tensile strength. The mechanical properties of collagen reach a maximum with maturation and begin to decrease with age (39). The collagen content of ligaments and tendons decreases as well. This loss of collagen results in a decrease in strength, stiffness, and the amount of deformation required to produce to failure (40). However, the overall biomechanical properties of tendon remain reasonably constant with age (41). The amount of time required for tissue repair and reconditioning (discussed previously) will also increase. Other physiologic factors, such as pregnancy, can also affect the biomechanical properties of ligaments and tendons (31,40).

SKELETAL MUSCLE

Skeletal Muscle Provides the Forces for Body Movement

Since a more complete description of muscle is given elsewhere in this volume, only those elements essential to understanding the biomechanical aspects of muscle tissue will be given here. Of the three types of muscle tissue, skeletal muscle is the most abundant tissue in the body, accounting for 40% of body weight (42). The forces necessary to provide movement to the body are provided by the contraction of skeletal muscles acting across joints. These contractions may produce dynamic work or participate in static maintenance of posture. While subcellular units known as *sarcomeres* are the source of muscle contraction, the basic contractile unit of skeletal muscle as a tissue is the *muscle fiber*. The fiber may range in size from 10 to 100 μm in diameter and between 1 and 30 cm in length (43). The metabolic and contractile properties of muscle fibers may differ according to the physiologic demands placed upon them as described subsequently.

Both Contractile Elements and Connective Tissue Contribute to the Biomechanical Properties of Muscle

Muscle may be histologically and mechanically described as bundles of contractile elements in a series of connective tissue sheaths (Fig. 5.11). The basic unit of the contractile/connective tissue relationship is an individual muscle fiber surrounded by a connective tissue sheath, the *endomysium*. This basic unit of skeletal muscle is then organized into fascicles or groups of fibers by a thicker connective tissue sheath, the *perimysium*. Finally, groups of muscle fascicles are organized into the entire muscle itself and covered by the epimysium, which surrounds the entire structure. The epimysium and loose connective tissue form the fascial planes between muscles. The connective tissue sheaths are continuous with each other and the muscle tendon and/or attachments to bone. Both connective tissue and the contractile elements contribute the biomechanical properties of muscle. The contractile elements provide active energy expending forces with some elastic and viscoelastic properties, while the connective tissue con-

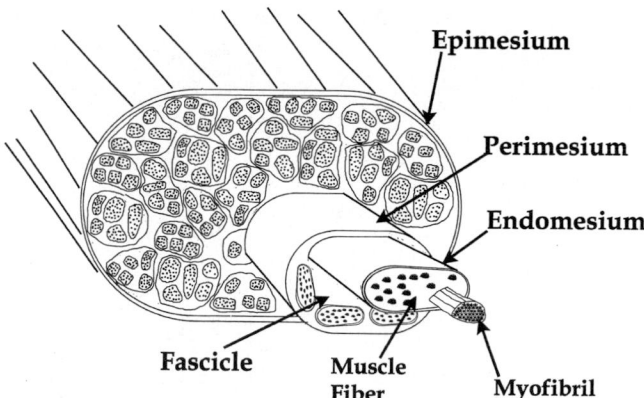

FIGURE 5.11. Schematic of the structural organization of a muscle. The basic subcellular unit of the muscle is the myofibril. Collections of myofibrils are present in muscle cells (muscle fibers). Muscle fibers are organized into fascicles and groups of fascicles make up the muscle. The connective tissue coverings of the muscle include the endomysium that surrounds muscle fibers, the perimysium surrounding muscle fascicles, and the epimysium surrounding the entire muscle.

tributes passive elastic and viscoelastic influences on the pattern of force transduction to the skeleton.

The Basic Relationship Between Nerve and Muscle Is Defined by the Motor Unit

Muscle fibers contract in response to acetylcholine released by motor nerves. An individual motor neuron, with the muscle fibers contacted by it, forms a motor unit. The size of motor units may vary dramatically between muscles and within the muscle itself. The motor neuron generates an action potential lasting 1 to 2 milliseconds that produces a contraction of all of the muscle fibers in a motor unit in an "on-off" fashion. The response of the motor unit to a single action potential is termed a *twitch*, the basic unit of recordable muscle activity. The time required for a motor unit to fully contract and then return to resting length is variable (from 10 milliseconds to 100 milliseconds) according to fiber type, but in all cases much longer than a nerve action potential. If additional nerve stimulation occurs before the contraction phase of the twitch has ended, contraction can be maintained and increased in a process called *summation*. The limit of summation, such that contraction is maintained and does not increase with a greater frequency of stimulation, is called *tetanic contraction* or *tetany*. The force of contraction of the muscle as a whole may be further regulated by increasing or decreasing the number of motor units used to produce the contraction, a process termed *recruitment*. In this way, the nervous system may control the force of muscle contraction by the size and number of motor units employed to produce the contraction and the frequency of activation of motor units.

Types of Muscle Contraction Are Defined by the Movements Occurring During Contraction

Dynamic muscle contractions in the processes of producing movement can be classified as *concentric* and *eccentric*. Concentric

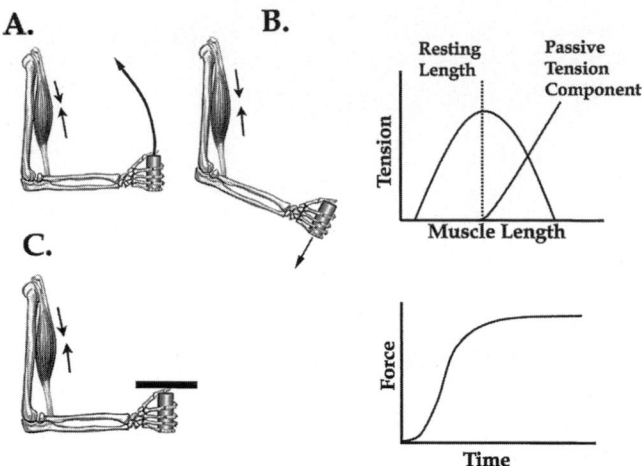

FIGURE 5.12. **Left:** Types of muscle contraction. **A:** Concentric. **B:** Eccentric. **C:** Isometric. **Right: (Top)** Muscle tension relationship to muscle length. The greatest active tension is near the muscle-resting length. The passive tension component from stretch of connective tissue increases beyond the resting length. **Bottom:** Force-time relationship of muscle contraction. The time lag in reaching maximum force is related to the elasticity of tissue components.

contractions produce movement in the direction of muscle contraction (Fig. 5.12), while eccentric contractions act to decelerate or resist movement, as in slowly placing an object down rather than letting it fall. Muscles also produce contractions without substantial movement, as in static posture against gravity. This type of contraction is termed *isometric,* as no change in muscle length occurs during contraction. Another term, *isotonic* contraction, refers to muscle contraction with a change in length under constant tension.

The Mechanical Properties of Contractile Elements and Their Connective Tissue in Muscle Is Described as a Musculotendinous Unit

The force production characteristics of a muscle as a whole are a combination of the material properties of its contractile components, the connective tissue that surrounds them (and the whole muscle), and the tendon of its insertion. From a mechanical viewpoint this combination is a *musculotendinous unit* (44). The contractile elements add a rapid tensile load on the connective tissue elements, which in turn respond according to their elastic and viscoelastic properties as described earlier. As with ligaments and tendons alone, this will mean that there is rapid component to stretch, produced in this case by contraction, followed by a slower change in length as the connective tissue elements reach equilibrium with the contracting force (Fig. 5.12).

The connective tissues surrounding the muscle and its tendon have elastic properties that can store energy with stretch like a rubber band. In the process of muscle contraction, the tendon and connective tissue are stretched. The energy is released by moving a body segment or by stretching the contractile elements as the muscle relaxes. The elasticity also helps to keep the muscle prepared for contraction by reducing slackening of contractile elements, preventing passive overstretch of muscle fibers, thereby reducing

the danger of injury. This energy storage also occurs as muscles are stretched under load. The muscle contractile elements may also have some elasticlike properties of energy storage (45,46).

The sum of the interaction of the contractile elements and elastic elements of muscle contraction can be demonstrated in the force-time curve of muscle contraction (Fig. 5.12). While the tension or force of contraction of the muscle fibers may reach maximum within a relatively short time, a much longer time is required for this tension to be transferred through the elastic components. Because of this time lag, the active contraction process must be long enough in time for the full transfer of tension to occur.

Many Factors, Such as Length, Load, and Temperature, May Affect the Force Produced by Muscle Contraction

The force of muscle contraction can be affected by various mechanical factors, including length-tension relationships, load-velocity, and force-time properties (43). Other significant factors may include temperature, muscle fatigue, and prestretching. The length-tension property of a muscle as a whole (Fig. 5.12) involves both the active contractile elements and the passive connective tissue elements (47). The maximum force or tension produced by contractile elements, such as the muscle fiber, is obtained at near its resting length. Contraction at lengths beyond or smaller than the resting length results in reduced tension production by the muscle fiber. This is a result of intrinsic properties of muscle fiber sarcomeres. For the muscle as a whole, reducing or increasing the muscle length from its resting position will reduce the tension produced by contractile elements. However, increasing muscle length will also produce a passive tension as a result of stretching the connective tissue elements, although the contractile force is reduced. The passive component of stretch, which is readily detectable by passively stretching a relaxed limb, will eventually become the dominant source of resistance or tension as muscle length increases, effectively protecting the muscle from overstretch. (Fig. 5.12).

Applied Loads Affect the Velocity of Muscle Contraction

The relationship of the load applied to a muscle and the velocity with which it contracts defines the load-velocity property of muscle contraction. The shortening of muscles contracting concentrically is most rapid with no external load and progressively slows with increasing external loads (48). The shortening velocity will reach zero as the load reaches the maximum contraction force of the muscle (isometric contraction) and then reverse to a lengthening velocity with eccentric contraction. As might be expected, eccentric contraction lengthening velocity increases with increasing external load.

A Rise in Temperature Can Increase the Efficiency of Muscle Contraction

In the process of contraction, muscle efficiency is usually no more than 20% to 25% in the translation of chemical energy into useful work, with the majority of the energy being dissipated as heat (42). Even so, the heat dissipation can have positive effects on muscle contraction properties by increasing temperature. As would be attained through a warm-up procedure, temperature increases usually arise from increased blood flow and the production of heat by the muscle itself from metabolic reactions and friction generated by the sliding of molecules past each other in the contractile and elastic elements. Within physiologic ranges, increases in temperature will increase the conduction velocity across the muscle fiber membrane (sarcolemma) (48), increasing the rate of contraction and increasing the rate at which the muscle can be stimulated. This can mean an increase in the production of muscle force. A rise in temperature can also increase enzymatic activity related to muscle metabolism and increase the efficiency of muscle contraction. The viscoelastic properties of the musculotendinous unit are also affected by rises in temperature, generally increasing the elasticity of the collagen, decreasing stiffness, and enhancing the extensibility of the unit. While these basic biomechanical properties of muscle tissue change with temperature to enhance the contractile properties of the musculotendinous unit, the effects from stretching or "warming up" prior to activity are much more complex and not completely understood (49,50). The physiologic aspects of stretch (or release) involve highly significant neural components and reflexes beyond the biomechanical properties of the tissues alone.

Muscle Fatigue Properties Are Affected by the Muscle Fiber Type(s) Comprising the Muscle

Fatigue of muscle with prolonged contraction activity results from the depletion of the nutrients and oxygen required to produce adenosine triphosphate (ATP) as an energy supply from either aerobic or anaerobic glycolysis. The result is a decrease in force production by the muscle eventually to total cessation (42). The rate at which a muscle will reach fatigue can vary according to the types of muscle fibers it contains. Muscle fiber types are distinguished by the rate at which ATP can be made available to the sarcomeres for contraction and the metabolic pathways through which ATP is generated. The rate of availability of ATP directly affects the rate of contraction or twitch time of a muscle fiber. Accordingly, muscle fiber types can be classified as slow or fast twitch. Two primary metabolic pathways involved to generate ATP (oxidative or glycolytic) further divides these two basic types of contractile behavior. Using these properties, three primary muscle fiber types are distinguished including type I or slow-twitch oxidative (SO) fibers, type IIA, fast-twitch oxidative-glycolytic (FOG) fibers, and type IIB, fast-twitch glycolytic (FG) fibers. These different fiber types have varying degrees of contraction time, resistance to fatigue, and a dependence on aerobic or anaerobic metabolism. As their names suggest, type I fibers have slower contraction rates, and, with a metabolism directed toward aerobic pathways, are resistant to fatigue. They are relatively small in diameter and produce a relatively low amount of tension per fiber. These properties make this fiber type well suited for prolonged low-intensity work (51). Type IIA fibers are fast contracting and rich in aerobic and anaerobic (glycolytic) enzymes with a moderate resistance to fatigue. They appear to be intermediate between type I and type IIB in their capacity for contractile force and resistance to

fatigue. Type IIB fibers are fast contracting, rely primarily on glycolytic pathways, and may fatigue rapidly. However, they have a large fiber diameter and can produce relatively large amounts of tension.

Muscles May Have Some Ability to Change Their Fiber Type According to Demand

Most muscles are of mixed fiber types with the proportion of fiber types determined by the nerve innervating the muscle (52,53). The overall distribution of muscle fiber types in the muscles of the body appears to have a strong genetic component (42,51,54). The fiber type can be changed with nerve stimulation (55), suggesting that patterns of activity may alter fiber metabolism. Some changes in fiber types may also occur with physical training, but much of this change is a result of increases in the cross-sectional area of the fiber type corresponding to the activity rather than an actual change in fiber type (54,56). The extent to which actual alterations in the type of muscle fiber occur as a result of activity demand therefore remains unclear.

Muscle Adapts to Physiologic Demands

Although the extent of fiber type change under physiologic conditions is unclear, muscle will clearly remodel according to the stresses placed upon it. Muscle atrophies with disuse and hypertrophies with increased use. Studies of muscle atrophy in both animal and clinical studies suggest that early dynamic motion after debilitating injury may be important in the minimization of atrophy, particularly of type I muscle fibers (57,58). Electric stimulation may also prevent some of this fiber loss (56). Hypertrophy of muscle with physical training is generally the result of increases in the cross- sectional area of all muscle fibers (58,59).

MUSCULOSKELETAL BIOMECHANICS

Primary Biomechanical Musculoskeletal Models Consist of Segments Moved by Muscles Across Joints

Biomechanical aspects of the skeleton involve contributions from all of the biomechanical aspects of the tissues described in the process of producing movement. As a simplistic model, it is easiest to consider the body as a series of segments (bones) containing muscles that are attached across the segments. Joints form the junctions between segments or bones and transfer the forces generated by muscles or from external sources between the segments. In the following simple models of movement, joints will be regarded as simple pivot points, moving in one plane (co-planar). The more complex considerations of joint movement and shape of articulation will be addressed in subsequent sections.

Force Moments Are Used to Describe Models of Musculoskeletal Movement

Using the simple model used for the descriptions of moments earlier in the chapter, a joint, such as the elbow (Fig. 5.13), becomes a rotation system with the flexor system and the extensors using the joint as a center of rotation to move the distal limb and any

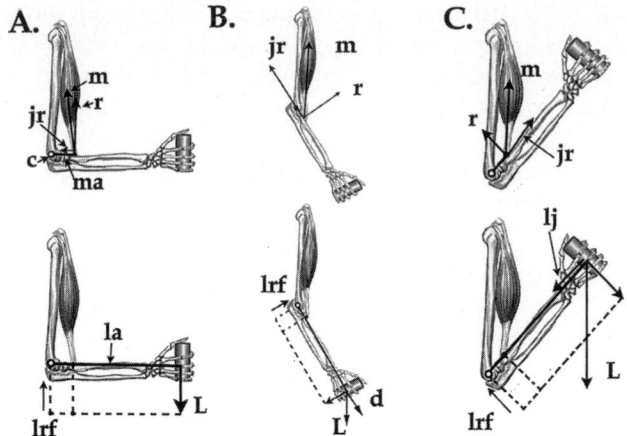

FIGURE 5.13. Schematic of basic joint moments and their variation with movement. Sections on top represent muscle contraction moments. Figures on the bottom show moments generated by the load. **A:** Right angle resistance to a load *(l)*. **Top:** Moments about the joint center *(c)* include the moment arm of the muscle *(ma)* that is moved by a resisting component *(r)* of the muscle contraction force *(m)*, this is resisted by the load **(bottom)** acting on a load moment arm *(la)*. Joint reaction forces include the portion of the muscle force directed into the joint *(jr)* and a moment generated from the load into the joint with a center of rotation about the muscle insertion *(lrf, dotted lines displaced)*. **B:** At extension, the angle of muscle pull directs more of the muscle force into the joint **(top)** and a portion of the load force *(l)* moment pulls out on the joint as a distracting force *(d)*. **C:** In a flexed position, the muscle moment **(top)** is divided into the resisting component *(r)* and a joint reaction distracting force away from the joint *(jr)*. A portion of the load force **(bottom)** now is directed into the joint *(lj)*.

load on the limb. In mathematical modeling of joint function, the description of such movements is a system of balanced moments produced by the load on the limb and muscle contraction forces. Characterizing movement in this way becomes particularly important as other aspects of joint function (non–co-planar movement, movement within the joint) and more mechanically complicated joint types are modeled.

As a distal segment moves relative to a more proximal segment, the distal segment will rotate about the instant center of the joint or center of rotation *(c,* Fig. 5.13). The effective distance from the center of the joint's rotation to where the force is acting (muscle insertion) is the *moment arm (ma)* for the muscle. The product of the force applied from the muscle and the moment arm (force × distance) is the *moment* (or torque) used to resist a load on the distal limb. For concentric contraction to occur, this moment of resistance must exceed the moment produced by the load (distance to the load from *c* × weight). In a more complete model, the weight of the limb must also be considered. Note also that if the load moment is resisted by the pull of the muscle, there is also a center of rotation created at the point of muscle insertion about which the load exerts a moment into the joint *(lrf,* Fig. 5.13). Together with the portion of the muscle contraction force directed into the joint (discussed subsequently), this becomes part of the *joint reaction force* which applies a stress to the joint during movement.

Muscle Moments Necessary to Resist a Load Vary with Joint Position

As can be seen from Fig. 5.13, although the length moment arm does not change, the proportion of muscle contraction force

(vector) that is applied to resist the load will vary as the limb is flexed. With the joint fully extended, most of the muscle contraction force vector is directed into the joint. This muscle component force also contributes to the joint reaction force and may be particularly important in the stabilization of load-bearing joints, such as the knee. The relative size of the joint reaction and load-resistive forces can be expressed by simple trigonometric functions in mathematical models, but it is sufficient here to be aware of how these forces change with joint position. In this model, the portion of the muscle contraction vector used to resist the load increases as the angle of tendon is closer to a right angle (Fig. 5.13, part A, orthogonal) to the forearm. Beyond this point, a portion of the load vector becomes directed into the joint (Fig. 5.13, part C) reducing the effective load on the muscle, but placing stress on the joint and more proximal segments. In the flexed position, the angle of pull by the muscle directs a portion of the muscle contraction force against this load into the joint.

Muscle Moments Are Also Transferred Across Joints by Tendons

Muscle forces are also conveyed to distal segments across joints by tendons. In joints associated with the knee, hands, and feet, tendons cross the joint(s) to produce a "pulley" effect (Fig. 5.14). In this arrangement, as in the knee, the distance between the center of rotation of the joint and the tendon defines the moment arm for the contracting muscle.

The wheel and axle mechanism (60) is an instructive related model used to achieve rotary movements (Fig. 5.14). In this case, muscle contraction forces are applied to the opposite sides of a segment to produce rotation about an axis. The length moment arm in this case is the distance to the center of rotation. This mechanism is used widely throughout the body to achieve rotation of limbs and the body, as in rotation of the head, torso, or shoulder. As with simple flexors and extensors, muscles producing rotational components work in pairs and significant clinical problems may arise from imbalances in function of the pair.

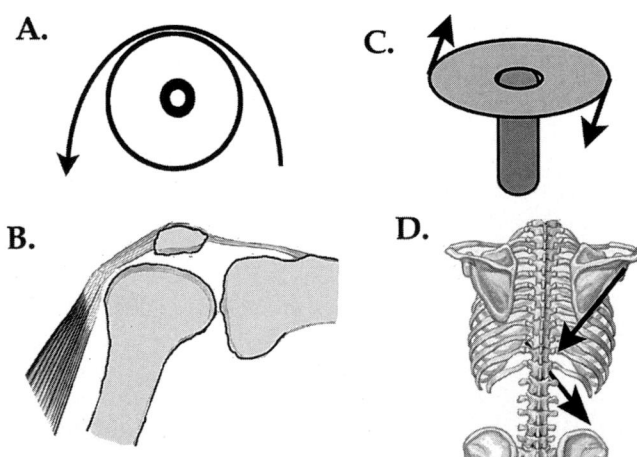

FIGURE 5.14. Strategies of muscles and tendons pulling across joints. **A:** A pulleylike mechanism in which the direction of pull is changed. **B:** A similar mechanism is used in knee extension. **C:** A wheel and axle mechanism in which co-active forces act to rotate an axle, such as the shoulders **(D)** relative to the spine.

Muscle Moments Generally Have a Low Mechanical Advantage

As suggested in the examples that have been given, the lever arrangement of muscle insertions and joints in limbs is such that a comparatively small distance of muscle contraction can produce a large displacement of the load at the expense of needing large muscle contraction forces. This is described as having a low mechanical advantage. The relative mechanical advantage is a function of the position of the muscle origin and insertion on the two bony segments relative to the joint. Because both the moment arm (distance, d) and contraction force (f) equally contribute to the moment (f × d) producing the movement or resistance, small differences in the moment arm can produce significant changes in the amount of muscle contraction required. As origins and insertions of muscles and segment lengths vary markedly between individuals, the ability to produce different types of movement using the same muscle contraction force will also differ.

While muscles must create large forces to produce movements at a low mechanical advantage, distally applied loads, such as to the hand acting through the elbow, have a comparatively large moment arm (Fig. 5.13) and require less force to produce large moments about the joint. This will be true of manipulative forces placed distally for purposes of applying passive stretch to muscles and joints. It is a useful principle, but must be approached with caution, since large, potentially damaging force moments can be generated.

Joint Structure Defines How Movements Can Occur Between Body Segments

Beyond movement models that regard joints as simple pivot points for the transfer muscle forces between body segments, the next level of modeling must consider the structure of these intersegmental contacts. In fact, the directions of movement that can occur between body segments are largely defined by the structure of the joints between them. Joints are classified according to the type of tissue they contain and their structure. On a tissue level, joints are classified into three primary types: fibrous, cartilaginous, and synovial. Fibrous joints are located in areas such as the articulations of the skull, while cartilaginous joints include the discs between vertebrae, and synovial joints are located in articulations of the limbs. The vast majority of body motion occurs across synovial and cartilaginous joints. The primary cartilaginous articulations will be described subsequently, with considerations of the spinal column. The remaining synovial joints have been divided into several categories according to the primary types of movements that occur across them. Anatomically, the major types are gliding, hinge, pivot, condyloid, saddle, and ball and socket (61). Other than the joints described later in this chapter, more detailed descriptions of these joint structures and their limitations on range of motion can be found in general anatomic texts.

Range of Motion Describes the Extent of Body Segment Movement Across Joints

Movements are usually described as occurring in one of the primary body planes (frontal, sagittal, or transverse). The extent of joint motion in a plane defines its *range of motion* in that plane, usually in degrees. Although all synovial joints may have some minor range of motion in all three planes, most joints in the extremities have a primary degree of freedom in one plane, such as in the knees, elbows, or fingers. Shoulder and hip joints are an exception, as they have significant ranges of motion in all three planes. Joints may also have a significant rotational component, usually expressed as range of motion of the distal rotated element, as in pronation and supination of the hand. In general, there is a trade-off between intrinsic structural stability of joints and range of motion, depending upon the physiologic demands placed upon the joint.

Joint Surfaces Have Several Different Types of Relative Movement

As body segments are moved through their range of motion, surfaces within the joint will also move relative to each other. This movement may contribute to various aspects of the motion produced. The relative motion of joint surfaces may include gliding, rolling, rotation, compression, or distraction (Fig. 5.15), or a combination of these movements. Gliding (also referred to as translation or sliding) represents a movement of one surface relative to another without a rotational component. In rolling, one surface of the articulation rolls over the other, like a ball rolling over a surface. Rotation (spinning) consists of one joint surface spinning on the surface of the other without a translational component. Compression represents force pushing the joint surfaces together, while distraction tends to pull the surfaces apart.

Movements between articular surfaces in a joint can occur in consistent combinations (coupled) such that, one type of motion is always accompanied by another. This motion coupling can occur for movements within the same articulation (see the upcoming example given under "The Knee") or in another joint that is part of an articulation complex (see the example given

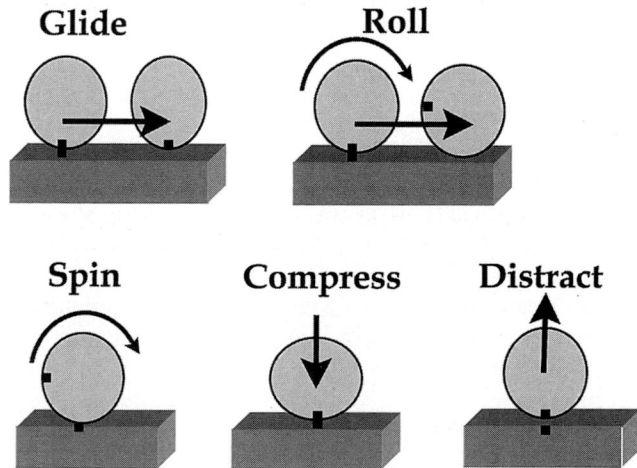

FIGURE 5.15. Intraarticular movement of joint surfaces relative to each other. In gliding (also referred to as sliding or translation), surfaces move without rotation. In rolling, one surface rotates and translates over the other at a distance equal to the arc of the rotating surface. In spinning, one surface rotates on the other without translation. Compression and distraction are opposing vertical forces on the joint.

with "The Elbow" later in the chapter) (62). A disruption of one part of a coupled motion will affect the other and can produce dysfunction of the joint or joint complex. An example of this is a coupling of the elbow complex where there is a coupling of the intraarticular motions of humeroulnar and humeroradial joints during flexion/extension movements (see "The Elbow"). Coupling of articular surface motions within the joint also depends upon which segment of the joint is mobile (62). An example of this difference is the articular surface movement of the knee during weight bearing versus swing phase (see "The Knee"). Significant alterations in the relative movements of joint surfaces can produce problems in joints, including abnormal wear and dislocation.

The Instant Center Defines the Center of Rotation of a Body Segment at Any Given Time

In order to study movement within a joint during functional movement, both the motion of the surfaces relative to each other and the shape of the articulating surfaces must be considered. As one segment moves in a joint such as the knee, the center of rotation located within the joint at any instant will have zero velocity. Because the femoral condyles and tibial plane are not spheric surfaces and translational movement can occur within the joint, the center of rotation of the leg will change as the leg is extended. To determine properties such as the length of the moment arm under these circumstances, the center of rotation must be redefined as *instant center* of rotation joint at any given time (63). The instant center can be defined clinically from sequential roentgenograms or other pictures of movement using the intersection of lines from defined points from the joint segments. This technique can be important for identifying abnormal joint movement. It should be noted, however, that displacement of the instant center can occur in all three dimensions simultaneously. Roentgenograms or other planar depictions of joint motion can be misleading. From a functional point of view, changes in the location of the instant center will change the relative magnitude of the contraction-force vectors of the muscle tendon acting across a joint. This can result in weakness or abnormal stresses within the joint.

SOME PROPERTIES OF SPECIFIC JOINT ARTICULATIONS

The previous discussions in this chapter have focused on the biomechanical properties of tissues and models of forces acting to create movements or stresses on body segments. We will now consider how these properties apply to some of the primary articulation systems in the body. The biomechanical aspects to be considered are not intended to be comprehensive.

THE KNEE

The knee joins two of the body's longest moment arms (the thigh and leg) in a joint consisting of two primary articulations, the tibiofemoral joint and the patellofemoral joint (Fig. 5.16).

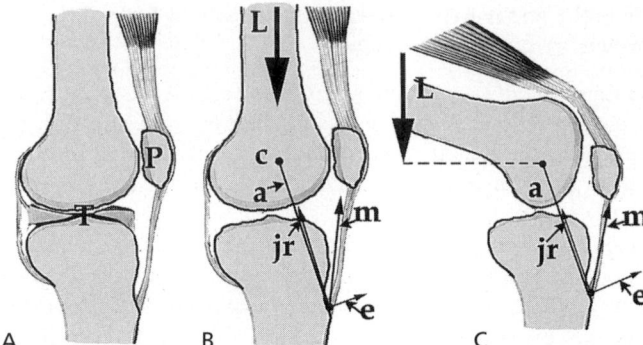

FIGURE 5.16. A: The knee joint consists of the tibiofibular *(t)* and patellofibular joints *(p)*. **B:** Moments produced by the load *(L)* of body weight require little muscle activity with the knee extended, but are maintained by a muscle contraction force through the patellar tendon *(m)*, which produces moments through a moment arm *(a)* to the instant center of rotation of the joint *(c)*. The moment is divided by the angle of muscle pull into a joint reaction force *(jr)* and an extending component *(e)*. **C:** With the knee flexed, the body weight produces a moment through the joint *(c)* that must be resisted by the extending component *(e)*. In this instance, the patella increases the distance of the tendon from the femur to provide a more advantageous angle for the muscle contraction force on the tibia. This increases the proportion of the extension moment. Note that the position of the center of rotation *(c)* has changed slightly.

Because of its location and weight-bearing properties, the knee sustains relatively high load forces and is particularly susceptible to injury. Stability of the knee is obtained from the internal and external ligaments, joint capsule, and muscles acting across the joint. The cartilage menisci act to distribute the compressive stresses between the condyles of the femur and the tibial plateau.

The Knee Has One Primary Range of Motion in the Sagittal Plane

Although the knee joint itself has some range of motion in all three planes of motion, its primary range of motion is in the sagittal plane where a range from full extension to full flexion is approximately 140 degrees (63). Motion in the transverse plane (internal and external rotation) and frontal planes (abduction and adduction) is dependent upon the positioning of the tibia relative to the femur. In the transverse and frontal planes, full extension of the knee precludes almost all motion due to an interlocking of the femoral and tibial condyles, while range of motion increases as the knee is flexed. Maximal internal and external rotation is possible with the knee flexed at approximately 90 degrees ranging from a neutral position to 45 degrees of external rotation and 30 degrees of internal rotation. In the frontal plane passive adduction and abduction is obtained at approximately 30 degrees of flexion, but it is only a few degrees in either direction (63).

Primary Muscle Forces Through the Knee Are Conducted Through the Hamstrings and the Patellar Tendon

The primary muscle forces through the joint occur through the quadriceps tendon and hamstrings. The hamstrings use the knee joint as a primary lever in flexing, while the quadriceps uses the patellar tendon system as a pulley with the center of rotation within the femoral condyles (Fig. 5.16). As with other hinge-type joints, in a basic biomechanical model, muscle contraction forces are divided primarily into a joint reaction force directed into the joint and a force moment that acts to move the mobile segment. In extension of the knee, the moment that acts to straighten the knee pulls on the leg through the patella and tendon. This will act to rotate the tibial plateau relative to the condyles of the femur. Presuming a constant muscle force, this component of moment decreases or mechanical advantage decreases in proportion to the joint reaction force as extension proceeds (Fig. 5.16). This decrease is to some extent compensated by the movement of the patella and the shape of the femoral condyles as described subsequently. With flexing a straightened knee, the opposite is true; the proportion of the flexor moment increases relative to the joint reaction force as the movement proceeds.

The Knee Must Withstand Very High Joint Reaction Stress Forces

In a load or weight-bearing model of the knee, the leg is considered stable, and muscle contraction forces and joint structure are used to resist gravity. The force exerted through the knee from the weight of the body is termed the *ground reaction force* (body mass × the acceleration of gravity). Note that both the ground reaction force and muscle contraction forces contribute to produce the *joint reaction force* or total force directed into the joint as described previously. These combined forces, along with the impact of landing from activities such as jumping, can produce very high compressive and other stress forces on the knee joint surfaces.

If the knee is fully extended, most of the ground reaction force is directed through the bone structure of the femur and tibia (a moment arm through the joint of almost zero), and minimal or no muscle contraction force is required to resist the ground reaction force. This changes as the knee is bent, and at 90 degrees of flexion, extensor muscle reaction forces must resist the ground reaction force consisting of the body weight acting at a distance of almost the entire length of the femur. At this angle, the extensor muscles have a relatively small moment arm. Accordingly, a very high muscle contraction force in excess of body weight must be exerted to resist a moment of this magnitude. The knee joint has several mechanisms to help compensate for the rather low mechanical advantage of muscle contraction forces in this situation.

The Application of Muscle Contraction Forces to Movement Across the Knee Is Affected by the Structural Properties of the Joints

Beyond the basic segment model, there are basic structural properties of the knee that change the mechanical advantage muscles across the joint. These primary structural properties include the patellofemoral joint and the shape and movement of the femoral condyles. The patella and tendon act to increase the moment arm for the quadriceps by increasing the effective distance of the tendon from the center of rotation of the joint, thereby increasing the component of the muscle contraction force vector acting to straighten the joint (Fig. 5.16). This adds mechanical advantage to the extensor muscle contraction forces in a partially flexed

knee. The gliding (sliding) motion of the patella between the medial and lateral femoral facets also alters the moment arm over the range of motion of the knee. Additionally, the patella acts to distribute this force over the surface of the femoral condyles.

The primary properties of the femoral condyles that affect the mechanics of movement include the noncircular shape of the condyles and their movement on the tibial plateau (Fig. 5.16). The shape of the femoral condyles is such that the center of rotation of the joint changes through the knee's range of motion, giving a greater moment arm to extensor forces as the knee is flexed. This can be important in resisting the high forces such as body weight with a partially flexed knee. In addition to a noncircular shape, the femoral condyles also have differences in their effective diameters with the medial being larger. This produces a coupling of flexion and extension with a rotational component to the knee (called the screw-home mechanism), such that flexion is accompanied by an internal rotation component and extension is accompanied by external rotation of the femoral condyles relative to the tibial plateau (64). This provides additional stability to the joint in certain circumstances.

The Intraarticular Movements of the Knee Depend Upon Which Surface Is Moving and Load Bearing

The femoral condyles also glide (slide, translate) on the tibial plateau as the knee is moved (described previously). These structural properties of the femoral condyles can act to change the center of rotation as the joint progresses through its range of motion and alter the effective moment arm length through which the muscle contraction forces are acting. The relative movements of the joint surfaces in the knee give an example of how motion coupling can depend upon the load status of the joint and which joint surface is mobile (62). In walking, as the leg swings forward (swing phase), the femoral condyles and tibial plateau are not under the compressive load of the body. The movement is a gliding motion of the tibial plateau coupled with a rolling of the tibia on the femoral condyles in the same direction. When the leg is placed on the ground with the knee partially flexed and then extended as the body is moved forward (see "Normal Locomotion (Gait) Employs the Entire Body for Efficiency of Movement" later in the chapter), the tibial plateau is stable relative to the femoral condyles. The motion of the joint surfaces now consists of a gliding and rolling of the femoral condyles on the tibia in opposite directions. This is an example of how compressive forces and segment stabilization change articular surface motion. This can have important implications in surface damage and dysfunction.

Knee Joint Structure and the Movement of Joint Surfaces Promote Efficiency of Movement

Through their structure and interaction during movement, the patellofemoral joint and femoral condyles contribute to the efficient use of muscle contraction forces for movement and joint stability by changing the moment arm (mechanical advantage) of the contracting muscles in the process of extending or flexing the knee. This has important consequences for movement through the knee and load bearing. The effective use of these structural properties is dependent upon internal joint movement and the joint stability provided by soft tissues. For this reason, soft-tissue injury or changes producing either a lack of or excess of internal "play" in the knee joint can contribute to serious problems with joint function.

THE HIP

The Hip Is a Load-Bearing Ball-and-Socket Joint with Ranges of Motion in All Three Planes

The relatively rigid ball-and-socket arrangement of the hip joint between the head of the femur and the acetabulum provides greater intrinsic stability compared to joints such as the knee. In addition to stability, the ball-and-socket structure of the hip allows greater range of motion in all three planes of body movement. Motion in the sagittal plane is greatest with approximately 140 degrees of flexion and 15 degrees of extension from a neutral position. The range of abduction is approximately 30 degrees and adduction 25 degrees. External rotation from a flexed position is approximately 90 degrees and internal rotation approximately 70 degrees. Rotation decreases with extension due to soft-tissue restrictions (65).

The Angular Alignment of the Articular Components Is Important for Normal Hip Function

The angular structure of the joint relative to the pelvis, femoral shaft, and knee joint can vary significantly between individuals and have a great influence on the biomechanics of the lower limb. In the relationship of the joint surface to the pelvis, the location of the acetabulum places the plane of its opening angled 40 degrees posterior to a sagittal plane and 60 degrees lateral to a transverse plane (Fig. 5.17). Both the femoral head and acetabulum have roughly spheric surfaces of contact. The relationship of the femoral head through its neck with the femoral shaft is important in the biomechanics of hip function and load-bearing

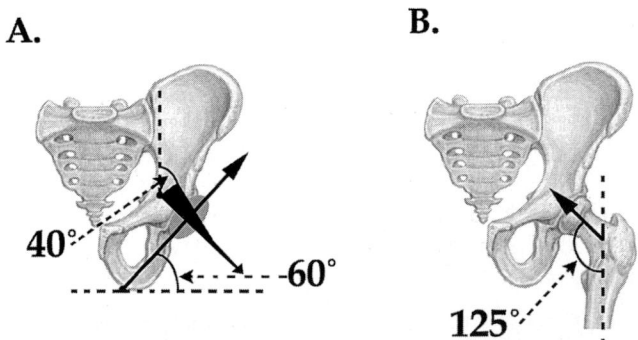

FIGURE 5.17. A: Angle of the opening of the acetabulum. The opening is oriented 60 degrees lateral to a transverse plane and 40 degrees posterior to a sagittal plane. **B:** The angle between the femoral neck and shaft is approximately 125 degrees.

stress on the neck. It is an important determinant of the effective moment arms of the muscles producing movement across the joint. The angle of inclination of the neck to the shaft (Fig. 5.17) is approximately 125 degrees, but may vary between 90 to 135 degrees. This angle offsets the femoral shaft from the pelvis laterally. The angle in a transverse plane between lines drawn through the femoral head and greater trochanter and between the medial and lateral condyles (angle of anteversion) determines the normal relationship of the primary plane of movement of the knee to the hip. It is normally about 12 degrees but can vary widely (65). An angle of greater than 12 degrees tends to produce internal compensatory rotation of the leg during gait, while an angle of less than 12 degrees produces an external rotation. These compensations are made to maintain the stability of the hip. They are common in children and usually outgrown (65).

Models of Hip Function Balance Ground Reaction, Joint, and Muscle Contraction Forces

Biomechanical models of the hip can be used to illustrate some of the important aspects of the structure-function relationship of the joint. Stability of the hip joint is maintained through the alignment of the body over the joint (Fig. 5.18), the joint capsule, and capsular ligaments and muscle contraction to counteract remaining ground force moments. The relative magnitude of forces applied into and across the hip joint can be considered through a model of a single leg stance with the body center of mass (or gravity) balanced (that is, located on an axis of alignment) over one hip joint (Fig. 5.18). In this balanced condition, little or no muscle contraction forces are necessary to maintain equilibrium,

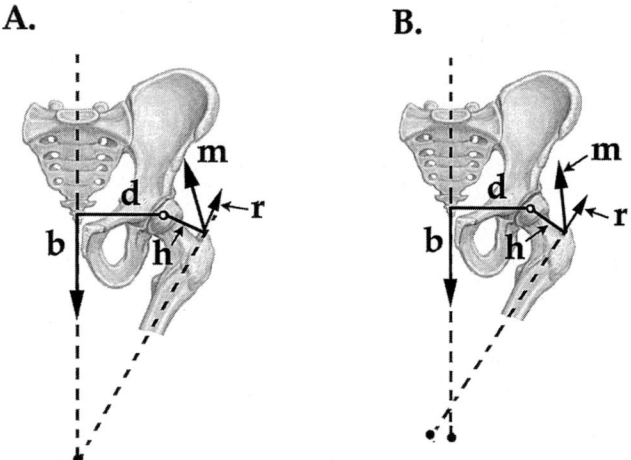

FIGURE 5.18. A simple co-planar model of a single leg stance moment in balance. **A:** In the balanced state, the body weight *(b)* is balanced over the foot (not shown), which would be at the intersection of the *dotted lines*. In this balance, the body weight *(b)* acts as a force applied on a moment arm *(d)* through the center of rotation in the femoral head to produce a body moment (b × d). This is balanced by the rotational component *(r)* of the muscle contraction force *(m)* acting over a moment arm through the femur *(h)* to produce a muscle contraction moment (r × h). For balance to be maintained (b × d) = (r × h). **B:** The balanced condition can be disturbed by a shift of the body and a slight change of the angle of pull by the muscle *(m)*. To restore balance, the moment *(r)* must be increased or altered so that the moments can be rebalanced.

as in the knee. The joint reaction force or force directed into the joint will equal the ground reaction force produced by the weight of the body above the hip. In an unbalanced state, the body center of mass is no longer directly over the bony structure and produces an unbalanced moment about the center of rotation of the hip joint. To restore equilibrium, the force of the contracting abductor muscles must generate an equal force moment across the hip in the direction opposite of the moment generated by the body weight. By measuring the length of the moment arms for muscle contraction in the body and knowing the body weight, the approximate resisting moment of muscle contraction can be calculated along with the joint reaction component produced.

Note that in this model, the angle of the femoral neck will affect the relative lengths of the moment arms (or the angle of pull) by muscles. This will directly influence the muscle contraction forces required to resist the body weight moment and the proportion of the contraction force directed into the joint. This is why an abnormal angle of the femoral neck can adversely affect hip function and the stresses on the joint.

Hip Joint Function Requires High Muscle Contraction Forces and the Ability to Withstand High Joint Reaction Forces

As with the knee, it can be seen that hip stability under load-bearing conditions can require high muscle contraction forces because of a relatively short moment arm though which the muscle forces are applied. As a combination of ground reaction force and the portion of the muscle contraction forces directed into the joint, the joint reaction forces are also high relative to the body weight. Calculations suggest that under these conditions, the muscle contraction force is approximately twice the body weight and the joint reaction force almost three times the body weight (66,67). Joint reaction forces are important in consideration of stresses on the hip joint itself in replacement or repair. Strategies to minimize the joint reaction force can also be important in subjects with arthritic pain in the hip joint. As suggested by the model given earlier, a reduction in joint reaction forces may be achieved by altering the angle of the hip by increasing the muscle moment arms. This can also be accomplished by using a support device, such as a cane on the opposite side, to reduce the opposing body weight moment.

THE ELBOW

The Elbow Is a Complex of Three Joints with Two Primary Ranges of Motion

The upper limb analogue of the knee is the elbow, which has adapted for increased mobility of the upper limb and a reduced load-bearing requirement. In achieving this, the joint has become a complex of three articulations, including the humeroulnar, the humeroradial, and the proximal radioulnar joints (Fig. 5.19). The joint complex allows two primary ranges of motion: flexion-extension and pronation-supination. Flexion and extension occur across the humeroulnar and humeroradial joints, which act as a hinged joint. The normal range of motion in flexion-extension is approximately 140 degrees, with limits established by the angular

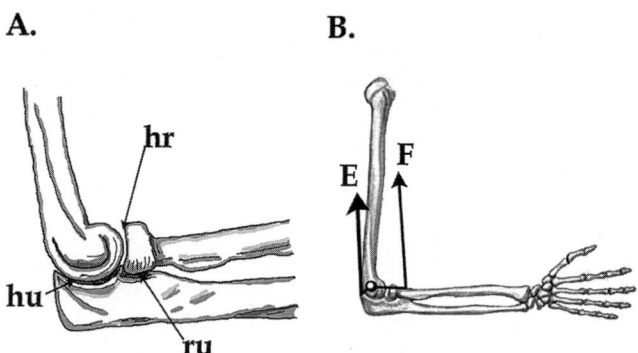

FIGURE 5.19. A: The elbow joint complex consists of the humeroulnar *(hu)*, humeroradial *(hr)*, and proximal radioulnar joints. **B:** The primary flexor *(F)* and extensor *(E)* moments across the joint.

characteristics of the bony components (68). The axis of motion passes through the middle of the trochlea and is principally a gliding motion (69) up to the last 5 to 10 degrees of flexion, where rolling occurs. Pronation and supination occur at the humeroradial and proximal radioulnar joint. The reported normal range of motion varies between studies (68) with the American Academy of Orthopaedic Surgeons (70) reporting an average of 70 degrees of pronation and 85 degrees of supination. The range of motion required for typical daily activities of both flexion-extension and pronation-supination can be performed between a much more limited range (71).

Much of the elbow joint's stability during normal use is supplied by the shape of the articulating surfaces. Of the three articulations, the humeroulnar articulation supplies the primary anterior-posterior stability, although the radiohumoral articulation can contribute to stability from posterior dislocation at flexion of 90 degrees or more. Beyond the bony stability of the joint, the ligaments and joint capsules around the elbow provide remaining stability and the interosseous membrane binds the radial and ulnar shafts together.

Basic Functions of the Elbow Can Be Described by Simple Joint Moments

The basic biomechanics of the elbow can be described largely as a system of simple levers or joint moments as suggested earlier in the section on basic mechanics of joint systems (Figs. 13 and 19). Muscle forces act at a low mechanical advantage to achieve a large movement. Due to disadvantageous vector angles through some of their range, relatively high muscle contraction forces are required. These muscle contraction forces typically generate large joint reaction force components that act through the bony elements to stabilize the elbow. These joint reaction forces may exceed body weight even during normal activities.

The Elbow Complex Provides an Example of Dysfunctions from the Coupling of Intraarticular Motion

As a joint complex, the elbow provides a reasonably simple example of coupling relationships of intraarticular joint motions that, when disrupted, can produce dysfunction. During flexion-extension movements, the humeroulnar joint has a primary gliding motion that is accompanied by a movement of the head of the radius on the capitulum of the humerus. This produces a smaller proximal and distal gliding of the proximal radius in the radial notch of the ulna (62). The extent of this latter movement is greatest when the joint is half-flexed. Although this motion is not a primary component of the segmental motion, its disruption can produce pain and dysfunction in the joint during movement. It is therefore important to understand the coupled movements of the complex as well as the individual articulations. More complicated examples can occur in more extensive joint chains such as in the spine and feet.

THE SHOULDER

The Shoulder Is a Complex of Four Joints with Different Properties

The shoulder consists of a complex of four articulations: the glenohumeral, acromioclavicular, sternoclavicular, and scapulothoracic articulations (Fig. 5.20). Of these, the scapulothoracic articulation is not a true articulation, but an indirect attachment of the scapula to the thoracic wall indirectly through muscles. The shoulder complex acts in concert with contributions from each joint to produce movement through greater than a hemisphere of range. The glenohumeral joint is a basic ball-and-socket joint, but has much less intrinsic stability than its lower limb analogue at the hip. The reduced stability is reflected by the structure of

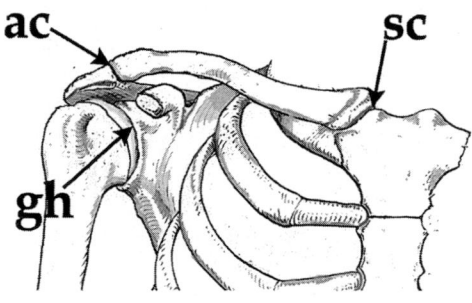

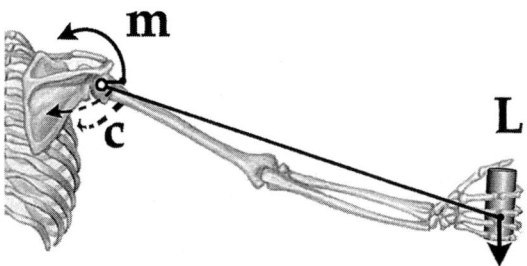

FIGURE 5.20. Top: Front view of the shoulder complex consisting of the glenohumeral *(gh)* acromioclavicular *(ac)*, and sternoclavicular *(sc)* articulations. The scapulothoracic junction is not a true articulation, but describes the relationship of the scapula and thorax as can be seen in the lower figure. **Bottom:** An example of the differences in the moment arms of shoulder muscles *(m)* and a load *(L)* in a lift with the shoulder abducted and arm extended. Co-contracting muscles *(c, dotted arrows)* are important to stabilize the shoulder complex during such tasks.

the articulating surfaces of the joint. The area of the glenoid fossa that contacts the humerus is only one-third to one-fourth the size of the joint surface of the humeral head (72). This allows a more circular range of motion relative to the scapula, but at the cost of intrinsic structural stability of the joint. Although some vertical structural support may be derived from the overlying acromion process and attached clavicle, the glenohumeral joint is reliant, to a great degree, on soft-tissue structures (ligaments, tendons, joint capsules, and muscles) for stability (73). During function, the glenohumeral joint primarily rotates, but rolling and translation may also take place. This translation may increase substantially with soft-tissue injury or dislocation.

The scapula attaches to the thoracic skeleton through a chain of two articulations, the acromioclavicular and sternoclavicular joints. The acromioclavicular joint between the clavicle and proximal acromion of the scapula has a meniscus of cartilage, a thick fibrous capsule, and supporting ligaments that stabilize the joint and allows the scapula motion in three planes (74). These planes include a vertical axis (protraction and retraction) and transverse axes in the frontal and sagittal planes. The proximal end of the clavicle (sternoclavicular joint) is stabilized by a fibrocartilage, meniscus-containing, articulation capsule and ligaments to the sternum and first rib. The joint allows protraction and retraction, elevation and depression, and rotation of the clavicle relative to the sternum.

The concept of a scapulothoracic articulation involves a description of the movement of the scapula relative to the thorax as limited by its muscular attachments and the clavicular chain. This structural arrangement allows a wide range of motion of the scapula including protraction retraction, elevation, depression, and rotation. Movement of the scapula involves the translocation of the entire glenohumeral joint, contributing substantially to the range of motion of the arm. A simple example is the contribution of scapular motion to the elevation of the arm. In this circumstance the scapula rotates to elevate the shoulder and the glenohumeral joint as the arm is raised.

Shoulder Range of Motion Is Usually Described for the Entire Joint Complex Rather than Individual Joints

With the complex interaction of the individual articulations, the range of motion of the shoulder is usually described for the complex as a whole. From a resting position at the side, the range of motion in the shoulder complex is typically described in the context of range of elevation of the shoulder or movement of the humerus away from the thorax in any of the three primary planes. Forward flexion and abduction are approximately 180 degrees, and in the plane of the scapula may exceed 180 degrees. Backward elevation or extension is approximately 60 degrees. Other motions including bringing the humerus in adduction beyond the midline limit of the body in an upward direction is approximately 75 degrees (70). Horizontal flexion in a transverse plane at 90 degrees of abduction is approximately 135 degrees, with horizontal extension of 45 degrees. Rotation about the long axis of the humerus varies with the degree of arm elevation, but in general, both internal and external rotation can be approximately 90 degrees, with a total range of 180 degrees (74).

The Glenohumeral Joint Depends upon Muscle Stabilizing Forces to Resist Distal Loads

Because of the relative lack of structural stability of the glenohumeral joint, soft-tissue connections through the joint must play a greater role in its stability. In addition to the joint capsule and ligamentous connections, muscle contraction forces that essentially hold the joint together become more important in resisting the loads placed on the distal upper limb. The use of force-coupling arrangements in the muscles of the rotator cuff is particularly important in this process. In force coupling, muscles of the rotator cuff act in concert to produce offsetting moments (a net joint reaction force) to stabilize the joint (Fig. 5.20) as elevation is produced. The actual calculations of joint reaction forces under these circumstances is difficult due to the large numbers of muscles involved in arrangements that will vary according to the plane of motion. Estimates of these forces suggest magnitudes near body weight (75). It is also important to note that the low mechanical advantage of muscles in the shoulder compared to the moment arm of a load in the hand of an extended arm requires very high contraction forces (Fig. 5.20). The low mechanical advantage of shoulder muscles under loading and the dependency of the joint on soft tissues for stability make the shoulder particularly vulnerable to injury.

THE SPINE

The spine as a whole represents an extremely complicated system of articulations and bony segments that act to protect the spinal cord while providing a basic support axis for the upper body. The structure and motion of spinal segments differs substantially over the spinal column. Due to this complexity and variation, only some basic principles of spinal biomechanics can be covered here.

Spinal Motion Segments Consist of Two Vertebrae and Associated Soft Tissues

The functional unit of the spine or motion segment consists of two vertebrae and their associated soft tissues (Fig. 5.21). The

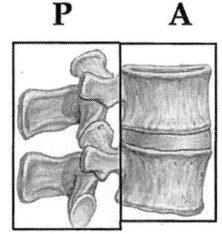 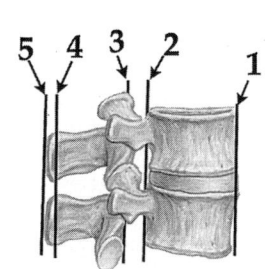

FIGURE 5.21. Left: A basic motion segment of the lumbar spine divided into anterior *(A)* and posterior *(P)* portions. The anterior portion contains the vertebral bodies, the spinal disc, and the anterior longitudinal *(1)* and posterior longitudinal *(2)* ligaments **(right)**. The posterior portion contains the vertebral canal, the bony segments associated with it, and associated ligaments including the ligamentum flavum *(3)*, the interspinous ligament *(4)*, and the supraspinous ligament *(5)*. Other soft-tissue structures (e.g., capsular ligaments, etc.) are not shown.

segment is functionally and physically divided into anterior and posterior segments. The anterior portion consists of the vertebral body, the disc between them, and the longitudinal ligaments (Fig. 5.21). The posterior segment consists of the vertebral arches, the articulations between the facets, the transverse and spinous processes, and the ligaments binding them together. Besides containing the spinal cord and associated structures, the architecture of the posterior segment acts to guide and limit the motion that can occur between the vertebrae of the segment. The anterior segment of the unit is the primary load-bearing section, with the vertebral bodies and the intervening disc increasing in size in the lower segments to sustain greater loading stress. Load bearing in the posterior segment can be significant when the spine is hyperextended (76) and during forward bending coupled with rotation (77).

The Bony Structure of the Spine Is Supported by an Intricate Arrangement of Soft Tissues

The soft-tissue support for the spinal column consists of the ligaments, joint capsules, and muscles that connect to the transverse and spinous processes of the vertebrae as part of the posterior motion segments. The primary ligaments include the anterior and posterior ligaments, the ligamentum flavum, the supraspinous and interspinous ligaments (Fig. 5.21), and the intertransverse ligaments, all of which provide intrinsic support for the spinal column. The capsular ligaments for the facet articulations also contribute to stability and limitation of motion. The ligaments have a high collagen content except for the ligamentum flavum, which has a high elastin content. The ligaments add stability and store energy during movement of the spinal column. For example, flexion primarily stretches the interspinous ligaments, capsular ligaments, and the ligamentum flavum. These store energy like an elastic band and can be used for subsequent recovery to a neutral position. Other ligaments similarly participate in lateral bending and rotation.

Intervertebral Discs Are Structured to Cushion and Distribute Stresses between Vertebrae

The intervertebral discs sustain and distribute primarily compressive loading of the vertebrae and restrict excessive motion. The disc consists of a tough outer covering of fibrocartilage, the annulus fibrosus, bounded above and below by a plate of hyaline cartilage adjacent to the vertebrae. The collagen fibers of the annulus fibrosus are arranged in concentric layers and differing orientations to the vertical axis of ±30 degrees in a cross-hatched arrangement. This covering encloses a gelatinous inner core, the nucleus pulposus, that acts to distribute and redirect stresses and store energy, similar to a partially inflated ball. The nucleus pulposus contains a water-binding glycosaminoglycan gel (80% to 88% water) (78) that becomes progressively less hydrated with age (79). This change can reduce the elasticity, ability to store energy, and stress loading distribution properties of the disc and make it less capable of resisting loads.

In the unloaded condition, longitudinal ligaments and the ligamenta flava exert pressure on the disc to create a pre-stress condition (80). Compressive stress on the disc through the vertebral bodies creates a circumferential tensile stress that is resisted by the annular fibers of the annulus fibrosus. During motions such as flexion bending, the vertebrae rotate forward, creating compression stress and some strain (bulging) on the anterior disc and tensile stress on the posterior portion of the disc (Fig. 5.4). Rotation produces torsional stress on the disc, which is also redistributed through its structure. These strain patterns allow vertebral movement under load, and redistribution of forces across the vertebral-disc interface, to minimize localized extremes in stress.

The Bony Structure of the Posterior Segment Is a Primary Determinant of Intervertebral Ranges of Motion

Aside from their connection through the vertebral bodies and the intervening disc, the vertebrae interact structurally through the facets of intervertebral joints in the posterior portion of the motion segment. Under most circumstances, vertebral movement is restricted by the orientation of these facets relative to the vertebral column and each other (Fig. 5.22). Exceptions include particular regions of the spinal column, where articulations with structures such as the skull, ribs, or sacrum may add additional constraints on vertebral movement. The orientation of intervertebral facets changes throughout the spinal column (81) and the actual angle of the facets may vary significantly between individuals. The orientation of intervertebral facets also acts to produce additional directional components (motion coupling, as described in the next section) in vertebral motion during basic movement, such as flexion, extension, rotation, and lateral flexion.

The primary variation in facet orientation can be defined in the transverse and frontal planes. A positive angle deviation from the transverse plane indicates that the facets are oriented above a hor-

izontal (transverse) plane through the body (Fig. 5.22). Positive deviation in the frontal plane effectively describes the orientation of the facet surfaces on each side of the vertebra relative to each other, although the angle is defined relative to a frontal plane (Fig. 5.22). The atlas and axis have facets that are almost parallel to the transverse plane, with the remaining facets of the cervical vertebrae oriented at a 45-degree angle to the transverse plane and parallel to the frontal plane (Fig. 5.22). The alignment of the C3-7 vertebrae allows flexion, extension, lateral flexion, and rotation (82). This can be compared to the facets of thoracic vertebrae that are oriented 60 degrees from the transverse plane and 20 degrees from the frontal plane. This allows lateral bending, rotation, and some flexion and extension. The lumbar vertebrae have facets oriented 90 degrees to the transverse plane and 45 degrees to the frontal plane. This allows almost no rotation, but flexion, extension, and lateral bending. The lumbosacral joints do allow more rotation (83), with facets oriented more obliquely to the transverse plane.

The Motion of the Spine Is a Composite of Small Movements in Individual Vertebrae and Coupling Between Vertebrae

The kinematic and kinetic considerations of spinal movements are particularly complicated, since overall movements are a composite of comparatively small movements of each vertebral segment. Each vertebra has some degree of rotation or translation in each of its transverse, sagittal, and longitudinal axes (or 6 degrees of freedom in movement). This movement is largely limited by the intervertebral joint facet orientations. These orientations vary markedly over the spinal column (81). Flexion-extension movements are greatest in the cervical, lower thoracic, and lumbar spine; rotation is greatest in the cervical and upper thoracic spine; and lateral bending is greatest in the cervical spine and more evenly distributed over remaining vertebrae.

It should be noted here that the convention in osteopathic medicine is to describe rotation of a vertebra as the direction in which the anterior part of the vertebral body or anterior segment rotates. In some biomechanical texts, rotation of the vertebra is described as the direction in which the posterior segment or spinous process rotates. Even though these conventions describe the same rotary motion, they are on opposite sides of the center of rotation and therefore the inverse of each other. This difference can become particularly confusing in relation to descriptions of motion coupling between vertebrae over the spine (discussed subsequently). The osteopathic convention will be used here, unless specific reference is made to the spinous process. Another caveat of the descriptions of vertebral movements given is that active, muscle contraction-based movement characteristics may or may not be similar to movements produced by external forces (e.g., manipulations). This should be taken into account in comparisons of these characteristics as described in the chapters on manipulation.

Physiologically normal movements of the spinal column in any of the primary directions (flexion-extension, lateral bending, rotation) produce additional motion vectors in the vertebrae as a consequence of the orientation of the intervertebral facets and other articulations (Fig. 5.23). This coupling may include

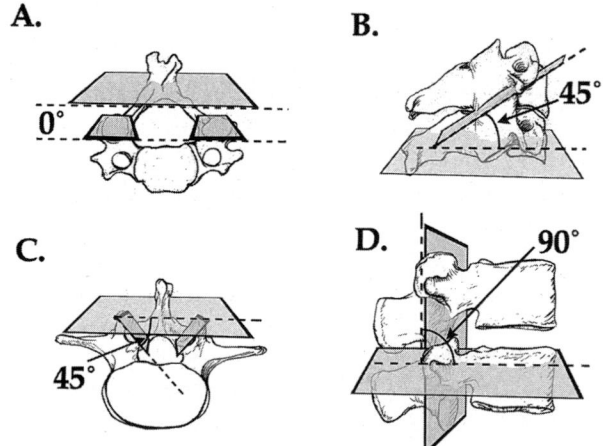

FIGURE 5.22. The orientation of intervertebral joint facets in the frontal and transverse planes relative to the spinal column. In the cervical vertebrae **(A, B)**, the surface of the facets on either side are parallel to each and to a frontal plane **(A)**, but inclined at 45 degrees above a transverse plane through a vertebra as viewed from the side **(B)**. In the lumbar spine **(C, D)**, the surfaces of the facets are oriented at 45 degrees to the frontal plane **(C)** and 90 degrees above a transverse plane as shown from the side **(D)**. The facet orientations restrict the mobility of intervertebral movement and define the motion-coupling characteristics.

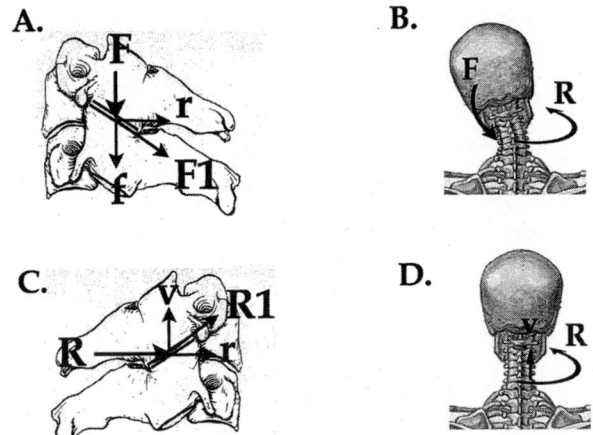

FIGURE 5.23. Motion coupling as influenced by the orientation of intervertebral facets in cervical vertebrae. **A:** A lateral flexing force *(F)* on the side of the vertebrae acting to move the upper vertebrae relative to the bottom will be redirected by the facets in a new direction *(F1)*. The divided moment will have a remaining flexing component *(f)* and a rotational component *(r)* that will add (couple) rotation *(R)* of the vertebrae to the flexing movement **(B)**. **C:** A rotational force *(R)* on one vertebra is redirected by the facets to glide in a new direction *(R1)*. R1 has both a vertical *(v)* and a remaining rotational component *(r)* (vectors). The vertical component will cause the side of the vertebra to lift upward and produces lateral flexion on the opposite side **(D)**. However, in isolated rotation movements, this flexing moment is restricted to produce vertical translation (telescoping) of the cervical spine, particularly at the C1-C2 joint.

motions of lateral bending (flexion), rotation, and translation in several axes simultaneously, although only major coupling relationships are typically noted as clinically significant. The coupling can differ markedly over the spine and only a limited description will be given here. In the thoracic region, rotation is coupled with lateral flexion. This is greatest in the upper thoracic region, with the vertebrae rotating toward the same side as the lateral flexion (81). In the lumbar spine, rotation is also coupled with lateral flexion, but the vertebrae rotate in a direction opposite the lateral flexion. Additional motion coupling in the cervical spine is described subsequently.

Overall Range of Motion of the Spine Varies Widely Between Individuals

The composite nature of spinal movements along with individual structural and soft-tissue differences help to explain a great variation in the range of motion in individuals. There are also significant variations in spinal range of motion with age and sex (84). This makes the listing of normal values without specification of these factors of little clinical significance. Difficulties in defining normal ranges of motion also derive from a large capacity of the spine to produce compensatory changes in movement to achieve a similar net movement. In this strategy, a limitation of movement that exists in the structural aspects of one area of the spinal column can be alleviated by a compensatory greater mobility in other areas (85). For example, the movement of the spinal column is also accompanied by motion in the pelvis. In body flexion, the initial 50 to 60 degrees of motion occurs in the lumbar spine with little contribution from the thoracic vertebra

due to the orientation of the facets and the rib cage. Additional flexion is accomplished by the tilting of the pelvis.

Restriction of movement in the lumbar spine can be replaced, to some extent, by greater and earlier tilting of the pelvis. The movement of the pelvis also contributes to lateral bending and rotation of the trunk, and may be used similarly to compensate for restrictions.

As in other multiple-articulation chains, movements of the spine are accomplished through complex interactions of agonist and antagonist muscle groups. Movement aspects are accomplished through the cooperative actions of antagonistic trunk and spinal muscles, some contracting to produce the movement, others co-contracting to provide stabilization.

Some Kinetic Considerations of Spinal Loading

Loading characteristics of the spine are similarly complex compared to movement. The loading of the spine includes body weight, muscle contraction, ligamentous pre-stressing, and externally applied loads. The natural kyphosis and lordosis of the spine add to the elastic resistance to load of the discs, again by redistributing compressive stress into bending stresses that can be resisted by muscle contraction (Fig. 5.24). The primary load-bearing region of the spinal column is in the lumbar spine. During normal standing, the center of gravity of the trunk passes near the center of the body of the fourth lumbar vertebra (86). This distribution and the static load on the spine can be altered appreciably by the angle of the pelvis. Tilting the pelvic angle (sacral angle) forward from its normal 30 degrees to the transverse plane accentuates the lumbar lordosis. Tilting backward from the normal angle flattens the lumbar lordosis. Both movements affect the lever arm of the body weight on the spine and require compensatory muscle activity to resist. This also creates greater loads

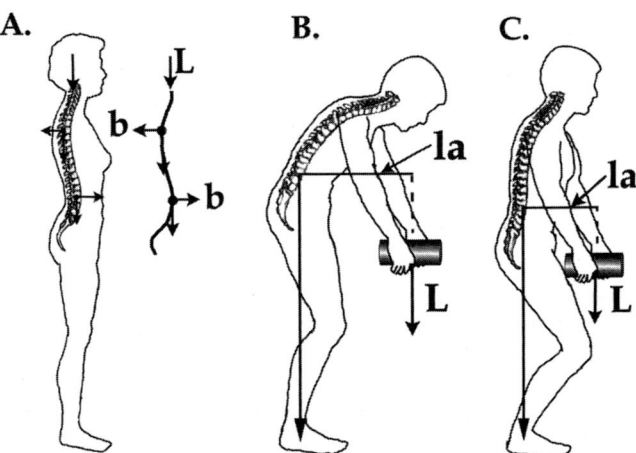

FIGURE 5.24. A: The normal curvatures of the spine *in situ* and in a model **(right)** will split vertical compression components into bending forces *(b)* that can be counteracted with muscle contraction. **B:** Force moments on the back are larger if an object is further from the vertebrae being compressed. The force moment is a product of the load *(L)* and the load arm *(la)*. This compressive force alone is not dependent upon the bending of the knees **(C)**, but bending of the knees can help to shorten the load arm.

on the lumbar spine during sitting versus relaxed standing (87). Reorientation of the spine from its normal curvature also produces stresses on the discs by changing the alignment of the vertebrae.

The Orientation of the Spine During Lifting Can Influence the Distribution of Stress on the Lumbar Spine

Lifting an object places added stress on the spine by creating an added load at a distance from the center of support in the spine (Fig. 5.24). The stress on the lumbar vertebrae by the load is primarily a function of the distance of the load from the vertebrae (moment arm or lever arm) and the weight of the load. Bending the body forward adds distance from the body, whether or not the knees are bent (82). Contraction of back muscles and to some degree, intraabdominal pressure must counterbalance the forward-bending forces. In consideration of posture in lifting, the lumbar spine has less resistance to bending compared to direct compressive forces (88) and lateral flexion or flexion combined with axial rotation (87) increases pressure on lumbar discs. This further suggests that a vertical lifting position of the spine is preferred to reduce pressures on lumbar discs.

The Cervical Spine Has Some Unique Structural Properties and Biomechanical Properties

The cervical spine and its articulation with the skull have some special biomechanical and structural properties that require special consideration. It has five of seven vertebrae that are described as more or less typical, except for the presence of the transverse foramen for the vertebral artery in C3 to C6. The grooving of the transverse process for the exit of the cervical nerves lends to further structural weakness. Both the presence of the vertebral artery and the comparative structural weakness of the transverse process suggest reason for caution with high-velocity manipulations of this region. This is particularly true for older adults in whom both soft tissue and bone biomechanical properties add weakness to this region. Other structural differences in the C3-6 vertebrae include more prominent uncinate processes and thinner intervertebral discs. Because of this, uncinate processes may also play a role in guiding and limiting cervical motion (89).

The Atlas and Axis Have Additional Structural Properties That Define Their Range of Movement

The atypical vertebrae (C1, C2) have unique bony structures that limit their mobility. The atlas (C1) has no true vertebral body or disc, but an anterior arch with an articulating surface for the dens of the axis (C2). The atlas articulates with the skull in two superior facets that have a semicircular shape. This limits the motion of the skull relative to the atlas to almost no rotation. The inferior facets of the atlas articulate with C2 almost parallel to the transverse plane. The axis, with its superior protrusion, the dens, provides an axis of rotation for C1. Posterior translation of the dens within the vertebral foramen is prevented by ligamen-

tous support from the cruciform ligament. It also contains two superior, convex-shaped facets for articulation, with two slightly convex-shaped articulations (62) of the atlas that affect motion coupling in rotation.

These structural properties help to make the cervical region the most mobile region of the spine. The range of motion at the atlanto-occipital articulation is approximately 10 to 15 degrees of flexion extension and 8 degrees of lateral bending (81,89). Axial rotation is largely precluded by the structure of the articulation, and is transferred to the C1-C2 articulation. The C1-C2 interface is the most mobile segment of the spine with about 47 degrees of axial rotation, or almost 50% of the axial rotation capability of the entire cervical spine (90). Flexion-extension is limited to 10 degrees, and little or no lateral bending occurs. Throughout the cervical spine, the combined range of motion is approximately 145 degrees of flexion-extension, 180 degrees of axial rotation, and 90 degrees of lateral flexion (89).

Motion Coupling of the Cervical Spine Includes Transverse and Vertical Translation and Rotation

Motion coupling of the cervical spine also has some important characteristics in addition to those mentioned earlier due to its unique anatomy. Flexion-extension is coupled with transverse translation, particularly at the C1-C2 interface (89,91). As discussed previously, lateral flexion (side bending) tends to rotate the spinous process away (vertebral body toward) from the direction of bending (Fig. 5.23) (81). Isolated rotation produces a vertical translation, or telescoping, of the cervical spine due to the orientation of the facets and restriction of flexor moments (Fig. 5.23).

Increased Mobility of the Cervical Spine Is Accompanied by Reduced Stability

The high range of motion in the cervical spine is accompanied by a lower intrinsic stability, but reduced load compared to the lumbar spine. This makes the cervical spine and associated soft-tissue support particularly vulnerable to excessive dynamic loading, with flexion-extension injuries the most common. As in other areas of the spine, restriction of movement in the cervical spine usually results in an increased compensatory mobility of other areas to achieve a functional range of motion. As a result restriction of motion at one level, due to injury or a brace, may produce increased motion (and increased stress) at other levels (83,92). This consideration can be important in the determination of symptom-cause relationships in the diagnosis of spinal dysfunction.

BIOMECHANICAL CONSIDERATIONS OF THE BODY AS A UNIT

Normal Locomotion (Gait) Employs the Entire Body for Efficiency of Movement

Motions of the body incorporate the individual biomechanical properties of soft and hard tissues and kinematic aspects of the

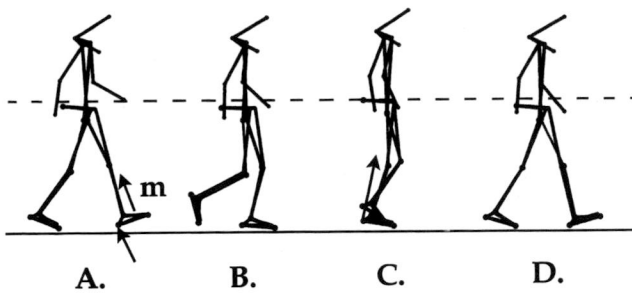

FIGURE 5.25. Basic gait patterns using computer-generated (Peak Performance Technologies, Inc., Englewood, CO.) stick figures of an individual in normal gait. The gait cycle arbitrarily begins with the contact of one heel with the floor **(A)**. The force of the body weight and motion on the heel *(arrow)* is decelerated by the anterior muscle group of the leg *(m, arrow)* through the ankle. **B:** Body weight is transferred to the supporting leg, which supports the body with slight knee flexion. **C:** The moving leg is swung forward and the supporting leg is slightly extended *(arrow)* to raise the body center of mass to its high point *(dotted line)*. **D:** The body is propelled forward by plantar flexion of the supporting leg to be "caught" with the heel strike of the moving leg and the cycle begins for the opposite side.

individual articulations into complicated movement processes. A particularly good example of this integration can be found in normal ambulation or gait (Fig. 5.25). Gait may be described as a controlled falling with propulsion. In this process, the center of mass of the body is subjected to relatively small vertical displacements. The actual energy expended is distributed over many muscle groups beyond the legs and by subtle, but significant movements. In normal gait, one leg is moved forward while the weight of the body is supported by the opposing leg (swing phase) (Fig. 5.25). In the swing phase of the leg, the foot goes from plantar flexion to dorsal flexion. The knee is flexed and then extended, the hip moves from extension to flexion, and the pelvis rotates and changes its tilt as muscles of the lower spine and trunk are used to generate power.

Swinging the opposing arm will assist in compensating balance and rotation moments through the trunk. The body is propelled forward and its center of mass moved slightly upward and then forward and down to be "caught" by the heel strike of the extended leg. As the heel hits a surface, the foot rocks down and is decelerated by the anterior muscle groups of the leg. The knee, which initially is almost completely extended, begins to flex and becomes progressively loaded as the body weight is transferred from the opposing leg. The opposing hip and pelvis are then rotated forward to begin the process for the opposite side. Small adjustments, such as increasing the tilt of the trunk and head in the direction of progression, bring the center of mass of the body forward and assist in increasing the rate of movement.

This basic process, grossly simplified here, can reflect one of the most frequently encountered examples of the ability of the body to adapt to injury or degenerative processes. Compensatory gait patterns can vary widely according to the underlying cause, but always have an underlying biomechanical rationale, even though these adaptations may themselves produce problems. In a typical example, an injury to the knee or foot on one side may produce a compensatory shift of the body center of mass over the opposing limb. This will produce pain, stress injuries, or palpable dysfunctions in the opposite knee, back, hip, or even neck, if body posture has been significantly affected. Some aspects of

these compensatory adjustments may survive the healing of the original injury, particularly if the recuperative process has been lengthy. This emphasizes the importance of the subject's history and careful observation and knowledge of mechanical body function in the diagnosis and treatment of somatic dysfunctions.

ACKNOWLEDGMENTS

The writing of this chapter has been supported by the New York College of Osteopathic Medicine (NYCOM) of the New York Institute of Technology, Old Westbury, NY.

The author wishes to acknowledge the helpful comments of Dr. Stanley Schiowitz, D.O., and other members of the NYCOM faculty and staff in the preparation of this chapter.

REFERENCES

1. Nordin M, Frankel VH. Biomechanics of bone. In: Nordin M, Frankel VH, eds. *Basic Biomechanics of the Musculoskeletal System*, 2nd ed. Philadelphia, PA: Lea & Febiger; 1989:3–27.
2. Dempster WT, Coleman RF. Tensile strength of bone along and across the grain. *J Appl Physiol.* 1960;16:355–360.
3. Reilly GC. Observations of microdamage around osteocyte lacunae in bone. *J Biomech.* 2000;33:1131–1134.
4. Siffert RS, Levy RN. Trabecular patterns and the internal architecture of bone. *Mt Sinai J Med.* 1981;48:221–229.
5. Sammarco J, Burstein A, Davis W, Frankel V. The biomechanics of torsional fractures: the effect of loading on ultimate properties. *J Biomech.* 1971;4:113–117.
6. Carter DR, Hayes WC. Compact bone fatigue damage. A microscopic examination. *Clin Orthop.* 1977;127:265–274.
7. Korpelainen R, Orava S, Karpakka J, et al. Risk factors for recurrent stress fractures in athletes. *Am J Sports Med.* 2001;29:304–10.
8. Wolff J. *The Law of Bone Remodeling,* Maquet P, Furlong R, trans. Berlin, Germany: Springer-Verlag; 1986, originally published in 1870.
9. Schneider VS, McDonald J. Skeletal calcium homeostasis and counter measures to prevent disuse osteoporosis, *Calc Tissue Int.* 1984;36[Suppl 1]:S141–S144.
10. Zerath E. Effects of microgravity on bone and calcium homeostasis. *Adv Space Res.* 1998;21:1049–1058.
11. Jenkins DP, Cochran TH. Osteoporosis: the dramatic effect of disuse of an extremity. *Clin Orthop.* 1969;64:128–134.
12. Kazarian LE, vonGierke HE. Bone loss as a result of immobilization and chelation. Preliminary results in Macaca mulatta. *Clin Orthop.*1969;65:67–75.
13. Huddleston AL, Rockwell D, Kulund DN, Harrison RB. Bone mass in lifetime tennis athletes. *JAMA.* 1980;244:1107–1109.
14. Woo SL, Kuei SC, Amiel D, et al. The effect of prolonged physical training on the properties of long bone: a study of Wolff's law. *J Bone Joint Surg Am.* 1981;63(5):780–787.
15. Morris FL, Naughton GA, Gibbs JL, et al. Prospective ten-month exercise intervention in premenarchal girls: positive effects on bone and lean mass. *J Bone Mineral Res.* 1997;9:1453–1462.
16. Burstein AH, Currey J, Frankel VH, et al. Bone strength. The effect of screw holes. *J Bone Joint Surg.* 1972;54A:1143–1156.
17. Smith EL, Gilligan C. Physical activity effects on bone metabolism. *Calcif Tissue Int.*1991;49[Suppl]:S50–54.
18. Wilmore JH. The aging of bone and muscle. *Clin Sports Med.* 1991;10:231–44.
19. Armstrong CG, Mow VC. Variations in the intrinsic mechanical properties of human articular cartilage with age, degeneration, and water content. *J Bone Joint Surg.* 1982;64A:88–94.
20. Poole AR, Kojima T, Yasuda T, et al. Composition and structure of articular cartilage: a template for tissue repair. *Clin Orthop.* 2001;391 [Suppl]:S26–33.

AUTONOMIC NERVOUS SYSTEM

FRANK H. WILLARD

KEY CONCEPTS

- The two components of the peripheral nervous system are: somatic and autonomic
- The somatic component provides innervation of the skeletal muscle; while the influence of autonomic portion, representing the predominant component, is seen on almost all other tissues in body
- Organization of the autonomic nervous system is similar to the somatic nervous system, including the following roles: receiving afferent fibers, processing information in central circuits, and forming output to connective tissue cells, smooth muscle cells, secretory cells, and immune cells
- The distinctive feature of the autonomic nervous system is the two-step output pathway involving centrally located preganglionic neurons and peripherally located ganglionic neurons
- There are two anatomically, biochemically, and functionally distinct divisions of the peripheral autonomic nervous system: sympathetic and parasympathetic, with dual effects on many organ systems
- Innervation of the visceral organs occurs through the great autonomic plexus that extends from the base of neck through the thorax, diaphragm, and abdomen and terminates in the pelvis
- The great autonomic plexus is supplied with parasympathetic fibers from the vagus and pelvic splanchnic nerves and sympathetic fibers from the thoracic, lumbar, and sacral splanchnic nerves
- The central origin and importance of sympathetic and parasympathetic innervation for organ systems in the head, neck, thorax, abdomen, and pelvis
- The origin and importance of sympathetic innervation for the peripheral vasculature
- The primary afferent innervation of organ systems is instrumental in controlling the output of the autonomic nervous system
- Neuropeptide markers in afferent nerve fibers and small-caliber, primary afferent fibers involved with detection of nociceptive stimuli

Our daily existence depends on the coordinated activities of our internal organ systems. A major factor in orchestrating the diverse functions of these internal structures is the autonomic nervous system. Through an extensive network of connections, the autonomic nervous system helps maintain the normal rhythm of activity in the visceral organs, adjusting their output to accommodate any external challenge. The limbic structures of the brain control the autonomic nervous system through the hypothalamus. The hypothalamus itself is closely integrated into a complex network involving the endocrine and immune systems. This conglomerate of interlocking systems, with its pervasive influence on our physiology and psychology, is called the neuroendocrine-immune network. This neuroendocrine-immune network is further described in Chapter 8.

The terminology used to describe the part of the nervous system usually not under voluntary control varies widely. Since the 18th century, different terms have been used by researchers in different countries. None of these terms refers to the exact same group of structures or functions. Examples include:

> Vegitive Nervensystem
> Grand symapathique
> Ganglionic nervous system
> Visceral nervous system

The two most commonly used terms are vegetative and autonomic nervous system. For a thorough discussion of the history of terminology concerning this system, see Clarke and Jacyna (1). The present chapter uses the term autonomic nervous system to refer to all components of the nervous system using preganglionic and ganglionic neurons as an efferent pathway. This definition excludes only the neuromuscular junctions between the ventral horn of the spinal cord (and a few cranial nuclei) and skeletal muscle.

The clinical importance of understanding the circuits of the autonomic nervous system cannot be overstated. Almost all communication between neurons in these circuits occurs via synaptic transmission. This process depends on the production, distribution, and recognition of specific neurochemicals. Most pharmaceutical agents, either as a desired first action or as an undesired side effect, affect these metabolic and stereologic events. Knowledge of nervous system structure, function, and chemistry is a necessity for the educated use of these substances and the intelligent approach to the maintenance of health.

The autonomic nervous system is sensitive to events occurring in somatic tissue such as cutaneous and musculoskeletal systems. The autonomic and somatic nervous systems are interlocked through numerous somatovisceral and viscerosomatic reflexes. Visceral symptoms may be the primary manifestations of somatic dysfunction and vice versa. This chapter examines the organization of the autonomic nervous system and its afferent component and emphasizes the pattern of innervation reaching the major organs of the thoracoabdominopelvic viscera and the segmental representation of these organs in the spinal cord.

ORGANIZATION OF THE AUTONOMIC NERVOUS SYSTEM

The autonomic nervous system has components in both the central and peripheral nervous systems (Fig. 6.1). The major autonomic components of the central nervous system (CNS) include:

Limbic forebrain
Hypothalamus
Several brainstem nuclei
Intermediolateral cell column of the spinal cord

The autonomic components of the peripheral nervous system (PNS) include numerous ganglia (collections of neuron cell bodies located outside of the central nervous system) and a network of fibers distributed to all tissues of the body with the exception of the hyaline cartilages, the centers of the intervertebral disks, and the parenchymal tissues of the central nervous system. This review focuses on the peripheral distribution of the autonomic nervous system.

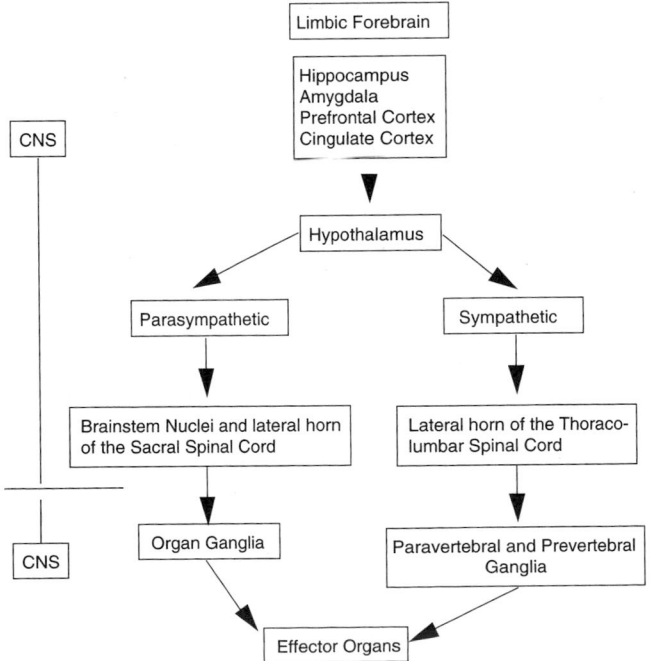

FIGURE 6.1. General organization of the autonomic nervous system. CNS, central nervous system; PNS, peripheral nervous system.

Peripheral Nervous Systems

The axons from neurons located in the CNS enter the periphery through spinal and cranial nerves. The peripheral portion of the nervous system can be divided into two fundamental parts based on the target structures of efferent fibers. Axons derived from the somatic component of the peripheral nervous system innervate skeletal muscle. Axons derived from the autonomic component of the peripheral nervous system enter the periphery and form complex interwoven plexuses containing clusters of cell bodies called ganglia. Neurons in these ganglia innervate all other targets, including:

Smooth muscle
Cardiac muscle
Glands
Connective tissue
Cells in the immune system

This fundamental division in the peripheral nervous system also reflects differential methods in cellular communication. The mechanism of transmission in the neuromuscular junction of the somatic system involves ionotrophic principles (2). This mechanism uses the ion-gated channels to quickly depolarize the cell membrane, a process referred to as fast transmission. Conversely, chemical signaling in the autonomic peripheral nervous system uses metabotrophic principles and volume transmission (3), the diffusion of transmitter substance away from axonal vesicles, as well as fast synaptic transmission. The metabotrophic methods of signaling usually involve a neuromodulator that binds to a membrane receptor, activating second-messenger pathways within the target cell. These methods are also called slow transmission and often lead to altered gene expression. To further understand the distinction between somatic and visceral peripheral nervous systems, compare the typical neural circuitry present in reflex arcs.

SOMATIC REFLEX ARC

Input and output for the peripheral somatic nervous system occur through spinal and cranial nerves. Fig. 6.2 diagrams a typical spinal nerve, illustrating the basic circuitry of the somatic reflex arc. In its simplest form, the reflex arc contains a primary afferent neuron in a ganglion and a centrally located motor neuron connected by a synaptic junction. Because only one synapse separates the input from the output, this circuit is called a monosynaptic reflex. The cell body of the primary sensory neuron is located in the dorsal root ganglia or in the peripheral ganglia of a cranial nerve. The peripheral process of the sensory neuron is directed outward along a spinal or cranial nerve to reach its target in the peripheral tissue. This process either acts as a receptor end organ itself or is attached to one located in skin, muscle, or connective tissue. Each sensory neuron also has a central process (axon) that extends into the dorsal horn of the spinal cord or into the brainstem.

Two fundamental types of primary afferent neurons are present in sensory ganglia. One class of sensory neuron features a large cell body with a myelinated process; this kind of cell forms the A-afferent or large-caliber fiber system and is involved

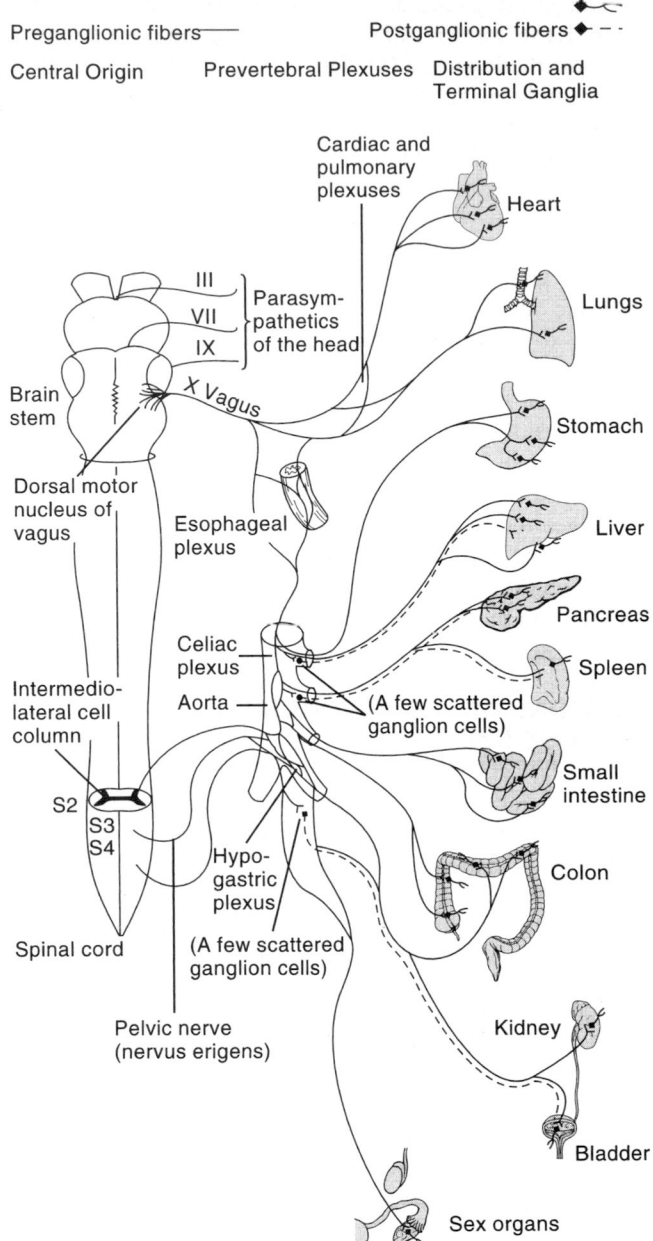

FIGURE 6.5. Parasympathetic division of peripheral autonomic system. From Chusid JG. *Correlative Neuroanatomy and Functional Neurology.* Los Altos, CA: Lange Medical Publishers; 1985, with permission.

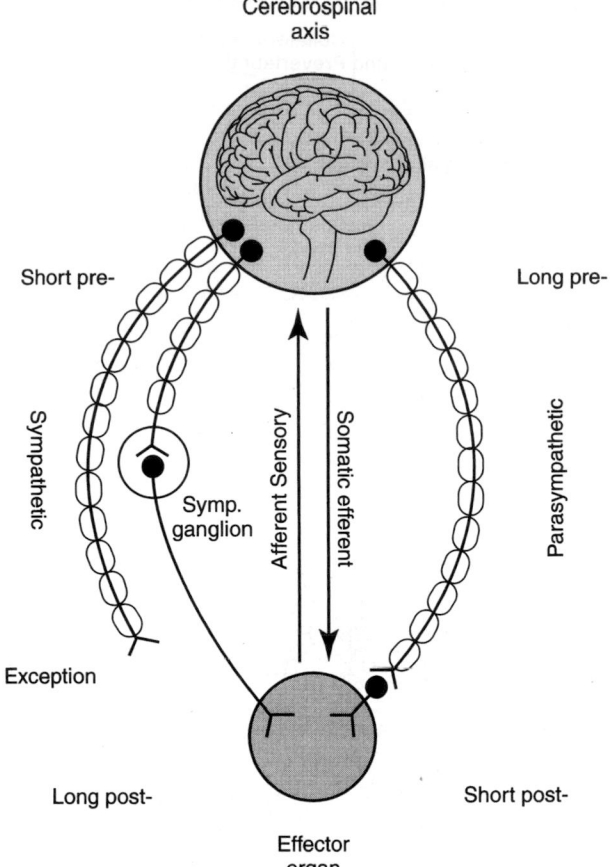

FIGURE 6.6. Major anatomical differences between sympathetic and parasympathetic divisions of autonomic system. From Harati Y. Anatomy of the spinal and peripheral autonomic nervous system. In: Low P, ed. *Clinical Autonomic Disorders.* Boston, MA: Little, Brown and Company; 1993, with permission.

parasympathetic system secrete acetylcholine and a wide variety of other neuron modulators such as the neuropeptides. Given that these two divisions of the autonomic nervous system can be differentiated on the basis of their anatomy and chemistry, it is not surprising that they have differing influences on their target organs.

Sympathetic Autonomic Nervous System

The sympathetic autonomic nervous system has two major components: vascular and visceral. The vascular component is associated with the spinal nerves and innervates:

Fascia
Smooth muscle of vasculature
Smooth muscle of hair follicles
Secretory cells in the sweat glands of the skin

The visceral component innervates:

Smooth muscle
Cardiac muscle
Nodal tissue
Glandular organs of the thoracic, abdominal, pelvic, and perineal viscera

sympathetic system arises from cholinergic preganglionic neurons located in the lateral horn of the thoracic and lumbar spinal cord; it is also called the thoracolumbar system. In general, the postganglionic neurons of the sympathetic system are adrenergic and secrete norepinephrine. However, there are important exceptions. For example, some cholinergic ganglionic neurons contribute to the innervation of the hair follicles and sweat glands as well as possibly innervating the vasculature in skeletal muscle (7). The parasympathetic system arises from cholinergic preganglionic neurons located in either cranial nerve nuclei of the brainstem or the lateral horn of the sacral spinal cord, and it is therefore called the craniosacral system. The postganglionic neurons of the

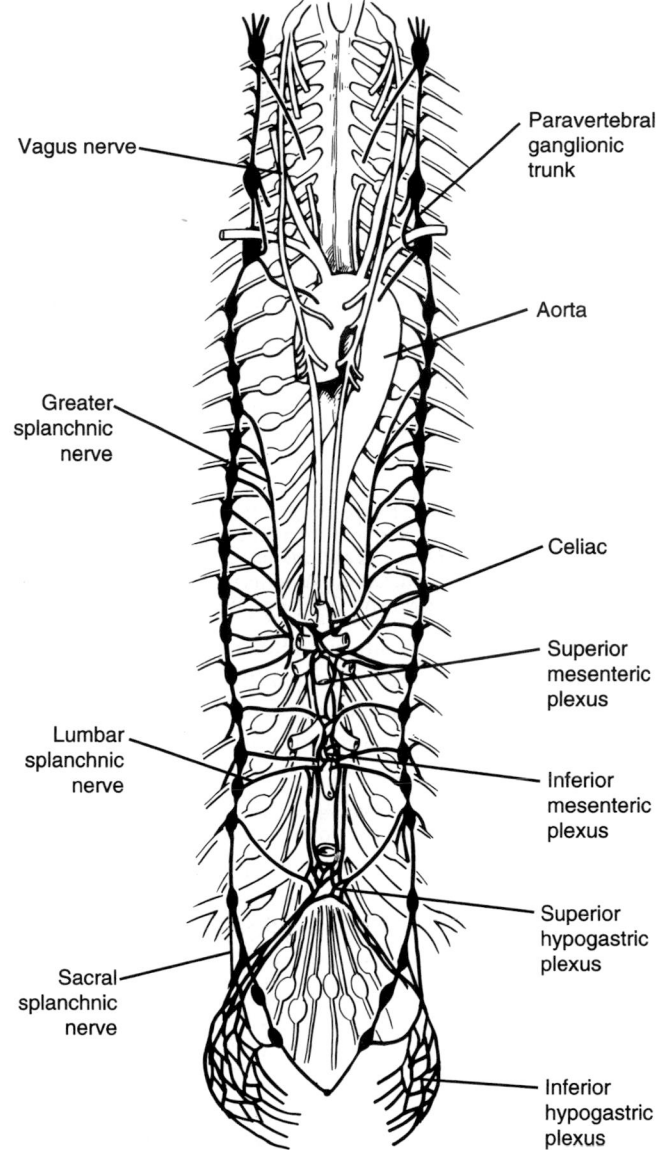

Vagus nerve

Paravertebral
ganglionic
trunk

Aorta

Greater
splanchnic
nerve

Celiac

Superior
mesenteric
plexus

Lumbar
splanchnic
nerve

Inferior
mesenteric
plexus

Superior
hypogastric
plexus

Sacral
splanchnic
nerve

Inferior
hypogastric
plexus

FIGURE 6.7. Paravertebral ganglia (sympathetic trunk) lying along median axis of body. From Rohen JW, Yokochi C. *Color Atlas of Anatomy.* New York, NY: Igaku-Shoin Medical Publishers; 1983, with permission.

tional small clusters of prevertebral ganglia are found scattered in the autonomic plexus of the pelvic basin.

The detailed organization of the sympathetic system is illustrated in Fig. 6.4. The following features are critical:

1. All preganglionic cell bodies are located in the lateral horn of spinal cord segments primarily between T1 and L2; however, they can extend as high as C7 and as low as L3. Their axons leave the spinal cord through ventral roots T1-L2 and course along the corresponding spinal nerves to reach white communicating rami (Fig. 6.8). The white rami carry the myelinated, preganglionic fibers from the spinal nerve directly into the paravertebral ganglia. They also carry sensory processes from the vasculature and viscera back to the spinal nerve.

2. The paravertebral ganglia are present on both sides of the spinal cord in the following distribution (8):
   - Three cervical segments (superior, middle, and stellate)
   - Ten to 12 thoracic segments
   - Four lumbar segments
   - At least four or five sacral segments

   Often the upper thoracic and lower cervical ganglia are fused to form the stellate ganglion. Only the ganglia between T1 and L2 receive white rami, because preganglionic fibers arise from only these segments.

3. Neurons in paravertebral ganglia located either above T1 or below L2 receive their innervation from preganglionic fibers arising in spinal segments T1-L2. These preganglionic axons enter the sympathetic trunk at their segmental level of origin and ascend or descend through the trunk to reach ganglia positioned above or below T1-L2.

4. Ganglionic neurons destined to innervate blood vessels, smooth muscles, and glands of the skin are found in all the paravertebral ganglia. Their postganglionic axons gain access to spinal nerves by passing over gray rami (Fig. 6.8). All paravertebral ganglia give rise to gray rami; each spinal nerve receives at least one gray ramus. The postganglionic axons follow the spinal nerves distally before shifting to assume a position in the fascia along the wall of a blood vessel.

5. Ganglionic neurons with axons innervating thoracic, abdominal, and pelvic viscera are found in the three cervical ganglia, the upper five thoracic paravertebral ganglia, and the prevertebral ganglia. These are the celiac and the superior and inferior mesenteric ganglia, as well as small scattered ganglia in the pelvic plexus. These prevertebral ganglia receive their preganglionic axons through thoracic, lumbar, and sacral splanchnic nerves. The term splanchnic refers to the viscera; splanchnic nerves are simply visceral nerves. Thoracic, lumbar, and sacral splanchnic nerves carry sympathetic fibers and pelvic splanchnic nerves carry parasympathetic fibers.

The sympathetic ganglia receive information from the central nervous system through the axons of the preganglionic neurons. A preganglionic axon of the sympathetic system has a number of options after passing through a white ramus between T1 and L2 to enter a paravertebral ganglion:

1. It can innervate a ganglionic neuron in the paravertebral ganglion at its spinal cord level of entry.

Also, portions of the sympathetic visceral system provide an innervation to the neurons of the parasympathetic ganglia in the walls of the visceral organs.

The ganglionic neurons of the sympathetic nervous system are located in two types of ganglia: paravertebral and prevertebral (Fig. 6.4). The paravertebral ganglia form two long chains called the sympathetic trunks, which are located on either side of the vertebral column (Fig. 6.7). Each sympathetic trunk extends from the upper cervical vertebrae along the heads of the ribs in the thorax, on the sides of the lumbar vertebral bodies in the abdomen, and along the ventromedial aspect of the sacroiliac joint in the pelvis. Inferiorly, the two trunks terminate by uniting to form the ganglion impar, a small neural structure on the ventral aspect of the coccygeal vertebrae. The three major prevertebral ganglia are found in clusters, embedded in the abdominal plexuses that surround the anterior branches of the aorta. Addi-

Histaminergic
Purinergic

In general, the adrenergic fibers function as constrictors, contracting smooth muscle in the tunica media and increasing the resistance in the peripheral vasculature. These norepinephrine-containing fibers arise from the paravertebral ganglia of the sympathetic nervous system and innervate all vasculature of the body. Cholinergic fibers are much fewer in number in most tissue, and are vasodilating in nature. These nerves are of mixed origin, and most often arise from the parasympathetic ganglia innervating the vasculature in the head and neck and the visceral organs of the thorax, abdomen, and pelvis. Cholinergic vasodilator fibers, innervating blood vessels in the extremities, arise in the sympathetic trunk of some mammals; however, the importance of this system is in humans is not known (16). Purinergic and histaminergic axons also mediate relaxation of vascular wall smooth muscle, but their origin and role in vasodilation are not clear (14).

The sympathetic innervation of blood vessels in muscle and skin is accomplished by preganglionic neurons located in the lateral horn of spinal segments T2 through L2-3. Their axons leave the spinal cord in the ventral roots and pass through white rami to innervate neurons located in the paravertebral ganglia (Fig. 6.8). Vasomotor neurons present in the paravertebral ganglia give rise to axons that leave the ganglia over the gray rami to rejoin the spinal nerves. In this way, they reach the somatic peripheral tissue where they innervate blood vessels, sweat glands, and hair follicles. A topographic map of the vasculature in the body is contained within paravertebral ganglia such that (17,18):

1. The vasomotor fibers to the head and neck come from spinal segments T1-4. Their axons travel superiorly in the sympathetic trunk to reach the cervical ganglia. Postganglionic axons follow the carotid vascular tree to reach the head and neck. Segments T1-2 provide innervation for the brain and meninges; T2-4 provides innervation to the vasculature of the face and neck.

2. The vasomotor fibers to the upper extremity come from spinal segments T5-7. Their axons course superiorly in the sympathetic trunk to reach the upper thoracic and lower cervical ganglia. Postganglionic axons join the spinal nerves of the brachial plexus to reach the vasculature of the upper extremity.

3. The vasomotor fibers to the lower extremity come from spinal segments T10 through L2-3. Their axons descend in the sympathetic trunk to reach the lower lumbar and sacral ganglia. Postganglionic axons join the spinal nerves of the lumbosacral plexus to reach the vasculature of the lower extremity.

Sympathetic fibers course along the outer border of the tunica media of the artery and secrete their neuroregulators into the extracellular fluids surrounding the vascular smooth muscle. Most sympathetic fibers release norepinephrine from small swellings along the terminal distribution of the axon. This neuromodulator interacts with its specific receptors on the vascular smooth muscle cell membranes. Both α- and β-adrenergic receptors are present on these plasma membranes (19). Activation of α-adrenoceptors leads to contraction of the smooth muscle cells and vasoconstriction, while activation of the β-adrenoceptors mediates relaxation of the muscle cell, resulting in vasodilatation.

In general, the α-adrenoceptors predominate on the smooth muscle of resistance vessels; therefore adrenergic stimulation yields vasoconstriction in skeletal muscle.

Additional control of skeletal muscle resistance arteries is accomplished through numerous endothelium-derived substances such as the vasodilator nitric oxide or the vasoconstrictors prostacyclin, endothelin, and angiotensin (20). The tone in the vessel wall is the product of a complex interaction of these vasoactive substances (21). Neurally mediated, active vasodilation of cutaneous capillary bed is well established in the literature (16). Sympathetic cholinergic fibers do not appear to innervate the cutaneous vascular tree; instead, a nonadrenergic, noncholinergic vasodilatory mechanism exists for these vessels (22). Neurally mediated, active vasodilation of skeletal muscle vascular beds appears to be doubtful and has recently been questioned (16).

Along with the efferent innervation of the vascular tree, afferent or sensory fibers also course in the walls of the blood vessels. Little is known of the sensory feedback to the spinal cord provided by these fibers. The nomenclature of these afferent fibers is confusing because it is not clear whether they are somatic or visceral afferent fibers. Jinkins and colleagues (23) have termed the vascular afferent fibers found in somatic tissue "somatosympathetic fibers" because they course through somatic tissue but are related to the autonomic nervous system. However, because these afferent fibers are generally small caliber and contain an array of neuropeptides such as substance-P, much of the information they carry is most likely related to nociceptive stimuli. The normal, baseline release of neuropeptides such as substance-P from these fibers may play an important role in maintaining vascular tone (24). Thus, the small-caliber, primary afferent fibers appear to have additional homeostatic functions in the peripheral tissue beyond that of nociception.

When irritated, some of these small-caliber, sensory axons can secrete quantities of substance-P (a proinflammatory, vasodilatory neuropeptide) into the surrounding tissue. This release of an inflammatory agent from a peripheral nerve terminal is involved in initiating the processes of neurogenic inflammation and edema (25). Neurogenic inflammation is a critical component in inflammatory joint disease, which suggests an important role for the small-caliber, primary afferent fibers in these diseases (26).

An interaction between sensory axons and sympathetic neurons appears to occur in the peripheral tissues. Sympathetic adrenergic terminals often end in close association with the peripheral processes of sensory neurons. Secretion of norepinephrine can increase the levels of prostaglandins E2 and I2 in the tissue (27). Prostaglandins are irritating to many small-caliber, primary afferent fibers. Sufficient sympathetic discharge therefore can result in a nociceptive input to the spinal cord. In addition, evidence strongly suggests that small-caliber, primary afferent fibers can become sensitized to sympathetic nervous system activity (27). This interaction between sympathetic efferent axons and primary afferent neurons is a possible mechanism for sympathetically dependent hyperalgesia such as that present in reflex sympathetic dystrophy (28).

Sweat Glands and Connective Tissue

Along with innervating the vasculature, the peripheral autonomic fibers also provide an innervation to sweat glands and fascia.

Sweat glands receive an exclusively cholinergic innervation from the sympathetic trunk ganglia; these fibers are termed the sympathetic cholinergic system (15). The cholinergic fibers stimulate secretory activity in the gland.

Small-caliber, neuropeptide-containing, primary afferent fibers innervate all forms of connective tissue. These fibers often course in close association with adrenergic sympathetic axons and blood vessels. A close relationship between these fibers and the connective tissue components of the fascia is seen in such tissue as the:

Cranial dura (29,30)
Gastrointestinal tract (31)
Synovium of diarthrodial joints (32)

In several locations, such as joints, these fibers have been demonstrated to play a role in modulating the cellular components (mast cells) of the connective tissue and to contribute to the maintenance of tissue integrity (32,33). Finally, the interaction of these two fiber types appears to play an important role in the maintenance of normal vascular tone in connective tissue (24).

Head and Neck

The autonomic innervation of the head and neck arises from two general sources: sympathetic and parasympathetic. The sympathetic innervation originates in the intermediolateral nucleus of the upper thoracic segments (T1-4) of the spinal cord, and their ganglionic neurons are located in the cervical sympathetic ganglia of the neck. Postganglionic fibers from the superior cervical ganglion enter the head following the course of the carotid and vertebral arteries and the jugular vein. The parasympathetic innervation originates from several nuclei in the brainstem, and the ganglionic neurons are located in these ganglia (Fig. 6.9):

Ciliary sphenopalatine
Otic
Geniculate

Recently, additional parasympathetic ganglia located on the walls of the internal carotid artery have been described (34–36). The autonomic innervation of the cranial viscera, the function of these nerves, and the neurology of their dysfunction are amply described elsewhere (17,37–40).

The third cranial nerve contains parasympathetic axons that arise in the Edinger-Westphal nucleus of the midbrain and innervate the ciliary ganglion of the eye (Fig. 6.9). These axons are responsible for constricting the pupil through the pupillary sphincter muscles and contracting the ciliary body to thicken the lens in the accommodation reflex. The facial (VII) cranial nerve carries parasympathetic preganglionic axons from the superior salivatory and lacrimal nuclei in the pontine region of the brainstem. These secretomotor and vasomotor axons course along the superficial petrosal nerve to reach the sphenopalatine ganglion. Postganglionic axons follow branches of the trigeminal nerve to reach the lacrimal gland and mucosal glands of the nasal and oral cavities. Preganglionic axons from the superior salivatory nucleus also follow the chorda tympani, a branch of the facial nerve, to reach the submandibular and sublingual ganglia. Postganglionic axons from these ganglia supply the salivatory glands on the floor

of the mouth. The glossopharyngeal nerve carries secretomotor and vasomotor axons from the inferior salivatory nucleus located at the pontomedullary border to the otic ganglion. These latter axons pass over the lesser petrosal nerve. Postganglionic axons from the otic ganglion extend to the parotid gland over branches of the third division of the trigeminal nerve.

Cranial nerve X, the vagus, is the largest of the parasympathetic nerves. It supplies preganglionic parasympathetic innervation of the viscera in the thorax and abdomen to the level of the splenic flexure in the transverse colon. Efferent vagal axons arise in the dorsal motor nucleus and nucleus ambiguous of the medulla. The vagus is largely a sensory nerve; afferent fibers outnumber efferent fibers in the mammalian vagus by more than 10:1 (41). These sensory fibers include the afferent innervation of the thoracoabdominal viscera and the general sensory innervation of the:

Pharynx
Larynx
Skin of the ear
External auditory meatus
External surface of the tympanic membrane

The cell bodies for these afferent fibers are located in the two nuclei of the vagus: the superior (jugular) ganglion and the inferior ganglion. Their central brainstem targets include the nucleus solitarius, nucleus ambiguous, and spinal trigeminal nucleus.

An area of much recent interest is the autonomic innervation of the vascular and dural systems in the head. Preganglionic sympathetic input to the cranial vasculature and dura arises in the upper thoracic spinal segments. Those controlling the vasculature of the brain and meninges are located in segments T1-2, and those involved with the vasculature of the face and neck are located in T2-4 (17). Ganglionic neurons are located in the superior cervical sympathetic ganglion and in small ganglia embedded in the fibers of the internal carotid nerve (18). Their axons course along the carotid arteries; those going to the cerebral vessels and dura form the well-developed internal carotid nerve. Within the dura, the adrenergic fibers diverge away from the vasculature to form a dense plexus within the connective tissue substrate of the dura itself (30). The extensive autonomic innervation may play a role in regulating the metabolic activity of the dural tissue. The sympathetic innervation of the dura and associated vasculature is of interest due to its proposed role in the cause of migraine headache (42).

Parasympathetic axons innervating the cerebral vasculature arise in these ganglia: sphenopalatine, otic, and internal carotid (36,43–45). Axons from the ganglia contain acetylcholine and neuropeptides such as vasoactive intestinal polypeptide and neuropeptide-Y, among others (35,46). The axons form a delicate plexus wrapped around cerebral arteries as they travel through the subarachnoid space. Primary afferent fibers containing neuropeptides such as substance-P and calcitonin gene–related polypeptide are also present in the plexus surrounding the cerebral vessels. These fibers arise in the ophthalmic and maxillary divisions of the trigeminal ganglion (47) and constitute the "trigeminovascular system" (48). Similar primary afferent fibers containing substance-P and calcitonin gene–related polypeptide have been described in the dura mater (30). Some of these fibers form free endings and are postulated to have trophic relationships with the connective tissue cells in the dura such as the fibroblast and mast cells. Release of these proinflammatory peptides has been indicated in the pathogenesis of certain inflammatory headaches such as the migraine and cluster varieties (49,50).

Thorax

A large autonomic plexus of fibers extends from the superior mediastinum inferiorly through the posterior mediastinum and continues into the abdominopelvic cavity, using the esophageal hiatus of the diaphragm as a conduit (Fig. 6.10). In total, this complex arrangement of fibers is best termed the thoracic plexus, although it has several regionally named components. The thoracic plexus is derived from the vagus nerve and its branches and from splanchnic branches from the paravertebral ganglia. The thoracic plexus is located near the midline and divided approximately into two parts: superior and inferior. Superiorly, this complex arrangement of fibers contains the interwoven cardiac and pulmonary plexuses that are distributed around the great vessels of the heart and the large airways. Inferiorly, it contains the esophageal plexus wrapped around the esophagus as it courses through the posterior mediastinum. Fig. 6.11 is a schematic

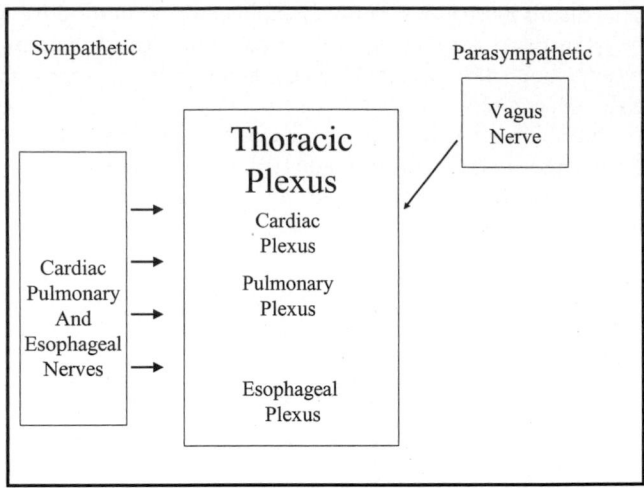

FIGURE 6.11. A schematic diagram illustrating the thoracic plexus and its associated systems. The thoracic, cardiac, pulmonary, and esophageal nerves are a source of sympathetic postganglionic fibers into the plexus. The vagus nerve is a source of parasympathetic preganglionic fibers to the plexus. Organ ganglia for the parasympathetic system will be found within the parts of the thoracic plexus.

diagram illustrating the thoracic plexus. Branches from this autonomic plexus in the thorax supply the following with afferent and efferent nerves:

Heart
Trachea
Bronchi
Lungs
Esophagus
Thoracic duct

Sympathetic innervation of the thoracic viscera arises in spinal cord segments T1 through T5 or T6. Axons from these preganglionic neurons synapse with ganglionic neurons in the superior, middle, and inferior cervical ganglia as well as in the sympathetic trunk ganglia T1 to T5-6. Sympathetic postganglionic axons from these paravertebral ganglia join the thoracic plexus via a series of small, delicate cardiac, pulmonary, and esophageal nerves. Within the thoracic plexus, sympathetic cardiac and pulmonary nerves descend through the superior mediastinum joining with similarly named parasympathetic branches from the vagus and recurrent laryngeal nerves. They form the complex cardiopulmonary plexus of fibers surrounding the great vessels of the heart (Fig. 6.12) and the vasculature and airway structures of the lungs (Fig. 6.13). The individual superior, middle, and inferior cardiac nerves of the sympathetic trunk and vagus are extremely inconsistent in actual form (51). The esophageal sympathetic nerves arise from the thoracic paravertebral ganglia and course diagonally downward across the thoracic vertebral bodies to reach the adventitial fascia surrounding the esophagus in the posterior mediastinum. Here, they join with the main trunks of the vagus nerve (parasympathetic) to form the esophageal plexus.

The mixing of parasympathetic and sympathetic axons begins in the most superior aspect of the thoracic autonomic plexus as it extends upward into the cervical region. Scattered communicating branches unite the vagus and recurrent laryngeal nerves

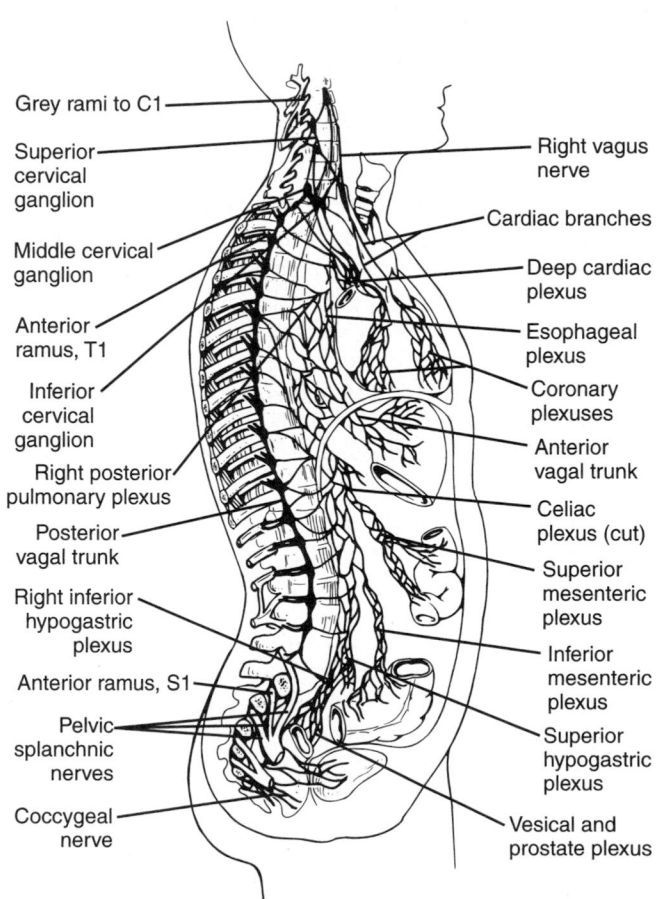

Grey rami to C1
Superior cervical ganglion
Middle cervical ganglion
Anterior ramus, T1
Inferior cervical ganglion
Right posterior pulmonary plexus
Posterior vagal trunk
Right inferior hypogastric plexus
Anterior ramus, S1
Pelvic splanchnic nerves
Coccygeal nerve

Right vagus nerve
Cardiac branches
Deep cardiac plexus
Esophageal plexus
Coronary plexuses
Anterior vagal trunk
Celiac plexus (cut)
Superior mesenteric plexus
Inferior mesenteric plexus
Superior hypogastric plexus
Vesical and prostate plexus

FIGURE 6.10. Great autonomic plexus extending from the lower cervical region through the thorax and abdomen to reach the pelvis. From Bannister LH, Berry MM, Collins P, et al, eds. *Gray's Anatomy.* New York, NY: Churchill Livingstone; 1995, with permission.

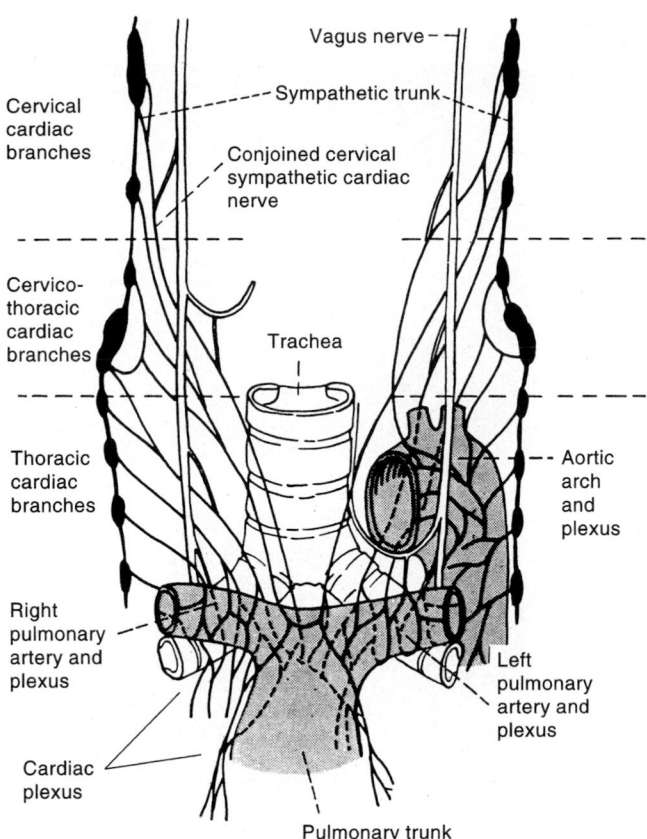

FIGURE 6.12. Nerve supply of heart. From Bonica JJ. General considerations of pain in the chest. In: Bonica JJ. *The Management of Pain.* Philadelphia, PA: Lea & Febiger; 1990, with permission.

with the sympathetic trunk. Therefore, even at the most superior aspect of the plexus, there are no pure sympathetic or parasympathetic nerves. Also, all fibers in the plexus contain a mixture of afferent and efferent axons, so the plexus cannot be considered a purely efferent structure either.

Cardiovascular Plexus

The cardiac plexus represents a region of the thoracic plexus closely related to the innervation of the heart. The cardiac plexus consists of a mixture of sympathetic and parasympathetic fibers (as well as afferent fibers) woven around the great vessels of the heart (Fig. 6.12). Sympathetic input to the cardiac plexus arises from preganglionic neurons located in the nucleus intermediolateralis of the lateral horn of the spinal cord extending from segments T1 to T5. This column of spinal cord neurons contains a topographic map of the heart. The ventricular innervation is represented in the higher thoracic segments, but the atrial representation is found in the lower segments (52). This inverted cardiac map results from the embryologic origin of the heart; the ventricular system forms superior to the atrial system (53). The preganglionic axons of the spinal cord neurons enter the sympathetic trunk by passing over white rami in the upper thoracic segments. Once in the trunk, most of these fibers ascend to reach their ganglionic neurons located primarily in the two to three cervical ganglia. Variable numbers of cervical and thoracic

sympathetic cardiac nerves leave the cervical and upper thoracic ganglia, course through the fascia of the mediastinum, and join the cardiac branches of the vagus to form the cardiac plexus. This plexus is primarily located on the walls of the pulmonary arterial tree (54).

The parasympathetic input to the cardiac plexus arises from preganglionic neurons in the dorsal motor nucleus of the vagus and the nucleus ambiguous of the medulla (55,56). These preganglionic axons leave the vagus nerve over its variable (one to three) cardiac branches beginning in the neck and extending into the superior mediastinum. The axons target a parasympathetic ganglion embedded in the cardiac plexuses, termed Wristberg's ganglion. Short cholinergic axons from these ganglia reach the sinoatrial and atrioventricular nodes and course in the myocardium of the ventricles. The parasympathetic innervation of the ventricular wall is much less dense than that of the sympathetic fibers (57).

From the cardiac plexus, sympathetic adrenergic and parasympathetic cholinergic, postganglionic axons form a rich network of fibers distributed along the coronary vasculature, coursing throughout the myocardium of the atria and ventricles, and reaching the sinoatrial and atrioventricular nodes (57). The innervation of the intrinsic nodal system of the heart is bilaterally asymmetric; the right side of the plexus favors the sinoatrial (SA) node but the left side of the plexus tends to target the atrioventricular (AV) node. Thus, stimulation of the sympathetic fibers on the left side accelerates cardiac output but is arrhythmogenic because it is directed to the AV node (58). A similar reaction is obtained by cooling the right sympathetic fibers, indicating that cardiac activity is influenced by the balance of activity between the two sympathetic inputs (58). Stimulation of the parasympathetic vagal fibers tends to stabilize heart rate. It appears that the balance of tonic neural activity occurring in the vagus and sympathetic systems influences, in part, heart rate and volume output.

Cardiac afferent nerves are an important consideration in understanding reflex control of the heart, patterns of referred cardiac pain, and patterns of cardiac facilitated segments. Small-caliber, primary afferent fibers are distributed throughout the (59–61):

> Myocardium
> Coronary vasculature
> Roots of its great vessel
> Parietal pericardium

There are at least two different pathways for these cardiac sensory fibers. Those coursing with the sympathetic nerves have their cell bodies located in dorsal root ganglia extending from C6 to T7, and their central processes terminate in the dorsal horn of the spinal cord (62,63). Sensory axons coursing with the parasympathetic nerves have cell bodies located in the nodose ganglion of the vagus nerve and central processes that terminate in the solitary nucleus of the medulla. In addition to the autonomic nerves supplying an afferent innervation of the pericardium, afferent fibers reach this structure over the phrenic nerve as well. These phrenic afferent fibers enter the spinal cord over segments C3-5.

Along with the dual origin of sensory nerves, there is a differential distribution of these two sensory pathways in the

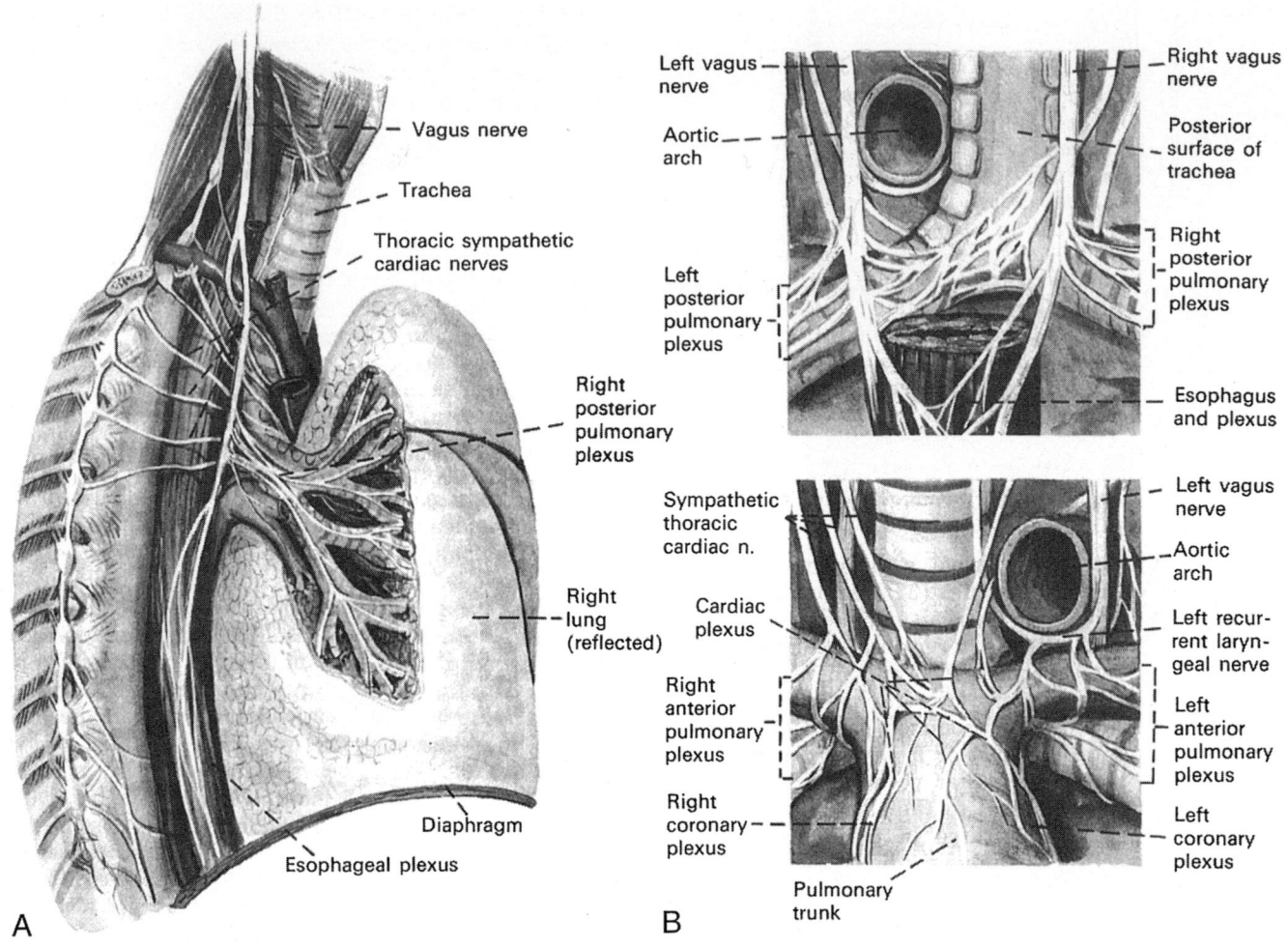

FIGURE 6.13. Innervation of lung. From Bonica JJ. General considerations of pain in the chest. In: Bonica JJ, ed. *The Management of Pain.* Philadelphia, PA: Lea & Febiger; 1990:981, with permission.

cardiovascular system. The afferent fibers of the vagus nerve terminate in the (61):

Ascending aorta
Aortic arch
Pulmonary trunk
Arterial walls
Atrial walls
Atrioventricular valve
Ventricular walls

The afferent fibers from the sympathetic nerves reach the (60):

Atrial walls
Pulmonary arteries
Atrioventricular and aortic valves
Parietal peritoneum

Afferent fibers from both systems reach the coronary arteries. Those from the vagus extend to a more distal level of the vasculature closer to the apex of the heart than do afferent fibers associated with the sympathetic nervous system. Both Aδ- and

C-afferent fibers are present in the heart (64). Many of these fibers contain neuropeptides such as substance-P or calcitonin gene–related polypeptide that are typical of small-caliber, primary afferent fibers. At least one population of these cardiac C-fibers has the physiologic properties of nociceptive axons.

In general, the afferent fibers coursing with the sympathetic nerves are involved with cardiac nociception, and those following the parasympathetic nerves are mainly involved in reflexogenic regulation of heart functions through their brainstem connection (62). Section of the sympathetic nerves to the heart can relieve cardiac pain in the chest, arms, and neck (65). These cardiac afferent fibers enter the spinal cord over a range of segments from C6 to T7, but the influence of these nerves can extend at least two segments below T7 (66). The signs of segmental facilitation due to cardiac disease can present in the vicinity of the cervicothoracic junction and extend downward through at least T9 (67). Importantly, the nociceptive afferent fibers reaching the dorsal horn of the spinal cord influence neurons with concomitant somatic receptive fields. This viscerosomatic convergence of nociceptive information provides an explanation for the referral of pain from cardiac structures to the body wall and extremity (68).

Respiratory Plexus

The airways of the respiratory system receive their innervation through the large pulmonary plexus that surrounds the pulmonary artery and extends onto the posterior surface of the trachea and bronchi (Fig. 6.13). Sympathetic preganglionic neurons that contribute to this plexus are located in the lateral horn of spinal segments T2-7, and their ganglionic neurons are located in the cervical and first four thoracic ganglia. Postganglionic axons from these ganglia course through cardiac and esophageal nerves from the sympathetic trunk to reach the pulmonary plexus. These adrenergic axons primarily target the glandular tissue surrounding the bronchi and bronchioles; little direct adrenergic innervation of the bronchial musculature has been noted. β-adrenergic receptors are present on the glandular cells and on bronchial smooth muscle cells. Stimulation of the β-adrenergic, sympathetic nervous system leads to bronchial dilation and the release of a more viscous secretion (69).

The vagus nerve is the source of parasympathetic innervation for the respiratory airways. After entering the thorax, the vagus shifts posteriorly in the mediastinum to pass behind the root of the lung. Anterior and posterior pulmonary branches are given off that contribute to the pulmonary plexus. Parasympathetic ganglia located in the walls of the airways receive preganglionic fibers from these vagal branches. Postganglionic parasympathetic fibers course in the arteriobronchial tree to terminate around bronchial smooth musculature, mucosal glands, and blood vessels. Stimulation of these cholinergic fibers causes (69):

Bronchoconstriction
Hypersecretion of a serous secretion
Vasodilation

The pulmonary plexus and ganglia contain intrinsic neurons, i.e., cells whose processes remain in the peripheral tissue and do not innervate the central nervous system. Such cells are called interneurons. Some of these cells produce a variety of neuropeptides, among which is vasoactive intestinal polypeptide, a potent bronchodilator (70). In addition, several neuropeptides corelease with norepinephrine from sympathetic terminals and with acetylcholine from parasympathetic terminals. These ubiquitous neuropeptides have recently gained considerable interest due to their role in controlling the diameter of the bronchial lumen and the initiation of bronchial wall inflammation (71).

Small-caliber, primary afferent fibers are also present in the pulmonary plexus. These fibers provide sensory information to the brainstem via the vagus and to the spinal cord via the sympathetic trunk. This information is involved in reflex arcs related to:

Sneezing
Coughing
Bronchospasms
Pulmonary congestion

Many of these fibers, and particularly the smallest of them, contain neuropeptides such as substance-P and calcitonin gene–related polypeptide, among others. Irritation of these sensory fibers results in the release of proinflammatory substances, leading to neurogenic edema and inflammation in the lung. Substance-P, released from these sensory axons into the pulmonary parenchyma, is a potent bronchoconstrictor, vasodilator, and secretagogue (72).

Activation of these primary afferent nociceptors can also facilitate segments in the spinal cord extending from the cervical region into the low thoracic cord (67). The extended range of activation most likely relates to the wide distribution of the central processes of these primary afferent fibers. Changes in spinal cord activity are seen in response to pulmonary afferent stimulation. Electrical stimulation of inflamed tracheobronchial mucosa produces a decrease in electrical skin resistance in the T2-5 dermatomes followed by cutaneous hyperalgesia hours later (65). Unlike the heart, pain from the lungs and bronchial tree is carried in the vagal fibers as well as in the spinal afferent fibers. Lung tumors can refer pain to the skin around the ear (73), which is a region of the head innervated by small cutaneous branches of the vagus nerve. Electrical stimulation of the laryngeal and tracheal mucosa refers pain to the neck, and similar irritation of the bronchial tree refers pain to the anterior chest wall. Section of the vagus nerve below the recurrent laryngeal branch ameliorates the pain (74), suggesting that the nerve is the conduit for this referred pain.

The costal parietal pleura receive an afferent innervation derived from the intercostal nerves of the thorax. The mediastinal pleura are innervated by sensory fibers from the phrenic nerve, and diaphragmatic pleura is innervated by twigs from the intercostal nerves (65). The parietal plural membrane is sensitive to noxious stimuli. The visceral pleura in the lungs receive sympathetic and sensory fibers from the autonomic plexuses surrounding the bronchi, but is insensitive to pain (65).

Esophageal Plexus

The esophagus extends from an upper sphincter region located at the inferior border of the pharynx to a lower sphincter region located at the border of the stomach. Along its route, the body of the esophagus is lodged in the loose connective tissues of the superior and posterior mediastinum.

The upper esophageal sphincter is mainly derived from the cricopharyngeus and thyropharyngeus muscles (together they compose the inferior pharyngeal constrictor), which receive their innervation from the pharyngeal plexus composed of the superior laryngeal and pharyngeal branches of the vagus nerve (75). The body of the esophagus is surrounded by a plexus of autonomic nerves derived from the inferior laryngeal branch of the vagus and esophageal branches of the sympathetic trunk (76). The superior portion of the esophagus is a mixture of skeletal and smooth muscle, although the lower portion is composed of smooth muscle only. The preganglionic parasympathetic innervation to the superior portion of the esophagus (skeletal muscle portion) is derived from the nucleus ambiguous. The smooth muscle of the esophagus is derived primarily from the dorsal motor nucleus of the vagus nerve (77). The left and right vagal trunks approach the esophagus at the root of the lung and form an elaborate plexus, which follows this structure through the esophageal hiatus in the diaphragm. The postganglionic parasympathetic neurons are contained in two intrinsic ganglia in the walls of the esophagus: Auerbach's, or the myenteric plexus, and Meissner's, or the submucosal plexus. Sympathetic preganglionic neurons are located in the intermediolateral nucleus of spinal cord segments ranging from T2-8 (78):

Cervical esophageal portion T2-4
Thoracic esophageal portion T3-6
Abdominal portion T5-8

The preganglionic axons synapse in the cervical and upper thoracic sympathetic ganglia. Small esophageal branches, derived from the cervical to fourth and fifth thoracic ganglia and carrying postganglionic sympathetic fibers, join the vagal plexus along the walls of the esophagus (78).

At rest, the cricopharyngeus and thyropharyngeus muscles maintain a tonic contraction driven by the vagal fibers from the nucleus ambiguous (75). During swallowing, the tonic vagal drive is inhibited and the upper esophageal sphincter relaxes. Peristalsis in the upper portion (skeletal muscle portion) of the esophagus is driven by the nucleus ambiguous of the vagus nerve (75), although that in the body and lower portion of the esophagus is driven by the dorsal motor nucleus of the vagus. The relaxation of the lower esophageal sphincter is accomplished by the nitrergic neurons in Aurbach's plexus driven by the dorsal motor nucleus of the vagus nerve (79).

Afferent fibers from the esophageal walls follow the vagus nerve back to the solitary nucleus of the medulla. They also follow the sympathetic fibers back to the dorsal horn of the upper segment of the spinal cord (80). Vagal afferent fibers ending in the solitary nucleus of the medulla contribute to a viscerovisceral reflex arc by synapsing on premotor neurons of the nucleus ambiguous and preganglionic neurons of the dorsal motor nucleus of the vagus nerve (75). The premotor neurons subsequently innervate the motor neurons of the nucleus ambiguous. The premotor neurons form the central pattern generator for organized movements of the esophagus such as swallowing (79). The spinal afferent fibers from the esophagus contribute to the referral of pain. These afferent fibers innervate spinal segments that also receive afferent information from the:

Heart
Pulmonary tree
Chest
Upper back and torso

Esophageal pain can refer substernally (heartburn) or posteriorly through the back into the area of the scapula (81). Referred pain from the esophagus has numerous patterns, the more common of which are gripping, pressing, boring, or stabbing (82).

Aortic Plexus

The thoracic aorta has an intimate relationship with both divisions of the autonomic nervous system. Sympathetic input and sensory fibers reach the superior thoracic aorta through cardiac and pulmonary nerves as well as by following direct branches from the sympathetic trunk. The inferior thoracic aorta receives branches of the thoracic splanchnic nerves. The preganglionic sympathetic axons arise in the upper five thoracic spinal segments and the postganglionic fibers arise from the upper five thoracic paravertebral ganglia. Once on the wall of the aorta, these fibers form an adrenergic plexus in the adventitial tissue. Afferent fibers

from this large, elastic artery follow the sympathetic nerves back to the upper five thoracic spinal segments (65). This observation accounts for the referral of pain from the thoracic aorta to the thoracic spinal segments, resulting in their subsequent facilitation. Vagal cardiac nerves traverse the walls of the aorta as they descend toward their targets. Small twigs from these branches provide afferent as well as parasympathetic efferent innervation (Fig. 6.14).

Thoracic Duct Innervation

The thoracic duct, located in the posterior mediastinum near the esophagus, receives an innervation similar to the vascular innervation elsewhere in the trunk. Its muscular walls receive cholinergic innervation from the vagus nerve and sympathetic adrenergic innervation from branches of the intercostal nerves in a segmental pattern. The eleventh thoracic ganglion and the left splanchnic nerve innervate the cisterna chyli, which is the origin of the thoracic duct (83). Norepinephrine and epinephrine act to increase the flow of lymph through the thoracic duct (84). The effect of these adrenergic compounds on lymph vessels appears to be mediated through α-receptors on the smooth muscle cells of the lymph vessel wall (85).

Abdominopelvic Region

The thoracic plexus passes through the diaphragm to continue inferiorly in the abdominopelvic cavity as the abdominopelvic plexus. This plexus is a massive network of fibers lying along the midline astride the aorta and extending from the abdominal diaphragm to the pelvic diaphragm.

At the level of the abdominal diaphragm, the plexus has two major components: parasympathetic and sympathetic. The two vagal trunks and their associated branches, representing the parasympathetic component, enter the abdomen riding on the walls of the esophagus. The sympathetic component (or thoracic splanchnic nerves) passes directly through the crura of the diaphragm or under the medial arcuate ligament to enter the abdomen. Once in the abdominal cavity, the vagal trunks and thoracic splanchnic nerves unite around the aortic prevertebral ganglia. The resultant abdominopelvic plexus of fibers follows the abdominal aorta to the pelvic brim and bifurcates slightly above the sacral promontory, and the resulting two divisions of the plexus descend into the pelvic basin (Fig. 6.15). Throughout the abdomen, the plexus contains both sympathetic and parasympathetic axons and also has numerous afferent fibers. Toward the inferior end of the abdominopelvic plexus, additional sympathetic contributions arise in the lumbar and sacral splanchnic nerves, although additional parasympathetic contributions come from the pelvic splanchnic nerves in the pelvic basin.

Like the thoracic plexus, the abdominopelvic plexus can be divided into several geographical regions. Along the abdominal aorta, the major prevertebral ganglia mark out differing territories:

Celiac
Superior mesenteric
Inferior mesenteric

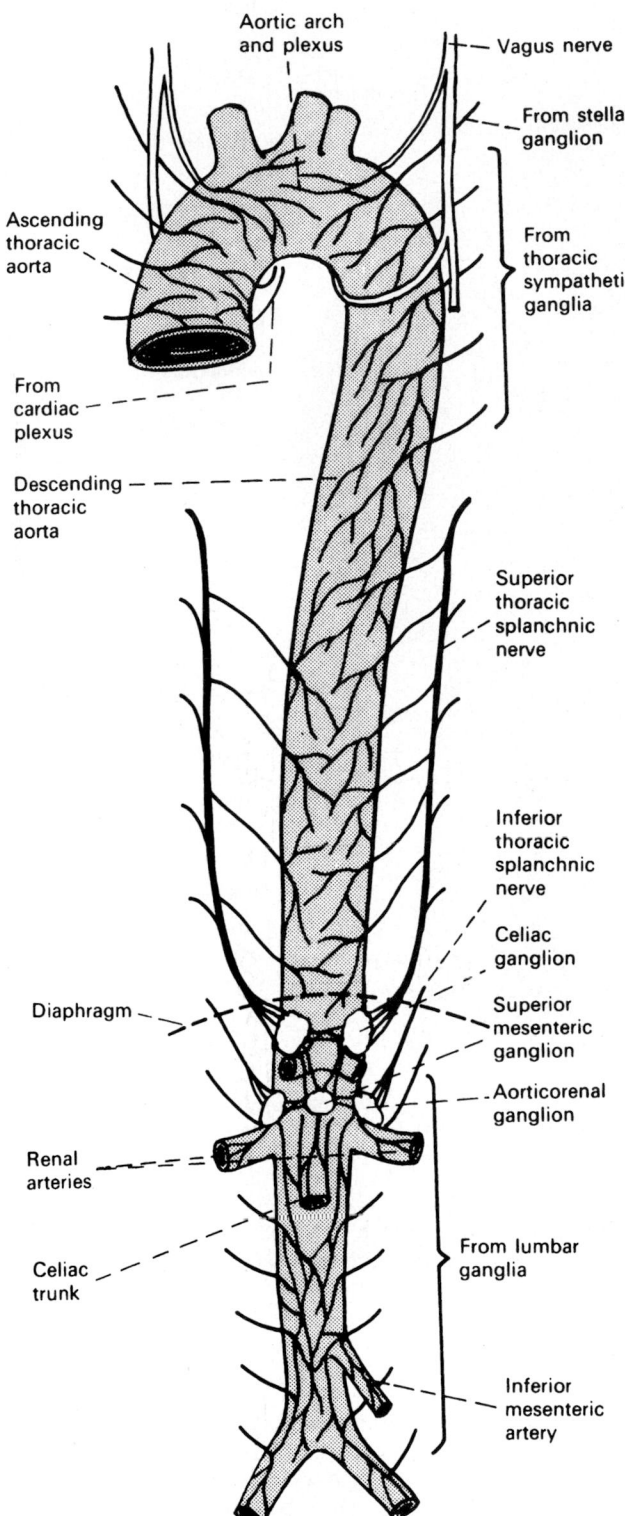

FIGURE 6.14. Innervation of thoracic and abdominal aorta. From Bonica JJ. General considerations of pain in the chest. In: Bonica JJ, ed. *The Management of Pain.* Philadelphia, PA: Lea & Febiger; 1990:979, with permission.

The superior hypogastric plexus lies between the inferior mesenteric plexus and the sacral promontory. Below the sacral promontory, the plexus splits to pass laterally around the pelvic organs. This region is called the inferior hypogastric plexus or, simply, the pelvic plexus. Frequently, the fibers of the superior hypogastric plexus unite into a few large cords in the region directly over the sacral promontory and just prior to bifurcation into the two inferior hypogastric plexuses. These cords are often referred to in the surgical literature as the presacral nerve (86). Although the abdominal autonomic nervous system has regional names, in reality the components blend together to form one great abdominopelvic plexus. The abdominal portion of this great plexus supplies efferent and afferent nerves to the organs of the abdominal cavity including the gastrointestinal organs, spleen, and kidneys. The pelvic portion of this plexus supplies the rectum, urinary organs, and reproductive organs. In addition to the organs, the abdominopelvic plexus also innervates the vasculature of the abdominopelvic cavity.

Gastrointestinal Tract

The gastrointestinal system receives a complex pattern of extrinsic innervation involving splanchnic nerves derived from the thoracolumbar and sacral portions of the spinal cord and the terminal portion of the vagus and pelvic splanchnic nerves (Figs. 6.4 and 6.5). These nerves form a complex network of fibers lying along the abdominal aorta and extending from the thoracoabdominal diaphragm to the pelvic diaphragm (Fig. 6.15). This elaborate plexus, like its visceral blood supply, can be divided into three zones based on embryologic partitions of the gastrointestinal system:

Celiac (foregut)
Superior mesenteric (midgut)
Inferior mesenteric (hindgut)

A complex network of intrinsic fibers and neurons called the enteric nervous system is found within the walls of the gut. The enteric or intrinsic neural system controls the activity of gut smooth muscle and glands. In turn, it is modulated by the extrinsic fibers from the central nervous system via the sympathetic and parasympathetic nerves. Numerous sensory feedback loops exist in the gastrointestinal system. Afferent fibers within the luminal surface and gut wall form short feedback loops within the enteric nervous system. Longer feedback loops connect the gut to the prevertebral ganglia, and still longer loops connect the gut with the spinal cord and brainstem (6,13,87–90). Figure 6.16 is a schematic diagram of the abdominopelvic plexus demonstrating its input from sympathetic and parasympathetic sources.

The gastrointestinal tract has a special pattern of sympathetic innervation that differs significantly from that of the thoracic viscera. Preganglionic fibers arise in the lateral horn of spinal segments T9-L2, but they do not terminate in the paravertebral ganglia. Instead they pass through a series of thoracic, lumbar, and sacral splanchnic nerves (branches off of the sympathetic truck) to reach the prevertebral sympathetic ganglia on the anterior wall of the abdominal aorta (Fig. 6.15).

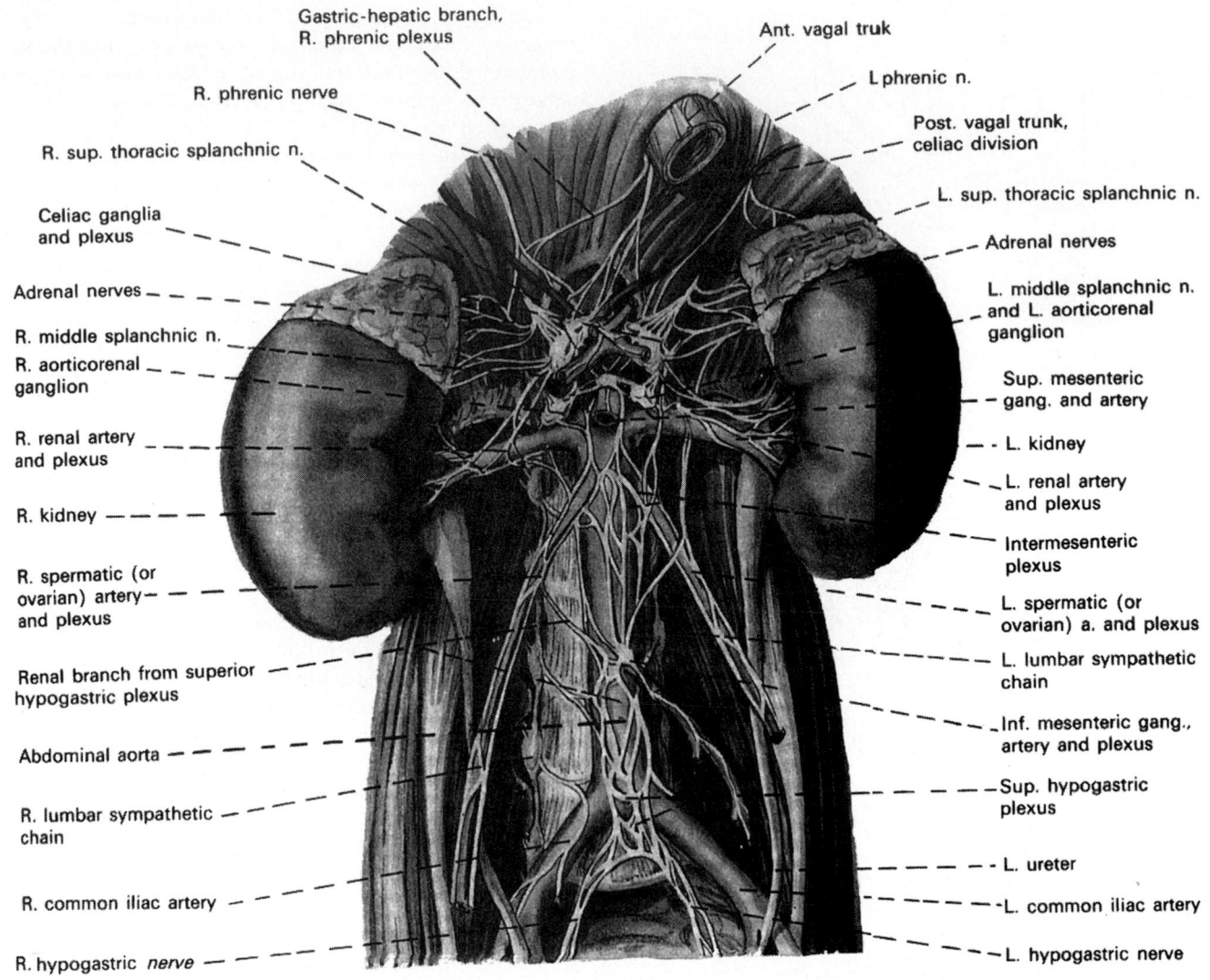

Gastric-hepatic branch,
R. phrenic plexus

R. phrenic nerve

R. sup. thoracic splanchnic n.

Celiac ganglia
and plexus

Adrenal nerves

R. middle splanchnic n.

R. aorticorenal
ganglion

R. renal artery
and plexus

R. kidney

R. spermatic (or
ovarian) artery
and plexus

Renal branch from superior
hypogastric plexus

Abdominal aorta

R. lumbar sympathetic
chain

R. common iliac artery

R. hypogastric *nerve*

Ant. vagal truk

L phrenic n.

Post. vagal trunk,
celiac division

L. sup. thoracic splanchnic n.

Adrenal nerves

L. middle splanchnic n.
and L. aorticorenal
ganglion

Sup. mesenteric
gang. and artery

L. kidney

L. renal artery
and plexus

Intermesenteric
plexus

L. spermatic (or
ovarian) a. and plexus

L. lumbar sympathetic
chain

Inf. mesenteric gang.,
artery and plexus

Sup. hypogastric
plexus

L. ureter

L. common iliac artery

L. hypogastric nerve

FIGURE 6.15. Position of major prevertebral sympathetic ganglia in great autonomic plexus of abdomen. From Bonica JJ. General considerations of pain in the chest. In: Bonica JJ, ed. *The Management of Pain.* Philadelphia, PA: Lea & Febiger; 1990:1157, with permission.

The major prevertebral ganglia are distributed around the three abdominal arteries:

Celiac
Superior mesenteric
Inferior mesenteric

Anatomical authorities subdivide the celiac ganglia into numerous parts based on its location about the celiac artery and aorta; however, from a practical perspective, it is simpler to consider it as one anatomical unit. Also, the celiac and superior mesenteric ganglia are often fused together into an inseparable mass surrounding the trunks of their two arteries. An older term for this arrangement is the solar plexus. Additional clusters of sympathetic ganglia neurons are found scattered in the hypogastric plexus as it enters the pelvic basin.

Neurons in each prevertebral ganglion give rise to postganglionic fibers that innervate abdominal and pelvic viscera. These axons travel to their target organs by hitchhiking on abdominal and pelvic arteries. Each prevertebral ganglion innervates a different region of the viscera.

Celiac Ganglia

The celiac ganglionic mass surrounds the celiac trunk. It is often fused to the superior mesenteric ganglia to form one large, complex mass. When carefully dissected, the precise shape of the ganglion complex is very irregular and defies meaningful classification (51). The celiac ganglia receive afferent fibers from the thoracic splanchnic nerves (T5-9). In turn, it supplies postganglionic sympathetic axons to the vascular territory of the celiac artery including the (Figs.6.17 and 6.18):

Distal esophagus
Stomach
Proximal duodenum
Liver
Gall bladder
Spleen
Portions of the pancreas

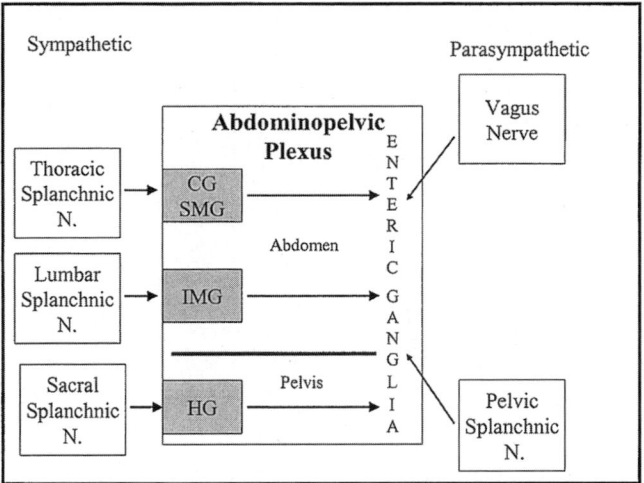

FIGURE 6.16. A schematic diagram of the abdominopelvic plexus illustrating its ganglia and sources of input. Thoracic, lumbar, and sacral splanchnic nerves for the sympathetic trunk carry sympathetic preganglionic fibers to the paravertebral ganglia located in the plexus. Postganglionic axons from the paravertebral ganglia target the intrinsic enteric ganglia of the organ walls. Parasympathetic fibers arise in the vagus nerve superiorly and the pelvic splanchnic nerves inferiorly. These fibers also target the intrinsic enteric ganglia located on the organ walls.

Superior Mesenteric Ganglia

This ganglion is found wrapped around the superior mesenteric artery. As mentioned above, it is often fused with the celiac ganglia. The superior mesenteric ganglia also receive preganglionic axons from the thoracic splanchnic nerves. Its distribution of postganglionic axons reaches the territory supplied by the superior mesenteric artery (Fig. 6.19):

> Distal duodenum
> Portions of the pancreas
> Jejunum
> Ileum
> Ascending colon
> Proximal two-thirds of the transverse colon

Inferior Mesenteric Ganglia

The most ventral of the three prevertebral ganglia, the inferior mesenteric ganglia, surrounds the abdominal artery of the same name. It receives axons from the three lumbar splanchnic nerves and supplies postganglionic axons to the vascular territory of the inferior mesenteric vessels, namely the (Fig. 6.18):

> Distal third of the transverse colon
> Descending colon
> Sigmoid colon
> Rectum

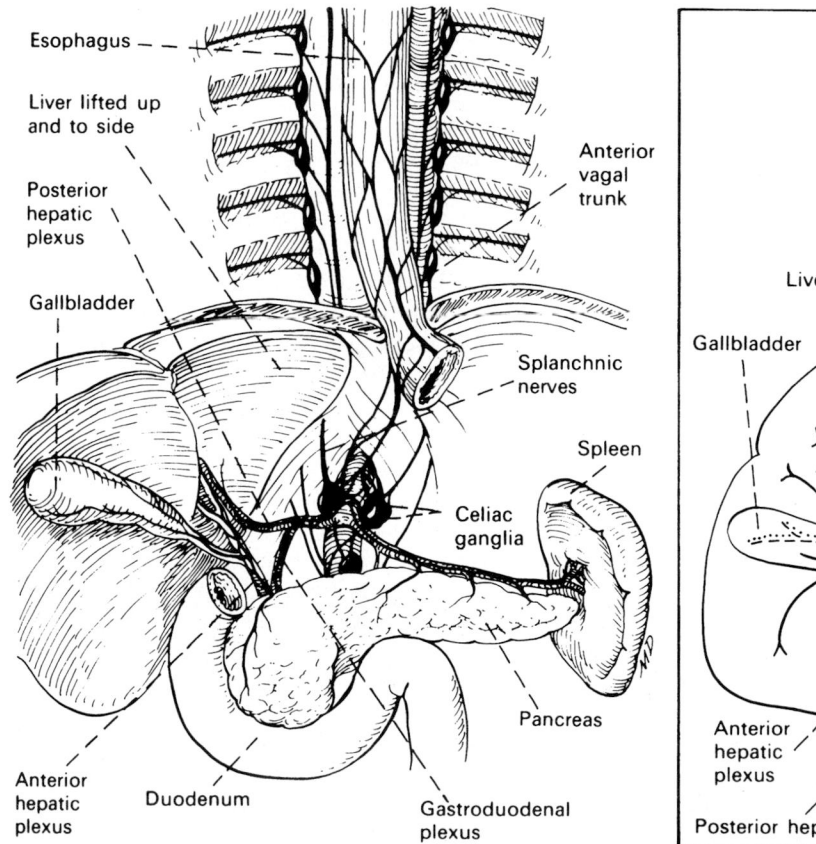

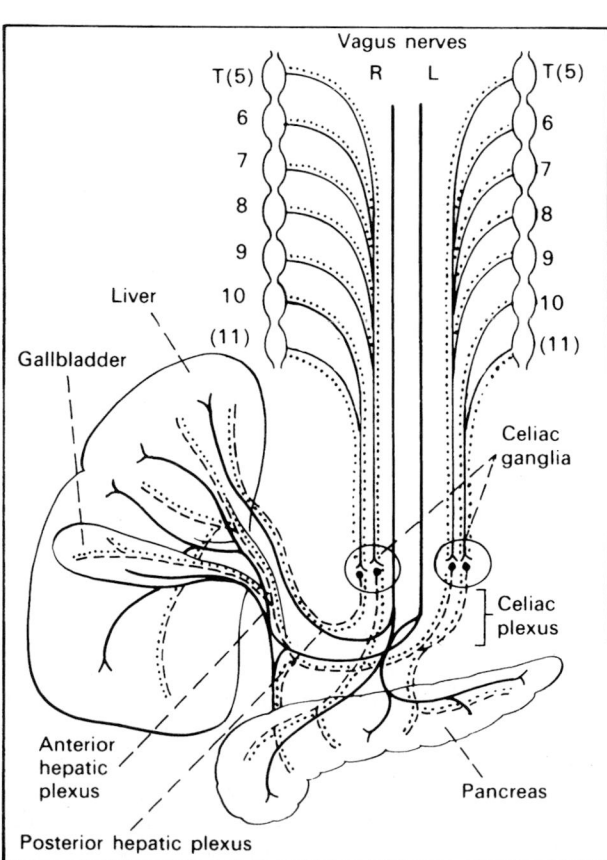

FIGURE 6.17. Connections of celiac ganglion and innervation of stomach. From Kimmey MB, Silverstein FE. Diseases of the gastrointestinal tract. In: Bonica JJ, ed. *The Management of Pain.* Philadelphia, PA: Lea & Febiger; 1990:1189, with permission.

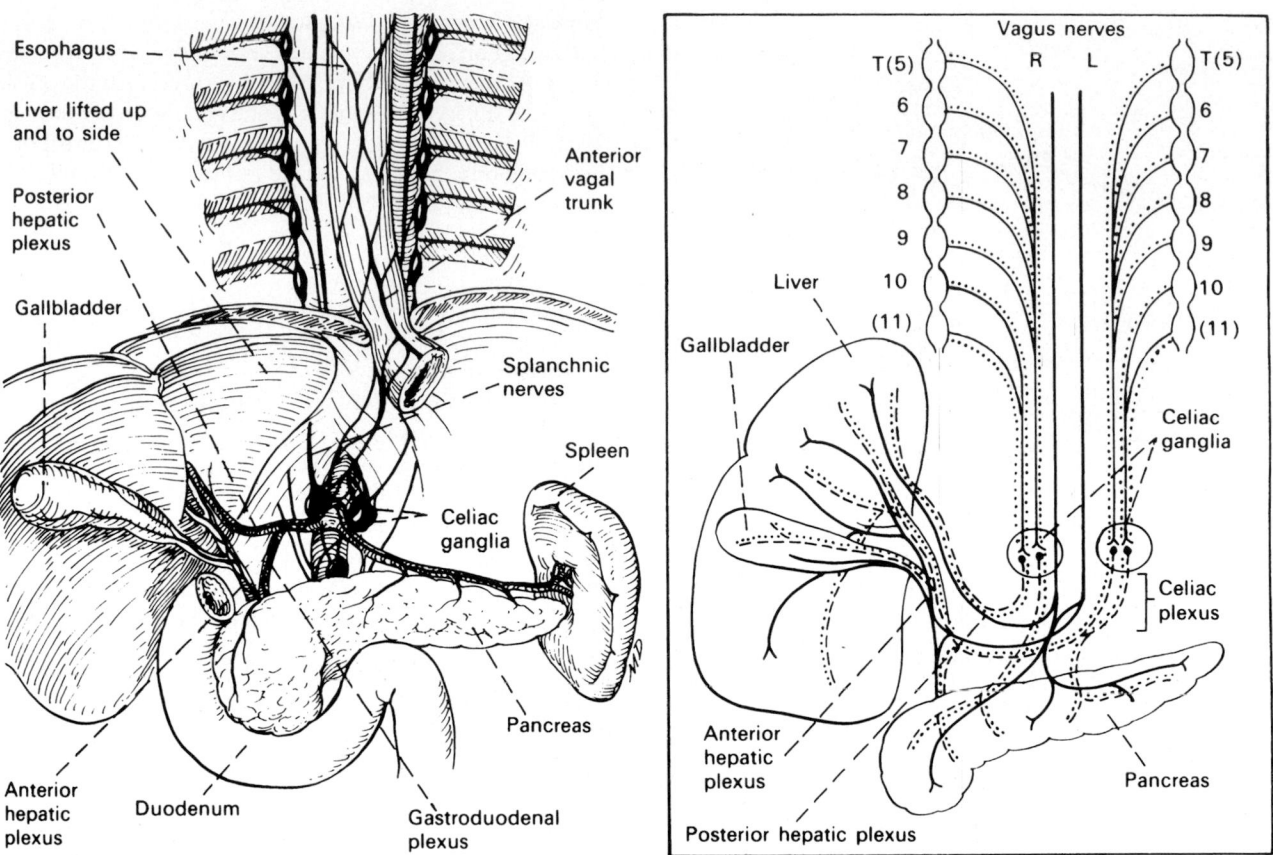

FIGURE 6.18. Connections of celiac ganglia and the innervation of the liver and biliary tree. From Mulholland MW, Debas HT. Diseases of the liver, biliary system, and pancreas. In: Bonica JJ, ed. *The Management of Pain.* Philadelphia, PA: Lea & Febiger; 1990:1215, with permission.

Postganglionic fibers from the prevertebral ganglia follow their specific blood supplies through the mesenteric ligaments to reach the specific organs. The termination of these noradrenergic fibers is primarily on the neurons in the enteric ganglia (91). Sympathetic fibers also terminate in the muscular coat of blood vessels, and an abundance of these fibers reaches the sphincter musculature of the enteric wall. Only scattered sympathetic fibers are present in the muscularis externa and submucosa of the gastrointestinal tract (92). There are almost no adrenergic cell bodies in the enteric plexus; therefore, most enteric adrenergic fibers are of external origin. In general, stimulation of the sympathetic fibers inhibits the activity of cholinergic neurons of the parasympathetic system and slows peristalsis and motility.

The parasympathetic innervation of the organs located below the thoracoabdominal diaphragm has a dual origin, which also segregates along vascular and embryologic divisions. The organs of the foregut and midgut, serviced by the celiac and superior mesenteric arteries, receive parasympathetic preganglionic fibers from the vagus nerve (Figs. 6.17 through 6.19). The vagus nerve follows the esophagus through the diaphragm to enter the abdominal cavity on the walls of the stomach. The esophageal hiatus of the diaphragm is the last place the vagus can be identified as a distinct nerve. Vagal axons, however, continue into the abdominal cavity, joining those of the sympathetic system in the celiac and superior mesenteric ganglia and forming mixed nerves, which

pass along celiac and superior mesenteric blood vessels eventually to reach the abdominal viscera. Vagal fibers are plentiful in the walls of the stomach and small bowel, and a few reach as far distally in the enteric plexus as the splenic flexure of the large colon. The preganglionic vagal axons terminate on neurons in enteric ganglia. Short postganglionic fibers from these neurons innervate the glands and course within the layers of smooth muscle of the alimentary canal. Cholinergic stimulation increases glandular secretions and peristaltic activity.

The organs of hindgut origin (transverse colon to anus) receive parasympathetic preganglionic innervation from the pelvic splanchnic nerves (Fig. 6.20). These nerves arise in the lateral horn of the S2-3 spinal cord segments and exit the spinal canal with the sacral nerve roots. As the roots pass along the pelvic wall on their way to the greater sciatic foramen, the delicate pelvic splanchnic nerves are given off. These thin nerves course through the endopelvic fascia to reach the inferior hypogastric plexus surrounding the walls of the rectum. Once in the hypogastric plexus, these parasympathetic preganglionic fibers can ascend to the origin of the inferior mesenteric artery. By hitchhiking along the branches of this artery, they reach upward to the splenic flexure of the large colon. Not all parasympathetic axons from the pelvis follow this route to reach the inferior abdominal organs. Some preganglionic fibers in the inferior hypogastric plexus gain access to the enteric plexus in the wall of the rectum and ascend

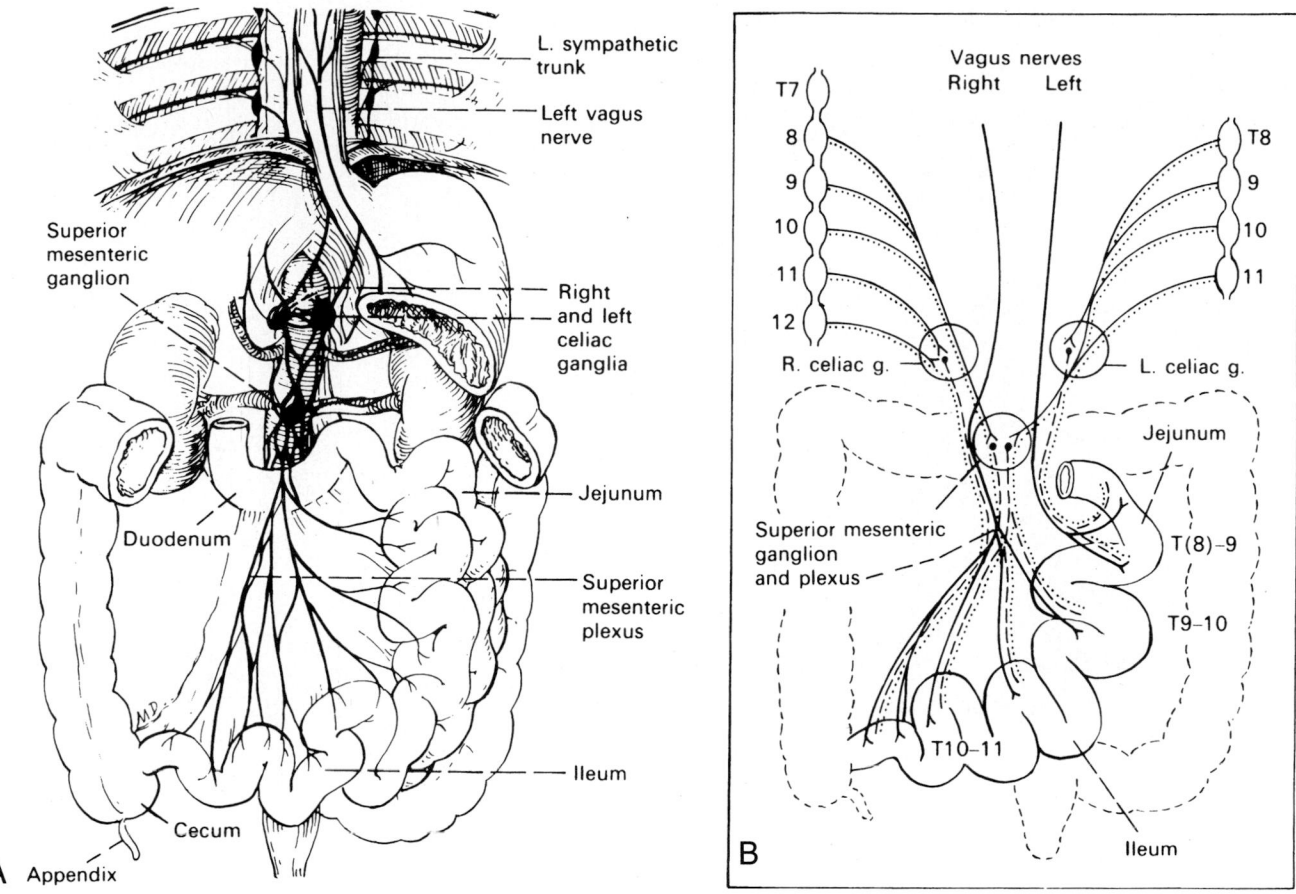

FIGURE 6.19. Connections of superior mesenteric ganglion and the innervation of the small bowel. From Kimmey MB, Silverstein FE. Diseases of the gastrointestinal tract. In: Bonica JJ, ed. *The Management of Pain.* Philadelphia, PA: Lea & Febiger; 1990:1198, with permission.

along the colon to reach more proximal levels of the hindgut. The preganglionic axons of the pelvic splanchnic nerves eventually terminate on the neurons of the enteric nervous system. Stimulation of the parasympathetic fibers increases gut peristalsis and mobility.

The enteric ganglia and plexus within the walls of the gut form a highly complex and elaborate network, often referred to as the third division of the autonomic nervous system. It exerts a major influence over all activities in the gut (6,93). The enteric nervous system is estimated to possess as many neurons as are found in the entire spinal cord (94). The enteric system is divided into two layers: The external layer is the myenteric plexus (Auerbach's) controlling the muscularis externa, and the internal layer is the submucosal (Meissner's) controlling the glandular and immune components of the submucosal layers. A full understanding of these structures requires a knowledge of the gastrointestinal histology and is beyond the scope of this review (95,96).

Numerous neurotransmitters and neuromodulators are found within enteric neurons, for example:

Acetylcholine
Serotonin
Purines
Gamma-amino butyric acid
Histamine

There are also many peptides such as:

Substance-P
Somatostatin
Vasoactive intestinal polypeptide
Enkephalins

Recently, nitric oxide has been described as a significant noncholinergic, nonadrenergic mechanism of neurotransmission in the enteric nervous system as well as elsewhere (97,98). Nitric oxide is synthesized from the amino acid arginine by neurons in the myenteric plexus and is a potent smooth muscle relaxing factor. For this reason, it is postulated to be important in dilation of the alimentary canal.

Three levels of sensory information processing are necessary for the proper regulation of gastrointestinal tract function (6,87). The first level features afferent neurons that form a short loop interconnecting the gut mucosa, submucosa, or muscle to the enteric ganglia only. These neurons are responsible for local reflexes along the gut wall. The second level of sensory information processing involved is arranged in a longer loop involving afferent neurons from the mucosa that project to the prevertebral ganglia along the aorta. These sensory neurons participate in intraabdominal reflex arcs coordinating various regions of the gastrointestinal system. Neither of these two sensory levels can

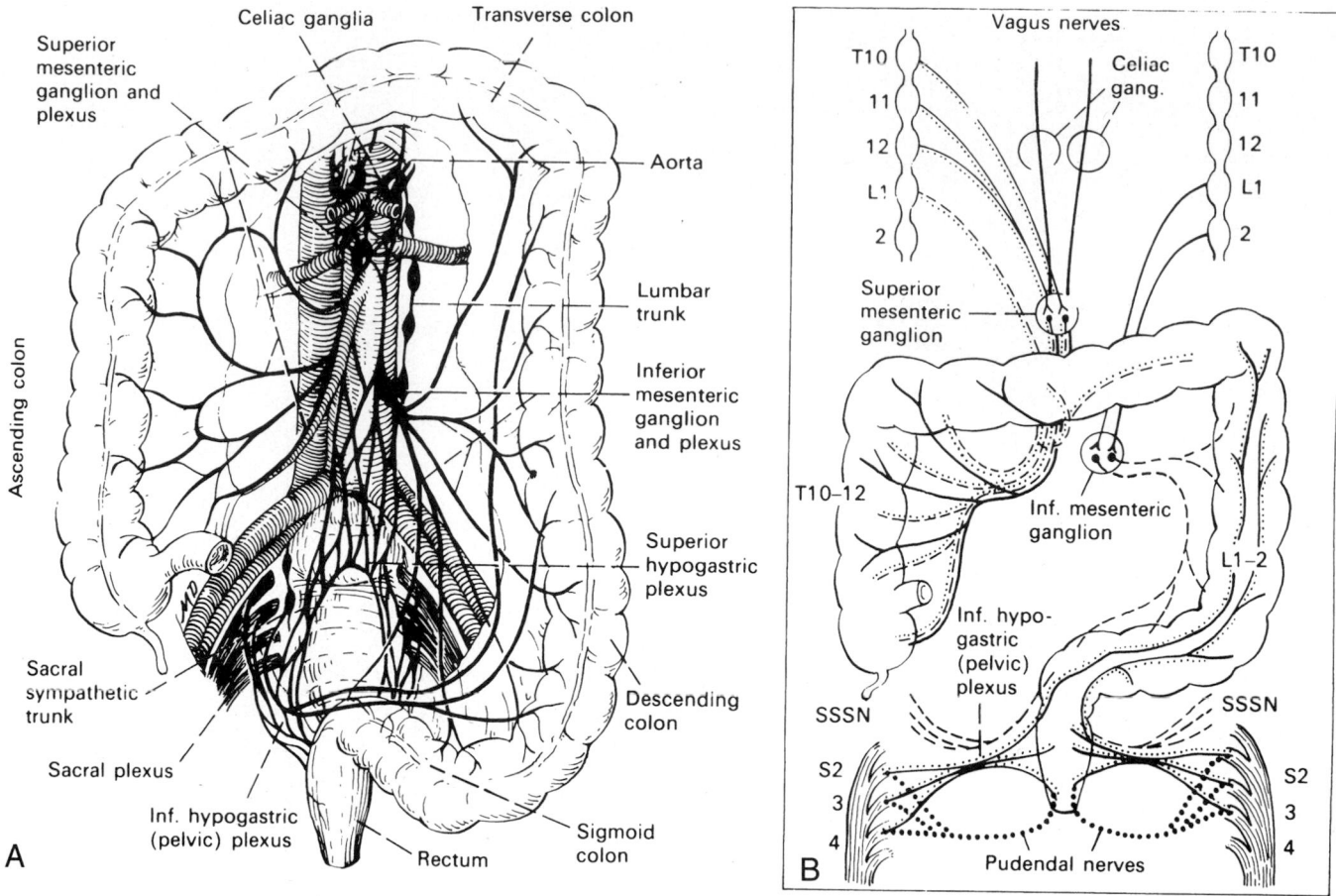

FIGURE 6.20. Connections of inferior mesenteric ganglion and the innervation of the large bowel and rectum. SSSN, sacral sympathetic splanchnic nerve. From Kimmey MB, Silverstein FE. Diseases of the gastrointestinal tract. In: Bonica JJ, ed. *The Management of Pain.* Philadelphia, PA: Lea & Febiger; 1990:1199, with permission.

reach consciousness, thus we are generally unaware of the reflex control activity occurring in the gut wall. Finally, the third level of sensory feedback loops involves afferent neurons that project from the gut wall to the brainstem via the vagus nerve or to the spinal cord via the thoracic, lumbar, and pelvic splanchnic nerves. These visceral afferent neurons assist the central nervous system in integrating the activity of the alimentary canal with that of external environmental conditions. Information in this third sensory level can, on occasion, reach consciousness.

There are significant differences in distribution, morphology, and neurochemistry between the visceral afferent fibers associated with sympathetic nerves and those coursing with the parasympathetic nerves. There are very few large, encapsulated nerve endings in the gut wall, most of which are related to axons from the parasympathetic vagus nerve. However, the majority of afferent terminals in the gut are small-caliber, naked nerve endings (87). In the vagus nerve, mechanoreceptive, chemoreceptive, and polymodal fibers have been described with their receptive fields in the mucosa and submucosa of the gut wall. At least in the stomach, very few of these vagal fibers contain calcitonin gene–related polypeptide, a neuropeptide typically related in nociceptive afferent fibers of the somatic tissue. However, some nociceptive information is carried in the vagus nerve because pain from a

hiatal hernia can be referred to the face (99) via the vagus nerve. Little is known of nociceptive function in vagal fibers below the level of the diaphragm. The visceral afferent fibers that follow the sympathetic nerves to the spinal cord are mechanoreceptive and chemoreceptive, and they tend to be distributed to the mesenteries and peritoneal ligaments of the gut and along its vascular system. In contrast to the vagal fibers, those projecting to the spinal cord are mostly of small caliber and are rich in calcitonin gene–related polypeptide, suggesting that they have a role in nociception. Their endings are commonly distributed within the mesentery and supporting ligaments of the abdominal organs (88). These nerve endings are frequently present near the branch points for the vasculature in the peritoneal lining. Few small-caliber nerve endings are present within the visceral organs themselves. (See additional comments concerning vagal activity in Chapter 8.)

Physiologic (68) and clinical studies support the general separation of regulatory information into the vagal system and nociceptive information into the spinal cord. Stimulating the greater thoracic splanchnic nerve at surgery elicits severe pain; however, blockade of the splanchnic nerve relieves pain (100). In addition, applying local anesthetic to the greater thoracic splanchnic nerve after abdominal surgery prevents the endocrine metabolic

**TABLE 6.1. VISCERAL ORGANS AND THEIR APPROXI-
MATE SPINAL CORD LEVEL FOR THE ORIGIN OF THEIR
PREGANGLIONIC NEURONS[a]**

Heart	T1–T5	
Stomach	T5–T9	
Liver and gall bladder	T6–T9	
Pancreas	T5–T11	
Small intestine	T9–T11	
Colon and rectum	T8–L2	S2–S4
Kidney and ureters	T10–L1	
Urinary bladder	T10–L1	S2–S4
Ovary and fallopian tube	T9–T10	
Testicle and epididymus	T9–T10, L1–L2	S2–S4
Uterus	T10–L1	
Cervix		S2–S4
Prostate	L1–L2	

[a] These levels create a viscerotopic map in the lateral horns of the spinal cord.

responses such as increased plasma cortisol and urinary adrenaline levels that are usually present in the early stages of recovery (101). The projection of the viscera afferent fibers through the sympathetic system creates a nociceptive map of the abdominopelvic organs on the dorsal horn of the spinal cord. This map has been demonstrated in humans by sectioning the white rami commicans during the surgical treatment of visceral pain [White and Sweet, as cited in Janig and Morrison (88)]. A summary of the organotopic map of the human viscera is presented in Table 6.1. The position of a specific organ in the visceral afferent organotopic map of the spinal cord coincides approximately with the origin of the sympathetic efferent system to that specific organ. The nociceptive input to the spinal cord over these visceral afferent fibers is not precisely mapped; instead, input from any one organ overlaps considerably with that from surrounding organs (88).

Hepatobiliary Tree and Pancreas

The vasculature and parenchyma of the liver and pancreas, as well as their associated ducts, receive innervation from both divisions of the autonomic nervous system (Fig. 6.18). In addition, these organs have an abundant supply of visceral afferent fibers that course in the vagus and thoracic splanchnic nerves. Preganglionic sympathetic innervation to these organs arises in thoracic segments at approximately T6 to T9-11 and approaches the abdomen through the thoracic splanchnic nerves. Sympathetic ganglionic neurons are located in the celiac ganglia. Their postganglionic axons reach the liver and pancreas by hitchhiking on the hepatic and pancreatic branches of the celiac trunk. Preganglionic parasympathetic axons, derived from the vagus nerve, pass through the fascia of the celiac region and follow the vasculature to the target organs. Little is known concerning the effects of autonomic nerve stimulation on liver function. However, in general, sympathetic activation drives the liver toward increasing the output of glucose (102).

A significant percentage of the axons in the vagus and thoracic splanchnic nerves traveling to the liver and pancreas are sensory in nature. Approximately 90 of the vagal axons and 50 of the splanchnic axons to the liver are visceral afferent fibers (103). These two afferent systems perform different functions (13).

Those afferent axons traveling with the vagus nerve respond to such stimuli as plasma glucose concentration, portal venous blood osmotic pressure, and temperature changes. The visceral afferent fibers associated with the splanchnic nerves are high-threshold mechanoreceptors and chemoreceptors located in the walls of the biliary system, among other places, and are responsive to stretch and bradykinin concentration. The evidence available to date suggests that all pain sensation from the liver and biliary tree is transmitted via the splanchnic nerves and not the vagus nerve.

Kidney and Urinary Tract

Kidney
Although the kidney is primarily controlled by endocrine mechanisms, it does receive significant innervation from the sympathetic adrenergic system that regulates, in part, the retention of sodium (Table 6.1) (104–107). Alterations in the neural activity in sympathetic fibers are involved in the generation of certain forms of hypertension (108). Very little vagal parasympathetic (cholinergic) input to the kidney has been reported. This organ does, however, receive neuropeptide-containing, primary afferent fibers that course along with the adrenergic fibers (Fig. 6.21).

The kidney receives most of its innervation from the thoracolumbar spinal cord. Preganglionic sympathetic neurons regulating the kidney are located in the lateral horn of the spinal cord extending approximately from segments T11 to L1. Their axons enter the abdominopelvic plexus over the lower thoracic and first lumbar splanchnic nerves (Table 6.1). The postganglionic sympathetic adrenergic fibers are derived from laterally positioned ganglia (sometimes called aorticorenal ganglia) in the celiac and superior mesenteric plexuses and course into the hilus of the kidney along the renal vasculature.

The adrenergic axons of the mammalian kidney terminate on the (109):

Afferent and efferent glomerular arterioles
Proximal and distal renal tubules
Ascending limb of Henle's loop
Juxtaglomerular apparatus

All portions of the cortical tubular nephron are under neural influence. The relative density of adrenergic fibers is greatest around the ascending limb of the loop of Henle, followed in decreasing relative density by the distal convoluted tubule and the proximal convoluted tubule (110,111). α-adrenoceptors have been located on the proximal convoluted tubule (112) as well as on the smooth muscle of the vasculature. Sympathetic innervation of the kidney is involved in the normal regulation of sodium retention, both by increasing the transport of sodium across the tubule walls and by directly increasing the release of renin from the juxtaglomerular apparatus (113,114). Studies have shown that there is increased activity in the renal sympathetic nervous system in essential hypertension in humans (108).

A dual sensory innervation of the kidney exists: afferent fibers follow the thoracic splanchnic nerves back to the spinal cord and the vagus nerve back to the brainstem. Within the kidney, peripheral endings of both mechanoreceptors and chemoreceptors are found in close association with ureteric blood vessels (arteries and veins) and in the walls of the pelvis of the ureter (115).

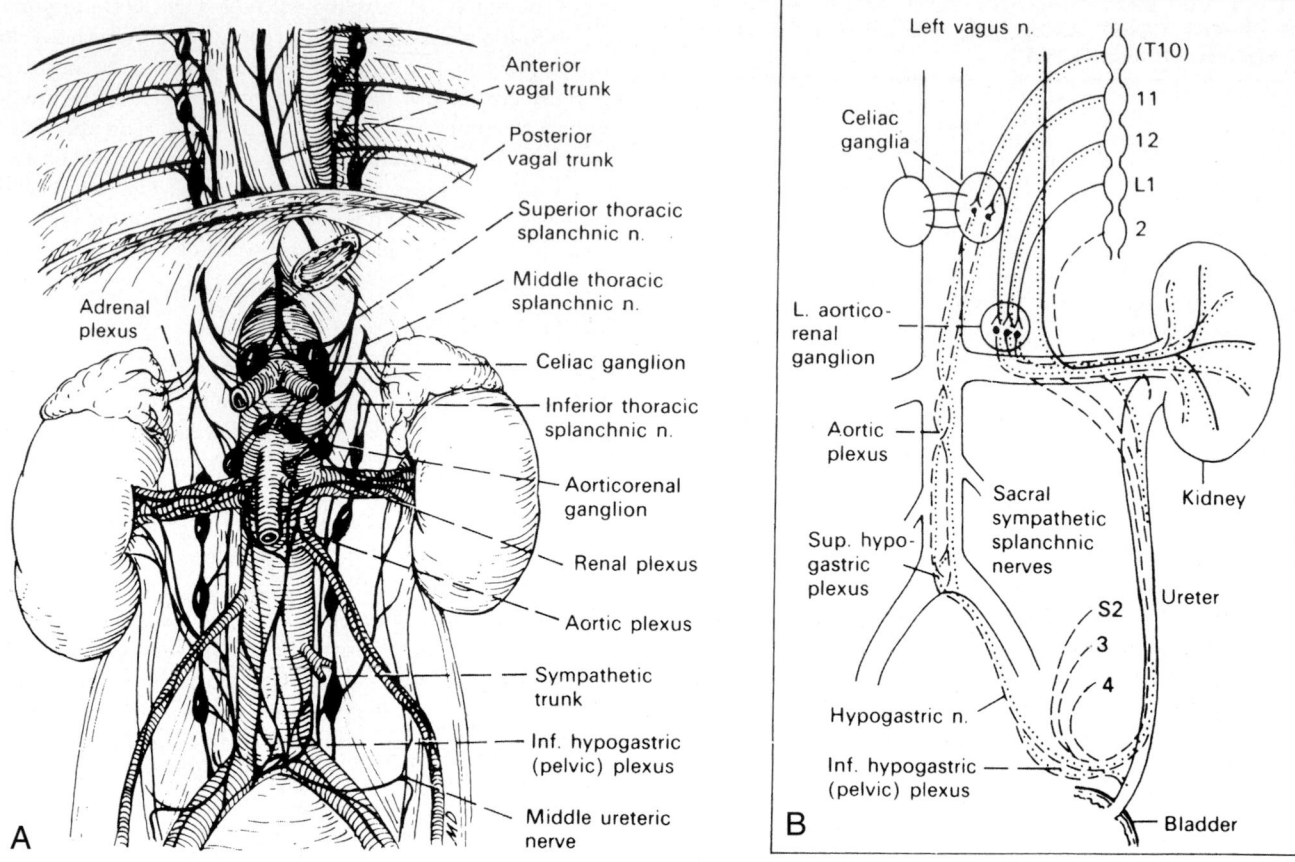

FIGURE 6.21. Innervation of the kidney. From Ansell JS, Gee WF. Diseases of the kidney. In: Bonica JJ, ed. *The Management of Pain.* Philadelphia, PA: Lea & Febiger; 1990:1233, with permission.

Their cell bodies are in the dorsal root ganglia located mainly in segments at the thoracolumbar junction (T10-L3), and their central processes terminate in the dorsal horn of the spinal cord. These afferent axons are classified as A and C-fibers. Vagal afferent fibers, both mechanoreceptors and chemoreceptors, play a role in renorenal reflexes. The mechanoreceptors are also involved in modulating cardiovascular reflexes, thus regulating blood pressure (115). Pain is the only detectable sensory perception that can be elicited from the kidney (13). This modality is carried in the visceral afferent fibers of the thoracic splanchnic nerves to reach the spinal cord and the spinothalamic tracts. In a study of the sympathetic renal afferent fibers in the primate, all spinothalamic tract cells excited by renal afferent fibers were also excited by somatic afferent fibers, indicating a powerful somatovisceral convergence on these cells (116). This convergence has been suggested as a mechanism to explain the referral of pain from the kidney out to somatic structures such as the flank of the body. In addition, this relationship may explain the changes in the tone of muscle innervated by the segments T10-L1 that accompany renal infection or inflammation.

Ureter

Primary function of the ureter is the unidirectional flow of urine from the kidney to the urinary bladder. Although it is richly invested with nerves (117), peristalsis in the ureter is primarily myogenic in nature, driven by specialized pacemaker cells (118).

The course of the ureter is retroperitoneal, lying along the posterior abdominal body wall and embedded in the transversalis fascia. The walls of the ureter consist of interlacing bundles of smooth muscle fibers woven into a theca muscularis. Individual smooth muscle cells interconnect via numerous gap junctions, making the muscularis a functional syncytium (119). Modified smooth muscle cells within the muscular layer serve as pacemakers, initiating peristaltic contractions (120). A plexus of efferent and afferent nerve fibers that are capable of regulating the pacemaker cells is wrapped around the muscularis (119).

The ureter receives its innervation in a segmental fashion. The upper portion is innervated by the lower thoracic and upper lumbar segments (T10-L1) and by the vagus nerve. The lower portion of the ureter is innervated by the upper lumbar segments (L1-2) and the pelvic splanchnic nerves (Table 6.1). The sympathetic innervation reaches the upper ureter through the lesser thoracic and lumbar splanchnic nerves. Ganglionic neurons are located in the celiac and associated renal and gonadal (testicular or ovarian) ganglia. The lower ureter receives its sympathetic innervation from lumbar and sacral splanchnic nerves that contribute to ganglia located in the superior and inferior hypogastric plexus (121).

Fibers containing tyrosine hydroxylase and neuropeptide-Y, markers for sympathetic axons, are in the outer muscle layers and the surrounding adventitia of the human ureter (122–124). Activation of α-adrenergic receptors increases ureter peristalsis and elevates luminal pressures; whereas activation of β-adrenergic receptors decreases ureter peristaltic frequency and lowers intraureter pressures (125). The actual role of the noradrenergic system in human ureter peristalsis has been questioned, and it appears that control over the surrounding vascular system is the dominant theme for the ureteric nerves (118).

Parasympathetic innervation for the upper portion of the ureter arises in the vagus nerve and reaches the ureter through the celiac and superior mesenteric plexus. The lower portion receives its cholinergic innervation from spinal segments S2-4. These pelvic splanchnic nerves communicate with the ureter via the inferior hypogastric plexus. Acetylcholine-containing neurons are present in the mural ganglia of the ureter, and fibers containing acetylcholine are present in the mammalian ureter. These fibers are of greatest density as the ureter enters the vesical wall. Stimulation of the ureter wall with acetylcholine results in an increased contractile activity and an increased basal tone of the mural smooth muscle (125,126). Acetylcholine also relaxes the ureter resistance arteries using a mechanism involving endothelium-derived nitric oxide (125).

Afferent fibers to the ureter are derived from dorsal root ganglia ranging from L2-3 to S1-2 (in guinea pigs) (127). Two classes of mechanoreceptors have been described in the ureter walls (128). One class has low thresholds and is responsive to peristaltic-type contractions of the ureteric smooth muscle. The other class of mechanoreceptor has higher thresholds of activation and is most likely related to nociception. Many of these primary afferent fibers contain neuropeptides such as substance-P and calcitonin gene–related polypeptide, thereby suggesting that they are involved in nociceptive activities.

Pain, presumably from these nociceptors, is the only sensory perception obtainable from the human ureter (13). In the thoracolumbar dorsal horn of the spinal cord, input from the ureter converges with somatic input from thoracolumbar spinal segments. Pain from distention of the ureter is often referred to the somatic body wall over a range of body segments. From the upper ureter, pain refers to the area from the anterior superior spine of the ileum anteriorly to the border of the rectus abdominis muscle (T11-12). From the middle ureter, pain refers to the area from the inguinal ligament anteriorly to the rectus abdominis muscle (T12-L1). From the lower ureter, pain refers to the suprapubic area (L1) and below into the scrotum or labia (L2) (121). This descending segmental pattern of primary afferent fibers from the ureter is responsible for the descending movement of facilitated segments as any obstructing material moves through the ureteric lumen.

Urinary Bladder

The muscular components of the urinary bladder can be divided into two anatomical and functional parts: the body (or detrusor urinae muscle) and the base (or the trigone muscle). The detrusor urinae muscle is the larger of the two parts and is active during expulsion of urine from the bladder. The trigone muscle surrounds the openings of the ureter in the base and the opening of the urethra in the neck of the bladder. It acts as an internal sphincter and, when contracted, helps to prevent the flow of urine from the bladder. The detrusor and the trigone tend to oppose each other in activity. Both detrusor and trigone muscles comprise multiple layers of smooth muscle fibers and receive an efferent innervation from the large autonomic pelvic plexus. A third muscle related to bladder function is located inferior to the trigone in the layers of the perineum. It is the deep transverse perineal muscle; the portion of this muscle that surrounds the urethra is called the sphincter urethra. Unlike the detrusor and trigone, this component of the perineal diaphragm is composed of skeletal muscle and innervated by branches of the pudendal nerve, a somatic nerve (S2-4).

The autonomic innervation of the urinary bladder is accomplished through the hypogastric plexus that is embedded in endopelvic fascia (Fig. 6.22). Parasympathetic preganglionic (cholinergic) fibers from the intermediolateral nucleus of spinal segments S2-4 enter the hypogastric plexus via the pelvic splanchnic nerves. These axons continue anteriorly into the vesicle plexus to terminate on ganglionic neurons located in the walls of the bladder. Their postganglionic (cholinergic and purinergic) axons supply motor innervation to all portions of the bladder wall. Stimulation of the parasympathetic system, which occurs during voiding, is excitatory to the detrusor muscle and inhibitory to the trigone muscle (129).

Sympathetic preganglionic fibers arise in the intermediolateral nucleus of spinal segments T11-L2 (Fig. 6.22). They leave the sympathetic trunk coursing on lumbar and sacral splanchnic nerves to enter the inferior hypogastric plexus, eventually targeting prevertebral ganglia (130). Sympathetic postganglionic (adrenergic) axons pass anteriorly through the inferior hypogastric plexus and ultimately contribute to the vesicle plexus in the bladder adventitia. Their major target is the smooth muscle cells of the trigone muscle with a much smaller contribution to the smooth muscle of the detrusor urinae. Sympathetic tone facilitates contraction of the trigone muscles and relaxation of the detrusor urinae muscle, which is necessary to allow expansion of the bladder while it is filling (130).

The vesicle plexus contains many ganglionic neurons traditionally associated with the parasympathetic system. However, it is now clear that these neurons also receive input from adrenergic axons in the sympathetic system. Thus, the sympathetic system can influence the activity of the parasympathetic system by modulating the activity of the ganglion cells. The ganglion cells innervating the trigone muscle have α-adrenoceptors on their membranes and respond to sympathetic stimulation with contraction. Conversely, ganglion cells innervating the detrusor muscle have β-adrenoceptors on their membranes and respond to sympathetic stimulation with relaxation. It is through this differential distribution of adrenoceptors that the sympathetic nervous system is capable of increasing the tone in the trigone while simultaneously relaxing the detrusor urinae (130).

The sphincter urethrae muscle, or external urethral sphincter, at the base of the bladder, is skeletal muscle; it receives its innervation from the perineal branches of the pudendal nerve (Fig. 6.22). This is a somatic nerve containing axons from motoneurons located in the ventral horn of the spinal cord (S2-4). The release of urine from the bladder requires an integrated viscerosomatic reflex involving:

1. Excitation of the parasympathetic system to activate the detrusor urinae muscle.

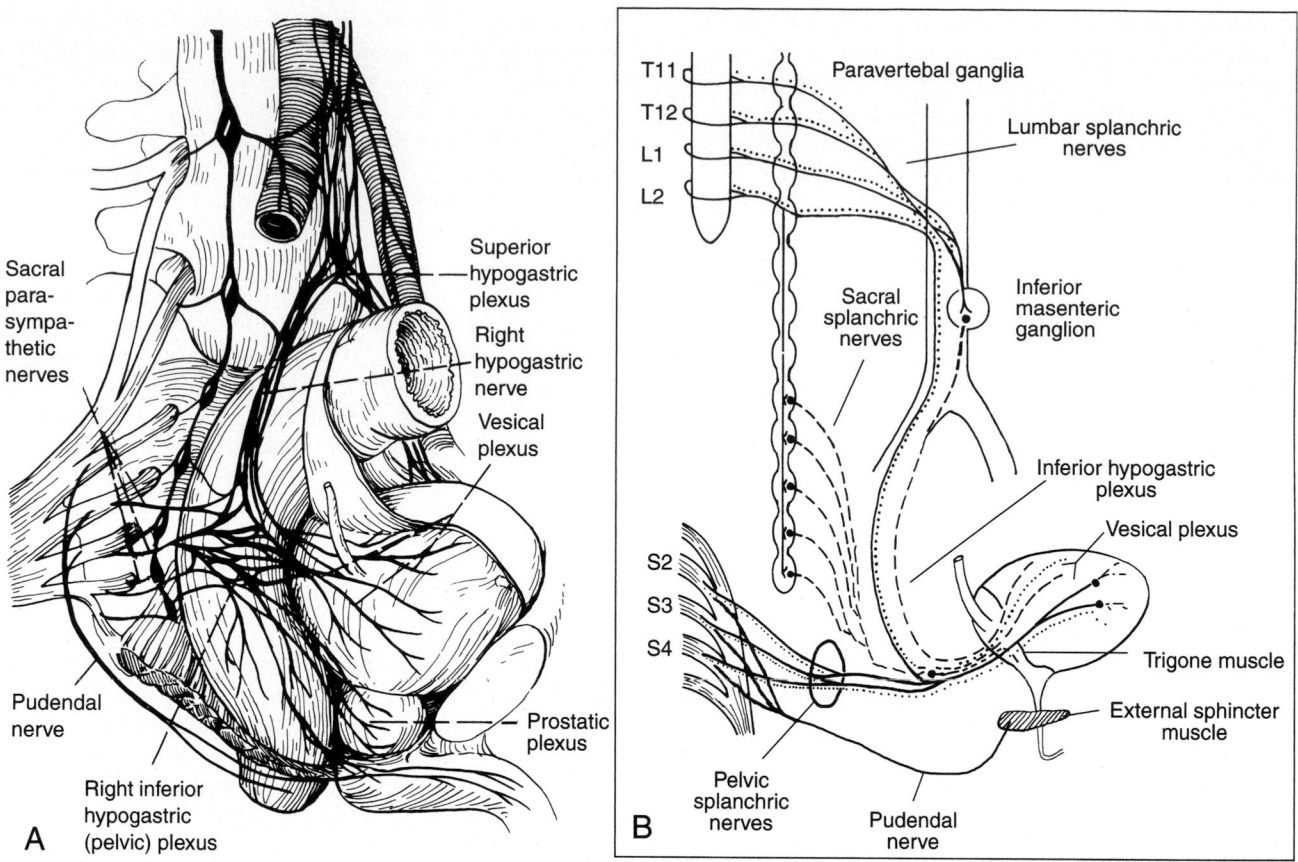

FIGURE 6.22. A: Inferior hypogastric plexus as it innervates the viscera of the pelvic basin. **B:** Somatic innervation of the urinary bladder and its external sphincter. From Gee WF, Ansell JS. Pelvic and perineal pain of urologic origin. In: Bonica JJ, ed. *The Management of Pain.* Philadelphia, PA: Lea & Febiger; 1990:1369, with permission.

2. Inhibition of the sympathetic system to relax the trigone and internal sphincteral muscles.

3. Subsequent inhibition of the pudendal nerve to relax the external sphincteral muscles.

Vesicle afferent fibers arise from mechanoreceptor endings in the connective tissue and epithelium of the vesicle mucosa and travel over the lumbar and pelvic splanchnic nerves as well as pudendal nerves to reach the cord at the L1-2 and S2-4 levels. Cell bodies for these nerves are present in the associated dorsal root ganglia. Many of these fibers contain neuropeptides such as those represented in the small-caliber, primary afferent fibers system (130). The afferent fibers reach only to the dorsal horn of the spinal cord near their segmental level of entry; however, a small number of these fibers enter the spinal cord and follow the ascending tracts rostrally to terminate in the lower regions of the medulla.

Sensory information from distension of the bladder initiates the reflexes involved in voiding. Initial filling of the bladder triggers low-level afferent volleys that increase the tone in the trigone muscle and external sphincter muscles and inhibit the tone in the detrusor urinae muscle, allowing the bladder to serve as a reservoir for urine. After a certain level of filling is reached, a higher intensity of afferent volleys from the bladder wall reverse these reflexes such that the detrusor urinae muscle tone is enhanced and the tone of the trigone and external sphincter is inhibited.

This reversal of reflexes prepares the bladder for voiding. The last step, relaxation of the external sphincter, requires cooperation of the suprasegmental control of the bladder musculature, allowing volitional control of voiding (130).

Reproductive Tract

The pelvic and perineal organs of the male and female reproductive systems receive both sympathetic and parasympathetic innervation through the complex abdominopelvic plexus (Fig. 6.23). This innervation targets the glandular cells and smooth muscle of the vasculature as well as the mural smooth muscle present in the tubular portions of these organs. The origin of this innervation varies according to the embryonic origin of the specific organs. The testis and ovary, which arise in the gonadal ridge of the posterior abdominal wall, receive their afferent and efferent supply from the abdominal portions of the abdominopelvic plexus. The remaining pelvic organs of reproduction are innervated from the pelvic portion of the plexus. Afferent fibers are present in each of these organs, and their input to the spinal cord is a key feature in the presentation of pelvic pain.

Testis and Ovary

Gonadal tissue receives sympathetic innervation from preganglionic neurons located in spinal segments T10 and T11. These

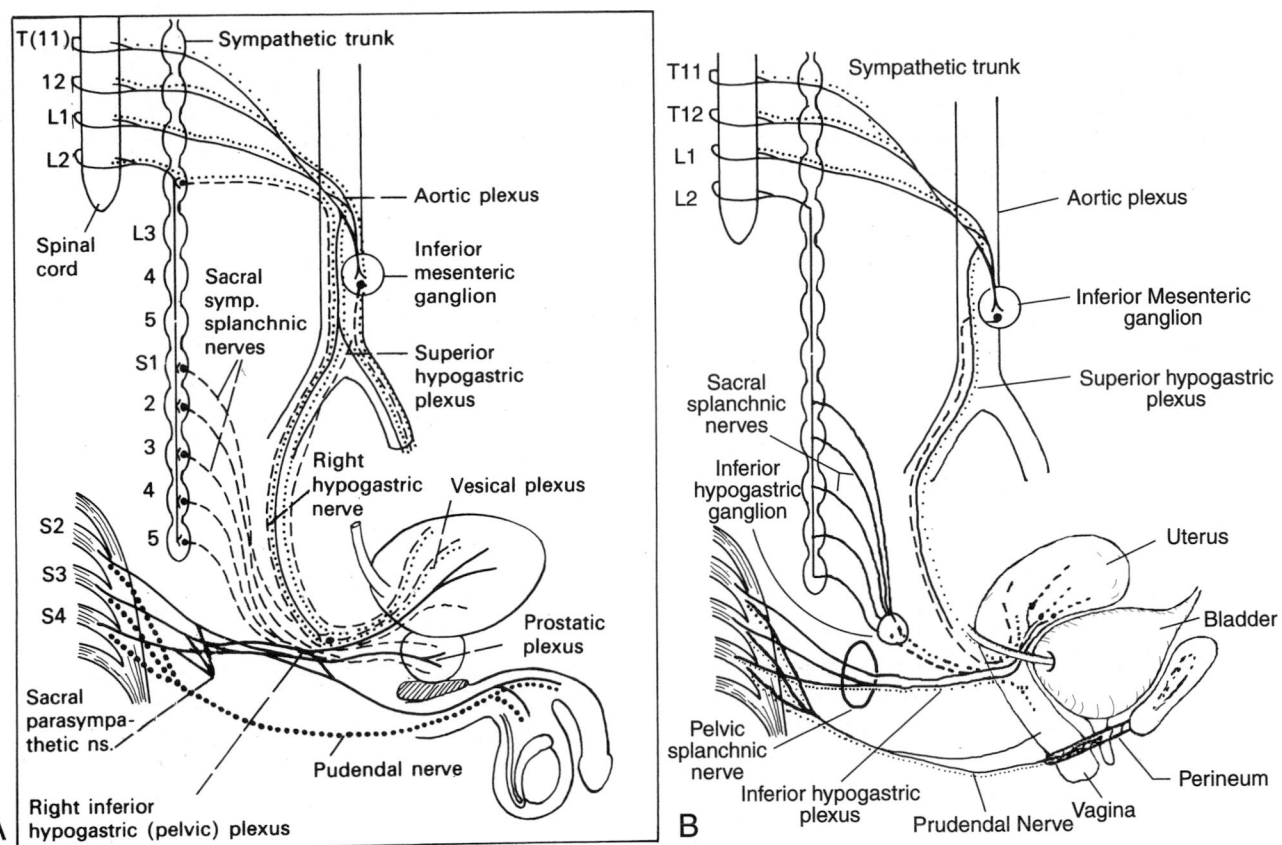

FIGURE 6.23. A: Innervation of the male reproductive organs. **B:** Innervation of the female reproductive organs. From Gee WF, Ansell JS. Pelvic and perineal pain of urologic origin. In: Bonica JJ, ed. *The Management of Pain.* Philadelphia, PA: Lea & Febiger; 1990:1369, with permission.

preganglionic axons target neurons in the celiac and superior mesenteric ganglia. The gonadal (spermatic or ovarian) plexus of fibers arises from these ganglia and follows the course of the gonadal arteries. Additional sympathetic postganglionic axons join the gonadal plexus from the superior hypogastric plexus in the lower abdomen. In females, the gonadal (ovarian) plexus innervates the ovary and extends on to reach the uterine tubes. In males, the gonadal (spermatic) plexus joins the spermatic cord with the vas deferens and proceeds through the inguinal canal to reach the scrotum. Adrenergic fibers in the testis are present around blood vessels and interstitial cells of the seminiferous tubules and in the tubules of the epididymis (125). Stimulation of the sympathetic nervous system initiates strong peristaltic waves in the vas deferens, which is responsible for the propulsion of sperm. Parasympathetic innervation of the gonadal tissue is less dense than that of the sympathetic fibers. Cholinergic fibers arise from the vesical plexus and join the gonadal plexus as it passes though the pelvis. These fibers primarily target the vas deferens and the seminal vesicles.

Afferent fibers from the testis, epididymis, and vas deferens extend through the gonadal plexus to reach the thoracolumbar spinal cord. Fibers arising in the testis target segment T10, those from the epididymis enter the spinal cord at T11 and T12, although those from the vas deferens enter at T10-L1 (131). Afferent fibers from the ovary also ascend in the gonadal plexus to enter the spinal cord at the T10 level. The return of afferent axons from the gonadal tissue to the lower thoracic level of the spinal cord is responsible for the referral of pain to the thoracolumbar junction and the facilitation of segments in this area consequent to irritation of the gonadal tissue.

Uterus, Uterine Tube, Cervix, and Vagina

The distal portion of the abdominopelvic plexus bifurcates as it descends over the sacral promontory to enter the pelvic basin. The pelvic portion of this complex neural structure is called the inferior hypogastric or pelvic plexus. This network of ganglia and fibers sweeps laterally along the pelvic walls to surround the midline organs of the female pelvis. As this plexus crosses over the transverse cervical ligament, its fibrous network thickens to form the elaborate plexus of Frankenhuser (a regional subset of the inferior hypogastric plexus). From here, autonomic axons accompany the uterine vessels medially along the transverse cervical ligament to gain access to the uterus, cervix, and vagina. The remainder of the inferior hypogastric plexus extends anteriorly to surround the bladder (this collection of fibers is often referred to as the vesical plexus).

Sympathetic preganglionic neurons capable of influencing the uterus and cervix are located in the T10-L2 spinal segments (Fig. 6.23). Their axons target neurons in the celiac ganglia and other prevertebral ganglia. Postganglionic fibers from these ganglia descend into the pelvic basin coursing in the superior and inferior hypogastric plexus to eventually reach the uterus. For the most part, these adrenergic fibers end on the vasculature of the uterus. Some axons terminate in the smooth muscle of the myometrium, particularly in the longitudinal layer (132) and among the glands of the endometrium. The parasympathetic input to the uterus and cervix arises in the intermediolateral nucleus of spinal segments S2-4. These axons target ganglia located in the plexus of Frankenhuser; whereas postganglionic (cholinergic) axons extend from this plexus into the uterus following the uterine artery. Most of the cholinergic input to the uterus is confined to the vascular supply with a small amount reaching the glands of the endometrium and a few fibers in the circular muscle layer of the myometrium (132). Beyond regulation of the vasculature, the function of this elaborate autonomic innervation of the uterus is not well known. Evidence suggests that stimulation of the adrenergic and cholinergic inputs can enhance the contraction of mammalian uterine myometrium (133). The number and size of adrenergic nerves appears to increase in the uterus during pregnancy (134), further suggesting a role for these fibers in the uterine contractions of labor and delivery.

The uterus, cervix, and vagina receive a complex afferent innervation that influences the referral of pain during parturition (135). Experimental studies in cats demonstrate that afferent fibers from the uterus and cervix enter the spinal cord over a range of levels (T12-S3) (136). The majority of fibers from the fallopian tubes have cell bodies in the dorsal root ganglia of the lumbar segments; whereas the majority of fibers from the cervix have cell bodies in the dorsal root ganglia of the sacral segments. Clinical studies suggest that the afferent fibers from the human uterus project to even higher levels of the spinal cord (T10) (135) and that the majority of pain fibers from the uterus enter the thoracolumbar spinal cord (137,138). Nociceptive fibers from the uterus pass upward through the superior hypogastric plexus and lumbar splanchnic nerves to enter the spinal cord over the white rami of the lower thoracic and lumbar segments. For this reason, the white ramus at L1 can be particularly large. The pathways handling sensory information from the female reproductive tract are split. Input from above the cervix ascends through the superior hypogastric plexus to the thoracolumbar junction although afferent fibers from the cervix and below descend into the sacral spinal cord (68). This arrangement of primary afferent fibers is responsible, in part, for the presentation of low-back pain late in pregnancy as well as accompanying facilitation of spinal segments around the thoracolumbar junction.

Erectile Tissue of the Penis and Clitoris

The sympathetic innervation of the vasculature and erectile tissue in the penis and clitoris has its origin in the intermediolateral cell column of spinal cord segments T11-L2 (Fig. 6.23). At least two routes exist through which these fibers reach the penis. One route involves preganglionic axons that arise in the thoracolumbar spinal cord and synapse in the associated paravertebral ganglia. From these ganglia, adrenergic postganglionic fibers join the hypogastric plexus to pass into the pelvic basin, eventually entering the penis at its root on the perineal diaphragm. The second route comprises sympathetic preganglionic axons from thoracolumbar segments that pass by the paravertebral ganglia to terminate in pelvic ganglia located deep in the pelvic plexus. Postganglionic adrenergic axons from these ganglia reach the root of the penis or clitoris by following the associated perineal vasculature.

Parasympathetic innervation of the vasculature and erectile tissue arises in the sacral (S2-4) spinal cord. Postganglionic axons from neurons in the scattered ganglia of the pelvic plexus join the sympathetic axons entering the penis or clitoris over its root. Nonadrenergic, noncholinergic axons, presumably from cells located in the pelvic ganglia, also innervate the erectile tissue. Somatic motor innervation of the clitoris and penis arises in Onuf's nucleus of the ventral horn of spinal cord segments S2-4. Their axons travel the course of the pudendal to the perineum where they innervate the following structures, all of which are composed of skeletal muscle:

> Bulbocavernosus muscles
> Ischiocavernosus muscles
> Superficial and deep perineal muscles
> External urethral sphincters
> Anal sphincters

The sex act requires coordinated viscerosomatic reflexes involving the organs and musculature of the pelvic and perineal region (130). Initially, somatic and/or emotional stimuli activate parasympathetic outflow from the sacral cord to the vasculature of the erectile tissue. The cholinergic fibers activate the release of nitric oxide from endothelial cells, which relaxes the vessel walls and results in increased perfusion of the tissue. Once the erectile tissue is engorged, additional stimuli initiate a sympathetic barrage from the thoracolumbar junction of the cord. This output results in contraction of smooth muscle in the vas deferens in the male and in the walls of the vagina in the female. Coordinated reflex activation of the perineal nerve subsequently results in contraction of the bulbospongiosus, ischiocavernosus, and transverse perineal muscles. The rhythmic contraction of these muscles assists in forcing the ejaculate along the urethra in the male and constricts the vestibule of the vagina in the female. Integration of these three efferent pathways (parasympathetic, sympathetic, and somatic) occurs in the circuitry of the sacral spinal cord segments and is necessary for successful completion of the sex act.

CONCLUSION

The autonomic nervous system is a major factor orchestrating the diverse functions of internal structures. Through an extensive network of connections, the autonomic nervous system helps maintain the normal rhythm of activity in the visceral organs as well as adjust their output to accommodate any external challenge. This conglomerate of interlocking systems, with its pervasive influence on our physiology and psychology, is called the neuroendocrine-immune network. This network is described in more detail in Chapter 8 and in Chapter 9 of the previous edition of this book (139).

REFERENCES

1. Clarke E, Jacyna LS. *Nineteenth-Century Origins of Neuroscientific Concepts.* Berkeley, CA: University of California Press; 1987.
2. McGeer PL, Eccles JC, McGeer EG. *Molecular Neurobiology of the Mammalian Brain.* New York, NY: Plenum Press; 1987.

3. Agnati LF, Bjelke B, Fuxe K. Volume transmission in the brain. *Am Sci.* 1992;80:362–373.

4. Prechtl JC, Powley TL. B-afferents: A fundamental division of the nervous system mediating homeostasis? *Behav Brain Sci.* 1990;13:289–331.

5. Wang FB, Holst MC, Powley TL. The ratio of pre- to postganglionic neurons and related issues in the autonomic nervous system. *Brain Res Brain Res Rev.* 1995;21(1):93–115.

6. Goyal RK, Hirano I. The enteric nervous system. *N Engl J Med.* 1996;334(17):1106–1115.

7. Renkin EM. Control of microcirculation and blood-tissue exchange. *Handbook of Physiology.* New York: Oxford University Press, 1984; Sect. 2, Vol. IV:627–687.

8. Harati Y. Anatomy of the spinal and peripheral autonomic nervous system. In: Low PA, ed. *Clinical Autonomic Disorders.* Boston, MA: Little, Brown and Company; 1993:17–37.

9. Freire-Maia L, Azevedo AD. The autonomic nervous system is not a purely efferent system. *Med Hypotheses.* 1990;32:91–99.

10. Dockray GJ, Sharkey KA. Neurochemistry of visceral afferent neurons. *Progress Brain Res.* 1986;67:133–148.

11. Schott GD. Visceral afferents: their contribution to "sympathetic dependent" pain. *Brain.* 1994;117:397–413.

12. Cervero F. Mechanisms of acute visceral pain. *Br Med Bull.* 1991;47:549–560.

13. Cervero F. Sensory innervation of the viscera: peripheral basis of visceral pain. *Physiol Rev.* 1994;74:95–138.

14. Vanhoutte PM, Shepherd JT. Autonomic nerves of the systemic blood vessels. In: Dyck PJ, Thomas PK, eds. *Peripheral Neuropathy.* Philadelphia, PA: W.B. Saunders; 1993:208–227.

15. Burnstock G. Cholinergic and purinergic regulation of blood vessels. *Handbook of Physiology.* New York: Oxford University Press, 1980; Sec. 2; Vol. II.:567–612.

16. Joyner MJ, Halliwill JR. Sympathetic vasodilatation in human limbs. *J Physiol.* 2000;526(3):471–480.

17. Bonica JJ. General considerations of pain in the head. In: Bonica JJ, ed. *The Management of Pain.* Philadelphia, PA: Lea & Febiger; 1990:651–675.

18. Mitchell GAG. The cranial extremities of the sympathetic trunks. *Acta Anat (Basel).* 1953;18:195–201.

19. Bevan JA, Bevan RD, Duckles SP. Adrenergic regulation of vascular smooth muscle. In: Bohr DF, Somlyo AP, Sparks HV, Geiger SR, eds. *Handbook of Physiology,* section 2, The Cardiovascular System: volume II, Vascular Smooth Muscle. Bethesda, MD: American Physiology Society; 1980:515–566.

20. Shepherd RFJ, Shepherd JT. Control of blood pressure and the circulation in man. In: Bannister R, Mathias CJ, eds. *Autonomic Failure.* Oxford, UK: Oxford Medical Publications; 1992:78–93.

21. Joyner MJ, Shepherd JT. Autonomic control of circulation. In: Low PA, ed. *Clinical Autonomic Disorders.* Boston, MA: Little, Brown and Company; 1993:55–67.

22. Kawarai M, Koss MC. Neurogenic cutaneous vasodilation in the cat forepaw. *J Auton Nerv Syst.* 1992;37:39–46.

23. Jinkins JR, Whittermore AR, Bradley WG. The anatomic basis of vertebrogenic pain and the autonomic syndrome associated with lumbar disk extrusion. *AJR Am J Roentgenol.* 1989;152:1277–1289.

24. Yonehara N, Chen J-Q, Imai Y, et al. Involvement of substance P present in primary afferent neurons in modulation of cutaneous blood flow in the instep of the rat hind paw. *Br J Pharmacol.* 1992;106:256–262.

25. Basbaum AI, Levine JD. The contributions of the nervous system to inflammation and inflammatory disease. *Can J Physiol Pharmacol.* 1991;69:647–651.

26. Kidd BL, Gibson SJ, O'Higgins F, et al. A neurogenic mechanism for symmetrical arthritis. *Lancet.* 1989;2:1128–1130.

27. Gonzales R, Sherbourne CD, Goldyne ME, et al. Noradrenaline-induced prostaglandin production by sympathetic postganglionic neurons is mediated by 2-adrenergic receptors. *J Neurochem.* 1991;57:1145–1150.

28. Levine JD, Fields HL, Basbaum AI. Peptides and the primary afferent nociceptor. *J Neurosci.* 1993;13:2273–2286.

29. Keller JT, Marfurt CF, Dimlich RVW, et al. Sympathetic innervation of the supratentorial dura mater of the rat. *J Comp Neurol.* 1989;290:310–321.

30. Keller JT, Marfurt CF. Peptidergic and serotonergic innervation of the rat dura mater. *J Comp Neurol.* 1991;309:515–534.

31. Stead RH, Dixon MF, Bramwell NH, et al. Mast cells are closely apposed to nerves in the human gastrointestinal mucosa. *Gastroenterology.* 1989;97:575–585.

32. Levine JD, Coderre TJ, Covinsky K, et al. Neural influences on synovial mast cell density in rat. *J Neurosci Res.* 1990;26:301–307.

33. Levine JD, Dardick SJ, Roizen MF, et al. Contribution of sensory afferents and sympathetic efferents to joint injury in experimental arthritis. *J Neurosci.* 1986;6:3423–3429.

34. Hardebo J-E. Activation of pain fibers to the internal carotid artery intercranially may cause the pain and local signs of reduced sympathetic and enhanced parasympathetic activity in cluster headache. *Headache.* 1991;31:314–320.

35. Suzuki N, Hardebo J-E. The cerebrovascular parasympathetic innervation. *Cerebrovasc Brain Metab Rev.* 1993;5(1):33–46.

36. Suzuki N, Hardebo J-E. Anatomical basis for a parasympathetic and sensory innervation of the intracranial segment of the internal carotid artery in man. Possible implication for vascular headache. *J Neurol Sci.* 1991;104(1):19–31.

37. Spalding JMK, Nelson E. The autonomic nervous system. In: Joynt RJ, ed. *Clinical Neurology.* Philadelphia, PA: JB Lippincott Co; 1986:1–58.

38. Williams PL. *Gray's Anatomy: The Anatomical Basis of Medicine and Surgery,* 38th ed. Edinburgh, Scotland: Churchill Livingstone; 1995.

39. Wilson-Pauwels L, Akesson E, Stewart P. Cranial Nerves: Anatomy and Clinical Comments. Toronto, Ontario, Canada: BC Decker Inc.; 1988.

40. Haerer AF. *DeJong's The Neurologic Examination,* 5th ed. Philadelphia, PA: JB Lippincott Co; 1992.

41. Grundy D. Speculations on the structure/function relationship for vagal and splanchnic afferent endings supplying the gastrointestinal tract. *J Auton Nerv Syst.* 1988;22:175–180.

42. Lance JW. Current concepts of migrane. *Neurol India.* 1993;43 (Suppl3):S11–S15.

43. Ruskell GL. The orbital branches of the pterygopalatine ganglion and their relationship with internal carotid nerve branches in primates. *J Anat.* 1970;106:323–339.

44. Suzuki N, Hardebo J-E, Skagerberg G, et al. Central origins of preganglionic fibers to the sphenopalatine ganglion in the rat. A fluorescent retrograde tracer study with special reference to its relation to central catecholaminergic systems. *J Auton Nerv Syst.* 1990;30(2):101–109.

45. Walters BB, Gillespie SA, Moskowitz MA. Cerebrovascular projections from the sphenopalatine and otic ganglia to the middle cerebral artery of the cat. *Stroke.* 1986;17:488–494.

46. Hardebo J-E, Suzuki N, Ekblad E, et al. Vasoactive intestinal polypeptide and acetylcholine coexist with neuropeptide Y, dopamine-beta-hydroxylase, tyrosine hydroxylase, substance P or calcitonin gene–related peptide in neuronal subpopulations in cranial parasympathetic ganglia of rat. *Cell Tissue Res.* 1992;267(2):291–300.

47. Suzuki N, Hardebo J-E, Owman C. Origins and pathways of cerebrovascular nerves storing substance P and calcitonin gene–related peptide in rat. *Neurosci.* 1989;31:427–438.

48. Moskowitz MA. The neurobiology of vascular head pain. *Ann Neurol.* 1984;16:157–168.

49. Diamond S. Head pain. *Clin Symp.* 1994;46(3):1–34.

50. Moskowitz MA. Basic mechanisms in vascular headache. *Neurol Clin.* 1990;8(4):801–815.

51. Pick J. *The Autonomic Nervous System.* Philadelphia, PA: JB Lippincott Co.; 1970.

52. Mitchell GAG. *Cardiovascular Innervation.* London, UK: E&S Livingstone; 1956.

53. Moore KL, Persaud TVN. *The Developing Human,* 6th ed. Philadelphia, PA: WB Saunders; 1998.

54. Mizeres NJ. The cardiac plexus of nerves. *Am J Anat.* 1963;112:141.

55. Standish A, Enquist LW, Schwaber JS. Innervation of the heart

and its central medullary origin defined by viral tracing. *Science.* 1994;263:232–234.

56. Standish A, Enquist LW, Escardo JA, et al. Central neuronal circuit innervating the rat heart defined by transneuronal transport of pseudorabies virus. *J Neurosci.* 1995;15(3):1998–2012.

57. Levy M, Martin PJ. Neural control of the heart. *Handbook of Physiology,* section 2: The Nervous System vol. 1. New York: Oxford University Press, 1979:581–620.

58. Talman WT. The central nervous system and cardiovascular control in health and disease. In: Low PA, ed. *Clinical Autonomic Disorders.* Boston, MA: Little, Brown and Company; 1993:39–53.

59. Baluk P, Gabella G. Some intrinsic neurons of the guinea-pig heart contain substance-P. *Neurosci Lett.* 1989;104:269–273.

60. Quigg M, Elfvin L-G, Aldskogius H. Distribution of cardiac sympathetic afferent fibers in the guinea pig heart labeled by anterograde transport of wheat germ agglutinin-horseradish peroxidase. *J Auton Nerv Syst.* 1988;25:107–118.

61. Quigg M. Distribution of vagal afferent fibers of the guinea pig heart labeled by anterograde transport of conjugated horseradish peroxidase. *J Auton Nerv Syst.* 1991;36:13–24.

62. Hopkins DA, Armour JA. Ganglionic distribution of afferent neurons innervating the canine heart and cardiopulmonary nerves. *J Auton Nerv Syst.* 1989;26:213–222.

63. Malliani A, Lombardi F, Pagni M. Sensory innervation of the heart. *Progress Brain Res.* 1986;67:39–48.

64. Foreman RD, Blair RW, Ammons WS. Neural mechanisms of cardiac pain. *Progress Brain Res.* 1986;67:227–243.

65. Bonica JJ. General considerations of pain in the chest. In: Bonica JJ, ed. *The Management of Pain.* Philadelphia, PA: Lea & Febiger; 1990:959–1000.

66. Ammons WS. Cardiopulmonary sympathetic afferent excitation of lower thoracic spinoreticular and spinothalmic neurons. *J Neurophysiol.* 1990;64:1907–1916.

67. Beal MC. Viscerosomatic reflexes: a review. *J Am Osteopath Assoc.* 1985;85:786–801.

68. Ruch TC. Pathophysiology of pain. In: Ruch TC, Patton HD, Woodbury JW, et al, eds. *Neurophysiology,* 2nd ed. Philadelphia, PA: WB Saunders; 1965:345–363.

69. Thurlbeck WM, Miller RR. The respiratory system. In: Rubin E, Farber JL, eds. *Pathology.* Philadelphia, PA: JB Lippincott Co.; 1988:542–627.

70. Barnes PJ, Baraniuk JN, Belvisi MG. Neuropeptides in the respiratory tract. Part II. *Am Rev Respir Dis.* 1991;144:1187–1198.

71. Barnes PJ. Neurogenic inflammation in the airways. *Respir Physiol.* 2001;125(1–2):145–154.

72. Drazen JM, Gaston B, Shore SA. Chemical regulation of pulmonary airway tone. *Annu Rev Physiol.* 1995;57:151–170.

73. Bindoff LA, Heseltine D. Unilateral facial pain in patients with lung cancer: a referred pain via the vagus? *Lancet.* 1988;1:812–815.

74. Morton DR, Klassen KP, Curtis GM. Clinical physiology of the human bronchi. I. Pain of tracheobronchial origin. *Surgery.* 1950;28:669.

75. Sivarao DV, Goyal RK. Functional anatomy and physiology of the upper esophageal sphincter. *Am J Med.* 2000;108(Suppl4a):27S–37S.

76. Richards WG, Sugarbaker DJ. Neuronal control of esophageal function. *Chest Surg Clin N Am.* 1995;5(1):157–171.

77. Collman PI, Tremblay L, Diamant NE. The central vagal efferent supply to the esophagus and lower esophageal sphincter of the cat. *Gastroenterology.* 1993;104(5):1430–1438.

78. Hightower NC. Applied anatomy and physiology of the esophagus. In: Bockus HL, ed. *Gastroenterology.* Philadelphia, PA: WB Saunders; 1974:127–142.

79. Goyal RK, Padmanabhan R, Sang Q. Neural circuits in swallowing and abdominal vagal afferent-mediated lower esophageal sphincter relaxation. *Am J Med.* 2001;111(Suppl8A):95S–105S.

80. Collman PI, Tremblay L, Diamant NE. The distribution of spinal and vagal sensory neurons that innervate the esophagus of the cat. *Gastroenterology.* 1992;103(3):817–822.

81. Pope CE. Heartburn, dysphagia, and chest pain of esophageal origin. In: Sleisenger MH, Fordtran JS, eds. *Gastrointestinal Disease: Pathophysiology, Diagnosis, Management.* Philadelphia, PA: WB Saunders; 1983:145–148.

82. Bennett J. ABC of the upper gastrointestinal tract: Oesophagus: Atypical chest pain and motility disorders. *BMJ.* 2001;323(7316):791–794.

83. Bulloch K. Neuroanatomy of lymphoid tissue: a review. In: Guillemin R, Cohn M, Melnechuk T, eds. *Neural Modulation of Immunity.* New York, NY: Raven Press; 1985:111–141.

84. McHale NG. Innervation of the lymphatic circulation. In: Johnston MG, ed. *Experimental Biology of the Lymphatic Circulation.* Amsterdam, The Netherlands: Elsevier Science; 1985:121–140.

85. Benoit JN. Effects of alpha-adrenergic stimuli on mesenteric collecting lymphatics in the rat. *Am J Physiol.* 1997;273(1 Pt 2):R331–R336.

86. Elaut L. The surgical anatomy of the so called presacral nerve. *Surgery, Gynecology and Obstetrics.* 1932;55:581–589.

87. Mayer EA, Raybould HE. Role of visceral afferent mechanisms in functional bowel disorders. *Gastroenterology.* 1990;99:1688–1704.

88. Jänig W, Morrison JFB. Functional properties of spinal visceral afferents supplying abdominal and pelvic organs, with special emphasis on visceral nociception. *Progress Brain Res.* 1986;67:87–114.

89. Paintal AS. The visceral sensations—some basic mechanisms. *Progress Brain Res.* 1986;67:3–19.

90. Cervero F, Tattersall JEH. Somatic and visceral sensory integration in the thoracic spinal cord. *Progress Brain Res.* 1986;67:189–204.

91. Wood JD. Physiology of the enteric nervous system. In: Johnson LR, ed. *Physiology of the Gastrointesinal Tract,* vol. 1. New York, NY: Raven Press; 1981:1–37.

92. Gabella G. Structure of muscles and nerves in the gastrointestinal tract. In: Johnson LR, ed. *Physiology of the Gastrointestinal Tract,* vol. 1. New York, NY: Raven Press; 1981:197–241.

93. Goyal RK, Crist JR. Neurology of the gut. In: Sleisenger MH, Fordtran JS, eds. *Gastrointestinal Disease.* Philadelphia, PA: WB Saunders; 1989:21–52.

94. Ottaway CA. Neuroimmunomodulation in the intestinal mucosa. *Gastroenterol Clin North Am.* 1991;20:511–529.

95. Schofield GC. Anatomy of muscular and neural tissues in the alimentary canal. In: Code C, ed. *Handbook of Physiology,* section 6, Alimentary Canal: volume IV, Motility. Bethesda, MD: American Physiology Society, 1968:1579–1627.

96. Fawcett D. *A Textbook of Histology,* 11th ed. Philadelphia, PA: WB Saunders; 1986.

97. Stark ME, Szurszewski JH. Role of nitric oxide in gastrointestinal and hepatic function and disease. *Gastroenterology.* 1992;103:1928–1949.

98. Sanders KM, Ward SM. Nitric oxide as a mediator of nonadrenergic noncholinergic neurotransmission. *Am J Physiol.* 1992;262:G379–G392.

99. Blau JN, MacGregor EA. Migraine and the neck. *Headache.* 1994;34(2):88–90.

100. Cervero F. Neurophysiology of gastrointestinal pain. *Bailliere's Best Pract Res Clin Gastroenterol.* 1988;2:183–199.

101. Shirasaka C, Tsuji H, Asoh T, et al. Role of the splanchnic nerves in the endocrine and metabolic response to abdominal surgery. *Br J Surg.* 1986;73:142–145.

102. Nonogaki K, Iguchi A. Role of central neural mechanisms in the regulation of hepatic glucose metabolism. *Life Sci.* 1997;60(11):797–807.

103. Mulholland MW, Debas HT. Diseases of the liver, biliary system, and pancreas. In: Bonica JJ, ed. *The Management of Pain.* Philadelphia, PA: Lea & Febiger; 1990:1214–1231.

104. Osborn JL. Relation between sodium intake, renal function, and the regulation of arterial pressure. *Hypertension.* 1991;17(1 Suppl):I91–I96.

105. DiBona GF, Wilcox CS. The kidney and the sympathetic nervous system. In: Bannister R, Mathias CJ, eds. *Autonomic Failure.* Oxford, UK: Oxford Medical Publications; 1992:178–196.

106. DiBona GF. Sympathetic neural control of the kidney in hypertension. *Hypertension.* 1992;19(1 Suppl):I28–I35.

107. DiBona GF, Jones SY. Analysis of renal sympathetic nerve responses to stress. *Hypertension.* 1995;25(4 Pt 1):531–538.

108. Hollenbreg NK. Renal vascular tone in essential and secondary hypertension. *Medicine.* 1975;54:29–44.

109. DiBona GF. Neural control of renal function: cardiovascular implications. *Hypertension.* 1989;13:539–548.

110. Barajas L, Powers K. Innervation of the renal proximal convoluted tubule of the rat. *Am J Anat.* 1989;186:378–388.

111. Barajas L, Powers K, Wang P. Innervation of the renal cortical tubules: a quantitative study. *Am J Physiol.* 1984;247:F50–F60.

112. Insel PA, Snavely MD, Healy D, et al. Radioligand binding and functional assays demonstrate postsynaptic alpha2-receptors on proximal tubules of rat and rabbit kidney. *J Cardiovasc Pharmacol.* 1985;7:S9–S17.

113. DiBona GF, Kopp UC. Neural control of renal function. *Physiol Rev.* 1997;77(1):75–197.

114. Gottschalk CW. Renal nerves and sodium excretion. *Annu Rev Physiol.* 1979;41:229–240.

115. Ammons WS. Renal afferent inputs to the ascending spinal pathways. *Am J Physiol.* 1992;262:R165–R176.

116. Ammons WS. Electrophysiological characteristics of primate spinothalamic neurons with renal and somatic inputs. *J Neurophysiol.* 1989;61:1121–1130.

117. Nemeth L, O'Briain DS, Puri P. Demonstration of neuronal networks in the human upper urinary tract using confocal laser scanning microscopy. *J Urol.* 2001;166(1):255–258.

118. Santicioli P, Maggi CA. Myogenic and neurogenic factors in the control of pyeloureteral motility and ureteral peristalsis. *Pharmacol Rev.* 1998;50(4):683–722.

119. Tahara H. The three-dimensional structure of the musculature and the nerve elements in the rabbit ureter. *J Anat.* 1990;170:183–191.

120. Weiss RM. Physiology and pharmacology of the renal pelvis and ureter. In: Walsh PC, Gittes RF, Perlmutter AD, et al, eds. *Campbell's Urology.* Philadelphia, PA: WB Saunders; 1986:94–128.

121. Ansell JS, Gee WF. Diseases of the kidney and ureter. In: Bonica JJ, ed. *The Management of Pain.* Philadelphia, PA: Lea & Febiger;1990:1232–1249.

122. Edyvane KA, Smet PJ, Trussell DC, et al. Patterns of neuronal colocalization of tyrosine hydroxylase, neuropeptide Y, vasoactive intestinal polypeptide, calcitonin gene–related peptide and substance P in human ureter. *J Auton Nerv Syst.* 1994;48(3):241–255.

123. Smet PJ, Edyvane KA, Jonavicius J, et al. Colocalization of nitric oxide synthase with vasoactive intestinal peptide, neuropeptide Y, and tyrosine hydroxylase in nerves supplying the human ureter. *J Urol.* 1994;152(4):1292–1296.

124. Edyvane KA, Trussell DC, Jonavicius J, et al. Presence and regional variation in peptide-containing nerves in the human ureter. *J Auton Nerv Syst.* 1992;39(2):127–137.

125. Stewart JD. Autonomic regulation of sexual function. In: Low PA, ed. *Clinical Autonomic Disorders.* Boston, MA: Little, Brown and Company; 1993:117–123.

126. Prieto D, Simonsen U, Martin J, et al. Histochemical and functional evidence for a cholinergic innervation of the equine ureter. *J Auton Nerv Syst.* 1994;47(3):159–170.

127. Semenenko FM, Cervero F. Afferent fibres from the guinea-pig ureter: size and peptide content of the dorsal root ganglion cells of origin. *Neuroscience.* 1992;47:197–201.

128. Cervero F, Sann H. Mechanically evoked responses of afferent fibres innervating the guinea-pig's ureter: an in vitro study. *J Physiol.* 1989;412:245–266.

129. De Groat WC. Anatomy and physiology of the lower urinary tract. *Urol Clin North Am.* 1993;20(3):383–401.

130. De Groat WC, Booth AM. Autonomic systems to the urinary bladder and sexual organs. In: Dyck PJ, Thomas PK, eds. *Peripheral Neuropathy.* Philadelphia, PA: WB Saunders; 1993:198–207.

131. Gee WF, Ansell JS. Pelvic and perineal pain of urologic origin. In: Bonica JJ, ed. *The Management of Pain.* Philadelphia, PA: Lea & Febiger; 1990:1368–1394.

132. Taneike T, Miyazaki H, Nakamura H, et al. Autonomic innervation of the circular and longitudinal layers in swine myometrium. *Biol Reprod.* 1991;45:831–840.

133. Bulat R, Kannan MS, Garfield RE. Studies of the innervation of rabbit myometrium and cervix. *Can J Physiol Pharmacol.* 1989;67:837–844.

134. Thilander G. Adrenergic and cholinergic nerve supply in the porcine myometrium and cervix. A histochemical investigation during pregnancy and parturition. *Zentralbl Veterinarmed A.* 1989;36:585–595.

135. Bonica JJ. The nature of pain in parturition. *Clin Obstet Gynecol.* 1975;2:499.

136. Kawatani M, Takeshige C, De Groat WC. Central distribution of afferent pathways from the uterus of the cat. *J Comp Neurol.* 1990;302:294–304.

137. Bonica JJ, McDonald JS. The pain of childbirth. In: Bonica JJ, ed. *The Management of Pain.* Philadelphia, PA: Lea & Febiger; 1990:1313–1343.

138. Bonica JJ, Chadwick HS. Labor pain. In: Wall PD, Melzack R, eds. *Textbook of Pain.* Edinburgh, Scotland: Churchill Livingstone; 1989:482–499.

139. Willard FH, Mokler DJ, Morgane PJ. Neuroendocrine-immune system and homeostasis. In : Ward RC, ed. *Foundations for Osteopathic Medicine.* Baltimore: Williams & Wilkins; 1997:107–135.

NEUROPHYSIOLOGIC MECHANISMS OF INTEGRATION AND DISINTEGRATION

MICHAEL M. PATTERSON
ROBERT D. WURSTER

KEY CONCEPTS

- The background of neurophysiologic research in osteopathic medicine
- The reflex and the interactions affecting reflex activity
- Types of reflex interactions and the importance of reflexes in body function
- Neural basis of reflex interaction and integration and how reflex integration is exhibited in cardiac control
- How spinal and higher nervous areas interact in reflex control
- Concept of the facilitated area or segment of the spinal cord and how it affects function
- Effects of nociception on peripheral tissues and how nerve fibers transmit materials to and from peripheral structures
- Central excitation changes and four stages of alteration of spinal neuron excitability
- What causes the changes of spinal neuron excitability and the time course of each
- Importance of trophic factors for normal function
- The implications of alterations in neural integrative function for health
- Importance of manipulative treatment in maintaining optimal function and health

The human body is a machine run by the unseen force called life, and that it may be run harmoniously it is necessary that there be liberty of blood, nerves, and arteries from the generating point to destination (1).

The foundations of the osteopathic profession, laid by its founder, Andrew Taylor Still, MD, DO, recognize that the state of health is a continuum from complete breakdown to perfect function. One of Still's basic beliefs about function was that the body was a totally integrated unit, its structures working together harmoniously to produce a state of health. Lacking that harmonious function, the body produced conditions promoting loss of health,

or disease. Implicit in these assumptions is the idea that the various parts of the body are functionally interconnected, allowing for necessary adaptations when demands on the body change. This view necessitates that the supply and maintenance organs, mainly the visceral structures, are functionally connected with the primary energy consumer of the body, the musculoskeletal system. This interrelationship has long been neglected in medical practice. The communicating systems of the body, including the immune, endocrine, and neural systems, provide this interconnectedness. When a problem develops in the integrating systems of the body, function cannot help but be compromised, and the stage is set for a lowered state of health, and eventually disease, to occur.

The field of neurophysiology is important to the physician. A thorough knowledge of anatomy and the structural relationships within the body are vital. The physician must also know how these structures function and relate to each other. He or she needs a basis for providing the patient with a rational course of treatment, especially manipulative treatment. The physician must be aware of what palpatory diagnosis is telling him or her about the underlying state of the body, and therefore of the person. Many excellent neurophysiology texts are available that outline the basics of the field.

This chapter does not attempt to give an overview of the entire field or all the areas of special interest to the osteopathic physician. It focuses on the integration of somatic and visceral function through the reflex pathways and relates these interactions to their specific neural basis. Functional alterations in reflex pathways that can disrupt integration are reviewed, along with the nonimpulse-based or trophic function of the nervous system, and how this provides a means of two-way communication within the body not dependent on the better understood neural impulse–based communication. These aspects of the integrative activity of the nervous system are important in the osteopathic clinical experience and the role of manipulative treatment in health care. As Still recognized before the turn of the century, proper function necessitates the free interaction and integration of all body systems. Rational treatment of functional problems likewise requires an understanding of how these interactions occur and what can alter their function.

NEUROPHYSIOLOGY IN THE OSTEOPATHIC PROFESSION

The search for mechanisms underlying the efficacy of osteopathic methods began with the founding of the osteopathic profession. Although Still did not pursue what we would call organized research, he certainly was a fine researcher. He constantly questioned his observations and searched for better ways to find health and ameliorate disease. His early students at the American School of Osteopathy soon began to actively investigate the basis for the treatments they were developing. Their observations resulted in the formulation of the concept of the osteopathic lesion (now known as the somatic dysfunction). The osteopathic lesion was a set of palpatory cues and signs that indicated a functional disturbance in the body that predisposed it to disease. The early pioneers of the profession believed that somatic dysfunctions were primary causes of clinical breakdowns that resulted in the many manifestations of disease, either by themselves or by allowing, through reduced function, microorganisms to overwhelm the body defenses. When viewed in this perspective, the statement by Still that "all diseases are mere effects, the cause being a partial or complete failure of the nerves to properly conduct the fluids of life" (1) is more meaningful.

Still believed that various types of diseases were not entities unto themselves but were the result of the body's efforts to regain optimal function in the face of adverse influences, which is a view that is becoming more strongly supported by the current idea of the "illness response" (2,3). Thus, the events that led to the disruption of the body's normal function became the primary events to treat in the osteopathic physician's efforts to remove the influences resulting in clinical illness. The osteopathic lesion was viewed as one of the primary factors influencing body function. In addition, the osteopathic lesion was amenable to physical manipulations. In addition, Still and his students realized that the body was of necessity an integrated unit; the visceral systems were tightly connected to the somatic systems. They felt strongly that visceral disturbances would cause manifestations in the somatic structures and that somatic disturbances would cause visceral dysfunctions. This reciprocal relationship became very important in the profession's thinking, clinical practice, and research endeavors.

Early research efforts in the profession largely aimed at providing evidence for the somatic problems identified as the osteopathic lesion and the effects of these dysfunctions on various aspects of function (4). In their efforts to find objective measures of the osteopathic lesion, researchers at the American School of Osteopathy used skiography, an early form of x-ray, to look at bony placement and circulatory function as early as 1898. Another early research thrust was the effects of somatic disturbances on visceral function. Louisa Burns began research in this area early in the 1900s with studies on dogs that showed that stimulation of the lower dorsal region increased muscle contraction in the stomach and intestines but that steady pressure for a time tended to inhibit such contractions (4). Burns eventually became head of the A. T. Still Research Institute in Chicago and produced a body of research suggesting that strains produced in the vertebral column would, over time, have definite and reproducible effects on visceral function and morphology. Aided later by Wilber Cole, effects of somatic strains on neural endplate

function controlling visceral organs were found and documented by neural stains. In addition, Cole was able to well delineate the pathways for the effects of somatic influences on visceral function (5). The early research efforts of the osteopathic profession by Burns, Cole, and others were attempts to describe the effects of somatic disturbances on visceral function and the effects of manipulative treatment on immune and general function, among other things. They established a firm interest in the profession on the interrelationships between somatic and visceral function.

Beginning in the late 1930s, a new era of research in osteopathic medicine began. In an effort to enhance the profession's reputation, J. S. Denslow began a program of research at the Kirksville College of Osteopathy and Surgery that was to span 40 years and add much to the understanding of the methods of manipulative treatment. With his colleagues, Denslow used the then cutting edge technology of electromyographic (EMG) recording to obtain objective evidence of specific alterations in somatic function that correlated almost exactly to palpatory findings (6). Joined by Irvin M. Korr in 1945, Denslow used the EMG technology to show that one of the underlying causes of palpatory findings was, indeed, altered muscle excitability. Korr then interpreted these findings in terms of neural function and the concept of the facilitated segment was developed as an underpinning of the osteopathic lesion (7). The research of the Kirksville group (see discussion later in this chapter) firmly placed the interactions between somatic and visceral structures in the forefront of the underpinnings of osteopathic clinical practice and philosophy. It became obvious that the interactions between visceral and somatic structures were important in health maintenance and disease processes. These interactions also provided an explanatory framework for the impact of manipulative treatment as not only influencing somatic function but also having a real and often vital effect on visceral function. Thus, this chapter will focus on the interactions between visceral and somatic structures and how they are organized. In addition, the alterations in spinal cord function that can occur with somatic input and its influence on visceral function will be discussed. Understanding these interactions and alterations, beginning with the organization of the basic reflex arc, is important in understanding the value of osteopathic treatment techniques and the neural basis of health.

THE REFLEX

In 1905, Charles Sherrington (8) published *The Integrative Action of the Nervous System*. This classic text represented current knowledge about the fundamental aspects of how the nervous system handled and integrated information. Over the ensuing years, considerably more has been learned about the function of the nervous system and how it integrates the many functions of the body. A great deal is known about how the basic structural unit of the nervous system, the neuron, interacts with other cells through synaptic structures and the release of neurotransmitters and neuromodulators. The billions of neurons and glial cells that make up the nervous system are organized into functional groups, often with widely differing structural and functional characteristics. Many of the neurons are involved in networks that respond to stimuli impinging on or even originating in the body, which results in commands to muscles and glands that produce activity or secretions. These networks, the reflexes, have been more fully analyzed in recent years. What were previously considered to be almost autonomous units of function are actually complex and interactive aspects of an organizational whole. The reflex has been found to be anything but a static unit of input/output relationships, but rather it is an active and ever-changing mosaic. The characteristics of reflex function are modulated by messages from other areas of the nervous system and by activity of the endocrine and immune systems. In fact, reflexes must not be viewed as separate entities but as parts of various programs that control motor and secretory actions. Thus, an individual reflex may serve differing functions depending on which control program is operating (9). However, for purposes of analysis, reflexes have usually been isolated for study, a practice that has erroneously led many students to view reflexes as simple and unchanging entities.

Structure

The common concept of the reflex is basically one of a relationship between an input stimulus to the body and an output action to either a muscle or a secretory organ. Sherrington viewed the reflex as an input/output relationship between information coming into the body and a response to that information. He viewed a reflex as always inherited and innately given (8). The concept of a reflex includes an afferent or incoming limb from a sensory receptor, which is a central component in the spinal cord or brain. It also includes an output (efferent) limb that is usually a motor component to either somatic (musculoskeletal) or visceral structures terminating in synaptic connections that may either activate or inhibit activity in these structures (Fig. 7.1).

The usual concept of the reflex suggests that the reflex limbs are fairly well defined and limited primarily to one input and one output channel, with little interaction with other reflex networks (Figs. 7.2 and 7.3). Almost all reflex networks can be influenced by a wide variety of other excitatory and inhibitory signals, including those coming from higher or lower levels of the central nervous system. The picture of a reflex as a simple message pathway from the patellar tendon that causes the quadriceps femoris muscle to contract, resulting in a knee jerk, is a vast oversimplification of the interactions that occur when a stimulus causes a response. The tendon tap reflex, exemplified by the patellar tap/knee jerk reflex activation, is, however, a prime example of the simplest reflex structure.

The tendon tap, or myotatic reflex, is a monosynaptic reflex. It is the only monosynaptic reflex present in the human. The stimulus of a tap to a tendon stretches the muscle attached to the tendon, which in turn stretches the muscle spindle organs in the muscle. Neural signals, or action potentials, are sent from the spindle organs to the spinal cord on the incoming, or afferent, limb of the reflex. In this case, the signals travel through the spinal cord on the axons from the spindles directly to the motoneurons that innervate the muscle that was stretched. They make synaptic contact with the motoneurons causing them to generate action potentials that travel over the efferent, or outgoing, limb of the reflex network back to the muscle, which causes it to contract.

It would be a simple picture if this was all that happened.

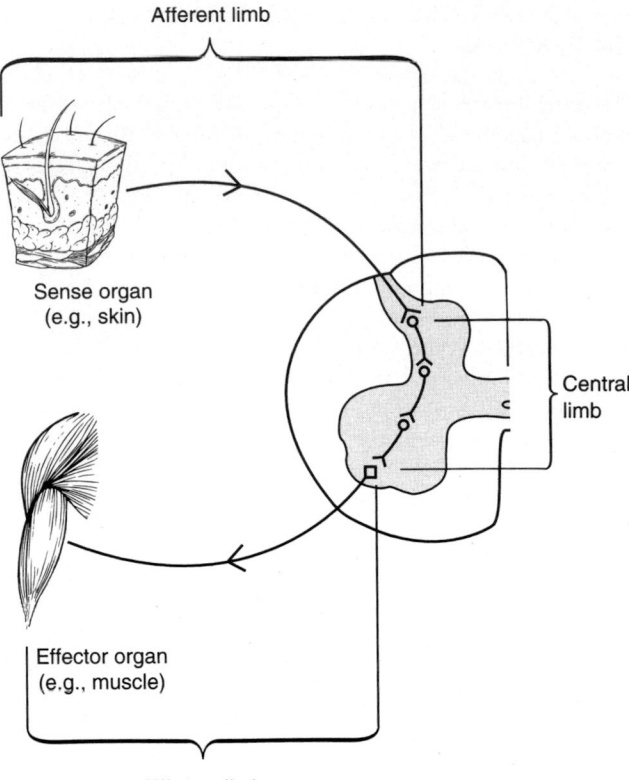

FIGURE 7.1. Schematic of reflex as it is usually envisioned, with afferent, central, and efferent limbs.

However, the incoming axons send off branches that go to other neurons in the spinal cord that, in turn, send axons to the motoneurons of the antagonist of the stretched muscle. These axons provide signals that inhibit the motoneurons innervating the antagonist muscle. When the stretched muscle contracts, the antagonist muscle is inhibited to allow a smooth movement to occur.

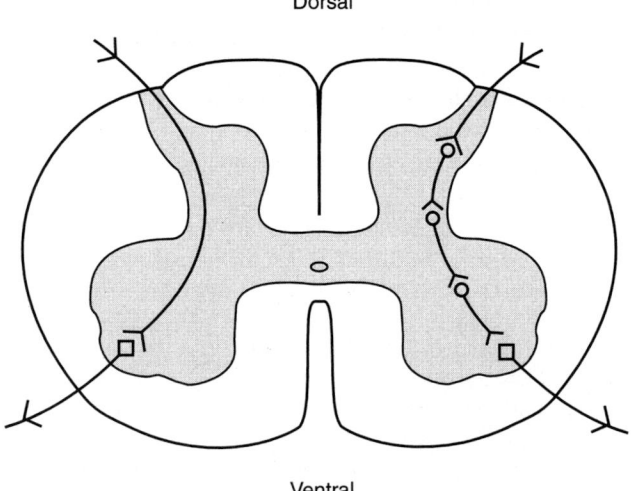

FIGURE 7.2. A common, mistaken concept of how a reflex is constructed. Afferent limb simply connects with central limb, which activates efferent limb. *Left,* monosynaptic reflex; *right,* polysynaptic reflex. Actual complexity is better represented in Fig. 7.3.

Dorsal

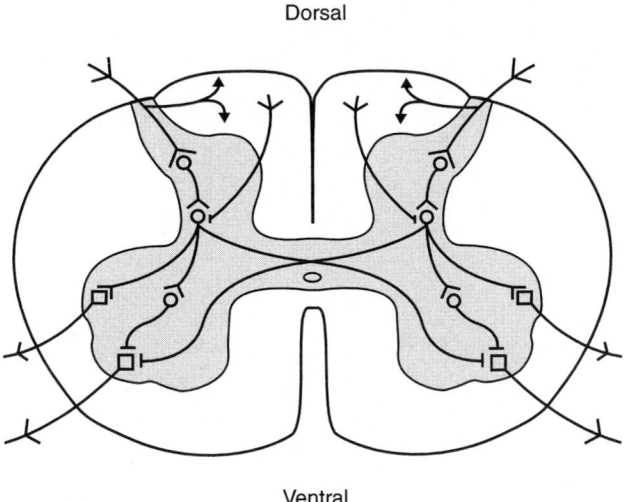

Ventral

FIGURE 7.3. Schematic of neural interactions at the spinal level, indicating the complexity of even simple reflexes. Input to the spinal cord sends collaterals up and down the cord and is acted on by ascending and descending influences, as well as input from the opposite side of the cord. Input courses through several synapses and interneurons before acting (in thoracolumbar cord) on both somatic and sympathetic motoneurons. In cervical and sacral cord areas, parasympathetic pathways are involved.

In addition, other branches from the incoming axons go up the spinal cord to other spinal areas (for example, to the arms if the patellar reflex was stimulated), to the brainstem, as well as down the spinal cord to lower spinal centers. What appeared to be a simple reflex network has become a complex set of pathways within the spinal cord and brainstem. In addition, pathways from both above and below the level of the input axons can directly influence the basic excitability of the motoneurons involved and, hence, alter the reflex activity observed when the tendon is tapped. Indeed, when elicited clinically, the tendon tap reflex is used as a porthole into the nervous system to see how it is functioning, and the clinician is not usually interested in that reflex per se. In fact, the main purpose of using the tendon tap reflex clinically is to test the excitability of the motoneurons, as a function of both local and distant influences.

SOMATO-SOMATIC

Although the tendon tap reflex is used a great deal clinically, the most familiar of the spinal reflexes are the defensive reflexes, such as the withdrawal movements of a limb to a noxious stimulus. These somato-somatic reflexes occur when some stimulus is applied to a somatic structure. This initiates a volley of neural activity (often nociceptive) through the afferent limb of the reflex to the spinal cord. The afferent input activity flows through synapses into the interneurons of the spinal cord central gray, and finally into the ventral horn motoneurons. These motoneurons then cause somatic muscle contraction. The reflexes have at least one interneuron between the sensory input in the dorsal horn of the cord and the motoneurons of the ventral horn (Fig. 7.3). They are named from the origin of the information and the locus of action, both somatic.

Many somato-somatic reflexes have been documented and studied. The simple somato-somatic reflexes are exemplified by defensive withdrawal actions such as when accidentally touching a hot object and the arm jerks back. Very complex activities, such as the righting reflexes that occur, for example, when a cat is dropped upside down and lands on its feet are also found, but even these reflexes do not occur in isolation; as with the myotatic reflexes, they are accompanied by a spread of activity throughout the nervous system.

VISCERO-VISCERAL

A second type of reflex is the viscero-visceral reflex, in which sensory input from a visceral structure causes activity in a visceral organ. These reflexes are involved, for example, in distention of the gut that results in increased contraction of the gut muscle. Viscero-visceral reflexes involve afferent activity flowing from the receptors into the spinal cord through interneurons to produce efferent or outflow activity within the sympathetic and/or parasympathetic motoneurons.

REFLEX INTERACTIONS

We might expect to find that afferent input from somatic structures has some influence on visceral organs and that input from visceral structures has some effect on somatic organs. Somato-visceral and viscero-somatic reflexes have been known for many years but, until recently, have received little attention from the research and medical community. However, these types of reflex interactions are very important for the practice and understanding of osteopathic palpatory diagnosis and treatment and for the integration of body function.

A familiar example of a viscero-somatic reflex is pain and muscle tightness in the left shoulder with onset of a myocardial infarction (MI). The nociceptive input from the compromised myocardium (a visceral structure) is exciting not only the pathways that are interpreted as shoulder pain (a somatic structure) but is also causing the motoneurons supplying the shoulder muscles to become active. In a classic study, Eble (10) showed several such reflexes by stimulating visceral structures and recording somatic muscle activity. He demonstrated that stimulation of various visceral structures produced somatic muscle activity.

Conversely, activity in a somatic structure can alter visceral function. In a number of studies over the last several years, Sato (11) clearly demonstrated the effect of somatic stimulation on various visceral functions, ranging from heart rate to adrenal output. These studies have also shown that some of these reflex interactions occur directly in the spinal cord. With others, the afferent activity from the somatic stimulation travels up the spinal cord to the brainstem, resulting in a cascade of activity from the brainstem back down to the spinal autonomic motoneurons.

In both viscero-somatic and somato-visceral reflex networks, activity resulting from the stimulation of a structure can have either an excitatory or inhibitory influence on the motoneurons involved. For example, stimulation of the belly skin usually results in inhibition of gut activity (a somato-visceral reflex) but increases heart rate.

In daily life, the body's somatic system is active. The skeletal muscles are the machines that carry out activities. The visceral organs are the means by which the energy demands and maintenance of the muscles are met and by which waste is disposed of. Without a continuous and highly integrated communication between these two systems, the body could not continue to achieve a balance among:

Its energy needs and supply
The amount of blood necessary to carry nutrients and waste and fulfill the demands of the muscles and bones
Supply and demand in general

The neural connections represented by these reflex systems are one of the primary ways this integration is carried out.

For the osteopathic physician, the viscero-somatic and somato-visceral reflexes are of extreme importance. When using palpatory diagnosis to detect subtle problems in function, whether it be tissue texture changes, motion characteristics, or temperature variations of the body, the physician is sensing clues from the musculoskeletal system, skin, muscles, and fascias. These clues reflect not only aspects of these tissues but also functional characteristics of the underlying visceral organs and tissues through the viscero-somatic reflex networks. When the physician uses manipulative treatment to correct somatic dysfunctions, underlying visceral function is affected through the somato-visceral reflex networks. Thus, for both palpation and treatment, an understanding of reflex function is necessary.

Neural Basis for Reflex Interactions

Evidence is accumulating about the neural basis of viscero-somatic and somato-visceral interactions. When a stimulus is applied, afferent input from either visceral or somatic structures flows into the spinal cord along the dorsal roots and enters the upper areas of the spinal gray matter. The spinal gray matter is commonly divided into ten layers, first documented on cytoarchitectural evidence by Rexed (12) (Fig. 7.4). Large-diameter, cutaneous afferent input that signals nonnociceptive stimuli enters the spinal gray of the dorsal horn and terminates primarily in layers III and IV. Nociceptive afferents from both somatic and visceral structures enter the cord and send branches rostrally and caudally in Lissauer's tract that runs along the apex of the dorsal horn. Branches of this nociceptive input then terminates in layers I, II, V, VII, and X. Layers I and V display an especially tremendous overlap of the input from somatic and visceral nociceptors (13).

It now appears that in most areas of the spinal cord, practically every interneuron that receives input from a visceral nociceptor also receives input from a somatic source. It also appears that almost 80% of interneurons that receive input from somatic structures also receive visceral input. Presently, there is no evidence for any ascending pathway that transmits only visceral sensory signals from the spinal cord to the brain. This raises the question of how an individual can distinguish visceral from somatic pain or sensation at all. In many cases, visceral pain is felt as a diffuse and poorly localized sensation and is referred to somatic structures. The overlap of somatic and visceral input explains the referral of visceral pain to somatic structures, which is designated as referred pain.

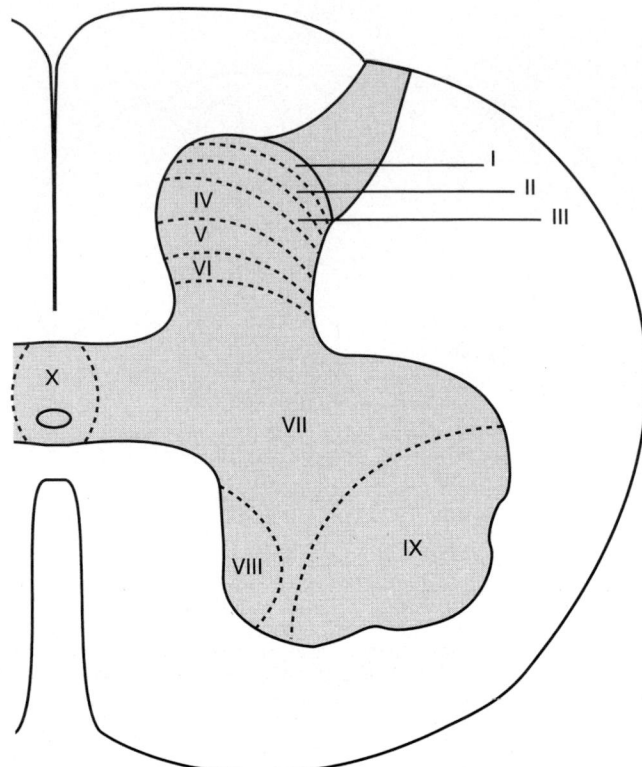

FIGURE 7.4. Rexed layers. Laminae at the L-7 segment of a cat spinal cord. From Rexed B. The cytoarchitectonic organization of the spinal cord in the cat. *J Comp Neurol.* 1952;96:415–495, with permission.

Impulses arriving from visceral structures and converging onto interneurons also receiving somatic afferents activate ascending pathways to the brain that result in the perception of pain in the somatic structure. In addition, more somatic than visceral input occurs because the viscera are much more sparsely innervated with sensory receptors. This suggests that visceral input has much more diffuse functional effects than the corresponding somatic afferents do. For example, it appears that many of the somatic C fibers terminate primarily in focal areas of layer II of the cord. Visceral C fibers extend for several segments and give off collaterals at regular intervals. Only about 10% of the inflow into the thoracolumbar spinal cord comes from visceral structures (14). This sparse innervation but wide distribution of visceral afferents may be the basis for the diffuse nature of most visceral pain. The evidence indicates that the widespread effects of visceral input is due more to functional (spread of activity through networks) than anatomic (many collateral branches) divergence (15). Figure 7.5 shows the afferent terminations of somatic and visceral afferent fibers in the various levels of the spinal cord.

The overlap of input onto common interneurons within the gray matter of the spinal cord is also the basis for the activation of somatic muscle activity seen with visceral disturbances. The excitatory drive provided onto common interneurons by visceral input activates not only sympathetic outflow back to visceral structures but also motoneurons (both alpha and gamma) that innervate skeletal musculature. The result is a tonic activation of skeletal muscles in the referral area of visceral input. This is the viscero-somatic reflex manifestation, or splinting, that is seen, for example, in appendicitis.

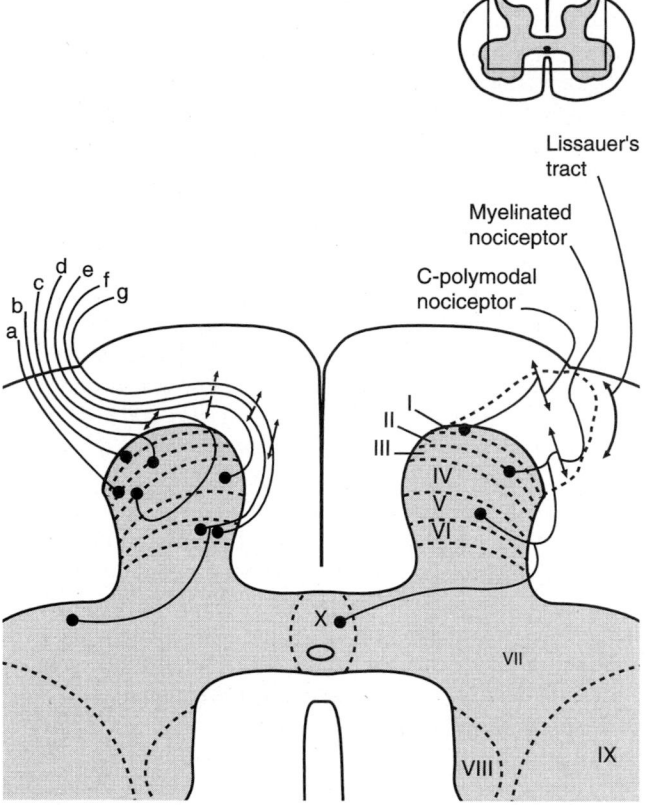

FIGURE 7.5. Terminal patterns of primary afferent collaterals in the transverse plane of spinal cord. *Left,* primary afferent terminations of axons not associated with nociception. *A,* C-low threshold mechanoreceptor; *B,* innocuous cooling receptor; *C,* A hair afferent; *D,* G-1 and G-2 hair receptors; *E,* slowly adapting type I and II afferents; *F,* primary and secondary muscle spindle afferents; *G,* Golgi tendon organ. The *arrow* indicates that the parent axon bifurcates and ascends and descends the spinal cord for 17 segments giving off collaterals along this course. *Right,* nociceptor afferents from both somatic and visceral structures. Both visceral and somatic A and C fiber nociceptor afferents terminate in Rexed lamina I, II, V, and to some extent in VII and X. Lamina are indicated on the right and outlined by *dotted lines.* From Light AR. *The Initial Processing of Pain and Its Descending Control: Spinal and Trigeminal Systems.* Basel, Switzerland: Karger; 1992:88, with permission.

These relationships also underlie the reverse phenomenon, that of the somato-visceral reflex, in which somatic input alters sympathetic and parasympathetic outflow. The data on the convergence of somatic and visceral input are beginning to explain the interrelations between visceral and somatic structures, especially when nociceptive input is activated.

There are descending influences on the activity of both somatic and visceral reflex pathways. In many of the reflex loops driven by both visceral and somatic input, there is a strong effect of descending pathways on the long-lasting excitability of the reflex outflow. These descending influences can maintain the excitability of the reflex for extended periods. They may account for some of the long-term increases in sensitivity, muscle contractions, and hyperexcitable sympathetic output seen especially with visceral disturbances. Likewise, the long-lasting descending influences can be inhibitory, resulting in lowered somatic or autonomic outflow. For example, the effects of rib-raising techniques (a somatic stimulation) on sympathetic outflow seems to be primarily inhibitory through the descending brain influences,

resulting in decreased vasoconstriction and better fluid flow in the thoracic area (16).

Although much of our information on the activation of sympathetic afferents by skeletal input has come from nociceptive input, there is evidence that sympathetic output can also be strongly driven independent of nociception by muscle proprioceptors. For example, Kaufman (17) has shown large effects on sympathetic outflow driven by alteration of proprioceptive input from muscles. Thus, the evidence for activation and control of sympathetic activity by somatic input strongly suggests a basis for musculoskeletal activity in the regulation of body function through somato-visceral reflexes. Likewise, recent research by Jou and Foreman (18) has shown that cardiac efferents can have dramatic influences on muscle activity, supporting the role of viscero-somatic reflex connections as underlying the effectiveness of palpatory diagnosis in visceral disease states.

CARDIAC CONTROL

We will now consider a model of viscero-somatic and somato-visceral interactions shown in cardiac control. Neural input from somatic structures may affect neural activity to both somatic and visceral structures. A good example of the interaction between somatic afferents and autonomic outflow is the control of the heart. As with most visceral structures, the heart receives its autonomic innervation from both sympathetic and parasympathetic nerves.

SYMPATHETIC INNERVATION OF THE HEART

Excitation of the cardiac sympathetic nerves (Fig. 7.6) causes these effects:

Increased heart rate
Increased atrial and ventricular contractility
Decreased conduction time from the atrium to the ventricle

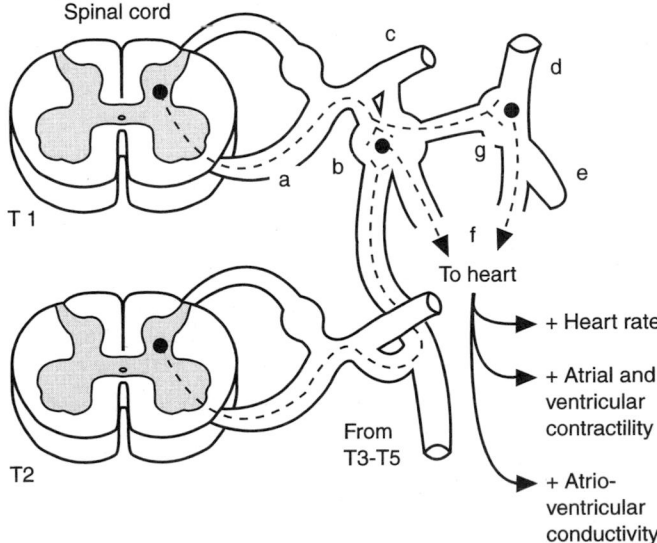

FIGURE 7.6. Sympathetic innervation of heart. *A,* ventral root; *B,* stellate ganglion; *C,* spinal nerve; *D,* vagosympathetic trunk; *E,* vagus nerve; *F,* cardiac nerves; *G,* middle cervical ganglion.

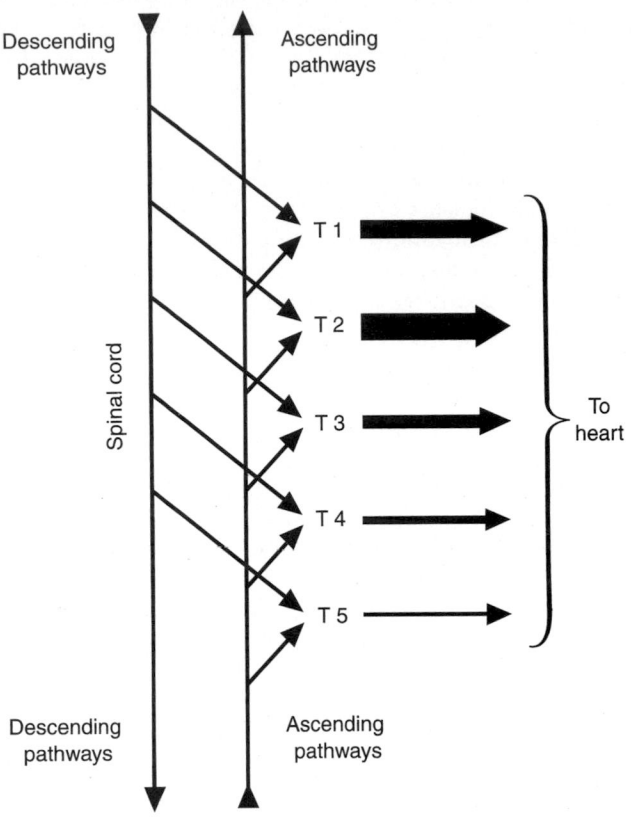

FIGURE 7.7. Spinal sympathetic innervation of the heart and related ascending and descending pathways. The heart receives spinal cord control via T1 to T5 spinal cord levels with T2 making the largest functional contribution. Lesions above T1 and below T5 block brain control of cardiac sympathetic activity and reflex responses to ascending afferent activation, respectively.

The heart's spinal innervation is associated with spinal cord levels from T1 to about T5, with T2 probably contributing the most (Fig. 7.7).

The preganglionic fibers leave the spinal cord via the ventral roots and course a short distance in the spinal nerves (Fig. 7.6). The preganglionic fibers then exit the spinal nerves to enter the adjoining sympathetic chain ganglia. Most preganglionic sympathetic fibers controlling the heart course though the stellate ganglion to the middle cervical ganglion. There, they excite ganglion cells that send their axons, the postganglionic fibers, via the cardiac nerves to innervate:

Pacemaker cells
Myocardium
Conductile system
Coronary arteries

The first paravertebral ganglion associated with the heart is the stellate ganglion, where some preganglionic axons excite ganglion cells whose axons also run directly to the heart (19).

Segmental-like innervation to different portions of the heart does not seem to occur (20). In other words, a particular spinal level (e.g., T4), sends its sympathetic influences to most areas of the heart, not to one area. One should be cautious in relating problems in one portion of the heart to problems associated with one spinal level. However, different spinal segmental levels innervate different organs, for example, heart versus lungs. Some degree of segmental-like innervation does occur.

Understanding the spinal cord levels that control the heart is helpful in understanding responses of spinal cord–injured patients (Fig. 7.7) (21,22). With spinal cord lesions above T1, the brain has no control of the heart via the spinal cord and sympathetic nerves, but it can still activate the parasympathetic pathways. However, marked cardiac alterations may occur via reflexes mediated by sensory input that enters the spinal cord below the C8 level. For example, input from the urinary bladder may cause markedly increased sympathetic activity to the heart. Patients with spinal lesions below T1 have some brain control of the heart via descending spinal pathways. Patients with lesions below T5 rarely show any spinal reflexes influencing the heart from the spinal afferents entering the cord below the lesion level. Specific levels of the spinal cord innervate specific visceral organs.

Sympathetic motoneurons located in both sides of the spinal cord and their corresponding sympathetic nerves innervate the heart. There are some quantitative differences in the regions of the heart that are innervated (20). For example, stimulation of sympathetic preganglionic nerves from both sides of the spinal cord causes increases in heart rate. The right side has a greater influence on heart rate and the sinoatrial node function. Both sides innervate the atrioventricular node, both ventricles, and atria. However, sympathetic output from the left spinal cord has a greater effect on cardiac output and myocardial contractility (20,22). Visceral organs receive asymmetrical autonomic control from the left and right sides of the spinal cord.

Several different descending spinal pathways can affect autonomic outflow from the spinal cord. Many of these pathways are located in the lateral funiculus of the spinal cord. Both anatomic (23) and physiologic (24) evidence suggests that the descending spinal pathways are organized according to a viscerotropic pattern. Localized lesions of the spinal cord, or portions of the descending spinal pathways, may result in loss of brain control of one particular visceral organ, which also suggests that the brain has the potential to separately control different visceral organs (Fig. 7.8).

PARASYMPATHETIC INNERVATION OF THE HEART

Parasympathetic innervation of the heart is via the vagus nerve that causes the following (Fig. 7.9):

Decreased heart rate
Slowed atrioventricular conduction

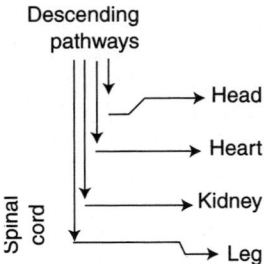

FIGURE 7.8. Viscerotropic organization of the descending spinal pathways controlling autonomic outflow.

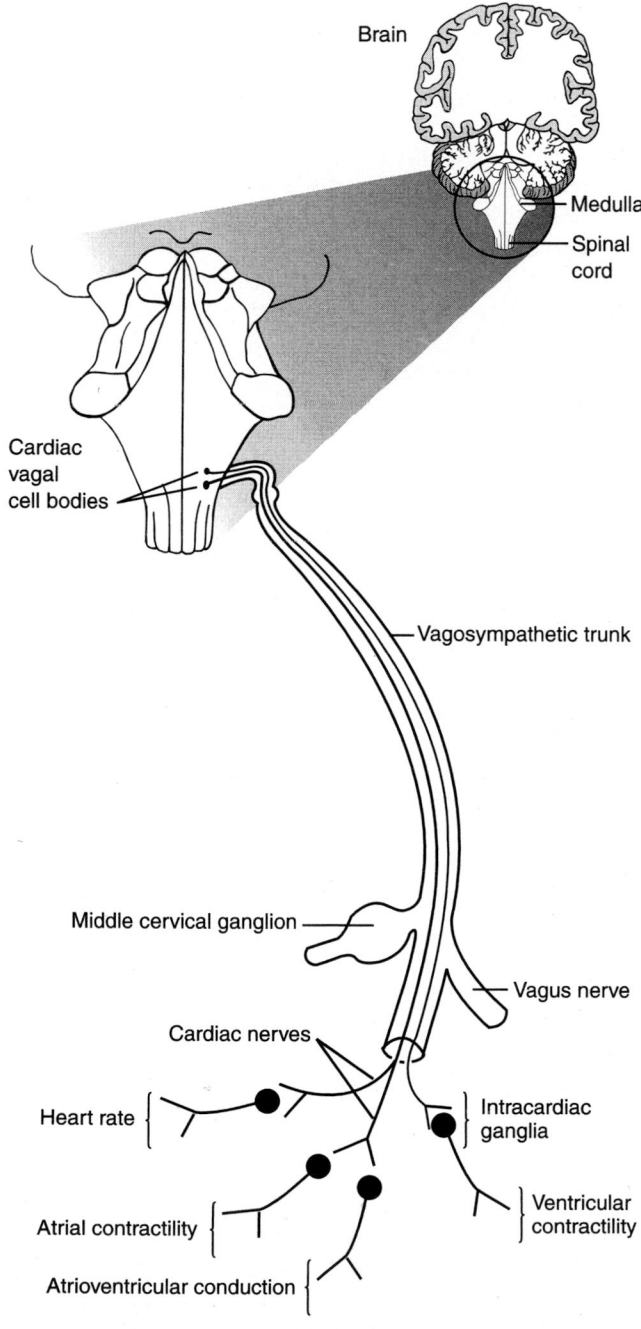

FIGURE 7.9. Parasympathetic innervation of the heart.

Decreased atrial contraction
Limited decrease of ventricular contractility

The cardiac vagal fibers travel in the cervical vagus nerve (vagosympathetic trunk) into the thorax where they separate from the vagus nerve to form the cardiac nerves. These cardiac vagal nerves have their cell bodies in the medulla, that is, the nucleus ambiguous and the dorsomotor nucleus (25–29).

These two medullary regions may subserve different cardiac functions. For example, the nucleus ambiguous may mediate heart rate while the dorsomotor nucleus regulates ventricular contractility (27). Not only are there regions of the brainstem controlling cardiac function that seem to be distinct from those controlling gastrointestinal function and other visceral organs but different brainstem regions may control separate cardiac functions.

VISCERAL FUNCTION CONTROL

Cardiovascular function can be reflexively controlled by somatic afferents via the somatosympathetic reflexes. These reflexes may be mediated at the spinal cord level or via suprasegmental connections. The spinal somatosympathetic reflexes demonstrate dependency on segmental organization. These sympathetic reflex responses at one segmental level are larger if the somatic afferent activity enters at the same spinal level than if it enters at adjoining levels (30,31). These reflexes also demonstrate laterality, because they are larger for ipsilateral reflexes than for contralateral reflexes (Fig. 7.10).

Visceral afferents can also influence somatic reflexes, and muscle tone may be altered by visceral input. Many of these reflex possibilities are very important for osteopathic palpatory diagnosis and treatment because they provide mechanisms for the use of muscle tone as an indicator of visceral disturbances. The work by Eble (32) showed activation of skeletal muscles with stimulation of visceral structures, and Schoen and Finn (33) reported EMG activity in shoulder muscles of the cat following experimental myocardial infarction. The cardiac viscero-somatic reflex has an influence on somatic musculature (18).

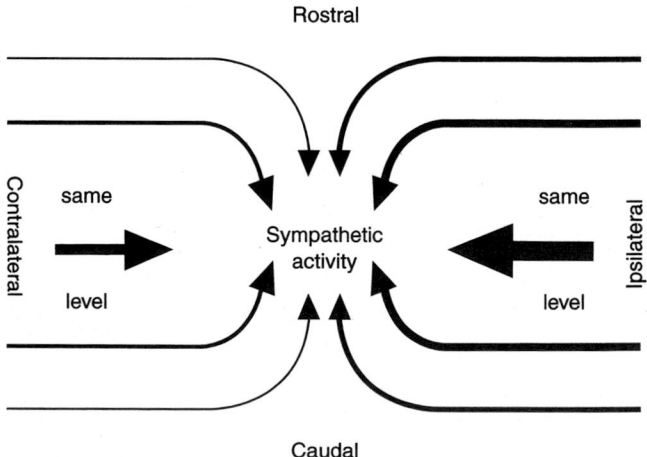

FIGURE 7.10. Laterality of cardiac sympathetic control and segmental organization of spinal sympathetic reflexes.

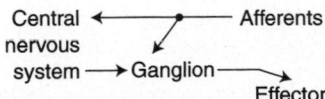

FIGURE 7.11. Afferent reflex control of autonomic effectors may be mediated via reflexes within peripheral autonomic ganglia as well as via central nervous system connections.

Not only can there be activity from somatic or visceral structures that influences the opposite structures, but another type of activity, independent of the brain or spinal cord, may also occur. Recently, neural activity has been recorded from *in vitro* sympathetic ganglion cells and intracardiac ganglion cells, demonstrating considerable action potential activity even when the neuronal connections to the central nervous system are severed (25,27–29). These observations suggest that the autonomic ganglia may function as little brains within peripheral ganglia and the heart. These ganglia may have the neural circuitry to act almost independently and have the ability to integrate intrinsic cardio-cardiac reflexes as well as information from the central nervous system. However, the functional roles of these peripheral nervous system interactions are presently unknown (Fig. 7.11).

The possibility of little brains within the autonomic ganglia presents many more possibilities. If visceral afferents have reflexes within the autonomic ganglia, somatic afferents could also have reflex connections within them. Some somatic afferent fibers pass through the autonomic ganglia. It is possible that somatic afferents influence sympathetic activity not only to the somatic structure but also to visceral structures such as the heart. Activation of somatic afferents might cause reflex alteration of cardiac function via direct ganglionic reflexes as well as via the central nervous system–mediated reflexes. Likewise, visceral afferents might activate sympathetic ganglion cells with axons supplying somatic structures (34–37). The therapeutic implications of reflexes within autonomic ganglia may be important.

INTERACTIONS OF SOMATIC AFFERENTS AND BARORECEPTOR CONTROL OF AUTONOMIC ACTIVITY

Blood pressure and cardiac function are reflexively controlled through alteration of autonomic activity mediated by arterial blood pressure afferent receptors called baroreceptors. Increased arterial blood pressure excites baroreceptor activity, which is carried to the brainstem via the glossopharyngeal and vagus nerves. In the brainstem, the baroreceptor afferent activity eventually

leads to excitation of the medullary cardiac vagal cell bodies. It also leads to inhibition of the sympathetic activity to the cardiovascular system via descending brainstem/spinal pathways (38). Baroreceptor reflexes involving the cardiac vagus nerves have parallel inhibitory effects on the sinoatrial node (slowing heart rate) and atrioventricular node (slowing atrioventricular conduction) (39).

Although these baroreceptor reflexes have powerful influences on cardiovascular function, they also interact with other spinal reflexes, especially from small, high-threshold, afferent fibers. With activation of these spinal afferents, reflex changes in sympathetic activity (somatosympathetic reflexes) occur at the spinal cord level and through suprasegmental reflexes involving ascending and then descending pathways to and from the brainstem (40,41).

Baroreceptor reflexes inhibit both spinal and supraspinally mediated somatosympathetic reflexes (42). Presumably, other visceral afferents that also mediate sympathetic reflexes are also inhibited by these powerful baroreceptor reflexes.

Somatic afferent activity can modulate baroreceptor reflex vagal control of the heart. Baroreceptor activation excites the cardiac vagus nerve activity. However, somatic afferent stimulation attenuates or blocks the baroreceptor influence of vagal cardiac nerves. Somatic afferents and baroreceptors compete for control of autonomic activity. The ascending and descending pathways for these reflexes have been localized in the dorsal portion of the lateral funiculus of the spinal cord (43–45).

Summation Characteristics of Somato-Visceral Reflexes

Somato-visceral reflexes demonstrate temporal and spatial summation as indicated by the wind-up phenomenon and the effect of input from different parts of the body. These somato-visceral reflexes do not reach their maximal activity immediately (46). Rather, when stimulated at a slow repetition rate, these reflexes exhibit wind-up. With each repetition of the stimulation up to about 20 times, the autonomic response increases in size (Fig. 7.12).

The wind-up, or as it has also been termed, sensitization phenomenon suggests that maximal effectiveness of therapeutic procedures involving somatic afferent influences on autonomic control may require frequent repetitions of the procedure to allow the response to build to its maximum. Furthermore, afferent input from different portions of the body can summate to activate autonomic responses (47). Accordingly, one would expect that a subliminal or noneffective stimulus to one part of the body might

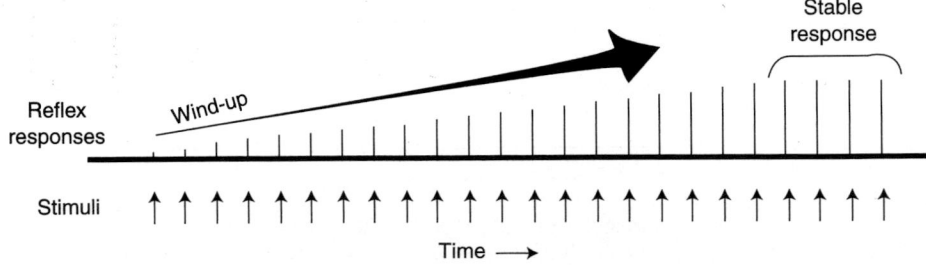

FIGURE 7.12. Wind-up or sensitization. When a stimulus is repeated at a rate of once every second or two, response to stimulus may continue to grow for 20 seconds or more. Finally, a stable response level is reached that can continue at an increased level as long as the stimulus is continued.

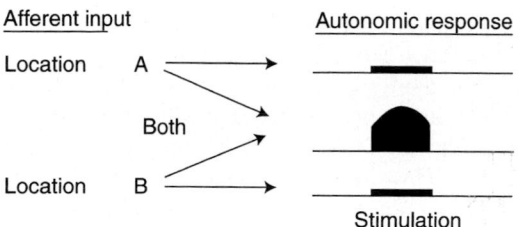

FIGURE 7.13. Summation of autonomic responses. Input from two different locations add together to produce a larger autonomic response than either input produces when it occurs alone.

actually have an effect if combined with stimulation to another area (Fig. 7.13).

The reflex system is truly a complex integrating network. Perhaps most important for the osteopath is the fact that somatic input can and does influence visceral function, just as input from the viscera causes changes in output to the somatic structures. This can often be felt as altered tissue tensions or changes in motion characteristics of joints. Maps have been published listing somatic areas that become abnormal to palpation with various visceral disturbances (48).

A corollary of this is that manipulation of the somatic structures can alter the function of visceral structures through the same pathways. The reflexes are not simple systems with only local influences, but interconnected networks that receive input from many sources and process that information for distribution to both local and distant areas of the body.

ALTERATION OF INTEGRATIVE FUNCTION

Input from each area of the body and from descending brain areas interacts on a highly overlapping and integrated neural network in the spinal interneurons. Afferent input from any source influences both visceral and somatic structures. For normal functioning of organs, muscles, fluid motion, and other body activities, these complex and interacting networks within the nervous system must act in concert. Should one area of the neural network respond either more or less than normal, the finely tuned balance necessary for normal and optimal physiologic function will be disturbed. Not only must the control mechanisms from the brain be normal for proper reflex function, but the networks of neurons that make up the reflexes must also be acting normally. Unfortunately, these networks themselves can be altered, resulting in a loss of proper function.

Although Sherrington postulated that reflexes are innately given, evidence is accumulating that the function of reflex networks can be influenced by many factors. They are subject to both short-term and long-term changes that can have consequences for the health of the individual.

In the early and mid-1940s, Denslow and colleagues (49–51) were among the first to show the results of changes in the integrative function of reflex networks in humans. They performed a series of studies on normal, young adult volunteers to determine whether the reflex excitabilities at various spinal levels of the body were stable and comparable. They measured how much stimulation it took to evoke muscle activity (EMG) in the

paraspinal muscles of the back at several levels of the thoracic spine.

They found that, on the average, reflex excitability to pressure on the spinous processes was highest in the upper thoracic area and lowest in the midlumbar area. Although decreased excitability from the upper thoracic to the lower lumbar areas was seen overall in the subjects studied, practically all individuals studied had areas that were very highly excitable, responding to small amounts of pressure on the spinous process at that spinal level. In normal areas, in contrast, even a fairly heavy pressure in the spinous processes did not produce any muscle activity in the associated muscles. The highly excitable areas were characterized by not only the increased muscle activity to pressure on the spinous process but also often by pain and tenderness in the area. The areas of increased sensitivity to stimulation were not uniform from individual to individual and were long-lasting (some cases remaining almost the same for years). In most cases, the individual did not realize that any change was present.

These long-lasting, low-threshold areas to afferent input could be activated not only by stimulating tissues at the same level of the spinal cord but also by stimulating other areas of the back or even by providing a psychological stress to the individual. With remote input, such as pressure on a spinous process four vertebrae away from the level of the low-threshold area, the muscles at the level of the input remained silent while those at the level of the low threshold became active. The same pattern occurred with psychological stressors. The normal areas remained silent, but the low-threshold areas showed muscle activity.

In later studies, Denslow and co-workers (52,53) found that not only was muscle activity affected but so were the activities of visceral organs through altered sympathetic output. Here, again, the interrelatedness of the somatic and visceral portions of the body was shown.

Although many otherwise normal subjects had low-threshold or high-excitability areas, it became evident from subject-to-subject variability, and from further data showing that the excitability increases often accompanied injury and disease, that the excitability changes were not a normal state. They represented areas of neural function that were operating out of synchrony with other areas of the neural system, causing the organs served by those neural supplies also to be out of synchrony with the total body function.

Korr (7) suggested that these low-threshold spinal reflexes represented pathways that were being held in a hyperexcited state, perhaps by continued bombardment of input. He termed these areas facilitated. He pointed out that they acted to magnify input to the area from any source and to cause a magnified outflow to the organs innervated by that level of the spinal cord. Thermographic studies were also conducted (52,53). Not only did the skeletal muscles respond in an exaggerated fashion in the low-threshold areas but the sympathetic outflow also increased. Such areas of abnormally increased excitability or decreased threshold within the otherwise normal areas of the spinal cord must act to decrease the overall integration of body function. No matter the source of input to a facilitated spinal area, the neural outflow would be exaggerated relative to the same response at other spinal levels. Such a situation lasting over time can have only undesirable consequences for total body function.

Beginning and Maintenance of Reflex Facilitation

The finding that facilitated or low-threshold areas could continue for long periods of time and the fact that these areas were not the same between individuals suggested that some process could occur that would establish these chronically hyperactive areas. Initial speculation suggested that the hyperexcitability was maintained by tonic afferent input. Most input from either somatic or visceral structures, however, decreases dramatically with activities such as sleep or other forms of relaxation. Why should the hyperexcitability continue even with the loss of afferent activity? What is the nature of the neural processing within the reflex pathways to afferent stimuli that might explain the appearance of regions of hyperexcitability? More recent studies have provided some answers that have a bearing on how changes in reflex excitability can at times be an adaptive process and at times a detrimental one.

ALTERATION OF REFLEX EXCITABILITY

The concept of the reflex as a simple, unchanging, static input/output relationship is oversimplified. Although he characterized reflex function as innately given, even Sherrington recognized that reflex excitability could be momentarily altered by influences such as signals from higher brain structures or by rapid and repeated use, which, he noted, caused reflex fatigue. The notion that reflexes are fundamentally unchanging, static input/output relationships is still widespread despite the fact that it is now clear that the excitability of spinal reflex pathways can be altered by many influences. These changes can range from short-lasting, fleeting changes to very long-lasting ones that may even become permanent. These long-lasting alterations may well be the basis for the changes shown by Denslow in his studies of human motoneuron excitability and for the facilitated state hypothesized by Korr. These threats to functional integration of the body may be related to the effects of nociceptive stimuli at the periphery.

ALTERATION OF NOCICEPTIVE STIMULI

Inflammation from strong stimulation of the skin or other peripheral somatic or visceral structures produces a set of changes in the sensory receptors of the organ that dramatically alters the amount of neural activity sent to the spinal cord (54). Most tissues are innervated by various sensory receptors, such as:

Touch
Temperature
Stretch
Nociceptors

The nociceptors are composed primarily of naked (unmyelinated) nerve endings that respond to potentially tissue-damaging stimuli. In the hollow visceral organs, they respond to stretch or dilation of the organ, for example. These receptors send impulses through thin myelinated (group III or A) or unmyelinated (group IV or C) fibers into the spinal gray matter, where they synapse primarily in Rexed layers I and V. When activity occurs in these pathways, the resulting sensation is usually discomfort or pain, although the input may be blocked (by other neural activity) from reaching the areas of the brainstem where they are appreciated as pain. However, even though a nociceptive input to the spinal cord does not reach the conscious level, it may affect the dynamics of the spinal pathways (55).

Once a stimulus sufficiently strong to activate nociceptive input begins, impulses travel into the spinal cord via the dorsal roots. At the branches of the peripheral neurons, the afferent impulses invade the afferent branches and are conveyed back out to the nerve terminals where they cause release of various peptides into the surrounding tissues. The sites of peptide release may be some distance from the original stimulus. The result of this release is the start of a cascade of events that leads to involvement of the sympathetic postganglionic nerve terminals and to the release of serum from the surrounding capillaries. Prostaglandins released from the sympathetic nerve terminals continue the serum release that leads to local inflammation.

This process begins the healing process, although it may be sufficiently severe that the healing process is retarded (56). The inflammation also produces dramatic changes in the characteristics of the local nociceptors in the area. Schmidt (54) demonstrated in the cat knee joint that the number of nociceptors responding to a stretch stimulation may be between 3,000 and 4,000 after inflammation. In contrast, even severe stretch of the normal joint may cause only 400 nociceptors to fire. Also, the receptive fields of the active nociceptors enlarge dramatically in the inflamed area, and the threshold to activation significantly decreases. The result of an inflammatory process (or a strong stimulus that produces tissue damage) will be to lower nociceptor thresholds and dramatically increase input to the spinal cord. Peripheral events can lead to dramatic changes in the amount of stimuli caused by changes in the peripheral receptors.

What happens to spinal reflex networks when stimulus input changes? In the normal reflex pathway, repeated activation of the pathway by a weak afferent input results in a temporary decrease in the output of the network. Sherrington described this short-term decrease in reflex pathway excitability as reflex fatigue. This process, now termed habituation, has been studied extensively and is a characteristic of polysynaptic reflex pathways in the spinal cord and brainstem.

Habituation is characterized by a decrease in output from a neural pathway that has repeated stimulus input of a mild to moderate intensity. A stimulus may initially produce a response of a certain magnitude, but if the stimulus is repeated several times, the response decreases. If the stimulus is then terminated, the response returns to its initial level in a matter of seconds to minutes (57). The process of habituation is a ubiquitous phenomenon, occurring in almost all animals and in all mammalian reflex pathways except the monosynaptic myotatic reflex. It is a necessary part of the neural integration, because it allows nonessential stimuli to be muted in their effects on the nervous system.

The opposite of habituation is an increase in reflex excitability. Earlier we described the phenomenon of wind-up, in which a stimulus repeated several times causes an increased number of neural firings. Wind-up has also been called sensitization in earlier studies (Fig. 7.12). In this process, a repetitive stimulus can cause an increase in output rather than a decrease. A stimulus causing habituation can cause sensitization simply by increasing its intensity. This causes more nociceptors to become active, or the same nociceptors to produce more impulses. Like habituation, sensitization can occur within a matter of seconds, and it can also dissipate in a matter of seconds when the stimulus is terminated (57).

Both habituation and sensitization have been extensively studied at the cellular level. In the mammal, both occur within the spinal central gray matter in the interneuron pathways. They are probably subserved by two different sets of interneurons, which then synapse on the motoneurons of both the sympathetic and somatic systems. Both sensitization and habituation are apparently presynaptic processes that either inhibit (habituation) or enhance (sensitization) the release of neurotransmitter with each activation of the presynaptic terminal (58). They are independent of descending influences from higher nervous centers. Both processes can be demonstrated in humans with spinal cord transections.

Habituation and sensitization are different processes but occur at the synaptic level and can occur over a few seconds of sensory input. Although the process of sensitization may not be a unitary one (because there may be more than one form of sensitization), when the initiating stimulus is terminated, both processes do appear to dissipate in a fairly short time.

Habituation allows the organism to damp the response to nonthreatening stimuli while sensitization allows the individual to respond more forcefully to a stimulus that is stronger and thus threatens tissue damage. These two processes are valuable in maintaining the organism in its everyday existence. Under normal conditions, the opposing processes of habituation and sensitization function to maintain a balance between overreaction and underreaction to normal stimuli. When the inflammation process occurs, whether it is a minimal or maximal inflammation, the balances of habituation and sensitization are disrupted. The normal damping effects of habituation are shifted toward the sensitization process. This is caused by the larger and more extreme responses of the peripheral receptors to what would usually be a nonthreatening stimulus. The result is a larger than normal motor output to both the visceral and somatic structures innervated by the affected reflex pathways and, thus, to an overresponse to stimuli. The process disrupts the normal integration of physiologic function.

Once the process of sensitization has begun, often over a few seconds of strong input, a secondary process begins to occur. Sensitization dissipates a few seconds or minutes after the stimulus is gone. A longer lasting process, termed long-term sensitization, begins to develop in the reflex pathways once sensitization has been in place for several minutes. This process precludes the excitability of the neural pathways from returning to normal for some time, often hours.

The effects of this process can often be seen in laboratory experiments when bursts of stimulation are given followed by an occasional stimulus pulse to test the responsiveness of the reflex system. After initial sensitization and the rapid decrease of reflex excitability after stimulus termination, the response being tracked does not return to its prestimulation baseline but remains a small but significant amount above the base level. This hyperexcitability does not decay for varying amounts of time depending on the time and strength of the stimulus. Unlike sensitization, long-term sensitization is thought to be a postsynaptic event, possibly involving the elaboration of proteins in the postsynaptic neuron that remain active for some time after the initiating event.

Recently, Mantyh and colleagues (59) have shown dramatic changes in the substance P receptors and even structural reorganization of the dendrites of spinal interneurons after nociceptive input. These changes could be the basis for long-term sensitization. Long-term sensitization involves a different mechanism than the short-term process does and can have effects that far outlast the originating stimulus.

Once a stimulus has acted on a reflex network for a longer time, the results can be even more dramatic. For many years, a process known as spinal fixation has been known but not fully recognized. First shown in anesthetized animals, spinal fixation was manifest as remaining active leg flexion after 3 to 4 hours of limb flexion secondary to a cerebella lesion. The lesion produced disrupted outflow from the postural centers in the cerebellum, resulting in sustained flexion of a leg. When the spinal cord was sectioned immediately after the lesion, the limb dropped to the usual flaccid paralysis of the animal. However, if the spinal cord was allowed to remain intact for 3 to 4 hours after the lesion and then transected, the limb remained flexed to some extent. The explanation was that the strong outflow from the injured cerebellum caused a hyperexcitability to develop in the target interneurons of the cord that remained active after spinal transection and resulted in continued motor activity.

In the mid-1960s, research showed that the minimal time necessary for the fixation of this excitability was approximately 45 minutes. Animals receiving the spinal transection within 35 minutes showed no remaining flexion, but those having 45 minutes between lesion and transection showed remaining flexion (60). This effect has now been shown to occur not only as a result of a cerebella lesion but also with stimulation of the skin of the hind limb, and it has also been shown to occur in either intact or animals with spinal transection (61–63). The change in the spinal reflexes produced by the cerebella lesion was caused not by pain or nociceptive input but by changes in outflow from the postural centers.

This, along with more recent research, shows that changes in the reflex functions can occur with both nociceptive and nonnociceptive input, although nociceptive input produces the changes more quickly than nonnociceptive input does. Reflex excitability changes can be influenced by many factors, including:

Stress prior to stimulation
Length and severity of stimulation
Whether the spinal cord is intact or sectioned

The changes have been traced for 3 to 7 days after only 45 minutes of fairly intense nociceptive stimulation and may last even longer. With intense stimulus input, the effect is seen after as little as 20 minutes of stimulation (64). Obviously, strong input, especially nociceptive in nature, can have rapid and long-lasting effects on the excitability of reflex circuits. Although the locus of the changes seen in fixation is not yet known, it seems likely that the alterations observed are processes akin to long-term sensitization but which last a much longer time. It appears that the fixation process is also dependent on the elaboration of proteins in the postsynaptic cells and that it would affect the responsiveness of those cells not only to the original input but also to all input to the cell.

Another line of evidence of long-lasting increases in reflex excitability comes from studies of peripheral inflammation that show that there are peripheral effects of inflammation on afferent input and receptive fields. Continued afferent input from peripheral inflammation produces dramatic changes in the responsiveness of spinal interneurons. Interneurons on which afferent fibers from affected nociceptors synapse begin to respond much more easily to input from a variety of sources, such as touch, pressure, and even the movement of distant muscles. These dramatic changes in excitability also last for long periods (days and weeks) and develop during the initial inflammatory episode (65,66).

Knowing something about the mechanisms of the changes may allow us to restore more normal function. Dubner, Ruda, and Gold (67,68) summarized a series of intracellular changes that are linked to the excitability alterations seen with the inflammation process. The cells activated by nociceptive input from inflamed peripheral structures begin to show enhanced activation of specific parts of the postsynaptic cell membrane called N-methyl D-aspartate (NMDA) receptors. When these receptors become more active, the excitability of the cell is increased. If cellular activation continues even longer, changes in the activity of genes within the neuron are seen. A class of genes called intermediate-early genes, c-fos, and c-jun, become more active, causing increased dynorphin release within the cell. Dynorphin is a substance that causes increased cell excitation. With more of it being produced, the cell is then held in a hyperexcitable state. Wolpaw provided strong evidence that excitability increases and decreases can be produced not only by nociceptive input to the spinal circuits, but also by nonnociceptive input (69). In Wolpaw's studies, both increased and decreased spinal reflex excitability were produced by long-term input that was nonnociceptive. Thus, it is beginning to appear that spinal circuits can be altered rapidly by nociceptive input, and more slowly by nonnociceptive input.

Other studies have begun to show that a fourth type of spinal circuit excitability alteration can occur. With heightened excitability over several days, a process begins to occur in the interneuron cell body that finally destroys the cell. Although both inhibitory and excitatory interneurons should theoretically both be affected by this process, it appears that inhibitory interneurons are affected primarily (70). Thus, after the long-term excitability increases of the fixation type are established, continued activation of the pathways may result in the loss of inhibitory interneurons. This is certainly an almost permanent event. However, it is apparently not the end of the story. In some cases where inhibitory interneurons have been lost, there may be new excitatory synapses actually formed to replace the lost inhibitory synapses (71). These two additional processes would further shift the balance of excitation in the spinal cord toward enhanced excitability, perhaps permanently.

We have outlined four steps that have been shown to occur in the spinal cord reflex circuitry to alter the excitability of those pathways:

Sensitization
Long-term Sensitization
Fixation
Loss of inhibitory interneurons/new excitatory synapse formation

These four overlapping and progressive stages in spinal excitability alterations are underlain by different neural processes, ranging from simple synaptic transmission alterations to complex changes in the genetic function of the cell. With increased understanding of the underlying processes involved, it may be possible to find ways to stop or even reverse them and, hence, reestablish normal excitability in an affected region. In addition, the restoration of normal input to an affected spinal area would have an ameliorative effect on the function. However, at present, little is known about how to reverse the effects of these excitability alterations.

These four steps are a progression from short-term to long-term and even permanent alterations of spinal excitability. It seems almost certain that these steps underlie the changes recorded by Denslow (49) and interpreted by Korr (7) as the facilitated segment. They saw these alterations as having widespread and often grave consequences for the patient. Although they had no way to understand the basis of the facilitated segment at that time, they rightly viewed these alterations in function as a real threat to the health and function of the patient. An area of spinal reflex pathways that are either temporarily or permanently in a state of increased excitability would respond to all input in an exaggerated way, with the result that the organs or tissues innervated by those areas of the spinal cord would receive exaggerated neural drive. Thus, the affected tissues, somatic or visceral, would be driven to respond in a fashion that was not in harmony with the rest of the body. Over time, this increased drive on the tissues would be expected to take a toll on the functional ability of the tissues and could result in premature breakdown or loss of normal function.

It is also evident that areas of increased spinal excitability would respond to central commands in an inappropriate way. This could be the reason why some people respond to stress with heart palpitations while others respond with gastric distress. The abnormally excitable area of the cord would be the one to respond with abnormal drive onto the innervated tissues, resulting in clinical manifestations not seen in other tissues. Thus, a clinical problem may be the result of a long-standing facilitated area of the spinal cord.

In addition to spinal circuit changes, it is now becoming apparent that nociceptive input may cause changes in the brainstem and even in the cortical areas that could account for many of the usual symptoms seen with chronic pain. Indeed, there is evidence that in the prefrontal cortex, cortical neurons analogous to the spinal inhibitory interneurons may be destroyed with some types of pain input (72). The probable result of these changes in the brainstem and even cortex that may be analogous to those seen in the spinal cord will be to alter the ability of the system to respond to environmental stress, and may predispose to disease, altered immune function, and depressive states (see Chapter 8 by Willard in this section for further discussion).

Thus, the spinal excitability alterations first seen by Denslow and Korr seem to be underlain by a series of progressively longer-lasting spinal circuit alterations that result in altered outflow to central brain areas and to both somatic and visceral tissues innervated by that area. As noted above, the restoration of normal input to the area from somatic and visceral tissues would almost surely help normalize the function of the affected areas in all but extreme cases. The restoration of normal tissue function by manipulative procedures would be expected to help restore normal function in the spinal circuits. Thus, given an altered reflex network, that area can no longer respond in concert with other networks, producing diminished functional integration, and beginning the loss of health associated with disease.

NONIMPULSE-BASED INTEGRATION

Neurons not only convey impulses throughout the body to integrate function but also a steady stream of material flowing from the neural cell body out the axon and dendrites. This flow is called axoplasmic flow. It transports materials from where they are manufactured in the cell body down a complex microtubular structure within the axon. Materials to supply rebuilding of the axon walls, to resupply the transmitter substances, and so forth are carried on this system. The most common clinical effects of the loss of this transport system can be seen when neural contact is withdrawn from an end organ, such as when a muscle is denervated by cutting its motor nerve (a relatively common occurrence). Not only does the muscle cease to contract but unless the nerve regrows again to contact the muscle, the muscle fibers eventually lose their ability to contract. They change their structure to that of noncontractile connective tissue. Likewise, if an end organ is damaged, its nerve supply often retracts and the synapses are lost. The end organ supplies something to the nerve that allows the synapses to remain viable.

A great deal of study has been done on the uptake of substances supplied by the end organ by nerve terminals. A family of substances known as nerve growth factor (NGF) is essential to continued nerve contact with an end organ and for continued viability of contacts between nerves higher up the chain. If the end organ does not supply NGF, the synaptic contact is lost.

This factor is also essential in development, allowing appropriate nerves to reach and establish contact with the appropriate end organs. Loss of appropriate NGF causes deterioration of the nerve and its contacts. NGF is elaborated in the end organ and taken up by the presynaptic membranes, where it is transported up the axon to the cell body, a process called retrograde transport. There, it regulates the function of the nerve and the nerve's ability to maintain synaptic contacts. Many other substances can be taken up and transported to the cell body, but not all of them are helpful to nerve function. The tetanus toxin, tetanospasmin, is made in peripheral structures after infection by the Clostridium tetani bacterium. The toxin is taken up by nerve terminals and transported to the central nervous system, where it affects neural function, causing the clinical signs of tetanus.

Many common nerve-tracing techniques rely on the ability of the neuron to take up substances and transport them from the periphery of the nerve to the cell body. For example, horseradish peroxidase is used as a nerve tracer by injecting it into the area of nerve terminals, where it is taken into the cell and transported up the axon, eventually filling the cell body and even dendrites. A fixative can then be used to turn the horseradish peroxidase a dark brown-black, providing an easily visualized portrait of the cell. Many other dyes and materials are commonly used in this way to visualize nerve cells.

Although much is known about the NGF family and some other substances and about the actual transport mechanisms within the axon, less is known about the delivery of substances to end organs through transport from cell body to axon (anterograde flow), such as what is delivered to keep a muscle functional. In 1967, Korr et al (73) published the results of a study that showed that amino acids placed on the cell bodies of the hypoglossal nucleus on the floor of the fourth ventricle were incorporated into the cell body and transported down the axon to the tongue muscle, where they were delivered into the muscle fibers. Later work showed that not only was the material transported but it was also transported at several different rates of flow. That study and others since have shown that flow rates within an axon vary from as slow as 0.5 mm/day to as fast as 400 mm/day. The observed rates are (74):

Slow (0.52 mm/day)
Medium (25 mm/day)
Fast (up to 400 mm/day)
Very fast (up to 2,000 mm/day)

Although much of the anterogradely transported materials are related to support of the neuron and synaptic functions (such as supply of neurotransmitter components), materials delivered by the nerve to its end organ are necessary for either its function or continued existence (75).

The nervous system is not only the network for rapid communications within the body, but it serves as a vast network for a far slower two-way communication between the central nervous structures and every part of the body. Disruption of this slow transport of materials has consequences for continued function that may not be immediately evident but that range from subtle to disastrous. Complete withdrawal of NGF or of the materials delivered by the nerve to its end organ may result in loss of function. Disturbance of the flow of materials in either direction results in less than optimal function of the organs involved.

Many questions remain about the two-way communication of axoplasmic flow. What substances are being delivered? How necessary are they? What do the materials transported from the periphery to the nerve cell bodies do to the function of the cell or of the entire CNS? Are there crucial times for delivery of nerve factors to end organs for proper development? However these questions are answered, it is important to recognize the vast integrating nature of the nonimpulse-based transport systems of the nervous system and the importance of proper function of this system.

Many things have been shown to affect the material flow within the nerve cells. Even small pressure on axons can impede proper axoplasmic flow. A sustained increased number of impulses carried by the neuron (as in those originating in facilitated areas of the cord) may decrease flow rates. Improper supplies of nutrients and oxygen to the cell body or axon alter the flow. The occurrence of the tissue tensions and fluid flow disturbances often associated with somatic dysfunctions can be factors in altering axoplasmic flows. The somatic dysfunctions treated with the use of manipulation would be expected to have a positive effect on the flow of materials in axons of the area and, hence, to improve body function and integration.

CONCLUSION

In the normal, integrative function of the nervous system, a great number of influences obviously act on any neural pathway. Afferent input activates reflex outflow. Descending activities from higher nervous centers modulate excitability of interneurons. Ascending influences from lower spinal areas increase or decrease activity. Psychological effects are played out on all levels of the neuraxis. The nerves deliver the materials necessary for normal function to their end organs while the end organs send the substances necessary for continued synaptic viability to the nerves.

These influences come together to determine the moment-to-moment excitability of any area of the central nervous system and to determine overall outflow to both somatic and visceral structures. If all of these influences are working in harmony, optimally integrated function can be expected from the various organs. If, however, one area is in a hyperexcitable state, the output from that area of the system will not be in harmony with the output of the other areas. In that case, the optimal function is disrupted and the individual becomes increasingly prone to loss of function and disease.

The long-term alterations in spinal reflex excitability (now well-demonstrated by various studies) seem almost certain to underlie the alterations demonstrated by Denslow and his colleagues. These breaks in the normal integration of the nervous system were shown to affect both visceral and somatic structures. The interaction between visceral and somatic input in the spinal cord provides the basis for that common effect. The changes shown in response to nociceptive input can easily account for the long-lasting nature of the facilitation identified in those studies. The facilitation was hypothesized by Korr to be the basis for the somatic dysfunctions long recognized by the osteopathic profession.

Because the neurons involved in the altered excitability are interneurons (the neurons on which a variety of different pathways synapse), the data also support the effects of excitability changes on both somatic and autonomic outflow. The input from both visceral and somatic structures ends on common interneurons. When the excitability of those interneurons is altered, the outflow to all structures innervated by motoneurons to which those interneurons connect is affected.

The reflex networks of the nervous system are not at all static, genetically determined entities. They are a vast network of highly interconnected pathways that are continually changing to meet local needs and to maintain integration of function. These processes allow the delicate moment-to-moment integration that

characterizes optimal functional capacity. The integration, however, can be turned against the very system it serves. When abnormal or very strong input occurs, the result can be a long-term disruption of the normal excitatory/inhibitory balances and a shift to excessive excitability (or in some cases, to excessive inhibition). The result, in either case, is the loss of functional integration and a decrease in functional capacity of the individual.

There are many factors that influence the total function of the individual, including their:

Accumulated effects of life
Habits
Living environment
Food
Psychological and spiritual makeup and state

The role of the state of the nervous system is but one of the factors influencing the total health of the person. Because it affects all organs and structures with which it communicates, an area of central excitation or facilitation delivers the effects of all other stressors on the individual to the end organs. In essence, it is the final common factor in communicating with the end organ. Most of the other stressors in life are difficult to change, and the osteopathic physician has little impact on or control over them. However, the physician can directly affect the course of the facilitation and its effects by recognizing that it occurs and by using modalities, especially manipulative treatment, that alter it.

Rational therapy dictates the normalization of afferent input as quickly as possible. In chronic situations, use methods to reduce the abnormal input to allow the body to restore normal balances of excitation and inhibition as fully as possible. In this way, the goal of total osteopathic treatment, to optimize each individual's function and to restore the individual's dynamic functional balance of optimal health, can be brought closer to reality.

REFERENCES

1. Still AT. *Autobiography of A. T. Still*. Kirksville, MO: Published by the author; 1897.
2. Watkins LR, Maier SF. The pain of being sick: Implications of immune-to-brain communication for understanding pain. *Annu Rev Psychol.* 2000;51:29–57.
3. Watkins LR, Maier SF. Implications of immune-to-brain communication for sickness and pain. *Proc Natl Acad Sci U S A.* 1999;96(14):7710–7713.
4. Northup GW, ed. *Osteopathic Research: Growth and Development*. Chicago, IL: American Osteopathic Association; 1987.
5. Cole WV. The osteopathic lesion syndrome. In: *American Academy of Osteopathy Yearbook*. Indianapolis, IN: American Academy of Osteopathy; 1951:149–178.
6. Denslow JS. *The Early Years of Research at the Kirksville College of Osteopathic Medicine*. Kirksville, MO: Kirksville College of Osteopathic Medicine Press; 1982.
7. Korr IM. The neural basis of the osteopathic lesion. *J Am Osteopath Assoc.* 1947;46:191–198.
8. Sherrington CS. *The Integrative Action of the Nervous System*. New Haven, CT: Yale University Press; 1905.
9. Wurster RD. Program control of circulatory behavior. *Behav Brain Sci.* 1986;9:305.
10. Eble JN. Patterns of response of the paravertebral musculature to visceral stimuli. *Am J Physiol.* 1960;198:429–433.

11. Sato A. Reflex modulation of visceral functions by somatic afferent activity. In: Patterson MM, Howell JN, eds. *The Central Connection: Somatovisceral/Viscerosomatic Interaction.* Indianapolis, IN: American Academy of Osteopathy; 1992;53–72.

12. Rexed B. The cytoarchitectonic organization of the spinal cord in the cat. *J Comp Neurol.* 1952;96:415–495.

13. DeGroat WC. Spinal cord processing of visceral and somatic nociceptive input. In: Patterson MM, Howell JN, eds. *The Central Connection: Somatovisceral/Viscerosomatic Interaction.* Indianapolis, IN: American Academy of Osteopathy; 1992:47–71.

14. Cervero R, Foreman RD. Sensory innervation of the viscera. In: Loewy AD, Spyer KM, eds. *Central Regulation of Autonomic Functions.* New York, NY: Oxford University Press; 1990.

15. Cervero F. Visceral and spinal components of viscero-somatic interactions. In: Patterson MM, Howell JN, eds. *The Central Connection: Somatovisceral/Viscerosomatic Interaction.* Indianapolis, IN: American Academy of Osteopathy; 1992:77–85.

16. Sato A. The somatosympathetic reflexes: Their physiological and clinical significance. In: Goldstein M, ed. *The Research Status of Manipulative Therapy.* Bethesda, MD: National Institutes of Health; 1975:163–172.

17. Hill JM, Adreani CM, Kaufman MP. Muscle reflex stimulates sympathetic postganglionic efferents innervating *triceps surae* muscles of cats. *Am J Physiol.* 1996;271(1 Pt 2):H38–H43.

18. Jou JC, Farber JP, Qin C, et al. Afferent pathways for cardiacsomatic motor reflexes in rats. *Am J Physiol Regul Integr Comp Physiol.* 2001;281:R2096–R2102.

19. Hopkins D, Armour J. Localization of sympathetic postganglionic and parasympathetic preganglionic neurons which innervate different regions of the dog heart. *J Comp Neurol.* 1984;229:186–198.

20. Norris J, Foreman R, Wurster R. Responses of the canine heart to stimulation of the first five ventral thoracic roots. *Am J Physiol.* 1974;227:912.

21. Wurster R, Randall W. Cardiovascular responses to bladder distension in patients with spinal transection. *Am J Physiol.* 1975;228:1288–1292.

22. Wurster R. Spinal sympathetic control of the heart. In: Randall WC, ed. *Neural Regulation of the Heart.* New York, NY: Oxford University Press; 1976:157–186.

23. Chung K, Chung J, LaVelle F, et al. The anatomical localization of descending pressor pathways in the cat spinal cord. *Neurosci Lett.* 1979;15:71–75.

24. Barman S, Wurster R. Visceromotor organization within descending spinal sympathetic pathways. *Circ Res.* 1975;37:209–214.

25. Geis G, Kozelka J, Wurster R. Organization and reflex control of vagal cardiomotor neurons. *J Auton Nerv Syst.* 1981;5:63–73.

26. Geis G, Wurster R. Horseradish peroxidase localization of cardiac vagal preganglionic somata. *Brain Res Brain Res Rev.* 1980;182:1930.

27. Geis G, Wurster R. Cardiac responses during stimulation of dorsal motor nucleus and nucleus ambiguus in the cat. *Circ Res.* 1980;46.606–611.

28. Kalia M, Mesulam M. Brainstem projections of sensory and motor components of the vagus complex in the cat. II: Laryngeal, tracheobronchial, pulmonary, cardiac, and gastrointestinal branches. *J Comp Neurol.* 1980;193:467–508.

29. Hopkins D, Armour J. Medullary cells of origin of physiologically identified cardiac nerves in the dog. *Brain Res Bull.,* 1982;8:359–365.

30. Beacham W, Perl E. Background and reflex discharge of sympathetic preganglionic neurons in the spinal cat. *J Physiol.* 1964;172:400–416.

31. Beacham W, Perl E. Characteristics of a spinal sympathetic reflex. *J Physiol.* 1964;173:431–448.

32. Eble JN. Patterns of response of the paravertebral musculature to visceral stimuli. *Am J Physiol.* 1960;198(2):429–433.

33. Schoen RE, Finn WE. A model for studying a viscerosomatic reflex induced by myocardial infarction in the cat. *J Am Osteopath Assoc.* 1978;78(1):122–123.

34. Amour J. Activity of in situ stellate ganglion neurons of dogs recorded extracellularly. *Can J Physiol Pharmacol.* 1986;64:101–111.

35. Amour J. Activity of in situ middle cervical ganglion neurons in dogs, using extracellular recording techniques. *Can J Physiol Pharmacol.* 1985;63:704–716.

36. Boznjak Z, Kampine J. Intracellular recordings from the stellate ganglion of the cat. *J Physiol.* 1982;324:273-283.

37. Gagliardi M, Randall W, Bieger D, et al. Activity of in vivo canine cardiac plexus neurons. *Am J Physiol.* 1988;255:789–800.

38. Terui N, Koizumi K. Responses of cardiac vagus and sympathetic nerve to excitation of somatic and visceral nerves. *J Auton Nerv Syst.* 1984;10:73–91.

39. O'Toole M, Wurster R, Phillips J, et al. Parallel baroreceptor control of sinoatrial rate and atrioventricular conduction. *Am J Physiol.* 1984;246:H149–H153.

40. Koizumi K, Brooks C. The integration of autonomic system reactions: Discussion of autonomic reflexes, their control and their association with somatic reactions. *Ergeb Physiol Biol Chem Exp Pharmakol.* 1972;67:168.

41. Sato A, Schmidt R. Somatosympathetic reflexes: Afferent fibers, central pathways, discharge characteristics. *Physiol Rev.* 1973;53:916–947.

42. Barman S, Wurster R. Interaction of descending sympathetic pathways and afferent nerves. *Am J Physiol.* 1978;234:H223–H229.

43. Geis G, Wurster R. Localization of ascending inotropic and chronotropic pathways in the cat. *Circ Res.* 1981;49:711–717.

44. Kozelka J, Christy G, Wurster R. Somato-autonomic reflexes in anesthetized and unanesthetized dogs. *J Auton Nerv Syst.* 1982;5:63–70.

45. Kozelka J, Chung J, Wurster R. Ascending spinal pathways mediating somato-cardiovascular reflexes. *J Auton Nerv Syst.* 1981;3:171–175.

46. Chung J, Webber C, Wurster R. Ascending spinal pathways for the somatosympathetic A and C reflex. *Am J Physiol.* 1979;237:H342–H347.

47. Chung J, Wurster R. Neurophysiological evidence for spatial summation in the CNS from unmyelinated afferent fibers. *Brain Res.* 1978;153:596–601.

48. Te Poorten BA. Spinal palpatory diagnosis of visceral disease. *Osteopathic Annals.* 1979:52–53.

49. Denslow JS, Korr IM, Krems AD. Quantitative studies of chronic facilitation in human motoneuron pools. *Am J Physiol.* 1947;105(2):229–238.

50. Denslow JS. The central excitatory state associated with postural abnormalities. *J Neurophysiol.* 1942;5(5):393–402.

51. Denslow JS. An analysis of the variability of spinal reflex thresholds. *J Neurophysiol.* 1944;7(July):207–215.

52. Korr IM, Thomas PE, Wright HM. Patterns of electrical skin resistance in man. *J Neural Transm.* 1958;17:77–96.

53. Wright HM. Local and regional variations in cutaneous vasomotor tone of the human trunk. *J Neural Transm.* 1960;22:34–52.

54. Schmidt RF. Neurophysiological mechanisms of arthritic pain. In: Patterson MM, Howell JN, eds. *The Central Connection: Somatovisceral/Viscerosomatic Interaction.* Indianapolis, IN: American Academy of Osteopathy; 1992:130–151.

55. Schmidt RF. Nociception and pain. In: Schmidt RF, Thews G, eds. *Human Physiology.* Heidelberg, Germany: Springer-Verlag; 1987.

56. Payan DG. Peripheral neuropeptides, inflammation, and nociception. In: Willard FH, Patterson MM, eds. *Nociception and the Neuroendocrine-Immune Connection.* Indianapolis, IN: American Academy of Osteopathy; 1994:34–42.

57. Groves P, Thompson R. Habituation: A dual-process theory. *Psychol Rev.* 1970;77(5):419–450.

58. Kandel ER, Brunelli M, Byrne J, et al. A common presynaptic locus for the synaptic changes underlying short-term habituation and sensitization of the gill-withdrawal reflex in aplysia. *Cold Spring Harbor Symposium on Quantitative Biology.* 1977;40:465–482.

59. Mantyh PW, DeMaster E, Malhotra A, et al. Receptor endocytosis and dendrite reshaping in spinal neurons after somatosensory stimulation. *Science.* 1995;268:1629–1632.

60. Chamberlain TJ, Halick P, Gerard RW. Fixation of experience in the rat spinal cord. *J Neurophysiol.* 1963;26:662–673.

61. Steinmetz JE, Cervenka J, Robinson C, et al. Fixation of spinal reflexes in rats by central and peripheral sensory input *J Comp Psychol.*1981;95:548–555.

62. Steinmetz JE, Patterson MM. Fixation of spinal reflex alterations in spinal rats by sensory nerve stimulation. *Behav Neurosci.* 1985;99(1):97–108.

63. Patterson MM, Steinmetz JE. Long-lasting alterations of spinal reflexes: A potential basis for somatic dysfunction. *J Am Osteopath Assoc.* 1986;2:38–42.

64. Patterson MM. Spinal fixation: Long-term alterations in spinal reflex

excitability. In: Patterson MM, Grau JW, eds. *Spinal Cord Plasticity: Alterations in Reflex Function.* Boston, MA: Kluwer Academic Publishers; 2001:77–100.

65. Willis WD. Mechanisms of central sensitization of nociceptive dorsal horn neurons. In: Patterson MM, Grau JW, eds. *Spinal Cord Plasticity: Alterations in Reflex Function.* Boston, MA: Kluwer Academic Publishers; 2001:127–162.

66. Coderre TJ. Noxious stimulus-induced plasticity in spinal cord dorsal horn: Evidence and insights on mechanisms obtained using the formalin test. In: Patterson MM, Grau JW, eds. *Spinal Cord Plasticity: Alterations in Reflex Function.* Boston, MA: Kluwer Academic Publishers; 2001:163–184.

67. Dubner R, Ruda MA. Activity-dependent neuronal plasticity following tissue injury and inflammation. *Trends Neurosci.* 1992;15(3):96–103.

68. Dubner R, Gold M. The neurobiology of pain. *Proc Natl Acad Sci U S A.* 1999;96(July):7627–7630.

69. Wolpaw JR. Spinal cord plasticity in the acquisition of a simple motor. In: Patterson MM, Grau JW, eds. *Spinal Cord Plasticity: Alterations in Reflex Function.* Boston, MA: Kluwer Academic Publishers; 2001:101–126.

70. Mayer DJ, Mao J, Holt J, et al. Cellular mechanisms of neuropathic pain, morphine tolerance, and their interactions. *Proc Natl Acad Sci U S A.* 1999;96(July):7731–7736.

71. Woolf CJ, Saler MW. Neuronal plasticity: Increasing the gain in pain. *Science.* 2000;288:1765–1768.

72. Grachev ID, Fredrickson BE, Apkarian AV. Abnormal brain chemistry in chronic back pain: An in vivo proton magnetic resonance spectroscopy study. *Pain.* 2000;89(1):7–18.

73. Korr IM, Wilkinson PN, Chornock FW. Axonal delivery of neuroplasmic components to muscle cells. *Science.* 1967;155(760):342–345.

74. Korr IM, ed. *The Neurobiologic Mechanisms in Manipulative Therapy.* New York, NY: Plenum Publishing; 1978.

75. Korr IM. The spinal cord as organizer of disease process: Axonal transport and neurotrophic function in relation to somatic dysfunction. *J Am Osteopath Assoc.* 1981;80(7):451–459.

8

NOCICEPTION, THE NEUROENDOCRINE IMMUNE SYSTEM, AND OSTEOPATHIC MEDICINE

FRANK H. WILLARD

INTRODUCTION

Somatic Dysfunction Represents a Critical Concept in Osteopathic Medicine

Paramount to the osteopathic concept of patient care is the notion that the health of the body—soma and viscera—has a direct influence of the ability of the patient to fend off disease states. Thus, a critical aspect of osteopathic evaluation involves a structural examination of the patient to locate and characterize somatic and visceral dysfunction. These dysfunctions, usually detected by palpation, have been described as manifesting with

1. changes in tissue texture,
2. increased sensitivity to touch, termed hyperalgesia,
3. altered ease or range of motion, and
4. anatomic asymmetry of the effected region (1).

As one can determine simply from the clinical manifestations, somatic dysfunction involves significant alteration in the underlying tissue; Denslow (1) was able to relate these changes to edematous and inflammatory processes using histopathologic investigation.

Somatic Dysfunction Results in Facilitation of the Spinal Cord

The physical process of somatic dysfunction releases signals leading to alteration of activity in the nervous system, endocrine system, and immune system. This chapter and several others in this text will review the changes occurring in the spinal cord segments consequent to somatic dysfunction. In the spinal cord, altered or enhanced neuronal activity is termed facilitation. The result of spinal facilitation is significant change in outflow over both somatic and autonomic routes from the spinal cord. Numerous manifestations of altered spinal outflow can be seen clinically in the target peripheral tissue.

Somatic Dysfunction, Spinal Facilitation, and General Health

Along with activating related spinal cord circuits, somatic dysfunction also releases humoral factors. Both the circulating humoral factors and the enhanced neural activity summate at the level of the brainstem to initiate general arousal and associated, protective endocrine and neural reflexes. Many aspects of this process relate to the general adaptive response of described by Selye (2). Although such neuroendocrine reflexes can be beneficial and protective in the acute situation, chronic exposure to this compensated state, termed allostasis (3) is pathologic. A significant portion of this chapter will focus on the drives initiating allostatic processes and the consequent inflammatory and degenerative injury chronic allostasis inflicts on body and mind. A major conclusion of the chapter will be that the osteopathic approach to patient care is aimed at helping the patient to restore a more natural homeostatic condition. This is accomplished by defacilitating allostatic drives, thereby creating a condition in which the person will be better capable of fending off diseases states.

NOCICEPTION AND SOMATIC DYSFUNCTION

Pathophysiology of Somatic Dysfunction

Biopsies of Palpable Lesions Reveal Signs of Inflammation and Edema

The term somatic dysfunction or osteopathic lesion has been used throughout osteopathic literature. Its effect on the activity of skeletal muscle was demonstrated by Korr and Patterson () in the 1950s and 1960s; but, until the 1970s, these terms still lacked a solid pathophysiologic basis. Using the four cardinal manifestations of somatic dysfunction as criteria to identify these lesions in volunteers, Denslow (1) biopsied the lesions and reported overt signs of inflammation and edema as underlying causes.

Inflammatory Events Signal the Spinal Cord Through Peripheral Nerves

Given that somatic dysfunction has an underlying inflammatory basis, we can now examine the events in the body initiated by the inflammatory process. Chemical mediators released from numerous types of cells in fascia act to stimulate wound repair and tissue growth. At the same time, these mediators also stimulate nociceptive nerve endings in the local tissue resulting in a signal being sent to the spinal cord (Fig. 8.1). The nature of this interaction

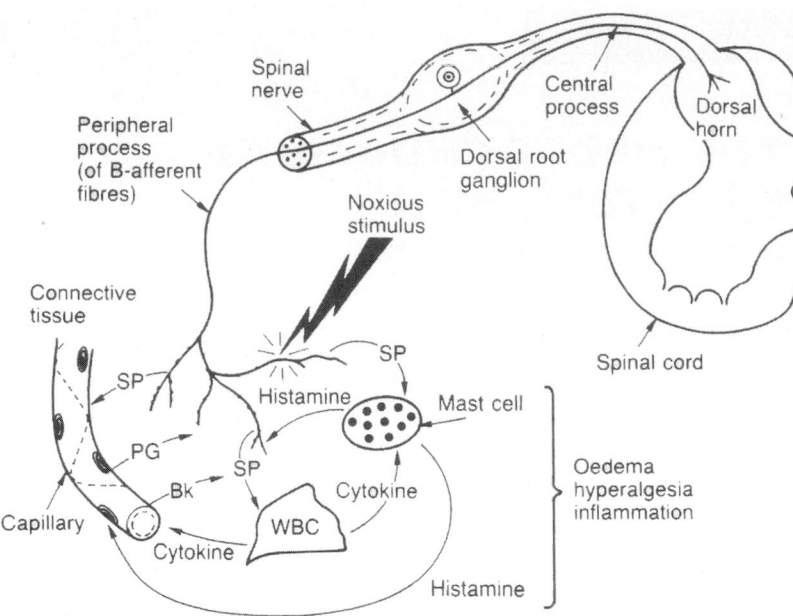

FIGURE 8.1. Interaction between neuropeptides and immunocytes: production of a feed-forward inflammatory cascade. The peripheral terminal of the primary afferent nociceptor (PAN) is illustrated and ends in connective tissue near a capillary. A noxious stimulus has triggered the release of neuropeptide (substance-P) from the PAN terminals. The substance P (SP) has triggered the release of histamine from the surrounding mast cells, prostaglandins from the capillary endothelial cells, and the formation of bradykinin from the plasma protein preprobradykinin. White blood cells migrate to the tissue and release proinflammatory cytokines. Many of these substances are capable of triggering increased activity of the PAN and further secretion of neuropeptides. Thus, a feed-forward situation is established, leading to edema in the local tissue with sensitization of the PAN. From Willard FH. Neuroendocrine-immune network, nociceptive stress, and the general adaptive response. In: Everett T, Dennis M, Ricketts E, eds. *Physiotherapy in Mental Health: A Practical Approach.* Oxford, UK: Butterworth-Heinemann; 1995:102–126, with permission.

in the peripheral nervous system is critical to the formation of spinal facilitation and its subsequent impact on body function.

The Peripheral Nervous System and Primary Afferent Nociceptors

The Peripheral Sensory Nervous System Can Be Divided Into Two Components

The neuronal processes (fibers) contained in peripheral sensory nerves (termed primary afferent fibers), whether they supply somatic or visceral tissue, can be divided structurally and functionally into two major categories: primary afferent fibers from large sensory neurons involved in detecting discriminative and proprioceptive events, and small, sensory neurons that are more typically involved in detecting general warnings of potential danger (4). Although numerous studies point to the small fiber system as being critical to the establishment of demonstrable spinal facilitation (5–7), once established, both large and small fiber systems can become major components in the relationship between somatic dysfunction and spinal facilitation (8).

Large Fiber System Provides Discriminative Touch and Proprioception

Characteristics of the Large Fiber System

The large-caliber primary afferent fibers typically are well-myelinated and rapidly conducting. They terminate in peripheral tissue with specialized, encapsulated endings such as Pacinian or Meissner corpuscles, Merkel discs, or Ruffini endings. Within the central nervous system, the large-caliber fibers ascend the spinal cord to terminate in the dorsal column nuclei of the caudal medulla. From the dorsal column nuclei, projections ascend to the thalamus and then to the somatic sensory cortex where they are precisely mapped with respect to body structure (9).

The large fiber system typically responds to low-level energy stimuli such as light touch, vibration, or tissue movements. Thus,

this system is involved in discriminative touch and proprioception. Under normal conditions, stimulating components of the large fiber system produce a perception that is very specific to the type of ending on the process and not sensitive to the source of stimulation. For example, stimulating a Pacinian corpuscle will produce the sensation of vibration regardless of how it is stimulated—either mechanically or electrically, or of how intensely it is stimulated (10).

Another major characteristic of the large fiber system is its adaptability. Under repeated stimulation, many of these fibers will adapt such that the number of action potentials generated diminishes (11). Thus, the large fiber system is best stimulated by novel activity and will tend to adapt to repetitive stimuli, thereby reducing its detection of this information.

Small Fiber System Provides Nociception and General Adaptation

Characteristics of the Small Fiber System

The small-caliber primary afferent fibers are typically unmyelinated or very lightly myelinated. They terminate in peripheral tissue with naked nerve endings, devoid of any encapsulation. Within the brain, information from the small-caliber system is distributed to numerous brainstem and thalamic areas before being sent to the cerebral cortex (9).

The small fiber system is capable of detecting high-energy stimuli such as that which is either damaging or potentially damaging to the surrounding tissue. Thus, major functions of this system involve protection and defense. Mapping of this information on the cerebral cortex is not as precise as that seen in the large-caliber fiber system. Not only does this system activate somatic sensory cortex, it also has projections reaching much of the limbic forebrain (12–14). Furthermore, the sensation obtained from intensely stimulating a small-caliber fiber often differs from that derived from low-level stimulation. Low-level stimulation can produce the sensation of crude touch or contact while intense activity in the fiber produces the sensation of pain. More importantly, intense activation of the small-caliber system initiates brainstem responses involving arousal and general adaptation. Thus the small fiber system is an important avenue into the arousal system of the brainstem. Activation of the arousal system serves to alter endocrine and immune functions throughout the body and represents the major focus of this chapter.

Finally, another major characteristic of the small fiber system is its ability to sensitize to repetitive stimuli (11). Under such stimulation, many of the neurons in the small fiber system will lower their thresholds of activation, thereby becoming sensitized to the stimulus.

Location of the Small Fiber System

Small-caliber, primary afferent fibers are distributed throughout the tissues of the body. They extend throughout the connective tissue of the dermis and enter the deep layer of the epidermis. Small fibers can be found coursing in the fascial wrappings of blood vessels and nerves and in the connective tissue support network throughout muscle, tendon, and ligament as well as in the capsules and synovial linings of joints. This includes the outer third of the intervertebral discs that are also innervated by components of the small-caliber fiber system. In addition, similar processes can also be found in the support ligaments and organ walls of the viscera. The meningeal layers of the central nervous system also contain small-caliber fibers that course along, and fan out from the meningeal blood vessels. The only tissues in the body that do not receive an innervation from the small fiber system are the articular and hyaline cartilages, nucleus polposus, and the parenchyma of the central nervous system.

Activation of the Small Fiber System

Because the small fiber system represents an important component of the arousal system, it is necessary to consider its activity. Three forms of energy are capable of activating components of the small fiber system: mechanical, thermal, and chemical. In understanding somatic dysfunction, mechanical and chemical forms of activation are of major concern. Mechanical energy appears to activate primary afferent fibers by distorting their membranes and opening associated ion channels, allowing depolarization of the fiber. Chemical energy works through a myriad of receptors located on the surface of the primary afferent fiber. Receptors are present for such chemicals as bradykinin, serotonin, histamine, norepinephrine, and a variety of neuropeptides (15). Importantly, the receptor composition of the primary afferent fiber is not static and can shift consequent to the condition of the tissue. Thus receptors for norepinephrine are not normally active on these fibers but sensitivity to sympathetic catecholamines can develop after tissue injury (16).

Nociception is the physical action of exciting small-caliber, primary afferent endings (whether by mechanical, thermal, or chemical means). Therefore, the small-caliber fibers that are sensitive to tissue damaging stimuli are often termed primary afferent nociceptors or PANs (15).

Human Perception of Small Fiber Activity

Primary afferent fiber activity can be studied using the technique of microneurography (17). From such studies, it has become clear that nociception can occur in the peripheral tissue and primary afferent nociceptors can be active without our knowledge of these events. Thus, low-level firing of PANs can occur without our perception, or at best, perhaps giving us the sensation of poorly localized touch. Conversely, we can perceive high-level or rapid firing of PANs as pain. Most critical, however, is the fact that high-level activity of the PANs can alter the properties and behavior of components of the surrounding large fiber system and, under these pathologic conditions, we then also perceive large fiber activity as pain (18).

Peripheral Sensitization of Primary Afferent Nociceptors

Primary Afferent Nociceptors Are Involved in the Process of Somatic Dysfunction and Spinal Facilitation

The observation that palpable somatic dysfunction involves the histologic signs of inflammation and edema opens the door for understanding the role of PANs in this type of lesion. PANs can be extremely sensitive to the chemical mediators of inflammation (15) and, in many situations, release proinflammatory neuropeptide mediators that will worsen the situation (Fig. 8.2). This condition is termed neurogenic inflammation (19).

Chemoreceptor Primary Afferent Nociceptors Respond to Proinflammatory Compounds

During an inflammatory event, vascular endothelial cells release prostaglandins and local mast cells release histamine. White blood cells are attracted into the tissue and release various cytokines such as interleukin-1, interleukin-6, and tumor necrosis factor. Within the area of inflammation, the pH drops indicating an increase in the concentration of protons, a condition known to

Neurogenic Inflammatory Cycle

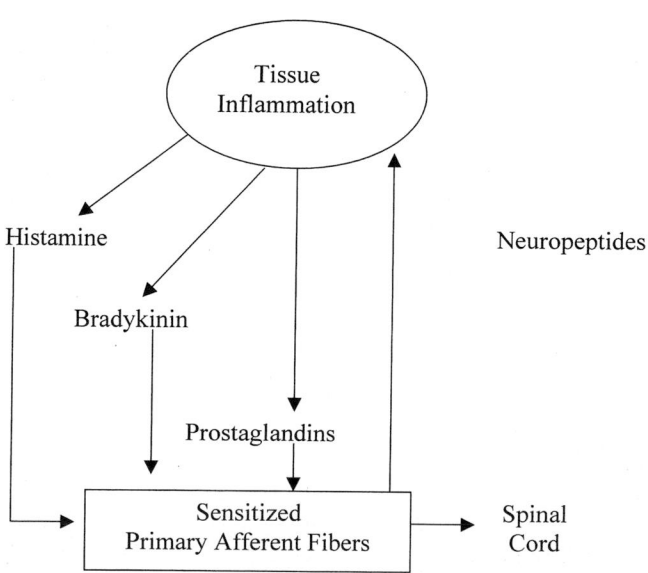

FIGURE 8.2. Summary diagram illustrating the tissue inflammatory cycle and the sensitization of primary afferent fibers.

activate PANs in human skin (20). In addition, the plasma protein preprobradykinin is unblocked to yield bradykinin. Receptors for most of these compounds are present on the PANs and these compounds have been demonstrated to increase the firing rate of the PANs. Furthermore, when the smallest of the PANs (the C fibers) become active, they not only carry an action potential toward the spinal cord but also release neuropeptides from their peripheral terminals (19). Typical neuropeptides released are substance-P, calcitonin gene–related polypeptide, and somatostatin among others. Not only are some of these peptides vasodilatory (creating neurogenic extravasation) but they also can stimulate mast cells to degranulate thereby releasing more histamine into the tissue. Finally, at least one of the secreted peptides, substance-P, is also capable of direct irritation of the PANs.

Alteration of Primary Afferent Nociceptor Phenotype by Inflammatory Chemicals

Normally, members of the large fiber system—such as the Aβ fibers—do not secrete peptide when activated. During the inflammatory process, however, the Aβ fibers have been observed to undergo a phenotypic change developing behaviors similar to the C fibers of the small fiber system including the secretion of neuropeptide (18). Not only does this finding demonstrate that the large fiber system can contribute to the inflammatory process, but it also demonstrates how plastic the peripheral nervous system can be in response to challenge.

Increased Responsiveness of Primary Afferent Nociceptors Results in Peripheral Sensitization

As PANs become active in an inflammatory situation, an important change manifests in their behavior. Under repetitive stimuli, there is a shift in their response properties such that they become much more sensitive to low thresholds of energy (Fig. 8.2). In this condition, a previously noxious stimulus now elicits a greater pain sensation. This condition is termed primary hyperalgesia (21). If the tissue is so sensitive that typically nonnoxious stimuli can elicit the sensation of pain, then the condition is termed allodynia—a special subset of the hyperalgesic condition. When PANs alter their thresholds to produce an area of primary hyperalgesia, they are said to have undergone a process of peripheral sensitization (22). Hyperalgesia that develops around the immediate area of noxious stimulation is termed primary hyperalgesia; whereas that which develops outside of the area of stimulation is termed secondary hyperalgesia. In some situations, the area of secondary hyperalgesia is not in continuity with the area of primary hyperalgesia (17).

Application to Understanding Somatic Dysfunction

Edematous Response Underlies the Tissue Texture Changes

The extravasation of fluid into the extracellular space during inflammation alters the tissue composition and changes its palpatory presentation. These observations account for the tissue texture changes that represent the first criterion for the diagnosis of somatic dysfunction.

Peripheral Sensitization Contributes to the Increased Sensitivity to Touch or Hyperalgesia

The lowered thresholds of the PANs contribute to the increased sensitivity to touch or hyperalgesia, representing the second of the four criteria for the diagnosis of somatic dysfunction. Thus, knowledge of the inflammatory process and the PAN response allows an understanding of the first two criteria used in diagnosing somatic dysfunction. In the next section, the response of the spinal cord to PAN activity will be examined in an effort to gain understanding of the last two criteria used in osteopathic palpatory diagnosis.

NOCICEPTION AND SPINAL FACILITATION

Termination and Activity of Primary Afferent Nociceptors in the Dorsal Horn

Based on the model of an inflammatory process, somatic dysfunction in the peripheral tissue produces inflammatory chemicals that irritate PANs; these fibers then relay action potentials into the dorsal horn of the spinal cord. Activity in the dorsal horn plays a crucial role in determining the outcome of the dysfunction. In one sense, the dorsal horn neurons can convert the nociceptive activity of primary afferent fibers into a signal that the brain can interpret as pain. Woolf and colleagues (23) divided the activity of the dorsal horn neurons into four functional states.

The Four Modes of Activity in the Dorsal Horn

In the first mode, which represents normal function, the input to the dorsal horn is balanced with the output; in essence, the output is in normal proportion to the input received by the dorsal horn neurons. This allows a given nociceptive input to be converted into an acute pain signal sent to the brainstem and forebrain. In the second state, the output of the dorsal horn is partially inhibited; therefore, the response to a given input is suppressed. This is also a normal mode and allows the brain to reduce the amount of pain that is experienced consequent to a given nociceptive stimulus. The third mode is the converse of the second and is also normal in function; here, the dorsal horn output to a given nociceptive signal is increased or facilitated. In this mode, the dorsal horn neurons have become sensitized to the nociceptive input and are generating an enhanced pain signal to the brain. This latter mode is considered to be a protective defense against further injury by usage. Finally, the fourth mode of dorsal horn activity is pathologic in nature. Here, the output from dorsal horn neurons is way out of proportion from the input; thus a stimulus, nociceptive or otherwise, produces an enlarged and prolonged output from the dorsal horn. Each of these modes will be considered briefly.

Mode One: Normal Input—Normal Output

Distribution of Central Terminals in the Dorsal Horn

The central processes of the PANs enter the dorsal horn from its dorsal surface and terminate primarily in the upper layers of the structure—laminae I and II. Some of these fibers also extend in

Mode 1 — Normal Transmission

Innocuous or noxious stimulation

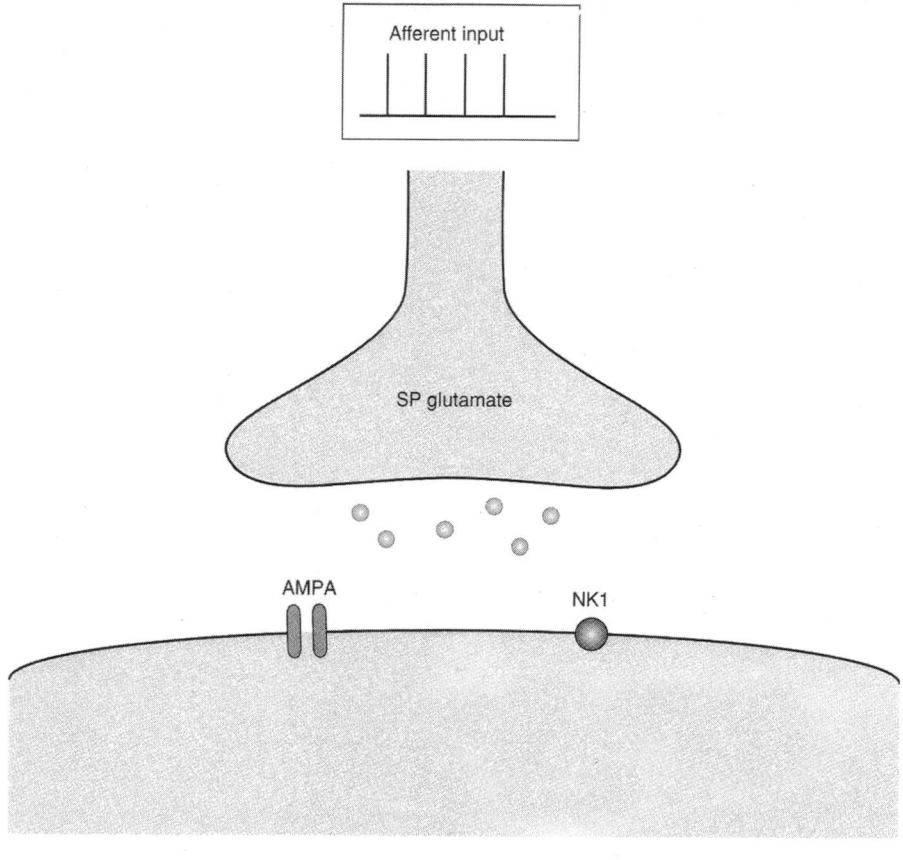

Normal Sensibility

FIGURE 8.3. Mode 1 demonstrating balanced input/output relations between the pre- and postsynaptic element. From Doubell TP, Mannion RJ, Woolf CJ. The dorsal horn: state-dependent sensory processing, plasticity and generation of pain. In: Wall PD, Melzack R, eds. *Textbook of Pain.* Edinburgh, Scotland: Churchill Livingstone; 1999:165–181, with permission.

to the deep portion of the dorsal horn, lamina V. In contrast, the central terminals of the large fiber system, such as the Aβ fibers, pass medially over the dorsal horn to enter the spinal cord along the margin of the dorsal columns. From here, the large-caliber fibers climb up the dorsal columns to reach the dorsal column nuclei at the base of the brainstem, from which information is passed onto thalamus and, eventually, the cerebral cortex. However, before ascending the spinal cord, many of these axons give off a collateral fiber that enters the dorsal horn synapsing in layers III and IV.

Chemistry of Primary Afferent Nociceptor Central Processes in the Dorsal Horn

Within the dorsal horn, all fibers appear to release amino acids, such as aspartate and glutamate, as neurotransmitters. Typically, these amino acids are released into the clefts of synapses on dorsal horn neurons. The PANs, however, also release a neuropeptide transmitter, substance-P, not necessarily into the synaptic cleft, but into the extracellular spaces of the dorsal horn. The neuropeptide then diffuses on to receptors on the membranes of surrounding dorsal horn neurons.

Normal Activity of the Dorsal Horn

The depolarization of PANs by a nociceptive stimulus activates the rapid release of excitatory amino acids into the clefts of synapses on dorsal horn neurons. The resultant firing (action potential) pattern of the dorsal horn neurons is directly related to the amount of transmitter released (Fig. 8.3). This is experienced in a healthy individual when, for example, their skin is pinched and they feel a quick sensation of pain that terminates shortly after the stimulus is ceased. The stimulus is noxious and can trigger rapid, protective reflexes, but has not damaged the tissue.

Mode 2 — Suppressed Transmission

Activation of segmental and descending inhibitory systems

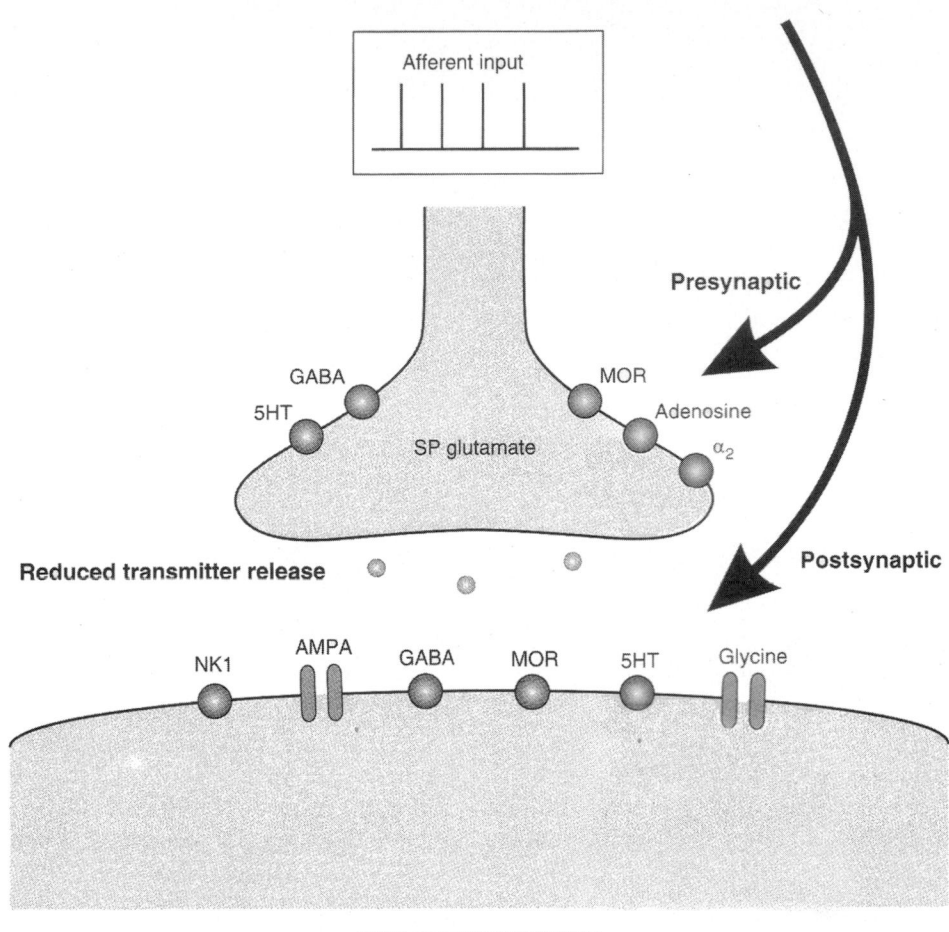

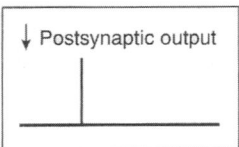

Reduced Sensibility

FIGURE 8.4. Mode 2 demonstrating the pre- and postsynaptic inhibition of activity resulting in the suppression of firing in the dorsal horn neuron. From Doubell TP, Mannion RJ, Woolf CJ. The dorsal horn: state-dependent sensory processing, plasticity and generation of pain. In: Wall PD, Melzack R, eds. *Textbook of Pain.* Edinburgh, Scotland: Churchill Livingstone; 1999:165–181, with permission.

Mode Two: Normal Input—Suppressed Output

Two Systems Combine to Suppress Dorsal Horn Activity

In the second mode, a normal nociceptive input generates a reduced output from the dorsal horn. In this condition, the dorsal horn neurons are being inhibited by two mechanisms (Fig. 8.4). From the periphery, through a complex mechanism, the large-caliber (Aβ) fibers whose collateral branches terminate in the middle layers of the dorsal horn trigger an inhibition of neurons in the upper layers of the structure. This represents the classic gate-control theory of Melzack and Wall (24). Additional suppression of dorsal horn neuronal activity comes from descending supraspinal pathways. These descending pathways allow the cerebral cortex and brainstem, especially its limbic or emotional components, to exercise control over the conversion of nociceptive input into pain signals by the dorsal horn. Using these endogenous pain control systems, the body can reduce the amount of pain it is experiencing. This can be useful in critical situations such as escape behavior where pain needs to be minimized.

Mode Three: Normal Input—Enhanced Output

In this mode, neural activity in the primary afferent fiber results in an enhanced response from the neurons in the dorsal horn (Fig. 8.5). This enhancement of activity represents a mode of spinal facilitation and is underwritten by a complex series of interactions.

Mode 3 — Facilitated Transmission

Increased excitation/reduced inhibition

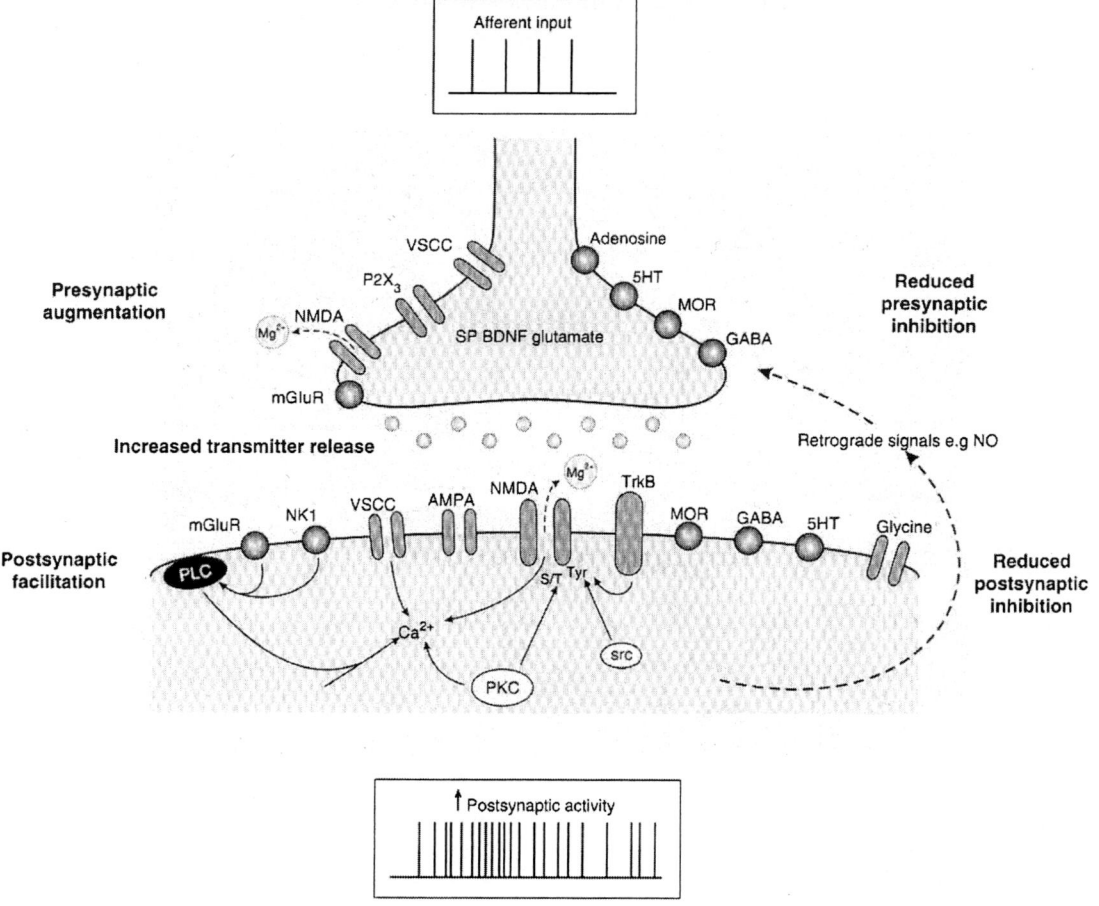

FIGURE 8.5. Mode 3 demonstrating the enhanced activity in the dorsal horn neuron indicating a state of sensitization. From Doubell TP, Mannion RJ, Woolf CJ. The dorsal horn: state-dependent sensory processing, plasticity and generation of pain. In: Wall PD, Melzack R, eds. *Textbook of Pain.* Edinburgh, Scotland: Churchill Livingstone; 1999:165–181, with permission.

Release of Peptide and Activation of Voltage-Gated Channels

Prolonged PAN stimulation results in the release of neuropeptide, such as substance-P, in the extracellular spaces of the dorsal horn. Responding to the neuropeptide signal, neurons trigger internal phosphorylation events that result in the opening of voltage-gated membrane channels for glutamate. These channels allow calcium influx to the cell. Events that are triggered by a change in the cell's voltage due to repeated firing are referred to as "activity-dependent."

Activity-Dependent Changes Lead to Altered Gene Expression and Protein Synthesis

The calcium influx from the voltage-gated channels is involved in gene induction. An example of an activity-dependent, induced gene expression is the gene encoding for dynorphin. A barrage of activity on the PANs can result in the induction of mRNA for dynorphin and, ultimately, its synthesis in numerous dorsal horn neurons. Dynorphin is known to increase the facilitation of neurons; therefore, it can increase the sensitivity of dorsal horn neurons. This is particularly interesting because it means that excessive activity in the PANs can result in a molecular change (involving altered gene expression) in the dorsal horn neurons.

Mode Four: Subnormal Input—Grossly Enhanced Output

In this mode, dorsal horn neurons have altered their membrane properties such that they overrespond to very minimal input, and in some cases, to no input at all. This hypersensitivity state is a pathologic condition that is most likely related to at least three conditions: the sprouting of processes from damaged nerves, the activation of dorsal horn glial cells, and cell death of overexcited inhibitory interneurons in the dorsal horn (Fig. 8.6).

Mode 4

Structural reorganization

Aberrant connections with facilitated transmission

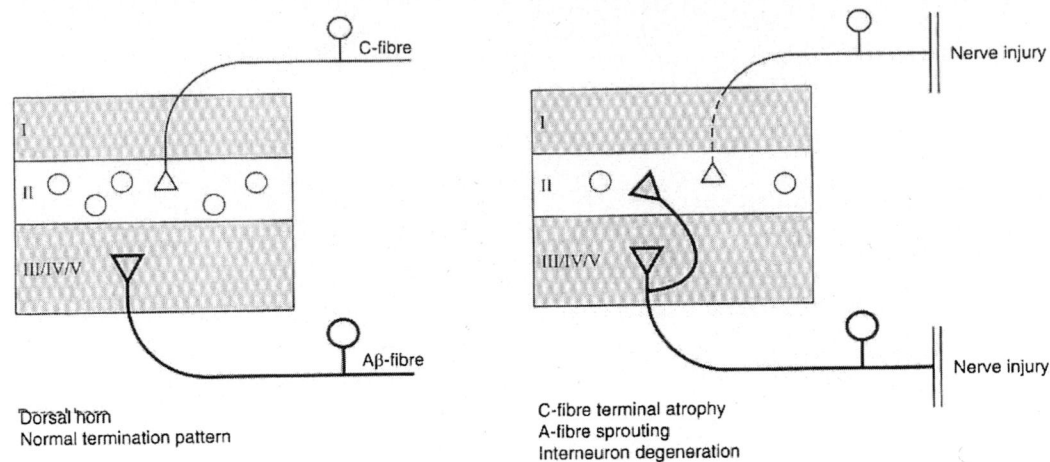

FIGURE 8.6. Mode 4 demonstrating pathologic changes in the loss of C fibers secondary to nerve injury and the sprouting larger fibers from the deeper levels of the dorsal horn. From Doubell TP, Mannion RJ, Woolf CJ. The dorsal horn: state-dependent sensory processing, plasticity and generation of pain. In: Wall PD, Melzack R, eds. *Textbook of Pain*. Edinburgh, Scotland: Churchill Livingstone; 1999:165–181, with permission.

The Central Terminals of Aβ Fibers in an Injured Nerve Sprout Within the Dorsal Horn

Damage to a peripheral nerve can lead to enhanced sprouting of peripheral and central fibers of dorsal root ganglion neurons. In addition, the damage of the small PAN fibers secondary to nerve injury will result in the withdrawal of their axons from lamina II of the dorsal horn. Sprouting from the central terminals of Aβ fibers in the deeper laminae can then invade the upper layers and replace these terminals by forming abnormal synaptic contacts with neurons in lamina II (25). In this condition, light touch, which is usually a nonnoxious stimulus, can result in Aβ fiber activity and the subsequent activation of upper level dorsal horn neurons whose activity typically encodes the signals for pain.

Excessive Primary Afferent Nociceptor Activity Can Activate Dorsal Horn Glial Cells

Recent studies have proposed an interesting role for glial cells in the development and maintenance of spinal facilitation (26,27). In this model, excessive release of neurotransmitters from the central terminals of PAN fibers results in the activation of dorsal horn astrocytes and microglial cells. This appears to be a receptor-mediated process. The activated glial cells respond by releasing proinflammatory cytokines, reactive oxygen species, nitric oxide, prostaglandins, excitatory amino acids, and adenosine triphosphate; all of which are compounds that can contribute to the excitation of dorsal horn neurons. Interestingly, blocking the metabolic activity of spinal glial cells or antagonizing the production or release of proinflammatory cytokines in the spinal cord prevents the development of hyperalgesic states consequent to viral antigens (28). Thus, glial activation appears exacerbate the ongoing activity of the PAN–dorsal horn neuron couple leading to the excessive activity states characteristic of spinal facilitation.

Excessive Neuronal Activity in the Dorsal Horn Can Result in Cell Death.

In situations involving tissue injury and subsequent PAN activity, such as chronic constriction injury to a nerve (29) or a surgical incision (30), damage occurs in the population of laminae I to III dorsal horn neurons. This damage is seen as darkened, pynotic neurons. It is proposed that they represent neurons dying through a process of excitatory toxicity due to excessive exposure to excitatory amino acids released from excessively active PANs. The facts that these dying neurons are typically the smaller neurons in the dorsal horn and that the dorsal horn loses inhibitory transmitter after nerve injuries suggest that the dying cells are inhibitory interneurons involved in modulating activity in the dorsal horn circuits (31). The loss of inhibitory neurons from a dorsal horn circuit would allow greater facilitation of pain pathways.

Central Sensitization of Spinal Cord Neurons

In modes three and four of dorsal horn operation, the primary input encounters a hypersensitive neuronal circuitry. The hyperactivity represents a form of central sensitization that is to be distinguished from sensitization of the peripheral terminals of the primary afferent fibers (23). In mode three, the central sensitization is related to phosphorylation events, altered membrane properties, and subsequent gene inductions. These activities have a reversible nature, unlike the situation in mode four. In this later mode, pathologic changes in the tissue such as terminal sprouting or neuronal cell death have indelibly altered the activity of the dorsal horn. Development of mode four in a patient underlies some of the changes experienced in shift from acute to chronic pain.

Spinal Facilitation and Altered Spinal Cord Output

Central sensitization in the spinal gray matter creates a condition of spinal facilitation. In this condition, circuits in the spinal cord have lowered thresholds of activation and can therefore be more easily engaged by the synaptic drive of the primary afferent fibers.

Spinal Facilitation Is the Product of Multiple Factors

Multiple events are involved in facilitation of the spinal cord. As previously outlined, primary afferent fibers release amino acid and peptide neurotransmitter, dorsal horn neurons undergo membrane property changes due to phosphorylation events, and gene induction occurs in the nucleus of these neurons, producing facilitatory compounds such as dynorphin.

Spinal Facilitation Suggests a Form of Spinal Memory

The facilitation of dorsal horn circuits secondary to intense PAN activity and the long-term to permanent nature of these changes suggest the existence of a spinal memory. This memory would allow the ingraining of old pain patterns and their reactivation by milder stimuli at a later date (5,32).

Spinal Facilitation Leads to Altered Output On the Ventral Root

Facilitation of the spinal cord by PANs results in altered activity in the ventral roots (33). Because the ventral roots contain somatic efferent axons innervating skeletal muscle, the outward manifestation of this activity involves altered muscle tone in the associated spinal segments. These changes in muscle tone suggest a neurophysiologic basis for the altered ease or range of motion present in patients with somatic dysfunction. Furthermore, the altered somatic muscle tone would be expected to create an anatomic asymmetry in the effected region of the body, thus explaining the third and fourth criteria for the diagnosis of somatic dysfunction.

The ventral root also carries visceral efferent fibers innervating glands and vascular and organ wall smooth muscle as well as associated fascia and immunocytes. Evidence suggests that spinal facilitation also alters the output of the visceral afferent fibers (34), thereby accounting for the vasomotor, sudomotor, and organ-specific changes often associated with somatic dysfunction.

Convergent Input to the Spinal Circuit and Spinal Facilitation

Finally, it is significant to point out that many of the dorsal horn neurons that receive afferent terminals from somatic PANs also have afferent terminals from visceral PANs (35). Thus, nociceptive activity converges on neurons in the spinal cord that are capable of responding to excessive input with facilitation. Using this model, it can be seen that either somatic or visceral (or both) dysfunction(s) can serve to facilitate the spinal cord. Once facilitated, input of somatic or visceral origin can function to activate spinal cord neurons, generating the subsequent somatic or visceral peripheral changes commonly associated with somatic dysfunction. These somatovisceral and viscerosomatic reflexes are further discussed in Chapter 7.

SUMMARY: THE NOCICEPTIVE MODEL OF SOMATIC DYSFUNCTION

The Role of the PANS

Primary Afferent Nociceptors Are Important in the Establishment of Spinal Facilitation

Spinal facilitation involves changes in cellular membrane properties, gene expression, and in the distribution of synaptic terminals in the spinal gray matter, as previously described. These structural and functional alterations in neurons depend on the excessive synaptic drive from the PANs. In fact, in experimental paradigms, outward manifestations of spinal facilitation are difficult or impossible to obtain without elevating the stimulus parameters to the level of activating the PANs (8).

Primary Afferent Nociceptors Are Not Necessary to Maintain Spinal Facilitation

Once spinal facilitation has been established, eliminating peripheral spinal input by section of the dorsal roots does not eliminate the outward signs of facilitation (8); instead, the increased muscle tone abates slowly with time. Thus although PANs are necessary to establish facilitation, they appear not to be necessary to maintain the facilitation.

Alterations in Spinal Interneurons Results in Long-term Memory of Circuit Facilitation

Spinal facilitation survives transection of the spinal cord, which suggests that it arises in the spinal gray matter itself and not from descending brainstem influences (8). These observations are in line with the above-cited literature that implicates the neurons and possibly the glial cells of the spinal gray matter as the main culprits in facilitation of the spinal cord (27). The emphasis placed on the PANs has given rise to the "nociceptive model of spinal facilitation" (36).

SPINAL FACILITATION AND THE BRAINSTEM AROUSAL SYSTEM

Ascending Spinal Pathways

Somatic dysfunction that occurs in peripheral tissue generates a signal carried by the PANs into the dorsal horn of the spinal cord. This nociceptive information is processed by spinal neurons and relayed upstream to the brainstem and thalamus en route to the cerebral cortex. Most of the ascending information is carried in the classically defined anterolateral system, which contains spinothalamic fibers, spinohypothalamic fibers, and spinoreticular tract.

Anterolateral System

The Spinothalamic Tract carries Information on Pain Localization to the Parietal Cortex

The spinothalamic tract extends from the segmental levels of the cord to the posterior and ventral portions of the thalamus. As it ascends, most of its fibers lie in the both the lateral and ventral regions of the anterolateral tract. The tract arises from neurons located in three clusters in the spinal gray: lamina I, laminae IV and V, and laminae VII and VIII (13). The target of this pathway is the contralateral thalamus, especially its lateral and posterior portions. Although the activities of the spinothalamic tract are complex and multifactorial, a major function of the structure appears to be the conduction of information on stimulus localization from the spinal cord through the lateral positions of thalamus to the somatic sensory areas of cerebral cortex (11) (Chapter 9).

The Spinohypothalamic Tract carries Nociceptive Information to the Limbic Forebrain

Projections from the spinal cord to the contralateral hypothalamus have been described in numerous studies (37). All of the neurons involved with this tract appear to be responsive only to noxious stimuli, strongly suggesting that the tract is involved in limbic response to nociceptive stimuli (38). Recent studies have also demonstrated trigeminohypothalamic tracts carrying noxious information from the orofacial region to the hypothalamus (39). Although functional studies of the trigemino- and spinohypothalamic tracts have yet to be done, they both appear to carry noxious information and they both are in a position to activate or influence neuroendocrine and emotional response.

The Spinoreticular Tracts carry Warning Information to the Brainstem and Prefrontal Cortex

Projections from spinal cord neurons to the brainstem form a complex system involved in autonomic regulation and protection of homeostasis. These pathways arise from spinal laminae I, V, and VII, and project to the reticular formation as well as to other regions of the brainstem such as the parabrachial nucleus, periaqueductal gray, hypothalamus, and amygdala (40). Additionally, projections from the spinal trigeminal nucleus into the brainstem reticular formation also exist (41). These pathways are predominantly contralateral in distribution; however, some of these fibers, especially those going to the lower brainstem, are bilateral. Ascending pathways from the reticular formation lead to the medial nuclei of the thalamus, from which fibers project to the prefrontal and anterior cingulate cortex. Thus, the spinoreticular tracts target the limbic forebrain, the major emotional component of the brain.

Information in the Spinoreticular and Spinal Hypothalamic Tracts Is of Both Somatic and Visceral Origin

Activity in the spinoreticular tracts is both somatic and visceral in origin and is typically of a nociceptive nature. The spinoreticular

pathways initiate protective, suprasegmental reflexes related to cardiovascular, respiratory, and endocrine control system as well as provide the affective and emotional components of pain (12). Taken together, this older and slower ascending system activates a brainstem arousal system that is protective in nature but that has a huge influence on the homeostatic mechanisms of the body.

Brainstem Reticular Formation

Anatomy

The reticular formation represents a broad column of cells and fibers extending through the center of the brainstem and arising from the spinal gray matter at the cervicomedullary junction and blending into the hypothalamus at the rostral end of the midbrain. The cranial nerve nuclei are embedded in the reticular formation (42). The reticular formation of the brainstem is a major target of ascending fibers carrying nociceptive information from either somatic or visceral dysfunctions.

The Reticular Formation Is the Integral Core of the Brainstem, Extending from the Medulla to the Thalamus

The reticular formation contains many of the phylogenetically oldest cell clusters of the brain and plays a major role in controlling the defense mechanisms for protecting homeostasis. The formation is divided functionally into caudal and rostral portions.

The Caudal Reticular Formation Contains Areas Controlling the Autonomic Nervous System

The caudal portion of the reticular formation is contained in the medulla and pons. It has cell clusters associated with cardiovascular and respiratory control located ventrally and laterally (41) and surrounding a central portion that influences posture by modulating skeletal muscle tone. Other regions of the caudal reticular formation are involved with modulating spinal facilitation. These regions receive significant input from the anterolateral fibers systems (nociceptive information) and, in turn, control several descending pathways that reach the dorsal and ventral horns. These descending brainstem–spinal projections can either inhibit or excite neurons in the spinal gray.

The Rostral Reticular Formation Contains Areas Controlling Attention and Arousal

The rostral portion of the reticular formation begins in the pons and extends through the midbrain into the caudal regions of the hypothalamus. A major component of the rostral brainstem is the arousal system (43). This system consists of two interconnected components. A medially positioned cluster of nuclei forms the reticular activating system that is capable of modulating cerebral cortical activity between states of sleep and wakefulness. More dorsal and laterally, monoamine-producing nuclei (such as the locus coeruleus) function to integrate the hormonal and autonomic nervous system components of the arousal response. Both aspects of the arousal system respond to nociception from somatic or visceral dysfunction. It is critical to consider how the arousal system works and its overall or long-term impact on body function.

Arousal System of the Brainstem

The Rostral Portion of the Brainstem Plays a Key Role in the Arousal System

Protection of the body from external or internal threat requires that the individual be awake and capable of focusing attention on the surrounding environment. The midbrain plays an essential role in this process. Projections extend into the generalized nuclei of the thalamus from the neurons in the reticular formation of the midbrain, which, in turn, form a diffuse projection to the neocortex. Long known as the reticular activating system, this circuitry is deeply involved in controlling the activity of cerebral cortex, determining such states as sleep and wakefulness (44). In addition to the reticular activating system, several monoamine pathways arise in the brainstem and innervate both thalamus and neocortex. Like the reticular activating system, the monoamine pathways modulate the activity of neocortical neurons in various ways. One system that arises from the locus coeruleus in the midbrain plays an important role in arousal (45). Fluctuations in the activity of coeruleus neuron are directly reflected in the activity of the cortical electroencephalogram. Together, the reticular activating system and the associated monoamine pathways control the attention and arousal states of the individual; this circuitry forms the basis for the arousal system.

The Arousal System Is Most Responsive to Novel, Unexpected, or Unwanted Stimuli

Any unexpected or unanticipated stimulus can activate the arousal system of the brainstem. This includes visual, acoustic, and somatic sensory stimuli. Nociceptive stimuli represent a particularly strong drive on the arousal system. Stimulation of the sciatic nerve at a level that activates its PANs results in increased neuronal activity in the locus coeruleus (46). Although the pathway from the spinal cord to the locus coeruleus is multisynaptic (47), the effect on the coeruleus is still very powerful.

Somatic Dysfunction and the Arousal System

Increased activity of PANs secondary to somatic dysfunction will be detected by the arousal system. Thus, somatic dysfunction can alter the state of arousal in the brain. This is most clearly seen in acute injuries. The peripheral nervous system becomes active either through mechanical irritation or through the release of proinflammatory cytokines. Spinal cord neurons respond with increased activity, and the individual becomes aware of the injury. Rapid adaptive changes, detailed below, also occur in the endocrine and autonomic nervous systems after activation of the midbrain arousal circuitry. In the short-term situation, these reflex responses are beneficial to survival of the individual. However, long-term exposure to these adaptive changes, such as chronic somatic or visceral dysfunction, can have pathologic consequences.

Visceral Dysfunction and the Arousal System

Visceral afferent fibers in the vagus nerve carry signals concerning visceral dysfunction to the solitary nucleus of the brainstem. Mechanical irritation, infection, or inflammation of visceral tissue results in the release of proinflammatory cytokines by macrophages, dendritic cells, and other immune cells, some of which occurs in the vicinity of the vagal nerve endings. Recent studies demonstrated that the proinflammatory cytokine, interleukin-1β interacts in various ways with the vagus nerve to activate its primary afferent fibers (48). These relationships have given rise to the concept of an "immunosensory system" (49). In this concept, dendritic cells and other antigen-presenting cells interact with foreign substances through immune-type receptors; the activated antigen-presenting cell releases proinflammatory cytokine that interacts with receptors on the vagal primary afferent fibers. Thus, the antigen-presenting cell is behaving as a highly variable receptor, capable of detecting the enormous range of stimuli typical of the immune system but then generating a common signal that peripheral nerves can understand. The activated vagal fibers transmit signals to the solitary nucleus of the brainstem from which immunosensory information ascends through the brainstem to the thalamus and limbic forebrain. The response to such information has been termed sickness behavior or the acute-phase response (50). Sickness behavior is characterized by physiologic changes: fever, increased sleep, alterations in blood chemistry; behavioral changes: decreased locomotion, decreased libido, decreased exploration and aggression, and decreased food and water intake; and by hormonal changes: activation of the sympathetic nervous system (SNS) and of the hypothalamic-pituitary-adrenal axis (50). Thus, the immune system and the nervous system combine their activity such that the immune system's amazing abilities to detect an infinite number of substances is coupled to the nervous system's abilities to generate a rapid adaptive and protective response.

Emotional Stimuli and the Arousal System

Not only does the arousal system respond to unexpected or unwanted sensory stimuli but it also is sensitive to emotional activity. Strong connections exist between the forebrain limbic system (the center of emotional activity in the brain) and the arousal system of the midbrain. For example, the amygdala nuclear complex in the medial aspect of the temporal lobe—a major component of fear or negative memory system—has a prominent descending projection to the area immediately surrounding the locus coeruleus in the brainstem (51). Viewed in this light, the arousal system of the brainstem is performing as a convergence point. It receives sensory stimuli (somatic, visceral, visual, and acoustic) and emotional stimuli and channels this warning information into a wide-ranging output circuitry that significantly alters activity in the nervous, endocrine, and immune systems.

AROUSAL AND THE NEUROENDOCRINE IMMUNE NETWORK

Output of the Arousal System Alters Hemostasis

Activation of the arousal system consequent to physical (somatic or visceral) or emotional stimuli has a profound impact on homeostatic mechanisms in the body. Initiating a strong systemic sympathetic response and triggering the release of the adrenal cortical steroid hormones to accomplish this effect. These two

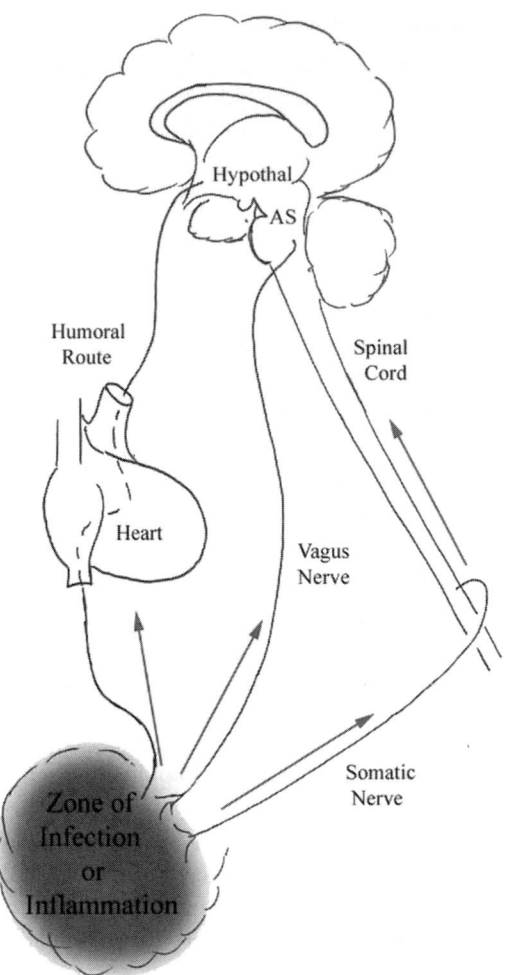

FIGURE 8.8. Diagram illustrating the neural and humoral route used in activating the arousal system of the brainstem. AS, arousal system.

The Neuroendocrine-Immune Network

Integration of a Neural-Endocrine-Immune Reaction

Two significant observations arise from the preceding sections. First, acting through the nervous system, somatic dysfunction relays an excitatory drive on the LC-NE and HPA axes of the midbrain and hypothalamus. Second, acting through humoral routes and the release of cytokines from inflammatory tissue, that same dysfunction also stimulates the HPA axis (Fig. 8.8). Studies inducing small, local inflammatory reactions similar to those seen in somatic dysfunction and examining the response of the HPA axis have verified these observations (76). The HPA axis has a biphasic response to an acute, local inflammatory event; the first phase is acute (less than an hour) and is followed by a second phase that develops more slowly (after 3 hours) and parallels the rise in the inflammatory event (69,76). The first phase is mediated via the peripheral nervous system whereas the second phase is mediated humorally through the release of cytokines. These, and similar studies, demonstrate a neuroendocrine-immune network that responds both acutely and in a more prolonged manner to threat or injury.

Output of the Neuroendocrine-Immune Network Is Protective

The major output chemicals of the neuroendocrine-immune axis are norepinephrine, cortisol, and a mixture of cytokines. The numerous interactions between these substances fostered the concept that communications in the neuroendocrine-immune network are "bidirectional" (77). Cells in each component of the network—neural, endocrine, and immune—contain receptors for the other's regulatory products. Thus, neural cells in the hypothalamus and other locations, as well as immunocytes throughout the body, can respond to hormones such as CRH, ACTH, and cortisol. Conversely, cells in the anterior pituitary and adrenal gland can respond to some cytokines and neurotransmitters. This concept has given rise to the term "bidirectional communication" between these systems (78). Clearly, the boundaries between these systems have been transcended and the network is functioning in a unitary manner. The neural and immune components serve as the sensory inputs to the network (79) (detecting external and internal signals) and the complex output of chemicals serves to regulate the homeostatic mechanisms of the body (3). The regulatory effect of the neuroendocrine-immune system on homeostasis is protective in nature, and has been termed allostasis, which means the "maintenance of stability through change" (80).

Allostasis

Homeostasis is Critical to Survival

Homeostasis includes the carefully controlled rhythms of parameters such as heart rate, blood pressure, fluid ionic balance, temperature, and plasma glucose levels. All of these values are in a state of constant flux; however, not only must the values for these items be maintained within narrow limits to be compatible with life, but many of these items must also be closely regulated with respect to each other. Any situation, of either external or internal origin, that threatens homeostasis is considered stressful (81). In a potentially threatening situation, the neuroendocrine-immune system is capable of rapidly modulating homeostatic rhythms in a coordinated manner, effecting the appropriate changes necessary for promoting the survival of the individual.

The Impact of Norepinephrine and Cortisol on the Body rearranges Its Homeostatic Rhythms Into a State Termed "Allostasis"

When threatened, the neuroendocrine-immune network is capable of responding with rapid release of an impressive list of chemicals that alter the normal homeostatic rhythms: norepinephrine, adrenal cortical steroids, and cytokines. This altered state of body function has been termed allostasis to distinguish it from the normal mechanism of homeostasis. Its feedback control is critical to proper function of the allostatic system. As the threat diminishes, the feedback control systems should suppress the levels of allostatic compounds, returning the body to its normal function. Disease processes all represent threats to the body and, as such, will activate the allostatic response. This has been demonstrated in studies of very ill patients; their body markedly shifts into excessive production of cortisol in a last effort chance at survival (82). If the individual survives the disease, the feedback control systems attempt to return the body to normal homeostasis.

The Allostatic State and Defense: Short-Term Gains, Long-Term Losses

Enhanced production of norepinephrine, cortisol, and cytokines can create a protective environment for rapid defense of the body against threat. The short-term gains of this system can be enormous because they can determine the very survival of the individual. However, recent studies have demonstrated that long-term exposure to this altered chemical milieu is cumulative and appears to be pathologic (3), giving rise to the term "allostatic load" to describe the accumulation of damage in the system due to prolonged activation of the allostatic mechanism.

Allostatic Load

Somatic, Visceral, and Inescapable Emotional Stimuli Are Strong Drives on the Allostatic Mechanism

Through the arousal system, most stressors can activate the SNS-HPA couple, which results in an allostatic response. Examples include emotional events acting through limbic forebrain connections as well as physical stressors acting via the spinoreticular and spinohypothalamic pathways. Physical stressors can be divided into somatic and visceral origins. Somatic stressors include any form of trauma or injury including somatic dysfunctions. Visceral stressors range from traumatic injury, infection, or inflammation of visceral organs to more subtle, diet-related events.

Long-Term Activation of the Allostatic Mechanism Results in Extensive Wear and Tear on the Organ Systems of the Body

Continual or repeated activation of the SNS-HPA couple creates an abnormal state that is stressful to the body. In this condition of repeated allostasis, organ systems are literally damaging one another with their activity (3). Evidence suggests that the exposure to allostatic substances (such as catecholamines and cortisol) is cumulative; that is, the effects of stressors add up progressively. This concept of the summating effects of stress exposure has been termed allostatic load (81). Thus, allostatic load represents the price paid for chronic (either continual or repeated) exposure to the stress-mediated neuroendocrine adaptations. Another effect of increased exposure to allostatic chemicals is the gradual loss of the effectiveness of feedback pathways meant to reestablish normal homeostasis (83). Specifically, long-term exposure to allostatic chemistry has been demonstrated to destroy hippocampal formation neurons that contain cortisol receptors and that function in a long-loop feedback pathway to the hypothalamus, which controls the secretion of corticotropin-releasing factor (84). Thus, the more the arousal system stimulates release of allostatic substances, the worse the body becomes at reestablishing homeostasis. Animal models are available to demonstrate this phenomena (83,85), but more recent evidence suggests that human situations,

TABLE 8.1. MARKERS ASSAYED TO DETERMINE ALLOSTATIC LOAD

Systolic blood pressure
Diastolic blood pressure
Waist to hip ratio
Total cholesteral-HDL ratio
Total glycosylated hemoglobin level
Urinary cortisol level
Urinary norepinephrine level
Urinary epinephrine level
HDL cholesterol level
Dihydroepiandrosterone

such as adult survivors of child sexual abuse, may also suffer from dysregulation of the arousal-allostatic response system (86,87).

Degenerative and Inflammatory Diseases May Have Their Roots in the Allostatic Mechanism

McEwen and co-workers devised a method for indexing allostatic load (88). In this study, they developed a list of markers that could be measured in an aging population. Their markers are listed in Table 8.1. Whether the person was in the high-risk category was determined for each parameter. Allostatic load was the sum of the number of categories in which the person exceeded high-risk level. Thus, each participant in the study received an index number indicating his or her allostatic load. The participants were then assessed for cognitive and physical functions and, based on this information, divided into three groups: high-, medium-, and low-functioning groups. When functional status was compared with allostatic load scores, the results were remarkable. The higher allostatic load score correlated with lower cognitive and physical functioning scores in a cross-sectional view of the population. Furthermore, higher allostatic load baseline scores predicted greater decline in cognitive and physical functions over a seven-year period of follow-up (89). These results strongly support the concept that long-term exposure to the allostatic chemical environment (catecholamines, cortisol, and cytokines) is damaging to organ systems.

The Consequences of Increasing Allostatic Load

Allostasis is the adaptive condition that results from activation of the arousal system of the brainstem. Evidence suggests that long-term exposure to the allostatic response is cumulative and results in the gradual destruction of organ systems. This section examines specific examples of systems breakdown that can be correlated to increased drive on the allostatic mechanism.

Allostasis Has Been Correlated to Increased Occurrence of Cardiovascular Disease

Evidence that prolonged activation of the allostatic system is detrimental to the cardiovascular system is extensive. Numerous studies demonstrate the effect of psychosocial and mental stress on increased blood pressure, obesity, enhanced activity of the fibrinogenic system, and increased atherosclerosis (3). A recent review (90) highlights the devastating effects of increased sympathetic tone on the cardiovascular system including congestive heart failure, left ventricular hypertrophy, hypertension, and atherosclerosis. It is instructive to look at some possible mechanisms by which these pathologies occur. Increased SNS activity has been correlated with essential hypertension (57). Factors contributing to increased SNS activity include psychosocial stress as well as somatic and visceral nociceptive activity. Acute and chronic pain from either somatic or visceral origins will increase the SNS output and influence cardiovascular function. Both acute and chronic somatic stimuli can elevate blood pressure (55,91,92). Increased cortisol levels promote insulin resistance at the tissue level (93). This results in increased production of insulin to counteract the resistance. Elevated levels of insulin secretion stimulate more SNS activity (94) and lead to enhance atherosclerosis. In addition, the insulin resistance serves to raise the level of plasma glucose, which increases the risk of infection and kidney damage (95).

Allostasis Has Been Related to Demise of the Central Nervous System

Memory loss and depression are two cardinal manifestations of the effect of allostasis on the nervous system (3). Cortisol uses portions of the brain, such as the hippocampus, as a feedback mechanism to control the production of corticotropin-releasing hormone from the hypothalamus (96). Long-term exposure to elevated levels of cortisol has been associated with significant damage to the hippocampal formation, ranging from reversible dendritic regression to the excitotoxic death of hippocampal neurons (the latter being a permanent event) (97,98). The hippocampal formation plays a central role in the memory process; cell loss from this structure underlies, in part, the notable memory loss reported clinically.

Allostasis Has Multiple, Complex Effects on the Immune System

The classic response of the immune system to long-term exposure to elevated cortisol and catecholamine levels is immunosuppression (99,100). Thus, in patients with chronic hypercorticism, one manifestation is immunosuppression (63,64). However, acute exposure to elevated cortisol levels can enhance certain immune system function (3). One mechanism for immunoenhancement following stress would be for allostatic chemicals to shift the balance of activity in the immune system from Th1 toward Th2 immunocytes by suppressing the Th1 cells (101). Corticosteroids and sympathetic stimulation are known to be inhibitory to Th1 cell activities and often are stimulatory to Th2 cytokines (102). Th1 lymphocytes are known to enhance cell-mediated forms of immunity, and Th2 lymphocytes are involved in enhancing antibody production from plasma cells (102). If the Th2 pathways are enhanced, more antibody-mediated autoimmune and allergic types of diseases would be expressed (102).

Allostatic Shifts Have an Impact on Numerous Other Systems

SNS activity plays a major role in the regulation of the kidney (103). Stressful situations that activated the sympathetic out-

flow resulted in increased water retention, retention of sodium, hypervolemia, and hypertension (104). Long-term pathologic consequences occur in the kidney secondary to exposure to elevated sympathetic activity (105). In the gastrointestinal system and skin, elevated cortisol and catecholamines increase the responsiveness of delayed-type hypersensitivity (95,106, 107).

SUMMARY: AROUSAL, ALLOSTASIS, AND ALLOSTATIC LOAD

Allostasis, the General Compensatory Response and Disease

The Healthy Body Has the Capability to Defend Against Disease

In health, the human body and mind have remarkable abilities to resist disease. These capabilities can be influenced by genetic background as well as environmental history.

The Concept of Allostasis Represents an Aspect of the General Compensatory Response

Allostasis is the body's attempt to compensate for a stressful situation in a protective way, whether the stress is physical or psychosocial in nature. Both forms of stressors activate the arousal system of the brainstem, leading to SNS and HPA responses, and the elevation of plasma catecholamines and cortisol (Fig. 8.9). In this manner, the SNS and HPA couple acts as the last common pathway through which multiple forms of a stressor may initiate the appropriate compensatory responses. The convergence of multiple, different pathways on a common mechanism also facilitate summation of differing drives to obtain a more intense response. Thus, somatic or visceral dysfunction can exacerbate the response of the arousal system in a person with an emotional dysfunction.

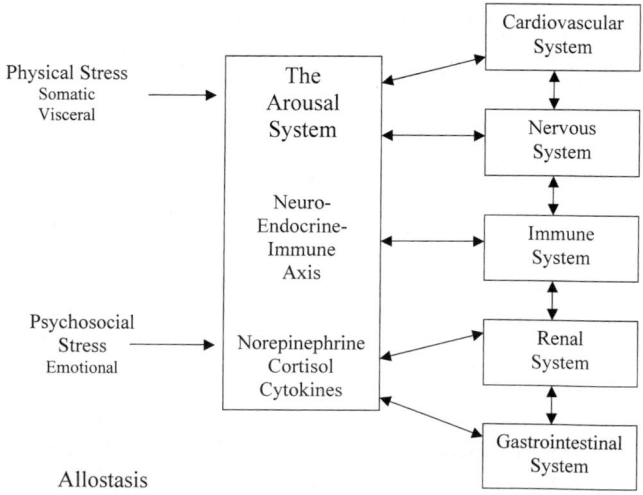

FIGURE 8.9. A diagram illustrating the allostasis-arousal system and its impact on the homeostatic mechanism of the body.

In the Compensated State, There Is Less Room for Further Adaptation

In this compensated state, the body is less capable of further adaptation to an increased stress or a new stressor. This is true whether the compensation is in the form of structural or metabolic change, or more typically, both.

Long-term Existence in the Compensated State Can Be Destructive

Long-term exposure to elevated levels of SNS-HPA output forces organ systems in the body to function abnormally and, literally, grind each other down (3). Neurons and endocrine cells operated in an excited state are susceptible to excitotoxic cell death; immune cells maintained in an excited state can be more responsive, attacking the wrong tissues, stimulating surrounding cells to proliferate creating plaques in inappropriate locations, or becoming repressed and improperly defending the body.

Many inflammatory, neoplastic, and degenerative processes that we accept as common occurrences of aging may, in fact, be the result of a compensated individual, unable to adequately stave off disease.

REEXAMINATION OF THE OSTEOPATHIC PHILOSOPHY OF MEDICINE

Events in Peripheral Tissue and at the Spinal Cord Level Suggest an Understanding of Somatic Dysfunction

This chapter began by examining the pathophysiology of a somatic dysfunction (edema and inflammation) and demonstrated that there are two routes by which this event can signal the spinal cord. The neural route is by far the best known; however, recent studies suggest that the mediators of inflammation can also reach the central nervous system through humoral routes. In the spinal cord, neural and humoral signals combine to produce short-term changes in dorsal horn neuronal activity. In situations of excessive or repeated injury, long-term (and in some cases, permanent) changes in spinal cord neural circuitry can occur, thus underlying various pain states. Altered segmental activity in the spinal cord leads to somatic responses that manifest as altered ease or range of motion in skeletal muscles and anatomical asymmetries in joint position. In addition, spinal cord sympathetic outflow can also change, thus accounting for clinically well-known somatovisceral reflexes.

Somatic Dysfunction Triggers the Arousal System of the Brainstem

The arousal system is composed of a complex neural circuitry expending from the medulla, pons, and midbrain. Its connections descend into the spinal cord to modulate spinal circuitry and ascend into the forebrain to trigger behavioral states. It is responsive to any kind of unexpected or unwanted stressor. Somatic dysfunction (stress) that works through ascending spinal cord tracts is but one drive on the arousal system. Others include visceral dysfunctions (stressors) signaling through ascending spinal cord tracts and both somatic and visceral dysfunctions using cytokines traveling through humoral routes to reach the hypothalamus and arousal system. Finally, descending connections from limbic forebrain structures such as the prefrontal cortex and amygdala provide a strong drive for emotional dysfunction (stress) on the arousal system.

The Arousal System of the Brain Stem is Coupled to the Allostatic Response

The arousal system is coupled to two major efferent pathways: the SNS and the hypothalamic-pituitary-adrenal axis (HPA). Increased drive on the arousal system leads to the release of catecholamines from the SNS and adrenal cortical steroids from the HPA. Norepinephrine and cortisol modify the production of numerous cytokines from the immune system. All three systems (neural, endocrine, and immune) function together in a network to alter homeostatic processes in to a protective state termed allostasis. The defensive compensation created by the allostatic response can be very beneficial to escape behavior and wound repair as well as the prevention or containment of infection.

Feedback Pathways Restore Homeostasis via Adequate Function of the Neural and Circulatory Systems of the Body

The allostatic response occurs in the face of a stressor. As the stressor abates, feedback pathways—both neural and humoral—function to restore natural homeostatic balance. Failure of the neural or humoral routes or excessive exposure to the allostatic chemistry can result in inappropriate feedback and failure to return to baseline homeostatic values; thus, the body exists in a chronic compensatory state.

Failure to Restore Homeostasis Exposes the Body to Increased Risk of Disease

Long-term exposure to the allostatic response forces organ systems to work with each other in unnatural or compensated states. In this condition, the organ systems literally grind each other down (3). Epidemiologic research has related this compensated situation to the chronic and insidiously progressive development of numerous degenerative and inflammatory diseases.

The Osteopathic Approach to the Patient Is Focused on Relieving the Drives on the Allostatic Mechanism

The osteopathic approach to the patient helps that person find his way back to baseline homeostatic condition. In this chapter, two major drives on the arousal-allostatic response have emerged: physical and psychosocial. Both are very capable of significantly altering baseline homeostasis. In the physical category, we find somatic dysfunction and visceral dysfunction; in the psychosocial category, we find emotional and cognitive sources. The important concept is that these drives, working through the common pathway of the arousal-allostatic system, appear to summate with each other to augment the allostatic impact on normal homeostasis. Thus, regaining health for the individual is dependent on reestablishing baseline homeostatic values by mitigating the drives on the arousal-allostatic system. In one sense, these drives represent the handles available for modulating the activity of the arousal-allostatic system. To best address the status of these handles, the osteopathic physician needs to consider the individual, not only in terms of their specific complaints but also in terms of the general status of their body (soma) and visceral functions, as well as their integration with their surrounding family, social, and work environments. The treatment plan is then based on a rational approach to normalizing these processes. The ability of the osteopathic physician (by virtue of his or her training) to assess the patient's somatic and visceral status as well as the specific complaint underscores the unique osteopathic approach to medicine.

REFERENCES

1. Denslow JS. Pathophysiologic evidence for the osteopathic lesion: the known, unknown, and controversial. *J Am Osteopath Assoc.* 1975;74:415–421.
2. Selye H. The general adaptive syndrome and the diseases of adaptation. *J Clin Endocrinol Metab.* 1946;6:117–173.
3. McEwen BS. Protective and damaging effects of stress mediators. *N Engl J Med.* 1998;338(3):171–179.
4. Prechtl JC, Powley TL. B-afferents: a fundamental division of the nervous system mediating homeostasis? *Behav Brain Sci.* 1990;13:289–331.
5. Coderre TJ, Katz J, Vaccarina AL, et al. Contribution of central neuroplasticity to pathological pain: review of clinical and experimental evidence. *Pain.* 1993;52(3):259–285.
6. Woolf CJ, Thompson WN. The induction and maintenance of central sensitization is dependent on N-methyl-D-aspartic receptor activation; implications for the treatment of post-injury pain hypersensitivity states. *Pain.* 1991;44:293–299.
7. Rossi A, Decchi B. Cutaneous nociceptive facilitation of Ib heteronymous pathways to lower limb motoneurons in humans. *Brain Res.* 1995;700:164–172.
8. Anderson MF, Winterson BJ. Properties of peripherally induced persistent hindlimb flexion in rat: Involvement of *N*-methyl-D-aspartate receptors and capsaicin-sensitive afferents. *Brain Res.* 1995;678:140–150.
9. Willard FH. *Medical Neuroanatomy: A Problem-Oriented Approach with Annotated Atlas.* Philadelphia, PA: JB Lippincott Co; 1993.
10. Kandel ER, Schwartz JH, Jessell TM. *Principles of Neural Sciences,* 4th ed. New York, NY: Elsevier Science; 2000.
11. Willis WD, Coggeshall RE. *Sensory Mechanisms of the Spinal Cord,* 2nd ed. New York, NY: Plenum Publishing; 1991.
12. Bonica JJ. Anatomic and physiologic basis of nociception and pain. In: Bonica JJ, ed. *The Management of Pain.* Philadelphia, PA: Lea & Febiger; 1990:28–94.
13. Craig AD, Dostrovsky JO. Medulla to thalamus. In: Wall PD, Melzack R, eds. *Textbook of Pain.* Edinburgh, Scotland: Churchill Livingstone; 1999:183–214.
14. Ingvar M, Hsieh J-C. The image of pain. In: Wall PD, Melzack R, es. *Textbook of Pain.* Edinburgh, Scotland: Churchill Livingstone; 1999:215–233.
15. Levine JD, Fields HL, Basbaum AI. Peptides and the primary afferent nociceptor. *J Neurosci.* 1993;13:2273–2286.
16. Sato J, Perl E. Adrenergic excitation of cutaneous pain receptors induced by peripheral nerve injury. *Science.* 1991;251:1608–1610.
17. Raja SN, Meyer RA, Ringkamp M, et al. Peripheral neural mechanisms of nociception. In: Wall PD, Melzack R, eds. *Textbook of Pain.* Edinburgh, Scotland: Churchill Livingstone; 1999:11–57.
18. Neumann S, Doubell TP, Leslie T, et al. Inflammatory pain hypersensitivity mediated by phenotypic switch in myelinated primary sensory neurons. *Nature.* 1996;384(6607):360–364.
19. Payan DG. Substance P: a neuroendocrine-immune modulator. *Hosp Pract (Off Ed).* 1989;24(2):67–80.
20. Steen KH, Issberner U, Reeh PW. Pain due to experimental acidosis in human skin: Evidence for non-adapting nociceptor excitation. *Neurosci Lett.* 1995;199(1):29–32.
21. Devor M, Seltzer Z. Pathophysiology of damaged nerves in relation to chronic pain. In: Wall PD, Melzack R, eds. *Textbook of Pain.* Edinburgh, Scotland: Churchill Livingstone; 1999:129–164.
22. Woolf CJ, Chong M-S. Preemptive analgesia—treating postoperative pain by preventing the establishment of central sensitization. *Anesth Analg.* 1993;77:362–379.
23. Doubell TP, Mannion RJ, Woolf CJ. The dorsal horn: state-dependent sensory processing, plasticity and generation of pain. In: Wall PD, Melzack R, eds. *Textbook of Pain.* Edinburgh, Scotland: Churchill Livingstone; 1999:165–181.
24. Melzack R, Wall PD. Pain mechanisms: a new theory. *Sci.* 1965 Nov.; 150(699):971–9.
25. Woolf CJ, Shortland P, Coggeshall RE. Peripheral nerve injury triggers central sprouting of myelinated afferents. *Nature.* 1992;355(6355):75–78.
26. Watkins LR, Milligan ED, Maier SF. Glial activation: a driving force for pathological pain. *Trends Neurosci.* 2001;24(8):450–455.
27. Watkins LR, Milligan ED, Maier SF. Spinal cord glia: new players in pain. *Pain.* 2001;93(3):201–205.
28. Milligan ED, O'Connor KA, Nguyen KT, et al. Intrathecal HIV-1 envelope glycoprotein gp120 induces enhanced pain states mediated by spinal cord proinflammatory cytokines. *J Neurosci.* 2001;21(8):2808–2819.
29. Sugimoto T, Bennett GJ, Kajander KC. Transsynaptic degeneration in the superficial dorsal horn after sciatic nerve injury: effects of a chronic constriction injury, transection, and strychnine. *Pain.* 1990;42(2):205–213.
30. Nachemson AK, Bennett GJ. Does pain damage spinal cord neurons? Transsynaptic degeneration in rat following a surgical incision. *Neurosci Lett.* 1993;162:78–80.
31. Dubner R, Ruda MA. Activity-dependent neuronal plasticity following tissue injury and inflammation. *Trends Neurosci.* 1992;15:96–103.
32. Patterson MM. Spinal fixation: long-term alterations in spinal reflex excitability with altered or sustained sensory inputs. In: Patterson MM, Grau JW, eds. *Spinal Cord Plasticity: Alterations in Reflex Function.* Norwell, MA: Kluwer Academic Publishers; 2002:77–100.
33. He X, Proske U, Schaible HG, et al. Acute inflammation of the knee joint in the cat alters responses of flexor motoneurons to leg movements. *J Neurophysiol.* 1988;59:326–340.
34. Sato A, Schmidt RF. Somatosympathetic reflexes: afferent fibers, central pathways, discharge characteristics. *Physiol Rev.* 1973;53:916–947.
35. Cervero F, Tattersall JE. Somatic and visceral inputs to the thoracic spinal cord of the cat: marginal zone (lamina I) of the dorsal horn [published erratum appears in *J Physiol.* 1987;393:777]. *J Physiol.* 1987;388:383–395.
36. Van Buskirk RL. Nociceptive reflexes and the somatic dysfunction: a model. *J Am Osteopath Assoc.* 1990;90(9):792–809.
37. Giesler Jr. GJ, Katter JT, Dado RJ. Direct spinal pathways to the limbic system for nociceptive information. *Trends Neurosci.* 1994;17(6):244–250.
38. Zhang X, Wenk HN, Gokin AP, et al. Physiological studies of spinohypothalamic tract neurons in the lumbar enlargement of monkeys. *J Neurophysiol.* 1999;82(2):1054–1058.
39. Malick A, Strassman RM, Burstein R. Trigeminohypothalamic and reticulohypothalamic tract neurons in the upper cervical spinal cord and caudal medulla of the rat. *J Neurophysiol.* 2000;84(4):2078–2112.
40. Nauta WJH, Kuypers HGJM. Some ascending pathways in the brain stem reticular formation. In: Jaspers HH, ed. *Reticular Formation of the Brain.* Boston, MA: Little, Brown and Company; 1958:3–29.

41. Stocker SD, Steinbacher Jr. BC, Balaban CD, et al. Connections of the caudal ventrolateral medullary reticular formation in the cat brainstem. *Exp Brain Res.* 1997;116(2):270–282.

42. Brodal A. *Neurological Anatomy: In Relation to Clinical Medicine.* New York, NY: Oxford University Press; 1981.

43. Blessing WW. *The Lower Brainstem and Bodily Homeostasis.* New York, NY: Oxford University Press; 1997.

44. Klemm WR. The behavioral readiness response. In: Klemm WR, Vertes RP, eds. *Brainstem Mechanisms of Behavior.* New York, NY: John Wiley and Sons; 1990:105–145.

45. Robbins TW, Everitt BJ. Arousal systems and attention. In: Gazzaniga MS, ed. *The Cognative Neurosciences.* Cambridge, MA: The MIT Press; 1995:703–720.

46. Chiang C, Aston-Jones G. Response of locus coeruleus neurons to footshock stimulation is mediated by neurons in the rostral ventral medulla. *Neuroscience.* 1993;53:705–715.

47. Aston-Jones G, Ennis M, Pieribone VA, et al. The brain nucleus locus coeruleus: restricted afferent control of a broad efferent network. *Science.* 1986;234:734–737.

48. Goehler LE, Gaykema RP, Nguyen KT, et al. Interleukin-1 beta in immune cells of the abdominal vagus nerve: a link between the immune and nervous systems? *J Neurosci.* 1999;19(7):2799–2806.

49. Goehler LE, Gaykema RP, Hansen MK, et al. Vagal immune-to-brain communication: a visceral chemosensory pathway. *Auton Neurosci.* 2000;85:49–59.

50. Watkins LR, Maier SF. The pain of being sick: implications of immune-to-brain communication for understanding pain. *Annu Rev Psychol.* 2000;51:29–57.

51. Van Bockstaele EJ, Peoples J, Valentino RJ. Anatomic basis for differential regulation of the rostrolateral peri-locus coeruleus region by limbic afferents. *Biol Psychiatry.* 1999;46(10):1352–1363.

52. Svensson T. Emerging aspects of the adrenergic nervous systems. *Acta Anaesthesiol Scand Suppl.* 1982;76:8–11.

53. Van Bockstaele EJ, Aston-Jones G. Integration in the ventral medulla and coordination of sympathetic, pain and arousal functions. *Clin Exp Hypertens.* 1995;17:153–165.

54. Chan-Palay V, Asan E. Quantitation of catecholamine neurons in the locus coeruleus in human brains of normal young and older adults and in depression. *J Comp Neurol.* 1989;287:357–372.

55. Allen GV, Pronych SP. Trigeminal autonomic pathways involved in nociception-induced reflex cardiovascular responses. *Brain Res Brain Res Rev.* 1997;754:269–278.

56. Esser MJ, Pronych SP, Allen GV. Trigeminal-reticular connections: possible pathways for nociception-induced cardiovascular reflex responses in the rat. *J Comp Neurol.* 1998;391(4):526–544.

57. Mancia G, Grassi G, Giannattasio C, et al. Sympathetic activation in the pathogenesis of hypertension and progression of organ damage. *Hypertension.* 1999;34:724–728.

58. Basbaum AI, Fields HL. Endogenous pain control mechanisms: Review and hypothesis. *Ann Neurol.* 1978;4:451–462.

59. Calogero AE, Gallucci WT, Chrousos GP, et al. Catecholamine effects upon rat hypothalamic corticotropin-releasing hormone secretion in vitro. *J Clin Invest.* 1988;82:839–846.

60. Elmquist JK, Scammell TE, Saper CB. Mechanisms of CNS response to systemic immune challenge: the febrile response. *Trends Neurosci.* 1997;20(12):565–570.

61. Breder CD, Dinarello CA, Saper CB. Interleukin-1 immunoreactive innervation of the human hypothalamus. *Science.* 1988;240:321–323.

62. Sapolsky RM, River C, Yamamoto G, et al. Interleukin-1 stimulates secretion of hypothalamic corticotropin- releasing factor. *Science.* 1987;238:522–524.

63. Gold PW, Goodwin FK, Chrousos GP. Clinical and biochemical manifestations of depression: relation to the neurobiology of stress. Part I. *N Engl J Med.* 1988;319:348–353.

64. Gold PW, Goodwin FK, Chrousos GP. Clinical and biochemical manifestations of depression: relation to the neurobiology of stress. Part II. *N Engl J Med.* 1988;319:413–420.

65. Ganong WF. The stress response—a dynamic overview. *Hosp Pract (Off Ed).* 1988;23(6):155–190.

66. Sapolsky RM, Romero LM, Munck AU. How do glucocorticoids influence stress responses? Integrating permissive, suppressive, stimulatory, and preparative actions. *Endocr Rev.* 2000;21(1):55–89.

67. Ganong WF. *Review of Medical Physiology,* 20th ed. New York, NY: McGraw-Hill; 2001.

68. Fleshner M, Nguyen KT, Cotter CS, et al. Acute stressor exposure both suppresses acquired immunity and potentiates innate immunity. *Am J Physiol.* 1998;275:R870–R878.

69. Turnbull AV, Rivier CL. Regulation of the hypothalamic-pituitary-adrenal axis by cytokines: actions and mechanisms of action. *Physiol Rev.* 1999;79(1):1–71.

70. Watkins LR, Maier SF. Implications of immune-to-brain communication for sickness and pain. *Proc Natl Acad Sci U S A.* 1999;96(14):7710–7713.

71. Marsh CB, Wewers MD. The pathogenesis of sepsis. Factors that modulate the response to gram-negative bacterial infection. *Clin Chest Med.* 1996;17(2):183–197.

72. Panos RJ, Baker SK. Mediators, cytokines, and growth factors in liver-lung interactions. *Clin Chest Med.* 1996;17(1):151–169.

73. Matuschak GM. Lung-liver interactions in sepsis and multiple organ failure syndrome. *Clin Chest Med.* 1996;17(1):83–98.

74. Olszewski WL, Pazdur J, Kubasiewicz E, et al. Lymph draining from foot joints in rheumatoid arthritis provides insight into local cytokine and chemokine production and transport to lymph nodes. *Arthritis Rheum.* 2001;44(3):541–549.

75. Tilg H, Dinarello CA, Mier JW. IL-6 and APPs: anti-inflammatory and immunosuppressive mediators. *Immunol Today.* 1997;18(9):428–432.

76. Turnbull AV, Rivier C. Corticotropin-releasing factor, vasopressin, and prostaglandins mediate, and nitric oxide restrains, the hypothalamic-pituitary-adrenal response to acute local inflammation in the rat. *Endocrinology.* 1996;137(2):455–463.

77. Carr DJJ, Blalock JE. Neuropeptide hormones and receptors common to the immune and neuroendocrine systems: bidirectional pathway of intersystem communication. In: Ader R, Felten DL, Cohen N, eds. *Psychoneuroimmunology.* San Diego, CA: Academic Press; 1991:573–558.

78. Weigent DA, Carr DJJ, Blalock JE. Bidirectional communication between the neuroendocrine and immune systems: common hormones and hormone receptors. *Ann N Y Acad Sci.* 1990;579:17–27.

79. Blalock JE. The immune system as a sensory organ. *J Immunol.* 1984;132:1067–1070.

80. Sterling P, Eyer J. Allostasis: a new paradigm to explain arousal pathology. In: Fischer S, Reason J, eds. *Handbook of Life Stress, Cognition and Health.* New York, NY: John Wiley and Sons; 1988:629–649.

81. McEwen BS, Stellar E. Stress and the individual. Mechanisms leading to disease. *Arch Intern Med.* 1993;153:2093–2101.

82. Parker LN, Levin ER, Lifrak ET. Evidence for adrenocortical adaptation to severe illness. *J Clin Endocrinol Metab.* 1985;60(5):947–952.

83. Sapolsky RM, Krey LC, McEwen BS. Stress down-regulates corticosterone receptors in a site-specific manner in the brain. *Endocrinology.* 1984;114:287–292.

84. Sapolsky RM, Uno H, Rebert CS, et al. Hippocampal damage associated with prolonged glucocorticoid exposure in primates. *J Neurosci.* 1990;10:2897–2902.

85. Sapolsky RM, Krey LC, McEwen BS. Prolonged glucocorticoid exposure reduces hippocampal neuron number: implications for aging. *J Neurosci.* 1985;5:1222–1227.

86. Lemieux AM, Coe CL. Abuse-related posttraumatic stress disorder: evidence for chronic neuroendocrine activation in women. *Psychosom Med.* 1995;57(2):105–115.

87. Heim C, Newport DJ, Heit S, et al. Pituitary-adrenal and autonomic responses to stress in women after sexual and physical abuse in childhood. *JAMA.* 2000;284(5):592–597.

88. Seeman TE, Singer BH, Rowe JW, et al. Price of adaptation—allostatic load and its health consequences. MacArthur studies of successful aging. *Arch Intern Med.* 1997;157(19):2259–2268.

89. Seeman TE, McEwen BS, Rowe JW, et al. Allostatic load as a marker of cumulative biological risk: MacArthur studies of successful aging. *Proc Natl Acad Sci U S A.* 2001;98(8):4770–4775.

This is caused by shear forces on endothelial cells that release nitric oxide.

■ Although the direct effect of stimulation of sympathetic nerves to the heart is coronary constriction, this is overwhelmed by the active hyperemia resulting from the increased metabolism of cardiac muscle.

■ Skin blood flow is influenced both by local and core body temperature.

■ The cutaneous response to injury includes a red line, a flare, and a wheal.

■ The red line is caused by release of paracrines.

■ The flare is caused by a local axon reflex, involving the release of substance P and calcitonin gene-related peptide.

■ The wheal is local edema resulting a combination of increased transport of plasma proteins into the interstitial space and is caused by substance P, histamine and bradykinin, and increased capillary hydrostatic pressure accompanying arteriolar vasodilatation.

A major role of the physician is to encourage the normal physiologic processes responsible for maintenance of a favorable environment for each cell of the body, and when necessary, to fight pathologic events that disrupt this environment (1). Each cell must meet its needs for energy by producing adenosine triphosphate (ATP) in sufficient quantities. In most cells, this is primarily done by oxidative phosphorylation. Oxidative phosphorylation requires a cellular environment that provides a steady supply of oxygen and substrate and a route for the disposal of the byproducts of cellular respiration, CO_2 and H_2O. Circulation of the blood plays a key role in maintaining the internal environment of cells. The circulation is the cell's connection to the outside world, bringing oxygen and substrates and removing the waste products of metabolism. This chapter discusses the regulation of cellular respiration and the local mechanisms that regulate circulation to maintain the internal environment.

REGULATION OF TISSUE RESPIRATION

ATP is the common intermediate that provides chemical energy for cellular function. Motility, pumping of ions, and metabolic pathways all use ATP as a source of energy (1). The cell makes use of ATP by enzymatically transforming ATP to adenosine 5'-diphosphate (ADP) and in the process capturing the chemical energy released. A cell needs a supply of ATP calibrated to meet its needs at a given time. In some cells, such as muscle fibers, energy requirements may vary greatly in just a few seconds, as the cells go from resting to high activity (2). When ATP is rapidly broken down, it must be resynthesized from ADP in a timely fashion.

In many cells, including skeletal and cardiac muscle, phosphocreatine provides a quick source of ATP by the following reaction (3):

$$ADP + PCr \longleftrightarrow ATP + Cr$$

The equilibrium constant for this reaction favors the formation of ATP, so that PCr falls to approximately 10% of its maximal value before a physiologically significant decrease in ATP occurs. Although phosphocreatine is a rapid means for replenishing ATP, the amount of ATP available via this pathway is limited. Cells must turn to other pathways for a more sustained supply of ATP.

Glycolysis, the breakdown of glucose to pyruvate is a rapid source of ATP, although not as quick as the phosphocreatine reaction. Glycolysis captures only a small fraction of the energy available in the glucose molecule for the formation of ATP, but it does this quickly and without requiring oxygen. In a few cell types, including red blood cells, glycolysis is the source of ATP. However, in most cells, glycolysis serves to provide ATP for a few seconds before oxidative phosphorylation begins to meet the steady-state requirements for ATP. When short bursts of energy are needed, or when the supply of oxygen is limited, glycolysis is a significant source of ATP (4).

Under most circumstances, in most cells, oxidative phosphorylation is the mainstay for the synthesis of ATP from ADP. Oxidative phosphorylation is capable of supplying ATP for a wide range of cellular energy requirements. As the rate of oxidative phosphorylation increases, the circulation must deliver an increasing supply of oxygen and substrates. Later, we will consider how this delivery is regulated. For the moment, let us assume that oxygen and substrate are available. If that is the case, ATP supply from oxidative metabolism exactly matches ATP use. The regulation of oxidative metabolism is our next topic.

The cellular controls that match ATP supply to ATP use are not fully understood, but recent studies involving the use of *in vivo* nuclear magnetic imaging have provided important clues. We will use the muscle cells of the heart as our example in discussing regulation of oxidative metabolism. This is a good choice because cardiac muscle cells exhibit a wide range of rates of oxidative phosphorylation. In addition, energy supply to cardiac cells is vital to survival and is the main issue in coronary artery disease, a major cause of morbidity and mortality in Western societies (2). Later we will return to a discussion of coronary blood flow to complete our consideration of energy supply of the myocardium.

The mitochondrion is the intracellular site of the events that make use of oxygen, substrate, ADP, and inorganic phosphate (Pi) to produce CO_2, H_2O, and ATP. Isolated mitochondria are stimulated to produce ATP by increased concentrations of ADP and Pi. One view is that this pertains directly to the regulation of mitochondria inside cells (5). According to this view, as ATP is used, cytosolic ADP and Pi concentrations rise. The mitochondria, bathed in the cytosol, respond to the increased ADP and Pi by producing more ATP. However, recent observations of mitochondrial function in intact heart and brain as well as other tissues demonstrate that there can be large changes in ATP synthesis by mitochondria without significant changes in the cytosolic concentrations of ADP and Pi. This raises the question of what regulates oxidative phosphorylation in the absence of changes in ADP and Pi.

At least two factors stimulate ATP synthesis independent of a change in ADP or Pi. First, nicotinamide adenine dinucleotide (NADH) is formed at a number of steps in the metabolism of substrates, most importantly in the citric acid cycle, and it is a thermodynamic driving force increasing the rate of oxidative phosphorylation (6). Second, an increase in cytosolic calcium ion concentration stimulates mitochondrial ATP synthesis (7). It appears that increased cytosolic calcium ion concentration raises the effectiveness of NADH in driving oxidative phosphorylation. This observation raises the possibility that in the presence of increased calcium concentration, minimal changes in ADP, Pi, and NADH may be adequate to drive oxidative phosphorylation. This view is compatible with the available information from the study of oxidative phosphorylation in intact hearts.

The view that calcium ions are integral to the normal regulation of oxidative phosphorylation puts this ion in a central role in both the synthesis and the use of ATP. For example, in cardiac muscle, increased cytosolic calcium ion concentration unleashes actomyosin cross bridge cycling and contraction. This event dramatically increases the hydrolysis of ATP. At the same time, the increase in cytosolic calcium ion concentration stimulates oxidative phosphorylation. In this scenario, a rise in ADP and Pi is not required for an increased rate of ATP synthesis. Instead, the same stimulus, cytosolic calcium ion concentration, is responsible for increasing ATP hydrolysis and also increasing ATP synthesis (7).

This discussion of the regulation of mitochondrial ATP synthesis brings us to the definition of oxygen demand. Oxygen demand is the net stimulus for oxidative phosphorylation. As we presently understand, it is dependent on the cytosolic concentrations of ADP, Pi, and calcium ion as well as NADH delivery to the mitochondrial respiratory chain. The next section discusses the factors that influence the supply of oxygen by circulation. Maintenance of the balance of supply and demand for oxygen is necessary if cells are to continuously carry out their functions.

REGULATION OF TISSUE CIRCULATION

Blood flow in tissue is determined by the pressure difference between the arterial and venous sides of its circulation and the resistance to flow offered by its own vasculature. The heart generates the pressure difference across a tissue. Elaborate control mechanisms adjust cardiac output and systemic vascular resistance to maintain adequate arterial pressure. Given an adequate pressure head, tissue blood flow is regulated by local mechanisms that allow precise regional adjustment of blood flow. The systemic control of arterial pressure and the regulation of the arterial partial pressure of O_2 and CO_2 by the lungs is beyond the scope of this chapter. In the following discussion, we will assume that arterial pressure and arterial blood gas composition is normal, unless otherwise specified. We will focus our attention on the local regulation of blood flow.

Blood vessels in systemic circulation can be categorized according to their function. The aorta and large arteries distribute blood to organs and tissues with a very small drop in pressure. Smaller arteries and arterioles are the main site of resistance to blood flow. Capillaries and small venules are the locus of exchange of substances between tissues and blood. Larger venules and veins hold the largest share of blood volume and therefore are said to have a capacitance function. These terms will be used below.

After discussion of the general mechanisms governing the local regulation of blood flow, two contrasting vascular beds will be considered in some detail. Regulation of coronary blood flow is dominated by the requirement to balance oxygen supply and demand. We will use this vascular bed as our example of local

regulation of flow in a tissue that undergoes large changes in respiration. Regulation of skin blood flow provides us with a contrast to coronary blood flow. Under most circumstances, skin receives sufficient blood flow to meet its metabolic needs. However, skin is the site of heat loss to the external environment. Blood flow to skin plays a major role in the extent of this loss, and its control reflects this fact. In addition, skin is juxtaposed to the external environment and is frequently injured. We will also discuss the changes in skin blood flow in response to injury.

GENERAL MECHANISMS GOVERNING LOCAL REGULATION OF BLOOD FLOW

Local regulation of blood flow occurs by means of three basic regulatory mechanisms: metabolic, myogenic, and paracrine. The control of blood flow in any one tissue can be understood as a particular application of these three mechanisms. A discussion of these mechanisms will serve as a background for the description of blood flow in particular tissues.

Metabolic regulation refers to changes in blood flow that occur in response to alterations in the ratio of blood flow to the metabolic requirements of tissues (8). It is mediated by vasodilator metabolites, including adenosine, potassium ions, CO_2, and hydrogen ions released from parenchymal cells. These vasodilators relax the smooth muscle of nearby arterioles. The resulting vasodilatation results in reduced resistance to flow and, in the presence of a constant arterial pressure, increased blood flow. Increased blood flow supplies more O_2 and other nutrients. The stimulus for release of vasodilator metabolites can be either increased metabolic activity of parenchymal cells or decreased PO_2 resulting from reduced O_2 supply relative to the use of oxygen. Tissue PO_2 decreases with increased use of O_2 relative to supply and under conditions when arteriolar wall PO_2 decreases, which contributes to vasodilatation. In general, if arterial PO_2 is normal, PO_2 of the arteriolar wall is normal. This is because O_2 diffuses readily from blood into the arteriolar wall. The relative importance of the various metabolic vasodilator mechanisms depends on the parenchymal cell in question, the mix of tissue activity, and blood supply.

A feedback loop describing metabolic regulation is shown in Figure 9.1. In this feedback loop, a decrease in arterial pressure reduces blood flow and the delivery of oxygen. The mismatch between O_2 supply and use lowers tissue PO_2. Lowered tissue PO_2 limits the formation of ATP and results in the release of vasodilator metabolites: adenosine, for example. Vasodilator metabolites raise flow toward normal. Alternatively, increased tissue metabolism leads to increased O_2 use and lowers tissue PO_2. Lowered PO_2 limits formation of ATP from ADP and increases the same vasodilator metabolites. Increased blood flow restores tissue PO_2. In Figure 9.1, tissue PO_2 is used as the error signal in the negative feed back loop. However, some metabolites are not ordinarily released in response to lowered tissue PO_2. A good example is K+, which is released with each action potential of the tissue. It acts as a feed-forward mechanism, initiating vasodilatation before the action potentials that release it have time to trigger the cellular events that will ultimately result in increased O_2 use.

Myogenic regulation refers to changes in the tone of resistance vessels in response to alterations in their transmural pressure. It

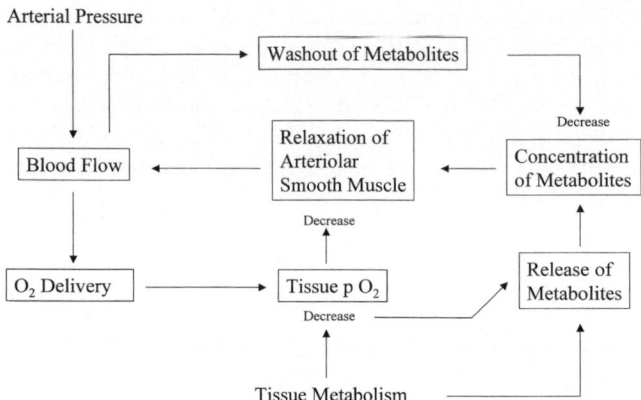

FIGURE 9.1. Metabolic regulation of blood flow. Either reduced arterial pressure or increased tissue metabolism reduces tissue PO_2. This leads to release of vasodilator metabolites, relaxation of arteriolar smooth muscle, and decreased vascular resistance. In the case of decreased arterial pressure, blood flow returns toward the original value (autoregulation). In the case of increased metabolism, blood flow increases (active hyperemia). Metabolic regulation of blood flow also plays a role in reactive hyperemia.

occurs when a change in transmural pressure results in increased or decreased stretch of the vascular smooth muscle of resistance vessels (Fig. 9.2). Increased stretch results in contraction of vascular smooth muscle. The myogenic response counteracts the influence of increased or decreased transmural pressure on resistance vessel diameter. For example, when we stand up, transmural pressure increases dramatically in the resistance vessels of the legs and feet. These resistance vessels are stretched and their response is to constrict. This response has at least two beneficial effects. First, it prevents the dilatation that would otherwise occur as a result of the increased transmural pressure. Second, constriction of the resistance vessels lessens the hydrostatic pressure transmitted to the capillaries of the legs and feet as a result of standing.

The error signal for myogenic regulation is stretch of vascular smooth muscle cells within the wall of resistance vessels (9). Stretch of vascular smooth muscle causes opening of stretch-

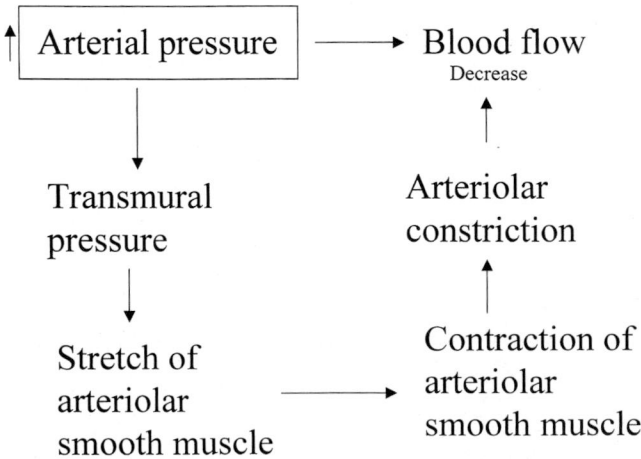

FIGURE 9.2. Myogenic regulation of blood flow results from a change in arteriolar tone in response to a change in stretch of arteriolar smooth muscle. Increased transmural pressure, (ordinarily the effect of increased arterial pressure) stretches the vascular wall, which causes contraction of arteriolar smooth muscle, arteriolar constriction, and a decrease in blood flow. Myogenic regulation plays a role in autoregulation of blood flow and reactive hyperemia.

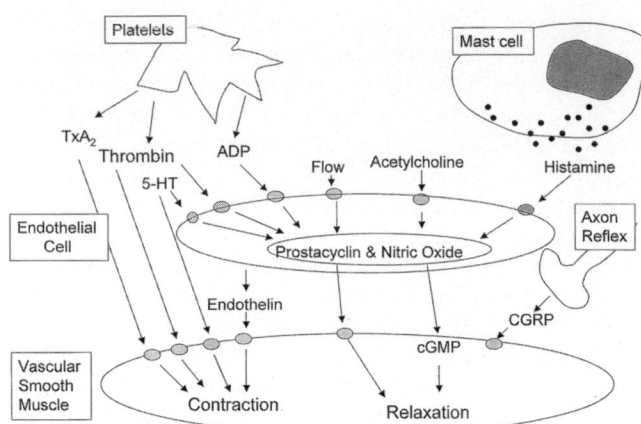

FIGURE 9.3. Paracrine regulation of blood flow results from mediators released from blood elements and endothelial cells. Platelets release thromboxane A_2, thrombin, and serotonin that, in the absence of intact endothelium, cause contraction of the underlying vascular smooth muscle. Thrombin, serotonin, and ADP cause release of nitric oxide and/or prostacyclin from endothelial cells, which results in vascular smooth muscle relaxation. Thus, activated platelets cause vasoconstriction only in the presence of locally disrupted endothelium. Histamine released from mast cells also causes vasodilatation via endothelial cells. Two elements of local control that are not paracrine are flow-induced vasodilatation and vasodilators released from collaterals of axons mediating nociception.

activated cation channels that carry Ca^{++} and initiate contraction (10). Stretch also activates signaling pathways involving phospholipase C and protein kinase C (11).

Paracrine regulation refers to the local release of chemical mediators that cause vasodilatation or vasoconstriction. Only a small fraction of these mediators will be mentioned. Many paracrines have effects on smooth muscle growth and/or apoptosis (in addition to their effects on tone), but only effects on tone will be considered here. Endothelial cells and platelets release mediators that influence vascular smooth muscle tone (12). In a number of cases, endothelial cells modify the effects of substances released from platelets. Serotonin, ADP, and thrombin released from platelets cause vascular smooth muscle relaxation in the presence of endothelium. But these agents act directly on vascular smooth muscle to cause contraction. Perhaps the most significant interaction is between thromboxane A_2 (TxA_2) and prostacyclin (PGI_2). Platelets release TxA_2, a vasoconstrictor, and this effect predominates when the endothelial layer of the blood vessel is damaged. However, normal endothelium releases PGI_2, a vasodilator, and it has the dominant effect in normal blood vessels (13).

Figure 9.3 shows two other phenomena that are not strictly paracrine, but are of significance. Flow-induced dilation (14) plays an important role in producing high flows in the heart during metabolic hyperemia. The axon reflex is also shown in this figure and will be described in the discussion of skin blood flow (15).

ELEMENTS OF LOCAL CONTROL OF BLOOD FLOW

The three mechanisms described above underlie in varying degrees four elements of local control of blood flow: active hyperemia (metabolic and paracrine regulation), reactive hyperemia (metabolic, myogenic, and paracrine regulation), autoregulation (metabolic and myogenic regulation), and the vascular response to injury (paracrine regulation).

Active hyperemia occurs when tissue metabolism is increased. This leads to release of vasodilator metabolites in proportion to the level of activity of the tissue. Paracrines such as prostaglandins are also released during increased metabolic activity, and as metabolic activity increases, so does tissue blood flow. In many tissues, including cardiac muscle, skeletal muscle, brain, and gut, there is a linear relationship between oxygen consumption and blood flow. In this way, oxygen supply, oxygen demand, and oxygen consumption are matched. The precise mix of metabolites and paracrines depends on the conditions of the increased metabolism, how well oxygen supply meets oxygen demand, and the tissue type.

Reactive hyperemia occurs when blood flow is stopped due to occlusion of the artery supplying the region. The occlusion can be caused by compression of the artery by external pressure or by thrombus formation in the lumen. In the case of reactive hyperemia, the time period of the occlusion is short enough so that, although there may be metabolic adjustments in the tissue in response to a lack of oxygen, there is no sustained cell injury or death. When the occlusion is removed, flow increases well above the level observed before the occlusion. It then returns to baseline with a time course dependent on the duration of the occlusion: the longer the occlusion, the longer the duration of the reactive hyperemia. The local vasodilatation responsible for reactive hyperemia is caused by three mechanisms: metabolic, paracrine, and myogenic regulation. When flow to the affected region is stopped and tissue PO_2 drops, vasodilator metabolites and paracrines are released. They accumulate in the tissue because there is no blood flow to wash them out. In time, they completely dilate the resistance vessels. The occlusion of the artery supplying a region of tissue lowers transmural pressure in the resistance vessels beyond the occlusion. This reduces stretch of the vascular smooth muscle and results in its relaxation. In general, the myogenic response dominates in occlusions of short duration when there is little time for the build-up of metabolites and paracrines. In longer occlusions, the paracrine and metabolic responses gain in importance.

Autoregulation of blood flow refers to the ability of tissues to maintain flow within a narrow range despite changes in arterial pressure. Most tissues including brain, heart, kidney, skin, and gut display autoregulation. Autoregulation depends on two mechanisms: metabolic and myogenic regulation. The reduction in flow accompanying a decrease in perfusion pressure allows the build-up of locally released metabolic vasodilators. These vasodilators decrease vascular resistance and restore flow. The converse happens when perfusion pressure is elevated. A fall in perfusion pressure also reduces transmural pressure in resistance vessels. The myogenic response leads to a reduction in vascular smooth muscle tone and a decrease in resistance to blood flow. Thus, both mechanisms tend to restore flow to its original level despite the reduction in perfusion pressure.

The vascular response to injury refers to the constellation of vascular changes after local tissue injury. In general, paracrines such as histamine, bradykinin, and prostanoids are released and cause dilatation of resistance and capacitance vessels as well as increased leakiness of exchange vessels to plasma proteins. The cutaneous circulation provides the prototypical vascular response to injury and this subject will be expanded in that context.

REGULATION OF BLOOD FLOW IN THE MYOCARDIUM

Coronary blood flow (16) is determined by the interactions of five factors: diastolic arterial pressure, myocardial compression, active hyperemia, endothelial function, and sympathetic nerve tone.

Because intramural vessels are compressed during cardiac contraction, perfusion of the myocardium is uniquely dependent on diastolic arterial pressure (17). The larger distributing coronary arteries run over the epicardial surface of the heart. Transmural branches penetrate the myocardium and deliver blood flow throughout the thickness of the wall. It is the transmural vessels and their branches within the myocardium that are subject to the compressive forces of each cardiac contraction. During systole, blood flow ceases in the myocardium near the subendocardium because myocardial compression completely closes the vessels supplying this region. Vessels supplying myocardium near the subepicardium are not occluded by cardiac contraction; therefore, this region has steady blood flow across the entire cardiac cycle. However, on the average, over the complete cardiac cycle, myocardial blood flow is as high or higher in the subendocardium. This is because very high flow during diastole balances the lack of flow during systole. The high flow during diastole can be viewed as reactive hyperemia in response to the cessation of flow with each systole. With stenosis of the distributing arteries on the surface of the heart (as occurs in coronary atherosclerosis), subendocardial flow is more threatened than subepicardial flow because more coronary reserve is used to provide adequate perfusion under normal conditions (see below).

Coronary flow stops at a diastolic arterial pressure well above zero. This is primarily because of the "waterfall" phenomenon (17). Coronary veins of the left ventricle are usually compressed by the relatively high tissue pressure that results from the ventricular cavity pressure present, even during diastole. Pressure upstream from the point of compression builds up until the vessels are forced open and flow proceeds to the coronary sinus. This is of consequence because the pressure head for an organ is the upstream (ordinarily mean arterial) pressure minus the downstream (ordinarily venous) pressure. We have already seen that in the case of the coronary bed, the upstream pressure is diastolic arterial pressure. The down stream pressure is just above tissue pressure, the pressure required to keep tissue pressure from collapsing coronary veins. Tissue pressure is close to diastolic ventricular cavity pressure. This number is ordinarily low compared with diastolic arterial pressure, and its effect can be ignored. However, in the presence of elevated diastolic pressure (as occurs with decreased diastolic ventricular compliance), the downstream pressure can become a significant factor in limiting coronary flow. This occurs, for example, with myocardial hypertrophy.

Active hyperemia (8,16) is the main determinant of coronary blood flow. Because three-fourths of arterial O_2 is extracted by the myocardium under resting conditions, significant increases in the requirement for O_2 must be served by higher blood flow. Physiologic increases in myocardial metabolism are almost always the result of increased sympathetic nerve activity to the heart. Depending on the circumstances, part of the increase in coronary blood flow may be provided by increased arterial (primarily diastolic) pressure. However, coronary arteriolar vasodilatation resulting

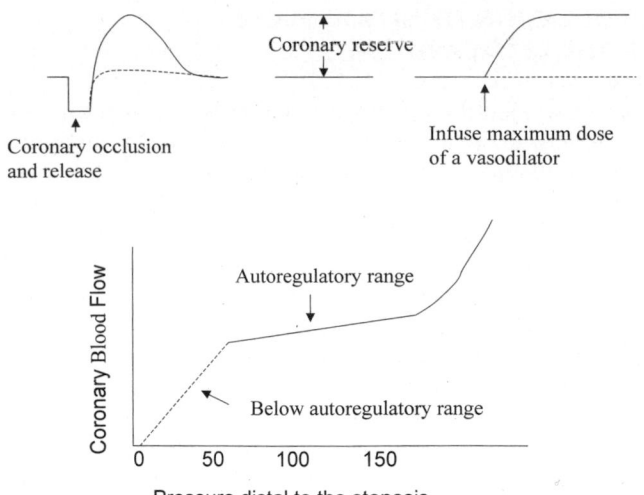

FIGURE 9.4. Coronary reserve refers to the ability of vessels downstream from a stenosis to dilate. It is manifested in the autoregulatory range by reactive hyperemia and/or increased flow in response to a vasodilator. Below the autoregulatory range, vessels downstream from a stenosis are completely dilated and so a vasodilator stimulus such as reactive hyperemia or a drug does not increase flow. Within the autoregulatory range, the magnitude of coronary reserve depends on how much downstream dilatation is necessary to compensate for an upstream stenosis; that is, more coronary reserve is found when the pressure distal to the stenosis is 100 mm Hg than when it is 75 mm Hg.

from release of vasoactive metabolites is usually required to provide adequate supply of O_2. In general, there is a linear relationship between coronary blood flow and myocardial metabolism. Flow-induced dilatation (see below) of epicardial-distributing arteries is necessary to maintain the full pressure gradient across the wall of the heart.

The concept of coronary reserve in the face of coronary artery stenosis is closely tied to active hyperemia and autoregulation (18). Stenosis of coronary arteries occurs in individuals with coronary atherosclerosis. Until a stenosis becomes quite severe, it has little or no effect on resting coronary blood flow. This is due to autoregulation of blood flow. Figure 9.4 shows coronary flow as a function of coronary perfusion pressure downstream from stenosis of a major epicardial coronary artery. The region of the curve where changes in pressure are accompanied by small changes in flow is the result of autoregulation. If the coronary circulation is within the autoregulatory range, reactive hyperemia can be elicited by briefly stopping flow. Furthermore, infusion of a vasodilator such as adenosine causes increased flow. Both of these responses require that the resistance vessels downstream from the stenosis are capable of dilating. The resistance vessels can respond to an added vasodilator stimulus to the extent that they are not maximally dilated to maintain resting flow in the face of an upstream stenosis. The remaining ability for resistance vessels to dilate in the face of an upstream stenosis is called coronary reserve. The magnitude of the increase in flow observed with reactive hyperemia or drug infusion gives an estimate of the coronary reserve.

If pressure distal to a stenosis falls below the autoregulatory range (Fig. 9.4), flow decreases in proportion to the drop in pressure. This is because the ability of the resistance vessels to

dilate (coronary reserve) has been completely exhausted. At this point, reactive hyperemia and increased flow in response to a vasodilator do not occur.

There is a third method for estimating coronary reserve. It can be observed by measuring the pressure drop across the stenosis during infusion of a vasodilator (18). This method relies on the assumption that the resistance across the stenosis does not change. In this situation, if increased flow occurs because of downstream resistance vessel dilatation, the pressure drop across the stenosis increases. If no change in the pressure drop across the stenosis is observed, the conclusion is that no increase in flow was possible and that coronary reserve is exhausted.

The issue of reduced flow caused by coronary stenosis is made more complex by the fact that if coronary flow is reduced, the myocardium quickly adjusts to this new situation. During a period of reduced flow that results in a reduced oxygen supply relative to myocardial demand, a rapid decrease in myocardial contractility is found in the region served by the reduced flow. After one or more periods of reduced oxygen supply relative to demand, myocardial contractility may be reduced for minutes to hours, despite a return to normal resting coronary blood flow. This is called myocardial stunning (19). The reduction(s) in the supply/demand ratio that causes myocardial stunning may be the result of either periods of reduced coronary blood flow or increased myocardial oxygen consumption. The cause of myocardial stunning appears to involve the liberation of oxygen free radicals and a decrease in the sensitivity of the contractile machinery to calcium ions (20).

After repeated bouts of myocardial stunning or after a sustained period of suboptimal blood flow, a chronic depression in myocardial contractility may ensue. This is called hibernation (19,21,22), and it is not the result of infarction of myocardium. At first, during *functional hibernation,* the causes may be similar to those of stunning. Hibernation of a more severe and/or longer nature is referred to as *structural hibernation* and involves rarefaction of contractile proteins, reduced mitochondria, and other later changes, including apoptosis. If normal flow is restored by coronary artery bypass or angioplasty, hibernating myocardium can return to normal function (23).

The myocardium is protected from stunning, hibernation, and infarction by previous short bouts of ischemia. This is called ischemic preconditioning (24). Ischemic preconditioning occurs in many organs, including brain, lung, liver, and skeletal muscle. Although there appear to be multiple mechanisms responsible for preconditioning, adenosine seems to play a central role.

Coronary endothelial cells are important in the regulation of coronary blood flow. The full development of active hyperemia is dependent on normal endothelial cell function. The primary event causing increased coronary blood flow during active hyperemia is dilatation of arterioles by local metabolites and paracrines. However, if the epicardial-distributing arteries do not participate in this dilatation, there is an increased pressure drop along their length. This means that the pressure available to drive blood flow across the wall through transmural coronary arteries is decreased and happens when endothelial communication with vascular smooth muscle is curtailed by atherosclerosis, hypertension, and other conditions. If the coronary endothelium is normal, increased flow velocity in distributing arteries causes release of nitric oxide from endothelial cells. Nitric oxide diffuses to vascular smooth muscle where it causes relaxation by elevating smooth muscle cyclic guanylic acid (GMP). The resulting increase in diameter of distributing arteries is sufficient to minimize the drop in pressure that would otherwise accompany the increased flow associated with active hyperemia (25).

Coronary endothelium also plays an important role in protecting vascular smooth muscle from the constrictor effects of a number of agonists in the blood. These include platelet-derived serotonin and thrombin (12,26). Coronary artery spasm is thought to occur in the absence of the normal vasodilator influences of nitric oxide, prostacyclin, and perhaps other substances that are released from normal endothelium.

Stimulation of the sympathetic nerves to the heart has two competing effects. Norepinephrine released from sympathetic nerves acts on α_1-adrenergic receptors to cause increased heart rate and contractility; these effects increase myocardial metabolism and result in active hyperemia. Norepinephrine also acts on β_1-adrenergic receptors to cause contraction of coronary smooth muscle. The net effect of these opposing effects of sympathetic nerve stimulation is to raise coronary blood flow in proportion to the increase in myocardial oxygen consumption. Coronary blood flow increases almost as much as it does in the absence of the α_1-adrenergic–mediated coronary constrictive effect (16).

REGULATION OF SKIN BLOOD FLOW

Skin has a low metabolic rate; therefore, its nutrient requirements are ordinarily met unless severe pathologic reductions in blood flow occur. For the most part, changes in skin blood flow are unrelated to changes in local metabolism. Skin blood vessels demonstrate impressive reactive hyperemia. This is evidenced by the erythema and increase in surface temperature that is commonly seen after a period of external compression.

Skin temperature both influences and is influenced by blood flow. Skin is crucial in the elimination of heat from the body by radiation, convection, and evaporation. As core body temperature increases, cutaneous blood flow rises (27,28). This is a result of at least two events (29); the first is withdrawal of sympathetic vasoconstrictor tone, and the second is release of a vasodilator from the sympathetic cholinergic nerve endings that stimulate sweat glands. The vasodilator has not been identified. A third possibility is that the bradykinin released from active sweat glands causes increased skin blood flow during sweating. The evidence currently available indicates that bradykinin may play a role, but it is not necessary to achieve maximum skin blood flow during body heating.

Local skin temperature also influences skin blood flow (30). At a given core temperature, placing skin in a warmer local temperature raises blood flow. This is because increased local temperature reduces sensitivity of cutaneous vessels to norepinephrine. At extremely high or low temperatures, other mechanisms come into play. At local temperatures over 45°C, the vascular response to injury occurs (see below). At local temperatures below 10°C, the phenomenon of cold vasodilatation is observed. At this temperature, vascular smooth muscle contraction fails and cutaneous vessels dilate; however, the increased blood flow warms the smooth muscle and it then contracts. Once it contracts, blood flow decreases and the temperature of the vascular smooth muscle drops again. The smooth muscle fails to contract and blood flow increases. This establishes periodic oscillations in skin blood flow.

The cutaneous response to injury (Fig. 9.5) is observed in response to many stimuli ranging from mechanical and thermal damage, to insect bites, to allergic reactions (31). With mechanical injury, a red line appears at the site of the insult. This is the result of local release of a number of vasodilators, including histamine, bradykinin, prostaglandins, and nitric oxide, all of which increase the filling of the subcutaneous venous plexus causing a

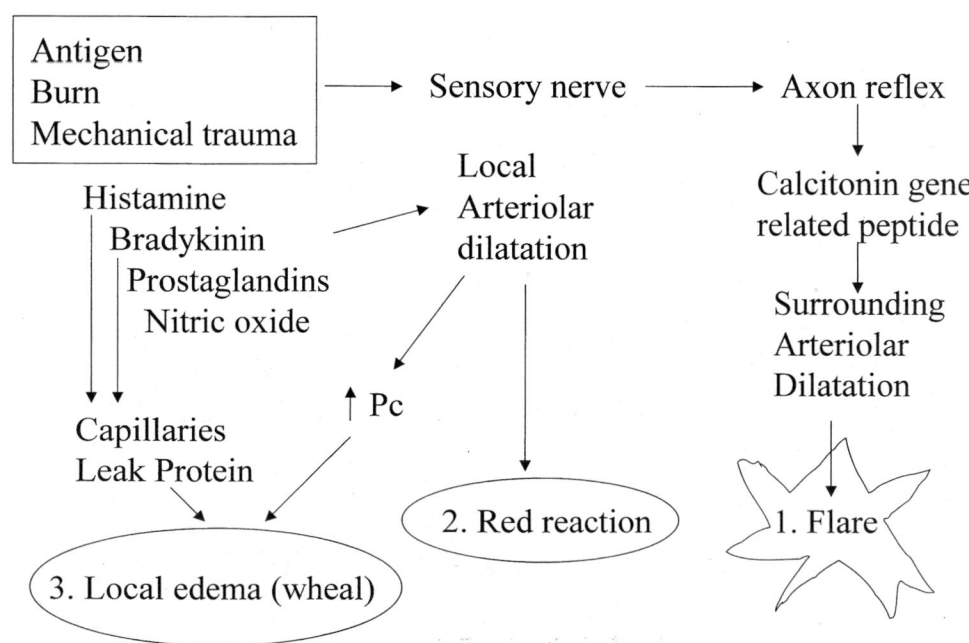

FIGURE 9.5. The cutaneous response to injury consists of three elements. Local dilatation at the site of the injury (red reaction) results from local release of a number of vasodilators, including histamine, bradykinin, prostaglandins, and nitric oxide. Edema results from a combination of increased transport of proteins across the capillary wall stimulated by histamine and bradykinin, and increased capillary hydrostatic pressure resulting from arteriolar dilatation. Collaterals of nociceptive C fibers that release calcitonin gene-related peptide and other vasodilators cause the flare around an injury.

red line. A nociceptive stimulus also activates pain fibers that give off collaterals that innervate the region near the sensory nerve endings (32). These collaterals arise directly from the sensory nerve axon without passing through a synapse. When the nerves are activated, they release a number of peptides, including substance-P and calcitonin gene-related peptide (CGRP) from the collaterals. This is called an *axon reflex.* CGRP causes dilatation around the injury: *a flare.* Finally, the combination of increased microvascular transport of plasma protein and increased capillary hydrostatic pressure causes local edema formation: *a wheal.* The increased transport of plasma proteins into the interstitial space is caused by substance-P, histamine, and bradykinin. The increase capillary hydrostatic pressure is caused by the vasodilators mentioned above.

SUMMARY

Tissue respiration is matched to the cellular requirements for ATP. In cardiac muscle, the regulation of the synthesis of ATP appears to be linked to the major cytosolic signal responsible the level of contractile activity, calcium ions. This links the use of ATP by contractile machinery to the supply of ATP by the mitochondria. The ability of the mitochondrion to supply ATP is dependent on the circulatory supply of O_2 and substrates. This is largely a matter of adjustment of blood flow to the active tissue by local mechanisms. Local mechanisms responsible for regulation of blood flow can be divided into three categories: metabolic, myogenic, and paracrine regulation. These basic mechanisms account for active hyperemia, reactive hyperemia, autoregulation of blood flow, and the vascular response to injury.

Coronary blood flow provides an excellent example of a tissue in which local regulation of blood flow is primarily concerned with matching oxygen supply to the demand created by oxidative phosphorylation. The heart also provides an illustration of the interaction between blood supply and function through consideration of myocardial stunning, hibernation, and preconditioning.

Skin blood flow is a counter example in which matching of metabolism and blood flow is not usually of great significance. Instead, regulation of skin blood flow is primarily concerned with temperature regulation and the local response to injury.

REFERENCES

1. Boyer PD. The ATP synthase—a splendid molecular machine. *Annu Rev Biochem.* 1997;66:717–749.
2. Korzeniewski B. Regulation of ATP supply in mammalian skeletal muscle during resting state to intensive work transition. *Biophys Chem.* 2000;83:19–34.
3. Sahlin K, Tonkonogi M, Soderlund K. Energy supply and muscle fatigue in humans. *Acta Physiol Scand.* 1998;162(3):261–266.
4. Hardie DG. Metabolic control: a new solution to an old problem. *Curr Biol.* 2000;10:R757–R759.
5. Chance B, Williams G. Respiratory enzymes in oxidative phosphorylation: I. Kinetics of oxygen utilization. *J Biol Chem.* 1955;217:383–393.
6. Moreno-Sanchez R, Hogue BA, Hansford RG. Influence of NAD-linked dehydrogenase activity on flux through oxidative phosphorylation. *Biochem J.* 1990;268:421–428.
7. Territo PR, Mootha VK, French SA, et al. Ca2+ activation of heart mitochondrial oxidative phosphorylation: role of the F0/F1-ATPase. *Am J Physiol Cell Physiol.* 2000;278:C423–C435.
8. Laughlin MH, Korthuis RJ, Duncker DJ, et al. Control of blood flow to cardiac and skeletal muscle during exercise. In: Rowell LB, Shepherd JT. *Handbook of Physiology Section 12: Exercise: Regulation and Integration of Multiple Systems.* New York, NY: Oxford University Press; 1996.
9. Davis MJ, Hill MA. Signaling mechanisms underlying the vascular myogenic response. *Physiol Rev.* 1999;79:387–423.
10. Jackson WF. Ion channels and vascular tone. *Hypertension.* 2000;35:173–178.
11. Bakker EN, Kerkhof CJ, Sipkema P. Signal transduction in spontaneous myogenic tone in isolated arterioles from rat skeletal muscle. *Cardiovasc Res.* 1999;41(1):229–236.
12. Vanhoutte PM. Endothelial dysfunction and inhibition of converting enzyme. *Eur Heart J.* 1998; Suppl J:J7–J15.
13. Ware JA, Heistad DD. Platelet-endothelium interactions. *N Engl J Med.* 1993;328:628–635.
14. Bevan JA. Shear stress, the endothelium and the balance between flow-induced contraction and dilation in animals and man. *Int J Microcirc Clin Exp.* 1997;17:248–256.
15. Owman C. Peptidergic vasodilator nerves in the peripheral circulation and in the vascular beds of the heart and brain. *Blood Vessels.* 1990;27:73–93.
16. Feigl EO. Coronary physiology. *Physiol Rev.* 1983;63:1–205.
17. Downey JM. Extravascular coronary resistance. In: Sperelakis N, ed. *Physiology and Pathophysiology of the Heart,* 2nd ed. Boston, MA: Kluwer Academic Publishers; 1989.
18. Pijls NH, De Bruyne B. Coronary pressure measurement and fractional flow reserve. *Heart.* 1998;80:539–542.
19. Camici PG, Dutka DP. Repetitive stunning, hibernation, and heart failure: contribution of PET to establishing a link. *Am J Physiol Heart Circ Physiol.* 2001;280(3):H929–H936.
20. Bolli R, Marban E. Molecular and cellular mechanisms of myocardial stunning. *Physiol Rev.* 1999;79(2):609–634.
21. Canty Jr. JM, Fallavollita JA. Chronic hibernation and chronic stunning: a continuum. *J Nucl Cardiol.* 2000;7(5):509–527.
22. Heusch G, Schulz R. The biology of myocardial hibernation. *Trends Cardiovasc Med.* 2000;10(3):108–114.
23. Rahimtoola SH. Concept and evaluation of hibernating myocardium. *Annu Rev Med.* 1999;50:75–86.
24. Ferrari R, Ceconi C, Curello S, et al. Ischemic preconditioning, myocardial stunning, and hibernation: basic aspects. *Am Heart J.* 1999;138:S61–S68.
25. Sparks HV, Wangler RD, Gorman MW. Control of the coronary circulation. In: Sperelakis N, ed. *Physiology and Pathophysiology of the Heart,* 2nd ed. Boston, MA: Kluwer Academic Publishers; 1989.
26. Fleming I, Busse R. NO: the primary EDRF. *J Mol Cell Cardiol.* 1999;31:5–14.
27. Rowell LB. *Human Circulation Regulation during Physical Stress.* New York, NY: Oxford University Press; 1986:177–178.
28. Rowell LB. *Human Cardiovascular Control.* New York, NY: Oxford University Press; 1993.
29. Joyner MJ, Halliwill JR. Sympathetic vasodilatation in human limbs. *J Physiol.* 2000;526(Pt 3):471–480.
30. Minson CT, Berry LT, Joyner MJ. Nitric oxide and neurally mediated regulation of skin blood flow during local heating. *J Appl Physiol.* 2001;91(4):1619–1626.
31. Borici-Mazi R, Kouridakis S, Kontou-Fili K. Cutaneous responses to substance P and calcitonin gene–related peptide in chronic urticaria: the effect of cetirizine and dimethindene. *Allergy.* 1999;54:46–56.
32. Sann H, Pierau FK. Efferent functions of C-fiber nociceptors *Z Rheumatol.* 1998;57(Suppl 2):8–13.

MICROBIOLOGIC CONSIDERATIONS AND INFECTIOUS DISEASES

LAURITZ A. JENSEN
JAMES B. JENSEN

KEY CONCEPTS

- Global and national significance of microbial diseases in terms of morbidity and mortality
- Germ theory of disease and its credence in osteopathic medicine
- Limitations of the germ theory of disease
- Microbial virulence and pathogenicity
- Structural and physiologic barriers and defenses; nonspecific and specific immunologic mechanisms
- Positive nutritional status and its role in tempering the immune response
- Therapeutic and antimicrobial considerations
- Vaccinations and other preventive measures to control infectious diseases

Life expectancy in the United States has increased significantly during the past century, from 47 years in 1900 to nearly 77 years (both sexes) in 2000. This tremendous improvement is due in part to a marked drop in the impact of infectious diseases. Four principal factors responsible for this dramatic betterment of the quality of human life are improved nutrition, improved personal and community hygiene, the development of antibiotics, and the development of vaccines. This chapter will discuss the role infectious diseases play on human morbidity and mortality and the impact of these four factors on the improvement of the human condition.

HAS THE WAR AGAINST INFECTIOUS DISEASE INDEED BEEN WON?

During the early days of the 20th century, Americans were terrified of infectious diseases, mainly because they did not understand how to prevent "catching" them and understood even less about how to "cure" them. The influenza A outbreak that emerged at the close of World War I is perhaps the supreme example of just how devastating and feared a disease could be. The

Spanish flu—so named because it was first reported in the Spanish newspapers—engulfed Europe within a few months, overwhelming public health services and killing millions of people who were otherwise healthy and in the prime of their lives. When General Pershing's troops returned home to America, they brought this influenza virus with them. Although Americans may have fared better than much of the affected world, the death toll was still staggering. Approximately 675,000 died (1), and more than 25% of the country suffered intense illness. Because this strain of virus was so lethal, many people died within 48 hours of onset of symptoms. At its height, thousands perished each week, prompting health officials to close public schools and forbid people from attending church services or theaters. Worldwide, between 20 and 40 million lost their lives (2).

The history of infectious diseases contains many grim tales, but medicine has come a long way since those early years of the 20th century. Just 51 years following the devastating pandemic of influenza, the United States Surgeon General, William H. Stewart, enthusiastically proclaimed that the war against microbes had been won and that it was time to "close the book on infectious diseases."

In 1969, this point of view seemed reasonable. Antibiotics could knock out almost any bacterial infection, smallpox had been eradicated in most regions of the world, the risk of tuberculosis (TB) was presumed to be in decline, and poliomyelitis and other scourges of children were being effectively controlled by hard-hitting immunization programs. In retrospect, however, Stewart was a bit optimistic. The rise of antibiotic resistance and the overflow of Third World disease problems into the United States—not to mention the emergence of new diseases and the reemergence of previously controlled diseases—were looming on the horizon. Physicians were about to be faced with many new and somewhat ominous challenges.

Worldwide Importance

Globally, microbial or infectious diseases are more destructive than malignancies or cardiovascular disease. One-third of the world is infected with the tubercle bacillus, and TB kills at least 2 million annually (3). In 2001, the Centers for Disease Control

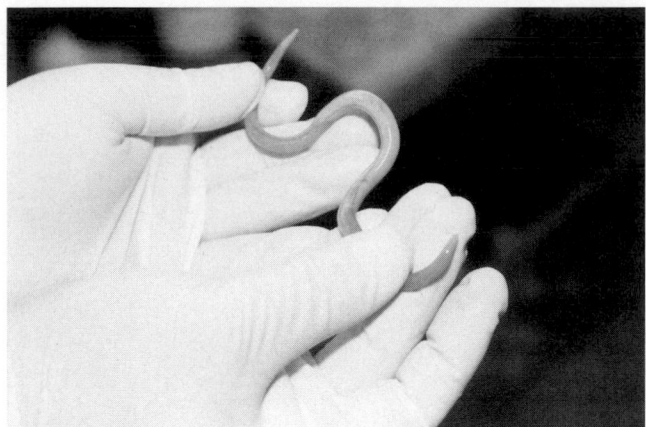

FIGURE 10.1. Ascarid worm passed by a Guatemalan child. (Photo courtesy of L.D. Goldsmith.)

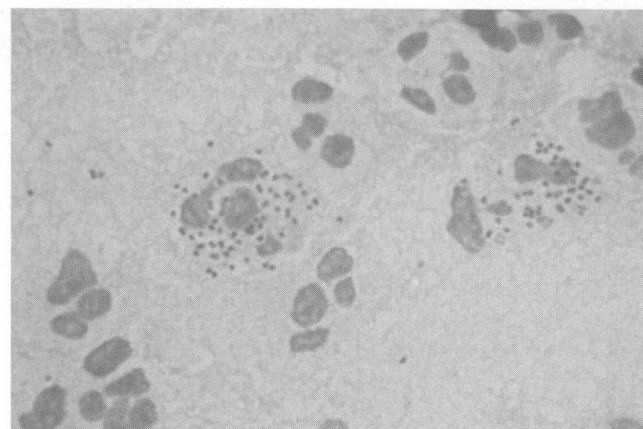

FIGURE 10.2. Positive Gram stain from a male patient with gonorrhea. (Photo by L.A. Jensen.)

and Prevention (CDC) reported that an estimated 36 million people are afflicted with the human immunodeficiency virus (HIV) (4). We are losing more people to malaria each year than we were 30 years ago; five children die of malaria in the world every minute. In Africa, this computes to the death of 1 million children each year (5). Surely these figures are conservative estimates. One of us (JBJ) has spent 18 years working on malaria in remote African villages and has personally witnessed hundreds of malaria deaths in children who were buried within an hour of passing. None of these deaths were ever reported. Worldwide, 2 billion people are infected with *Ascaris* (Fig. 10.1), another 1.3 billion with whipworm and hookworms, 120 million with lymphatic filariasis, and 200 million with schistosomes (6). What these data do not reflect is the toll these infections extract in human well being, creative energy, and vitality (7).

National Importance

In the United States, infectious diseases pose a real threat to people of all age groups. Each year, 2 to 3 million cases of community-acquired pneumonia—*Streptococcus pneumoniae* being the usual agent—are identified. Approximately 110,000 Americans are hospitalized annually because of influenza or influenza-related complications. Sadly, about 20,000 of these people will die (8). Older Americans are particularly vulnerable, as microbes account for one-third of all deaths (9). Strep throat, although ordinarily not as debilitating as pneumonia and mostly involving children or young adults, ranks third on the list of common complaints to the office-based physician (10). Probably 6 million Americans have periodontal disease—not usually thought of as an infectious disease—but because of its polymicrobial etiology, it is rightfully placed in this category. Recent studies have even shown a positive connection between unhealthy dentition and cardiovascular disease (11). The number of cases of sexually transmitted disease (STD) reported nationally is not only striking, but seems to be increasing. Surveillance data in recent years indicate that at least 15 million STD infections occur annually, with genital warts, genital herpes, gonorrhea (Fig. 10.2), chlamydia, and trichomoniasis being commonly reported in young, sexually active Americans (12).

Other microbial diseases of significance included in the year-to-date or cumulative reports are hepatitis A, legionellosis, Lyme disease (Fig. 10.3), hemorrhagic *Escherichia coli* infections, invasive *Haemophilus influenzae,* meningococcal disease, and pertussis. Outbreaks of Norwalk-like virus account for 23 million cases of gastroenteritis each year (13). Furthermore, foodborne bacterial pathogens, including *Campylobacter* and gram-negative enterobacterial organisms, produce an estimated 13.8 million cases of gastrointestinal (GI) disease annually (14). *Giardia,* the most commonly detected intestinal protozoan parasite in the United States, is responsible for up to 2.5 million cases of diarrhea each year—a prevalence equal to that of *Salmonella* and *Shigella* combined (15). Not only do treatable infectious diseases present substantial health challenges by themselves, but the emergence of antibiotic-resistant organisms, such as methicillin-resistant *Staphylococcus aureus* (16), vancomycin-resistant enterococci (17), multidrug-resistant strains of *Streptococcus pneumoniae* (18), and *Mycobacterium tuberculosis* (19), threaten to overturn years of progress in antimicrobial therapy. Moreover, genetically engineered antibiotic-resistant bacteria, if intentionally released as biological warfare agents—similar to the anthrax-laced letters that resulted in the contamination of U.S. government buildings,

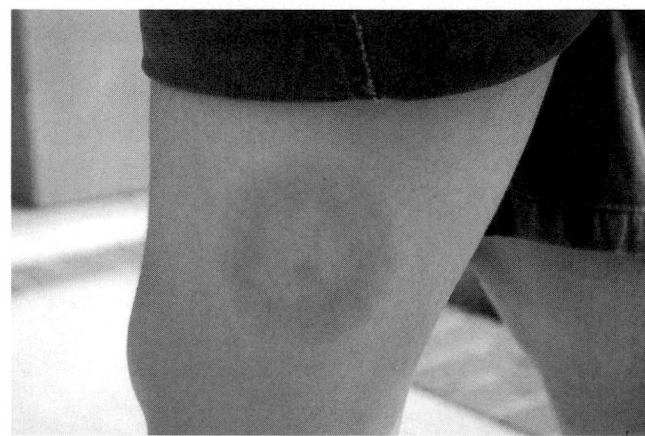

FIGURE 10.3. Lyme disease from a patient in the Midwestern United States. (Photo by L.A. Jensen.)

media offices, and postal facilities in the fall of 2001, could have catastrophic consequences. In addition to these old and familiar infectious scourges, we face fresh enemies in that more than 22 newly recognized diseases that have emerged since 1973, including acquired immunodeficiency syndrome (AIDS), rotavirus infections, Ebola virus, Lyme disease, Hantaan virus infections, and others (20). And so it goes. A century ago, Americans were terrified of infectious disease. Today bacteria, viruses, and parasites are still making us sick—even killing us—and infectious disease specialists are not sanguine about the future. Indeed, as one scientist remarked: "The war has been won . . . by the other side" (21).

GERM THEORY OF DISEASE: KOCH'S POSTULATES AND THEIR LIMITATIONS

The Origin and Early History

The German physician Robert Koch changed forever the way we look at communicable diseases by his elegant demonstration in 1876 that the endospore-forming bacterium *Bacillus anthracis* was the etiologic agent of splenic fever, otherwise known as anthrax. His 1882 paper to the Berlin Physiological Society is universally considered by microbiologists as a signature moment in medical science and the cornerstone of the germ theory of disease, although many scientists laid the foundation for Koch's seminal studies. The thought process likely began with the German anatomist Jacob Henle, Koch's mentor. It was Henle who put forth the idea of a "parasite" or contagium as the inducer of certain diseases (i.e., disease communicability). But Henle did not know how to prove this. It was Koch's genius to develop methods of pure culture so that only one species of bacterium at a time could be examined for its ability to induce disease. In 1884, Koch outlined his methods as a series of rules—later to be called Koch's postulates—that he developed during his studies on the etiology of tuberculosis. In fact, within 20 years of the publication of Koch's classic papers, the agents of most of the major bacterial diseases were discovered by carefully following his postulates (22,23). Along with the French bacteriologist Louis Pasteur, Koch is recognized as the co-founder of medical microbiology (24). Although some of Koch's postulates cannot be applied experimentally (these exceptions will be discussed subsequently), they represent the keystone in the history of infectious diseases. These postulates are succinctly stated in the 1890 paper given at another scientific forum—the Tenth International Congress of Medicine. The translation that follows is by T.M. Rivers (25):

> However, if it can be proved: first that the parasite occurs in every case of the disease in question, and under circumstances which can account for the pathological changes and clinical course of the disease; secondly, that it occurs in no other disease as a fortuitous and nonpathogenic parasite; and thirdly, that if, after being fully isolated from the body and repeatedly grown in pure culture, can induce the disease anew; then the occurrence of the parasite in the disease can no longer be accidental, but in this case no other relation between it and the disease except that the parasite is the cause of the disease can be considered.

A fourth condition dealing with reisolating the parasite (microorganism) from the experimental infection was eventually

added, which only strengthened belief in Koch's blueprint of causality.

Undoubtedly, Koch's research on anthrax, published in 1876, kindled his interest in defining a standard for disease causation. It is possible that anthrax transmission as the paragon for the germ theory may have been one of the reasons why the medical community in the U.S. initially fought against the premise. Even in the 1800s, anthrax was a disease primarily of domestic animals. It seemed to have little relevance to the U.S. physician. Koch's work on the tubercle bacillus was somewhat more compelling but only because of its diagnostic value. No useful therapy to effectively combat tuberculosis existed in those days, and furthermore, the newly developed isolation and culture techniques in clinical bacteriology had no practical application in the art of healing for the average practitioner. In his historical vignette on medicine in the United States, King gives a clear account of the circumstances and prevailing medical beliefs (e.g., miasmatic-contagious origin of disease, attitudes of physicians) of the era (26).

Osteopathy and the Germ Theory of Disease

In the first decade of the 20th century, osteopathic physicians gradually recognized microorganisms as potential causative agents for various diseases. In 1906, McConnell and Teall espoused strong views on good hygiene and sanitary practices (27). To their credit, they confessed that the germ theory was a correct principle, plainly acknowledging that a bacillus was the "exciting cause" of typhoid fever. Other diseases like scarlet fever, diphtheria, and malaria also were believed to have direct microbial links, but usually microorganisms were considered to be of secondary importance only. Viral diseases were obviously ill-defined, being impossible to identify in that era. Hulett, in 1903, had a similar view (28):

> These [Pasteur, Klebs, and Koch], with others, placed the theory upon fairly sure ground in showing by methods to which no objections could be raised that in certain cases there is such a definite relationship between the pathologic condition and the presence of the microorganism. *The question is not yet entirely settled as to the nature of that relation. Is the disease as it exists responsible for the presence of the micro-organism or do the bacteria produce the pathologic condition?* [The italics are the author's.]

He further suggested that because the healthy person often harbors "so-called" pathogenic bacteria, their presence in the sick patient may not be sufficient proof of a causal relationship but merely an incidental finding (28). The limitations with regards to causality were quite apparent in Hulett's day.

Health care professionals still have many of the same questions a century later. Is merely bringing the host and the microbe together sufficient to cause disease or are there other issues that should be factored into the equation to answer the question? Perhaps certain strains of microbes are less virulent and require a larger infective dose to produce infection and illness. Host–parasite relationships and innate abilities to resist active disease likely produce the carrier state or result in subclinical infections. And what about adaptive immune responses? It is clear that disease results from complex interactions between pathogens and their hosts, and many such interactions, remain ill-defined even today.

Constraints of the Germ Theory of Disease When Attempting to Show Causality

In many respects, the basic premise of "cause and effect" is viewed as a working theory; hence, it is constantly being refined. With this in mind, Fredricks and Relman (29) point out some obvious encumbrances with Koch's postulates. Sometimes all the postulates cannot possibly be fulfilled. For example, chlamydiae, rickettsiae, viruses, and many eukaryotic parasites do not grow in pure culture, but require elaborate cell culture and similar techniques for successful *in vitro* propagation. Furthermore, pathogenic strains of the syphilis spirochete cannot be indefinitely transferred in conventional media or in tissue culture. Polymicrobial causation is even more perplexing. Hepatitis D virus cannot complete its life cycle and produce disease unless it coexists with hepatitis B. Often, bacteria will secrete exotoxins, whose site of cellular or tissue damage is located far from the site of bacterial colonization. The historical example of this is diphtheria, where the bacteria colonize only the nasopharynx, but the disease results in notable damage to the heart, kidney, and tissues of the central nervous system. Moreover, staphylococcal food poisoning and *Aspergillus* aflatoxicosis are not infections at all, but are diseases due to the ingestion of toxins produced in foods. As such, they are classified as intoxications, and one would not find the causative organism in the body of the host during the clinical presentation. Finally, using genotype-based microbial identification, such as hybridization and amplification (PCR or polymerase chain reaction) technology, a high degree of sensitivity and specificity and can provide persuasive evidence of a cause-and-effect association sufficient for a laboratory diagnosis without the specific identification of the actual organism. Thus, it can be seen that Koch's postulates are not totally satisfied when identifying microorganisms that may be the cause of disease. In summary, Fredricks and Relman state it this way: "A microbe that fulfills Koch's postulates is most likely the cause of the disease in question. A microbe that fails to fulfill Koch's postulates may still represent the etiologic agent of disease or may be a simple commensal" (29).

So, what makes one microorganism a fierce pathogen while a closely related strain of the same species is nothing more than a harmless commensal? The short answer, at least from the perspective of the microbe, is the acquisition and phenotypic expression of one or more virulence factors.

VIRULENCE AND PATHOGENICITY: MICROBIAL WEAPONRY AND WARFARE AT THE CELLULAR LEVEL

Attributes of the Microbe That Contribute to Disease

What constitutes a pathogen has been an issue that microbiologists have wrestled with for more than a century. Before this question can be answered, basic definitions for terms like pathogenicity, virulence, and virulence factors must be explained. Classically defined, these terms focus only on the microbe. Furthermore, pathogen refers to a microbe that is capable of producing disease, pathogenicity as the microbe's capacity to cause infection or disease, and a virulence factor as a microbial component that

contributes to pathogenicity (30). Recently, however, Casadevall and Pirofski refined the overall concept of pathogenicity, along with subordinate terms. Accordingly, a pathogen is a microorganism that damages a host directly or as a result of an immunologic response, and pathogenicity refers to the organism's ability to cause damage to host cells. Virulence pertains to the relative capacity of a microorganism to damage the host, and a virulence factor is a bacterial component that damages the host (31). These new definitions are not microbe centered as such, but reflect a combined effort of both the pathogen and host to produce a disease state. In other words, disease is a multifactorial process. To ignore the complexity of the human host by focusing solely on the pathogen produces an incomplete picture of the disease. Fortunately, these definitions also take into account the variant nature of host–pathogen interactions (e.g., opportunistic pathogens producing disease in the immunodeficient host, degree of host specificity by the pathogen, specificity of tissue involved).

Host Peculiarities and Disease

Sometimes, a classic pathogen like *Salmonella* produces overt disease in one person but is asymptomatic in another. Subclinical infections are always a concern since they serve as reservoirs for the spread of pathogens to others, whose infections are likely to be symptomatic. Typhoid Mary (Fig. 10.4), a somewhat pejorative nickname given to an immigrant Irish cook in New York City, represents the classic example of the carrier state. Although Mary Mallon, her real name, never presented with symptoms (at least denied ever being ill), she repeatedly tested positive for *Salmonella* (32). Over the course of her career as a cook, she infected 47 people with typhoid fever, three of whom died (33). But the point is this: harboring the microbe does not necessarily mean that the person will present with overt disease. The complexities of the host–pathogen interaction including genetic makeup, variations in physiology, and innate and adaptive immunity, all must be considered—and not all of these factors are well understood.

Some persons are genetically predisposed to resist specific infections. In the case of falciparum malaria, sickle cell heterozygotes typically have low parasite counts in the bloodstream. A single amino acid substitution (valine in place of glutamic acid)

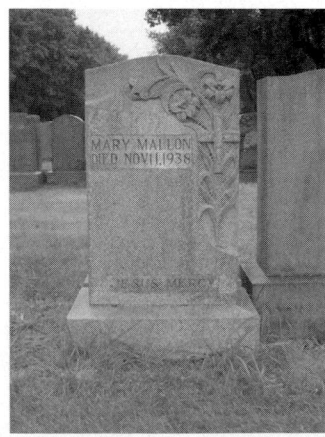

FIGURE 10.4. Grave of Typhoid Mary, Bronx, N.Y. (Photo by L.A. Jensen.)

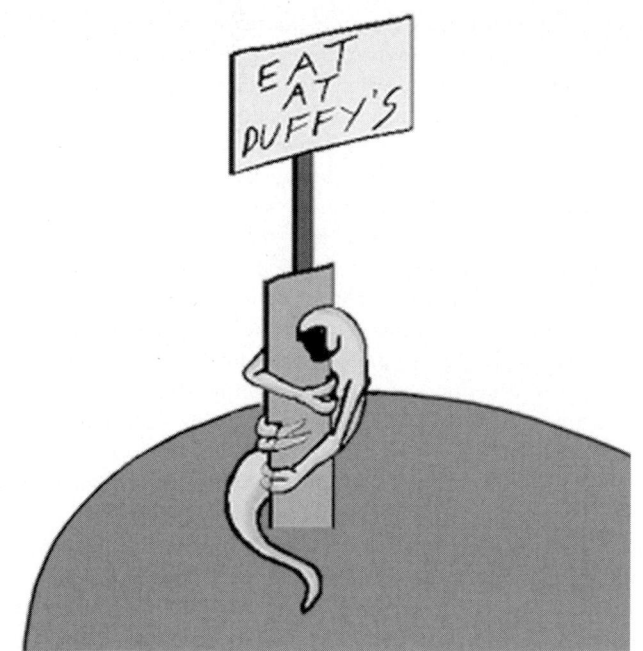

FIGURE 10.5. Eat at Duffy's cartoon. (Illustration by K.L. Rhodes, DO.)

in the β-polypeptide chain of hemoglobin accounts for the difference. People with the homozygous condition usually die early in adulthood, but a heterozygous genome provides protection for individuals living in areas where malaria is prevalent. The pathologic mechanism is still unclear; it has been suggested that sickling encourages increased destruction of parasitized erythrocytes by the reticuloendothelial system or it may be that the reduced oxygen blood levels are deleterious to the *Plasmodium* parasite. Regardless of the exact mechanism, people of African heritage are more likely to carry this abnormal gene, and as such, have a selective advantage against the lethal form of malaria (34).

Another form of inherited resistance to malaria, specifically to *Plasmodium vivax,* is centered around a cytokine receptor on the erythrocyte. The site is referred to as the Duffy antigen or glycoprotein (named after a patient who received transfusion for hemolysis in 1950), which normally serves as the receptor for proinflammatory cytokines (e.g., interleukin-8). But, it also functions as the merozoite receptor in *P. vivax* infections (Fig. 10.5), so erythrocytic cells that are Duffy negative are less likely to carry the parasite. Since West Africans lack this antigen, they ordinarily are resistant to vivax malaria (35).

Specific Examples of How Microorganisms Make Us Sick

In order for microorganisms to cause disease they must penetrate the host's natural barriers (skin, mucous membranes, etc.), then colonize the tissues—generally by specific attachments—and eventually begin to reproduce (36). To accomplish this they must also avoid the host's immune response. Pathogenic organisms have developed an astonishing array of molecules to assist them with cellular penetration, colonization, and immune avoidance. If, as is often the case, such molecules are injurious to the host or augment colonization, they are called virulence

factors (sometimes referred to as virulence determinants, traits, or mechanisms). An ordinary characteristic involved with some housekeeping chores, like the fermentation of glucose, is not generally classified as a virulence factor (30). Again, virulence factors are linked to the microbe's capacity to produce disease. Examples include structural elements (e.g., pili, pneumococcal or cryptococcal polysaccharide capsule, influenza virus hemagglutinins) that contribute to cellular adherence and colonization, and secreted products, such as those that directly injure cells and tissues—perhaps to provide nutrients for the bacteria or allow the microbes to penetrate to other areas of the body.

Sometimes these determinants work in concert to elicit disease. Case in point, in order to be pathogenic, *Bacillus anthracis* must possess genes capable of expressing a potent tripartite toxin as well as genes for a polyglutamyl capsule. A toxigenic strain of *B. anthracis* that fails to assemble a capsule and thus avoids the immune response, is incapable of inducing disease (37). Conversely, a strain of *B. anthracis* that produces a polyglutamyl capsule but not the toxin is nonvirulent as well. Hence, in order to be pathogenic, both virulence factors must be expressed (38).

Many population and evolutionary biologists have questioned the notion that pathogenesis is simply an artifact of a recent association between the microparasite and the host (39). Virulence mechanisms likely afford the causative agent a competitive advantage in terms of perpetuation, dispersal, and survival in a parasitic niche. Malignant pests they are, but only because they are "sophisticated opponents" or "artful contenders" struggling to make a living at our expense (40). Many successful parasites have evolved clever means of avoiding the immune response. For example, *Trypanosoma brucei,* the causative agent of African sleeping sickness, is the "artful dodger" of the microbial world, hiding from the host by perpetually switching its surface glycoproteins (i.e., antigenic switching). The bait-and-switch scheme renders the host powerless to mount an effective immunologic defense. Schistosomes (blood flukes) employ a slightly different strategy to conceal themselves from the host. By disguising themselves with a coating of blood antigens, the body defenses are easily warded off (35). *Staphylococcus aureus* avoids antibody responses because of the surface component, protein A, which binds immunoglobulin G (IgG) in reverse. *Neisseria* spp. (agents of gonorrhea and spinal meningitis) actually destroy immunoglobulin A (IgA) found on mucosal surfaces with IgA proteases (41). Molecular mimicry, undermining and nullifying the killing effects of neutrophils and macrophages, and manipulation of host physiology during an infection (e.g., bloody diarrhea, excessive sneezing) are comprehensible and sensible strategies only when viewed through the lens of natural selection. These responses are not merely accidental accompaniments or incidentals of disease. To clarify this concept further, other examples follow.

The bacterium *Legionella pneumophila* naturally infects the free-living soil amoeba *Acanthamoeba.* When it is phagocytosed, the bacterium will prevent phagolysosome development (42). In fact, the bacillus is also capable of multiplying within the phagosome of alveolar macrophages if a bountiful supply of iron (also cysteine) is available. The cytoplasm of the macrophage, however, is normally an iron-poor environment. Legiobactin, a siderophore or iron-chelating compound, provides the means to overcome this obstacle. The result is intracellular replication and

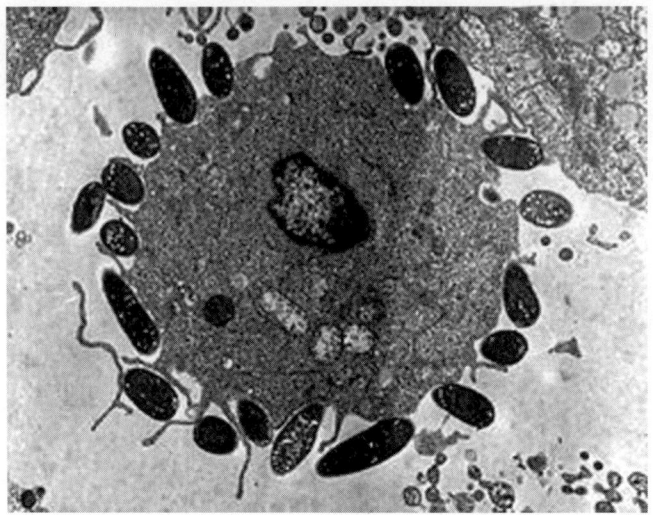

FIGURE 10.6. *Yersinia* injecting virulence proteins into the host cell cytoplasm. (Courtesy of ASM News, 2000.)

increased virulence (43). Another advantage of the intracellular niche is that the microbe, *Legionella* in this case, is able to hide from specific immune mechanisms.

Yops (*Yersinia outer membrane proteins*) are a series of plasmid-mediated virulence proteins that prevent phagocytic destruction of these organisms. Essentially the phagocyte (Fig. 10.6) is hijacked, paralyzed, and disarmed because Yops prevent phagocytic oxidative bursts and inhibit the release of proinflammatory cytokines. The *Yersinia* organism will then be disseminated deeper into the body (e.g., lymph nodes, liver, spleen) and eventually elicit a phagocytic apoptosis (44).

Sometimes a bacterial or viral component elicits exaggerated immunologic responses. Virulence factors that induce these altered immune responses are called superantigens, such as the staphylococcal enterotoxin, the most common cause of food poisoning, and toxic shock syndrome toxin-1, which induces the often fatal toxic shock syndrome. Such superantigens nonspecifically activate T lymphocytes, producing a nondirected cytokine cascade, leading to multiple organ and tissue dysfunctions expressed as fever, nausea, vomiting, and desquamation (45).

The mechanisms and strategies that microbes employ are seemingly endless and beyond the scope of this presentation. Suffice it to say that a better understanding of the nature of a pathogen is crucial when contemplating antibiotic, antiinflammatory, and other therapeutic options to control the pathogenesis caused by microorganisms.

IMMUNITY-BORDER INCURSIONS AND THE BODY'S "TOP GUNS"

The Historical Perspective and General Principles

The word immunity comes from the Latin, *immunis,* which means exempt. The term was coined in recognition of the observation that many people who experienced a disease were often "exempt" from suffering the same malady in the future. In 1890, von Behring and Kitasato introduced the concept of humoral immunity by showing that serum from laboratory animals immunized against the toxigenic diseases of tetanus or diphtheria would neutralize the effects of the respective disease (46,47). This innovative work actually followed the studies by Elie Metschnikoff, who in 1884, noted that certain white blood cells regularly "eat" or phagocytose disease-producing microorganisms (48). This principle became known as cellular immunity. For decades the field of immunology was sharply divided into what appeared to be irreconcilable factions—cellular versus humoral immunity. These seemingly opposing views were finally reconciled in the 1950s when it became clear that both humoral and cellular immunity were collective effects of the multiple functions of the lymphocytes.

The capability to resist invasion and pathogenic insults by microbes is divided into two categories of immunity—innate or nonspecific and adaptive or specific immunity. There is some overlap between the two. By definition, innate immunity includes those mechanisms of resistance that basically remain the same regardless of previous experience with microbes. In other words, such mechanisms have no immunologic memory and, thus, are not "boosted" by subsequent exposures. On the other hand, adaptive or specific immunity improves with experience and often results in a profound resistance to an otherwise highly virulent disease agent. Innate immunity can be divided into four domains: anatomic, physiologic, endocytic, and inflammatory. In essence, these four domains are barriers to invasion by pathogenic microorganisms.

Barriers That Limit the Success of Microbes

Anatomic barriers include the skin, which has several unique protective properties. Skin is made up of two major components. The inner component, the dermis, is richly vascularized and contains sebaceous glands, which secrete sebum (an oily secretion or coating), and accommodates immense numbers of macrophages and other phagocytic cells. The outer portion, the epidermis, is nonvascular and layered. The outermost layer is dead at maturation, contains the waxy protein keratin, and is constantly being shed. This shedding or desquamation prevents the excessive accumulation of bacteria. Furthermore, the epidermis is salty and acidic, due in part to the sebum. (Similarly, the antibacterial properties of cerumen protect the auditory canal.) Lysozyme is another antibacterial substance that is found on the skin (it is also found in tears and other body secretions). Lysozyme attacks the peptidoglycan layer of the prokaryotic cell wall, which results in lysis of many types of bacterial cells. Truly, this is an inhospitable place for the survival and multiplication of most pathogens; however, many types of bacteria, which are benign in that they normally do not produce disease, have become adapted to the skin and other body surfaces. These so-called friendly bacteria are known as normal flora, and their mere presence affords the host protection since they out compete or crowd out pathogenic organisms. The low pH of the skin is due in part to metabolic by-products of normal bacterial flora.

In spite of these defenses, a few pathogens are able to colonize the skin. The anaerobic bacterium *Propionibacterium acnes*

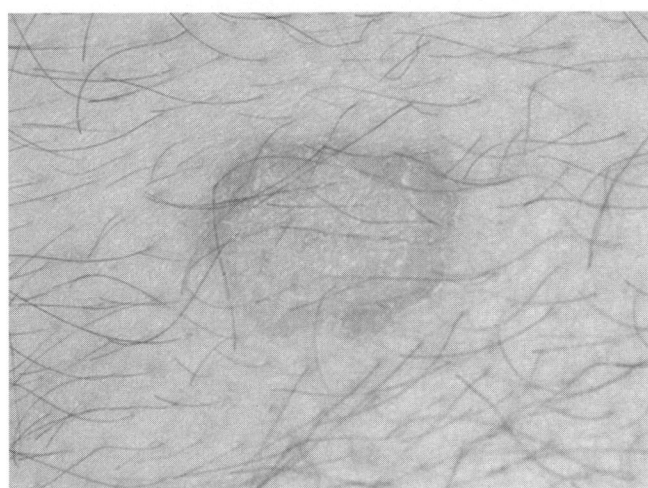

FIGURE 10.7. Tinea corporis, or ringworm of the body, on the leg of a college student. (Photo by L.A. Jensen.)

readily multiplies in hair follicles and crevices, producing acnes vulgaris—an inflammatory condition that is the nemesis of many adolescents. Cutaneous mycoses, like those that cause ringworm in prepubescent children (Fig. 10.7) or athlete's foot in young adults (Fig. 10.8), are ordinarily confined to keratinized surfaces and tissues such as skin, nails, and hair. What is more, pathogens are only rarely capable of penetrating intact skin. The spirochete *Treponema pallidum* and infective stages of some helminths (e.g., schistosome cercariae, filariform hookworm larvae) are notable exceptions and easily pass through the epidermal barrier, even if it is undamaged.

Like the epidermis, the mucosal layer of the GI tract is a nonspecific defensive barrier. The stomach's acidic environment destroys sizable numbers of microbes, but a few pathogens are acid-tolerant, such as *Shigella dysenteriae* and *Helicobacter pylori,* and other organisms are spared because they are evidently insulated in chunks of food. Progressing down the alimentary canal, the number of bacteria increases until the intestinal content contains 25% to 30% bacterial load by dry weight. The intestinal mucosa is prime real estate, so to speak, and certain types of

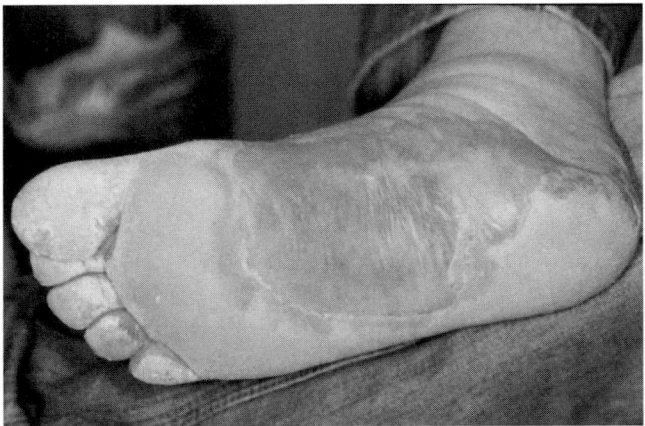

FIGURE 10.8. A severe case of tinea pedis, or athlete's foot, in a homeless man. (Photo courtesy of A.H. Dekker.)

microorganisms compete vigorously for space. Like the skin flora, these organisms are generally not pathogenic. They are highly adapted to specialized GI niches and, as such, control pathogenic organisms. In short, the indigenous microbiota out compete would-be pathogens for space and nutrients.

Mucous membranes, such as those that line the respiratory and urogenital tracts, possess numerous innate defenses (e.g., mucus, ciliated epithelial cells, lysozyme). In the case of the respiratory tract, mucous secretions effectively bog down would-be invaders, and the resident ciliated epithelial cells, located deep in the system, constantly sweep the mucous-trapped microbes, dust, and pollen into the pharynx where they are swallowed into the stomach. The outer third of the urinary tract contains some resident bacteria, but the outward flow of acidic urine helps keep the upper system sterile. The female genital tract has its own microflora, composed in part of acidophilic streptococci and lactobacilli. During their initial attempt to get a foothold in the vaginal canal, many invading pathogens are overwhelmed by these microorganisms, possibly as a result of the low pH and again, simply by being crowded out. When microorganisms do pervade these physical and chemical barriers, they encounter billions of phagocytes, such as macrophages and neutrophils, which attempt to destroy the invaders.

Inflammation and Other Nonspecific Defenses

From time to time, regardless of the physical barricades and patrols of white blood cells, violations do occur and microbial pathogens are successful in colonizing a site in the body. This incursion will generally lead to the initiation of inflammatory responses. Inflammation consists of a highly complex series of events that sometimes acts as a two-edged sword, killing or restraining microbes on the one hand and exacerbating disease conditions on the other. Inflammation means "setting on fire" and represents a series of events that have been recognized since ancient times. The Roman physician Celus aptly described inflammation as "*rubor et tumor cum calore et dolore*" which means *redness* and *swelling* with *heat* and *pain*. The events behind this description are complex and difficult to thoroughly describe within the context of this chapter, and thus will only be briefly described. When microbial invasion occurs (also, sprain and contusion), released inflammatory mediators like histamines, prostaglandins, and cytokines induce vasodilation and increased blood flow to the compromised or injured tissue site. This influx of blood not only results in erythema (*rubor*) but also raises the local temperature (*calore*). These mediators also increase the permeability of the dilated blood vessels, allowing for the escape of plasma components and circulating leukocytes. Localized edema (*tumor*) follows, and an accumulation of fibrin prevents the spread of the invaders. Finally, to help protect the already damaged tissues from further insults, these mediators of inflammation upregulate pain receptors (*dolore*). The clotting components of the escaped plasma form a fibrin barrier to restrict further invasion, and other intrinsic antimicrobial blood components (e.g., complement) begin to destroy the pathogens. Finally, the neutrophils and macrophages clear out the microbial invaders. Hence, innate immunity represents a collection of preventive measures, blocking the incursion and colonization of pathogenic organisms. Such nonspecific mechanisms are generally not influenced by repeated experience with pathogens.

Under certain conditions, inflammation may have systemic impacts such as fever (the cardinal symptom) and shock. Fever occurs when certain exogenous pyrogens, such as the bacterial cell wall components, peptidoglycan and lipopolysaccharide (LPS), arouse macrophages and other immunologic cells that release proinflammatory cytokines, such as tumor necrosis factor (TNF), interleukin-1 (IL-1), and IL-6. These cytokines, described as endogenous pyrogens, provoke the hypothalamus to increase the body temperature above the normal 37°C set-point (49). Fever is a defensive measure of the host—not simply an incidental consequence of disease. In theory, a febrile temperature will damage the pathogen. Fever evidently subdues certain temperature-sensitive pathogens, such as *T. pallidum*. This was the driving principle that inspired Julius Wagner-Jauregg, an Austrian physician in the early 1900s, to employ malariotherapy as a means to ameliorate the devastating sequelae of neurosyphilis (50). Thus, fever-suppressing therapy like aspirin and ibuprofen might aggravate the infection; however, a fever that is excessively high must obviously be dealt with aggressively. Furthermore, febrile temperatures are believed to enhance phagocytic capacities and activation of the alternative complement pathway. Also, a slightly higher than normal temperature has a positive influence on specific T-lymphocyte–mediated cytotoxicity (51). Hence, the production of fever, although nonspecific, is an effective way to retard pathogenic growth.

Another nonspecific defensive strategy that checks the growth of many pathogens—organisms like streptococci, legionellae, shigellae, yeasts, intestinal amoebae, and malaria sporozoans—involves the tying up of free iron in the human body. Many pathogenic species require iron to reproduce. Iron-binding proteins, such as lactoferrin and transferrin, which are found in breast milk, tears, respiratory mucus, and GI and reproductive tract secretions, inhibit these pathogens (30). High levels of free iron—perhaps from supplements—will exacerbate TB and amoebic dysentery, and children afflicted with cerebral malaria will probably get better faster when therapeutic measures include iron-binding drugs. Good evidence suggests that the practice of providing iron therapy to a patient with an infection who is also experiencing an apparent transitory iron-deficiency anemia might actually be counterproductive (21). On the other hand, a true iron-deficient anemia could depress the immune system by decreasing lymphoid cell development and IL-1 production (52). Undoubtedly, it is a matter of degree.

Other nonspecific protective mechanisms include coughing, sneezing, pain, and diarrhea. People who are unable to remove bacterial-laden mucus from their respiratory tract have a good chance of dying of pneumonia (21). Diarrhea and vomiting are important as clearing mechanisms for diarrheagenic bacterial or viral toxins. A bout of diarrhea will aid healing by decreasing the contact time between the invasive bacterial pathogen (e.g., *Shigella*) and the intestinal mucosal surface. Antimotility therapy, therefore, is generally not recommended for shigellosis and salmonellosis (53). Of course, some of these mechanisms induced by microbes have undesired consequences—at least from the human perspective—like the enhanced spread of disease through aerosolization or contamination of food and water.

Specific Immunologic Mechanisms

Unlike the innate or nonspecific immune mechanisms, adaptive or specific immunity becomes more focused, more profound, and more efficient at dealing with microbial pathogens (especially repeat microbial experiences). Specific immunity has four characteristics: specificity, diversity, memory, and the ability to differentiate self from nonself. Specificity is determined by the molecular configuration of the pathogens—structural components known as antigens which are loosely defined as molecular sequences that evoke immune responses. Amazingly, the immune system can differentiate between two proteins that vary only by a single amino acid. Moreover, it can recognize billions of separate antigens. These characteristics are due to the fact that leukocytes, known as lymphocytes, recognize and respond only to the specific antigen to which they are committed. Thus, in each person there exists billions of unique lymphocytes, each dedicated to a given antigen providing the immune response its incredible diversity. The seminal event of immunity is called immunologic memory. This means that once the lymphocytes respond to a given antigen, any subsequent appearance of the same antigen will elicit a rapid, profound, and highly focused reprisal. Finally, the immune system has the ability to differentiate most proteins, as well as all cells that belong to an individual, from molecules and cells derived from other living things, including viruses, bacteria, fungi, and parasites.

The immune system is second to the central nervous system in complexity and, as such, simple explanations as to how it works are challenging, to say the least. Nonetheless, the key participants in specific immunity are the lymphocytes and a group of cells known as antigen-presenting cells (APCs) and their products. Lymphocytes are derived from pluripotent stem cells in the bone marrow. Some lymphocytes develop in the bone marrow before being released into the bloodstream—these are the B lymphocytes or B cells. Other lymphocytes are derived in the bone marrow but are further altered in the thymus gland, becoming thymus-derived lymphocytes or T cells. Both B and T lymphocytes have specific antigen recognition molecules on their surfaces, called antibodies on B cells and T-cell receptors (TCR) on T cells. Thus, for each antigen that a person can react to, there are specific lymphocytes already committed to that antigen. The activation of the lymphocyte triggers the specific immune response and requires an intimate interaction between the antigen and its corresponding lymphocyte. As a means of differentiating self from nonself, each individual has a unique molecular code that annotates every nucleated cell in the body. This unique code comes from a gene complex called the major histocompatibility complex (MHC). Thus, each individual has a particular MHC molecular complex; only identical twins have the same set of MHC markers. These MHC markers or proteins are classified into MHC class I and MHC class II. MHC class II markers are found only on certain cells of the immune system (APCs), whereas all nucleated cells express MHC class I markers on their plasma membranes. Several immune system cells act as APCs, but generally these are the macrophages, B lymphocytes, and dendritic cells.

Before lymphocytes interact with their antigens they are known as naive lymphocytes. Naive lymphocytes do not undergo the cell cycle, but after leaving the bone marrow or thymus as B cells they circulate for a period of time and, unless activated by their respective antigens, undergo apoptosis and are replaced by other identical cells from the bone marrow stem cells. The B cells can react directly with their antigens by means of their antibody surface receptors. The binding of antigen to the surface antibody, along with receipt by the B cell of other signals delivered from T-helper cells, stimulates the B cell to undergo a reproductive process called clonal expansion, which results in numerous identical cells. Plasma cells and memory B cells are the products. The plasma cells are generally short-lived, but they produce copious quantities of antibody—up to 2,000 antibody molecules per second. These antibody molecules circulate throughout the body in blood and tissue fluids and react only with the antigen that initiated its production. The memory B cells constitute a major component of recall of the immune system. Following the initial antigenic stimulation, far more memory B cells than naive B cells of the same specificity will be found. Moreover, these memory B cells remain viable for long periods of time to guard against subsequent infections. If the antigen reappears at a later time, generally as a reinfection, the memory B cells swing into action and undergo another round of clonal expansion, rapidly producing new antibody-secreting plasma cells and new memory B cells. Thus, the memory or secondary response is faster, more profound, and more focused than the initial reaction. Such antibody responses are known as humoral immunity and were the basis of von Behring and Kitasato's initial observations, discussed earlier (46,47).

Antibodies are only part of the immune response. Cellular immunity resides principally with the T lymphocytes. These lymphocytes are classified according to protein surface markers. T cells with CD4 markers are called CD4 lymphocytes, whereas those with CD8 markers are referred to as CD8 lymphocytes.

Although the CD4 and CD8 cells are committed to react with specific antigens, naive T cells do not recognize their antigens unless the antigen has been processed and binds in the peptide-binding groove of the MHC molecules. Such antigen processing, in association with the MHC self-markers, is the primary means of preventing the immune system from reacting against one's own cells. Antigen receptors on CD4 cells will only recognize antigen presented to them in association with class II MHC molecules. This means that APCs must first phagocytose and break down the antigen into strings of amino acids (referred to as antigen processing), complex it with MHC class II molecules, and then present it to CD4 lymphocytes. Once this happens, the activated CD4 cells will differentiate into either T_H1 or T_H2 cells. Briefly, armed T_H1 cells are responsible for inflammatory-type reactions in that they secrete various proinflammatory cytokines and are involved in defending against intracellular pathogens. T_H2 cells are involved with B-cell activation, and like T_H1, produce a variety of cytokines. Also, some of the members of the expanded clone of CD4 cells become memory T cells.

Like the CD4 cells, CD8 lymphocytes cannot recognize antigens unless the antigen has been presented in association MHC markers of the class I, rather than the class II variety. Antigens that are processed in this manner arise within somatic cells. Thus, antigens from intracellular pathogens, cancer cells, and foreign cells (organ transplants), are the primary targets of CD8-cell responses. Once the CD8 cells have been stimulated by their respective antigens in association with MHC class I markers, they too undergo clonal expansion to produce cell-specific cytotoxic T lymphocytes (CTLs) and appropriate CTL memory cells. These CTLs do not produce antibodies like the B cells. They are, however, killers of cancer cells and foreign tissue cells, such as organ transplants and cells which harbor intracellular pathogens. CTLs destroy their target cells by secreting a substance called perforin that lyses the target cell membrane. Thus, the antibodies from the B cells (plasma cells) generally target extracellular pathogens, bacteria, parasites, or viruses found in blood or body tissues.

The initial appearance of a pathogenic organism will require activation of the naive lymphocytes through antigen recognition and clonal expansion to produce the effector cells, plasma cells, T helper cells, and CTLs and their respective effector molecules—antibodies, cytokines, and perforin. This primary immune response requires 5 to 12 days before it can make a significant impact on the pathogenic microbe, and this time lag often has fatal consequences. However, once the memory cells have been put in place by the primary response, a subsequent appearance of the pathogen triggers a rapid secondary immune response in 1 to 3 days. Such expeditious protective immunity is the basis for vaccines that implement a primary immune response, generally without the pathogenic consequences, and set up the immunologic memory mechanisms for a rapid and intense protective secondary response. Humoral immunity in women can partially protect their neonates by passive transfer of antibody via the placenta and through breast milk. Thus, effective vaccination or previous exposure to pathogens may offer vertical protection between generations by way of these passive immune mechanisms.

The *New England Journal of Medicine* recently published several review articles on basic science and clinically relevant topics in immunology that physicians and medical students will find especially useful (54–69). The series has an easy-to-read style with colorful illustrations, and can be downloaded from the Internet (*www.nejm.org*).

NUTRITIONAL AMMUNITION: PLEASE PASS THE VITAMINS AND MINERALS

The Importance of a Healthy Diet

The pathogenesis of many infectious diseases (e.g., pneumonia, diarrhea, measles, TB) are notably magnified by malnutrition (70). This negative impact on infectious diseases is due chiefly to its effects on immunity. Cell-mediated immunity, the complement system, the phagocytic response, and cytokine and antibody production are all adversely affected (50). Vitamin A deficiency is associated with impaired phagocytosis and reduced humoral and cellular immunity, and it is believed to worsen measles in children, which in some African countries kills more children than malaria. Likewise, nutritional deficiency noticeably increases the risk of respiratory and diarrheal illnesses (70). A vitamin E deficiency impedes T-cell function, whereas a lack of calcium is linked to a low fibrinogen level, exacerbating numerous bacterial infections. Finally, a zinc deficiency adversely affects cytokine production and is a predisposing factor for a variety of infections (50).

In addition to the negative impact that malnutrition has on immunity, a healthy diet plays a more direct role in modulating the devastating effects of infectious disease. Furthermore, it is obvious that microbes are capable of compromising a person's nutritional status. In their monograph on nutrition, el Lozy and co-workers describe this concept as a synergy of malnutrition and infection (71). To illustrate this concept further, Koski and Scott point out that heavy *Ascaris* infections will likely have a deleterious effect on the nutritional status of the infected person and, concomitantly, malnutrition is believed to increase or intensify susceptibility to other parasitic infections (72). They appropriately describe this as the "negative spiral." In our experience in Africa and Latin America, children with pathogenic bacterial or parasitic infections often present to clinics with loss of appetite as the most predominant symptom. This finding seems somewhat predictable, however, since a sick child, especially one who is vomiting profusely or suffering from severe diarrhea, will probably be anorexic. The duodenal protozoan *Giardia lamblia* usually produces watery diarrhea and malabsorption in children. Sometimes an infection will, in time, spontaneously clear. If a chronic infection does occur however, there is a risk of long-term growth retardation (73).

Intestinal helminths may also negatively impact the nutritional status of the host. *Necator americanus* and *Ancylostoma duodenale,* the two human hookworm species, are linked to iron-deficiency anemia. Hookworms apparently are avaricious feeders and if the worm burden is heavy enough, appreciable blood loss will result (35). To a more serious extent, the chronic loss of serum protein markedly worsens protein malnutrition, common in rural tropical regions where hookworm infections are abundant. Another example, well known to students of parasitology, is tapeworm pernicious anemia, a potential complication resulting from an infection with the broad fish tapeworm *Diphyllobothrium latum.* The condition, characterized by the presence of megaloblastic anemia, is directly linked to a deficiency of vitamin B_{12}. Apparently, the tapeworm simply sops up this important vitamin, producing a marked deficiency. Ingestion of the dried pulverized worms, expelled in the person's feces, was once believed to be a useful remedy to reverse the anemia (74).

THERAPY AND ANTIMICROBIALS: THE ENDLESS BATTLES

The Osteopathic Approach in Treating Influenza Patients in 1918

During the 1918 influenza epidemic most American physicians, DOs and MDs alike, understood the benefits of isolating their sick patients, instituting appropriate hygiene measures, and diligently regulating adequate fluid intake. According to Gevitz, these were fundamental and universal concepts in medicine at the time (75). But instead of prescribing calomel (a mercury compound) and Dover powder (ipecac and opium mixture) to the patient with influenza for the purpose of relieving pain and inducing perspiration, the unswerving osteopathic practitioner rejected the orthodox pharmaceutical regimen completely. The results proved to be remarkable, especially for patients with pneumonia. While 12% to 15% of the patients treated by MDs died, only 1% of those treated by DOs succumbed. It was a defining period in osteopathic medicine, and patients inevitably came to realize that DOs had the medical skills not only to manage chronic diseases but to provide additional treatment choices for acute illnesses like influenza and bacterial pneumonia (76).

The Principles of Chemotherapy and Present-Day Worries

Admittedly, the treatment of influenza and other infectious diseases during the 1918 flu pandemic was primitive by today's standards. In recent years, the pharmaceutical industry has provided many options to battle influenza and its complications. There are neuraminidase inhibitors—an effective medication that, if started early enough, will reduce the number of days a person is symptomatic (77)—and several antibiotic choices to fight the deadly bacterial pneumonia that often accompanies influenza-weakened lungs. Without question, the use of antibiotics—those antimicrobial agents developed from natural effusions of certain bacteria and fungi—has made a significant impact on human health by reducing malaise, attenuating postinfectious sequelae, and often curtailing mortality. But there are qualifiers and issues to be reckoned with in future years. The antibiotic age we live in is a fallacious utopia. The continual emergence of new antibiotic-resistant strains of pathogenic organisms (e.g., staphylococci, pneumococci, enterococci, mycobacteria) is an alarming but not unexpected consequence of natural evolution, coupled with unwise overuse of these powerful tools. Now we face multiple-drug resistance, the ultimate equalizer from the microbe's perspective. All this, of course, raises concerns about human prospects and medical practices in a postantimicrobial era (78).

Antibiotics (microbial by-products) did not evolve for the benefit of humans. Antibiotics evolved because they enhance leverage in the struggle for space and nutrients with other microbial species. This should come as no surprise since microbes have competing interests. A toxic substance secreted by one species may provide the necessary competitive advantage for colonization by keeping the other species at bay (Fig. 10.9). Humankind is merely an unintended benefactor of this microbial struggle for survival. In this vein, many microorganisms have evolved countermeasures—mechanisms that impede antibiotic efficacy. Unfortunately these mechanisms also undermine modern medical uses of these therapeutic agents. Most of these *anti*-antibiotics are enzymes like β-lactamase and other antibiotic-destroying enzymes. The genes for these enzymes are often located on plasmids, self-replicating extragenomic DNA circles that are often transferable to other bacteria, even if the species is unrelated (79). Conjugative transfer of vancomycin-resistant genes from a strain of *Enterococcus faecalis* to *S. aureus* has been demonstrated in the laboratory (80). The significance of this suggests that "superbugs"

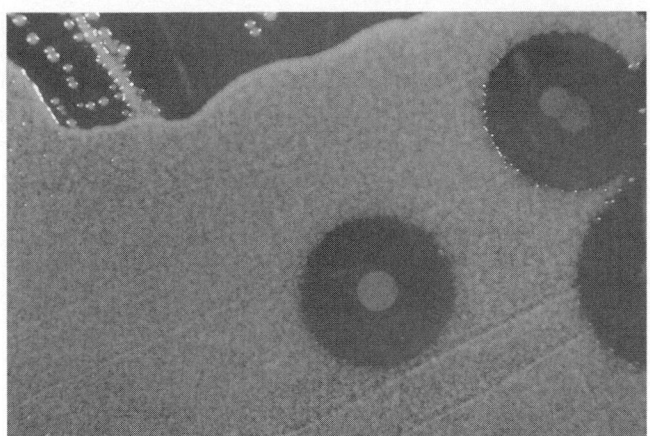

FIGURE 10.9. An example of competitive inhibition. Note the zone of inhibition. (Photo by L.A. Jensen.)

or bacteria that are resistant to all known antimicrobials will be a reality in the future.

Mechanisms by which bacteria resist antimicrobial drugs include:

1. *Loss of antibacterial activity.* Beta-lactamases hydrolyze the β-lactam ring of penicillin and cephalosporins and other enzymes that destroy aminoglycosides.
2. *Loss or modification of a receptor.* An altered receptor of penicillin-binding proteins (PBPs) in the methicillin-resistant *S. aureus* (MRSA) and an altered receptor on the 50S ribosomal subunit.
3. *Bacterial permeability changes.* Bacterial resistance to tetracyclines and polymyxins are represented in this category.
4. *Altered metabolic pathways.* Some organisms that are resistant to the sulfonamides are able to utilize preformed folic acid and do not require *p*-aminobenzoic acid (PABA).
5. *Altered enzyme function.* Some bacteria with resistance to trimethoprim have reduced dihydrofolic acid reductase inhibition (79).

Many reasons exist as to why antibiotics should be used with caution and discretion. Antibiotics, especially broad-spectrum drugs, often eliminate the normal microbiota—collateral damage of sorts—creating secondary problems, such as oral or vaginal candidiasis. The yeast replaces the normal flora. More serious is the potentially life-threatening diarrhea of pseudomembranous colitis, caused by a marked overgrowth of *Clostridium difficile* after robust and prolonged antibiotic use. For some infections, antibiotic therapy has absolutely no relevance and may actually hinder clearance of the pathogen (80). Case in point, antibiotics are generally contraindicated for uncomplicated cases of intestinal salmonellosis or campylobacteriosis. These infections almost always resolve without treatment, and the use of antibiotics would only disrupt the normal flora, allowing an unrestrained proliferation of the pathogen. Furthermore, the possibility always exists that inappropriate use—possibly based solely on faulty empiric assessment—will hasten the development of drug resistance.

The responsibility of prudent use of antimicrobials, of course, does not rest with physicians alone—dentists, nurse practitioners, and other medical professionals compound the problem. Moreover, there is a critical problem of patient self-medication. Often patients fail to comply with the regimen prescribed because of a lack of understanding of their responsibilities. It is incumbent that physicians and midlevel health care providers also function as health educators. Many patients horde medications to be used without medical approval in the future. The unfortunate tendency is to avoid the physician whenever possible, even borrowing medicines, or clandestinely purchasing them via the Internet or just over the U.S. border in Mexico, where many medications can be obtained without prescription. Of course, the long-term stockpiling of antibiotics is pointless and may even be counterproductive since most drugs will lose potency if stored improperly, and many (e.g., penicillins) have short shelf lives. The patient should at least be informed of the problems associated with these practices.

One of the most serious influences on the emergence of antibiotic-resistance involves the use of antimicrobials as growth promoters in animal feed. Penicillins, cephalosporins, tetracyclines, fluoroquinolones all have been used for this purpose. It has been estimated that 50% of the antimicrobials produced in the U.S. are used for subtherapeutic purposes in animals (81). The possibility exists that vancomycin-resistant enterococci, associated with avoparcin (a glycopeptide), have already evolved in livestock; circumstantial evidence points to this conclusion in Europe (82). Furthermore, ground meats (poultry, pork, and hamburger) are potential sources for antibiotic-resistant salmonellae (83). Similarly, other resistant pathogens that normally reside in animals (e.g., *Campylobacter jejuni,* hemorrhagic *E. coli*) are often passed to humans in foods. In conclusion, the feeding of antibiotics to healthy domestic animals for growth promotion is an unsound practice, one that will only complicate therapeutic options for people in the future. Likewise, indiscriminate use of antibiotics in any form will most assuredly lead to an increase in resistant organisms.

CONTROL EFFORTS: KEEPING A SAFE DISTANCE

The Importance of Hygiene

Several years ago, one of us (LAJ) observed a surgeon examining a patient for an inguinal hernia. The physician was not wearing gloves during the examination and did not immediately wash his hands when he left the room to check a postsurgical case. Undoubtedly, a basic medical school lesson was forgotten. Maybe handwashing seems just too simple a procedure to be of any value to the average physician (84), but, the fact still remains, handwashing prevents the transmission of disease. It is the principal means of preventing nosocomial infections and to reduce the spread of antibiotic-resistant organisms from one patient to another (85). It is simply the cardinal rule: physicians must wash their hands between patients. Such has been the case since the 1840s when the Hungarian physician Ignaz Semmelweis, in an effort to control puerperal fever (*S. pyogenes*) in the maternity ward of a Vienna hospital, required that all medical students and student midwives wash their hands before examining obstetric patients (86). Correspondingly, diligent handwashing by food handlers after using the toilet prevents the spread of GI viral and bacterial foodborne pathogens (87). Caregivers who wash their hands between diaper changes will prevent the spread of *Shigella* in day care centers (88), and salmonellosis can be averted if children will wash their hands after playing with pet reptiles (89) and chicks or ducklings (90). Another important control procedure includes the changing of gloves between patients. Gloves protect both the patient and the health care worker. Moreover, wearing latex gloves should not be considered a substitute for proper hand hygiene. Physicians and nurses should wash their hands whether they wear gloves during procedures or not (84).

It has been proven that in countries where personal hygiene and community public health practices—like the inspection foods, sanitation of waste, and filtration of drinking water—are regularly practiced, there are considerably fewer problems with infectious diseases than in countries where food and water sources are microbiologically suspect. It has even been suggested that the purification of drinking water is the most important preventive measure for intestinal disease in humans and saves more lives than antimicrobial therapy and immunizations combined (22).

The History of Vaccines and the "Snuffing Out" of Smallpox

As mentioned throughout this chapter, our present era of relative good health has been due to improvements in nutrition, personal and community hygiene, antibiotics, and vaccines. The basis for vaccines has been underscored in the discussion on immunity. However, the chronicles of vaccination begin in the occult history of smallpox, a disease so dreaded that even the founder of osteopathic medicine, Dr. A.T. Still feared contracting it and referred to smallpox as his "dread by day and by night" (91). Over recorded time and probably long before, smallpox was one of the most feared and detestable of all diseases. Not only was its death toll appallingly high, but survivors were often horribly scarred.

The normal portal of entry for the variola virus, the etiologic agent of smallpox, is the respiratory tract, but it was discovered that a cutaneous route was not nearly as lethal (mortality rate of 1%) and conferred complete protection against any future assault. This technique was referred to as variolation (the practice of introducing purulent matter extracted from an open smallpox lesion into the skin of another person). It was employed in India prior to 1000 B.C. It was a dangerous practice since too deep a scarification would result in a full-blown smallpox attack. Nonetheless, it became widely practiced, and since variolation required a fresh source of infectious pus, some enterprising "professional" variolators would pick scabs from smallpox patients and grind them into a powder. The material could be stored for months in quills. These early practitioners would travel from village to village just ahead of predicted epidemics and offer the powdered smallpox scabs as a snuff to the fearful public for a price. This practice was especially harmful because the normal route of transmission of the virus was through the nasal mucosa and, as one would expect, it led to far more epidemics than it prevented.

In 1796, the English physician Edward Jenner discovered a safer way to prevent smallpox. Jenner noted that milkmaids often had sores resembling smallpox on their hands and rarely, if ever, contracted smallpox. Interestingly, they were often enlisted to nurse those with the disease. He surmised that the sores on the milkmaid's hands, which came from similar lesions found on the udders of cows, provided protection. He extracted pus from a cowpox lesion on the hand of a dairymaid and inoculated it just under the skin of an 8-year-old boy (parental consent was obtained). Complete immunity evidently resulted because, when challenged with "variolous matter" (i.e., variolation), smallpox or isolated pox lesions at the inoculation site did not develop (92–94). Jenner reconfirmed these results several times. The word "vaccination" (after *vacca* for cow, a Latin etymology) was originally coined by Jenner to describe this procedure, although Pasteur later enlarged the basic meaning to include all like protective measures for infectious diseases.

Jenner's remarkable success led to the development of a large-scale vaccination program for the prevention of smallpox. The last known case of naturally acquired smallpox occurred in Somalia in 1977, but just 10 years earlier, 2 million people had died from the disease (93). Smallpox has now been eradicated; thus, vaccination, with all its potential side effects is no longer relevant. If only humankind could be as lucky with other infectious diseases. With regard to smallpox, the war has almost been won. Elimination of the variola virus will be completed when remaining stocks maintained by the United States, the Russian Federation, and possibly other countries are totally destroyed—not before (95). As it stands now, the victory is incomplete. Intentional release of the smallpox virus, considering that most people currently lack immunity, could be disastrous. An *MMWR* editorial noted in 1997: "Some things need be done only once in the entire history of the world" (96). The smallpox virus as a biological warfare threat is real.

Modern-Day Vaccines and Safety Issues

The vaccine used by Jenner was made from pus and lymph from infected cows, an impure concoction by modern standards. Also, arm-to-arm vaccination was often employed. Human-to-human vaccination was convenient but it was not without risk. Sometimes, presumably because of a co-infection, the variola virus was transmitted to the unwitting vaccinee. Poxviruses are antigenically related and, therefore, immunity induced by Jenner's cowpox virus was protective against variola—at least for a while. The cowpox vaccine was different from the traditional vaccines of today. Lived-attenuated or chemically inactivated microbes and microbial components (e.g., capsular polysaccharide conjugated with protein and bacterial toxoids) currently employed provide a much purer and safer product. The hepatitis B recombinant-DNA vaccine, for example, is based on a surface antigen.

With regard to safety issues of vaccines, serious adverse reactions associated with licensed vaccines are rare. Some serious complications of the vaccinia vaccine (for smallpox) are eczema vaccinatum, generalized vaccinia, progressive vaccinia, and postvaccinial encephalitis. These occur more often among primary vaccinees than revaccinees. Fatal complications, as a result of postvaccinial encephalitis or progressive vaccinia, occur at a rate of 1 death per 1 million primary vaccinations or 1 death per 4 million revaccinations. As with other live-viral vaccines, vaccinia is contraindicated for pregnant women (97). Rare adverse complications of other vaccines occur, including intussusception for rotavirus, demyelinating encephalopathy for measles, Guillain-Barré syndrome for influenza, and paralysis for oral poliovirus. Anaphylaxis, of course, is always a possibility with any injectable preparation (55). Many present-day vaccines are currently being redesigned as subunit or even DNA-based vaccines that reduce potential complications even further. With regard to vaccinations, a moderate and a conservative approach is probably best.

SUMMARY

Although some infectious diseases have been virtually contained or eradicated altogether because of aggressive vaccination and control programs, newly identified microbes, antibiotic-resistant strains, and reemerging pathogens represent formidable challenges for physicians and midlevel health care providers. For a microbe to be classified as a pathogen, virulence determinants—factors of toxicity and invasiveness—must be expressed. These factors, which evolved for the singular purpose of giving the microbe a selective advantage, oftentimes work in conjunction with inflammatory mechanisms to produce morbidity. As a result, cells and tissues are damaged and the patient experiences clinical symptoms like fever and diarrhea. Evidence suggests that a positive nutritional health status will strengthen the immune system (nonspecific and adaptive immunity) and mitigate the effects of disease. And finally, to avoid encouraging the evolution of resistant microbes, antibiotics and antimicrobial agents should be employed only when other therapeutic options do not otherwise exist.

ACKNOWLEDGMENTS

We wish to thank Douglas R. Rushing, professor of biochemistry at The University of Health Sciences (UHS), for reviewing the manuscript. We also grateful for the suggestions on the immunology sections by Bonnie A. Buxton, associate professor of microbiology (UHS).

REFERENCES

Note: *Because of the immenseness of the literature in microbiology and understanding the time constraints of the average reader, we have elected to cite many secondary and review articles, edited translations of foreign publications, and even a few textbooks.*

1. Taubenberger JK. Seeking the 1918 Spanish influenza virus. *ASM News.* 1999;65:473–478.
2. Kolata G. *Flu: The Story of the Great Influenza Pandemic of 1918 and the Search for the Virus That Caused It.* New York, NY: Farrar, Straus and Giroux; 1999.
3. World Health Organization. Tuberculosis. *WHO Fact Sheet* 2000; no 104.
4. Centers for Disease Control. The global HIV and AIDS epidemic, 2001. *MMWR.* 2001;51:434–439.
5. Phillips RS. Current status of malaria and potential for control. *Clin Microbiol Rev.* 2001;14:208–226.
6. Crompton DWT. How much human helminthiasis is there in the world? *J Parasitol.* 1999;85:397–403.
7. Colley DG, LoVerde PT, Savioli L. Medical helminthology in the 21st century. *Science.* 2001;293:1437–1438.
8. Centers for Disease Control. Updated recommendations from the advisory committee on immunization practices in response to delays in supply of influenza vaccine for the 2000–01 season. *MMWR.* 2000;49:888–892.
9. Mouton CP, Bazaldua OV, Pierce B, Espino DV. Common infections in older adults. *Am Fam Physician.* 2001;63:257–268.
10. Ebell MH, Smith MA, Barry HC, et al. Does this patient have strep throat? *JAMA.* 2000;284:2912–2918.
11. Loesche WJ, Grossman, NS. Periodontal disease as a specific, albeit chronic, infection: diagnosis and treatment. *Clin Microbiol Rev.* 2001;14:727–752.
12. Cates W Jr. Estimates of the incidence and prevalence of sexually transmitted diseases in the United States. American Social Health Association Panel. *Sex Transm Dis.* 1999;26:[4 Suppl]:S2–7.
13. Fankhauser RL, Noel JS, Monroe SS, et al. Molecular epidemiology of Norwalk-like viruses in outbreaks of gastroenteritis in the United States. *J Infect Dis.* 1998;178:1571–1580.
14. Mead PS, Slutsker L, Dietz V, et al. Food-related illness and death in the United States. *Emerg Infect Dis.* 1999;5:607–625.
15. Centers for Disease Control. Giardiasis. Surveillance United States, 1992–1997. *MMWR.* 2000;49(SS-7):1–17.
16. Neu HC. The crisis in antibiotic resistance. *Science.* 1992;257:1064–1073.
17. Cetinkaya Y, Falk P, Mayhall CG. Vancomycin-resistant enterococci. *Clin Microbiol Rev.* 2000:13:686–707.
18. Whitney CG, Farley MM, Hadler J, et al. Increasing prevalence of multidrug-resistance *Streptococcus pneumoniae* in the United States. *N Engl J Med.* 2000;343:1917–1924.
19. Pablos-Méndex A, Raviglione MC, Laszlo A, et al. Global surveillance for antituberculosis-drug resistance, 1994–1997. *N Engl J Med.* 1998;338:1641–1649.
20. Satcher D. Emerging infections: getting ahead of the curve. *Emerg Infect Dis.* 1995;1:1–6.
21. Nesse RM, Williams GC. Evolution and the origins of disease. *Sci Am.* 1998;279:86–93.
22. Brock TD. *Robert Koch: A Life in Medicine and Bacteriology.* Washington, DC: ASM Press; 1999.
23. De Kruif P. *Microbe Hunters.* San Diego, CA: Harcourt Brace and Company; 1996.
24. Dubos R. *Pasteur and Modern Science.* Washington, DC: ASM Press; 1998.
25. Rivers TM. Viruses and Koch's postulates. *J Bacteriol.* 1937;33:1–12.
26. King LS. Germ theory and its influence. *JAMA.* 1983;249:794–798.
27. McConnell CP, Teall CC. *The Practice of Osteopathy,* 3rd ed. Kirksville, MO: Journal Printing Company; 1906.
28. Hulett GD. *A Text Book on the Principles of Osteopathy.* Kirksville, MO: Journal Printing Company; 1903.
29. Fredricks DN, Relman DA. Sequence-based identification of microbial pathogens: a reconsideration of Koch's postulates. *Clin Microbiol Rev.* 1996;9:18–33.
30. Salyers AA, Whitt DD. *Bacterial Pathogenesis: A Molecular Approach,* 2nd ed. Washington, DC: ASM Press; 2002.
31. Casadevall A, Pirofski L. Host-pathogen interactions: redefining the basic concepts of virulence and pathogenicity. *Infect Immun.* 1999;67:3703–3713.
32. Leavitt JW. *Typhoid Mary.* Boston, MA: Beacon Press; 1996.
33. Bourdain A. *Typhoid Mary.* New York, NY: Bloomsbury Publishing; 2001.
34. Hill AVS, Weatherall DJ. Host genetic factors in resistance to malaria. In: Sherman IW, ed. *Malaria: Parasite Biology, Pathogenesis, and Protection.* Washington, DC: ASM Press; 1998:445–455.
35. Roberts LS, Janovy J. *Gerald D. Schmidt & Larry S. Roberts' Foundations of Parasitology,* 6th ed. Boston, MA: McGraw-Hill Companies; 2000.
36. Falkow S. What is a pathogen? *ASM News.* 1997;63:359–365.
37. Barbieri JT, Pederson KJ. Bacterial toxins in disease production. In: Brogden KA, Roth JA, Stanton TB, eds. *Virulence Mechanisms of Bacterial Pathogens,* 3rd ed. Washington, DC: ASM Press; 2000:163–174.
38. Dixon TC, Meselson M, Guillemin J, Hanna PC. Anthrax. *New Engl J Med.* 1999;341:815–826.

39. Levin BR. The evolution and maintenance of virulence in microparasites. *Emerg Infect Dis.* 1996;2:93–102.

40. Nesse RM, Williams GC. *Why We Get Sick: The New Science of Darwinian Medicine.* New York, NY: Vintage Books; 1994.

41. Brooks GF, Butel JS, Morse SA. *Jawetz, Melnick, and Adelberg's Medical Microbiology,* 22nd ed. New York, NY: Lange Medical Books/McGraw-Hill; 2001.

42. Harb OS, Kwaik YA. Interaction of *Legionella pneumophila* with protozoa provides lessons. *ASM News.* 2000;66:609–616.

43. Viswanathan VK, Cianciotto, NP. Role of iron acquisition in *Legionella pneumophila* virulence. *ASM News.* 2001;67:253–258.

44. Ruckdeschel K. *Yersinia* species disrupt immune responses to subdue the host. *ASM News.* 2000;66:470–477.

45. Janeway CA, Travers P, Walport M, Shlomchik MJ. *Immunobiology: The Immune System in Health and Disease,* 5th ed. New York, NY: Garland Publishing; 2001.

46. von Behring E, Kitasato S. The mechanism of immunity in animals to diphtheria and tetanus. In: Brock TD, ed. *Milestones in Microbiology: 1546 to 1940.* Washington, DC: ASM Press; 1999:138–141.

47. von Behring E. Studies on the mechanism of immunity to diphtheria in animals. In: Brock TD, ed. *Milestones in Microbiology: 1546 to 1940.* Washington, DC: ASM Press; 1999:141–144.

48. Metschnikoff E. A disease of daphnia caused by a yeast. A contribution to the theory of phagocytes as agents for attack on disease-causing organisms. In: Brock TD, ed. *Milestones in Microbiology: 1546 to 1940.* Washington, DC: ASM Press; 1999:132–138.

49. Dinarello CA. Cytokines as endogenous pyrogens. In: Mackowiak PA, ed. *Fever: Basic Mechanism and Management,* 2nd ed. Philadelphia, PA: Lippincott-Raven Publishers; 1997:87–116.

50. Stolley PD. Fever therapy: lessons from the history and efficacy of malariotherapy. In: Mackowiak PA, ed. *Fever: Basic Mechanism and Management,* 2nd ed. Philadelphia, PA: Lippincott-Raven Publishers; 1997:331–336.

51. Hasday JD. The influence of temperature on host defenses. In: Mackowiak PA, ed. *Fever: Basic Mechanism and Management,* 2nd ed. Philadelphia, PA: Lippincott-Raven Publishers; 1997:177–196.

52. Meydani SN, Han SN. Nutrient regulation of the immune response: the case of vitamin E. In: Bowman BA, Russell RM, eds. *Present Knowledge in Nutrition,* 8th ed. Washington, DC: ILSI Press; 2001:449–462.

53. DuPont HL, Hornick, RB. Adverse effect of Lomotil therapy in shigellosis. *JAMA.* 1973;226:1525–1528.

54. Ada G. Vaccines and vaccination. *N Engl J Med.* 2001;345:1042–1053.

55. Buckley RH. Primary immunodeficiency diseases due to defects in lymphocytes. *N Engl J Med.* 2000;343:1313–1324.

56. Busse WW, Lemanske RF. Asthma. *N Engl J Med.* 2001;344:350–362.

57. Davidson A, Diamond B. Autoimmune disease. *N Engl J Med.* 2001;345:340–350.

58. Delves PJ, Roitt IM. The immune system: first of two parts. *N Engl J Med.* 2000;343:37–49.

59. Delves PJ, Roitt IM. The immune system: second of two parts. *N Engl J Med.* 2000;343:108–117.

60. Kamradt T, Mitchison NA. Tolerance and autoimmunity. *N Engl J Med.* 2001;344:655–664.

61. Kay AB. Allergy and allergic diseases: first of two parts. *N Engl J Med.* 2001;344:30–37.

62. Kazatchkine MD, Kaveri SV. Immunodulation of autoimmune and inflammatory diseases with ultravenous immune globulin. *N Engl J Med.* 2001;345:747–755.

63. Klein J, Sako A. The HLA system. *N Engl J Med.* 2000;343:702–709.

64. Lekstrom-Himes JA, Gallin JI. Immunodeficiency disease caused by defects in phagocytes. *N Engl J Med.* 2000;343:1703–1714.

65. Medzhitov R, Janeway C. Innate immunity. *N Engl J Med.* 2000;343:338–344.

66. von Andrian UH, MacKay CR. T-cell function and migration: two sides of the same coin. *N Engl J Med.* 2000;343:1020–1034.

67. Walport MJ. Complement: first of two parts. *N Engl J Med.* 2001;344:1058–1066.

68. Walport MJ. Complement: second of two. *N Engl J Med.* 2001;344:1140–1144.

69. Zinkernagel RM. Maternal antibodies, childhood infections, and autoimmune diseases. *N Engl J Med.* 2001;345:1331–1335.

70. Whitney EN, Rolfes SR. *Understanding Nutrition,* 9th ed. Belmont, CA: Wadsworth/Thomson Learning; 2002.

71. el Lozy M, Herrera MG, Latham MC, et al. *Nutrition: A Scope Publication.* Kalamazoo, MI: The Upjohn Company; 1980.

72. Koski KG, Scott ME. Gastrointestinal nematodes, nutrition, and immunity: breaking the negative spiral. *Annu Rev Nutr.* 2001;21:297–321.

73. Adam RD. Biology of *Giardia lamblia. Clin Microbiol Rev.* 2001;14:447–475.

74. von Bonsdorff B. *Diphyllobothriasis in Man.* London, England: Academic Press; 1977.

75. Gevitz N. *The D.O.'s: Osteopathic Medicine in America.* Baltimore, MD: John Hopkins University Press; 1982.

76. Gevitz N. The sword and the scalpel—the osteopathic 'war' to enter the military medical corps: 1916–1966. *JAOA.* 1998;98:279–286.

77. Laver WG, Bischofberger N, Webster RG. Disarming flu viruses. *Sci Am.* 1999; 280:78–87.

78. Cohen ML. Epidemiology of drug resistance: implications for a postantimicrobial era. *Science.* 1992;257:1050–1055.

79. Jawetz J. Antimicrobial drugs: mechanisms and factors influencing their action. Kagan BM, ed. *Antimicrobial Therapy.* Philadelphia, PA: WB Saunders Co; 1980:3–10.

80. Noble WC, Virani Z, Cree RGA. Co-transfer of vancomycin and other resistance genes from *Enterococcus faecalis* NCTC 12201 to *Staphylococcus aureus. FEMS Microbiol Lett.* 1992;93:195–198.

81. Gorbach SL. Antimicrobial use in animal feed—time to stop. *N Engl J Med.* 2001;345:1202–1203.

82. Murray BE. Vancomycin-resistant enterococcal infections. *N Engl J Med.* 2000;342:710–721.

83. White DG, Zhao S, Sudler R, et al. The isolation of antibiotic-resistant salmonella from retail ground meats. *N Engl J Med .* 2001;345:1147–1154.

84. Pittet D, Boyce JM. Hand hygiene and patient care: pursuing the Semmelweis legacy. *Lancet Infect Dis.* 2001;April:9–20.

85. Simmons B, Bryant J, Neiman K, et al. The role of handwashing in prevention of endemic intensive care unit infections. *Infect Control Hosp Epidemiol.* 1990;11:589–594.

86. Semmelweis I. Lecture on the genesis of puerperal fever (childbed fever). In: Brock TD, ed. *Milestones in Microbiology: 1546 to 1940.* Washington, DC: ASM Press; 1999:80–82.

87. Centers for Disease Control. Outbreaks of Norwalk-like viral gastroenteritis—Alaska and Wisconsin, 1999. *MMWR.* 2000;49:207–211.

88. Centers for Disease Control. Shigellosis in child day care centers—Lexington-Fayett County, KY. *MMWR.* 1992;41:440–442.

89. Centers for Disease Control. Reptile-associated salmonellosis—selected states, 1996–1998. *MMWR.* 1999;48:1009–1013.

90. Centers for Disease Control. Salmonellosis associated with chicks and ducklings—Michigan and Missouri, spring 1999. *MMWR.* 2000;49:297–299.

91. Still AT. *Osteopathic Research and Practice.* Kirksville, MO: AT Still; 1910:454.

92. Behbehani AM. The smallpox story: life and death of an old disease. *Microbiol Rev.* 1983; 47:455–509.

93. Tucker JB. *Scourge: The Once and Future Threat of Smallpox.* New York, NY: Atlantic Monthly Press; 2001.

94. Jenner E. An inquiry into the causes and effects of the variolae vaccinae, a disease discovered in some of the western counties of England, particularly Gloucestershire, and known by the name of the cow pox. In: Brock TD, ed. *Milestones in Microbiology: 1546 to 1940.* Washington, DC: ASM Press; 1999:121–125.

95. Maurice J. Virus wins a stay of execution. *Science.* 1995;267:450.

96. Centers for Disease Control. Smallpox surveillance—worldwide. *MMWR.* 1997;46:990–994.

97. Centers for Disease Control. Vaccinia (smallpox) vaccine: recommendations of the advisory committee on immunization practices (ACIP), 2001. *MMWR.* 2001;50(RR10):1–25.

ENDOCRINE SYSTEM AND BODY UNITY: OSTEOPATHIC PRINCIPLES AT A CHEMICAL LEVEL

RONALD PORTANOVA

KEY CONCEPTS

A review of the general chemical types of hormones (amines, peptides/proteins, and steroids) and for each chemical type of hormone a discussion regarding:

- Biosynthesis, storage, and release
- Characteristics of transport in the blood
- Mechanism of action (receptor, signal transduction, and effector mechanisms)
- Metabolism/degradation
- "Classic" endocrine glands, the hormone(s) secreted, the mechanisms that control the rate of hormone secretion, including feedback (positive, negative) mechanisms, and the principal biologic action(s) of the hormone(s)

A review of the integration of hormone action with regard to the regulation of:

- Reproduction
- Growth and development
- Energy management
- Preservation and stabilization of the internal environment
- Intimate relationship between the principles that underlie endocrinology and the principles that guide the study and practice of osteopathic medicine

---

The endocrine system is a whole-body communications system. Endocrine information is transmitted in the form of structurally specific chemical messengers, the hormones, and received by equally specific chemical structures, the cell receptors. The endocrine system participates in the control and integration of bodily processes that are fundamental to human life:

- Reproduction, growth, and development
- Energy management
- Preservation and stabilization of the internal environment

ENDOCRINOLOGY

Terms and Definitions

The traditional view of hormones and endocrine glands dates from the work of Baylis and Starling in the early part of the 20th century. A hormone is an information-carrying molecule, secreted in small amounts by a specific gland and transported in the blood to a distant site, where it exerts its biologic effect. These ideas pertain to what might be called the traditional or classic hormones and endocrine glands. It is now clear that certain hormones and hormonelike substances (e.g., prostaglandins, various growth factors) do not fit this description. These nonclassic hormones have two key characteristics:

1. They are produced in organs not normally thought of as endocrine glands; for example, atrial natriuretic peptide (ANP) is secreted by the heart. The kidney produces renin, erythropoietin, and the hormonally active metabolite of vitamin D $(1,25\text{-}[OH]2\text{-}D3)$.
2. They may act locally, without transport in the blood, on contiguous cells or even on the cells that produce them, functions that are referred to, respectively, as paracrine and autocrine.

Chemical Structure of Hormones

Endocrine information is encoded in specific chemical structure. Every hormone is structurally unique; seemingly minor differences in chemical structure can dramatically affect the activity of the molecule. Nevertheless, chemically, all of the hormones considered below fall into one of three broad structural categories (Table 11.1):

1. Amino acid derivatives
2. Peptides and proteins
3. Steroids

These structural categories are associated with typical physical and chemical characteristics that have important functional implications.

TABLE 11.1. CLASSIC ENDOCRINE GLANDS AND HORMONES BASED ON STRUCTURE[a]

Chemical Structure	Gland	Hormone	Major Target and/or Function
Amines	Adrenal medulla	Epinephrine, norepinephrine	Whole-body adaptation to stress, including regulation of cardiovascular system (CVS) and energy flux
	Thyroid	Thyroxine (T_4), triiodothyronine (T_3)	Whole-body including central nervous system (CNS); growth and development, organ system performance, energy metabolism
Peptides and proteins	Neurohypophysis	Vasopressin (AVP, antidiuretic hormone [ADH])	Nephron, water metabolism; CVS, regulation of blood flow/pressure
		Oxytocin	Smooth muscle; milk let down, uterine motility
	Hypophysis, pars intermedia	Melanocyte-stimulating hormone (MSH)	Melanocytes in lower vertebrates; however, role in humans unknown
	Adenohypophysis	Adrenocorticotropic hormone (ACTH), corticotropin	Adrenal cortex; regulation of growth and functional status (especially steroidogenesis)
		Prolactin (PRL)	Mammary; growth of gland and milk synthesis
		Growth hormone (GH) (somatotropic hormone [STH], somatotropin)	Whole body; growth and development, organic metabolism
		Thyroid-stimulating hormone (TSH, thyrotropin)[b]	Thyroid; regulation of growth and functional status (especially thyroid hormone secretion)
		Follicle-stimulating hormone (FSH)[b] Luteinizing hormone (LH)[b]	Gonads; regulation of reproduction including gamete production and development and gonadal steroidogenesis
	Hypothalamus	Corticotropin-releasing hormone (CRH) Thyrotropin-releasing hormone (TRH) Gonadotropin-releasing hormone (GnRH, FSH/LH-releasing hormone) Growth hormone-releasing hormone (GH-RH, somatocrinin) Growth hormone-inhibiting hormone (somatostatin)	Adenohypophysis, regulation of adenohypophysial hormone secretion; also found at other sites (extrahypothalamic regions of CNS, pancreas, others) and may serve neurotransmitter, neuromodulation, or other local (paracrine) functions
	Blood (via hepatic precursor), CNS	Angiotensin	Adrenal cortex; regulation of steroidogenesis (aldosterone); CNS, neurotransmission/modulation
	Parathyroids	Parathyroid hormone (PTH, parathormone)	Bone/kidney; regulation of calcium and phosphate metabolism
	Pancreatic islets, β-cells	Insulin	Liver, adipocyte, muscle, other; regulation of energy metabolism, plasma levels of glucose and other metabolites; widespread anabolic actions
	Pancreatic islets, α-cells	Glucagon	Liver, adipocyte, regulation of energy metabolism, mobilizes glucose and other oxidative substrates
	Thyroid, C cells	Calcitonin	Bone, calcium metabolism
Steroids	Adrenal cortex, zona fasciculata	Cortisol	Liver, adipocyte, muscle, other; energy metabolism, widespread catabolic actions; adaptations to a wide variety of whole-body noxious insults (stresses)
	Adrenal cortex, zona glomerulosa	Aldosterone	Nephron, sweat glands, salivary glands, other; promotes sodium retention and potassium loss
	Ovary	Estrogens (E_2, E_3)	Reproductive tract, mammary; regulation of growth, development, function; tissue-specific anabolic effects
		Progesterone	Reproductive tract, mammary; regulation of reproduction, lactation

(continued)

TABLE 11.1. (*continued*)

Chemical Structure	Gland	Hormone	Major Target and/or Function
	Testes T-sensitive tissues (via T as precursor)[c]	Testosterone (T) Dihydrotestosterone (DHT)	Reproductive tract; regulation of growth, development, function; tissue-specific and general somatic anabolic effects

[a]The information contained in this table is not intended to be all-inclusive. A given hormone may be produced at multiple sites and may be known by additional synonyms. Certainly, with regard to hormone-responsive targets and function, the information summarized here is grossly incomplete; many targets and biologic actions, indeed important biologic actions, are not included. It must also be stressed that only those glands and substances "classically" recognized as primarily endocrine in nature are included. Indeed, a comprehensive tabulation of the large and growing list of hormones (or hormonelike substances) would include, at least, the following: the pituitary endorphins and lipotropins, the placental hormones (human chorionic gonadotropin [hCG] and human placental lactogen [hPL]), additional pancreatic and gastrointestinal hormones (gastrin, vasoactive intestinal peptide [VIP], pancreatic polypeptide, cholecystokinin [CCK], gastric inhibitory peptide [GIP], and secretin), as well as a number of hormones produced in organs traditionally considered to be nonendocrine, such as heart (atrial natriuretic peptides [ANPs], kidney (cholecalciferol metabolites, erythropoeitin [ESF], renin), lymphocytes (interleukins), liver (insulinlike growth peptides [IGPs, somatomedins]), platelets (growth or transforming factors, including platelet derived growth factor [PDGF] and tumor growth factor [TGF-β]), and other sites (various growth and/or transforming factors, including epidermal growth factor [EGF] and TGF-α).
[b]TSH, FSH, and LH contain a carbohydrate moiety attached to the protein component and are thus glycoproteins.
[c]Testosterone is converted to DHT in various peripheral tissues; both metabolites, T and DHT, are biologically active.

ENDOCRINOLOGY AND OSTEOPATHY

This chapter discusses the basic elements of endocrine physiology. The information is presented in summary form and is meant to serve as a guide for further study.[1] The information is organized with reference to principles that guide the study and practice of osteopathic medicine. This arrangement is didactic and natural since body unity is the focus of endocrinology and osteopathy.

STRUCTURE AND FUNCTION

Structure and function are not only interrelated but are inseparably linked at all levels of the biologic spectrum.

The interdependence of structure and function, a basic principle of osteopathic medicine, is also a fundamental principle of endocrinology. Indeed, the specific biologic activity of a hormone originates in the structural characteristics of the molecule. Endocrine physiology is most usefully studied and understood in terms of molecular structure. In the following discussion the interrelation of hormone structure and function is considered in relation to endocrine processes that underlie the actions of all hormones. In this regard, it is useful to view the hormone as part of a simple endocrine system (Fig. 11.1), consisting of the following:

1. An endocrine gland and the hormone it produces
2. A transport system to deliver the hormone from its site of production to its site(s) of action
3. An effector organ (target) that undergoes a biologic change in response to the hormone

The biochemical events that occur in the endocrine gland are referred to as cellular processing. They include the biosynthesis, storage, and release of the hormone. Transport of the hormone in the plasma depends on the physical and chemical characteristics of the hormone. The nature of the transport process is an important determinant of the metabolism of the hormone and

its rate of removal from the plasma, that is, the metabolic clearance rate (MCR) of the hormone. The biochemical events that account for the biologic change in the target are referred to as the mechanism of action of the hormone. These three fundamental components of an endocrine system—cellular processing, transport, and mechanism of action—are considered in the following sections with reference to the inexorable link between structure and function.

Cellular Processing

The cellular and subcellular events involved in the biosynthesis, storage, and release of hormones are generally differentiated and grouped on the basis of the chemical structure of the hormone (peptide/protein, steroid, and amine).

Peptides and Proteins

The biosynthesis of peptide and protein hormones is basically consistent with the typical pattern of eukaryotic protein synthesis. That is, specific messenger RNAs are transcribed in the nucleus on DNA and carry the genetic message to the cytoplasm, where it is translated into the specific sequence of amino acids that constitute the hormone. In the case of proteins to be exported from the cell, including hormones, peptide bond formation occurs on membrane-bound ribosomes, that is, the rough endoplasmic reticulum (RER). As peptide bond formation occurs, the polypeptide is extruded through the lipid membrane of the endoplasmic reticulum, sequestered within the lumen of the RER, and transported to the Golgi apparatus, where it is packaged into secretory vesicles. During this entire process, the polypeptide is effectively segregated from other cellular proteins and constituents of the cell cytosol. This feature has the

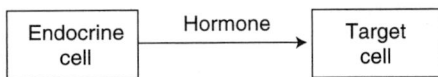

FIGURE 11.1. A simple endocrine system consisting of the endocrine cell and the hormone it produces, the transport system to deliver the hormone from its site of production to its site of action, and the target (effector) cell that undergoes a biologic change in response to the hormone.

---

[1]In this text, the reader will find Chapters 7 (by Patterson and Wurster), 8 (by Willard), 9 (by Sparks), and 10 (by Jensen and Jensen) especially useful.

advantage of simultaneously protecting and concentrating the nascent polypeptide.

The molecule that is initially synthesized on the RER is not the hormone per se, but rather one of two larger precursor molecules, referred to as a prohormone or a pre-prohormone. The authentic (mature) hormone is formed by sequential proteolytic cleavages of the precursor as it is transported through the RER and packaged into secretory vesicles in the Golgi apparatus. In response to an adequate stimulus, the secretory vesicles fuse with the cell membrane and release their contents, including the hormone, into the extracellular perivascular space. This bulk transport process is known as exocytosis, or reverse pinocytosis, and characteristically involves these processes:

- Expenditure of energy (adenosine triphosphate)
- Mobilization of calcium ion
- Participation of the contractile microtubular system

In most cases, as a means of rapidly responding to demands for increased hormone secretion, polypeptide hormone-secreting cells store ample amounts of hormone-filled secretory vesicles. That is, the hormone has been presynthesized and prepackaged and is held in the cell in a form ready for release.

Steroids

Just as polypeptide hormone-secreting cells are able to respond rapidly to circumstances that require increased secretion of the hormone, so too are cells that secrete steroid hormones. The strategy employed by these cells is different from that already described. The cells that secrete steroid hormones (adrenocortical, ovarian, testicular) all originate from a common embryologic site, the primitive urogenital ridge. As such, it is not surprising that these functionally distinct cells are not only structurally similar but also employ basically similar pathways for steroid hormone biosynthesis (steroidogenesis).

In all cases, steroid hormones are produced from a common precursor, cholesterol, via sequential enzymatic modifications of the steroid nucleus. The steroid-secreting cells store large amounts of esterified-cholesterol (in the form of fat droplets). The intracellular pool of the precursor is maintained by cholesterol biosynthesis in the cell and also by taking up preformed cholesterol from the blood. Ring modifications to the steroid nucleus are catalyzed by enzymes associated with specific subcellular structures (e.g., mitochondria, endoplasmic reticulum). The enzyme profile of the cell determines the nature and location of the ring modifications. In so doing, it determines whether the final steroid product is cortisol, aldosterone, androgen, or estrogen. Steroid hormones are highly lipid-soluble and are released from the cell by simple diffusion across the plasma membrane. Unlike peptide and protein hormones, the steroids are not packaged into secretory vesicles and are not stored within the cells in significant amounts. Increasing the rate of steroid synthesis meets demands for increased secretion of the hormones.

Amino Acid Derivatives

The amine-type hormones are secreted by the adrenal medulla (catecholamines, including epinephrine and norepinephrine) and the thyroid gland (triiodothyronine and thyroxine). In both glands, the active hormones are derived from a precursor, the amino acid tyrosine, supplied via the blood. Once formed, the catecholamines are packaged into secretory granules and stored within the cell. Release of the hormones occurs by means of an exocytotic process similar to that described for peptide and protein hormones.

The biosynthesis and release of the thyroid hormones is closely tied to the metabolism of a large glycoprotein, thyroglobulin. Thyroid hormones are derived from the iodination and linkage of two residues of the amino acid tyrosine. During the entire biosynthetic sequence, however, the tyrosine molecules are not free within the cell but instead are incorporated into thyroglobulin via peptide bonds. After the thyroid hormones are formed, they remain covalently linked to thyroglobulin. This macromolecule, thyroglobulin with its attached hormones, comprises the major constituent of a gelatinous material known as the thyroid colloid. Large amounts of the colloid are stored in the lumen of the thyroid follicle, that is, outside of the thyroid follicular cell.

Release of the thyroid hormones involves the exquisite interplay of several subcellular organelles. In brief, follicular cells take up droplets of colloid (by endocytosis). In the cell, lysosomes (containing hydrolytic enzymes) merge with the colloid droplets, and proteolysis of the thyroglobulin molecule frees the active thyroid hormones that then diffuse across the cell membrane and enter the bloodstream. It is difficult to imagine that A.T. Still would not consider the subcellular ballet involved in production and release of the thyroid hormones to be a graphic representation of the interrelationship of structure and function.

Transport and Metabolism

Once the hormone is released at its site of production, it is transported in the blood to a distant target site, where it produces a biologic change. The magnitude of the change in the target, the biologic response, is proportional to the concentration of the hormone in the blood. This, in turn, is a function not only of the rate at which the hormone enters the blood (rate of secretion), but also of the rate at which it is removed from the blood, that is, the MCR. The characteristics of a particular hormone's transport process have a significant effect on the MCR and therefore on the biologic action of the hormone.

In general, hormones circulate in the blood in one of two ways, depending on the chemical structure and solubility characteristics of the molecule. Amine and polypeptide hormones are readily soluble in the aqueous phase of the plasma and circulate in a free, unbound form. In contrast, steroid and thyroid hormones are hydrophobic and travel in the blood in association with carrier proteins. The carrier, or transport, protein may be a specific plasma globulin with high-affinity binding sites for a particular hormone (e.g., testosterone-binding globulin, or TeBG). It can also be a nonspecific plasma protein (e.g., albumin) that associates loosely with a number of hormones.

Several aspects of the binding of hormones to carrier proteins are of particular importance and again underscore the notion that form indeed gives rise to function. First, only the free, unbound fraction of the hormone is biologically active. Functionally, the transport protein-hormone complex serves as a circulating hormone reservoir that can be used to augment or replenish the free, biologically active, hormone pool.

Second, changes in plasma levels of binding proteins occur both physiologically (e.g., cortisol-binding globulin levels increase during pregnancy) and pathologically (e.g., liver disease). Such changes are reflected in the total (bound plus free) hormone concentration, but not necessarily in the concentration of free, biologically active hormone. This is of practical importance to the osteopathic physician, since diagnostic procedures may measure total plasma hormone, an unreliable index of the actual activity of the hormone.

Third, the MCR of a circulating hormone is directly related to its binding characteristics. Hormones that are tightly bound to carrier proteins have a longer lifetime in the plasma than hormones that circulate in a free or loosely bound form (e.g., respectively, thyroxine, days versus vasopressin, minutes).

Mechanism of Action

The mechanism of action of a hormone refers to the sequence of chemical and morphologic events that mediate the specific biologic action of the molecule on a particular target tissue. At minimum, these intermediary processes must account for certain general characteristics of hormone action. That is, hormones are distributed (via the blood) indiscriminately throughout the body, but only certain tissues (targets) respond to the hormone. A particular tissue may respond to only one hormone or to several different hormones. Some hormones act on only a single tissue or tissue type, whereas other hormones act at numerous, distinct sites. Finally, a particular hormone may elicit widely differing responses in different target tissues.

Hydrophilic Hormones

Peptide hormones and catecholamines act on target cells through a four-stage process.

Stage 1. Hormone Receptor Interaction: Signal Generation

Stage 1 occurs when the interaction of the hormone with a specific, high-affinity receptor on the cell membrane signals the initiation of the response sequence. It is the presence or absence of the receptor that determines whether the cell responds to the hormone. A particular cell may have receptors for one or more hormones. Fasciculata cells in the adrenal cortex respond selectively to adrenocorticotropic hormone (ACTH), whereas adipose cells respond to several hormones, including glucagon, epinephrine, ACTH, and vasopressin. Both the number of receptors and the affinity of the receptors are physiologically regulated and significantly affect the biologic response. Moreover, abnormal receptor structure and/or function is an important component of the pathophysiology of endocrine disorders (e.g., diabetes mellitus).

Stage 2. Signal Transduction

In stage 2, signal transduction, hormone receptor interaction influences the guanine nucleotide-sensitive components of the cell membrane, G-proteins, which, in turn, regulate (increase or decrease) the generation of substances referred to as second messengers.

Stage 3. Second Messengers

Stage 3 is that of the second messengers. The hormone (first messenger) initiates the biologic response, but the response is mediated by intracellular second messengers. Cyclic adenosine monophosphate (cAMP) was the first of the intracellular mediators to be recognized, but it is now clear that other substances also fill this role, including, for example, cyclic guanosine monophosphate (cGMP), calcium ion, and phospholipid metabolites such as diacylglycerol and inositol triphosphate.

Stage 4. Biologic Response

Stage 4 occurs when the second messenger interacts with the chemical machinery of the cell to produce the biologic response. The interaction normally involves a change in the activity of a protein, often an enzyme. It is this protein (enzyme) that determines the characteristics of the biologic response. For instance, in the hepatocyte, cAMP generated in response to glucagon stimulates the phosphorylase enzymes and glycogen breakdown. In the adipocyte, glucagon increases the production of cAMP, activation of an enzyme known as hormone-sensitive lipase, and the hydrolysis of triglyceride.

One characteristic feature of peptide and protein hormones requires further discussion. A particular hormone may elicit widely differing responses in different target tissues. For example, the same posterior pituitary hormone that produces antidiuresis in the nephron produces vasoconstriction in the vasculature and thus is known, respectively, as antidiuretic hormone (ADH) and vasopressin. In the case of the parathyroid hormone (PTH), even a partial list of biologic actions and respective targets would include:

- Phosphaturia and bicarbonaturia in renal proximal tubules
- Increased calcium reabsorption in renal distal tubules
- Bone resorption in osteoblasts
- Increased thymidine incorporation in osteocytes

The presence of multiple distinct biologic actions within a single molecule gives rise to the notion that some hormones may contain multiple distinct structural features (amino acid sequences); that is, that some hormones are in fact polyhormones.

Lipophilic Hormones

Steroid hormones and thyroid hormones enter the target cell and bind to specific receptor proteins, localized primarily within the nucleus. The hormone-receptor complex regulates the transcription of specific genetic segments in DNA and ultimately the synthesis of specific messenger RNAs and cellular proteins. In contrast to the hydrophilic hormones that regulate the activity of existing cellular proteins (enzymes), the response to lipophilic hormones is mediated by changes in the amount of new protein (enzyme). The final biologic response is characterized by the chemical activity (function) of the protein(s) synthesized in response to the hormone. It can range from the increased synthesis of a particular enzyme or functionally related group of enzymes, such as increased hepatic synthesis of gluconeogenic enzymes in response to cortisol, to cellular differentiation and tissue growth, such as prostate hypertrophy in response to androgens.

THE BODY FUNCTIONS AS A WHOLE

The body functions as a whole. It is regulated, coordinated, and integrated through multiple interactive systems.

Hormones play a major role in the orchestration of body unity. In this endeavor, the endocrine system does not operate in isolation but is interdependent with other body systems. The following discussion deals with the interrelation of endocrine, cardiovascular, and neural function.

Cardiovascular System

Endocrine function is dependent on cardiovascular function. This is most obvious in that hormones rely on the cardiovascular system (CVS) as a means of transport to distant sites. The transport function of the CVS usually involves the systemic circulation, but other specialized vascular networks are also employed to great advantage (discussed subsequently). The circulatory system also participates in controlling the secretion of hormones and in determining the magnitude of their effect at the site of action (target). That is, alterations in blood flow to the endocrine gland contribute to alterations in secretion rate. For example, hyperemia often accompanies increased secretion, and changes in blood flow to the target affect the rate of delivery and the effect of the hormone. Commensurate with the role of the CVS in endocrine function, endocrine glands are typically highly vascularized. For example, throughout the mammalian kingdom, blood supply to the pituitary (mL per mg of tissue weight) is greater than that of any other tissue. In the adrenal gland, cells of the zona fasciculata are arranged in bicellular columns separated by capillaries; that is, each cell is in direct contact with a capillary.

While the endocrine system clearly depends on cardiovascular function, hormones have a major influence on the CVS:

Catecholamines have well-known actions on the heart and vasculature.

Adrenergic cardiac fibers influence myocardial contractility and rhythm.

Adrenergic vasoconstrictor fibers are a dominant influence on systemic vascular resistance.

Catecholamines of adrenal medullary origin and a number of other hormones also influence the CVS:

Vasopressin and angiotensin are vasoconstrictors.

Thyroid hormones affect heart rate.

Thyroid hormones and aldosterone increase the force of ventricular contraction.

In addition to these direct actions, endocrine mechanisms (the renin-angiotensin-aldosterone system, antidiuretic hormone, ANPs) are an important component in the regulation of whole-body fluid and electrolyte metabolism, the extracellular fluid (ECF) and blood volume and, indirectly, cardiovascular function. The endocrine mechanisms serve to maintain fluid homeostasis and cardiovascular function under normal conditions and to protect cardiovascular function against the consequences of challenges such as water deprivation or hemorrhage.

Nervous System

A wide variety of external stimuli, or changes in the external environment, alter the activity of the endocrine system by means of multisynaptic neural pathways. For example, auditory stimuli activate the hypothalamic-pituitary axis and increase cortisol secretion. Light cycles influence endocrine rhythms, and groups of females living together may develop synchronous periods of gonadotropin secretion and ovarian function. Changes in the internal environment, such as the chemical composition of the blood, directly affect hormone secretion without the necessity of neural intervention (discussed subsequently). Nevertheless, even in cases like this, neural influences may play a role. Insulin secretion is a typical example: Although glucose and other metabolites stimulate release of the polypeptide, β-cell innervation (sympathetic and parasympathetic) modulates the secretory response.

Just as the nervous system influences endocrine activity, hormones have significant effects on neural activity. The endocrine effects can range from actions on single neurons to alterations of complex mental activity and behavior.

Peptides

A number of peptide hormones have been found to alter central nervous system (CNS) activity. For example, vasopressin acts in the CNS to decrease body temperature and to improve memory. In some cases, peptide hormones have been found not only to act in the CNS but also to be produced in the CNS. Examples of these hormones include the ANPs and angiotensin, which, respectively, inhibit and stimulate the sensation of thirst.

Steroids

Gonadal and adrenocortical steroids affect the activity of the hypothalamic neurons that control the anterior pituitary. They thus play a major role in regulating pituitary-gonadal and pituitary-adrenocortical activity. Moreover, both types of steroids influence complex patterns of neural activity; for example, androgens stimulate libido (sex drive) in both males and females. Cortisol deficiency (adrenal insufficiency, Addison disease) is accompanied by an abnormal electroencephalographic pattern and behavioral and emotional disturbances, including anxiety and depression. The cortisol deficiency is corrected by administering the steroid, but caution must be exercised since cortisol excesses also lead to behavioral disorders.

Amines

The actions of the thyroid amines on the development and function of the CNS are especially profound. Thus, infantile hypothyroidism (cretinism) is associated with retarded mental development. The earlier the condition appears and the longer it goes untreated, the more severe the effects, culminating in irreversible damage to the brain. Congenital hypothyroidism is a current leading cause of preventable mental deficiency. Even after the developmental period, thyroid hormones influence neural activity. In the adult, thyroid status is related to gross behavior such as alertness, mental acuity, and irritability.

In some cases the interaction of endocrine and neural function is so complete that the distinction between the two systems is in fact blurred. Nowhere is this more evident than in the hypothalamic-pituitary complex, where neural and endocrine activity are combined in the same neuroendocrine cell. The peptide hormones oxytocin and vasopressin are secreted by neurons having their cell bodies located in the hypothalamus and sending their axons into the neurohypophysis (posterior pituitary). Instead of ending on another nerve or effector, such as a muscle, the neuroendocrine cells terminate on pituitary capillaries and release their hormones into the systemic circulation. Another group of hypothalamic neuroendocrine cells deliver their hormones not to the systemic circulation, but rather to a specialized (portal) vascular system that supplies blood to the adenohypophysis (anterior pituitary). These cells, referred to as hypophysiotropic neurons, regulate the secretory activity of the anterior pituitary.

Final Common Path

Neural influences predominate in the regulation of anterior pituitary hormone secretion. It is well known that ACTH secretion is related to photoperiod. Growth hormone secretion is associated with sleep stages. Light, odor, auditory, and tactile stimuli as well as emotional disturbances influence gonadotropin secretion and reproductive function. For a time, the relationship between anterior pituitary and CNS function presented a conceptual difficulty, since the adenohypophyseal secretory cells are not innervated. (The anterior pituitary is innervated by vasomotor fibers.) Indeed, the (older) endocrine literature refers to the anterior pituitary as a gland under neural control, but lacking a nerve supply.

The physical link between the CNS and the anterior pituitary is not neural but vascular, consisting of a specialized arrangement of vessels, alternatively known as the pituitary portal vessels or the hypothalamic-hypophyseal portal vessels. In brief, the anterior pituitary is regulated by neurohormones that are produced in the hypothalamus and transported to the pituitary in the portal venous blood. The portal vessels originate in a capillary network (primary plexus) located in the hypothalamus. The capillaries coalesce to form the pituitary portal veins, which enter the anterior pituitary and give rise to a secondary capillary plexus. The hypothalamic neurohormones, hypophysiotropic hormones, are produced by neurons that terminate in the hypothalamus in close contact with the primary capillary plexus. The neurohormones enter the portal venous blood and are delivered to the anterior pituitary. This exquisite interrelationship of neural, vascular, and endocrine function is sometimes referred to as the final common path.

Sir Geoffrey Harris postulated the functional significance of the pituitary portal vessels about 40 years ago. It is a credit to A.T. Still that he recognized the importance of such relationships almost half a century earlier.

SELF-REGULATING, SELF-HEALING

The body is inherently self-regulating and self-healing. Responses to internal and external events are modulated through feedback mechanisms with homeostasis of the internal environment, the internal milieu, as a major goal.

Homeostasis of the internal environment is a primary goal of endocrine physiology. To accomplish this goal, the rate of hormone secretion is modulated according to changes in the internal environment. The relationship between hormones and the internal environment is completely interactive: Changes in the internal environment affect hormone secretion, and changes in hormone concentration influence the composition of the internal environment.

Regulation of Hormone Secretion

The rate of hormone secretion is controlled by specific chemical signals that increase or decrease the rate of hormone biosynthesis and release. The chemical signals include neural transmitters (e.g., acetylcholine, norepinephrine), supplied at a synaptic junction, and numerous constituents of the blood and extracellular fluid, such as:

- Various substrates (e.g., glucose, amino acids)
- Ions (e.g., sodium, potassium, calcium)
- Other hormones

Regardless of the chemical nature of the signal(s), in all cases the rate of hormone secretion is tightly coupled to demands for the hormone. This is in response to changes in the internal environment, which in turn are, of course, responsive to changes in the external environment. The control mechanisms are designed to ensure that the rate of hormone secretion is, in fact, appropriate to environmental conditions. When these mechanisms succeed, as they usually do, the hormone plays a vital role in the self-regulating and self-healing aspects of the body. On the other hand, failure of these mechanisms leads to hormone imbalances and the creation of an internal environment hostile to the health, well being, and even the very survival of the individual.

Control Mechanisms

The secretion of a hormone is typically controlled by a self-regulating servomechanism designed to match circulating concentrations of the hormone to the momentary needs of the individual. Two essential features of the control scheme are readily apparent. First, the systemic concentration of the hormone, or of some variable related to the hormone, such as a metabolite, must be monitored. Second, this information must be returned or fed back to the endocrine organ. The secretion of the hormone is adjusted up or down according to the nature of the information returned: inhibitory, negative feedback or stimulatory, positive feedback.

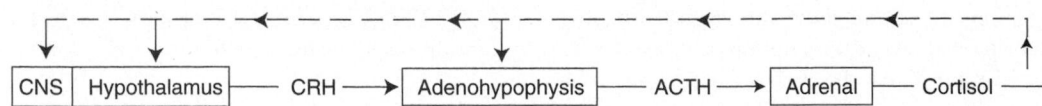

FIGURE 11.2. Cortisol feeds back at several sites to dampen activity of hypothalamic-pituitary-adrenal axis and ultimately to limit its own secretion. *CNS,* central nervous system; *CRH,* corticotropin-releasing hormone; *ACTH,* adrenocorticotropic hormone; *solid arrow,* stimulates; *dashed arrow,* inhibits.

Negative feedback mechanisms are more common than positive feedback mechanisms throughout the endocrine system. Negative feedback mechanisms are inherently self-limiting. In their most basic form they operate as follows:

1. The hormone produces a response in a target cell.
2. Some feature of that response acts back on the cell that produces the hormone to decrease (limit) its secretion.

For example, the adenohypophysis secretes ACTH, which then acts on fasciculata cells in the adrenal cortex to stimulate the production of cortisol. Cortisol has widespread effects throughout the body. One important action of the steroid is to act back on the adenohypophysis to inhibit ACTH secretion.

This closed-loop information pathway is diagrammed in Fig. 11.2 as one component of a multifaceted control scheme that regulates the hypothalamic-pituitary-adrenocortical axis. This complex control scheme includes several hormones and multiple negative feedback loops. The first hormone, corticotropin-releasing hormone (CRH), is produced in the hypothalamus and delivered to the pituitary in the portal venous blood. The hypothalamic peptide stimulates the secretion of a second hormone, ACTH, that enters the systemic circulation, and activates the adrenocortical secretion of still another hormone, cortisol. The adrenal steroid feeds back on the anterior pituitary, the hypothalamus, and on other sites in the CNS. Negative feedback effects at these several loci all contribute to dampen the activity of the hypothalamic-pituitary-adrenal axis and ultimately to limit the secretion of cortisol. Since negative feedback mechanisms are inherently self-limiting in nature, it is perhaps not apparent that this mechanism is equally important as a means of increasing hormone secretion. For example, inadequate circulating levels of cortisol are accompanied by decreased negative feedback that leads to activation of the hypothalamic-pituitary-adrenal axis and increased secretion of the steroid.

As noted, positive feedback mechanisms are also employed to control endocrine systems. Here, two hormones (or other variables) change in the same direction, so that an initial increase in the activity of the system leads to further increased activity. This type of mechanism does not limit, but rather, amplifies the magnitude of the effect and produces an abrupt, explosive change in the activity of the system.

Although positive feedback mechanisms are rather uncommon, they nevertheless play a vital role in regulating certain aspects of endocrine function. A particularly noteworthy example is the role of positive feedback in regulating reproductive function. The pituitary gonadotropins, follicle-stimulating hormone and luteinizing hormone (FSH and LH, respectively), stimulate the production of estrogen. The steroid acts back on the ovary to promote growth and development of the ovarian follicle and additional estrogen secretion. As a consequence, plasma concentrations of estrogen rise dramatically. Near the midpoint of the menstrual cycle, the high-circulating levels of steroid trigger a sudden, marked increase in LH secretion, which, in turn, induces ovulation. Ovulation depends on the preovulatory LH surge, and LH secretion is driven by the positive feedback effects of estrogen at two primary sites: the ovary and the pituitary. The importance of these events to normal reproductive function is underscored by the fact that contraceptive steroid regimens are expressly designed to create steroid imbalances that prevent the preovulatory LH surge.

Temporal Patterns

As described, the rate of hormone secretion is tightly controlled and responsive to physiologic demands. Although it is clear that secretion rate (the amount of hormone delivered to the blood per unit time) influences the circulating concentration and activity of the hormone, hormone activity is not a simple function of concentration. That is, the temporal pattern of changes in secretory rate and circulating concentration of the hormone also influence hormone activity. Many, perhaps all, endocrine glands secrete hormones in a repetitive stop-and-go fashion, a quiescent period followed by a burst of secretory activity. This leads to small but physiologically significant oscillations in plasma hormone concentrations. This secretory pattern, referred to as pulsatile or episodic secretion, has two important characteristics:

1. The rate of hormone secretion (amount/time) is the product of the frequency (episodes/time) and amplitude (amount/episode) of the secretory episodes.
2. Changes in secretory rate are produced by corresponding changes in both parameters; for example, negative feedback signals decrease both the frequency and amplitude of the secretory episodes.

Episodic secretion is characteristically associated with high-frequency oscillations in secretory activity: Release episodes are separated by only brief intervals of time (minutes). In some cases the high-frequency secretory episodes are superimposed upon other lower frequency temporal patterns or rhythms having periodicities of hours, days, or even months. For example, ACTH and the pituitary gonadotropins are secreted episodically and display high-frequency oscillations in plasma concentration. At the same time, plasma levels of ACTH (and also cortisol) are well known to cycle on a daily basis, in the classic diurnal rhythm. In reproductively competent females, pituitary gonadotropins (and also the gonadal steroids) cycle rhythmically within approximately a 1-month period.

The cellular and molecular mechanisms that generate patterned or rhythmic hormone secretion are not well understood. The implication of phasic hormone release also requires further study. Nevertheless, it is clear in a few cases that the oscillations are physiologically significant. For example, inadequate secretion of hypothalamic luteinizing hormone-releasing hormone (LH-RH) leads to reproductive failure. This condition is corrected by administration of the peptide, but only if the LH-RH is given in a pulsatile fashion that approximates normal endogenous secretion.

Processes Regulated by Hormones

Hormones are involved in regulating the most fundamental aspects of human life. Indeed, hormones play a vital role with regard to the survival of the species. That role includes:

- Reproduction
- Growth
- Development to reproductive maturity

Hormones also play a vital role with regard to the survival of the individual:

- Maintenance of the internal environment
- Energy metabolism

Reproduction

Hormones produced by the hypothalamus (gonadotropin-releasing hormone, or GnRH), the pituitary (FSH, LH, prolactin (PRL), growth hormone), and the gonads (androgens, estrogens, progestogens) interact to regulate reproductive function. Reproductive competence requires the ability to produce gametes (ova, sperm) and the ability to unite the gametes by attracting and mating with members of the opposite sex. There are several aspects of this process:

- Gamete formation (e.g., spermatogenesis, oogenesis)
- Mating ability (e.g., growth, development, maintenance of the reproductive tract)
- Mutual attractiveness (e.g., male and female phenotype, pattern of sexual behavior)

All are influenced by or totally depend on the reproductive hormones. After conception, maternal support for the developing fetus (pregnancy) is hormone-dependent, and in mammals, even after birth, hormones continue to play a role in nurturing the infant during lactation.

Growth and Development

The regulation of intrauterine growth is poorly understood. Surprisingly, hormones that have dramatic effects on the neonate (growth hormone, thyroid hormone) appear to have little influence on fetal growth. Somatomedins and other growth factors undoubtedly play a role in prenatal growth, but much research must be done to clarify that role.

The regulation of postnatal growth is better understood. In addition to a number of nonhormonal factors, such as nutrition, hygiene, and general health, normal growth and development depend on the interplay of several hormones, including:

- Growth hormone and the somatomedins
- Thyroid hormone
- Insulin
- Cortisol
- Gonadal steroids

Imbalances in the secretion of these hormones, excesses as well as deficiencies, dramatically affect growth, especially if the imbalance occurs during the normal growing period. For example, hyposecretion of growth hormone produces dwarfism. Hypersecretion of the hormone leads to giantism. Thyroid-hormone deficit impairs growth of the body and also has devastating effects on the development of the CNS and mental capacity. Cortisol or the gonadal steroids in excess slow or even arrest growth and lead to short adult stature.

Internal Environment

Many, and in a broad sense all, hormones participate in the defense of the internal environment. Although no aspect of the internal environment is unimportant to health and well being, certain features are regulated and guarded especially closely by functional groups of hormones. These include:

1. Ionic composition ($Na+$, $K+$, and $H+$) of the body fluids, most notably the blood and cerebrospinal fluid (the renin-angiotensin-aldosterone system, ANP, insulin, and other hormones)
2. Volume of the body fluids, especially the ECF volume and the blood volume (ADH, the renin-angiotensin-aldosterone system, ANP, cortisol, and others)
3. Plasma level of calcium and phosphate ions (PTH, 1,25-[OH]2-D3), calcitonin, and others)
4. Structural integrity and function of body tissues, including bone, muscle, and adipose tissue (growth hormone and the somatomedins, PTH, 1,25-[OH]2-D3, gonadal steroids, insulin, glucagon, cortisol, and others)
5. Direction and rate of flow of metabolic energy

Energy Metabolism

The hormonal regulation of energy metabolism allows the body to meet its need for a constant supply of energy in spite of the intermittent intake of food. Even at rest, vital bodily processes must be maintained. There is a significant metabolic "cost of living," the basal metabolic rate. On the other hand, the intake of energy (calories contained in food) is sporadic; the consumption of excess food (caloric intake exceeds momentary needs) is interspersed with periods of fasting. To resolve this problem, excess energy is stored in a form that is readily mobilized and available for use when necessary. The metabolic flow in both directions, storage and retrieval, is directed and controlled by hormones.

During the period when exogenous fuels are available, insulin is of primary importance. The polypeptide stimulates the uptake and metabolism of glucose (glycolysis) and promotes the storage of small metabolites in their respective macromolecular forms (i.e., glucose as glycogen, amino acids as protein, and free fatty acids as triglyceride). When exogenous fuels are not available, several hormones, most notably glucagon and cortisol, collaborate to mobilize energy from endogenous storage sites. Glucagon stimulates the hydrolysis of glycogen (glycogenolysis) and triglyceride (lipolysis). It increases the formation of new glucose from noncarbohydrate sources (gluconeogenesis). Cortisol stimulates gluconeogenesis and mobilizes amino acids (gluconeogenic precursors) from protein depots. The precise physiologic role of newly (since the previous edition of this text) discovered hormones, such as ghrelin and leptin—shown to influence energy balance, fuel utilization, and body weight—remains to be determined.

The importance of the hormonal controls is dramatically illustrated in clinical conditions such as diabetes mellitus and Addison disease (cortisol deficiency). The absence of insulin leads to a metabolic profile that in many respects resembles that seen in long-term food deprivation (starvation) and, if left untreated, death. In the absence of cortisol, gluconeogenesis is so seriously impaired that short periods of food deprivation, even an overnight fast, pose a serious threat to life.

CONCLUSION

This chapter reviews the endocrine system with reference to osteopathic philosophy and concepts. The picture that emerges is that osteopathy embraces endocrine physiology. The principles that direct the study and practice of osteopathic medicine might well have been formulated on the basis of a through understanding of endocrine physiology. Yet A.T. Still never studied endocrinology, for this is a new science, evolving entirely during the 20th century. Almost all of the endocrine information presented here is a product of the last few years of research and virtually none of this

information was available at the time osteopathy came into being. The future surely holds still more, and even unexpected, information concerning not only endocrinology but all body systems. However, the conclusion is inescapable: Osteopathic philosophy is so deep-rooted in an understanding of the fabric of life that this new information, too, will be embraced.

SUGGESTED READINGS

Friedman JM, Halaas JL. Leptin and the regulation of body weight in mammals. *Nature.* 1998;395:763–770.

Frohman LA, Felig P. Introduction to the endocrine system. In: Felig P, Frohman LA, eds. *Endocrinology and Metabolism.* New York. NY: McGraw-Hill; 2001:3–17.

Greenspan FS, Gardner DG, eds. *Basic and Clinical Endocrinology,* 6th ed. New York, NY: Lange/McGraw-Hill; 2001.

Griffin JE, Ojeda SR, eds. *Textbook of Endocrine Physiology,* 4th ed. New York, NY: Oxford University Press; 2000.

Horvath TL, Diano S, Sotonyi P, et al. Ghrelin and the regulation of energy balance—a hypothalamic perspective. *Endocrinology.* 2001;142:4163–4169.

Kahn CR, Smith RJ, Chin WW. Mechanism of action of hormones that act at the cell surface. In: Wilson JD, Foster DW, Kronenberg HM, Larsen PR, eds. *Williams Textbook of Endocrinology.* Philadelphia, PA: WB Saunders Co; 1998:55–94.

Kelly RB. Pathways of protein secretion in eukaryotes. *Science.* 1985;230:25–28.

Min-Jer T, Clark JH, Schrader WT, O'Malley BW. Mechanism of action of hormones that act as transcription-regulatory factors. In: Wilson JD, Foster DW, Kronenberg HM, Larsen PR, eds. *Williams Textbook of Endocrinology.* Philadelphia, PA: WB Saunders Co; 1998:55–94.

Molitch ME. Neuroendocrinology. In: Felig P, Frohman LA, eds. *Endocrinology and Metabolism.* New York, NY: McGraw-Hill; 2001:111–171.

Sayers G, Portanova R. Regulation of the secretory activity of the adrenal cortex: cortisol and corticosterone. In: Greep RO, Astwood EB, eds. *Handbook of Physiology, Section 7: Endocrinology.* Vol 2. Baltimore, MD: Williams & Wilkins; 1975:4153.

Themmen APN, Huthaniemi, IT. Mutations of gonadotropins and gonadotropin receptors: elucidating the physiology and pathophysiology of pituitary-gonadal function. *Endocr Rev.* 2000;21:551–583.

Theofilopoulos AN. The basis of autoimmunity. Part 1: Mechanisms of aberrant self-recognition. *Immunol Today.* 1995;16:90–98.

PHARMACOLOGIC AND OSTEOPATHIC BASIC PRINCIPLES

ROBERT J. THEOBALD, JR.

KEY CONCEPTS

- Appreciate the development of pharmacology as a biomedical discipline, its importance in the history of medicine, and its relevance to A.T. Still's position on drug use
- Appreciate similarities between basic pharmacologic concepts and the basic principles of osteopathic medicine
- Understand and explain the differences of a reductionist view and a holistic view of biomedical science
- List several intrinsic and extrinsic factors that influence drug responses of an individual
- Be able to list and describe the pharmacologic phases of drug responses

This chapter is designed to provide the reader with appreciation of the relationship between the biomedical science of pharmacology and osteopathic medicine. The foundation of all medicine is a solid basic science education in which medical students learn the fundamental concepts of biomedical science. These concepts allow them to build on this foundation with clinical courses and training. During their basic science education, and while students learn about the concepts of osteopathic philosophy, structure-function relationships, and the importance of homeostasis and body unity, they should begin to realize that the concepts of pharmacology and the concepts of osteopathy are similar. These concepts complement each other and other medical modalities. The concepts of osteopathy are concepts crucial to the practice of good medicine, to making sound clinical decisions, and to the integration of basic science and clinical science in the treatment of patients.

For the reader to have a perspective of the relationship of pharmacology and osteopathic medicine, it is necessary to provide some historical background of both disciplines and definitions of some basic terminology. The detailed history of both pharmacology and osteopathic medicine would be better found in other volumes. References to both can be found in any library in any osteopathic medical school, or by visiting the website for the Kirksville College of Osteopathic Medicine (*www.kcom.edu*) and the American Society for Pharmacology and Experimental Therapeutics (ASPET, *www.aspet.org*). Pharmacology is a biomedical science that encompasses the study of substances that have potential therapeutic and/or toxicologic activity in biological systems. There are subsets of the discipline of pharmacology in which studies are focused on specific classes of substances, such as chemotherapeutic agents, or on specific arenas, such as pharmacokinetics. Pharmacokinetics is the study of how an organism affects substances, including absorption, distribution, biotransformation, and excretion of the substance. Pharmacodynamics is the study how drugs affect an organism, how the drugs interact with receptors and second messengers, mechanisms of action, and other parameters of drug-organism interaction. Pharmaceutics is the science of drug preparation, including factors such as physical and chemical characteristics of a specific chemical entity.

The scientific discipline of pharmacology is relatively new when considering the history of disciplines such as anatomy and physiology. The use of various plants and other natural substances in the treatment of disease has been occurring for millennia; however, an organized study of pharmaceutical agents by a discipline was an important advance. Historically, discovery and development were based on folklore or observation, but today new drugs are mainly developed by organic chemists working with pharmacologists using basic knowledge of molecular targets. Early scientists laid the groundwork for modern pharmacologic studies. A more complete listing is available on the Internet from ASPET.

Among those notable scientists listed on the website are:

Rudolph Bucheim (1820–1879), who established the first laboratory dedicated to experimental pharmacology in Dorpat (now renamed Tartu, Estonid);

Oswald Schmeideberg (1838–1921), who set up an institute of pharmacology in Strasbourg, France;

J.N. Langley (1852–1925) and Sir Henry Dale (1875–1968), two scientists in late 19th century England, who pioneered pharmacology using a physiologic approach; and

John J. Abel (1857–1938), who established the first chair of pharmacology in the United States in 1891 at the University of Michigan. Abel, known as the "Father of American Pharmacology", trained many U.S. pharmacologists.

Modern research in pharmacology was accelerated during World War II, when the U.S. government established several programs, such as the wartime antimalarial program, and the initiation of strong analytical and synthetic chemical approaches in the discipline. Since then, biomedical science has expanded to encompass studies in many other areas, including neuropharmacology and cardiovascular pharmacology.

In the era of medicine when A.T. Still was formulating and implementing his philosophy and principles of osteopathic medicine, the use of pharmaceuticals was routinely irrational and heroic. Mercurial compounds, quinine, and many other toxic compounds were commonly used for treatment of a variety of diseases with little or no basis in science (1). Still's distrust and disdain for drugs was a decision of safety and preservation for his patients because, in many instances, the treatments used were worse than the disease. As pharmacologic advances occurred, based on scientific study and thought, Still embraced therapy based on these studies and allowed a course in pharmacology to be presented in the osteopathic curriculum (1).

As stated earlier, the basic concepts or tenets of osteopathic medicine are the foundations of the practice of good medicine. These tenets were recently readdressed in the Louisa Burns Lecture presented by Felix Rogers, DO, at the 2001 American Osteopathic Association Convention (2). In his presentation, Dr. Rogers restated the tenets as follows:

1. A person is the product of dynamic interaction between body, mind and spirit;
2. An inherent property of this dynamic interaction is the capacity of the body to maintain health and recover from disease;
3. Many forces, both intrinsic and extrinsic to the person, weaken this inherent capacity and contribute to the onset of disease; and
4. The musculoskeletal system significantly influences the body's ability to maintain this inherent capacity and to resist disease processes.

From these Dr. Rogers espoused four principals of patient care. These principals revitalize and reemphasize the basic concepts of osteopathic medicine, refocusing them on the holistic approach to patient care. It is not in the scope of this chapter to provide a forum for discussion of the restatement of Still's basic tenets; therefore, this chapter will restrict focus to the original basic tenets of osteopathic medicine.

Still's original basic concepts of osteopathic medicine were discussed in a paper by Korr (3) in the 1990s, in which he emphasizes the need to redirect basic biomedical research from a reductionist view to a view more suited to investigation of the body as a whole unit. Korr states, "the reductionist paradigm is not unproductive . . . but it is incomplete" and "reductionist, mechanistic medical research fails to see that when illness occurs, whatever the affected part, it is illness of the person" (3). The logical corollary to this is the need for clinical medicine to treat the whole person, not just the diseased part. Korr further states that this "mechanistic biomedical philosophy" believes "that the way to understand anything, including humans, their illnesses, and the origins of their vulnerability, is to take them apart; that is, to reduce them to their components, and to study these and their interactions as

minutely as possible" (3). The major problem with this view is the lack of appreciation of the effect of illness and treatment of illness on the whole organism, the total human body. This reductionist view, held by many practicing clinicians, is contrary to basic concepts of pharmacology, and to the concepts of osteopathy. As Korr's paper implies, whatever the physician does to any part of the patient, the physician also does to the whole body because the body is a unit whose parts respond to anything done to any part.

The osteopathic principles, body unity, homeostasis, and the relationship of structure and function, are mutually supportive of the basic principles of pharmacokinetics and pharmacodynamics. These pharmacokinetic and pharmacodynamic principles provide the basic foundation of our understanding of how the body deals with these drugs and how drugs work in the body. These principles complement osteopathy and the role of osteopathic manipulative treatment (OMT) similar to the way they complement other medical modalities. Use of drugs to treat an illness does not, and should not, preclude the use of OMT any more than it should preclude the use of other modalities, such as surgery. The role of the physician is to orchestrate the use of all appropriate interventions to the best advantage of the patient, always basing decisions on fundamental principles of osteopathy and of all good medicine. This chapter focuses on the basic principles of pharmacology, providing a basis for the student's understanding of the similarities of pharmacology and osteopathy, and how pharmacology, OMT, and other medical modalities can be mutually complementary. This chapter also discusses the interaction of these principles, illustrating that they are intertwined and must be considered together during any decision-making process.

The most important pharmacologic concept to remember when considering the use of drugs is that of individualization of therapy. A major point in this concept is that physicians treat people, whole people, and whatever they do to any part of a person, they also do to the whole person. The body, as a unit, is comprised of many components and factors, some of which are intrinsic and some extrinsic, which affect responses to drugs and other medical interventions. To individualize drug therapy, one must be fully aware of these factors, both intrinsic and extrinsic, that are part of each person and influence any response to drugs. The intrinsic factors include characteristics such as age, sex, genetics, health, race, and other factors inherent in a person's makeup. The extrinsic factors include characteristics such as occupation, lifestyle (smoking, alcohol consumption, physical activity, etc.), diet, home environment, and other factors that may be altered, if necessary. These factors, found in Table 12.1, determine who the

TABLE 12.1. FACTORS THAT INFLUENCE DRUG RESPONSES

Intrinsic Factors	Extrinsic Factors
Body weight and size	Diet
Age	Smoking
Sex	Occupation
Body composition	Lifestyle
Genetic factors	Physical activity level
Somatovisceral factors	Home environment
Physical health	
Psychological health	

patient is and influence how the patient will respond to any drug prescribed. These are the factors a physician must consider when choosing medication for any patient because that person is the composite of the extrinsic and intrinsic factors. In other words, the body is a unit (one osteopathic principle) made up of these factors, each of which will be affected by whatever the physician does to the patient.

A second osteopathic principle states that the body has inherent self-regulatory, defensive, and recuperative powers. This principle is very similar to the phenomenon called homeostasis. Homeostatic mechanisms are a system of control mechanisms that use feedback loops to maintain stability of bodily functions. These mechanisms help the body self-regulate, provide defense against anything that triggers an untoward response, and help maintain a stable internal environment in which injured tissues can utilize the natural recuperative powers inherent in the body, described so well by Still (4). Many diseases, in fact probably all diseases, may be considered disruptions of homeostasis; that is, they are disruptions of the stability of activity or function of some system in the body. Discussion of homeostatic mechanisms is vital to understanding the effects of many drugs on the systems of the body. Drugs produce many effects throughout the body, changing levels of activity in organ systems; changes that stimulate reflex responses in the body, or sometimes blunt these responses. Drugs can also alter the environment in which an organ functions such that the body's reflex mechanisms, homeostatic mechanisms, can reclaim control of a malfunctioning system, reinforcing the concept of body unity.

The third osteopathic principle states that structure and function are reciprocally related. This principle is analogous to the structure activity relationship described for many drugs. In the mid-19th century an English physician, James Blake, established the principle that the chemical structure of drugs determines their effect on the body (5). Fraser, another English physician, and Brown, a chemist, further defined the relationship between functional groups of drugs and the characteristics of the drugs (5). The concept of structure-activity relationships for drugs and their effects is vitally important to the understanding of the pharmacokinetics and pharmacodynamics of a drug, including administration, distribution, biotransformation, excretion, and effect at specific receptor sites. The processes occurring with the administration of a drug and the production of effects in a living system can be divided into three phases: (a) the pharmaceutical phase, (b) the pharmacokinetic phase, and (c) the pharmacodynamic phase. These phases are shown in Table 12.2.

The pharmaceutical phase is the study of the relationship between the nature and intensity of the biologic effects observed and the different factors related to the nature of the drugs, such as the physical state, particle size, which salt is used, and so forth. These factors are important and affect the dissolution and disintegration of a drug after oral administration. In order to be absorbed into the body from the gastrointestinal (GI) tract, a drug must be dissolved in the aqueous contents of the stomach. For this to occur it must disintegrate from the tablet or capsule form. The importance of this area for pharmacology involves the assumption that drugs dissolve completely in the GI tract upon oral administration. The validity of this assumption involves consideration of differences in various commercial preparations. This factor must

TABLE 12.2. DRUG ADMINISTRATION AND EFFECTS

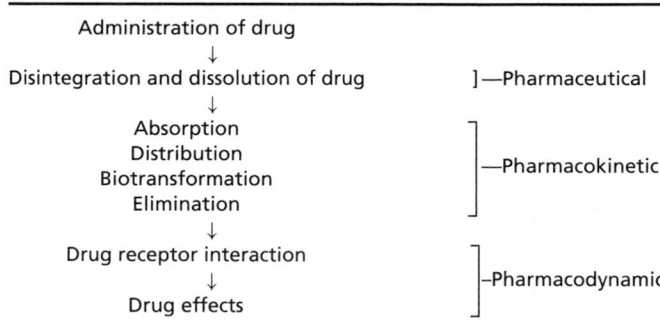

be considered when choosing preparations for administration to patients. It is important in determining bioavailability of drugs that can be critical in certain clinical situations.

Pharmacokinetics is the study of factors that determine the *amount of drug* at sites of biologic effect at various times after application of the drug to a biologic system. These factors deal with the concentration of drugs in the body as a function of time. Phenomena of absorption, distribution, biotransformation (metabolism), and elimination are considered by pharmacokinetics; in other words, *what the body does to the drug*. In order to have any effect on the body, a drug must have access to the body and appropriate sites of action within the body, usually receptors. It must be absorbed in sufficient amounts to produce effective concentrations at the sites of action. Age, diet, blood flow through the site of administration, and pH of body fluids at the site of administration are some of the factors influencing absorption. Distribution of the drug from the site of administration to the site of action is influenced by factors such as structure of the drug, binding of the drug to plasma proteins, pK_a, and other factors. One important fact to remember is that only the portion of drug that is *free* (not bound to or stored in some biological tissues, such as plasma proteins) is active and capable of producing an effect, of distributing and equilibrating in the body, of being biotransformed and excreted. Termination of drug effects in the body occurs several ways, through redistribution to nonsites of action, biotransformation, and/or excretion. Remember that just because the effects of a drug are no longer apparent, the drug is not necessarily excreted from the body, and that the clinical manifestation of effects that are expected are not the only effects of the drug.

Pharmacodynamics is the study of biochemical and physiological effects of drugs as they interact with the body at various levels of organization and systems in the body. Attention is focused on the characteristics of drugs; in other words, *what a drug does to the body*. The effects of a drug are the consequence of the interaction of the drug with structures in the body called receptors. This interaction occurs through the attachment of the drug to the receptor via some type of chemical binding, such as hydrogen or ionic or covalent binding. The interaction can occur because the structure of any given drug determines if it will bind to a specific receptor and if it binds, what type of effect it will have—agonistic or antagonistic. An agonist is a drug whose structure allows it to bind to its receptor and produce some action or effect. An agonist is said to possess intrinsic activity. An antagonist is a drug whose structure allows it to bind to its receptor without producing an action or effect; it possesses no intrinsic activity. This phenomenon of drug-receptor interaction exemplifies the osteopathic principle of structure-function relationships. The structures of the drugs and receptors determine their function. The student should also remember that many drugs are structural analogues of endogenous substances that have been isolated from the body and identified. Still strongly encouraged this when he said in his autobiography, "Man should study and use the drugs compounded in his own body" (6). In effect, that is what has been done. Structural analogues of endogenous substances have been synthesized and altered to have agonist or antagonist effects on specific receptors. Alteration of structure, for example, addition of an OH group or a methyl group, can produce an altered function, again exemplifying the basic osteopathic principle that structure and function are intimately related. Recent examples of this include immunologic agents, such as the interferon analogues, and the prostaglandin-based antisecretory/cytoprotective agent, misoprostol.

Most drug effects, but not all drug effects, are mediated through receptors. Receptors are proteins or protein-related structures in membranes that link drugs to intracellular functional systems through signal transduction mechanisms. The interaction of receptors and signal transduction mechanisms are varied and include receptors coupled to ion channels, receptors coupled to G-proteins, receptors linked to tyrosine-kinase, and intracellular steroid receptors interacting with specific target DNA elements. Nonreceptor-mediated drug actions include mechanisms such as drug interaction with small molecules (e.g., chelation, or gastric acid neutralization) and inhibition of enzymes (e.g., inhibitors of angiotensin-converting enzyme). It is important to remember that although drugs are classified by a major mechanism of action, such as α-adrenergic receptor antagonists, drugs may have other mechanisms of action and *all drugs have multiple effects.*

It may be best to address the interactions of osteopathic and pharmacologic principles individually. For example, when considering treatment for a patient with a central nervous system (CNS) disorder that requires medication that will enter the CNS, the physician must consider the structure-function relationship of the tissues involved and the structure-activity relationship of any drug being considered. The blood–brain barrier, a barrier that restricts polar molecules from entering the brain readily, protects the brain from severe toxic effects of drugs like penicillins or tubocurarine. The structure of the cerebral capillaries has an essentially continuous layer of endothelial cells with tight gap junctions that form the barrier. The blood–brain barrier is neither absolute nor invariable. Very large doses of drugs, such as penicillin, will cross the barrier. In addition, inflammation of the barrier lessens its effectiveness. Also by knowing that the barrier allows small molecules and lipid-soluble molecules to enter the CNS much more readily, the physician can choose a drug with those characteristics. A drug like succinylcholine, a neuromuscular blocking agent used as an adjuvant in surgery, possesses a charged ion in its structure, is not very lipid soluble, and therefore, does not readily cross the blood–brain barrier. However, a drug like thiopental, a barbiturate that is highly lipid soluble, enters the CNS so rapidly that it produces effects within seconds after an intravenous administration of sufficient dose. Subsequently, because of its lipid solubility, thiopental rapidly leaves the CNS and sequesters in other lipid tissues that are not sites of action, such as

adipose tissue. This termination of effects is due to redistribution of the drug away from the site of action.

Structure-activity relationships are also important when considering drugs that readily sequester in certain tissues for clinical effect. In treating a patient with a lower urinary tract infection, several factors must be considered when choosing an appropriate antimicrobial agent. First, the antimicrobial agent must be effective against the infecting organism. Second, and of key importance here, any pharmacologic agent used must concentrate in the urine in large enough levels to provide adequate antimicrobial activity. Structural characteristics of pharmacologic agents influence mechanisms of termination of effects and clearance of the drug from the plasma. Agents such as sulfonamides and trimethoprim are rapidly cleared into the urine, providing ample concentrations in the urine for antimicrobial activity. Drugs such as minocycline and doxycycline do not concentrate in the urine and therefore would not be appropriate choices for treatment of lower urinary tract infections.

Considering the interactions of osteopathic and pharmacologic principles in this manner should help the student understand the interrelationship; however, the student should remember that these principles need to be integrated so that as a physician, one can provide a comprehensive approach to caring for each individual patient. It is the intention of the author that the following discussion of hypertension will provide an example of the interrelationships of the principles.

The etiology of primary hypertension, although not clearly understood, apparently involves an initial increase in cardiac output (7). This increase in cardiac output increases blood flow to tissues, which, in turn, causes a compensatory autoregulation at the tissue level. The autoregulation involves a twofold action; a functional autoregulation produces a vasoconstriction that will decrease flow to the tissue while a structural autoregulation causes hypertrophy of the vessel wall that amplifies any vasoconstrictor activity or stimulus, such as sympathetic nerve stimulation. The structural change, hypertrophy, contributes and amplifies the functional change, vasoconstriction, producing an even greater elevation of blood pressure (8). This interaction of structure as an amplification of the functional change provides support for the osteopathic tenet involving structure and function relationships.

The structural change, vascular hypertrophy, is not solely responsible for the elevation of blood pressure, but it is an important contributor and, in fact, may be the autoregulatory component responsible for the chronic elevation of blood pressure seen in hypertension (7). Understanding this chronic role of hypertrophy may lie in consideration of the concept of down-regulation of receptors that are under chronic neurotransmitter stimulation. However, that may be a tangential issue here. The basic concept is that some trigger, unknown perhaps, creates a change that produces a structural/functional alteration in vascular smooth muscle resulting in an abnormal homeostatic level of blood pressure.

Treatment of hypertension with pharmacologic agents alters this abnormal state and attempts to return blood pressure to a "normal" level, that level which would be maintained by the body's own homeostatic mechanisms, if they were functioning properly. The pharmacologic intervention provides several benefits. During the time of pharmacologic maintenance of blood pressure, there is some evidence that the hypertrophy of vascular smooth muscle regresses, leading to a decrease in blood pressure

(7). This again supports the osteopathic tenet that structure and function are related. A decrease in muscle mass leads to a decrease in muscle tension and a decrease in blood pressure. Evidence is also emerging that after some period of time, pharmacologic intervention may be decreased or stopped completely because the patient's own homeostatic mechanisms become capable of normal regulatory control of blood pressure, eliminating the need for pharmacologic intervention. Therefore, treating hypertension with pharmacologic agents is not in contrast to the osteopathic tenet that describes the body's self-healing potential, it actually supports this and may provide benefit similar to OMT, where a treatment regimen, in addition to other benefits, provides an opportunity for the body to heal itself. In this instance, the body's homeostatic mechanisms are allowed to regain proper control of blood pressure because the pharmacologic agents maintain blood pressure at the appropriate level while the self-healing actions of the body occur; in this instance, the decrease in vascular smooth muscle mass. Additionally, OMT has been shown to decrease hypersympathetic tone, decrease total peripheral resistance, and affect the renin-angiotensin-aldosterone system (9). Therefore, appropriate OMT in conjunction with pharmacologic therapy could hasten the return of normal function of the body's autoregulatory systems.

Prior to initiation of pharmacologic treatment of hypertension, several points must be considered in light of the principles of viewing the body as a unit and individualization of therapy. First, the cause of the hypertension should be fully investigated, determining if the hypertension is primary or secondary. If any factors are present that tend to raise blood pressure, such as smoking, then these factors should be eliminated or at least modified to lessen their influence. Second, when treating very high blood pressure, treatment should begin without delay; however, overaggressive treatment may be risky and should be done with extreme care. It is important in treating patients with very high blood pressure to lower blood pressure gradually so that hypotension does not result. Third, treatment of hypertension requires a long-term, perhaps lifelong, relationship between the patient and the physician. Physicians need to reassess patients periodically to determine if pharmacotherapy is still necessary and, if so, is still effective. The reassessment should be an evaluation of the total patient, with the aim being to find a therapeutic regimen, including a drug or combination of drugs, that lowers blood pressure effectively, that is not contraindicated in any way, and that may be positively helpful in other ways. These points have been adapted from F.O. Simpson's chapter on hypertensive disease in *Avery's Drug Treatment* (10).

Drugs used to treat hypertension fall into several classes, including diuretics, β-adrenergic receptor blocking drugs, α-adrenergic receptor blocking drugs, adrenergic neuron blocking drugs, centrally acting α-adrenergic agonists, calcium-channel blocking drugs, direct acting vasodilators, angiotensin-converting enzyme inhibitors, and ganglionic blocking agents. Choice of which agent to use depends upon fully evaluating the patient, including all factors listed here. For example, use of a β-adrenergic receptor blocking drug, such as propranolol, would be effective in lowering blood pressure. However, consideration must be given to other factors, such concurrent diseases. Blockade of β-adrenergic receptors can exacerbate symptoms of other diseases, such as congestive heart failure, peripheral vascular disease, bronchial asthma, or chronic obstructive pulmonary disease. Some of these agents could also interfere with the control of diabetes because of blockade of β_2-adrenergic receptors, while other agents with intrinsic sympathomimetic activity could aggravate anginal symptoms or increase risk for patients with a previous myocardial infarction. These agents are also known to cause sexual dysfunction in some men. This indicates the need to consider sex and age factors in clinical decisions, as well as making counseling available prior to and during the use of these agents in male patients. Other antihypertensive agents, such as the adrenergic neuron-depleting agent, reserpine, cross the blood–brain barrier and can cause CNS side effects like depression and sedation. Consideration of lifestyle must be made when agents such as these are part of the clinical armamentarium. If a patient lives alone and must be self-sufficient, such as in the case of many older adult patients, then agents that cause depression and sedation may be particularly dangerous. Prescribing other agents with no or less CNS side effects would be a better choice. It should be apparent that in making pharmacologic decisions, the total patient must be considered. The physical, mental, and spiritual aspects of the patient must be known because the physician does *not* treat just the hypertension, the physician treats the whole patient. The intrinsic and extrinsic factors listed in Table 12.1 are just a checklist, a beginning for total patient evaluation.

In summary, the physician must remember that pharmacologic therapy does not preclude therapy with other modalities, especially osteopathic modalities, and can be effectively integrated into an osteopathic approach for the treatment of disease and dysfunction. It must be understood that the principles of osteopathy and pharmacology are mutually supportive and are, in reality, very similar. Individualization of therapy and understanding body unity, should be the framework of all clinical decisions. Do what is best for the patient, the whole patient, and remember that whatever drug you give, or treatment you apply to any part of the body, you are administering to the whole body.

REFERENCES

1. Lane MA. In: *A.T. Still Founder of Osteopathy.* Kirksville, MO: The Journal Printing Company; 1926:7–8;52.
2. Rogers, FJ. Building on tradition. Louisa Burns Lecture, October 23, 2001.
3. Korr IM. Osteopathic research: the needed paradigm shift. *JAOA.* 1991;91(2):156–171.
4. Still AT. In: Schmucker RV, ed. *Early Osteopathy in the Words of A.T. Still,* 36. Kirksville, MO: Thomas Jefferson University Press, Northeast Missouri State University; 1991.
5. Levine RR. *Pharmacology: Drug Actions and Reactions,* 4th ed. Boston, MA: Little, Brown and Co; 1990:12.
6. Still AT. *Autobiography of Andrew T. Still.* Published by the author, Kirksville, MO; 1908:89. Reprinted 1981, by American Association of Osteopathy, Indianapolis.
7. Onrot J, Rangno RE. Treatment of cardiac disorders: hypertension. In: Melmon KL, Morrelli HF, Hoffman BB, Nierenberg DW, eds. *Melmon and Morrelli's Clinical Pharmacology: Basic Principles in Therapeutics* New York: McGraw-Hill, 3rd ed. 1992:52–83.
8. Folkow B. Early structural changes. Brief historical background and principale nature of process. *Hypertension.* 1984;6[Suppl 3]:1–3.
9. Mannino JR. The application of neurologic reflexes to the treatment of hypertension. *JAOA.* 1979;79(10):225–231.
10. Simpson FO. Hypertensive disease: In: Speight TM, ed. *Avery's Drug Treatment,* 3rd ed. Oxford: Blackwell, 1987:676–731.

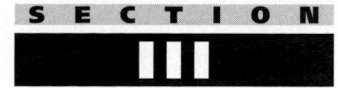

SECTION III

OSTEOPATHIC CONSIDERATIONS IN THE BEHAVIORAL SCIENCES

INTRODUCTION

JOHN A. JEROME

During the last century, the leading causes of death were diseases such as influenza, tuberculosis, pneumonia, diphtheria, and gastrointestinal infections. "*Since then, the yearly death rate from these diseases per 100,000 people has been reduced from 580 to 30!*" (1). Today the major causes of premature death and disability result from behavioral factors, such as accidents and violence, or long-standing habits, such as smoking, high-fat diets, lack of routine exercise, stress, and alcohol abuse (2). The World Health Organization and Harvard School of Public Health both predict that by 2020, in the developing countries where four-fifths of our planet's people will live, seven out of ten deaths will be traced to lifestyle factors setting the stage for ischemic heart disease, depression, and chronic obstructive pulmonary diseases. In fact by 2020 tobacco alone is expected to cause more premature death and disability than any single disease (3). Future improvements in health will come from managing the effects of unhealthy behaviors (4).

From an osteopathic perspective, the behavioral sciences are the clinical and scientific application of biophysical knowledge to the understanding and treatment of health and illness. Signs and symptoms of various types represent behavioral and physiologic imbalances and breakdowns in a patient's effort to adapt to and cope with change. Osteopathic philosophy is deeply rooted in the belief that balances of physical, mental, and social systems are necessary for health. When one system is stressed or altered, the structure and function of other systems are stressed and altered as well. The primary care physician sees the repercussions from this imbalance as the signs and symptoms of physical and behavioral illness. Somatic dysfunction and neuromusculoskeletal changes are common examples.

All patients with physical illness of any kind have an emotional reaction to the illness. Over half of all patients in the United States with emotional problems are treated solely by a primary care provider (5). During treatment, they use approximately twice as much routine medical care as those without psychological problems.

The goal of this section on behavioral sciences is to add clinical and scientific knowledge to the understanding and treatment of the patient as a unit of body, mind, and spirit. These chapters present some behaviorally based strategies for helping patients manage their physical health, thinking patterns, emotional condition, and levels of functioning in relationships within the context of the patients' social and cultural environment.

Osteopathically oriented patient care bases part of its philosophy on the understanding that these biophysical factors are interrelated and interdependently linked with disease and illness; a patient's health should be an optimal balance of physical, mental, emotional, and spiritual well being. This balance is achieved through a collaborative partnership based on trust and active communication.

REFERENCES

1. Centers for Disease Control and Prevention. *Ten Leading Causes of Death in the United States, 1977.* Washington, DC: Government Publishing Office; 1994.
2. National Center for Health Statistics. *Health of the United States.* Hyattsville, MD: Public Health Service; 1990.
3. World Health Organization. Murray JL, Lopez AD, eds. *The Global Burden of Disease and Global Health Statistics.* Cambridge, MA: Harvard University Press; 2000:389–940.
4. Shapiro S, Skinner EA, Kessler LG, et al. Utilization of health and mental health services: three epidemiologic catchment area sites. *Arch Gen Psychiatry.* 1984;41:971.
5. Hankin J, Oktay JS. *Mental Disorder and Primary Medical Care: An Analytic Review of the Literature.* Rockville, MD: Government Printing Office; 1979. National Institute of Mental Health, Series D No. (ADM) 78–661.

13

HEALTH PROMOTION AND MAINTENANCE

GERALD G. OSBORN

KEY CONCEPTS

- Impact of lifestyle and behavior on health and illness
- The importance of nutrition and health, including food pyramid
- Physical activity, and effects on disease and weight
- Obesity and disease, weight control and fitness
- Substance use, abuse, and treatment, including tobacco, alcohol, and illegal drugs
- Personal safety, especially in automobiles and homes
- Safe sexual practices
- Healthy families and work satisfaction
- Stress anticipation and self-regulation
- Importance of personal support systems
- Doctor–patient relationship, and strategies for communication and change

Historians of medicine describe in detail the dramatic changes that have taken place in medical education, practice, research, and technology in the 20th century. All agree that these changes in our system of health care have traded short-term mortality for long-term morbidity. It is ironic, however, that our modern high-technology advances in acute medical care have done little to improve overall human survival.

At the beginning of the 20th century the average life expectancy was 47 years. By 1994, life expectancy dramatically increased to 71.4 years for men and 78.4 years for women (1). A recent epidemiologic study, the Global Burden of Disease (GBD), based upon a very sophisticated analysis and more egalitarian principles, sets life expectancy standards at 82.5 years for women and 80 years for men (2). These increases are mostly attributable to a drastic reduction in infant mortality. Overall mortality has decreased because of effective public health measures aimed at disease prevention for large populations, not because of high-technological medical procedures aimed at individuals. These fundamental preventive measures include those that provide us with clean air and water, high-quality affordable food, and safer work environments. Adding to this increased survival expectancy is a pharmaceutical industry providing us with immunizations to prevent the most common acute infectious diseases and with antibiotics to treat those infections we fail to prevent. Further strides in improving the long-term health of our patients depend on understanding the major impact of lifestyle and behavior on health and illness. This involves educating our patients, encouraging their active participation in and cooperation with health maintenance, and motivating them to make choices that promote healthy, vigorous, and enjoyable lives. Aging is inevitable, but for most people, ill health is not.

Assisting patients to live long and live well does not mean emphasizing prevention while neglecting high technological research and practice. Research and the development of new technologies are permanent and vital components in the continuum of health care. Helping patients to live longer and better does mean, however, that new preventive health care must be given at least equal status in the medical education and practice of the future if osteopathic physicians are to make a significant difference in the overall health of the population.

The GBD represents the most current and profound study surveying health, injury, and illness worldwide. This investigation is a long-term collaborative effort by the Harvard School of Public Health, the World Health Organization, and the World Bank Group. Mortality data are very important but epidemiologists have always known that mortality statistics alone provide an incomplete picture of the impact of illness. Mortality is easy to define and measure; morbidity is not. The GBD study has come closest to providing the more complete picture health policy planners need by developing the concept of "Disability-Adjusted Life Years" (DALY). This manner of studying the impact of illness goes beyond the factors that contribute to death and adds a method to determine which illnesses rob people of fulfilling and productive lives. The GBD identifies and confirms a number of startling and dramatic shifts in the patterns of disease worldwide, allowing clear comparisons to be made between mature market-economy "developed" and developing nations. Since the GBD's data sets begin in 1990 and project to 2020 and its current data are so accurate, it provides a reliable road map into the future. One of the surprising trends clearly shows that developing nations are moving more toward the patterns of developed ones today. Noncommunicable diseases such as depression and heart disease are eclipsing past threats like infectious disease and malnutrition. Considering disability as well as mortality, the GBD also demonstrates the formerly underestimated burden of mental illness. Even back in 1990, the data show that psychiatric conditions (unipolar depression, alcoholism, bipolar disorder, schizophrenia, and obsessive-compulsive disorder) accounted for five of the top ten leading causes of disability worldwide. The burden of mental illness is even higher in developed nations and the trends continue in an alarming direction. It is also striking to note the complex interlocking nature of behavioral risk factors and many diseases. The most common behaviors involved with disease and ill health are tobacco use, alcohol use, and unsafe sexual practices. The GBD predicts that by 2020 the burden of illness by tobacco use alone will out weigh any single disease. Complicating things further, some diseases predispose to others (e.g., hypertension and diabetes increase the risk of heart disease and peripheral vascular disease).

These noncommunicable diseases are highly influenced by lifestyle and health habits. Osteopathic physicians committed to comprehensive care must place more focus upon effective behavioral change to improve upon the health care we deliver. Genetic therapies offer exciting possibilities to correct basic defects involved with noncommunicable diseases, but these treatments remain far into the future. For the foreseeable future we must continuously improve our present model of treatment, and this includes lifestyle alterations. We simply must pay more attention to self-imposed behavioral risks. Focusing upon "the basics" proven by compelling data will assist our patients to live long and live well.

NUTRITION

Science verifies Oscar Wilde's aphorism: *"You are what you eat."* Issues regarding nutrition need not generate the controversy and confusion so often portrayed in the popular media. Although controversies do exist, scientific nutritionists agree far more often than they disagree about what constitutes a healthy diet. Research consistently demonstrates that what people choose to eat is key to their general well being as well as to specific illnesses, especially cardiovascular disease, neoplastic disease, diabetes, and osteoporosis (3,4) (Tables 13.1 and 13.2). A diet consisting of the most currently determined proportions of protein, carbohydrate, and fat can radically improve one's overall level of health.

TABLE 13.1. THE LEADING CAUSES AND PERCENTAGES OF ALL DEATH IN THE UNITED STATES

1. Heart disease	32.1%
2. Cancer	23.5%
3. Stroke	6.8%
4. Bronchitis and emphysema	4.5%
5. Accidents	3.9%
6. Pneumonia and influenza	3.6%
7. Diabetes mellitus	2.4%
8. HIV infection	1.6%
9. Suicide	1.4%
10. Chronic liver diseases	1.1%

Reprinted with permission from *The United States Surgeon General's Report on Nutrition and Health,* 1994.

TABLE 13.2. CHANGE IN THE RANK ORDER OF DISEASE BURDEN FOR 15 LEADING CAUSES, WORLDWIDE 1990–2020

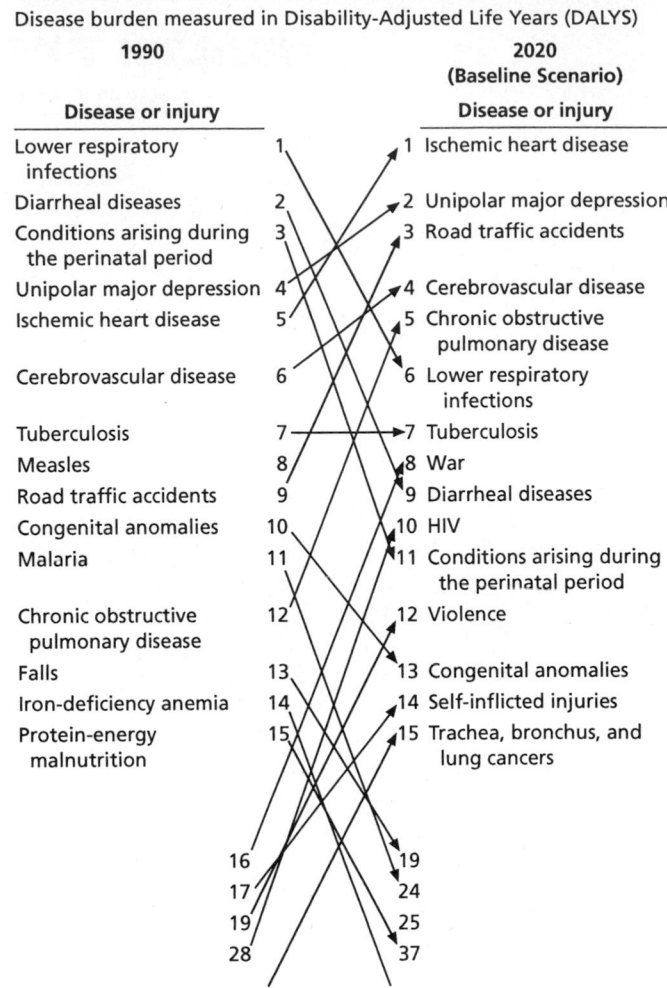

More useful than the former "Four Food Groups," which most patients learn in elementary school, is the more up-to-date "Food Pyramid" (Fig. 13.1). The food pyramid helps clarify the newer and healthier proportions of proteins, carbohydrates, and fats in a more understandable visual construct. The typical American diet after World War II has been about right in the amount of protein, overly generous in simple carbohydrates and fats, and too meager in complex carbohydrates. The food pyramid helps guide patients toward these newer and healthier proportions (Table 13.3).

A simple readjustment of these proportions to current recommended levels offers significant protection from the development of cardiovascular disease and neoplastic illness (5). Further readjustment, encouraging foods lower in sodium and richer in calcium and potassium, offers protection against osteoporosis and hypertension.

Even patients who develop hypertension despite following these dietary recommendations experience better control with multimodal treatment, which includes becoming more aerobically fit and moderating alcohol use, along with the most current pharmacologic care (6).

Food Guide Pyramid
A Guide to Daily Food Choices

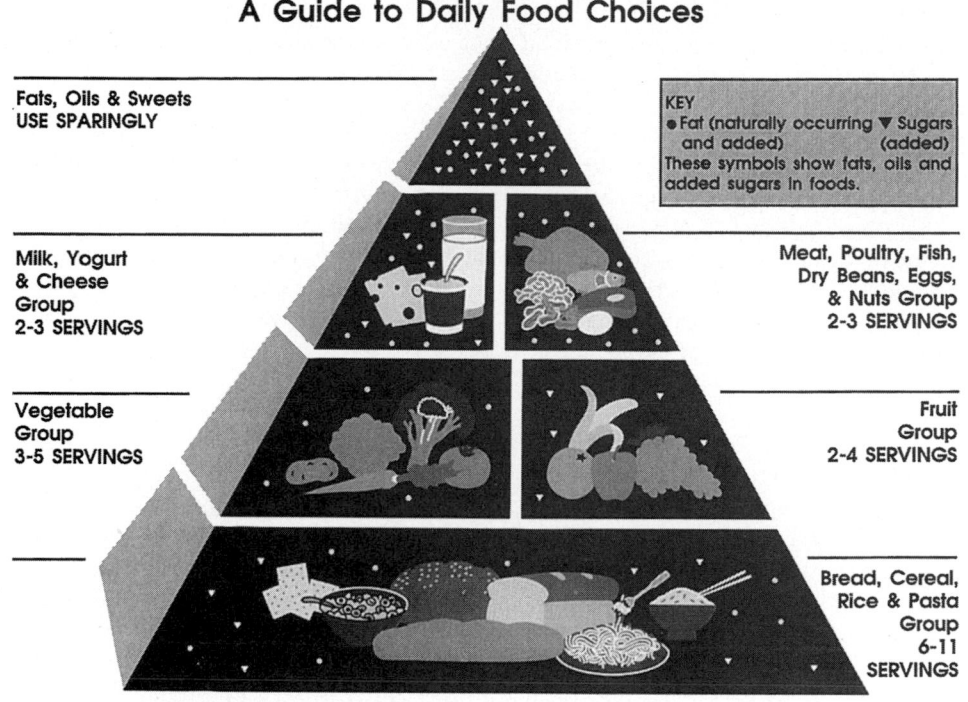

Fats, Oils & Sweets
USE SPARINGLY

KEY
• Fat (naturally occurring ▼ Sugars and added) (added)
These symbols show fats, oils and added sugars in foods.

Milk, Yogurt & Cheese Group
2-3 SERVINGS

Meat, Poultry, Fish, Dry Beans, Eggs, & Nuts Group
2-3 SERVINGS

Vegetable Group
3-5 SERVINGS

Fruit Group
2-4 SERVINGS

Bread, Cereal, Rice & Pasta Group
6-11 SERVINGS

FIGURE 13.1. *Use the Food Guide Pyramid to help you eat better every day . . . the Dietary Guidelines way. Start with plenty of Breads, Cereals, Rice, and Pasta; Vegetables; and Fruits. Add two to three servings from the Milk group and two to three servings from the Meat group. Each of these food groups provides some, but not all, of the nutrients you need. No one food group is more important than another—for good health you need them all. Go easy on fats, oils, and sweets, the foods in the small tip of the pyramid.* (Reprinted with permission from U.S. Department of Agriculture. Human Nutrition Information Service, August 1992. Leaflet No. 572.)

PHYSICAL ACTIVITY

Modern science consistently shows that a healthy life is an active life. Although the popular media provide many stories about people who compulsively exercise, these stories teach us nothing beyond the obvious consequence of fanaticism in any health endeavor. Health researchers in this area agree that higher levels of physical activity delay all-cause mortality primarily because of lower rates of cardiovascular disease and cancer. Their research also shows that physical activity is inversely associated with morbidity as well as mortality. A comprehensive prospective study of physical activity and its relationship to health and specific illnesses demonstrates that the risk of all-cause and cause-specific mortality declines across physical fitness quintiles from the least fit to the most fit in both sexes (7). These trends remain even after statistical adjustment for factors such as age, smoking, cholesterol levels, parental history of heart disease, and follow-up intervals.

TABLE 13.3. PERCENTAGE OF DAILY CALORIES CONSUMED

	Typical American Diet (%)	Recommended Diet (%)
Protein	15	15
Complex carbohydrates	20	40
Simple carbohydrates	25	15
Unsaturated fats	25	10
Saturated facts	15	20

Adapted from Pfeiffer GJ. *Taking Care of Today and Tomorrow. A Resource Guide for Aging and Long-Term Care.* Reston, VA: The Center for Corporate Health Promotion, 1989.

Like nutrition, the basic principles of exercise are straightforward and easy to understand for most people. Becoming more fit through exercise provides many benefits, which include reducing risk of cardiovascular disease, osteoporosis, and noninsulin-dependent diabetes. General benefits of regular moderate exercise also include a reduction in feelings of anxiety and depression and even improvement in immune responses.

The most important principle to emphasize regarding exercise is fun and enjoyment. If all physicians would encourage their patients to pursue enjoyable physical activities, these activities would more likely become a component of a healthier lifestyle. Most people find exercise more enjoyable when paired with a social activity. Therefore, physical activities that can be shared with family, friends, and colleagues are more likely to be continued as a part of ordinary social lives. The other important general principles include common sense, balance, and variety. The most systemically healthful types of physical activity are those that are aerobic. Aerobic exercise generally involves sustained, comfortable, submaximal effort as opposed to anaerobic, short-burst, quickly exhausting, "sprint style" activities.

Patients beginning an exercise program are encouraged to start slowly, regardless of initial level of fitness, and then increase their activity gradually. Most patients do not need cardiac stress tests or expensive, highly technical sports medicine evaluations prior to starting an exercise regimen. Patients should begin at a comfortable point consistent with their age and overall fitness level. They should then gradually increase to their self-determined level of maximal fun and enjoyment. Gentle stretching before warming up and after cooling down will prevent injury, speed up post-exercise recovery, and decrease the probability of delayed muscle soreness. It will also increase the likelihood of patients continuing their fitness programs.

Americans spend approximately $8 billion per year on health spas and exercise clubs (10). While this may add to their social enjoyment, becoming more fit need not be expensive. The most important expenses for any exercise program involve having proper shoes and safety equipment (such as a helmet for bicycling and wrist braces and elbow and kneepads for inline skating) recommended for the patients' selected activity. Careful attention must be paid to clothing when exercising in hot or cold weather. This is especially true for older patients because of the increased risk of heat stroke, heat exhaustion, and hypothermia. Functional and protective clothing are essential. Style is optional. Other protective equipment important for safety involves protection from the sun. Good quality sunglasses and sun block should be a part of most outdoor exercise equipment kits. Likewise, adequate hydration is extremely important. For aerobic exercise lasting less than one hour, cool water is generally sufficient. For longer periods of exercise or in hot, humid conditions, any of the popular "sports drinks" provide important additional glucose and electrolyte replacement, preventing dehydration and speeding up postexercise recovery.

OBESITY

It is ironic that, along with the current emphasis on health and fitness, an increasing number of Americans are obese (11). Health researchers and physicians engage in vigorous debate over the relative risks of being mildly to moderately overweight. They agree, however, that as patients become increasingly overweight, their health risks also increase. Both cross-sectional and cohort studies show associations between obesity and hyperlipidemia, hypertension, and hyperinsulinemia. These lead to the increased prevalence of coronary artery disease and noninsulin-dependent diabetes mellitus (12–15). Some types of cancer, degenerative joint disease, sleep apnea, gout, and gallbladder disease also more prevalent with increasing obesity (16–18).

An additional irony is that the caloric-restriction dietary treatments for obesity so often recommended are ineffective over time. Surveys of current literature indicate that dietary treatments alone do not work; some are detrimental and even dangerous. Recent surveys illustrate the complexity of the dilemma (10–19). The definitive criteria for a risk/benefit analysis of the risk of obesity and the risks of weight loss diets are yet to be determined. The current approach to the problem is to suspend the singular concern for weight alone and focus on the overall level of fitness regardless of weight.

When patients ask about weight loss, the physician should include a complete discussion about physical fitness. The detrimental and ultimately ineffective results of caloric-restriction diets should also be emphasized. Patients should be frequently reminded that nutritious food in the proportions shown in the food pyramid is the necessary fuel for healthy physical activity and basic body functions. Healthy eating, not caloric restriction, and daily aerobic activity are the cornerstones of living long and living well. In the U.S., weight-loss industry estimated at nearly $30 billion is supported more by the widespread American social stigma toward obesity rather than by a concern for health. Confronting our own aesthetic prejudices and those of our patients is an excellent place to start when it comes to weight management. The aesthetic ideal most often promoted by the advertisement and fashion industries is simply unrealistic for most people (10).

Following scientifically corroborated principles related to fitness is the best advice for the foreseeable future. Exciting research into the genetic controls involved in hunger, satiety, and lipid metabolism continues, but new clinically applicable treatments remain far in the future (20). In the meantime, physicians who deemphasize weight and emphasize fitness will serve their patients best. Literature written by exercise physiologists for laypeople emphasizes these points and is available to augment physicians' advice and counsel (21).

SUBSTANCE USE AND ABUSE

Popular media attention and rancorous political debate tend to focus on illegal substance abuse. Yet two legal substances, tobacco and alcohol, contribute more to the misery and ill health of our patients than do all the illegal substances combined. Focusing on those legal substances that constitute the most significant health hazards to our patients is central to primary care practice. Public health research on the matter is clear, despite political debate clouding the issues about the dangers of substance abuse.

Tobacco

The 1989 *United States Health and Prevention Profile,* published by the Centers for Disease Control (CDC), does not equivocate: "*Cigarette smoking is the single most preventable cause of death in our society.*" The first *Surgeon General's Report on Smoking* was published in January 1964. It created instantaneous, justifiable worldwide shock. The second report was issued in January 1979. What the Secretary of Health, Education, and Welfare, Joseph Califano, wrote in that report's preface was even more forceful: "*[T]his document reveals with dramatic clarity, that cigarette smoking is even more dangerous—indeed, far more dangerous—than was supposed in 1964.*" Smoking cessation is so critically important that the predictions of the GBD need to be repeated here. "By 2020 tobacco is expected to kill more people than any single disease, surpassing even the HIV epidemic." The message to our patients must be clear, consistent, and firm: "If you don't smoke, please don't ever start; if you do, *please stop!*"

This is clearly more easily said than done, but acting as an agent of change to promote smoking cessation among our patients, might be the best thing we, as physicians, ever do for our patients and their families. The vast majority of those who have stopped smoking have done so on their own, without formal or professional help of any kind (mostly by the "cold turkey" technique). The rest have required some level of professional guidance or a specific program. The following are some useful methods the physician can suggest to help patients stop smoking (22).

1. Declare a date to stop and make it public. A written statement, including a request for the support and encouragement of family, friends, and co-workers, is a good idea. An advertisement

declaring one's intent to stop smoking can even be taken out in a local newspaper.

2. Prepare to quit by making efforts to minimize stress, eat healthier than before, and begin a gradual and systematic program of physical fitness.

3. Attend to nicotine withdrawal by smoking fewer cigarettes per day, or only smoking a portion of each cigarette before extinguishing it; switching to a different low-tar and nicotine brand of cigarettes after each pack; never buying more than one pack at a time; and continuing the gradual weaning process.

4. Stop learned smoking behavior patterns by waiting at least 10 minutes before lighting up when the craving begins; distracting attention from the craving to light up by using only the nondominant hand to hold a cigarette and setting the cigarette down between puffs; lock up the pack of cigarettes between smokes.

5. Think in terms of one-day-at-a-time. Rather than thinking that smoking will *never* again be an option, concentrate simply on *not smoking for one day*. One day is easier to manage than a lifetime.

6. Stay positive and think of the endeavor as life enhancing rather than as a sacrifice.

On the quitting date and thereafter:

1. Make sure all cigarettes are gone.

2. Build in rewards: money that would have been spent each week on smoking can be placed into a special savings account. Spin-off savings can be banked, too, if one considers the replacement/repair costs of clothes, furniture, and car interiors damaged by cigarettes. The cost of at least one visit to the doctor for a smoking-related health problem can also be added to the account.

3. Prepare for times of craving by keeping substitutes handy, such as sugarless gum, sliced fruit, carrot or celery sticks.

4. Increase fluid intake.

5. Keep a calendar or diary of the day-to-day progress.

Even with physician advice, some patients may require medications to assist their smoking cessation program. Medications useful for attenuating nicotine craving and the effects of withdrawal include nicotine polacrilex chewing gum and nicotine transdermal patches. Other medications include doxepin, a tricyclic antidepressant, bupropion, a newer antidepressant, and clonidine, a centrally acting antihypertensive agent (23,24). Other agents under investigation include corticotropin and citric acid aerosols (25,26).

The most current comprehensive metaanalysis of smoking cessation interventions reveals that the most effective programs employ more than one modality for motivating behavioral change and involve both physicians and nonphysicians in an individualized face-to-face effort. These programs also provide a motivational message on multiple occasions, over the longest possible time period (27).

Smokers have a death rate 30% to 80% higher than nonsmokers, and they consume a disproportionate share of health care resources. In 1985, the direct health care costs of smoking-related illnesses exceeded $16 billion. Calculations for the indirect costs, such as lost productivity and earnings from excess mortality, disability, and premature death, totaled more than $37 billion. Promoting smoking cessation for patients is one of the most important primary prevention efforts physicians can undertake.

Alcohol

The excessive use of alcohol accounts for a wide spectrum of health and social problems. Alcohol plays a casual or contributing role in deaths resulting from accidents, homicides, and suicides, as well as diseases such as cirrhosis and cancer. Beyond the negative effects on individuals with alcoholism, the disorder also has been estimated to negatively affect the lives and health of many other people. Alcohol abuse is implicated in 50% of all divorces, in 45% to 68% of spouse abuse cases, and in up to 38% of child abuse cases. Alcohol abuse is especially harmful during pregnancy. Fetuses can be seriously harmed by alcohol. Fetal alcohol syndrome is now one of the three leading causes of prenatal mental retardation in the United States, and it is completely preventable.

A person who abuses alcohol rarely changes this maladaptive behavior without strong, consistent, systematic, and long-term treatment. The first step involves accurate diagnosis so that the appropriate treatment can follow. A number of useful examiner and self-administered questionnaires are available, but the most useful diagnostic screen consists of four simple questions. The screen's acronym, CAGE, comes from the critical word in each question (28):

1. Have you ever tried to *Cut* down on your drinking?
2. Are you *Angry or Annoyed* when people ask you about your drinking?
3. Do you ever feel *Guilty* about your drinking?
4. Do you ever take a morning *Eye* opener?

One positive response suggests the possibility of alcoholism and merits further exploration. Two positive answers make the likelihood extremely high. Three positive responses to questions 1 through 3, or a single positive response to question 4, is most likely diagnostic. The helpful features of these questions are their simplicity, sensitivity, and efficiency. These questions take under two minutes to ask and they should be included in every initial ambulatory and hospital admission workup. One of the most recent surveys of treatment options for alcoholism indicates that compulsory inpatient treatment followed by close monitoring for incipient relapse yields the best results (29).

Alcohol abuse often is a symptom of psychiatric illness, most commonly anxiety and mood disorders. The ubiquity, social acceptance, and relative low cost of alcoholic beverages make drinking an effective short-term and maladaptive long-term manner of self-medication. If the alcohol problem is a primary disorder (alcohol-related disorder, *Diagnostic and Statistical Manual of Mental Disorders, Fourth Edition* [DSM-IV]) (30), substance abuse treatment alone suffices. If the alcohol problem is secondary to a psychiatric disorder (dual-diagnosis), specific attention to the underlying illness must be addressed simultaneously with the substance abuse disorder. The most useful recent method to diagnose psychiatric disorders efficiently and accurately in an ambulatory care setting is the Prime-MD (Primary Care Evaluation of Mental Disorders) (31). Prime-MD is a well-validated and highly reliable questionnaire that screens for psychiatric disorders. Patients fill out a questionnaire and the physician then follows up any positively endorsed target symptoms. It is specific for the most common psychiatric disorders presenting to primary care practice, including mood, anxiety, somatoform concerns, and alcohol-related problems.

If a psychiatric disorder is coexistent with alcoholism, referral for psychiatric consultation and co-management is strongly recommended.

Illegal Substance Abuse

The effects of illegal substance abuse range from harmful to deadly; prevention is paramount. Efforts must be made on a spectrum of fronts, from governmental to personal, to discourage illegal substance use. Early diagnosis is imperative and in most cases treatment involves a lifelong recovery process. Self-help groups are useful and the most successful therapy usually involves multimodal treatment efforts by a multidisciplinary team. The primary care physician generally is the coordinator of the team-oriented treatment program.

PERSONAL SAFETY

Attending to personal and family safety is a major component of a preventive health program. Educating patients by providing the best and most current information is key. Addressing personal safety issues can be incorporated into new patient screening and provided for current patients in the form of pamphlets. Some safety videos are also available.

Automobiles

Approximately 50,000 people in the United States die every year in automobile accidents. The automotive industry has made significant strides in making cars safer with the advent of air bags and antilock brakes. Laws that make the use of seat belts mandatory and call for infants and small children to be secured in the rear seats in protective seating have also helped reduce deaths from automobile accidents. Physicians can help patients better understand automobile safety issues by encouraging patients to:

- Purchase vehicles with the latest safety devices (i.e., air bags, antilock brakes)
- Keep automobiles safer through proper maintenance, especially of brakes and tires
- Obey speed limits and all traffic regulations
- Follow all regulations when operating recreational vehicles
- Wear an approved helmet and protective clothing when operating a bicycle, moped, or motorcycle
- Avoid driving while taking sedative medications
- *Never* drink alcohol before driving

Home

Provide patients with information on how to maintain a safe environment in their home. The following list is not inclusive

of all issues; rather it represents significant areas where simple attention can make a major difference in household safety. The general nature of these recommendations do not minimize their importance for the health of patients.

- Keep medicines, harmful chemicals, and cleaning products secure and especially out of reach of children.
- Prevent fires by judicious use of auxiliary home heating devices and by proper use of electrical appliances and outlets.
- If fire should occur, minimize danger and damage by the use of smoke detectors and fire extinguishers.
- Develop and practice an escape plan from the home in the event of fire or other disaster (i.e., earthquake, hurricane, tornado). Most local fire departments and electric companies will inspect your home and make safety recommendations at little or no cost.
- Patients who choose to own guns should keep them in a secure place, unloaded, with appropriate locking mechanisms on the triggers. Likewise, ammunition should be kept in a secure place, separate from the weapons.
- Keep power tools and lawn care equipment in good repair, especially their safety guards, and wear safety glasses and ear plus during their operation.
- Falls are a major cause of injury to older adults. Keep bathrooms and stairways free of obstacles and install appropriate lighting, handles, and banisters. Secure the edges of throw rugs to minimize trips and falls.
- In winter, keep sidewalks and outdoor stairs clear of snow and ice. This can be a component of a family's fitness plan.

The home health checklist in Table 13.4 was specifically developed for older adult patients (32).

SEXUALITY

Sexual behavior is a central component of healthy human functioning and a source of pleasure, comfort, and intimacy. Unfortunately, lack of knowledge about human sexuality can result in more than an unwanted pregnancy; it can result in illness and death. As well as providing the best possible counsel and information about contraception and family planning, physicians must also inform sexually active patients about safe sex practices. Female patients suffer far more than male patients in the area of sexually transmitted diseases (STDs) due to their more complicated and lengthy reproductive roles. Again, ironically, ill health, disability, and death from unhealthy sexual practices are almost completely preventable. High-risk practices should immediately be curtailed. These include:

- Sex with an intravenous substance abuser
- Sex with a prostitute, stranger, or person whose sexual history is unknown
- Sex without the use of a condom
- Sex with any person who engages in any of the above behaviors

Further, patients should be advised that abstinence or maintaining a mutually monogamous relationship with one partner are the best methods for preventing all types of STDs. For many

TABLE 13.4. HOME HAZARD CHECKLIST

Stairs
  Adequate illumination
  Top and bottom steps painted
  Nonskid treads
  Handrail: detached, graspable, end of rail shaped to signify bottom
    of stairway
  Risers painted in easily visible color

Living areas—Carpets
  Edges tacked down completely
  Wall-to-wall with thick, shock-absorbent pads
  No throw rugs

Living areas—Floors
  No highly polished floor surfaces
  Nonskid wax
  Thresholds removed
  No extension cords
  Access pathways free of low-lying furniture or other objects
  Baseboard lighting in halls

Other
  Emphasis on control of pets and small children to avoid causing trips
  No low couches, sharp-cornered furniture, or chairs on casters
  Light switches easily accessible to door or room
  Lighted switches

Bathroom
  Nonskid rubber mats in shower or bath
  Handrails in bath and by toilet
  Adequate lighting in bath and night light on access path
  Water temperature regulated at 43°C (110°F) or lower
  Clearly marked hot and cold faucets, preferably with separate controls
  Seat in tub

Kitchen
  Adequate illumination
  Stove controls large and clearly marked
  Large, easily grasped, protected handles on pots and pans
  Stored items easily accessible

Miscellaneous
  Smoke detectors with regularly checked, working batteries
  Adequate access and escape doors and windows
  Consider personal alarm system keyed to emergency system to be
    worn by high risk patient

Reprinted with permission from Snipes GE. Accidents in the elderly. *Am Fam Physician.* 1982;26:117–22.

people, however, this advice is not acceptable. In such cases, the physician should instruct patients to minimize high-risk behaviors. Although not 100% effective, consistent and correct use of condoms and other barrier contraceptives decrease risk of pregnancy and STDs and should be encouraged. Studies reveal that using contraceptives containing the spermicide nonoxynol-9 with condoms offers further projection if the barrier should fail.

FAMILY AND WORK

A healthy family life has long been known to be a source of comfort, joy, and inspiration. The family is the basic unit of society and needs the support of all. Fragmented, blended, or single-parent families need even more support. Families experiencing problems or who are in turmoil should be encouraged to seek help, whether it be support from caring relatives and friends, support groups, or professional family therapy. The primary care osteopathic physician should engage patients in constructive discussions about family health. A recent guide for health and long-term care (4) lists five qualities shared by healthy families:

- A clear understanding of each member's role and responsibilities
- An equitable distribution of power
- Support and encouragement
- Effective communication
- A shared system of values or beliefs

It should become routine in osteopathic, family-oriented health care to inquire about these characteristics in medical history taking and to promote them at every therapeutic opportunity.

Doing work that one finds meaningful is a source of pride and personal fulfillment. The most tragic work situation is for one to feel trapped in a work circumstance one despises. Many people, however, fail to take the steps necessary to make their work more meaningful or to prepare themselves to change jobs or careers. If patients find that, despite their best efforts, they are unhappy in their work, they should be encouraged to survey their situation and develop a plan of change. Opportunities for alternative education and training are more abundant and accessible now than ever before. Even in the most difficult economic circumstances, education is the best investment a person can make.

Many people unhappy with their work never take full advantage of what the situation offers. Most large employers have tuition-reimbursement plans for educational courses that go unused by employees. Patients should also be encouraged to cultivate friendships at work. If a workplace does not provide activities, patients can become agents of change who organize and develop work-related social or sports activities. Work need not be daily tedium and loathing and even planning for a change can be the activity that lifts a patient's spirits and gives them hope and comfort. Work should not be a constant endeavor of joyless striving, but rather an undertaking that provides meaning and satisfaction.

STRESS

No life is without stress. There are, however, adaptive and maladaptive manners of coping, even under the most stressful circumstances. Although there are many events that can happen in our lives that are completely unexpected, many of life's difficulties can be anticipated and managed effectively. Many people accept high levels of stress in their lives but do not appreciate the high price they pay. Medical research has shown that a life lived in chronic stress can trigger and activate psychophysiologic disorders such as hypertension, peptic ulcer disease, and coronary artery disease (33). More recent research in psychoneuroimmunology shows a relationship between stress and attenuation of immune responses (34). Mental health researchers have long known that stress plays a strong role in various forms of anxiety and depressive disorders, as well as in many forms of substance use and abuse.

TABLE 13.5. SOCIAL READJUSTMENT SCALE

Life Events	Holmes Points
1. Death of spouse	100
2. Divorce	73
3. Marital separation	65
4. Jail term	63
5. Death of close family member	63
6. Personal injury or illness	53
7. Marriage	50
8. Fired from job	47
9. Marital reconcilation	45
10. Retirement	45
11. Change in health of family member	44
12. Pregnancy	40
13. Sex difficulties	39
14. Having a baby	39
15. Business readjustment	39
16. Change in financial state	38
17. Death of close friend	37
18. Change to different line of work	36
19. Change in number of arguments with spouse	35
20. Mortgage large in relation to income	31
21. Foreclosure of mortgage or loan	30
22. Change in responsibilities in work	29
23. Son or daughter leaving home	29
24. Trouble with in-laws	29
25. Outstanding personal achievement	28
26. Spouse begins or stops work	26
27. Begin or end school	26
28. Change in living conditions	25
29. Change in personal habits	24
30. Trouble with boss	23
31. Change in work hours or conditions	20
32. Change in residence	20
33. Change in schools	20
34. Change in church activities	19
35. Change in recreation	19
36. Change in social activities	18
37. Small mortgage in relation to income	17
38. Change in sleeping habits	16
39. Change in number of family get-togethers	15
40. Change in eating habits	13
41. Vacation	13
42. Christmas	12
43. Minor violations of the law	11

Reprinted with permission from Holmes TH, Rahe RH. The social readjustment rating scale. *J Psychosom Res.* 1967;7:17–20.

Most recently, stress has been conceptualized as an organism's nonspecific response in an attempt to adapt to demands. Those demands can cover the spectrum of psychological, social, and physiological functioning. Even ordinary day-to-day events, whether seen as positive or negative, involve adaptation to change. The concept of adaptation to change now dominates current thinking about stress. In 1967, Holmes and Rahe verified the stress of adaptation (35). They developed a scale and assigned points to 43 common life events to develop a stable and objective point of reference. They were not concerned with how people interpreted or felt about these events but merely with whether they happened. They demonstrated that the greater number of points a person scored over a 1-year period, the greater the probability of illness occurring within the next 2 years. The preventive implications are clear. Although a number of stress scales are now available, the Holmes & Rahe Social Readjustment Scale remains one of the most highly validated and widely used (Table 13.5) (35). This scale can be easily incorporated into medical practice and used liberally to help patients judge their own vulnerabilities and develop increasingly effective anticipatory coping strategies.

Stress can also be self-generated. The "type A personality" first described by Friedman and Rosenman has now become a household word (36). Although it has been argued excessively as to whether the "type A personality" is a feature of coronary artery disease, the adaptive style of a person with type A characteristics can hardly be envied. Research beyond Friedman and Rosenman's seminal work indicates that competitiveness, impatience, and difficulty dealing with anger and hostility are the core characteristics of people prone to coronary artery disease. It might be difficult to completely alter these maladaptive styles, but counseling and education can modify them to the point where a patient's risks are significantly lowered (37).

SUPPORT SYSTEMS

One of the major factors attenuating stress is an effective system of psychosocial support. The physician should conceptualize a patient's support system as a network of expanding concentric circles with the patient's closest confidant at the center. The importance of having person(s) in whom we can confide cannot be overemphasized in buffering the effects of life stress. Most times this central confidant is a spouse or best friend, or it could be anyone who demonstrates care, concern, and respect for feelings and opinions. This confidant serves the preventive role of ensuring that all burdens and troubles can be shared. A system of support ranges from the confidence of having trusted advice available when planning a predicted transition to the comfort and nurturing of friends, neighbors, and community during an unforeseen tragedy. Confidants also help professionals, such as the clergy or physicians, to provide assistance. Last, but certainly not least, religious faith provides the opportunity for a spiritual confidant. Patients for whom a spiritual dimension to life is important derive great comfort and benefit from their belief in power and meaning beyond what can be known in life in the world. Physicians should not underestimate the positive healing power of spiritual belief systems.

DOCTOR–PATIENT RELATIONSHIP

The doctor–patient relationship remains the single most powerful healing tool of the physician. Technology is obviously important, but the power of the doctor–patient relationship allows "high-tech" medicine to be used most wisely and to the greatest benefit. Primary and secondary prevention are two of the most important goals of the osteopathic physician, especially those in primary care practice. Physicians can do the most to encourage patients to become partners in their health care by using the power inherent in the doctor–patient relationship.

Most physicians agree that counseling is one of their most important tasks; paradoxically, most feel ineffective in this role.

Many physicians feel generally pessimistic about their ability to motivate patients toward positive change. This pessimism exists partly due to a lack of effective training about behavioral change during medical school and in postgraduate medical education. Physicians generally underestimate the difficulty in changing behavior, even their own. Most wrongly believe their only duty is to provide information and end up preaching to or lecturing their patients, rather than informing them. Because this approach alone usually fails, physicians can become discouraged and stop trying to change patient behavior or begin to provide information in a cursory manner, never really expecting patients to cooperate.

Behavioral scientists investigating change as a process have proposed both general and specific approaches that are realistic, practical, and broadly applicable in health care settings. One of the most helpful models is that proposed by Prochaska and DiClemente (38,39). This approach divides the process of change into stages. The duty of osteopathic physicians is then to assist their patients to identify the stage they are in and to move successfully into the next. This approach is useful in three important ways because it:

1. Acknowledges that change is difficult and requires planning.
2. Minimizes discouragement on the part of patient and physician.
3. Continually encourages positive work toward lasting or permanent change.

The stages of change include:

1. *Precontemplation:* In this first stage patients are unaware of or perhaps deny the negative consequences of their behavior. This can include, for example, rationalizations like: "I know lots of people who smoke who are healthy." The task of the physician in this stage is to make patients aware of the fallacy of such rationalizations by providing good information and/or by introducing therapeutic tension into the patient's belief systems.
2. *Contemplation:* At this stage, patients spend variable lengths of time reflecting on their behaviors and assessing both negative consequences of continuing a behavior and the probable benefits of positive change.
3. *Preparation:* Patients acknowledge that change is desirable. The physician's task is to negotiate a plan aimed at the higher likelihood of success.
4. *Action:* The patient and physician implement the plan for behavioral change with clear outcome measures to monitor progress.
5. *Maintenance:* Patients have experienced the reinforcing effects of their action plan to the point where the change becomes an ordinary part of their life.

The Prochaska/DiClemente model allows for the possibility and probability relapse, especially with difficult changes like smoking cessation. If or when relapse occurs rather than abandoning the process, the physician and patient move back to a prior stage to troubleshoot the problem before moving ahead again. Continuous attention and incremental improvement are far superior in the long run to giving up in frustration or demoralization.

TABLE 13.6. COMMUNICATION STRATEGIES FOR BEHAVIOR CHANGE ENCOUNTERS

Informing a patient
  Establish a baseline
  Explain and instruct
  Be clear, avoid jargon
  Check understanding

Obtaining a commitment to behavior change
  Make clear statement about desired behavior
  Explore readiness for change
  Obtain a commitment

Negotiating and tailoring regimen
  Identify congruence between physician's and patient's expectations
  Work toward plan that patient can agree to
  Tailor plan to patient's circumstances; disrupt routines minimally
  Consider a written contract

Attending to emotional responses
  Ask about and label feelings
  Legitimize feelings
  Support and encourage patient
  Be nonjudgmental
  Generate respectful statements

Reprinted with permission from Stoffelmayr B, Hoppe RB, Weber N. Facilitating patient participation: the doctor–patient encounter. *Primary Care.* 1989;16:265–278.

A review of doctor–patient relationship literature proposes four specific sequential strategies for motivating patient cooperation and encouraging patients to take more personal responsibility for their health (40). These strategies are grounded in the patient compliance literature and have been expanded and integrated to include relevant social influences and psychotherapy research. A major contribution of this research has been the identification of the patient's health beliefs as a powerful predictor of cooperation with treatment. The review focuses on the critical importance of the doctor–patient relationship and interaction and then expands to the patient's relationship with the entire integrated primary care health team.

Patients who are not clear about what they are expected to do are unlikely to follow recommendations. A number of studies show major patient dissatisfaction with not receiving enough information from physicians! Dissatisfied patients are less likely to cooperate and may not even return (Table 13.6) (40).

Strategy 1: Informing the Patient

The physician should never make assumptions about a patient's knowledge and understanding, regardless of socioeconomic class or level of education. A confident level of baseline knowledge should first be established. The physician can implement this by allowing the patient time to explain their understanding of health problems and then identify any incorrect or idiosyncratic perceptions. The cultural belief system of patients should also be explored. Verbal instructions should be clear and can be supplemented with pictures and printed materials if necessary. The physician should avoid jargon whenever possible. The physician can check the patient's level of understanding by asking the patient to repeat instructions or demonstrate how they might share the instructions with a third party.

TABLE 13.7. PRIMARY CARE-BASED HEALTH PROMOTION

Activity	Outcome	Agent	Adjunct
Screening	Identification of risky behavior	Physician Nurses Other staff	Questionnaires Interactive Computer
Informing (Table 13.6)	Knowledge	Physician Nurse Health educator	Written materials Video station
Counseling (Table 13.6)	Commitment to behavior change	Physician	Written contract
Training/education	Skills to make short-term behavior change	Physician Nurses Other staff Health educator Nutritionists	Written materials
Emotional support	Motivation	Entire PHCO team	Telephone calls/letters
Plan adjustment/motivation	Long-term	Entire PHCO team	Telephone calls/letters Biologic measurement

Reprinted with permission from Stoffelmayr B, Hoppe RB, Weber N. Facilitating patient participation: the doctor–patient encounter. *Primary Care.* 1989;16: 265–278.

Strategy 2: Obtaining Commitment from the Patient

This involves the use of referent power, social power bestowed on a significant figure whose acceptance and approval are highly regarded and desired. The use of this referent power involves making direct and clear statements about a desired behavior change and eliciting the patient's commitment to cooperate. Using the example of smoking, this would involve stating in a nonjudgmental but direct and authoritative manner the detrimental effects of smoking, and then asking the patient directly for a commitment to stop. Physicians' success in eliciting this commitment is revealed in higher patient smoking cessation rates.

Strategy 3: Negotiating and Tailoring a Regimen

All treatment recommendations require a change from the patient's ordinary lifestyle. The more complex the changes recommended, the more difficult for the patient to cooperate. The goal of negotiation is to arrive at an agreement. Through negotiation and exploration of lifestyle and belief system issues, a regimen can be tailored to the individual life circumstance of each patient. When the negotiated agreement is written up as a mutually binding contract, it is more likely to be kept. A verbal agreement may also suffice.

Strategy 4: Attending to the Patient's Emotional Responses

The quality of the doctor–patient relationship is crucial at this point. Patients often complain, even bitterly so, about not being listened to or not having the opportunity to tell their story. Stories abound about technically competent but cold and aloof physicians. Research into doctor–patient relationships has shown that patients' judgments about physicians are made on the basis of the physician's ability to recognize and respond to emotional concerns. Positive behavior change occurs more often in the presence of a high-quality doctor–patient relationship. Patients in distress

and suffering anxiety are not in the best condition to attend to the cognitive components of their instructions. When physicians attend to a patient's emotions and set the patient at ease, they facilitate and promote the patient's understanding and cooperation.

Physicians also need to communicate their interest and concern for their patients nonverbally. Several tactics communicate care and interest including smiling, sitting down, using appropriate eye contact, and not appearing to be rushed.

The osteopathic physician has a distinct advantage over other health care professionals through the medium of touch and "the laying on of hands." Through the integrated verbal and nonverbal communication of care, trust is promoted, cooperation is maximized, and the doctor–patient relationship is further strengthened.

The use of the integrated primary care team in this process is summarized in Table 13.7 (40).

CONCLUSION

Most of the task of providing the highest quality, cost-effective care involves teaching and motivating patients. The place to begin in creating the desired behavior we wish to see in our patients is to make them clearly reflected in our own. Many physicians have been successful in altering their personal health behavior habits for the better, but there is always room for improvement. Doctor means teacher, and the old maxim remains sounds: "Example isn't the best way to teach, ultimately it is the only way to teach."

REFERENCES

1. National Center for Health Statistics. *United States Health and Prevention Profile.* Hyattsville, MD: U.S. Department of Health & Human Services; 1994. Public Health Service. (All statistics cited in this chapter are taken from this source unless otherwise indicated.)
2. Murray CJL, Lopez AD. *The Global Burden of Disease, a Comprehensive Assessment of Mortality and Disability from Diseases, Injuries, and Risk*

Factors in 1990 and Projected to 2020. Cambridge, MA: Harvard University Press; 2000.

3. *The United States Surgeon General's Report on Nutrition and Health, 1988.* Washington, D.C.: U.S. Department of Health and Human Services, 1988.

4. Pfeiffer GJ. *Taking Care of Today and Tomorrow: A Resource Guide for Aging and Long-Term Care.* Reston, VA: The Center for Corporate Health Promotion; 1989.

5. Willett WC. Diet and cancer. *The Oncologist.* 2000;5(5):393–404.

6. Joint National Committee on Prevention, Detection, Evaluation and Treatment of High Blood Pressure and the National High Blood Pressure Education Program Coordination Committee. Sixth Report. *Arch Intern Med.* 1997;157:2413–2446.

7. Blair SN, Kohl WH III, Paffenbarger RC Jr. Physical fitness and all-cause mortality. *JAMA.* 1989;262:2395–2401.

8. Shin Kai S, et al. Aging, exercise training, and the immune system. *Immunol Rev.* 1997;3: 68–95.

9. Pyne DB, et al. Training strategies to maintain immunocompetence in athletes. *Int J Sports Med.* 2000;May 21[Suppl 1]:551–560.

10. Garner DM, Wooley SC. Confronting the failure of behavioral and dietary treatments for obesity. *Clin Psychology Rev.* 1991;11:729–780.

11. Kuczmarski RJ. Prevalence of overweight and weight gain in the United States. *Am J Clin Nutr.* 1992;55:4955–5025.

12. Atkinson RL, et al. Weight cycling. National Task Force on the prevention and treatment of obesity. *JAMA.* 1994;272(15):1196–1202.

13. National Institutes of Health. Health implication of obesity: consensus development conference statement. *Ann Intern Med.* 1985;103:1073–1077.

14. Hubert HB, Feinlaub M, et al. Obesity as an independent risk factor for cardiovascular disease: a 26-year follow-up of participants in the Framingham heart study. *Circulation.* 1983;67:968–977.

15. Andres R, et al. Long-term effects of change in body weight on all-cause mortality. *Ann Intern Med.* 1993;19(7):737–743.

16. Hubbard VS. *Overview of obesity and its health implications.* Nashville, TN: Health Implications of Obesity Series; 1992;5:1–13. Meharry Medical College.

17. Van Itallie TB, Lew EA. *Assessment of Morbidity and Morality Risk in the Overweight Patient. Treatment of the Seriously Obese Patient.* New York, NY: Guilford; 1992:3–32.

18. Willit WC. *Assessment of Morbidity and Morality Risk in the Overweight Patient. Treatment of the Seriously Obese Patient.* New York, NY: Guilford; 1992.

19. Brownell KD, Rodin J. The dieting maelstrom. Is it possible and advisable to lose weight? *Am Psychologist.* 1994;49(9):781–791.

20. Zhang Y, et al. *Nature.* 1994;372:425–432.

21. Bailey C. *Smart Exercise, Burning Fat, Getting Fit.* Boston, MA: Houghton-Mifflin Co; 1994.

22. Sees KL. Cigarette smoking, nicotine dependence, and treatment. *West J Med.* 1990;152:578–584.

23. Edwards NB, Murphy JK, et al. Doxepin as an adjunct to smoking cessation: a double-blind pilot study. *Am J Psychiatry.* 1989;146(3):373–376.

24. Franks P, Harp J, Bell B. Randomized controlled trial of clonidine for smoking cessation in a primary care setting. *JAMA.* 1989;262(21):3011–3013.

25. McElhancy JL. Repository corticotropin injection as an adjunct to smoking cessation during the initial nicotine withdrawal period: results from a family practice clinic. *Clin Ther.* 1989;11(6):854–861.

26. Rose JE, Hickman CS. Citric acid aerosol as a potential smoking cessation aid. *Chest.* 1987;92(6):1005–1008.

27. Kottke TE, Battista RN, et al. Attributes of successful smoking cessation interventions in medical practice. A meta-analysis of 39 controlled trials. *JAMA.* 1988;259(19):2883–2889.

28. Ewing JA. Detecting alcoholism, the CAGE Questionnaire. *JAMA.* 1984;252:1905–1907.

29. Walsh DC, Higson RW, et al. A randomized trial of treatment options for alcohol abusing workers. *N Engl J Med.* 1991;325:775–782.

30. American Psychiatric Association. Alcohol-related disorders. In: *Diagnostic and Statistical Manual of Mental Disorders,* 4th ed.. Washington, DC: American Psychiatric Association; 1994:194–205.

31. Spitzer RL, Williams JBW, et al. Utility of new procedure for diagnosing mental disorders in primary care. *JAMA.* 1994;272(22):1749–1756. (PRIME-MD materials are available from Dr. Robert Spitzer, Biometrics Research Department, New York State Psychiatric Institute, Unit 74, 722 W. 168th St., New York, NY 10032.)

32. Snipes GE. Accidents in the elderly. *Am Fam Physician.* 1982;26:117–122.

33. Kiecolt-Glaser JK, Glaser R. Psychosocial factors, stress, disease, and immunity. In: Glaser R, ed. *Psychoneuroimmunology.* New York, NY: Academic Press; 1991:849–867.

34. Cohen S, Tyrell DAJ, Smith AP. Psychological stress and susceptibility to the common cold. *N Engl J Med.* 1991;325:606–612.

35. Holmes TH, Rahe RH. The social readjustment rating scale. *J Psychosom Res.* 1967;7:17–20.

36. Friedman M, Rosenman RH. *Type-A Behavior and Your Heart.* New York, NY: Knopf; 1973.

37. Friedman M, Ulmer D. *Treating Type-A Behavior and Your Health.* New York, NY: Knopf; 1984

38. Prochaska JO, DiClemente CC, Norcross JC. In search of how people change: applications to addictive behaviors. *Am Psychologist.* 1992;47:1102–1104.

39. Prochaska JO, DiClemente CC. Stages of change in the modification of problem behaviors. In: Hersen, M, Eisler, RM, Miller PM, eds. *Progress in Behavior Modification.* Sycamore, IL: Sycamore; 1994:183–218.

40. Stoffelmayr B, Hoppe RB, Weber N. Facilitating patient participation: the doctor–patient encounter. *Primary Care.* 1989;16:265–278.

14

INTRODUCTION TO PSYCHONEUROIMMUNOLOGY

DAVID A. BARON

KEY CONCEPTS

- The effects of stress on health and disease, and the field of psychoneuroimmunology
- The role of the hypothalamic-pituitary-adrenal (HPA) axis in stress medicine
- Conceptualization of the brain and immune functioning as an interactive system
- Integration and similarity of the functioning of the central nervous, immune, and neuroendocrine systems
- Historical perspective of mind–body medicine
- Altered immune function with mood disorders
- The relationship between emotional stress and altered immune response
- Differentiating the biomedical and biopsychosocial models

PSYCHONEUROIMMUNOLOGY

This chapter introduces the field of psychoneuroimmunology (PNI). PNI conceptualizes the brain and immune functioning as an interactive system. As Rubinow (1) points out, the immune, neuroendocrine, and central nervous systems are stimulus-response systems that are similar in the functions they subserve and tightly integrated in their actions. The reciprocal regulatory effects of these systems provide a basis (but not proof) for the belief that brain-immune interactions are clinically relevant and not reducible to characteristics of component systems.

Research

Research from the past decade confirms the tightly integrated and surprising similarities between the functioning of the central nervous, immune, and neuroendocrine systems. Pert and colleagues (2) suggest that the intimate integration of these three systems warrants their consideration as a single system. All three systems can function as sensory and effecter organs, recognizing foreign antigen (immune) or incoming physiologic signals (endocrine or nervous). All three transmit signals and information as part of their basic function. Specifically, the immune response can be modulated by input from the nervous and neuroendocrine systems. The high degree of similarity and integration between the immune, central nervous, and neuroendocrine systems is teleologically sensible due to the fact they have a common task, to persevere homeostasis and assure the consistency and integrity of body cells and tissues, for which integration and regulatory redundancy is an obligation (1).

In many ways, this hypothesis is similar to osteopathic philosophy. In addition to musculoskeletal integrity, it emphasizes the importance of total body homeostasis in maintaining health and treating disease. The basic principles of PNI, like Engle's (3) biopsychosocial model, stress the interconnectedness, or hard wiring, of emotions to the body's physiologic functions.

Despite centuries of interest, clinical observation, and anecdotal reports, research on the complex interactions between the central nervous system (CNS) and the immune system has only taken place in modern medicine. This in part, is due to the lack of understanding of the complexities of immune functioning and the limited availability of biologic probes to observe and measure the impact of one system on another. George F. Solomon, MD coined the term psychoimmunology as recently as 1964, in his classic paper, "Emotions, Immunity, and Disease: A Speculative Theoretical Integration" (4). In this paper, Solomon offers a theoretical explanation of how emotional states can diminish immunocompetence, ultimately resulting in physical disease. These speculations were of significant interest to the mental health community, particularly psychologists and psychiatrists. However, they did not enjoy a similar level of acceptance by the medical community at large, and especially not by immunologists. Without data derived from well-controlled research studies, the consensus was that something as imprecise and variable as emotion could not have an impact on a seemingly hard-wired physiologic response like immune functioning. No reasonable explanation existed regarding how these systems could communicate with each other. There was no reason why they should.

Despite repeated reports of illness following a significant emotional stressor, nothing more substantial than observational or anecdotal reports existed to convince the nonbelievers. It was Ader's (5) accidental finding that immunosuppression could be classically considered in mice, by pairing taste aversion (saccharin) with an immunosuppressive medication (cyclophosphamide), that ignited research interest in PNI. For the first time, direct evidence demonstrated the potential for external manipulation of the immune system. Intriguing questions followed. If immunologic response could be behaviorally conditioned to turn off, could it be conditioned to turn on? Could this help explain why the patient who, shortly after giving up the will to live, dies, or conversely, why some patients refuse to succumb and ultimately defy the odds to survive life-threatening illnesses. These and related questions stimulated human PNI research.

In the early 1980s, Kiecolt-Glaser published a series of prospective studies examining the effects of emotional stress on the function of the immune system. Kiecolt-Glaser (6) measured natural killer (NK) cell activity, γ-interferon (IFN-γ) production by lymphocytes, stimulated with concanavalin A (Con A), and mitogen responses in medical students prior to important examinations. The results of this study demonstrated that emotional stress did in fact have a measurable negative effect on the immune system. In an important follow-up study, students who were taught relaxation training had a significant increase in NK cell activity compared to students who had not received stress-reduction training. This was the first well-controlled clinical human study that demonstrated evidence of immune enhancement resulting from a psychological intervention (6). Not only did stress reduction improve immune response; students who were not taught stress-reduction techniques self-reported an increase in infectious illness symptoms around exam time (7). These provocative experiments clearly demonstrated an effect in otherwise healthy subjects. Would the results be similar in a study of patients with underlying chronic illness?

Castes and colleagues (8) conducted a prospective study of 35 asthmatic children to evaluate the impact of a psychosocial intervention (PSI) on immune functioning. The immune measures studied included NK cell number and activity, interleukin (IL)-2, (9) and leukocyte affinity for immunoglobulin E (IgE) receptors (an important marker related to asthmatic attacks). Clinical outcomes assessed included the number of asthmatic attacks, use of bronchodilators, and overall pulmonary function. The psychosocial intervention consisted of a 6-month training program in self-relaxation, guided imagery, and enhanced self-esteem. The results of the study demonstrated a significant reduction in the number of asthmatic attacks, decreased used of bronchodilator medications, and overall improvement in pulmonary functioning during the psychosocial interventions, as compared to the 6 months before entry into the study. In fact, surface markers for IgE in the children receiving the PSI became similar to nonasthmatic children. Smyth and colleagues (10) report similar findings in adults with asthma and rheumatoid arthritis. These well-designed clinical trials offer preliminary data supporting the hypothesis that psychosocial stress can, and does, affect immune functioning and ultimately wellness.

Mood Disorders

A merry heart doeth good like a medicine but a broken spirit dries the bones.
—*Galen*

In addition to stress-induced immune suppression, altered immune functioning has been reported in patients with mood dis-

orders. The Greek physician, Galen, reported the relationship between clinical depression and physical illness in the 2nd century c.e. He observed that melancholic (depressed) women were especially susceptible to breast cancer. In an effort to replicate and further explain this observation, Levy and colleagues (11) measured NK cell activity (a measure of immune competence) and psychological stress in women with breast cancer. They found NK activity to be a reliable and valid predictor of the patient's prognosis relative to their lymph node status. In a separate study, these same authors reported that 51 of baseline NK activity changes could be accounted for by assessing a patient's adjustment to diagnosis, depressive symptoms, and perceived lack of social support. They concluded, based on multiple clinical trials, that differences in NK activity and overall prognosis could be predictably determined by assessing baseline stress as measured by emotional adjustment, depression or fatigue, and lack of social supports.

A more recent review of the relationship between PNI and cancer by Kiecolt-Glaser (12) reports: "substantial evidence from both healthy populations under stress as well as individuals with cancer associated psychological stress for immune deregulation and that stress may also enhance carcinogenesis through alterations in DNA repair and or apoptosis." The study concluded that psychological and behavioral factors could influence the incidence and progression of cancer through psychosocial influences on immune function. Other studies over the past decade have explored the relationship between emotional stress and altered immune response. Stein (13) reports behavioral pathology and neuropsychiatric impairment of patients with autoimmune and viral conditions associated with systemic lupus erythematosus (SLE) and multiple sclerosis (MS). Early studies in the 1970s reported an increase in the prevalence of herpes simplex virus in patients with a psychotic depression when compared with age-matched nondepressed controls. Unfortunately, these studies did not monitor any specific immune parameters.

Schleifer and colleagues (14) demonstrated that depressed patients have a decreased number of peripheral T cells compared with those of nondepressed control subjects. Their data suggest that the functional activity of lymphocytes, as well as the number of circulating immunocompetent cells, is reduced in patients with clinical depression. They also speculate that the altered immune functioning in patients with depression might be related to the severity of their depressive symptoms.

Implications for Medical Education

The primary goal of medical educators in the United States is to train medical students to diagnose and treat organic pathologic conditions. Much of what takes place in the practice of clinical medicine and surgery is based on conventional wisdom and long-standing patterns of practice. Mental health issues are often ignored and viewed as unimportant for treating physically ill patients. Too often psychiatrists are considered experts only in mental illness, rather than medical specialists. In the biopsychosocial model, psychosocial issues are seen as separate and distinct from biologic concerns. Yet consider the following facts:

- Emotionally distressed patients visit the doctor and are hospitalized more often than nondistressed patients.

- People with emotional distress commonly visit their doctors with physical symptoms and complaints (dizziness, headaches, fatigue, pain, etc.) and never report mood symptoms.
- Nearly two-thirds of all physician visits fail to confirm a biologic diagnosis.
- Medical illness can precipitate emotional distress, which complicates medical treatment and increases medical costs.
- Emotional distress often goes unrecognized and untreated in medical encounters.
- Appropriate mental health treatment reduces emotional distress, medical utilization, and costs.
- Savings from reduced medical costs can offset the cost of providing mental health treatment and stress-reduction training, which may result in lower overall health care costs.

Unfortunately, these facts are often ignored, leading to a striking mismatch between the true needs of patients and the health care services offered. The result is often less effective care, frustration for both patient and physician, and the waste of ever-shrinking health care resources. If nothing else, PNI research underscores the need to assess patients' emotional distress. Eliciting information on stress levels and recommending appropriate stress-reduction strategies might have a positive impact on a patient's overall health. For patients suffering from ongoing illness, attending to these issues may improve response to other somatic treatments.

Treatment Recommendations

The physician should emphasize the importance of lifestyle alterations such as cutting down on caffeine, maintaining a healthy diet, quitting smoking, and exercising regularly. Other stress-reduction strategies can be tailored to the patient's lifestyle and can be a key component in disease prevention. It is the responsibility of physicians to educate their patients about the importance of maintaining a healthy lifestyle. Make patients aware of target organs and areas particularly vulnerable to stress, such as the heart, kidney, gastrointestinal tract, and musculoskeletal system. Osteopathic physicians with special training in musculoskeletal dysfunction are likely to encounter a disproportionate number of patients with stress-induced musculoskeletal complaints. The education process should include protecting patients from claims of miracle cures or unsound, potentially dangerous interventions, such as unproven megavitamin therapies. The physician should be cautious not to overinterpret or overgeneralize clinical observations. A laboratory finding demonstrating a decrease in an immune parameter does not necessarily predict a change in health status.

THE EFFECTS OF STRESS ON HEALTH AND DISEASE

The arrival of a good circus consisting of clowns is a greater benefit upon the health of a town than that of twenty Asses laden with drugs.
—*Dr. Thomas Sydenham*

Throughout history, medical researchers and clinicians have observed and reported the effects of stress on health and disease.

Despite the general acceptance of this concept by health care providers, it is difficult to define stress, let alone the impact it has on disease and wellness. Early concepts focused on stress being a force of universality, acting on a passive body, with all people reacting in a similar way to a disruption. The modern concept emphasizes that stress is not what happens, but rather how a person reacts to a stressful event.

Distress arises when a person perceives that imposed demands (stress) have exceeded their ability to cope with them. There is a physiologic response to stress. This response involves activation of the hypothalamic-pituitary-adrenal (HPA) axis; it is modulated by the autonomic nervous system (ANS). The ANS maintains balance through its two primary components, the sympathetic branch, regulating arousal, and the parasympathetic branch, inducing relaxation. How stress and other noninfectious stimuli affect the body's defenses against disease are not yet completely understood. Although significant advances have been made (15–17), key questions need to be answered to better understand the clinical implications of stress on health and disease. These include:

- How does everyday emotional stress affect the immune system?
- What are the actual health consequences of stress-induced immunologic changes?
- Does chronic psychological stress promote long-term deregulation of the immune function?
- Can stress management and alteration of immunologic and endocrine effects alter or cure disease?
- Is there, to some extent, well-controlled, valid, and reliable research that can address these clinical questions? (18)

CONCLUSION

Our understanding of the intricate complexity of immunology and neuroscience is growing rapidly. Since the first edition of this text (1997), significant advances have been made in understanding the basic molecular mechanisms of PNI. Early clinical observation is rapidly becoming scientifically proven fact. As with osteopathic concepts, the key to continued acceptance in the medical community, and ultimately the enhancement of the welfare of patients, is adherence to the principles of methodologically sound scientific research. PNI researchers can be proud of their accomplishments to date. Research has demonstrated that the CNS is in direct and constant communication with the immune system. The goal of future investigation is to better understand their "language" and how to manipulate it to promote health. The challenge to the next generation of osteopathic researchers and clinicians is to continue, and to expand on, the work in progress in this exciting and important field.

REFERENCES

1. Rubinow DR. Brain, behavior and immunity: an interactive system. *J Natl Cancer Inst.* 1990;(monograph no.10):7982.
2. Pert CB, Ruff MR, Weber RJ, et al. Neuropeptides and their receptors: a psychosomatic network. *J Immunol.* 1985;135:820–826.
3. Engel GL. The need for new medical model: a challenge for biomedicine. *Science.* 1977(Apr 8);196:129–136.

4. Solomon GF, Moos RH. Emotions, immunity, and disease. *Arch Gen Psychiatry*. 1964;11:657–674.

5. Ader R, Cohen N. Behaviorally conditioned immunosuppression. *Psychsom Med*. 1975;37:333–340.

6. Keicolt-Glaser, JR. Stress, personal relationships, and immune function: health implications. *Brain Behav Immun*. 1999;13:61–77.

7. Keicolt-Glaser JR, Garner W, Speicher C, et al. Psychosocial modifiers of immunocompetence in medical students. *Psychsom Med*. 1984;46: 714.

8. Castes M, Hagel I, Palenque M, et al. Immunological changes associated with clinical improvement of asthmatic children subjected to psychosocial intervention. *Brain Behav Immun*. 1999;13:1–13.

9. Glaser R, Kennedy S, Lafuse W, et al. Psychological stress-induced modulation of IL-2 receptor gene expression and IL-2 production in peripheral blood leukocytes. *Arch Gen Psychiatry*. 1990;47:707–712.

10. Smyth M, Stone A, Hurwitz A, et al. Effects of writing about stressful experiences on symptom reduction with asthma or rheumatoid arthritis, a randomized trial. *JAMA*. 1999;281:1304–1309.

11. Levy SR, Lippman M, d'Angelo T. Correlation of stress factors with sustained depression of natural killer cell activity and predicted prognosis in patients with breast cancer. *J Clin Oncol*. 1987;5:348–353.

12. Kiecolt-Glaser J, Glaser R. Psychoneuroimmunology and cancer: fact or fiction? *Eur J Cancer*. 1999:35(11):1603–1607.

13. Stein M. Future directions for brain, behavior, and the immune system. *Bull NY Acad Med*. 1992;68(3):390–410.

14. Schleifer SJ, Keller SE, Siris SG, et al. Depression and immunity. *Arch Gen Psychiatry*. 1985;42:129–133.

15. Hassed, C. Psychoneuroimmunology: A platonic view of the immune system. *Austral Fam Physician*. 1999;28 (9):950–951.

16. Watkins A. *Mind-Body Medicine: A Clinician's Guide to Psychoneuroimmunology*. London, England: Churchill Livingstone; 1997.

17. Keicolt-Glaser J, Glaser R, Gravestein S, et al. Chronic stress alters the immune response to influenza virus vaccine in older adults. *Proc Natl Acad Sci*. 1996;93:3042–3047.

18. Trilling, JS. Psychoimmunology: validation of the biopsychosocial model. *Fam Pract*. 2000;17(1):90–93.

SUGGESTED READINGS

Ader R, Felton DL, Cohen N, eds. *Psychoneuroimmunology*. San Diego, CA: Academic Press; 1991.

Trilling JS. Psychoneuroimmunology: validation of the biopsychosocial model. *Fam Pract*. 2000;17(1):90–93.

Watkins A. *Mind-Body Medicine: A Clinician's Guide to Psychoneuroimmunology*. London, England: Churchill Livingstone; 1997.

PAIN MANAGEMENT

JOHN A. JEROME

KEY CONCEPTS

- History and theories of pain management
- Different types of pain, including acute and chronic
- Areas of information flow with chronic pain, central control process cognitive/emotional appraisals
- Use of medications and anesthetics in pain management
- Osteopathic approach to pain management

Pain is the most common complaint for which individuals seek medical attention (1). Persistent pain is associated with large decrements in psychological health and daily functioning (2). When successful, pain treatment that relies on the traditional medical model can be gratifying for both physicians and patients. Relief of discomfort can be accomplished safely and easily with nonprescription medications and/or osteopathic manipulation. However, effective treatment using this model depends on two factors:

1. Clearly identifiable and correctable biologic mechanisms underlying the pain
2. A straightforward treatment strategy that interrupts the pain signal

Unfortunately, only a small subset of pain cases meets these criteria. For the vast majority of patients the pain persists and becomes chronic. The underlying causes cannot be clearly identified or medically corrected and numerous attempts to surgically or biochemically decrease the pain signal fail to provide significant long-term relief.

The founding principles of osteopathic medicine are based on the observations that the body possesses a natural healing power and that there are inherent recuperative, restorative, and rehabilitative powers. As Irvin Korr writes in Chapter 1 of this text:

We recover from illnesses, fevers drop, blood clots and wounds heal, broken bones reunite, infections are overcome, skin eruptions clear up, and even cancers are known to undergo spontaneous remission.

Chronic pain is unique in that the organized, integrated unity and collaboration of body components are not functioning in a restorative manner. The person in pain has a wonderfully evolved endogenous opioid system built to relieve pain, and yet this natural ability to adjust and adapt has somehow failed in the patient with chronic pain. Such pain problems are so remarkably resistant to conventional medical therapies that chronic pain is one of the most frequent causes of disability in the United States today (2).

For the osteopathically trained physician, the musculoskeletal system is the primary means of pain expression. In the musculoskeletal system, unique sensory, affective, and evaluative expressions of pain and its related behavior are made possible by the coordinated contractions and relaxations of striated muscles. It is inevitable that continuous or chronic pain causes both structural and functional disturbances in the musculoskeletal system. In turn, chronic pain causes repercussions elsewhere in the body and has an impact on the total functioning of the person.

The osteopath recognizes that the person in pain is more than a biologic event. He or she is a thinking, feeling problem solver. That person, when confronted with pain, actively seeks information, makes decisions, and attempts to put forth his or her best effort possible in adapting to the painful condition. Osteopathic treatment is aimed at *the person in pain*, not the pain in the muscle or the pain in the head. The dualistic separation of mind and body, which currently is universally rejected in osteopathic philosophy, is still unfortunately the basis of much clinical medical practice and biomedical research (3).

HISTORY OF PAIN THEORY

The modern history of pain theory began with Descartes (1596–1650), who considered the brain, rather than the heart or some other organ, as the site where pain sensation was recognized. He described the sequence of a pain event in three stages:

1. Onset of tissue damage
2. Movement of a signal up a transmission line
3. Conscious experience of, and behavioral response to the pain

Descartes wrote (Fig. 15.1):

If for example fire (A) comes near the foot (B), the minute particles of this fire, which as you know move with great velocity, have the power to set in motion the spot of the skin of the foot which they touch, and by this means pulling upon the delicate thread (c, c) which is

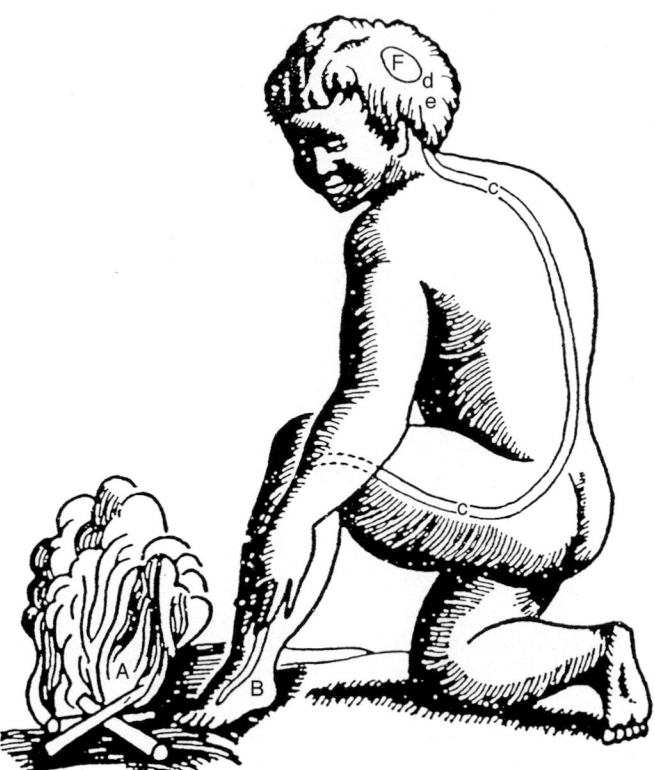

FIGURE 15.1. Descartes' (1664) concept of pain pathway. Fire **(A)**, foot **(B)**, thread **(c, c)**, pore **(d, e)**. (From Melzack R, Wall PD. Pain mechanisms: a new theory. *Science*. 1965;150:971, with permission.)

attached to the spot of the skin, they open up at the same instant the pore (d, e) against which the delicate thread ends, just as by pulling at one end of a rope makes to strike at the same instant a bell which hangs at the other end.

Continuous pain that could not be linked to such a tissue-damaging event was considered a mystery, a punishment, or a mental problem.

As a result, the first systematic studies of pain did not take place until the early 19th century, when physiology emerged as a true experimental science. These early studies provided evidence that Descartes' theory of pain transmission lines and other mechanisms responsible for adverse pain signals were overly simplistic. Since that time, rather than focusing on the unity of mind and body, pain research has focused instead on mapping and describing the pain transmission (nociceptive) pathways. Consequently, the evolution of pain theory has closely paralleled the increasing knowledge of sensory physiology. Since current concepts of pain management are based on historical transmission theories, a brief outline of those theories follows.

Specificity Theory

Specificity theory asserts that pain is an independent sensation. Pain has its own specialized sensory transmission apparatus that is associated with touch and temperature, which conveys information from the sensory organ to the brain center responsible for that sensation.

Specificity theory argues that pain results from *excessive* stimulation of touch sensors. It asserts that any sensory stimulus is capable of producing pain if it reaches sufficient intensity.

Pattern Theory

Pattern theory suggests that all nerve endings at the periphery are fundamentally alike. A particular pattern of impulses produces pain through the overstimulation of sensory nerves.

Central Summation Theory

Central summation theory asserts that *reverberatory* activity in the spinal cord, which projects signals to brain mechanisms, is the process underlying the perception of pain in response to intense stimulation or tissue damage.

Fourth Theory of Pain

The "fourth theory of pain" proposes that pain can be separated into two components: perception of pain and psychologic reaction to pain. It assumes a one-to-one relationship between the intensity of the incoming noxious signal and the resultant experience of pain. The psychologic reaction to the pain is assigned a minor role. This theory is another version and refinement of the earlier specificity and summation theories of pain. It differs from earlier theories in that the psychological perception of pain is recognized as a component of the pain experience.

Sensory Interaction Theory

The sensory interaction theory identifies the existence of two transmission systems involved in the movement of pain and other sensory information:

1. A slow system that involves the thinly myelinated fibers
2. A fast system that involves the large myelinated fibers

According to this theory, both systems transmit signals into the spinal cord. The cord sums the inputs and produces a neural pattern that is transmitted to the brain, where it is perceived as pain.

Gate-Control Theory

The gate-control theory of pain (4,5) blends the scientifically agreed on elements of the earlier signal transmission theories and emphasizes signal modulation at the spinal cord. This theory predominates today. The model is heuristic and incorporates evidence of subcortical information processing mechanisms that can influence the experience of pain. This includes specialization, central summation, patterning, and modulation of inputs (Fig. 15.2). These mechanisms were all cornerstones of earlier theories. The gate-control theory also includes the influence of psychological events on the perception of pain.

A limitation of the gate-control theory of pain is that psychological events are not defined or differentiated from each other. All the brain's mechanisms and psychosocial factors involved in pain perception are placed under the umbrella term "central control

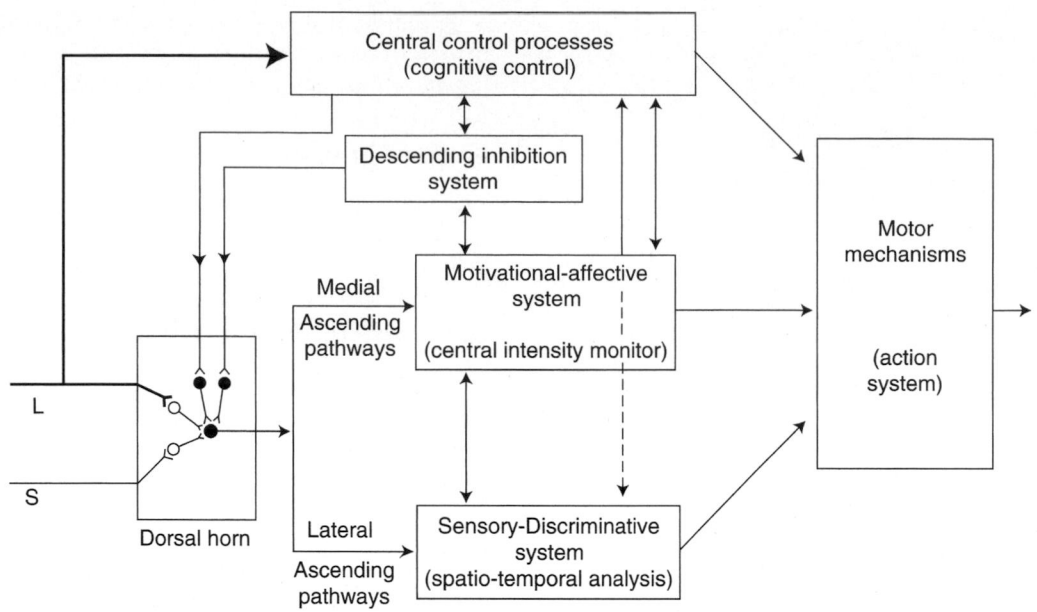

FIGURE 15.2. Conceptual model of sensory, motivational, and central control determinants of pain according to Melzack and Casey. Output of T cell in the dorsal horn projects to the sensory-discriminative system via the lateral ascending system, and to the motivational-affective system via the medial ascending system. Central control "trigger" is represented by the *heavy line* running from the large system to the central control processes. Interaction between motivational-affective and sensory-discriminative systems is indicated by *arrows*. (Slightly modified from Bonica JJ, sec. ed. *The Management of Pain, I*. Philadelphia, PA: Lea & Febiger, 1990:90.)

processes." Since the advent of gate theory, research on the spinal thalamic tracts and gating mechanisms in the spinal cord has increased and added to the development of this theory.

PSYCHOLOGICAL COMPONENTS

Signal transmission is the main focus of all these earlier pain theories. The consequence of this preference for transmission models of pain is that the central control processes become an inconsequential repository for the mind and the psychosocial factors associated with the experience of pain. The psychological factors includes:

- Memory for pain
- Attention and distraction
- Cognition and affect
- Meaning of the pain
- Personality traits and disorders
- Early pain experiences and learning
- Social context and cultural background
- Information-processing style
- Mind and conscious awareness

The organization, let alone function, of the central control processes must be at least as complex as the physiologic pain transmission systems studied thus far (4).

Bonica took a significant step toward incorporating psychological components into chronic pain models. He included the brainstem pain inhibitory systems into the evolving blueprints of pain signal transmission within the brain. According to

Bonica (5), one structure of the descending inhibitory system, the periaqueductal gray, "receives important input from such rostral structures as the frontal and insular cortex and other parts of the cerebrum that are involved in cognition." As understanding of the brain's involvement in pain perception grows, a complete blueprint of the transmission system must include a description of how the conscious human mind processes pain information.

For the osteopathic physician, the mind and body are inseparable. Osteopathic philosophy is rooted the belief that the experience of pain as displayed in the musculoskeletal system is influenced by:

- Genetics
- Lifelong learning and conditioning
- Use and abuse of the body
- Social and cultural factors that shape the individual's perception of pain

DEFINING PAIN

In 1979, the Subcommittee on Taxonomy of the International Association for the Study of Pain redefined pain by integrating both physiological and psychological components. This modification was published in *Pain* (International Association for the Study of Pain) (6) as well as in the *Proceedings of the 3rd World Congress on Pain* (7).

> Pain: An unpleasant sensory and emotional experience associated with actual or potential tissue damage, or described in terms of such damage.

Note: Pain is always subjective. Each individual learns the application of the word through experiences related to injury in early life. Pain is the experience that we associate with actual or potential tissue damage. It is always unpleasant and therefore an emotional experience. Many people report pain in the absence of tissue damage or any pathophysiological cause; usually this happens for psychological reasons. This definition avoids tying pain to the stimulus. Activity induced in the nociceptor and nociceptive pathways by noxious stimulus is not pain, which is always a psychological state.

Acute Pain

Acute pain is usually associated with a well-defined biologic cause and a rapid onset. It vanishes after healing has occurred. Acute pain follows an injury to the body and implies a natural healing process of short duration. It is only expected to persist as long as the tissue pathologic condition itself. Acute pain is also often, but not always, associated with objective physical signs of:

- Increased cardiac rate
- Increased systolic and diastolic blood pressure
- Increased pupillary diameter
- Striated muscle tension
- Decreased gut motility
- Decreased salivary flow
- Decreased superficial capillary flow
- Changes in bronchiole diameter
- Releases of glycogen, adrenaline, and noradrenaline

These changes in dynamic activity are assumed to be roughly proportional to the intensity of a noxious stimulus. The enormous biologic value of acute pain is a rapid orientation to the noxious stimulus and reaction to minimize or escape the damage being done by the noxious stimulus. Some acute pain during the healing process fosters rest, protection, and care of the injured area and thereby promotes healing and recuperative processes.

The overall behavioral signs of acute pain are agitation and the emerging flight-or-fight reaction. Patients with acute pain are anxious about the pain's intensity, meaning, and impact on themselves and their lifestyles. Drug therapy and allowing the natural healing processes to occur are the mainstay of treatments for the management of acute pain.

Chronic Pain and Suffering

Unfortunately, and rather often, pain persists after healing. It also persists after all conventional medical treatments and drugs have been tried. A constant barrage of erratic nociceptive impulses into the brain provide no new or useful information, but the adverse signal continues to reach consciousness. As an example, a patient with a failed back surgery 2 years postoperatively does not need to experience pain every time he moves his spine to remind him that he has scar tissue, adhesions, and functional changes in the structure of his back. Since he is no longer in the acute healing phase, the information provided by this type of repetitive noxious stimulation leads to center sensitization, neuroendocrine abnormalities, and abnormalities of regional cerebral blood flow.

At the biochemical level, when noxious stimulation of muscle afferent C fibers is *prolonged* and persistent, excitatory amino acid and peptide neurotransmitters are released in greater amounts and for longer periods (8). The resulting activation of N-methyl-D-aspartate (NMDA) receptors and the release of substance P leads to hyperexcitability of central nervous system (CNS) neurons and expansion of the size of the painful area beyond the original site of damage. This central sensitization and enlargement of peripheral pain receptor fields (9) allows nonnoxious sensations such as light touch to be experienced as painful (allodynia) and noxious stimuli to be perceived as more painful (hyperalgesia) (10).

These biochemical changes add to the suffering and misery associated with chronic pain. A pattern of objective signs also emerges as the patient in chronic pain now reports:

- Sleep disturbance
- Decreased libido
- Irritability
- Depression
- Decreased activity level
- Deterioration in interpersonal relationships
- Change in work status
- Increased preoccupation with health and physical function

Over time, patients in chronic pain become hypervigilant to all incoming stimuli, their behavior regresses, and they demand pain control from the medical community at any cost. The environment around the patient in chronic pain also often reinforces these ongoing pain behaviors. The pain behaviors are expressed through the musculoskeletal system and are integrated into the patient's lifestyle. The result is that pain becomes the focal point of the individual's life. This leads to demoralization and suffering. The outcome of these structural and functional disturbances is the refractory, enduring pain experience commonly referred to as the "chronic pain syndrome."

The person in pain expresses all these structural changes, functional disturbances, thoughts, feelings, and pain behaviors through the musculoskeletal system. Much visceral, metabolic, and endocrine activity is also responding to the moment-by-moment changes of the musculoskeletal system in response to prolonged pain. With this rich afferent input of the musculoskeletal system into the CNS, it is inevitable that continuous redundant pain has profound consequences to the patient's mind, body, and spirit.

NEUROPATHIC PAIN

Convincing arguments exist for the stance that chronic pain in some cases is caused, or at least set in motion, by chronic pathologic conditions and/or damage to the CNS. Neuropathic pain mechanisms that can be self-sustaining produce complex, erratic nociceptive data that continually activate the biological and psychological systems involved in the perception and expression of pain (5). Examples include:

1. An abnormal neural hypersensitivity that results from prolonged nociception, such as when wide dynamic range neurons (WDRNs) of the dorsal horn are activated in response

to repeated intense stimulation. Once activated, the WDRNs will respond to nonnoxious stimuli as strongly as they had to noxious stimuli.

2. Tonic sensory inputs that originate in scar tissue, damaged nociceptive fibers, collateral sprouting, and peripheral neuropathies.

3. Phasic sensory inputs that are brief, fast-rising (i.e., quickly reaching maximal intensity), intense, novel, or complex.

4. Visceral and sympathetically maintained somatosensory and nociceptive inputs.

5. All other sensory end-organ inputs, particularly thermal-sensory and mechanical-sensory inputs that have become conditioned stimuli through repeated pairing with nociception.

6. A lack of descending inhibitory tonic and phasic down-flow from the brain.

NOCICEPTORS

Pain begins when a potentially tissue-damaging stimuli activates specialized sensory receptors called nociceptors. These nociceptors are found mostly in the skin, subcutaneous tissue, and muscle fascia and joints. When activated, nociceptors, like other end-organ receptors generate impulses that are transmitted along peripheral fibers to the CNS. Some characteristics that differentiate nociceptors from other somatosensory receptors are:

1. Small receptive fields
2. High-response thresholds
3. Relatively persistent discharges without rapid adaptation
4. Location restricted to the endings of small afferent fibers

NOCICEPTION

Nociception is a neurochemical process by which a noxious stimulus creates a pain signal that is transmitted from the periphery to the brain. It begins with noxious stimulus that distorts or damages tissue releasing the endogenous inflammatory chemical by-products of tissue damage such as prostanoids, serotonin, cytokines, histamine, and bradykinin.

These chemical by-products of tissue damage activate two classes of peripheral nociceptors that cause subjectively different noxious inputs. The Aδ fibers produce sharp, well-localized, distinct pain associated with the injury itself. In contrast, C fibers produce a dull, poorly localized, surprisingly persistent signal that evolves after injury. At the time of injury, pain is first created by Aδ fibers, and later by unmyelinated C fibers. Activation of these primary afferent neurons leads to a release of excitatory amino acids, such as glutamine and asparagine, which act on NMDA receptors. Substance P is then released (11) which leads to *long-lasting* depolarization of the cell membrane and initiates continuing transmission of the noxious signal straight to the brain, which explains why pain may continue long after injury.

The final subjective pain experience is only weakly correlated with the degree of injury, the extent of damage, the number of receptors affected, or the energy of the noxious stimulus that provoked them. It is not the noxious input itself but rather how it is interpreted by the brain and conscious mind that determines an individual's unique pain perception and behavior.

SPINOTHALAMIC PATHWAYS

The spinothalamic system consists of two parts: the neospinothalamic tract and the paleospinothalamic tract. Both contribute in different ways to the perception of pain.

In addition to nociception, other sensory information is transmitted along these pathways, contributing to the information and raw data entering the brain in response to nociception. The neospinothalamic tract rapidly delivers noxious impulses that give rise to the perception of sharp, well-localized pain, and an immediate warning of possible progressive injury.

The slower paleospinothalamic tract is composed of both long and short fibers projecting to the thalamus, insula, and cingulate and prefrontal cortices. Its pain perception is one of dull, aching, poorly localized pain sensations. Impulses arriving from the paleospinothalamic pathways synapse with neurons that reach the limbic forebrain structures. They then profusely project to many other parts of the brain. This pathway transports large amounts of general information that produce the long-term motivational and emotional dimensions of pain.

Although the spinothalamic transmission systems appear to correlate well with Aδ- and C-fiber pain, one cannot assume that these structures simply represent subjective dimensions on a one-to-one basis. There are many interactions and feedback loops between them. Nor should it be assumed that the Aδ and C fibers contribute solely to neospinothalamic and paleospinothalamic pathways, respectively. Pain transmission can be closely approximated by such a model, but it is a comparatively simple transmission schematic.

Although nociceptors can faithfully detect, transduce, and signal tissue injury, the afferent barrage is modulated at all levels of the nervous system by a multitude of neurochemical processes, spinal cord excitability, and brain reorganization. Long-term changes in sensory neurons create self-perpetuating neuronal activity even before the noxious stimuli reach higher brain centers. Much of this modulation is activated by sympathetic and somatic efferent neurons, which cause vasoconstriction and skeletal muscle spasm. In the brain, the synthesis of a complex pain perception from the incoming sensory information is further modified by anxiety and brain chemical changes following persistent noxious input. Functional brain imaging studies indicate that there are brain chemical abnormalities in chronic pain patients and that pain perception is linked to specific neurochemical changes resulting in long-term cortical reorganization (12). Specifically, there is a depletion of N-acetyl aspartate and glucose in prefrontal cortex. N-acetyl aspartate is localized within the neurons and involved in synaptic processes and functions as a neural axonal marker (13). More important, the breakdown of N-acetyl aspartate has been documented in various conditions of neuronal cell damage and losses including stroke, multiple sclerosis (MS), Alzheimer disease, and epilepsy (14). Persistent noxious input alters brain chemistry in the prefrontal cortex, which is important to sensory learning (15). Changes in prefrontal cortex chemistry also disrupts overall cognitive processes

(16) contributing to the suffering experienced with continuous noxious sensory input (17,18).

Functional imaging studies also support the idea that pain is processed and experienced within a distributed and interconnected network or neuromatrix of cortical and subcortical structures. This complex synthesis of chemical and biopsychosocial factors into a network of interconnected causal agents helps to explain why chronic pain often persists. It also explains why the osteopathic emphasis on the musculoskeletal system and treating the whole person is critical to the effective management of chronic human pain.

Central Control Processes (the Mind)

Central control processes is the term for the brain's mental transformation of a nociceptive signal into cognitions, emotions, and behavior responses. The patient's responses to pain also are either reinforced or punished by the environment. That information is then fed back through the central control processes. This synthesis of nociceptive information across a series of cognitive and emotional appraisals allows the individual to survive, adapt, and learn. The suffering associated with chronic human pain reflects ongoing challenges to the pain information-processing system. The suffering and agony occurring in the patient's mind is often a consequence of prolonged and erratic noxious stimulation. The end product is the patient's inability to integrate additional incoming noxious data into adaptive information-processing routines or to elicit effective strategies for coping with pain. For the osteopathic physician, already well versed in the philosophy and practice of manual medicine, the realization comes quickly that the patient in pain has a mind (or central control processes) inseparable from the body and that the patient actively thinks and has feelings about their pain. Becoming versed in how the pain information is psychologically organized in the human mind allows the osteopath to bring their medical practice to fruition.

PAIN INFORMATION FLOW AND THE MIND

Information flow implies that humans have the capacity to identify and incorporate potentially useful stimuli, to translate and transform the information received from the stimuli into meaningful patterns, and to use these patterns in forming an optimal response (19,20). The pain information contained in Aδ-fiber input immediately accesses and activates precise central control processes, which then rapidly and efficiently respond to a potential tissue-damaging stimulus. In contrast, C-fiber pain information supplies an ongoing status report after the injury and brings into focus all conditions that surround the injury.

As the individual thinks about the particulars of the tissue-damaging event, learning takes place. The individual anticipates damaging events and makes adjustments to optimize their chances for adaptation, learning, and long-term survival (21). Historically, the basic need to anticipate and avoid potential tissue-damaging events has set the stage for considerable complex higher-ordered thinking and innovative problem solving. Through evolution, humans have become good at anticipating, avoiding, or minimizing pain. When these skills are augmented

with the ability to create symbols for communication, and to use language, reasoning, and abstract thinking, the result is the capacity for maximal adaptation.

Persistent pain can lead to spinal cord excitability, brain reorganization, and self-perpetuating neuronal activity. The cellular and neurobiologic consequences are anxiety, depression, and reduction in quality of life (21). Behaviorally, the patient continually seeks medical attention in search of treatment that will either interrupt the pain signal or help manage the impact of the pain on lifestyle. As a result, the patient begins to suffer, and the suffering continues until the threat has passed. Information processing models of pain assert that a specific series of mental events occurs at the central control level, following prolonged noxious stimulation (19). Figure 15.3 illustrates the flow of somatosensory data through an interconnected network or cortical and subcortical structures, as a noxious stimulus is transformed into information that facilitates pain perception, cognitive-emotional appraisals, and musculoskeletal/behavioral responses. The consequences of these responses are remembered and fed back through the central control processes. This results in a dynamic-plastic system; dynamic in that the information-processing systems *continually respond* to nociception, and plastic in that they also *continually change* as a result of nociception. The synthesis of pain information, coupled with the cognitive-emotional appraisals, allows individuals to survive, learn, and adapt.

The osteopathic profession has a historic opportunity to help suffering patients because of its philosophy of whole-person, health-oriented care. Osteopathic physicians already recognize the relationship between the musculoskeletal system and pain expression. Osteopathic physicians understand and expect the interaction of mind and body systems. Osteopathic physicians know that systems both influence and are influenced by mental information-processing systems, the manifestation of which—a patient's pain and suffering—is shaped by a history of learning experiences, pain perceptions, and appraisals.

Pain Perception

The noxious sensory input is initially directed to the medial and lateral thalamus, anterior cingulate cortex, somatosensory, and perifrontal cortex. The noxious stimulus is consciously registered along with many other sensory inputs surrounding the painful event. Conscious attention is directed quickly toward noxious, damaging, or threatening sensory events. The mind's central control processes scan this pain information for recognizable patterns in an effort to attach meaning, affect, and (eventually) a label to the nociceptive event. The ability to focus selectively on noxious stimuli in the perceptual field, while ignoring others, is extremely important. If human beings did not quickly focus on pain, we would be overwhelmed by the many extraneous events present at the point of the tissue-damaging event and not protect ourselves, fight, run, or tend to the wound.

If the noxious signal is very intense or the damage very serious, the central control processes will stop the pain processing to devote all resources to coping and survival. We are built to survive first and have pain second. Descending pain inhibitory pathways from the brain modulate the transmission of the nociceptive signals to form an endogenous, anti-nociceptive system.

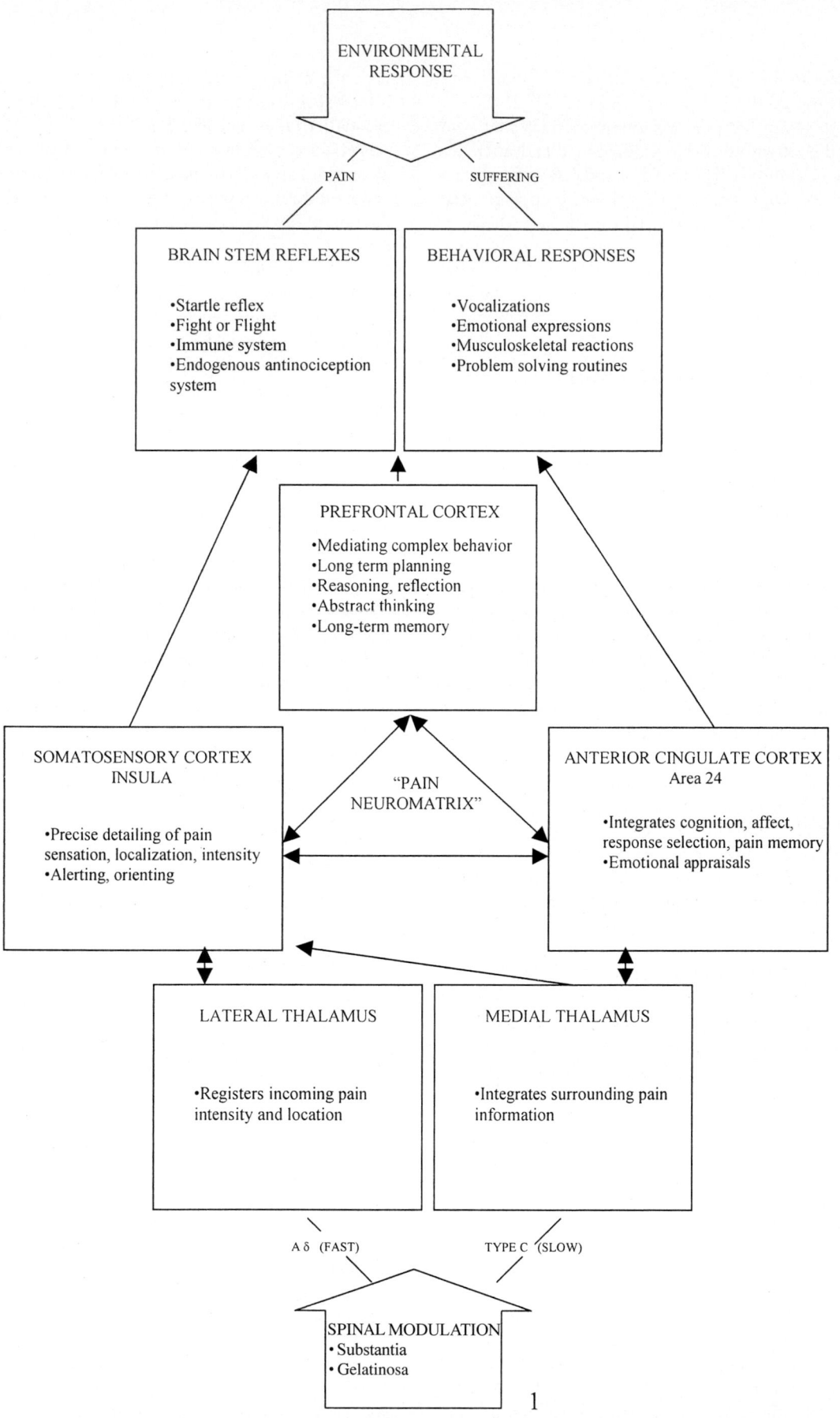

FIGURE 15.3. Central control flowchart for the series of cortical activations and mental events that occur following noxious sensory input. Pain and suffering are an emergent property of the human brain as the noxious stimulus is processed in an interconnected, parallel neuronetwork ("pain neuromatrix") composed of cortical and subcortical brain structures.

Components of this system are found in the midbrain periaqueductal gray matter, the nucleus raphe magnus, and the locus caeruleus. The chemical spinal mediators involved in descending anti-nociception include serotonin, norepinephrine, and acetylcholine 8. When activated, these brain systems can dampen pain sensation and inhibit behavior reactions typically evoked by noxious stimuli (22).

Cognitive/Emotional Appraisals

When the nociceptive signal reaches higher brain centers and true consciousness, thoughts, feelings, and words are put to the event, memories form, and plans of action are made. The cognitive/emotional appraisals occur at the anterior cingular cortex, particularly the Brodmann areas (23,24). The anterior cingulate cortex is an extensive area of the limbic cortex overlying the corpus callosum which is involved in the integration of cognition, affect, and response selection. Projections to the prefrontal cortex activate thinking about the pain and review of past memories of pain (24).

Continuous pain and activation of pain memories encourage the assignment of global labels to pain experiences, lumping a large variety of pain experiences into a single pain construct. Memories that are associated with the nociceptive signal are stored to form an expansive network, or *neuromatrix,* of pain-related information (25). A pain neuromatrix can be thought of as a cognitive structure that forms the basis for all future beliefs about pain and for the problem-solving strategies employed in response to pain.

As pain becomes chronic, the pain neuromatrix expands and becomes more rigid in a self-perpetuating process. In trying to find a way to cope with the pain, individuals begin focusing more on the pain, ignoring information or explanations that do not fit the pain neuromatrix. Over time, pain memories and appraisals are revised to fit the pain neuromatrix, further expanding and solidifying it. Emotional appraisals of the noxious stimulus become "hot" or emotionally charged when the current pain event is perceived as having a significant personal impact. A number of appraisal steps are involved in this process. The outcome of each appraisal can set the stage for the next appraisal. The entire appraisal process triggers significant emotional linkages to the pain.

The emotional appraisal process begins with orienting and startle reflexes, and subsequent feelings of *surprise* or interest, preparing the individual to engage in more focused detailing. For example, further appraisals might determine that the noxious stimulus is harmful, generating *fear* and hypervigilance. If the noxious stimulus is appraised as damaging, the individual would feel *anxious* and likely avoid the stimulus. If the noxious stimulus is appraised as benign, the individual might experience some interest or curiosity and even decide to approach and learn more about the noxious input.

In either case there is generalized autonomic arousal and motor responses, such as those that would be called on to fight or flee. If a person is unable to take any action, they often feel *anger* when their actions are blocked or sadness from a sense of loss of control. Over time, the loss of control over the noxious stimulus leads to *depression.* The patient begins to report feeling trapped, helpless, or frustrated with the inability to overcome pain.

Eventually the patient makes a global appraisal in an effort to understand the painful event, especially why it happened and its long-term impact. Emotions attached to the outcome of global appraisal include *shame,* fostered by a sense that one has failed to reach an ideal standard for mastering and living with chronic pain. Emotions also include *guilt,* fostered by a sense that one has transgressed personal, family, and/or cultural expectations for adequately coping with pain. As a result of these perceptual and appraisal processes, behaviors are selected, emotions are labeled and linked to painful musculoskeletal sensations, and the experience of pain and suffering reaches full expression, often through the musculoskeletal system.

Pain Information-Processing Summary

Processing the pain information contained in a noxious stimulus requires that a person:

1. Selectively review all information at the onset of pain.
2. Retain various aspects of the information to be analyzed and organized into meaningful patterns (i.e., "pain neuromatrix").
3. Compare this noxious stimulus information to pain information already catalogued in memory.
4. Transmit recognized pain patterns to specific pain information appraisal systems, including those responsible for attaching affect and meaning to the experience, and those responsible for translating the pain information into behaviors, musculoskeletal reactions, and problem-solving routines.
5. Selecting and executing various problem-solving strategies in an effort to adapt and cope with pain and learning. These pain strategies both influence and are influenced by the patient's musculoskeletal environment. A major player in the patient's musculoskeletal environment is the osteopathic physician, who often only sees the end product of musculoskeletal reactions, pain behaviors, and the patient's demand for immediate pain management.

PAIN MANAGEMENT

Conventional treatment of chronic pain is often complicated by a patient's beliefs about medical science and the expectations that they consequently place on physicians. For example, many patients believe that complete pain relief is not only obtainable but is their right, and they expect physicians to provide that relief. Unfortunately, the underlying biopsychosocial mechanisms of chronic pain are not fully understood. As a result, conventional treatments fail, leading to frustration for the patient, whose expectations are unfulfilled, and for the physician, whose goals are blocked.

A large part of a physician's practice involves treating patients who have chronic pain. Treatment begins with a biopsychosocial pain history. A simple mnemonic for that history is found in Table 15.1. Conventional approaches to pain treatment rely primarily on:

1. Medications
2. Anesthetic blockade

TABLE 15.1. SIMPLE MNEMONIC TO COLLECT BIOPSY-CHOSOCIAL PAIN HISTORY

P	Palpatory evidence; motion that provokes pain
A	Area (location, radiation, dermatomes)
I	Intensity (0–10 score)
N	Name (how it feels in sensory, affective, and evaluative terms)
S	Suffering and stress (pain's impact on quality of life, mood, relationships, and family)

3. Physical therapies
4. The osteopathic mission to restore function

Medications

Medications are an important management strategy, particularly for acute pain. The three main categories of medications are:

1. Nonopioid analgesics: aspirin, salicylate salts, acetaminophen, and nonsteroidal antiinflammatory drugs (NSAIDs)
2. Opioid analgesics
3. Analgesic adjuvants

These drugs are prescribed according to the World Health Organization's analgesic ladder. It involves choosing among these three groups based primarily on pain intensity. Many mild-to-moderate acute pains readily respond to nonopioid analgesics alone; they are the obvious first choice. Some moderate-to-severe pains may require combining the nonopioid analgesics with a low-dose opioid preparation, the second step in the analgesic ladder. The third step is the addition of a high-dose, time-released opioid preparation to the nonopioid analgesics. At any of these three steps, analgesic adjuvants might also be useful.

The American Pain Society (APS) and the International Association for the Study of Pain (IASP) outline a number of important concepts to remember when choosing drugs to manage pain:

1. Individualize route, dosage, and schedule
2. Administer analgesics on a regularly predetermined time schedule
3. Recognize and treat side effects
4. Do not use placebos to assess nature of pain
5. Watch for development of tolerance
6. Use analgesic adjuvants
7. Block pain transmission

These organizations are a constant source of updated information on the rapidly changing pharmacologic knowledge base regarding pain control with drugs. See the "Resources" section at the end of this chapter for contact information.

INDIVIDUALIZATION

The oral route of medication administration is optimal because of its convenience, safety, flexibility, and the relatively steady blood levels produced. It is especially optimal when compared with the intermuscular route, which has the disadvantages of painful administration, fluctuations in the absorption from muscle, an up to 60-minute lag to peak effect, and a rapid fall-off. Intravenous bolus administration provides the most rapid onset, with shorter time to peak effect. Repeated boluses can be used to load concentrations providing pain relief, followed by maintenance infusion for severe pain. Continuous infusions provide steady blood levels with fewer side effects.

Patients can also be given active responsibility and a sense of control over their medication by self-administering an analgesic bolus with a microprocessor controlled by infusion pump. The opioids can also be administered intraspinally (epidural or intrathecal). Described as patient-controlled analgesia (PCA), the patient can activate a demand switch that delivers a preset dose of opioid into an intravenous line, if a predetermined time (often called the "lock out" interval) has elapsed since the previous dose. In some of the most severe and long-term chronic pain cases, the entire system can also be implanted in the individual and programmed to deliver medication across a preset daily schedule. An implanted morphine pump is for severe, long-term chronic pain cases, such patients with cancer or who are terminally ill, or when all other treatments have failed.

Another advance in the route of administration is transdermal patches that allow the medication to be absorbed through the skin. These patches provide continuous opioid infusion without pumps, needles, or internally implanted devices. Children, in particular, would rather endure pain than have a shot or painful procedure. Fortunately, opioids in lollipops, nasal sprays, and rectal suppositories are now available. New, longer-acting topographical preparations such as a lidocaine patch are also available and can be applied to the skin an hour before a painful injection.

It is crucial not to create pain during the attempt to relieve pain. The old adage that "something has to hurt or taste bad to work" is archaic. Painful injections and procedures run the risk of provoking inflammation and muscle spasm in the vicinity of the injection, thereby generating central sensitization and even more pain. Similarly, sympathetic reflexes can occur, which decrease microcirculation in the injured tissue and adjacent muscle, producing some degree of ischemia and smooth muscle spasm. Because pain is a complex perception, many painful procedures performed to relieve pain can, over time, alter how pain information is processed mentally. This can lead to pain avoidance behaviors such as inactivity and/or fear in anticipation of pain leading to excessive autonomic arousal and analgesic use.

ANALGESICS

When pain medications are given on an as-needed basis, it can take several hours and higher doses of opioids to relieve pain, leading to a cycle of undermedication alternating with periods of overmedication and drug toxicity. Administering opioids on a *scheduled, around-the-clock basis* leads to fewer side effects. Although morphine is a strong opioid and often is a drug of choice, it is important to be familiar with the dose and time course of a variety of opioids. Patients must be followed closely, particularly when beginning or changing an analgesic regimen. Monitoring pain relief and side effects frequently, and adjusting the regimen accordingly, is crucial.

SIDE EFFECTS

The most common side effects of opioids include sedation, constipation, nausea, vomiting, itching, and respiratory depression. These side effects can escape recognition unless the patient is asked directly about them. Several ways to treat side effects are to:

1. Change the dose, regimen, or route on the same drug
2. Try a different opioid
3. Add another drug that counteracts the adverse effect
4. Use a route of administration that minimizes drug concentrations at the site producing the side effect

When choosing drugs, one should also be aware of the potential hazards of mixed agonist-antagonists.

PLACEBOS

The analgesic effect from intramuscular saline (or another placebo) provides little if any useful information about the genesis or the mechanisms of pain. In fact, many patients who have a documented organic basis for their pain obtain temporary relief from saline injection. A recent systematic review of 130 studies involving 3,795 patients with physical pathology indicated a consistent reduction in pain intensity for those assigned to placebo groups (25). There are many sufficient biochemical and psychological reasons to explain a person's favorable response to placebos. The brain produces a variety of morphinelike peptide substances, the most prevalent of which are enkephalins and endorphins. Derivatives of these compounds, metencephalon and endorphin, are derived from pituitary-lipotropin and have opioid-agonist properties. Binding of enkephalins to specific receptors appears to inhibit the transmission of noxious impulses via peripheral unmyelinated fibers to the higher centers of the brain. These endogenous opioids have also been found in higher centers of the CNS, such as the hypothalamus, periaqueductal gray matter, and nucleus raphe magnus. Pain-relieving, morphinelike peptides are produced in response to a person's feelings and beliefs about the treatment. These naturally occurring peptides act like morphine, with the exceptional advantage of being produced endogenously. A positive placebo response simply speaks to the strength of an individual's central control processes (i.e., mind) to recruit their descending inhibitory system to block pain. The osteopathically trained physician knows that pain relief occurs both in the mind and in the body.

PHYSICAL TOLERANCE/DEPENDENCE

Tolerance means that a larger dose of medication is required to maintain the original effect. This is an especially common occurrence in patients in all age groups who regularly use opioid analgesics. To delay the development of tolerance, and to provide effective analgesia for the tolerant patient, opioids can be combined with nonopioids or switch can be made to an alternate opioid. Be aware of the development of physical dependence. Physical dependence means that an abrupt cessation of the opioid will lead to withdrawal symptoms. Opioid use is limited by legitimate concerns such as misuse, addiction, and possible diversion for nonmedical uses (26).

PSYCHOLOGICAL ADDICTION

It is difficult to compete with morphine for its analgesic efficacy. Opioids are very reinforcing as they relieve pain. Morphine, like alcohol or caffeine, easily passes through the blood–brain barrier and goes directly to the brain. Behaviors on the patient's part that secure a continuous flow of opioids are quickly reinforced. Addictive behaviors, including excessive medication demands or prescription misuse, are often determined and shaped by the reinforcement, or consequences of the patient's request for pain-relieving drugs and the powerful relief they bring. In addition drugs that appear to stimulate brain reward mechanisms, such as opioids, sedatives, stimulants, anxiolytics, and cannabinoids, are particularly prone to addictive behaviors. The patient in chronic pain exhibiting drug-seeking behaviors and becoming overwhelmingly involved with using and procuring pain-relieving drugs may be demonstrating learned addictive behaviors, some of which are inadvertently learned in the doctor–patient relationship. In the usual medical setting, these learned behaviors take the form of:

1. Missed office appointments with subsequent off-hour calls for prescription renewals
2. Forgery of prescriptions, or solicitation of prescriptions from multiple physicians
3. Securing drugs from other patients, family members, or off the street
4. Loss of control, craving, and compulsive use despite negative consequences
5. Novel dosing, timing, or route of administration, such as oral to mucosal or intravenous

It is important to be alert to these cues. Remember, the patient with physical pathology who is undermedicated will also be exhibiting addictive behaviors, and the diagnosis in that case will be "pseudo-addiction." Patients with legitimate chronic pain will respond to opioids administered on a scheduled around-the-clock basis.

ANALGESIC ADJUVANTS

A number of other classes of drugs can either enhance the effect of opioids or aspirinlike drugs, have independent analgesic activity in certain situations, or counteract the side effects of analgesics. The most common of these are the tricyclic antidepressants and the newer serotonin reuptake inhibitors (SSRIs). In controlled trials, these drugs have relieved pain related to neuropathy, postherpetic neuralgia, and chronic pain syndromes, regardless of whether the patient was depressed. The analgesic effect of tricyclics begins at lower doses. In animal studies, tricyclics potentiate opiate analgesia, possibly by blocking the reuptake of serotonin and norepinephrine at CNS synapses. However, there is no evidence to support the use of tricyclics in acute pain treatment. Interestingly, tricyclic antidepressants, which block the reuptake of norepinephrine and serotonin, are largely used for the treatment of neuropathic pain. Noradrenergic-2 agonists are popular but they can produce side effects, especially hypotension and sedation. They are primarily limited to patients with long-term chronic pain. The following have all been prescribed as analgesic adjuvants with varying and limited degrees of success:

- NSAIDs
- Cyclooxygenase (COX)-2 inhibitors
- Antihistamines
- Benzodiazepines
- Hypnotic agents
- Muscle relaxants
- Steroids
- Opioid agonist/antagonists/extenders/antiemetics
- Anticonvulsants

As with all medications prescribed as analgesic adjuvants, these should provide an opportunity for:

- Increasing activities of daily living
- Participating in physical therapy
- Decreasing pain behaviors
- Developing long-term behavioral changes and pain-coping strategies

The patient given drugs for pain control should be actively participating in rehabilitation aimed at restoring functioning. Goals should be outlined for the patient that include a *pharmacologic interruption of the pain to allow behavioral changes* and new cognitive and behavioral strategies for pain control. Discuss treatment goals with the patient *prior to* and continuously during the administration of any drugs for pain control.

PAIN TRANSMISSION BLOCKING

To control acute pain, anesthetic blockade of neural transmission to virtually any part of the body can temporarily be achieved by direct application of local anesthetics (nerve blocks), such as procaine, lidocaine, tetracaine, or bupivacaine. In some severe cases, substances that destroy neural tissue can be injected (neurolytic block) in an effort to permanently obliterate the neural transmission mechanisms.

Diagnostically, nerve blocks determine specific pathways to aid in the differential diagnosis of the site or transmission mechanisms of a given pain. Prognostically, they partially predict the probable effectiveness of neurolytic or neurosurgical procedures. Interestingly, the pain-relieving effects of local anesthetics can often exceed the duration of the chemical blockade of neural transmission. The reason for this is not completely understood. It might be a result of decreasing sympathetic reflexes and skeletal muscle tension. Perhaps it results from the creation of pain-free time during which the patient can restructure the pain information-processing routines or learn new behavior

patterns that help in coping with the pain. There are several anesthetic blockades that attempt to intercept the noxious input and thereby prevent its entry into the perceptual field. These include:

Facet Injection:	temporarily decreases small fiber afferent activity by injection of a local anesthetic into the articular branches of Luschka, which innervate the zygoapophyseal joint capsules.
Facet rhizotomy:	eliminates small fiber afferent activity through thermocauterization of the articular branches of Luschka.
Dry needling of trigger points:	produces a volley of small fiber afferent activity that causes brainstem inhibition of the ascending spinoreticular, spinothalamic, and spinocortical pathways.
Local infiltration of trigger points with anesthetics:	causes a biphasic effect that initially decreases pain by the same mechanism as dry needling. Infiltration of the anesthetic decreases small fiber input from the trigger sites and central facilitory states. This decreases afferent activity associated with pain.

Counter Irritants

Counter irritants flood the perceptual field with many complex somatosensory stimuli, preventing the noxious input from being fully recognized and channeled into the higher levels of the central control processes. These treatments, prescribed by the physician, are often carried out by a physical therapist sensitive to the osteopathic model of treating the biopsychosocial aspects of pain.

Hot Packs

Hot packs promote local and reflexive decreases in sympathetic tone. Locally, this increases blood flow and washes out nociceptive metabolites. In general, it decreases segmental reflexes and sympathetic tone, decreasing afferent activity and promoting muscle relaxation.

Transcutaneous Nerve Stimulation

Transcutaneous nerve stimulation (TNS) involves peripheral nerve stimulation with small amounts of electric current. The mechanisms underlying the therapeutic effect are not clearly understood, but three theories have been proposed:

1. Electrical stimulation preferentially activates large myelinated fibers in the spinal cord, interfering with pain perception and increasing pain tolerance.
2. Electrical stimulation results in local axonal fatigue of Aδ fibers, reducing small fiber afferent (nociceptive input) activity.
3. Electrical stimulation activates the descending inhibitory system, which is involved in endogenous opioid production.

Ice

Ice causes a sudden increase in small fiber activity that floods the afferent pathways, causing the brainstem to inhibit further nociceptive input from the affected area.

Vibration

Vibration differentially stimulates large proprioceptive afferent fibers. This action is thought to interfere with pain perception.

Ethyl Chloride

Ethyl chloride floods the ascending nerve pathways with small fiber input. When intense, it can result in supraspinal descending inhibition of small fiber afferents.

OSTEOPATHIC PAIN MANAGEMENT

Current osteopathic thinking is far more than structural diagnosis and pharmacologic management. The mission of osteopathic pain management is to restore both physiologic and psychological function through multiple avenues of intervention (27). The magnitude and vision of treatment must go beyond the conventional medical models of obstructing and/or flooding nociceptive pathways. The art and science of osteopathic medicine is best expressed in the treatment of the musculoskeletal system. Osteopathic manipulative diagnosis and treatment are extensively reviewed in Section VII. The focus in this chapter is on other medical and psychological restorative treatments that complement the structural and functional management of the musculoskeletal system.

Stretching

Poorly conditioned muscles tend to be sore after exercise. Stretching produces relaxation of hypertonic muscles by increasing Golgi tendon-organ discharge and reflex inhibition. Stretching the hypertonic muscles causes an increase in γ-afferent discharge that elicits brainstem- descending inhibition, thereby facilitating muscular relaxation. Simple stretching exercises reduce both the number and intensity of myofascial trigger points (28).

Strengthening

Strengthening exercises hypotonic muscles. Muscle activity increases blood flow and produces a trophic response. Patients are encouraged to begin a regular fitness program of simple flexion and extension exercises with the ultimate goal of establishing a maintenance program of walking, running, or aquatic exercise to achieve muscle conditioning and cardiovascular endurance.

Cardiovascular Fitness

Research indicates that more that 80% of patients with muscular pain are not physically fit, as determined by maximal oxygen uptake (28). Cardiovascular fitness training decreases subjective and objective pain measurements in patients with fibromyalgia (29). Increased aerobic activity can also reduce headache (30).

Proprioceptive Neuromuscular Facilitation

Proprioceptive neuromuscular facilitation (PNF) involves the use of dynamic and static muscular contractions in the reacquisition of joint mobility and general flexibility. PNF stimulates proprioceptive and efferent impulses that promote more efficient muscle use, relaxation, and nutrition through improved neurocirculatory effects. PNF range-of-motion exercises use reciprocal inhibition concepts to relax muscles. The goal is to rehabilitate muscle groups and reinforce appropriate motor unit patterning.

Gait Training

Patients in pain will develop limps and move in guarded ways to obtain short-term pain relief. Gait training is used to improve patterned motion behaviors (gait) through synergistic muscular activities that improve complex motor behavior.

Biofeedback and Muscular Relaxation

Biofeedback therapy trains the patient to modify physiologic processes that are monitored by some instrument or device. Tension headaches appear to originate with sustained contraction of the musculature of the neck and possibly the scalp. Investigators have developed biofeedback techniques for tension headache therapy using electromyography to evaluate tension in frontalis and other muscles. For pain relief, the patient is also taught general relaxation techniques, such as diaphragmatic breathing and progressive relaxation. Patients are taught how to relax their muscles and to manage insomnia and anxiety associated with chronic pain. Relaxation techniques alter sympathetic activity as indicated by decreased respiratory and heart rate, oxygen consumption, and blood pressure.

Counseling

Counseling uses interpretation to identify unrecognized factors underlying maladaptive pain-processing routines. Some patients might unearth early traumas that are played out in their chronic pain experiences. For example, an individual might begin to understand that pain perceptions are triggered or amplified by feelings that originated in childhood but that later came to be labeled as pain. Counseling also actively reinterprets the associations between pain and other feelings—especially depression, shame, and guilt that sometimes arise out of the experience of pain itself. The primary purpose of counseling is to foster coping mechanisms through conscious awareness of feelings, behaviors, and consequences.

Behavior Modification

Behavior modification includes classic and operant conditioning, desensitization, and direct reinforcement for modifying pain behavior to alter the patient's perception and report of pain. For example, children and adolescents who are reinforced to attend school, despite having a headache, not only maintain their class progress, but have a significant reduction in their headache activity (31). The osteopathic physician strongly reinforces pain-coping strategies.

TEACHING PAIN COPING STRATEGIES

Osteopathic physicians encourage adaptive coping mechanisms and mature defense mechanisms that are common among the mentally healthy.

Distraction: redirecting attention to reduce subjective distress associated with nociception.

Sublimation: indirectly solving a problem by doing something else that gives you pleasure.

Suppression: a conscious decision to postpone paying attention to nociception and its consequences.

Problem solving: anticipating future dangers linked to nociception and setting strategies in motion to deflect the danger.

Humor: which permits continuing emotional expression without individual discomfort or unpleasant effects on others.

Volunteerism: being altruistic involves getting pleasure from giving and supporting others, rather than being a victim to pain.

SUPPORT GROUPS

Pain support groups rely on developing a strong therapeutic alliance among group members and the physician or psychologist leading the group. These groups are an extremely powerful and low-cost strategy for managing large numbers of patients with chronic pain (32). The goal is to help patients cope with and adjust to their pain and condition. In support groups, patients reconceptualize the meaning of their pain, their cognitive and emotional appraisals, and problem-solving strategies. They review how their pain impacts themselves and their lifestyle and identify the events in the environment that reinforce their pain behaviors and musculoskeletal reactions. If not taught in a group therapy model, the following concepts form at least an outline for teaching coping strategies within the doctor–patient relationship. These concepts are also the foundational ideas for the advice given to the pain patient on how to think about and manage their pain (20).

1. My pain is real. I will reject any notion that what I am feeling is all in my head.

2. I accept that I might need outside help to control my pain, and I refuse to quit or give in to the pain and the deterioration it causes.

3. At times my pain has had an overwhelming influence on my life, but I believe that I can choose how I react to it.

4. My best efforts and those of the medical community have not stopped my pain. This is not necessarily a fault of mine or

a shortcoming of medicine. I will no longer fight with myself about this or blame medicine. No fight, no blame.

5. I will start by taking an inventory of the price I pay for pain, and the rewards I get from pain. This inventory must be done honestly and without fear of the findings. I will recognize some aspects of my coping with pain that I am doing well, and will also admit to myself mistakes that I have made in trying to cope with the pain.

6. I will forgive myself unconditionally for the past mistakes I have made while trying to adjust to the pain, and forgive others whom I perceive are responsible for my pain and troubles.

7. I will discuss my pain-driven behaviors, feelings, and thoughts openly with those I trust and when appropriate, be willing to make amends for any harm that I might have done.

8. I will hold two ideas in my head: (a) something might come along to relieve my pain and (b) at this time, I have to cope with the pain I have. I will accept myself as a worthwhile and fallible person who is living with pain at this point in my life. I will then move forward, with hope and courage, toward my primary goals of intimacy, bonding with others, and healthy interpersonal relationships.

9. I can choose to seek additional help at each step by developing a spiritually based program directed toward acceptance of my pain. I can then live by whatever spiritual principles promote wellness.

10. After gaining a reasonable level of functioning and pain control, I will recognize that there is still more to life than a constant struggle to live with pain. Then, I will gradually separate myself from my pain management program or doctor, with the complete understanding that I may return at any time. I understand that I have more important primary goals in life, and that coping with pain is a secondary issue—something I do to get to these primary goals.

CONCLUSION

Pain management options run along a continuum from noninvasive and low-risk to invasive and high-risk alternatives. Low-risk choices center on the osteopathic philosophy of compassionate care regarding the whole person in pain, with the primary emphasis on factors originating in the musculoskeletal system. In addition to osteopathic manipulative treatments, further low-risk choices include:

- Medications
- Exercise
- Relaxation training and biofeedback
- Counseling and support groups

Mild-risk options incorporate nerve blocks, and nonopioid and opioid analgesics. Moderate-risk alternatives include implantable therapies, particularly spinal cord stimulation and intraspinal drug-infusion systems. The high-risk treatments consist of surgeries and nerve-destroying procedures. The most prudent overall treatment starts out and stays low-risk and noninvasive. Fortunately, osteopathic manipulative treatments and the other low-risk pain management options are also the most cost-effective and the most user-friendly to the patient. Patients in pain can be sedentary, deconditioned, overweight, tense, underexercised, and depressed. With encouragement from the physician, they can become physically fit, receive osteopathic manipulative treatment, be trained in relaxation training, and be enrolled as members of a chronic pain support group that will likely lead to adjustment to the pain condition.

Most patients with chronic pain can be managed effectively when the treating physician uses a combination of these low-cost, conservative treatments. For the most difficult cases, nerve blocks and/or opioid analgesics might be necessary. With a pain that is severe and disabling, implantable therapies and neurodestructive procedures are always the last resort. They should only be carried out in consultation with other physicians and psychologists, as an orchestrated team effort. The choice of invasive therapeutic intervention for pain is determined largely by the severity of the patient's pain problem, resources available, comparative risk of the procedures under consideration, and emotional and physical state of the patient (33).

Finally, it is of great importance for osteopathic physicians to distinguish between acute and chronic pain in their daily practice. Chronic pain can continue in an unrelenting fashion without ongoing evidence of tissue damage. Its persistence does not necessarily mean that the original organic damage has failed to heal or that the patient has significant psychiatric problems. Chronic pain behavior might reflect:

- Allodynia
- Hyperalgesia
- Spinal cord excitability
- Sleep disturbance
- Depression or anxiety
- Brain reorganization as a result of continuous noxious input
- Preoccupation with health and physical function
- Personality disorder
- Job stress
- Dysfunctional family environment

Such high-risk chronic pain patients require psychological and social management in addition to medical care. There are a variety of traps (34) into which the well-intentioned but unwary primary care physician can fall when managing high-risk chronic pain patients. Such patients should be referred to a multidisciplinary pain service when a complex problem is encountered. These complex problems are more often the exception than the rule, and the vast majority of patients with chronic pain can be treated easily by using the least invasive, conservative treatments (35,36).

In summary, the physician's goal is to restore both physical functioning and adaptive musculoskeletal responses through the simultaneous use of physiological and psychological interventions (37). When managing chronic pain, it is routine to use osteopathic manipulative techniques (38), medications. and psychological counseling.

Combining these elements into a comprehensive treatment approach increases the chances of a successful outcome (39). Intervention strategies, which simultaneously address the biological, psychological, and social factors of chronic pain, are more likely to succeed and modify chronic pain perception and behavior (40).

Pain is the most common element in the symptoms presented to physicians. But as so eloquently stated by John Loeser (41):

It is suffering, not pain, that brings patients into doctor's offices in hopes of finding relief. Astounding developments in our understanding of the mechanisms of nociception should not cause us to lose sight of our patients' goals. Chronic pain is far more than a sensory process. We must maintain the biopsychosocial model of chronic pain if we are to provide effective health care to our patients. Understanding the components of pain facilitates this goal. Suffering is an emergent property of the human brain and is dependent upon consciousness. It too is worthy of study by scientists and of concern to clinicians.

Successful management of chronic pain depends on much more than knowledge. Knowledge must be teamed with keen observation, patience, and compassion. Many physicians have come to believe that treating chronic pain and suffering, with all its biopsychosocial elements, reflects both the true art and the true science of osteopathic medicine.

REFERENCES

1. Schappert M. National Ambulatory Medical Care Survey: 1992 summary, Washington, DC: National Center for Health Statistics, 1992.
2. Elliott AM, Smith BH, Penny KI, et al. The epidemiology of chronic pain in the community. *Lancet* 1999;354:1248–1252.
3. Jerome JA. Theory leads: statistics follow. *Am Pain Soc J.* 1995;(Fall);4(3).
4. Melzack R. The gate control theory 25 years later: New prospectives on phantom limb pain. In: Bond MR, ed. *Proceedings of the 6th World Congress on Pain.* New York, NY: Elsevier; 1991.
5. Bonica JJ. *The Management of Pain,* 2nd ed. Philadelphia, PA: Lea & Febiger; 1990.
6. International Association for the Study of Pain. Pain terms: a list with definitions and notes on usage. *Pain.* 1982;14:205.
7. Mersky H. Development of a universal language of pain syndromes. In: Bonica JJ, Lindblom U, Iggo A, eds. *Advances in Pain Research and Therapy, V.* New York, NY: Raven Press; 1983:37–52.
8. Urban MB, Gebbart GF. Central mechanisms in pain. *Med Clin North Am.* 1999;83(3)585–596.
9. Allemer SR, Bradley LA, Crofford LJ, et al. The neuroscience and endocrinology of fibromyalgia. *Arthritis Rheum.* 1997;40(11):1928–1939.
10. Bennett RM. Emerging concepts in the neurobiology of chronic pain: evidence Abnormal sensory processing in fibromyalgia *Mayo Clinic Proc.* 1999;74(4):385–398.
11. Lu H, Mantyh PW, Basbaum AL. NMDA-receptor regulation of substance P release from primary afferent nociceptors. *Nature.* 1997;386(6626):721–724.
12. Grachev ID, Fredrickson BE, Apkarian AV. Abnormal brain chemistry in chronic pain: an in vivo proton magnetic resonance spectroscopy study. *Pain,* 2000;15:89(1)7–18.
13. Castillo M, Kwock L, Scatliff J, Mulkedi S. Proton MR spectroscopy in neoplastic and non neoplastic brain disorders. *Magn Reson Imaging Clin North Am.* 1998;6:1–20.
14. Salibi N, Brown MA. *Clinical MR Spectroscopy: First Principles.* New York, NY: Wilcox, 1998.
15. McIntosh AR, Rajah MN, Lobaugh NJ. Interactions of pre frontal cortex in relation to awareness in sensory learning. *Science.* 1999;284:1531–1533.
16. Grachev ID, Fredrickson BE, Apkarian AV. Chronic pain is associated with abnormal brain chemistry. *Soc Neurosci Abstr.* 1999;25:141.
17. Talbot JD, Maret S, Evans AC, et al. Multiple representations of pain in human cerebral cortex. *Science.* 1991;251:1355–1358.

18. Casey KL, Monoshima S, Berger KL, et al. Positron emission tomographic analysis of cerebral structures activated specifically by repetitive noxious heat stimuli. *J Neurophysiol.* 1994;2:802–807.
19. Jerome JA. Information processing theory of chronic pain [Bulletin]. *Am Pain Soc J.* 1992;1:7–10.
20. Jerome JA. Life after pain. *Clin J Pain.* 1991;7:167–168.
21. Hunt SP, Manyh, PW. The Molecular dynamics of pain control. *Nat Rev Neurosci.* 2001;2(2)83–91.
22. Davidoff RA. Trigger points and myofascial pain: toward understanding how they affect headaches. *Cephalgia.* 1998;18:436–448.
23. Vogt BA, Derbyshire S, Jones AKP. Pain processing in four regions of the human cingulate cortex localized with coregistered PET and MR imaging. *Eur J Neurosci.* 1996;8:1461–1473.
24. Devinsky O, Morrell MJ, Vogt BA. Contributions of anterior cingulate to behavior. *Brain.* 1995;118:279–306.
25. Hrobjartsson A, Gotzsche PC. An analysis of clinical trials comparing placebo with no treatment. *N Engl J Med.* 2001;344(21): 1594–1602.
26. Savage S, Covington EC, Heit HA. Definitions related to the use of opioids for the treatment of pain. *Consensus document. Am Acad Pain Med, Am Pain Soc, Am Soc Addict Med.* 2001.
27. Elkiss M, Jerome J. Chronic pain syndrome: an analysis of current therapies. *Mich Osteopath J.* 1978;43:8.
28. Bennett RM, Clark SR, Goldberg, et al. Aerobic fitness in patients with fibrositis. A controlled study of respiratory gas exchange and 133 xenon clearance from exercising muscle. *Arthritis Rheum.* 1989;32(4):454–460.
29. McCain GA, Bell DA, Mai FM, Halliday PD. A controlled study of the effects of a supervised cardiovascular fitness training program on the manifestations of primary fibromyalgia. *Arthritis Rheum.* 1988;31(9):1135–1141.
30. Lockett DM, Campbell JF. The effects of aerobic exercise on migraine. *Headache.* 1992;32:50–54.
31. Lake AE III. *Behavioral and Nonpharmacological Treatments for Headache.* Philadelphia, PA: WB Saunders; 2001.
32. Turk DC, Meichenbaum D, Genest M. *Pain and Behavioral Medicine: A Cognitive Behavioral Perspective.* New York, NY: Guilford; 1983.
33. Turk DC, Melzack R. *Handbook of Pain Assessment.* New York, NY: Guilford; 1992.
34. Hartwick CT. Tutorial 17: how to manage a difficult pain patient. *Pain Digest.* 1995;5:93–95.
35. Wall PD, Melzack R. *Textbook of Pain,* 3rd ed. New York, NY: Churchill Livingstone; 1994.
36. Acute Pain Management Guideline Panel. *Acute Pain Management: Operative or Medical Procedures and Trauma. Clinical Practice Guideline.* Rockville, MD: Agency for Health Care Policy and Research, Public Health Service; February 1992. U.S. Dept. of Health and Human Services publication 92-2.
37. Aranoff GM. *Pain Centers—A Revolution in Health Care.* New York, NY: Raven Press, 1988.
38. Anderson GB, Lucente T, Davis AM, et al. A comparison of osteopathic spinal manipulation with standard care for patients with low back pain. *N Engl J Med.* 1999;341(19):1426–1431.
39. Seaman DR, Cleveland C. Spinal pain syndromes: nociceptive, neuropathic, and psychologic mechanisms. *J Manipulative Physiol Ther.* 1999;(7):458–472.
40. Jerome JA. Transmission or transformation? Information procession theory of chronic human pain. *Am Pain Soc J.* 1993;2(3):160–171.
41. Loeser JD. Pain and suffering. *Clin J Pain.* 2000;16[Suppl 2]:S2–6.

RESOURCES

International Association for the Study of Pain (*www.iasp-pain.org*)
Headquarters Office
909 NE 43rd Street, Suite 306
Seattle, WA 98105-6020 USA
Phone: 206-547-6409
Fax: 206-547-1703
E-mail: *iaspdesk@juno.com*

American Pain Society (*www.ampainsoc.org*)
Corporate Office
4700 West Lake Avenue
Glenview, IL 60025-1485
Phone: 847-375-4715
Fax: 877-734-8758 (toll free)
E-mail: *info@ampainsoc.org*

16

LIFE PHASES AND HEALTH

JED MAGEN

A useful definition of development is "a sequential increase in the structural or functional complexity of a system" (1). Historically, the understanding of human development has also led from the less to the more complex. For example, infants were once thought of as being almost "blank slates." Early environmental experiences, especially with the primary caretaker, were assumed to result in the formation of the personality, and biologic influences were discounted. Individual development was thought of as a smooth upward reaching line that had a somewhat inevitable progression. The logical extension of this model was that very early experiences and behavior should predict later behavior. In fact, early experiences do not seem to predict later behavior in any simple way (2). Instead, it appears that human development is characterized by periods of time when behaviors change radically, then relative stability until the next period of change. This discontinuous view of human development along with rapid advances in the neurosciences has helped to alter our clinical approaches to behavior disorders in both children and adults. It is now as important to understand how the central nervous system responds to various environmental inputs as it is to understand behavioral responses. Maternal depression and child abuse and neglect are the best-studied examples of adversity in humans and other primates. These phenomena will be used throughout this chapter as paradigms for understanding neurobiologic responses to adversity.

CONTINUITIES AND DISCONTINUITIES IN DEVELOPMENT

Considerations of the process of development must take into account biologic influences, environmental effects, and the paradigm of discontinuous development. It appears that rather than shifting smoothly from one phase to another, transitions are characterized by "biobehavioral shifts" (3). These times of transition involve fairly sudden reorganizations of the biologic, cognitive, affective, and social characteristics of the organism. The end result is new, more complex behaviors (4). The timing and genesis of these shifts relates to repression and derepression of genes, both due to internal timing factors and to environmental influences. Furthermore, it is becoming apparent that the organism is busily attempting to manipulate the environment in ways beneficial to the organism. The move

from childhood to adolescence is a particularly cogent example of a biobehavioral shift. Puberty is associated with an upsurge in sexuality with very different behaviors toward the opposite sex, an increase in aggression, and striking physical changes (5). Teenagers develop very different relationships with parents and peers than were present as children. The epidemiology of various disorders changes. For example, the sex ratio for depression changes from 1:1 to a large predominance in females. These kinds of shifts in behavior are characteristic of growth and development.

PRENATAL PERIOD

Brain growth and development in utero and in infants and children proceeds from the brainstem to the cortex (6). Infants in utero respond to environmental influences in terms of both physical and behavioral development. A long list of factors can influence intrauterine growth and development (7). Cigarette smoking and malnutrition are associated with decreased fetal growth. Alcohol use can result in fetal alcohol syndrome. The effects of these and other substances on later development are much less clear. The literature on later effects of intrauterine exposure to substances of abuse reveals no compelling evidence that illicit substances result in long-term deficits. Rather, it appears this risk is probably related to the adverse environmental circumstances to which many of these children are exposed (8).

Just as the fetus grows and develops, the mother and other family members are likely to go through developmental steps in preparation for childbirth and caring for a new child. Mothers specifically are said to become more preoccupied with the self and with the neonate, especially after perceiving fetal movement. Fathers may also experience a beginning attachment when movement is palpable through the abdomen. When this developmental process is not allowed to proceed to completion, parents may not be ready to interact with their infant in helpful ways. For example, parents of very premature infants may not be ready to feed, nurture, and otherwise care for their infant. They may have difficulty in feeling as if the baby is responding to them in any way. This may lead to further difficulties with growth and development. Thus, various behavioral difficulties may have their genesis in this period.

INFANCY

At birth, the brainstem is almost fully functional. However, forebrain limbic structures are very immature (9). Infants come into the world with certain preprogrammed capabilities that have evolved to help maximize their chances for survival. For those who wonder why human infants do not come into this world with more developed capabilities, consider that there is a limit to the capacity of the female pelvis to accommodate an infant head. Given this limit on brain size, infants are equipped with only those capacities needed for survival. Rooting, sucking, grasping, and the Moro reflex are all adaptive in that they help the infant feed or maintain contact with the primary caretaker. Less obvious capabilities are also present. It turns out that newborns engage in complex visual activities. They scan patterns by means of eye movements going back and forth across edges (10). By the age of 1 to 4 months, they are able to discriminate many speech sounds (11). These innate preprogrammed behaviors and capabilities are critical to the ability of the infant to develop and participate in the dyadic interaction between it and the primary caretaker, a phenomenon often termed "attachment." Attachment can also be defined as "an enduring emotional bond uniting one person with another" (12). In their very influential work, Bowlby and Ainsworth (13) suggest that all of these preprogrammed behaviors and predispositions serve to help develop a secure attachment between the infant and caretaker so that optimal psychosocial development can take place. In fact, a secure base for attachment has at least three characteristics:

1. it is reliable,
2. it shields the infant from environmental threats, and
3. it is sustaining and provides the infant with resources (13).

Klaus and Kennell (14) used the term "bonding" for the first manifestation of this phenomenon because it occurs immediately after birth. They theorized that infants who were separated from their mothers and cared for in the newborn nursery did not bond as well as infants who were allowed to stay with their mothers. Although this particular notion has not been substantiated, a *process* of bonding does take place and is promoted by a variety of behaviors in which infants and parents engage. Holding infants at a distance that maximizes face-to-face contact, exaggerated greeting behaviors, and parental imitation of newborn facial and vocal expressions are all part of this process (15). For the newborn's part, eye contact with the primary caretaker, vocalizations, and the appearance of a social smile at about eight weeks are all behaviors that will engage the caretaker and help promote reciprocal interaction. These behaviors that elicit stimulation from caretakers are incredibly important for brain growth and development. The human brain grows more through the first year of life than at any other time. Glucose use by the cerebral cortex rises from birth to 4 years; at age four, it is twice that of adults. There is also tremendous growth and proliferation of neurons and the production of axons, dendrites, and synapses during the first 2 years of life. These networks are actually pruned as time goes by based, in part, on how active they are (16). This "use it or lose it" phenomenon partly accounts for the smaller brain growth seen in deprivation. Failure to thrive is a diagnosis made in infants who do not grow and who do not achieve developmental milestones such as the development of a social smile. This is often the direct result of the failure to achieve a relationship with a caretaker when they rarely handle or interact with the infant. There is experimental evidence that touch, in part, operates as a soothing mechanism in animals by activating brain opiates (17). This mechanism may be operative in the therapeutic effect of osteopathic manipulative therapy. In summary, human infants are born with predispositions and tendencies to grow and learn in particular directions. This selective seeking of specific types of activities promotes brain growth and development. Evidence in rodents shows that rats raised in complex group environments have 20% to 25% more synapses per neuron in the upper visual cortex than rats reared socially or individually in standard cages (18). This same phenomenon is likely operative in humans.

A further issue of importance is that of adaptability. The ability to modulate and change behaviors to match what might be happening in the environment is an important attribute. For instance, a parent who is unable to become calm and to sooth an irritable, cranky infant is likely to have an infant who is, in fact, irritable and crying much of the time. The situation, sometimes labeled as colic, may be the result of a mismatch between what a parent is able to provide and what a particular child needs. Given at least average parenting ("the ordinary devoted mother"), most infants are able to obtain the stimulation and nurturance needed from the environment to progress developmentally (19). Competent caretakers are able to modulate their infant's arousal caused by displeasure, fear, or frustration by calming the infant and returning him or her to a tolerable emotional state (18). A large and rapidly growing literature now exists documenting the interaction between neurobiology and environment in infants and children. Clearly, infants respond to their environment behaviorally and their central nervous systems respond as well. Decreases in the normal expected amount of stimulation can have profound effects. For instance, infants whose mothers are depressed exhibit dysregulated neurobiologic rhythms including elevated norepinephrine and cortisol levels, decreased vagal tone, and increased right frontal EEG activation. They show lower scores on the Bayley scale of infant development and growth delays up to the age of 12 months (20).

AGES ONE TO FIVE

Many changes occur during the ages of one to five. Brain growth and development continues. As noted previously, the number of synapses in the one- to two-year-old is greater than the number in the adult brain. Around the age of one, children begin to walk. A sense of one's own body also begins to emerge in a coherent way. Gender identity seems to be set by about age two and a half (21). Expressive language becomes evident. Babbling is present from about age 6 months to age 18 months. Words first appear between 8 and 18 months, after which there is rapid acquisition of words (22). Receptive language usually exceeds expressive language until the age of four to five. With increasing independence and a developing ability to understand and evaluate social situations comes the appearance of behavior different than that desired by parents. Some parents will begin to have oppositional battles with their suddenly not so compliant two- to three-year-old. Talking with parents about consistent and calm limit-setting will often help parents through these difficult times.

Other common problems in this age group include toilet training and problems with the birth of siblings. Most children will become interested in toilet training between two and a half and four years of age. There are many good texts and videos available on this subject. It is important not to develop battles of will around this issue. The birth of siblings is a time when children will feel displaced by a new intruder. They will often oscillate between excitement and anger at the new arrival. Opportunities to be with parents without the sibling and to engage in pleasurable activities are helpful, as are opportunities to vent anger in protected settings. A child who begins to throw dolls around the room after a new sibling arrives home is expressing anger in a way that will not hurt the sibling. Some regressive behavior can also be expected. Bedwetting, thumb sucking, or more oppositional behavior might be seen.

Children who are abused and/or neglected in early life do suffer long-term behavioral and neurobiologic consequences. At a minimum, they appear to have increased vulnerability for psychiatric disorders (18). Abuse is correlated with a host of behavior and psychiatric difficulties in young children including interpersonal and academic difficulties, aggression, suicidal behavior, risk taking, and diagnosable psychiatric disorders (23). A variety of studies demonstrate that children who are abused and/or neglected have either hyperreactive or blunted hypothalamic-pituitary-adrenal axis responses to various stressors (24–29). Persistent changes in corticotropin releasing factor neuronal systems are seen in many primates who experience stress, as well as in depressed humans (30–32). Overall, there is a great deal of evidence for long-lasting changes in the central nervous systems of individuals who have been abused and neglected in childhood.

SCHOOL-AGE CHILD

Generally, children from kindergarten to puberty are considered to be school age or latency-age children. The major tasks of this period are cognitive development and socialization. Cognitively, young school-age children are said to be dominated by "centration." They tend to view events as happening to them or in some way being affected by them. For example, children in this age group who experience parental divorce usually think that they, in some way, caused the divorce. It is not unusual to see increases in depression, oppositional and angry behavior, and declines in school performance as a result. Objects also tend to be measured and defined by only a few of several possible dimensions and may be classified in idiosyncratic ways. Children may measure the volume of a column of water exclusively by its height or width without taking into account changes in both parameters (33). Cognitive psychologist Jean Piaget (33) termed this preoperational thinking. When the school-age child achieves the ability to conserve, that is, to recognize constant qualities or quantities of material even when the material undergoes changes in shape or color, he is said to have achieved the concrete operational level (33).

School is a central experience for children. For some, this is the first time they spend the majority of the day with other children.

School may be the first experience with adults other than parents in authority roles. Thus, a premium is placed on the ability to interact in socially appropriate ways with other children and adults. Rapid advances in interaction abilities take place. Children begin to learn strategies for continuing interactions and for reengaging after rejection and failure in groups. The development of self-concept as well as further internalization of a self-identity is heavily dependent on these early experiences in school.

Many children are likely to have daycare experiences either beginning in the preschool or early school years. Although this is a controversial subject because non-parental daycare can certainly be harmful, high-quality, non-parental daycare is very likely to be beneficial. The most important variable is probably the quality of care, which is highly dependent on the sensitivity and warmth of the caretakers (34). Much more research needs to be done on this subject to understand optimal types, length of care, and how such care interacts with parental care.

Pediatricians and family practitioners are likely to see children with common problems such as aggressive behavior, separation anxiety when going to school, academic problems, and the appearance of attention-deficit hyperactivity disorder. Because school is a central experience and the family is still a center of activity, in order to evaluate these difficulties, physicians will need information from the parents, child, and the school.

ADOLESCENCE

As noted previously, adolescence marks a time of profound biobehavioral shift with reorganization of cognitive, emotional, and biologic functioning. Adolescence generally coincides with the onset of puberty. In females, breast budding precedes menarche by about 1 year (35). In males, the onset of puberty is marked by pubic hair and penile growth. Hormonal increases tend to begin before these secondary sexual characteristics appear (35). One of the triggers for the pubertal process may be related to a particular fat to lean body mass ratio (36).

Cognitive and social-emotional changes are extremely important during this time period. Cognitively, in Piagetian terms, the adolescent moves from the stage of concrete operations to formal operational processes (33). The individual begins to grasp highly abstract concepts and to manipulate them. The ability to formulate hypotheses and the use of deductive reasoning are formal operational processes that have obvious applications in school.

Perhaps the hallmark of adolescence is the process of separation-individuation (37). During this period, it is said that the "final" crystallization of the adult personality is taking place along with a gradual separation from the family of origin. Many factors contribute to and interact in this developmental process. Cognitively, the adolescent can now conceive of a larger world and others outside the family as having importance and relevance. The peer group begins to overtake parents in importance regarding matters of dress, opinion, and in numerous other areas. Relationships with the same and the opposite sex become of overwhelming concern. In short, the adolescent uses these relationships and the ability to think independently in order to separate from the family, build an increasingly independent lifestyle, and develop a character structure capable of self-regulation and independent action. Some conflict with parents seems to be an inevitable result of and may enhance this process to some extent. However, the traditional view of adolescence as a developmental period of turmoil does not seem to be true for a substantial number of adolescents. Offer and colleagues (38) documented a large group of male adolescents who seemed to go through this period of time in a "continuous growth" mode. Little evidence of conflict or turmoil with family members was found, and this group was able to integrate various experiences of adolescence and to accept cultural and societal norms without conflict.

Adolescents may also choose to separate in maladaptive ways. Individuals who engage in delinquent acts may be choosing an alternate path of separation from the family. In a chronic disease situation such as diabetes, adolescents may need more care and may not be able to become as independent as their peers. In reaction, they may become neglectful of diets or insulin injections. The adolescent diabetics with repeated ketoacidotic episodes might be engaging in a maneuver to express independence in the only effective way they know.

The opposite also occurs; that is, adolescents who never really separate and remain childish and enmeshed with parents. In Western and especially American culture, adolescence is prolonged. College and professional education can extend into the late 20s or early 30s with continuing financial dependence on parents. This pattern may be particularly pertinent to medical students who undergo long periods of training, at first without any and then with minimal remuneration.

Other patterns of progression through adolescence do occur. That which we consider normative is, in part, culture-bound. In some cultures, preadolescent and early adolescent male homosexuality is normative and does not seem to result in large numbers of homosexual adults. In a number of cultures, a sharp demarcation takes place between adolescence and adulthood with rites of passage.

Hamburg (39) comments that the fundamental requirements for healthy adolescent development are:

1. finding a valued place in a constructive group,
2. learning how to form close, durable human relationships,
3. feeling a sense of worth as an individual,
4. achieving a reliable basis for making informed choices,
5. knowing how to use the support systems available to them,
6. expressing constructive curiosity and exploratory behavior,
7. believing in a promising future with real opportunities,
8. finding ways to be useful to others,
9. learning to live respectfully with others in circumstances of democratic pluralism, and
10. cultivating the inquiring and problem-solving skills that serve lifelong learning and adaptability.

For practitioners caring for adolescents, it is important to be supportive of the normal developmental process of the age group. Seeing the adolescent with parents for at least part of the medical visit is helpful, but teenagers will often have concerns about confidentiality that will need to be discussed and respected.

ADULTHOOD

Although some personality development and change continues to occur in adulthood, for the most part, research in this area demonstrates that personality is fairly stable (40,41). Based on this viewpoint, drastic personality changes in adulthood or old age should be viewed with a high index of suspicion. Similarly, cognitive changes should not be attributed to "aging" but should be investigated as a sign of possible pathology (42). As he did for childhood and adolescence, Erik Erikson (37) outlined a series of stages, including young adulthood, adulthood, and old age. He assigned a number of developmental tasks to each stage. In young adulthood, he contrasts competing drives of intimacy and isolation. Intimacy involves the development of a sharing mutual relationship; whereas, isolation is a sense of being separate and unrecognized. The most important relationships are those that develop with potential partners. Developing a sharing, intimate relationship is of paramount importance.

In adulthood, the core task is generative, meaning creativity, procreativity, and productivity. There is a drive to have children, to succeed at one's career, and to be productive. One of the driving forces of adulthood is that of caring for and raising children. Passing on values and resources is a prime motivation.

However, as a consequence of increasing life spans, a competing dynamic seen in increasing frequency is that of the need to care for aging parents. Middle-aged adults may find themselves responsible for the financial and perhaps physical care of elderly parents as well as their own children (43). The stress and burden of this kind of situation can be significant.

Clinically, younger and middle-aged adults may present with depressions and anxiety disorders. Even more common, somatic symptoms as an expression of various stressors are seen.

ELDERLY

In most cultures, advanced age has been highly regarded but rarely encountered (44). Improved medical care is resulting in lengthening life spans. Formerly lethal disorders may now result in longer-term chronic illnesses with morbidity and disability. It is appropriate that Erikson (37) has included a stage of old age in his schema. In old age, the competing drives are said to be integrity vs. despair. Despair and depression can be related to the knowledge that the life span is increasingly limited and to the loss of a spouse, friends, and career. Erikson does propose the competing drive of integrity, a sort of wisdom and perspective that comes with experience. In the Berkeley older generation study, when asked what periods of their lives brought them the most satisfaction, "right now" was named most often (45). This set of coping mechanisms will be extremely helpful in old age when changes occur in many areas of social and individual functioning.

As individuals age, they may begin to expect to slow down and to develop some infirmities and disabilities. If expected, these problems may be taken in stride without too much upset or turmoil. Dietz (46) reports that older adults generally experience higher levels of self-efficacy and self-esteem compared with younger individuals. This finding may be explained by a continuing process of maturation in older age in which elders begin to look inward for a sense of meaning and accept their accomplishments in life as adequate. On the other hand, unexpected or catastrophic life events are especially stressful and less likely to be handled well (47).

In many cultures, the elderly are viewed as carriers of culture and memory and repositories of wisdom and judgment. This viewpoint comes close to the Eriksonian concept of an ideal old age. However, old age can degenerate into despair over continual losses of function, spouse, and friends. Good health is particularly important for good morale and coping skills (48).

Thus, one of the primary concerns of elderly individuals is the quality of the physical and psychological care they receive. They may be increasingly demanding of health care professionals for care that promotes the best possible functioning. Among the problems becoming more frequent in the very old is dementia. The Swedish Centenarian Study estimated that at least 27% of their cohort of individuals aged 100 had symptoms of dementia (44). Older individuals have a justified concern with the quality of their final days. The avoidance of discomfort and long, drawn-out deaths while attached to various life support devices creates concern and should become a topic of discussion. Physicians are often not comfortable with talking about death and will actively try to avoid such discussions. Pain especially deserves particular attention, not least because the Joint Commission on Accreditation of Health Care Facilities require health care facilities to

1. recognize the right of patients to appropriate assessment and management of pain,
2. identify pain in patients during their initial assessment and reassessments,
3. document acceptable outcomes of treatment, and
4. educate providers, patients and their families about pain management (49).

Pain scales are a useful means of measuring pain severity. Quality, location, duration, and phenomena that might increase or decrease pain are also important to assess.

A number of sources discussing medication approaches to pain relief are available. In general, mild pain may be treated with aspirin, acetaminophen, or nonsteroidal, antiinflammatory drugs. Moderate pain may be treated with these agents plus opiates such as codeine or oxycodone. More severe pain is treated with morphine and similar opiates plus other analgesics.

End-of-life care is not truly complete without the components of advance care planning, clear discussions of palliative care, and the use of hospice care with its team approach. Finally, relatives and others close to dying individuals also need care and often need help with grieving.

CONCLUSION

The course of human development is characterized by an ever-increasing level of complexity with a series of biobehavioral shifts to new levels of organization. Although individual early experiences are important, it is not likely that any single incident will produce a radical alteration in personality. What seems to be important is consistent parenting and an adequate environment in which the individual can grow and develop. What is carried forward, what is continuous, is the pattern of consistent relationships that develops. Human development is a complex process that has no singular determinant of behavior or disorder. Development is truly a biopsychosocial process.

REFERENCES

1. Yates TT. Theories of cognitive development. In: Lewis M, ed. *Child and Adolescent Psychiatry: A Comprehensive Textbook.* Baltimore, MD: Williams & Wilkins; 1991.
2. Kagen J. Continuity and change in the opening years of life. In: Emde RN, Harmon RJ, eds. *Continuities and Discontinuities in Development.* New York, NY: Plenum Publishing; 1984:15–39.
3. Zeanah CH, Anders TF, Seifer R, et al. Implications of research on infant development for psychodynamic theory and practice. *J Am Acad Child Adolesc Psychiatry.* 1989;28(5)657–668.
4. Emde RN, Easterbrooks MA. Assessing emotional availability in early development. In: Frakenbert WK, Emde RN, Sullivan JW, eds. *Early Identification of Children at Risk.* New York, NY: Plenum Publishing;1985.
5. Rutter M. Continuities and discontinuities in socio-emotional development: Empirical and conceptual perspectives. In: Emde RN, Harmon RJ, eds. *Continuities and Discontinuities in Development.* New York, NY: Plenum Publishing;1984:41–68.
6. Nelson A, Bloom E. Child development and neuroscience. *Child Dev.* 1997;68:970–987.
7. Smotherman WP, Robinson SR. Prenatal influences on development: behavior is not a trivial aspect of fetal life. *J Dev Behav Pediatr.* 1987;8(3):171–176.
8. Hans S. Prenatal drug exposure: behavioral functioning in late childhood and adolescence. *NIDA Res Monogr.* 1996;164:261–276.
9. Joseph R. Environmental influences on neural plasticity, the limbic system, emotional development and attachment: a review. *Child Psychiatry Hum Dev.* 1999;29(3):189–208.
10. Haith MM. *Rules that babies look by.* Hillsdale, NJ: Erlbaum; 1980.
11. Eimas PD, Siquelend ER, Josczyk P, et al. Speech perception in infants. *Science.* 1971;171:303–306.
12. Thompson RA. Attachment theory and research. In: Lewis M, ed. *Child and Adolescent Psychiatry: A Comprehensive Textbook.* Baltimore, MD: Williams & Wilkins; 1991:100–108.
13. Kraemer GW. Psychobiology of early social attachment in rhesus monkeys. *Ann N Y Acad Sci.* 1997;807:401–418.
14. Klause MH, Kennell JH. Mothers separated from their newborn infants. *Pediatr Clin North Am.* 1970;17:1015–1037.
15. Emde RN. Development terminable and interminable: innate and motivational factors from infancy. *Int J Psychoanal.* 1988;69:23–42.
16. Singer W. Development and plasticity of cortical processing architectures. *Science.* 1995;270:758–764.
17. Kuhn CM, Schanberg SM. Responses to maternal separation: mechanisms and mediators. *Int J Dev Neurosci.* 1998;16(3–4):261–270.
18. Glaser D. Child abuse and neglect and the brain—a review. *J Child Psychol Psychiatry.* 2000;41(1):97–116.
19. Winnecott DW. *Primitive Emotional Development.* New York, NY: Basic Books; 1945.
20. van der Kolk B, Fisler R. Childhood abuse and neglect and loss of self regulation. *Bull Menninger Clin.* 1994;58:145–168.
21. Money J, Hampson JG, Hampson JL. An examination of some basic sexual concepts: the evidence of human hermaphroditism. *Johns Hopkins Hospital Bulletin.* 1995;97:301–319.
22. Baker L, Cantwell DP. The development of speech and language. In: Lewis M, ed. *Child and Adolescent Psychiatry: A Comprehensive Textbook.* Baltimore, MD: Williams & Wilkins; 1991:100–108.

For example, catecholamines and corticosteroids secreted by the adrenal medulla and cortex, respectively, can be measured from urine and plasma levels. The secretion of catecholamines reflects sympathetic arousal because the adrenal medulla is innervated by the sympathetic nervous system.

Secretions of epinephrine and norepinephrine are also part of the sympathetic arousal process. The secretion of catecholamines leads to systemic reactions in the body such as increased cardiovascular reactivity and changes in cognitive, emotional, and behavioral functioning. These changes are often expressed as chronic muscle tension. Little doubt exists in the mind of the osteopathically trained physician that stress is reflected in the musculoskeletal system (4,5).

By considering function along with structure, osteopathic concepts emphasize the role of the body's communication systems (nervous, circulatory, and endocrine) in facilitating somatic dysfunction caused by stress. The term facilitation means the enhancement or reinforcement of otherwise subthreshold neuronal activities that stimulate effector units to inappropriately carry out whatever action they normally do (6). Examples of effector sites are:

Muscle bundles
Muscle groups
Viscera
Other neural units and networks

Osteopathic treatment is designed to raise stimulus thresholds so that stressors are less likely to induce or maintain somatic dysfunction-related problems.

THEORIES OF STRESS

In 1932, Cannon (7) was the first to write that the release of catecholamines and musculoskeletal arousal initially facilitate adaptation. Being aroused by stress provides a biologic advantage that enables the individual to rapidly respond to danger. Historically, these stress-related increases of catecholamines enhanced survival and adaptive responses. We ignored a pain, fought back, ran to safety on broken bones, and scrambled to the top of the food chain. We have survived as a species, but now survival depends on how we relate to our cortically driven society. That first described in Cannon's early work as our "fight-or-flight" strategy no longer serves us adequately in our ambiguous and increasingly complex world. Now we internalize the stressors and become distressed. We experience somatic dysfunction then present ourselves to the primary care physician requesting treatment for symptoms and problems.

Damaging stress levels are reached when perceived threats or dangers upset the biopsychosocial balance. When prolonged stress reaches critical levels, chronically increased concentrations of antiinflammatory corticosteroids and proinflammatory prostaglandins can negatively alter immune responses, with increased vulnerability to immune-related problems. Damaging stress levels are reflected in the neuromusculoskeletal system as disruption of the body's homeostasis that exhausts the patient. Chronic diseases, impairments, and disabilities are apt to follow under certain circumstances.

Osteopathic philosophy teaches that structure and function are interdependent; that form follows function. Thoughts, emotions, and behaviors in response to stressors are in a blended and complex relationship that can affect both anatomy (structure) and physiology (function).

Selye (8) first described the interdependent processes of responding to stress as the general adaptation syndrome (GAS). Selye believed that our response to stress was a specific syndrome following certain patterns and affecting specific organs. Stress itself could be induced by a variety of internal or external stimuli.

When patients are continually stressed, they move through three response stages. First, there is a startle response and orienting reflex as the patient becomes aware of the stress and is biologically alarmed. Adrenal, cardiovascular, respiratory, and musculoskeletal functions increase.

Next is an attempt to cope and problem-solve biologically, psychologically, and socially. The patient mobilizes all resources to meet and resist the stressor. If the patient is successful, mastery and learning occur. If the patient fails, he or she becomes exhausted physiologically, mentally, and emotionally.

The third stage, exhaustion, is what the osteopathic physician sees clinically as a variety of dysfunctional signs and symptoms affecting any and all organ systems, including the neuromusculoskeletal network. As coping responses fail, the exhaustion depletes adaptive reserves and resistance disappears. Common consequences of this failure to adapt include:

Fatigue
Depression
Anxiety
Insomnia
Musculoskeletal complaints
Drug-seeking behaviors

When emotional and biologic reserves become depleted, patients often seek medical attention. Careful questioning is needed to uncover such problems as:

Family disruptions
Job dissatisfaction
Chronic overstimulation
Feeling overwhelmed
Poor nutrition
Lack of exercise
Abuse—physical, emotional, verbal, sexual

Inquiries to the primary care physician are not about coping with stress, but more often requests for a quick fix:

"I need something for my stomach."
"Can I have some time off work?"
"I need something for depression."
"Give me something to sleep."
"What should I do about my teenager?"

Because osteopathic theory emphasizes the interdependence of body structure and its overall function, osteopathic physicians commonly use palpatory diagnosis and osteopathic manipulative treatment in the primary care setting to help diagnose and manage somatic components of this syndrome.

Clinically, two approaches are possible:

1. Change the stressor.
2. Help the patient respond in healthy ways to the stress.

Change Stressor

Before seeking medical treatment, the patient probably has already tried to change the stressor without much success. More quick advice usually doesn't work. Many studies illustrate that compliance with physician advice is low (7), particularly in the current climate of health care delivery where the pace is hectic and often impersonal. As patients shift between physicians and insurance plans in a managed care environment, the personal relationships once forged between physician and patient disappear. Trusting relationships are difficult to establish under these circumstances, increasing the likelihood that professional advice will go unheeded.

Many patients who come to a primary care setting are looking for help with stress-related symptoms. A primary care osteopathically oriented approach assesses all the disturbing psychosocial and organic problems, including the neuromusculoskeletal elements, so that a long-term treatment strategy can be developed. In such cases, after a detailed history is taken and complete physical examination, the treatment strategy incorporates all elements of the osteopathic philosophy. It includes:

Palpatory diagnosis
Manipulative treatment
Exercise, diet, smoking, alcohol, drug cessation
Appropriate medication
Coping strategy education

When hands-on procedures are used to identify stress-induced somatic dysfunction, the experienced osteopathic practitioner can determine whether the observed pattern of somatic dysfunction is associated with primary neuromusculoskeletal dysfunction, contribution from somatovisceral or viscerosomatic components, or a more complex behavioral dysfunction. Directing all aspects of treatment toward modifying the biopsychosocial causes and maladaptive responses to stress is important. The primary care physician must constantly be aware that clinically evident stress reflects two realities:

1. A patient's immediate response to stress-inducing environmental events produces biopsychosocial consequences.
2. A patient's long-term stress management style is an important process in which the physician must intervene for long-term adaptive change.

Change Response to Stress

As previously mentioned, stress-related conditions are found in at least 20% of primary care outpatients (9–11). By changing the response to stress, one immediately treats some of the autonomic components of stress-related somatic dysfunction and their antecedents. Success is more likely when physicians educate patients, guide and mentor their adaptation, and teach them coping and stress-mastery skills. In a primary care practice, diagnosis begins by accurately reviewing four of the most common behavioral consequences of stress (12,13):

Depression
Anxiety
Substance abuse
Insomnia

When the exact diagnosis is made, carefully inform the patient and then guide him or her through a process of problem identification and problem-solving designed to either relieve or cope with the stress. The remainder of this chapter reviews these four stress-induced problem areas from a cognitive behavioral standpoint. Emphasis is on rapid techniques for diagnosis and on specific strategies to be employed within the doctor-patient relationship.

DEPRESSION

Feeling "down" is a universal experience. Being sad or "blue" accompanies disappointments, setbacks, or losses in life. The depressed mood usually lasts a short time and passes. For some people, however, the sadness becomes intense and long lasting, coloring every aspect of their existence. The future seems hopeless. They feel:

Powerless
Consumed by their helplessness
Overwhelmed
Unable to concentrate, sleep, or solve the routine problems of life

In the United States, clinical depression results in the hospitalization of 6% of all women and 3% of all men (14,15), with 15% of all who are severely clinically depressed eventually committing suicide (16).

The *Diagnostic and Statistical Manual of Mental Disorders,* Fourth Edition (DSM-IV) (17) and the Guidelines for Detection and Diagnosis in Primary Care (18,19) categorize mental health diagnoses. The word depression refers to a syndrome in which a variety of signs and symptoms occur. Typically, there is a change from previous adequate emotional functioning to a depressed mood and a loss of pleasure in life's usual activities. The depressed person feels sad or empty most of the time and often experiences impairment in interpersonal, social, or occupational functioning.

Associated symptoms include:

Fatigue
Feelings of worthlessness
Excessive guilt
Agitation
Diminished abilities to problem solve or concentrate
Indecisiveness
Insomnia or hypersomnia
Possible suicidal thoughts

If five or more of these symptoms are present for more than 2 weeks, a diagnosis of major depressive disorder is considered. If over the last 2 years the patient reports having felt these symptoms and says that for more than half of that time it was hard to work, take care of simple things at home, or get along with people, the diagnosis is dysthymia.

Measurement of Depression

There are many self-administered inventories, such as the Zung Depression Scale (20,21), the Beck Depression Inventories (22,23), and the MMPI Depression Scale (24,25). These inventories provide reliable and valid measures of the severity of depression. The patient can initially be tested for a baseline measure and then repeatedly tested with the same instrument to measure progress. More recently developed structured interviews such as the PRIME-MD (26,27) allow one to quickly (i.e., in 8.4 minutes) determine the presence of pivotal signs and symptoms (Table 17.1). Medical disorders with intrusive symptoms of depression must be ruled out (Table 17.2). Depression has also been reported as a serious adverse effect of more than 100 commonly prescribed drugs (Table 17.3).

Tricyclic antidepressants and serotonin reuptake inhibitors are the gold standards for initiating management of many serious, possibly organic, depressions (28,29). Recoveries are often dramatic as the patient reverts to predepression levels of functioning. Primary care physicians are exposed to a tremendous amount of publicity and marketing from drug companies to manage the symptoms of depression with various pharmacologic products.

TABLE 17.1. STRUCTURED INTERVIEW QUESTIONS FOR DEPRESSION[a]

For the last 2 weeks, have you had any of the following problems *nearly every day?*

1. Trouble falling or staying asleep, or sleeping too much?	YES	NO
2. Feeling tired or having little energy?	YES	NO
3. Poor appetite or overeating?	YES	NO
4. Little interest or pleasure in doing things?	YES	NO
5. Feeling down, depressed, or hopeless?	YES	NO
6. Feeling bad about yourself, or that you are a failure or have let yourself or your family down?	YES	NO
7. Trouble concentrating on things, such as reading the newspaper or watching television?	YES	NO
8. Being so fidgety or restless that you were moving around a lot more than usual? If No: What about the opposite—moving or speaking so slowly that other people could have noticed?	YES	NO
9. In the last 2 weeks, have you had thoughts that you would be better off dead or of hurting yourself in some way? (Tell me about it.)	YES	NO

SCORING: If five or more of #1 to #9 are yes, one of which is #4 or #5, then consider *major depressive disorder.* If the condition has persisted over the last 2 *years* and the patient reports that it was hard to do their work, take care of things at home, or get along with other people, then consider *dysthymia.*

[a]Primary care evaluation for mental disorders (Prime-MD). From Spitzer RL, Williams JB. *PRIME-MD Clinical Evaluation Guide.* New York, NY: Biometrics Research, New York State Psychiatric Institute; 1994, with permission.

TABLE 17.2. MEDICAL ILLNESSES AND CONDITIONS WITH INTRINSIC SYMPTOMS OF DEPRESSION

Parkinson disease
Normal pressure hydrocephalus
Multiple sclerosis/stroke
Brain tumors (temporal lobe)
Adrenal insufficiency syndrome
Hyperparathyroidism
Vitamin B_{12} or iron deficiency
Serum sodium or potassium reductions
Hypercalcemia
Cancer
Metal (thallium, mercury) intoxication
Chronic pain and disease (i.e., fibromyalgia, diabetes mellitus)
A common symptom in geriatric populations
20%–24% of medical inpatients
Neurologic disorders (i.e., related to abnormal catecholamines or indoleamine metabolism)
Cardiac disease
Serious medical injury (i.e., spinal cord, end-stage renal disease)
Dementia, head trauma, seizure disorders

From Derogatis LR, Wise TN. *Anxiety and Depressive Disorders in the Medical Patient. Clinical Practice No. 4.* Washington, DC: American Psychiatric Press; 1989:121, with permission.

TABLE 17.3. DRUGS WITH KNOWN PROPENSITY TO INDUCE CLINICAL DEPRESSION

Antihypertensives
 Reserpine
 α-methyldopa
 Guanethidine
 Clonidine
 Propranolol
 Hydralazine

Hormones
 Corticosteroids
 Progesterone
 Estrogen

Central nervous system depressants
 Benzodiazepines
 Barbiturates
 Alcohol

Neuroleptics
 Haloperidol
 Fluphenazine

Cardiovascular agents
 Digitalis
 Procainamide

Anti-parkinsonian drugs
 L-Dopa
 Amantadine

Antimicrobials
 Cycloserine
 Gram-negative agents
 Sulfonamides

From Derogatis LR, Wise TN. *Anxiety and Depressive Disorders in the Medical Patient. Clinical Practice, No. 4.* Washington, DC: American Psychiatric Press; 1989:125, with permission.

The belief is that as the symptoms are relieved, the patient's physical complaints and general adaptation will improve. More commonly, however, problems do not subside entirely. When this is the case, other interventions can be used. General osteopathic care uses multiple strategies, such as:

Counseling
Drug therapy
Exercise
Osteopathic manipulative treatment designed to decrease the effects of stress-related disorders and somatic dysfunction

Cognitive Behavioral Factors in Depression

Depression can be understood in many ways within the framework of learning theory (30,31). Deficits in social skills can set the stage for unrewarding social, vocational, and personal relationships causing subsequent feelings of depression. Studies with animals and humans exposed over time to inescapable stress have shown that the subjects failed to demonstrate simple behaviors to escape or avoid the stress and subsequent punishment (32). In a laboratory setting, when exposed to inescapable electric shock, dogs and humans felt helpless and both suffered from naturally occurring depression. Human and animal groups showed similar response patterns of:

Passivity
Slowed learning
Impaired problem solving
Loss of appetite

Their inability to stop the stressor or to escape from the stressor initiates cognitive processes that lead to a sense of powerlessness. Victims of inescapable stress lower their future expectations for control over stress and have measurably lower self-esteem and lower motivation (33–35).

Beck (23,30) describes negative schemas as a learned maladaptive thinking process that often leads to depression. When faced with stressful events, some patients routinely employ negative views of themselves and their abilities (i.e, negative schemas) and are dominated by themes of failure and personal inadequacies. They have learned to expect their performance to be worse than that of others (36,37), and view the world as an overwhelming place, laden with burdens, and filled with excessive demands and daily defeats (38).

Over time, negative depression schemas become stable, long-standing thought patterns. People with these patterns both organize experiences as depressing and selectively direct attention to the negative aspects of current and future stressors. These depression-prone personalities perceive the present as depressing, remember the past the same way, and respond to the future in a fixed, negative manner, independent of what occurs in their environments.

There are six basic cognitive errors in logic that a patient learns over time (Table 17.4). Insight into these faulty reasoning patterns is helpful for some depressed patients. Osteopathically trained physicians routinely work with their patients' cognitive coping styles in addition to pharmacologically managing their depressive symptomatology. Obviously, drug therapy and cognitive behavioral treatments augment and complement one another. With major clinical depression, administering these strategies simultaneously often yields a superior result (39,40).

TABLE 17.4. FAULTY REASONING PATTERNS NOTED IN DEPRESSION-PRONE PATIENTS

Arbitrary inference–drawing a specific conclusion in the absence of evidence to support the conclusion.
Selective abstraction–drawing a conclusion based on a detail taken out of context.
Overgeneralization–drawing a broad, global conclusion on the basis of one or more isolated pieces of information.
Magnification and minimization–exaggerating the significance of negative events and minimizing the significance of positive events.
Personalization–relating external events to oneself when there is no realistic basis for making such a connection.
Absolutistic, dichotomous thinking–placing all experiences in one of two opposite categories.

From Beck, AT, Rush AJ, Shaw BF, Emery G. *Cognitive Therapy of Depression: A Treatment Manual.* New York, NY: Guilford: 1979, with permission.

ANXIETY

Chronic anxiety is a generalized state of fear or apprehension in response to a perceived threat. The chronically threatened individual will eventually begin to experience anxiety and distress in everyday situations that would not normally have elicited such reactions in the past. An anxious reaction is a basic, genetically programmed human response to a real or imagined threatening stressor. The biologic changes elicited by an anxious reaction have specific adaptive survival value. They represent alertness and arousal responses for better behavioral and biologic focusing and coping with the threat.

An anxious reaction represents one of several built-in stress programs that patients can use to adapt to and cope with new threats in their environment. Physically, anxiety is a generalized state of fear with especially strong manifestations in the hypothalamic, sympathetic, autonomic, adrenal, and reticular neuroendocrine networks. Physiologically, the symptoms reflect heightened autonomic arousal, including:

Elevated heart rate
Occasional heartbeat irregularities
Blood pressure changes
Sweating
Intestinal distress
Blood sugar changes
Generalized muscle tension
Decreased pain tolerance

The last two are readily observed during an osteopathically oriented examination of the musculoskeletal system. Anxious individuals also report general symptoms such as:

Insomnia
Excessive worrying
Forgetfulness
Irritability
Difficulty concentrating

Experienced osteopathic physicians soon learn that chronic exposure to anxiety-inducing scenarios without adequate coping strategies often involve irrational cognitive appraisals of threats that, in turn, can lead to further and commonly excessive anticipatory anxiety.

Anxiety disorders occur in 15.4% of the patient population and account for 11% of all physician visits (13). A study of 350 primary care physicians rated anxiety disorders as the most common psychiatric problem seen in their clinical practice (41). Anxiolytic benzodiazepines are among the most commonly prescribed medications in the United States, and primary care physicians write 85% of these prescriptions. The diagnosis of anxiety is complicated by the fact that anxiety is often not the patient's chief complaint. Rather, patients experiencing anxiety generally complain of physical problems. Primary care physicians often focus exclusively on physical symptoms, failing to note that the patient's complaints are really created by unreported or unrecognized anxiety and chronic autonomic arousal including disturbed sleep-wake cycles. Hypervigilance is apparent with expressions of apprehensive expectations and generalized unfocused fears. Remember that there are medical problems that magnify anxiety. Table 17.5 lists medical disorders and conditions associated with high amounts of anxiety.

Anxiety is also identified by diffuse and often severe panic attacks and general agitation that might not be related to any one particular situation or immediate stressor. The panic usually lasts anywhere from a few seconds to more than an hour. These dreaded feelings of being overwhelmed and out of control appear suddenly and climb to high intensities. The attacks are accompanied by intense feelings of apprehension over some presumed or pending distress or catastrophe. During panic attacks, one will experience:

Sweating
Trembling
Choking
Shortness of breath
Chest pain
Heart palpitations
Dizziness
Paresthesia

TABLE 17.5. MEDICAL DISORDERS AND CONDITIONS ASSOCIATED WITH DISPROPORTIONATELY HIGH AMOUNTS OF ANXIETY

Hyperthyroidism
Cardiac disease (e.g., arrhythmias, paroxysmal tachycardias)
Mitral valve prolapse
Pernicious anemia
Respiratory disease
Endocrine disorders (e.g., hypoglycemia)
Porphyria
Depressive illness
Pre-senile or senile dementias
Effects of drug or alcohol use/withdrawal
Caffeine/tobacco use
Hypoglycemia
Pheochromocytoma
Epilepsy

Measurement of Anxiety

Anxiety inventories such as the state-trait anxiety inventory (STAI) (42) and anxiety subscales of the MMPI-2 (24,25) measure individual differences in anxiety susceptibility and the patient's tendency to perceive a wide range of situations as threatening. The inventories also measure the patient's reported response to these situations with associated activation and arousal of the autonomic nervous system. Physiologic measurements of anxiety focus on:

Skin conductance
Heart rate
Blood pressure
Respiratory rate
Gastric motility symptoms
Pupillary diameter
Muscle tension

These measurements can also be routinely collected in the primary care setting. Structured interview questions to elicit information from the anxious patient seen in family practice settings are another tool (Table 17.6).

Anxiety Treatments

An osteopathically oriented approach for managing anxiety involves treating both the physical symptoms of chronic arousal and the mechanisms of learned and reinforced maladaptive arousal in response to prolonged stress. Benzodiazepines can be prescribed

TABLE 17.6. STRUCTURED INTERVIEW QUESTIONS FOR GENERALIZED ANXIETY DISORDER[a]

1. Have you felt nervous, anxious, or on edge on more than half the days in the last month?   YES   NO

In the last month, have you *often* been bothered by any of these problems?

2. Feeling restless so that it is hard to sit still?	4. Muscle tension, aches, or soreness?	6. Trouble concentrating on things, such as reading a book or watching TV?
3. Getting tired very easily?	5. Trouble falling asleep or staying asleep?	7. Becoming easily annoyed or irritated?

8. Are three or more of #2 to #7 checked?   YES   NO
9. In the last month, have these problems made it hard for you to do your work, take care of things at home, or get along with other people?   YES   NO
10. In the last 6 months, have you been worrying *a great deal* about *different things,* and has this been on more than half the days in the last 6 months? (Count as yes only if yes to both.)   YES   NO
11. When you are worrying this way, do you find that you can't stop?   YES   NO
12. These current anxiety symptoms *are not* due to the biologic effects of a physical disorder, medication, or other drug?   YES   NO

SCORING: Yes to 1, 8, 9, 10, 11, and 12 constitutes a probable diagnosis of *generalized anxiety disorder.*

[a]Primary Care Evaluation for Mental Disorders (PRIME-MD).
From Spitzer RL, Williams JB. *PRIME-MD Clinical Evaluation Guide.* New York, NY: Biometrics Research, New York State Psychiatric Institute, 1994, with permission.

to reduce the paralyzing anxiety associated with a clear external stressor. These are most effective if prescribed on a temporary emergency basis with the goal of preventing dependence and iatrogenic withdrawal anxiety when medications are stopped. One should avoid chronic use. Physical symptoms can also be controlled by relaxation, controlled diaphragmatic breathing, and biofeedback (43,44). Anxiety-generating thoughts can be identified and techniques to counter them explored. These treatments attempt to reduce anxiety by enhancing coping abilities, providing interpersonal support, and training the patient to reduce learned anxiety associated with environmental stimuli.

All of these treatment modalities can be effectively used together or separately according to patient needs. Also, general measures to improve coping ability such as a healthy diet, moderate exercise, weight control, and mobilizing a support system of family and friends can set the stage for effective long-term anxiety management (45). Positive outcomes of the proposed treatment will result when the primary care physician enters collaborative management relationships with anxious patients. The goal of these relationships is to alleviate overly aroused patients' fears as they learn new coping styles.

ALCOHOL USE AND DEPENDENCE

Medical care for alcohol abuse has become routine work in primary care practice. The use of alcohol as a coping strategy is uniquely human. As our society becomes more complex and ambiguous, more patients use and alcohol to manage stress. The reported use and abuse of intoxicating chemicals that alter the physiology of the body and the central nervous system dates back to the ancient Egyptian papyri and the Greek amphitheater at Delphi. Alcohol abuse and dependency have become a self-medication strategy for stress that is socially tolerated and modeled for our children.

Alcohol abuse adversely affects the lives of 10 million Americans and their families, and is involved in 10% of all deaths in the United States. Alcohol abuse and dependence are often prevalent in both partners where spousal and child abuses occur (46,47). Physicians in primary care settings recognize only about half the problem drinkers they encounter and are even less likely to identify problems in women and the elderly (48–51).

At one end of the drinking spectrum, alcohol is used in moderation without adverse consequences. At the other end of the spectrum are those drinkers who suffer medically, vocationally, and psychosocially from repeated abuse of alcohol. Most of the drinkers with varying consumption patterns and risks of alcohol-related problems lie in the middle. Only 5% of the three-fourths of all Americans who drink acquire the disorder of alcoholism (48). Many people drink while under stress to anesthetize themselves and to experience the numbing effects of alcohol as a strategy for managing their anxiety or depression. Excessive problem drinking, in and outside the work place, costs U.S. industry approximately $15 billion a year (49). Besides the significant economic consequences, alcohol also presents a significant health hazard and challenge to the osteopathic physician attempting to help his or her patients manage stress. Alcohol overuse is both a response to stress and a cause of further stress.

Alcohol as Response to Stress

It is important to distinguish between the effects of alcohol and the disease of alcoholism. Alcoholism is the consequence of the overuse of alcohol in people who are predisposed to addiction by genetic, physiologic, psychological, sociologic, and other factors. The disease of alcoholism, regardless of the cause or whether the onset is acute or insidious, will eventually take over the life of the patient and his or her family.

In low concentrations, alcohol depresses the brain's neuronal and synaptic transmission systems, including inhibitory centers (52). These depressant effects create three self-reinforcing psychological and behavioral patterns (53):

Euphoriant effects
Disinhibiting effects
Anxiety-relieving effects

Initial euphoriant effects reflect central nervous system sedation, temporarily increasing self-esteem, courage, and confidence. To the alcoholic, these disinhibiting and anxiety-relieving effects seem almost magical. For example, alcohol's effects often allow a person to:

Talk to the opposite sex
Speak up at school or parties
Interact with the boss
Have fun playing with the children
Dance well
Be less sexually inhibited

As with any mood-altering drug, the magic ends and the individual returns to previous functional levels after he or she stops drinking.

A clear understanding of the drinking pattern is necessary to detect whether the problem is harmful or abusive or represents alcohol dependency. The DSM-IV (17) is the most widely used diagnostic framework for alcohol-related disorders. Questions used in the PRIME-MD structured interview for alcohol use are also useful (Table 17.7). The CAGE questionnaire (54) is another simple diagnostic screen that consists of four questions:

1. Have you ever tried to **C**ut down on your drinking?

2. Are you **A**nnoyed when people ask you about your drinking?

3. Do you ever feel **G**uilty about your drinking?

4. Do you ever take a drink as a morning **E**ye opener?

Positive answers on three or four questions are diagnostically significant.

Alcohol as Cause of Further Stress

Once alcohol use becomes a primary stress management strategy, further stress follows (Table 17.8). Alcohol might have been initially used to manage stress, but disruption in work, personal, and social relationships, and isolation are the final consequences. The urgent need to drink concentrates the patient's remaining energies on securing and ingesting alcohol. Denial, minimization, and self-deception are used to explain the alcoholic's deterioration, especially when discussing alcohol use with the primary care physician. When the patient's self-esteem or prominence in the

TABLE 17.7. STRUCTURED INTERVIEW TO ELICIT INFOR-MATION ON PROBABLE ALCOHOL ABUSE/DEPENDENCE[a]

Opening Inquiries:

Have . . . . you thought you should cut down on your drinking? Why?
Has . . . . someone complained about your drinking? Who? Why?
Do . . . . you feel guilty or upset about your drinking? Why?
Have . . . . you had five or more drinks in a single day in the past month? How often have you had that much to drink in the past 6 months? Has that caused any problems?

1. Has a doctor ever suggested that you stop drinking because of a problem with your health? (Count as yes if patient has continued to drink in the last 6 months after doctor suggested stopping.)	YES	NO

Have any of the following happened to you *more than one time* in the last 6 months?

2. Were you drinking, high from alcohol, or hung over while you were working, going to school, or taking care of other responsibilities?	YES	NO
3. What about missing or being late for work, school, or other responsibilities because you were drinking or hung over?	YES	NO
4. What about having a problem getting along with other people while you were drinking?	YES	NO
5. What about driving a car after having several drinks or after drinking too much?	YES	NO

SCORING: Yes to most questions. (Consider responses to opening inquiries and other information known about the patient, such as information obtained from a family member.)

[a] Primary Care Evaluation for Mental Disorders (PRIME-MD).
From Spitzer RL, Williams JB. *PRIME-MD Clinical Evaluation Guide.* New York, NY: Biometrics Research, New York State Psychiatric Institute; 1994, with permission.

community is at risk, lying, evasion, and other manipulative behaviors emerge as strategies to avoid admitting the problem to the primary care physician and to others. At the point of threatened or actual loss of job, family, home, or health, the physician may intervene and encourage the patient to enter an alcohol treatment program.

Primary care physicians normally refer patients with alcoholism to specialized treatment programs. Alcohol abuse is a chronic, relapsing disease, and these patients often require more consistent and involved treatment than primary care physicians can provide (55). The recovering alcoholic will need a physician's guidance and family support to learn to face life's stressors without the use of intoxicants. With support from the physician, the family, and a peer support group, the patient can change his or her maladaptive stress management style and abstain from alcohol.

TABLE 17.8. ALCOHOL-RELATED STRESS-INDUCED FACTORS AFFECTING SOMATIC DYSFUNCTION

Increased central nervous system excitability
Associated vitamin and nutritional deficiencies
Cirrhosis
Wernicke-Korsakoff syndrome
Alcoholic dementias
Functional gastrointestinal changes with and without gastrointestinal bleeding
Pancreatitis
Esophageal varices
Blackouts; brief amnesic periods
Ataxia and poor coordination

The tasks of the physician are to:

Develop a strong relationship built on trust
Make the diagnosis of alcoholism compassionately
Elicit the support of family and friends
Refer the alcoholic to a recognized recovery program
Reinforce the stress management techniques

STRESS MANAGEMENT TECHNIQUES

Social Support

The most powerful tool in the management of the patient's stress is his or her support network. This social network gives a person the feeling that he or she is valued and cared about. The idea that people need to be surrounded by groups of people who provide love and a sense of belonging is not new. The patient needs help to identify mentors and significant others in his or her environment whom he or she can trust and with whom he or she can share feelings. The osteopathic physician assumes an important role by providing this help and counseling the stressed patient. Referrals to self-help groups in the community such as Alanon and Recovery, Inc. can help to reduce the patient's self-absorption. Participation in these groups also leads to the development of outside interests that are compatible with a lifestyle free of addictions.

Spiritual Support

For patients undergoing elective open heart surgery for coronary artery disease, those experiencing strength or comfort from their spiritual feelings are three times more likely to survive than are those without spiritual support. Those who participate in social and community groups (such as local school programs, senior centers, historical societies, etc.) also have three times the survival rate of those who do not take part in social activity. A 1995 study (56) involving 232 patients over age 55 found that seniors who had both "protective factors," i.e., spiritual and social support, enjoyed a 10-fold increase in survival. The amount or type of spiritual or social activity did not matter as much as the *participation, comfort, and support derived from the activity* (56). Why and how spiritual feelings and social support extend life after open heart surgery is not understood. There are over 200 studies corroborating this health-enhancing, life-prolonging effect in a variety of circumstances and population groups. It is well documented, for example, that Mormons (both clergy and devout members) have extremely long life expectancies. The physiologic mechanisms behind longevity, health, and social support are not well understood, however.

Sense of Control

A sense of control is a powerful mitigator of stress. Patients can be given a sense that they can cope by learning to anticipate a potential stressor. The perception that a stressor can be accurately anticipated or stopped increases one's range of problem-solving possibilities and consequent feelings of control. By giving a patient information about stressors before the patient's exposure to them, researchers have reduced the threatening appraisals made when the stressor is experienced. Studies have determined that the stress of surgery or of common medical procedures can be reduced by giving patients accurate expectations, particularly in terms of pain and recovery time.

Perceptions of Risk

Assessment of risk is influenced by certain biases and perceptions brought into the stressful situation by the patient and the health care provider. Many patients need to construct simplified models of the complex interaction of stressful factors in their environment to effectively cope with stress. The physician must provide the patient with simplified models of how the world works and which risks must be taken to put the patient at ease. Many patients like to use simple models to increase their understanding of health problems and the subtle and complex factors surrounding the risks posed by a stressor. Setting the stage for decreased anxiety and adaptive coping is as easy as taking a moment to listen to the patient's conceptual model of the stressors in his or her life. From there, the physician can offer concrete explanations of the stressors and the risks imposed on the patient. One example is telling a patient with back pain that he or she has degenerative disc disease and osteoarthritis. This can sound intimidating and hopeless. To help the patient understand the diagnosis, the physician can describe the condition from the patient's perspective. In this example, the patient's diagnosis could be described as "an aging back with stiffness that can be treated in many ways."

Observational Learning

Observational learning occurs without any apparent direct reinforcement. Many coping behaviors for stress can be learned if the patient observes another person modeling the behavior. Learning occurs without the individual patient making a response or receiving tangible external reinforcement for the behavior. This suggests the importance of our internalizations and cognitive abilities, which allow us to transform what has been observed into many new patterns of behavior.

Encourage your patient to become involved in settings and groups of people who are coping with stress. This can lead to new patterns of coping behaviors. For example, patients with intractable pain fear physical movement. Having them attend a group aquatic exercise program lets them observe others, perhaps older or in poorer health than themselves, moving without damage or injury. This vicarious learning lessens the patient's apprehension when the painful area is moved.

Progressive Relaxation

Progressive relaxation is based on the premise that muscle tension is closely related to anxiety. Individuals feel a significant reduction in experienced anxiety as their tense muscles are made to relax. The teaching of progressive muscular relaxation skills follows a standard procedure. The individual practices muscle relaxation after he or she decides which muscle groups are tense. For example, tell an individual to tighten his or her jaw and notice a pattern of feeling strain in these muscles. After maintaining the tension for approximately 10 seconds, tell the subject to let the muscle group completely relax, and then to notice a difference in sensation as the places that were previously tense and strained relax. After a few minutes of relaxation, repeat the sequence. The main goal of the training program is to teach individuals what it feels like to relax each muscle group and to provide practice in achieving greater relaxation. Once the individual can discriminate the pattern of tension in a particular muscle group, omit the instruction to tense before relaxing. Instead, the individual must relax the muscle from the present level of tension. The original relaxation procedure required months of training with hundreds of trained muscle sites. Clinical practice employs a much more abbreviated form of training and is easy to teach to the patient in a primary care setting.

Systematic Desensitization

This treatment procedure employs a graded hierarchy of stressful scenes and images. It incorporates the patient's perception of the least stress-provoking situations to the most stress-provoking situations. Using imagery, the individual is first taught to relax individual muscles. When the imagery and muscle relaxations are mastered, work begins on an increasingly complex hierarchy of imagery and learning that moves gradually from low- to high-stress situations. Successful deep muscle relaxation inhibits stress-inducing anxiety as both nonthreatening and threatening scenarios are imagined. As skills improve, instruction helps the learner tolerate increasingly difficult scenes during the relaxation process. As tolerance increases for anxiety-related imagery, the patient learns tolerance for anxiety-induced life situations. The therapeutic effectiveness of systematic desensitization has been shown with many anxiety-related disorders, such as phobias (including medical procedures), insomnia, and stress-related psychophysiologic disorders such as ulcers, asthma, and hypertension (57).

Behavioral Rehearsal

Allowing individuals to act out or role-play their problem-solving strategies of behavior is a method used in many different forms in primary care settings. The physician observes, listens to, and models or encourages the appropriate behaviors the patient might try.

The physician often teaches assertiveness and problem-solving techniques. These techniques are most effective with individuals who experience stress as a result of difficulties in self-expression. A lack of appropriate interpersonal skills exacerbates stress-related physical symptoms. For example, an overwhelmingly demanding boss or spouse is a common cause of stress-related symptoms and health care seeking in a primary care setting. By teaching verbal strategies to more effectively deal with excessive and unfair demands, patients learn new and more effective coping behaviors.

Cognitive Restructuring

In cognitive restructuring, the physician determines and challenges specific thoughts or self-verbalizations that contribute to the stress-related disorder. Treatment is designed to help the patient modify negative, self-doubting statements by replacing them with self-enhancing declarations (58). One cognitive restructuring method is called thought stopping. Thought stopping is used when patients experience distress because of obsessive thoughts about stressors they have difficulty controlling. This also occurs with insomniacs, who cannot stop thinking long enough to fall asleep. The patient is asked to concentrate on the anxiety-induced thought and, after a short period, the physician suddenly and emphatically says, stop. After this procedure has been repeated several times, the patient will report that the thoughts were interrupted by the word stop. The physician then shifts control back to the patient. Specifically, the client is taught to utter a subvocal stop whenever he or she begins to engage in a self-defeating rumination.

Biofeedback

Using physiologic monitoring equipment, the patient can be taught to influence physiologic processes such as:

Blood pressure
Heart rate
Sweat gland activity
Skin temperature
Neuromuscular activity
Sphincter control
Penile tumescence

By receiving auditory or visual feedback, one learns about the close relationship between mind and body. The availability of sensitive recording devices for home use has made it possible to work on these skills in a more organized and regular manner. There is a lack of systematic and well-controlled outcome studies that conclusively show the clinical effectiveness of some new monitoring devices. However, supportive literature for biofeedback-related muscle relaxation is slowly and cautiously appearing. Temperature biofeedback, which is also receiving positive support in the literature, has been shown to control Raynaud's phenomena and migraine headaches. From an osteopathic perspective, biofeedback makes it possible to extend voluntary control over some elements of somatic dysfunction by decreasing arousal responses affecting somatic and viscerosomatic reflex activities. Learning to master these responses helps develop a sense of control and improves confidence in one's self-healing abilities.

Psychophysiologic Insomnia Management

In the United States, approximately 10 million people consult their health care provider annually for sleep disorders, with half receiving prescriptions for sleeping medications (59). Epidemiologic studies suggest that 20% to 35% of respondents describe sleep problems as severe or constant for as long as 14 years; however, other health problems are commonly identified as the primary complaint (60). Persistent insomnia is not life threatening. When compared with good sleepers, however, insomniacs

experience more (61,62):

Hospitalizations
Anxiety
Depression
Fibromyalgia
Propensity for alcohol and other substance abuse

An inability to remain asleep is most common, followed by difficulty falling asleep, and abnormal early morning awakening. Contributing factors appear divided among the following (60):

Psychiatric (35)
Psychophysiologic (15)
Drug and alcohol dependency (12)
Periodic limb movements (12)
Medical, toxic, environmental (4)
Various other (15)

Typically, insomniacs are chronically aroused autonomically (anxious), or cognitively depressed and unable to stop thinking and worrying at bed time. They worry about not getting to sleep and then are too aroused at bedtime to sleep. This worrying leads to fears that they will have poor daytime performance if they cannot make themselves sleep. Insomnia begets more insomnia and leads to poor learned sleep habits and routines. Insomnia lasting more than 3 weeks requires specific behavioral strategies to counteract the learned aspects of the insomnia. It also requires relaxation techniques and, if needed, intermittent use of sedatives or hypnosis.

Insomnia can be managed effectively by teaching sleep habit techniques that employ a variety of strategies (Table 17.9). These techniques form the foundation for the guidance that the osteopathically trained physician gives to the patient. When sleep is restored, the patient feels more alert, and there are fewer vegetative and clinical signs of depression and anxiety during waking hours. Patients practicing good sleep habits report improved concentration, better problem solving, and more effective management of their stress.

Augmenting sleep habit strategies with medication for sleep during short intervals is another method used to manage insomnia. A prescription for exercise and a muscular relaxation

TABLE 17.9. GOOD SLEEP HABITS

Get up about the same time every day, regardless of when you go to bed.
Go to bed only when sleepy.
Establish relaxing pre-sleep rituals.
Exercise regularly and keep active.
Organize your day around regular times for eating and outdoor activities with regular exposure to bright light, which synchronizes circadian cycles.
Avoid caffeine, nicotine, alcohol, excessive warmth, and hunger at bed time.
If you nap, try to nap at the same time every day.
When laying down to sleep, relax all your muscles, particularly your face and jaw, and breath slowly and evenly.
If you don't fall asleep in 20 minutes, get back up and return to bed when sleepy.

training tape to be used in the evening hours will also promote better sleep. All this, coupled with encouragement by the physician who functions both as educator and guide, will alleviate insomnia.

CONCLUSION

The osteopathically trained physician has many available tools to employ a broad approach to stress-related problems, including varieties of somatic dysfunction. Anxiety, depression, insomnia, and drug and alcohol abuse are common symptoms seen in primary care offices. Osteopathic management can be practiced in three ways:

1. By treating symptoms as they are reported and observed.
2. By giving advice on managing stressors.
3. By guiding and mentoring stress-related responses toward positive coping behaviors and strategies (the most rewarding).

Successful diagnosis depends on understanding the interactions of the biopsychosocial factors that lead to stress-induced problems. Successful treatment depends on giving clear explanations so that the patient understands the mechanisms that perpetuate his or her distress. The long-term goal is to assist the patient toward self-mastery and self-healing.

REFERENCES

1. Centers for Disease Control. *Ten leading causes of death in the United States.* Washington, DC: Government Publishing Office; 1980.
2. Surgeon General's Office. *Healthy people.* Washington, DC: Government Printing Office; 1979.
3. Surgeon General's Office. *Report on nutrition and health.* Washington, DC: Government Printing Office; 1988.
4. Korr IM. The sympathetic nervous system as mediator between somatic and supportive processes. In: *American Academy of Osteopathy Yearbook.* Indianapolis, IN: American Academy of Osteopathy;1970:170–175.
5. Korr IM. Sustained sympathicotonia as a factor in disease. In: *American Academy of Osteopathy Yearbook.* Indianapolis, IN: Amcrican Academy of Osteopathy;1978:207–221.
6. Ward R. Manual healing methods. In: *Report to the National Institutes of Health on Alternative Medical Systems and Practices in the United States,* pub. no. 1294;1995:113–119.
7. Cannon WB. *The Wisdom of the Body.* New York, NY: Norton; 1932.
8. Selye H. *The Stress of Life,* rev. ed. New York, NY: McGraw-Hill; 1976.
9. Anderson SM, Harthorn BH. The recognition, diagnosis and treatment of mental disorders by primary care physicians. *Med Care.* 1989:27;869–886.
10. Schulberg HC, Burns BJ. Mental disorders in primary care: epidemiologic, diagnostic, and treatment research directions. *Gen Hosp Psychiatry.* 1988:10.
11. Barrett JE, Barrett JA, Oxman RE, et al. The prevalence of psychiatric disorders in a primary care practice. *Arch Gen Psychiatry.* 1988;45:1100–1106.
12. Robins LN, Regier DA, eds. *Psychiatric Disorders in America.* New York, NY: Free Press; 1991.
13. Schurman RA, Kramer PD, Mitchell JB. The hidden mental health network: treatment of mental illness by nonpsychiatrist physicians. *Arch Gen Psychiatry.* 1985;42:8994.
14. Secunda R, Friedman RJ, Schuyler D. *The Depressive Disorders.* Washington, DC: Government Printing Office; 1973.
15. Beck AT. *Depression: Clinical, Experimental, and Theoretical Aspects.* New York, NY: Harper & Row; 1967.
16. Copas JB, Robin A. Suicide in psychiatric patients. *Br J Psychiatry.* 1982;141:503–511.
17. American Psychiatric Association. *Diagnostic and Statistical Manual of Mental Disorders,* Rev. 4th ed. Washington, DC: American Psychiatric Association; 1987.
18. Depression Guideline Panel. *Depression in Primary Care. I. Detection and Diagnosis. Clinical Practice Guideline No. 5.* Rockville, MD: US Dept of Health and Human Services, Public Health Service, Agency for Health Care Policy and Research publication 93–0550; April 1993.
19. American Psychiatric Association. *Diagnostic and Statistical Manual of Mental Disorders. Primary Care Version.* Washington, DC: American Psychiatric Association; 1996.
20. Zung WWK. A self-rating depression scale. *Arch Gen Psychiatry.* 1965;12:6370.
21. Zung WWK. A rating instrument for anxiety disorders. *Psychosomatics.* 1971;12:164–167.
22. Beck AT. *Depression: Clinical, Experimental and Theoretical Aspects.* New York, NY: Harper & Row; 1967.
23. Beck AT. *Cognitive Theory and the Emotional Disorders.* New York, NY: International Universities Press; 1976.
24. Hathaway SR, McKinley JC. *MMPI Manual.* Minneapolis, MN: Psychological Corp; 1943.
25. Dahlstrom WG, Welsh GS. *An MMPI Handbook.* Minneapolis, MN: University of Minnesota Press; 1972.
26. Spitzer RL, Williams JB, et al. *PRIME-MD Clinical Evaluation Guide.* New York State Psychiatric Institute, Biometrics Research Dept. 722 West 168th Street, Unit 74. New York, NY; 1994.
27. Spitzer RL, Williams JB. Utility of a new procedure for diagnosing mental disorders in primary care. *JAMA.* 1994;272(22): 1749–1756.
28. Cameron OG. *Presentations of Depression.* New York, NY: John Wiley and Sons; 1987.
29. Nezu AM, Nezu CM. *Problem-Solving Therapy for Depression.* New York, NY: John Wiley and Sons; 1989.
30. Beck AT, Rush AJ, Shaw BF, et al. *Cognitive Therapy of Depression: A Treatment Manual.* New York, NY: Guilford; 1979.
31. Overmier JB, Seligman MEP. Effects of inescapable shock upon subsequent escape and avoidance learning. *J Comp Psychol.* 1967;64:2333.
32. Seligman MEP, Maier SF. Failure to escape traumatic shock. *J Exp Psychol.* 1967;74:19.
33. Abramson LY, Sackheim HA. A paradox in depression: uncontrollability and self-blame. *Psychol Bull.* 1977;84:835–851.
34. Abramson LY, Seligman MEP, Teasdale J. Learned helplessness in humans: critique and reformulation. *J Abnorm Psychol.* 1978;87:4974.
35. Seligman MEP. *Helplessness: On Depression, Development, and Death.* San Francisco, CA: Freeman; 1975.
36. Hollon SD, Beck AT. Cognitive therapy of depression. In: Kendall PC, Hollon SD, eds. *Cognitive-Behavioral Interventions: Theory, Research and Procedures.* New York, NY: Academic Press; 1979:153–204.
37. Hollon SD, Kendall PC. Cognitive self-statements in depression: development of an automatic thoughts questionnaire. *Cognit Ther Res.* 1980;4:383–395.
38. Funabiki D, Calhoun J. Use of a behavioral-analytic procedure in evaluating two models of depression. *J Consult Clin Psychol.* 1979;47:183–185.
39. D'Zurilla TJ. *Problem-solving Therapy: A Social Competence Approach to Clinical Intervention.* New York, NY: Springer-Verlag; 1986.
40. D'Zurilla TJ, Nezu AM. Development and preliminary evaluation of the social problem-solving inventory (SPSI). Paper presented at the meeting of the Association for the Advancement of Behavior Therapy. New York, November 1988.
41. Noyes R, Roth M, Burrows GD. *The Treatment of Anxiety, IV.* New York, NY: Elsevier Science; 1990.
42. Spielberger CD, Gorsuch RC, Lushene RE. *Manual for the state-trait anxiety inventory.* Palo Alto ,CA: Consulting Psychologists; 1970.
43. Keabie D. *The Management of Anxiety.* New York, NY: Churchill Livingstone; 1989.

44. Kennerley H. *Managing Anxiety.* Oxford, UK: Oxford University Press; 1990.
45. Morris CG. *Psychology: An Introduction.* Englewood Cliffs, NJ: Prentice Hall; 1993.
46. West LJ, Cohen S. Provisions for dependency disorders. In: Hollant WW, Detels R, Knox G, eds. *Oxford Textbook of Public Health.* New York, NY: Oxford University Press; 1985;9:2.
47. Rankin JG, Ashley MJ. Alcohol-related health problems. In: Last JM, Wallace RB, eds. *Public Health and Preventative Medicine,* 13th ed. East Norwalk, CT: Appleton & Lange; 1992:43.
48. Cleary PD, Miller M, Bush BLT, et al. Prevalence and recognition of alcohol abuse in a primary care population. *Am J Med.* 1988;85:4664–4671.
49. Buchsbaum DG, Buchanan RG, Poses RM, et al. Physician detection of drinking problems in patients attending a general medicine practice. *J Gen Intern Med.* 1992;7:517–521.
50. Curtis JR, Geller G, Stokes EJ, et al. Characteristics, diagnosis and treatment of alcoholism in elderly patients. *J Am Geriatr Soc.* 1989;37:310–316.
51. Dawson NV, Dadheech G, Speroff T, et al. The effect of patient gender on the prevalence and recognition of alcoholism on a general medical service. *J Am Intern Med.* 1992;7:3815.
52. Kissin B. The pharmacodynamics and natural history of alcoholism. In: Kissin B, Begleiter H, eds. *The Biology of Alcoholism, III: Clinical pathology.* New York, NY: Plenum Publishing; 1974.
53. Grenell RG. Effects of alcohol on the neuron. In: Kissin B, Begleiter H, eds. *The Biology of Alcoholism, II: Physiology and behavior.* New York, NY: Plenum Publishing; 1978.
54. Ewing JA. Detecting alcoholism. The CAGE questionnaire. *JAMA.* 1984;252:1905–1907.
55. Saunders JB, Aasland OG, Amundsen A, et al. Alcohol consumption and related problems among primary health care patients: WHO collaborative project on early detection of persons with harmful alcohol consumption. I. *Addiction.* 1993;88:349–362.
56. Oxman TE. Lack of social participation or religious strength and comfort as risk factors for death after cardiac surgery in the elderly. *Psychosom Med.* 1995;57:681–689.
57. Gatchel RJ, Baum A. *An Introduction into Health Psychology.* New York, NY: Random House; 1983.
58. Meichenbaum D, Turk D. The cognitive-behavior management of anxiety, anger and pain. In: Davidson PO, ed. *The Behavior Management of Pain.* New York, NY: Brunner/Mazel; 1976.
59. Lacks P, Morin CM. Recent advances in the assessment and treatment of insomnia. *J Consult Clin Psychol.* 1992;60:586–594.
60. Rosekind MR. The epidemiology and occurrence of insomnia. *J Clin Psychiatry.* 1992;53(suppl 6):46.
61. Lesch DR, Spire J-P. Clinical electroencephalography. In: Thorpy MJ, ed. *Handbook of Sleep Disorders.* New York, NY: Marcel Dekker Inc; 1990:1331.
62. Buysse DJ, Reynolds III CF. Insomnia. In: Thorpy MJ, ed. *Handbook of Sleep Disorders.* New York, NY: Marcel Dekker Inc; 1990:375–433.

18

OSTEOPATHIC PSYCHIATRY

RONALD H. BRADLEY
GERALD G. OSBORN
JOHN A. JEROME
MARY C. WILLIAMS

KEY CONCEPTS

- History of osteopathic psychiatry
- Psychiatric diagnosis and multiaxial assessment
- Depression, anxiety, and somatoform disorder identification and care
- Considerations when treating various psychotic disorders and substance abuse disorders
- Assessment and management of personality disorders

Osteopathic philosophy and its practices are organized around the belief that everyone is basically healthy and that the disease processes are superimposed. We also know that genetic and constitutional variables deeply affect these processes. In this context, the goal of structural diagnosis and osteopathic manipulative treatment is to correct neuromusculoskeletal changes in such a way that natural homeostatic mechanisms become more efficient at maintaining health. Importantly, this belief system affects the way osteopathic psychiatrists work with patients. Collaborative care that respects an individual's natural restorative processes is a core concept.

As a specialty, osteopathic psychiatry systematically integrates individual, biologic, psychological, and social elements to better understand mental health and illness. Fundamentally, its area of expertise is to care for the mentally ill. In contemporary terms, osteopathic psychiatry believes that mental illness arises from complex interactions among genetic and constitutional vulnerabilities as influenced by interpersonal, environmental, and societal stressors. An objective multiaxial diagnostic and reporting system is used to communicate investigational and treatment information to patients, their families, and professional colleagues. Comprehensive treatment plans focus on the whole person—*mind, body, and spirit.* The origins of osteopathic psychiatry begin early in the 20th century with the establishment of the Still-Hildreth Sanitarium in Kirksville, Missouri (see below).

EPIDEMIOLOGY

Current United States population studies estimate that approximately 20% of the U.S. population is affected by mental disorders during any given year. In total, about 26% have either a mental or addictive disorder. Six percent have addictive disorders and 7% to 10% suffer from a variety of depressive syndromes. Many deal with more than one disorder at the same time (1–4). Importantly, these individuals are more likely to experience a variety of chronic, long-term physical and psychiatric illnesses.

In 1996, the direct cost of mental health services in the U.S. totaled $69 billion. This figure represents approximately 7.3% of total health care spending during that fiscal year. An additional $17.7 billion was spent on Alzheimer's disease and $12.6 billion on substance abuse disorders (5).

History of Osteopathic Psychiatry

Psychiatry became one of the earliest osteopathic specialties. A.T. Still strongly believed his methods were most beneficial when used to treat the whole person—body, mind, and spirit. He worked diligently for the establishment of the first osteopathic sanatorium and kept a close eye on its progress. Shortly before his death in 1917, his last dictated note to members of the osteopathic profession was:

> Dear Boys and Girls,
> I know you are keeping your eyes on the progress that is being made at Macon, Mo., in the treatment of mental and nervous diseases. We have a great deal of experience. My personal experience covers a period of something over fifty years in the treatment of mental cases, but until Arthur and the boys Charlie, and Harry, became interested in Macon sanatorium, we never had a place where we had a chance to look after this class of patients. I have always contented that a majority of the insane patients could be treated successfully by osteopathy, and the success that the boys have been having in the last three and one-half years bears out my faith, and I am very anxious for the entire profession to know of the work that is being done.'

The above message was enclosed with the following letter from Dr. Charlie Still:

The above is the Christmas Greeting that Father intended sending out to all of the boys and girls in the field practicing osteopathy. He has been so interested in the work at Macon; he felt that it was the crowning sheaf in his life's work. He, however, had a stroke of paralysis that terminated fatally before the greeting was sent.

A.G. Hildreth, D.O., Charles E. Still, D.O., and Harry M. Still, D.O., founded what was to become the Still-Hildreth Sanatorium. A.G. Hildreth served as its president and superintendent until his death in 1941 (6). Shortly after opening, they hired Lynn van Horn Gerdine D.O., M.D., who was the first chief psychiatrist. When the Still's approached him with their offer, he was already teaching physiology at Harvard medical school under the guidance of the renowned Walter Cannon, M.D. Dr. Gerdine taught psychiatry, osteopathic therapeutics, pathology, and physical diagnosis at the American School of Osteopathy in Kirksville from 1903 until 1914.

Dr. Gerdine obtained his A. B. from Johns Hopkins in 1895 where he studied political science under Woodrow Wilson. He received his master's degree from Harvard University in 1899 during its "golden age" when William James, Ph.D., the father of modern psychology, was achieving fame. Dr. James encouraged Dr. Gerdine to seek his training in osteopathic medicine at the Massachusetts College of Osteopathy. He did so, obtaining his D.O. degree in 1901 and his M.D. degree from Rush medical school in Chicago in 1908. Subsequently, he spent his entire career practicing as an osteopath and was the only clinician at Still-Hildreth Sanitarium with formal postdoctoral training in psychiatry.

Sanitarium patients were a diverse group, both as to diagnosis and time spent in the hospital. Some came for diagnostic evaluation while others stayed for months. In general, a firm diagnosis was not fully established until the patient had been there for at least 6 weeks. Prior to arrival, many had been diagnosed elsewhere and were found to be beyond hope of recovery (6).

These early osteopaths noted that psychiatric patients had considerably less freedom of cranial suture motion, especially around the cranial base and temporal bones. They also reported less cranial vault resiliency. Diagnostically, there seemed to be more inherent movement restrictions involving the following:

- Occipital sites in schizophrenia
- Sphenobasilar symphysis in manic-depressive cases
- Frontosphenoid articulations in "involutional dementias" (6)

In the 1950s, Floyd Dunn, D.O., a professor of psychiatry at both the Philadelphia College of Osteopathy, and later at the Kansas City College of Osteopathy and Surgery, spoke of the association of autonomic dysfunction with psychiatric disorders. He cited data from 1,000 psychiatric patients. More than 50% demonstrated palpable sites of somatic dysfunction at C2 and T4-6 paravertebral regions of the spine (7). Far in advance of his peers, his classroom lectures routinely connected neuroendocrine activities with a variety of mental disorders.

Of several osteopathic sanitariums, the Still-Hildreth operation opened first and stayed open the longest. Several similar operations emerged during the early 1900s. These included the Dufur Osteopathic Hospital in Ambler, PA, which opened in 1921, Merrill Osteopathic Sanatorium in Venice, CA, in 1923, the Edgehill Sanatorium in Knoxville, TN, in 1924, and the Brooklawn Osteopathic Sanatorium and Clinic in Syracuse, NY, in 1932.

The American College of Neuropsychiatry, now called the American College of Osteopathic Neurologists and Psychiatrists, was founded in 1939. Many of its early members combined neurology, psychiatry, and internal medicine. Some practiced each specialty separately while others combined their work with internal medicine. Grover Gillum, D.O., a founding member of the College, and professor of internal medicine and neurology at the Kansas City College of Osteopathy and Surgery, was a prominent example. Another example was Wilbur Cole, D.O., who combined neurology and basic science research. Among his many accomplishments was the 1940s publication of his discovery of motor end plates on striated muscle.

The Still-Hildreth Osteopathic Sanatorium's holistic practices, first instituted by Arthur Grant Hildreth, D.O., initially emphasized nutrition and diet along with its neuromusculoskeletal osteopathic work. Consuming large quantities of milk was a central tenet because it was considered a "natural food." The institutional environment was upbeat and socially positive, a marked contrast to the stark and punitive atmospheres of most other psychiatric institutions. For example, patients were encouraged to use the boathouse, beaches, music room, and library, as well as many other social activities (6).

MENTAL HEALTH AND ILLNESS: "THE BRAIN-BODY DILEMMA"

Most themes of modern osteopathic psychiatry began with ancient Greeks. Almost 3,000 years ago, Homer marveled at the range of personality and emotional variables. He stated that "to one man a god has given deeds of war, to another the dance, to another the lyre and song, and to another the wide-sounding Zeus puts a good mind." The Greeks treated depression as something the body could overcome by using strong emetics, purges, rest, and counsel. Hippocrates, the father of medicine, wrote that mental illness had natural causes and that the brain was the seed of emotions and thought. Much of modern science and psychiatry amplifies Aristotle's assertions that the human brain is capable of reason and moral choice (i.e., mental health).

What distinguishes the human brain from other brains is the relative size of the cerebral cortex, the one-fourth inch thick covering of gray matter on the lobes and hemispheres of the cerebrum. Only in human beings is the cerebral cortex so large in relation to general body size. Its many folds and convolutions, the gyri, which increase the surface area of the brain and allow the body to pack a maximal amount of neural tissues inside the skull, further distinguish the human cortex.

Scientists today agree that the unique abilities of the human mind are directly attributable to the cerebral cortex. These abilities go hand in hand with thinking, observing, analyzing, and integrating experiences and feelings to solve problems and plan ahead. Within this biophysical context, the mind, body, and spirit are tightly integrated. This has led to the development and evolution of *the biopsychosocial model,* developed by George Engel, which emphasizes the *unity of mind, body, and spirit* within the context of one's social and cultural environment. Clinically, complex interactions among these areas influence both the patient's level of distress and mental health, as well as disease and illness-related responses.

EARLY TREATMENT HURDLES: ASYLUMS

In the Middle Ages, European psychiatric treatment took a huge step backwards when mental illness was generally viewed as "possession by the devil," a penalty for moral depravity or as punishment for wrongdoing. Asylum inmates were routinely restrained and treated like dangerous animals. Some were tortured, beaten, or burned at the stake. Skulls were analyzed to look for lunacy stones. Asylum keepers often thought that a sudden shock would restore reason. As a result, inmates were commonly dropped without warning into tanks of icy water or strapped into chairs and rotated rapidly to induce shock. Bloodletting was also a favorite treatment. Abandoning both adults and children whose intelligence or behavior did not measure up to society's standards was common. This was often a death sentence. In rare cases, the mentally disturbed were treated well. This was particularly true when they were seen as divinely blessed and spiritually enlightened.

The idea of humane therapy began several centuries later when Phillippe Pinel (1745–1826) became director of the Bicetre Asylum in Paris. He rejected the notion that the mentally ill were possessed by demons. He set new precedents by unchaining inmates and beginning programs of "kindness, reassurance, and counsel." His therapies included discussions with patients about their problems. His radical and "enlightened" acts helped lay the foundation for modern psychiatry as a branch of medicine.

In the 1860s, Charcot became interested in patients displaying neurologic deficits without organic findings. Routinely, these patients were dismissed as hysterical and malingering. Insightfully, Charcot understood that these patients were truly suffering and treated them with combinations of hypnosis and counseling. Since then, patient care has steadily improved through combinations of expanding psychological and behavioral knowledge coupled with better understanding of cultural and fundamental humanitarian concerns for the rights and feelings of the mentally ill.

LACK OF UNIFORM DESCRIPTIONS AND NOMENCLATURE: A MAJOR PROBLEM

An early major and fundamental communication hurdle was a lack of uniform descriptions for mental disorders and their treatment. This changed in 1883 when the German psychiatrist Amil Kraepelin published the first uniform classification of mental illnesses. He created categories based on the onset, symptoms, development, and outcome of illness. Over the next 40 years, Kraepelin expanded and revised his lists. Eventually, his system

became the foundation for later psychiatric taxonomies and an indispensable guide for the diagnosis and treatment of mental illness through the first half of the 20th century.

Since the 1950s, the American Psychiatric Association has published additional diagnostic guidelines referred to as the *Diagnostic and Statistical Manual of Mental Disorders* (DSM). The DSM-IV is the current revision (8). The manual describes and categorizes more than 200 mental conditions. It is beginning to look at outlines and protocols for the use of specific medications and counseling techniques.

DOCTOR/PATIENT RELATIONSHIPS

One of the most important clinical tasks that any osteopathic physician, including a psychiatrist, should perform is a meaningful biopsychosocial history. When done well, this foundation becomes a framework for insightful diagnosis.

After developing essential demographic data, the reason for seeking psychiatric help is explored. For example, ask the patient "why are you seeking (psychiatric) treatment right now?" Understanding that most people are resistant to ask for help, the physician needs to empathize with the patient's plight. Three important interview characteristics are essential: *clinical congruence, empathic understanding, and unconditional positive regard* for the patient. When done well, these characteristics create a safe, nonjudgmental clinical environment that allows the patient to speak freely.

Clinical congruence demonstrates a clear, consistent, and organized way of probing, inquiring, and sorting out issues, signs, and symptoms. *Empathic understanding* implies genuine acceptance of all of the patient's feelings and concerns about his or her situation. *Unconditional positive regard* means the clinician is nonjudgmental, regardless of how self-defeating or irrational particular behaviors appear to be.

A chronologic narrative history of events leading to the first visit are explored using the *who, what, when, and where* inquiry model. As the process unfolds, family members and other treating sources are gleaned for essential information. This includes obtaining previous medical and mental health records.

PAST PSYCHIATRIC HISTORY

Past history includes exploration of psychological and biologic vulnerabilities, including environmental and social factors. Examples are substance abuse history and evidence of previous illegal or illicit activities. Previous pathologic diagnoses are documented and should include presenting symptoms, extent of incapacity, type of treatment, and names of treating physicians and hospitals.

PSYCHIATRIC DIAGNOSES, DATA COLLECTION, AND MEDICAL RECORDKEEPING

The DSM-IV is an official international numerical coding system that classifies mental disorders. The system facilitates data collection and reporting procedures for insurance carriers, as well as both governmental and nongovernmental organizations.

Diagnostically, the multiaxial assessment system evaluates five axes using the following:

DSM-IV Classification

Axis I	Clinical Disorders and other conditions identified as primary focus of clinical attention
Axis II	Personality Disorders and Mental Retardation—developmentally longstanding and typically predate onset of Axis I symptoms
Axis III	General Medical Conditions that are linked to presenting somatic dysfunction
Axis IV	Psychosocial and Environmental Problems that may affect diagnosis, treatment, and prognosis
Axis V	Global Assessment of Functioning across all areas of biopsychosocial functioning

This multiaxial system approach forms a systematic structure for organizing, reporting, and conveying clinical information. Each axis represents a simplified assessment for that particular area. Selected common Axis I disorders, signs, symptoms, and treatment options are described below.

AXIS I DIAGNOSIS

Depression and Anxiety Disorders

Major depressive disorders (MDD) and anxiety disorders commonly occur together (9). Fifty percent to 60% of individuals with MDD over a lifetime also report one or more anxiety disorders. The anxiety disorder predates depression in the majority of cases (10). The combined evidence of several studies demonstrates that co-morbid depression and anxiety disorders are associated with greater symptom severity and persistence, more severe social impairment, increased help-seeking behavior, and higher incidence of suicidal thinking and attempts (11–13). Multidimensional treatment is generally more effective than single interventions alone. In general, they combine pharmacologic approaches with psychotherapy, cognitive restructuring, and, in some cases, social effectiveness and relaxation training (14,15). Factors affecting both neurophysiologic and pharmacokinetic principles are important to successful treatment. For example, a working knowledge of serotonin, norepinephrine, and dopamine systems is essential.

Many patients who are anxious or depressed report great comfort and tension relief from basic osteopathic manipulative techniques. Simply being touched and thoughtfully cared for is very powerful treatment. As osteopaths, we know that much emotional tension is stored in muscles. Releasing that tension is at the core of treating anxiety and musculoskeletal symptoms.

Bipolar Disorders

Bipolar disorder is a recurrent mood disorder. More than 90% of the individuals who have a single manic episode have future occurrences. A manic episode is characterized by periods of abnormally and persistently expansive and irritable moods that last at least 1 week.

The manic episode needs to be sufficiently severe to cause marked impairment in social or occupational functioning or to require hospitalization, and may be characterized by the presence of irrational behaviors and speech. The episode must not be due to the direct physiologic effects of drug abuse, a prescribed medication, or somatic treatments for depression (e.g., electroconvulsive therapy, light therapy, or toxin exposure). The episode must not be due to the direct physiologic effects of a general medical condition (e.g., multiple sclerosis, brain tumor). Manic speech is typically pressured, loud, rapid, and difficult to interrupt. Individuals often talk nonstop, sometimes for hours on end without regard for others' wishes to communicate. Speech is sometimes characterized by joking, punning, and amusing irrelevancies. Theatrical behavior with dramatic mannerisms and singing is not unusual. Thoughts may race, often at a rate faster than can be articulated. Distractibility is evidenced by an inability to screen out irrelevant external stimuli (e.g., the interviewer's tie, background noises, conversations, or furnishings in the room).

Goal-directed activities involve excessive planning and disproportionate participation in wide-ranging multiple activities (e.g., sexual, occupational, political, and religious). Increased sexual drive, fantasies, and behavior are often present.

Decreased need for sleep is a hallmark. Early waking and feeling full of energy is common. Sometimes the sufferer goes sleepless for days without feeling tired.

Treatment for bipolar disorder requires long-term medication management and supportive counseling. Osteopathic manipulative therapies alone have not proved helpful. Lithium carbonate, carbamazepine, and valproic acid are medications used to treat acute mania. Lithium's effects are usually delayed for up to 1 to 2 weeks, but 85% of patients usually respond well. Because of lithium's slow response, antipsychotics and benzodiazepines are also important in the initial treatment (16–18). Lithium also has been used in the strategy to treat resistant depression. Carbamazepine may be used in rapid-cycling bipolar illness if either lithium or valproate is ineffective or poorly tolerated. As of this writing, carbamazepine therapy is not approved for acute mania by the Food and Drug Administration (FDA). The FDA approved valproic acid as an alternative for nonresponders to carbamazepine or lithium.

GENERAL ANXIETY DISORDER

General anxiety disorder (GAD) is a very common DSM-IV diagnosis in primary care. Essential features are excessive anxiety and worry (apprehensive expectation) occurring more days than not for at least 6 months. The individual finds it impossible to control worry, which is accompanied by at least three additional symptoms: restlessness, easy fatigability, difficulty concentrating, irritability, muscle tension, and disturbed sleep.

Benzodiazepines are a frequently over-prescribed treatment mainstay. Antidepressants for GAD are also surprisingly effective because co-morbid relationships occur with depression in approximately 95% of this population (19–21). Antidepressants have a real advantage because of their lower potential for abuse and dependency. In general, they are also better tolerated than benzodiazepine for long-term use.

A most striking and prominent symptom of GAD is a full-blown panic attack (8). The essential feature of a panic attack is a discrete period of intense fear or discomfort that is accompanied by at least four of 13 somatic or cognitive symptoms. Too often needless laboratory testing and unnecessary treatment goes into chasing down the biology of these symptoms when GAD is the real underlying mechanism. Symptoms include:

1. palpitations or pounding heart/accelerated heart rate
2. sweating
3. trembling or shaking
4. sensations of shortness of breath or smothering
5. feelings of choking
6. chest pain or discomfort
7. nausea or abdominal distress
8. dizziness or lightheadedness
9. derealization or depersonalization
10. fear of losing control or "going crazy"
11. fear of dying
12. parasthesias (numbness or tingling sensation)
13. chills or hot flashes

The hallmark of osteopathic treatment should include relaxation training, breathing exercises, establishing a thorough differential diagnosis, reassurance, and routine osteopathic manipulative therapy (OMT) for the musculoskeletal display of emotional tension. Pharmacologic treatments for panic attacks include combinations of selective serotonin release inhibitors (SSRIs) such as paroxetine and serotonin-norepinephrine release inhibitors (SNRIs) such as venlafaxine. Symptom relief is almost immediately obtained with high-potency benzodiazepines such as alprazolam (22,23). Antidepressants are the first-line agents because of their documented efficacy, safety, and tolerability before use of long-term benzodiazepines. Sometimes high doses of alprazolam (up to 10 mg/day) are needed to relieve the initial anxiety. Low doses should be used initially (alprazolam 0.5 mg two or three times daily) with subsequent dose increases as needed (24).

Somatoform Disorders

The essential features of somatoform disorders are patterns of vague, expansive, and recurring multisystem somatic complaints. A somatic complaint is clinically significant if it results in medical treatment (e.g., taking medication) or causes significant impairment in social, occupational, or other important areas of functioning. Multiple somatic complaints cannot be fully explained by any known general medical condition or the direct effects of a substance (8). These patients typically overuse emergency room visits, osteopathic and chiropractic treatment, massage therapy, or other similar systems.

Multiple somatic complaints generally begin before age 30 and occur over several years. Importantly, symptom reports cannot be fully explained by any known medical, genetic, constitutional, or drug-related diagnosis.

At least *four different sites* (e.g., head, abdomen, back, joints, extremities, chest, rectum) or *functions* (e.g., difficulties with menstruation, sexual intercourse, urination) are needed to establish the diagnosis. At least two gastrointestinal symptoms other than pain must be present.

Most sufferers also report chronic nausea, abdominal bloating, diarrhea, or constipation. Gastrointestinal complaints (sometimes caused by medications taken to treat other symptoms) can lead to frequent x-ray examinations. Sometimes inappropriate abdominal surgery occurs if clinicians are not alert. Irregular menses, menorrhagia, and vomiting throughout pregnancy are common. Men often experience erectile or ejaculatory dysfunction.

Often conversion symptoms suggest *a neurologic condition,* such as impaired coordination or balance, paralysis, localized weakness, difficulty swallowing, aphonia, urinary retention, numbness, dimming vision, blindness, hearing impairment, unexplained seizures, amnesia, or loss of consciousness other than fainting.

The adages of "first do no harm" and "don't make a thick chart out of a thin chart" are particularly appropriate when working with somatoform disorder patients. Management should employ insight-oriented psychotherapy, appropriate osteopathic manipulative care (to relieve symptoms), support groups, and exercise physiologist training programs.

Schizophrenia

Schizophrenia is a psychotic disorder characterized by disturbed thinking, blunted/flattened affect, poor concept of self, and psychomotor agitation/retardation. Conceptually, the term is defined as the loss of ego boundaries and gross impairment in reality testing, with accompanying loss of one's sense of self. Both auditory and visual hallucinations and delusions are prominent (8).

Because of their presentation, delusions are sometimes difficult to judge, especially across cultures. In general, however, when poor psychosocial functioning appears in the history, it is related to unusual thinking patterns. Some are relatively unimpaired in their subculture, interpersonal relations, and occupational roles. Others exhibit substantial impairments, including deteriorating occupational functions and social isolation. Usually, their families seek help before the patient does.

Brief Psychotic Disorder

Brief psychotic disorder is a disturbance involving the sudden onset of at least one of the following positive psychotic symptoms: delusions, hallucinations, or disorganized speech (e.g., frequent incoherence, grossly disorganized, or catatonic behavior). *A typical episode lasts at least 1 day, but less than 1 month. Recovery to prior levels of functioning is the rule* (8).

Both schizophrenia and brief psychotic disorders respond well to antipsychotic medications. Typical antipsychotics depress or reduce maladaptive behavioral responses and emotional tension. They also decrease auditory hallucinations and delusions. In some, they induce generalized sedation. They are not universally effective and many have significant side effects involving one or more organ systems, which tends to limit patient compliance. Osteopathic manipulative therapies are of limited value with these primary brain chemistry/organization conditions. Even when stabilized on medications, touch is often confusing and misinterpreted.

SUBSTANCE ABUSE

The first step to effectively treating substance abuse or dependence is to conduct a complete biopsychosocial evaluation to be sure there is not an underlying medical or psychiatric problem contributing to the situation.

Even when medical and psychiatric problems are identified and managed, outpatient treatment for substance abuse is often indicated for a minimum of 2 years. This should include long-term support groups for relapse prevention and 12-step recovery model programs such as Alcoholics Anonymous (AA) or Narcotics Anonymous (NA). Continuing drug screens on an outpatient basis and overall psychiatric monitoring are essential. Managing somatic complaints with OMT is often beneficial once the addictive behaviors are stabilized.

Substance abuse related disorders include:

1. disorders related to the taking of a drug of abuse, including alcohol
2. misuse of prescribed medications
3. over-the-counter medications taken improperly or excessively

The diagnosis is made by biopsychosocial history and urine drug screen. Differentiation should be made between tolerance, pseudotolerance, physical dependence, addiction, and pseudoaddiction.

■ Tolerance is the need for an increased dosage of a drug to produce the same level of analgesia that previously existed. Tolerance also occurs when a reduced effect is observed with a constant dose.
■ Pseudotolerance is the need to increase dosage that is not due to tolerance, but due to other factors such as disease progression, new disease, increased physical activity, lack of compliance, change in medication, and drug interaction.
■ Physical dependence can be described as the occurrence of withdrawal symptoms after drug use is stopped or quickly decreased without titration. It is not addiction. Physical dependence "... is not a clinical problem if patients are warned to avoid abrupt discontinuation of the drug and a tapering regimen is used."
■ Addiction is "psychological dependence on the use of substances for their psychic effects and is characterized by compulsive use ..." Addiction should be considered if patients no longer have control over drug use and continue to use the drugs despite harm.
■ Pseudoaddiction is drug-seeking behavior that seems similar to addiction but is due to unrelieved pain. This behavior stops once that pain is relieved, often through an increase in opioid dose. "Misunderstanding of this phenomenon may lead the clinician to inappropriately stigmatize the pain patient with the label 'addict.' In the setting of unrelieved pain, the request for increases in drug dose requires careful assessment, renewed efforts to manage pain, and avoidance of stigmatizing labels."

Neither tolerance nor withdrawal is necessary or sufficient for a diagnosis of substance dependence. Some individuals show a pattern of compulsive use without signs of tolerance or withdrawal. Some use larger quantities for longer periods than intended, and virtually all daily activities revolve around the substance and great amounts of time spent obtaining, using, and recovering from its effects.

COCAINE ADDICTION

Cocaine is one of the most commonly abused pharmacologic agents. Table 18.1 outlines use patterns for various cocaine preparations.

Addiction is the most common complication of cocaine use. Because the drug "high" is so pleasant, compulsive drug seeking quickly takes over the victim's life. Family, social, work, and recreational withdrawal is the rule rather than an exception. Chronic use results in tolerance of its many effects. This is particularly likely to occur with usage at high doses or in conjunction with binges. Because of its alleged ability to produce prolonged and intense orgasms, early cocaine use is often linked with compulsively promiscuous sexual activity. In the long term, however, reduced sexual drive and complaints of sexual problems are common. Table 18.2 outlines some of the effects.

There is no standard protocol or recognized pharmacologic treatment for cocaine dependency at the present time. Substance abuse treatment discussed earlier yields mixed results at best. Osteopathic medicine is truly challenged by this chemically induced, often total, breakdown in mind, body, and spirit (Table 18.3).

Benzodiazepine Abuse

Benzodiazepines are the most widely prescribed medications for anxiety disorders and insomnia in the United States (25,26). Actions of each type are listed in Tables 18.4 and 18.5, and withdrawal is very difficult.

The most common treatment approach is slow withdrawal over 6 to12 weeks. To prevent seizures, phenobarbital is sometimes used to control the clinical course. The phenobarbital approach calls for assessment of the total amount of daily benzodiazepine use that is then converted to a phenobarbital equivalent. Carbamazepine is another useful agent (27–29).

TABLE 18.1. EFFECTS OF COCAINE BASED ON TYPE AND ROUTE OF ADMINISTRATION

Cocaine Preparation	Route of Administration	Onset of Action	Peak Effect
Cocaine	Intranasal	2–3 min	30–45 min
Hydrochloride (powder)	Intravenous	30–45 s	10–20 min
Crack cocaine (alkaloidal, free base)	Inhalation (smoking)	8–10 s	5–10 min

TABLE 18.2. EFFECTS OF COCAINE AT VARYING DOSES

Low doses
  Heightened sense of well-being, alertness, energy, and
    self-confidence
  Modest elevation in heart rate and blood pressure
  Enhanced performance on mental and physical tasks

Increasing doses
  Intense euphoria, agitation, impulsivity
  Heightened aggressive and sexual behavior
  Paranoia
  Headache
  Chest pain

Severe overdoses
  Hallucinations
  Delirium
  Seizures
  Severe hypertension
  Tachycardia
  Cardiac arrhythmia
  Hyperthermia
  Coma
  Respiratory arrest
  Death
  Seizures and intense muscle activity contributing to hyperthermia;
    and rhabdomyolysis resulting in acute renal failure

Protocols for the withdrawal process can be found in many references. Table 18.6 outlines phenobarbital/benzodiazepine equivalencies. Recovery, lapse, and relapse are common elements of substance abuse rehabilitation. Benzodiazepines are no exception.

Recovery in the initial stage of abstinence is affected by many factors, including:

a. patient's motivational level,
b. severity of abuse,
c. related medical, psychiatric, and psychosocial problems,
d. age, gender, and ethnicity,
e. social support (30).

Because detoxification alone is rarely adequate, many relapse without suitable aftercare. Relapse prevention should be part of the long-term plan. Steps that help maintain abstinence include:

a. supportive individual psychotherapy,
b. joining a self-help recovery group,
c. joining a 12-step program,
d. anxiety management techniques such as biofeedback and exercise,
e. learning to anticipate, identify, and cope with risks that increase relapse risks. (31,32).

TABLE 18.3. DETERMINANTS OF HOSPITALIZATION FOR COCAINE ABUSE

Chronic crack smoking or intravenous use
Concurrent dependency on other addictive drugs or alcohol
Serious concurrent medical or psychiatric problems
Severe impairment of psychological functioning
Insufficient motivation for outpatient treatment
Lack of family and social support
Failure in outpatient treatment

TABLE 18.4. CATEGORIES OF BENZODIAZEPINES BY HALF-LIFE

Ultrashort-acting	Short- or Intermediate-acting	Long-acting
Estazolam	Alprazolam	Chlordiazepoxide
Midazolam	Lorazepam	Clonazepam
Temazepam	Oxazepam	Clorazepate
Triazolam		Diazepam
		Flurazepam
		Prazepam
		Quazepam

ALZHEIMER'S DISEASE

Symptoms of Alzheimer's disease include memory loss that affects everyday living and overall quality of life, difficulty performing familiar tasks such as naming common objects, getting lost easily in familiar places, poor and decreased judgment abilities, problems with abstract thinking, frequently losing or misplacing items, a general loss of interest, and changes in mood, behavior, and personality (8).

Patients are often symptomatic for as long as 5 years before a clear diagnosis is made. Three stages characterize Alzheimer's disease (33).

1. Stage one is mild and usually lasts 2 to 4 years. During this stage, the victim often says the same thing over and over, gets lost easily, and loses interest in previously enjoyable activities. As time passes, personality changes are clearly evident.

2. Stage two usually lasts 2 to 10 years. This stage is characterized by increasing difficulty dealing with recent events, dressing, feeding, and personal hygiene. With progression, argumentativeness, paranoia, and assaultive behavior are increasingly common.

3. Stage three usually lasts 1 to 3 years. At this point, the victim is no longer physically or mentally capable of speech or cognition, and general coordination steadily deteriorates. Loss of bladder and bowel function is common (34).

There is no cure for this devastating problem. At the time of this writing, two or three brain-selective pharmacologic agents are available. Donepezil hydrochloride is the oldest of the group and has been shown to slow the deterioration processes by several months. Osteopathic care centers provide active planning and supportive counseling for both the family and caregivers who themselves suffer the musculoskeletal and emotional stress of this disease.

DELIRIUM

Delirium may occur in individuals with normal brain functioning, but it is actually more common in those with underlying brain disease, such as dementia. It is more common in the elderly, probably due to changes in neurotransmitters because of age and disease-related loss of neural tissues.

Delirium may be due to primary brain disease or diseases elsewhere in the body that affect the brain. Metabolic, toxic, structural, or infectious processes are most common. Physiologically,

TABLE 18.5. BENZODIAZEPINE WITHDRAWAL SYNDROMES

Syndrome	Signs/Symptoms	Time Course	Response to Reinstitution of Benzodiazepine
High-dose withdrawal	Anxiety, insomnia, nightmares, major motor seizures, psychosis, hyperpyrexia, death	Begins 1–2 days after a short acting benzodiazepine is stopped; 3–8 days after a long-acting benzodiazepine is stopped	Signs and symptoms reverse 2–6 hours following a hypnotic dose of a benzodiazepine
Low-dose withdrawal (slow taper)	Anxiety, agitation, tachycardia, palpitations, anorexia, blurred vision, muscle cramps, insomnia, nightmares	Signs and symptoms emerge 1–7 days after discontinuation of the benzodiazepine or after	Signs and symptoms reverse 2–6 hours following a sedative dose of high-potency benzodiazepine

arousal mechanisms of the thalamus and reticular activating systems of the brainstem are physiologically impaired. Sleep disruption and superimposed stress often worsen symptoms.

Symptoms of delirium fluctuate rapidly, often within a matter of minutes and worsening late in the afternoon to early evening, which is commonly called sun downing. Consciousness clouds with increasingly prominent disorientation as to time, place, and person. Attention deficits are the rule, with frequent confusion regarding day-to-day events and daily routines.

Personality changes and altered affect are common. Symptoms include irritability, inappropriate behavior, fearfulness, or overtly psychotic features, such as delusions, hallucinations, or paranoia. Some may be withdrawn, quiet, or apathetic. Others become hyperactive, excitable, and physically restless (35,36).

ADULT ATTENTION DEFICIT DISORDER

Adult attention deficit disorder (ADHD) is a common but controversial syndrome characterized by inappropriate hyperactivity, impulsivity, and inattention dating from childhood (8). It is characterized by excessive physical and mental activity. Limited abilities to control daily behaviors are the rule, even when adjusted for age.

The most prominent childhood and adolescent symptoms and signs are poor social performance, hyperactivity, tantrums, drug and alcohol use, antisocial personality, depressed mood, and general anxiety. Significant controversies surround the best treatment strategies. Combinations of centrally acting stimulants such as methylphenidate along with lifestyle education and support group activities are commonly used.

TABLE 18.6. DETERMINING BENZODIAZEPINE/PHENO-BARBITAL EQUIVALENCIES

Benzodiazepine	Dose Equivalent of 30 mg Phenobarbital (mg)
Alprazolam	1
Chlordiazepoxide	25
Clonazepam	2
Clorazepate	15
Diazepam	10
Flurazepam	30
Lorazepam	1
Oxazepam	30
Temazepam	30
Triazolam	1

AXIS II DIAGNOSES
Personality Disorders

The term *personality disorder* refers to longstanding patterns of disordered (often chaotic) behavior and emotional activities. Learning the behavioral features of personality disorders can improve management and treatment planning. Primary care physicians are apt to miss the diagnosis, particularly if unaware of Axis II disorders, because the disorder often underlies persistent chronic illness. Importantly, personality disorders are persistent, develop early, and endure for life. In stressful situations, underlying genetic and environmental stressors often express themselves through personality disorders. Frequent reactions are reports of vague, nonspecific whole-body pain, intrapsychic and emotional pain, worsening of preexisting problems, and reporting the life-long effects of physical, verbal, sexual, and psychological abuse.

1. *Cluster A: asocial personality cluster* consisting of paranoid, schizoid, and schizotypal personality disorders.
2. *Cluster B: dramatic/emotional personality disorder cluster* consisting of borderline, histrionic, and narcissistic personality disorders.
3. *Cluster C: Anxious personality disorder cluster* consisting of avoidant, dependent, obsessive-compulsive, and passive-aggressive personality disorders

Assessment of Axis II Personality Disorders

The most common assessment tool is the Minnesota Multiphasic Personality Inventory-2 (MMPI-2) (37,38). Over 50 years old, it is one of the oldest and research-validated personality evaluation tools, and it is often used to evaluate fundamental personality characteristics associated with chronic physical and mental disorders. From an osteopathic perspective, it is important to know that the MMPI-2 results are valid. Only valid testing delineates patients who present with ambiguous functional and organic neuromuscaloskeletal complaints (39–41).

Of the three clusters, patients fitting into cluster B (dramatic/emotional) are the most troublesome for the primary care physician. This is because borderline histrionic and narcissistic personality disorders represent a pervasive pattern of instability in interpersonal relationships, affecting self-image and affective/emotional relationships. Patients with musculoskeletal complaints that defy treatment spend a lot of time visiting many primary care physicians.

These cluster B individuals show marked *impulsivity* beginning in early adulthood. Four psychosocial areas are affected:

1. Continual efforts are made to avoid real or imagined abandonment by the physician or his staff.
2. Patterns of unstable and intense interpersonal relationships are characterized by alternating extremes of idealization and devaluation of the doctor/patient relationship.
3. Typically, there is a persistent identity disturbance with markedly disturbed and/or distorted self or body image.
4. Persistent impulsivity also occurs in at least two outside areas that are potentially self-damaging:
   a. spending
   b. sexual activities
   c. reckless driving
   d. substance abuse
   e. binge eating
   f. recurrent suicidal behavior, gestures, and threats
   g. affective instability, particularly strikingly apparent mood shifts and overreactivity
   h. chronic feelings of loneliness and emptiness
   i. inappropriately intense anger and lack of control over anger
   j. transient-related paranoid ideation or severe dissociative symptoms

Behaviorally, cluster B personality disorder patients enter your office in the following ways:

1. They think you're wonderful and claim that all other physicians before you did not understand them.
2. They 'make scenes to fill needs' for attention, disrupting both your practice schedule and private life.
3. They fight with the staff and are never satisfied.

Typically, they are demanding, and treatment failure or regression is the rule. Negative counter-transference complexities are also common. In some, self-mutilation tendencies and manipulative suicidal efforts occur. They also demonstrate abandonment, engulfment, and annihilation concerns that do not respond to medications.

The most difficult differential diagnosis is sorting out personality disorder and its many manifestations from depressive disorder. Depressive disorder is characterized by pervasive guilty feelings, agitation, suicidal tendency, remorse, and withdrawal. Stable (as contrasted with unstable) relationships are present along with more severe vegetative signs.

Personality disorders, on the other hand, speak of loneliness and emptiness. Repeated suicidal gestures, persistent rage, creation of demanding relationships, and delusionary self-sufficiency are other traits.

The best way to treat personality disorders includes concurrent treatment with a psychiatrist or psychologist. The goal is to help strengthen ego and self-concept defenses so the patient can more effectively tolerate anxiety while gaining greater control over counterproductive impulses and manipulative counter transferences.

Counter-transference effects are common with these patients. Typically, they want frequent visits, cannot tolerate separation,

and are easily angered with you and your staff. Boundaries must be set between you, your staff, and the patient. Manipulative behavior, such as missing appointments, must be addressed immediately in order to establish a stable treatment framework. A passive therapeutic approach is counterproductive with these patients. Osteopathic manipulative therapies are always misinterpreted, never productive, and complicate an ever-increasing complex doctor/patient relationship. Instead, the active approach is confronting self-destructive behaviors, establishing connections between feelings and actions, and setting limits while maintaining focus on the here and now.

IMPORTANCE FOR PRIMARY CARE PHYSICIANS

The need for the primary care physician to understand and use this multiaxial diagnosis system is of utmost importance in developing an overall treatment plan that sets realistic and obtainable goals. A multiple biopsychosocial approach is apt to be most effective. Medication, psychotherapy, and healthy lifestyle modifications that focus on strengthening mind, body, and spiritual aspects are fundamental management strategies. Important "here-and-now" considerations are diet, exercise, focusing on healthy relationships, and use of appropriate osteopathic manipulative care.

CONCLUSION

Thoughts, feelings, and behaviors are influenced by complex combinations of genetic inheritance and cultural influences. Realistic and reasonable diagnostic and treatment planning should always incorporate these complexities within the capacity of the patient. At best, this is a difficult task. This chapter describes a widely accepted, multiaxial diagnostic system that identifies treatable Axis I behavioral/psychological problems. It also focuses on the Axis II personality disorders that complicate routine treatments of Axis I and a myriad of Axis III general medical disorders. Osteopathic manipulative techniques covered elsewhere in this text address the musculoskeletal management of many psychiatric signs and symptoms. The patient needs to experience a nonthreatening environment that encourages open self expression and long-term mental health.

Osteopathic psychiatry is based on the assumption that people have within themselves the resources to understand their thoughts, feelings, and the environmental forces surrounding them. With that understanding and physician support, they can change their behavior and mood. Empathic understanding, nonjudgmental acceptance, and genuine caring about the patient are an osteopathic hallmark for psychiatry.

REFERENCES

1. Regier DA, Narrow WE, Rae DS, et al. The de facto mental and addictive disorders service system. Epidemiologic Catchment Area prospective 1-year prevalence rates of disorders and services. *Arch Gen Psychiatry.* 1993;50(2):85–94.
2. Kessler RC, Nelson CB, McGonagle KA, et al. Comorbidity of DSM-III-R major depressive disorder in the general population: results from

the US National Comorbidity Survey [see comments]. *Br J Psychiatry Suppl.* 1996 Jun;(30):17–30.

3. Kessler RC, Sonnega A, Bromet E, et al. Posttraumatic stress disorder in the National Comorbidity Survey. *Arch Gen Psychiatry.* 1995;52:1048–1060.

4. Kessler RC, Stang PE, Wittchen HU, et al. Lifetime panic-depression comorbidity in the National Comorbidity Survey. *Arch Gen Psychiatry.* 1998;55:801–808.

5. Rice DP, Miller LS. The economic burden of schizophrenia: conceptual and methodological issues, and cost estimates. In: Moscarelli M, Rupp A, Sartorious N, eds. *Handbook of Mental Health Economics and Health Policy, Volume 1: Schizophrenia.* New York, NY: John Wiley and Sons; 1996:321–324.

6. Still FM. Dementia praecos. *J Am Osteopath Assoc.* 1933;40:534–536.

7. Dunn FE. Osteopathic concepts in psychiatry. *J Am Osteopath Assoc.* 1950;49(7):354–357.

8. American Psychiatric Association. *Diagnostic and Statistical Manual of Mental Disorders,* 4th ed. Washington, DC: American Psychiatric Association; 1994.

9. Kessler RC, McGonagle KA, Zhao S, et al. Lifetime and 12-month prevalence of DSM-III-R psychiatric disorders in the United States. Results from the National Comorbidity Survey. *Arch Gen Psychiatry.* 1994;51:8–19.

10. Breier A, Charney DS, Heninger GR. Agoraphobia with panic attacks. Development, diagnostic stability, and course of illness. *Arch Gen Psychiatry.* 1986;43(11):1029–1036.

11. Fava GA, Sonino N. Psychosomatic medicine: emerging trends and perspectives. *Psychother Psychosom.* 2000;69(4):184–197.

12. Fava M, Kendler KS. Major depressive disorder. *Neuron.* 2000; 28(2):335–341.

13. Matthews JD, Fava M. Risk of suicidality in depression with serotonergic antidepressants. *Ann Clin Psychiatry.* 2000;12(1):43–50.

14. Richelson E. Biological basis of depression and therapeutic relevance. *J Clin Psychiatry.* 1991;52(6, suppl):4–10.

15. Baldessarine RJ. Drugs and the treatment of psychiatric disorders. II. Drugs used in the treatment of disorders of mood. In: Gilman AG, Rall TW, Nies AS, et al, eds. *Goodman and Gilman's The Pharmacological Basis of Therapeutics,* 8th ed. New York, NY: Pergamon Press; 1990:404–423.

16. Licht RW, Vestergaard P, Rasmussen NA, et al. A lithium clinic for bipolar patients: 2-year outcome of the first 148 patients. *Acta Psychiatr Scand.* 2001;104(5):387–390.

17. Sachs GS. Bipolar mood disorder: practical strategies for acute and maintenance phase treatment. *J Clin Psychopharmacol.* 1996;16 (2 Suppl 1):32S–47S.

18. Compton MT, Nemeroff CB. The treatment of bipolar depression. *J Clin Psychiatry.* 2000;61(Suppl 9):57–67.

19. Gulley LR, Nemeroff CB. The neurobiological basis of mixed depression-anxiety states. *J Clin Psychiatry.* 1993;54(Suppl):16–19.

20. Ressler KJ, Nemeroff CB. Role of serotonergic and noradrenergic systems in the pathophysiology of depression and anxiety disorders. *Depress Anxiety.* 2000;12(Suppl 1):2–19.

21. Weiss JM, Stout JC, Aaron MF, et al. Depression and anxiety: role of the locus coeruleus and corticotropin-releasing factor. *Brain Res Bull.* 1994;35:561–572.

22. Blier P, de Montigny C. Current advances and trends in the treatment of depression. *Trends Pharmacol Sci.* 1994;15:220–226.

23. Owens MJ, Nemeroff CB. Role of serotonin in the pathophysiology of depression: focus on the serotonin transporter. *Clin Chem.* 1994;40:288–295.

24. Smith DE, Wesson DR. Benzodiazepines and other sedative-hypnotics. In: Galanter M, Kleber H, eds. *American Psychiatric Press Textbook of Substance Abuse Treatment.* Washington, DC: American Psychiatric Press; 1994:179–190.

25. Wesson DR, Smith DE, Seymour RB. Sedative-hypnotics and tricyclics. In: Lowinson JH, Ruiz P, Millman RB, et al, eds. *Substance Abuse: A Comprehensive Textbook,* 3rd ed. Baltimore, MD: Williams & Wilkins; 1997:271–279.

26. O'Brien CP. Drug addiction and drug abuse. In: Hardman JG, Limbird LE, eds. *Goodman & Gilman's The Pharmacological Basis of Therapeutics,* 9th ed. New York, NY: McGraw-Hill; 1996:557–577.

27. Klein E, Uhde TW, Post RM. Preliminary evidence for the utility of carbamazepine in alprazolam withdrawal. *Am J Psychiatry.* 1986;143:235–236.

28. Ries RK, Roy-Byrne PP, Ward NG, et al. Carbamazepine treatment for benzodiazepine withdrawal. *Am J Psychiatry.* 1989;146:536–537.

29. Pages KP, Ries RK. Use of anticonvulsants in benzodiazepine withdrawal. *Am J Addict.* 1998;7:198–204.

30. Daley DC, Marlatt GA. Relapse prevention: cognitive and behavioral interventions. In: Lowinson JH, Ruiz P, Millman RB, et al, eds. *Substance Abuse: A Comprehensive Textbook,* 3rd ed. Baltimore, MD: Williams & Wilkins; 1997:533–542.

31. Daley DC, Salloum I. Relapse prevention. In: Ott PJ, Tarter RE, Ammerman RT, eds. *Sourcebook on Substance Abuse.* Needham Heights, MA: Allyn & Bacon; 1999:255–263.

32. Alling FA. Detoxification and treatment of acute sequelae. In: Lowinson JH, Ruiz P, Millman RB, et al, eds. *Substance Abuse: A Comprehensive Textbook,* 3rd ed. Baltimore, MD: Williams & Wilkins; 1997:402–415.

33. Morris JC. Differential diagnosis of Alzheimer's disease. *Clin Geriatr Med.* 1994;10:257–276.

34. Small GW, Rabins PV, Barry PP, et al. Diagnosis and treatment of Alzheimer's disease and related disorders: consensus statement of the American Association for Geriatric Psychiatry, the Alzheimer's Association, and the American Geriatrics Society. *JAMA.* 1997;278:1363–1371.

35. Wise MG. Delirium due to a general medical condition, delirium due to multiple etiologies, and delirium not otherwise specified. In: Gabbard GO, ed. *Treatment of Psychiatric Disorders,* 2nd ed., volume 1. Washington, DC: American Psychiatric Press; 1995:423–443.

36. Marcantonio ER. Delirium. In: Rakel RE, Bope ET, eds. *Conn's Current Therapy.* Philadelphia, PA: WB Saunders; 2001:1144–1147.

37. Dahlstrom WG, Welsh GS, Dahlstrom LE, eds. *An MMPI Handbook. Volume 1: Clinical Interpretation,* revised ed. Minneapolis, MN: University of Minnesota Press; 1960.

38. Hathaway SR, McKinley J. *Minnesota Multiphasic Personality Inventory.* Minneapolis, MN: University of Minnesota Press; 1930.

39. Hanvik LJ. MMPI profiles in patients with low back pain. *J Consult Clin Psychol.* 1951;15:350–353.

40. McCreary C, Turner J, Dawson E. Differences between functional versus organic low back pain patients. *Pain.* 1977;4:73–78.

41. Sternbach RA, Wolf SR, Murphy RW, et al. Traits of pain patients: the low-back "loser." *Psychosomatics.* 1973;14:226–229.

OSTEOPATHIC CONSIDERATIONS IN CLINICAL PROBLEM SOLVING

■ Four approaches
  including patterr
  method, problem
  decision analysis
■ Problem-solving p
  musculoskeletal pa
  and medication,
  thinking
■ Osteopathic approa

... in the long term, the
principles never die. They m
will emerge again, stronger
day in patient care to show h

This chapter discusses cl
pathic primary care persp
ferent approaches to clini
each can be incorporated
tification and explanatio
section discusses case vigr
into osteopathic practitior
cesses. That inquiry is the
used throughout this cha
case illustrating applicatio
cal problem solving.

EXAMPLE CASE

Consider the following case
The setting is the office o
family practitioner. Mr. Jo
see the physician. At the ti
looks at the chart and notes
the office. One-half hour ha
Based on preliminary exami
entered in the chart:

STOP: In our presentation of Mr. Johnson's case, we have intentionally placed the clinician in a listening rather than questioning role. In a scenario portraying the physician as an active hypothesis tester, he or she asks numerous questions to elicit information specifically relevant to the hypotheses under consideration. Furthermore, the physical examination could have focused on only the region of the complaint and on those regions that would yield data positive or negative for favored hypotheses. That pattern of data gathering is not usually functional for the osteopathic primary care physician, so we have elected not to emphasize it here.

Now we have a reasonably complete preliminary data set for Mr. Johnson. A thorough evaluation of his illness is in order. The two major possible mechanisms for his presenting problem are chest pain atypical for angina with secondary musculoskeletal pain (probably as a result of coronary artery disease), and primary musculoskeletal pain.

The first explanation has the strongest support. The patient's pain could likely be of cardiac origin. It is a heavy, aching pain that is brought on by exertion and relieved by rest. It is not reproduced by direct pressure on or movement of the affected area. It does not seem to be related to eating (i.e., exacerbated by certain foods, or associated with gas or bloating), or breathing (e.g., brought on by taking a deep breath). The patient has many health risk factors for coronary artery disease. He is male, age 55, has a sedentary stressful job, does not exercise, is overweight, and smokes. Although the patient has few pertinent physical findings, those you did elicit are telling: elevated systolic and diastolic blood pressure, femoral artery bruits, and tenderness and tissue texture abnormalities at T2-5, which have been shown to be associated with viscerosomatic reflexes from coronary artery disease (17,18).

There are four characteristics used to establish a diagnosis of typical angina pectoris:

1. Chest discomfort brought on by exertion and/or stress.

2. Location substernal or anterior chest wall.

3. Pain feels heavy, like pressure or squeezing.

4. Pain is soon (10 minutes or less) relieved by rest, or immediately with nitroglycerine.

This patient has three of the four characteristics. Last, a normal chest x-ray film and ECG do not rule out coronary artery disease.

At this point, you can assign approximately 70% likelihood to a diagnosis of coronary artery insufficiency, with the diagnosis of primary musculoskeletal problem at a 20% likelihood, and other diagnostic possibilities combined in the remaining 10% probability range. You are now able to develop a management plan for the patient.

CONCLUSION

As we leave Mr. Johnson, consider what we have learned from his case and the many other brief cases presented here that could comprise an osteopathic approach to clinical problem solving.

Osteopathic problem solving is loosely couched in the four basic precepts of

Body unity
Structure-function interrelationship
Self-regulation
Rational therapy

The application of those precepts by any given clinician problem solver to any given patient problem is not only idiosyncratic to the patient but also to the problem solver. The following considerations seem to be fundamental to osteopathic problem solving.

In considering a patient's problem, the osteopathic physician must be able to perceive the problem as evolving from a compromise in the body's ability to maintain a healthy dynamic equilibrium or homeostatic state. Under circumstances of adequate nutrition, exercise, and physiologic and anatomic balance, the body's normal state is one of health. Whether they are amenable to labeling as disease processes, health problems constitute deviations from that normal state of health. The goal of osteopathic problem solving is to ascertain the nature and source of the deviation from health.

The major problem solving models articulated here, which, in various forms, comprise most of what we know about clinical problem solving, can be considered to represent a subset of osteopathic problem solving. The problem-solving models and the osteopathic approach are far from being mutually exclusive. Rather, the osteopathic problem solver is seen as calling on the more restricted, reductionistic models to incorporate into his or her more global, holistic, conceptualization of health and illness, to achieve a more complete understanding of a patient's problem.

Not all osteopathic primary care physicians use osteopathic problem solving or are even cognizant of it. Therefore, it would be inaccurate to say that osteopathic problem solving is just what osteopathic physicians do. It is more than that. With further understanding and investigation, we can characterize osteopathic problem solving to the point of articulating a model that is as applicable and teachable as the more allopathic models we have now.

REFERENCES

1. Astell L. Reflections and a forecast. *The DO.* 1981;21(5):155–159.
2. Groen GJ, Patel VL. The relationship between comprehension and reasoning in medical expertise. In: Chi MTH, et al., eds. *The Nature of Expertise.* Hillsdale, NJ: Erlbaum; 1988:287–310.
3. Patel VL, Groen GJ, Norman GR. Reasoning and instruction in medical curricula. *Cognition and Instruction.* 1993;10:335–378.
4. Schmidt HG, Norman GR, Boshuizen HPA. A cognitive perspective on medical expertise: theory and implications. *Acad Med.* 1990;65:611–621.
5. Norman GR, Brooks LR, Allen SW, et al. The development of expertise in dermatology. *Arch Dermatol.* 1989;125:1062–1065.
6. Brooks LR, Allen SW, Norman GR. Rule and instance-based inference in medical diagnosis. *J Exp Psychol Gen.* 1991;120:278–287.
7. Schmidt HG, Boshuizen HPA. Encapsulation of biomedical knowledge. In: Evans D, Patel VL, eds. *Advanced Models of Cognition for Medical Training and Practice.* New York, NY: Springer-Verlag New York; 1993.
8. Hunter KM. *Doctors' Stories: The Narrative Structure of Medical Knowledge.* Princeton, NJ: Princeton University Press; 1991.
9. Eistein AS, Shulman LS, Sprafka SA. *Medical Problem Solving: An Analysis of Clinical Reasoning.* Cambridge, MA: Harvard University Press; 1978.
10. Weed LL. *Your Health Care and How To Manage It.* Essex Junction, VT: Essex Publishing Co; 1975.

sl
te

EST

Patie
treat
chroi
prob
patte
patte
the p
comp
probl
for th
given
answ
patie

MU!

Ostec
probl

1. Tl
   th
   pa
2. Tl
   pa
   fui
3. Tl
   gir
   is a
   sto
   mt

UNU

At the
patter
forme
even l
cumst
which
some (
viral il
(i.e., a
provid
Refere
drome
and ot
tern of
physic
nized.
awaren

CLINICAL PROBLEM SOLVING

SARAH A. SPRAFKA

KEY CONCEPTS

- Four approaches to data gathering and synthesis, including pattern recognition, hypothetico-deductive method, problem-oriented perspective, and clinical decision analysis
- Problem-solving practices, including therapeutic touch, musculoskeletal pain, osteopathic manipulative treatment and medication, patient as a whole, and integrative thinking
- Osteopathic approach to clinical problem solving

... in the long term, the osteopathic concept will survive because true principles never die. They may be averted, submerged, even denied, but they will emerge again, stronger than ever. They have only to be applied every day in patient care to show how fundamental and timeless they are (1).

This chapter discusses clinical problem solving from an osteopathic primary care perspective. It begins by looking at four different approaches to clinical problem solving and discussing how each can be incorporated in the osteopathic family doctor's identification and explanation of a patient's problem. The second section discusses case vignettes to report and analyze an inquiry into osteopathic practitioners' self-reported problem solving processes. That inquiry is the source for the illustrative quotations used throughout this chapter. The third section summarizes a case illustrating application of the osteopathic approach to clinical problem solving.

EXAMPLE CASE

Consider the following case. It is a Wednesday in mid-November. The setting is the office of A.B. Martin, DO, an osteopathic family practitioner. Mr. Johnson has made an appointment to see the physician. At the time of the patient's visit, Dr. Martin looks at the chart and notes that this is the patient's first visit to the office. One-half hour has been allocated for the appointment. Based on preliminary examination, the following data have been entered in the chart:

Personal Data

Name: Richard Johnson
Age: 55
Ethnicity: White
Reason for visit: "I was raking leaves on Sunday and I got an aching sensation in my left shoulder. It still bothers me today."

Vital Signs

Height: 6' 1"
Weight: 203 lbs.
Blood Pressue: 160/110 mm Hg
Pulse: 75 regular
Respirations: 16

Discussion

If you were Dr. Martin, what might you be thinking? At this point you have just the slightest bit of information about Mr. Johnson. He complains of shoulder pain. His weight is high relative to his height. You picture a large man. His blood pressure is elevated.

At this stage of your interaction with this patient (you have not met him yet), your first priority is clearly to conduct a thorough history and physical examination including a diagnostic palpatory examination, and to become acquainted with the patient as a person. As you plan for what you would like to learn from Mr. Johnson, you begin to consider some possible mechanisms for his presenting problem. These may be wide-ranging and include trauma to the shoulder or somatic dysfunction in the shoulder. He may have viscerosomatic reflex activity associated with cardiovascular and/or pulmonary disease.

At this point we leave the actual visit with Mr. Johnson, and consider some approaches you might take with this patient:

How you organize your data gathering and data synthesis
How you view this patient as an individual and as a member of a group
How you plan a short-term as well as longer-term strategy for your interaction with Mr. Johnson

STOP: In our presentation of Mr. Johnson's case, we have intentionally placed the clinician in a listening rather than questioning role. In a scenario portraying the physician as an active hypothesis tester, he or she asks numerous questions to elicit information specifically relevant to the hypotheses under consideration. Furthermore, the physical examination could have focused on only the region of the complaint and on those regions that would yield data positive or negative for favored hypotheses. That pattern of data gathering is not usually functional for the osteopathic primary care physician, so we have elected not to emphasize it here.

Now we have a reasonably complete preliminary data set for Mr. Johnson. A thorough evaluation of his illness is in order. The two major possible mechanisms for his presenting problem are chest pain atypical for angina with secondary musculoskeletal pain (probably as a result of coronary artery disease), and primary musculoskeletal pain.

The first explanation has the strongest support. The patient's pain could likely be of cardiac origin. It is a heavy, aching pain that is brought on by exertion and relieved by rest. It is not reproduced by direct pressure on or movement of the affected area. It does not seem to be related to eating (i.e., exacerbated by certain foods, or associated with gas or bloating), or breathing (e.g., brought on by taking a deep breath). The patient has many health risk factors for coronary artery disease. He is male, age 55, has a sedentary stressful job, does not exercise, is overweight, and smokes. Although the patient has few pertinent physical findings, those you did elicit are telling: elevated systolic and diastolic blood pressure, femoral artery bruits, and tenderness and tissue texture abnormalities at T2-5, which have been shown to be associated with viscerosomatic reflexes from coronary artery disease (17,18).

There are four characteristics used to establish a diagnosis of typical angina pectoris:

1. Chest discomfort brought on by exertion and/or stress.
2. Location substernal or anterior chest wall.
3. Pain feels heavy, like pressure or squeezing.
4. Pain is soon (10 minutes or less) relieved by rest, or immediately with nitroglycerine.

This patient has three of the four characteristics. Last, a normal chest x-ray film and ECG do not rule out coronary artery disease.

At this point, you can assign approximately 70% likelihood to a diagnosis of coronary artery insufficiency, with the diagnosis of primary musculoskeletal problem at a 20% likelihood, and other diagnostic possibilities combined in the remaining 10% probability range. You are now able to develop a management plan for the patient.

CONCLUSION

As we leave Mr. Johnson, consider what we have learned from his case and the many other brief cases presented here that could comprise an osteopathic approach to clinical problem solving.

Osteopathic problem solving is loosely couched in the four basic precepts of

Body unity
Structure-function interrelationship
Self-regulation
Rational therapy

The application of those precepts by any given clinician problem solver to any given patient problem is not only idiosyncratic to the patient but also to the problem solver. The following considerations seem to be fundamental to osteopathic problem solving.

In considering a patient's problem, the osteopathic physician must be able to perceive the problem as evolving from a compromise in the body's ability to maintain a healthy dynamic equilibrium or homeostatic state. Under circumstances of adequate nutrition, exercise, and physiologic and anatomic balance, the body's normal state is one of health. Whether they are amenable to labeling as disease processes, health problems constitute deviations from that normal state of health. The goal of osteopathic problem solving is to ascertain the nature and source of the deviation from health.

The major problem solving models articulated here, which, in various forms, comprise most of what we know about clinical problem solving, can be considered to represent a subset of osteopathic problem solving. The problem-solving models and the osteopathic approach are far from being mutually exclusive. Rather, the osteopathic problem solver is seen as calling on the more restricted, reductionistic models to incorporate into his or her more global, holistic, conceptualization of health and illness, to achieve a more complete understanding of a patient's problem.

Not all osteopathic primary care physicians use osteopathic problem solving or are even cognizant of it. Therefore, it would be inaccurate to say that osteopathic problem solving is just what osteopathic physicians do. It is more than that. With further understanding and investigation, we can characterize osteopathic problem solving to the point of articulating a model that is as applicable and teachable as the more allopathic models we have now.

REFERENCES

1. Astell L. Reflections and a forecast. *The DO.* 1981;21(5):155–159.
2. Groen GJ, Patel VL. The relationship between comprehension and reasoning in medical expertise. In: Chi MTH, et al., eds. *The Nature of Expertise.* Hillsdale, NJ: Erlbaum; 1988:287–310.
3. Patel VL, Groen GJ, Norman GR. Reasoning and instruction in medical curricula. *Cognition and Instruction.* 1993;10:335–378.
4. Schmidt HG, Norman GR, Boshuizen HPA. A cognitive perspective on medical expertise: theory and implications. *Acad Med.* 1990;65:611–621.
5. Norman GR, Brooks LR, Allen SW, et al. The development of expertise in dermatology. *Arch Dermatol.* 1989;125:1062–1065.
6. Brooks LR, Allen SW, Norman GR. Rule and instance-based inference in medical diagnosis. *J Exp Psychol Gen.* 1991;120:278–287.
7. Schmidt HG, Boshuizen HPA. Encapsulation of biomedical knowledge. In: Evans D, Patel VL, eds. *Advanced Models of Cognition for Medical Training and Practice.* New York, NY: Springer-Verlag New York; 1993.
8. Hunter KM. *Doctors' Stories: The Narrative Structure of Medical Knowledge.* Princeton, NJ: Princeton University Press; 1991.
9. Eistein AS, Shulman LS, Sprafka SA. *Medical Problem Solving: An Analysis of Clinical Reasoning.* Cambridge, MA: Harvard University Press; 1978.
10. Weed LL. *Your Health Care and How To Manage It.* Essex Junction, VT: Essex Publishing Co; 1975.

11. Walker HK, Hurst JW, Woody MF. *Applying the Problem-Oriented System.* New York, NY: Medcom Press; 1973.
12. Sox Jr HC, Blatt MA, Higgins MC, et al. *Medical Decision Making.* Boston/London: Butterworth's; 1988.
13. Sackett DL, Haynes RB, Tugwell P. *Clinical Epidemiology: A Basic Science for Clinical Medicine,* 2nd ed. Boston/Toronto/London: Little, Brown and Company; 1991.
14. Schappert S. *National Ambulatory Medical Care Survey: 1990 Summary.* Hyattsville, MD: US Department of Health and Human Services, Public Health Service, Centers for Disease Control, National Center for Health Statistics; 1992.
15. Special committee on osteopathic principles and osteopathic technic of the Kirksville College of Osteopathy and Surgery. An interpretation of the osteopathic concept: tentative formulation of a teaching guide for faculty, staff, and student body. *Journal of Osteopathy.* October 1953:8–10.
16. Sprafka SA, Ward RC, Neff D. What characterizes an osteopathic principle? Selected responses to an open question. *J Am Osteopath Assoc.* 1981;81(2):29–33.
17. Beal MC. Viscerosomatic reflexes: a review. *J Am Osteopath Assoc.* 1985;85(12):786–801.
18. Kuchera M, Kuchera WA. *Osteopathic Considerations in Systemic Dysfunction.* Kirksville, MO: KCOM Press; 1990.
19. Sackett DL, Rosenberg WMC, Muir Gray JA, et al. Evidence-based medicine: What it is and what it isn't. *http://cebm.jr2.ox.ac.uk/ebmisisnt.html.*

APPENDIX TO CHAPTER 19

Section 1. Statistical Properties of Stress ECG as it Relates to Coronary Artery Disease

Diagnostic statistics for the stress ECG: a common method for displaying statistics is shown in Table 19.1 below, known as a 2-by-2 table.

We can analyze the table step by step as follows. Imagine that we conducted an experiment on a sample of 500 patients. Furthermore, imagine that half (250) of our patients had CAD as determined by the gold standard, an objective verification of the presence or absence of the disease in our patient sample. That is our defined disease prevalence for this purpose. It is clearly unrealistically high; a change in prevalence to a more realistic level can change what we learn from test results. We have now established the values at the bottom of our "CAD present" and "CAD absent" columns. Now, say all 500 of our patients underwent a stress ECG. We would find that approximately 172 of them had positive test results and that test results for 328 of our patients would be normal. That would establish the values for the "Stress ECG +" and "Stress ECG −" rows of our table. We would also learn that, of the patients who had CAD, approximately 150 had a positive stress test result. Those are our true positives. Furthermore, approximately 228 of our healthy patients would have normal test results (true negatives). Clearly, the test is not perfect, but it does identify a fair number of true positives and a large proportion of true negatives. To allow us to

generalize from this study of 500 patients to other populations, we convert the number of true positives and true negatives to a proportion. In the first instance, we divide true positives by total number of patients with CAD (150/250 = 0.60). That gives a statistic expressing the probability that a patient with CAD will have a positive stress ECG result, which is called the true positive rate or sensitivity of the test. Similarly, we divide the true negatives by the total of non-CAD patients (228/250 = 0.91). That statistic tells us the probability that a patient with no CAD will have a normal stress ECG result, which is the true negative rate or specificity of the test. Sensitivity and specificity remain constant for a test over time and with changes in disease prevalence. They would only change if, for example, the quality of the test changed to increase or decrease its association with the presence or absence of this disease process.

Two other values of even greater interest to physicians than sensitivity and specificity are positive predictive value and negative predictive value. Those are the values that tell us for a known disease prevalence what the probability is of the disease being present given a positive test result (positive predictive value) and, conversely, what the probability is of a patient being disease free given a normal test result (negative predictive value). In our example above, these can be found as follows:

Positive predictive value = True positives/All positives
or 150/172 = .87

Negative predictive value = True negatives/All negatives
or 228/328 = .70

Thus, in a patient population where approximately half of the patients actually have coronary artery disease, any given patient with a positive stress ECG result will have an 87 probability of having the disease, and a patient with a normal stress ECG result will have a 70 probability of being disease free. However, unlike sensitivity and specificity, positive and negative predictive values are strongly affected by changes in disease prevalence. Consider the following example in Table 19.2.

As in the first example, we have a total patient sample of 500. However, we have revised the disease prevalence to 10, or 50 out of 500 patients who have CAD, a level much more likely to be seen by the primary care physician. We know that the true positive rate or sensitivity of the stress ECG is 0.60, so we can establish that for this patient population, 30 of our patients who have CAD by the gold standard will have a positive stress ECG result. We also know that the true negative rate or specificity of our test is 0.91, so we can establish that approximately 430 of our healthy patients in this group will have a normal stress ECG result. Now, what if a patient in this group whose health status we didn't know had a positive stress test result? How sure could we be that he or she had CAD? We can ascertain that as

TABLE 19.1. DIAGNOSIS OF CORONARY ARTERY DISEASE

	Present	Absent	Total
Stress ECG +	150	22	172
Stress ECG −	100	228	328
Total	250	250	500

TABLE 19.2. DIAGNOSIS OF CORONARY ARTERY DISEASE

	Present	Absent	Total
Stress ECG +	30	40	70
Stress ECG −	20	410	430
Total	50	450	500

follows:

> Positive predictive value = True positives/Total positives
> or 30/70 = .43

Note how strongly the positive predictive value is affected by prevalence of the problem. In our previous examples where we arbitrarily decided that half of the patients had the target disease, our stress ECG had a positive predictive value of .87. However, if we decrease the disease prevalence to a more realistic level of 10, we find that the positive predictive value of the test decreases also, to just over half of what it was in the previous example. Let us look at what happens to negative predictive value:

> Negative predictive value = True negatives/All negatives
> or 410/430 = .95

Thus, the negative predictive value of the stress test is also strongly affected by change in disease prevalence, only in the opposite direction. Its predictive power improves.

Section 2. Revising probabilities: Bayes theorem

The formula version of Bayes theorem we use in the example reads as follows:

$$p(D/t) = \frac{p(D) \times p(+|D)}{\{p(D) \times p(+|D)\} + \{p(\sim D) \times p(+|\sim D)\}}$$

What does it all mean? First, a brief introduction to the symbols we have used

Symbol	Meaning	Example
p	Probability	$p(A)$ = probability of A
~	Not	$P(\sim A)$ = probability of not A
|	Given	$P(A|B)$ = probability of A given B

Looking first at the equation's numerator:

$p(D|+)$ This is what we are trying to find. For this example, it reads the probability of the diagnosis given a positive test result. Or, what is the probability that Mr. Johnson has CAD given that he has a positive test result? Conceptually it is the same as the positive predictive value, and could be calculated using a 2-by-2 table. In this instance, it is being applied to a specific case rather than a patient population, and we are calculating it using Bayes theorem.

$p(D)$ The probability of the diagnosis. In this case, consider a 70 probability of CAD for Mr. Johnson.

$p(+|D)$ The probability of a positive test result given the diagnosis. We also know that. It is the sensitivity of the test, equal to 0.60 for the stress ECG.

In the denominator of the equation, we repeat the numerator (the probability of disease times the true positive rate) and add the following:

$p(\sim D)$ Probability of no disease, or our subjective probability that Mr. Johnson's chest pain is not the result of coronary artery disease.

$p(+|\sim D)$ Which reads "the probability of a positive test result given no disease" that we determined earlier was the false-positive rate.

How do we determine the appropriate numbers to fill into Bayes theorem for Mr. Johnson?

a. We have settled on a tentative diagnostic probability of coronary artery insufficiency of 0.70 for Mr. Johnson. So, for us, $p(D) = 0.70$

b. We know the sensitivity or true positive rate of the test to be 0.60. $p(+|D) = 0.60$

c. By subtracting, we can establish the probability that Mr. Johnson's pain does not result from CAD: $p(\sim D) = 1\ p(D)$ or, in our case, $1-.70$ or 0.30.

d. Last, we can look back at Table 19.1 and find the false-positive rate of our test to be 22/250 or 0.09. $p(+|\sim D) = 0.09$.

Substituting the numbers in the formula, we obtain the expression:

$$p(D|+) = \frac{0.7 \times 0.6}{(0.7 \times 0.6) + (0.3 \times 0.09)}$$
$$= \frac{0.42}{0.42 + 0.027}$$
$$= 0.94$$

Then using Bayes theorem and starting with a diagnosis to which a probability of 0.70 was assigned (called the prior probability) and knowing the sensitivity and specificity of the stress ECG, we have learned that we can improve our prediction of CAD for this patient from 70 to 94 if the result of the stress test is positive. Another way of saying this is the posterior probability of CAD for this patient is 94. That is a reasonable improvement, and many diagnosticians would probably justify asking the patient to undergo the test.

Section 3. A Firefighter in his 50s with Chest Pain

In sections 1 and 2, we obtain the necessary values for our formula. First, we try to determine the probability that the patient has the disease given a negative test result (or the negative predictive value of the test). To do that, we use a combination of the following elements:

The probability that he does have the disease; [P(D)] which, given the strength of his risk factors, we could set rather high, like at 0.90 (or 90% probability).

The probability of a negative test result given the disease (or the false-negative rate), which in this case is 1 − the sensitivity, or 0.40

The probability that we think the patient does not have the disease, which is 1 − the probability that he does, or 0.10.

The specificity of the test, which we know to be 0.91.

Putting those numbers in our formula, we get the following expression:

$$p(D|-) = \frac{p(D) \times p(-|D)}{\{p(D) \times p(-|D)\} + \{p(\sim D) \times p(-|\sim D)\}}$$

$$= \frac{0.9 \times 0.4}{(0.90 \times 0.4) + (0.1 \times 0.91)}$$

$$= 0.798$$

We see from this illustrative analysis that our physician's intuition was correct. Going through the formalities of probabilistic reasoning for a patient whom we are so sure has a diagnosis of coronary artery disease that we can assign a probability of 90% tells us that a negative stress ECG result only reduces our probability for that diagnosis to just below 80%. In fact, for this patient, we probably did not need the stress test to establish the diagnosis.

several of the unique focuses of family medicine: (a) longitudinal care; (b) care of the individual in the family and social context; and (c) care of multiple generations of the same family. In fact these longitudinal, holistic, patient-oriented aspects of osteopathic family medicine more easily lend it to the application of classic osteopathic principles than possibly any other specialty area of medical practice.

It is in these contexts that this chapter will evaluate osteopathic family medicine. Many of the concepts to be explored are shared by the other osteopathic primary care specialties and as well by nonosteopathically trained family physicians. It is beyond the scope of this chapter to evaluate all components of family practice in detail. Textbooks of family medicine are available for the reader who wishes to pursue this subject in depth (4,5). This chapter is intended to provide a general overview of the nature of family medicine in an osteopathic context and, where appropriate, emphasize those aspects of osteopathic family medicine that are distinctive in contemporary medicine.

THE WHOLE PERSON AND DISEASE

> To find health should be the object of the doctor. Anyone can find disease (2).
> —A.T. Still, *Philosophy of Osteopathy*

A tendency to consider disease the appropriate focus of health care exists in both popular thinking and in the generally used medical model. While some attention is given to "preventive medicine," the focus is on the diagnosis, treatment, and management of disease. It is as if disease were the natural state of human beings. In the general osteopathic model and in osteopathic family medicine the focus is on the development and maintenance of health. In the osteopathic model the normal, balanced, and integrated human organism can generally avoid infection, even though pathogenic organisms colonize the body. A person can avoid most other disease as well, and those illnesses that cannot be avoided often can be recuperated from readily, provided a healthy environment is maintained and stressors are controlled in the context of structural integrity and balance.

Disease, when it occurs, is considered to be a disturbance of the innate dynamic balance of health. Genetic predisposition, inappropriate immune response, dietary insufficiencies or indiscretions, emotional upheavals, familial-social-economic stress, environmental stress, and/or musculoskeletal disturbances can perturb the body's dynamic balance. Many of these factors can coexist. Disease occurs when such perturbations, particularly those of a long-term nature, overwhelm the body's natural compensatory mechanisms.

The body's ability to compensate is such that most individuals maintain what they would characterize as "good health" for most of the time, even in the presence of chronic disease. It is the objective of the physician to restore and maintain the patient's balance of health. The primary care objectives of the osteopathic family physician extend beyond acute episodes and interventions into the longitudinal maintenance of health and stabilization of disease where it cannot be eliminated.

It is clear that most disease has widespread effects. Although it may be convenient to classify a particular disease as being focused in a particular organ, it is rare that a disease does not have effects throughout the body. An obvious example is seen in cardiovascular disease where effects are found from the smallest capillaries to the heart itself, thereby affecting the whole body. A similar example is seen in diabetes where an endocrine disorder has vascular, neural, renal, and immunologic effects.

A less obvious example that will further illustrate this point can be seen in pharyngitis. Typically, pharyngitis produces both local pain in the throat and a more generalized body ache and malaise. These symptoms require both nociceptive neural activation and a general alteration of central and autonomic neural activity. Inflammation arises due to localized and systemic immune activation, with altered macrophage, lymphocyte, and monocyte responses. Fever develops from altered temperature control mechanisms as a method of weakening the invading organism. Fatigue and loss of appetite are mediated by glucose-insulin, glucocorticoid, and tumor necrosis factor activity. Local pharyngeal pain and inflammation is associated with congestion and lymphedema of the pharyngeal and anterior cervical soft tissues. Neural reflex mechanisms mediated through the trigeminal and sympathetic nerves produce viscerosomatic reflexes in the upper cervical and upper thoracic regions (8,9). Similar to this example, based upon the experience of generations of osteopathic physicians, there is local, general, and segmentally related spinal musculoskeletal involvement in virtually all disease.

OSTEOPATHIC DIAGNOSIS AND TREATMENT OF DISEASE

Despite the impressive strides that have been made in the past 60 years, contemporary medical methods of diagnosis and therapeutics remain significantly less than perfect. Modern laboratory studies and noninvasive imaging have significantly improved our ability to diagnose disease. Yet, false positives and equivocal results continue to raise questions as to the correct diagnosis. The best diagnostic tools are often very expensive or the diagnostic alternatives are too diverse for the patient or the health care system to be able to afford all of the tests available. Established traditional methods of history taking and physical examination still provide the best foundation for clinical decision making and often allow the physician to limit the number of additional procedures necessary to attain a diagnosis.

Traditionally, the best treatment plan was based on patterns learned from mentors and/or one's experience with patients. The current move toward what is termed "evidence-based medicine" would appear to be a useful additional tool in as much as it provides some guidance as to what is or is not an effective treatment for a specific disease. On the other hand, even in the face of the most rigorous diagnostic criteria and a treatment plan based on the most rigorous scientifically proven data, patients continue to confound us with their individual variation in response and tolerance to our treatments and their side effects. Therefore experienced family physicians often use multiple strategies. Osteopathic family physicians have a special advantage when using palpatory diagnosis and manipulative treatment.

specialist generally
On the other hanc
tient from birth to
the great mobility
for the osteopathic
the patient, and ye
this can provide a
family physician w
but also with chrc
longitudinal care a
chosocial and med
family and its imm
understanding fam
the family functio

Osteopathic far
variety of minor s
and gynecologic p
preferences will de
perform. Most are
now being termed
joint injections, lc
procedures that cc

Finally, when
it is the primary
end-of-life counse
pathic family phy:
and knows the pa
more natural for
sensitive manner,
subsequent suppo
omy and beliefs.

PREVENTIVE
MAINTENAN(

All diseases and d
anatomic, genetic
discussed in Sectic
cluding sprains, s
from traumatic is
Genetic problems
lifestyle and self-d
influenced behav
ple possibilities fo
maintenance inte
family physicians

As noted previ
ventive medicine
health (4,5). Thi:
concept that dise
compensatory m
ment. This conce
is best effected by
and balance, whil
son's environmer
preventable, mak
role to help patier

THE ROLE OF PALPATORY DIAGNOSIS AND MANIPULATIVE CARE

A basic osteopathic principle states that the neuromusculoskeletal system is functionally and inextricably linked with all body systems. A corollary of this concept is the explicit statement that disease and musculoskeletal dysfunction are also inextricably linked. This is the fundamental principle behind somatic dysfunction. Somatic dysfunction is functional impairment with its primary manifestation in the neuromusculoskeletal and fascial systems. Although somatic dysfunction may exist in the presence of pathology, it is not in itself pathology. As noted in Section II, the basic science section of this text, somatic dysfunction has the potential for negatively affecting both the immune and endocrine systems as well.

When treating a patient with any health problem, one can determine how to integrate the treatment of somatic dysfunction into the therapeutic protocol by asking the following questions:

1. How is musculoskeletal dysfunction affecting the ability of the person to function? Whether one is dealing with activity restrictions as the result of pain or gait and other body use disturbances, this is the most obvious manifestation of somatic dysfunction and the one that becomes the occasion for almost universal musculoskeletal treatment by osteopathic physicians.

2. How are musculoskeletal and fascial dysfunctions affecting the patient's ability to respond to disease processes? The mechanical component of somatic dysfunction results in restriction of motion. The compromising effect of thoracic cage somatic dysfunction upon the patient with chronic obstructive pulmonary disease is an example.

3. How is circulatory stasis affecting the patient? Efficient movement of the thoracic inlet, thoracic cage, abdominal diaphragm, mesenteries, and pelvic diaphragm is necessary for optimal low-pressure fluid (lymphatic and venous) dynamics and tissue perfusion. Inefficiency of this mechanism further adds to the tendency for tissue congestion. Somatic dysfunction of the extremities can compromise arterial, venous, and lymphatic flow.

4. What sympathetic somatovisceral mechanisms are present? Spinal facilitation associated with thoracic and upper lumbar somatic dysfunction results in increased sympathetic tone to segmentally related structures.

5. What parasympathetic somatovisceral mechanisms are present? Spinal facilitation associated with high cervical and sacral somatic dysfunction results in increased parasympathetic tone to segmentally related structures.

6. What organ level dysfunctions are manifesting in musculoskeletal and fascial restrictions and tissue texture changes?

The first three questions address predominantly the mechanical effect of somatic dysfunction upon the patient. The fourth and fifth questions deal with the impact of somatovisceral reflexes upon the patient. The sixth question relates to what have been termed the viscerosomatic reflexes.

Each of the first five questions focuses on direct effects of primary somatic dysfunction on the general functional level of the individual. Each represents part of the most obvious clinical manifestation of the effects of the musculoskeletal system on the function of the body as a whole. All five of these questions are

considered valid reasons for treating the musculoskeletal system. While it may be tempting to restrict musculoskeletal treatment to only those manifestations oriented around the first question, the other four are equally valid.

Thus OMT is indicated for the specific treatment of the neuromusculoskeletal manifestations of somatic dysfunction. OMT is used to increase available motion, modify activity of the nervous system, and increase tissue perfusion. The experience of the osteopathic profession is that OMT is often sufficient for recovery from a variety of conditions, including many that are not specifically musculoskeletal in nature. Part of this effect is undoubtedly due to the interactive effects of the musculoskeletal system on the fascia, circulation, and the autonomic nervous system. Diseases are often the result of structural disorders relating to both the viscera and the somatic system. In current terms, there is close interleaving of visceral, autonomic, neural, immunologic, and musculoskeletal systems (see Chapters 7, 9, 10, and 13). As first propounded by A.T. Still with the founding of the profession, the key to restoration of health is to enable the body's own restorative mechanisms (2,3). For example, based on the experience of the osteopathic community in the 1918 influenza epidemic (10), and on the general experience of osteopathic physicians over the past 100 years, OMT should have some added benefit in the recovery from at least some viral illnesses (11–18). However, it should be noted that formal outcome studies supporting the use of OMT in the treatment of nonmusculoskeletal disease is sparse (13–22).

Finally there is the viscerosomatic relationship between dysfunctions in the viscerae and the musculoskeletal system. Palpatory evaluation of viscerosomatic reflexes has been used as a diagnostic tool by the osteopathic profession for at least a century. As demonstrated both clinically and in the laboratory (8,12,13–32), viscerosomatic reflexes are present with a wide variety of disease. They develop in response to visceral pathology. Although there is considerable overlap in the presentation of these reflexes for various viscera, they can help the osteopathic physician distinguish between various potential diagnoses (Table 1). Viscerosomatic reflexes are identifiable as tissue texture abnormality and tenderness in the dermatomes and myotomes that are embryologically and neurologically related to the viscera that stimulate them. They are most easily palpable in the paravertebral soft tissues. A pure viscerosomatic reflex, without concomitant mechanical spinal somatic dysfunction, generally will demonstrate tissue texture abnormality and tenderness proportionate to the degree of visceral pathology in the absence of definitive restriction of motion. The tissue texture abnormality may or may not demonstrate left/right asymmetry, but there will not be vertebral positional asymmetry.

One of the dilemmas of osteopathic musculoskeletal medicine is the differentiation between a viscerosomatic reflex and primary somatic dysfunction. Johnston and Golden, however, have recently suggested that there are significant differences in the patterns that can help distinguish the two (33). Viscerosomatic reflexes, like primary somatic dysfunction, cause muscle spasm, tissue tenderness, and pain. For instance, the pudendal nerve (S2-4), a branch of the pelvic splanchnic nerves, innervates the pelvic diaphragm. Pain in the pelvic floor may be viscerosomatic (pelvic parasympathetic) in origin, or it may simply be the result

bronchitis, as we
lymphatic funct
see also Chapter
tunity for the p
to stop smokin
and that of his
lead to a diagno
long-term impl

These three
erational care, ;
aspects of disea
term restoratio
cian must ofte
and social expc
of the care proj
times religious
the physician.

**PHARMAC(
OSTEOPATI**

Early in its h
drugs. At tha
of toxic, ineff
calomel, mor
credit, Dr. Sti
His own exp
the day convi
teopathy was
that restoratic
ance would p
ery from dise
could resort
included app
tion, and phy

During th
attitude amc
peutics shifte
ing and medi
tics was bein
pharmacolog
offered in th

Today, m
ican osteopa
limitations
in the case
drugs to inc
from both
pathic fami
moves struc
normal abil
ications wh

Much of
21st centur
the sympto
pathologic
symptoms (

eye that cannot completely close and a smooth forehead. There is often an associated CN VI palsy with lateral rectus weakness and nystagmus. Nerve entrapments like these can be treated with cranial OMT (22–25). Residual dysfunctions can have serious consequences in relation to neurobehavioral development.

Sphenobasilar lateral strain patterns produce the appearance of a "parallelogram"-shaped head. Sphenobasilar and intracranial membranous strains can cause abnormal tension on the tentorium cerebelli. Cranial somatic dysfunction affecting CN III, CN IV, and CN VI is thought to play a role in disorders of abnormal position and movement of the eye. Cranial OMT has been noted empirically to facilitate restoration of normal eye position and movement (21,22). Some strain patterns are believed to affect brainstem functions and respiratory drive. Apnea and bradycardia can be manifestations of these somatic dysfunctions (22). Cranial strain patterns in children do not necessarily manifest as neurologic deficits. Patients may be asymptomatic or have generalized complaints, ranging from allergies to severe head pain. The most common presentation is the child with chronic or recurrent upper respiratory tract disorders (discussed later in this chapter).

Research into the effects of cranial somatic dysfunction is in its infancy. Though there are as yet no prospective randomized clinical trials investigating this clinically apparent relationship, expert panels of osteopathic physicians recommend that cranial somatic dysfunction in the neonate or infant, whether symptomatic or asymptomatic, warrants OMT (26).

Treatment of cranial traumatic birth injuries involves rib raising at delivery to calm the sympathetic nervous system and improve efficiency of breathing and body fluid movement, O-A and condylar decompression, sacral traction, and affected cranial bone decompression. Treatment involves releasing the restrictions as soon as the infant is physiologically stable. The sacrum is treated with gentle traction and can facilitate release of intracranial membranous strain patterns. The O-A and condylar parts are decompressed with gentle posterolateral traction. Treatment of each restriction involves gentle, but firm direct action OMT that involves distracting and guiding the cranial bones into their respective restrictive motion barriers and maintaining them in that position until a release is felt. This requires very little force.

Costal Cage

Costal cage somatic dysfunction may be the result of a direct traumatic force to the area or an indirect result of muscle imbalance or spasm secondary to a nonrhythmic breathing mechanism. The history may reveal asthma or chronic cough, but particularly, an episode of severe coughing or wheezing related to this incident is most common. In normal breathing, air movement is accomplished by unrestricted movement and mobility of the diaphragm. The coordinated contraction of the diaphragm is mediated via the phrenic nerve and nerve fibers that exit from the midcervical area (C3-5). Thus, cervical or thoracic somatic dysfunction can predispose to rib dysfunction.

It is rare for children to sustain rib fractures since their ribs are flexible and well calcified with good cartilaginous articulations. Infants with posterior rib fractures should always be suspected of having suffered abuse. Fractured ribs have nodular calcified areas at the costotransverse articulation adjacent to the spinal column. Radiographically, the fractures are often at various stages of calcification. Posterior rib fractures are the result of the infant being held and shaken. The cartilage absorbs the force anteriorly, but posteriorly the ribs have bony articulations with the transverse processes and are relatively inflexible. Such infants present with severe to moderate pain with breathing. They have tenderness and fullness over the affected rib that becomes worse with either inhalation or exhalation. The upper ribs are best palpated anteriorly and the lower ones are best palpated in the midaxillary regions. There are usually associated thoracic segmental somatic dysfunctions that need to be treated.

Children with cystic fibrosis or α-1-antitrypsin deficiency are at the greatest risk for rib somatic dysfunction. These children present with severe chest pain that is worse with inhalation. Children and adolescents with scoliosis and asthma are predisposed to developing rib somatic dysfunctions as well. These children should be screened and treated after a thorough structural examination at each visit. First, the physician should relieve muscle spasm with inhibition, counterstrain, or muscle energy OMT. Next, the segment/rib is treated with indirect OMT. The physician monitors the rib movement while the child takes a deep breath, then moves the rib further into the direction of ease of movement. Attempting direct positioning often elicits guarding due to aggravation of the intercostal muscle spasms. High velocity/low amplitude (HVLA) is a useful technique with the patient supine or sitting. The child will immediately be able to breathe without pain, although some residual tenderness to palpation will remain. The physician must remember to also relieve any associated diaphragm motion restrictions.

Vertebral Spine

Torticollis ("wry neck") can present shortly after birth or at any time during childhood. It is defined as shortening or contracture of the SCM on one side with the head tilted toward and rotated away from that side. There may be irritation of the spinal accessory nerve (CN XI) from somatic dysfunction of the cranial base affecting the jugular foramen and its contents. In congenital cases, the SCM becomes shortened and ropy. In acute cases, a lymph node may be irritating the SCM or trauma has occurred that results in SCM spasm. In acute torticollis, the SCM is exquisitely tender. The differential diagnosis includes a cervical dislocation of the vertebra or spinal cord tumor which would have other structural and neurologic findings including sensory deficits. In chronic torticollis, there is often a pattern of long-standing O-A dysfunction with a cranial lateral and possibly vertical strain patterns. These are the result of abnormal intrauterine positioning or an abnormal birth event/position. There may be a history of a shoulder dystocia at birth. The differential diagnosis of chronic torticollis includes a cervical malformation or Klippel-Feil anomaly.

The best treatment outcomes are obtained by addressing the underlying cranial and cervical somatic dysfunction. These children respond to indirect, followed by direct, action OMT procedures. The physician should begin with inhibition of tender points via counterstrain and indirect techniques. This requires good communication and a level of understanding that, unfortunately, many children have not yet achieved. In these cases, the techniques must be modified so that the area is positioned until a tense fascial area of palpation softens. Indirect muscle energy techniques (reciprocal inhibition) can also be helpful. In some cases, the use of antiinflammatory medication and muscle relaxants may be necessary, with the child returning in 24 to 48 hours for definitive OMT. Muscle energy, with infants and children, works well and can be devised like a game. Addressing other related vertebral and sacral dysfunctions is often necessary as well. The physician can teach parents techniques to stretch the SCM and the child is seen and treated on several visits over a period of weeks.

Scoliosis is most often first diagnosed in childhood. It can show up in the neonatal period but is rare. Congenital scoliosis is caused by anomalies of the spine involving fusion or abnormal development of the spine. These infants may have other organ involvement.

Scoliosis seen in childhood is defined as an abnormal curvature of the spine in the coronal and sagittal planes. It is categorized as structural or nonstructural. The structural curves have an axial rotation on forward bending. Definitive diagnosis is by standing postural radiographs. Nonstructural scoliosis is the result of poor posture, muscle spasms, or a short leg. In the instance of structural curves, the spinous process rotates toward the concavity and is seen as a prominence of either the ribs or paraspinal muscles on that side with forward bending. The etiology of most abnormal spinal curves is idiopathic. Patients must be managed with careful observation, sequential radiographs, balanced muscle strengthening/fascial mobilization, and bracing.

Many curves classified as idiopathic are actually secondary to "short leg syndrome." These children present with scoliosis, chronic lumbar or sacral somatic dysfunction, and/or hip pain. Standing postural radiographs show unequal iliac crest heights and sacral base and femoral head heights that are not level. The lumbar convexity is toward the short leg side often with a compensatory curve in the opposite thoracic side. Correction of the short leg with a heel or sole lift (orthotic device) along with OMT, leads to improvement or alleviation of the scoliosis.

Lumbosacral somatic dysfunction is often symptomatic if induced from a fall or hyperextension injury. It can be the result of "overuse" with a preexisting structural problem, such as a short leg, scoliosis, or spondylolysis/spondylolisthesis. Patients present with pain in the low back or hip. They complain of pain with forward bending and experience a "catch" in their low back or hip. Palpatory findings include L5-S1 side-bending somatic dysfunction associated with a sacral rotation or shear. Children with lumbosacral dysfunction will have a positive standing flexion test on the affected side. When neurologic findings are present, radiographs should be taken and must include oblique lumbar views. When the x-ray results are available and normal, treatment is begun and directed toward relieving the acute problem. Initial relaxation of muscle spasm using counterstrain, soft-tissue relaxation, trigger-point inhibition. and muscle energy will allow definitive treatment.

Physiological sacral nutation (anterior movement of the sacral base) occurs along a transverse axis at S2. The sacrum may engage a restriction with rotation around an axis or shear. The sacrum undergoes nutation, then counternutation during the birthing process. There is a torsion component as well, since the occiput presents anterior or posterior and undergoes rotation in the birthing process. When the toddler sits and then ambulates, the sacrum assumes the normal position. Toddlers have an accentuated lumbar lordosis due to inadequate abdominal musculature. This induces bilateral sacral nutation. As growth and develop-

ment continue into adolescence, the sacrum undergoes unusual stresses secondary to rapid phases of growth and physical activities. Lumbar dysfunction and restriction of motion of the ilium affect sacral motion. Conversely, there is often an iliac rotation to compensate for the sacral imbalance. This is corrected using muscle energy and positioning. Sacral and lumbar somatic dysfunctions respond well to both direct and indirect OMT procedures. An associated pubic shear may be present that can be treated using muscle energy technique. When the child has recurrent problems, exercises and stretching can help. Unequal leg lengths also affect sacral mechanics. Consider a lift for the short leg in the older adolescent to prevent sacral somatic dysfunction from recurring.

Upper Extremity

Shoulder dystocia and fractured clavicles from a traumatic birth are common in the newborn period. Motion testing will reveal crepitance, with palpation over the clavicle. There may be an associated brachial (Erb) palsy with the arm lying extended by the side and hand internally rotated. This is the result of injury to C5-6 nerve roots. A rarer injury occurs to C7-8 and T1 nerve roots. These infants will have additional paralysis of the hand and ipsilateral ptosis and miosis. Prognosis is better if the upper arm is involved and, unless the nerves are severed, 90% resolve spontaneously within the first year. These are treated with gentle handling, avoidance of placing the infant on the fractured side, and splinting the hand in physiologic position when the lower arm is affected. Indirect manipulation of spinal somatic dysfunction may help, but direct HVLA should be avoided.

Children are at increased risk of injury of their extremities secondary to increased range of motion of joints, growth plates, participation in competitive activities and, due to their immaturity, relative inability to make safe decisions. Because the child's long bones are in the process of mineralization during this highly competitive period, they may suffer from overuse injuries.

Shoulder injuries include strains of the rotator cuff, clavicle fractures, and acromioclavicular separation or strain. Rotator cuff injuries involve overuse tendonitis or forces of torque on the forearm. These may occur to such an extent that an avulsion fracture occurs at the tendon insertion site. The child presents with pain and aching with rotation of the arm, particularly when the forearm is bent 90 degrees at the elbow. Acromioclavicular and clavicle fractures result from blunt injuries to the lateral aspect of the shoulder. Rotator cuff and acromioclavicular injuries are treated with counterstrain, ice, and nonsteroidal antiinflammatory medication.

Physicians must remember to consider underlying visceral disease in patients with persistent shoulder pain, pain unexplained by the structural findings, or in those patients who do not respond to treatment. Referred pain to the right shoulder occurs with gallbladder disease. Duodenal inflammation refers pain to the left shoulder. Tender points found over the anterior shoulder could be a manifestation of Chapman reflexes from upper respiratory tract infections and can be treated with inhibition.

Clavicle fractures are diagnosed with a defect to the lateral aspect of the clavicle, with palpable crepitance upon elevation of the shoulder. These fractures are treated initially with immobilization in a clavicle restraint, then after 3 to 4 weeks, range of motion (Spencer technique) and counterstrain. Children rarely function and maximize circulation to the joints. Keeping lymph flow going via lymphatic pumps, and gentle joint pumping, will maximize the circulation of nutrients to the joints and the removal of waste. Balancing the sympathetics and parasympathetics via CV4 and rib raising will ensure good circulation to the joints and the synovial membranes that are already inflamed. HVLA should be avoided since the joints are inflamed, but muscle energy and the use of indirect or counterstrain work well and are tolerated. Maintaining range of motion to T2-8 and T10-L2 will help reduce associated visceral symptoms from facilitated segments associated with upper and lower extremity involvement. Diaphragm mobility and removal of restrictions at the O-A junction will optimize fluid mobilization. Remember that ankylosing spondylitis can be associated with joint pain and is experienced as pain in the sacroiliac joint, hip, and back. The inflammation of the spine over time results in a rigid spine and starts in the lumbar spine and works its way up. This is opposite of JRA, which starts in the cervical spine. Treatment includes OMT to maintain range of motion, good posture, and maximizing circulation of nutrients to and removal of wastes from the joint spaces. Untreated, the spine becomes stiff and immobile with loss of the normal curves. OMT can help to maintain segmental mobility but should be gentle. Indirect muscle energy and counterstrain techniques are most helpful.

Children with JRA should be encouraged to maintain activities including non–weight-bearing activities such as swimming. Pain can be relieved by treatment of trigger points with inhibition and positioning. Special attention should be given to relieving any fascial restrictions to promote maximum range of motion and circulation. Daily CV4 cranial technique has been helpful in controlling symptoms.

RESPIRATORY SYSTEMIC DYSFUNCTION

Mechanics of Pediatric Respiratory System

An infant or small child is not a miniature adult in respiratory terms. The upper airway and nose account for the majority of airway resistance in adults. In children younger than 5, the lower airway resistance is 2.5 times greater, accounting for the greater threat to infants and young children from viral infections of the lower airway.

Infant tissues are softer and the tissue planes are looser and more compressible than those in the adult. An infant with difficulty breathing may recruit accessory muscles of the neck, thoracic cage, and abdomen to aid breathing. The increase in force may cause airway collapse. Changes in airway resistance play a major role in pediatric pulmonary diseases such as asthma, pneumonia, and bronchiolitis. Because the muscles in the small airways are incompletely developed during the first years of life, young infants may be less responsive to bronchodilator therapy. Their sympathetic nervous system is well developed however, and they respond well to rib-raising techniques.

The genioglossus muscle is innervated by the hypoglossal nerve and is the principal muscle maintaining the patency of the upper airway. It pulls the base of the tongue and hyoid bone anterior when it contracts, dilating the upper airway and opposing the negative pressure exerted by the diaphragm. Suppression

of upper-airway muscle activity may occur with sleep or severe esophageal reflux. Compared to adults, the thoracic volume of a child is small due to short, narrow airways. Therefore, mucosal edema profoundly decreases the radius of the airway and increases the resistance.

The cartilaginous ribs of the infant and young child are twice as compliant as the bony ribs of the older child or adult. Infants' ribs are oriented in a more horizontal direction than those in adults because they articulate linearly with the spinal column and sternum. There is anterior-posterior displacement during inspiration. The intercostal muscles primarily stabilize the chest wall in the first years of life because they do not have the leverage to lift and expand the ribs. Therefore, though the diaphragm is the chief muscle of respiration in all patients, it is especially important in the child for its role in generating changes in tidal volume. The diaphragm muscle fibers insert horizontally on the inner surfaces of the ribs in the infant instead of obliquely as in the adult. Ideally, breathing, vigorous crying, and nursing re-expand the overlapping cranial bones. If this does not occur as nature planned, freeing any restrictions in the newborn's body helps establish optimal respiration. An infant who suffers more severe birth trauma, or other insult, may not have the vitality to self-correct.

Newborn Diaphragm Dysfunction

A restriction or twist in the thoracic diaphragm, which can be caused by the rotation of the baby passing through the birth canal or by *in utero* positioning may also cause problems. Respiration may be irregular and the infant may be irritable or prone to the hiccups. For example, a twin who was in a transverse lie throughout pregnancy continued to have irregular breathing and grunting in his 3rd month of life. In addition, he was quite irritable and never smiled. Examination showed a twist through the thoracolumbar area and thoracic diaphragm. He also had marked lumbosacral compression, restricted temporal bones, and an O-A compression. Though he was born via cesarean section, the tight quarters of the uterus shared with his brother caused marked compression throughout his body. As he was treated and his diaphragm released, he began to visibly relax. His breathing became more regular and within a week he began to smile. His parents were thrilled to have a happier, more relaxed baby.

Newborn Temporal Bone Somatic Dysfunction

At birth, the neonate's first breath must overcome the resistance of the lungs and the surface tension of the fluid in the lungs. The first forceful contraction of the inspiratory muscles must be deep and accompanied by large transpulmonary pressures to overcome the surface and viscous forces. If the neonate has suffered trauma, infection, or the effects of drugs, the first breath may not contain the force needed to establish effective respiration. Infants with respiratory difficulties have a higher incidence of temporal bones that are not moving in a symmetric, physiologic pattern. This type of strain may most commonly result from unilateral compression of the condylar parts, or the occipital-mastoid area or the frontal-sphenoid area. When the temporal bones have restricted or asymmetric motion, the newborn or infant may have poor respiratory effort or uneven respiration. This may occur when the sphenobasilar symphysis is compressed due to birth trauma as is seen in cephalopelvic disproportion. Release of restricted temporal bones and condylar decompression can aid the development of quiet, easy respiration, emphasizing once again the importance of structure and function.

Osteopathic Approach to the Pediatric Patient with Respiratory Tract Infections

An injury, lack of sleep, poor nutrition, and/or social stress can predispose a child to be more susceptible to viral infections. Symptoms often start with activation of the immune system. In the upper respiratory tract, there would be signs of erythema, fever, or cough, signaling an immune response to a presumed infection and can also include wheezing, rales, retractions of accessory muscles of respiration, nasal flaring, and an increased respiratory rate. Treatment may include OMT, a variety of pharmacologic agents, fluids, and in the case of airway swelling, home treatment with warm steam for about 10 minutes, cool outside air, and oxygen mist, if hospitalized.

Otitis Media

Otitis media is the most common reason for a child to visit a pediatrician in the first 5 years of life. It is the most prevalent disease after respiratory illness in children, affecting nearly 20% of all infants in the United States. It is responsible for nearly 30 million physician visits per year.

Acute otitis media is characterized by the sudden onset of inflammation of the middle ear, which is accompanied by fever, pain, and irritability. There is a loss of anatomic landmarks, erythema, and bulging of the tympanic membrane.

Chronic otitis media with effusion is a chronic inflammation of the inner ear that persists for 3 or more months. In this condition, the middle ear may be frequently retracted or concave and the child may present without signs of acute infection.

Since the early 1950s, the mainstay of medical treatment of middle ear infections has been antimicrobial therapy. Although antimicrobial therapy is shown to be about 20% more effective than placebo, studies show that once therapy is initiated the likelihood of reinfection is high. Bacterial organisms most commonly involved in otitis media infection include *Streptococcus pneumoniae, Haemophilus influenza,* and *Moraxella catarrhalis.* However, these organisms are rarely cultured from the middle ear even in acute infections. Pathogenic bacteria can be cultured from the middle ear in only 11% to 22% of children presenting with acute infection. Viral etiology may play a role and is found in about 20% of symptomatic children. Thus, it is important to remember that any infection is a result of a combination of influences: degree of virulence and quantity of an infecting agent, along with host susceptibility. The osteopathic approach favors measures that improve host resistance and recovery concurrent with weakening, or eradicating the infecting agent.

Allergens also seem to be important in both chronic and acute infection. It has long been known that exposure to tobacco smoke, wood-burning stoves, and airborne allergies are associated with increased frequency of otitis media. However, in recent years, food allergies have also been implicated. The most prevalent of these are allergies to dairy, wheat, and egg white.

Regardless of the source, nearly all authorities on the subject refer to the key role the eustachian tube plays in the development of otitis media. The eustachian tube is a short canal found on the lateral wall of the pharynx connecting the middle ear to the nasopharynx. Like the respiratory tract, it is lined with ciliated epithelial cells. These cells function to move secretions from the middle ear to the nasopharynx. The tube also functions to equilibrate middle ear pressure with atmospheric pressure. The child who is less than 3 years of age has a relatively short eustachian tube and it is prone to collapse, especially during swallowing. At birth to about 3 to 4 years of age, the eustachian tube has a horizontal orientation. This changes to a more downward slant in children over the age of 4 and accounts for the dramatic decreased incidence of otitis media after this stage of development.

When one approaches otitis media from a structural point of view, it is clear that any structure placing tension on the eustachian tube will increase the likelihood of obstruction. Certainly hypertonicity of the posterior pharyngeal muscles, especially the medial pterygoid, the digastric muscles, and dysfunction of the hyoid bone, may play an important role in eustachian dysfunction. Yawning, sucking, and swallowing aid the eustachian tube in equilibrating atmospheric pressure with middle ear pressure. However, uncoordinated, inefficient sucking and swallowing may worsen eustachian tube dysfunction and cause reflux. Irritation of the glossopharyngeal (CN IX) and the hypoglossal (CN XII) nerves resulting from compression of the jugular foramen and hypoglossal canal are the most common osteopathic findings associated with sucking and swallowing difficulty.

This may also be yet another benefit of breast-feeding. It is well known that infants who are breast-fed have a much lower incidence of otitis media. The immunologic makeup of breast milk certainly plays a major role. However, the actual sucking process itself may also be involved. Infants who are breast-fed use an entirely separate muscular sequence compared to those who are bottle-fed. Breast-fed infants tend not to tongue thrust and therefore widen the arch of the hard palate. Bottle-fed infants, on the other end, tend to tongue thrust, pushing the rigid bottle nipple superiorly which results in a narrow hard palate reducing the relative space between the eustachian tube and the adenoids in the fossa of Rosenmüller. This predisposes the eustachian tube to reflux and obstruction. The use of pacifiers and chronic thumb sucking essentially causes the same process and may account for the increased rate of otitis media reported in these children.

Perhaps the most common structural finding in children with otitis media, however, is the association with impaired mobility of the petrous portion of the temporal bone. Prior to birth, the temporal bone is in three developmental parts, each of which moves physiologically relative to the others. The petromastoid portion, which develops in the cartilaginous cranial base, contains the structures of the middle and inner ear. The squamous portion, developing in membrane, forms a large part of the lateral wall of the skull. The tympanic portion, resembling a tiny horseshoe applied laterally to the petromastoid-squamosal junction, progressively develops after birth into the external auditory canal.

In the healthy child the temporal bones have a slight internal and external rotation movement, about 8 to 14 times per minute. This physiologic motion aids in mucociliary transport and drainage of the middle ear. If this motion is impeded, then drainage of the middle ear will be impaired. The resulting fluid stasis may result in middle ear fluid accumulation and inflammation. When the temporal bone is internally rotated and its motion is restricted from moving into external rotation, eustachian tube blockage can occur. This can be further complicated by a hypertonic sternocleidomastoid muscle (SCM), which will pull the petrous portion of the temporal bone into internal rotation and prevent its motion into external rotation. A primary cause of such a restriction is direct trauma to the temporal bone from birth trauma or from a blow to the head. Birth trauma resulting in cranial somatic dysfunction predisposes the infant to otitis media.

Hypertonicity of the SCM may also result from direct trauma, impaired mobility secondary to impaired diaphragmatic respiration, or hyperirritability of the spinal accessory nerve. The spinal accessory nerve exits though the jugular foramen at the base of the occiput. As has previously been discussed, this area is a common area of birth trauma.

The goal of OMT is to obtain unimpeded physiologic motion of the temporal bones, diaphragm, and lymphatic system along with a coordinated, efficient swallowing cycle that allows appropriate drainage of middle ear fluid through the eustachian tube. OMT addresses somatic dysfunction found in the surrounding myofascial structures including the medial and lateral pterygoid muscles, the digastric muscles, and the SCM on the side of the dysfunction. The O-A area should be addressed and any specific cranial strain patterns should be ameliorated. Several specific treatments can be used to address temporal bone motion dysfunction.

Pharyngitis

Pharyngitis is one of the most common complaints of children, representing about 5% of all pediatric visits. These children may present with inflammation of the pharynx, adenoids, and tonsils. The lymphoid ring in the posterior pharynx, known as the Waldeyer ring, serve as a defense against infections of the mouth and throat.

The most common cause of pharyngitis is susceptibility to a viral pathogen, primarily rhinovirus. Adenovirus, which often additionally presents with rhinitis and a posterior cervical lymph node, is another common virus.

Less commonly, bacterial etiology is an infectious agent, accounting for less than 15% of cases. Group A β-hemolytic *Streptococcus* is the most common bacterial pathogen. The tonsils may be covered with an exudate and the child may present with high fever, strawberry tongue, and scarlatiniform rash. If a bacterial pathogen is suspected, a culture and rapid antigen test should be obtained. Culture-positive disease requires antibiotic treatment to prevent rheumatic fever. Therapy must be initiated within 9 days of the start of the symptoms. Therapy, however, does not decrease incidence of poststreptococcal glomerulonephritis.

Structurally, there is inflammation of the posterior pharyngeal muscles. The hyoid may be markedly restricted in motion on one side. There may be cervical lymphadenopathy and posterior cervical somatic dysfunction. The medial pterygoid may be hypertonic. The child may have a narrow arched palate, which may be related to pacifier use, chronic thumb sucking, and mouth breathing.

Restriction in the physiologic motion of the clavicles, thoracic outlet, and diaphragm may result in decreased lymphatic drainage. This may be accompanied on the side of the dysfunction by hypertonicity of the SCM and elevation of the first rib.

Treatment. It is important to increase fluids, and a wholesome diet free of processed, mucous-forming foods, especially dairy and sugar, should be encouraged. The underlying structural issues must be addressed. The clavicle and first ribs should be free in their motion and the diaphragm should be released if restricted. Somatic dysfunction of the anterior cervical fascia, the medial pterygoid muscles, and the hyoid bone should also be addressed. Last, techniques to enhance to the body's own inherent immunity should be used. This may include lymphatic and splenic pump, compression of the fourth ventricle, and lymphatic drainage techniques. Anterior cervical fascial release and muscle energy techniques can be very beneficial.

OMT can be helpful in the resolution of pharyngitis. A simple, noninvasive manual procedure is anterior cervical fascia stretching as outlined below:

- The patient lays supine.
- The hands are placed beneath the cervical spine while the thumbs are gently introduced posterior to the SCM between the anterior fascial planes.
- Extremely gentle stretching of the soft tissue is performed until free motion is restored to the area.

Muscle energy OMT can be used to release tense pharyngeal musculature as follows:

- The child is in a sitting position.
- The cornu of the hyoid bone is held by the thumb and index finger, while the opposite hand stabilizes the cervical spine.
- The hyoid is grasped and moved to the right side and the left side, away from the midline.
- The hyoid is then held away from the midline on the side of greatest ease, while the child swallows several times.
- The procedure is then repeated on the opposite side.
- This results in relaxation of the pharyngeal musculature and often provides significant relief from pain.

Croup

OMT is a great help in alleviating symptoms in children suffering from an illness such as croup. Physicians who are skilled with their hands can hasten comfort and recovery in mild croup and often eliminate the need for hospitalization in moderate to moderately severe croup. Croup (acute laryngotracheal bronchitis) is common in young children and results from a viral infection of the subglottic area of the upper airway that causes acute inflammation and edema. Because a child's airway is small and the cartilage of the trachea soft, upper airway narrowing during inspiration occurs more often in children than adults. The narrowest segment of a child's airway is the solid cricoid cartilage in the subglottic region, the origin of the characteristic hacking cough and often a hoarse voice. If there is a greater degree of airway obstruction, children may have inspiratory stridor and respiratory distress. Occasionally, respiratory distress is so severe that endotracheal intubation is needed.

Accurate diagnosis from history and physical examination is the first step. Croup is a viral illness that must be differentiated from several more serious bacterial infections such as bacterial tracheitis, acute epiglottis (supraglottis), and retropharyngeal abscess.

Osteopathic treatment of children with croup is directed at supporting normal physiologic processes and counteracting deleterious pathophysiologic processes. Because of the inflammation and the edema, stimulating the sympathetic nervous system will help. In contrast to the airway edema found in asthma due to bronchoconstriction, in croup, it is the vasodilation. Vigorous stimulation of the sympathetic chain ganglia in the upper thoracic region will aid vasoconstriction.

Drug therapy follows a similar approach. Nebulized epinephrine rapidly ameliorates moderate to severe symptoms, but because its effects last only 1 to 2 hours, it is usually only used when a child is admitted to the hospital.

Bronchiolitis

Bronchiolitis is an acute viral infection of the lower respiratory tract in children up to age 2. It can cause mild to severe respiratory distress. The organism invades the epithelial cells of the bronchioles causing sloughing of the cells, edema, and increased mucus. Narrowing and overdistention of the small airways, uneven air trapping, and the mismatching of ventilation and blood flow (ventilation perfusion mismatch) can lead to hypoxemia. The diagnosis is based on clinical presentation, age of the child, and the time of year (28).

The incidence of bronchiolitis increases in winter and spring and can be caused by a number of viruses. The most common cause is respiratory syncytial virus (29). Other viruses include parainfluenza, adenovirus, rhinoviruses, influenza viruses, and *Mycoplasma*. Some symptoms may be more prominent depending on the viral cause. Each virus can cause different signs of dysfunction. For instance, rhinovirus can cause much nasal congestion. With influenza virus, cough, diarrhea, and myalgias may be more prominent symptoms. Adenovirus may cause erythema and congestion in the pharynx. *Mycoplasma* can cause bullous myringitis (air behind the tympanic membrane).

In children under 5 years, lower airway resistance is 2.5 times greater than in adults. These changes in airway resistance make bronchiolitis a challenge in the young infant. In addition, the muscles in the small airways in very young infants and children may not be developed enough to make bronchodilator therapy helpful. However the sympathetic nervous system is well developed, making osteopathic techniques, such as rib raising, effective. As the heads of the ribs are raised, it is postulated that the thoracic sympathetic chain ganglia are stimulated. In T1-6 this stimulates efferent activity to the airways, which includes the release of epinephrine. Along the same lines, nebulized epinephrine has been found in some studies to be helpful in infants hospitalized with bronchiolitis (30). In a child not needing hospitalization, stimulating the body's own supply of epinephrine avoids the possible rebound effect of the drug epinephrine. How long this effect lasts depends on the severity of the illness and the effectiveness of the physician performing OMT.

In using OMT to enhance effective physiology in any condition, one must treat the physical findings of that particular patient. Somatic areas important to assess for somatic dysfunction and treat with OMT in patients with bronchiolitis include:

1. *Cervical region:* The phrenic nerve (C3, C4, C5) provides motor innervation to the thoracic diaphragm. Parasympathetic innervation to the vagus nerve can be addressed at the O-A and atlantal-axial (A-A) junction. Techniques include O-A decompression and myofascial release.

2. *Rib cage:* The work of breathing can be reduced by assuring that the thoracic cage has free motion. Optimizing rib cage motion will facilitate blood flow to and from lungs as well as enhance lymphatic drainage, improve immune response, and prevent accumulated bronchial secretions. Techniques include rib raising, scapula release, intercostal fascial release, thoracic diaphragm release, and clavicular release. Rib raising in an infant or small child can be done by encircling the rib cage with both hands; the fingerpads are placed bilaterally on the posterior-inferior rib angles. Lateral and cephalad traction are applied. Be sure to note that the ribs are more horizontal in children than in adults.

3. *Sympathetic nervous system:* The sympathetic nervous system can be addressed at the costovertebral junction. Rib raising initially stimulates sympathetic outflow, but ultimately will reduce sympathetic outflow.

4. *Thoracic diaphragm:* Free diaphragm motion is important in generating changes in tidal volume. Note the more horizontal insertions in infants. A seated or prone diaphragm release can be used in infants and small children. The posterior crural attachments can be treated with lateral traction of the heads of ribs 11 and 12.

5. *Sacrum:* Free motion is essential for efficient functioning of the respiratory system because of the dural tube which attaches at the foramen magnum, C2, and second sacral segment. In an infant or small child the sacrum can be gently decompressed; the physician places two fingers under the sacrum and uses caudal traction.

6. *Temporal bones:* Respiration is influenced through the tentorium cerebelli attaching to the petrous portion of the temporal bones. If the temporal bones are restricted in internal rotation, breathing will be shallower. The temporal bones are balanced to free motion.

The sooner osteopathic treatment is initiated, the faster the response. The respiratory rate can be counted before and after treatment to assess the effectiveness of treatment. The lungs should be auscultated before and after treatment to assess the changes to see if secretions have cleared, whether or not there are fewer rhonchi and wheezes, and if the airflow has improved. Parents can be taught to do rib raising at home to continue treatment. Rib raising can be done once or twice a day for a mild illness, and more often if indicated.

Certainly, much research needs to be done to document the efficacy of OMT in infants with upper respiratory tract viral illnesses. The parents in our practice know the effectiveness of OMT in respiratory illnesses. Belcastro and colleagues developed a research protocol for bronchiolitis (31). The initial respiratory score was based on respiratory rate, retractions/nasal flaring, and cyanosis. The OMT included scapular release, rib raising, intercostal fascial release, anterior and posterior diaphragm release, and cervical fascial release. Although the study was inconclusive due to a small number of patients and extremely short treatment time (60 to 90 seconds), it provides a useful model.

Infants and children develop respiratory problems for a number of reasons. As noted earlier, children's airways are smaller, magnifying distress caused by foreign invasion or structural issues. The following is a case history of a child with both issues. The patient was initially seen at 2 weeks of age. Labor began spontaneously 10 days early. Maternal medications included oxytocin, pain medication, and epidural anesthesia. There was some bradycardia. After a spontaneous vaginal delivery, the baby was gray and the cord was wrapped around his neck three times. Apgar scores were 3 and 7, and the newborn's muscle tone was low. He had a pectus excavatum with much drawing in of the chest with breathing. Upon examining him the following day, sacral compression, temporal bones held in internal rotation, and tight periscapular and intercostals muscles were noted. Using direct action myofascial release OMT, the sacral compression was released, and temporal bones were released so they could move freely in external and internal rotation. Scapulae and intercostal muscles were released. Feeding improved after the first treatment. The baby received soy formula and fed well without any problems. At 8 weeks of age he developed nasal congestion without fever, and a cough. Upon auscultation a few diffuse expiratory wheezes were heard. The infant's rib cage showed mild retractions but there was no nasal flaring. He was alert and feeding well despite a respiratory rate of 60.

Due to his age, the season (winter), and the presentation of the illness, this child's distress was most likely related to a viral infection and diagnosed as bronchiolitis. Osteopathic structural examination found a restricted costal cage and upper thoracic spine, especially at T2-4 on the left, including restriction of the left second to fourth ribs. OMT to address restricted areas including rib raising was done initially on a daily basis for 2 days, then every 2 to 3 days until the baby's illness resolved. This infant avoided hospitalization as a result of OMT and reliable parents who knew how to count his respiratory rate and look for signs of respiratory distress. He continued to receive regular osteopathic treatments directed at improving compliance of his musculoskeletal system and quality of motion of respiratory structures (i.e., sacrum, ribs, spine, cranium), and by 6 months, his pectus excavatum was significantly reduced. He had one other episode of wheezing before he was a year old. The child is now 7 years old and has not gone on to develop reactive airway disease.

Because bronchiolitis may lead to recurrent airway obstruction symptoms and many pharmacologic agents have limited effectiveness, the search continues for the most effective treatment (32). The osteopathic approach of addressing the pathophysiology and somatic dysfunction can be of great assistance to patients with bronchiolitis. The authors (SC, MAM) have found that infants and children treated aggressively with osteopathic manipulation improve their respiratory status faster and are less likely to develop reactive airway disease.

Osteopathic Approach to the Pediatric Patient with Asthma

Asthma is the most common chronic disease in children and the most frequent admitting diagnosis in children's hospitals. The incidence of childhood asthma has dramatically increased in the last decade. Many external causes have undoubtedly contributed:

increased environmental and chemical toxins, subclinical nutritional deficiencies from processed diets and devitalized soil lacking trace minerals in commercial farming, in addition to assaults on the human immune system. Asthma is a lung disease characterized by (a) airway obstruction or narrowing that is usually reversible, (b) airway inflammation, and (c) bronchial hyperresponsiveness.

Asthma is a prevalent disease in children that favors boys (10% to 15%) over girls (7% to 10%)—a number that equalizes in adolescence as boys tend to outgrow their asthma more quickly than girls. Eighty to ninety percent of children who develop the disease are symptomatic by 5 years of age and 30% are symptomatic as early as 1 year.

A number of factors may precipitate an asthma attack:

- emotional stress including anxiety, fear, anger, and suppressed feelings that may be caused by such factors as a dysfunctional family
- exercise
- gastroesophageal reflux
- inhaled and ingested allergens (e.g., pollens, mold, spores, house dust, mites, animal dander, food)
- inhaled irritants (e.g., tobacco, smoke, air pollution, aerosol sprays, strong odors)
- medication (e.g., aspirin, nonsteroidal antiinflammatory drugs, βblockers)
- poor diet or mucogenic foods (e.g., dairy products)
- viral respiratory infections
- weather changes (including wind and changes in temperature and humidity)

Additionally, mechanical injuries can precipitate an asthma attack. This is especially true of injuries to the head or sacral regions. The authors (SC, MAM) have found that a hard fall on the sacrum will often precipitate an asthma attack. It is essential to be sure the sacrum is fully released. One patient who had many hospitalizations for asthma had been under good control for several years, with the need for only occasional medication, suffered an exacerbation when he ran head-on into a railing, hitting his nose and bruising his face. When the effects of the injury were removed, his symptoms subsided.

The clinical manifestations of asthma—wheezing, dyspnea, cough–are the result of airway obstruction that may develop gradually or abruptly. The diameter of the airway lumen determines the amount of obstruction and is influenced by a number of factors including airway smooth muscle contraction and hypertrophy. Bronchial smooth muscle is innervated by the vagus nerve (CN X) and vasovagal reflexes can cause bronchoconstriction. Therefore, in asthma bronchial spasm and increased bronchial secretions can be caused by overactivity of the bronchial branches of the vagus nerve. On a cellular level many changes also take place. Action of the sympathetic nerves innervating the bronchi are diminished and the normal equilibrium with the vagus nerve is disturbed.

Physical Examination

Though wheezing is a characteristic breath sound in asthma, it may not be heard in the most severe cases in which all breath sounds will be markedly reduced. The physician should look for

TABLE 22.2. PHYSICAL SIGNS OF POTENTIAL AIRWAY OBSTRUCTION

A prolonged forced exhalation phase	Decreased mobility of the thoracic cage, especially during exhalation
Whispering or inability to talk signals severe respiratory distress	Nasal polyps, rhinitis, sinusitis, tonsillitis
Evidence of lung hyperinflation (barrel chest)	Increased kyphotic spinal curve
Use of accessory muscles (e.g., intercostals, scalenes, and sternocleidomastoid muscles)	Mouth breathing, malocclusion, drooling
Pectum excavatum or carinatum	Allergic shiners, nasal crease
Agonal or anxious facial expression	Eczema, often in flexor creases

the signs and symptoms outlined in Table 22.2 when examining the patient. To optimize the effects of OMT these specific areas should always be checked for evidence of somatic dysfunction:

1. Upper thoracic vertebrae, ribs, and sternum.
2. T1-5 to address sympathetic innervation to the lungs.
3. O-A junction and the course of the vagus nerve to address parasympathetic responses.
4. Accessory muscles of respiration.
5. Anterior cervical fascia.
6. Thoracic diaphragm (used in all phases of breathing, the pumping action of the diaphragm also assists the adrenal glands. The phrenic nerve from the cervical plexus [C3-5] enervates the diaphragm. Its mobility is influenced by the lower six ribs, L1-2, and the sternum.).
7. Chapman reflexes for the lungs, sinuses, and adrenal glands.
8. Evaluate the cranial-sacral mechanism. Is there a sphenobasilar compression? Treat the sacrum and temporal bones to enhance the primary respiratory mechanism.
9. T10-L2 (significant for the relationship with the kidneys, adrenal glands, diaphragm, and ribs 11 and 12).

In considering the differential diagnosis in patients with signs and symptoms of obstructive airway disease, search for the underlying cause (Table 22.3).

TABLE 22.3. DIFFERENTIAL DIAGNOSIS OF AIRWAY OBSTRUCTION IN INFANTS AND CHILDREN

Obstruction of Large Airway	Obstruction of Large and Small Airways
Foreign body in trachea, bronchus, or esophagus	Asthma
Vascular rings	Viral bronchiolitis
Laryngotracheomalacia	Bronchopulmonary dysplasia
Enlarged lymph nodes or tumor	Aspiration from swallowing mechanism dysfunction or gastroesophageal reflux
Laryngeal webs	Vascular engorgement
Tracheostenosis or bronchostenosis	Pulmonary edema
	Croup
	Tuberculosis
	Pneumonia

Osteopathic Management of Patients with Asthma

The most effective approach toward treating the child with asthma is multifaceted and involves treating the underlying pathophysiology and structural restrictions, medications, diet, environmental control, breathing exercises, emotional support, and allergen reduction. It is evident that for health, there must be a balance of the sympathetic and parasympathetic nervous systems. During an acute attack, it is important to reassure and calm the child and the mother. Shortness of breath is very frightening. Acute treatment of asthma includes beta-sympathomimetic drugs to bronchodilate constricted bronchioles. In addition, osteopathic manipulation can aid the body in producing similar chemicals. The physician should focus on vigorous stimulation of the sympathetic nervous system, particularly T1-6, to aid in bronchodilation and rib raising to ease breathing.

When a patient is too uncomfortable to lie down, initial treatment can be performed with the patient seated or standing. After an acute attack, it is important to treat all aspects of the primary and secondary respiratory system. For healing, the imbalance in the nervous system must be corrected.

The hands-on osteopathic approach involves the following: (a) aiding the body in balancing the parasympathetic and sympathetic response of the nervous system; (b) optimizing blood flow to and from the lungs; (c) lymphatic drainage; (d) maintaining adrenal and glandular function; and (e) assisting in free motion of the rib cage, diaphragm, sacrum, temporal bones, etc., based on the physical findings.

OMT of children with asthma has several objectives. The most important is correcting the structural component of the illness. Often this addresses the underlying pathophysiology and leads to reduction of medication as well as a reduction of the frequency of asthma attacks. The patient and their parents also benefit from an increased awareness of the body's ability to heal itself, leading to earlier, wiser, and more constructive intervention. The authors (SC, MAM) have found that most children who receive early and regular osteopathic care, and whose parents are compliant with a healthy diet and early intervention, do not require maintenance medication.

A.T. Still had great success relieving asthma and hay fever. He attributed his success to correcting spinal somatic dysfunctions, especially of the third and fourth thoracic vertebrae (2,3). The presence of somatic dysfunction at this spinal segment is most likely due to a viscerosomatic reflex. It is also one of the spinal segments from which the sympathetic nervous system innervates the lungs.

The most useful techniques for treating asthma patients include: thoracic stimulation while the patient is either seated or lying down; rib raising; scapula release; diaphragm release; lymphatic pump via the feet and thoracic cage; evaluation and treatment of the sacrum and head; and cervical, thoracic, and lumbar manipulation with myofascial release, muscle energy, counterstrain, or HVLA, if appropriate for the patient's age. A child unable to lie down can be treated in a seated position. The entire body should always be examined, as a somatic dysfunction in a distant extremity may be the cause of a fascial strain affecting the thorax or elsewhere. It has been our experience (SC and MAM) that if a child can receive a vigorous OMT within 12 hours of the onset of an asthma attack, the attack can often be broken without the use of medication.

Medications for Asthma

Drug therapy for asthma focuses on treating the bronchospasm and inflammatory components of asthma. Many new drugs are being developed to address specific receptor sites. However as an osteopathic physician, we must not overlook the underlying pathophysiologic cause of the problem. Bronchial asthma is presently regarded as a chronic inflammatory disorder with reversible airway obstruction and increased airway responsiveness to many stimuli. This suggests there is an altered response of the target organ and not a single inflammatory process (33).

It is important to be aware of all side effects of any medication prescribed. Although inhaled corticosteroids are far safer than systemic steroids, 80% of the inhaled steroid passes through the gastrointestinal tract. Steroids adversely affect the normal flora of the intestine, contributing to "leaky gut" syndrome. This intensifies allergic tendencies, which are usually already present. A diagnosis of asthma or allergy presupposes a stress on the adrenal gland. This stress is compounded by the use of steroids, which suppress adrenal function. When antiinflammatory medications are used, probiotic support for the intestinal tract is needed as well as nutritional support for the adrenal gland. Steroids are lifesaving and should be used when needed. However, they can cause side effects such as immune suppression, shortened stature, weakened bones, and cataracts. The physician must search deeper for causes and not rely on constant medication. Popular medications to treat asthma include:

- Beta-agonists
- Mast cell stabilizers
- Corticosteroids (inhaled or systemic)
- Theophylline
- Anticholinergics
- Antibiotics (if bacterial infection)
- Leukotriene inhibitors

Environmental Concerns

Parents should be instructed on how to reduce dust, especially in the child's bedroom. Allergy covers should be used on mattresses and pillows. If carpets cannot be removed, they can be treated for dust mites. Sheets should be 100% cotton and washed in hot water. Decorating that encourages dust collection should be avoided. In a damp climate, a dehumidifier may be needed. In a dry climate, a humidifier can be helpful; however, it must be kept clean and free of mold. The use of toxic chemicals, cleaners, and pesticides near the child should be avoided.

Diet

When parents want to change the health of their child, it is essential that they understand, quite simply, that we are what we eat. Parents must be to sustain a healthy diet for their child. Such a diet consists primarily of fresh vegetables, fruits, nuts (if tolerated) and seeds, brown rice, and whole grains. They must take a firm stand against their child's desire to indulge in fast foods, sweets, processed foods, and artificially flavored, preserved, or colored products. The importance of fresh foods to avoid chemicals, allergens, and trans-fats routinely cannot be overemphasized. Parents should be taught to read labels on all foods because food colorings, sulfites, preservatives, and other modifications of food can trigger allergic reactions and asthma. For instance "modified wheat starch," a thickener used in many processed foods, is "modified" by six different chemicals, all of which can trigger asthma and allergic reaction. A "hypoglycemic diet" should be followed. Sufficient protein is important. Mucous-producing foods, such as milk, ice cream, excess cheese, white flour, and sugar, should all be avoided.

It is important to support adrenal gland health with adequate vitamin C plus bioflavonoids and a natural source of B vitamins. Patients with asthma with a high dietary intake of magnesium have better lung function and a reduction in wheezing. Magnesium deficiency increases the amount of histamine released in the blood. Encouraging breast-feeding exclusively in the first 3 months of life decreases the incidence of children developing reactive airway disease (34).

Breathing Exercises

Breathing is the only subconscious vital function that can be raised to a conscious level. Proper breathing helps the nervous system relax while shallow, spasmodic breathing signals alarm (35). Breathing exercises help strengthen peripheral and accessory muscles that aid breathing. Many breathing exercises can be adapted into games for children. Games are more fun than "exercise" or "therapy." Since asthma is an air-trapping disease, expiratory exercises are useful. For instance, a game can be created out of blowing a ping pong ball across a table. Many children with respiratory problems use their diaphragm incorrectly, raising it with inspiration instead of allowing it to descend. With the physician's hands cupped around the costal margins, the child "pushes the hands away" with a deep breath; the diaphragm is then allowed to rise on exhalation.

The osteopathic approach to asthma provides a unique and effective treatment opportunity that addresses the structural component of the illness, which reduces the need for medication and the frequency of attacks. In addition, OMT increases awareness of the body's ability to heal itself and therefore encourages timely, more effective intervention. OMT is designed to balance the sympathetic and parasympathetic responses, reduce mechanical impediments to optimal thoracic cage motion, enhance lymphatic and venous drainage, improve arterial blood supply, and optimize the primary respiratory mechanism. In addition, the osteopathic physician can use such tools as medication, environmental change, breathing exercises, nutrition, and psychological support to enhance the effects of OMT. Parents and patients alike need to be taught to act immediately at the first sign of an impending illness or asthma attack. Most children with a history of asthma who are on a wholesome diet and receive excellent osteopathic manipulative medicine management do quite well with reduced or no medication.

The Pediatric Gastrointestinal System

The gastrointestinal system is one of the most important systems in physiologic maintenance of health in children. It is fundamental for proper growth and development. Gastrointestinal complaints are among the most common reasons a child is seen by a pediatrician. A.T. Still and the early osteopathic physicians regarded the gastrointestinal system second only to the brain in its importance in well functioning of the body. In fact, it was often referred to as the second brain or abdominal brain. The enteric nervous system parallels the central nervous system in density and quantity of neurons. The system can be surgically separated from the central nervous system and still maintain physiologic function. Still attributed many childhood diseases to dysfunction of this system (3).

Gastroesophageal-Reflux Disease

Gastroesophageal-reflux disease (GERD) presents as frequent emesis shortly after feeding associated with failure to thrive, apnea and bradycardia, or wheezing. These children may have significant increase in their gag reflex. They often have a history of abnormal delivery events including vacuum extraction, augmentation with oxytocin, and prolonged labor. Somatic dysfunctions found include sphenobasilar lateral strain or torsion, O-A compression, and sacral torsions. These infants may have compression of the fourth ventricle due to foramen magnum asymmetry. These somatic dysfunctions produce abnormal stimulation of CN IX, CN X, and CN XI. The increased vagal tone is responsible for bronchospasm, bradycardia, and delayed gastric emptying. This is best treated by releasing the O-A restriction but may require treating the sacral base restriction simultaneously. The clinician should place the pads of the middle fingers over the condyles at the base of the skull, then apply gentle traction in an outward and upward direction until the tissue softens. Gentle sacral traction may help facilitate release of the O-A somatic dysfunction.

Constipation

Constipation in young children is a common complaint and responds readily to OMT. An appropriate history and physical examination is an essential first step in all cases. The history should especially focus on the dietary intake including noncomplex carbohydrates, and water intake. Psychosocial issues should be addressed in older children.

Osteopathically, the physician should be careful to examine for autonomic imbalance and pay close attention to the A-A and O-A joints as vagus nerve involvement can contribute to autonomic imbalance. Both the pelvic and abdominal diaphragms should be examined and treated since ptosis of the viscera may be a problem. The patient assumes the prone knee-to-chest position and the practitioner gently lifts the intestines from the pelvis, thus restoring free unimpeded motion and blood flow. This often brings immediate results. Treating the child with fascial release of the colon can be extremely helpful.

Diarrhea

Diarrhea in the infant and child is common and responds to OMT. The underlying cause must first be addressed. Acute diarrhea, most often caused by viruses, must be differentiated from chronic diarrhea, which could have multiple causes. Infectious diarrhea should be differentiated from the noninfectious type. Regardless of cause, somatic dysfunction is often found.

Decreasing hyperparasympathetic activity may be very beneficial. The use of deep inhibitory pressure from T10 to the sacrum is indicated. Deep pressure over the sacrum may result in decreased tenesmus. Correction of lumbar somatic dysfunction and rib raising will also be helpful.

NEUROLOGIC DYSFUNCTION IN CHILDREN

The nervous system of the child is a dynamic, expanding, and integrated system that ultimately affects all other vital systems of the child's body. Function of this system is dependent upon an unimpeded, physiologic, and integrated structure. This structure includes the osseous case that surrounds the brain and spinal cord, the delicate fascial and membranous coverings that lie beneath the osseous covering, the arterial, venous, and lymphatic channels, and the ligamentous and articular structures that check and allow motion. Impairment of this delicate structure will impair function.

Evaluation of children from a neurodevelopmental approach can give valuable clues in developing a management plan, including the utilization of OMT. It can serve as a guide to evaluate the success of treatment of developmentally delayed children undergoing osteopathic treatment. In some instances, restoration of lost reflexes to cultivate integrated arm, leg, and head movement and visual tracking may be needed. These exercises, when part of an overall osteopathic treatment program, can be very beneficial.

Sensory neural developmentalists refer to neurologically disorganized children as those children who are inefficient in their ability to receive, process, store, and utilize information through their five senses. They may exhibit hyperesthesia or hypoesthesia. Hyperesthesia is defined as an abnormal increased response to sensory stimulation. Hypoesthesia is defined as an abnormal decreased response to sensory stimulation. For example, a child with tactile hypoesthesia may have an extremely increased pain threshold, may exhibit self-mutilating behavior in order to receive tactile pain stimulation, may constantly run their hands across the carpet to receive deep joint stimulation, and may seek and be contented with various forms of vibration. Children with tactile hyperesthesia may refuse to wear certain types of clothing, exhibit extreme irritability from tags on clothing, may refuse certain textured food or in some cases all solid food, and may be adverse to any type vibratory stimulation.

These developmental inefficiencies are thought to be the result of a disorganized nervous system. A number of studies show that brain growth and development occur at predetermined chronologic ages. These predetermined times of rapid growth occur between 3 months of fetal life to about 2 to 3 years postnatally. The fundamental cause of neurologic disorganization results from a child ineffectively passing through or missing milestones at certain critical stages of neurologic and neuronal development. This may occur if there is prolonged interruption of normal infant development and stimulation.

As an osteopathic physician it is especially important to evaluate children who have known somatic dysfunction for problems related to neurologic disorganization. Neural disorganization can be from organic or external causes. A child who is seriously ill (i.e., a serious bacterial illness, seizures, chronic illness) during a time of rapid neuronal growth may not receive adequate sensory-motor stimulation in a given area. Myofascial strain and somatic dysfunction may also be a causative factor in limiting the child's active range of motion and opportunity for sensory stimulation and development. The child never reaches the specific developmental milestone, yet the myelination associated with that milestone continues to develop. The neural pathway is developed but the neurologic skill is never realized. External causes include forced deprivation as seen in orphan children placed in cribs until late infancy with little social or intellectual stimulation or the so-called border babies who are housed in inner city hospital nurseries and do not receive normal parent-child bonding and stimulation.

In neurologically compromised children manipulation directed toward the autonomic nervous system may positively affect the sensory responses and disorganization of the central nervous system. Both neurologically compromised and uncompromised children show marked improvement in standard neurodevelopmental profiles upon receiving OMT compared with a control group (36). Osteopathic treatment may improve the functional restrictions or disability, but because that functional restriction has been present during crucial periods of development, neurologic disorganization may occur. In these cases it may be necessary to re-pattern the specific neurologic sequences that may have been missed. This is the focus of neurodevelopmental therapy. Although osteopathic manipulation appears to help in overall neurologic development, if a child, because of functional disability, does not receive adequate neurologic stimulation, disorganization will often persist.

Disorganization is the result of discrepancies in motor-sensory organization and the level or age of neuronal development. The child may progress from a sitting position to standing position or walking without ever crawling. The vestibular stimulation from side-to-side turning of the head, ventral tactile stimulation, ocular-foveal far and near vision stimulation, acoustic spatial stimulation, and cross-lateral hemispheric stimulation of the central nervous system that occur as the child crawls is never experienced. Without this previous stimulation the child walks. However, the child may have deficits in coordination. The gait cycle may be abnormal. The child may have difficulty with depth perception and orientation in space. Because of the disparity between neuronal growth and developmental stimulation and depending on the child's age and which level or levels of the brain are involved, the child may exhibit a number of problems in areas of learning, socializing, and behaving.

Four principles govern sensory neural development. First, development is a continuous process that proceeds in a caudad-cephalad direction. Therefore, the infant will initially present with the most primitive reflexes at the level of the medulla and spinal cord, such as the startle reflex, Babinski reflex, and light reflex. As neuronal development proceeds, the well-organized newborn will initially have an atonic neck reflex and fencing pose (1 to 4 months), which will lead to the ability of the infant to roll back to front at 5 months. From 6 to 8 months, as progressive neuronal development occurs, the infant will begin to first crawl, and then creep. The myelination and developmental stimulation

in the areas of the pons and midbrain mediate this. Standing and walking begins at 9 to 12 months as the cortex develops. Second, the sequence of development is the same in all children. However, the rate of development may vary. Developmental rate is referred to as superior, average, or slow. If given proper stimulation and neurologic feedback, slow children may increase their rate. Third, primitive reflexes must be extinguished before corresponding voluntary movements can be obtained. This is particularly important in children who present with developmental delay and neurologic disorganization. Persistent reflexes and persistent hypersensitivity or hyposensitivity must be overcome before proper neurologic organization can occur. Fourth, the rate of milestone development in one area may not parallel the rate in another area. This is especially apparent in children who are neurologically disorganized.

It is important that every child receive a developmental screening (Table 22.4). Those with suspected neurologic or developmental issues may benefit from a more detailed profile of development. The presence of primitive reflexes such as the startle, rooting, Perez-Galant, and atonic neck reflexes should be evaluated even in those children who are older and do not appear to have gross neurologic damage. Children with significant deficits can be given an exercise program that effectively re-patterns the nervous system leading to improved neurologic organization.

Neidner worked with children who had muscular dystrophy. He developed an effective myofascial OMT procedure beneficial to many children with this disease (Table 22.5). From the osteopathic point of view, structural integrity permits freedom of physiologic motion allowing the inherent therapeutic capacity of the nervous system to stimulate neurologic development, integration, and organization. Even a slight change in this structural integrity may alter function.

Osteopathic treatment of the neurologic system involves diagnosis and treatment of the whole body since ligamentous, membranous, or fascial strain within any part of the body can affect any other part. We do not assume or confine treatment to the cranium but evaluate the body as a unit focusing on areas that impair inherent physiologic motility.

Colic

Colic, irritability, and sleeplessness present with lateral and vertical strain patterns (parallelogram heads). They exhibit impingement of the accessory nerve (CN XI). This occurs in the foramen magnum but may be the result of the torsion of the falx and tentorium. These infants often have significant membranous restrictions with poor cranial motion. They may have sacral base restriction. They have obvious abnormally shaped heads with one eye appearing "more shallow" than the other, and placed inferiorly. They may have a torticollis (tilt their head and rotate to the same side). These infants respond best to release of the sacral restrictions, then treatment of the strain patterns, the vertical then lateral. The strains are treated by direct, gentle remolding of any parietal and frontal abnormalities, and carrying the greater wings of the sphenoid into normal position. The O-A should be decompressed. Treatment of any trigger points on the SCM is by palpation of tight fascial areas with the head bent to the side and rotation until the area softens.

TABLE 22.4. DEVELOPMENTAL PROFILE

Scale/Age Range	Mobility	Language	Manual
Excellent: 36 mos Average: 72 mos Satisfactory: 96 mos	Able to do skilled activities, evidences laterality	Uses first-grade vocabulary with good sentence structure	Writes on first-grade level
Excellent: 22 mos Average: 48 mos Satisfactory: 67 mos	Walks and runs in cross-pattern	Speaks five- to eight-word sentences with good articulation	Performs bimanual tasks efficiently
Excellent: 13 mos Average: 24 mos Satisfactory: 45 mos	Walks with arms held below waist	Speaks 25 words and uses several two-word couplets	Capable of cortical opposition bilaterally and simultaneously
Excellent: 8 mos Average: 12 mos Satisfactory: 26 mos	Walks unassisted without pattern for ten steps, arms elevated	Spontaneously uses words	Capable of cortical opposition, either hand
Excellent: 4 mos Average: 8 mos Satisfactory: 13 mos	Creeps in cross-pattern	Makes meaningful, and goal-directed sounds with good tonality	Has volitional prehensile grasp
Excellent: 1 mo Average: 2.5 mos Satisfactory: 4.5 mos	Crawls in cross-pattern	Consistently has vital cry in response to threatening sounds or events	Able to release grasped object
Birth	Randomly moves arms and legs	Birth cry present	Reflexly able to grasp object

(Adapted from "Profile of Development." American Academy for Human Development. Piqua, OH; 1989.)

Apnea

In children with apnea, there is a marked reduction in the primary respiratory motion. They may have a cranium held in extension. Their head may appear long, from front to back, and narrow, from side to side. This is commonly seen in infants who were born prematurely who tend to have a high, arched palate. The temporal bones are fixed in internal rotation. The sphenoid is fixed in extension. The foramen magnum is narrowed and the fourth ventricle is compressed. The brainstem modulation of homeostasis is abnormal which results in high vagal tone causing apnea and bradycardia.

Treatment includes release of any cranial base dysfunction with restoration of the parasympathetic tone. This is accomplished with release of cranial base restrictions and any intraosseous restrictions in the sphenoid, if present. Associated sacral restrictions must be released. The major focus of treatment is to restore physiologic brainstem activity.

Closed Head Injuries

Injuries to the head and neck tend to be sudden acceleration/deceleration injuries and to involve the soft tissue. Children have flexible necks and relatively large heads. Their neurologic system is still developing and the membranes are highly vascular. Inertial injuries can result in concussion and whiplash. They present with the history of a blow to the head or a sudden change in directional forces, resulting in a brief period of loss of consciousness or disorientation, with or without neck pain. The palpatory findings include cervical spasm and somatic dysfunction, cranial dysfunction, and a greatly diminished primary respiratory mechanism. These are treated with counterstrain or indirect/muscle energy OMT to the cervical somatic dysfunctions. This is followed by cranial OMT for correction of any abnormalities and a CV4 to enhance the primary respiratory mechanism. The younger the child, the more significant the potential for cranial dysfunction due to the susceptibility to strain of the membranous attachments.

Learning Disorders/Hyperactivity

Learning disorders are increasingly common among children of all ages with few long-term or effective treatments. In one study, 209 children between the ages of 4 and 14 diagnosed with learning difficulty were evaluated by osteopathic structural examination (12). Seventy-two percent of the children with a learning difficulty diagnosis had a significant past history of birth trauma compared to only 28% in the control group. Labor lasting more than 24 hours was highly associated with learning difficulty. Eye-motor coordination and visual perception imbalances were highly associated with children experiencing difficulty.

Lateral strains of the sphenobasilar symphysis may be especially implicated in oculomotor disturbances. These dysfunctions may be a result of intrauterine pressure or early postnatal or perinatal trauma displacing the axis of the orbit. This can cause

TABLE 22.5. NEIDNER TECHNIQUE

William Neidner, DO, recognized that in health, viewing the human body from above the head, there is a clockwise fascial rotation. This is a profoundly relaxing treatment and should be considered at the conclusion of a treatment program after more local strain patterns have been resolved.

1. **Patient Supine**
   - Stand at the head of the patient with a hand over each shoulder, the fingers spread over clavicles and upper ribs.
   - Test the ease of diagonal motion anterior and inferior of right shoulder and then left shoulder.
   - In the counter-clockwise pattern the right shoulder will move more freely.
   - Apply a direct fascial release (i.e., attempt to carry the left shoulder anterior to the patient's right shoulder and inferior while restraining the right shoulder posteriorly).
   - Hold until the release occurs, and the left moves freely.
   - At the moment of release the resistance to the anterior-inferior motion of the left shoulder melts away.

2. **Stand on the Left Side of the Table for All of the Following Five (2–6) Steps**
   - Take patient's left arm, abduct it at the shoulder about 75°, flex it at the elbow 90°.
   - The operator slips their right arm posterior to the patient's left upper arm and rests their right hand on the patient's forearm.
   - Encourage internal rotation of the shoulder girdle by slightly lifting the upper arm toward the ceiling and depressing the forearm toward the floor.
   - Wait for release and ease of motion to occur.

3. **Place Each Hand on Either Side of the Lower Half of the Thoracic Cage**
   - Spread the fingers to encompass as wide an area as possible.
   - Evaluate ease of rotation: counter-clockwise (right hand will carry right thoracic cage anteriorly and inferiorly more easily) clockwise when left thoracic cage moves anteriorly to right and inferiorly more freely.
   - Apply direct action into the restrictive barrier until left side moves more freely anteriorly and inferiorly.

4. **Assess Pubic Tubercles**
   - In counter-clockwise pattern, left tubercle will be superior to right.
   - Apply direct action fascial release to move the left side inferiorly.

5. **Place Hands over the Innominate Bones Bilaterally with Thumbs over Anterior Superior Iliac Spine**
   - Test for anterior-inferior medial motion of each side.
   - If counter-clockwise, right side will move more freely.
   - Apply direct action fascial release to bring left side into anterior, right, and inferior directions.

6. **Left Lower Extremity**
   - Flex hip about 45° and knee about 80°, adduct, internally rotate, and hold the thigh until there is fascial release of pelvic girdle into direction of clockwise motion.

7. **Patient Prone with Face Turned to the Right**
   - Stand at the head of the table with hands placed over the shoulders. The fingers are spread over the scapulae.
   - If counter-clockwise motion predominates the operator's right hand will carry the patient's left shoulder posteriorly, inferiorly, and medially more easily than the operator's left hand will move the right shoulder posteriorly, inferiorly, and medially.
   - Apply direct fascial release through the left hand (i.e., to the patient's right shoulder, until the softening and ease of motion occurs).

8. **Stand on the Left Side of the Table (i.e., the right side of the patient for all the following steps)**
   - Take the patient's right shoulder to 80° of abduction and external rotation by lifting the hand toward the ceiling, and elbow with the upper arm posteriorly, medially.
   - Turn to face toward the patient's feet. Grasp the lower thoracic cage with both hands spreading the fingers over the ribs and laying the thumbs beside the vertebral column.
   - In counter-clockwise motion the physician's right hand will move the patient's left rib cage posteriorly, medially, and inferiorly more easily than is possible on the opposite side.
   - Apply direct action fascial release to move the right rib cage (i.e., the operator's left hand posteriorly, medially, inferiorly).
   - Hold until softening and melting of the resistance occurs.

9. **Facing the Child's Feet from the Head of the Table, Place Both Hands on the Iliac Crests, Thumbs toward the Posterior Superior Iliac Spine**
   - If counter-clockwise motion predominates, the operator's right hand will carry the patient's left innominate bone more easily into posterior, medial, inferior direction.
   - Apply direct fascial release into the restrictive barrier.
   - Hold the pressure until release is palpated.

10. **Place Right Hand over the Sacrum with the Heel of the Hand at the Base and Fingertips over the Coccyx**
    - Reinforce with the left hand.
    - To encourage clockwise motion apply direct fascial release to the sacrum inferiorly on the patient's right side (i.e., with the operator's thumb) and anteriorly on their left side (i.e., with operator's little finger).
    - Hold the pressure until release is palpated.

11. **Stand beside the Right Lower Extremity Facing toward the Head**
    - With right hand under the knee and the left hand on the ankle, carry the hip to 45° of flexion with external rotation and abduction.
    - To encourage clockwise motion lift the knee toward the ceiling with a posterior, inferior motion while depressing the foot toward the floor.
    - Hold this direct fascial release until the softening and increased freedom of motion occurs.

changes of tension in extraocular eye muscle resulting in eye muscle imbalance. These distortions would also change membranous, fascial, neural, and venous relationships.

Children with attention deficit with hyperkinesis often present with findings similar to those with learning issues. Visual tracking and lateral strains of the sphenobasilar symphysis are often seen. However, the child with hyperactivity often has more severe findings. Compression of the sphenobasilar symphysis is often an issue. The occipital condyles and the foramen magnum are often compressed, resulting in pyramidal and autonomic disturbances. Cranial dysfunction may arise in these children from sacral compression or other distant areas of the body. Frequently, condylar decompression and release of basilar compression will result in immediate and dramatic improvements in symptomatology.

Clearly, regardless of diagnosis, treatment of the underlying cause of the child's symptoms is essential. Certainly, attention to diet and a nutrition program that is wholesome (in its whole state), unprocessed, and free of pesticides and insecticides can be helpful. In some cases neurodevelopmental therapy or developmental optometric training may be necessary once the underlying somatic dysfunctions are corrected.

CONCLUSION

New challenges are arising in pediatrics. More infertility issues have led to a myriad of interventions. The number of multiple births has risen, producing challenges that result from two or more fetuses sharing the small space in the uterus. The next decade will continue to produce new challenges for the osteopathic physician working with children. In addition to infectious disease, autistic spectrum disorders and developmental delay, learning difficulties and behavioral issues, and environmental and lifestyle-related diseases are all on the rise. Major adult diseases, such as atherosclerosis, coronary artery disease, and hypertension, likely have roots in childhood. Improving the health and well being of the general population requires attention during the earliest years of life.

Osteopathic structural diagnostics and OMT used for children can be significant modalities for primary, secondary, and tertiary prevention. In general, children respond well to direct action, articulatory treatments, such as myofascial release, and mobilization. Older children also respond to a combination of muscle energy and mild thrust or HVLA. Cranial OMT is invaluable in the newborn period and throughout childhood. Counterstrain techniques are helpful if there are tender points related to the somatic dysfunction. Somatic dysfunctions related to acute injury often respond to indirect techniques. In many instances children are flexible enough for somatic dysfunctions to resolve spontaneously.

Relieving mechanical stresses and strains palpable throughout the body with OMT has benefited children with neurologic and behavior problems, academic and perceptual problems in school, an increased susceptibility to disease, such as ear infections, frequent colds, reactive air disease, and gastrointestinal problems. Unfortunately, little research on these modalities has been attempted. Osteopathic pediatrics provides a complete discipline

of health care for children; the future requires the expertise of osteopathic pediatric specialists conducting scientifically based, randomized, and blinded clinical trials.

The future of pediatrics will focus heavily on primary care and preventive medicine. As a primary care discipline, the pediatrician is in an ideal position to affect health and well being. Lifestyle diseases that affect the majority of the population can be prevented or minimized by providing anticipatory guidance, especially during adolescence, in epidemiologically important areas such as:

- Dietary counseling for control of obesity and hypercholesterolemia
- Drug, alcohol, and tobacco avoidance
- Accident prevention

Osteopathic pediatricians are responsible for systematically investigating and documenting applications of osteopathic concepts and principles during the early stages of child development. Early introduction of osteopathic care can affect and improve neurodevelopmental outcome significantly. Osteopathic treatment of the child will continue to be comprehensive, including osteopathic manipulation, nutrition counseling, strengthening and stretching exercises, and anticipatory guidance and prevention.

REFERENCES

1. Bomboy RP. *The Golden Anniversary History of the American College of Osteopathic Pediatricians, 1940–1990.* Trenton, NJ: American College of Osteopathic Pediatricians; 1990.
2. Still AT. *Autobiography of A. T. Still.* Indianapolis, IN: American Academy of Osteopathy; 1908.
3. Still AT. *Osteopathy: Research and Practice.* Seattle, WA: Eastland Press; 1992. Originally published in Kirksville, MO: Journal Printing Co; 1910.
4. Millard FP, ed. *Poliomyelitis.* Kirksville, MO: Journal Printing Co; 1918.
5. Watson JO, Percival, EN. Pneumonia research in children at Los Angeles County Osteopathic Hospital. A preliminary report. *JAOA.* 1939;39(3):153–159.
6. Arbuckle BE. Effects of Uterine Forces Upon the Fetus. *JAOA.* 1954;53:499–508. Also in *The Selected Writings of Beryl E. Arbuckle, D.O., F.A.C.O.P.* The National Osteopathic Institute and the Cerebral Palsy Foundation; 1977:121–141. (Original reference: Little WJ. On the influence of abnormal parturition, difficult labors, premature births, and asphyxia neonatorum, on the mental and physical conditions of the child, especially in relation to deformities. *Trans Obstet Soc* [London]. 1862;3:293–344.)
7. Whiting L. Can the length of labor be shortened by osteopathic treatment. *JAOA.* 1913:917–921.
8. King HH. Osteopathic manipulative treatment in prenatal care: evidence supporting improved outcomes and health policy implications. *AAOJ.* 2000;10:25–33.
9. Arbuckle BE. *The Selected Writings of Beryl E. Arbuckle, D.O., F.A.C.O.P.* The National Osteopathic Institute and the Cerebral Palsy Foundation; 1977.
10. Barnes M. Osteopathic treatment of infants. *JAOA.* 1941;40:242–243.
11. Upledger JE. The relationship of craniosacral examination findings in grade school children with developmental problems. *JAOA.* 1978;77:738–754.
12. Frymann VM. Learning difficulties of children viewed in the light of the osteopathic concept. *JAOA.* 1976;60–61.

13. Woods R. A physical finding related to psychiatric disorders. *JAOA.* 1961;60:988–993.

14. Woods R. Structural normalization in infants and children with particular reference to disturbances of the central nervous system. *JAOA.* 1973;72:903–908.

15. Wales AL, ed. *Teachings in the Science of Osteopathy. Transcribed Lectures of William Garner Sutherland, D.O.* Portland, OR: Rudra Press; 1990.

16. Frymann VM. Relation of disturbances of craniosacral mechanisms to symptomatology of the newborn: study of 1250 infants. *JAOA.* 1966;65:1059–1075.

17. King H, ed. *The Collected Papers of Viola M. Frymann, DO: Legacy of Osteopathy to Children.* Indianapolis: IN. American Academy of Osteopathy; 1998.

18. Behrman RE, Kliegman RM, Jenson HB, eds. *Nelson Textbook of Pediatrics,* 16th ed. Philadelphia, PA: WB Saunders; 2001.

19. Greenman PE. Structural abnormalities of children. *JAOA.* 1971;71:157.

20. Magoun HI Sr. Osteopathic approach to dental enigmas. *JAOA.* 1962;62:110–118.

21. Frymann, VF. The expanding osteopathic concept. *AAO Yearbook,* 1967;67:50–62. Reprinted in King HH, ed. *The Collected Papers of Viola M. Frymann, DO: Legacy of Osteopathy to Children.* Indianapolis: IN. American Academy of Osteopathy; 1998.

22. Magoun HI, ed. *Osteopathy in the Cranial Field*, 3rd ed. Kirksville, MO: Journal Printing Co; 1976.

23. Magoun HI Sr. Entrapment neuropathy in the cranium. *JAOA.* 1968; 67:643–652.

24. Magoun HI Sr. Entrapment neuropathy of the central nervous system, part II. Cranial nerves I-IV, VI-VIII, XII. *JAOA.* 1968;67:779–787.

25. Magoun HI Sr. Entrapment neuropathy of the central nervous system, part III. Cranial nerves V, IX, X, XI. *JAOA.* 1968;67:889–899.

26. Educational Council on Osteopathic Principles Core Curriculum. Washington, DC: American Association of Colleges of Osteopathic Medicine; 1988.

27. Beal MC. A review of the short-leg problem; and the short leg problem. In: Peterson B, ed. *Posture Balance and Imbalance.* Newark, NJ: American Academy of Osteopathy; 1983:26–42.

28. Panitch HB. Bronchiolitis in infants. *Curr Opin Pediatr.* 2001;Jun 13(3):256–260.

29. Oski FA, DeAngelis CD, Feiginm RD, et al, eds. *Principles and Practice of Pediatrics,* 2nd ed. Philadelphia, PA: JB Lippincott Co; 1994.

30. Bertrand P, Aranibar H, Castro E, Sanchez I. Efficacy of nebulized epinephrine versus salbutamol in hospitalized infants with bronchiolitis. *Pediatr Pulmonol.* 2001;31(4):284–288.

31. Belcastro MR, Backes CR, Chila AG. Bronchiolitis: a pilot study of osteopathic manipulative treatment, bronchodilators, and other therapy. *JAOA.* 1984;83(9):672–676.

32. Kattan M. Epidemiologic evidence of increased airway reactivity in children with a history of bronchiolitis. *J Pediatr.* 1999;135(2 Pt 2):8–13.

33. Brusasco V, Crimini E, Pellegrino R. Airway hyperresponsiveness in asthma: not just a matter of airway inflammation. *Thorax* 1998;53:992–998.

34. Gdalevich M, Mimouni D, Mimouni M. Breast-feeding and the risk of bronchial asthma in childhood: a systematic review with meta-analysis of prospective studies. *J Pediatr* 2001;139(2):261–265.

35. Firshcin RN. *Reversing Asthma.* New York, NY: Warner Books; 1996.

36. Frymann VM, Carney RE, Springall P. Effect of osteopathic medical management on neurological development in children. *JAOA.* 1992;92:729.

TABLE 23.1. (continue

Age-Relat

Aging Musculoskeletal Syste
  Loss of muscle mass
  Loss of bone mineral dens

  Osteoarthritis

Aging Hematologic System
  Decreased lymphocyte pro
  Decreased bone marrow ce
  Decreased hematopoietic f

Aging Endocrine System
  Impaired glucose tolerance
  Increased insulin resistance
  Decreased estrogen

Aging immune System
  Decreased T-cell function
  Decreased antibody produc
  Increased autoantibodies

Aging Gastrointestinal System
  Decreased gastric HCl prodi
  Colonic motility diminished
  Decreased calcium absorptic
  Decreased hepatic biotransf
  Decreased hepatic albumin

Aging Genitourinary System
  Decreased bladder capacity
  Alterations in pelvic support
  Enlarged prostate gland
  Diminished vaginal and cerv
  Decrease in sexual response

during metabolism into sup
and hydroxyl radicals causes
proposed that antioxidants, :
free radicals, thus slowing th
to show that antioxidants s
average life span in animal
aging include the error theor
linkage theory (3,4).

Physiology of Aging

The aging process itself is ch
vidual variation, manifested
versus physiologic age. Thus
logic age of 75 but a physiolog
of physiologic aging is that tl
occurring at the same rate o
cumulative and actually begin
decade. As such, an 80-year-ol
old but has the cumulative eff
or four decades (Table 23.1).

Later sections in this chapte
found clinical impact. Under
structure and function, and t
altered homeostasis are vital t
vanced age the body compositi

GERIATRICS

THOMAS A. CAVALIERI

KEY CONCEPTS

- Historical perspective on geriatric medicine
- Theories and physiology of aging
- Comprehensive geriatric assessment, including medical, functional, psychological, and social components
- Special clinical concerns with the elderly: confusion, urinary incontinence, falling, and iatrogenesis
- Special contribution of osteopathic medicine to the elderly

The elderly require a special approach in medical care and treatment; they are not just older adults. Elderly individuals have needs stemming from aging physiology, the psychosocial impact of aging, and age-related diseases. The approach to the care of the elderly must be multidisciplinary and holistic; it must be driven by the goals of health maintenance and optimizing function. Osteopathic medicine is ideally suited to provide an approach to clinical care of the elderly aimed at achieving these goals.

HISTORICAL PERSPECTIVE

The National Institute of Aging promulgated the geriatric imperative in the 1970s and 1980s. It called for health care professions to respond to unmet clinical needs of the elderly (1), and offered academic, attitudinal, demographic, and economic reasons to justify this concept. Academic reasons for the geriatric imperative centered on the absence of clinically relevant information on geriatrics and gerontology in the curricula of health professional schools and training programs. Attitudinal reasons for the geriatric imperative focused on negative stereotypes on aging believed to result in prejudice against the elderly and thought to be commonplace in our health care system.

Demographic and economic aspects of the geriatric imperative focused on the rapidly rising number of people who were 65 years and older in the United States and the impact of this population on health care costs. Representing over 12% of the total U.S. population today, this group is projected to increase to more than

18% of the population by the year 2030. The mean life span by the year 2040 will continue increasing and is projected to be well into the eighth decade of life for both sexes. The "old old," those over age 85, are the most rapidly growing segment of the U.S. population. By the year 2040 it is projected that there will be 1 million centenarians in the United States. With the elderly as the highest users of health care resources, these demographic changes will have an impact on the cost of health care (2).

The past two decades have witnessed the impact of the geriatric imperative on the development of geriatric medicine in this country. While it is generally believed that we are still far from meeting the health care needs of the elderly, the geriatric imperative has succeeded in spawning much-needed research in geriatrics and gerontology, influenced changes in medical education, and significantly altered our approach to the clinical care of the elderly. Osteopathic medicine has contributed greatly to the development of geriatrics in the United States.

AGING PROCESS

The aging process itself is far from being completely understood. Recognizing the interrelationship among structure, function, and homeostasis with regard to the aging process is critical to the clinical care of the elderly. While aging and disease are distinctly different, the effects of the aging process on various organ systems are believed to reduce the organ's capacity to respond to increased demand. This has been called impaired homeostasis; it has significant clinical impact.

Theories of Aging

Various theories of aging have been proposed. The immunologic theory for aging attributes the decline in organ reserve seen with aging to the diminishing effects of the immune system. Thus, the thymus gland might be the master gland of the aging process, beginning with its involution at a young age. Numerous cellular theories of aging are still actively being investigated. The transcription theory attributes aging to the cell's limited ability to repair errors in transcription that occur in all cells.

The oxidative stress theory is a widely acceptable explanation of the aging process. This theory claims the oxygen converted

TABLE 23.1. PHYSIC...

Body Composition and C
  Decreased height
  Decreased lean body r
  Decreased body water
  Increased body fat

Aging Skin
  Thinning and sparsene
  Hair follicles produce l
  Thin, fragile, wrinkled
  Capillary fragility
  Decreased subcutaneo
  Atrophy of sweat glan
  Decreased response to

Aging Eyes
  Loss of elasticity of len
  Increased density of le
  Change in aqueous kir
  Decreased pupillary siz
  Sluggish light reflex
  Decreased color vision
  Increased glare sensitiv

Aging Mouth and Teeth
  Loss of lingual papillae
  Poor taste sensation
  Atrophy of olfactory bi

  Resorption of gum and

Aging Ears
  Decrease in cerumen gl
  Atrophy of cochlear ha
  Loss of auditory neuror

Aging Cardiovascular Syst
  Increase in blood press
  Aorta and large arterie
  Decreased barorecepto
  Calcification and sclero
  Calcification and sclero
  Altered cardiac output
  Decreased heart rate

Aging Respiratory System
  Calcification of costal ca
  Decline in alveolar surfa
  Alteration in pulmonar
    Decreased vital capac
    Decreased maximum
    Increased residual vol
    Decreased Pao2

Aging Renal System
  Progressive loss of renal
  Decrease in renal blood
  Decrease in tubular funct
  Decrease in creatinine c

Aging Nervous System
  Decrease in brain weigh
  Alteration in CNS neuro
  Decrease in memory
  Decreased reaction time
  Altered sleep with decre
  Decreased vibratory sen
  Decreased righting refle
  Increased postural instal
  Altered gait

TABLE 23.8. DIFFERENTIATING DELIRIUM FROM DE-MENTIA

	Delirium	Dementia
Onset	Sudden	Insidious
Consciousness	Reduced	Clear
Attention	Globally disordered	Normal
Cognition	Globally disordered	Globally impaired
Hallucinations	Usually visual	Often absent
Delusions	Fleeting, poorly systemized	Often absent
Psychomotor activity	Increase or decrease	Usually normal
Speech	Often incoherent	Word-finding difficulty
Involuntary movements	Asterixis or coarse tremor	Often absent
Physical illness/drug toxicity	Present	Often absent

the problems of the patient with dementia span the dimensions of medical, behavioral, nursing, ethical, and social needs, management should be multidisciplinary. The physician must be an effective team leader to access and implement the plan of care. Osteopathic physicians, with their emphasis on holistic primary care, are well suited for this role. Skillful management can contribute significantly to the well being of the patient and their family (17).

While the precise cause of Alzheimer disease is still unknown, recent clinical and basic science research have expanded our understanding of this devastating disorder. Data suggest a genetic link to Alzheimer disease probably related to chromosome 14, 19, or 21. Diagnosis requires careful clinical assessment and the exclusion of other causes for dementia. Cholinesterase inhibitors are now available as cognitive enhancing agents for the treatment of Alzheimer disease. Donepezil is most widely used. These agents are best used for mild and moderate disease. Their long-term effect is still being studied. Other agents being assessed as possible cognitive enhancers include estrogen, nonsteroidal anti-inflammatory agents, gingko biloba, and vitamin E (18,19).

Urinary Incontinence

Urinary incontinence is a common disorder that is referred to as a hidden illness in the elderly because it is often overlooked by clinicians and because the elderly often do not report it out of fear of institutionalization. In fact, urinary incontinence is often the last event to occur before nursing home placement. This problem afflicts approximately 10% of the community-dwelling elderly, 30% of the elderly in acute care settings, and approximately 50% of nursing home residents. Its impact is seen in the psychological effects of isolation and depression, the potential for skin breakdown and infection, and the economic impact of institutionalization and costs of care. Although incontinence can occur acutely as a result of drugs or infection, the focus here is on persistent incontinence. An understanding of normal micturition is essential to understand the mechanisms and management of this problem. There are four types of persistent urinary incontinence:

- Urge
- Stress
- Overflow
- Functional

Urge incontinence, the most common type in the elderly representing approximately 65% of cases, is the result of an unstable bladder with uninhibited bladder contractions. Patients with this type of incontinence have the sudden urge to void but simply cannot make it to the bathroom in time. It is commonly the result of CNS conditions such as stroke, dementia, and multiple sclerosis. It can be successfully treated with anticholinergic drugs to relax bladder contractions and biofeedback to aid in bladder relaxation.

Stress incontinence occurs primarily in women and accounts for 15% of cases. It is manifested by incontinence with coughing or laughing and is related to weakness of the pelvic musculature and urethral incompetence. Treatment can be accomplished by estrogen cream to enhance the integrity of the urethra, exercise, biofeedback to improve strength and tone of the pelvic musculature, and beta-adrenergic agonists to improve urethral tone. At times, surgical intervention is needed.

Overflow incontinence represents approximately 10% of cases and is often described as being associated with a diminished stream and leakage of small amounts of urine. It might be the result of urethral obstruction because of prostatic enlargement or a urethral stricture. It might also be the result of a distended acontractile bladder such as occurs in diabetes mellitus or as a complication of anticholinergic drugs. A urologic evaluation is essential to rule out obstruction. Cessation of anticholinergic medications is important, and if obstruction is ruled out, a trial of cholinergic agonists may be initiated.

Functional incontinence accounts for the remaining 10% of cases. This type is the result of the patient's physical inability to reach the toilet in time. It is usually a result of a problem with mobility, such as advanced arthritis, muscle weakness, or strokes. Treatment centers on making toilet facilities more readily available or obtaining a bedside commode.

The role of the primary care physician in the recognition and management of this incontinence is essential, and particularly involves coordinating the involvement of the multiple disciplines of nursing, social work, and urology (20). An indwelling Foley catheter should be avoided except in rare circumstances, such as with the presence of severe pressure sores. Significant advances have been made in clinical research in the treatment of incontinence. Once believed to be a disorder surgically treated by the urologist with little success, new data suggest that modalities initiated by the primary physician, coupling medical treatment with exercise and behavioral management, can result in improvement of most community-dwelling, cognitively intact elderly individuals with incontinence (21). While many osteopathic clinicians report increased efficacy when manipulative management is added to this regimen, studies are underway to document its efficacy.

Falling

Gait disorders and instability often result in falls in the elderly, and have a profound impact on the clinical care of older individuals.

Accidents are the fifth leading cause of death in the elderly; approximately 70% of accidents result from falls. Considering the decrease in bone mineral density with age, fractures of the hip, femur, wrist, and humerus are not uncommon. Hip fractures lead to hospitalization, complications of surgery, and complications of immobility. There is a significant risk of institutionalization after hip fracture; some clinicians report mortality rates as high as 20%. Until recently, little attention has been focused on why the elderly fall and what measures can be taken to prevent falls and their consequences. Changes in postural control such as a decrease in proprioception and muscle tone, a slower righting reflex, and an increase in postural sway are all thought to contribute to falls. The increased incidence of various disorders with age, such as degenerative joint disease, strokes, peripheral neuropathy, muscle weakness, and impaired vision, are all believed to contribute to the increased frequency of falls. The causes for falls in the elderly are classified as either extrinsic or intrinsic. Extrinsic causes account for approximately 50% of falls and are largely a result of environmental factors such as poor lighting, throw rugs and frayed carpets, unstable furniture, and inappropriate bed or toilet heights. Intrinsic causes for falls include such problems as syncope, drop attacks, cardiac dysrhythmias, strokes, transient ischemic attacks, seizures, Parkinson disease, and orthostatic hypotension (Table 23.9) (22). Drugs such as antihypertensives, sedatives, antipsychotics, and hypoglycemics are also common causes of falls in the elderly.

Evaluation of the falling patient should include a careful history of prior falls, a review of the patient's medical status, and a list of all current medications. The review of systems should include questioning the patient regarding symptoms suggesting transient ischemic attack, dysrhythmia, seizure, and so on. A careful physical examination should include supine and standing blood pressures for orthostasis, an assessment of visual acuity, evidence of joint or limb deformity, disorders of the feet, and evidence of muscle weakness or sensory deficits found in the neurologic examination. Gait should also be observed. A careful structural examination can reveal musculoskeletal abnormalities that might be contributory. Depending on the results of the history and physical, various laboratory studies such as a complete blood count, electrolytes, and blood urea nitrogen might be in order. Other studies that might be appropriate include an electroencephalogram, CT of the head, electrocardiogram, 24-hour Holter monitor, or carotid Doppler. An evaluation by a physical therapist and a home environmental assessment for hazards by a visiting nurse or occupational therapist are often necessary.

Management consists of treating the primary underlying disorder if discovered. Physical therapy for gait training and use of an assistive device such as a walker or cane might be in order. Environmental manipulation such as improving lighting, increasing toilet height, and installing safety bars might also be necessary. The team approach to care of the falling patient, incorporating the nurse, physical therapist, occupational therapist, and others, can contribute significantly to the outcome. Recent research has revealed that this approach can reduce the frequency of falling for elderly individuals who have a high risk of falling by 30% (23).

Research is under way to demonstrate the impact of osteopathic manipulative treatment (OMT) on prevention of falls in the elderly. Specialized assessment programs for falls have

TABLE 23.9. INTRINSIC CONDITIONS LEADING TO FALLS AMONG OLDER ADULTS

Condition	Symptoms Along with Fall
Orthostatic hypotension	Lightheadedness with postural change
	Palpitation or postural sway along with postural change
Diabetes mellitus	Reduced sensation of lower extremities
Vitamin B$_{12}$ deficiency	Reduced proprioception
Cardiac arrhythmia	Palpitation, shortness of breath, dizziness, or syncope
Transient ischemic attack or cerebrovascular accident	Unilateral weakness, visual disturbance, or speech changes
Seizure	Aura, urinary or bowel incontinence, or syncope
Osteoarthritis of hips or knees	Weakness in quadriceps or knees (or both)
Hyperthyroidism/ hypothyroidism	Proximal muscle weakness of lower extremities
Polymyalgia rheumatica	Pelvic girdle weakness or quadricep muscle weakness (or both)
Normal pressure hydrocephalus	Ataxic gait, urinary incontinence, and dementia
Central nervous system lesion	Mental status change
	Focal neurologic deficit
Ménière's syndrome, labyrinthitis, or benign positional vertigo	Poor balance, ataxia, vertigo, dizziness
Hypoglycemia	Acute onset of mental status change, tremors, dizziness, weakness, or diaphoresis
Alcohol intoxication	Ataxic gait, mental status change, slurred speech

(From Cavalieri TA, Gray-Miceli D. Evaluating and preventing falls among the elderly population. *JAOA.* 1994;94(7):610–614, with permission.)

contributed to much needed clinical research relevant to this important clinical syndrome in the elderly (24).

Iatrogenesis

The elderly are particularly prone to iatrogenic disorders. Altered homeostasis coupled with the failure of physicians to recognize the special needs of the elderly contribute to the increased frequency of iatrogenesis in this age group. Common iatrogenic problems in the elderly include polypharmacy, immobility, and unnecessary hospitalization. The elderly have a high frequency of adverse drug reactions; studies show that the incidence of adverse drug reactions increases significantly with age. It has been reported that approximately 40% of hospitalized elderly patients develop an adverse drug reaction. Studies have also demonstrated that approximately 3% of all hospital admissions are the result of drug-induced disease, and the majority of these patients are elderly. Studies show that adverse drug reactions increase with the number of medications taken. These observations are believed to occur because of a decrease in the therapeutic window with age. Both pharmacokinetic and pharmacodynamic changes occur that predispose the elderly to adverse drug reactions. Changes in body composition, such as a decline in serum albumin, altered hepatic metabolism, a decline in renal function, and changes in absorption, all contribute to the pharmacokinetic alterations.

Changes in receptors with age result in altered sensitivity to certain drugs. All of these changes are compounded by the problem of polypharmacy, common with the elderly. Elderly people take approximately four to five medications; nursing home patients average eight medications. It is estimated that approximately 25% of medications prescribed for the elderly are unnecessary. Reflex drug prescribing has led to unnecessary medications. Appropriate and rational drug prescribing for the elderly is essential. Effective nonpharmacologic treatment modalities, such as OMT, are particularly preferred for the care of the elderly when indicated.

Unnecessary bed rest and immobility are common iatrogenic problems for the elderly patient, particularly in hospitals and nursing homes. Physicians often fail to recognize the complications of immobility for their patients and neglect orders such as appropriate ambulation, rotating the patient, or physical therapy consultations. Consequences of prolonged immobility and bed rest include:

- Pressure sores
- Pneumonia
- Venous thromboembolism
- Constipation
- Contractures
- Urinary incontinence

Manipulative treatment might prevent many of the complications experienced by immobile geriatric patients. The rib-raising technique is easily performed and has a beneficial effect on the circulatory, respiratory, and nervous systems. The integral relationship of structure and function is the osteopathic concept most applicable to the consequences of immobility. Musculoskeletal activity is essential to maintain homeostatic mechanisms.

Admission to the hospital can result in significant dangers to the health of the elderly, unnecessary hospitalization should be avoided. Aside from the potential complications of medication and bed rest, hospitalized patients experience increased hazards as a result of diagnostic and therapeutic procedures and nosocomial infections. Diagnostic procedures that incorporate contrast media, such as arteriography, cardiac catheterization, or intravenous pyelography, are potentially risky procedures for the elderly because of a higher incidence of contrast-induced renal disease in the aged kidney. Elderly patients with diabetes mellitus and dehydration have an even greater risk of developing contrast-induced renal disease. Hospitalized elderly patients are also at high risk of developing virulent nosocomial infections as a result of potential immunosuppression related to their underlying illness as well as age-related changes in immune function. Microorganisms such as *Staphylococcus* or Gram-negative rods rapidly colonize the oropharynx, skin, or urinary tract and predispose the elderly to hospital-acquired pneumonias, urinary tract infections, and wound infections. The physician treating geriatric patients should consider every attempt to avoid hospitalization of the patient in their management approach. Specialized acute care for the elderly units have been shown to be more effective for the management of elderly patients requiring admission to the hospital. Management is provided by a multidisciplinary team of health care professionals specially trained in the care of the elderly

patient. Beneficial outcomes have included:

- Decrease in medication use
- Avoidance of nursing home placement
- Improvement in functional status
- Improved survival rate

More research is needed to determine the effectiveness of geriatric units in acute care hospitals (9).

GERIATRICS AND OSTEOPATHIC MEDICINE

The past few decades have seen enormous growth and development of the discipline of geriatric medicine in the United States. This has been an outgrowth of recognized unmet needs of the elderly within our health care system. Osteopathic principles and practice mesh nicely with basic concepts of geriatric medicine and offer osteopathic medicine a unique role in the growth and development of geriatrics in this country.

Incorporation of manipulative treatment into the clinical care of the elderly is an important modality of treatment that osteopathic physicians have as part of their therapeutic approach. Physicians often approach these patients with the use of pharmacologic treatment and fail to incorporate other modalities of treatment such as physical therapy or manipulative treatment. Medications such as nonsteroidal antiinflammatory agents often have adverse effects on the elderly, heightening the importance of including nonpharmacologic means of treatment. Manipulative techniques are beneficial to the elderly; as with any therapeutic modality, there might be a need to adjust certain approaches to fit the special needs of the elderly patient. The increased frequency of osteoporosis and decline in bone mineral density with age should discourage the use of certain high-thrust, high-velocity techniques in the elderly. Soft-tissue manipulation using muscle- and fascia-stretching techniques is particularly effective for many of the musculoskeletal complaints of the elderly.

Range of motion, respiratory, muscle energy, and craniosacral techniques are all beneficial approaches for geriatric patients. Although OMT is a valuable tool in the management of geriatric patients, controlled, randomized studies are under way to document its efficacy and expand its acceptance (25).

CONCLUSION

Many principles that have guided osteopathic medicine for decades are the same principles that are at the heart of geriatric medicine. The whole-person approach of osteopathic medicine is essential to geriatric care and involves a multidisciplinary, multidimensional approach to the evaluation and management of the elderly that considers the medical, socioeconomic, psychological, and functional aspects of the patient. The primary care setting is the best forum in which to implement this comprehensive care program. Primary care, stressing health maintenance, has been a true strength of osteopathic medicine and is vital to holistic geriatric care. The integral relationship of structure to function has been at the core of osteopathic medicine and is epitomized in the philosophy of geriatric medicine that has as its goal the maintenance of function. Osteopathic physicians are uniquely qualified to meet the health care needs of the elderly.

REFERENCES

1. Butler RN. Geriatrics and internal medicine. *Ann Intern Med.* 1979;91: 903–908.
2. National Center for Health Statistics. Health, United States, 1999, with Health and Aging Chartbook. Hyattsville, MD: US Department of Health and Human Services, 1999; DHHS Pub. no. (PHS) 99–1232.
3. Yates FE. Theories of aging: biological. In: *Encyclopedia of Gerontology,* vol. 2, 1996:545–555.
4. Hayflick L. *How and Why We Age.* New York, NY: Ballantine Books; 1994.
5. Kenney A. *Physiology of Aging.* Chicago, IL: Year Book Medical Publishers; 1989.
6. National Institutes of Health. Geriatric Assessment Methods for Clinical Decision-Making. National Institutes of Health Consensus Development Conference Statement. Bethesda, MD: US Department of Health and Human Services. Public Health Service; October 1987;6(23).
7. Cavalieri TA, Chopra A, Gray-Miceli D, et al. Geriatric assessment teams in nursing homes: do they work? *JAOA.* 1993(Dec);93(12).
8. Cavalieri TA, Chopra A, Bryman P. When outside the norm is normal: interpreting lab data in the aged. *Geriatrics.* 1992;47(5):66–70.
9. Kane R, Ouslander J, Abrass I. *Essentials of Clinical Geriatrics.* New York, NY: McGraw-Hill Co; 1999.
10. Kane RA, Kane RL. *Assessing the Elderly: A Practical Guide to Measurement.* Lexington, MA: Lexington Books; 1981:46–49.
11. Schor EL, Lerner DJ, Malspeis S. Physician's assessment of functional health status and well-being. The patients' perspective. *Arch Intern Med.* 1995;155(3):309–314.
12. Folstein MJ, Folstein S, McHugh PR. Mini-Mental State: a practical method for grading the cognitive state of patients for the clinician. *J Psychiatr Res.* 1975;12:189–198.
13. Yeasavage JA, Brink TL. Development and validation of a geriatric depression screening scale: a preliminary report. *J Psychiatr Res.* 1983;17(1):37–49.
14. *Diagnostic and Statistical Manual of Mental Disorders,* 4th ed. Washington, DC: American Psychiatric Association; 1994.
15. Cavalieri TA. Acute confusional states in the geriatric population. *JAOA.* 1984;83(11):801–805.
16. Barry PP, Moskowitz MA. The diagnosis of reversible dementia in the elderly. *Arch Intern Med.* 1988;148:1914–1917.
17. Cain T, Jurivich DA. Primary care guidelines for the evaluation of confusion in the elderly. *JAOA.* 1994;94(7):601–605.
18. Small GW. Treatment of Alzheimer's disease: current approaches and promising developments. *Am J Med* 1998;104(4A):32S–38S.
19. Small GW, Rabins TV, Barry PP, et al. Diagnosis and treatment of Alzheimer disease and related disorders. Consensus statement of the American Association for Geriatric Psychiatry, the Alzheimer's Association, and the American Geriatrics Society. *JAMA* 1997;278:1363–1371.
20. Burgio KL, Locher JL, Goode PS. Combined behavioral and drug therapy for urge incontinence in older women. *J Am Geriatr Soc* 2000 Apr;48(4):370–374.
21. Scientific Committee of the First International Consultation on Incontinence. Assessment and treatment of urinary incontinence. *Lancet* 2000;355:2153–2158.
22. Cavalieri TA, Gray-Miceli D. Evaluating and preventing falls among the elderly population. *JAOA.* 1994;94(7):610–614.
23. Tinetti ME, Baker DL, McAvary G, et al. A multifactorial interaction to reduce the risk of falling among elderly people living in the community. *N Engl J Med.* 1994;331(13):821–827.
24. Close J, Ellis M, Hooper R, et al. Prevention of falls in the elderly trial (PROFET): a randomised controlled trial. *Lancet* 1999;353:93–97.
25. Dodson D. Manipulative therapy for the geriatric patient. *Osteopath Ann.* 1979;7(3):115–119.

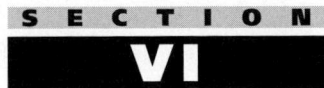

SECTION

VI

OSTEOPATHIC CONSIDERATIONS IN THE CLINICAL SPECIALTIES

INTRODUCTION

MICHAEL A. SEFFINGER

Although predominantly primary care oriented, osteopathic physicians have engaged in a wide variety of specialty disciplines since the early years of the profession. Included among these are general and orthopedic surgery, ophthalmology, otorhinolaryngology, and obstetrics and gynecology. Barred from allopathic hospitals, early DOs founded their own hospitals and specialty training programs (see Chapter 2).

Several mixed staff U.S. institutions offer both American Osteopathic Association (AOA) and Accreditation Council for Graduate Medical Education (ACGME) accreditation. Graduates of these programs are eligible to sit for both the osteopathic and allopathic specialty boards, and become members of each organization.

As of 2000, AOA records indicate the following:

62% of its membership list themselves in a primary care field
29% are in nonprimary care specialties, including subspecialty internal medicine
3% practice obstetrics and gynecology
0.85% list themselves as osteopathic manipulative medicine (OMM) specialists

This edition of *Foundations for Osteopathic Medicine* presents a number of changes in this section. Both geriatrics and pediatrics are now linked with the Primary Care section (Section V). Three chapters—nephrology, hypertension, gastroenterology—were dropped, chapters on emergency medicine, neuromusculoskeletal medicine and osteopathic manipulative medicine have been added, and chapters devoted to physical medicine and rehabilitation, sports medicine, and surgery have been expanded.

CARDIOLOGY

Chapter 24 has been updated and expanded. Felix Rogers uses a more current interpretation of osteopathic tenets that includes osteopathically oriented patient care guidelines for commonly occurring cardiovascular problems, including angina pectoris, coronary artery disease, and congestive heart failure.

OSTEOPATHIC MANAGEMENT OF EAR, NOSE, AND THROAT DISEASES

In Chapter 25, Harriet and Michael Shaw offer osteopathic approaches, including manipulative treatment, to the most common ear, nose, and throat (ENT) problems such as sinusitis, otitis media, and pharyngitis. Anatomy and physiology of the head and neck structures and associated pathophysiologic changes are concisely reviewed.

OSTEOPATHIC MEDICINE IN THE PRACTICE OF EMERGENCY MEDICINE

Peter Adler-Michaelson, Bernadette Peters, and Raul Garcia provide this new chapter (Chapter 26) with an osteopathic perspective for patients seen in the emergency department (ED). Although emergency care is fairly well standardized, the potential benefit associated with assessments of mechanically related neuromusculoskeletal problems is not commonly addressed either diagnostically or therapeutically. This is particularly true for problems that respond well to osteopathic manipulative treatment. In this offering, the authors use common chief complaints of patients presenting to the ED, such as, head, chest, or abdominal pain, to highlight ways in which osteopathically oriented thinking and management can make a real difference.

GENERAL SURGERY

In the first edition of this text, Sydney Ross covered the history of the general surgery discipline, the osteopathic approach to chest and abdominal surgery, and the appropriate use of osteopathic manipulative treatment (OMT) in treating and preventing postoperative complications. In this edition, Chapter 27 has been expanded by Constance Cashen to include selected examples of osteopathically oriented surgical evaluation and management of patients presenting with acute abdominal pain. As the author discusses a variety of interdependent relationships among visceral, neuroanatomic, and pathophysiologic processes, she also presents the use of adjunctive OMT for the prevention of postoperative ileus and atelectasis.

GYNECOLOGY AND OBSTETRICS

Melicien Tettambel has updated and refined her excellent chapters (Chapters 28 and 31) from the first edition. Women's health care has always been integral to the philosophy of osteopathy. These two chapters are intended to illustrate the application of osteopathic principles to some of the more common health care issues of women, including their neuromusculoskeletal components (see Chapter 1).

NEUROMUSCULAR MEDICINE AND OSTEOPATHIC MANIPULATIVE MEDICINE

Raymond J. Hruby has contributed this new specialty chapter (Chapter 29). Osteopathic palpatory diagnosis and manipulative treatment are the hallmarks of the osteopathic physician. The osteopathic physician who specializes in neuromuscular medicine and osteopathic manipulative medicine (NMM/OMM) is uniquely qualified to manage primary care problems or consult as a specialist on both hospitalized and ambulatory patients. Dr. Hruby presents an excellent overview of this new field.

NEUROLOGY

Unchanged from the first edition, in Chapter 30 Mitchell Elkiss and Louis Rentz look at the common neurologic disorders of headache, various spinal disorders, entrapment neuropathies, carpal tunnel syndrome, and chronic pain syndrome in light of osteopathic evaluation and management, including the use of OMT.

ONCOLOGY

First edition authors Michael Opipari, Augustine Perrotta, and David R. Essig-Beatty have updated and reorganized their material, emphasizing an osteopathically oriented, patient-centered approach for this large patient population (Chapter 32). Physicians need to be aware of musculoskeletal manifestations of primary tumors and metastasis. It is particularly important for the osteopathic physician who uses palpatory diagnosis and manipulative treatment to recognize manifestations of cancer and the potential benefits and risks of applying manual procedures to patients with oncologic disease. A discussion of appropriate utilization of OMM in this patient population in the light of common sense, experience, and evidence-based research literature review makes this chapter especially valuable.

ORTHOPEDICS

Richard Scott, Michael Kuchera, and Jeff Patterson expanded Chapter 33 to include osteopathic orthopedic approaches to the patient with shoulder instability, including concepts and principles of orthopedic medicine and prolotherapy. This complements the examples included in the first edition of osteopathic orthopedic approaches to common problems of the knee, hip, and lower back.

PULMONOLOGY

Gilbert D'Alonzo and Samuel Krachman have made Chapter 34 a definitive treatise on the osteopathic approach to patients with problems of the pulmonary system. An excellent discussion of the mechanics of pulmonary function is presented. The authors provide a thorough review of the osteopathic research literature on palpatory diagnosis and OMT for patients with pulmonary dysfunction as published in the *Journal of the American Osteopathic Association* over its 100-year history. They concisely summarize the evidence in support of osteopathic manipulative methods applicable to this patient population.

OSTEOPATHIC PHYSICAL MEDICINE AND REHABILITATION

In a rewritten and expanded chapter (Chapter 35), Michael Wieting and James Lipton focus on the OMM aspects of osteopathic physical medicine and rehabilitation (OPM&R). A concise history of the discipline is offered along with a review of the current evidence-based research literature related to manipulative medicine. Rehabilitation of the patient with common musculoskeletal problems, such as chronic low back pain, carpal tunnel syndrome, and sports injuries are used to demonstrate an osteopathic approach in evaluation and management.

RHEUMATOLOGY

Chapter 36 has been updated and expanded by Michael Finley, who provides considerable review of pertinent literature related to a modern osteopathic approach to rheumatologic problems and clearly defines the role of OMT in this patient population. He also provides a clear and concise osteopathic history and physical evaluation process for the patient suspected of, or already diagnosed as having a rheumatologic disease. In addition to highlighting osteopathic principles integral to the treatment of rheumatic diseases, the chapter provides a general overview of the knowledge and advances in treatment developed since the first edition of this text.

SPORTS MEDICINE

As specialists in the care of the musculoskeletal system, osteopathic physicians have been held in high regard by athletes for more than a century. Per Gunnar Brolinson, Kurt Heinking and Albert Kozar have rewritten and expanded Chapter 37 to give a comprehensive osteopathic perspective on the discipline of sports medicine. Included is osteopathic evaluation and management of the injured athlete, sideline care as a team physician, pathologic mechanics of sports and exercise-related injuries, and appropriate utilization of OMT.

INTRODUCTION TO THE FIRST EDITION

FELIX J. ROGERS

Osteopathic medicine is a comprehensive, integrated approach to patient care. Although the traditional strength of osteopathic medicine has been in primary care medicine, osteopathic physicians now provide health care within all specialties and most subspecialties of medicine and surgery.

The chapters that follow focus on dimensions of clinical practice that characterize or elucidate aspects of osteopathic philosophy or practice. Each chapter also reviews current and past research within the osteopathic profession. In some cases, additional scientific literature is incorporated because it directly pertains to issues central to osteopathic medicine. Each chapter provides a brief overview of the field of medicine described or discusses pertinent topics within the field; none are intended to represent a comprehensive description of the discipline.

DEFINING DISTINCTIVENESS

This section has 14 chapters representative of the clinical disciplines. Many subjects are not included, especially in the subspecialty areas of medicine and surgery. The topics included were chosen as examples of the manner in which osteopathic principles have been applied to these clinical areas. Other fields of study may not be included because of a paucity of osteopathic research in that area, because the implementation of osteopathic tenets is more complex or difficult to express, or because the osteopathic approach is so similar to another field that its inclusion would be redundant.

Medicine functions as a mix of clinical experience, expert opinion, and scientific evidence. Yesterday's expert opinion is regularly overturned by today's scientific evidence. More precise scientific evidence supersedes more general scientific evidence. Sometimes scientific evidence catches up with accepted clinical practice. It would be pleasant to think that we could define as scientific what we do every day in patient care, but this is not the case.

Osteopathic medicine, as a minority profession with certain philosophic emphases, is especially pressured to prove itself in the scientific arena. There are inherent difficulties in this endeavor, however, because of the global nature of osteopathy's philosophic emphases. It is hard to define even small, measurable hypotheses to test such tenets as structure-function interrelationships, or the full nature of viscerosomatic or somatovisceral reflexes.

At the same time, osteopathic medicine is obligated to define its distinctiveness. One aspect of our profession is that we have defining characteristics; we endeavor as a group to establish guiding principles to represent a philosophic and scientific basis for health care. The following chapters describe the extent to which these principles can be applied to the practice of medicine in the

clinical specialties. Other distinctive features of the osteopathic profession include:

Characteristics of students selected for admission to medical schools
The osteopathic educational process
An emphasis on primary care, especially in underserved areas
An orientation to clinical service as opposed to research and academic growth
A reliance on the patient–physician relationship as a key element in health care

These distinctive features are addressed in other sections of this textbook.

OSTEOPATHIC MANIPULATIVE TREATMENT AND CLINICAL PRACTICE

Osteopathic specialists must consider how osteopathic manipulative treatment (OMT), a modality distinct in this profession, might fit in with current clinical practice. Several clinical outcomes and related basic science research projects have suggested how and under what conditions manipulative interventions might work, but more extensive study is needed.

Because all medical practice is based on a significant proportion of clinical experience and expert opinion, osteopathic thought and, when appropriate, manipulative treatment are included in this introductory survey of clinical specialty correlations.

The chapters in this section represent a variety of approaches to osteopathic specialty practice and are different from one another. Each represents one or more tenets of traditional osteopathic philosophy: structure-function interrelationship, self-healing, and integration of systems. Some disciplines involve more obviously musculoskeletal problems than others; in other chapters other tenets are emphasized.

In practice, osteopathic medicine is a method of health care delivery implemented by an individual physician's approach to patient–physician relationships. In some cases, the relationship concentrates on the musculoskeletal system, either as the primary expression of disease or because of its integral relationship to health and/or a disease process. In this case, musculoskeletal palpatory diagnosis and OMT represent issues of such central importance that they are both necessary and sufficient for patient care. Other circumstances within the field of medicine are such that, while the musculoskeletal system might play a role in the patient's well being, the application of palpatory diagnosis and OMT might be considered adjunctive rather than primary.

For example, in obstetrics, sports medicine, psychiatry, and pain management, there are clear indications for OMT that allow for the most complete expression of comprehensive patient care management. Conversely, although OMT can be significantly beneficial in the treatment of the patient during pregnancy, labor, and delivery, the indications for OMT might be less frequently found in a general gynecology practice or in some of the medical specialties.

Recognizing the central role of the neuromusculoskeletal system in disease and health maintenance, osteopathic physicians have used OMT as a means to implement their philosophic principles. Remember that OMT is a tool for applying a philosophy, not the philosophy itself. Various approaches are now used to intervene with the neuromusculoskeletal system, including exercise, yoga, biofeedback, transcutaneous electrical nerve stimulation, acupuncture, and tai chi. Because each of these modalities, including manipulation, is used by health care practitioners outside the osteopathic profession, one might conclude that a defining characteristic of osteopathic medicine is not found in practice patterns that are in exclusive use. The key feature is the philosophic orientation behind the application of these methods of health care, with an emphasis on the role of the neuromusculoskeletal system.

The evolution of medicine in the 20th century has also changed the way in which OMT is used. With the development of new technologies, including imaging techniques, new pharmacologic agents, and the growth of molecular medicine, palpatory diagnosis and OMT might play a proportionately smaller role in some fields than they did in the recent past. These facts do not deny their historical or present importance. If OMT did in fact save tens of thousands of lives during the influenza epidemic after World War I (1), we would concede that it represented the best therapy available at that time. If genetic engineering were to provide a breakthrough to create specific antiviral agents to treat a similar influenza epidemic, we would all rejoice that more effective therapy is now available.

The development of effective antihypertensive agents has moved OMT to an adjunctive role in the treatment of hypertension, in contrast to a legitimate interest in studying the effectiveness of this modality a few decades ago. Ironically, the technological advances in heart transplantation might be seen as causing the opposite reaction. When patients on the waiting list for a heart transplant are enrolled in a program of cardiac rehabilitation exercise, a significant number show such improvement in their functional status that they are removed from the transplant list. This is because of enhanced musculoskeletal function, not because of a change in their cardiac status.

In those clinical sciences in which highly technical developments have come to the forefront, the osteopathic physician might have the greatest relevance because they can provide the comprehensive perspective and integrated philosophies that characterize the best of medical care. For example, diagnostic methods and therapies for patients with heart disease have proliferated dramatically in recent years. Unfortunately, so has the general tendency to apply all methods to all patients, even without scientific rationale. A clinical management strategy based on concepts of the unity of body, structure-function relationships, and the intrinsic ability of the body to heal still constitutes the most rational means of diagnosis and therapy as described in the following chapters.

The degree to which palpatory diagnosis and OMT are applied in each specialty varies considerably depending on the nature of that specialty, the applicability of manual medicine, and the scientific research to support use of these methods. Nonetheless, each chapter is based on the basic tenets of osteopathic medicine as defined more than 100 years ago.

CONCLUSION

Both the generalist and the specialist are obliged to use the best information available for the care of the patient. In some instances, this remains clinical experience, the tradition that has worked for osteopathic physicians throughout the profession's history. To make the best use of this experience, we rely on expert opinion. When scientific evidence is directly or indirectly available, it should be used. All three types of authority are reflected in these chapters. Each author has attempted to make clear the strength of the scientific evidence that underlies recommendations for treatment. The goal is always that of whole patient care, in itself one of the traditional values of the osteopathic profession.

REFERENCES

1. Smith RK. One hundred thousand cases of influenza with a death rate of one-fortieth of that officially reported under conventional medical treatment. *JAOA*. 1920;21:172–175.

AN OSTEOPATHIC PERSPECTIVE ON CARDIOLOGY

FELIX J. ROGERS

KEY CONCEPTS

■ It is appropriate to consider the cardiovascular system in terms of a modern interpretation of the basic tenets of osteopathic medicine and principles for patient care.

■ The growth of technology and scientific discovery in the field of coronary atherosclerosis has led to two contrasting developments. On the one hand, acute coronary syndromes are now understood in terms of local cellular and molecular mechanisms, for which highly specific, technical interventions are appropriate. On the other hand, the vast majority of cases of coronary heart disease are preventable, since the cause of coronary atherosclerosis is primarily related to diet and lifestyle.

■ The muscle hypothesis represents a model for heart failure that supplements the traditional approaches to heart failure and highlights the emphasis of the osteopathic profession on the musculoskeletal system.

■ A comprehensive approach to the patient with cardiovascular disease requires the incorporation of evidence based guidelines and an emphasis on primary and secondary disease prevention through lifestyle modification. The osteopathic profession has an historical mandate to provide emphasis to both components.

Cardiology represents the largest component of internal medicine, and heart disease is the leading cause of mortality in the United States. Screening for heart disease is an essential component of every comprehensive evaluation performed by a family practitioner, surgeon, anesthesiologist, or internist. The components of a cardiovascular screening evaluation are the history, physical examination, electrocardiogram (ECG), and chest x-ray film. In this chapter, these components are starting points for the evaluation of patients with ischemic heart disease and congestive heart failure. These two categories represent more than 75% of the patients with heart disease that practicing osteopathic physicians see. The pathophysiology of these disease processes is discussed along with the natural history, diagnosis, and therapy. The goal

of this chapter is to present a brief review of these two parts of the field of cardiology to clarify the application of osteopathic concepts; important subjects such as arrhythmias, valvular heart disease, hypertension, and congenital heart disease are not discussed.

It is appropriate to consider the cardiovascular system in terms of a modern interpretation of the basic tenets of osteopathic medicine and principles for patient care (1). Because this is a textbook primarily aimed at medical students, each of these tenets and principles will be listed in the overview, to provide a context for the discussion of pathophysiology and natural history and treatment of coronary heart disease and heart failure. It is hoped that medical students will incorporate these tenets and principles as benchmarks against which they can evaluate the medical literature in a critical manner, assess the relevance of osteopathic principles, and verify the applicability of the material that they read and study.

OVERVIEW

Tenet I: A Person Is the Product of Dynamic Interaction between Body, Mind, and Spirit

The heart is a remarkable organ. It can be removed from one person and transplanted into another and it still maintains its basic function and rhythmic activity. In fact, isolated strips of heart muscle can be placed in a physiologic bath, and these characteristics prevail. However, the optimal function of the heart occurs when it is in its appropriate context, in an intact person, with a complex control system and multiple inputs. There are an astounding array of interactions for the heart, including autonomic control of the heart, the hypothalamic-pituitary-adrenal axis, hormonal modulation, and interactions between the heart and the brain, cognitive and neuropsychiatric function, and circadian and ultradian function.

Consider further that the heart needs to pump every minute of every day and every year. It needs to respond appropriately to the activities of daily living, to sleep, and to sudden strenuous exertion. It needs to participate in instantaneous control of the blood pressure in spite of challenges of posture, temperature, and psychological stress.

Heart disease is the most common cause of death in United States, and chronic heart failure and coronary heart disease

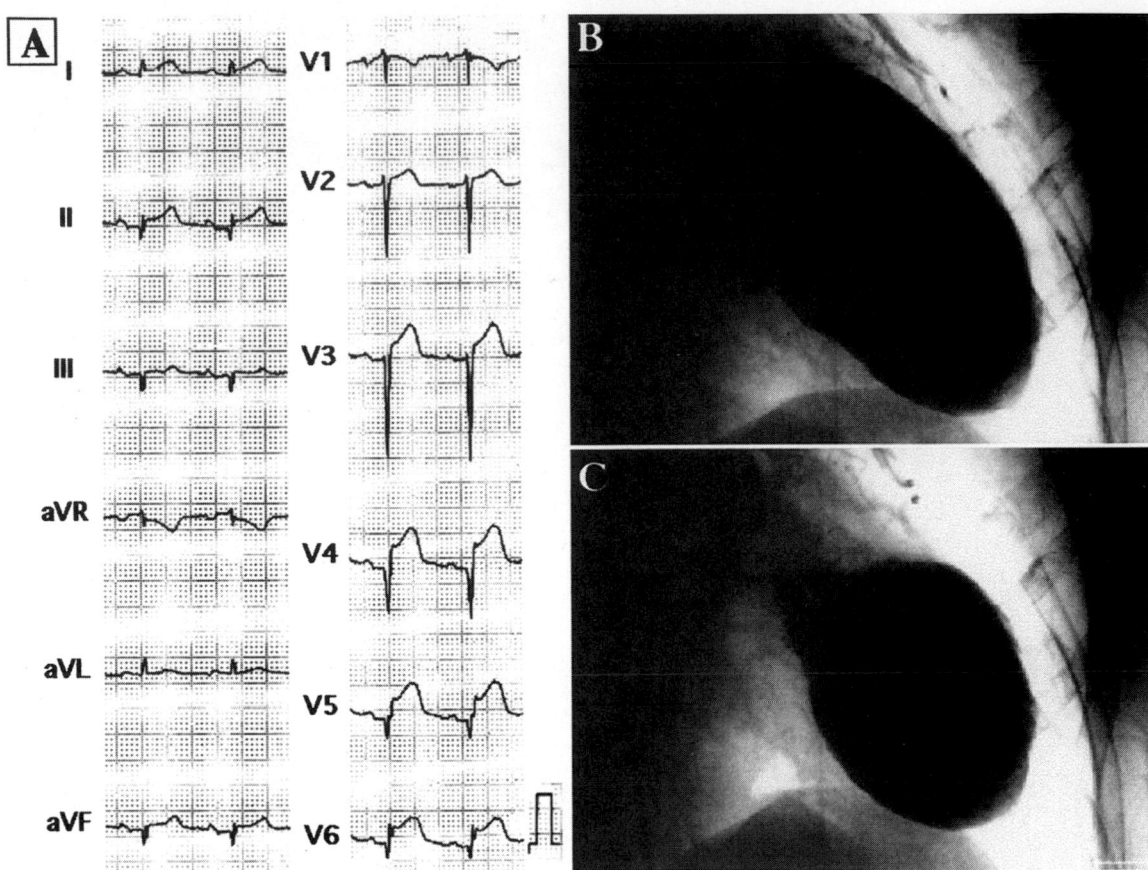

FIGURE 24.1. This patient presented with subdural hematoma and was shown to have evidence of acute anterior wall myocardial infarction on electrocardiogram (**Panel A**). Subsequently, cardiac catheterization showed normal coronary arteries. Left ventriculography demonstrated a large area of apical akinesia that is most evident when the diastolic (**Panel B**) and systolic (**Panel C**) images are compared. The wall motion abnormality resolved completely within 3 days. (From Ohtsuka T, Hamada M, Kodama K, et al. Neurogenic stunned myocardium. *Circulation* 2000;101:2122–2124, with permission.)

represent two of the most common chronic diseases in our society, especially in the geriatric population. Although it may be a chronic, slowly progressive disorder, cardiac deaths occur suddenly, and approximately one-fourth of all cardiac deaths occur without any warning or any premonitory signs.

The heart is well innervated and participates in a broad range of reflexes (2–12), including the viscerosomatic reflexes that are a major feature of classic osteopathic theory. The heart has extrinsic efferent (sympathetic and parasympathetic) and afferent innervation and also possesses an intrinsic (intracardiac) nerve supply (13–15). The extrinsic and intrinsic nerve supplies interact with one another and this intrinsic nervous system may even function as a "mini-brain" within the heart, to provide a "fine-tuning" of cardiac dynamics (13). The classic transmitters are adrenergic and cholinergic, but other important neurotransmitters coexist with these in the same nerve fibers, including adenosine, cardiac neuropeptides, somatostatin, and nitric oxide (13).

As we have all experienced, our emotional state is accompanied by alterations of heart rate and blood pressure. Anger and stress have been associated with the occurrence of cardiac disorders like sudden death, arrhythmias, and myocardial infarction (MI). Cardiovascular activity is regulated by a system comprised of various tightly connected diencephalic, midbrain, brainstem, and

spinal structures, in which the hypothalamus is functioning as the highest level of command (16). Regional damage to the central nervous system may also affect emotions and the functioning of the cardiovascular system. Figure 24.1 shows an example of extensive myocardial stunning that occurred in a patient with normal coronary arteries and a subdural hematoma (17).

A definite circadian pattern of onset of MI was demonstrated in the Myocardial Infarction Limitation Study (18). The increase in morning incidence of acute ischemic coronary events has been attributed to an increase in catecholamines and sensitivity of vascular receptors, increasing coronary vasomotor tone, and an increasing myocardial oxygen demand, all of which lower the threshold for ischemia (19).

The autonomic nervous system is also organized according to circadian influences, and important physiologic changes occur in the levels of circulating corticosteroids, vasopressin, and other components of the hypothalamic-pituitary-adrenal axis as well (20). Other biologic rhythms have also been demonstrated for cardiovascular events. For example, the likelihood of MI is greater on a Monday than any other day of the week (21). More MIs occur in the winter than in the summer. This holds true for areas in which it is warm in the winter (the southern United States) as well as those areas with a cold winter. This increase in winter mortality occurs in infants and dogs as well, and in both the Northern and Southern hemispheres. The common denominator appears not to be the stress of cold or the holidays, but the shorter days of winter, mediated by decreased daylight which is sensed by the suprachiasmic nucleus (22).

There are other well-defined examples of the interaction of the heart with other systems of the body. These include the cardiovascular response to stress, the hypothalamic-pituitary-adrenal system and the heart (23), the renin-angiotensin-aldosterone system (24) and systemic inflammation in patients with coronary artery disease (CAD) (25). Some of these will be discussed in more detail in the subsequent sections of this chapter.

The link between the heart and spirit goes back thousands of years. In Hebrew psychology, the heart is primarily the seat of the mind and will, together with a whole range of cyclical emotions (Hebrew *rŭah*, Greek *pneuma*, Latin *spiritus*) (26). Our language still contains many expressions in which the heart is used as a metaphor to express emotion, even though Western culture places emotional life in the brain, and not in the heart. Several non-Western societies place emotions in the heart (27,28).

Religion and spirituality are among the most important cultural factors that give structure and meaning to human values, behaviors, and experiences. Spirituality is a concept broader than religion and is primarily a dynamic, personal, and experiential process. One survey found that 94% of patients regard their spiritual health and their physical health as equally important (29). The implications of this for clinical practice have recently been reviewed (30). Studies have found that religious involvement is associated with less cardiovascular disease. Of 16 studies examined in a 2001 review (31), 12 found that religious involvement was associated with less cardiovascular disease or cardiovascular mortality. Religious involvement is associated with health-promoting behaviors, such as more exercise (32), proper nutrition (33), regular seat belt use (34), smoking cessation (32), and greater use of preventive services (35). The role of intercessory prayer on cardiac patients is less clear: A randomized, controlled trial conducted on 799 coronary care unit patients showed no significant effect (36).

Apart from the field of CAD, research in the last two decades demonstrates the complex nature of neural regulation of cardiovascular function and the components of the systemic effects mediated by cardiac receptors. Integration of cardiovascular function and interactive mechanisms with other body systems is modulated by local and systemic neuro-effector, humoral, and immunologic responses (37–42). Research has shown that these features have clinical significance in congestive heart failure (43–48). As well, research in therapy focuses on neuroendocrine modulation through exercise (49–52) and pharmacologic therapy (53–63) as an intermediate outcome, in addition to assessing health-related outcomes, such as functional status and mortality.

Tenet II: An Inherent Property of This Dynamic Interaction Is the Capacity of the Individual for the Maintenance of Health and Recovery from Disease

As physicians care for patients with heart disease over a period of years, they observe that the natural history of heart disease is quite different than other disease processes. Unlike chronic renal failure, diabetes, or metastatic cancer, in which there appears to be a relentless deterioration in the patient's condition, the clinical course of many patients with heart disease is characterized by exacerbation and remission. Many patients return to a virtually normal functional status, even after catastrophic experiences with MI or decompensation of left ventricular dysfunction.

CAD provides a clear example of inherent self-regulating and self-healing properties (64,65). A century ago, the rule of the artery was supreme. The dramatic role of revascularization therapy for acute MI makes this rule no less true today. The mechanism of atherosclerosis and the regulation of vascular smooth muscle tone are best understood in terms of the natural ability of the human organism to resist and combat harmful influences in the environment. Knowledge of self-regulation and self-healing forces at the arterial and arteriolar level forms the rational basis for the treatment of MI, angina pectoris, and congestive heart failure, as discussed in the following sections.

As more information is gathered about the pathophysiology of coronary atherosclerosis, and of left ventricular dysfunction, physicians are encouraged to adopt a long-term strategy of reversal, remodel, and regenerate. The past two decades have seen research that demonstrates lifestyle modifications, with or without medications to lower cholesterol, can halt or reverse the progression of atherosclerosis (66–68). It appears that the level of exercise intensity (69), diet (70), and antioxidants (71) are variables independent of serum cholesterol, which can have favorable effects on coronary events or regression of atherosclerosis. Patients with CAD and normal serum cholesterol gain significant benefit from further lowering of serum cholesterol (72). The evolving nature of this knowledge is shown by a recent study that found the combination of simvastatin plus niacin led to regression of coronary atherosclerosis, but this effect was attenuated when antioxidant vitamins were added to this treatment (73). In most studies, the rapid reduction in coronary events clearly precedes regression of atherosclerosis and is believed to represent a reestablishment of normal endothelial function (74–76).

Other dynamic aspects of arteries include angiogenesis and remodeling in response to the development of atherosclerosis. Although the development of collateral blood vessels (77) and the recannulation of occluded arterial segments have a beneficial effect in terms of improving blood flow, angiogenesis itself has been broadly linked to cancer (78,79). The neovascularization of proliferating vasa vasorum has been postulated to be a possible cause of plaque rupture (80).

Vascular remodeling is the phenomenon of compensatory enlargement in the presence of atherosclerosis to preserve near normal lumen diameter (Fig. 24.2). Initially described in monkeys fed an atherogenic diet, this biologic response has now been demonstrated in human coronary (81), carotid (82), and femoral (83) arteries. Functionally important lumen stenosis may be delayed until the lesion occupies 40% of the internal elastic lamina area. The preservation of a nearly normal lumen cross-sectional area should be taken into account in evaluating atherosclerotic disease with angiography (81). Lack of remodeling may be a major determinant in whether a person with coronary atherosclerosis develops any complications (84). The clinical application of intravascular ultrasound (IVUS) has provided clinicians with a

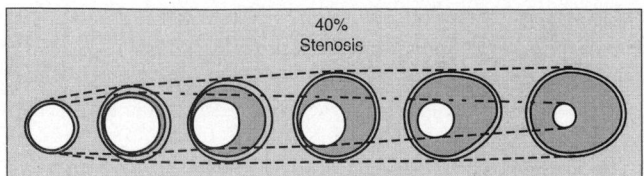

FIGURE 24.2. Possible sequence of changes in atherosclerotic arteries leading eventually to lumen narrowing. Artery enlarges initially (*left to right in diagram*) in association with plaque accumulation. (From Glagov S, Weisenberg E, Zarins CK, et al. Compensatory enlargement of human atherosclerotic coronary arteries. *N Engl J Med.* 1987;316:1371–1375, with permission.)

practical tool to study coronary arterial remodeling, in addition to the benefit it provides in terms of precise assessment of atherosclerotic plaque (85).

Remodeling is also a critical component in the management of the patient with left ventricular dysfunction. In some patients, the cause of primary left ventricular muscle dysfunction may be spontaneously reversible, such as peripartum cardiomyopathy, alcoholic cardiomyopathy, or viral myocarditis. In patients with ischemic heart disease, while the left ventricular dysfunction itself may be irreversible, therapy may halt or retard the progression of coronary atherosclerosis and the subsequent development of additional myocardial damage. Further, the use of angiotensin-converting enzyme (ACE) inhibitors may prevent or retard deleterious left ventricular remodeling (86) and thereby reduce mortality and morbidity (87,88). A recent report demonstrates the surprising result that left ventricular myocytes can in fact regenerate following acute MI (89). While the clinical significance of this is presently uncertain, it raises the hope that gene therapy may be able to take advantage of this process, with the ultimate outcome of significant myocyte regeneration following acute MI.

Tenet III: Many Forces, Both Intrinsic and Extrinsic to the Person, Can Weaken This Inherent Capacity and Contribute to the Onset of Illness

A useful perspective on CAD comes from the history of the homeopathic profession in the first systematic study of nitroglycerin in the United States. By using selected individuals as "provers," nitroglycerin was evaluated for its efficacy in treating headaches and palpitations. However, in spite of a very careful, systematic approach, it was never learned that nitroglycerin could be beneficial for the treatment of angina pectoris. Medical historian W. Bruce Fye (90) concluded that there simply were not enough people in the U.S. who had coronary heart disease for this diagnosis even to be considered. As recently as the 1896 *Textbook of Internal Medicine* by Sir William Osler, angina pectoris was considered to be rare. We might therefore view CAD as an epidemic confined to the 20th century and to the early part of this century. The prevalence of ischemic heart disease peaked around 1967 and has been falling ever since. The death rate from heart disease has dropped by an astounding 60% in just the past 30 years (91). The National Heart, Lung and Blood Institute called for a further 20% reduction in coronary heart disease deaths over the

TABLE 24.1. RISK FACTORS FOR CORONARY ATHEROSCLEROSIS

Major Independent Risk Factors
  Cigarette smoking
  Elevated blood pressure
  Elevated serum total (and LDL) cholesterol
  Low serum HDL cholesterol
  Diabetes mellitus
  Advancing age
  Obesity[a]
  Physical inactivity

Predisposing Risk Factors
  Abdominal obesity[b]
  Family history of premature CAD
  Ethnic characteristics
  Psychosocial factors

Conditional Risk Factors
  Elevated serum triglycerides
  Small LDL particles
  Elevated serum homocysteine
  Elevated serum lipoprotein(a)
  Prothrombotic factors (fibrinogen, etc.)
  Inflammatory markers (e.g., C-reactive protein)

[a]Obesity is a body mass index >30 kg/m^2.
[b]Abdominal obesity is defined by waist circumference: men >102 cm (40″), women >88 cm (35″).
(Modified from Grundy SM, et al. Assessment of cardiovascular risk by use of multiple-risk-factor assessment equations. *Circulation* 1999;100:1481–1492.)

2000–2010 decade (92). Clearly, the vast majority of heart attacks and manifestations of ischemic heart disease are preventable, since the cause of coronary atherosclerosis is largely extrinsic to the person. Table 24.1 lists the standard risk factors for CAD. The major modifiable risk factors are cigarette smoking, diet, obesity (and subsequent type 2 diabetes), and a sedentary lifestyle. Only one, family history, might be considered to be an intrinsic risk factor.

The most common conditions associated with heart failure in the United States are CAD and hypertension. Since CAD is preventable, and hypertension is imminently treatable, most cases of heart failure are potentially preventable. Figure 24.3 depicts the prevalence of certain conditions associated with heart failure by gender, while Table 2 lists the precipitating causes of heart failure.

Molecular genetics offers the possibility of a new paradigm for cardiology and medicine. Despite our knowledge of diagnosis and treatment, we seldom know the etiology or the specific molecular defect responsible for disease. Over the next few years, when the Human Genome Project is completed, there will be thousands of etiologies and specific molecular defects to be linked with their respective disease. Prevention will become the key to future success and represent the major initiative for the 21st century. The field of pharmacogenomics will evolve rapidly in the next decade, and individualization of therapy (the antithesis of health maintenance organizations and managed care) will be the norm (93,94). For example, ACE inhibitors may be more effective than angiotensin 1 (AT-1) receptor blockade for the hypertensive patient who has expressed a vulnerable polymorphism in the ACE, whereas the latter might be more appropriate for

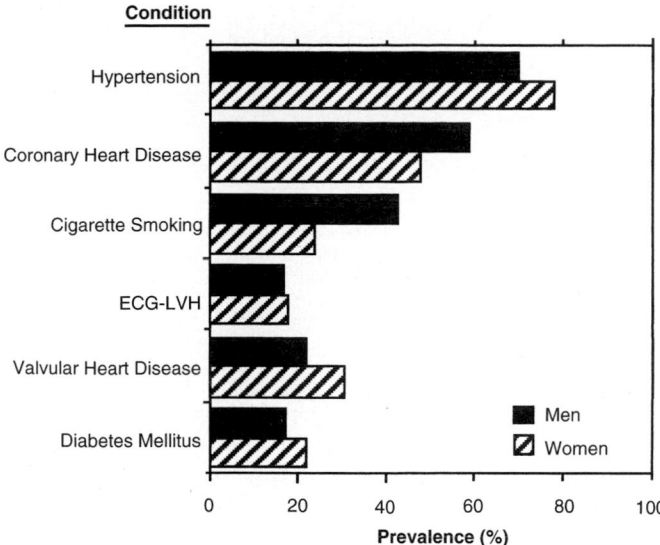

FIGURE 24.3. Prevalence of certain conditions among Framingham Heart Study subjects with congestive heart failure, by gender. *ECG-LVH*, electrocardiographic left ventricular hypertrophy. (From Ho KK, Pinsky J, Kanne LWB, Levy D. The epidemiology of heart failure; the Framingham Study. *J Am Coll Cardiol.* 1993;22[Suppl A]:6A–13A, with permission.)

those with an expressed vulnerable polymorphism in the AT-1 receptor. Familial hypertrophic cardiomyopathy was the first primary cardiomyopathy to be defined in terms of a genetic linkage (95).

The early practitioners of osteopathic medicine believed that the body produced its own medicine for healing, especially if there was normalization of structural abnormalities that affected circulation, the lymphatics, and nerve function. In cardiology, the challenge is to determine when the production of endogenous substances is beneficial and needs to be supported, or when it is deleterious. A few decades ago, physicians believed that the

TABLE 24.2. PRECIPITATING CAUSES OF HEART FAILURE

Acute myocardial ischemia or infarction
Nonadherence to therapy
   inappropriate reduction in medications
   noncompliance with dietary sodium restriction
Systemic hypertension
Arrhythmias, especially atrial fibrillation
Systemic infection
Anemia
Thyrotoxicosis
Infective endocarditis
Myocarditis
Physical, emotional, or environmental stress
Burden of new unrelated illness
   renal failure
   volume overload following surgery
Cardiac-depressant or salt-retaining drugs
Cardiac toxins
   alcohol
   cocaine
   anti-cancer chemotherapy
Pregnancy

endogenous neurohumoral mechanisms activated during heart failure played an advantageous, supportive role, and they were advised not to interfere with these compensatory mechanisms (96). It is now believed that systemic vasoconstriction will decrease left ventricular systolic performance and accelerate the progression of heart failure. Consequently, neurohumoral blockade with ACE inhibitors and β-blockers represent the standard therapy in heart failure management. In contrast, B-type natriuretic peptide is synthesized in the ventricular myocardium and released into the circulation in response to ventricular dilation and pressure overload (97). The serum level of brain natriuretic peptide (BNP) has now been shown to have diagnostic and prognostic value. Intravenous infusion of BNP in pharmacologic amounts represents an effective form of vasodilator therapy for patients with decompensation of heart failure (98).

Tenet IV: The Musculoskeletal System Significantly Influences the Individual's Ability to Restore the Inherent Capacity to Maintain Health and Therefore to Resist Disease Process

A sedentary lifestyle was elevated to the status of a primary risk factor for CAD in 1994 (99). To a large degree, this risk may accrue because of the rising importance of type 2 diabetes as a major risk for the development of CAD (100,101). The musculoskeletal system plays a major role in the predisposition of patients to develop type 2 diabetes, because of the interrelationship between insulin resistance (which largely resides in the musculoskeletal system), obesity, a sedentary lifestyle, and lack of physical fitness. The National Heart, Lung and Blood Institute has identified smoking, obesity, and physical inactivity to be the greatest threats to cardiovascular health in this decade (92).

Fitness and exercise capacity represent an important prognostic marker for the general population (102), patients with heart failure (103), and patients with coronary heart disease (104). As described subsequently, the muscle hypothesis is a new model of heart failure that proposes that the signs and symptoms of heart failure are often related to the abnormal activation of muscle ergoreceptors, which causes an increase in ventilation and resultant sensation of breathlessness. For as many of one-fourth of patients with heart failure, functional limitations are caused by the musculoskeletal system, and not by diminished cardiac output. The intervention of cardiac rehabilitation exercise provides an increase in exercise capacity that is twice that achieved with ACE inhibitor therapy.

The specific challenges to osteopathic medicine in the field of cardiology are many. The musculoskeletal system manifests subtle changes in response to chronic CAD (105) or acute MI (106), which may be detected by a focused palpatory examination. These basic observations give rise to additional questions. Can palpatory examination be used in a longitudinal manner to learn more about the natural history of patients with CAD? Will an emphasis on the role of the musculoskeletal system in health and disease contribute to the effective treatment of patients with coronary heart disease or heart failure? Will the osteopathic physician's traditional role as primary caregiver lead to improved therapy or more effective approaches to the prevention of heart disease?

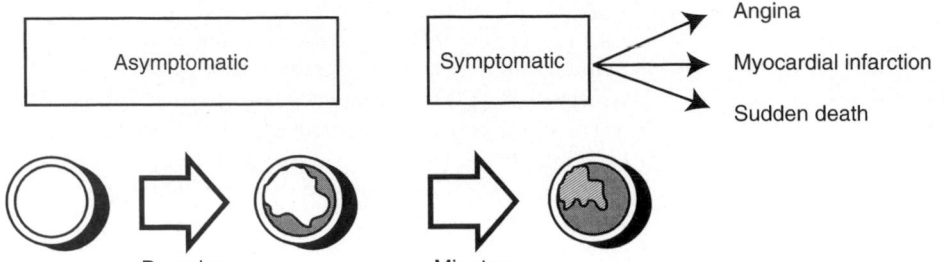

FIGURE 24.4. Natural history of coronary heart disease.

CORONARY ARTERY DISEASE

Pathophysiology and Natural History

The pathophysiology of CAD has been investigated extensively on both sides of the Atlantic for the last century. The literature now clearly defines the pathophysiologic processes that underlie the development of the atherosclerotic lesion, from its beginnings as a fatty streak to the complex obstructive lesion that characterizes ischemic heart disease (107–110). Similarly, cross-sectional and longitudinal epidemiologic surveys have clearly identified the role of risk factors in the development of coronary atherosclerosis, which have been summarized in various reports (111–113).

One of the most important clinical characteristics of ischemic heart disease is shown in Fig. 24.4. Atherosclerotic lesions can progress slowly for decades before they become symptomatic. Then, in a matter of moments, the lesions become symptomatic, with three manifestations: angina pectoris, MI, and sudden cardiac death. Angina is the only symptomatic presentation of ischemic heart disease in which there is neither permanent morbidity nor mortality, giving the physician the greatest opportunity to do the most good for the patient.

Epidemiologic studies of ischemic heart disease have concentrated on risk factors for coronary atherosclerosis, the early detection of asymptomatic disease, and the role of primary and secondary risk factor modification for the prevention or amelioration of heart disease. Physicians are now calling for an investigation into the triggers that transform the atherosclerotic plaque from an asymptomatic lesion into a symptomatic lesion. The histopathologic events associated with the transformation of stable atheroma into one of the acute coronary syndromes are now well defined from autopsy, cardiac catheterization, and intravascular ultrasound studies. The interrelationship of five vascular mechanisms causing acute myocardial ischemia is shown in Fig. 24.5.

Recently, Braunwald proposed an etiologic approach to management of unstable angina (114). He described five different, but not mutually exclusive, causes of angina:

1. Nonocclusive thrombus on preexisting plaque
2. Dynamic obstruction (coronary vasoconstriction)
3. Progressive mechanical obstruction
4. Inflammation and/or infection
5. Secondary angina pectoris (unstable angina precipitated by conditions extrinsic to the coronary vascular bed, such as thyrotoxicosis, anemia, hypotension, etc.)

This chapter will focus only on those acute coronary syndromes that share in common the pathophysiologic features of plaque fissure and/or rupture, and the subsequent development of thrombus on preexisting plaques. This type of unstable angina represents approximately 75% of those patients described in the Braunwald classification (114).

Vascular Biology of Acute Coronary Syndromes

The acute coronary syndromes represent a spectrum of conditions that hold in common the presence of plaque fissuring, which has been described as the cause of acute MI and unstable angina, as well as sudden ischemic death (115). The disruption of a formed plaque is a complex process that is the central feature of the initiation of the acute coronary syndromes. The sudden total or near total occlusion of a coronary artery usually occurs at the site of stenosis that was previously not hemodynamically significant, or at least not critical (116). The arterial lesion of unstable angina and MI is a complex eccentric plaque angiographically, which histologically represents a ruptured plaque with superimposed thrombus.

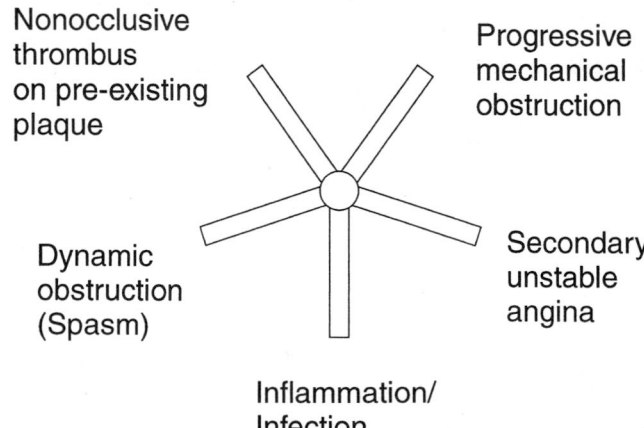

FIGURE 24.5. A framework for expressing the contribution of five pathophysiologic mechanisms that may cause unstable angina. Each component may contribute to the clinical picture in varying degrees. The most common occurs when atherosclerotic plaque causes moderate obstruction and acute thrombus overlying the plaque causes very severe narrowing. A common form of Prinzmetal angina occurs when the spasm is superimposed upon mild atherosclerotic obstruction. (Modified from Braunwald E. Unstable angina. An etiologic approach to management. *Circulation.* 1998;98:2219–2222.)

There are two main components to the vulnerable atherosclerotic plaque: the lipid-rich core, and the meshwork of extracellular-matrix proteins that form the fibrous cap. The vulnerable atherosclerotic lesion, although not necessarily stenotic at angiography (117) may be prone to disruption because of its softness caused by a high lipid content and macrophage-dependent chemical properties.

Chronic minimal injury to the arterial endothelium is physiologic and is often the result of a disturbance in the pattern of the blood flow at bending points and near bifurcations in the arterial tree. In addition to these local shear forces, endothelial dysfunction occurs because of hypertension, hypercholesterolemia, advanced glycation end products from diabetes, chemical irritants in tobacco, circulating vasoactive amines, immune complexes, and perhaps infections.

Passive plaque disruption occurs most often where the fibrous cap is the most thin, where it is most heavily infiltrated by foam cells and therefore weakest, and at sites of mechanical stress.

Active disruption of atherosclerotic plaques may be initiated by proteinases that are secreted by macrophages which then enzymatically degrade the fibrous cap by phagocytosis or secretion of proteolytic enzymes. These enzymes include plasminogen activators and matrix metalloproteinases. In addition to degradation of the matrix of the fibrous cap, shedding of membrane microparticles leads to a potent procoagulant activity. These shed particles account for almost all the tissue factor activity present in plaque, and may be a major contributor in the initiation of the coagulation cascade after plaque disruption. Following plaque disruption, local thrombosis results from complex interactions between the lipid core, smooth muscle cells, macrophages, and collagen.

Over the past 35 years the view has evolved that the acute coronary syndromes are caused by plaque rupture and formation of a platelet thrombus. Greater platelet stability and transmural infarction have been attributed to more severe or extensive plaque rupture. Unstable angina and non-Q wave infarction were believed to be due to less extensive, and less stable platelet thrombi that caused less severe, less extensive ischemia and/or infarction. However, more recent clinical findings have refined this viewpoint (118). The occlusive thrombi causing Q-wave MI contain more fibrin than the thrombi found in other acute coronary syndromes that are characterized by more platelets and less fibrin. The higher fibrin content of thrombi causing Q-wave infarction explains their higher stability. Further, this higher fibrin content suggests that the coagulation cascade is activated to a greater degree during Q-wave infarction than during non–Q-wave infarction, in which platelets play a more dominant role. This pathophysiologic feature defines the therapeutic role of thrombolytic agents for patients with ST-segment elevation MI, and the use of antiplatelet agents (aspirin, heparin, platelet glycoprotein IIb/IIIa receptor blocking agents) in non–Q-wave MI.

In about one-third of patients with acute coronary syndromes, and particularly in acute sudden coronary death, there is no disruption of a fairly small lipid-rich plaque, just a superficial erosion of a markedly stenotic and fibrotic plaque (119). Thus, complicated thrombi may well be dependent on a hypercoagulable state triggered by systemic factors. Evidence continues to evolve that circulating monocytes and white blood cells may be involved in tissue factor expression and thrombogenicity. Further, the predictive value for coronary events of high titers of C-reactive protein may be a manifestation of such systemic phenomena (120–122). Hypercholesterolemia, a high catecholamine drive, and perhaps infection may also be triggers of such hypercoagulable phenomena.

Up until recently, the embolization of plaque content and of platelet-thrombus into the distal microvasculature was thought to be uncommon. However, recent studies indicate that microvascular embolization is not only common, but carries an adverse prognosis (123). Histologic studies have confirmed platelet thrombus as part of occlusive material in the downstream microvasculature, and atherosclerotic particulate material has been identified as well. In addition, endothelial cells have been found to be present in the circulation with a higher frequency in patients with acute coronary syndrome compared with control patients, or those with stable effort angina. The benefits of short-term platelet glycoprotein IIb/IIIa-receptor blocking agents appears to be related to a decrease in microvascular obstruction from embolization with a subsequent decrease in myocardial necrosis and decrease in risk for malignant arrhythmias. These agents do not decrease the embolization of atherosclerotic lipid and matrix constituents. The embolic events may also reflect significant inflammation in the diseased artery.

In summary, for patients with chronic, stable CAD, angina or silent ischemia commonly results from increases in myocardial oxygen demand that outstrips the ability of stenosed coronary arteries to supply the needed blood flow. In contrast, in acute coronary syndromes, there is an abrupt reduction in coronary flow. In unstable angina, a relatively small erosion or fissuring of an atherosclerotic plaque may lead to an acute change in plaque structure and a reduction in coronary blood flow, resulting in exacerbation of angina. Transient episodes of thrombotic vessel occlusion at the site of plaque injury may occur, leading to angina at rest. This thrombus is usually labile and results in temporary vascular occlusion, perhaps lasting only 10 to 20 minutes. In non–Q-wave MI, more severe plaque damage would result in more persistent thrombotic occlusion, perhaps lasting up to 1 hour. Resolution of vasoconstriction may also be pathologically important in non–Q-wave MI. Therefore, spontaneous thrombolysis, vasoconstriction resolution, and the presence of collateral circulation are important in preventing the development of Q-wave infarction by limiting the duration of myocardial ischemia. In Q-wave MI, larger plaque fissures may result in the formation of a fixed and persistent thrombus, which is rich in fibrin.

DIAGNOSIS

The process of screening patients for heart disease involves the use of the history, physical examination, ECG, and chest roentgenogram. The diagnosis of ischemic heart disease is most easily accomplished with patients who are symptomatic. When more attention was given to annual health screening evaluations, treadmill stress tests were often employed as part of executive physical examinations. Testing for asymptomatic CAD is not generally considered to be a fruitful endeavor however, except in

TABLE 24.3. LIKELIHOOD OF DEFINING CORONARY ARTERY DISEASE AFTER STANDARD TREADMILL EXERCISE TESTING ACCORDING TO AGE, SEX, AND SYMPTOMS IN A GROUP OF PATIENTS WITH 1–1.5 Mm ST SEGMENT DEPRESSION

Age	Asymptomatic		Nonanginal Chest Pain		Atypical Angina		Typical Angina	
Years	Men	Women	Men	Women	Men	Women	Men	Women
30–39	3.9	0.6	10.4	1.7	37.7	8.5	83.0	42.4
40–49	11.0	2.1	25.8	5.8	64.4	24.5	93.6	72.3
50–59	18.5	6.5	36.7	16.3	75.2	50.4	96.1	89.1
60–69	22.9	14.7	45.3	32.6	81.2	71.6	97.2	95.3

(From Diamond GA. Analysis of probability as an aid in the clinical diagnosis of coronary artery disease. *N Engl J Med.* 1979;300:1350–1358, with permission.)

selected circumstances such as before noncardiac vascular surgery or in patients with multiple cardiovascular risk factors.

Diagnostic studies for patients with suspected or proven CAD fall into two general categories. The first consideration involves establishing the diagnosis of CAD. The history is the central element in this diagnosis. Numerous studies over the past three decades have validated Bayes theorem, clarifying that virtually every cardiovascular study performed has little meaning by itself but is properly understood in the context of the patient's clinical presentation (124) (Table 24.3). In patients with established heart disease, the second diagnostic consideration is to stage the severity of the disease process, and to define the patient's position on the continuum of stable or unstable coronary atherosclerotic syndromes described previously.

A high correlation exists between the clinical impression of stable angina, accelerated angina, resting angina, and acute MI with the findings demonstrated on angiography (125) and angioscopy (126). The initial evaluation should distinguish between those patients at low risk for MI who can be further evaluated on an outpatient basis and those patients for whom immediate hospitalization is required (127).

The evaluation of patients presenting with chest pain continues to be challenging. This is in spite of new advances in our understanding of the pathophysiology of acute coronary syndromes, new biochemical markers for cardiac injury, and insights from large, randomized controlled trials that provide important data on risk stratification and appropriate algorithms for patient management. The assessment of chest pain represents the starting point for evaluating the possibility that a person might have an acute coronary syndrome. The pertinent features of this evaluation are equally important for the primary care physician, emergency room physician, cardiologist, or house officer. The critical components of the evaluation include the history, physical examination, and ECG. There are several implications that arise from this apparently simple precept. Evaluation of the patient for chest pain cannot be conducted by telephone. An individual who telephones their primary care physician with a description of chest pain must be referred to a clinical setting where an ECG can be performed. Some of these patients will be shown to have acute MI, when it is appropriate for immediate restoration of flow through thrombolytic agents or direct angioplasty. Since the only hint that would reveal the urgency for this action is the description of chest pain, quality assurance programs for the evaluation of patients with acute coronary syndrome should not just look at door-to-needle time for thrombolysis. Rather, an

assessment needs to include door-to-ECG interpretation time, door-to-cardiac marker result time, and door-to-initiation of general treatment time (Fig. 24.6).

The general category of diagnostic studies for cardiovascular disease includes imaging techniques, tests of myocardial function, and physiologic assessments of cardiac performance. The new imaging techniques (magnetic resonance imaging, conventional or rapid sequence computed tomography, and ECG studies) are expensive compared with plain chest x-ray films and cardiac fluoroscopy. Many tests (such as treadmill exercise stress testing) provide functional data; they may be supplemented by imaging techniques such as postexercise myocardial perfusion imaging or postexercise ECG. Pharmacologic stress testing with dobutamine or dipyridamole is increasingly being substituted for exercise stress testing. Some studies provide physiologic information alone, such as radionuclide ejection fraction.

The development of such a wide array of tests forces decision making. Using all noninvasive studies is cost-prohibitive. If only a small number are to be used, they have to be carefully tailored to the patient's clinical state. These simple questions should be answered: Is this study being performed to establish the diagnosis

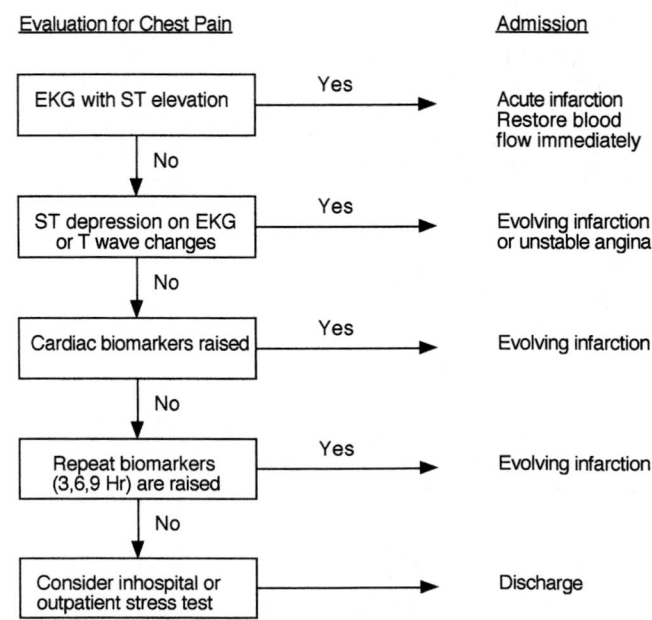

FIGURE 24.6. Stepwise evaluation of patients presenting with chest pain.

of heart disease or to stage known heart disease? Will the study provide useful information concerning the patient's prognosis? Is the study necessary to determine the best form of therapy for a patient, to assess the benefits of previously performed procedures, or to risk-stratify for noncardiac surgery? Which test is the safest and the most feasible to perform and yields the most information, with the least possibility of confounding information? Each of these issues is widely discussed in the medical literature (128–131). Clinical experience and thoughtful judgment are the most important features of decision making in this area.

DISTINCTIVE CONSIDERATIONS IN THE APPROACH TO THE PATIENT WITH CORONARY HEART DISEASE

The history is a critical feature of the evaluation of patients suspected of having CAD. From the start, as J. Willis Hurst points out, the physician interview with the patient has a dual purpose: to obtain important medical information and to establish a bond between the patient and the physician (132). Since the management of CAD involves lifestyle changes recommended by the physician, the initial history may also be considered as the first step in establishing the foundation for later risk factor modification programs.

Physicians should recall that the history of chest pain typical for angina pectoris may be present in a minority of patients with ischemic heart disease. Unusual somatic representation of chest pain to a site of previously experienced somatic pain may occur because of facilitation, convergence, or other mechanisms at the spinal level (133,134). Until recently, episodes of angina were thought to be synonymous with myocardial ischemia, and chest pain was considered to be a reliable indicator of ischemia. Several reports have since demonstrated that episodes of asymptomatic myocardial ischemia are common in patients with known CAD (135–137). Similarly, the Framingham Study has shown that unrecognized MIs are common, responsible for at least one out of every four infarctions. Half of the unrecognized infarctions are silent; the remainder are so atypical that neither the patient nor the physician entertains their possibility (138).

Clinical studies on the manifestations of pain have been performed in a variety of cardiac conditions. At the opposite end of the spectrum from silent ischemia are patients with a sensitive heart (139) or syndrome X (140), in whom an abnormal cardiac pain perception is a fundamental component of the clinical presentation.

The relationship between the myocardial locus of ischemia or infarction and the distribution of angina has been studied in several clinical circumstances. The distribution of cardiac pain during different locations of intracoronary stimulation by local injection of adenosine was experienced in the same body area by a majority of patients (141). For all patients with Q-wave MI, pain location, radiation, duration, and severity were similar, although gastrointestinal symptoms were more common with inferior wall MI (142). For the same group of patients, a second MI with a different location of pain was highly predictive of ischemia in a different cardiac region. In a study of palpatory findings of musculoskeletal changes with MI, abnormalities of paraspinal soft-tissue texture were more often associated with anterior than with inferior MI (143).

Clinical observations since the time of Sir William Harvey are consistent with the idea that myocardial nociceptors are sufficiently sparse that a certain mass of myocardium must be affected for pain to be perceived (144–147). A prospective radiographic study that showed a higher incidence of cervical osteochondrosis in patients with painful ischemia compared with painless ischemia proposed summation of pain input from a musculoskeletal reflexogenic zone as a possible mechanism to explain pain perception in these patients (148). (Osteophytic lipping of the lower thoracic spine has been shown to be more common in patients with coronary disease than in control patients (149), but this study did not distinguish patients with painful and silent ischemia.)

Because cardiac pain is transmitted to the spinal cord by sympathetic afferent nerves, osteopathic physicians have examined the paraspinal musculature and soft tissue for a segmental somatic expression of this visceral disturbance. Beal (150) reviewed the osteopathic literature, noting a preponderance of changes in the areas of T1-5. It should be noted that an examination of the entire axial skeleton was performed only in two studies in which the status of the coronary arteries was defined by angiography (105,106). In the study of patients with acute MI (107), the palpatory examination was restricted to the 12 thoracic segments.

In approximately one-third of patients who present with chest discomfort, no cardiac cause is found, and these patients are labeled as having noncardiac chest pain. In most of these patients, the pain is attributed to the esophagus on clinical grounds (151), but typical investigations do not identify the cause of the pain. One research group (152) has hypothesized that central sensitization, an activity-dependent amplification of sensory transfer in the central nervous system, is underlying visceral pain hypersensitivity and noncardiac chest pain. On the other hand, "linked angina" is a clinical situation in which esophageal acid stimulation causes anginal attacks and significantly reduces coronary blood flow in patients with CAD by a viscero-visceral reflex. The lack of any significant effect in heart transplant recipients with heart denervation suggests a neural reflex (153). This reflex mechanism only becomes important in the presence of an impaired coronary flow reserve, endothelial dysfunction, or significant coronary stenoses.

To date, clinical protocols for the assessment of patients with chest pain have not yet included palpatory findings as a prospective aid for the diagnosis of coronary disease. The reproduction of chest discomfort by palpation is part of an algorithm for the evaluation of chest pain in the emergency room (154). Because somatic factors can coexist with cardiac disease, and spinal segmental facilitation may augment the severity of chest wall pain (155), the osteopathic profession could make a contribution to clinical medicine by a study of palpatory musculoskeletal findings in patients with chest pain.

THERAPY

The ideal approach to patients with potential ischemic heart disease is primary prevention, so symptomatic or significant coronary atherosclerosis never develops. A holistic approach to the patient with coronary heart diseases recognizes that a multifactorial disease process requires a comprehensive therapeutic plan.

At least 25% of coronary patients have sudden death or nonfatal MI without any prior symptoms (156). Therefore, the search for the coronary patient with subclinical disease who could potentially benefit from intensive primary prevention efforts is critically important. A recent American Heart Association (AHA) conference (157) addressed ways to identify more patients who are asymptomatic and clinically free of coronary disease, but are at sufficiently high risk for future events to justify a more intensive risk reduction effort. Key findings from that report have been incorporated into an office-based approach to screen all patients, to better define their coronary event risk (158) (Fig. 24.7). Asymptomatic adults are stratified as low risk (about 35% of patients). They are reassured of this status by their physician and then retested in about 5 years. A second category is high-risk (about 25% of patients). They are candidates for intensive risk factor intervention. Noninvasive testing is not needed to determine treatment goals. Intermediate-risk patients may benefit from noninvasive testing for further risk assessment. Tests would include the ankle-brachial blood pressure index (159), electron-beam computed tomography (EBCT) (160), and exercise stress testing (161). While each patient deserves the benefit of a multifactorial risk factor modification program, the intensity of that program and the goals set for ideal cholesterol levels, and so forth, vary according to the patient's risk for subsequent cardiac events. The components of a multifactorial program include regular progressive aerobic exercise, weight loss where appropriate, control of hypertension and diabetes, cessation of cigarette smoking, education about cardiovascular disease, reduction of serum cholesterol, dietary modification of cholesterol and fats, and control of stress and hostility. Emotional and psychological support are key features in successful risk factor modification programs.

Patients with diabetes develop accelerated CAD and are 10 to 20 times overrepresented among those suffering from acute MI.

Mortality in the year following infarction is up to twice that of nondiabetics, and CAD remains the most common single cause of death in diabetic patients. Accordingly, the American Diabetes Association has set goals for the treatment of cardiovascular risk factors in diabetic patients that are so stringent they presume the existence of significant coronary heart disease. Treatment guidelines for diabetic dyslipidemia call for lowering the low-density lipoprotein (LDL) cholesterol to less than 100 mg per dL, raising high-density lipoprotein (HDL) to more than 45 mg/dL, and lowering triglycerides to less than 200 mg per dL (162). Most experts recommend a target blood pressure of 130/85 mm Hg. The target glycosylated hemoglobin value is 6.0.

Exercise is a particularly important component of a risk factor modification program. Exercise is recommended for healthy people, patients identified at risk for CAD, patients with defined ischemic heart disease, and patients following MI or revascularization (163). The type of program a patient enters depends on their physiologic state and cardiovascular status at the time of enrollment. Many patients enter rehabilitation while hospitalized and continue in a phase II posthospital program that is monitored and supervised. Others begin with a phase III maintenance program that is supervised but not monitored. Strength development through circuit weight training is both safe and feasible in selected patients with CAD (164). The primary goals of cardiac rehabilitation include a return to full functional status, resumption of previous occupation, and improved quality of life. Exercise itself has important additional benefits in terms of promoting the reduction of other cardiovascular risk factors such as obesity, hypertension, diabetes, and dyslipidemias (163). A meta-analysis of cardiac rehabilitation programs demonstrates a decrease in mortality for participants (165). It is important to recall the mechanism whereby cardiac rehabilitation works is not through improvement of coronary collaterals or myocardial blood flow but rather through enhancement of musculoskeletal efficiency. Because striated muscle represents the largest potential demand for cardiac output, improved functioning of this primary machinery of life has a significant effect on cardiovascular status.

Coronary Heart Disease Risk Assessment in Asymptomatic Patients: Selective Use of Noninvasive Testing following Office-Based Risk Assessment

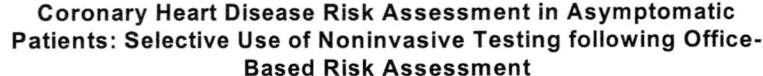

STEP 1	Initial Office-Based Assessment in all Asymptomatic adults using Multiple Coronary Disease Risk Factors / Global Risk Assessment

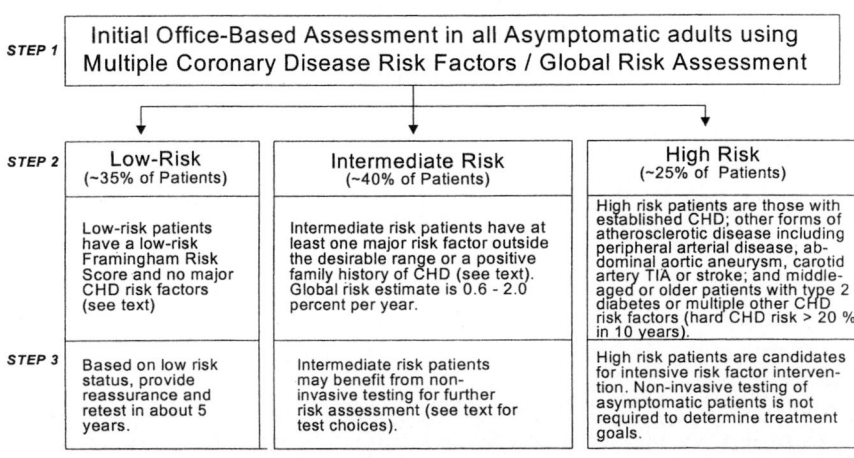

STEP 2	Low-Risk (~35% of Patients)	Intermediate Risk (~40% of Patients)	High Risk (~25% of Patients)
	Low-risk patients have a low-risk Framingham Risk Score and no major CHD risk factors (see text)	Intermediate risk patients have at least one major risk factor outside the desirable range or a positive family history of CHD (see text). Global risk estimate is 0.6 - 2.0 percent per year.	High risk patients are those with established CHD; other forms of atherosclerotic disease including peripheral arterial disease, abdominal aortic aneurysm, carotid artery TIA or stroke; and middle-aged or older patients with type 2 diabetes or multiple other CHD risk factors (hard CHD risk > 20 % in 10 years).
STEP 3	Based on low risk status, provide reassurance and retest in about 5 years.	Intermediate risk patients may benefit from non-invasive testing for further risk assessment (see text for test choices).	High risk patients are candidates for intensive risk factor intervention. Non-invasive testing of asymptomatic patients is not required to determine treatment goals.

FIGURE 24.7. A selective use of noninvasive testing for the detection of coronary artery disease in asymptomatic individuals, following office-based risk assessment. (From Greenland P, Smith SC, Grundy SM. Improving coronary heart disease risk assessment in asymptomatic people. Role of traditional risk factors in non-invasive cardiovascular tests. *Circulation.* 2001;104:1863–1867, with permission.)

All patients with ischemic heart disease should also have their spouse and family involved in this risk factor modification program. Family can be a significant source of support for the patient. Often, other family members have the same needs in terms of education, exercise, smoking behavior, and other risk behaviors. Last, ischemic heart disease is a frightening proposition. Even with an exercise program, many patients remain unable to break through the barrier of fear and return to fully functional lives. They represent clear examples of individuals who need psychological, social, and spiritual support as they cope with their illness.

ANGINA PECTORIS

Patients with chronic, stable angina pectoris are fortunate that a large number of effective pharmacologic agents are now available to them (166,167). Unless this benefit is turned to the curse of polypharmacy, certain guiding principles should be followed. First, a therapeutic agent should be selected based on the pathophysiology of the disease state, especially related to coexisting disease processes, and on other cardiovascular characteristics. Although β-blocking agents, nitrates, and calcium entry blockers all represent effective first-line agents for treating angina, some drugs may be superior to others in certain situations. Because the pathophysiology of ischemic heart disease involves healing of the intimal disruption in unstable angina, patients started on antianginal therapy during the acute phase of their illness may not require that medication indefinitely. A time should be selected to withdraw these drugs unless their continued use can be shown to be associated with a decreased risk of cardiovascular mortality, as is true with a β-blocking agent (Fig. 24.8).

The pathophysiology of acute coronary syndromes indicates that aspirin is appropriate for all patients with defined ischemic heart disease. Many physicians also advocate aspirin use for currently healthy individuals at risk, even without any evidence of CAD.

UNSTABLE ANGINA

Unstable angina has three possible presentations: (a) symptoms of angina at rest (usually prolonged for more than 20 minutes); (b) new onset (less than 2 months), exertional angina of at least Canadian Cardiovascular Society Classification (CCSC) III in severity; or (c) recent (less than 2 months) acceleration of angina reflected by an increase in severity of at least one CCSC class to at least CCSC III (127) (Table 24.4).

Aspirin and anti-anginals
Beta-blocker and blood pressure
Cholesterol and cigarettes
Diet and diabetes
Education and exercise

FIGURE 24.8. The ABCs of guidelines for the management of stable angina, as recommended by the American Heart Association. Ten areas of intervention for each patient.

TABLE 24.4. GRADING OF ANGINA PECTORIS BY THE CANADIAN CARDIOVASCULAR SOCIETY CLASSIFICATION SYSTEM

Class	Description of Stage
Class I	Ordinary physical activity does not cause angina, such as walking, climbing stairs. Angina [occurs] with strenuous, rapid, or prolonged exertion at work or recreation.
Class II	Slight limitation of ordinary activity. Angina occurs on walking or climbing stairs rapidly, walking uphill, walking or stair climbing after meals, or in cold, or in wind, or under emotional stress, or only during the few hours after awakening. Walking more than two blocks on the level and climbing more than one flight of ordinary stairs at a normal pace and in normal condition.
Class III	Marked limitations of ordinary physical activity. Angina occurs on walking one to two blocks on the level and climbing one flight of stairs in normal conditions and at a normal pace.
Class IV	Inability to carry on any physical activity without discomfort—anginal symptoms may be present at rest.

(Reprinted with permission from Campeau L. Grading of angina pectoris by the Canadian cardiovascular society classification system. *Circulation.* 1976; 54:522–523, with permission.)

The major treatment goals for patients with unstable angina are to control chest discomfort, relieve ischemia, and prevent the development of acute MI. Guidelines for the diagnosis and treatment of angina have been developed by an expert panel, based on scientific and clinical evidence (127) and recent review (168).

MYOCARDIAL INFARCTION

The treatment of MI today represents a combination of public health efforts, medical technology, and the application of molecular and cellular biology to patient care issues. Standard therapeutic interventions, including β-blockers, thrombolytic agents, ACE inhibitors, balloon angioplasty, and the coronary care unit itself, have all been developed only in the last few decades. Although controversy continues over specific issues related to optimal treatment, international multicenter trials and metaanalysis have established strong scientific evidence to support recommendations for therapy for MI (169–175). In the last decade, the strategy to treat MI has shifted from an approach to prevent or manage malignant arrhythmias to efforts to reduce the extent of infarction, prevent reinfarction, and protect against deleterious effects of ventricular remodeling. Fig. 24.9 summarizes the management of patients with MI.

The role of early ambulation and cardiac rehabilitation is important to avoid complications of MI and to maintain cardiovascular fitness before it is lost because of bed rest. Cardiac rehabilitation takes advantage of the patient being receptive to this intervention at this time, and it can be a part of a risk factor modification program that is begun in the hospital.

CHALLENGES

The foremost challenge in the management of patients in regard to CAD involves a change in mindset. Because CAD is the

Pharmacologic therapy

Medication	First 24 Hours	Discharge
Aspirin	Chewed in ED	81mg indefinitely
Reperfusion for ST elevation MI	Thrombolytics or Primary PTCA	
Heparin (UFH)	IV 60 U/kg bolus, infusion 12U/kg/hr	Coumadin for 3-6 mo if LV thrombus; chronically for AF
Low molecular weight heparin	Alternative to UFH	
Beta-blocker	IV metoprolol (up to 15 mg in 3 divided doses) or atenolol IV (10 mg in 2 divided doses)	Oral daily indefinitely
ACE inhibitor	Captopril, or lisinopril	Oral daily indefinitely
GP IIb/IIIa	Eptifibitide or tirofiban	
Nitroglycerin	IV for 24-48 hours if no contraind.	Oral for residual ischemia
Statins		Indefinitely if LDL > 100 mg/dl

Non-Pharmacologic Therapy

Dietary Advice		Recommend low-fat diet
Smoking	Reinforce cessation	Refer to smoking cessation class
Exercise	Education	Recommend regular aerobic exercise
Pre-discharge Stress Test	Plan for day 4-5 if uncomplicated MI	Cath patients with significant ischemia
Measure LVEF		
Cardiac Rehabilitation		Refer to rehab program near their home

FIGURE 24.9. Management of acute myocardial infarction (MI). This figure summarizes the pharmacologic and nonpharmacologic therapy for the management of the patient with acute MI, emphasizing treatment in the first 24 hours, and recommendations at the time of hospital discharge. (Modified from Ryan TJ. ACC/AHA guidelines for the management of patients with acute myocardial infarction: 1999 update. *Circulation.* 1999;100:1016–1030.)

most common cause of death in the United States, most people presume it to be inevitable, and medical schools, hospitals, and physicians devote much of their energy to the diagnosis and treatment of the various manifestations of this disease. We need to adopt the attitude that most, if not all heart attacks are preventable. While this has been promoted in the popular press (176), there is considerable scientific support for this paradigm shift. As one example, the Nurses' Health Study (177) followed 84,129 women who were free from diagnosed cardiovascular disease, cancer, and diabetes in 1980. Low-risk subjects were defined as those who were currently not smoking, had a body-mass index under 25, consumed at least one half a drink of an alcoholic beverage daily, engaged in moderate-to-vigorous physical activity for at least 30 minutes daily, and consumed a heart healthy diet.

At 14 years' follow-up, this low-risk cohort had a relative risk of cardiac death and nonfatal heart attack of 0.17 (95% confidence intervals 0.07 to 0.41) compared with all the other women. Eighteen percent of the coronary events that occurred in the study cohort could be attributed to lack of adherence to this low-risk pattern. A similar analysis of 84,941 women in the same Nurses' Health Study showed that 91% of the subjects who developed type 2 diabetes over a 16-year follow-up had habits and behaviors that did not conform to this same low-risk pattern (178).

A second challenge is to recognize that coronary artery bypass graft (CABG) surgery and percutaneous transluminal coronary angioplasty (PTCA) do not prevent MI (179). Because of the prominent position given to these interventions, and the importance of these services to building a high-visibility cardiology program, most patients and many physicians assume that revascularization will protect against subsequent MI. In fact, the vessels that undergo revascularization have high-grade stenosis, but generally represent stable atheromatous plaque. The "vulnerable" plaque typically is of borderline hemodynamic significance and would not be a target for CABG or PTCA. What does prevent MI? Plaque stabilization and risk factor modification with diet, exercise, cholesterol-lowering therapy, and control of coexisting conditions such as hypertension, diabetes, and obesity. As one example, the Atorvastatin vs. Revascularization Treatment (AVERT) trial (180) enrolled patients with chronic stable angina and 70% to 90% stenosis of one or two coronary vessels. The patients were randomized to receive PTCA or the lipid-lowering agent atorvastatin. The study was halted prematurely because of the superiority of lipid-lowering therapy. Finally, the magnitude of survival benefit of CABG surgery is a small fraction of the benefit of lipid-lowering therapy, ACE inhibitors, and aspirin use.

Just as PTCA and CABG gain attention as interventions over "ordinary" medical management, the immediate treatment of acute MI receives much more attention than the hospital discharge and posthospital management. The gap between accepted guidelines and treatment compliance is so great that the American College of Cardiology (ACC) established an initiative in 2000 to enhance quality care through a multidisciplinary program. The Guidelines Applied in Practice (GAP) project (181) is designed to provide tools that hospital-based caregivers can utilize to improve adherence to guidelines (166). Even so, with a hospital length of stay for MI at 3 to 5 days, and unstable angina at 1 to 2 days, it should be clear that the responsibility for implementing these risk factor modification programs falls to the outpatient cardiologist and primary care physician.

A third paradigm shift is to recognize that consensus statements and guidelines not only reflect scientific evidence, but also the personal opinions of the individuals who craft these documents, and a subtle or overt influence from major medical centers and the pharmaceutical industry. For example, in the ACC/AHA guidelines for unstable angina and non–ST-segment elevation MI, the weight of evidence is ranked as:

Highest (A), if the data are derived from multiple, randomized clinical trials involving large numbers of patients.

Intermediate (B), if the data are derived from a limited number of randomized trials involving small numbers of patients or from careful analysis of nonrandomized studies or observational registries.

Low (C), if expert consensus is the primary basis for the recommendation.

In those guidelines (168) the large majority of recommendations were a level of evidence of B or C. As another example, because of broad advertising, including direct-to-consumer ads, it is now widely known that cholesterol-lowering drugs in the statin class reduce the risk of cardiac events. However, consumption of nuts (182–186) will reduce cardiac events by a similar order of magnitude. Consumption of nuts is a major part of the Mediterranean diet, the only diet proven to reduce the risk of MI (187). It is clear who promotes statins for cardiac patients. But who is promoting

the Mediterranean diet and consumption of nuts? This author believes that the osteopathic tenets and principles for patient care (1) represent a clear mandate for this to fall in the domain of osteopathic medicine.

Osteopathic manipulative therapy (OMT) has been advocated on the basis that it reduces somatic dysfunction, interrupts the viscerosomatic reflex arcs, influences the viscus through stimulation of somatovisceral efferents, and reduces the potential preconditioning effect of somatic dysfunction to body stressors (150). OMT has been recommended for the treatment of coronary heart disease based on a presumed mechanism to favorably alter autonomic nervous system function (188).

There is a significant need for skilled practitioners of osteopathic palpatory diagnosis and manipulative therapy in hospitals. Specialists in osteopathic manipulative medicine often aid in the diagnosis of patients with chest pain atypical for angina. In those patients for whom MI is ruled out, OMT is especially useful for those with chest wall pain. In patients with proven MI, OMT has been safely employed in the coronary care unit and the stepdown unit, with favorable clinical responses. Those patients who receive the benefit of routine OMT following open-heart surgery often have dramatic responses to treatment. Unfortunately, these clinical observations have not been studied in controlled trials. Even a systematic recording of observations on a longitudinal or case-control basis would be of significant interest. The following quartet of clinical vignettes provides a glimpse of how an osteopathic perspective influences the management of patients with heart disease.

A QUARTET OF CLINICAL VIGNETTES

1. A 72-year-old man (Patient No. 1) with heart failure complains of excessive fatigue and dyspnea with exertion. He is already on a full program of maximal medical therapy, which meets all consensus guidelines. When he sees the osteopathic physician, an inventory of his activities of daily living and exercise habits indicate a very sedentary lifestyle with significant limitation in performing routine activities. *You enroll him in a program of cardiac rehabilitation exercise while he continues on the same pharmaceutical therapy. Six weeks later, his functional aerobic capacity has increased 25%, and he is pleased with the significant improvement in his symptoms during activities of daily living.*

2. An 80-year-old woman (Patient No. 2) with known three-vessel CAD and hypertension presents to the emergency department with pain in the lower anterior chest. The ECG shows left ventricular hypertrophy with repolarization changes. She is admitted to the cardiology service to rule out MI and is started on heparin and intravenous platelet inhibitors. The next day there is no objective evidence of MI, but the hemoglobin has dropped 3 g and the stool occult blood test is positive. The gastroenterology service is reluctant to perform endoscopy in the setting of possible unstable angina. The patient continues to experience anterior chest discomfort. *The patient is seen by the consultant in osteopathic manipulative medicine (OMM), who obtains a history not recorded by the house staff or specialist. The patient has had low back pain for 3 weeks and took over-the-counter nonsteroidal antiinflammatory agents for pain relief. The OMM consultant identifies and treats*

musculoskeletal abnormalities that account for the chest pain and the patient obtains relief of her symptoms.

3. A 62-year-old man (Patient No. 3) has end-stage ischemic heart disease. He has had open-heart surgery twice, and four coronary angioplasty procedures. He now has severe ischemic dilated cardiomyopathy and is not a candidate for revascularization. In spite of the severity of his heart disease, what he complains about most is pain in his neck and shoulders. An empiric trial of nitroglycerin is not beneficial. Somatic dysfunction is noted on physical examination. He is sent for further osteopathic evaluation and manipulative treatment. *The OMM consultant finds somatic dysfunction in multiple regions. The most symptomatic is the left trapezius counterstrain tender point. He also has clear abnormalities in the left shoulder, left costosternal area, sacrum, and innominate. However, after three encounters, he experienced little improvement. The OMM specialist attributed this to the effects of stress related to an ongoing custody battle with his ex-wife over their mentally impaired daughter. He was further managed through counseling and stress management education.*

4. A 58-year-old woman (Patient No. 4) with type 2 diabetes presents with unstable angina pectoris. Cardiac catheterization demonstrates 90% stenosis of the left anterior descending coronary artery. The patient undergoes coronary angioplasty with placement of a stent. She is discharged home on aspirin, clopridogrel, a β-blocker, and an oral agent for diabetes mellitus. She sees you, the osteopathic physician in follow-up. Neither the cholesterol nor glycosylated hemoglobin had been evaluated at the cardiac intervention center. When the patient presents to your office, she is pleased to be completely symptom-free and anxious to return to her work as a secretary. Her weight is 50 lbs above ideal, she has not been instructed in a diabetic diet, and she has stage I systemic arterial hypertension. *You enroll her in a supervised, but unmonitored program of cardiac rehabilitation exercise. She meets with the dietitian to learn about a low-fat weight loss diet patterned for a diabetic. Baseline cholesterol profile and hemoglobin (Hgb) A1C levels are obtained. Six weeks later she returns and reports an improvement in her exercise tolerance and weight loss of 8 lbs. She indicates that she is enjoying her new diet. However, her LDL cholesterol levels are above target values. You add a statin agent to lower cholesterol. You arrange for follow-up evaluation to include a repeat cholesterol profile, liver enzyme studies in 6 weeks. A repeat HgbA1C is evaluated in 3 months.*

Besides involving a component of cardiovascular disease what key features are incorporated in each of these clinical vignettes? First of all, it should be clear that the osteopathic physician utilizes the best clinical research and evidence-based treatment protocols in patient care management. One distinctive feature of each of these cases is an emphasis on the role of the musculoskeletal system. In Patient No. 2, abnormalities of the musculoskeletal system in fact represented the primary cause of the patient's presenting symptoms, but were several steps removed from the presenting complaint. It may be that an orientation toward the role of the musculoskeletal system led the OMM consultant to inquire more specifically about musculoskeletal symptoms. Certainly, the expertise of the specialist in manipulative medicine was critical in identifying musculoskeletal abnormalities that

explained the patient's symptoms that were subsequently relieved by manipulative treatment.

Another focus of the intervention in each case was an emphasis on lifestyle, behavior, and diet in addition to the usual pharmacologic support. In Patient No. 4, modifications of diet and lifestyle were major components of the treatment plan. In Patient No. 3, the patient's behavioral response to significant stress in his life elucidated the difficulty in obtaining a satisfactory treatment response to pharmacologic therapy and OMT.

In Patient No. 1 and Patient No. 4 the intervention directed to the musculoskeletal system was cardiac rehabilitation exercise. In heart failure patients, the improvement in functional capacity gained by exercise is twice the improvement demonstrated with pharmacologic support in the form of agents such as ACE inhibitors.

Finally, the solution to problems may take more than one perspective. Treatment for patients is often multifaceted and needs to be specifically tailored to each individual. Patient No. 4 did not achieve target LDL cholesterol levels with a program of diet, exercise, and weight loss and therefore a cholesterol-lowering medication was added.

HEART FAILURE

Pathophysiology and Natural History

Heart failure is a clinical syndrome or condition characterized by (a) signs and symptoms of intravascular and interstitial volume overload including shortness of breath, rales, and edema, or (b) manifestations of inadequate tissue perfusion such as fatigue or poor exercise tolerance (189). Patients may have one or both of these features. The term "heart failure" has been recommended instead of the term "congestive heart failure" because many patients with heart failure do not manifest pulmonary or systemic congestion (189).

It is estimated that more that more than 5 million U.S. citizens have heart failure and approximately 500,000 new cases are diagnosed annually. It accounts for 12 to 15 million office visits and 1.5 million hospital days each year (190). In the last 10 years, the number of patients hospitalized annually has increased from 550,000 to 900,000 when heart failure is a primary diagnosis and from 1.7 to 2.6 million when heart failure is a primary or secondary diagnosis (191). Nearly 300,000 patients die from heart failure being a primary or contributory cause each year. The number of deaths has increased steadily, even though there has been a reduction in mortality due to coronary heart disease and systemic arterial hypertension (192), which represent the two most common causes of heart failure.

Heart failure is primarily a disease of older adults (193). Approximately 6% to 10% of people older than 65 years of age have heart failure and approximately 80% of patients hospitalized with heart failure are more than 65 years old (191). Heart failure is the most common Medicare diagnosis-related group, and more Medicare dollars are spent for the diagnosis and treatment of heart failure than for any other diagnosis (194).

A recent practice guideline from the ACC/AHA (195) suggests a new approach to the classification of heart failure that emphasizes both the evolution and progression of the disease. This describes four stages of heart failure.

- Stage A identifies the patient who is at high risk for developing heart failure, but has no structural disorder of the heart.
- Stage B refers to a patient with a structural disorder of the heart, but who has never developed symptoms of heart failure.
- Stage C denotes the patient with past or current symptoms of heart failure associated with underlying structural heart disease.
- Stage D designates the patient with end-stage disease who requires specialized treatment strategies such as mechanical circulatory support, continuous inotropic infusions, cardiac transplantation, or hospice care.

Only the latter two stages qualify for the traditional clinical diagnosis of heart failure for diagnostic or coding purposes. This classification system is intended to complement but not to replace the New York Heart Association (NYHA) functional classification. Fig. 24.10 shows how these stages of heart failure are used to define treatment approaches to patients.

The clinical syndrome of heart failure may result from disorders of the pericardium, myocardium, endocardium, or great vessels, but the majority of patients with heart failure have symptoms due to an impairment of left ventricular function. In the United States, the most common cause of heart failure due to muscle damage is coronary heart disease; the most common etiology of heart failure due to pressure overload of the heart is systemic arterial hypertension (196). In South America, Chagas disease is the most common cause of heart failure because of left ventricular damage; in Third World countries, volume overload because of rheumatic heart disease remains an important cause of heart failure. Often the disease entity is multifactorial, including features of hypertension, ischemic heart disease, and volume overload. Typically, heart failure involves systolic dysfunction with depression of contractile performance leading to depressed ejection fraction and cardiac output, and, frequently, ventricular chamber dilation. Diastolic dysfunction is increasingly recognized as a significant feature in a minority of patients with heart failure (197). This term implies impaired left ventricular filling and normal left atrial pressures, resulting in pulmonary and systemic venous congestion with little or no systolic dysfunction. Diastolic dysfunction is especially common in patients with systemic arterial hypertension, ventricular hypertrophy, or infiltrative disease.

It should be emphasized that heart failure is not equivalent to cardiomyopathy or to left ventricular dysfunction. These latter terms describe possible structural reasons for the development of heart failure. Instead, heart failure is a clinical syndrome that

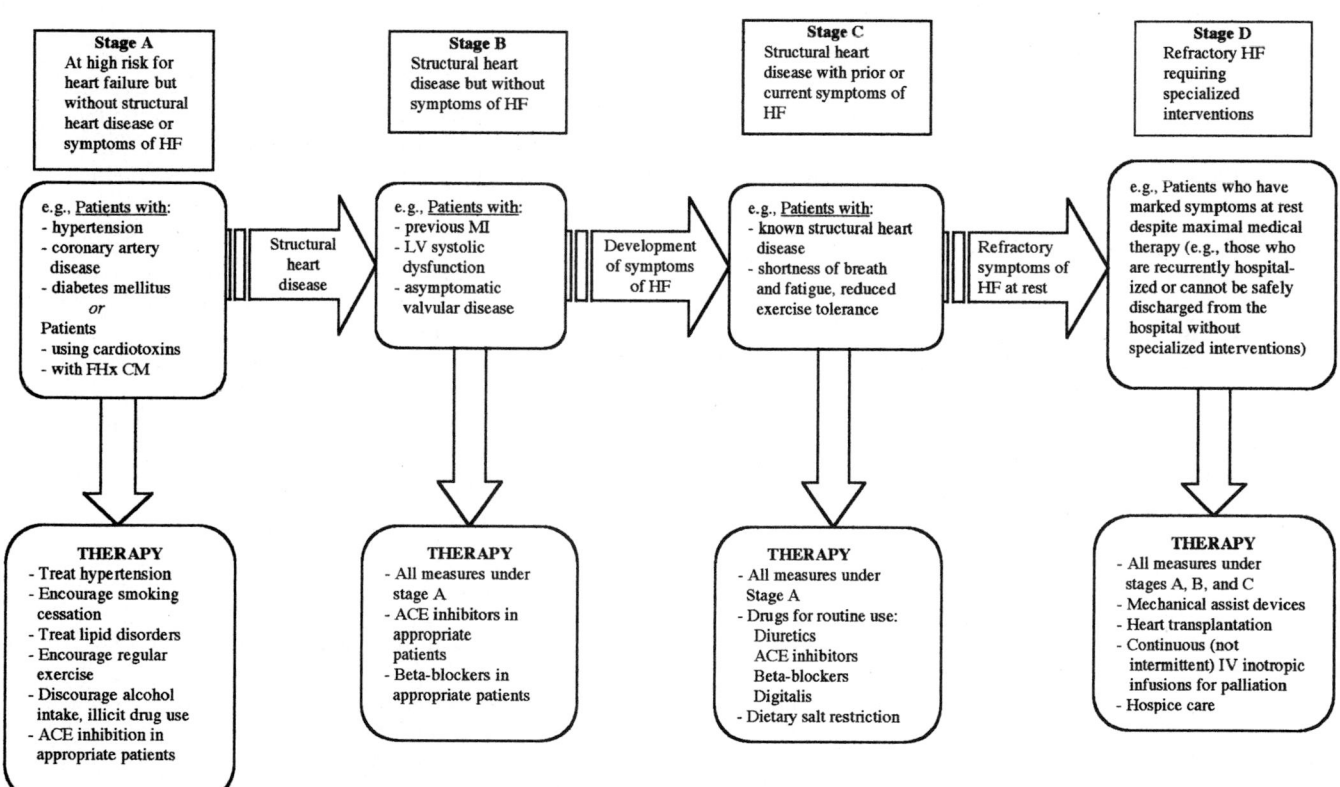

FIGURE 24.10. New model of four stages of heart failure as recommended by the American College of Cardiology and the American Heart Association. Stage A refers to individuals at high risk for heart disease, but without structural heart disease. Stage B represents patients with structural heart disease, but without symptoms of heart failure. (Modified from Hunt SA, Baker DW, Chin MH, et al. ACC/AHA guidelines for the evaluation and management of chronic heart failure in the adult: Executive Summary. *Circulation* 2001;104:2996–3007.)

is characterized by specific symptoms (dyspnea and fatigue) and signs (fluid retention). There is no diagnostic test for heart failure because it is largely a clinical diagnosis that is based on a careful history and physical examination (195).

Clinically significant left ventricular dysfunction activates neurohormonal mechanisms that promote fluid retention and that may perpetuate or worsen heart failure. Typically, these represent examples of compensatory mechanisms that are an exaggerated long-term response of a mechanism designed for short-term control. For example, the immediate hemodynamic response to hypotension caused by blood loss is intense vasoconstriction, elevation of systemic vascular resistance, and salt and water retention by the kidneys. The neurohumoral activation in heart failure includes alterations in the autonomic nervous system, including baroreceptor and peripheral adaptation (37,44,198,199), adrenergic receptors (200,201), renin-angiotensin-aldosterone system (202), atrial natriuretic factor (203,204), and endothelial function (205,206).

The degree of activation of neurohormonal mechanisms appears to depend on the severity and acuteness of cardiac impairment as well as the status of extracellular fluid volume (207). Local autocrine and paracrine systems in blood vessels and myocardium may also contribute to the long-term regulation of vascular tone and play a role in the pathogenesis of ventricular remodeling, dilation, and progressive heart failure (47). Besides these neurohormonal effects, heart failure also affects the kidneys, gastrointestinal system, and skeletal muscle.

Heart failure is a symptomatic disorder that occurs as a consequence of multiple influences on a patient with structural heart disease. Decompensation of heart failure is a clinical consideration of considerable relevance to the management of the patient with heart failure; it often occurs because of progressive worsening of structural heart disease. Sometimes decompensation of heart failure can be attributed to extracardiac features such as depression (208), malnutrition (209), anemia (210), and socioeconomic status (211). The most common cause of decompensation leading to re-admission to the hospital is non-adherence to recommendations in regard to diet and medications (212,213) (Table 24.2).

Natural History

The natural history of heart failure is affected primarily by the underlying disease process that causes left ventricular dysfunction. In some cases, this is idiopathic and irreversible. Some causes of primary muscle dysfunction may be spontaneously reversible, such as peripartum cardiomyopathy, alcoholic cardiomyopathy, or viral myocarditis. In other cases, the relentless deterioration of function may be interrupted by therapy for the underlying condition. For example, the treatment of systemic arterial hypertension, especially with ACE inhibitors, may not only control hypertension but also enhance cardiac performance and lead to regression of left ventricular hypertrophy. In the case of ischemic heart disease, although left ventricular dysfunction may be irreversible, therapy may halt or retard the progression of coronary atherosclerosis and the subsequent development of additional myocardial damage. Furthermore, ACE inhibitors may prevent or retard deleterious left ventricular

remodeling (86), and thereby reduce mortality and morbidity (87,88).

Typically, heart failure is a progressive disorder, even without a new identifiable source of cardiac damage. The most common manifestation of this progression is a deterioration in left ventricular geometry, associated with chamber dilation, hypertrophy, and an alteration in ventricular shape to become more spherical. These myocardial changes increase the hemodynamic stress on the wall of the heart, and also decrease its mechanical performance; this increases the magnitude of functional mitral regurgitation. In addition, fibrosis of the extracellular cardiac matrix has major adverse effects on the heart's electrical and mechanical function and coronary vasodilator reserve, which can be prevented by the administration of spironolactone (214).

Patients with heart failure have a poor prognosis, with average mortality rates of at least 10% at 1 year and 50% at 5 years. The important predictors of survival are: (a) the cause of heart failure, (b) patient's symptomatic and functional status, (c) hemodynamic and pathologic findings, (d) neurohumoral activity, and (e) the presence of cardiac arrhythmias (215).

Diagnosis

The standard screen of history, physical examination, ECG, and chest radiograph are helpful to establish the diagnosis of congestive heart failure. These modalities are best used to develop a composite assessment of the patient's status because pulmonary rales, jugular venous distension, and peripheral edema may be present in a minority of patients (216). Likewise, the ECG is usually nonspecific (217). In addition, complete blood count, serum electrolytes, creatinine, albumin, liver function tests, and urinalysis should be performed for all patients with suspected or clinically evident heart failure (189). Thyroxine and thyroid-stimulating hormone levels should be checked in all patients older than 65 years of age with heart failure and no obvious cause and in patients who have atrial fibrillation or other signs and symptoms of thyroid disease (189).

To assess the patient's status, more specific data are needed concerning left ventricular systolic and diastolic function. Two-dimensional ECG imaging with Doppler is the diagnostic method of choice to assess patients with suspected heart failure. These studies provide the most information about the heart, including left ventricular size and wall motion and function, in addition to providing information about the cardiac valves, atrial chambers, right ventricle, and pericardium (218). An estimation of ejection fraction is also possible from an ECG study. The diagnosis of left ventricular diastolic dysfunction has been well established using Doppler ECG criteria (219,220). Exercise testing is an emerging modality used to define the functional status of patients with heart failure (221).

Brain natriuretic peptide (BNP) is a cardiac neurohormone secreted from the cardiac ventricles as a response to ventricular volume expansion and pressure overload. BNP levels have been shown to be elevated in patients with left ventricular dysfunction and correlate with the NYHA classification as well as prognosis (222,223). A rapid point-of-care test for BNP has recently been shown to be beneficial for the diagnosis of heart failure in an urgent care setting (224,225).

Because heart failure is the end point in a diverse group of clinical disorders, effort should always be made to establish a specific diagnosis. The cause is often reversible or treatable. It is unacceptable simply to use heart failure as the final diagnosis without reference to possible causes. Approximately two-thirds of patients with heart failure have underlying CAD.

Treatment

Goals of therapy for heart failure are to enhance survival, improve the quality of life, and improve symptoms. These therapies have been well described in important practice guidelines and consensus statements (189,195,226).

Heart failure is the epidemic of largest magnitude within the field of internal medicine and the most important cardiovascular entity from a health care and economic standpoint. Therefore, the appropriate perspective is to identify those conditions and behaviors that are associated with an increased risk of heart failure *before* patients show any evidence of structural heart disease (stage A). Because early modification of these factors can often reduce the risk of heart failure, working with patients on these risk factors provides the earliest opportunity to reduce the impact of heart failure on public and individual health (195). Specific risk factor modification should be directed to the treatment of hypertension and diabetes, and the management of atherosclerotic disease. Increased systolic or diastolic blood pressure is a major risk factor for the development of heart failure (227,228). The presence of diabetes markedly increases the likelihood of heart failure in patients without structural heart disease (229) and adversely affects the outcome of patients with established heart failure (230,231). In patients with diabetes, the target level of blood pressure should be 130/85, lower than that of nondiabetic patients. Patients with known atherosclerotic disease are likely to develop heart failure, and physicians should control risk factors for atherosclerosis in these patients. Other conditions that cause cardiac injury include cigarette smoking, alcohol or cocaine use, cardiotoxic anticancer chemotherapy, and prolonged tachycardia (232,233).

The most common situation to diagnose left ventricular dysfunction in patients who do not have symptoms of heart failure (stage B) is in the setting of MI. These patients are at considerable risk of developing subsequent heart failure. They should all receive treatment with an ACE inhibitor and β-blocking agent. Patients with a history of MI and preserved left ventricular function will also benefit from an ACE inhibitor (234). Patients with severe valvular heart disease should typically undergo valve surgery before symptoms occur, especially with regurgitation of the aortic and mitral valves.

Patients with left ventricular systolic dysfunction and current or prior symptoms (stage C) are routinely managed with a combination of four types of drugs: a diuretic, an ACE inhibitor, a β-adrenergic blocker, and (usually) digitalis. The value of these drugs has been established in numerous large-scale clinical trials. Even if a patient symptomatically improves with diuretics alone, the clinical evidence clearly indicates that both an ACE inhibitor and a β-blocker should be given and maintained in all patients who tolerate them. In particular, physicians are encouraged to use β-blocking agents in the management of patients with heart failure, even though these drugs were previously thought to be relatively contraindicated in heart failure management. Three major clinical trials demonstrate the efficacy of these agents in patients with moderate and severe heart failure (235–237).

One new approach to the patient with heart failure looks not only at the enhanced activation of endogenous vasoconstrictor neurohormonal substances (such as the renin-angiotensin system) but also looks at inadequate response to endogenous vasodilator systems, such as kinins and natriuretic peptide. Current investigation is under way regarding vasopeptidase inhibitors that block not only the ACE, but also the neutral endopeptidase, which leads to enhanced activities of endogenous vasodilators. One vasopeptidase inhibitor, omapatrilat, is being developed for the treatment of hypertension and for the treatment of heart failure (238). Nesiritide, a BNP produced by recombinant gene technique, has beneficial hemodynamic effects in patients with decompensated heart failure (239).

Patients with end-stage, refractory heart failure (stage D) typically have symptoms at rest or with minimal exertion, and cannot perform most activities of daily living. They represent the most advanced stage of heart failure and should be considered for specialized treatment strategies such as mechanical circulatory support, continuous intravenous positive inotropic therapy, referral for cardiac transplantation, or hospice care (195). They will need meticulous control of fluid status, and they should receive ACE inhibitors and β-blockers given with caution.

Exercise and Heart Failure

The mechanisms responsible for the exercise intolerance of patients with chronic heart failure have not been clearly defined. Many studies show a poor relation between cardiac performance and the symptoms of heart failure. Patients with a very low ejection fraction may be completely asymptomatic, and patients with preserved left ventricular systolic function may have severe disability. The apparent lack of agreement between the severity of systolic dysfunction and the degree of functional impairment is not fully understood. It may be related to alterations in ventricular diastolic function, valvular regurgitation, pericardial restraint, and right ventricular function. In ambulatory patients, noncardiac factors may contribute to exercise intolerance. These include changes in peripheral vascular function, skeletal muscle physiology, pulmonary dynamics, and neurohormonal and reflex autonomic activity. These noncardiac factors may explain why the hemodynamic improvement produced by therapeutic agents in patients with chronic heart failure may not be immediately or necessarily translated into clinical improvement. Although pharmacologic interventions may produce rapid changes in hemodynamic variables, signs and symptoms may improve slowly over weeks or months, or not at all.

The Muscle Hypothesis

The "muscle hypothesis" proposes the possibility that abnormal skeletal muscle in heart failure results in activation of muscle ergoreceptors, which in turn leads to an enhanced signal to ventilation, and results in sympathetic activation (Fig. 24.11) (51). The afferents from skeletal muscle are sensitive to metabolic effects of muscular exercise. They then modulate hemodynamic,

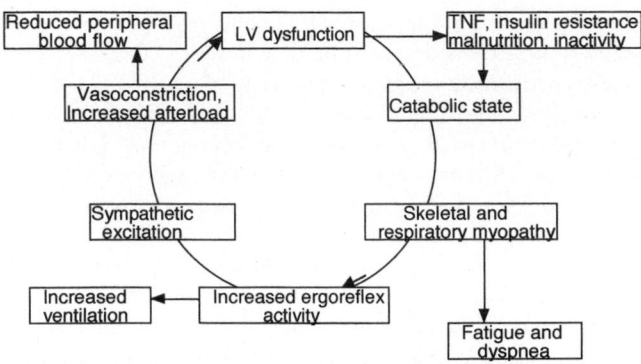

FIGURE 24.11. The muscle hypothesis. (Modified from Coats AJS, Clark AL, Piepoli M, et al. Symptoms and quality of life in heart failure: the muscle hypothesis. *Br Heart J.* 1994;72[Suppl]:S36–S39.)

ventilatory, and autonomic responses. These are small myelinated and unmyelinated afferents, of group III and IV afferents. They arise from "free" or "naked" nerve terminals, associated with collagen structure and skeletal muscles or with blood and lymphatic vessels. They are presumed to be engaged in feedback control, where muscle work regulates energy supply. The central reflection of these pathways is in the ventral lateral medulla, including the lateral reticular nucleus. These receptors are overactive during exercise, and play a larger role in responses to exercise in patients with chronic heart failure with respect to control subjects. The overactivated muscle signal in heart failure due to abnormalities in exercising muscle causes an increased ventilatory drive (239).

The muscle afferents are histologically inseparable from pain fiber afferents, so they may serve sensory as well as reflex function, mediating the sensation of fatigue and the exaggerated ventilatory and cardiovascular responses to exercise (240). This system could mediate a sympatho-excitatory and vasoconstrictor response to exercise. However, the subnormal blood flow response to exercise and pharmacologic vasodilation is complex, and may include persistent vasoconstrictor drive, edema of resistance vessel walls, a relative paucity of peripheral blood vessels, a deficient nitric oxide vasodilator, and enhancement of the vasoconstrictor endothelin (241).

The neural link to explain the muscle hypothesis of exercise intolerance in chronic heart failure was investigated in 92 stable patients with heart failure, compared to 28 age-matched controls. Exercise tolerance was measured by bicycle ergometry; the ergoreflex activity was evaluated with two dynamic handgrip tests. Three minutes of local circulatory occlusion was used during the second study, to isolate the neural component to the ergoreflex (as opposed to circulating metabolites). Isometric handgrip was associated with a prolonged increase in systolic and diastolic blood pressure, an increase in ventilation, and increase in leg vascular resistance. The intensity of the reflex was higher in NYHA class II and III heart failure patients than in class I patients (242).

The Role of Exercise Training in Chronic Heart Failure

It is estimated that at least one-fourth of patients with chronic heart failure are limited by skeletal muscle changes rather than decreased cardiac output and underperfusion. This may explain

why certain patients do not respond to inotropes or vasodilators, and establishes the role of cardiac rehabilitation exercise in patients with heart failure.

Randomized, controlled trials have assessed the effects of exercise training in patients with symptomatic heart failure (243–250). Studies have demonstrated improvement in exercise capacity (measured by peak exercise duration or peak oxygen consumption) (243–250) and also show favorable changes in autonomic nervous system function (249), regional blood flow (246), endothelial function (251), and skeletal muscle function (252,253).

During long-term moderate exercise training, heart failure patients randomized to the exercise group experience an increase in their peak exercise oxygen consumption and an improvement in the myocardial thallium score. Measures of their quality of life improved parallel to the increase in peak oxygen consumption (250). Exercise training has also been shown to lead to attenuation of the harmful process of left ventricular remodeling in postinfarction patients, perhaps through a chronic decrease in sympathetic nervous system tone (254).

With exercise training of 1 to 6 months, a significant increase in exercise duration has been demonstrated in the trained subjects. The observed increase of 26% to 37% is almost double that which has been reported with ACE inhibitors or digoxin (255,256). The improvement with exercise is additive to the benefits of ACE inhibitors and β-blockers (246,257). Some of the skeletal abnormalities are due to deconditioning, and they are partly reversed by exercise training. Training has also been shown to reduce the exaggerated ergoreflex activity, thereby improving the response to exercise (258).

The exercise prescription for patients with heart failure is similar to other types of heart disease—the patient should engage in aerobic activity that allows them to accumulate 30 minutes of exercise three times each week. Often these patients do not tolerate their first week of exercise well. They may need additional rest or may need to delay other household or leisure time activity. Because of co-existing disease, or exacerbation of symptoms, patients with heart failure may experience interruption of their exercise program. The patient should be encouraged that the person who is most unfit has the most to gain from an exercise program (Fig. 24.12).

An expert panel of the Agency for Health Care Policy and Research recommends exercise for patients with heart failure (163). Exercise needs to be incorporated into a comprehensive program of outpatient management for heart failure. Today, such a program includes more than the standard therapy of ACE inhibitors, diuretics, digitalis, β-blockers, and spironolactone. Additional components of a comprehensive program include diet instruction, salt restriction, nurse-directed telemedicine follow-up, and occasionally freestanding heart failure clinics.

Osteopathic Implication

Since the muscle hypothesis of chronic heart failure places a central role on peripheral mechanisms (51), especially involving muscle ergoreceptors, this model of heart failure is appropriate for evaluation and testing by members of the osteopathic profession.

The obvious question that arises is: what is the most appropriate intervention into the derangements of musculoskeletal

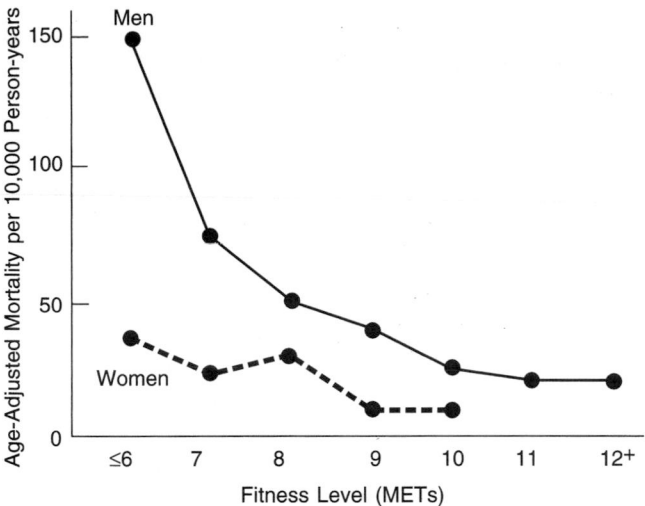

FIGURE 24.12. Age-adjusted, all-cause mortality per 10,000 person-years of follow-up by physical fitness level (METs) achieved during maximal treadmill exercise testing. Survival advantage of an improved fitness level is greatest at the lowest level of physical fitness: Unfit persons have the most to gain from exercise programs. (Modified from Blair SN, Kohl HW III, Barlow CE, et al. Changes in physical fitness and all-cause mortality. A prospective study of healthy and unhealthy men. *JAMA* 1989;262:2395–2401).

function associated with chronic heart failure? The obvious answer is those interventions that are most effective! Although it would be attractive to say that the most appropriate is to apply OMT, at the present time, the intervention with proven efficacy is cardiac rehabilitation exercise training and localized muscle group training as described above. On a theoretical basis, other interventions into the musculoskeletal system such as yoga, tai chi, and dietary approaches are worthy of study.

It is intriguing to consider the possibility that OMT could play a role in the management of patients with chronic heart failure. Very few studies have been conducted (259). However, the developing literature concerning the muscle hypothesis of heart failure and the effects of exercise training provide a road map that could lead to the development of a conceptual model for testing the efficacy of OMT. Manipulative treatment would be directed at the paraspinal musculature, the appendicular system, and the respiratory diaphragm. The magnitude of effect of OMT would be compared to other interventions such as cardiac rehabilitation exercise. The intermediate outcomes would be changes in palpatory findings of the musculature, the peak oxygen consumption with exercise, exercise duration, the slope of ventilation to carbon dioxide production, and measurements of autonomic nervous system tone such as heart rate variability. The health outcomes would be improved quality of life, NYHA classification, and functional status. Because of the delayed time course of improvements in musculoskeletal function in response to intervention, the response to OMT would have to be followed over an interval of 4 to 8 weeks, or possibly longer.

REFERENCES

1. Rogers FJ, D'Alonzo GE, Glover J, et al. Osteopathic tenets and principles for patient care. *JAOA*. 2002;102:63–65.

2. Linden RJ. Reflexes from the heart. *Prog Cardiovasc Dis.* 1975;18:201–221.

3. Paintal AS. Vagal sensory receptors and their reflex effects. *Physiol Rev.* 1973;53:159–227.

4. Malliani A, Peterson DF, Bishop VS, Brown AM. Spinal sympathetic cardiovascular reflexes. *Circ Res.* 1972;30:158–166.

5. Malliani A, Lombardi F, Pagani M. Functions of afferents in cardiovascular sympathetic nerves. *J Auton Nerv Syst.* 1981;3:231–236.

6. Mark AL. The Bezold-Jarisch reflex revisited: clinical implications of inhibitory reflexes originating in the heart. *J Am Coll Cardiol.* 1983;1:90–102.

7. Wurster RD. Cardiac autonomic control interaction of somatic and visceral afferents. In: Patterson MM, Howell JN, eds. *The Central Connection: Somatovisceral/Viscerosomatic Interaction. 1989 International Symposium.* Athens, OH: American Academy of Osteopathy, University Classics; 1989:266–276.

8. Lown B, Malliani A, Prosdocimi M, eds. *Neural Mechanisms and Cardiovascular Disease.* Fidia Research Series. Vol 5. Padova, Italy: Liviana Press, Springer-Verlag; 1986.

9. Hainsworth R, Kidd C, Linden RJ. *Cardiac Receptors.* Oxford, England: Cambridge University Press; 1979.

10. Abboud FM, Fozzard HA, Gilmore JP, Reis DJ. *Disturbances in Neurogenic Control of the Circulation.* Baltimore, MD: Williams & Wilkins; 1981.

11. Schwartz PJ, Brown AM, Malliani A, Zanchetti A, eds. *Neural Mechanisms in Cardiac Arrhythmias. Perspectives in Cardiovascular Research.* Vol 2. New York, NY: Raven Press; 1978.

12. Kobilka B. Adrenergic and muscarinic receptors of the heart. In: Roberts R, ed. *Molecular Basis of Cardiology.* Boston, MA: Blackwell Scientific Publications; 1993:193–209.

13. Crick SJ, Sheppard MN, Anderson RH. Neural supply of the heart. In: Ter Horst GJ, ed. *The Nervous System and the Heart.* Totowa, NJ: Humana; 2000:3–54.

14. Armour JA, Murphy DA, Yuan BX, et al. Gross and microscopic anatomy of the human cardiac nervous system. *Anat Rec.* 1997;247:289–298.

15. Wharton J, Polak JM, Gordon L, et al. Immunohistochemical demonstration of human cardiac innervation before and after transplantation. *Circ Res.* 1990; 66:900–912.

16. Ter Horst GJ. Emotions and heart-activity control: neurocircuitries and pathway interactions. In: Ter Horst GJ, ed. *The Nervous System and the Heart.* Totowa, NJ: Humana; 2000:55–115.

17. Ohtsuka T, Hamada M, Kodama K, et al. Neurogenic stunned myocardium. *Circulation.* 2000;101:2122–2124.

18. Muller JE, Stone PH, Turi ZG, et al. Circadian variation in the frequency of the onset of acute myocardial infarction. *N Engl J Med.* 1985;313:1315–1322.

19. Rocco MB. Timing and triggers of transient myocardial ischemia. *Am J Cardiol.* 1990;66:18G–21G.

20. Smolensky MH, D'Alonzo GE, Portman R. Chronobiology and chronotherapeutics: New concepts in cardiovascular medicine. *JAOA.* 1998;98[Suppl July]:S6–S16.

21. Gnecchi-Ruscone T, Piccaluga E., Guzzetti S, et al. Morning and Monday: Critical periods for the onset of acute myocardial infarction. The GISSI 2 Study experience. *Eur Heart J.* 1994;15:882–887.

22. Spencer FA, Goldberg RJ, Becker RC, Gore JM. Seasonal distribution of acute myocardial infarction in the second National Registry of Myocardial Infarction. *J Am Coll Cardiol.* 1998;31:1226–1233.

23. Bohus B, Korte SM. Stress, the hypothalamo-pituitary system, and the heart. In: Ter Horst GJ, ed. *The Nervous System and the Heart.* Totowa, NJ: Humana; 2000:241–264.

24. Reagan LP. The central renin-angiotensin system in cardiovascular regulation. In: Ter Horst GJ, ed. *The Nervous System and the Heart.* Totowa, NJ: Humana; 2000:415–465.

25. de Jongste MJL, Ter Horst GJ. Mediators of inflammation in patients with coronary artery disease. In: Ter Horst GJ, ed. *The Nervous System and the Heart.* Totowa, NJ: Humana; 2000:467–487.

26. Gehman HS. *The New Westminster Dictionary of the Bible.* Philadelphia, PA: Westminster Press; 1970:901–902.

27. Leff J, ed. *Psychiatry Around the Globe.* London, England: Gaskell; 1988.

28. Kleinman A, Kleinman J. Somatization: the interconnections in Chinese society among culture, depressive experiences and the meanings of pain. In: Kleinman A, Good B, eds. *Culture and Depression.* Berkley, CA: University of California Press; 1985:429–491.

29. King DE, Bushwick B. Beliefs and attitudes of hospital in patients about faith healing and prayer. *J Fam Pract.* 1994;39:349–352.

30. Mueller PS, Plevak DJ, Rummans TA. Religious involvement, spirituality, and medicine: implications for clinical practice. *Mayo Clin Proc.* 2001;76:1225–1235.

31. Koenig HG, McCullough ME, Larson DB. *Handbook of Religion and Health,* New York, NY: Oxford University Press; 2001.

32. Strawbridge WJ, Shema SJ, Cohen RD, Kaplan GA. Religious attendance increases survival by improving and maintaining good health behaviors, mental health, and social relationships. *Ann Behav Med.* 2001;23:68–74.

33. Wallace JM Jr, Forman TA. Religion's role in promoting health and reducing risk among American youth. *Health Educ Behav.* 1998;25:721–741.

34. Oleckno WA, Blacconiere MJ. Relationship of religiosity to wellness and other health-related behaviors and outcomes. *Psychol Rep.* 1991;68:819–826.

35. Comstock GW, Partridge KB. Church attendance and health. *J Chronic Dis.* 1972;25:665–672.

36. Aviles JM, Whelan E, Hernke DA, et al. Intercessory prayer and cardiovascular disease progression in a coronary care unit population: a randomized controlled trial. *Mayo Clin Proc.* 2001;76: 1192–1198.

37. Malliani A, Pagani M, Lombardi F, Cerulti S. Cardiovascular neural regulation explored in the frequency domain. *Circulation.* 1991;84:482–492.

38. Dzau VJ, Krieger JE. Molecular biology of hypertension. In: Roberts R, ed. *Molecular Basis of Cardiology.* Boston, MA: Blackwell Scientific Publications;1993:325–353.

39. Korr IM. The spinal cord as organizer of disease processes: the peripheral autonomic nervous system. *JAOA.* 1979;79:82–90.

40. Zucker IH, Gilmore JP, eds. In: *Reflex Control of the Circulation.* Boca Raton, FL: CRC Press; 1991.

41. O'Rourke ST, Vanhoutte PM. Vascular pharmacology. In: Loscalzo J, Creager MA, Dzau VJ, eds. *Vascular Medicine: A Textbook of Vascular Biology and Diseases.* Boston, MA: Little, Brown and Company; 1992:133–155.

42. Corti R, Burnett JC, Rouleau JL, et al. Vasopeptidase inhibitors. A new therapeutic concept in cardiovascular disease? *Circulation.* 2001;104:1856–1862.

43. Zelis R, Flaim SF. Alterations in vasomotor tone in congestive heart failure. *Prog Cardiovasc Dis.* 1982;24:437–459.

44. Eckberg DL, Drabinski M, Braunwald E. Defective cardiac parasympathetic control in patients with heart disease. *N Engl J Med.* 1971;285:877–883.

45. Levin TB, Francis GS, Goldsmith SR, et al. Activity of the sympathetic nervous system and renin angiotensin system assessed by plasma hormone levels and their relation to hemodynamic abnormalities in congestive heart failure. *Am J Cardiol.* 1982;49:1659–1666.

46. Cody RJ. Neurohormonal influences in the pathogenesis of congestive heart failure. *Cardiol Clin.* 1989;7:73–86.

47. Dzau VJ. Contributions of neuroendocrine and local autocrine-paracrine mechanisms to the pathophysiology and pharmacology of congestive heart failure. *Am J Cardiol.* 1982;62:76E–81E.

48. Cohn JN, Levine TB, Olivari MT, et al. Plasma norepinephrine as a guide to prognosis in patients with chronic congestive heart failure. *N Engl J Med.* 1984;311:819–823.

49. Drexler H. Reduced exercise tolerance in chronic heart failure and its relationship to neurohumoral factors. *Eur Heart J.* 1991;12[Suppl C]: 21–28.

50. Uren NG, Lipken DP. Exercise training as therapy for chronic heart failure. *Br Heart J.* 1992;67:430–433.

51. Coats AJS, Clark AL, Piepoli M, et al. Symptoms and quality of life in heart failure: the muscle hypothesis. *Br Heart J.* 1994;72[Suppl]:S36–S39.

52. Francis GS, Goldsmith SR, Cohn JN. Relationship of exercise capacity to resting left ventricular performance and basal plasma norepinephrine levels in patients with congestive heart failure. *Am Heart J.* 1982;104:725–731.

53. Cleland JGF, Oakley CM. Vascular tone in heart failure: the neuroendocrine therapeutic interface. *Br Heart J.* 1991;66:264–267.

54. Tuininga YS, van Veldhuisen DJ, Brouwer J, et al. Heart rate variability in left ventricular dysfunction and heart failure: effects and implications of drug treatment. *Br Heart J.* 1994;72:509–513.

55. Gheorghiade M, Ferguson D. Digoxin. A neurohormonal modulator for heart failure? *Circulation.* 1991;84:2182–2186.

56. Mark AL. Sympathetic dysregulation in heart failure: mechanisms and therapy. *Clin Cardiol.* 1995;18[Suppl I]:I3–I8.

57. Cody RJ. The effect of captopril on postural hemodynamics and autonomic responses in chronic heart failure. *Am Heart J.* 1982;104:1190–1196.

58. Rouleau J-L, Packer M, Moyé L, et al. Prognostic value of humoral activation in patients with acute myocardial infarction: the effect of captopril. *J Am Coll Cardiol.* 1994;24:583–591.

59. Cody RJ, Franklin KW, Kluger J, Laragh JH. Sympathetic responsiveness and plasma norepinephrine during therapy of chronic congestive heart failure with captopril. *Am J Med.* 1982;72:791–797.

60. Kluger J, Cody RJ, Laragh JH. The contributions of sympathetic tone and the renin-angiotensin system to severe chronic congestive heart failure: response to specific inhibitors (prazosin and captopril). *Am J Cardiol.* 1982;49:1667–1674.

61. Flapan AD, Nolan J, Neilson JMM, et al. Effect of captopril on cardiac parasympathetic activity in chronic heart failure secondary to coronary heart disease. *Am J Cardiol.* 1992;69:532–535.

62. Waagstein F, Caidahl K, Wallentin I, et al. Long-term β-blockade in dilated cardiomyopathy: effects of short- and long-term metoprolol treatment followed by withdrawal and readministration of metoprolol. *Circulation.* 1989;80:551–563.

63. Heilbrunn SM, Shah F, Bristow MR, et al. Increased β-receptor density and improved hemodynamic response to catecholamine stimulation during long-term metoprolol therapy in heart failure from dilated cardiomyopathy. *Circulation.* 1989;79:483–490.

64. Forrester JS, Litvack F, Grunfest W, Hickey A. A perspective of coronary disease seen through the arteries of living man. *Circulation.* 1987;75:505–513.

65. Davies MJ, Thomas A. Thrombosis and acute coronary lesions in sudden cardiac ischemic death. *N Engl J Med.* 1984;310:1137–1140.

66. Ornish DM, Brown SE, Scherwitz LW, et al. Can lifestyle changes reverse coronary atherosclerosis? The Lifestyle Heart Trial. *Lancet.* 1990;336:129–133.

67. Haskell WL, Alderman EL, Fair JM, et al. Effects of intense multiple risk factor reduction on coronary atherosclerosis and clinical cardiac events in men and women with coronary artery disease: the Stanford Coronary Risk Intervention Project (SCRIP). *Circulation.* 1994;89:975–990.

68. Pitt B, Mancini GBJ, Ellis SG, et al. Pravastatin limitation of atherosclerosis in the coronary arteries (PLAC I). Reduction in atherosclerosis progression and clinical events. *J Am Coll Cardiol.* 1995;26:1133–1139.

69. Hambrecht R, Niebauer J, Marburger C, et al. Various intensities of leisure time physical activity in patients with coronary artery disease: effects on cardiorespiratory fitness and progression of coronary atherosclerotic lesions. *J Am Coll Cardiol.* 1993;22:468–477.

70. Verschuren WMM, Jacobs DR, Bloemberg BPM, et al. Serum total cholesterol and long-term coronary heart disease mortality in different cultures. Twenty-five year follow-up of the Seven Countries Study. *JAMA.* 1995;274:131–135.

71. Hodis HN, Mack WJ, LaBrec L, et al. Serial coronary angiographic evidence that antioxidant vitamin intake reduces progression of coronary artery atherosclerosis. *JAMA.* 1995;273:1849–1854.

72. Jukema JW, Bruschke AVG, van Boven AJ, et al. on behalf of the REGRESS Study Group. Effects of lipid lowering by pravastatin on progression and regression of coronary artery disease in symptomatic men with normal to moderately elevated serum cholesterol levels. The

Regression Growth Evaluation Statin Study (REGRESS). *Circulation.* 1995;91:2528–2540.

73. Brown BG, Zhao X-Q, Chait A, et al. Simvastatin and niacin, antioxidant vitamins, or the combination for the prevention of coronary disease. *N Engl J Med.* 2001;345:1583–1592.

74. Pearson TA, Marx HJ. The rapid reduction in cardiac events with lipid lowering therapy: mechanisms and implications. *Am J Cardiol.* 1993;72:1072–1073.

75. Treasure CB, Klein JL, Weintraub WS, et al. Beneficial effects of cholesterol-lowering therapy on the coronary endothelium in patients with coronary artery disease. *N Engl J Med.* 1995;332:481–487.

76. Anderson TJ, Meredith IT, Yeung AC. The effect of cholesterol-lowering and anti-oxidant therapy on endothelium-dependent coronary vasomotion. *N Engl J Med.* 1995;332:488–493.

77. Factor SM, Bache RJ. Pathophysiology of myocardial ischemia. In: Schlant RC, Alexander RR, eds. *The Heart, Arteries, and Veins.* New York, NY: McGraw-Hill; 1994:1036–1037.

78. Braunwald E. On future directions for cardiology. The Paul D. White Lecture. *Circulation.* 1988;77:13–32.

79. Isner JM. Cancer and atherosclerosis. The broad mandate of angiogenesis. *Circulation.* 1999;99:1653–1655.

80. Barger A, Beeuwkes IR, Lainey L, Silverman K. Hypothesis: vasa vasorum and neovascularization of human coronary arteries. *N Engl J Med.* 1984;310:175–177.

81. Glagov S, Weisenberg E, Zarins CK, et al. Compensatory enlargement of human atherosclerotic coronary arteries. *N Engl J Med.* 1987;316:1371–1375.

82. Steinke W, Els T, Hennerici M. Compensatory carotid artery dilatation in early atherosclerosis. *Circulation.* 1994;89:2578–2581.

83. Lasordo DW, Rosenfeld K, Kaufman J, et al. Focal compensatory enlargement of human arteries in response to progressive atherosclerosis. In vivo documentation using intravascular ultrasound. *Circulation.* 1994;89:2570–2577.

84. Clarkson TB, Prichard RW, Morgan TM, et al. Remodeling of coronary arteries in human and non-human primates. *JAMA.* 1994;271:289–294.

85. Schoenhagen P, Ziada KM, Vince DG, et al. Arterial remodeling and coronary artery disease: the concept of "dilated" vs. "obstructive" coronary atherosclerosis. *J Am Coll Cardiol.* 2000;38:297–306.

86. Pouleur H, Rousseau MF, van Eyll C, et al. for the SOLVD Investigators. Cardiac mechanics during development of heart failure. *Circulation.* 1993;87[Suppl IV]:IV–14IV–20.

87. Pfeffer MA, Braunwald E, Moyé LA, et al. on behalf of the SAVE Investigators. Effect of captopril on mortality and morbidity in patients with left ventricular dysfunction after myocardial infarction: results of the survival and ventricular enlargement trial. *N Engl J Med.* 1992;327:669–677.

88. The SOLVD Investigators. Effect of enalapril on mortality and the development of heart failure in asymptomatic patients with reduced left ventricular ejection fractions. *N Engl J Med.* 1992;327:685–691.

89. Beltrami AP, Urbanek K, Kajstura J, et al. Evidence that human cardiac myocytes divide after myocardial infarction. *N Engl J Med.* 2001;344:1750–1757.

90. Fye WB. Nitroglycerin: a homeopathic remedy. *Circulation.* 1986;73:21–29.

91. Thom TJ, Kannel WB, Silbershatz H, D'Agostino RB, Sr. Incidence, prevalence and mortality of cardiovascular diseases in the United States. In: Alexander RW, Schlant RC, Fuster V, et al, eds. *Hurst's the Heart.* New York, NY: McGraw-Hill; 1998:3–17.

92. Healthy People 2010. Available at: www.nhlbi.nih.gov/health/prof/heart/other/hm_sp00/fedgov.htm. Accessed April 30, 2002.

93. Roberts R. A perspective: the new millennium dawns on a new paradigm for cardiology—molecular genetics. *J Am Coll Cardiol.* 2000;36:661–667.

94. McKusick VA. The anatomy of the human genome. A neo-Vesalian basis for medicine in the 21st century. *J Am Med Assoc.* 2001;286:2289–2295.

95. Jarcho JA, McKenna W, Pare JAP, et al. Mapping a gene for familial hypertrophic cardiomyopathy to chromosome 14q1. *N Engl J Med.* 1989;321:1372–1378.

96. Gaffney TE, Braunwald E. Importance of adrenergic nervous system in support of circulatory function in patients with congestive heart failure. *Am J Med.* 1963;34:320–324.

97. Yoshimura M, Yasue H, Okumura K, et al. Different secretion patterns of atrial natriuretic peptide and brain natriuretic peptide in patients with congestive heart failure. *Circulation.* 1993;87:464–469.

98. Colucci WS, Elkayam U, Horton D, et al. Intravenous nesiritide, natriuretic peptide in the treatment of decompensated congestive heart failure. *N Engl J Med.* 2000;343:246–253.

99. Fletcher GF, Balady G, Blair SN, et al. Statement on exercise: benefits and recommendations for physical activity programs for all Americans: A statement for health professionals by the Committee on Exercise and Cardiac Rehabilitation of the Council on Clinical Cardiology, American Heart Association. *Circulation.* 1994;89:1329–1445.

100. Lotufo PA, Gaziano JM, Chae CU, et al. Diabetes and all-cause and coronary heart disease mortality among U.S. male physicians. *Arch Intern Med.* 2001;161:242–247.

101. Manson JE, Colditz GA, Stampfer MJ, et al. A prospective study of maturity-onset diabetes mellitus and the risk of coronary heart disease and stroke in women. *Arch Intern Med.* 1991;151:1141–1147.

102. Blair SN, Kohl HW III, Barlow CE, et al. Changes in physical fitness and all-cause mortality. A prospective study of healthy and unhealthy men. *JAMA.* 1995;273:1093–1098.

103. Bittner V, Weiner DH, Yusuf S, et al. for the SOLVD Investigators. Prediction of mortality and morbidity with a 6-minute walk test in patients with left ventricular dysfunction. *JAMA.* 1993;270:1702–1707.

104. Mark DE, Shaw L, Harrell FE Jr, et al. Prognostic value of a treadmill score in outpatients with suspected coronary artery disease. *N Engl J Med.* 1991;325:849–853.

105. Cox JM, Gorbis S, Dick L, et al. Palpable musculoskeletal findings in coronary artery disease. Results of a double blind study. *JAOA.* 1983;82:831–836.

106. Beal MC. Palpatory testing for somatic dysfunction in patients with cardiovascular disease. *JAOA.* 1983;82:822–831.

107. Nicholas AS, DeBias DA, Ehrenfeuchter W, et al. A somatic component to myocardial infarction. *Br Med J.* 1985;291:13–17.

108. Schwartz SM, Campbell GR, Campbell JH. Replication of smooth muscle cells in vascular disease. *Circulation Res.* 1986;58:427–444.

109. Geer JC. Fine structure of human aortic intimal thickening fatty streaks. *Lab Invest.* 1965;14:1764–1783.

110. Fuster V, Badimon L, Badimon JJ, Chesebro JH. The pathogenesis of coronary artery disease and the acute coronary syndromes. *N Engl J Med.* 1992;326:242–250, 310–318.

111. Ross R. Atherosclerosis—an inflammatory disease. *N Engl J Med.* 1999;340:115–126.

112. Summary of the second report of the National Cholesterol Education Program (NCEP) Expert Panel on the detection, evaluation, and treatment of high cholesterol in adults (adult treatment panel II). *JAMA.* 1993;269:3015–3023.

113. Grundy SM. National Cholesterol Education Program: second report of the Expert Panel on detection, evaluation, and treatment of high blood cholesterol in adults. *Circulation.* 1994;89:1329–1445.

114. Expert Panel on Detection, Evaluation and Treatment of High Blood Cholesterol in Adults. Executive summary of the third report of the national cholesterol education program (NCEP) expert panel on detection, evaluation, and treatment of high blood cholesterol in adults (Adult Treatment Panel III). *JAMA.* 2001;285:2486–2497.

115. Braunwald E. Unstable angina. An etiologic approach to management. *Circulation.* 1998;98:2219–2222.

116. Davies MJ, Thomas AC. Plaque fissuring: the cause of acute myocardial infarction, sudden ischemic death, and crescendo angina. *Br Heart J.* 1985;53:363–373.

117. Ambrose JA, Winters S, Stern A, et al. Angiographic morphology and the pathogenesis of unstable angina pectoris. *J Am Coll Cardiol.* 1985;5:609–616.

118. Rentrop KP. Thrombi in acute coronary syndromes. Revisited and revised. *Circulation.* 2000;101:1619–1626.

119. Farb A, Burke AP, Tang AL, et al. Coronary plaque erosion without rupture into a lipid core: a frequent cause of coronary thrombosis in sudden coronary death. *Circulation.* 1996;93:1354–1363.

120. Morrow DA, Rifai N, Antman EM, et al. C-reactive protein is a potent predictor of mortality independently of and in combination with troponin-T in acute coronary syndromes: a TIMI IIa substudy. *J Am Coll Cardiol.* 1998;31:1460–1465.

121. Biasucci LM, Liuzzo G, Grillo RL, et al. Elevated levels of C-reactive protein at discharge in patients with unstable angina predict recurrent instability. *Circulation.* 1999;99:855–860.

122. Ridker PM, Hennekens CH, Buring JE, Rifai N. C-reactive protein and other markers of inflammation in the prediction of cardiovascular disease in women. *N Engl J Med.* 2000;342:836–843.

123. Topol EJ, Yadav JS. Recognition of the importance of embolization in atherosclerotic vascular disease. *Circulation.* 2000;100:570–580.

124. Diamond GA, Forrester JS. Analysis of probability as an aid in the clinical diagnosis of coronary artery disease. *N Engl J Med.* 1979;300:1350–1358.

125. Ahmed WH, Bittl JA, Braunwald E. Relation between clinical presentation and angiographic findings in unstable angina pectoris and comparison with that in stable angina. *Am J Cardiol.* 1993;72:544–550.

126. Sherman CT, Litvak F, Grundfest W, et al. Coronary angioscopy in patients with unstable angina pectoris. *N Engl J Med.* 1986;315:913–919.

127. Braunwald E, Mark DB, Jones RH, et al. *Unstable Angina: Diagnosis and Management.* Clinical Practice Guidelines No. 10. Rockwell, MD: Agency for Health Care Policy and Research and the National Heart, Lung and Blood Institute; March 1994. Public Health Service. US Department of Health and Human Services. AHCPR publication 94-0602.

128. Shub C. Stable angina pectoris, 2. Cardiac evaluation and diagnostic testing. *Mayo Clin Proc.* 1990;65:243–255.

129. Fletcher GF, Schlant RC. The exercise test. In: Schlant RC, Alexander RW, eds. *The Heart, Arteries, and Veins.* New York, NY: McGraw-Hill; 1994:423–440.

130. Marcus MI, Schelbert HR, Skorton D, et al. *Cardiac Imaging. A Companion to Braunwald's Heart Disease.* Philadelphia, PA: WB Saunders; 1991.

131. Moss AJ, Goldstein RE, Hall WJ, et al. Detection and significance of myocardial ischemia in stable patients after recovery from acute coronary event. Multicenter Myocardial Ischemia Research Group. *JAMA.* 1993;269:2379–2385.

132. Hurst JW, Morris DC. The history: symptoms and past events related to cardiovascular disease. In: Schlant RC, Alexander RW, eds. *The Heart, Arteries, and Veins,* 8th ed. New York, NY: McGraw-Hill; 1994:205.

133. Ruch TC. Pathophysiology of pain. In: Ruch TC, Patton HD, eds. *Physiology and Biophysics. The Brain and Neural Function,* 20th ed. Philadelphia, PA: WB Saunders; 1979:305–316.

134. Henry JA, Montuschi E. Cardiac pain referred to the site of previously experienced somatic pain. *Br Med J.* 1978;2:1605–1606.

135. Deanfield JE, Ribiero P, Oakley K, et al. Analysis of ST-segment changes in normal subjects: implications for ambulatory monitoring in angina pectoris. *Am J Cardiol.* 1984;54:1321–1325.

136. Deanfield JE, Maseri A, Selwyn AP, et al. Myocardial ischemia during daily life in patients with stable angina: its relation to symptoms and heart rate changes. *Lancet.* 1983;1:753–758.

137. Deanfield JE, Shea M, Kensett M, et al. Silent myocardial ischemia due to mental stress. *Lancet.* 1984;2:100–111.

138. Kannell WB, Cupples LA, Gagnon DR. Incidence, precursors, and prognosis of unrecognized myocardial infarction. *Adv Cardiol.* 1990;37:202–214.

139. Cannon RO III. The sensitive heart. A syndrome of abnormal cardiac pain perception. *JAMA.* 1995;273:883–887.

140. Chauhan A, Mullins PA, Thuraisingham S, et al. Abnormal cardiac pain perception in syndrome X. *J Am Coll Cardiol.* 1994;24:329–335.

141. Crea F, Gaspardone A, Kaski JC, et al. Relation between stimulation site of cardiac afferent nerves by adenosine and distribution of cardiac pain: results of a study in patients with stable angina. *J Am Coll Cardiol.* 1992;20:1498–1502.

142. Pasceri V, Cianflone D, Finocchiaro ML, et al. Relation between myocardial infarction site and pain location in Q-wave acute myocardial infarction. *Am J Cardiol.* 1995;75:224–227.

143. Rosero HO, Greene CH, DeBias DA. A correlation of palpatory observations with the anatomical locus of acute myocardial infarction. *JAOA.* 1987;87:119.

144. White JC. Cardiac pain: anatomic pathways and physiologic mechanisms. *Circulation.* 1957;16:644–655.

145. Gettes LS. Painless myocardial ischemia. *Chest.* 1974;66:612–613.

146. Chierchia S, Lazzari M, Freedman B, et al. Impairment of myocardial perfusion and function during painless myocardial ischemia. *J Am Coll Cardiol.* 1983;1:924–930.

147. Shakespeare CF, Karitis D, Crowsher A, et al. Differences in autonomic nerve function in patients with silent and symptomatic myocardial ischemia. *Br Heart J.* 1994;71:22–29.

148. Sakalnikas RG, Gradauskas L. Cervical osteochondrosis and angina pectoris. In: Bluzas J, ed. *Ischemic Heart Disease. Diagnosis, Clinical Manifestations, and Presentation.* Kaunas, Lithuania: Institute of Cardiology Publishers; 1993:139–142.

149. Cox JM, Gideon D, Rogers FJ. Incidence of osteophytic lipping of the thoracic spine in coronary heart disease: results of a pilot study. *JAOA.* 1983;82:832–836.

150. Beal MC. Viscerosomatic reflexes: a review. *JAOA.* 1985;85:781–801.

151. Richter JE, Castell DO. Esophageal disease as a cause of chest pain. *Adv Intern Med.* 1988;33:311–335.

152. Sarkar S, Aziz Q, Woolf CJ, et al. Contribution of central sensitisation to the development of non-cardiac chest pain. *Lancet.* 2000;356:1154–1159.

153. Chauhan A, Mullins PA, Taylor G, et al. Cardioesophageal reflex: a mechanism for "linked angina" in patients with angiographically proven coronary artery disease. *J Am Coll Cardiol.* 1996;27:1621–1628.

154. Goldman L, Cook EF, Brand DA, et al. A computer protocol to predict myocardial infarction in emergency department patients with chest pain. *N Engl J Med.* 1988;318:797–803.

155. Kuchera ML, Kuchera WA. *Osteopathic Considerations in Systemic Dysfunction,* 2nd ed. Columbus, OH: Greyden Press; 1994:57.

156. Myerburg RJ, Kessler KM, Castellanos A. Sudden cardiac death: epidemiology, transient risk, and intervention assessment. *Ann Intern Med.* 1993;119:1187–1197.

157. Smith SC, Greenland P, Grundy SM. AHA Conference Proceedings: Prevention Conference V: Beyond secondary prevention: identifying the high-risk patient for primary prevention: executive summary. American Heart Association. *Circulation.* 2000;101:111–116.

158. Greenland P, Smith SC, Grundy SM. Improving coronary heart disease risk assessment in asymptomatic people. Role of traditional risk factors in non-invasive cardiovascular tests. *Circulation.* 2001;104:1863–1867.

159. Criqui MH, Langer RD, Fronck A, et al. Mortality over a period of ten years in patients with peripheral vascular disease. *N Engl J Med.* 1992;326:381–386.

160. Arad Y, Spadaro LA, Goodman K, et al. Prediction of coronary events with electron beam computed tomography. *J Am Coll Cardiol.* 2000;36:1253–1260.

161. Gibbons LW, Mitchell TL, Wei M, et al. Maximal exercise test as a predictor of risk for mortality from coronary heart disease in asymptomatic men. *Am J Cardiol.* 2000;86:53–58.

162. American Diabetes Association. Management of dyslipidemias in adults with diabetes [Position statement]. *Diabetes Care.* 2001;24[Suppl 1]:S58–S61.

163. Wenger NK, Froelicher ES, Smith LK, et al. *Cardiac Rehabilitation.* Clinical Practice Guidelines No. 17. Rockville, MD: Agency for Health Care Policy and Research and the National Heart, Lung, and Blood Institute; October 1995. Public Health Service. US Department of Health and Human Services. AHCPR publication 96–0672.

164. Butler RM, Rogers FJ, Palmer G. Circuit weight training in early cardiac rehabilitation. *JAOA.* 1992;92:77–89.

165. Oldridge NB, Guryatt GH, Fischer ME, Rimm AA. Cardiac rehabilitation after myocardial infarction. Combined experience of randomized clinical trial. *JAMA.* 1988;260:945–950.

166. Smith SC Jr, Blair SN, Bonow RO, et al. AHA/ACC guidelines for preventing heart attack and death in patients with atherosclerotic cardiovascular disease: 2001 update. A statement for health care professionals

from the American Heart Association and the American College of Cardiology. *J Am Coll Cardiol.* 2001;38:1581–1583.

167. Gibbons RJ, Chatterjee K, Daley J, et al. AHA/ACC/ACP-ASIM guidelines for the management of patients with chronic stable angina. *J Am Coll Cardiol.* 1999;33:2092–2197.

168. Braunwald E, Antman EM, Beasley JW, et al. ACC/AHA guidelines for the management of patients with unstable angina and non-ST-segment elevation myocardial infarction: Executive summary and recommendations: A report of the American College of Cardiology/American Heart Association Task Force on Practice Guidelines (Committee on Management of Patients with Unstable Angina). *Circulation.* 2000;102:1193–1209.

169. LaFeuvre C, Yusuf S, Flather M, Farkouh M. Maximizing benefits of therapies in acute myocardial infarction. *Am J Cardiol.* 1993;72:145G–155G.

170. Yusuf S, Sleight P, Held P, McMahon S. Routine medical management of acute myocardial infarction. Lessons from overviews of recent randomized controlled trials. *Circulation.* 1990;82[Suppl II]:II-117–II-134.

171. The GUSTO Investigators. An international randomized trial comparing four thrombolytic strategies for acute myocardial infarction. *N Engl J Med.* 1993;329:673–682.

172. ISIS-3 (Third International Study of Infarct Survival). Collaborative Group. ISIS-3: a randomized comparison of streptokinase versus tissue plasminogen activator versus anistreplase and of aspirin plus heparin versus aspirin alone among 41,299 cases of suspected acute myocardial infarction. *Lancet.* 1993;339:753–750.

173. Gruppo Italiano per lo Studio della Sopravivenza nell'Infarto Miocardico. GISSI-3: Effects of lisinopril and transdermal glycerol trinitrate singly and together on 6 week mortality and ventricular function after acute myocardial infarction. *Lancet.* 1994;343:1115–1122.

174. Ball SG, Hall AS, Murray GD. Angiotensin-converting enzyme inhibitors after myocardial infarction: indications and timing. *J Am Coll Cardiol.* 1995;25[Suppl]:42S46S.

175. Rogers WJ, Dean LS, Moore PB, et al. Comparison of primary angioplasty versus thrombolytic therapy in acute myocardial infarction. *Am J Cardiol.* 1994;74:111–118.

176. Mogadam M. *Every Heart Attack is Preventable: How to Take Control of the 20 Risk Factors and Save Your Life.* Washington, DC: Lifeline Press; 2001.

177. Stampfer MJ, Hu FB, Manson JE, et al. Primary prevention of coronary heart disease in women through diet and lifestyle. *N Engl J Med.* 2000;343:16–22.

178. Hu FB, Manson JE, Stampfer MJ, et al. Diet, lifestyle, and the risk of type 2 diabetes mellitus in women. *N Engl J Med.* 2001;345:790–797.

179. Forrester JS, Shah PK. Lipid lowering vs. revascularization: an idea whose time (for testing) has come. *Circulation.* 1997;96:1360–1362.

180. Pitt B, Waters D, Brown WV, et al. For the Atorvastatin vs. Revascularization Treatment Investigators. Aggressive lipid-lowering therapy compared to angioplasty in stable coronary artery disease. *N Engl J Med.* 1999;341:70–76.

181. American College of Cardiology. Acute myocardial infarction. Guidelines applied in practice. GAP Project. Available at: http://www.acc.org/gap/gap.htm. Accessed April 30, 2002.

182. Hu FB, Stampfer MJ, Manson JE, et al. Frequent nut consumption and risk of coronary heart disease in women: prospective cohort study. *Br Med J.* 1998;317:1341–1345.

183. Prineas RJ, Kushi LH, Folsom AR, et al. Walnuts and serum lipids. *N Engl J Med.* 1993;328:603–607.

184. Hu FB, Stampfer MJ. Nut consumption and risk of coronary heart disease: a review of epidemiologic evidence. *Curr Atheroscl Rep.* 1999;1:204–209.

185. Spiller GA, Jenkins D, Gragen LN, et al. Effective of a diet high in mono unsaturated fat from almonds on plasma cholesterol and lipoproteins. *J Am Coll Nutr.* 1992;11:126–130.

186. Sabate J, Fraser GE, Burke K, et al. Effects of walnuts on serum lipid levels and blood pressure in normal men. *N Engl J Med.* 1993;328:603–607.

187. de Longeril M, Salen P, Martin JL, et al. Mediterranean diet, traditional risk factors and the role of cardiovascular complications after myocardial infarction. Final report of the Lyon Diet Heart Study. *Circulation.* 1999;99:779–785.

188. Rogers JT, Rogers JC. The role of osteopathic manipulative therapy in the treatment of coronary heart disease. *JAOA.* 1976;76:71–81.

189. Konstam M, Dracup K, Baker D, et al. *Heart Failure: Evaluation and Care of Patients with Left Ventricular Systolic Dysfunction.* Clinical Practice Guidelines No. 11. Rockville, MD: Agency for Health Care Policy and Research; June 1994. Public Health Service. US Department of Health and Human Services. AHCPR publication 94-0612.

190. O'Connell JB, Bristow M. Economic impact of heart failure in the United States: Time for a different approach. *J Heart Lung Transplant* 1993;13:S107–S112.

191. Haldeman GA, Croft JB, Giles WH, Rashidee A. Hospitalization of patients with heart failure: National Hospital Discharge Survey, 1985 to 1995. *Am Heart J.* 1999;137:352–360.

192. National Heart, Lung, and Blood Institute: Morbidity and Mortality Chartbook on Cardiovascular, Lung, and Blood Diseases/1992. Rockville, MD: US Department of Health and Human Services; 1992.

193. Kannel WB, Belanger AJ. Epidemiology of heart failure. *Am Heart J.* 1991;121:951–957.

194. Massie BM, Shah NB. Evolving trends in the epidemiologic factors of heart failure: rational for preventive strategies and comprehensive disease management. *Am Heart J.* 1997;133:703–712.

195. Hunt SA, Baker DW, Chin MH, et al. ACC/AHA guidelines for the evaluation and management of chronic heart failure in the adult: executive summary. A report of the American College of Cardiology/American Heart Association Task Force on Practice Guidelines (Committee to revise the 1995 guidelines for the evaluation and management of heart failure.) *Circulation.* 2001;104:2996–3007.

196. Ho KK, Pinsky J, Kanne LWB, Levy D. The epidemiology of heart failure: the Framingham Study. *J Am Coll Cardiol.* 1993;22[Suppl A]:6A–13A.

197. Stauffer JC, Gaasch WH. Recognition and treatment of left ventricular diastolic dysfunction. *Prog Cardiovasc Dis.* 1990;32:319–332.

198. Creager MA. Baroreceptor reflex function in congestive heart failure. *Am J Cardiol.* 1992;69[Suppl]:10G–15G.

199. Ferguson DW, Abboud FM, Mark AL. Selective impairment of baroreflex-mediated vasoconstrictor responses in patients with left ventricular dysfunction. *Circulation.* 1984;67:451–460.

200. Bristow MR, Ginsburg R, Minobe W, et al. Decreased catecholamine sensitivity and beta-adrenergic receptor density in failing human hearts. *N Engl J Med.* 1982;307:205–211.

201. Anderson FL, Port JD, Reid BB, et al. Myocardial catecholamine and neuropeptide Y depletion in failing ventricles of patients with idiopathic dilated cardiomyopathy: correlation with beta-adrenergic receptor down regulation. *Circulation.* 1992;85:46–53.

202. Lee WH, Packer M. Prognostic importance of serum sodium concentration and its modification by converting enzyme inhibition in patients with severe chronic heart failure. *Circulation.* 1986;73:257–267.

203. Cody RJ. Atrial natriuretic factor in edematous disorders. *Annu Rev Med.* 1990;41:377–382.

204. Wei CM, Heublein DM, Perrella MA, et al. Natriuretic peptide system in human heart failure. *Circulation.* 1993;88:1.

205. Treasure CB, Alexander RW. The dysfunctional endothelium in heart failure. *J Am Coll Cardiol.* 1993;22[Suppl]:129A–134.

206. Stewart DJ, Cernacek P, Costello KB, et al. Elevated endothelin-1 in heart failure and loss of normal response to postural change. *Circulation.* 1992;85:510–517.

207. Benedict CR, Johnstone DE, Weiner DH, et al. for the SOLVD Investigators. Relation of neurohormonal activation to clinical variables and degree of ventricular dysfunction: a report from the registry of studies of left ventricular dysfunction. *J Am Coll Cardiol.* 1994;23:1410–1420.

208. Vaccarino V, Casal SV, Abramson J, Krumholz HM. Depressive symptoms and risk of functional decline and death in patients with heart failure. *J Am Coll Cardiol.* 2001;38:199–205.

209. Witte KKA, Clark AL, Cleland JGF. Chronic heart failure and micronutrients. *J Am Coll Cardiol.* 2001;37:1765–1774.

210. Kannel WB. Epidemiology and prevention of heart failure: Framingham Study insights. *Eur Heart J.* 1987;8 [Suppl F]:F23–F29.

211. Philbin EF, Dec W, Jenkins PL, DiSalvo TG. Socioeconomic status as an independent risk factor for hospital readmission for heart failure. *Am J Cardiol.* 2001;87:1367–1371.

212. Opasich C, Rapezzi C, Lucci D, et al, on behalf of the Italian Network on Congestive Heart Failure (IN-CHF) Investigators. Precipitating factors and decision-making processes of short-term worsening of heart failure despite "optimal" treatment (from the IN-CHF Registry). *Am J Cardiol.* 2001;88:382–387.

213. Happ NB, Naylor MD, Roe Prior P. Factors contributing to rehospitalization of elderly patients with heart failure. *J Cardiovasc Nurs.* 1997;11:75–84.

214. Weber KT. Aldosterone in congestive heart failure. *N Engl J Med.* 2001;345:1687–1697.

215. Edwards BS, Rodeheffer RJ. Prognostic features in patients with congestive heart failure and selection criteria for cardiac transplantation. *Mayo Clin Proc.* 1992;67:485–492.

216. Harlan WR, Oberman A, Grimm R, et al. Chronic congestive heart failure in coronary artery disease: clinical criteria. *Ann Intern Med.* 1977;86:133–138.

217. Stapleton JF, Segal JP, Harvey WP. The electrocardiogram of myocardiopathy. *Prog Cardiovasc Dis.* 1970;13:217–239.

218. Echeveria HH, Bilisker MS, Myerburg RJ, et al. Congestive heart failure: echocardiographic insights. *Am J Med.* 1983;75:750–755.

219. Nishimura RA, Abel MD, Hatle LK, et al. Assessment of diastolic function of the heart: background and current applications of Doppler echocardiography, II. Clinical studies. *Mayo Clin Proc.* 1989;64:181–204.

220. Nishimura R, Tajik AJ. Evaluation of diastolic filling of the left ventricle in health and disease: Doppler echocardiography is the clinician's Rosetta stone. *J Am Coll Cardiol.* 1997;30:8–18.

221. Lipkin DP, Scriven AJ, Crake T, et al. Six-minute walking test for assessing exercise capacity in chronic heart failure. *Br Med J.* 1986;292:653–655.

222. Madda K, Takayoshi T, Wada A, et al. Plasma brain natriuretic peptide as a biochemical marker of high left ventricular end-diastolic pressure in patients with symptomatic left-ventricular dysfunction. *Am Heart J.* 1998;135:825–832.

223. Clerico A, Iervasi G, Chicia M, et al. Circulating levels of cardiac natriuretic peptides (ANP and BNP) measured by highly sensitive and specific immunoradiometric assays in normal subjects and in patients with different degrees of heart failure. *J Endocrinol Invest.* 1998;21:170–179.

224. Dao Q, Krishnaswamy P, Kazanegra R, et al. Utility of B-type natriuretic peptide in the diagnosis of congestive heart failure in an urgent-care setting. *J Am Coll Cardiol.* 2001;37:379–385.

225. Cheng V, Kazanegra R, Garcia A, et al. A rapid bedside test for B-type [natriuretic] peptide treatment outcomes in patients admitted for decompensated heart failure: a pilot study. *J Am Coll Cardiol.* 2001;37:386–391.

226. Packer M, Cohn JN, on behalf of the Steering Committee and Membership of the Advisory Council to Improve Outcomes Nationwide in Heart Failure. Consensus recommendations for the management of chronic heart failure. *Am J Cardiol.* 1999;83[Suppl 2A]:1A–38A.

227. Levy D, Larson MG, Vasan RS, et al. The progression from hypertension to congestive heart failure. *JAMA.* 1996;275:1557–1562.

228. Wilhelmsen L, Rosengren A, Eriksson H, Lappas G. Heart failure in the general population of men—morbidity, risk factors and prognosis. *J Intern Med.* 2001;249:253–261.

229. He J, Ogden LG, Bazzano LA, et al. Risk factors for congestive heart failure in US men and women: NHANES I epidemiologic follow-up study. *Arch Intern Med.* 2001;161:996–1002.

230. Krumholz HM, Chen YT, Wang Y, et al. Predictors of readmission among elderly survivors of admission with heart failure. *Am Heart J.* 2000;139:72–77.

231. Shindler DM, Kostis JB, Yusuf S, et al. Diabetes mellitus, a predictor of morbidity and mortality in the Studies of Left Ventricular Dysfunction (SOLVD) Trials and Registry. *Am J Cardiol.* 1996;77:1017–1020.

232. Peters KG, Kienzle MG. Severe cardiomyopathy due to chronic rapidly conducted atrial fibrillation: complete recovery after restoration of sinus rhythm. *Am J Med.* 1988;85:242–244.

233. Grogan M, Smith HC, Gersh BJ, Wood DL. Left ventricular dysfunction due to atrial fibrillation in patients initially believed to have idiopathic dilated cardiomyopathy. *Am J Cardiol.* 1992;69:1570–1573.

234. Yusuf S, Sleight P, Pogue J, et al. Effects of an angiotensin-converting-enzyme inhibitor, Ramipril, on cardiovascular events in high-risk patients. The Heart Outcome Prevention Evaluation Study Investigators. *N Engl J Med.* 2000;342:145–153.

235. Packer M, Bristow MR, Cohn JN, et al. The effect of carvedilol on morbidity and mortality in patients with chronic heart failure. *N Engl J Med.* 1996;334:1349–1355.

236. MERIT-HF Study Group: Effect of metoprolol CR/XL in chronic heart failure: metoprolol CR/XL randomized intervention trial in congestive heart failure (MERIT-HF). *Lancet.* 1999;353:2001–2007.

237. Packer M, Coats AJS, Fowler MB, et al. Carvedilol Prospective Randomized Cumulative Survival Study Group. Effect of carvedilol on survival in severe heart failure. *N Engl J Med.* 2001;344:1651–1658.

238. McClean DR, Ikram H, Garlick AH, et al. Clinical, cardiac, renal, arterial and neurohormonal effects of omapatrilat, a vasopeptidase inhibitor, in patients with chronic heart failure. *J Am Coll Cardiol.* 2000;36:479–486.

239. Piepoli M. Central role of peripheral mechanisms in exercise intolerance in chronic heart failure: the muscle hypothesis. *Cardiologia.* 1998;43 (9):909–917.

240. Abboud FM, Heistad DD, Mark AL, Schmid, PG. Reflex control of the peripheral circulation. *Prog Cardiovasc Dis.* 1976;18:371–403.

241. Drexler H. Reduced exercise tolerance in chronic heart failure and its relationship to neurohormonal factors. *Eur Heart J.* 1991;12[Suppl C]:21–28.

242. Piepoli M, Ponikowski P, Clark AL, et al. A neural link to explain the "muscle hypothesis" of exercise intolerance in chronic heart failure. *Am Heart J.* 1999;137:1050–1056.

243. Jetté M, Heller R, Landry F, Blumchen G. Randomized 4-week exercise program in patients with impaired left ventricular function. *Circulation.* 1991;84:1651–1667.

244. Koch M, Doward H, Brouset J-P. The benefit of graded physical exercise in chronic heart failure. *Chest.* 1992;101:231S–234S.

245. Kostis JB, Rosen RC, Cosgrove NM, et al. Nonpharmacologic therapy improves functional and emotional status in congestive heart failure. *Chest.* 1994;106:996–1001.

246. Hambrecht R, Niebauer J, Fiehn E, et al. Physical training in patients with stable chronic heart failure: effects on cardiorespiratory fitness and ultrastructural abnormalities of leg muscles. *J Am Coll Cardiol.* 1995;25:1239–1249.

247. Kiilavuori KM, Toivonen L, Naveri H, Leinonen H. Reversal of autonomic derangements by physical training in chronic heart failure assessed by heart rate variability. *Eur Heart J.* 1995;16:490–495.

248. Keteyian SJ, Levine AB, Brawner CA, et al. A randomized controlled trial of exercise training in patients with heart failure. *Ann Intern Med.* 1996;124:1051–1057.

249. Giannuzzi P, Tavazzi L, Temporelli PL, et al. Long-term physical training and left ventricular remodeling after anterior myocardial infarction: results of the exercise in anterior myocardial infarction (EAMI) trial. *J Am Coll Cardiol.* 1993;22:1821–1829.

250. Belardinelli R, Georgiou D, Cianci G, Pucaro A. Randomized, controlled trial of long-term moderate exercise training in chronic heart failure. *Circulation.* 1999;99:1173–1182.

251. Hambrecht R, Fiehn E, Weigl C, et al. Regular physical exercise corrects endothelial dysfunction and improves exercise capacity in patients with chronic heart failure. *Circulation.* 1998;98:2709–2715.

252. Gordon A, Tyni-Lenné R, Persson H, et al. Markedly improved skeletal muscle function with local muscle training in patients with chronic heart failure. *Clin Cardiol.* 1996;19:568–574.

253. Ohtsubo M, Yonezawa K, Nishijima H, et al. Metabolic abnormality of calf skeletal muscle is improved by localized muscle training without changes in blood flow in chronic heart failure. *Heart.* 1997;78:437–443.

254. Gianuzzi P. Attenuation of unfavorable remodeling by exercise training in post infarction patients with left ventricular dysfunction: Results of

the Exercise in Left Ventricular Dysfunction (ELVD) Trial. *Circulation.* 1997;96:1790–1797.

255. Meyer TE, Casadel B, Coats AJS, et al. Angiotensin-converting enzyme inhibition in physical training and heart failure. *J Int Med.* 1991;230:407–413.

256. Riegger GAJ. The effects of ACE inhibitors on exercise capacity in the treatment of congestive heart failure. *J Cardiovasc Phamacol.* 1990;15[Suppl 2]:S41–S46.

257. Meyer K, Schwaibold M, Westbrook S, et al. Effects of exercise training and activity restriction on 6 minute walking test performance in patients with chronic heart failure. *Am Heart J.* 1997;133:447–453.

258. Piepoli M, Clark AL, Volterrani M, et al. Contribution of muscle afferents to the hemodynamic, autonomic, and ventilatory responses to exercise in patients with chronic heart failure. Effects of physical training. *Circulation.* 1996;93:940–952.

259. Rogers FJ, Glassman J, Kavieff R. Effects of osteopathic manipulative treatment on autonomic nervous system function in patients with congestive heart failure. *JAOA.* 1986;86:605(abst).

OSTEOPATHIC MANAGEMENT OF EAR, NOSE, AND THROAT DISEASE

HARRIET H. SHAW
MICHAEL B. SHAW

KEY CONCEPTS

- Structure and function of the ear, nose, and throat (ENT) region
- Pathophysiology, diagnosis, and treatment options for common ENT problems seen in primary care settings, including sinusitis, allergic rhinitis, otitis media, and acute tonsillitis and pharyngitis
- The osteopathic approach to the diagnosis and treatment of ENT problems

The ears, nose, and throat are not a system unto themselves; they are parts of at least three different systems. Their grouping together as a specialty is likely due to their sharing of several factors, including having a respiratory mucosal lining, containing organs of special senses, having internal connections to each other, and being located in the head and neck. The nose, paranasal sinuses, mouth, and throat function in the respiratory system as passageways for inspired and expired air. In addition, the nose and paranasal sinuses play an important role in conditioning and filtering the inspired air. Olfaction is the special sense of the nose. The special senses of hearing and balance are housed in the ears. The mouth and throat function as part of the digestive system in chewing, swallowing, and the special sense of taste. The throat and mouth also aid in speech.

Due to the diverse nature of this area, numerous and very different clinical problems are associated with treating the ears, nose, and throat. They range from infectious processes to vertigo to difficulty swallowing or talking. Preventing and treating many of these problems depend on an appreciation of the physiologic functions and anatomical relationships that exist.

Several problems of the ear, nose, and throat are commonly encountered in the primary care setting. These include allergic rhinitis, sinusitis, otitis, and tonsillitis. Treating this area from an osteopathic perspective uses the basic concepts of structure-function relationship and the body's inherent healing capacity.

These common problems serve as examples of how to approach the ENT patient osteopathically.

The respiratory system demonstrates the remarkable health maintenance systems within the body. With an understanding and appreciation of normal anatomy and function, the physician can effectively treat ENT patients to enhance the ability for recovery and the natural resistance to disease. It is the responsibility of the osteopathic physician to consider the specific needs of the patient and design a management plan deemphasizing intervention in favor of promoting the body's ability to regulate itself toward health.

Patient education plays an important role in the treatment and prevention of ENT problems. Increasing patient awareness of medication abuse, pollutants, humidification, and allergies is a critical aspect of management.

Osteopathic manipulative treatment has been used empirically to treat ENT problems commonly encountered in primary care (1,2,3). This treatment is based on the musculoskeletal system's impact on circulatory flow to and from all the tissues of the body and its effects on physiologic function by way of the autonomic nervous system. Promoting lymphatic circulation plays an important role in reducing swelling and inflammation, as well as in stimulating the immune system. Studies have shown physiologic function of various organs to be affected by noxious somatic afferent stimulation (4,5). Clinical experience has shown that incorporation of musculoskeletal treatment in the management of ENT patients improves recovery time and reduces incidence of recurrence and complications (6,7).

Medical intervention can be accomplished in the most beneficial way when consideration is made of the natural forces at work to maintain homeostasis. Medications, surgery, and allergy desensitization can be most effective when based on specific diagnoses and combined with patient education and appropriate musculoskeletal treatment.

General knowledge of myofascial anatomy, lymphatic circulation, and autonomic nervous supply to the head and neck can enhance osteopathic treatment of patients with ear, nose, and throat problems. Specific attention to each organ's unique aspects of anatomy, built-in mechanisms for health, and predisposing factors for disease will enhance treatment of specific conditions.

MYOFASCIA OF THE HEAD AND NECK

As in other areas of the body, connective tissue forms covering and padding around the structures in the neck. It is denser immediately next to organs and muscles and looser between organs. The looser areas form potential spaces where fluid may collect, including infection, swelling, and blood.

Fascial relationships become important because of the structures that transverse or are enclosed by fascia and because of the location of fascial spaces. It is characteristic of fascia to split to surround muscles or organs and unite again on the other side. In places, it attaches firmly to bone as it blends into periosteum. This creates a situation of unlimited connectedness and relationship to various and distant structures. Fascia serves both a compartmentalizing and connecting function. It defines muscles, muscle bundles, and organs while connecting them to each other. It limits the spread of infection and swelling but allows it to follow the channels of fascial spaces. Fascial sheaths form around nerves and vessels, providing passageways for neural supply, blood, and lymph flow.

As in many other areas of the body, fascia in the head and neck is identified in layers (Fig. 25.1). The **superficial fascia** encircles the neck and contains variable amounts of fat but, unlike other parts of the body, encloses voluntary muscles, such as the platysma and the muscles of facial expression. Several arrangements of deeper fascia are deep to the superficial layer. **Prevertebral fascia** encloses the vertebral column and associated muscles, forming a vertebral compartment. Bilateral neurovascular compartments, the **carotid sheaths,** are formed by fascia surrounding and enclosing the great vessels and vagus nerve. In the anterior neck, the visceral compartment, formed by the **pretracheal fascia,** contains the trachea, esophagus, and associated structures.

The superficial layer of fascia attaches to the hyoid bone. Inferior to the hyoid, it courses downward and attaches both to the anterior and posterior surfaces of the sternum and the clavicle. Above the hyoid, the superficial fascia passes below the muscles of the floor of the mouth, around the submandibular and parotid glands, and encloses the masseter and medial pterygoid muscles; it then attaches to the mandible, pterygoid plate, and the zygomatic arch.

The prevertebral layer begins on the cervical spinous processes and ligamentum nuchae, forms a circle around the back muscles deep to the trapezius, and then courses around the transverse processes of the cervical vertebrae and in front of the vertebral bodies. In some places, it lies in direct contact with the superficial fascia, and in others, it separates from it to provide passage for nerves and vessels. The prevertebral fascia specifically follows the scalene muscles and forms a sleeve for the brachial plexus and the axillary artery. Near the transverse processes, the prevertebral fascia embeds the cervical sympathetic trunk.

The pretracheal fascia encircles the trachea, esophagus, and thyroid gland. It is continuous with the superficial layer of cervical fascia that encloses the infrahyoid muscles. Following these muscles inferiorly behind the sternum, it fuses with the fibrous pericardium in the superior mediastinum. Superiorly, the pretracheal fascia fuses to the hyoid bone and the thyroid cartilage. Above the hyoid bone, this fascia remains well developed around the esophagus and the pharynx.

LYMPHATIC CIRCULATION IN THE HEAD AND NECK

The lymphatic system of the neck consists of numerous lymph nodes connected by lymphatic channels that eventually end in the thoracic and right lymphatic ducts. The thoracic duct receives drainage from the left side of the head and neck while the right lymphatic duct drains the right side. Each empties independently into the junction of the internal jugular and subclavian veins on their respective side of the body (Fig. 25.2).

Cervical lymph nodes are generally divided in groups—submandibular, submental, superficial cervical, deep cervical, and paratracheal (Fig. 25.3). The submandibular and submental nodes are intimately connected with the superficial fascia covering

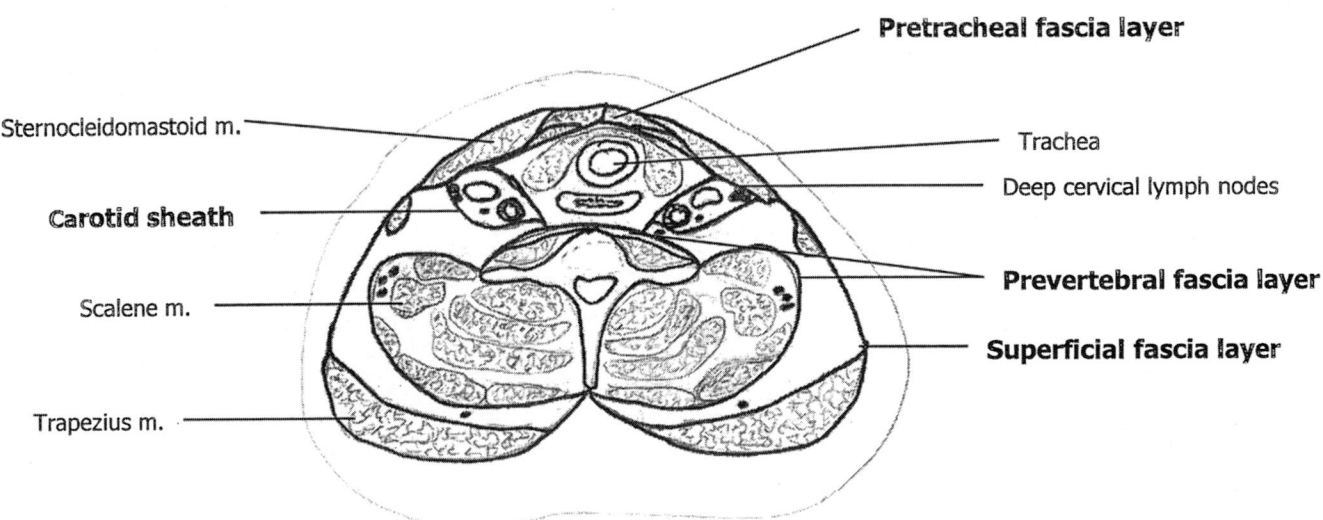

FIGURE 25.1. Fascial layers of neck.

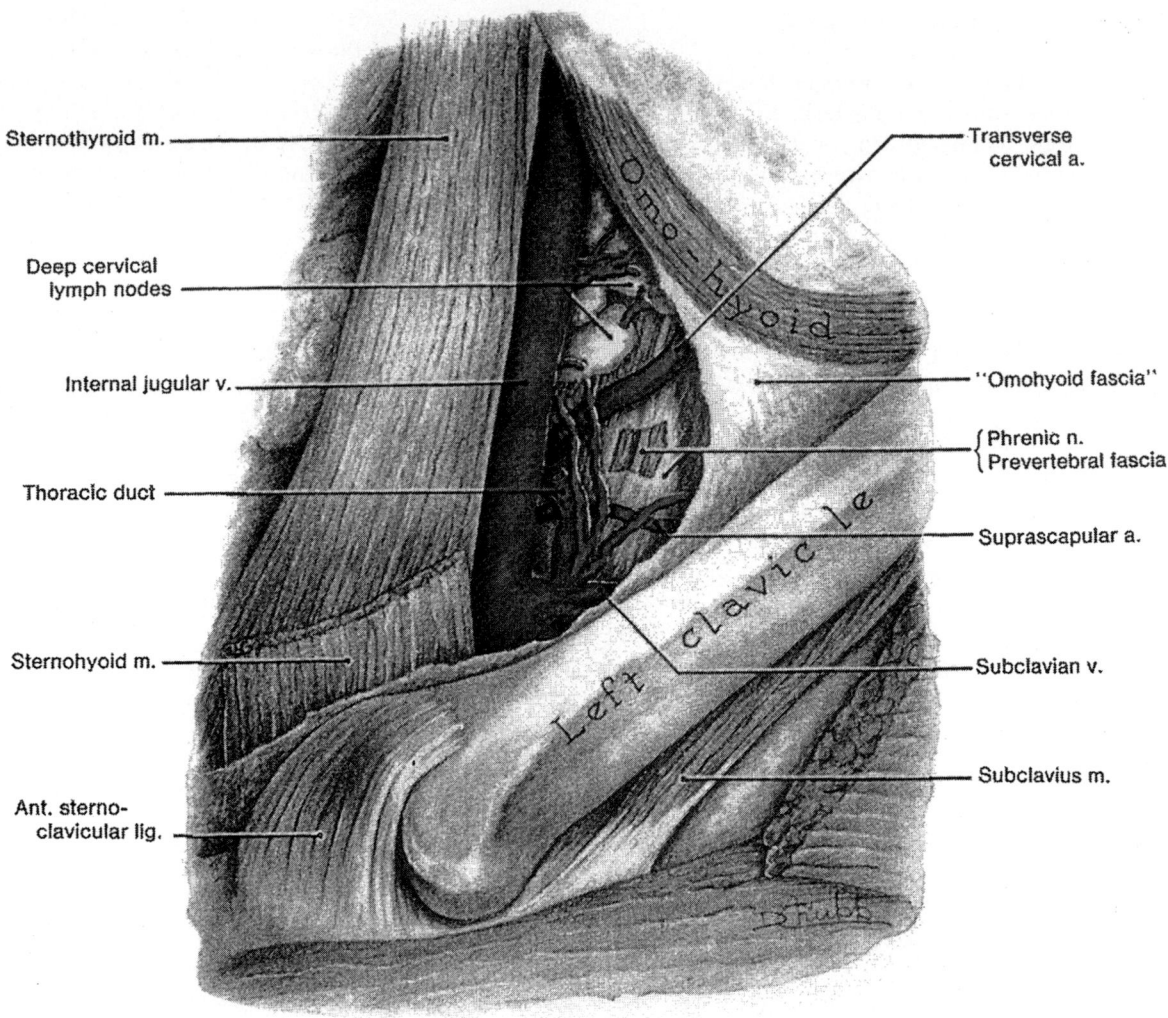

FIGURE 25.2. Deep cervical lymphatics. (From Moore KL. *Clinically Oriented Anatomy,* 2nd ed. Baltimore, MD: Williams & Wilkins; 1985, with permission.)

the digastric and mylohyoid muscles. The superficial cervical nodes lie along the external jugular vein and on the external surface of the sternocleidomastoid muscle. The paratracheal nodes are irregularly located and, as do all the aforementioned groups of nodes, drain into the deep cervical lymph nodes. These prominent, deep nodes form a chain embedded in the connective tissue of the carotid sheath around the internal jugular vein (Fig. 25.1).

The intimate association of the lymphatic channels to the myofascial structures in the neck makes lymphatic flow particularly susceptible to changes in myofascial tone. Hypertonia in the cervical myofascial tissues can impede lymphatic flow. Freedom of motion in muscles of normal tone improves lymphatic circulation.

AUTONOMIC NERVOUS SUPPLY IN THE HEAD AND NECK

Sympathetic fibers to the head arise from the upper thoracic segments of the spinal cord (Fig. 25.4). Preganglionic fibers ascend from there to the superior cervical ganglion in the upper

cervical area, where they synapse. Postganglionic fibers from the superior cervical ganglion join the internal carotid plexus. Sympathetic supply to the nose and paranasal sinuses passes through the sphenopalatine ganglion, which lies posterior to and slightly above the posterior end of the middle nasal concha (usually below the floor of the sphenoid sinus). Sympathetic fibers from the carotid plexus also reach the ear, by inferiorly penetrating the tympanic cavity. Sympathetic fibers are presumably vasomotor and are most often vasoconstrictors. Somatic influence on the sympathetic nervous supply to the head and neck, in the form of somato-visceral reflexes, would most likely occur in the upper thoracic area, where the sympathetic fibers originate, or the upper cervical area, related to the superior cervical ganglion.

Parasympathetic supply to the nose is from the facial nerve (cranial nerve VII). Its preganglionic fibers form part of the greater petrosal nerve, synapsing in the sphenopalatine ganglion. These include both vasodilator and secretory fibers. Postganglionic fibers are distributed from the sphenopalatine ganglion with the sensory and sympathetic fibers. The glossopharyngeal nerve (cranial nerve IX), which exits the cranium with the vagus and accessory nerves through the jugular foramen, also carries

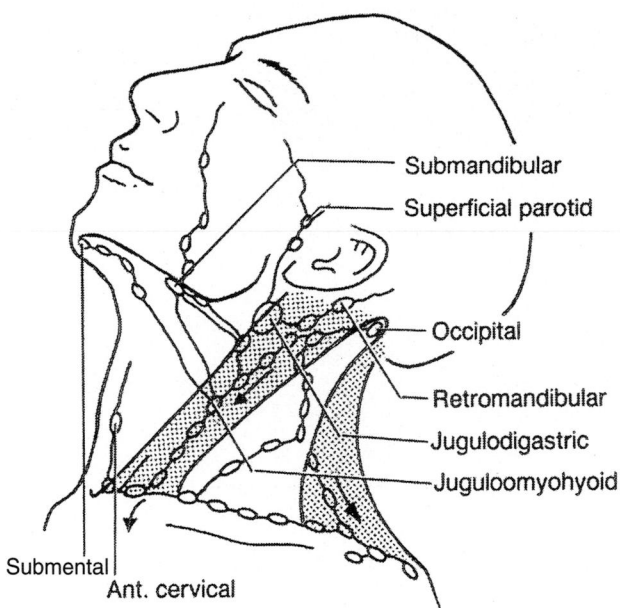

FIGURE 25.3. Superficial cervical lymph nodes. (From Moore KL. *Clinically Oriented Anatomy,* 2nd ed. Baltimore, MD: Williams & Wilkins; 1985, with permission.)

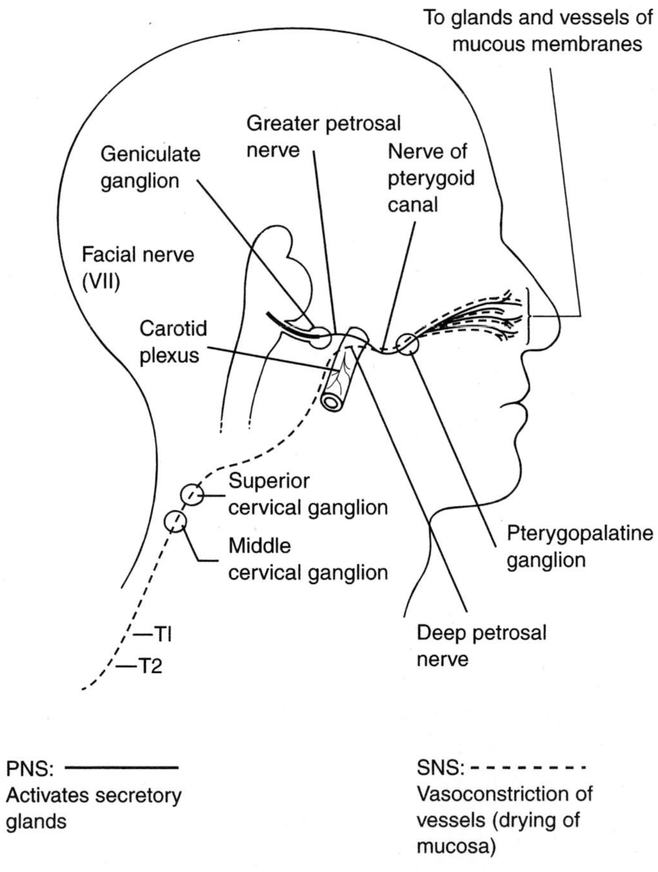

some parasympathetic fibers. These synapse in the otic ganglion and mostly supply the parotid gland.

NOSE AND PARANASAL SINUSES
Healthy Structure and Function

The nose, an organ of respiration and olfaction, functions to filter, humidify, and regulate the temperature of inspired air. The paranasal sinuses in the maxillary, frontal, sphenoid, and ethmoid bones are air-filled extensions of the nasal cavities and serve similar functions to that of the nose. Regardless of the temperature of outside air, the temperature of inspired air is changed to approximate body temperature during its passage through the nose. Similar changes are made in moisture content of inspired air so that it reaches the trachea at almost ambient humidity. The superior, middle, and inferior turbinates, or conchae, are elevations on the lateral nasal walls. Heavily endowed with blood vessels, they help control the temperature of the inspired air. The nose filters particulate matter in the air: Much of the smoke, dust, pollens, and bacteria are trapped and removed before the air enters the lungs. The nasal septum and the turbinates help create an air flow pattern in the nose that can maximize the air-conditioning function of the nose and paranasal sinuses.

The nasal cavity and paranasal sinuses are covered by pseudostratified, columnar, ciliated epithelium. Goblet cells and submucosal glands contribute to the mucous blanket that covers and protects the epithelium. This mucous film has two layers. The cilia beat within the inner, serous (sol phase) layer. The outer, more viscous (gel phase) layer is moved by synchronized ciliary action (Fig. 25.5). Secretions from the sinuses pass into the nasal cavity through the various ostia or openings in the sinuses. The outer layer of mucus traps dust and other particles and moves

FIGURE 25.4. Autonomic nerve supply to upper respiratory tract.

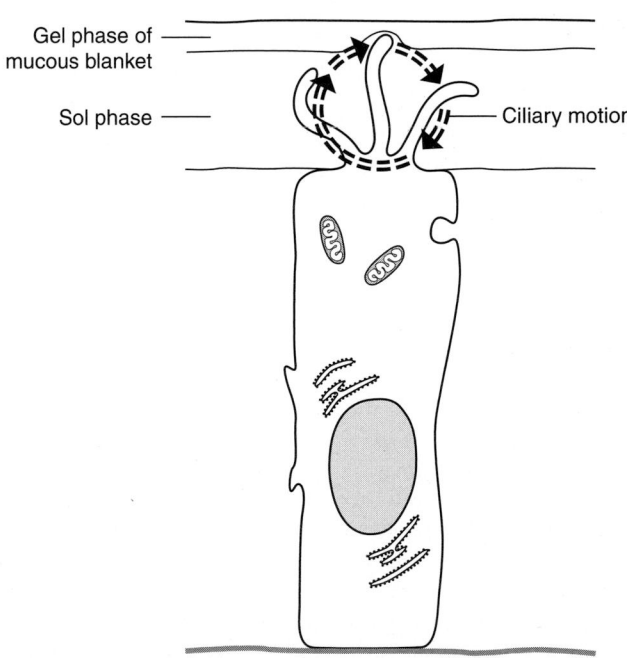

FIGURE 25.5. Ciliated respiratory epithelium.

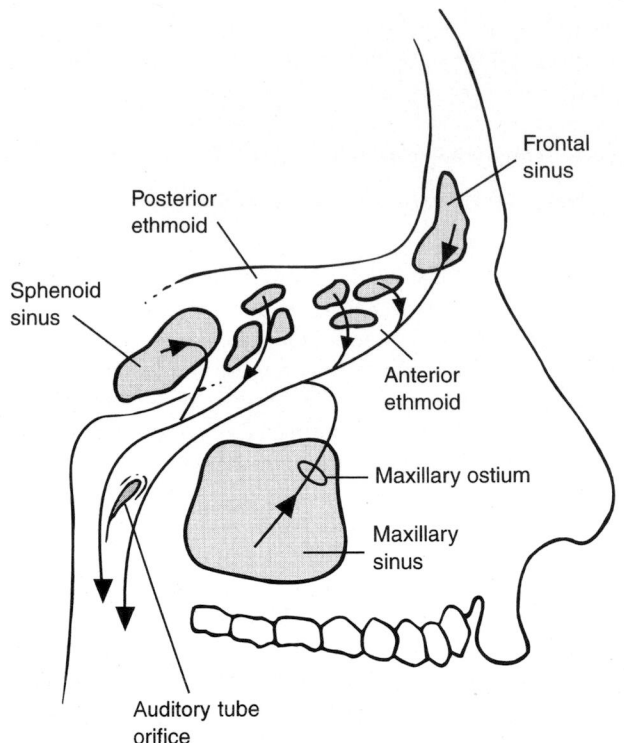

FIGURE 25.6. Paranasal sinus drainage patterns.

them through the ostia into the nasal cavity, where mucus is transported into the nasopharynx and swallowed. The process is referred to as mucociliary clearance. Pathogens may be incorporated into the cells of the mucosa or destroyed by lysozymes and secretory immunoglobulin A within the mucus.

Normal function of the paranasal sinuses depends on the effectiveness of mucociliary clearance. There are two basic drainage patterns of the sinuses. The anterior ethmoid, frontal, and maxillary sinuses are part of the anterior pattern draining to the ostiomeatal unit under the middle turbinate. The posterior ethmoid and sphenoid sinuses are in the posterior pattern and drain to the sphenoethmoid recess (Fig. 25.6). The ostiomeatal unit is located superior to much of the maxillary sinus, making it necessary to actively move the mucous blanket "uphill" for effective drainage. This nondependent drainage situation exists with the sphenoid and, in some instances, with the ethmoid sinus as well. Conditions that create obstruction to the normal flow of air and mucus predispose the sinuses to disease and are described in standard ENT references.

The lymphatics from the anterior portion of the nose drain into the lymphatics of the skin. Of the larger, posterior lymphatics, some drain directly to the deep cervical nodes, but most drain behind the throat to the retropharyngeal nodes before continuing to the deep cervical nodes.

Proper balance of the autonomic nervous system is necessary for healthy mucosal function. Blood supply to the nasal mucosa is regulated through the sympathetic nervous system. Sympathetic preganglionic fibers arise from the T1-4 cord level, and postganglionic fibers from the superior cervical ganglia join the internal carotid plexus. Fibers reach the sphenopalatine ganglion *via* the deep petrosal nerve and the nerve of the pterygoid canal.

TABLE 25.1. COMMON DISORDERS OF THE NOSE AND PARANASAL SINUSES

Disorder
Epistaxis
Nasal fractures
Acute rhinitis
Allergic rhinitis
Non-allergic vasomotor rhinitis
Atrophic rhinitis
Polyposis
Deviated nasal septum
Unilateral nasal discharge
Foreign body
Choanal atresia
Malignancy
Head trauma
Sinusitis

Unopposed sympathetic stimulation leads to vasoconstriction accompanied by drying of the mucosa. Nasal mucus production is predominantly regulated by parasympathetic nerve fibers, but sympathetic fibers also reach the glands. Stimulation of parasympathetic fibers generally increases goblet cell secretions. The parasympathetic, secretomotor innervation comes from the facial nerve (cranial nerve VII) and synapses in the sphenopalatine ganglion (Fig. 25.4). Tobacco smoke and other pollutants adversely affect mucus flow by inactivating cilia (8). The quantity and composition of the mucus is influenced by various factors, such as temperature, humidity, oxygen concentration, pollution, and irritants. Neuromediators, such as substance P, also appear to influence the function of the mucosal glands (9).

Common Pathophysiology

Inflammation is a common cause of disease in the nose and paranasal sinuses (Table 25.1). The inflammatory process can be initiated by infections (viral or bacterial), allergies (food or inhalants), and irritants (chemical or mechanical). Inflammation is accompanied by swelling of the mucosa, excessive mucus production, and decrease of ciliary motility. Symptoms include obstructed breathing, pain, rhinorrhea, and sometimes epistaxis. Prolonged inflammation predisposes to recurrent infection and changes, such as thickening of the mucous membranes and inhibition of cilia. These conditions impede the normal airflow and functioning of the mucosa. Poor venous and lymphatic circulation from the area can cause inflammatory mediators to remain in the tissues longer and prolong the inflammatory reaction.

Nasal obstruction and abnormal airflow may be due to venous and lymphatic congestion causing engorgement of the mucosa, as occurs with allergic rhinitis or upper respiratory infections. It may also be caused by structural defects, such as polyps or a deviated septum. Changes in the mucosa and in airflow patterns have an adverse effect on the cleaning, humidifying, and temperature control of the air, as well as on the oxygen concentration in the sinuses. Sinusitis may result from prolonged derangement of airflow.

Obstructions due to mucosal changes are responsive to activities that alter sympathetic nerve discharge. Vigorous physical exercise has been shown to improve nasal function for up to

60 minutes by reducing nasal airflow resistance and nasal blood flow (10). In a group of 12 subjects serving as their own controls, osteopathic manipulation resulted in significant improvement of nasal function, as measured by nasal pressure curves (11). Addressing somatic dysfunction with osteopathic manipulation adds to patient comfort and aids the normal healing process (6,7). Tissue changes in the upper thoracic and upper cervical areas would be expected to accompany sympathetic motor dysfunction of the nose and paranasal sinuses. Chronic conditions and progression of disease can be prevented by decreasing congestion and promoting good airflow.

SINUSITIS

Diagnosis

Acute sinusitis is one of the common manifestations of inflammation and obstruction in the upper respiratory tract. Patients often present with nasal congestion, pain in the face or head, a feeling of fullness around the eyes, and, occasionally, fever. Other signs and symptoms include a foul taste or smell, postnasal drainage, and fatigue. Physical examination reveals tenderness to percussion over the sinuses. Nasal mucosa is often red and congested with either clear or purulent drainage. Structural abnormalities, such as septal deviation or hypertrophied turbinates, are sometimes noted. Transillumination of the sinuses may reveal decreased light transmission, but is not a definitive test. Edema and tenderness are frequently evident in the periorbital area. Numerous studies describe accompanying cervical soft tissue hypertonia with varying degrees of motion dysfunction (1,12,13). Localized, small areas of tenderness and tissue tension corresponding to Chapman's reflex points have been noted in the suboccipital area and inferior to the clavicle, over the first rib (14). Various other somatic dysfunctions occur unique to the individual patient. Computed tomography (CT) of the sinuses is replacing standard x-ray films for evaluation of sinusitis. In recurrent sinusitis, CT can delineate an anatomic blockage at the ostiomeatal complex, which suggests the need for functional endoscopic surgery.

Chronic sinusitis can develop if the cause of inflammation is not removed and steps are not taken to restore the conditions favoring good physiologic function. It is important to determine whether infectious agents, allergens, or irritants are the primary etiology. Local structural deformities causing poor aeration of the sinuses may be predisposing to persistent infection. Decreased venous and lymphatic return can contribute to continued congestion and poor healing.

Treatment/Management

Treatment falls under several categories—patient instruction/participation, musculoskeletal, medical, and surgical. Once the underlying pathophysiologic process has been determined, management in the four areas can be tailored to the patient's particular needs, keeping in mind the general goals of reducing edema and inflammation, promoting sinus drainage, and controlling infection (15).

In all cases, promoting mucociliary clearance is essential to the overall treatment and prevention of complications. Patients should be instructed to drink warm, clear fluids to hydrate the mucous membranes and increase mucociliary clearance (10). Milk is believed to thicken secretions and is not recommended. No controlled clinical trials of antihistamines in sinusitis exist, nor is histamine known to play a role in this disease (10). Antihistamine side effects of overdrying the mucosa and slowing ciliary motion should be considered before use of these medications. For patients with concomitant allergic disease, the availability of nonanticholinergic antihistamines, such as astemizole and terfenadine, has made it possible to avoid some of these complications. Mucoactive agents, such as guaifenesin, hypertonic saline, and saturated solution of potassium iodide (SSKI), that alter the character, production, or movement of mucus may be helpful (10).

When medications are used, they should be selected for specific reasons. Inflammation due to infection should be treated with appropriate antibiotics. The most common pathogens involved in sinusitis are *Streptococcus pneumoniae*, *Haemophilus influenzae*, and *Moraxella catarrhalis*. In chronic sinusitis, *Staphylococcus aureus* may also be encountered. Oral decongestants may be helpful in treating congestion and swelling, but they are not usually recommended in children. Topical decongestants are often overused and lead to rebound swelling of the mucosa, which is known as rhinitis medicamentosa; therefore, they should be used short term in acute sinusitis. Topical corticosteroids may be helpful in reducing edema and inflammation, thus promoting sinus drainage. They are not, however, considered first-line therapy in sinusitis.

The rationale for the use of osteopathic manipulation in sinus disease is to affect myofascial constraint on venous and lymphatic flow and to alter somato-visceral reflexes to the sinuses (15). Muscle activity is a recognized mechanism of increasing lymphatic flow. Osteopathic manipulative treatment (OMT) to the neck, specifically those techniques involving muscle action (such as muscle energy and myofascial techniques), should contribute to increased lymphatic flow from the head. Because lymphatic channels are embedded in the cervical fascia, soft tissue technique treatment (see Chapter 54) to the cervical area may also serve to promote lymphatic circulation. The expected result would be reduced swelling of the sinus and nasal mucosa. Direct and indirect pressure techniques over the sinuses and sphenopalatine ganglion are described for assisting drainage of the sinuses (16). With some of the lymphatic drainage leaving the nose and entering the lymphatics of the skin, direct pressure in this area would be expected to encourage lymphatic circulation. Rhythmic motion of the cranial bones as part of the cranial rhythmic impulse may be a significant factor in promoting sinus drainage. Following this line of thinking, treatment of dysfunctional motion patterns, particularly involving the maxillae, sphenoid, ethmoid, and frontal bones, should be part of sinusitis treatment (see Chapter 62).

Ultimately, lymphatic fluid from the head and neck must enter the central circulation in the area of the subclavian and internal jugular veins. Somatic dysfunction of the structures in this area, including the upper ribs, upper thoracic spine, and clavicles, should be considered as a potential impediment to lymphatic flow (Fig. 25.7).

The observation of somato-visceral reflexes by Sata and Schmidt (4,5) suggests the modulation of visceral function with

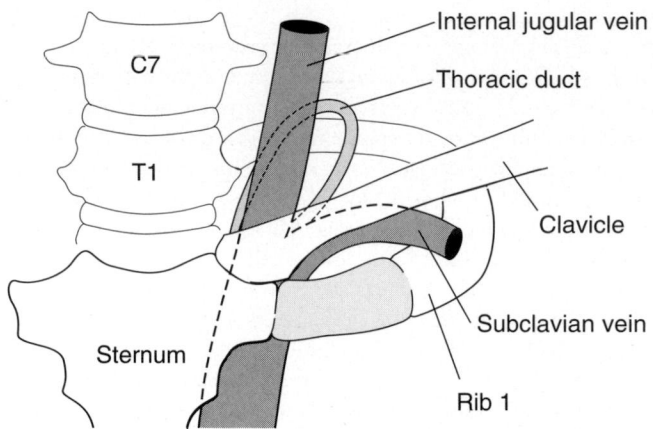

FIGURE 25.7. Thoracic inlet and lymphatic relationships.

various somatic stimuli. Somatic stimuli associated with somatic dysfunction of cervical and upper thoracic areas could impact the sympathetic vasomotor tone to the sinus area. One of the goals of OMT to this area would be to improve blood flow by altering the somatic component of this somato-visceral reflex.

Chemical irritants (tobacco smoke as the most prevalent) also cause inflammation of the respiratory mucosa. Smokers suffer from frequent inflammatory conditions of the nose and paranasal sinuses. Children living in a home where tobacco smoke is present are at high risk for developing respiratory disorders (17). Patient education is essential and often needs to be ongoing. Judicious use of nicotine supplements and smoking cessation programs are helpful for some patients. History is helpful in identifying patients with hypersensitivity or overexposure to common chemicals, such as formaldehyde and petroleum products. Increasing awareness of potential exposure is often sufficient treatment; however, some cases require substantial lifestyle and occupation changes.

Obstruction due to local structural abnormalities may exist and needs to be evaluated on physical examination and, at times, with further diagnostic tests (CT and endoscopy). In the presence of structural abnormalities, such as deviated septum, nasal polyps, enlarged turbinates, or obstruction of the sinus ostia, if conservative therapy fails to control recurrent infections, a surgical approach may be indicated.

ALLERGIC RHINITIS

Diagnosis

Symptoms of rhinorrhea, sneezing, itchy eyes, and watery eyes are associated with allergic rhinitis. This condition usually shows seasonal variation and recurrence. On physical examination, it is characterized by engorgement of the turbinates, which appear pale or violaceous rather than erythematous, as in viral rhinitis. Nasal polyps are sometimes present and appear as yellowish, boggy masses of mucosa. It is also common to see signs of chronic rhinorrhea and postnasal drainage.

Treatment/Management

Inflammation due to allergy, associated with allergic rhinitis, can be treated with antihistamines, steroids (inhaled or systemic),

cromolyn sodium, hydration, and manipulative techniques that aid circulation. Reducing swelling by promoting venous and lymphatic circulation and decreasing the concentration of chemical, inflammatory mediators in the interstitial tissues is particularly important. Antihistamines are useful in countering the inflammation and vasomotor symptoms associated with allergic disease. Their anticholinergic side effects, particularly mucosal drying, may complicate the treatment. Many patients do not tolerate the drowsiness associated with traditional antihistamine therapy. Selective H1 antihistamines (nonanticholinergic) minimize these side effects and offer a safer option for treating the allergic component of ENT problems (10). Nasally inhaled antihistamine preparations with minimal anticholinergic effect are also available. The inhaled steroids are effective in reducing the local inflammation and associated symptoms, and they are also indicated for preventing recurrence of nasal polyps. They may require from 3 days to 2 weeks of regular use for symptomatic improvement. Systemic steroids should be used cautiously and reserved for severe and/or resistant cases. Sodium cromoglycate (cromolyn sodium) serves as a mast-cell stabilizer and has a suppressive effect on other inflammatory cells. It is best used prophylactically for allergic rhinitis and may also require regular use over 1 to 2 weeks for benefits to become apparent (18).

Addressing the specific allergic cause is essential to effective and lasting treatment. Responsible allergens may be foods or inhalants (dusts, pollens, molds, animal dander). History is helpful in determining the offending allergens. Year-round symptoms that are worse indoors suggest animal dander, dust, or dust mite allergy. Pollens are most common in the spring, grasses in the summer, ragweed in late summer and fall. Allergy testing and elimination diets are often necessary for specific diagnosis and treatment. Environmental control, particularly for dust, molds, and animal dander, is an important part of treating ENT disease with an allergic etiology. This requires educating and encouraging the patient who may become discouraged with the demanding lifestyle changes.

EARS

Healthy Structure and Function

The ear is a complex organ of hearing and balance (Fig. 25.8). The temporal bone houses or provides attachment for all parts of the ear. The external ear consists of the pinna and external meatus. The pinna collects and localizes sound. The meatus is an air-filled tube through which sound waves travel to reach the middle ear.

The middle ear contains the tympanic membrane and three bones, or ossicles—malleus, incus, and stapes. The middle ear is air-filled and transmits sound from the air media to the liquid media of the inner ear. It is lined by ciliated, respiratory mucosa. The inner ear consists of the liquid-filled cochlea for auditory sense and the vestibular system for the sense of equilibrium.

Also lined by respiratory mucosa, the auditory or eustachian tube connects the middle ear to the nasopharynx. The lateral one-third of the auditory tube lies in the temporal bone, and the medial two-thirds is cartilaginous, opening only with swallowing or yawning. Air enters or leaves the middle ear cavity through this

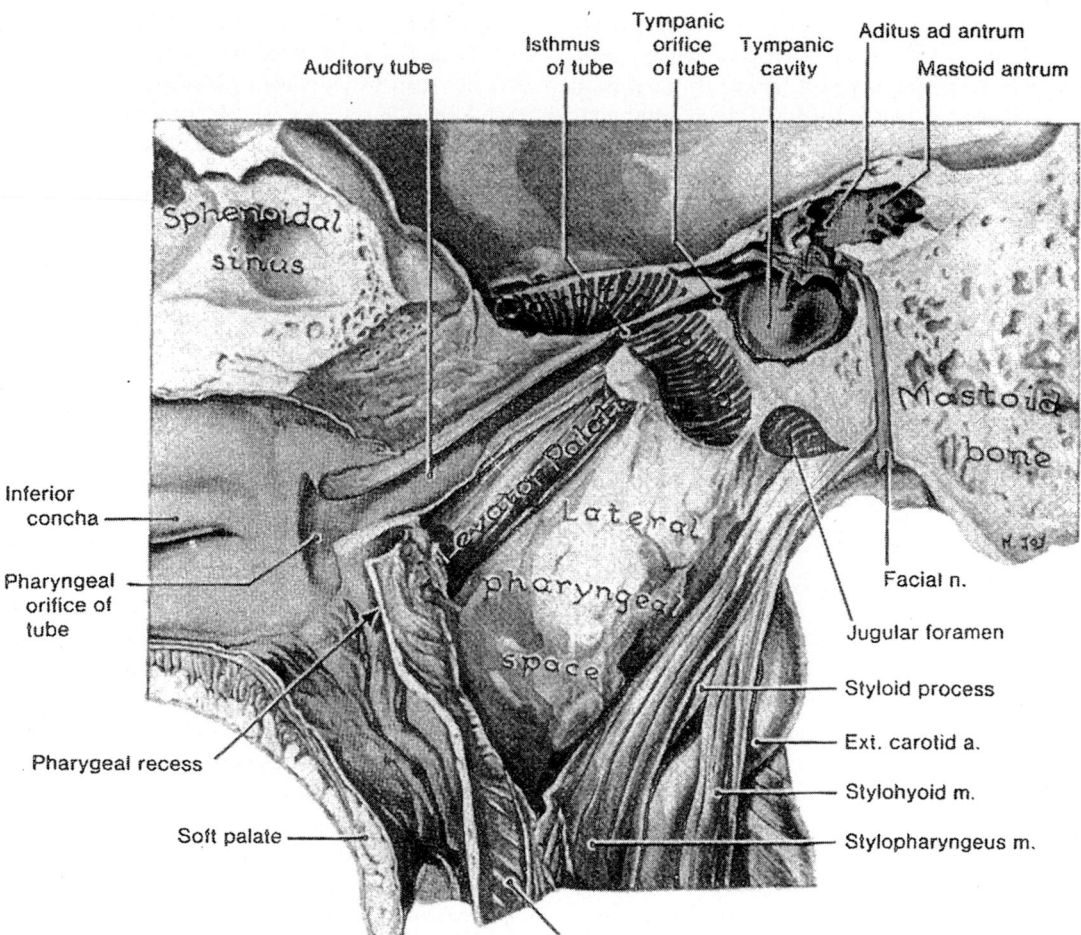

FIGURE 25.8. Structures of the ear. (From Moore KL. *Clinically Oriented Anatomy,* 2nd ed. Baltimore, MD: Williams & Wilkins; 1985, with permission.)

tube, providing balanced pressure between the atmosphere and middle ear. Loss of this connection due to obstruction, which can occur with swelling of the mucosa or hyperplasia of the adenoids, results in poor functioning of the auditory system. The result is fluid accumulating in the middle ear and subsequent infection. Children are often susceptible to middle-ear infections. Their auditory tubes are short and horizontal, and the supporting tensor veli palatini muscle is less efficient than in adults.

The blood vessels and lymphatics supplying all the structures in the head are contained in the cervical fascia. The deep cervical lymph nodes lie in the reflection of the cervical fascia. The prevertebral fascia that invests many of the muscles of the neck lies over the sympathetic chain. The superficial lymphatics, as well as the external jugular vein, pierce the superficial fascia as they pass to join deeper structures. Along with lymph from the nose and upper pharynx, the lymph drainage from the middle ear forms a plexus in front of the auditory tube before going to the retropharyngeal nodes. Obstruction of this plexus is believed to be one of the causes of serous otitis media. The intimate relationship of myofascial structures to the blood vessels, lymphatics, and ganglia serving the ear are evident (19). The influence of musculoskeletal manipulation in the treatment of ear problems is believed to exert some of its effect through these relationships (1,16,20).

Common Pathophysiology

The ear is subject to numerous types of disorders involving the external, middle, or inner ear (Table 25.2). It can be affected by infection and inflammation, and by neurologic and vascular problems. Pain, hearing loss, vertigo, and tinnitus are some symptoms

TABLE 25.2. COMMON DISORDERS OF THE EAR

Disorder
Hearing loss
Sensorineural
Conductive
External canal obstruction
Impacted cerumen
Exostoses/chondromas
Foreign bodies
External otitis
Bacterial
Fungal
Otitis media
Acute
With effusion
Mastoiditis
Tinnitus
Vertigo/Dizziness

associated with these processes. Because the sensory innervation to the ear is derived from the trigeminal, facial, glossopharyngeal, vagal, and upper cervical nerves, otalgia is frequently a result of referred pain from other areas of the head and neck. Temporomandibular joint dysfunction and cervical dysfunction are common causes of ear pain.

The external ear is subject to infections, especially if persistently exposed to a moist environment. The vestibular function of the inner ear can be disturbed as a result of infection or of neurologic or vascular impairment. Hearing loss can be due to various disturbances in the middle ear or to neurologic deficits. Chronic exposure to loud noise contributes to hearing loss (sensorineural) by traumatic damage to the receptors in the cochlea. Infectious and inflammatory processes in the auditory tube and middle ear are common causes of temporary hearing loss and ear pain.

Upper respiratory infections and allergy, with mucosal inflammation and lymphoid hyperplasia, may lead to auditory tube dysfunction. Persistent obstruction of the auditory tube pressure-equalizing system results in increasing negative pressure and decreased ventilation in the middle ear. Under these conditions, nasopharyngeal secretions could be aspirated into the middle ear and drainage impaired. The lowered PAO_2 impedes granulocyte formation, and bacterial colonization frequently results. Factors such as enlarged adenoids can aggravate the pooling of secretions in the middle ear. Reflux of nasopharyngeal contents into the middle ear is more likely when swallowing occurs in the supine position. Bottle feeding has been associated with increased incidence of otitis media, but evidence does not seem to warrant avoidance of bottle feeding (21). Evidence has been found that attendance at day-care programs and exposure to tobacco smoke increase the risk of middle ear infections (22).

Middle ear effusion can accompany acute infections and persist over several weeks or months. It is usually associated with temporary hearing loss and, when present over extended periods, may lead to delays in receptive and expressive language development (23).

OTITIS MEDIA

Diagnosis

Otitis media (infection of the middle ear) is among the most common childhood diseases encountered in primary care. The incidence may be increasing with larger numbers of children attending day-care centers. Acute otitis media often follows an upper respiratory infection. The patient presents with earache, fever, and hearing loss. Small children who are unable to clearly communicate these symptoms may present with irritability, insomnia, or tugging at the ear. With the presence of pus in the middle ear, the tympanic membrane appears bulging and erythematous, and has decreased mobility with pneumatic otoscopy.

After resolution of the acute infection, effusion may persist in the middle ear. Patients complain of painless hearing loss. The tympanic membrane may appear dull, and is often retracted in chronic cases. Evidence of fluid can be observed in the middle ear as bubbles or an air-fluid level; however, even though an effusion exists, these signs are not always present.

Auditory tube dysfunction, often accompanying middle ear disease, may manifest as tenderness just below the pinna near the angle of the jaw. Evidence of inflammation of the mucosa of the nasopharynx accompanied by postnasal drainage may also be noted in patients with otitis media. Lymphadenopathy and tenderness in the cervical soft tissues are also common findings. Examination should include evaluation for cervical and upper thoracic somatic dysfunction. Cranial dysfunction, particularly involving the temporal bones, is frequently seen (2,24).

Treatment/Management

Informing patients and families about practices that predispose to ear problems is part of total patient care. In the well-baby examination, the opportunity often exists to discuss infant feeding and avoidance of bottle feeding in the supine position. It is appropriate to encourage parents to protect their children from passive tobacco smoke.

There are conflicting views regarding treatment of acute otitis media (25). It is generally held that prolonged hearing loss, especially in certain developmental stages, is detrimental to development of language and, possibly, reading skills. Therefore, attention needs to be paid to otitis media that becomes chronic or recurrent. Guidelines have been published by the U.S. Department of Health and Human Services for uncomplicated otitis media with effusion in children ages one to three (21). The recommendations for the first 6 weeks of the condition are observation or oral antibiotics, as well as environment risk control. At 3 months, if significant hearing loss is present, tympanostomy with tube placement is an additional treatment option. If the condition has been present for 4 to 6 months with hearing loss, tube placement is indicated. According to the report, treatment in this age group should not include decongestants, antihistamines, or oral steroids.

Decreasing the edema in and around the auditory tube creates an environment for healthy function. Several manipulative techniques have been described to specifically address improved lymphatic and venous drainage from the head and neck (12,16,20).

Osteopathic manipulative technique, such as Galbreath mandibular drainage, is easily performed and may provide considerable benefit in reducing the congestion that leads to a chronic condition (16,20). Normalizing cervical muscle tone by treating specific cervical somatic dysfunction or using soft tissue techniques may allow for improved lymphatic drainage from around the auditory tube. Infectious processes benefit from improved blood flow, which is necessary for healing and delivery of medications. Arterial blood flow to the ears should be optimized by addressing the effect of somatic dysfunction in the upper thoracic and cervical areas on vasomotor tone. Techniques such as rib raising and lymphatic pump can provide a more general approach to increasing lymphatic circulation and reducing congestion and inflammation in the ears. Treatment of specific rib dysfunctions may offer a longer lasting improvement in lymphatic flow. Treatment of temporal bone dysfunction can allow for normal exit of the auditory tube from that bone. Recent studies provide evidence of clinical improvement in children with acute otitis media regarding decreased use of antibiotics, decreased number of infections, decreased need for surgical tube placement, and improved tympanograms (31). Osteopathic manipulation for the treatment of respiratory infections should include techniques to increase lymphatic flow, address viscerosomatic and somato-visceral reflexes, and improve thoracic cage motion (27).

Recognizing causes of auditory tube dysfunction may be critical to the treatment and prevention of otitis media. Allergic manifestations, such as red, itchy eyes and persistent, clear nasal discharge, suggest further allergic workup. Dietary questions regarding food intolerances or infant colic may suggest the influence of food sensitivities. Control of the allergic aspect of inflammation needs to be considered and discussed with the patient or the patient's family. Enlarged tonsils or adenoids are a cause of poor auditory tube drainage. Swallowing and chewing open the auditory tube and can be suggested as exercises for patients to help clear middle ear effusion (26). Allergy, as well as infection, may play a role in the enlargement of these lymphoid organs. If acute bacterial infection is the cause, it should be appropriately treated with antibiotics, considering the common pathogens— *S. pneumoniae, H. influenzae,* and *Streptococcus pyogenes.*

THROAT/PHARYNX

Healthy Structure and Function

The pharynx is divided into the nasopharynx, which includes the portion above the soft palate; the oropharynx, from the soft palate to the hyoid bone; and the laryngopharynx, from the hyoid bone to the lower border of the cricoid cartilage. The oral cavity lies immediately anterior to the oropharynx. The oral cavity and oropharynx are lined by squamous epithelium, whereas the nasopharynx and laryngopharynx are lined by pseudostratified ciliated columnar (respiratory) epithelium. A collection of lymphoid tissue, referred to as the Waldeyer ring, is located in the pharynx and plays an important role in immunity, especially in the first few years of life. The tongue and other structures in the oral cavity have important functions in digestion and speech.

The palatine (faucial) tonsils are masses of lymphoid tissue located on either side of the posterior oropharynx. The adenoids (pharyngeal tonsil) are found on the upper and posterior walls of the nasopharynx. The tonsils and adenoids comprise the major portion of the lymphoid tissue of the Waldeyer ring encircling the pharynx. These structures, together with the lingual tonsil, an aggregate of lymph nodules on the posterior aspect of the tongue, and scattered lymphoid nodules beneath the mucous membranes of the pharyngeal wall, are the sites for B and T lymphocyte activity (Fig. 25.9). All major classes of immunoglobulins are produced here by the B lymphocytes while the T lymphocytes participate in cell-mediated immunity. With high demands for immune function placed on these lymphoid organs, hyperplasia can occur. Secondary obstruction of airflow through the nasopharynx and auditory tubes results from significant lymphoid hyperplasia.

Blood supply to the tonsils is supplied by the external carotid system. Several arterial branches (typically three) go to the tonsils from the facial and lingual arteries. Venous drainage is accomplished by a plexus around the tonsillar capsule, which drains into the tonsillar branch of the lingual vein and connects with the pharyngeal plexus (28). The pharyngeal mucosa is rich in lymphatics. Lymphatic drainage of the tonsils goes to the submandibular nodes and to the superficial and upper deep cervical nodes. A node behind the angle of the mandible is especially associated with increased lymphatic activity from the tonsils (29).

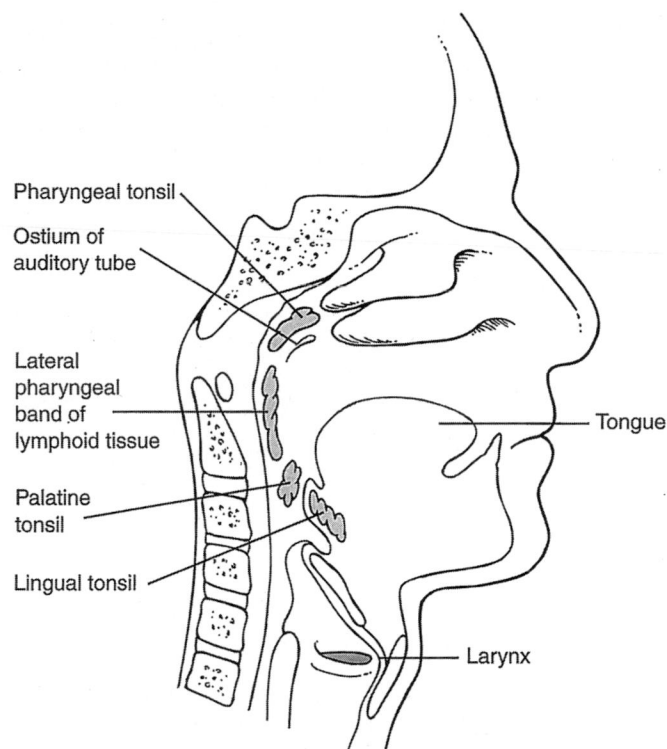

FIGURE 25.9. Lymphoid tissue in the pharynx.

Common Pathophysiology

A variety of pathologic processes can occur in the pharynx (Table 25.3), but infection is the most common. Group A beta-hemolytic streptococci and viruses are the common infectious agents. *Neisseria gonorrhoeae, Mycoplasma,* and *Chlamydia trachomatis* are also considerations. Viral infections may cause ulcerative lesions of the tongue, lips, or buccal mucosa. Herpes simplex virus is responsible for herpes labialis or cold sores. Oral candidiasis (thrush) is commonly encountered in denture wearers, patients on corticosteroids or broad-spectrum antibiotics, diabetics, and those immunocompromised, as by acquired immunodeficiency syndrome, chemotherapy, or local radiation.

ACUTE TONSILLITIS/PHARYNGITIS

Diagnosis

Sore throat is a common complaint, particularly in children. Edema, pain, and inflammation are usually associated with

TABLE 25.3. COMMON DISORDERS OF THE THROAT

Disorder
Pharyngitis
Tonsillitis
Epiglottiditis
Infectious mononucleosis
Thrush
Peritonsillar abscess
Laryngitis

pharyngitis. Often accompanied by fever, odynophagia, and tender adenopathy, it is difficult to differentiate viral from bacterial infection on inspection. Bacterial infection is typically exudative. Hoarseness, cough, rhinorrhea, and coryza are more often associated with viral infection. The appropriateness of using certain tests to identify group A beta-hemolytic streptococci infections is being questioned (30). Latex agglutination antigen tests and solid-phase enzyme immunoassays (ELISA) provide quick, but only moderately sensitive, screens for streptococcal infection. Although more sensitive, throat cultures take longer for results to become available. Because all group A beta-hemolytic streptococcal pharyngitis cases should be treated to prevent more serious sequelae, individual decisions for diagnosis and treatment should take into account the local prevalence of resistant streptococcal infections, patient history, potential for compliance, and the availability and reliability of the laboratory. Differential diagnosis includes infectious mononucleosis, diphtheria, fungal infections, and pharyngeal manifestations of systemic disease.

Treatment/Management

Group A beta-hemolytic streptococcal pharyngitis requires a 10-day course of oral antibiotics or a single intramuscular dose of Benzathine Penicillin G. Penicillin V potassium and cephalosporins are effective. Erythromycin or azithromycin are reasonable alternatives for individuals who are allergic to penicillin. Ancillary treatment to control symptoms and make the patient more comfortable includes analgesics, antiinflammatory agents, saltwater gargling, and osteopathic manipulation. Viral infections require only symptomatic treatment.

Osteopathic manipulation to reduce swelling and improve lymphatic flow (probably stimulating the immune response) can be particularly helpful in providing symptomatic relief (7,27). The Galbreath technique of mandibular drainage reduces tonsillar congestion and may offer pain relief and reduce the chance of lymphatic congestion around the auditory tube (Fig. 25.10). Improving lymphatic circulation by addressing any somatic dysfunction of the upper ribs, clavicle, cervical, and upper thoracic areas not only reduces swelling but also stimulates the immune response. Removing inflammatory mediators from the site of infection by promoting venous and lymphatic circulation allows for a more favorable healing environment. Healing may also be enhanced by addressing sympathetic, vasomotor control affected by somatic dysfunction of the upper thoracic and upper cervical (superior cervical ganglion) areas. Presumably, improved arterial flow would also increase the tissue levels of prescribed antibiotics or other medications.

MUSCULOSKELETAL APPROACH TO THE EAR, NOSE, AND THROAT PATIENT

The major principles to consider in treating ENT patients in terms of the musculoskeletal component of health and disease are:

1. assisting venous and lymphatic circulation,
2. promoting arterial flow,
3. normalizing spinal reflexes affecting function of the ear, nose, and throat, and
4. relieving pain.

It is reasonable to expect that the use of musculoskeletal diagnosis and treatment in these patients will help the patient feel better, assist in healing, and improve their overall resistance to disease.

As a guide, evaluate and treat somatic dysfunction from central body areas to the periphery, allowing for free flow of venous and lymphatic fluids. The rationale for treating somatic dysfunction in the upper thoracic and cervical spine is to decrease somatic stimulation in the area of the sympathetic outflow and ganglia supplying the head and neck. Improving venous and lymphatic flow also provides the rationale for osteopathic manipulative treatment to the cervical and thoracic inlet areas. An attempt is made to decrease myofascial tension in the

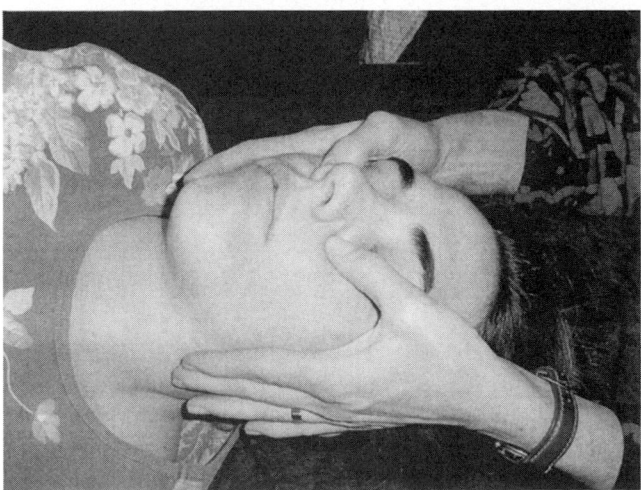

FIGURE 25.10. Superficial sinus drainage technique.)

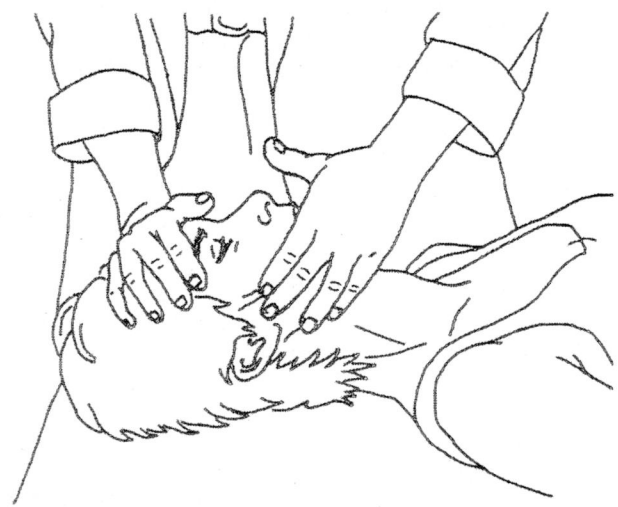

FIGURE 25.11. Galbreath technique for mandibular drainage. (From Shaw HH, Dyer RR. *One-Minute Osteopathic Techniques for the Busy Clinician,* 1st ed. Tulsa, OK: Oklahoma State University College of Osteopathic Medicine; 1997, with permission.

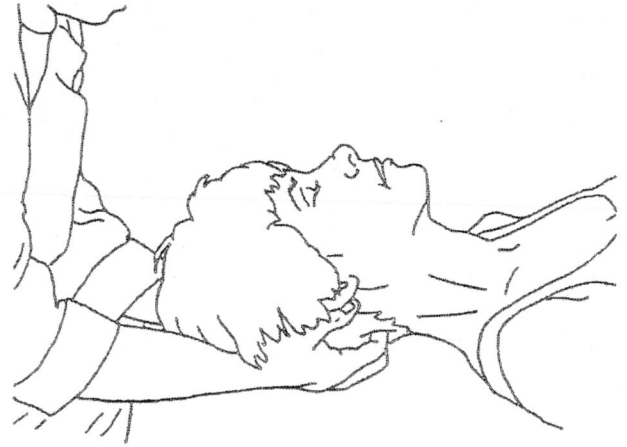

FIGURE 25.12. Suboccipital inhibitory pressure/cranial base release technique. (From Shaw HH, Dyer RR. *One-Minute Osteopathic Techniques for the Busy Clinician,* 1st ed. Tulsa, OK: Oklahoma State University College of Osteopathic Medicine;1997, with permission.)

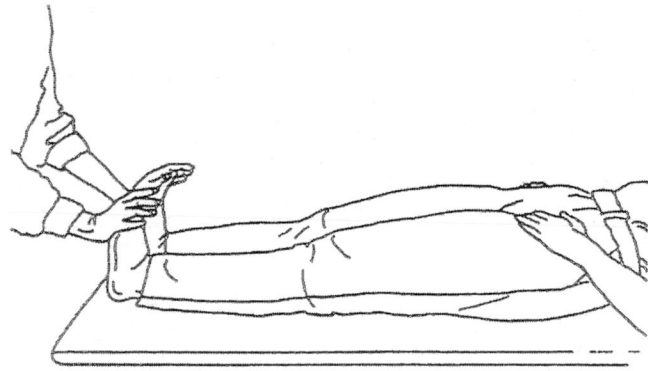

FIGURE 25.14. Pedal lymphatic pump technique. (From Shaw HH, Dyer RR. *One-Minute Osteopathic Techniques for the Busy Clinician,* 1st ed. Tulsa, OK: Oklahoma State University College of Osteopathic Medicine; 1997, with permission.)

osteopathic literature regarding treatment of infectious disease (15,16,27).

areas through which lymphatic and venous vessels pass from the head to where they enter the central circulation at about the level of the first rib. Superficial drainage techniques (effleurage) applied to the face from medial to lateral decrease tissue congestion in the anterior sinus regions (Fig. 25.11). The mandibular drainage technique described by Galbreath (20) is an effective lymphatic drainage procedure for the ear, auditory canals, and throat (Fig. 25.10). Chapman reflexes are small, nodular, and tender areas that have been observed in relationship to inflammatory diseases of visceral structures. Used for diagnosis and treatment, they are believed to represent viscerosomatic reflexes and have been shown to be responsive to a rotary pressure technique (14) (See chapter on Chapman reflexes). Cranial treatment, including suboccipital inhibitory pressure, is especially indicated in sinus disease and middle- and inner-ear conditions (Fig. 25.12). Lymphatic pump techniques are intended to stimulate general lymphatic flow by affecting intrathoracic pressures (Figs 25.13 and 25.14). Their use is described in the

REFERENCES

1. Blood HA. Infections of the ear, nose and throat. *Ost Ann.* 1978; 6(11):14–18.
2. Woods DE. Management of ENT problems. *Ost Ann.* 1980;8(5):31–41.
3. Moser RJ. Sinusitis, the effective osteopathic manipulative procedures in the management thereof. *Yearbook of Selected Papers.* Academy of Applied Osteopathy; 1953:15–16.
4. Sato A. Reflex modulation of visceral functions by somatic afferent activity. *The Central Connection: Somatovisceral/Viscerosomatic Interaction.* Proceedings of 1989 American Academy of Osteopathy International Symposium: 53–72.
5. Sato A, Schmidt RF. The modulation of visceral functions by somatic afferent activity. *Jpn J Physiol.* 1987;37:1–17.
6. Pintal WJ, Kurtz ME. An integrated osteopathic treatment approach in acute otitis media. *J Am Osteopath Assoc.* 1989;89(9):1139–1141.
7. Schmidt IC. Osteopathic manipulative therapy as a primary factor in the management of upper, middle, and pararespiratory infections. *J Am Osteopath Assoc.* 1982;81(6):382–388.
8. Wasserman SJ. Ciliary function and disease. *J Allergy Clin Immunol.* 1984;73:17–19.
9. Wagenmann M, Naclerio RM. Anatomic and physiologic considerations in sinusitis. *J Allergy Clin Immunol.* 1992;90:419–423.
10. Zeiger RS. Prospects for ancillary treatment of sinusitis. *J Allergy Clin Immunol.* 1992;90:478–495.
11. Kaluza CL, Sherbin M. The physiologic response of the nose to osteopathic manipulative treatment: preliminary report. *J Am Osteopath Assoc.* 1983;82(9):654–660.
12. Harakal JH. Manipulative treatment for acute upper-respiratory diseases. *Ost Ann.* 1981;9(7):30–37.
13. Hoyt WH. Current concepts in management of sinus disease. *J Am Osteopath Assoc.* 1990;90(10):913–919.
14. Owens C. *An Endocrine Interpretation of Chapman's Reflexes.* Academy of Applied Osteopathy; 1963.
15. Shrum KM, Grogg SE, Garton P, et al. Sinusitis in children: the importance of diagnosis. *J Am Osteopath Assoc.* 2001;101(5):S8–S13.
16. Cathie AG. The sino-bronchial syndrome. *Yearbook of Selected Papers.* Academy of Applied Osteopathy; 1968:9–11.
17. Charlton A. Children and passive smoking: a review. *J Fam Pract.* 1994;38(3):267–277.
18. Naclerio RM. Allergic Rhinitis. *N Engl J Med.* 1991;325(12):860.
19. Greenman PE. Fascial considerations in treatment of the head and neck. *Ost Ann.* 1975;3(2):34–42.

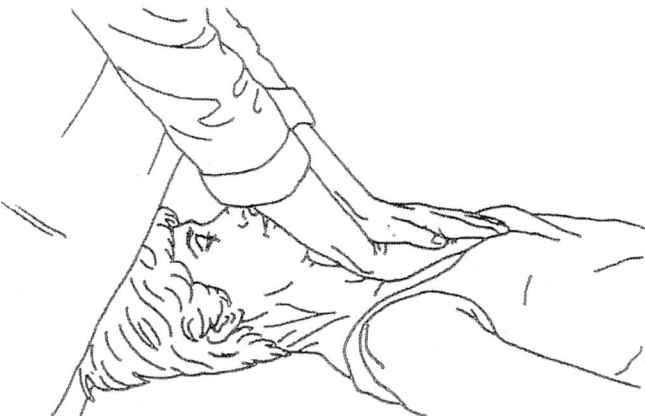

FIGURE 25.13. Thoracic lymphatic pump technique. (From Shaw HH, Dyer RR. *One-Minute Osteopathic Techniques for the Busy Clinician,* 1st ed. Tulsa, OK: Oklahoma State University College of Osteopathic Medicine;1997, with permission.)

20. Galbreath W. Manipulative structural adjustive treatment in middle ear deafness. *J Am Osteopath Assoc.* 1925;24:741.

21. U.S. Department of Health and Human Services. Managing otitis media with effusion in young children. *Arch Otolaryngol Head Neck Surg.* 1994;120:793–796.

22. Froom J, Culpepper L. Otitis media in daycare children. A report from the International Primary Care Network. *J Fam Pract.* 1991;32:289–294.

23. Updike C, Thornburg JD. Reading skills and auditory processing ability in children with chronic otitis media in early childhood. *Ann Otol Rhinol Laryngol.* 1992;101:530–537.

24. Magoun H. *Osteopathy in the Cranial Field.* Journal Printing Company; 1976:213–215.

25. Browning G, Bain B. Childhood otalgia: acute otitis media. *BMJ.* 1990;300:1005–1007.

26. Honjo I, Okazake N. Opening mechanism of the eustachian tube. *Ann Otol Rhinol Laryngol.* 1980;89(3):25–27.

27. Rumney IC. Osteopathic manipulative treatment of infectious diseases. *Ost Ann.* 1974;2:29–33.

28. Krmpotic-Nemanic J, Draf W. *Surgical Anatomy of Head and Neck.* New York: Springer-Verlag; 1988.

29. Hollinshead WH. *Anatomy for Surgeons: The Head and Neck.* Harper & Row; 1968.

30. Wegner DL, Witte DL. Insensitivity of rapid antigen detection methods and single blood agar plate culture for diagnosing streptococcal pharyngitis. *JAMA.* 1992;267(5):695–697.

31. Mills MV, Henley CE, Barnes LLB, Carrero JE. The use of osteopathic manipulative treatment (OMT) as adjunctive therapy for acute otitis media in children. Submitted for publication, June 2002.

OSTEOPATHIC MEDICINE IN THE PRACTICE OF EMERGENCY MEDICINE

PETER ADLER-MICHAELSON
BERNADETTE BRANDON
RAUL GARCIA

KEY CONCEPTS

- The history of the profession of osteopathic emergency medicine
- The philosophy of the profession of osteopathic emergency medicine
- The logistics and demographics of emergency medicine
- The application of the osteopathic philosophy and assessment in the Emergency Department (ED)
- The application of osteopathic philosophy, principles, palpatory diagnosis, and manipulative treatment in the ED

HISTORY AND DEVELOPMENT OF EMERGENCY MEDICINE AS A PROFESSION

Emergency medicine (EM), in one form or another, has existed since the beginning of time. However, as a medical specialty in the United States, it officially began in 1968 when a group of eight physicians formed the American College of Emergency Medicine (1). It grew out of the realization that many of the clinical lessons that had been learned in the Korean and Vietnam wars could also be applied in peace time and could help many patients. A year later, these eight physicians held the first Scientific Assembly in Emergency Medicine in the United States (1). In 1970, at the University of Cincinnati, the first residency in emergency medicine was started (1). At first, EM was regulated as a subspecialty under a coalition of the American Board of Family Practice, the American Board of Internal Medicine, the American Board of Obstetrics and Gynecology, the American Board of Otolaryngology, the American Board of Pediatrics, the American Board of Psychiatry and Neurology, and the American Board Surgery. In 1979, a separate, sovereign regulatory board, the American Board of Emergency Medicine (ABEM) was recognized by the American Board of Medical Specialties and the American Medical Association as the 23rd medical specialty (2). In 1980, the first emergency

physicians received their ABEM board certification (1). This was (and still is today) a 3-year training program leading to board eligibility. ABEM board certification is issued after passing the written and oral examination. Until 1988, the so-called "practice category" or "grandfather clause" by which one could become board eligible and likewise certified after having worked many years within the field of emergency medicine was also recognized (2). MDs and DOs alike were (and still are) accepted for board eligibility and certification by the ABEM. Today there are 125 medical schools, both allopathic and osteopathic, that have formal departments of EM producing roughly 600 board-eligible physicians each year (2).

HISTORY AND DEVELOPMENT OF OSTEOPATHIC EMERGENCY MEDICINE AS A PROFESSION

Like its allopathic counterpart, the American College of Osteopathic Emergency Physicians (ACOEP) was founded by physicians working in the field who felt this emerging specialty needed its own voice. In 1975, a small group of emergency osteopathic physicians sent a letter of intent to the American Osteopathic Association (AOA) seeking affiliate status within that organization. At the following AOA convention, the first officers were elected. The college was formally recognized in 1978 and held its first scientific assembly that year. Since that time, the ACOEP has grown to become the second largest specialty college within the AOA, second only to the American College of Osteopathic Family Practitioners (3).

In 1980, noting the growth and future of EM, the AOA created an osteopathic board to regulate the specialty of EM within the osteopathic profession, the American Osteopathic Board of Emergency Medicine (AOBEM) (3). Eligibility now requires completion of a 3-year residency program. Until 1997, there was also a practice category by which one could become AOBEM board eligible. Certification requires the successful completion of written, oral, and clinical examinations (parts I, II & III) (3). The first osteopathic emergency medicine residency was established in 1979 at the hospital of the Philadelphia College of Osteopathic Medicine (3). Presently there are 27 residency training programs in osteopathic emergency medicine in this country, graduating roughly 150 EM board-eligible osteopathic physicians each year (3).

PHILOSOPHY OF OSTEOPATHIC EMERGENCY MEDICINE

The osteopathic philosophy, which is discussed in more detail in Chapter 1 of this text, can be described as the application of the osteopathic principles of:

1. the unity of body, mind, and spirit,
2. the self-healing capacity of the body,
3. the interrelatedness of the structure and function within the body, and
4. the creation of a sensible treatment plan based on the first three principles that most appropriately leads patients back toward their best achievable level of homeostasis.

From the osteopathic perspective, the patient in the ED has experienced a breakdown in some aspect of their body-mind-spirit unity (e.g., fractures, lacerations, other trauma, fear, anxiety, depression, abuse, psychosis, drug or alcohol abuse, chronic disease, loneliness, alienation), has lost their innate ability to heal and self-regulate, (e.g., poor nutrition, chronic stress, chronic disease, aging, alienation within society), and has a disruption of the structure-function interrelatedness principle, such that they present with a variety of functional or structural dysfunction that makes up their symptomatology.

As described above, in the last 25 years, emergency medicine has developed into a separately regulated medical specialty for both the allopathic and osteopathic professions. The philosophy of EM is the application of the principles of emergency medicine: diagnosing and treating emergent and urgent conditions, using a primary assessment to quickly recognize life-threatening conditions, treating appropriately to stabilize the patient, completing a more detailed secondary assessment of the patient, and arranging definitive care to create an overall treatment plan that will assure the best outcome.

The synthesis of these two philosophies and practices is what osteopathic emergency medicine is about, and it provides a wonderful opportunity for us to help patients in emergent and urgent situations.

Osteopathic treatment in the emergency room is not much different than in other clinical situations. The goal is to assist the patient to regain their body-mind-spirit unification, to regain or optimize their self-healing capacities, and return to a more effective structure-function interrelatedness.

One distinctly osteopathic approach that helps accomplish this goal is the application of osteopathic palpatory diagnosis and treatment modalities. Many osteopathic students and physicians feel that it must be difficult to apply palpatory diagnostic skills and manipulative treatment modalities in the ED.

This is far from the truth. The main goal of this chapter is to provide an overview and some helpful guidelines as to when and how osteopathic philosophy, principles, palpatory diagnosis, and manipulative treatment modalities can be appropriately employed in the ED.

Of course, the priority in the ED to stabilize any potentially life-threatening illnesses takes temporal priority over the actual application of osteopathic manipulative medicine (OMM). There are periods of time in the ED when the osteopathic physician will not have the time or the inner peace necessary to apply OMM. There are, however, times when it is relatively quiet and the application of OMM is possible. The problem is that it is impossible to know this ahead of time in order to schedule OMM treatments, which can be frustrating for physician and patient.

The specific aspects of osteopathic assessment and treatment for a number of common presentations to the ED will be discussed later in this section. We will focus on the specific additional aspects of osteopathic assessment and treatment modalities that can be very helpful in the ED.

There was a time when ultrasound examination was not used very often in the ED. Later, after many of us became trained and competent in this assessment modality or had in-house staff able to do these examinations, it was hard to imagine not having ultrasound to assist in the evaluation of the patient. Osteopathic assessment and treatment is much the same. Many of us have become very comfortable with this important form of assessment and treatment and cannot imagine not having this modality as an option in the ED.

"EXTENT OF THE PROBLEM" IN OSTEOPATHIC EMERGENCY MEDICINE

Logistics and Demographics within Emergency Medicine

Table 26.1 shows the breakdown by category of chief complaints leading to visits to the ED (4). Cases of upper respiratory infection, low back pain, and other musculoskeletal disorders are the most common complaints with which patients present to the ED (4). These conditions provide excellent opportunities to apply OMM (5). Chest pain, asthma, abdominal pain, pelvic pain, and, of course, other musculoskeletal complaints, such as joint pain and extremity disorders, are just a few other very common ED presentations for which OMM can and should be implemented either in the ED or later in the primary care setting (5).

The prevalence of musculoskeletal disorders in this country is enormous and growing. Table 26.2 shows a breakdown of the chief musculoskeletal complaints presenting to the ED (6).

The financial burden on society of all musculoskeletal conditions has increased from an estimated $126 billion in 1988 to an estimated $215 billion in 1995 (6). In 1997 and again in 1998, the annual cost to treat the more than 3.8 million ED visits due to musculoskeletal sports injuries in the 5 to 24 year age range alone has been estimated to be $680 million (7). We have shown that there are many patients presenting to the ED that have a primary musculoskeletal complaint. For these patients, the application of OMM is often one of the most appropriate treatments (5). The

TABLE 26.1. NUMBER AND PERCENT DISTRIBUTION OF EMERGENCY DEPARTMENT VISITS WITH CORRESPONDING STANDARD ERRORS, BY PRIMARY DIAGNOSIS: UNITED STATES, 1999

Major disease category and ICD–9–CM code range[a]		Number of visits (in thousands)	Standard error (in thousands)	Percent distribution	Standard error of percent
All visits		102,765	4,493	100.0	—
Infectious and parasitic diseases	001–139	2,866	194	2.8	0.2
Neoplasms	140–239	346	63	0.3	0.1
Endocrine, nutritional and metabolic diseases, and immunity disorders	240–279	1,779	138	1.8	0.1
Mental disorders	290–319	2,903	215	2.9	0.2
Diseases of the nervous system and sense organs	320–389	5,863	388	5.8	0.2
Diseases of the circulatory system	390–459	4,397	273	4.4	0.2
Diseases of the respiratory system	460–519	12,991	765	12.9	0.4
Diseases of the digestive system	520–579	5,947	366	5.9	0.2
Diseases of the genitourinary system	580–629	4,372	249	4.3	0.2
Diseases of the skin and subcutaneous tissue	680–709	2,826	220	2.8	0.2
Diseases of the musculoskeletal system and connective tissue	710–739	5,578	359	5.5	0.2
Symptoms, signs, and ill-defined conditions	780–799	16,377	888	16.2	0.5
Injury and poisoning	800–999	29,586	1,322	29.3	0.6
Fracture	800–829	3,676	216	3.6	0.2
Sprains	840–848	6,290	354	6.1	0.2
Intracranial	850–854	281	47	0.3	0.0
Open wounds	870–897	7,296	405	7.1	0.3
Superficial	910–919	1,601	134	1.6	0.1
Contusion	920–924	4,458	234	4.3	0.2
Foreign bodies	930–939	635	78	0.6	0.1
Burns	940–949	574	75	0.6	0.1
Complications	958–959	1,587	134	1.5	0.1
Poisoning and toxic effects	960–989	953	102	0.9	0.1
Other injury	—	2,235	147	2.2	0.1
Supplementary classification	V01–V82	3,865	238	3.8	0.2
All other diagnoses[b]	—	1,732	127	1.7	0.1
Unknown[c]	—	1,338	288	1.3	0.3

— Category not applicable.
0.0 Quantity more than zero but less than 0.05.
[a]Based on the *International Classification of Diseases, Ninth Revision, Clinical Modification* (ICD–9–CM) (21).
[b]Includes diseases of the blood and blood-forming organs (280–289); complications of pregnancy, childbirth, and the puerperium (630–676); congenital anomalies (740–759); and certain disorders originating in the perinatal period (760–779).
[c]Includes blank diagnoses, uncodable diagnoses, and illegible diagnoses.
Note: Numbers may not add to totals because of rounding.
Source: Centers for Disease Control and Prevention, National Center for Health Statistics.

TABLE 26.2. NEW PROBLEM VISITS TO PHYSICIANS IN OFFICE-BASED PRACTICE FOR MUSCULOSKELETAL CONDITIONS, BY PATIENT'S MOST FREQUENTLY MENTIONED PRINCIPAL REASON FOR VISIT: UNITED STATES, 1995[a]

Reason for Visit Code[b]		Visits (in thousands)		
		Male	Female	Total
S905	Back symptoms	1,757	1,942	3,700
S925	Knee symptoms	1,538	1,821	3,359
S940	Shoulder symptoms	1,075	1,469	2,544
S935	Foot and toe symptoms	901	1,477	2,378
S910	Low back symptoms	869	1,259	2,128
S900	Neck symptoms	750	1,218	1,968
S960	Hand and/or finger symptoms	780	720	1,500
S955	Wrist symptoms	401	825	1,226
S920	Leg symptoms	676	547	1,224
S050	Chest pain or related symptoms	430	668	1,098
S930	Ankle symptoms	532	466	998
S945	Arm symptoms	434	527	961
S950	Elbow symptoms	397	374	771
S055	Pain, other specified sites	497	219	716
I570	Finger/hand injury, unspecified	366	320	686

[a]Reason for visit mentioned by patients with a musculoskeletal condition diagnosis.
[b]Codes are based on Schneider D, Appleton L, McLemore T: A Reason for Visit Classification for Ambulatory Care.
National Center for Health Statistics, Vital and Health Statistics 2, 1979.
Source: National Center for Health Statistics. National Ambulatory Medical Care Survey, 1995.

osteopathic emergency physician is uniquely able to provide this kind of treatment as time allows in the ED.

Theoretical Aspects of the Osteopathic Medicine Approach to the Patient in the Emergency Department

It may seem that EM and osteopathic medicine are mutually exclusive. This is far from the truth. Through many years in EM, I (Adler-Michaelson) have used osteopathic principles and practices during every emergency medicine shift I have ever worked. The unity of spirit, mind, and body, as well as the interrelatedness of structure and function, is as evident in the ED as it is in an office or hospital practice. The body's capacity and attempts at self-regulation and self-healing are, at times, even more apparent in the emergency department than in an office or hospital practice. I know of no presentation to the ED for which there were no osteopathic considerations that could be helpful to the patient.

For example, in the assessment and treatment of headaches, viral upper respiratory infections (URIs), sinusitis, whiplash injury, chest pain, abdominal pain, pneumonia, pyelonephritis, kidney stone, cystitis, obstetrical complications, pelvic inflammatory disease, arthritides, trauma to an extremity, and so on, applications of distinctly osteopathic principles and treatment modalities can considerably assist the patients' recovery (8).

One important aspect of EM that is also helpful in osteopathy is the need to always consider the larger picture, to be aware of the patient's primary illness or injury, and to move toward specific details as time allows. This is essentially the same as assessing the patient osteopathically to determine the *key somatic dysfunction* or the primary restriction, treating this, and knowing that the secondary somatic dysfunction will subside (see Chapter 29).

Patient *history* is imperative. Listening carefully to the patient's description of the pain or discomfort will often give important clues as to the cause. The concept of *typical patterns of referred pain* from various structures in the body is a crucial concept in all of medicine. For example, gallbladder disease often refers pain to the tip of the right scapula (9). Heart disease with ischemia or infarction typically refers pain up into the jaw, down the inside of the left arm, or into the midepigastrium (10). The typical pain described by the patient suffering from pancreatitis is a midepigastric pain that radiates straight through to the back (10). This same concept applies when the problem is a somatic dysfunction of a myofascial structure. For example, the psoas muscle will typically cause pain in the low back and anterior groin areas on the side of the dysfunction (11). A right psoas somatic dysfunction will often present together with a left piriformis somatic dysfunction: the so-called psoas syndrome (12). A piriformis muscle dysfunction typically causes buttock and/or posterior thigh pain due to its origin and insertion and proximity to the sciatic nerve. Knowing these "typical" symptom distribution patterns for various disease states or somatic dysfunction allows the physician to more readily and reliably arrive at the correct diagnosis.

A screening structural examination that is done quickly and efficiently and that includes lymphatic, myofascial, cranial, and somatic aspects can help the osteopathic emergency physician find the key lesions that, when treated, will provide the most assistance to the patient in regaining homeostasis. This examination is performed during the secondary survey and after any life-threatening condition has been addressed. See the "Practical Considerations" section below for an example.

The concept of *facilitation* can also help the emergency physician with his or her diagnosis in the ED. A visceral disease process will commonly cause facilitation of spinal segments in a specific pattern. For example, significant coronary artery disease (CAD) facilitates to the spine in the T1-6 region and often causes typical somatic changes: bogginess or ropiness of the paraspinal tissues and more diffuse palpatory changes (usually without hyperemic skin changes). The segments often follow Fryette type 2 mechanics, i.e., T_2 FR_L S_L (8). This is an example of viscerosomatic reflex activity.

Another important aspect of osteopathic medicine is the use of Chapman reflex points, which can indicate the presence of visceral disease and can be very helpful in the assessment of the ED patient (13). To use the example of the patient with CAD, he or she will display significantly painful reflex points bilaterally in the 2nd intercostal space close to the sternum ventrally and between the 2nd and 3rd transverse processes dorsally. We will give further examples of the application of these later in the section. For more details on Chapman reflex points, see Chapter 67.

Another important consideration of osteopathic medicine that applies to every patient regardless of setting is improvement in the function of the lymphatic system. In acute ureteral obstruction, it has been shown that renal hilar lymph flow can increase up to three times their original capacity in an attempt to compensate for the illness (14). In addressing this very important self-regulatory system, whether through techniques to eliminate or reduce obstructions to lymphatic flow, techniques to actually increase the flow of lymphatic fluid, or both, we can significantly help the patient move toward homeostasis. Several examples of the application of these techniques are described later in the section. For more details on the structure and function of the lymphatic system, see Chapter 68.

In essentially every presentation to the ED, it is possible to address the imbalance within the autonomic (sympathetic and parasympathetic) nervous system. Achieving or moving toward balance will greatly assist the body in its self-regulatory mechanism, regardless of the patient's complaint (8). Several examples of the application of these techniques are given later in this section. For more details on the structure and function of the autonomic nervous system (ANS), see Chapter 6.

Especially in emergency medicine, it is important to be aware of the possibility of *atypical presentations* in patients. For example, chest pain with normal laboratory values, normal electrocardiogram, and even subjective improvement after an OMM treatment can still be due to unstable angina or even a myocardial infarction. This is one example of why the missed or incorrectly diagnosed acute myocardial infarct (AMI) is the highest malpractice payment situation in emergency medicine. Table 26.3 shows the leading causes of malpractice suits by category in the ED (14). The present medical-legal climate in this country, especially in the ED, is such that an emergency physician is constantly aware of possible "traps" in assessment and treatment and of situations where a missed diagnosis or incorrect treatment could have grave consequences. As shown later in the section, using several of the concepts described in this chapter gives the osteopathic

TABLE 26.3. MALPRACTICE CLAIMS MADE, PAID, AND AVERAGE PAYOUT

Reason	Total Claims Made Since 1985	Number of Claims Paid	Average Payout($)
Breast cancer	2,986	1,039	204,436
Brain-damaged infant	2,613	934	449,486
Pregnancy	1,953	530	128,978
Heart attack	1,770	563	190,347
Intervertebral-disc displacement	1,662	402	172,041
Lung cancer	1,639	504	149,823
Appendicitis	1,296	368	83,100
Femur fracture	1,290	365	85,255
Cataracts	1,151	269	96,603
Sterilization	1,119	349	46,770

Source: "The Cutting Edge: Vital Statistics." *Washington Post,* 12 September 1995, p. 5.
Data are for the period 1985 through 1995 derived from Physician Insurers Association of America data. The organization insures 25% of the nation's doctors.

emergency physician a significant advantage over his or her allopathic counterpart.

PRACTICAL OSTEOPATHIC CONSIDERATIONS IN EMERGENCY MEDICINE DIAGNOSIS AND TREATMENT

A number of important, practical osteopathic considerations in emergency medicine diagnosis and treatment are presented, followed by an example of how to do a musculoskeletal screening examination in the ED and a case example.

Several important considerations in osteopathic medicine can be specifically helpful in diagnosing and treating patients in the ED. Signs of *viscerosomatic reflex activity:* typical tissue/segmental changes of facilitation and/or the presence of Chapman reflex points are important diagnostic signs.

In addition, addressing *lymphatic system* considerations and attempting to balance the *autonomic nervous system* will further assist the patient in his/her self-regulatory mechanisms.

Viscerosomatic Activity

An important sign of *viscerosomatic activity* is finding bogginess or ropiness of the paraspinal tissues on osteopathic palpatory examination, more diffuse palpatory changes, and usually less warmth without hyperemic skin changes in a spinal segment area appropriate for the organ(s) in question (37). These somatic dysfunction changes usually affect one or two segments, often in a Fryette type 2 orientation (i.e., T_2 FR_L S_L) in cardiac disease states (8).

A second important sign of *viscerosomatic activity* is the presence of Chapman reflex points (13). In the above cardiac patient, the presence of anterior and/or posterior Chapman reflex points in the second intercostal space on the left, just lateral to the sternal border ventrally and between the transverse processes of T2 and T3 on the left dorsally, would be excellent support for the diagnosis of significant heart disease. Research is currently under way to determine the diagnostic and therapeutic reliability of these points (Adler-Michaelson and Crow, unpublished research). Treatment of these points, through a firm circular mas-

saging motion until the tissues begin to soften, was found by Chapman nearly 100 years ago to improve function and relieve clinical symptoms (13).

The Lymphatic System

A quick but effective way of assessing the lymphatic system is to check for signs of fluid congestion in key points on the body that correspond to larger body areas, e.g., supraclavicular area, posterior axillary folds, midepigastrium, on so on. Based on the osteopathic physician's knowledge of the flow of lymphatic fluid in the body, the practical considerations involving the *lymphatic system* are to first eliminate any myofascial restrictions to the lymphatic flow (release all diaphragms) and then to increase the flow from the area in question, as appropriate for the patient. See Chapter 68 for specific lymphatic techniques.

The Autonomic Nervous System

Attempting to normalize the *autonomic nervous system* is an important goal of osteopathic medicine. The majority of ill patients present in a hypersympathetic state. It is tempting to think in terms of decreasing the sympathetic tone or increasing the parasympathetic tone, but in true osteopathic fashion (believing that the body has self-regulatory faculties), it is more appropriate to think in terms of normalizing the two aspects of this very important homeostatic system: the sympathetic and parasympathetic nervous systems. Techniques applied to the craniosacral and upper cervical areas will tend to normalize the parasympathetic system. Techniques applied to the thoracic and lumbar areas will tend to normalize the sympathetic system. See Chapter 6 and Chapters 48 through 50 for specific techniques.

The Screening Examination

There are many forms that the screening examination in the ED can take, depending on the skills of the particular osteopathic physician and the time available. One form described here has been tested over many years of practice. This screening examination can be completed in approximately 10 to 15 minutes. The physician may not need to perform all of the following steps during the assessment of every patient.

First, the *presenting complaint* will often suggest the problem. It is therefore important (as mentioned above) to know the typical distribution or patterns of pain that most patients describe with various dysfunctions (11). Knowing the typical pain distribution patterns present in musculoskeletal dysfunction, whether due to the primary underlying disease processes or only secondary changes, helps the physician to more quickly and correctly arrive at the appropriate diagnosis.

Second, evaluation of the patient in the ED, especially one with a musculoskeletal complaint or component, should begin with *observation* of:

- the patient walking (observe asymmetries in the gait cycle),
- the patient standing (static tests: gross asymmetries from the anterior, posterior, and lateral perspectives, a short leg, scoliosis, congenital abnormalities, etc.; motion tests: standing flexion and hip-drop tests),
- the patient seated (static tests: gross asymmetries, scoliosis, congenital abnormalities; motion tests: seated flexion test, trunk sidebending and rotation tests, cervical spine flexion, sidebending, and rotation tests).

These observations and tests will often give important clues as to the location of the patient's primary restriction.

The screening examination should then include visual and palpatory *examination of the skin.* The patient should be evaluated for changes in temperature (warmer in areas of acute somatic dysfunction, cooler in areas of chronic somatic dysfunction), moisture (may be increased in areas of acute somatic dysfunction), oiliness (may be increased in areas of acute somatic dysfunction), texture (may be rougher or have obvious skin changes, such as pimples, cafe-au-lait spots, rough or heavy hair growth patterns in areas of somatic dysfunction or congenital anomalies), and turgor or congestion (may be increased in areas of acute or chronic somatic dysfunction).

Next, a *fascial listening* sequence, based on the observations of Zink and Lawson (15) (see Chapter 41), may give valuable information as to the presence of compromised homeostatic mechanisms in the body. Assessing the body's fascial preferences, especially at the four transition zones (craniocervical, cervicothoracic, thoracolumbar, and lumbosacral), allows the osteopathic physician to determine where, if at all, the patient is decompensated. In a healthy person, there will either be no identifiable preference or there will be a pattern of alternating preferences (L,R,L,R, or R,L,R,L) called compensatory patterns. Areas of decompensation (non-alternating pattern) correlate well with areas of somatic dysfunction in the body.

Next, a more focused examination of specific muscle groups or individual muscles suspected, from the earlier evaluation, to be in somatic dysfunction can then be performed using the well known muscle *trigger points.*. Travell and Simmons (11) have shown that the presence of extremely painful, well-demarcated areas in predescribed locations within a specific muscle correlates well with somatic dysfunction of that muscle. In just a few seconds, the knowledgeable osteopathic physician can determine which muscles or muscle groups are in dysfunction by using this method.

Examination of the strain/counterstrain "tender points" discovered by Jones (16) (see Chapter 63) can contribute valuable information about the body's state of balance/imbalance (see Chapter 63 for more on strain/counterstrain).

Next, the *lymphatic system* can be quickly assessed by examining the following areas for signs of bogginess or congestion within the tissues: the supraclavicular space, the posterior axillary fold, the midepigastric area, the popliteal space, the inguinal region, the wrist area, the antecubital fossa, and the Achilles tendon area. Congestion in these areas can be an important clue to dysfunction of the lymphatic system in the related body areas.

At an appropriate time in the screening examination sequence, the craniosacral mechanism can be assessed for rate, vitality, and quality of the cranial rhythmic impulse (CRI) and for the motions of flexion, extension, and internal and external rotation of the bones of the skull and sacrum (see Chapter 62).

Another appropriate screening examination in the osteopathic assessment of the patient is the assessment of the abdominal collateral ganglia, and the celiac, superior, and inferior mesenteric ganglia. The celiac ganglion innervates the stomach, duodenum, liver, gallbladder, pancreas, and spleen. The superior mesenteric ganglion innervates the jejunum, ileum, the proximal half of the colon, the kidneys, adrenals, and the gonads. The inferior mesenteric ganglion innervates the distal half of the colon and the pelvic organs (except the gonads). If a subjective report of tenderness or an objective sense of restriction is noted in the area examined, this can be a clue to visceral dysfunction in organs related to that ganglion (8).

As time allows, a focused assessment of the patient for further signs of viscerosomatic reflex activity can be quickly performed. Appropriate segmental levels and the presence of Chapman reflex points can be helpful in confirming the presence of visceral disease (13).

Last, a focused assessment of spinal segments in dysfunction is completed while looking for tenderness, asymmetry, range of motion differences, and tissue texture changes (the TART criteria for somatic dysfunction).

A good osteopathic structural examination should be a part of every patient visit to the ED, especially as part of the secondary survey for those with musculoskeletal complaints. That is, following the primary assessment survey with any necessary initial stabilization and completion of any more urgent priorities.

A case example helps to show the application of the above principles.

A 34-year-old female presents to the ED with sudden onset, excruciating, right low back, flank, and groin pain, as well as left buttock pain, for the last 2 hours accompanied by nausea and vomiting. Her pulse is 110 beats/min and her respirations are 14 per min. Her vital signs are otherwise normal. She is unable to walk back to the examination area (no observation possible) and is unable to find a comfortable position in which to lie (typical situation for a kidney stone or gallstone). She continues to vomit in the ED and is screaming in pain. She is pale, sweaty and begins feeling faint. She receives an i.v. with normal saline and oxygen at 100%. The cardiac monitor shows sinus tachycardia. Blood is drawn and sent to the laboratory along with a urine sample (screened for stones) for a urinalysis. She is given an analgesic and an antiemetic by vein and becomes quieter. Her personal and family medical/surgical history is negative. Her blood work is all within normal limits. Urine shows gross blood and no signs of infection. She is feeling much better after the medication, which allows a screening structural examination.

1. The nature of her pain and presentation is classic for kidney stone. Low back pain and groin pain can also indicate psoas dysfunction, a common complication of a passing kidney stone (the ureter passes directly over the psoas muscle).

2. Static and motion tests reveal only a sidebending and rotation to the right in the lumbar area.

3. Examination of the skin reveals only diffuse cool, sweaty changes consistent with her hypersympathetic state (secondary to pain) on presentation.

4. Fascial preference examination reveals an decompensated L,R,R,R pattern (there could be a problem in the thoracolumbar region).

5. Evaluation of her trigger points shows positive findings in the upper lumber paraspinal musculature on the right.

6. Evaluation of the counterstrain tender point shows dysfunction of the right psoas and iliacus muscles, as well as the left piriformis muscle (psoas syndrome).

7. Evaluation of her lymphatic system shows no abnormalities.

8. Craniosacral evaluation shows only slightly increased rate, normal vitality, and normal cranial bone motion.

9. Examination of her superior mesenteric ganglion is painful and shows significant restriction (the kidney is supplied by this ganglion).

10. She has painful Chapman reflex points for the right kidney (anterior: 2 cm cephalad and 2 cm lateral-right of the umbilicus; posterior: between the right transverse processes of L1 and L2), as well as boggy, cool, mildly swollen tissue in the T12-L3 area.

11. We find the TART criteria for L1-2 FR_R S_R segmental somatic dysfunction.

The diagnosis is nephrolithiasis with secondary psoas and piriformis muscle somatic dysfunction and viscerosomatic lumbar spine somatic dysfunction.

The patient receives additional, small doses of the narcotic analgesic and stabilizes well. As the ED is relatively quiet, she receives OMM for her psoas, piriformis, and lumbar spine dysfunction, as well as fascial release for her superior mesenteric ganglion, and Chapman reflex point treatment for the kidney. She feels better and prefers to not wait the 2 hours for the intravenous pyelogram (IVP) to be done (the radiology technician is busy with other emergencies), but rather to go home with medications and instructions to screen her urine, get the IVP in the morning (scheduled), and to see her family practitioner (an osteopathic physician) the next day. The next day she does not present for the IVP but delivers the stone to her family practitioner, who continues the OMM for the remaining somatic dysfunctions. She is seen 4 days later and again 8 days later, at which time she is pain free.

This case shows the use of the osteopathic screening examination leading to an integrated osteopathic management approach to the patient. As mentioned above, not all steps must be completed in each patient. There are certainly cases where not all

steps will provide additional or even consistent information. With enough pieces of the puzzle in place, however, we will be able to see the picture clearly!

As in all areas of medicine, one has to be cognizant of the situations in which OMM is relatively or absolutely contraindicated. A patient with extremely low vitality will often not tolerate OMM. A patient who refuses to allow you to touch them (i.e., a case of rape or molestation, or post traumatic stress syndrome) will be difficult to treat with OMM. As it is impossible to know which patient is immunocompromised or contagious at any one time, it is important to always take precautionary measures when handling body tissues, fluids, and contacting patients in the ED setting. In acute trauma cases, the use of gentle, indirect OMM treatment techniques is indicated. In the osteoporosis patient, avoid high-velocity, low amplitude (HVLA) techniques.

PATIENT-ORIENTED CLINICAL SCENARIOS

The goal in this section is to present the distinct aspects of the application of osteopathic principles and practices regarding diagnosis and treatment that apply to given body regions or presenting complaints. A more detailed discussion of the underlying specific pathology or description of the application of specific osteopathic manipulative medicine (OMM) techniques is referred to in the various sections and can be found in other areas of this text.

The Osteopathic Approach to the Patient with Complaints in the Head and Neck Regions

The emergency physician encounters a variety of pathophysiologic processes in the head and neck region. Up to 50% of the injuries to the body occur in the head, and this is the leading cause of death in persons younger than 45 years of age (10).

Symptoms, Pathophysiology, and Epidemiology

Cephalgia
Cephalgia is a very common chief complaint encountered in emergency medicine, and it carries great potential for serious, adverse effects (17). Studies have shown that 69% of patients with subarachnoid hemorrhage reported headache on presentation to the ED (18). Evaluation of the severe headache can be difficult. Many patients that look generally ill do not frequently have life-threatening illness (18).

Eye Pain
Three percent of patients presenting to the ED have an eye-related chief complaint, and most of these patients can be treated by the emergency physician without consulting an ophthalmologist (19). Otitis media is the most common diagnosis made in this country for children younger than 15 years of age (19). This is caused, in large part, by developmental factors of the eustachian tube. In adult patients, tinnitus and vertigo are frequently seen in the ED, as is ear trauma (20). Inflammatory processes, infection, foreign bodies, and ototoxic drugs contribute significantly to a list of common etiologic factors leading to ear complaints in the ED. Cranial somatic dysfunction can play a role in the etiology

of secondary vertigo and tinnitus (20). Direct ear trauma can be caused by a number of mechanisms, such as blast injury, chemical or thermal exposure, acoustic trauma, and blunt trauma (20).

Nosebleeds/Upper Respiratory Infection
Epistaxis is seen in 15 out of every 10,000 patient visits requiring medical care, and more than 10% of these require hospital admission (19). Upper respiratory infection (URI) and sinusitis are, by far, the most common processes in this part of the body that are seen in the ED. Sinusitis has been reported to affect 14% of the general population (10).

Neck Pain
Neck pain is a symptom arising from a large number of etiologic factors, including trauma (watch out for abuse situations), degenerative disorders, infection, neoplasm, inflammatory processes, as well as musculoskeletal injury (10). Acute trauma to the cervical spine commonly follows automobile and motorcycle accidents, and falls of all kinds, as well as abuse situations (19). Pharyngitis and URI frequently cause neck pain as part of their symptomatology (through viscerosomatic activity). Peritonsillar and retropharyngeal abscesses are infectious processes presenting with neck pain that can quickly lead to airway compromise and death. Infections, such as meningitis, frequently present with neck pain and stiffness due to meningeal irritation. The knowledgeable physician will recognize that muscles will often be hypotonic immediately after trauma, only to become significantly hypertonic several hours later. Furthermore, trauma that is severe enough to tear muscle or ligament tissue or to break bone will certainly be significant enough to cause concomitant somatic dysfunction locally, as well as elsewhere in the body. In cases of trauma, rarely are chief complaints focusing on the neck isolated. The so-called "whiplash of the neck" involves inertial forces that affect the entire body, particularly the cervical region but also having key sites in the sternum and pelvis. Long-term cervical problems typically will be associated with compensatory somatic dysfunction in these areas, as well as elsewhere in the body.

Diagnosis

Cephalgia
Cephalgia may occur as a result of many disease processes that fall under the categories discussed above. Three major groups of pathologic conditions affect the pain-sensitive structures of the head and neck (19). They emanate from a vascular, tension, or inflammatory process. Tension leads the list of etiologic factors for headaches, followed by vascular origin and inflammatory processes (19). The osteopathic physician must be astute and recognize that the cephalgia may be referred from other structures in the head (eyes; ears; nose; intracranial, subarachnoid, subdural, epidural bleeds; mass lesions; hypertensive emergency; meningitis; toxic exposure). A careful neurologic emphasis in the clinical evaluation is critical in the diagnosis process (18). A neurologic deficit can warn the physician of a fast, potentially lethal process that must be reversed in order to bring that patient's body toward its homeostatic state. The osteopathic clinical evaluation may also include assessment of the articular mobility of the cranial bones. The primary respiratory mechanism can be assessed to help find

the root of the pathologic process. The physician should evaluate the eyes, nose, ears, and throat, as well as the muscles within the face and neck area.

Eye
Trauma, foreign bodies, infections, inflammatory processes, and sequestration of fluids in the eyes are commonly seen. Osteopathic physicians must first rule out worse possible disease process (e.g., acute angle glaucoma, acoustic exposure, central artery occlusion, retinal detachment, ruptured globe). Osteopathic palpatory skills will assist in the diagnosis of processes like an increase in intraocular pressure. With the exception of a splash injury that needs immediate copious irrigation, the initial step in all eye evaluations is the assessment of visual acuity (21). Every emergency physician should be familiar with diagnostic instruments, such as the slit lamp, tonometer, and ophthalmoscope (10). The evaluation of cranial bone movement and tissue texture changes in the orbits, maxillae, and vomer is also important in ophthalmologic presentations. Secondary causes of eye disease process like URI/sinusitis must be entertained. Sinusitis is the most common cause of orbital cellulitis (22).

Ear Pain
A foreign body must always be considered in children presenting with ear complaints (23). Foreign bodies in adults usually present immediately after the entry of the foreign body as opposed to children (where the foreign body may have been self-inserted), and the time to presentation can be prolonged (23). The assessment of cranial somatic dysfunction can assist the osteopathic emergency physician in the complete assessment of the patient presenting with an ear complaint. The temporal bone plays a vital role in ear problems, especially in children. The distal part of the eustachian tube lies on the temporal bone, and tissue texture changes or abnormal movement of the temporal bones can lead to eustachian tube problems. Temporal bone dysfunction, occipitomastoid suture dysfunction, medial pterygoid muscle spasm, and cranial torsions have also been implicated to cause ear symptoms (8,11). Additionally, otalgia may be referred from other structures, such as teeth, tongue, tonsils, the esophageal area, and the temporomandibular joint (24).

Nosebleeds/Upper Respiratory Infection
Blunt trauma to the nose frequently produces nasal fractures and epistaxis. Epistaxis can be separated into anterior and posterior varieties, based on the location of the bleed. There is a long list of causes of epistaxis. Infection, foreign bodies, trauma, allergic rhinitis, hypertension, tumors, and hereditary coagulopathies are several common etiologies (10). Sinus mucosal obstruction is the most common cause of sinusitis. Cranial somatic dysfunction can also play a large role in the etiology of sinusitis. Frontal and maxillary bone fixations are believed to impair drainage from the sinuses by obstructing blood circulation, as well as maxillary sinus drainage pathways (24). Physicians must be quick to recognize emergent processes, such as nasal trauma, epistaxis, and cerebrospinal fluid (CSF) rhinorrhea, that may warrant immediate ear, nose, and throat (ENT) and neurosurgery consults. Children frequently insert foreign bodies in the nasal cavity (10). Patient assessment is augmented by the use of osteopathic palpatory skills

to examine for an increase in pain or tension over specific sinuses or over the exit sites of the supraorbital and infraorbital branches of the trigeminal nerves, and for cranial bone restrictions. Correcting secondary causes of the nasal disease process, such as otitis media, should also be considered.

Neck Pain

Emergent problems, such as airway compromise and acute neck injury secondary to trauma, must be considered. Musculoskeletal hyperactivity from torticollis, "whiplash," somatic dysfunction, or other cervical strains and sprains are common problems that the osteopathic emergency physician can diagnose and treat. A strain or sprain diagnosis should not be made before obtaining a good history and physical examination that includes an osteopathic structural examination and necessary radiographic studies to rule out more serious processes. Myofascial trigger points are frequently the result of overuse or trauma, and their evaluation can assist the ED physician in diagnosis.

Integrated Osteopathic Treatment

Cephalgia

The American College of Emergency Physicians' clinical policies for adolescents and adults presenting with headaches serve as a guide to objectives of treatment (17). The four goals are:

1. To provide effective treatment for primary headache syndromes.
2. To diagnose and effectively treat patients with generally benign and reversible secondary headache causes.
3. To appropriately select patients for emergency investigation and treatment of suspected critical secondary headache causes.
4. To provide appropriate disposition and follow-up for all discharged patients.

With the suspicion of vascular headaches, the occipitomastoid release, which is considered to be a jugular venous congestion release technique, will be very helpful. The jugular veins and vagus nerves pass through the jugular foramen that is located between the occipital bone and the petrous portion of the temporal bones (26). Eighty-five percent of the venous drainage in the head passes through the jugular foramen (8). Occipitoatlantal decompression is also thought to enhance the parasympathetic nervous system by normalizing vagus nerve function (8). Compression of the fourth ventricle (CV4) technique, used to dissipate cerebral spinal fluid and normalize the vagus nerve function, is another craniosacral technique useful in this setting (24). As most of these patients will have a hypersympathetic tone, normalization of the segments T1-4 will help to balance the sympathetic supply to the head and neck area. Once sympathetic and parasympathetic systems are normalized, thoracic inlets can be released, and venous return from the head can be further enhanced. Thoracic lymphatic pump techniques may then be used to further the elimination of metabolic waste products and other by-products of the underlying pathophysiology through the thoracic duct. Chapman reflex points can be used as a further adjunct in the therapy of cephalgia. These and other reflex points can also be shown and taught to the patient for self-treatment.

Medications are often used in conjunction with other treatment modalities to enhance rapid recovery. The use of appropriate analgesics to shorten the time to pain resolution and muscle relaxants to enhance the patient's recovery from muscular spasms may be warranted. However, the need for medication is often decreased with the application of OMM. Improvement of sleeping pattern and nutrition, correction of postural imbalance, relaxation and relief of stress, control of caffeine, alcohol, or other drug intake, and home stretching exercises could enhance recovery. Timely educational reinforcement by the emergency physician of the importance of ongoing care by their primary care physician enhances future patient compliance in these often simple, yet important, adjunctive measures.

Eye Pain

Acoustic exposure, splash injury, and central arterial occlusion warrant immediate treatment prior to complete clinical evaluation (19). The physician must first rapidly take charge of and control any emergency, order necessary therapies and medications, and/or secure an ophthalmology consult as required. Primary or adjunctive use of OMM is again directed toward enhancing the patient's ability to self-heal. Healing from processes of infectious or inflammatory etiologies require optimal ANS, lymphatic, structural, and immune system function. Improving venous and lymphatic drainage with familiar techniques (see above) will help to accomplish this. Normalization of the sympathetic and parasympathetic nervous system function will also assist the patient. Ophthalmologic lymphatic pump consists of light percussion over the affected eye's closed eyelid. This has been shown to be beneficial in decreasing intraocular pressure in patients with chronic open-angle glaucoma (8). This is not recommended for patients with acute closed-angle glaucoma who need medicinal treatment within 3 to 5 days to prevent blindness (8). Muscle energy of extra ocular muscles can be used to balance the myofascial tensions in this region (8). Avoidance of a cigarette smoke environment that will irritate the eyes is warranted. Glaucoma patients should avoid sudden changes between dark and bright environments.

Ear Pain

With regard to ear pain, the treatment priorities in the ED are immediate reversal of any life-threatening pathologic process, repair of trauma, immediate removal of foreign bodies, and addressing the etiology of a sudden hearing loss. A foreign body that is irremovable in the ED should prompt an ENT referral. It is unclear whether pharmacologic treatment of otitis media is warranted because evidence-based documentation shows that over 80% of the cases resolve spontaneously (27). However, the use of antibiotics has greatly reduced the risk of complications from bacterial infection processes (27). Inflammatory processes may be treated with an appropriate antiinflammatory agent. Correcting cranial somatic dysfunction greatly benefits recovery by increasing circulation to the area and normalizing structure of nerves and venous/lymphatic return (24). Inhibition or intermittent traction to the medial pterygoid muscle, ear lobe traction, or hyoid bone release may be employed to enhance eustachian tube drainage (8,11,28). The "Muncie technique," referring to Curtis H. Muncie, who originally described the procedure in the

1920s, can also be used. The technique requires the physician to intraorally place a finger posteroinferior to the tonsillar pillar, and to gently pump in the Rosenmuller fossa in a cephalad direction to release the obstructed eustachian tube (29). Lifestyle changes can also enhance recovery from ear problems. Avoiding cigarette smoke environments that may increase frequency of disease processes like otitis media is indicated (8). Be alert for disease process breakouts in school or day-care.

Nosebleeds/Upper Respiratory Infection

Racemic epinephrine can be used to decongest the nasal mucosa and loosen a stuck foreign body (10). Inability to remove foreign objects in the ED should prompt ENT referral. Displaced nasal fractures warrant plastic surgery referral (10). Epistaxis should be tamponaded with anterior and posterior packing. Antibiotics, antihistamines, and topical steroids are the mainstream therapy for sinusitis. Modifying autonomic balance (parasympathetic stimulation causes a thin mucus to be produced and sympathetic stimulation a thick mucus) to affected tissues can improve important self-regulatory mechanisms in the patient. Another goal of OMM is to assist in reducing pain symptomatology resulting from the disease process. This can be accomplished by normalizing the ANS (hypersympathetic tone is usually present), improving lymphatic drainage (reducing local congestion contributing to pain), and balancing the musculoskeletal structures involved in the pathology. The release of the upper cervical somatic dysfunction and the cervicothoracic junction has been empirically shown to create better circulation and improved venous/lymphatic drainage (30). Other manipulative treatments can be implemented to directly reduce tissue edema and facilitate sinus drainage, as well as to decrease mucus viscosity (31). Intraoral stimulation of the sphenopalatine ganglia, inhibition of lateral pterygoid muscle trigger points, and CV4 and trigeminal nerve stimulation techniques will produce parasympathetic stimulation and production of thin nasal secretions (8,11). Frontal, maxillary, and nasal bone restrictions should be released for significant improvement of sinus drainage (24). The most direct drainage enhancement is achieved through sinus drainage techniques that create gentle intermittent pressure over the sinuses (32). Lifestyle changes may lead to faster recovery. Avoidance of allergens is beneficial. Discussion of controlling alcohol consumption and other drug use that may decrease immune system response is warranted in the ED to reinforce the importance of patient involvement and compliance.

Neck Pain

Any signs of airway compromise should be promptly treated with early airway management and anesthesia consultation. Neurosurgery consultation should be obtained if unstable cervical spine injury is suspected. Infectious processes may be treated with incision and drainage, antibiotics, or both. Systemic steroids can be used to decrease inflammation. Secondary causes of pharyngeal disease, such as otitis media and sinusitis, must be considered, assessed, and treated as appropriate. After assessment, treatment of any painful myofascial trigger points with a variety of manual or medical means (pressure, spray, injection) can play a significant role in improving the subjective pain of the patient. Musculoskeletal neck pain, even in an acutely painful

presentation, can often be effectively treated with counterstrain using cervical tender points (16), indirect myofascial release to muscles and fascia of the neck and anterior cervical region, facilitated positional release (FPR), or even gentle muscle energy techniques (30). Acute torticollis is often responsive to a rhythmic muscle energy protocol first described by Ruddy (33) and designed to decongest the swelling in the involved cervical muscle bellies.

The Osteopathic Approach to the Patient with Chest Pain

Any physician who has treated a patient presenting with chest pain knows that the large component of fear and anxiety from the patient regarding their symptoms can significantly compound the problem. Nearly everyone in our society has either known someone or heard a story about someone who had a heart attack and died or was seriously debilitated as a result. The patient often presents with tachypnea, tachycardia, mydriasis, and a cold sweat—all clear signs of a hypersympathetic state that, in most patients, will negatively impact the delicate supply and demand of perfusion balance to the myocardium.

The first priorities in the evaluation and treatment of the chest pain patient are the potentially life-threatening conditions: e.g., unstable angina, acute myocardial infarction (AMI), aortic dissection, pulmonary embolism, spontaneous pneumothorax, and esophageal rupture (Boerhaave syndrome) (10).

An unstable patient must first be stabilized by the best methods available at the time. This usually means administering oxygen, starting an intravenous (IV) line and giving appropriate fluids, monitoring the patient for heart rhythm disturbances, and giving appropriate additional medications to treat his/her pain, anxiety, dysrhythmia, and any hemodynamic instability. A primary survey is then completed where any life-threatening problems are identified and treated. After this, a secondary survey is performed with a head-to-toe examination and fingers or tubes in every orifice as appropriate. A structural examination is completed during this secondary survey. When this is completed, definitive care is then planned for the patient and undertaken. Please refer to an emergency medicine textbook for more detailed information on these interventions (*ACLS Textbook*, *ATLS Textbook*, refs. 10 and 19).

Diagnosis

When the patient is stable, the osteopathic approach to the chest pain patient should include such issues as detailed family and social history, identification of risk factors for coronary artery disease (CAD), strategies for reduction of alterable risk factors (table showing risk factors) (34; see also Chapter 13), medications presently being taken (or not taken), nutrition, exercise patterns (or lack thereof), and OMM considerations.

There are many common musculoskeletal conditions, such as scoliosis, increased or decreased kyphosis, and so on, that can have a negative impact on the function of the cardiovascular system—either as a primary problem or as a compensatory mechanism for other ailments. There are a number of congenital conditions, for example Marfan syndrome, with obvious musculoskeletal findings that are known to also have congenital cardiac anomalies present.

An inspection of the patient to determine if any of these conditions are present is an important first step. A leg length discrepancy, for example, that leads to compensatory postural changes and facilitation of the upper thoracic segments can lead to compromise of cardiovascular function.

Regional range of motion abnormalities and uncompensated fascial patterns (15) in the cervicothoracic area can be a further sign of a compromised homeostatic mechanism, and might be creating somato-visceral reflex activity that potentially weakens the cardiovascular system. In the case of the cardiovascular system, the T1-6 area is often facilitated.

An additional example of a somato-visceral connection is the right pectoralis major trigger point that Travell (11) describes as causing or contributing to supraventricular dysrhythmias. (An arrhythmia is the absence of a rhythm, whereas a dysrhythmia is an abnormal rhythm.) This point overlies the right fifth intercostal space one-half the distance from the sternum to the nipple. If this point is active and apparently playing a role in the generation or maintenance of the dysrhythmia, then treating this point (pressure, spray, injection, etc.) can help eliminate the problem.

As mentioned above and shown by Schwarz and Stone (35), there is usually a hypersympathetic tone present in chest pain patients. Rosero (36) has shown, however, that there are situations where hyperparasympathetic tone is found, especially with inferior wall ischemia and infarction with hypotension and/or bradycardia. Both situations of abnormal ANS function are inappropriate responses and need to be addressed.

Assessment of the lymphatic system is also important. This is accomplished by first assessing the key areas of the body (e.g., supraclavicular space, posterior axillary folds, midepigastrium) for signs of fluid congestion, and then appropriately treating any somatic dysfunction in the following areas, for the given reasons:

1. The T1-2 spinal area and the ribs 1-2 left and right (these are important for the proper function of the thoracic inlet and the entire lymphatic system);
2. The thoracic inlet (the first very important central lymphatic diaphragm);
3. The iliopsoas muscle group, the thoracolumbar spinal area, the quadratus lumborum muscle, as well as the lower ribs (all important for the proper function of the respiratory diaphragm);
4. The respiratory diaphragm (the second very important central lymphatic diaphragm);
5. The piriformis muscle, innominate, and sacral areas (all important for the proper function of the pelvic diaphragm);
6. The pelvic diaphragm (the third very important central lymphatic diaphragm).

If you are treating a patient that displays recurring somatic dysfunction in the upper thoracic area despite appropriate OMM, you should consider the possibility of cardiovascular pathology (or pathology in other viscera that facilitates to these segments). In addition, the Chapman reflex points can be helpful in clarifying whether there is viscerosomatic reflex activity. The anterior

Chapman reflex points for the heart overlie the second intercostal space bilaterally near the sternum, and the posterior points are between the second and third thoracic vertebrae bilaterally just lateral to the spinous processes.

In the patient with chest pain, we must be aware of the fact that the pain may be of musculoskeletal origin, of cardiovascular origin, or both. We must realize that the presence of apparent chest wall syndrome based on appropriate history, physical (including structural examination), and negative laboratory/x-ray/EKG findings, even with significant improvement after an OMM treatment, does not rule out cardiovascular disease nor the need for further cardiovascular workup. Costosternal syndrome, thoracic outlet syndrome, costochondritis, and intercostal neuritis are common presentations that can mimic chest pain of cardiac origin (10).

Integrated Osteopathic Treatment

Rogers and Rogers (37) showed significant improvement in symptoms in patients with coronary insufficiency after the application of OMM. The goals of the application of OMM for the chest pain patient are to maximally support the body's own self-regulatory, self-healing mechanisms through improving the perfusion of oxygenated blood to the tissues at risk and improving venous and lymphatic return from these tissues. When both structural and functional elements related to the cardiovascular system are normalized, the body will be in a position to find its own best level of homeostasis.

The form, timing, and manner of application of OMM will depend on the history, present status of the patient, and the diagnostic and therapeutic plan for the patient.

The key concepts in achieving these goals are addressing any somatic structural abnormalities with facilitation of spinal segments, normalizing the autonomic nervous system function as much as possible, improving the lymphatic system function, and addressing the issues of viscerosomatic reflexes with facilitation of spinal segments.

The most appropriate concept for the treatment of the ANS in the chest pain patient is that of normalizing the two components, the sympathetic and parasympathetic nervous systems. See Chapter 6 for the common ANS effects on the various organ systems.

This is accomplished by examining and appropriately treating any somatic dysfunction in the following areas, for the given reasons:

■ The T1-6 region: normalizing sympathetic distribution to the heart (38).
■ The ribs in this same region: "rib raising" technique to inhibit the dorsal chain ganglia and reduce hypersympathetic tone; the T10-11 segments: sympathetic distribution to the kidneys and adrenals; the craniosacral, C0-2 region: normalizing parasympathetic distribution to the heart.
■ The C3-5 region: diaphragmatic irritation due to inferior wall pathology, by way of the phrenic nerve, can facilitate to these segments.

The most appropriate concept for the treatment of the lymphatic system in the chest pain patient is that of first removing any blockages to the appropriate flow of lymphatic fluid, and then to specifically increase this flow as the patient is able to tolerate it. In this way, we can best support the patient in homeostatic self-regulation. See Chapter 68 for more detail regarding lymphatic function.

After the release of any somatic dysfunction and normalization of the functions of the above structures, any number of the following techniques can be applied in order to improve the general flow of lymphatic fluid in the body:

- Miller thoracic pump
- Other thoracic pump variations
- Pectoral traction technique
- Abdominal pump techniques and variations
- Splenic and liver pump techniques
- Specific extremity techniques
- Pedal pump technique and variations

Treating these points with either light vibratory pressure or firm massaging pressure until the tissue softens will assist the body in healing.

An example from my (Adler-Michaelson) ED practice may further encourage the reader to maintain an open mind regarding an integrated treatment approach.

A 50-year-old male was brought into the ER after driving into a tree at about 45 mph. His vital signs were unstable, he was moaning in pain, and he showed apparent supraventricular cardiac dysrhythmias on the EKG monitor. He had a bleeding facial laceration and a significant thoracic contusion with ecchymoses; active bleeding had been controlled by the paramedics. With oxygen delivery, fluid resuscitation, bleeding control, and moderate pain control, the patient stabilized. The laboratory results came back showing elevated muscle enzyme levels. X-rays were negative, and the cardiac dysrhythmias remained nonlethal, requiring no further specific treatment. The patient was admitted for monitoring with the diagnosis of thoracic/cardiac contusion, and facial contusion and laceration secondary to the motor vehicle accident (MVA). The next day, the patient was able to add the very important history that he had excruciating chest pain while driving and felt faint before waking up in the ambulance on the way into the hospital. His enzyme levels stayed elevated and followed the typical pattern for an AMI. He continued to do well and was discharged to cardiac rehabilitation. In all probability, his MVA was a direct result of his cardiac chest pain and AMI. In medicine we have to always be able to think beyond the obvious!

By addressing, evaluating, and treating to normalize the somatic structural aspects, autonomic nervous system aspects, lymphatic system aspects, and viscerosomatic aspects of the patient, we can best assist the patient in reestablishing his or her best possible level of homeostasis. In this way, we are truly putting into practice the best of our osteopathic knowledge and wisdom.

The Osteopathic Approach to Disorders of the Cardiopulmonary System

The emergency physician is called on everyday to examine, diagnose, and treat patients who complain of difficulty breathing. The trained emergency physician is well prepared to determine the etiology of dyspnea and provide timely and appropriate treatment.

For the most critical patients, the emergency physician must always be ready to intervene and take control of ventilation and respiration through the use of artificial means.

Community-acquired pneumonia accounts for several million visits to physicians and hundreds of thousands of hospitalizations each year. It is the sixth leading cause of death, and it is often more severe in those patients at the extremes of age.

There are numerous reports detailing the success of osteopathic treatment of pneumonia in the pre-antibiotic era, with the most famous being the great difference in morbidity and mortality between those patients treated with OMM versus those treated medically in the influenza pandemic of 1918 (39). More recently, a clinical trial showed that older adults with pneumonia who were treated with OMM had a significantly shorter duration of intravenous antibiotic treatment and a shorter hospital stay when compared with patients who did not receive manipulation (40).

Congestive heart failure (CHF) is a syndrome of abnormal fluid retention secondary to the loss of the normal contractile strength of the myocardium and manifested primarily by shortness of breath (10). The osteopathic emergency physician must be familiar with the multiple etiologies of heart failure and be prepared to begin standard medical treatment with oxygen, diuretics, nitrates, and other therapies, as indicated by the underlying cause. Aggressive airway management should be anticipated and performed if necessary.

In CHF, the lymphatic load is increased. If the thoracic inlet is restricted or if there is somatic dysfunction of the thoracic cage or the respiratory diaphragm with a reduction of the usual pressure gradient between the intrathoracic and intraabdominal cavities, lymphatic pumping will be reduced and flow will be impeded. OMM to these structures and lymphatic pump techniques will improve lymphatic fluid mobilization and assist in the clinical improvement of the patient (8). The astute physician must realize, however, that the ability of the CHF patient to deal with this extra fluid load (mobilized lymphatic fluid) is limited. It is detrimental to further overload the already overloaded heart, and so how much lymphatic fluid the patient can handle must be carefully considered.

Diagnosis

The ANS innervation to the lungs comes from the vagus nerves—cranium, C0-2 levels (parasympathetic), and the T1-6 thoracic trunks (sympathetic). The right and left vagus nerves descend and pass through the thoracic inlet on their respective sides, and each divides and branches to form part of the right or left pulmonary plexus. The thoracic sympathetic trunks are contributed from the posterior mediastinum and complete each pulmonary plexus. The fibers then form on the root of each lung and spread out along bronchial subdivisions (41).

Pulmonary dysfunction and mucosal irritation result in increased visceral afferent impulses to the spinal cord, primarily in the T1-6 levels. The painful Chapman reflex points for the lungs can be palpated in the third or fourth intercostal spaces anteriorly and at the T3-4 vertebrae posteriorly (8).

Patients presenting with an acute exacerbation of asthma typically demonstrate one or more of a triad of symptoms, including coughing, wheezing, or dyspnea (42). The diagnosis of a reactive airway state is usually obvious with the history and physical examination of the patient, but the osteopathic emergency physician must exclude other causes of dyspnea that present with cough and/or wheezing. The mobility of the thoracic cage must also be addressed. Viscerosomatic reflexes can lead to thoracic vertebral somatic dysfunction, and vigorous coughing can produce multiple areas of exhalation rib somatic dysfunction, especially at the third or fourth rib (8). Assessment of thoracic inlet and respiratory diaphragm functions are critical in the context of pulmonary disease processes. Prior to releasing the thoracic inlet itself, the upper thoracic segments, upper ribs bilaterally, and the sternum are important structures to assess and treat if in dysfunction. Before releasing the respiratory diaphragm, the thoracolumbar junction is equally important to assess and treat if in dysfunction. If the C3-5 region is in dysfunction, it should be assessed and treated to optimize the phrenic nerve function in support of the respiratory diaphragm function.

Clinically, pneumonia may present with obvious features, such as tachypnea, chest pain, rigors, inspiratory rales, bronchial breath sounds, rhonchi, and/or wheezing. Atypical pneumonia may present with any or none of the above symptoms, or with a variety of extra-pulmonary signs and symptoms. Some older patients may present with only a change in mental status (without respiratory complaints) (10). A recent, as yet unpublished study by T. Crow, et al. showed a good correlation between Chapman reflex points in the 3rd and 4th intercostal space anteriorly and on T3-4 posteriorly and the diagnosis of pneumonia. This knowledge can assist the osteopathic physician in both making the diagnosis of pneumonia and in beginning a helpful therapy.

Integrated Osteopathic Treatment

The osteopathic treatment plan for the acutely ill patient does not need to be elaborate or extensive. In fact, some believe that too much manipulation early in a patient's course of illness would be detrimental (8). The osteopathic emergency physician should begin standard medical treatment for asthma with oxygen, beta agonists, and steroids as indicated. With the medical management begun, the osteopathic emergency physician can address the ANS, lymphatic, viscerosomatic, and structural components of the disease process. Initially, the thoracic sympathetics in the area of the first six thoracic vertebrae may be stimulated for a bronchodilator response. The vagus nerve function can be normalized at the occipitoatlantal junction, the cervical spine, and the thoracic inlet. However, the osteopathic emergency physician must remember that these segments are probably already facilitated and care should be given not to over treat them. It might be preferable to treat the parasympathetic innervation to normalize the vagus nerve function. Consequently, rib raising and general lymphatic techniques can then be applied to improve rib motion, pulmonary function, and lymphatic function.

It is important to remember that many of these structural lesions are viscerosomatic in origin and probably do not respond well to high-velocity, low-amplitude techniques, so more gentle techniques, perhaps with activating forces, are likely to be more efficacious (8).

Treatment of asthma, pneumonia, or CHF can include, for example, the ANS, lymphatic, immune, viscerosomatic, and

structural musculoskeletal systems in order to reduce congestion, reduce sympathetic hyperactivity, and mobilize the thoracic cage (8). OMM to the thoracic spine, rib cage, and diaphragm will improve the actual mechanics of breathing. Lymphatic flow can then be improved by applying myofascial techniques to the thoracic inlets and then by using a pectoral lift or lymphatic pump technique to mobilize the lymph fluid. As mentioned above, treatment of the C3-5 region in advance of normalizing the respiratory diaphragm function will also greatly assist the patient.

Osteopathic Considerations in Patients with Abdominal/Pelvic Pain

Abdominal pain is a common presenting complaint among ED patients (43). Potentially life-threatening events, such as ruptured abdominal aortic aneurysm or ischemic bowel, do often present with abdominal pain, so a high level of suspicion must be maintained. More commonly, the patients presenting to the ED have a benign cause for their abdominal pain, but often an extensive workup occurs before that determination can be made (44). Approximately 20% of patients presenting to the ED with abdominal pain may require admission for observation or further workup.

Diagnosis

There are some historic clues that can help the osteopathic emergency physician determine the etiology of pain. Pain in the right upper quadrant may originate from hepatitis or cholecystitis. Pain in the epigastrium is typical for gastric irritation from gastritis or peptic ulcer disease, but may also be seen with intrathoracic pathology, such as a lower lobe pneumonia or cardiac ischemia. Pancreatitis may also present with epigastric or left upper quadrant pain. Pain in the left lower quadrant may indicate colitis, diverticulitis, or in a female, problems with the fallopian tube or ovaries. Right lower quadrant pain suggests appendicitis, Meckel diverticulitis, or, again, fallopian tube or ovarian disease. Pain described as coming from the back or the side and radiating into the groin is typical of nephrolithiasis, but when abdominal aortic aneurysms are misdiagnosed, it is commonly as a kidney stone (45). Psoas spasm/dysfunction also frequently presents as pain in the flank or midabdomen radiating into the lower quadrants or groin area. Dysfunction in the lower extremities, especially the hip, may also present as abdominal pain. This is particularly true in children. Males with testicular pathology may present with lower abdominal pain as well.

The quality and onset of the pain can also give some clues to the diagnosis. Appendicitis typically develops over 1 to 2 days. The pain is described as dull, achy, beginning in the periumbilical region, and slowly moving to the right lower quadrant. The viscera of the abdomen respond to distension by producing discomfort in the associated soma; so inflammation and distension of the appendix produces pain in the tenth thoracic nerve distribution—the periumbilical region. As the inflammation increases, the peritoneum also becomes irritated. The peritoneum does have pain fibers, so at that time, the patient senses pain at the region of irritation—the right lower quadrant. Pain originating from other hollow viscous presents similarly; a patient with small bowel obstruction or diverticulitis may initially complain of an achy midline pain. Only as direct peritoneal inflammation develops will they localize to the area of real pathology. These patients may also complain of waves of pain, often referred to as "colic," which are produced by the normal peristalsis against a fixed obstruction, such as a stone. Pain described as burning is typically associated with peptic ulcer disease.

Abdominal pain in a female patient includes several other diagnostic possibilities, including ectopic pregnancy, salpingitis, mittelschmerz, ovarian torsion, or cyst. Any female of childbearing age who presents with abdominal pain must have a pregnancy test. Although a negative pregnancy test does not completely rule out ectopic pregnancy, in the absence of other compelling symptoms it effectively does. If the patient with abdominal pain is pregnant, physical examination alone is not an adequate determinant of whether the pregnancy is in the uterus. An ultrasound and a serum quantitative β HCG should also be performed.

Certain conditions are more likely to occur at different ages. In a young, otherwise healthy individual, aortic abdominal aneurysm or ischemic bowel is unlikely, but these must certainly be entertained in the older population. In young children with abdominal pain, intussusception should be considered if the clinical picture of intermittent severe pain, progression to depressed mental status, and the late finding of "currant jelly" stool are present. Other conditions are more common in certain age groups, but certainly can occur any time in life. These include peptic ulcer disease (perhaps with perforation), volvulus, intestinal obstruction, or appendicitis. Ectopic pregnancy is more often a disease of young women, but can occur in any woman of childbearing age.

Assessment of the abdominal collateral ganglia and the celiac, superior, and inferior mesenteric ganglia can assist the osteopathic physician in arriving at a diagnosis. The celiac ganglion innervates the stomach, duodenum, liver, gallbladder, pancreas, and spleen. The superior mesenteric ganglion innervates the jejunum, ileum, proximal half of the colon, kidneys, adrenals, and gonads. The inferior mesenteric ganglion innervates the distal half of the colon and the pelvic organs (except the gonads). If a subjective report of tenderness, or an objective sense of restriction is noted in the area examined, this can be a clue to visceral dysfunction in organs related to that ganglion (8).

The assessment of the fascial envelopes of the organs in the abdominal area can assist the osteopathic emergency physician in making a diagnosis. Restriction of fascial motion in a region of the abdomen or around a specific organ is a clue to the loss of compensatory mechanisms in this area.

Assessment for the presence of asymmetrically painful Chapman reflex points is a clue to the presence of viscerosomatic activity, indicating the likelihood of visceral disease in the related organs of the body. The facilitation of specific spinal segments due to visceral organ pathology can tell the astute osteopathic physician which organ or organ system might be decompensated, that is, where the body's self-regulatory capacity has been overwhelmed. Assessment of the spine with this knowledge in mind will assist in the overall assessment of the patient.

As with abdominal pain, in any patient presenting with pelvic pain, the life- or organ-threatening conditions, such as ectopic pregnancy, ovarian or testicular torsion, or pelvic inflammatory

disease must be considered first. A common cause of pelvic pain is pelvic inflammatory disease. A patient may present in a fairly typical position that has been sometimes referred to as the "PID shuffle": a gait with the hip flexed and the lumbar spine extended. The intimate connection between the iliopsoas muscle complex and the pelvic organs makes this quite understandable.

Integrated Osteopathic Treatment

To normalize the sympathetic nervous supply to the gastrointestinal system in order to improve excursion of the rib cage (Chapter 49), assess and treat any somatic dysfunction in the thoracic and thoracolumbar areas, as well as in the rib cage. To free-up and improve the function of the lymphatic system, release restrictions and improve the function of the respiratory diaphragm. The pressure gradients between the thoracic and abdominal cavities are a primary driving force in the lymphatic flow within the body. Improving the function of the respiratory diaphragm also improves the mobility of and stimulation to the abdominal organs.

Specific osteopathic abdominal/lymphatic techniques include visceral techniques, such as the treatment of the above-mentioned ganglia to free-up restrictions in the fascial sheaths around the abdominal organs, mesenteric release technique, colonic stimulation technique, and techniques like the pedal pump that assist in lymphatic drainage.

Chapman reflex points for the abdominal area can be assessed for asymmetrical tenderness and treated to assist the osteopathic physician in diagnosis and to assist the body in homeostasis. Splenic and liver pump techniques can release important humoral and cellular agents into the circulation to assist the immune system.

Non life-threatening causes of pelvic pain, such as dysmenorrhea, may be greatly helped by the addition of OMT to patient treatment. Improved motion at the pelvic and thoracic diaphragms acutely decreases pelvic congestion, and these women would also greatly benefit from referral to an osteopath for longer-term treatment.

Treatment of the psoas would be beneficial in patients with primary muscle problems, as well as visceral problems causing somatic reaction. Treatment of the psoas should focus on release at both the origin and insertion. The psoas arises from the lateral aspect of T12 and the lumbar vertebra. Its fascia thickens to form the medial arcuate ligaments, a site of attachment for the diaphragmatic crura (46). The psoas continues its descent in the posterior abdominal wall; its fibers mesh with the iliacus muscle, which arises from the iliac fossa and lateral sacrum (46). The iliacus and psoas converge deep to the inguinal ligament and femoral vessels and insert into the anteromedial aspect of the femur (46). Treatment with facilitated positional release (Chapter 64), counterstrain, or muscle energy (Chapter 63) techniques can be particularly effective in this area. An indirect myofascial release method may also be used as follows: With the patient supine, the 12th rib/vertebral complex is carried inferiorly and slightly anteriorly. The insertion of the iliopsoas is then palpated at the lesser trochanter of the femur, just inferior to the inguinal ligament, which is usually a tender point for the patient. The hip may then be flexed and slightly externally rotated, or the muscle simply released between the treating hands (H. Ettlinger, personal communication).

Patients with spasm of the piriformis muscle and compression of the sciatic nerve often present with low back or buttock pain, but may complain of inguinal, pelvic, or lower abdominal pain. Facilitated positional release (Chapter 64) is particularly useful in the emergency department because of its rapid result, but if time allows, counterstrain, muscle energy, or myofascial release techniques may also be employed.

SUMMARY

We have described some of the important steps and dates in the history and development of the profession of allopathic and osteopathic EM. Important philosophical considerations in the field of osteopathic emergency medicine have been discussed, and a number of theoretical and practical insights into the use of osteopathic principles and practices in EM have been given. Several of the more important case scenarios in EM have been presented, and concrete examples of how osteopathic principles and practices can be safely and effectively applied have been given.

The practices of osteopathy and EM are not inconsistent; in fact, they lend themselves very nicely to a cooperation or synthesis of assessment and treatment in the ED. Obviously, there are times in a busy ED when OMM cannot be applied as one would in an OMM practice. The specific osteopathic form of assessment and treatment, including observation, skin assessment, palpatory structural examination, referred pain patterns, facilitation of spinal segments, assessment of abdominal collateral ganglia, trigger points, tender points, ANS balance issues, lymphatic assessment and treatment techniques, and the use of Chapman reflex points can significantly help the osteopathic emergency physician in the diagnosis and treatment of the patient. The osteopathic treatment, given with the correct indication and applied in a gentle and respectful fashion, can and will, sometimes dramatically, improve the patient's ability to self-regulate and achieve their most appropriate homeostatic level. These will often be applied as an adjunct measure in the ED and, when done correctly, will assist in significantly decreasing the patient's morbidity.

REFERENCES

1. Vukich D. *Emergency Medicine: Coming of Age. Jacksonville Medicine.* March; 1999.
2. American Board of Emergency Medicine. What is ABEM? Available at: http://www.abem.org. Accessed 2001.
3. American Osteopathic Board of Emergency Medicine. Available at: http://www.aobem.org. Accessed 2001.
4. Centers for Disease Control. The National Center for Health Statistics. Available at: http://www.cdc.gov/nchs/. Accessed July, 2001.
5. Paul F, Buser B. Osteopathic manipulative treatment applications for the emergency department patient. *J Am Osteopath Assoc.* 1996; 96(7).
6. The Economic Burden of Musculoskeletal Complaints to the ER. National Center for Health Statistics. National Ambulatory Medical Care Survey. Atlanta: National Center for Health Statistics, 1995.
7. Emergency visits for sports related injuries. *Ann Emerg Med.* 2001; 37:3.
8. Kuchera ML, Kuchera WA. *Osteopathic Considerations in Systemic Dysfunction,* 2nd ed. Columbus, OH: Greyden Press; 1994.
9. Goroll AH, May LA, Mulley Jr AG. *Primary Care Medicine.* Philadelphia, PA: JB Lippincott Co; 1995:328.
10. Tintinalli. *Emergency Medicine: A Comprehensive Study Guide.* New York: McGraw-Hill; 1985.
11. Travell JG, Simmons DG. *Myofascial Pain and Dysfunction: A Trigger Point Manual.* Baltimore: Williams & Wilkins; 1983.
12. Psoas syndrome. In: Ward R, ed. *Foundations for Osteopathic Medicine,* Baltimore: Williams & Wilkins; 1997.
13. Owens C. *An Endocrine Interpretation of Chapman's Reflexes.* American Osteopathic Association; 1937.
14. Malpractice suits by category, "The Cutting Edge" Vital Statistics, *The Washington Post,* 12 September, 1995.
15. Zink G, Lawson WB. An osteopathic structural examination and functional interpretation of the soma. *Osteopath Ann.* 1979; December.
16. Jones L. *Strain/Counterstrain Tender Points.* AAO; 1961.
17. American College of Emergency Physicians. Clinical Policy for the Initial Approach to Adolescents and Adults Presenting to the Emergency Department with a Chief Complaint of Headache. *Ann Emerg Med.* 1996:6:.
18. Shesser R. Headache caused by serious illness. Evaluation in an emergency setting. *Postgrad Med.* 1987;81:3.
19. Rosen P. *Emergency Medicine, Concepts and Clinical Practice,* 4th ed. St. Louis: Mosby-Year Book; 1998.
20. Turbiak T. Ear Trauma. *Emerg Med Clin North Am.* 1987;5:2.
21. Garcia GE. Management of ocular emergencies and urgent eye problems. *Am Fam Physician.* 1996;53:2.
22. Melanson SW. Clinical pearls, headache and eye pain. *Acad Emerg Med.* 1996;3:9.
23. Fritz S. Foreign bodies of the external auditory canal. *Emerg Med Clin North Am.* 1987;5:2.
24. Magoun HI. *Osteopathy in the Cranial Field.* Kirksville, MO: The Journal Printing Company; 1976.
25. Deleted in page proofs.
26. Moore KL. *Anatomy,* 3rd ed. Washington, D.C.: Library of Congress; 1985.
27. Hoyt WH. Osteopathic manipulation in the treatment of muscle-contraction headache. *J Am Osteopath Assoc.* 1979;78:5.
28. Pintal W. An integrated osteopathic treatment in acute otitis media. *J Am Osteopath Assoc.* 1989;89.
29. Pratt-Harrington D. Galbreath technique: A manipulative treatment for Otitis media revisited. *J Am Osteopath Assoc.* 2000;100.
30. Frank P. Osteopathic manipulative treatment applications for the emergency department patient. *J Am Osteopath Assoc.* 1996.
31. Graig TJ. State of the art therapy for sinusitis. *J Osteopath Assoc.* 1998.
32. Digiovanna E. *An Osteopathic Approach to Diagnosis and Treatment,* 2nd ed. Philadelphia, PA: Lippincott-Raven Publishers; 1997.
33. Ruddy TJ. Osteopathic rhythmic duction therapy. In: Barnes MW, ed. *Yearbook of Academy of Applied Osteopathy.* Indianapolis, IN: AAO; 1961.
34. Heart Disease Risk Factors. Dallas: American Heart Association; 1998.
35. Schwarz PJ, Stone HL. The role of the autonomic system in sudden coronary death. *Ann N Y Acad Sci.* 1982;382.
36. Rosero H, et al. Correlation of palpatory observations with anatomic locus of acute myocardial infarction. *J Am Osteopath Assoc.* 1987; 87.
37. Rogers JT, Rogers JC. The role of osteopathic manipulative therapy in the treatment of coronary heart disease. *J Am Osteopath Assoc.* 1976; 76.
38. Beal MC. Viscerosomatic reflexes: a review. *J Am Osteopath Assoc.* 1985;85.
39. Riley GW. Osteopathic success in the treatment of influenza and pneumonia. *J Am Osteopath Assoc.* 2000;100:5.

40. Noll DR, Shores JH, Gamber RG, et al. Benefits of osteopathic manipulative treatment for hospitalized elderly patients with pneumonia. *J Am Osteopath Assoc.* 2000;100:12.

41. Moore KL, Dalley AF. *Clinically Oriented Anatomy,* 4th ed. Philadelphia: Lippincott Williams & Wilkins; 1999.

42. Cullison B, Emerman C. The clinical challenge of acute asthma: diagnosis, disposition and outcome-effective management: Year 2001 update. *Emerg Med Rep, Am Health Consult.* 2001;22:11.

43. Ciccone A, Allegra JR, Cochrane DG, et al. Age-related differences in diagnosis within the elderly population. *Am J Emerg Med.* 1998; 16.

44. Gold M, Azevedo D. The content of adult primary care episodes. *Public Health Rep.* 1982;97.

45. Bessen HA. Abdominal aortic aneurysms in emergency medicine. Rosen, Barkin, eds. *Emergency Medicine: Concepts and Clinical Practice,* 4th ed. St. Louis: Mosby-Year Book, 1998.

46. Clemente CD. *Anatomy: A Regional Atlas of the Human Body,* 3rd ed. Baltimore, MD: Urban & Schwarzenberg; 1987. Fig 225.

GENERAL SURGERY

CONSTANCE CASHEN
SYDNEY P. ROSS

KEY CONCEPTS

- Foundations of osteopathic concept in surgery
- Osteopathic principles in abdominal and chest wall surgery
- The relationship of neuroanatomy and pathophysiology in the evaluation of acute abdominal pain
- Diagnosis of the most common causes of acute abdominal pain requiring surgical treatment
- Management of postoperative complications using osteopathic methods
- Somatic dysfunction and the alimentary tract
- The use of osteopathic manipulative treatment as an adjunct in the prevention and treatment of postoperative ileus and atelectasis

One chapter representing the field of general surgery is necessarily selective; therefore, this chapter will provide a brief review of the development of general surgery as a discipline in osteopathic medicine. It will then focus on the essential area of diagnosis and treatment in general surgery, the acute abdomen, taking an integrative view to highlight relevant osteopathic concepts.

The practice of surgery is almost as old as humanity. With the use of tools, Neolithic men and women became craftspeople. They might have also used implements for surgical purposes, because examples of trepanation (removal of a segment of bone from the skull) have been discovered in France dating to the Neolithic period. Signs that skull wounds healed indicate that a fair proportion survived the operation (1). Surgical procedures were highly developed among some of the pre-Columbian peoples. Wounds were cleaned and closed with an astringent vegetable concoction or egg substances from diverse birds and then covered with feathers or bandages made of skin. Among the Incas and other pre-Columbian peoples, the surgeon was often a separate practitioner who looked after wounds and performed bloodletting and other lesser surgical procedures (2). The ancient Egyptians employed cauterization and the fire drill as surgical tools. They made a type of adhesive tape by impregnating gums into linen strips used to pull gaping wounds together (3).

In the early years of the 19th century, the principal therapies open to European and American physicians were general regimens of:

Diet
Exercise
Rest
Baths and massage
Bloodletting
Scarification
Cupping
Blistering
Sweating
Emetics
Purges
Enemas
Fumigations

Many plant and mineral drugs were available, but only a few rested on sound physiologic or even empirical foundations. For the most part, practitioners permitted illnesses to run their course without interference; careful observers noted little benefit from the therapies available. When anesthesia became commonplace and the limitations of pain disappeared, surgical procedures multiplied in number and complexity. The potential benefits of surgery were overshadowed, however, by the frequent, devastating infections that often resulted in death. Only when the bacterial origin of infectious disease was discovered and the necessity for keeping germs away from the operative field was proved (notably by Lister) could surgery safely enter the interior regions of the body (4).

Surgery has been included in the training of osteopathic physicians since the first school of osteopathy opened in 1892. Andrew Taylor Still addressed the field of surgery and reflected appropriate concern regarding this training in the following statement from 1901:

How much surgery should be taught in an osteopathic school is a very important inquiry, and should be answered positively to the point. We claim under our charter to teach surgery, and if we fail to teach that branch we have not lived up to our promise, and we have failed to honor our obligation to the student. We have a chair of surgery filled by a professor whose learning and practice have made him an able judge of the importance of this branch. In answer to reason for urgent surgical consultation. Four of the most common causes include acute appendicitis, acute cholecystitis, diverticulitis, and small bowel obstruction. These entities share common mechanisms of pathophysiology. To appreciate the evolution of symptoms and physical signs, understanding these mechanisms is essential.

In each of these diseases, the initiating factor is the obstruction of a hollow viscus or duct structure. This results in luminal distention and stasis of organ contents. Because venous and lymphatic supply form low-pressure networks, the increasing back pressure causes obstruction of these outflow networks resulting in organ wall edema. This progresses to arterial inflow obstruction and ischemia. "The law of the artery is supreme"—ischemia leads to wall gangrene, perforation, and peritonitis.

Because the gastrointestinal tract is colonized with varying levels and types of bacteria, the stasis described above causes bacterial overgrowth. Transmural infection of the compromised viscus results and contributes to the peritonitis caused by gangrene and perforation. Bacterial liberation of endotoxins and the release of inflammatory mediators result in the systemic septic response. Left untreated, the systemic inflammatory response syndrome of multiple organ failure occurs with high levels of co-morbidity and mortality.

We will consider some individual case studies, reviewing historic and physical findings, laboratory and imaging studies, and principles of treatment.

Case One

A 28-year-old African-American male presents to the emergency department (ED) with progressive abdominal pain occurring over the last 8 hours. Previously well, he noticed mild pain in the periumbilical area that became progressively worse, was unrelieved by antacids, and is now more intense and focused in the right lower quadrant (RLQ). He has eaten no unusual foods, but is nauseated and has vomited once since admission to the ED. He denies urinary complaints. Previous medical history is negative. He is married and works as a bank teller.

Physical examination reveals a temperature of 99.8° F, pulse of 95 beats/min and blood pressure (BP) of 110/70. Neurologic, cardiovascular, and pulmonary examinations are negative.

Abdominal examination demonstrates a nondistended abdomen with decreased bowel sounds. Light palpation reveals cutaneous hypesthesia in the T10-12 dermatome on the right. Tenderness at McBurney point and localized rebound are noted. Rovsing, psoas, and obturator signs are positive. Rectal examination is negative and no inguinal hernias are appreciated. Structural examination reveals tissue texture changes and tenderness at T11-12 on the right, and right rib 12 tip tenderness. CBC shows a leukocytosis of 13,000/mm^3. Urinalysis and acute abdominal series are negative.

What differential diagnoses are suggested by this clinical picture? Does the testing verify the likely cause?

The temporal pattern and quality of the pain provide important clues. As stated previously, the visceral component of acute abdominal pain causes initial vague discomfort pointing to an organ derived from one of three embryologic gut segments based on neurovascular supply. In this case, the periumbilical location

suggests an organ supplied by the superior mesenteric vasculature and ganglion (small bowel, right colon, appendix).

The subsequent somatic component localizes the pain, suggesting the right lower quadrant position of the appendix. In particular, McBurney point tenderness (located one-third of the distance from the anterior superior iliac spine to the umbilicus) reveals the localized peritonitis of progressive appendicitis. Rovsing sign (palpatory pressure of the left lower quadrant causing RLQ pain), a positive psoas sign (RLQ pain with straight-leg raising on the right), and obturator sign (RLQ pain with passive internal rotation of the flexed right thigh) confirm the peritoneal irritation.

Somatosensory structural findings are consistent with the innervation level of the appendix (T11-12), and other associated symptoms (e.g., nausea and vomiting following the occurrence of pain) strengthen the diagnosis.

The list of differential diagnoses for appendicitis is long and is well presented in standard surgical textbooks (also, see Emergency Medicine, Chapter 26). History and physical examination are the cornerstones of confirming or discarding this diagnosis, but certain tests that strengthen the clinical impression are generally obtained.

Leukocytosis of 10,000 to 18,000 per mm^3 with a left shift is common but not absolute. Other laboratory studies, such as urinalysis, liver function studies, and amylase, may be obtained if the clinical picture is unclear. Elevated C-reactive protein with neutrophilia substantiates the diagnosis.

Imaging studies are useful in equivocal cases, especially with pediatric, older patients, and some female patients. Plain films of the abdomen are generally nonspecific, but may reveal an isolated loop of adjacent small bowel ("sentinel loop") or an appendicolith (10% to 20%). Ultrasound showing a noncompressible appendix is diagnostic in about 90% of cases. Computerized tomography (CT) changes, including a dilated appendix and/or periappendiceal/cecal inflammation or mass, are 90% to 100% sensitive and 95% specific for appendicitis. A strong clinical picture obviates the need for these studies and they should not be ordered on a routine basis.

Appendicitis remains the most common surgical emergency, affecting 7% of the population, both male and female, and peaking between ages 10 to 30. Treatment is straightforward and consists of appendectomy, performed laparoscopically or via open technique.

Preoperative antibiotic coverage for the usual bacteria in this area (Gram-negative aerobes, such as *Escherichia coli* and *Klebsiella,* and Gram-positive aerobes, such as *Streptococcus faecalis,* and anaerobes, specifically *Bacteroides fragilis*) is routine. Recovery is generally rapid (discharge in 24 to 48 hours) but may be delayed in cases of perforation and abscess.

Case Two

A 44-year-old Hispanic female presents with complaints of upper abdominal pain, nausea, and vomiting. She states the pain started last evening after a fast food meal. It began in the epigastric region, accompanied by bloating. Because she has suffered similar mild "indigestion" recently, she generally avoids fried foods. She took an over-the-counter H-2 blocker and went to bed only to be awakened by progressively severe upper quadrant abdominal pain, which was continuous and radiated to the right shoulder and subscapular area.

She is a multiparous female with a positive family history of gallstones in two sisters and her mother. She works as a school counselor and "watches her diet" because she is mildly overweight. Her history is otherwise negative.

Physical examination reveals a healthy-appearing female in moderate distress from abdominal pain. She intermittently changes position and grips her right subcostal area. Vital signs show a temperature of 100.1° F, pulse of 110 beats/min and BP of 140/85. Neurologic and cardiopulmonary examinations are negative.

Abdominal examination reveals a rounded abdomen, which is silent on auscultation. Palpation confirms acute tenderness in the right upper quadrant (RUQ) with a palpable fullness and positive Murphy's sign (inspiratory arrest with RUQ palpation). TART changes at T7-9 on the right, and tenderness over the medial right seventh intercostal space (Chapman reflex) are noted.

Laboratory studies show a moderate leukocytosis of 15,000. Bilirubin, alkaline phosphatase, serum glutamic-oxaloacetic transaminase (SGOT), and amylase are mildly elevated.

Ultrasound confirms gallstones with a thickened gallbladder wall (greater than 4 mm). HIDA scan indicates cystic duct obstruction with nonfilling of the gallbladder after 4 hours.

This patient presents with the classic picture of acute calculus cholecystitis. Her symptoms are directly correlative to the pathophysiology of this disease.

The early onset of epigastric pain is consistent with the gallbladder's foregut origin. Due to cystic duct obstruction by the offending calculus, mucus hypersecretion ensues, causing progressive gallbladder distention. Increasing wall tension results in small-vessel ischemia and wall edema. The other critical mechanism involves the toxic effects of altered, supersaturated bile (lysolethicin and platelet-activating factor are thought to be involved) in patients with cholelithiasis.

The resultant inflammation of the adjacent subcostal peritoneum (innervated by T7-8) explains the progression of clinical findings, i.e., focused RUQ pain and tenderness and the positive Murphy's sign. The referred pain pattern of the right subscapular area (T7-8) and shoulder (C4), as well as the viscerosomatic reflex changes at T7-9 on the right, are predictable based on the nociceptive anatomy of the biliary system and adjacent diaphragmatic surface (innervated by the phrenic nerve, C4).

Laboratory and imaging studies are routinely ordered to confirm the diagnosis. The pattern of findings discussed above is typical. Ultrasound accuracy exceeds 95% in detecting cholelithiasis; hence, it is the study of choice to confirm the diagnosis. A positive ultrasound and consistent clinical picture generally obviate the need for a HIDA scan, but its accuracy (greater than 90%) is excellent and it is useful if the impression of acute versus chronic cholecystitis or other acute disease is unclear. CT is also used if the diagnosis is equivocal, because it can demonstrate gallbladder distention, wall thickening, and pericholecystic fluid, though not with the accuracy of ultrasound.

About 20% of patients with symptomatic cholelithiasis will develop acute cholecystitis. Females exceed males three to one in the development of gall stones, though this drops by half above

age 50. Other risk factors include obesity, multiparity, and a positive family history of gallstones.

The indicated therapy for acute calculus cholecystitis is cholecystectomy. Treatment has historically questioned the value of early (within 48 to 72 hours) versus delayed surgery (medical treatment to resolve the acute episode with an "interval" cholecystectomy in 6 to 8 weeks). With the increasing expertise in laparoscopic cholecystectomy (the preferred surgical technique), the early approach is favored. Conversion to an open procedure is increased in cases of perforation, abscess, or extreme edema.

Antibiotic coverage for typical gut pathogens is routine, but cultures of the bile are frequently negative.

Uncomplicated acute cholecystitis treated in this manner generally results in rapid recovery and discharge in 24 to 48 hours. Complicated disease (perforation, abscess, emphysematous cholecystitis) or severe co-morbid disease can be approached with vigorous medical therapy with or without cholecystostomy (drainage of the gallbladder), and eventual cholecystectomy when the patient's medical condition permits.

Case Three

A 50-year-old white female is evaluated for diffuse abdominal pain and bloating that began 2 days ago. She states it began as intermittent cramping pain with nausea and two episodes of diarrhea. She thought it was the flu. However, the colicky pain became more continuous and was accompanied by recurrent episodes of vomiting, initially described as bilious but now feculent. She has had no further stools and her abdomen is "swelling."

Her past history is positive for a hysterectomy 6 months ago and for anemia due to recurrent uterine bleeding from uterine fibroids. She is an accountant who recently moved her office to a new location and was consequently moving heavy boxes.

Based on the history, what aspects of the physical examination would corroborate a diagnostic impression of small bowel obstruction?

On examination, vital signs are stable, but she is obviously uncomfortable. Inspection of the abdomen confirms moderate distention. Bowel sounds are high-pitched and peristaltic rushes are heard. Palpation reveals generalized tenderness with minimal rebound in the mid to lower abdomen. A lower midline surgical scar is evident. No hernias or abdominal masses are appreciated. Pelvic and rectal examinations reveal no masses. Structural examination demonstrates paraspinal muscle spasm and tenderness at T8-10 bilaterally.

Laboratory studies include complete blood cell count (CBC), basic chemistry profile, and urinalysis. A mild leukocytosis, and elevated blood urea nitrogen (BUN) and urine specific gravity are noted. Serum potassium is slightly decreased. Amylase is normal.

An acute abdominal radiograph series is performed. Findings include dilation of the small bowel, absence of gas in colon and rectum, and multiple air-fluid levels in a "stairstep" pattern. CT scan is negative for free air but confirms a small bowel obstruction with dilated, slightly thickened loops of small bowel.

These findings are consistent with acute mechanical small bowel obstruction. The most likely cause is postoperative adhesions (up to 70%) from the prior hysterectomy. Hernias and neoplasm are next in frequency for causing obstruction.

The characteristic diffuse pattern of pain indicates a prominent visceral component of nociception in most patients presenting with small bowel obstruction. Development of more localized continuous pain with prominent somatic signs (e.g, rebound, guarding, and rigidity) signal the development of ischemia and gangrene at the site of obstruction. Fever and leukocytosis strengthen this possibility and mandate early surgical intervention. Still, it should be noted that none of these signs either alone or in combination can absolutely identify strangulated bowel. Metabolic acidosis and hyperamylasemia also suggest compromised bowel.

Fluid and electrolyte abnormalities are common. Dehydration, as evidenced by elevated BUN and urine specific gravity, occurs due to fluid losses through vomiting and sequestration in the obstructed bowel loops. Nasogastric suction to decompress the bowel and repletion of the fluid and electrolyte losses is critical. Surgery is often delayed for several hours in cases of severe volume depletion until vital signs and urine output are improved.

Antibiotic coverage of gut bacteria is given perioperatively in cases of simple mechanical obstruction requiring surgery.

Patients showing signs of incomplete obstruction, such as small amounts of colonic air on abdominal films or contrast passing slowly into the colon on CT scan, are treated with nasogastric decompression and observation. Up to 80% will resolve spontaneously, with obvious improvement in 24 to 48 hours.

Operative treatment of small bowel obstruction includes release of the obstructing element (e.g., adhesive band, hernia entrapment, resection, or bypass of neoplasm). Judging viability of an ischemic portion of bowel requires experience, but can be assisted by Doppler studies and fluorescein staining. Resection of all nonviable bowel is mandatory. If question remains, a second-look operation in 24 hours should be performed.

With these strategies, the morbidity and mortality historically associated with small bowel obstruction have been markedly decreased. Continued efforts to prevent further adhesion formation, such as the application of barrier agents (such as a bioresorbable membrane), will be the key to reducing the incidence of small bowel obstruction in the future.

Case Four

A 70-year-old white male is seen after presenting with lower abdominal pain, which began 4 days ago and is primarily in the LLQ with radiation to the left lumbar area. The patient has not suffered from nausea or vomiting, but has no appetite and some fever and chills. He has been constipated for the last 3 days and states that he usually has a bowel movement every 2 days. He denies any rectal bleeding. He has had somewhat similar symptoms on one or two occasions in the past, but felt that this was simply due to constipation. He has no urinary tract complaints.

His history is positive for mild hypertension, for which he takes a β-blocker. He underwent an appendectomy at age 16. Medical history is otherwise negative. He is retired and lives with his wife.

If this patient were seen in the physician's office, what physical findings would prompt you to consider hospitalization?

Examination of the patient demonstrates a well-nourished, well-developed 70-year-old white male with noticeable abdominal discomfort. Vital signs show a blood pressure of 152/87, pulse of 80 beats/min and a temperature of 101° F. Cardiopulmonary examination is noncontributory.

Abdominal examination demonstrates mild distention. A RLQ scar is evident. Bowel sounds are present but diminished. Marked localized tenderness in the LLQ is present with a palpable mass. Rebound tenderness and guarding are noted in this area. Mild tenderness is present in the RLQ and left upper quadrant (LUQ). Some left flank concussion tenderness is noted. Rectal examination demonstrates a nonnodular, slightly enlarged prostate, no rectal masses, and a borderline positive hemoccult study.

Structural examination reveals increased tissue texture changes with tenderness in the L1-2 level on the left. Tenderness is also noted along the superior third of the iliotibial band of the left leg—the area of Chapman reflex for the sigmoid colon.

Laboratory studies demonstrate a leukocytosis of 18,000. Electrolyte and chemistry profiles are within normal limits. Acute abdominal series is performed. Findings of mild, nonspecific small bowel distention are noted. Gas is seen in the colon. The psoas stripe on the left is obscured. No free air is evident. CT scan demonstrates marked inflammatory change in the sigmoid colon with a pericolic abscess.

This patient presents with acute perforated diverticulitis, a complication of diverticulosis. Diverticulosis affects greater than 50% of people over the age of 60, and 75% by age 85. Fortunately, only about 10% to 25% will develop diverticulitis.

The cause of diverticulosis is related to the American low-fiber diet (10 to 15 grams per day), which creates firm stool that requires high colonic pressure to propel. This particularly affects the sigmoid colon with its intrinsically smaller lumen. Continued contraction against firm stool promotes circular muscle hypertrophy, which causes further luminal narrowing. The law of Laplace predicts that transmural pressure increases as the radius of a cylinder decreases, so the weak points of the colonic wall, where nutrient vessels penetrate, develop the small herniations of mucosa and muscularis that we call diverticulosis.

Obstruction of the neck of the diverticulum by inspissated feces with resultant ischemia and perforation leads to varying degrees of pericolonic inflammation and abscess. This spreading process can result in a reflex ileus or entrap adjacent small bowel (10% to 30%) and cause obstruction. In either case, nausea and vomiting result. Erosion into the bladder or vagina, causing fistulas (5% to 10%) is a long-term sequelae that causes pneumaturia and chronic infection.

Evaluation of diverticulitis routinely involves CT scan, which is 90% to 95% sensitive and greater than 70% specific. Barium enema and colonoscopy should not be performed due to the risk of perforation.

The Hinche classification of clinical progression of diverticulitis is helpful in planning treatment. Stage I (pericolonic inflammation) often responds to medical therapy (70% to 80%), i.e., intravenous antibiotics to cover normal colonic bacteria, hydration, and bowel rest.

If fever, leukocytosis, and LLQ pain do not improve within 24 to 48 hours, surgery is indicated. Sigmoid resection with primary anastomosis is possible in contained disease. Otherwise, the use of resection with end colostomy and closure of the rectal stump (Hartmann procedure) is performed. This "two-stage" procedure requires repeat laparotomy in 6 to 12 weeks for reanastomosis of the colon.

Stage 2 (pericolic abscess) may be drained with CT-guided aspiration and then treated as stage 1 disease if the abscess collection is accessible (70% to 90%). Otherwise, a Hartmann procedure is required. Stage 3 (generalized purulent peritonitis), and stage 4 (fecal peritonitis) are routinely treated with a Hartmann procedure.

MANAGEMENT OF POSTOPERATIVE COMPLICATIONS

Atelectasis

Major surgical procedures that involve the abdominal wall have a relatively high morbidity. Table 27.1 lists the serious complications that can occur after a variety of major surgical procedures. Sabiston (8) stated that pulmonary complications can occur in 57 of all major surgeries performed with general anesthesia. The incidence of complications can double in abdominal surgery, triple for smokers, and quadruple for patients with chronic obstructive pulmonary disease. Atelectasis, a collapse of alveoli that renders them unable to be involved in gas exchange, is the most frequent pulmonary complication after surgery. This complication generally sets the framework for subsequent pulmonary infections.

In considering the problem of atelectasis, an appreciation of respiratory mechanics after abdominal surgery is required. Respiratory motion depends full diaphragmatic excursion, as well as unencumbered rib motion (see Chapter 49, Regional Examination and Treatment: Rib Cage, for detailed discussion). Unfortunately, the natural response of the patient with incisional pain is abdominal wall splinting and shallow breathing, which increases the risk for this complication. Without this pumping action, full alveolar expansion, especially in the lung bases, does not occur. Because oxygen exchange in these areas is greatly diminished, an environment is created that encourages the development of pneumonia (a dreaded postoperative complication that inevitably lengthens hospital stay and can precipitate other organ dysfunction in vulnerable patients).

In the United States, an incentive spirometer is the most popular mechanical method used for prevention of postoperative atelectasis. It is used extensively because it encourages deep breathing and requires minimal supervision and personnel to administer (9,10). The beneficial effects of incentive spirometry in the prevention of postoperative complications have recently been challenged, however (11,12), because changing the angle of the patient's recumbency from 60 to 30 altered the effectiveness of postoperative incentive spirometry. This finding suggests features other than just lung mechanics involving the major airways. One suggestion for the alteration in airflow with a change in recumbency is fluctuating diaphragmatic motion (13). In the presence of diaphragmatic dysfunction, incentive spirometry can have little effect on improving gas exchange. The change in recumbency angle alone is believed to result in an improved diaphragmatic link tension relationship and a shift in compartment compliance as the patient reclines (14,15).

The earliest osteopathic physicians incorporated their understanding of viscerosomatic and somatovisceral reflexes into their management of patients in the postoperative period. The visceral motor, visceral sensory, and visceral tropic reflexes that arise from stimuli originating in the lungs appear to manifest themselves in tissue supplied by nerves arising in most of the cervical segments; the reflexes are most marked in those tissues supplied by neurons arising in the third to fifth cervical segments. Pottinger (16) stated that the visceral motor reflex caused by inflammation in the lungs shows itself in the contraction of the fibers of those muscles that receive their origin from the cervical portion of the cord and particularly from the third to fifth cervical segments. This manifests clinically as an increased tone or spasm in the paraspinal tissues involved.

Osteopathic surgeons have presumed that this viscerosomatic reflex might be clinically significant and could have important implications for the possibility that modifying a somatovisceral reflex could be beneficial in the postoperative state (17–22). In 1963, Henshaw (23) published the results of an interventional trial of surgical patients. A total of 1,031 surgical patients were studied from 1961 to 1963. Of this total, 109 (10.6%) had preexisting somatic dysfunction at the level of the third, fourth, and fifth cervical vertebra before surgery. This cohort formed the study group for investigation. Seventy-five of the 109 patients were given osteopathic manipulative treatment (OMT) for these somatic dysfunctions. In this group, three patients (4%) developed postoperative pulmonary complications. In the 34 patients who had cervical spine somatic dysfunction but did not receive OMT, 29 (85%) developed some form of pulmonary complication.

Unfortunately, the external validity of such a study is diminished in our era because the patients were not randomized. In addition, the definition of pulmonary complications was so broad that a high percentage of the defined entities (emphysema, pulmonary edema, cough) are of such sufficiently vague end points that they do not represent meaningful outcomes. There would be considerable interest in knowing the outcome of the 922 patients who had surgery in the absence of preexisting cervical spine somatic dysfunction.

The Henshaw study was conducted according to research methods and employed statistical methodology that was typical for that time period. Although the study does not withstand modern scientific scrutiny, the described results are so impressive that a current study to replicate these findings is warranted.

TABLE 27.1. POSTOPERATIVE COMPLICATIONS OF MAJOR SURGICAL PROCEDURES

Wound infections
Intraabdominal sepsis (peritonitis)
Subphrenic and subhepatic abscess
Empyema
Mediastinitis
Pneumonia
Acute respiratory insufficiency [including adult respiratory distress syndrome (ARDS)]
Renal failure
Postoperative jaundice
Postoperative ileus
Bowel obstruction
Acute gastric hemorrhage
Multiple organ failure
Myocardial infarction

Another form of OMT that is described as effective in the prevention of atelectasis in the postoperative period is the thoracic lymphatic pump (TLP). The TLP is a ventilator-assist technique that uses passive and active rib excursion. The TLP technique is reported to have reduced the mortality from the 1918 influenza outbreak from 5% in the general population to 0.25% in 100,000 treated patients (24).

A recent study indicated that TLP can be equally as effective as incentive spirometry in reducing the postoperative occurrence of atelectasis (25). This study also indicated that patients treated with the TLP had an earlier recovery and faster return to preoperative values for both the forced vital capacity and forced expiratory volume at 1 second (FEV1) compared with patients who did not receive TLP. OMT has been recommended in the postoperative median sternotomy patient to promote faster return to normal chest and diaphragmatic dynamics (26). This is particularly important because there are more than 250,000 patients annually undergoing coronary bypass grafting through a median sternotomy incision.

The postoperative addition of rib raising provides a means of directly assessing and enhancing respiratory motion. This articulatory technique is well described in Chapter 55, Articulatory Techniques, and can be easily applied to the hospitalized patient.

VISCEROSOMATIC AND SOMATOVISCERAL REFLEXES

Many osteopathic physicians believe that treating the somatic component of a viscerosomatic reflex can improve a visceral pathologic condition. The diagnosis of a viscerosomatic reflex is based on a documentation of visceral disease and the objective findings of somatic dysfunction on palpatory examination. The finding of somatic dysfunction should lead to a review of the patient's clinical status to determine whether symptoms of a visceral disorder can be elicited.

Beal (27) defines the somatic component of a viscerosomatic reflex as having the following findings:

- Two or more adjacent spinal segments that show evidence of somatic dysfunction located within the specific autonomic reflex area
- A deep confluent muscle reaction
- Resistance to segmental joint motion
- Skin and subcutaneous tissue changes consistent with the acuity or chronicity of the reflex

However, the predictive value of palpatory findings in the differential diagnosis of visceral disease has not been established for clinical practice. The results can be variable, depending on interobserver differences or issues related to the interpretation of musculoskeletal findings. At the same time that the clinical utility of musculoskeletal findings is incompletely defined, the effectiveness of manipulative treatment for somatic manifestations of chronic organ disease has not been established. Many osteopathic physicians have advocated manipulative treatment as part of the treatment regimen for organic problems of the heart and gallbladder. Although postoperative manipulative treatment has been recommended as promoting a shorter, smoother con-

valescence from the effects of visceral disease, prospective studies have not been conducted to test this hypothesis.

PRE- AND POSTOPERATIVE SOMATIC DYSFUNCTION

The process of surgery, i.e., lying on the rigid table under anesthesia, can result in postoperative back pain and cephalgia. Similarly, many patients have chronic areas of somatic dysfunction that become exacerbated during a surgical illness. Despite the surgical treatment of the visceral dysfunction, the somatic component may persist and even mimic a recurrence of the original condition, such as causing a variant of post-cholecystectomy syndrome in cases of continued somatic dysfunction at T7.

Ileus

One of the major postoperative problems that can affect any type of surgery is postoperative ileus. Ileus is defined as the functional inhibition of propulsive bowel activity, regardless of the pathogenic mechanism. This is differentiated from motility disorders resulting from structural abnormalities, which is called a mechanical bowel obstruction. Ileus after surgery is further classified into postoperative and paralytic ileus. Postoperative ileus is the uncomplicated ileus that occurs after surgery and resolves spontaneously within 2 to 3 days. It most likely results from the temporary inhibition of extrinsic motility regulation and is more severe in the colon. In contrast, postoperative paralytic ileus lasts for more than 3 days after surgery. It affects all segments of the bowel and probably results from further inhibition of local, intrinsic contractile systems. Patients who have this disorder accumulate gas and secretions in the intestinal system, leading to bloating, distension, emesis, and pain.

Despite major advances in many areas of medicine, relatively few improvements have been made in the understanding of ileus. The most important advance was made over a century ago, in 1884, with the introduction of nasogastric suction (28). The earliest studies of bowel motility focused on mechanisms for reduction and stimulation of intestinal contractions. Early in this century, the role of inhibitory sympathetic reflexes mediating ileus was recognized. With the inhibitory reflex efferent limb clearly established, investigators searched for the afferent system. Many possibilities exist, including peritoneal or cutaneous stimulation, release of inhibitory humoral agents, inhibition of smooth muscle by inflammation, or muscle or nerve inhibition by anesthetic agents.

Parasympathetic fiber stimulation increases motility, and stimulation of sympathetic fibers inhibits it. Vagal nerve section in animals does not alter small intestinal motility, whereas splanchnic nerve division increases contractility. Sympathetic chronic inhibitor control predominates in the gut. Sympathetic activation occurs with stress and surgery and is thought to significantly alter bowel motility during the postoperative period.

The treatment for ileus has changed little in the last 100 years. Nasogastric intubation and suction is the only proven effective therapy. The medical regimen is modified so that medications diminishing motility are minimized. Intravenous hydration is necessary until the ileus resolves and the alimentary tract can be used. Total parenteral nutrition may be necessary in cases of prolonged ileus.

In 1968, Herrmann (29) reported the results of a study in which he performed a chart review of 317 consecutive patients undergoing major surgery who received routine postoperative OMT compared with a subsequent series of 92 patients who did not receive postoperative OMT. In this study, the description of adynamic ileus used the following criteria:

i. Absence of bowel sounds
ii. Abdominal distension
iii. Tympany to percussion of the abdomen
iv. Absence of flatus being passed per rectum

For those patients in whom adynamic ileus was diagnosed, OMT was then performed in the following manner. With the patient supine, intermittent pressure was applied to the paravertebral tissues of the lumbar and lower thoracic spine, producing extension of those areas, in addition to deep pressure. This was done for approximately 2 minutes. The treatment was repeated every 2 hours. Each patient was periodically reexamined to observe the effect, if any, that the treatment had on the criteria used for the diagnosis of postoperative adynamic ileus.

Only one case of ileus was noted in the series of 317 patients who received OMT postoperatively. This represents an incidence of 0.3. Seven patients (7.6%) in the group of 92 patients who did not receive postoperative OMT developed ileus. In these seven cases, the age range was from 9 to 73 years. After the administration of OMT, six of these patients showed improvement, as manifest by a resumption of bowel sounds or passage of flatus. This study was not a controlled, randomized trial, and the report provides scant details of the study design and methodology. It suggests that postoperative OMT aids in prevention of postoperative ileus. Because this viewpoint is widely held by practitioners of OMT, a randomized trial is warranted to investigate its efficacy in the treatment of this and other postoperative complications.

OMT has been used in the management of postoperative ileus for years. It addresses the sympathetic effects on gut motility. Inhibition of sympathetic hyperactivity allows the natural return of intestinal function as the balance with parasympathetic stimulation is restored. Manipulative treatment of ileus is directed toward influencing sympathetic outflow through the paravertebral ganglia (sympathetic chain) of T5-11. The following are a few of the OMT techniques that are used in treating postoperative ileus:

i. Gentle inhibition of hypertonic thoracic and lumbar paravertebral muscles to the point of tissue relaxation (2 to 5 minutes total time); this is most effectively directed toward spinal segments that are associated with the surgical site via supplying sympathetic innervation to the involved viscera.
ii. Indirect method fascial release manipulation of the diaphragm, thoracic inlet, and mid-cervical spine.
iii. Treating Chapman reflex points along the outer thigh and paravertebral regions (30).
iv. Thoracolumbar counterstrain tender points can also be treated to facilitate recovery (31).

CONCLUSION

Osteopathic principles are widely implemented in the surgical treatment of patients today. The formal development of this process began with the establishment of regular surgical training programs in the osteopathic profession in 1926. The primary focus has centered on the osteopathic concepts of:

i. The interrelationship between structure and function.
ii. The need to treat the patient as a regulated, integrated, and coordinated unit

The first precept represents the rationale for the application of osteopathic manipulative treatment in the preoperative or postoperative period. The second precept is expressed in the surgeon's approach to the patient, the patient's family and social support, and the patient's psychological state as critical features related to the overall outcome of any surgical procedure.

Understanding the approach to the surgical patient requires an appreciation of anatomy, with regard to both organ function and nociception. The anatomic structure of the autonomic nervous system and the pathophysiology of organ dysfunction determine the nature of pain expression and clinical presentation. This was further explored by presenting four cases of acute abdominal pain. Surgery for these and any major illness can result in postoperative complications, most commonly atelectasis and ileus. An osteopathic approach can contribute to the prevention and resolution of these problems. The osteopathic approach to the surgical patient uses the diagnostic information provided by structural examination, as well as the added treatment dimension provided by manipulative care.

The addition of osteopathic manipulative treatment to the postoperative care of the surgical patient is therapeutic and greatly appreciated by the patient. All patients should be routinely screened for somatic dysfunction as part of the basic surgical examination. Although the acutely ill patient often cannot comply with a full musculoskeletal examination in three positions, an appropriate screening examination can be integrated into the physician's usual approach to these patients. An excellent example with diagrams is described in Chapter 44, Musculoskeletal Examination for Somatic Dysfunction.

Attention to possible viscerosomatic reflexes and assessing Jones and Chapman tender points (see Chapters 63 and 67, respectively) can provide valuable information in formulating the surgical diagnosis and can indicate areas to be included in a manipulative treatment plan. Comparative assessment in the postoperative patient and attention to the patient's structural complaints will guide an appropriate treatment program.

Osteopathic manipulative treatment is underused in the treatment of surgical patients. The challenge for the osteopathic surgeon is to translate years of clinical experience with osteopathic palpatory diagnosis and treatment into research protocols that determine the effectiveness of these methods for the surgical patient. Specific areas for investigation include the possibility that thoracic lymphatic pump or other techniques might reduce the overall incidence of pulmonary atelectasis, or that OMT might reduce postoperative adynamic ileus.

REFERENCES

1. Lyons AS. Prehistoric medicine. In: Lyons AS, Petrucelli RJ, eds. *Medicine, An Illustrated History.* New York, NY: Harry N. Abrams; 1978:27.
2. Bosch J, Petrucelli RJ. Medicine in the pre-Columbian Americas. In: Lyons AS, Petrucelli RJ, eds. *Medicine, An Illustrated History.* New York, NY: Harry N. Abrams; 1978:50–55.
3. Lyons AS. Ancient Egypt. In: Lyons AS, Petrucelli RJ, eds. *Medicine, An Illustrated History.* New York, NY: Harry N. Abrams; 1978:98.
4. Lyons AS. The beginning of modern medicine. In: Lyons AS, Petrucelli RJ, eds. *Medicine, An Illustrated History.* New York, NY: Harry N. Abrams; 1978:523–533.
5. Schnucker RV, ed. *Early Osteopathy in the Words of A. T. Still.* Kirksville, MO: The Thomas Jefferson University Press; 1991.
6. *Dorland's Medical Dictionary.* Philadelphia, PA: WB Saunders; 1981.
7. Minutes of the meeting of the Board of Governors of the American College of Osteopathic Surgeons; October, 1983. Also, American College of Osteopathic Surgeons, General Surgery Discipline Bylaws, Article II, 1988.
8. Sabiston Jr. DD. *Essentials of Surgery.* Philadelphia, PA: WB Saunders; 1987.
9. Dohi S, Gold MI. Comparison of two methods of postoperative respiratory care. *Chest.* 1978;73:592–595.
10. Jung R, Wight J, Nusser R, et al. Comparison of three methods of respiratory care following upper abdominal surgery. *Chest.* 1980;78:31–35.
11. Schweiger I, Gamulin Z, Forster A, et al. Absence of benefit of incentive spirometry in low risk patients undergoing elective cholecystectomy. *Chest.* 1986;89:652–656.
12. Stock MC, Downs JB, Gauer PK, et al. Prevention of postoperative pulmonary complications with C-pap, incentive spirometry, and conservative therapy. *Chest.* 1985;87:151–157.
13. Froese A, Bryan AC. Effect of anesthesia and paralysis on diaphragmatic mechanics in man. *Anesthesiology.* 1974;41:242–255.
14. Braun NMT, Aurora NS, Rochester DS. Force length relationship of the normal human diaphragm. *J Appl Physiol.* 1982;53:405–412.
15. Sharp JT, Goldberg NB, Druz WS, et al. Relative contribution of the rib cage and abdomen to breathing in normal subjects. *J Appl Physiol.* 1975;39:608–618.
16. Pottinger FF. *Essentials of Surgery,* 5th ed. St. Louis, MO: Mosby; 1938.
17. Brock WW. Osteopathy and surgery. *J Osteopathy.* April 1905:111–113.
18. Downing WJ. Osteopathic manipulative treatment of nonsurgical gallbladder. *Academy of Applied Osteopathy Yearbook.* Carmel, CA: American Academy of Osteopathy; 1965:196–199.
19. Koogler P. Osteopathic care of surgical cases. *J Osteopathy.* April 1949:21–24.
20. Larson NJ. Manipulative care before and after surgery. *Osteopath Med.* 1977:41–49.
21. Stiles ET. Osteopathic treatment of surgical patients. *Osteopath Med.* September 1976:21–23.
22. Young GS. Postoperative osteopathic manipulation. *Academy of Applied Osteopathy Yearbook.* Carmel, CA: American Academy of Osteopathy; 1970:77–82.
23. Henshaw RE. Manipulation and postoperative pulmonary complications. *The DO.* September 1963:132–133.
24. Smith RK. 100,000 cases of influenza with a death rate 1/40th of that officially reported under conventional medical treatment. *J Am Osteopath Assoc.* January 1920:172–173.
25. Sleszynski SL, Kelso AF. Comparison of thoracic manipulation with incentive spirometry in preventing postoperative atelectasis. *J Am Osteopath Assoc.* 1993;93:834–835.
26. Dickey JL. Postoperative osteopathic manipulative management of median sternotomy patients. *J Am Osteopath Assoc.* 1989;89:1274–1277.
27. Beal MC. Viscerosomatic reflexes: a review. *J Am Osteopath Assoc.* 1985;85:787–801.
28. Livingston EH, Passaro EP. Postoperative ileus. *Dig Dis Sci.* 1990;35:121–132.
29. Herrmann E. Precepts and practice. *The DO.* 1965:163–164.
30. Kuchera ML, Kuchera, WA. *Osteopathic Considerations in Systemic Dysfunction,* 2nd ed. Columbus, OH: Greyden Press; 1994:96–97.
31. Schwartz HR. The use of counterstrain in an acutely ill in-hospital population. *J Am Osteopath Assoc.* 1986;86:433–442.

RECOMMENDED READING

1. Cameron JL, ed. *Current Surgical Therapy,* 7th ed. St. Louis, MO: Mosby; 2001.
2. Fischer JE, Nussbaum MS, Chance WT, et al. Manifestations of gastrointestinal disease. In: Schwartz SI, ed. *Principles of Surgery.* New York, NY: McGraw-Hill; 1999:1033–1041.
3. Glasgow RE, Mulvihil SJ. Abdominal Pain, Including the Acute Abdomen. In: Feldman M, Scharschmidt BF, Sleisenger MH, eds. *Sleisenger and Fordtran's Gastrointestinal and Liver Disease.* Philadelphia, PA: WB Saunders; 1997:80–89.
4. Guyton AC, Hall JE. *Textbook of Medical Physiology.* Philadelphia, PA: WB Saunders; 2000:720–727.
5. Klein KB, Mellinkoff SM. Approach to the Patient with Abdominal Pain. In: Yamada T, ed. *Textbook of Gastroenterology.* Philadelphia, PA: JB Lippincott Co; 1994:660–664.
6. Netter FH. *Atlas of Human Anatomy,* 2nd ed. East Hanover, NJ: Novartis; 1999.
7. Sorkin LS, Wallace MS. Acute Pain Mechanisms. *Surg Clin North Am.* 1999;79: 213–229.

GYNECOLOGY

MELICIEN TETTAMBEL

KEY CONCEPTS

- Anatomy of the pelvis
- Somatic dysfunction and pelvic pain
- Osteopathic evaluation of pelvic pain
- Osteopathic approach to the treatment of pelvic pain

What diseases does woman have that man does not have? Such diseases as belong to the womb and its appendages . . . It matters not whether the cause is far remote or in close proximity to the uterus; we must find it, or we will be found in the antediluvian tribe of speculum cranks of all the blind female doctors' ages. —A. T. Still (1)

The osteopathic obstetrician-gynecologist has the opportunity to integrate the influences of the musculoskeletal system into the management of a variety of health care concerns experienced by female patients. Knowledge of anatomy and physiology of the reproductive system is key to osteopathic management of related somatic dysfunction. Palpatory expertise of the female pelvis and its contents is a prerequisite for ancillary testing and patient management. Because of the broad scope of gynecology, this chapter does not address all diagnostic and treatment topics involving the female reproductive system. Instead, it focuses on two common women's health care issues frequently encountered by primary care providers—pelvic pain and pelvic organ disorders.

PELVIC PAIN

Anatomy

Evaluation of pelvic pain requires extensive knowledge of the anatomy and physiology of the female pelvis. Although standard references (2–4) completely discuss the anatomy of the female pelvis, salient points helpful to osteopathic physicians are summarized here to illustrate possible causes of somatic dysfunction.

The pelvic floor consists of the levator ani muscles and pelvic diaphragm complex (5). It contains the visceral pelvic fascia and pelvic diaphragm, and the urogenital anal triangles with superficial and deep genital muscles. The sphincters of the urethra are also included.

The levator ani group forms the deepest layer of striated muscles and is laterally bordered by the arcus tendineus, the piriformis muscle, and the obturator internus muscle. The fascia of this group is continuous with these pelvic diaphragm muscles. The anterior pubic portion of the levator ani muscles includes the pubococcygeus, with the puborectalis and pubovaginalis portions. The iliococcygeus forms the posterior iliac portion. The ischiococcygeus muscle lies adjacent but more superior to the levator ani group and assists the levator ani in its supportive function.

The perineum can be divided into the urogenital triangle regions and the anal triangle regions (6) (Tables 28.1 and 28.2). Superficial external genital muscles form a figure eight around the vagina and urethra and around the anus (Fig. 28.1). Deeper in the urogenital triangle is the urogenital diaphragm. It is anterior to and more superficial than the pelvic diaphragm. It is also incorporated transversely with muscle and fascia that span bilaterally across the ischiopubic rami. The urogenital diaphragm consists of the striated urogenital sphincters.

The female urethral sphincters include the striated sphincter urethrae and distal intrinsic and external sphincters. The levator ani and the compressor urethrae muscles assist the sphincters in urethral closing (7).

The pelvic floor performs three important functions: supportive, sphincteric, and sexual. The pelvic floor, in conjunction with the pelvis bones, muscles, and connective tissues, provides support of the pelvic organs against gravity and any increases in abdominal pressure. Support and tone for vaginal walls are also provided. Sphincteric function aids in control of perineal openings. Pelvic floor muscles prevent incontinence by increasing intraurethral pressure and stabilizing endopelvic fascia during sphincter contraction. The muscles also relax for defecation and contract to control flatus. They help prevent fecal incontinence by keeping the anorectal angle closed (8). A functional pelvic floor stabilizes the proximal urethra, improves severe lower tract symptomatology, and assists in the ability to delay urination via bladder reflex inhibition (8). The sexual function consists of contraction of perivaginal muscles during coitus to enhance sexual activity. The muscles also respond reflexively during orgasm. Decreased pubococcygeal strength and awareness impede sexual response (9).

The striated muscles of the vaginal introitus and skin of the perineum receive somatic motor and sensory fibers from the had a hysterectomy. Extensive metabolic and psychological studies have yet to identify a specific abnormality, but serotonergic neurotransmission dysfunction has been implicated (40). Treatment options have included:

- Medication to suppress cyclic ovarian activity
- Psychotherapy to develop coping skills
- Diuretics to reduce bloating
- Diets with reduced fat, caffeine, or salt to reduce irritability or water retention
- Dietary or food supplements (pyridoxine or primrose oil), which may interfere with prostaglandin synthesis to lessen cramps (41,42)
- Osteopathic manipulative treatment (43)

Endometriosis

Endometriosis is a benign condition in which endometrial glands and stroma are present outside the endometrial cavity. Other locations include the ovary, bowel, bladder, peritoneum, and sites outside the pelvic boundaries. Endometriosis is a challenge to gynecologists because it is a diagnostic and surgical enigma (44). More than 15% of women have some degree of the disease. It is noted in approximately 20% of gynecologic surgical procedures and half the time, endometriosis is an unexpected finding (45).

The characteristic triad of symptoms associated with endometriosis is dysmenorrhea, dyspareunia, and dyschezia. Secondary dysmenorrhea first appears or escalates in the late 20s or early 30s. If the endometriosis is associated with obstructive genital anomalies, severe dysmenorrhea may occur at menarche (46).

Dyspareunia is generally associated with deep coitus, which can irritate the endometrial implants located in the cul-de-sac, the uterosacral ligaments, or in portions of the posterior vaginal fornix. On pelvic examination, the cul-de-sac may feel gritty and be exquisitely tender to the touch (47).

Dyschezia is experienced with uterosacral, cul-de-sac, and rectosigmoid colon involvement. As stool passes between the uterosacral ligaments, the patient experiences pain. This symptom is highly characteristic and is more common with endometriosis than with chronic salpingo-oophoritis, a condition sometimes otherwise mistaken for endometriosis (48).

If the ovarian capsule is involved with endometriosis, ovulatory pain and midcycle vaginal bleeding are reported by the patient. However, the nature of pelvic pain caused by endometriosis is variable. Some investigators have found that the degree of pain is inversely proportional to the extent of the disease (45). Minimal endometriosis in the cul-de-sac may be more painful than a large ovarian endometrioma that can expand freely into the abdominal cavity. Frequently, pelvic examination yields no signs of endometriosis.

The diagnosis of endometriosis should be suspected in an afebrile patient with the previously mentioned characteristic endometriosis symptom triad: a firm, fixed, tender adnexal mass and tender nodularity in the cul-de-sac and uterosacral ligaments. Pelvic ultrasound may indicate an adnexal mass of complex echogenicity. The definitive diagnosis is made by the characteristic gross findings of "blueberry" spots, chocolate cysts, or

"powder burns," or by histologic findings of endometrial tissue at laparoscopy or laparotomy (49,50).

Management of endometriosis depends on the following considerations (30):

- Certainty of the diagnosis
- Severity of symptoms
- Extent of the disease
- Preservation of fertility
- Compromised function of the gastrointestinal and/or urinary tracts

If reproductive capacity is not a concern, total abdominal hysterectomy with bilateral salpingo-oophorectomy should be considered. Menopause can be managed with hormone replacement therapy. If future fertility is a consideration, pursue conservative surgery, including resection of the disease, lysis of adhesions, ovarian resection, or ablation of small lesions (49).

Medical therapy may be considered if the endometriosis is minimal in extent and the symptoms are tolerable. NSAIDs or COX-2 inhibitors are recommended to address dysmenorrhea. Oral contraceptive pills or hormonal manipulation may decrease the intensity and duration of dysmenorrhea and menses. Temporary suppression of menstruation and endometrial implant formation can be achieved through short-term use of danocrine or GnRH agonists (51). Fertility is preserved by involution of implants. However, when a palpable endometrioma is present, the likelihood of a complete response to medical therapy is small (51).

Osteopathic treatment considerations for menstrual disorder pain include "rocking" of the sacral base for parasympathetic inhibition (34) and treatment of somatic dysfunction of the thoracolumbar spine, particularly T10-L2. Mobilization of the respiratory diaphragm should improve respiration and circulation of body fluids. Treatment of the pelvic diaphragm relieves pelvic congestion and edema of the lower extremities. Because the menstrual cycle is controlled by neuroendocrine system feedback, cranial base or vertebral strain may interfere with endocrine function.

Ovarian Pain

Ovarian cysts are usually asymptomatic, but pain may occur as a result of rapid distension of the ovarian capsule. Some women may develop recurrent hemorrhagic ovarian cysts that apparently cause pain and dyspareunia. Impaired blood supply to the ovaries has been implicated, especially after previous pelvic surgery, such as partial oophorectomy or hysterectomy (52). Bimanual examination reveals an adnexal enlargement with tenderness. Ultrasound may determine whether the cystic structure is complex or contains clear fluid. Resultant cyst formation may become painful. An ovary or ovarian remnant may become retroperitoneal secondary to inflammation or previous surgery (53).

Osteopathic treatment considerations for ovarian pain include treatment of somatic dysfunction of the thoracolumbar junction, assessment of sacral imbalance and leg length discrepancy, and identification of Chapman reflex areas. Mobilization of the spine addresses aberrant somatovisceral reflex pathways. Additional treatment of the sacral base and leg length discrepancies may mechanically affect and improve blood supply to the ovaries and the pelvis. Chapman reflex areas identify possible related somatic dysfunction of the reproductive system and gastrointestinal tract.

Uterine Pain

Pelvic pain is not usually the result of variations in uterine position in the pelvis. Deep dyspareunia may occasionally be associated with retroversion, whereby the pelvic nerves are irritated by stretching of the uterosacral ligaments, and pelvic veins become congested from uterine heaviness and position (54).

A tender uterus that is noted on pelvic examination to be fixed in retrogression should arouse suspicions of other intraperitoneal pathology, such as endometriosis or pelvic inflammatory disease. Laparoscopy is indicated to evaluate all pelvic structures. Pelvic heaviness and low back pain may be present with advanced degrees of uterine prolapse. Before deciding on hysterectomy as a course of treatment, some of these symptoms may be remedied by use of a pessary. Low back pain may respond to osteopathic treatment of the pelvic diaphragm or myofascial trigger points in the vaginal floor or rectum. Application of deep inhibitory pressure may relieve back or pelvic pain in addition to identifying and treating pelvic and lower extremity somatic dysfunction (55). Under normal conditions, the chief characteristic of uterine support is its mobility, and any loss of this mobility or changes associated with altered positional relationships are important diagnostic signs. The structures involved in uterine support are the levator muscle and fascia of the pelvic floor, the paracervical and paravaginal tissues, which extend outward from the vagina to the pelvic walls and which include the cardinal and uterosacral ligaments, and the round ligaments, which assist in holding the uterus in its anterior position. Of these, the cardinal ligament is the most important. This structure consists of a loose meshwork of connective tissue, which cannot be palpated when it is relaxed, but which forms a very firm ligament when the area is under tension.

The concept of pelvic congestion syndrome has a variety of proponents. This syndrome has been described in multiparous women who have pelvic vein varicosities and congested pelvic organs (54). Pain is worse premenstrually and is aggravated by fatigue, standing, and sexual intercourse. In the clinical examination, the uterus is mobile, usually retroverted, soft and boggy, and slightly enlarged. There may be associated menorrhagia and urinary frequency (56). Dilated veins may be seen on venographic studies (57). Additional and independent factors other than venous congestion may be involved, as some women with pelvic varicosities have no pain. Surgery is not usually beneficial for this condition (58). There have been some uncontrolled observations of similar symptoms of pain and metrorrhagia occurring after tubal ligation, but no prospective studies have been performed (35). Structural and postural evaluation with palpatory examination of somatic dysfunction of the lumbar spine and pelvis may elucidate areas for osteopathic treatment to relieve muscle distress and improve circulation to the pelvis.

Uterine leiomyomas (fibroids) are smooth muscle tumors of the uterus that are the most common indication for major surgery in women. Twenty percent of women develop uterine fibroids by age 40 (3). Fibroids have the potential to grow to an enormous size but have low malignant potential. The majority cause no symptoms and may require no treatment other than careful ob-

servation. Occasionally, the patient may become aware of a lower abdominal fullness or mass above the pubic symphysis. Symptoms develop insidiously as the fibroid competes with neighboring organs for space in the pelvis. Symptoms include:

- Pressure
- Congestion
- Bloating
- Urinary frequency or retention
- Dysmenorrhea

Other causes of pain are the result of fibroid infarction with degeneration, torsion on the fibroid's pedicle, or compression of pelvic nerves. Occasionally, a submucous leiomyoma may attempt to protrude through the cervix, causing pain akin to that of vaginal childbirth.

Management of this condition includes addressing the patient's desire for preserving future fertility, along with careful observation. Myomectomy may be performed to maintain the uterus for future pregnancy. Uterine curettage or endometrial ablation may control menorrhagia. GnRH agonists have been used to shrink myomas to enhance fertility, as well as reduce intraoperative blood loss. Oral contraceptives also reduce menstrual flow, preserve fertility, and control dysmenorrhea. Hysterectomy is reserved for the symptomatic patient for whom reproductive capability is not an issue.

Adenomyosis may cause dysmenorrhea and menorrhagia, but rarely does it cause chronic intermenstrual pain. Adenomyosis is defined as the extension of endometrial glands and stroma into the uterine musculature. Approximately 15% of women develop varying degrees of adenomyosis in their late 30s and early 40s, and they may have associated endometriosis (35). Patients express that their dysmenorrhea is of a colicky nature. In 30% to 40% of patients with adenomyosis, the disease is an unexpected pathologic finding in a hysterectomy patient who did not experience menorrhagia or uterine enlargement (45). In the case of a large adenomyoma, pressure on the bladder or rectum may be reported by the patient. On pelvic examination, the uterus is symmetrically enlarged, but occasionally the uterus may enlarge asymmetrically, suggesting the presence of a fibroid. However, the adenomyomatous uterus is softer than a uterine myoma. Treatment depends on the specific symptoms and on the exclusion of other uterine pathologic conditions. Menorrhagia and dysmenorrhea, if not too severe, may be treated palliatively with NSAIDs, COX-2 inhibitors, oral contraceptives, or GnRH agonists (29). Osteopathic management consists of treating somatic dysfunction of the lumbar spine and pelvis, pelvic diaphragm, and muscles of the anterior abdominal wall that may be influenced by posture. Otherwise, hysterectomy may be indicated. The ovaries may be preserved if they are normal and if the patient is not menopausal.

Pelvic Inflammatory Disease

Pelvic inflammatory disease (PID) comprises a constellation of inflammatory disorders of the upper genital tract, including:

- Endometritis
- Salpingitis

- Tubo-ovarian abscess
- Pelvic peritonitis

The two most common conditions of PID in the nonpregnant patient are salpingo-oophoritis and tubo-ovarian abscess. The diagnosis of acute salpingo-oophoritis is often made inappropriately (59,60). The patient usually presents with lower quadrant abdominal pain that is frequently bilateral. She may have recently started her menstrual period. Additional symptoms may include nausea, dysuria, and purulent vaginal discharge. Abdominal examination reveals generalized tenderness without palpable masses. Bimanual examination reveals cervical motion tenderness and bilateral adnexal tenderness. Usually there are no adnexal masses. Differential diagnoses must include (60):

- Acute appendicitis
- Urinary tract infection
- Adnexal torsion
- Endometriosis
- Hemorrhagic corpus luteum cyst
- Ectopic pregnancy

The definitive diagnosis is confirmed by laparoscopy or laparotomy, especially when the patient is unresponsive to antibiotic therapy. If surgery is not indicated, empirical treatment with broad-spectrum antibiotics may be initiated on an outpatient or inpatient basis until the infectious agent is identified (61). Medication alterations are then based on laboratory results. Patients with acute tubo-ovarian abscess experience:

- Severe pain in the low abdomen/pelvis
- High fever
- Nausea and vomiting
- Impending septic shock

Abdominal examination reveals marked tenderness with muscular rigidity, a pelvic mass, and rebound tenderness. Bimanual pelvic examination is extremely difficult because of the abdominal pain. An adnexal mass may be discovered. It may be easier during a rectal examination to recognize a pelvic mass that may be directed into the cul-de-sac.

Differential diagnosis may include the following:

- Septic incomplete abortion
- Uterine rupture
- Acute appendicitis with possible rupture
- Peritonitis with or without abscess formation
- Diverticular abscess (in left-sided pain)
- Adnexal torsion
- Perforated peptic ulcer
- Pancreatitis
- Mesenteric artery thrombosis

Laboratory results of any vaginal cultures confirm the infectious cause. Sonography may demonstrate adnexal pathology or cul-de-sac flocculation.

The treatment plan includes hospitalization with intravenous hydration, analgesics, and systemic antibiotics. Abscesses may resolve without need for acute surgical intervention. Timing of surgical intervention requires clinical judgment. Should the patient not respond to 72 hours of multiagent broad-spectrum antibiotics and have persistent spiking fevers, urgent surgery may be necessary to remove affected pelvic organs that have become infected by the ruptured abscess. Drainage and lavage of the peritoneal cavity may conserve pelvic organs.

Chronic PID may cause pain because of recurrent exacerbation that requires antibiotic therapy or because of hydrosalpinges and adhesion formation around the tubes, ovaries, and intestines. Endometriosis is the most frequently encountered differential diagnosis, particularly if there is no well-documented history of acute infection. Before ascribing pain symptoms to adhesions, one should note adhesions specifically in the area of pain localization. Some patients with extensive pelvic adhesions may be asymptomatic. Laparoscopy or laparotomy may be required to identify the adhesions.

Osteopathic considerations for treatment of PID include evaluation and treatment of somatic dysfunction at T11-L2 to improve circulation, and at the sacrum and related pelvic bones to balance the nervous system, as well as improve body fluid circulation/lymphatic drainage.

Pelvic Floor Dysfunction

Pelvic floor muscle dysfunction can contribute to many conditions, including:

- Urinary stress incontinence
- Fecal incontinence
- Sexual dysfunction
- Pelvic relaxation
- Levator ani syndromes

These problems are underreported, embarrassing, and undertreated (62). Symptoms of these problems may limit a woman's activities of daily living. Pelvic floor dysfunctions are often preventable; emphasis should be placed on prevention through education and exercise before problems arise (63).

Women are twice as likely as men to be incontinent (64). Denial is common because many patients believe that it is an inevitable result of childbirth and aging. Involuntary loss of urine during physical activity is called stress incontinence. Nygaard et al. (65,66) studied the relationship between exercise and incontinence and found that 47% of regularly exercising women experience some degree of incontinence. Of 326 women, 22% were nulliparous. High-impact exercises (running and jumping) resulted in even more episodes of incontinence than did low-impact activities. Women who frequently exercised addressed their incontinence by wearing protective pads, staying close to a toilet, and limiting fluid intake (67).

Urogynecologic dysfunctions have multifactorial causes that require medical evaluation and urodynamic testing. When an evaluation indicates muscle dysfunction, an osteopathic physician may gain additional insight from understanding interrelationship between structure and function of the pelvic structures. Successful manipulative treatment and exercise depend on the condition of the sensory and motor system of the patient. A routine pelvic examination may identify poor performance of pelvic floor musculature. Further examination should include visual inspection of the perineum during a pelvic floor contraction to note whether the proper muscles are contracting and relaxing, and digital palpation to detect muscle strength or pain. Note any cystocele, rectocele, or poorly repaired episiotomies. Uterine or vaginal prolapse should be noted.

Pelvic relaxation with decrease in normal pelvic floor support can occur with congenital or developmental weakness of the supportive structures, or when pelvic structures (especially the pudendal nerve) are damaged during childbirth (68). Even if the pelvic floor muscles are not damaged in vaginal delivery, the muscles must accommodate the passage of the fetus through the pelvis. Scar tissue may limit muscle contractility (69). Postpartum patients are often afraid to recondition the perineum because of pain, and they usually fail to perform the Kegel exercises taught in childbirth classes (70,71). Manipulative treatment can be very beneficial in improving muscle tone and general nervous and circulatory function; particularly in correcting associated postural imbalance. Nervous system dysfunction may be affected by uterine displacement and sacral base dysfunction (54).

The fascia and support structures are also influenced by menopause and aging (72). Changes in the pelvic floor from chronic constipation and straining during defecation can lead to anorectal incontinence with outstretched perineum and sphincter denervation (73). Chronic cough also strains the muscles of the pelvic floor (74). Kegel exercises, developed in the 1950s, were meant to address early stages of pelvic relaxation, not to prevent the need for surgery (70). Although the mechanism by which these exercises alleviate dysfunction is not fully understood, the patient benefits from regular contraction and relaxation of isolated muscle groups to increase motor recruitment abilities.

Hypertonus dysfunctions of musculoskeletal and urogynecologic systems are known as the levator ani syndrome (75). Poorly localized pain is the primary symptom. The pain may be located in perivaginal or perirectal areas, in lower abdominal quadrants, and in the pelvis. Vulvar or clitoral burning may sometimes be present. Pain can also be located in suprapubic or coccyx regions, even down the posterior thigh. More specific symptoms reported by women with hypertonus dysfunction include (76):

- Dysmenorrhea
- Dyspareunia
- Sexual dysfunction
- Voiding difficulty
- Urinary frequency/urgency

Tension myalgia of the pelvic floor is a spectrum of diagnoses of various syndromes of pelvic musculature, including piriformis syndrome, levator ani syndrome, coccygodynia, and vaginismus (77). Other diagnoses with a component of hypertonus dysfunction include (78,79):

- Chronic low back pain
- Endometriosis
- Chronic pelvic pain with negative surgical findings
- Interstitial cystitis
- Urethral syndrome
- Sphincter dyssynergia

Chronic pelvic pain is the second most common complaint in gynecologic practice. Musculoskeletal postural dysfunction has been implicated and can lead to levator ani syndrome by maintaining inefficient holding patterns of muscles that contribute to the persistence of pain (79–81). Somatic dysfunction of the pelvis, if untreated, may cause hypertonus as a result of restriction of motion of pelvic joints and their related structures. Myofascial pain syndromes create pain, tenderness, and autonomic phenomena from myofascial trigger points. Travell and Simons (82) have identified trigger points in these muscles:

- Coccygeus
- Levator ani
- Obturator internus
- Adductor magnus
- Piriformis or oblique abdominals

These pelvic muscle somatic dysfunctions may be treated with bimanual relaxation of muscle contractions. The vaginal palpating digits may apply inhibitory pressure, or use principles of counterstrain or myofascial technique to achieve release of tension or spasm. Identification of Chapman reflex points may also direct the osteopathic physician to treat related somatic dysfunction within the pelvis (83).

OTHER ORGANIC CAUSES OF PELVIC PAIN

Because the uterus and fallopian tubes share the innervation of the lower intestinal tract, pelvic pain can be nongynecologic in origin. Gastrointestinal sources of pelvic pain include:

- Penetrating neoplasms of the GI tract
- Irritable bowel syndrome
- Partial bowel obstruction
- Inflammatory bowel disease
- Diverticulitis
- Hernia formation

Osteopathic consideration for treatment involves addressing somatic dysfunction of the thoracolumbar spine, pelvis, and lower extremities to improve circulation and enhance lymphatic drainage. Chapman reflex areas aid with differential diagnosis (83). Counterstrain tender point treatment relieves the somatic dysfunction component of GI pain.

Low back pain of neuromuscular origin usually increases with activity and stress. Chronic low back pain without lower abdominal pain is seldom of gynecologic origin (84). Occasionally, a pelvic mass accompanied by neuromuscular symptoms may be revealed during surgical exploration to be a neuroma or bony tumor (85).

CONCLUSION

Although gynecologists are trained to perform surgery on female patients, osteopathically trained gynecologists develop an appreciation of the architecture and engineering of the pelvis. Through use of skilled palpatory evaluation of a patient's internal and external body structure, they have the opportunity to both diagnose and prevent dysfunction that has been influenced by the musculoskeletal system. Appropriately used osteopathic manipulative treatment offers relief of gynecologic pain that is not available by surgery or pharmacology.

REFERENCES

1. Still AT. *The Philosophy and Mechanical Principles of Osteopathy.* Kansas City, MO: Hudson-Kimberly Publishing Co; 1902.
2. Clemente CD. *Gray's Anatomy,* 30th ed. Philadelphia, PA: Lea & Febiger; 1985.
3. Scott JR, DiSaia P. *Danforth's Obstetrics and Gynecology,* 7th ed. Philadelphia, PA: JB Lippincott Co; 1994:105–128.
4. Mattingly RF, Thompson JD. *Te Linde's Operative Gynecology.* Philadelphia, PA: JB Lippincott Cop; 1985.
5. DeLancey J, Richardson AC. Anatomy of genital support. In: Benson JT, ed. *Female Pelvic Floor Disorders.* New York, NY: WW Norton; 1992.
6. Moore KL. *Clinically Oriented Anatomy,* 3rd ed. Baltimore, MD: Williams & Wilkins; 1992:342–349.
7. Mostwin J. Current concepts of female pelvic anatomy and physiology. *Urol Clin North Am.* 1991;18:175–195.
8. Spence-Jones C, Kamm MA, Henry MM, et al. Bowel dysfunction: A pathogenic factor in uterovaginal prolapse and urinary stress incontinence. *Br J Obstet Gynaecol.* 1994;101:147–152.
9. Graber B, Kline-Graber G. Female orgasm: Role of pubococcygeus muscle. *J Can Psychiatry.* 1979;40:348–351.
10. Beal MC. Viscerosomatic reflexes: A review. *J Am Osteopath Assoc.* 1985;185:786–801.
11. Walker E, Katon W, Harrop-Griffiths J, et al. Relationship of chronic pelvic pain to psychiatric diagnoses and childhood sexual abuse. *Am J Psychiatry.* 1988;145:75–80.
12. Smith RP. Identifying the causes of pelvic pain. *The Female Patient.* 1993;18:41–51.
13. Scialli AR. Evaluating the patient with chronic pelvic pain. *OBG Management.* 2000;February:7–11.
14. Glintner KP. Chronic pelvic pain. *J Am Osteopath Assoc.* 1974;74:335–340.
15. Gambone JC, Lench JB, Slesinski MJ, et al. Validation of hysterectomy indications and the quality assurance process. *Obstet Gynecol.* 1989;73:1045–1049.
16. Reiter RC, Milburn A. Exploring effective treatment for chronic pelvic pain. *Contemp OB/GYN.* 1994:84–89.
17. Perez-Stable EJ, Miranda J, Munoz RF, et al. Depression in medical outpatients: Under-recognition and misdiagnosis. *Arch Intern Med.* 1990;150:1083–1089.
18. Harrop-Griffith J, Katon W, Walker E. The association between chronic pelvic pain, psychiatric diagnosis, and childhood sex abuse. *Obstet Gynecol.* 1988;71:589–594.
19. Clemons J, Arya LA, Myers DL. Diagnosing interstitial cystitis in women with chronic pelvic pain. *Obstet Gynecol.* 2001;97:S7–S8.
20. Barbieri RL. Evaluating pelvic pain using Barbieri's Triad. *OBG Management.* 2000;12:26–39.
21. Barbieri RL, Propst AM. Physical examination findings in women with endometriosis: Uterosacral ligament abnormalities, lateral cervical displacement, and cervical stenosis. *J Gynecol Techniques.* 1999;4:1–3.
22. Propst AM, Storti K, Barbieri RL. Lateral cervical displacement is associated with endometriosis. *Fertil Steril.* 1998;70:568–570.
23. Rapkin AJ, Reading AE. Chronic pelvic pain. *Curr Probl Obstet Gynecol.* 1991;49:99–106.
24. Burrows EA. Disorders of the female reproductive system. In: Hoag JM, Cole WV, Bradford S, eds. *Osteopathic Medicine.* New York, NY: McGraw-Hill; 1969:676–684.
25. Wood DP, Wiesner MG, Reiter RC. Psychogenic chronic pelvic pain, diagnosis, and management. *Clin Obstet Gynecol.* 1990;33:179–195.
26. Pickles VR. A plain muscle stimulant in the menstruum. *Nature.* 1957;180:1198–1199.
27. Rosenwaks Z, Seegar-Jones G. Menstrual pain: Its origin and pathogenesis. *J Reprod Med.* 1980;25:207–212.
28. Barbieri RL. Stenosis of the external cervical os: An association with endometriosis in women with chronic pelvic pain. *Fertil Steril.* 1998;70:571–573.
29. Minjarez DA, Schlaff WD. Update on the medical treatment of endometriosis. *Obstet Gynecol Clin North Am.* 2000;27:641–651.
30. Boesler D, Warner M, Alpers A, et al. Efficacy of high velocity, low amplitude manipulative techniques in subjects with low back pain during menstrual cramping. *J Am Osteopath Assoc.* 1993;93:203–214.
31. Hitchcock ME. The manipulative approach to the management of primary dysmenorrhea. *J Am Osteopath Assoc.* 1976;75:109–118.
32. Chapman JD. Progress in scientifically proving the benefits of OMT in treating symptoms of dysmenorrhea. *J Am Osteopath Assoc.* 1993;93:196.
33. Lapp T. ACOG issues recommendations for the management of endometriosis. American College of Obstetricians and Gynecologists. *Am Fam Physician.* 2000;62:1431–1434.
34. Kuchera M, Kuchera W. *Osteopathic Considerations in Systemic Dysfunction.* Columbus, OH: Greyden Press; 1994:139–142.
35. Hacker N, Moore JG. *Essentials of Obstetrics and Gynecology.* Philadelphia, PA: WB Saunders; 1996.
36. Frank RT. The hormonal causes of pre-menstrual tension. *Arch Neurol Psychiatry.* 1931;26:1053–1064.
37. Greene R, Dalton K. The pre-menstrual syndrome. *BMJ.* 1953;1:1007–1009.
38. Steiner M, Born L. Diagnosis and treatment of PMDD: An update. *Int Clin Psychopharmacol.* 2000;3:S5–S17.
39. Frackiewicz EJ, Shiovitz TM. Evaluation and management of premenstrual syndrome and premenstrual dysphoric disorder. *J Am Pharm Assoc (Wash).* 2001;41:437–447.
40. Steiner M, Romano SJ, Babcock S, et al. The efficacy of fluoxitine in improving physical symptoms associated with premenstrual dysphoric disorder. *BJOG.* 2001;108:462–468.
41. Herbal treatment for PMS? *Harv Womens Health Watch.* 2001;8:7.
42. Khoo SK, Monroe C, Battistutta D. Evening primrose oil and treatment of premenstrual syndrome. *Med J Aust.* 1990;153:189–192.
43. Starzinski M. Pre-menstrual syndrome: Update and osteopathic approach to treatment. *Osteopath Ann.* 1987;14:39–42.
44. Perry CP. Criteria that indicate endometriosis is the cause of chronic pelvic pain. *Obstet Gynecol.* 1999;93:473.
45. Adamson G. Diagnosis and clinical presentation of endometriosis. *Am J Obstet Gynecol.* 1990;162:568–569.
46. Wolfman WL, Kreutner K. Laparoscopy in children and adolescents. *J Adolesc Health.* 1984;5:261–265.
47. Wellbery C. Diagnosis and treatment of endometriosis. *Am Fam Physician.* 1999;60:1767–1768.
48. Moore JG, Binstock MA, Growdon WA. The clinical implications of retroperitoneal endometriosis. *Am J Obstet Gynecol.* 1988;158:1291–1298.
49. Ranney B. Endometriosis I: Conservative operations. *Am J Obstet Gynecol.* 1970;107:743–753.
50. Revised American Fertility Society classification of endometriosis. *Fertil Steril.* 1985;43:351–352.
51. Prentice A, Deary AJ, Goldbeck-Wood S, et al. Gonadotrophin-releasing hormone analogues for pain associated with endometriosis. *Cochrane Database Syst Rev.* 2000;CD000346.
52. Dicker RC, Greenspan JR, Strauss LT, et al. Complications of vaginal and abdominal hysterectomy in the United States. The collaborative review of sterilization. *Am J Obstet Gynecol.* 1982;144:841–848.
53. Pettit PD, Lee RA. Ovarian remnant syndrome: Diagnostic dilemma and surgical challenges. *Obstet Gynecol.* 1988;71:580–583.
54. Taylor HC. Vascular congestion and hyperemia: Their effect on structure and function of the female reproductive system: Parts I and II. *Am J Obstet Gynecol.* 1949;57:211–221.
55. Taylor HC. Pelvic pain based on a vascular and autonomic nervous system disorder. *Am J Obstet Gynecol.* 1954;57:1177–1182.
56. Mathis BV, Miller JS, Lukens ML, et al. Pelvic congestion syndrome: A new approach to an unusual problem. *Am Surg.* 1995;61:1016–1018.

57. Harris RD, Holtzman SR, Poppe AM. Clinical outcome in female patients with pelvic pain and normal pelvic US findings. *Radiology.* 2000; 216:440–443.

58. Duncan CH, Taylor HC. A psychosomatic study of pelvic congestion. *Am J Obstet Gynecol.* 1952;64:1–8.

59. Stones RW, Mountfield J. Intervention for treating chronic pelvic pain in women (Cochrane Review). *Cochrane Database Syst Rev.* 2000; CD000387.

60. Toth A. Alternative causes of pelvic inflammatory disease. *J Reprod Med.* 1983;28:699–702.

61. American College of Obstetricians and Gynecologists (ACOG). *Technical Bulletin 153: Antimicrobial therapy for gynecological infections.* Washington, DC: The American College of Obstetricians and Gynecologists; 1991.

62. Physicians hear about incontinence [editorial]. *JAMA.* 1990;264:2381–2382.

63. Pope CS, Rabin J. Urinary incontinence: Evaluation and non-surgical management. *The Female Patient.* 2001;26:41–47.

64. Urinary Incontinence Guideline Panel. *Urinary Incontinence in Adults. Clinical Practice Guidelines.* Rockville, MD: United States Department of Health and Human Services; 1992.

65. Nygaard I, DeLancey JO, Arnsdorf L, et al. Exercise and incontinence. *Obstet Gynecol.* 1990;75:848–851.

66. Nygaard I, Thompson FL. Urinary incontinence in elite nulliparous athletes. *Obstet Gynecol.* 1994;84:183–187.

67. Wallace K. Female pelvic floor functions, dysfunctions, and behavioral approaches to treatment. *Clin Sports Med.* 1994;13:459–481.

68. Sampselle CM, Miller JM, Mims BL. Effect of pelvic muscle exercise on transient incontinence during pregnancy and after birth. *Obstet Gynecol.* 1998;91:406–412.

69. Fitzpatrick M, O'Herlilhy C. The effects of labour and delivery on the pelvic floor. *Baillieres Best Pract Res Clin Obstet Gynaecol.* 2001;15:63–79.

70. Kegel A. Early genital relaxation: New technique of diagnosis and non-surgical treatment. *Obstet Gynecol.* 1956;8:545–550.

71. Morkved S, Bo K. The effect of post-partum pelvic muscle floor exercise in the prevention and treatment of urinary incontinence. *Int Urogynecol J.* 1997;8:217–222.

72. Fantl JA, Bump RC, Robinson D. Efficacy of estrogen supplementation in the treatment of urinary incontinence. *Obstet Gynecol.* 1996;88:745–749.

73. Halligan S, Bartram CR. Evaculation, proctography, combined with positive contrast peritoneography to demonstrate pelvic floor hernias. *Abdom Imaging.* 1995;20:442–445.

74. Swami SS, Abrahams P. Urge incontinence. *Urol Clin North Am.* 1996;23:417–425.

75. Salvati E. The levator syndrome and its variant. *Gastroenterol Clin North Am.* 1987;16:71–78.

76. Clock SC. Female sexuality and sexual counseling. *Curr Probl Obstet Gynecol Fertil.* 1993;16:107–139.

77. Sinaki IM, Merritt J, Stillwell GK. Tension myalgia of the pelvic floor. *Mayo Clin Proc.* 1977;52:717–722.

78. Benson JT. *Female Pelvic Floor Disorders: Investigation and Management.* New York, NY: WW Norton; 1992.

79. King PM. Musculoskeletal factors in chronic pelvic pain. *J Psychosom Obstet Gynaecol.* 1991;12:87–98.

80. McCandless S, Mason G. Physical therapy as an effective change agent in the treatment of patients with urinary incontinence. *J Miss State Med Assoc.* 1995;36:2714.

81. Cammu H, Nylan MV. Pelvic floor exercises in genuine urinary stress incontinence. *Int Urogynecol J.* 1997;8:297–300.

82. Travell J, Simons D. *Myofascial Pain and Dysfunction: The Trigger Point Manual, Volume 2: The Lower Extremities.* Baltimore, MD: Williams & Wilkins; 1992.

83. Owens C. *An Endocrine Interpretation of Chapman's Reflexes,* 2nd ed. Chattanooga, TN: Chattanooga Printing & Engraving Co; 1937.

84. Holley R, Richter H, Wang L. Neurologic disease presenting as chronic pelvic pain. *South Med J.* 1999;92:1105–1107.

85. Malinak LR. Operative management of pelvic pain. *Clin Obstet Gynecol.* 1980;23:191–200.

29

NEUROMUSCULOSKELETAL MEDICINE AND OSTEOPATHIC MANIPULATIVE MEDICINE

RAYMOND J. HRUBY

KEY CONCEPTS

- The development of the earned fellowship in the American Academy of Osteopathy
- The evolution of certification in neuromusculoskeletal medicine and osteopathic manipulative medicine
- The development of the hospital-based osteopathic manipulative medicine consultation and treatment service
- The role of the osteopathic manipulative medicine specialist
- The examination and treatment of acutely ill hospitalized patients
- The osteopathic manipulative medicine consultation in the hospital
- Recording structural diagnosis and treatment of hospitalized patients
- A case study in critical thinking for the osteopathic manipulative medicine specialist

Osteopathic principles and philosophy (OPP) and the practice of osteopathic manipulative treatment (OMT) are part of the education of every osteopathic physician. These elements are incorporated into the everyday practice of osteopathic medicine. Like other areas of medicine, over time a need developed for osteopathic physicians with special expertise in these distinctive elements of osteopathic medicine. Thus, the specialist in osteopathic manipulative medicine (now called neuromusculoskeletal medicine, or NMM) and OMT was born. These specialists are primarily responsible for the further expansion of osteopathic concepts and methods, and they contribute this expanded knowledge to the profession through teaching, writing, and specialized clinical practice. The need to recognize this special expertise in NMM and OMT led to the development of a primary certification in this area through the American Osteopathic Association and to the development of an earned fellowship through the American Academy of Osteopathy.

In 1958, a meeting was held by a committee comprised of representatives from the Academy of Applied Osteopathy (AAO, now called the American Academy of Osteopathy) and the American Osteopathic Association (AOA). This committee met to study and to establish the fellowship program of the Academy of Applied Osteopathy (FAAO). The program was to recognize doctors of osteopathy (DOs) with special expertise in manipulative skills and to encourage other DOs to improve their skills. In 1959, the following paragraph appeared in the directory of the Academy of Applied Osteopathy:

> A proposal was presented to the Board of Governors of the Academy, and to a special committee of the Advisory Board for Osteopathic Specialists for the formation of a new certifying board called the American Osteopathic Board of Manipulative Arts and Sciences. The proposal was made by a group of osteopathic physicians headed by Dr. T. F. Schooley, Phoenix, Arizona. Proposals for certification in the field of manipulative therapy have been studied for several years with no success in reaching agreement relative to the propriety and value of such a program. Those favoring such a step contend that there must be established a means of recognizing and accrediting the members of the profession who have developed a high degree of knowledge and skill in the field, and whose practices are based principally upon the structural approach. Those opposed to certification in the field contend that the manipulative application of osteopathic principles is basic to every osteopathic physician's approach to the problems presented by his patients, and certification of this basic and fundamental aspect of osteopathy would be improper and would limit the profession. All who have studied the matter are in agreement that a means must be established for recognizing ability in the field (1).

In 1960, the committee presented detailed recommendations for the functioning of the Board on fellowship, which was adopted by the Academy's Board of Governors and the AOA's Board of Trustees. The fellowship was described as an "earned" fellowship because it required certain prerequisites, a 5,000 word written thesis, and oral, written, and practical examinations. The FAAO process was thus established.

In 1971, a joint committee of representatives from the AAO and the AOA met to discuss the steps necessary to convert the FAAO process to certification in osteopathic manipulative medicine. A resolution to this effect was presented to the AOA Board of Trustees but was not approved. However, in 1977, the AOA Board of Trustees did approve certification for the FAAO. The Board on Fellowship now became an AOA board directly responsible to the Board of Trustees. Residency programs in osteopathic manipulative medicine were developed by the American Osteopathic Board on Fellowship in the American Academy of Osteopathy (AOBFAAO).

Over the years, the AOBFAAO underwent several name changes. In 1983, the AOA asked for a name change for the board, and the Academy submitted the name "American Board on Osteopathic Manipulative Medicine." This was approved by the AOA Board of Trustees in July 1984, but because of subsequent opposition to this name by other constituents of the profession, the name was later returned to the AOBFAAO. In 1989, to parallel similar processes in other AOA specialty colleges, the AOA requested that the combined processes of certification in OMM and conferring of the FAAO be separated. This was accomplished with the FAAO now being adjudicated by a Committee on Fellowship within the AAO. A new certifying board was formulated and named the American Osteopathic Board on Special Proficiency in Osteopathic Manipulative Medicine (AOBSPOMM). The AOBSPOMM was a certifying board directly responsible to the AOA Board of Trustees. In 1999, the AOBSPOMM was changed to the "American Osteopathic Board on Neuromusculoskeletal Medicine and Osteopathic Manipulative Medicine." Osteopathic physicians who successfully pass this Board's examination are issued certificates indicating that they are certified in neuromusculoskeletal medicine and osteopathic manipulative treatment. Tables 29.1 and 29.2 describe the current requirements for certification in NMM and OMT, and the requirements for achieving the FAAO, respectively.

THE DEVELOPMENT OF THE HOSPITAL-BASED OSTEOPATHIC MANIPULATIVE MEDICINE CONSULTATION AND TREATMENT SERVICE

As osteopathic hospitals were developed in the early years of the profession, OMT was an essential part of the treatment of hospitalized patients. With the development of specialties and subspecialties within the osteopathic profession, it became more difficult for these DOs to provide regular OMT to their hospital patients, due to increasing patient loads, time constraints, and the overall demands of specialty practices. As a result, DOs who had more extensive training in OMT and who dedicated much of their patient care to the use of distinctive osteopathic methods were called on to provide consultation and treatment for hospital patients. These DOs were viewed as specialists in OMM.

This type of practice gained further impetus and an expanded role with the development of a unique program at the Waterville Osteopathic Hospital in Waterville, Maine, in 1973. This hospital established the position of Director of Osteopathic Medicine, a full time osteopathic physician hired by the hospital to provide the basis for a consultation and treatment service in the areas of OMT and OPP. The first director of this service was Edward G. Stiles. His successful leadership of this program led

other osteopathic hospitals to provide similar services. In addition, Dr. Stiles did much to establish the role of the OMM specialist in such a setting. He described the elements of this role as follows:

> As developed by Waterville Osteopathic Hospital, the duties of the director of osteopathic medicine are as follows:
>
> i. The director is to provide clinical consultation services for referred patients and to document properly the osteopathic diagnosis and treatment utilized.
> ii. The director is to be an educator and to increase the staff's expertise and awareness of the applications and indications for osteopathic care. Creating a service of osteopathic medicine in a hospital setting provides a tremendous educational potential. The following educational tools can be utilized: (a) consultation reports; (b) courses in technique and principles; (c) committee reports on utilization of osteopathic manipulation; (d) departmental educational meetings; and (e) staff educational meetings. Each of these tools provides an opportunity to increase the awareness of the staff of the implications, applications, and indications for utilization of osteopathic care in a hospital environment. This naturally increases the awareness of the staff as to the types of patients who should be referred to this service and offers a challenge to staff members to improve their own levels of expertise in the delivery of health care.
> iii. The director of osteopathic medicine is to fill a public relations role for the hospital (2).

Doctor Stiles also made note of the research potential afforded by such a hospital-based service.

In recent years, a number of smaller osteopathic community hospitals in the United States have closed because of changes brought about by managed care and economic conditions. Other osteopathic hospitals have merged with allopathic institutions. Despite these changes in the health care climate, a few hospital-based osteopathic medicine services are still in operation.

THE ROLE OF THE OSTEOPATHIC MANIPULATIVE MEDICINE SPECIALIST

Today those DOs who have chosen to specialize in NMM and OMM continue to serve in expanded roles beyond those described above. Some of these roles include:

i. Providing outpatient consultation and treatment services.
ii. The private practice of NMM and OMM.
iii. Serving as medical and legal experts in NMM and OMM.
iv. Teaching at colleges of osteopathic medicine, either as full-time or part-time faculty.
v. Serving in administrative positions, such as department chairs or deans, in colleges of osteopathic medicine.
vi. Directing residency programs in NMM and OMM.
vii. Participating in research projects in NMM and OMM.
viii. Teaching in postgraduate training programs and in continuing education programs.
ix. Participating in international programs on manual medicine.
x. Writing scholarly works for journals and textbooks.

TABLE 29.1. CERTIFICATION AS A DIPLOMATE OF THE AMERICAN OSTEOPATHIC BOARD OF NEUROMUSCULOSKELETAL MEDICINE (AOBNMM)

A Doctor of Osteopathy may be certified by the Board of Trustees of the American Osteopathic Association in recognition of his/her proficiency in neuromusculoskeletal medicine and the use of osteopathic structural and palpatory diagnosis and manipulative treatment in the total health care of patients. Osteopathic physicians who have completed a residency in neuromusculoskeletal medicine may establish board eligibility. Until December 31, 2005, osteopathic physicians, whether in general practice or in any specialty practice, can also be so certified by fulfilling the appropriate eligibility requirements.

Minimum Requirements

I. The applicant must be a graduate of a college of osteopathic medicine approved by the American Osteopathic Association.

II. The applicant must be licensed to practice in a state, territory, province or country.

III. The applicant must be able to show evidence of conformity to the standards set in the Code of Ethics of the American Osteopathic Association.

IV. The applicant must have been a member in good standing of the American Osteopathic Association or the Canadian Osteopathic Association for a continuous period of at least 2 years prior to the date of certification.

V. The applicant must have completed satisfactorily an internship of at least 1 year in a hospital approved for intern training by the American Osteopathic Association.

VI. The applicant must have completed by AOBNMM application deadline:

    A. At least 2 years of an AOA-approved residency in neuromusculoskeletal treatment and osteopathic manipulative medicine and meet the AOA's criteria for board eligibility.

    B. Completion of the residency plus 1 year of neuromusculoskeletal medicine residency training option and who meets the AOA's criteria for board eligibility.

    C. If the board eligibility of a candidate who is a graduate of an neuromusculoskeletal residency program—either a 2-year AOA-approved residency program or if a residency plus 1 year of neuromusculoskeletal medicine residency training program has expired, the Academy will recognize the candidate as an applicant under the 5-year practice requirement under section D as follows:

    D. Until December 31, 2005, osteopathic physicians who graduated from AOA-approved colleges of osteopathic medicine prior to December 31, 1999, may qualify via a "practice track", i.e., they must complete 5 years of practice, which may include an AOA-approved residency in other than a neuromusculoskeletal medicine residency. This training shall include active experience in the use of structural diagnosis and manipulative management in osteopathic medicine, with CME documentation:

        1. Five years CME credits based only on the last 5 years from an AOA printout, average of 50 hours per year (minimum of 250 hours total) and of these.

        2. 150 hours (category 1-A only) must be programs sponsored by the American Academy of Osteopathy, or approved by the AOBNMM certifying board.

    E. Four years of practice plus a college of osteopathic medicine approved pre-doctoral fellowship in osteopathic manipulative medicine. The continuing medical education requirements as stated in D1 & 2 above are applicable; or

VII. The applicant must document his or her qualifications in the formal application.

VIII. The applicant must prepare and submit three case histories suitable for publication which document understanding of osteopathic sciences and their application in health and disease as it relates to his/her practice discipline. These cases should demonstrate breadth of knowledge, understanding and skills in various techniques, and paradigms, as well as will be expected on the written, oral and practical aspects of the certification exam. If a candidate's case(s) is(are) not approved, the candidate must submit an entirely new case(s) for the board's review.

IX. The board shall establish individual eligibility of the candidate for examination.

X. A written, oral, and practical examination will be required of each applicant.

(From information posted on the American Academy of Osteopathy website at *http://www.academyofosteopathy.org/certif.htm,* with permission.)

THE OSTEOPATH MANIPULATIVE MEDICINE SPECIALIST'S OSTEOPATHIC EXAMINATION OF THE HOSPITALIZED PATIENT

History Taking and Data Gathering

Begin the osteopathic history of the hospitalized patient with a review of the medical record, paying close attention to factors affecting or affected by the neuromusculoskeletal system. Next, take the patient's history. If the patient is unable to give the history because of age, neurologic damage, intubation, or other causes, ask a family member to provide the history. The history for the neuromusculoskeletal evaluation includes the routine medical and surgical history, in addition to questioning the patient or family member about previous injuries and structural abnormalities. Typically, the following are included in the patient's history:

Head trauma
Motor vehicle accidents
Pratfalls
Fractures

Episodes of loss of consciousness
Presence of known short leg
Scoliosis
Previous experience with osteopathic manipulative treatment (OMT)
Previous experience with other manual medicine modalities
Response to previous treatments

The historic data assist the physician in deciding which musculoskeletal areas might contain primary somatic dysfunction and/or which might contain secondary somatic dysfunction produced by somatovisceral reflexes from related visceral dysfunction. The history also assists in deciding which manipulative techniques are most appropriate.

Physical Examination

Begin the examination with a review of the patient's original radiographs. This is extremely important because bony and fascial abnormalities significant to the patient's disease process may not

TABLE 29.2. REQUIREMENTS FOR FELLOWSHIP IN THE AMERICAN ACADEMY OF OSTEOPATHY (FAAO)

Only AAO members may apply to the Fellowship Committee for examination pursuant to the earned Fellowship in the American Academy of Osteopathy (FAAO). Fellowship is awarded by the Academy's Board of Governors only upon the recommendation of the Fellowship Committee following successful completion of examination.

Purposes

1. To recognize continued and special achievement in the preservation and use of osteopathic principles and practices.
2. To acknowledge ability and service to the Academy and to the profession. Emphasis on the "categories" of activity as a gauge of achievement.
3. To maintain a group of leaders to encourage high standards of osteopathic medical practice with special emphasis on manipulative diagnosis and treatment, and to work for the integration of osteopathic concepts into all areas of practice. For this reason, physicians in other areas of practice or specialties are encouraged to qualify for this Fellowship.

Such leaders would serve as resources and inspiration for the entire profession, but especially for those who have sought certification in manipulative medicine under the requirements of the American Osteopathic Association.
Fellowship shall represent a second stage of high achievement in no way denigrating the importance of the first step which is Certification by the American Osteopathic Board of Special Proficiency in Osteopathic Manipulative Medicine or the American Osteopathic Board of Neuromusculoskeletal Medicine. It will represent an "earned" degree.

Requirements

1. Certification is a prerequisite, either in Special Proficiency in Osteopathic Manipulative Medicine or Neuromusculoskeletal Medicine and Osteopathic Manipulative Medicine.
2. Evidence of continued good standing in the American Osteopathic Association or the Canadian Osteopathic Association.
3. Membership in the American Academy of Osteopathy for a period of 5 years prior to application and to maintain Fellowship.
4. Practice requirement: Ordinarily, the practice requirements will be satisfied by the achievement of certification. At least 3 years of practice should intervene between the Certification and Fellowship application in the case of resident-trained candidates.
5. Scientific Paper/Thesis requirement: A Scientific Paper/Thesis (primary author) suitable for publication is required. Such papers shall not have been part of any qualification for another degree. The scientific paper/thesis will hopefully reflect originality and make some contribution to the body of osteopathic literature. A topic heading and brief outline and tentative bibliographyt (approximately 1–3 pages in length with appropriate explanatory statements) shall be approved prior to the writing of the scientific paper/thesis.
6. CME requirements shall include at least 30 hours of AAO-sponsored or Committee-approved training of each 50 hours per year as required by the AOA. The candidate will give evidence of this for the previous 3 years via the AOA CME printout. (There may be overlap here with the AOBSPOMM requirement.)
7. Case histories: ten case histories (not to include material supplied for certification) will be required.
8. Categories of service: the candidate shall supply evidence of fulfilling at least four of the six categories below:
   a. Contribution to osteopathic literature (specific publication, etc., should be listed).
   b. Development of osteopathic theory and/or manipulative method or procedure.
   c. Research related to osteopathic theory and practice.
   d. Contributions in the field of osteopathic education:
      Faculty (college, AAO, cranial, etc.)
      Visiting clinician
      Visiting scientist
      Preceptorship activity
      Clinical and/or hospital supervision and/or consultation
   e. AAO organizational activity (boards, committees, etc.)
   f. Public relations
      Community activity
      School physician
      Sponsor of health activity
      Public health service
      Other

Examinations

No written examination will be given, but in-depth oral and practical examinations will be required.

(From information posted on the American Academy of Osteopathy website at *http://www.academyofosteopathy.org/certif.htm*, with permission.)
CME, continuing medical education.

have been mentioned in the radiology report. Only after review of the chart and the original radiographs, and recording of an integrated history is the physician prepared to perform a physical examination of the patient. As with the history, integrate the osteopathic palpatory examination into the routine medical examination of the patient. The history and chief complaint dictate that some areas of the body must be more thoroughly investigated than others. It is generally easier to use a standard approach to the patient that can be modified slightly to fit each individual

patient's needs. Follow routine body fluid contamination procedures during the examination of all patients.

The following protocol is suggested, although alterations are necessary depending on the patient's needs and the physician's preference. This protocol is based primarily on the respiratory, circulatory, and neurologic models of osteopathic evaluation and treatment (4,5). Emphasize the major diaphragms of the body that impede normal fluid flow, and the bony and fascial attachments of those diaphragms. Emphasize rib function because of

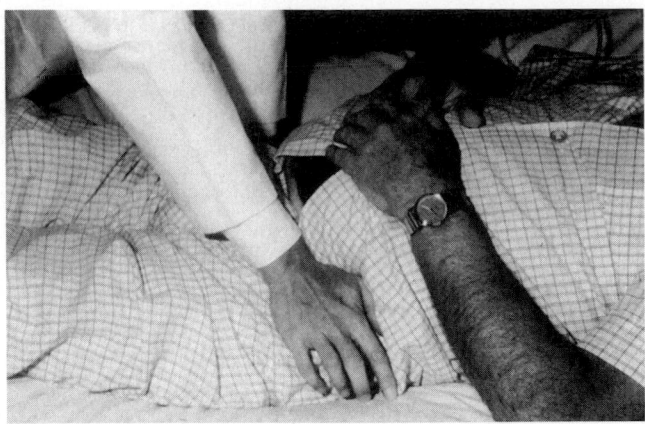

FIGURE 29.1. Anterior superior iliac spine compression test.

its relationship both to fluid movement within the body and to reflexes mediated by the sympathetic nervous system via the chain ganglia that lie anterior to the rib heads. Emphasize the paraspinal myofascial elements of the suboccipital, sacral, and thoracolumbar areas because of their involvement with autonomic reflexes that manifest in these areas.

If the patient is ambulatory, the musculoskeletal examination is not significantly different from an outpatient structural evaluation. However, the routine outpatient musculoskeletal examination is not appropriate for acutely ill patients. A bedside osteopathic evaluation in the supine position is necessary. A suggested examination begins with bilateral compression of the anterior superior iliac spines (ASISs), the ASIS compression test. This test indicates restrictions in iliosacral mobility that interfere with sacral and pubic motion, and pelvic diaphragm tension (Fig. 29.1).

Evaluate and treat the sacrum and lumbar areas from the patient's side. Generally, the patient is lying on an absorbent pad over a draw sheet and fitted mattress sheet. The sacrum and lumbar areas are easily approached by slipping the hands under the patient, palms up, between the draw sheet and the fitted mattress sheet. This is made easier by loosening the draw sheet from under the mattress and rolling it up parallel to the patient on either side of the bed (Fig. 29.2). This rolled-up draw sheet serves as a sling with which the patient can be gently lifted and rolled away, enabling the physician to place a hand under the pelvic or lumbar area without any effort required by the patient. Although this treatment procedure requires palpating and treating through the thickness of the absorbent pad and draw sheet, it becomes easy with practice. This approach also protects the patient's modesty, and the physician is less likely to come into contact with any discharge, drainage, urine, or feces in the bed.

Next, place the fingertips of one hand at the inferolateral angle of the sacrum and the fingertips of the other hand at the ipsilateral sacral base (Fig. 29.3). Exert alternate pressure in an anterior direction with the fingertips, ascertaining the ability of the sacrum to rock on its L-shaped articulation. This procedure reveals sacral motion restrictions.

Next, place one or both hands under the patient's lumbar spine, and assess the tissue texture changes and motion restrictions of the lumbar spine according to the protocol suggested by Larson (3). This is carried out by pressing anteriorly on the paraspinal elements. First note tissue texture changes, then note any ease in

rotatory motion induced by using an alternating anterior pressure on the transverse processes. The characteristic texture changes resulting from viscerosomatic referral are most easily discerned with the patient supine, and with the examiner executing anterior palpatory pressure. With the patient relaxed as much as possible, estimate the degree of lumbar lordosis.

If the patient is not in the immediate postoperative period after abdominal or pelvic surgery, palpate the abdomen for visceral dysfunction. Assess restrictions of the thoracoabdominal diaphragm by placing one hand under the patient at the T10-L2 area posteriorly, and the other hand anteriorly, just inferior to the xiphoid process. One hand gently twists the underlying fascia clockwise while the other hand twists counterclockwise; then, reverse the direction of testing. The abdominal diaphragm dysfunction is named according to the direction of preferred fascial movement sensed by the abdominal hand.

Assess the excursion of the lower and upper ribs by having the patient breathe deeply. Lightly palpate the rib cage at the midaxillary line for the lower ribs. Palpate over the midclavicular line lateral to the sternum for the upper ribs. If the patient has a chest tube in place or is on a respirator, follow the motion present by lightly resting hands on the rib cage. Gently rest the palpating hand on the sternum and follow its motion, noting any fascial pulls and any costosternal articular restrictions (Fig. 29.4). Perform a screen of the anterior Chapman (6) and Jones points (7) in the thoracic and abdominal areas. Note any specific rib restrictions so that they can be treated later. Note the symmetry of the thorax and tension of the accessory muscles of respiration.

Adjust the bed to place the patient in the Fowler position (approximately 15 degrees of head elevation), elevating the mattress until it is even with the top of the headboard. Move to the head of the bed and remove the patient's pillow. This positioning allows treatment with minimal stooping and without removing the headboard. If the Fowler position is contraindicated, the entire bed may be elevated. The bed may need to be pushed away from the wall to permit access to the head of the bed. Be careful not to disturb peripheral and central lines, suction tubing, urinary catheters, and other bedside obstacles. Follow this same procedure in the intensive care unit as well. If the patient is on a respirator, treat him or her in the position dictated by the life support systems.

Standing and leaning over the head of the bed, place a hand on each side of the patient's head, palms facing upward, and glide them between the draw sheet and the bed, or between the bed sheet and the mattress, down to the T12-L2 area of the patient's back (Fig. 29.5). With elbows leaning on the head of the bed for support, place the fingertips over the transverse processes. Push anteriorly with the fingertips of both hands, first assessing the tissue texture changes. Then, push alternately to assess the rotatory motion of the paraspinal elements. This is the same assessment used for the lumbar area. Move the hands more cephalad and repeat the process until the entire thoracic spine has been evaluated. Also note fascial restrictions of the thorax and further define rib somatic dysfunction noted on the rib motion screening examination. Place the fingertips of the anterior hand against the costochondral junction, and those of the posterior hand at the rib head of the same rib (Fig. 29.6).

Next, evaluate the thoracic inlet for fascial restrictions (Fig. 29.7). If the patient has any central venous lines, the hand

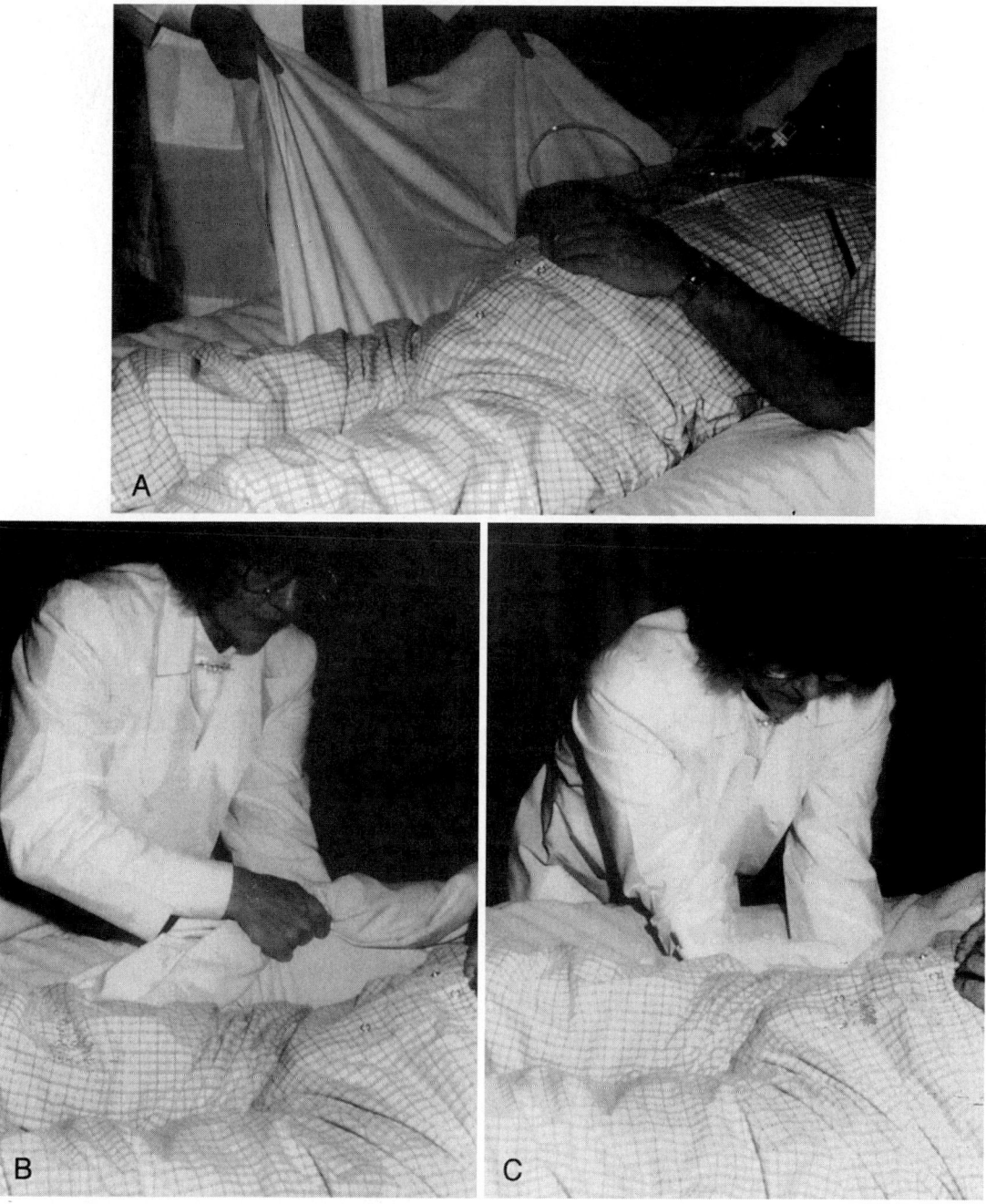

FIGURE 29.2. Draw sheet sling for posterior palpation and treatment of the patient. **A:** Loosen draw sheet from under the mattress. **B:** Roll draw sheet parallel to the patient. **C:** Place hands between the draw sheet and the mattress to contact lumbar areas.

on that side must be placed more laterally, near the acromioclavicular joint. The presence of these lines does not contraindicate evaluating and treating this area but makes it even more imperative that it be evaluated. Evaluate the cervical area for the presence of somatic dysfunction.

Assess the suboccipital area for condylar compression and occipito-atlantal (O-A) and atlanto-axial (A-A) somatic dysfunction (Fig. 29.8). Gently cradle the head and upper cervical area with the fingertips and hands. If craniosacral diagnosis is to be performed, the cranium is now palpated for somatic dysfunction. The cranium can be evaluated with many hand positions. In one position (Fig. 29.9), the palms and fingertips gently rest on the

head with thumbs at the vertex or off the head, index fingers at the area of the great wing of the sphenoid bone, middle and ring fingers on either side of the ear, and little fingers on the occiput. The bed is in Fowler position, and the physician is resting his or her elbows on the head of the bed for support.

At this point, the neuromusculoskeletal system of the patient has been assessed, including:

i. Sympathetic nervous system: Evidence of somatic dysfunction associated with the sympathetic nervous system is indicated by palpation of the thoracic and upper lumbar area (spinal levels of origin of the sympathetic nervous system)

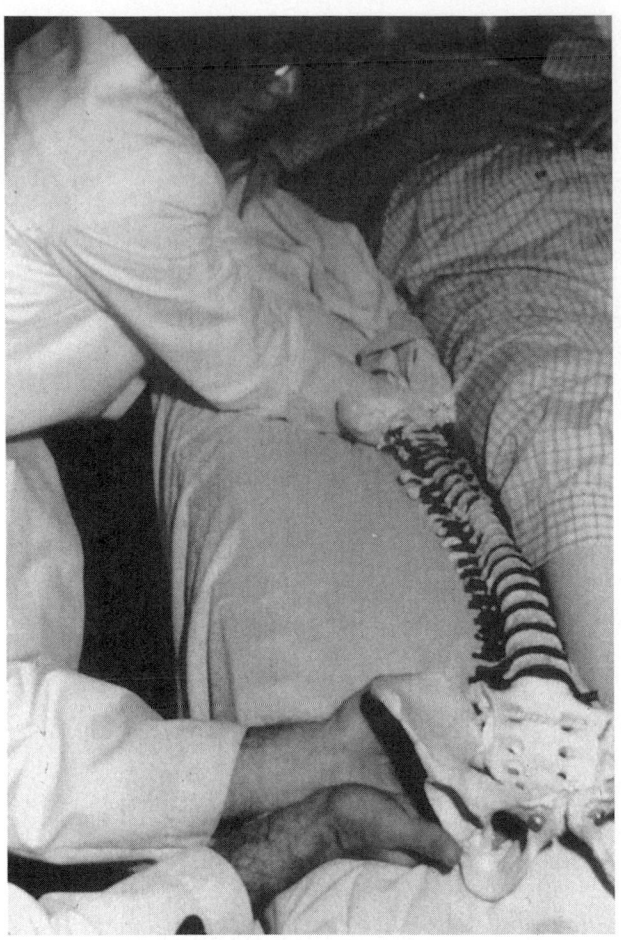

FIGURE 29.3. Sacral rocking.

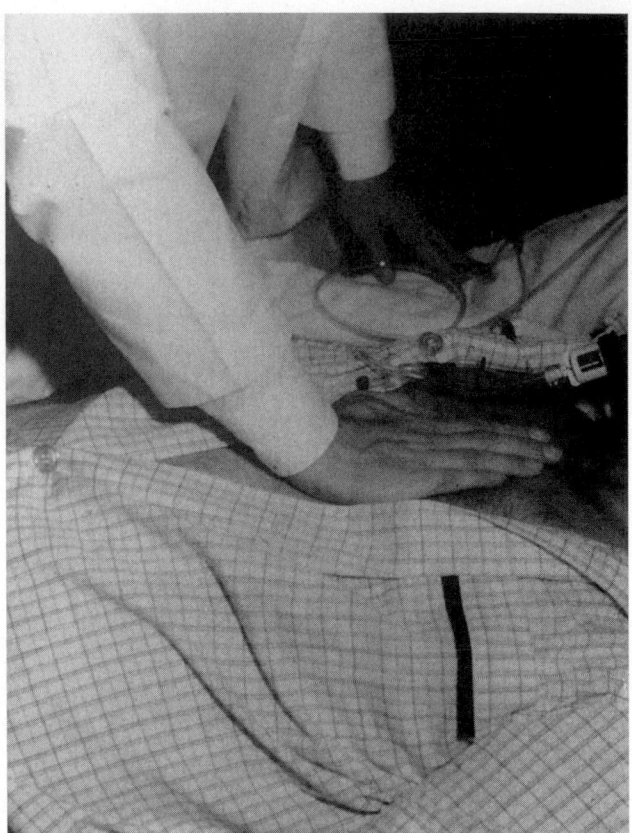

FIGURE 29.4. Sternal palpation.

for viscerosomatic and articular restrictions, and palpation of the rib cage for restrictions affecting or being affected by the sympathetic chain ganglia.

ii. Parasympathetic nervous system: Evidence of somatic dysfunction associated with the parasympathetic nervous system is indicated by palpation of the sacral, suboccipital, and cranial areas (its central nervous system site of origin).

iii. Lymphatic system: Evidence of dysfunction affecting lymphatic flow is indicated by assessing the four major diaphragms of the body (pelvic, thoracoabdominal, thoracic inlet, and foramen magnum) and rib motion.

iv. Visceral dysfunction: Visceral dysfunction is reflected by positive anterior Chapman points, visceral palpation (when possible), and spinal somatic dysfunction that may be related to facilitated segments.

v. Structural component: Asymmetries and abnormalities of the cervical, thoracic, rib, and pelvic areas affect optimal functioning of the autonomic and lymphatic systems.

TREATMENT OF THE HOSPITALIZED PATIENT

General Considerations

When treating the hospitalized patient, remember that the patient is acutely ill. The treatment goal is to promote homeostasis

and the body's ability to heal itself. Each intervention performed requires energy from that patient to incorporate the changes induced into their body by the manipulation. Therefore, treat only those dysfunctions that impede the homeostatic processes. Leave long-standing or unrelated problems for outpatient care. There

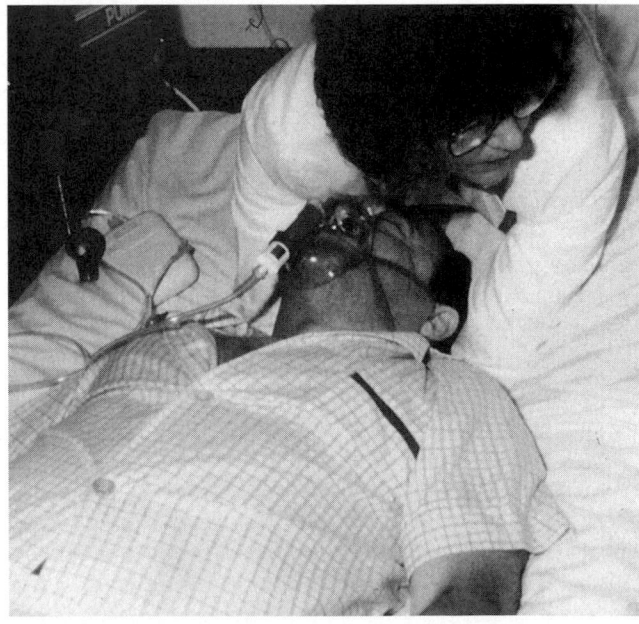

FIGURE 29.5. Palpation of posterior thoracic area.

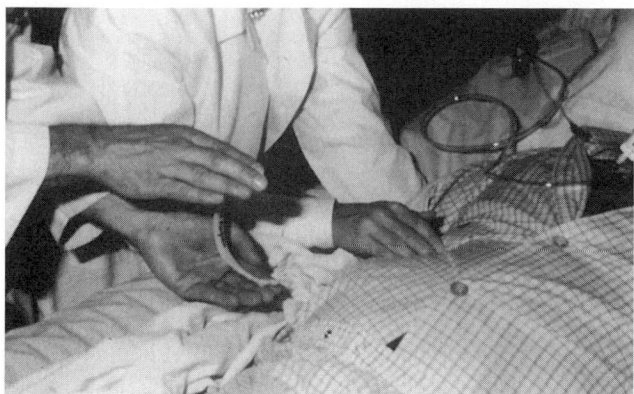

FIGURE 29.6. Individual rib evaluation and treatment position.

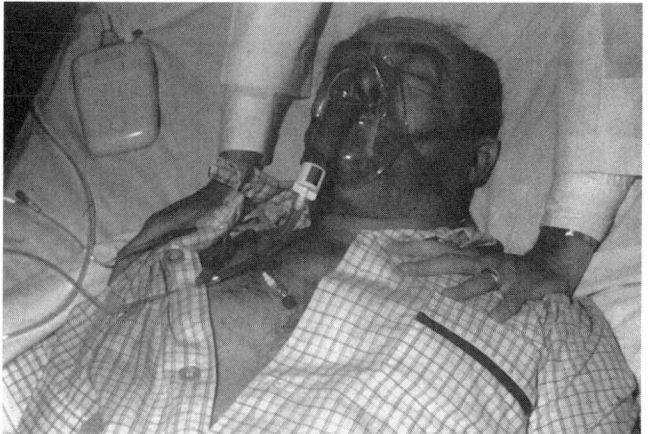

FIGURE 29.7. Thoracic inlet evaluation and treatment position.

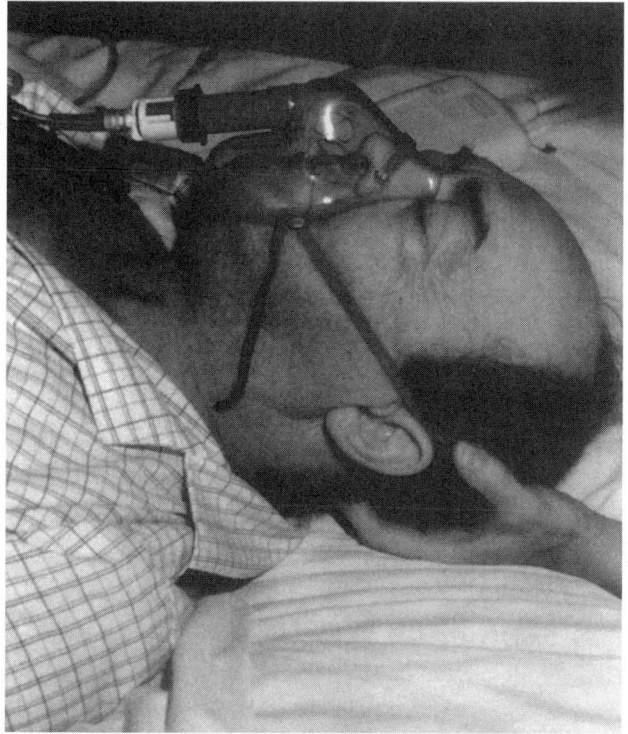

FIGURE 29.8. Suboccipital evaluation and treatment position.

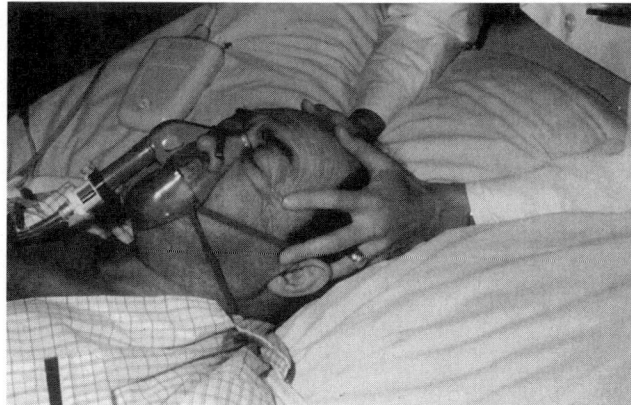

FIGURE 29.9. Cranial evaluation with vault hold position.

is consensus among experts in hospital OMT that the acutely ill patient may only be able to tolerate short periods of treatment at any given time, so manipulative efforts may need to focus on areas of the body that require immediate attention. For example, a short leg and mild functional scoliosis may not need to be addressed during a hospitalization for pneumonia unless they contribute to impaired homeostasis during the acute illness. The short leg, though it may be a contributing factor in lowering the patient's resistance to infections and trauma, can usually be evaluated after recovery from the acute incident.

Alterations in tissue texture changes are helpful in following the patient's medical progress. The presence of new tissue texture changes at a given level alerts a physician to possible early organ dysfunction. Likewise, resolution of the viscerosomatic reflex indicates improved health in that area. One notable exception occurs when treating extremely compromised patients. The severely ill patient whose vital resources or immune system has been exhausted will fail to show tissue texture changes that should, in fact, be present considering the site of the organ dysfunction. In these patients, the presence of new tissue texture change in areas that are appropriate for that patient's illness may be a favorable sign.

When formulating a manipulative prescription (8) for an inpatient osteopathic treatment, determine the frequency and duration. This varies according to the patient's condition. In general, for very ill patients, it is better to provide frequent treatments over short time intervals and to use less forceful techniques. This usually means treating the patient once daily, although some literature suggests more frequent application (9,10,11). As the patient improves, the interval between treatments and the treatment duration may be lengthened if needed. The patient may also be able to tolerate the use of more direct techniques. Treat only those areas most likely to impair the recovery process, considering both lymphatic flow and autonomic balance. When a hospitalized patient can tolerate 3 or 4 days between treatments, the manipulative treatments may essentially be provided on an intensive outpatient schedule. Psychiatric inpatients and those in drug and alcohol inpatient treatment programs may require a different schedule and are discussed separately.

If the patient is unfamiliar with osteopathic treatments, especially those given at the bedside, briefly explain the philosophy and reason for the OMT. A simple explanation seems to work best, such as: "There are nerves from your spine that go to both the back muscles and the organs inside. When an internal organ is sick, a reflex is created that causes your back muscles to get tense. By treating your back, the reflex is calmed so that the organs can heal faster." Or you might say: "When you have pneumonia (or congestive heart failure, etc.), the fluids in your body pool in your lungs, making your illness worse. Your ribs don't move normally either, making it more difficult to get rid of this fluid. The osteopathic treatment will help your ribs work more normally, and help pump the fluids out of your lungs."

Further answers may be provided if the patient expresses an interest. Usually, however, the patient simply relaxes with the physician's soothing touch, and no further explanations are needed.

For any medically ill, hospitalized patient, the presence of somatic dysfunction in areas that impede normal autonomic or lymphatic functioning can and should be treated. The patient's disease process dictates the areas to treat and the techniques to use.

Treatment Protocol

Decide which areas most impair the patient's homeostatic balance, which techniques are best suited for the patient, and how much treatment the patient can tolerate. In other words, create a manipulative prescription (5). A general rule of thumb is to select at least one or two principle areas for treatment that are most relevant to the patient's recovery. Additional areas may be added, depending on the response of the patient. In this way, the patient is not overtreated, and no important areas are missed. One should give consideration to treatment approaches that would improve any or all of the following:

Autonomic nervous system function
Lymphatic flow
Respiratory excursion
Biomechanics
Visceral function

Using this approach, important autonomic, lymphatic, visceral, and structural components relevant to the patient's recovery are evaluated and treated.

Some manipulative techniques appropriate in one situation may not be appropriate in another. For example, for a patient with fractures, avoid any treatment positioning that could destabilize the fracture site. A patient in the intensive care unit with a myocardial infarction generally should not receive techniques using isometric patient contractions. The decision of where and why to treat the patient lies with the physician and is part of the medical decision-making process.

Special Considerations
Acquired Immunodeficiency Syndrome Patients

Persons with acquired immunodeficiency syndrome (AIDS) who are hospitalized should be treated manipulatively with the same rational and systemic approach as all hospitalized patients. The nature of the disease process for which they have been hospitalized dictates which areas should be treated manipulatively, as well as the intensity, duration, and frequency of the treatment. As with

all patients, routine body fluid precautions should be taken. If the patient is in isolation, special precautions are necessary, as discussed below.

Drug and Alcohol Detoxification and Rehabilitation Patients

During drug or alcohol detoxification, the patient is not usually responsive to OMT. After the detoxification has been completed, OMT has been noted by experts to be helpful in aiding the recovery process. Most patients undergoing drug or alcohol treatment have a long history of trauma and/or abuse. OMT should address the lasting effects of that trauma on the musculoskeletal, emotional, and cranial systems. Any medical or surgical conditions are treated according to the guidelines described earlier.

OMT in the inpatient psychiatric or drug/alcohol treatment setting seems to be generally more effective than treatment of the same patient as an outpatient. Presumably, the intensive setting, where nutrition, medication, exercise, peer support, situation control, and counseling are structured into the patient's existence, allows an increased recovery rate in the entire person (mind, body, and spirit). Experts have reported that OMT is extremely effective in this optimal setting.

Intensive Care Unit and Respirator Patients

When moving a patient in the bed or changing the bed position, request assistance so as not to endanger the stability of any drainage, intravenous, arterial, endotracheal, or feeding tubes. Patients on respirators can and should be treated manipulatively. Avoid techniques that interfere with the respiratory rate, such as the pedal pump or classic lymphatic pump.

Isolation Patients

If the patient has been placed in some form of isolation, requirements for gloves, gown, and mask must be followed. Palpatory examination and OMT with gloves are not ideal, but protection is necessary. For patients with profuse secretions, it is wise to use gloves even if no isolation protocols are ordered. During the treatment, position yourself and the patient in a manner that will reduce your chances of becoming infected.

Pediatric Patients

Newborns occasionally need treatment in the nursery for cranial entrapment neuropathies that result in colic and feeding disorders (12). These conditions can often be relieved by simple, gentle, condylar decompression.

Treatment of pediatric patients for medical illnesses (such as pneumonia) and postoperative OMT for infants involve the same processes used for treating adults. The techniques recommended, however, are usually articular, balanced ligamentous tension, balanced membranous tension, or myofascial approaches. One treatment for children described by Max Gutensohn (personal communication) enables the physician to simultaneously articulate vertebral levels and encourage lymphatic flow while seemingly playing a game with the child. This is especially nice for assisting recovery from respiratory disease. The child is held in the air with the physician's hands encircling the child's chest under the axillae.

The legs are then gently swung in a circle, thereby mobilizing the area just distal to the hands on the torso. To articulate other areas, hold the child higher or lower on the torso. Gentle rib raising and spinal articulatory procedures in the lateral recumbent, supine, or seated positions are also well tolerated.

Postoperative or Posttrauma Patients

When treating postoperative patients who are in the hospital, avoid excessive jiggling and overhead arm techniques. Some techniques, such as the lymphatic pump with arms overhead or vigorous pedal pump, may endanger the stability of the operative site or injury.

Psychiatric Patients

The osteopathic premise states that the body is a unit, with mind, body, and spirit as interwoven parts of one being. This supports the concept of treating a patient with psychiatric illness to improve functioning of the rest of the body. If the psychiatric patient is hospitalized for a medical or surgical condition, he or she is treated for that condition following the guidelines described earlier. Patients who are hospitalized for their psychiatric disease also deserve an osteopathic structural evaluation and manipulative treatment if indicated.

The structural examination should closely evaluate the cranial sacral mechanism and the upper thoracic regions, looking for evidence of somatic dysfunctions that could be produced by autonomic reflexes. Older literature makes a strong case for dysautonomia as a significant factor in psychiatric disease, based in part on clinical observations at the Still-Hildreth Osteopathic Sanitorium. Dunn (13) discusses the association of autonomic dysfunction with psychiatric disease and supports this association with data from 1,000 psychiatric patients. More than 50 of these patients demonstrated palpable somatic dysfunction at C2 and T4-6 paravertebral regions of the spine. In 2,288 examinations, Woods (14) demonstrated an altered rate of the cranial rhythmic impulse in various psychiatric diseases, as compared with controls.

In addition to affecting autonomic reflexes, OMT appears to have a calming effect on the psychiatric patient. Psychiatric patients generally do not tolerate high-velocity/low-amplitude techniques well. Use a soothing treatment approach and a slow, gentle touch (15). When psychiatric patients are receiving electroconvulsive shock treatments (ECTs), OMT within 24 hours of a treatment event does not appear to be productive. Providing OMT on the day after ECT, however, has been observed to be extremely effective. Osteopathic treatment of the cranial and pelvic areas is especially important for these patients (16).

OMT may be contraindicated for some psychiatric patients. A paranoid schizophrenic patient may interpret a hands-on treatment modality as threatening and usually does not tolerate it well. Touch may be misinterpreted by patients having difficulty differentiating fantasy from reality. For patients with a history of abuse, the manipulative treatment may be seen as a sexual advance or assault. In rare cases, the physician may decide against the manipulative treatment because of concerns of personal safety.

As with all patients, the benefits of osteopathic treatment for psychiatric patients must be weighed against its potential adverse outcomes. Most psychiatric patients in inpatient settings tolerate the treatment extremely well and quickly respond to treatment.

Recording Osteopathic Diagnosis and Treatment on the Hospital Chart

After a session with a patient, the following must be recorded in the hospital chart:

> History
> Physical examination (including the osteopathic diagnoses)
> Treatment plan
> Treatment provided

A protocol for adequately recording an osteopathic structural examination is outlined by the American Osteopathic Association in the Accreditation Requirements for Acute Care Hospitals (17) and is used in hospital credentialing. Each hospital may also have individual guidelines for the recording of osteopathic structural examinations. The American Osteopathic Association has also approved a standardized form for use in recording neuromusculoskeletal examination findings on hospitalized patients (Fig. 29.10). In general, the following should be included in the recorded neuromusculoskeletal examination:

> Position(s) in which the patient was examined
> Notation of asymmetries of the spine, ribs, head, shoulders, and extremities noted by visual examination or palpation
> Results of screening the range of motion of the spine and extremities
> Location of tissue texture changes
> Any other relevant positive or negative findings from the neuromusculoskeletal examination, as described above
> Correlation of the musculoskeletal examination with the chief complaint(s)

Follow-Up Evaluation and Treatment

Begin the follow-up examination with a review of any new radiographs, followed by a review of the medical record since the last evaluation. Take an interval history. Perform the physical examination following the protocol described above, noting any changes in response to the previous treatment or in the disease process.

The areas to be treated may change at every visit and are determined by the interval history and physical examination. The tolerance for a longer treatment generally increases as the patient improves. The intervals between treatments are also usually increased as the patient improves.

THE OSTEOPATHIC CONSULTATION

All osteopathic physicians are trained to provide osteopathic diagnosis and treatment for their patients. Some osteopathic physicians, with additional training and skill, elect to provide this service on a consultation basis for other physicians. In this case, the physician becomes a consultant in osteopathic manipulative medicine (OMM) to the patient's attending physician. Most hospitals require that physicians serving as consultants go through

Osteopathic Musculoskeletal Examination of the Hospitalized Patient

Examiner: (print) ______________________

Chief Complaint: ______________________

Required

Ant./Post. Spinal Curves:

	I	N	D
Cervical Lordosis	▯	▯	▯
Thoracic Kyphosis	▯	▯	▯
Lumbar Lordosis	▯	▯	▯

I = increased; N = normal; D = decreased.

Scoliosis (Lateral Spinal Curves)

- ▯ None
- ▯ Functional
- ▯ Mild
- ▯ Moderate
- ▯ Severe

- sitting ▯
- standing ▯
- prone/supine ▯
- lat. recumb. ▯
- unable to examine ▯

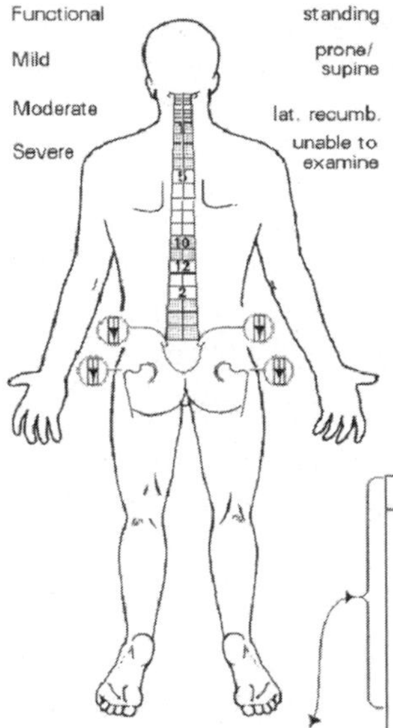

For Coding Purposes Only

Assessment Tools:

- ▯ T = Tenderness
- ▯ A = Asymmetry
- ▯ R = Restricted Motion
  - ▯ Active
  - ▯ Passive
- ▯ T = Tissue Texture Change

Severity Key:

- ⓿ = No SD or background (BG) levels
- ❶ = Minor TART more than BG levels
- ❷ = TART obvious (R & T esp) +/− symptoms
- ❸ = Symptomatic, R and T very easily found, "key lesion"

Optional Worksheet

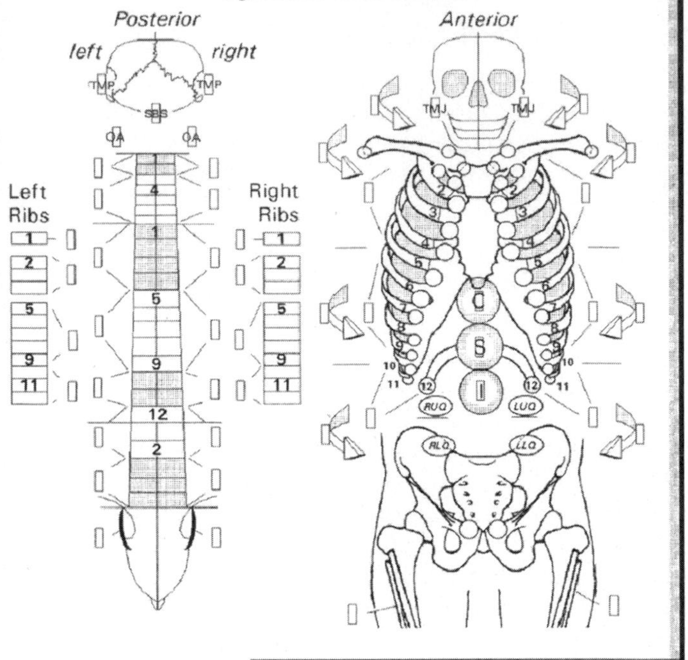

Abbreviation Key:

- OA Occipitoatlantal joint
- Sympathetic ganglia:
  - C Celiac
  - S Superior Mesenteric
  - I Inferior Mesenteric
- TMJ Temporo-mandibular Jnt.
- TMP Temporal bone
- SBS Sphenobasilar symphysis

Region Evaluated		Severity 0	1	2	3	Specific of Major Somatic Dysfunctions
Head		▯	▯	▯	▯	
Neck		▯	▯	▯	▯	
Thoracic T1-4		▯	▯	▯	▯	
T5-9		▯	▯	▯	▯	
T10-12		▯	▯	▯	▯	
Lumbar		▯	▯	▯	▯	
Pelvis/Sacrum		▯	▯	▯	▯	
Pelvis/Innominate		▯	▯	▯	▯	
Extremity (lower)	R	▯	▯	▯	▯	
	L	▯	▯	▯	▯	
Extremity (upper)	R	▯	▯	▯	▯	
	L	▯	▯	▯	▯	
Ribs		▯	▯	▯	▯	
Other / Abdomen		▯	▯	▯	▯	

Major Correlations with:

▯ Traumatic	▯ Rheumatological
▯ Orthopedic	▯ EENT
▯ Neurological	▯ Cardiovascular
▯ Viscero-somatic	▯ Pulmonary
▯ Primary Ms-Skeletal	▯ Gastrointestinal
▯ Activities of daily living	▯ Genitourinary
▯ Other ______	▯ Congenital

Other: ______________________

Signature of the examiner: ______________________ *Date of Examination:* ______________

Signature of the examiner(s): ______________________ *Date of Examination:* ______________

FIGURE 29.10. Recommended neuromusculoskeletal examination form for hospitalized patients.

a credentialing process and be granted privileges in their area of specialty. This credentialing also applies to OMM.

The Consult

The OMM consultant becomes involved with a patient's care when the attending physician writes an order requesting an OMM consult. The order should state the reason for the consult, specifying either the specific patient complaint (e.g., headache) or the organ system or disease to be evaluated. This order may be written as a consultation only, or as an order to consult and treat manipulatively as indicated ("Consult regarding left lower lobe pneumonia with OMT as indicated"). If the order does not also specify for the consultant to treat the patient if indicated, the consultant provides only an examination and recommendations for treatment. In most cases, the attending physician also specifies that treatment is requested. The attending physician may sometimes specify a certain number of treatments, essentially dictating part of the manipulative prescription. However, the consultant is the one performing the procedure (OMT), and the burden of actually formulating the manipulative prescription is the responsibility of the consulting physician.

As in the process described earlier, the OMM consult begins with a review of the patient's radiographs and medical record, with special notation of findings that relate to the neuromusculoskeletal, fascial, and visceral systems. The osteopathic physician then evaluates the patient for the presence of somatic dysfunction of the neuromusculoskeletal, fascial, and visceral systems, and determines its relevance to the disease process for which the patient has been hospitalized. If the attending physician does not request treatment, the consultant is ready to write the consultation. If the attending physician also orders treatment if indicated, the consultant is obliged to determine if treatment is indicated. If so, the consultant proceeds with the OMT of the patient, following the treatment protocol described earlier.

After the examination and treatment (if ordered and indicated) are completed, a consult is written in the medical record. Usually, a specially designated sheet is provided for the consultant's written summary, which includes impressions and recommendations. A summary is written so that it can be immediately used by the attending physician, and the full report is then dictated. A written note should also be made in the progress note section stating that a consult was completed, including the date and time. If the results of the examination or treatment indicate a clinical need for immediate information, the consultant should also contact the attending physician directly and discuss the patient's case.

The dictated OMM consultation should contain the following:

   i. Date and time of the consult.
  ii. Name of the attending physician, reason for consult request, and whether the patient's chart and radiographs were reviewed.
 iii. Statement that a history was taken from the patient (or family member), and a written summary of those findings.
  iv. Statement of the positions in which the patient was examined (was examined in the sitting, supine, and lateral recum-

bent position, or examined in the supine position only due to presence of an endotracheal tube), and the results of the patient's physical examination.
   v. Impressions. Generally, the consultant limits his or her diagnoses to somatic dysfunctions. Also include any other diagnoses that are directly related to the somatic dysfunction and the disease process, and the viscerosomatic and somatovisceral reflexes. The consultant is functioning as an OMM specialist, not assuming other parts of the patient's medical management.
  vi. Recommendations. This includes the manipulative prescription if OMT is indicated, and recommendations for radiographs, further evaluations, and treatment modalities relevant to the consult.
 vii. Treatment given, if any. Areas treated, techniques used, and the patient's response to treatment are recorded here. Use standard nomenclature as defined in the Glossary of Osteopathic Terminology (see Glossary).
viii. Follow-up recommendations.
  ix. An expression of thanks to the requesting physician for the consult.
   x. Request that the original consult be placed in the medical chart and that photocopies of the consult be sent to the attending and consulting physicians.

Follow-Up

Follow-up consultations are performed at the request of the attending physician or if the consultant feels that a reevaluation is indicated. The protocol is essentially the same as the initial consultation, with the exception that radiograph and chart reviews are only necessary from the date of the initial consultation.

Follow-up treatment is provided at the consultant's discretion if he or she has been asked to participate in the patient's care. In this case, the consultant is then seeing the patient as an established patient and no longer as a consultant. The protocol for follow-up treatment is described in the Follow-Up Evaluation and Treatment section above.

A CASE STUDY IN CRITICAL THINKING FOR THE OSTEOPATHIC MANIPULATIVE MEDICINE SPECIALIST

The following case study (18) provides an example of how the specialist in NMM and OMM applies osteopathic theory, methods, and thought processes in the care of the patient.

Case Presentation

A 48-year-old man was admitted to the hospital with a diagnosis of acute myocardial infarction (MI) and congestive heart failure. At this time, he states he is worried about his outcome. He complains of slight chest pressure and slight nausea.

He has a history of hypertension and hypercholesterolemia. He has known coronary artery disease from electrocardiogram (ECG) and stress treadmill evaluations, as well as angina on exertion, but refuses invasive studies or treatments and agrees to take medications for chest pain, hypertension, and hypercholesterolemia. Present medications are aspirin, atenolol, atorvastatin, and p.r.n. use of sublingual nitroglycerin for chest pain. He had been shoveling snow, developed chest pain, left arm pain, and then nausea that did not respond to sublingual nitroglycerin. The chest pain persisted, but he waited 16 hours before telling his wife. He had emergent medical care on admission to the emergency room that included aspirin, oxygen administration, heparin, and application of nitropaste on the chest. He was stabilized and admitted to the hospital.

The NMM and OMM specialist is asked to do a structural evaluation and provide appropriate osteopathic manipulative treatment (OMT) for this patient.

Physical Findings

He is 6 feet tall, and weighs 230 pounds. He appears anxious, pale, and slightly diaphoretic and is resting in the bed in a semi-Fowler position. A nasal cannula is in place, a large-bore i.v. is infusing into left forearm, and a right subclavian line has been placed. A cardiac monitor is attached. He is having slight chest pressure, but no respiratory distress. There is an S3 gallop rhythm, rales in the lungs, the liver is enlarged and soft, and there is grade 2 pretibial edema. Osteopathic evaluation reveals:

OA FS_LR_R
A-A rotated left
Left first rib elevated
T1 ERL_LS_L
T2-4 NS_RR_L with tissue texture abnormalities in paraspinal soft tissues along T2-4 left, inclusive of the rib angles
T7-10 NS_LR_R
Diaphragm motion restriction on the left with ribs 7-10 exhalation restriction (inhalation somatic dysfunction)

Diagnostics

The ECG shows ST segment elevation, and laboratory results reveal that CK enzyme (MB fraction) is elevated. Troponin-1 is elevated. Chest radiograph is reported as normal.

Given the above information, the NMM and OMM specialist considers the following questions:

i. Of all the specific structural findings listed above, which are the most significant ones? Which are the next most significant ones?
ii. What is the rationale for why each of the somatic dysfunctions listed above might be related to this patient's condition?
iii. What would be the goals for providing osteopathic manipulative treatment (OMT) for this patient?
iv. Will the structural examination need to be modified for this patient? If so, how?
v. Are there manipulative techniques that would be appropriate for each of the somatic dysfunctions listed above? Will they need to be modified to be applied in this case? If so, how?
vi. Are there any OMT techniques that are contraindicated in this patient?
vii. What is the evidence base for the use of OMT in conditions like this? Where would such information be found?

viii. Our osteopathic principles state that the body is a unit and that the body has self-healing and self-regulatory capabilities. Does doing OMT address these principles? What other things might be considered for this patient that would demonstrate that he is being treated holistically and being helped to "self-heal" and improve his health?

The NMM and OMT specialist would consider the following points about the patient's pathophysiology:

i. He has both backward and forward cardiac failure.
ii. Coronary thrombosis secondary to platelet aggregation with antecedent coronary artery disease is the most common mechanism.
iii. Compensatory responses include increased sympathetic tone, increased blood pressure and heart rate, increased myocardial contractility, and increased myocardial work load.
iv. These mechanisms contribute to a "supply and demand" imbalance for perfusion of the myocardium.
v. Arrhythmias are commonly associated with heart disease and myocardial ischemia. Sympathicotonia encourages tachyarrhythmias and inappropriate increased parasympathetic tone encourages bradyarrhythmias and heart blocks.
vi. Visceral facilitation of the spinal cord from the visceral afferent fibers from the myocardium in the region of the myocardial infarction facilitates its spinal cord segments and produces the deep severe pressure. This then refers to the corresponding somatic efferents and enhances the palpable tissue texture changes.

Certain points about functional anatomy are also considered. This includes knowledge of structure and physiology necessary to properly carry out the osteopathic manipulative treatment support:

i. Chronic viscerosomatic tissue changes are palpable in the paraspinal deep soft tissues of related spinal cord segments (i.e., T1-5). Chronic segmental somatic dysfunction, acting over time, can produce a hyperexcitable or "facilitated" spinal segment. This irritable segment responds abnormally (usually excessively) to minimal stimuli and can cause an increase in the sympathetic outflow to related visceral organs, e.g., the heart and coronary arteries.
ii. Research studies have documented viscerosomatic reflexes in the left upper thoracic area of patients with myocardial infarction.
iii. Some osteopathic physicians describe the cardiac reflex as sidebent left and rotated right (group mechanics) in the upper thoracic spine. This long-term positional change is produced by chronic hypertonicity of the left upper thoracic muscles.
iv. Somatic dysfunction at T1-2 is often associated with patients that develop tachyarrhythmias.
v. A *right* pectoralis major trigger point has been associated with some cardiac arrhythmias, many of which are resistant to antiarrhythmic drugs.
vi. Scientists have identified dorsal root ganglion cells with a visceral projection to the heart and a somatic projection to the left arm. A single cell has two projections: one to the periphery, and one to the viscera. This cell reports to the

spinal cord. The central nervous system is not accustomed to the nociceptive input from the heart, so the pain is interpreted as coming from the arm.

vii. Initial pain from an MI is visceral in nature and is usually a severe deep pressure feeling. This then often begins to disappear, but is followed by development of severe sharp chest pain with arm and neck referral as the viscerosomatic reflex takes over.

Goals for osteopathic manipulative management include a general plan for manipulative treatment of this patient and a discussion of treatment options, contraindications, and plans for follow-up evaluation and treatment.

Initial Management

i. Treat viscerosomatic reflexes with inhibitory pressure or release techniques directed toward upper thoracic and O-A somatic dysfunctions.

ii. This reduces viscerosomatic chest pain.

iii. Improvement of chest pain relieves anxiety, which reduces central nervous system facilitation.

iv. Treat the musculoskeletal (O-A, cervical, upper thoracic, rib) components associated with arrhythmias. This reduces detrimental somatic influence to the facilitated segment and the heart.

v. For tachyarrhythmias, treat the upper thoracic somatic dysfunctions that encourage inappropriate sympathetic outflow to the heart. These areas are usually located at T1-2 and their corresponding ribs.

vi. For bradyarrhythmias and heart block, normalize the vagal response. This includes treatment of O-A/A-A and cervical region somatic dysfunctions. Some useful techniques for this include suboccipital inhibition and indirect approaches to cervical somatic dysfunction.

Long-Term Management

i. Treat chronic motion restrictions of the upper thoracic region if present. This type of treatment is best performed once the patient is ambulatory.

ii. Treat as necessary to maintain proper diaphragmatic function. Technique selection may involve direct or indirect methods, such as myofascial release or thoracoabdominal diaphragm release using the indirect method.

iii. Treat the cervical spine with suboccipital inhibition and relieve any midcervical somatic dysfunction. This may help with diaphragm function via the phrenic nerve.

iv. Use thoracolumbar soft tissue release, articulatory treatment, or myofascial release; all can improve diaphragm function.

v. Normalize fascias at the thoracic inlet and re-dome a flattened thoracoabdominal diaphragm. Congestion of the myocardium has been associated with an increased amount of myocardial damage from similar coronary artery blockage.

Contraindications and cautions regarding treatment:

i. Do not use forceful direct method treatments.

ii. Do not overtreat and tire the patient.

iii. Do not put the patient in treatment positions that restrict respiratory efforts.

iv. Liver pump, liver flip, and classic thoracic pumps may be too vigorous for this patient. The liver and spleen may be friable, so be careful to avoid undue sudden compression or decompression changes in the abdomen or undue abdominal pressure

v. Continue to treat to provide optimal lymphatic flow to reduce the amount of scarring from the healing process.

Further Thoughts

This man had significant antecedent heart problems. One would, therefore, expect to find chronic upper thoracic changes (usually left). Often, this type of patient would have a group upper left thoracic curve (type I). It usually takes about 24 hours for a cardiac viscerosomatic reflex to develop, so this should be present in this patient by now. As the viscerosomatic reflex takes over, the chest pressure becomes sharper in nature. A viscerosomatic reflex change develops at the T3-T5 region unless the infarct is posterior. In a posterior MI, the reflex is usually at T5, and this usually spills over into the stomach area producing GI symptoms in the patient. This viscerosomatic visceral reflex begins to affect upper GI sympathetic innervation. Upper GI symptoms are also influenced through the C2 connection with the vagus nerve. Nausea, vomiting, or other upper GI complaints are a common clinical problem.

There are two basic rhythm problems:

i. Bradyarrhythmias and heart block are likely if vagal nerve irritation dominates. Somatic dysfunction in these patients is usually found in the neck. Right-sided O-A and C2 somatic dysfunctions are more likely to initiate or predate cardiac bradyarrhythmias. Left-sided O-A and C2 somatic dysfunction are more likely to initiate or predate cardiac bradyarrhythmias or heart blocks.

ii. Tachyarrhythmias are likely if sympathicotonia dominates the clinical picture and T1-2 is the usual site of the somatic dysfunction

Initial OMT

This involves initial use of paraspinal inhibitory pressure and myofascial release technique to the T1-2 region and then treatment of the T3-5 regions. Clinical experience has shown that if C3-5 is treated first before inhibition of the T1-2 and T4-5 regions, arrhythmias increase. Apparently the treatment of C3-5 further facilitated the cord segments at the T1-2 region.

Somatic dysfunctions at the O-A, A-A, C2, and/or the occipitomastoid suture are treated to reduce or eliminate inappropriate vagal cardiac response.

If there is a tachyarrhythmia, check for a right pectoralis muscle trigger point and if tender, spray and stretch to relieve it. This type of tachyarrhythmia is often unresponsive to antiarrhythmic drugs. If this trigger point is etiology of the arrhythmia, the arrhythmia responds almost instantaneously.

The patient must be treated in a comfortable position in bed unless the cardiologist allows the patient to sit up. Be careful not to disturb the patient's tubes, i.v. lines, and other monitoring equipment.

CONCLUSION

The specialist in neuromusculoskeletal medicine and osteopathic manipulative medicine is a valuable addition to the osteopathic profession. The role of this important specialist is to provide clinical expertise when requested, and to expand the ever-evolving osteopathic concept. The NMM and OMM specialist plays a crucial role in the development and application of osteopathic theory and practice in the areas of education, research, and service.

ACKNOWLEDGMENTS

The author wishes to express appreciation to John P. Goodridge, DO, FAAO, for his valuable advice and information regarding the development of the certification process for NMM and OMT and the FAAO, and to Karen M. Steele, DO, FAAO, for the use of material regarding hospital evaluation and treatment. In addition, the following acknowledgements from the previous version of this chapter are gratefully extended: Mr. Lowell Jackson for allowing photography of an actual inpatient osteopathic treatment for educational purposes; Richard Koss, DO, for assisting in the treatment and photography; Ross Carlson, DO, for his assistance in the research and writing of this chapter; and William A. Kuchera, DO, FAAO, for his invaluable critique of this chapter.

REFERENCES

1. Eggleston, A. President's Report. *Academy of Applied Osteopathy Directory.* Indianapolis, IN: American Academy of Osteopathy; 1959.
2. Stiles EG. Osteopathic manipulation in a hospital environment. *J Am Osteopath Assoc.* 1976;76:17–32.
3. Larson N. Summary of site and occurrence of paraspinal soft tissue changes in the intensive care unit. *J Am Osteopath Assoc.* 1976;75:840–842.
4. Hruby RJ. Pathophysiologic models: aids to the selection of manipulative techniques. *J Am Acad Ostoepath.* 1991;1(3):8–10.
5. Zink JG. Respiratory and circulatory care: the conceptual model. *Osteopath Ann.* 1987;10:108–111.
6. Owens C. *An Endocrine Interpretation of Chapman's Reflexes.* Carmel, CA: American Academy of Osteopathy; 1963.
7. Jones L. *Strain Counterstrain.* Newark, OH: American Academy of Osteopathy; 1981.
8. Kuchera WA, Kuchera ML. *Osteopathic Principles in Practice,* 2nd ed. Columbus, OH: Greyden Press; 1994:297–302.
9. Herrmann EP. Postoperative adynamic ileus: Its prevention and treatment by osteopathic manipulation. *The DO.* Precepts & Practice. 1965;(October):163–164.
10. Young GS. Post-operative Osteopathic Manipulation. *Academy of Applied Osteopathy Yearbook.* Colorado Springs, CO: American Academy of Osteopathy; 1970:77–82.
11. Rumney IC. Osteopathic manipulative treatment of infectious disease. *Osteopath Ann.* 1974;(July):29–33.
12. Magoun HI. *Osteopathy in the Cranial Field,* 2nd ed. Kirksville, MO: Journal Printing Co; 1966:234, 263.
13. Dunn FE. Osteopathic concepts in psychiatry. *J Am Osteopath Assoc.* 1950;49(7)March:354–357.
14. Woods JM, Woods RH. A physical finding related to psychiatric disorders. *J Am Osteopath Assoc.* 1961;60:988–993.
15. Bradford, SG. Role of osteopathic manipulative therapy in emotional disorders: A physiologic hypothesis. *J Am Osteopath Assoc.* 1965;64:484–493.
16. Upledger JE, Vredevoogd JD. *Craniosacral Therapy.* Seattle, WA: Eastland Press; 1983:268.
17. *Accreditation Requirements, Acute Care Hospitals.* Chicago, IL: American Osteopathic Association; 1992:75–76.
18. Adapted from: Kearns C, ed. *Clinical Osteopathically Integrated Learning Scenarios.* Chevy Chase, MD: The Educational Council on Osteopathic Principles, A Council of the American Association of Colleges of Osteopathic Medicine; 2001.

NEUROLOGY

MITCHELL L. ELKISS
LOUIS E. RENTZ

KEY CONCEPTS

- Overview of neurologic structures
- Headaches, including migraine, cluster, and tension-type
- Treatment for headache
- Spinal disorders
- Peripheral nerve entrapments, including carpal tunnel syndrome and chronic pain syndrome

The specialty of neurology deals with the structure, function, disease, and dysfunction of the neuromusculoskeletal system. The neuromusculoskeletal system includes the brain, spinal cord, and peripheral and autonomic nervous systems, as well as the muscular system. The early development of osteopathic medical concepts emphasized the role of the nervous system as an integrator of function between the various systems of the body (1).

This chapter provides an overview of neurology as practiced by osteopathic physicians, focusing on some common neurologic disorders in which the application of osteopathic concepts is straightforward. The syndromes of headaches, spinal disorders, peripheral nerve entrapments, and chronic pain are described in more detail.

OVERVIEW

The central nervous system (CNS) is particularly unique in the human animal. It allows us the potential to pursue rational thought, experience the deepest emotional states, perform complex motor functions with little or no conscious attention, and have mechanisms for integrating a multitude of bodily functions. The system includes segmental mechanisms for regulating sensory and motor functions. It includes primitive brain centers responsible for posture and locomotion, more evolved systems of personality and feeling, and the most evolved system of the capacity for human mindfulness. All functions of the human organism are under some form of neural control; therefore, the maintenance of normal nervous system activity is essential for health. Relevant to the osteopathic physician is the intimate relation between the nervous system and manifestations of somatic dysfunction (2). As we dissect the nervous system into its component parts, we must remember that the subtotal of nervous system activity is a complex of electrophysiologic and neurochemical phenomena, demonstrating features of instability superimposed on tonic activity at multiple levels of the nervous system and resulting in the complex neurobiology of humans.

The structure of the nervous system can be clinically divided into reasonably circumscribed areas that correspond to specific neurologic functions. For purposes of discussion, these divisions are the:

Brain, including the cerebral cortex, basal ganglia, cerebellum, and brainstem
Spinal cord
Peripheral nerves and muscles

These areas are discussed more comprehensively in other texts (3).

The cerebral cortex contains the primary motor system for the initiation of conscious motor activity, the primary sensory system for the appreciation of conscious sensory input, and the centers for memory, speech, and visuospatial integration. Lesions in these areas produce contralateral defects in motor and sensory functions. Compromise of the dominant hemisphere disturbs speech and language functions while nondominant hemispheric disruption influences visuospatial processing and the potential for visual imagery.

The basal ganglia are intermediate nuclear structures that act as relay stations between the other sensorimotor control systems. The primary clinical functions of the basal ganglia include the inhibition of segmental reflexes, such that resting muscles can remain at rest. They control automatic and associated movements that occur without conscious processing (e.g., swinging the arms while walking, or smiling while talking). Disorders of the basal ganglia typically produce tremors at rest, rigidity, loss of associated movements, and posture disturbances.

The cerebellum functions to match proprioceptive input (state of the muscles and joints) with cortical output (motor intent) to control muscles during movement to ensure smooth motor transitions and to maintain posture and balance. Clinical disorders of the cerebellum manifest as tremor during movement, postural abnormalities, imbalance, and ataxia.

The brainstem acts as a connection between the cerebral cortex, the basal ganglia, the cerebellum, and the spinal cord. Through it, all impulses traveling into or out of the CNS are transmitted to the spinal segmental level. The brainstem also contains the nuclei of the cranial nerves and the autonomic centers.

The spinal cord extends in segments from the brainstem. The segments exist in relation to each nerve root and contain the anterior horn cells from which the peripheral motor nerves arise and the dorsal horns where sensory neurons enter. In essence, the motor roots supply all the muscles related to that segment (myotome) and similarly receive the sensory input from that segment (dermatome). The peripheral nerves transmit impulses to the muscles for movement and contain the sensory fibers for pain, temperature, touch, and proprioception.

The autonomic nervous system, sympathetic and parasympathetic, controls the visceral functions of the body. With rapidity and intensity, the autonomic nervous system can influence visceral functions. Each autonomic pathway comprises a preganglionic and postganglionic neuron. Preganglionic sympathetic neurons originate in the intermediolateral column of the thoracolumbar spinal cord and exit through the ventral roots and spinal nerve to pass into one of the chain ganglia. There they either synapse or pass through to one of the outlying sympathetic ganglia. From the sympathetic chain ganglia or the outlying ganglia, postganglionic neurons originate and course to their organ of destination. The parasympathetic division originates in the brainstem and the sacral cord. Their preganglionic neurons pass uninterrupted to the organ that is to be controlled. The postganglionic neurons are located in the wall of the target organs.

These summary descriptions of the anatomy of the nervous system illustrate that each of these systems is interdependent and exerts its ultimate effect in either the facilitation or inhibition of the spinal cord segments (4). The nervous system continually receives information about the organism's internal and external environment through the afferent sensory system arising from the musculoskeletal system and the viscera. This information is processed centrally, transmitted in the CNS in some form, and stored as learned or retained information. The nervous system output is transmitted through the efferent limb to the somatic and visceral compartments of the body. It is through the motor unit that the dominant effects of the motor system are manifest and through the peripheral autonomic system that efferent nervous functions are played out on the viscera. Through this process, the neuromuscular system helps to preserve and maintain total body functional integrity.

Practically speaking, the assumption of the upright stance involves an intricate interaction of the basic neurologic centers, with particular reference to the descending supraspinal pathways, the cooperation of the basal ganglia and cerebellum, the limbic system, and the lobes of the neocortex. This evolutionary accomplishment frees the human hands for manipulation of its environment and for further development. Biomechanical dysfunction can be a consequence of an imperfect adaptation to a continually changing center of gravity in the upright stance. The neuromusculoskeletal system provides the human with its behavioral repertoire; dysfunction of the neuromusculoskeletal system results in the clinical phenomenon of somatic dysfunction.

The next section elaborates on the concept of the osteopathic lesion and common neurologic disorders that illustrate osteopathic concepts in the genesis of symptoms and signs, as well as in therapeutic management.

CONCEPT OF SOMATIC DYSFUNCTION

Theoretical mechanisms of the interrelationship between the spinal cord and musculoskeletal abnormalities known as somatic dysfunction are largely based on the concept of segmental facilitation. J. Stedman Denslow originally defined this concept in the early 1940s using a new investigational technique of the time: electromyography. The concept of segmental facilitation, as described by Denslow (5), was that motor neuron pools in spinal cord segments related to areas of somatic dysfunction were maintained in a state of facilitation. That is, they were chronically hyperirritable and therefore hyperresponsive to impulses reaching them from any source in the body. The source of input included proprioceptive and nociceptive stimuli from the periphery under the influence of the supraspinal centers described above. Denslow (6) went on to conclude that muscles innervated from these segments are, therefore, kept in a state of hypertonus much of the day with inevitable impediment to spinal motion and with structural and functional consequences to the muscle and person over a period of time.

Stated another way, the facilitated segments are believed to be related specifically to somatic dysfunction such that areas of localized pain, tenderness, increased muscle tension, or limitation of motion in a spinal segment influence that part of the nervous system to which they are connected. Conversely, the musculoskeletal phenomena can be influenced by the segmental nervous system behavior itself, which can be produced by facilitation originating from peripheral, central, and visceral pathways (7).

The concept of segmental facilitation is an extension of general concepts of neuronal facilitation. In segmental facilitation, a spinal segment receives exaggerated input from either a somatic or visceral structure. The efferent motor and autonomic components of the spinal segment are maintained in a state of excitement, such that further stimulation results in additional activation with somatomotor and sympathetic manifestations that are clinically recognizable. The segment is hyperirritable and, like a lens, shows qualities of focusing the input. In this way, ascending or descending input tends to converge and locally increase the activity at the facilitated segment. A decreased threshold to stimuli is applied above or below the segment and can result in increased efferent somatic (muscle contraction) and autonomic (sweat, vasomotor) activity at this level. In this way, the spinal cord can be seen as an organizer and active participant in the disease process (8–11). The involved muscles can be maintained in a hypertonic state and thereby affect spinal motion, contributing to the restrictive musculoskeletal pattern typical of somatic dysfunction. Likewise, excess sympathetic segmental efferent activity can affect related somatic and visceral structures. The pathophysiologic consequences of local sympathetic hyperactivity are documented (12) and could play a role in the signs and symptoms of somatic dysfunction.

Segmental dysfunction of the neuromusculoskeletal system becomes visible when it manifests signs of somatic and/or sympathetic hyperactivity. Afferent stimuli from internal and external sources are organized by spinal cord mechanisms and manifest clinical features unique to the individual. Individuals have uniquely different responses to a general increase in psychic or physical stress. The common presence of increased somatic and sympathetic activity results in tissue texture abnormalities (TTA), one of the cardinal features of osteopathic palpatory diagnosis (13). It is the pattern of somatic dysfunction and its relationship to visceral disease that becomes particularly relevant as a diagnostic tool (14,15). Manipulative treatment influences the neural mechanisms responsible for the aforementioned reactive tissue changes; therapeutic success can be assessed through changes in these same factors.

Impulse-based electrical activity is not the only mechanism whereby the nervous system can influence bodily functions. The presence of trophic substances produced by the nerve cell and transported along its axon and microtubular structures are critical in maintaining the vitality of the organism (16). These substances transsynaptically affect a variety of target end organs. The antegrade and retrograde flow of axoplasm suggests that the communication is bidirectional. This normal axoplasmic flow is disturbed by primary disease of the neuron (motor neuron disease) or in those conditions that produce mechanical deformation of the nerve by entrapment, stretch, angulation, or pressure (17).

Perceptions and feelings can influence the state of the body's muscular activity, autonomic activity, and the capacity of its homeostatic mechanisms to respond to exogenous influences—including the ability to respond to osteopathic manipulative treatment (OMT). Neuroendocrine mechanisms allow the affective tone of individuals, their feeling state, and their personality to have an impact on their neuromusculoskeletal system. These mechanisms can be localized to the limbic system, the hypothalamus, the pituitary gland, and the neuroendocrine circuits.

In the early stages, continued afferent barrage (nociceptive, proprioceptive, autonomic) and a widening zone of involvement maintains the state of chronic facilitation. With chronic somatic dysfunction, a more lasting mechanism must be at work. Sustained patterns of excitability and synaptic transmission become learned behavior in the spinal cord and brain (18). The facilitated segment is the focus of efferent neuronal hyperexcitability. Metaphorically speaking, the zone of somatic dysfunction continues to represent the squeaky wheel. Additional local or general afferent stimulation results in an increased somatic and sympathetic efferent outpouring to those tissues innervated through the facilitated segment, manifesting as increased signs and symptoms of somatic dysfunction. See also Chapters 7, 8, and 73.

The osteopathic point of view considers wellness or health a positive state. It appreciates the organizational unity, inherent healing capacity, and self-regulating ability of the human body. Concern for the interrelationship between structure and function is crucial.

HEADACHES

Headaches are one of the most frequent presenting complaints to both the general practitioner and the neurologist. Table 30.1 represents the current International Headache Society classification of headaches (19). This classification is useful for establishing a clinical diagnosis of headache type; good scientific models exist for only some of the headache types, and there could be overlap

TABLE 30.1. INTERNATIONAL HEADACHE SOCIETY CLASSIFICATION OF HEADACHES

1. Migraine
2. Tension-type headache
3. Cluster headache and chronic paroxysmal hemicrania
4. Miscellaneous headaches unassociated with structural lesion
5. Headache associated with head trauma
6. Headache associated with vascular disorders
7. Headache associated with nonvascular intracranial disorder
8. Headache associated with substances or their withdrawal
9. Headache associated with noncephalic infection
10. Headache associated with metabolic disorder
11. Headache or facial pain associated with disorder of other facial or cranial structures
12. Cranial neuralgias, nerve trunk pain, and deafferentation
13. Headache not classifiable

(From International Headache Society. Classification of headaches. *Cephalgia.* 1988;8(suppl 7), with permission.)

between categories of headache in a given patient. Most headaches are mixed tension-type and migraine. This presentation is complicated by the multifactorial nature of headache, including these features:

Physical
Psychological
Familial
Ethnic
Cultural

The osteopathic physician is uniquely situated to evaluate the headache patient and to manage diagnostic and therapeutic resources.

Pain can result from noxious stimulation of the eyes, ears, mouth, and nasal cavities. Pain-sensitive intracranial structures include the venous sinuses and their tributaries, the dura (particularly at the base of the brain), and the arteries of the piaarachnoid and dura mater. Some extracranial structures are also pain sensitive, including the:

Skin
Subcutaneous tissues
Fascia
Muscles
Arteries
Cranial periosteum
Regional articulations

Acute head pain is often the result of dysfunction, displacement, or encroachment on one of the above structures. Cranial nerves V, VII, IX, and X, and upper cervical nerve roots II and III convey impulses from the head and face. The afferent signal is carried along A and C fibers of the peripheral nervous system, predominantly with the cells in the spinothalamic and trigeminal spinal tracts in laminae I, II, V, and X. The nociceptor fibers transmit synaptically using glutamate, substance P, and other neuropeptides (20).

A description of the quality and location of the headache is useful in establishing a cause. Investigate these questions:

■ Does it pound like a vascular headache or squeeze like a tension headache?

■ Does it localize to the region of the extracranial arteries, sinuses, teeth, tendinomuscular attachments, temporomandibular joint, or cervical vertebrae?
■ What are the severity and the time course of the pain?
■ Is there an acute, severe onset, as is typically seen in subarachnoid hemorrhage?
■ Is it chronic and nagging, more typical of tension-type headache?
■ Does it tend to reoccur like migraine?
■ Is it a once in a lifetime event like most CNS infections?

For example, migraines often occur in the morning and rarely last more than a day or two. Cluster headaches typically occur at night and rarely last for more than 30–120 minutes. Tension headaches can last for weeks or months.

The associated features of a headache include its relation to:

Menstruation
Activities
Head position
Time of day
Exercise
Sleep habits
Environmental toxicity
Food and drink intake

It is important to know the age of onset, relevant family history, and exacerbating and relieving factors. A psychosocial assessment and thorough history and physical examination can reveal the symptoms and signs of anxiety, depression, and anger that can increase and heighten pain awareness.

The physical examination of these patients includes a thorough general examination and a comprehensive neurologic examination, including:

Mental state
Cranial nerves
Strength
Reflexes
Coordination
Sensation
Appropriately detailed musculoskeletal assessment

The musculoskeletal assessment is most rewarding for patients with chronic or acute recurring headache.

The neuromusculoskeletal assessment includes active and static body analysis. Observe and palpate the facial and mandibular attachments, the temporomandibular joints, and the temporalis, masseter, occipito-frontalis, buccinator, and pterygoid muscles, evaluating levels of muscle contraction and local tenderness with direct superficial and deep cervical palpation from the skin to the synovial joints. Assess rotational characteristics of the head, cervical, and upper thoracic regions, as well as the basioccipital attachments at the atlas for anterior, lateral, and posterior asymmetry. In addition, carry out a screening of the total musculoskeletal system. The screening can include evaluation of:

Leg length and lower extremity symmetry
Sacropelvic base analysis
Cranial rhythmic activity
Suture mobility analysis

In clinical practice, the relationship between symptoms and signs and the ability to reproduce the painful symptoms during the examination are helpful in clinical localization. This is particularly true for the biomechanical syndromes, such as (21–23):

Temporomandibular joint syndrome
Malocclusive dental syndromes
Cervical spine syndromes (spondylosis, disc degeneration, facet dysfunction)
Cranial neuralgias
Cranial suture syndrome
Short leg syndrome
Nerve encroachment syndrome
Myofascial pain syndromes

This type of evaluation supplies information that can be essential to formulating comprehensive therapeutic objectives.

Therapeutic success can be optimized by multimodality evaluation and treatment. The psychosocial model can suggest whether cognitive, behavioral, or psychotherapeutic intervention is needed. The pharmacologic model attempts to describe the problem neurochemically and offers a logical interventional protocol based on differential pharmacotherapeutic profiles (such as serotonergic, dopaminergic, noradrenergic, GABA-ergic, cholinergic). The biomechanical model provides a rational basis for choosing among manipulative treatment methods (i.e., direct action, indirect action, or myofascial techniques).

Furthermore, therapies directed at enhancing the self-healing capacities of an individual are important in the overall therapeutic formulation. These therapies include nutritional evaluation and counseling, evaluation and education in sleep hygiene, instruction and prescription of appropriate relaxation and stress reduction therapies, the use of therapeutic exercise, and the promotion of a positive attitude through education about the nature of headaches, the realistic objectives of management, and the use of positive visual imagery (24).

Migraine Headaches

In migraine headaches, disordered neurogenic control of the craniocerebral circulation accompanies the attack (25). The trigeminal vascular system (the trigeminal neuron whose unmyelinated axon surrounds a cephalic blood vessel) functions in pain transmission and in promoting inflammation in the affected blood vessels via the neurochemical activity of substance P (26). Cerebral, meningeal, basilar, and vertebral arteries can be affected through the trigeminal, vagal, and upper cervical axons, which all converge in the trigeminal nucleus caudalis of the brainstem (27,28). The inflammatory response is associated with norepinephrine and serotonin release of brainstem origin, and histamine, adenosine, and bradykinin of local origin.

When the migraine is triggered, the intrinsic brainstem noradrenergic system (from the locus ceruleus) is activated and triggers enhanced neuronal firing in the susceptible cerebral cortex. This firing in the cerebral cortex originates a spreading wave of cortical depolarization that ultimately reaches pain-sensitive blood vessels, resulting in depolarization of the associated trigemino-vascular axon. This depolarization triggers a sterile inflammatory reaction through the release of substance P and the activation of mast cells and prostaglandin synthesis (25,26).

Migraine can be accompanied by an aura consisting of neurologic changes, typically in a vascular distribution, lasting from 10 to 90 minutes, that mimics and sometimes results in transient cerebral ischemia. In rare cases, the neurologic aura resolves and the migraine becomes complicated as the patient suffers cerebral infarction. The most common auras are ocular and can involve scintillating scotomata or flashing lights, often occurring in jagged lines—the so-called fortification spectrum (29). The visual phenomena can be multicolored and typically changes size, shape, and distribution during the evolving aura. The aura usually precedes the actual headache but can occur during and even after. On occasion, the aura is separate from the headache component or the headache can be absent (30).

Multifocal neurologic symptoms can occur in the basilar artery distribution (the Bickerstaff syndrome) and include (31):

Cranial nerve changes
Dysarthria
Facial paresthesia
Ataxia
Vertigo

In the middle cerebral artery distribution, migraine can have manifestations of hemiparesis, hemisensory loss, or aphasia. In general, the aura presents with visual phenomena, atypical for cerebrovascular insufficiency. A clue to migraine symptoms is a gradual progression of symptoms, unlike the rapid march of a focal seizure or the sudden onset of cerebral vessel thrombosis or embolism.

Migraine can begin in childhood, adolescence, or adulthood. In women, it can be associated with hormonal fluctuation. Migraine is typically a throbbing pain, following a vascular distribution of the superficial or deep cerebral vessels and lasting for several hours. It is often associated with nausea or vomiting, and sensitivity to bright lights, loud noises, or strong smells. For some patients, tenderness, tightness, pain, and limitation of motion in the suboccipital and cervical musculature accompanies migraine. Characteristically, migraine is relieved by sleep.

On initial presentation of migraine, it is not always possible to be certain of the diagnosis, and a well-designed differential diagnostic process is appropriate (Table 30.2). Although the risk of aneurysm, brain tumor, arteriovenous malformation, or vasculitis is slight, enhanced brain computed tomography, magnetic resonance imaging (MRI), or cerebral angiography is useful to exclude these possibilities and should be used if the diagnosis is uncertain (32).

Migraine can acutely respond to vasoactive drugs, such as sumatriptan, other triptans, dihydroergotamine, ergotamine, isometheptene, and even caffeine. The serotonin 1-d receptor agonists (sumatriptan, dihydroergotamine) are particularly effective in aborting a migraine. Simple agents like aspirin or acetaminophen are often combined with barbiturates and/or narcotics. Other nonsteroidal antiinflammatory drugs (NSAIDs) are also used with variable success. The parenteral use of phenothiazines is helpful; but unfortunately, they are frequently associated with unacceptable side effects (33).

When migraine headaches are frequent or severe, the prophylactic use of medications is indicated. Medications used regularly to help prevent migraines include beta-blockers (e.g., propranolol), calcium channel blockers (e.g., verapamil), tricyclic antidepressants (e.g., amitriptyline), serotonin antagonists (e.g., cyproheptadine, fluoxetine), ergot derivatives (e.g., methysergide), and anticonvulsants (e.g., valproic acid).

Nonpharmacologic approaches, including OMT, are often valuable. Osteopathic management of migraine can include OMT. In the active phase of migraine, vigorous treatment can, theoretically, increase blood flow to an already inflamed vascular bed, thereby explaining the clinical exacerbation that can follow treatment. Gentle therapy with indirect techniques, and venous and lymphatic drainage techniques are likely more helpful during the attack. Because of the prominent autonomic involvement, evaluate and treat at the sympathetic sites of lower cervical and upper thoracic vertebrae, associated ribs, and myofascial attachments. Treatment can be directed at joints of the head and neck, muscles, and myofascial restrictions of the head, neck, and shoulders. Behavioral techniques like biofeedback, relaxation therapy, and programs that teach stress reduction and coping skills have also been successfully used to reduce the frequency and severity of migraine attacks (34). For some patients, musculoskeletal triggers or prodromes exist for their migraines (35,36).

The possible role of musculoskeletal triggers is further suggested in posttraumatic migraine. In such cases, trauma to the skull, cervical spine, or myofascial elements is followed by a unilateral, throbbing migraine (21,37). These headaches can recur for days, weeks, and months. OMT can be used in an attempt to modify triggers that arise from bony, ligamentous, and myofascial structures. In practice, OMT is especially useful between migraine events, when the patient is more tolerant of manipulation.

Applications of local heat, cold, massage, acupressure, trigger point therapy, acupuncture, traction, or local anesthetic blockade can be used in these regions that typically harbor tender points referring pain to the headache zone. These applications might help to decrease the afferent activity from the painful site and reduce the primary and secondary muscle spasms.

Cluster Headaches

Cluster headache is a distinctive vascular syndrome characterized by attacks that tend to occur daily for weeks at a time only to vanish again for months or years. Approximately 20% of patients develop a chronic form, called chronic paroxysmal hemicrania or hemicrania continua (38). Clinicians believe that cluster headaches are the result of neurogenic inflammation affecting the vascular plexus of the cavernous sinus, its tributaries, and its autonomic nervous supply (39,40). The headaches tend to occur at certain times of the day; most notably, they develop 2–3 hours after going to sleep. Like migraine, cluster headaches often occur when the individual is switching from rapid eye motion (REM) sleep to non-REM sleep. This is accompanied by a shift from parasympathetic, cholinergic activity to sympathetic, aminergic (catecholamine, serotonin, and norepinephrine) activity (41).

TABLE 30.2. HEADACHES RESULTING FROM SYSTEMIC DISEASE OR PRIMARY NEUROLOGIC DISORDER

Disorder	Pathophysiology	Clinical Features	Paraclinical Features (lab, x-ray, etc.)	Treatment
Glaucoma (61)	Increased intraocular pressure	Dilated pupil, disturbed vision, general headache	Abnormal tonometry	Medication, surgery
Cerebral aneurysm, ruptured or unruptured (62)	Berry aneurysm, hypertension	Explosive headache, nuchal rigidity, abnormal neurologic signs	Blood in the CSF, abnormal angiogram	Neurosurgery
Temporal arteritis (63)	Inflammation	Throbbing headache, >55 years old, tender temporal artery, blurred vision, jaw claudication	Elevated ESR, positive biopsy for arteritis	Glucocorticoids
Optic neuritis (64)	Inflammation, demyelination	Orbital pain, loss of vision, worse with eye motion, papillitis	Abnormal visual evoked response, abnormal MRI	Glucocorticoids
Dissection of carotid or vertebral arteries (65–67)	Drugs, trauma	Severe, local pain, tender artery, Horner syndrome	Angiogram, ultrasound, MRI, MRA	Surgery, anticoagulants
Temporomandibular joint syndrome, internal derangement, myofascial (68)	Joint degeneration, muscular imbalance	Pain in jaw, click in joint, locking of joint, pain with lateral or vertical movement, tight muscles	Abnormal MRI	Dental, physical therapy, exercise
Trigeminal neuralgia (69)	Irritation of CN-5, vascular loop, mechanical	Sharp, stabbing pain in trigeminal zone, triggers: wind, eating, chewing	Rarely abnormal MRI	Medication (anticonvulsants), neurosurgery
Herpes zoster trigeminalis cervicalis	Infection	Burning pain hypersensitive rash/vesicles	Virus identification	Antiviral therapy
Meningitis encephalitis	Usually infection bacterial viral, etc.	Nuchal rigidity acute headache, fever, signs of infection	(+)CSF pleiocytosis, low glucose, high protein	Antibiotics, corticosteroids, supportive therapy
Sinusitis, facial osteomyelitis (70)	Infection	Nasal obstruction, tender bone, fever	Leukocytosis, abnormal CT/MRI	Antibiotics
Intracranial hypertension from a mass	Traction, displacement of painful structures, block of CSF, hydrocephalus	Recent onset, headache, worse at rest papilledema	Abnormal CT/MRI	Glucocorticoids, furosemide, mannitol, neurosurgery
Benign intracranial hypertension (71)	Altered CSF dynamics	Young, female, obesity, hormone fluctuating, sight papilledema	Increased CSF pressure, small ventricles, enlarged blind spot	Glucocorticoids, acetazolamide, CSF removal, neurosurgery
Exertional headache, strain, lift, cough, exercise, coitus (72)	Posterior fossa mass, Chiari malformation, migraine variant	Abrupt, severe, lasts 15–20 minutes, men > women	CT/MRI	If no mass, precede activity with NSAIDs
Normal pressure hydrocephalus	Communicating, block in CSF absorption	Ataxia, incontinence, dementia	Hydrocephalus, cisternography	Ventricular shunt, CSF removal
Myofascial pain syndrome (23)	Trauma	Bands, nodules, trigger points, poor sleep	—	OMT, spray/stretch, needling

CSF, cerebrospinal fluid; ESR, erythrocyte sedimentation rate; MRI, magnetic resonance imaging; CT, computed tomography; NSAIDS, nonsteroidal antiinflammatory drugs; OMT, osteopathic manipulative treatment.

Cluster headaches tend to be periorbital in location and characteristically develop rapidly and reach severe intensity within minutes. They are associated with autonomic vasomotor features including:

Ptosis
Miosis
Conjunctival injection
Unilateral lacrimation
Rhinorrhea
Nasal stuffiness

Distinct from migraine, cluster headaches are much more common in men. They can occur several times a day and can even awaken the sufferer from sleep. Cluster headaches can be seen after trauma and, at times, can refer pain to the cervical and upper thoracic paraspinal region, as well as to the suprascapular region (42,43).

The carotid-cavernous vasculature is involved along with its autonomic innervation. This includes the pterygopalatine ganglion and the cervical sympathetic ganglia. Patients often have a tender carotid artery, called carotidynia. Attempts to anesthetize the pterygopalatine ganglion with cocaine or lidocaine have been somewhat successful. Cluster headaches might respond acutely to parenteral sumatriptan or dihydroergotamine, both of which are serotonin 1-d receptor agonists (44). Many respond to inhaled oxygen via facial mask (5–7 L/minute for 5–10 minutes). Prophylactically, beta-blockers, calcium channel blockers, and tricyclic antidepressants are used along with short courses of high-dose steroids or NSAIDs. For the more chronic cluster, lithium is a potent therapy. Not surprisingly, OMT is best directed to the upper ribs, the cervicothoracic spine, the associated soft tissues, and the relevant craniofacial structures.

Tension-Type Headaches

Tension-type headaches are classified by the International Headache Society as episodic or chronic. They are further divided by the presence or absence of involvement of the pericranial muscles. Involvement can be demonstrated by electromyography or palpation (45,46).

Tension-type headache is the most frequent headache type. It is characterized by mild-to-moderate intensity pain, described as pressing or tightening, typically bilateral, and usually occipital in location. In distinction from migraine, it is not aggravated by exercise or routine physical activity. Like migraine, it runs in families, is more common in women, and can be affected by hormonal cycles. It is episodic if it occurs less than half the days of the month and chronic if it occurs more than half the days of the month (47).

The International Headache Society distinguishes between tension-type and migraine headaches. Many believe, however, that these headache types are related disorders. In fact, most patients with migraines have tension-type headaches, and many patients with tension-type headaches have migraines. Both migraine and tension-type headaches might be the result of abnormalities in central pain control mechanisms, as well as trigeminal neuronal hypersensitivity. Both might be associated with muscle tenderness, electromyographic abnormalities, and abnormal platelet serotonin levels. When severe, they both can be associated with depressed cerebrospinal fluid; β-endorphins (47).

Clinicians theorize that there might be a vascular, supraspinal, and myogenic integrated model for migraine and tension-type headache (48). The trigeminal nucleus caudalis is a major relay nucleus for head and neck pain. Nociceptive input from the pericranial muscles and the cephalic arteries converge at this nucleus, which has excitatory and inhibitory output. When the afferent nociceptive signal is intense, sensitization of the entire pain pathway, peripheral and central, can occur. This facilitation creates a painful sensitivity to typically nonnoxious stimuli. In the migraine, the nociceptors are vascular and the nonnoxious stimuli are vascular pulsations. In the tension-type headache, the nociceptors are myofascial and the nonnoxious stimuli are muscle contractions. In either case, supraspinal facilitation is likely to be present and neuronal sensitization can occur.

Some neurologists would modify the classification of the International Headache Society to include chronic daily headache, which is further differentiated as a daily or near-daily type of headache with superimposed migraine. Patients with chronic headaches are prone to overusing multiple drugs and have a high rate of treatment failure. The headaches can be primary, as a transformed migraine, a chronic tension-type headache, a new daily headache, or hemicrania continua. Secondary causes of chronic daily headache can exist, including posttraumatic headache, cervical spine dysfunction, vascular disorders, and nonvascular intracranial disorders (35,49–51). Frequently, an episodic problem becomes chronic as a result of analgesic medication overuse.

Treatment begins with a close look to identify any medication overuse, drug dependency, or depression, which require specific intervention. Inquire for a past history of emotional, physical, or sexual abuse and incorporate that information into the treatment rationale. Every effort is made to identify and eliminate potential sources for triggers, such as the:

Teeth
Jaw
Sinuses
Cranial and cervical bones
Joints
Ligaments
Associated myofascial structures

These, too, demand specific interventions. Physical, psychological, and pharmacologic therapies can operate concurrently (52).

Treatment

In headache management, the presence of somatic dysfunction is systematically identified and handled with OMT. Cervical vertebral segmental disorders, focal and regional myofascial disorders, and craniosacral disorders are common (53,54). Exercise particular care with regard to manipulation of the cervical spine. Infrequently, cervical manipulation has been reported to aggravate a herniated intervertebral disc or a spinal cord injury (55); most critically, cervical manipulation has been associated with vertebral artery laceration, intimal dissection, thrombosis, and thromboembolic infarction in the vertebrobasilar distribution of the posterior circulation (56–58). Most of the complications have been seen with hyperextension and hyperrotation of the upper craniocervical segments, often in the course of a thrusting technique (59).

Pharmacologic therapy is best served with a clearly limited (symptomatic) regimen to prevent drug-induced headaches. Preventive therapy is usually begun with a tricyclic antidepressant, especially useful when there is an associated sleep disturbance. More recently, sodium valproate has been found to have prophylactic value in chronic daily headache.

Nonpharmacologic therapies are also prescribed. Patients can be evaluated and educated regarding proper sleep hygiene. A therapeutic exercise program should be customized to the patient. Nutritional evaluation and recommendations can be given. Relaxation strategies and visual imagery techniques can be taught to each patient. It is important to involve the patient as an active participant in his or her own therapy.

Being able to assess the patient more completely permits a more comprehensive diagnosis. Multifactorial problems allow the formulation of a more thorough and multifaceted treatment program, increasing the potential for success. The osteopathic approach offers a successful model for an integrated multidimensional treatment with the patient as the focus and the physician as the facilitator (60).

In addition to primary headache syndromes, a wide variety of neurologic and systemic disorders present with headache. These disorders must be considered when evaluating the patient en route to establishing a working and differential diagnosis, before proceeding with any therapeutic intervention. Table 30.2 is a collection of some of those conditions, highlighting clinical, diagnostic, and therapeutic features.

In general, less specific symptoms indicate a greater suspicion that something more than benign headache is present. Consider further diagnostic studies, MRI, computerized tomography, electroencephalography, cerebral angiography, blood and cerebrospinal fluid analysis, and neurologic consultation when the patient does not respond promptly and appropriately to osteopathic medical management.

SPINAL DISORDERS

The practice of neurology frequently involves problems affecting the spine. This can involve the spinal column and its structural elements (spondylopathy), the nerve roots (radiculopathy), and even the spinal cord (myelopathy).

The spinal column includes the vertebral body, the intervertebral disc, the facet joints, the ligaments, and the myotendinous structures. The pathophysiology of spinal column disorders often involves a degenerative process, such as spondylosis (osteoarthritis) of the vertebral body, which is frequently seen in association with degeneration of the intervertebral disc. The degeneration ultimately affects the adjacent related facet joints and results in strain in ligaments and myotendinous structures. Trauma commonly underlies this process (73).

The spinal column can also be affected by malignancy arising in the bone or, more commonly, from secondary metastasis of systemic cancer. Infection of the spinal column can result from systemic infection, such as mycobacterial, fungal, or bacterial sepsis. Spinal pathologic conditions can also occur with osteoporosis and other metabolic abnormalities of bone, or from less common arthritic diseases, such as ankylosing spondylitis or rheumatoid arthritis. Disease processes adjacent to the spine can also result in spinal column destruction, including paraspinal tumors and abscesses (74–77).

A common pathophysiologic process affecting the spinal column is the process of somatic dysfunction. Somatic dysfunction can affect single segments or multiple spinal segments and accompany any of the aforementioned spinal column pathologies.

The spinal nerve roots are affected by their location within the spinal canal. They are exposed to trauma from (78–80):

Extruding discs
Fractured bone fragments
Spinal and paraspinal tumors
Degenerative changes in the vertebral elements
Intraspinal ligaments
Frank avulsions

In addition, the nerve roots lack the tight endothelial junction of the blood–brain barrier; the result is lowered protection from infection (e.g., herpes zoster, syphilis), neoplastic invasion, inflammatory demyelination (e.g., Guillain-Barré syndrome), or toxic exposure to chemotherapy agents, myelographic contrast agents, or anesthetic agents. The nerve roots are also suscepti-

ble to vascular insufficiency in the form of vasculitis, diabetes mellitus, and radiation exposure (81).

Spinal cord syndromes can result from an intrinsic pathologic condition or from injury to the spinal cord from extrinsic compression. Intrinsic spinal cord pathologic conditions include myelitis, typically as a result of a virus, vasculitis, or multiple sclerosis, and neoplasms of the glial elements of the cord. Nutritional deficiencies can also result in degeneration of the spinal cord—typically subacute combined degeneration from cobalamin deficiency. CNS degenerative diseases affecting the spinal cord include motor neuron disease and multisystem degeneration. The spinal cord is vulnerable to ischemia if there is disruption in the anterior spinal artery circulation. Severe spinal trauma can result in hemorrhage or laceration of the spinal cord. Extrinsic compression of the spinal cord can result from the same conditions that cause nerve root compression, typically tumors that are primary or metastatic in the spinal canal, and from epidural infection or hematoma. Compression fractures of the vertebral bodies can result in subluxation and spinal cord compression. When the spinal cord is compressed from epidural tumor or infection, the spinal cord symptoms are preceded by vertebral pain (82–85).

The symptom of vertebral bone or ligament disease is usually pain. Typically, patients complain of deep and aching pain in the affected region of the spine. Often, the pain is worse in certain positions or with certain activities. For example, patients with intervertebral disc disease commonly complain that their back pain is worse with prolonged sitting or standing, whereas acute problems are made worse with activity and improved with rest. The pain can refer locally to paraspinal segments. This referral pattern most likely has to do with nociceptors converging on a common dorsal horn projection neuron (86). In the cervical region, the pain can involve the upper arm, shoulder, and scapulothoracic region. In the lumbar region, it involves the low back, hip, and upper leg. Numbness, weakness, and other neurologic symptoms are notably absent when only the bone and ligamentous vertebral elements are affected.

Patients with radiculopathy might complain of pain, numbness, tingling, or other sensations that typically are described as radiating from proximal to distal. In the cervical region (C-2–T-2), the radiation is in a dermatomal pattern in the posterior cranial region, neck, upper torso, and upper extremity. In the lumbosacral region (L-1–S-5), it is in a dermatomal pattern in the low back, buttock, and low extremity. In the thoracic region, the radiation is in a dermatomal pattern in the chest or abdomen. Because the pain is generated in the nerve root, patients describe a variety of pain sensations, including electric, burning, stabbing, dull, sharp, or tearing pain. Patients also describe impulses of pain with coughing, sneezing, lifting, or moving the bowels. The pain is often worse with positions that either compress the nerve root (side-bending of the spine) or stretch the nerve root (forward bending of the spine). The pain can be relieved by maneuvers that take the pressure or stretch off of the nerve root. Spinal stenosis can produce radicular symptoms on the basis of intermittent ischemia to the nerve roots, typically related to walking.

When the motor fibers are affected, patients with radiculopathy can complain of weakness localized to the muscles innervated. In the lumbosacral region, the nerves supplying bladder, bowel, and sexual function can be affected; patients might complain of urinary hesitancy or retention, constipation, or impotence.

The pain of spinal tract origin is diffuse and referred several segments below the level of the lesion. The location of motor and sensory complaints depends on the area of the spinal cord involved. Unilateral lesions of the spinothalamic tract cause contralateral numbness to pain and temperature, whereas lesions of the posterior columns cause ipsilateral loss of position sense, light touch, and vibration. Bilateral lesions of the sensory fibers result in bilateral sensory disturbances below the level. Limb weakness results when there is an abnormality in the anterior horn cells or corticospinal tracts. The weakness can be accompanied by atrophy if it is in the lower motor neurons or spasticity if in the upper motor neurons. Bladder, bowel, and sexual functions are often compromised.

On physical examination, test sensation with pain, temperature, and touch. With radiculopathy, the sensory loss is dermatomal, and the margins of sensory loss might not be as demarcated, as seen in peripheral nerve lesions. The motor deficits are in muscle groups with a common myotomal innervation. The weakness of individual muscles is usually partial rather than complete. Because the ventral roots contain the lower motor neurons, radicular weakness is often associated with fasciculations, decreased muscle tone and bulk, and decreased reflexes. In the upper extremities, the root innervation is checked by the deep tendon reflexes of the biceps (predominantly C-5), brachioradialis (predominantly C-6), triceps (C-7), and the finger flexors (C-8). In the lower extremities, the root innervation is checked by the deep tendon reflexes of the quadriceps (predominantly L-4), biceps femoris (L-5), and gastrocnemius (predominantly S-1). Unilateral sacral root lesions can cause numbness but usually do not affect muscle control. However, when bilateral sacral roots are involved, the rectal sphincter becomes weak. Test muscle strength for all of the major muscle groups of the upper and lower extremities.

Provocative maneuvers can be of great diagnostic value in patients with radiculopathy. In cervical or lumbar nerve root compression syndromes, side-bending of the involved spine can narrow the intervertebral foramina and increase radicular complaints (Spurling sign). Conversely, applying manual traction to the cervical or lumbar region usually offers relief. Stretching the nerve roots of the sciatic nerve with straight leg raising can provoke radicular symptoms (Lasègue sign). Manual compression of the external jugular veins can cause an increase in intraspinal pressure. Compression aggravating radicular symptoms in either the upper or lower extremity (Naffziger sign) can be a sign of nerve root compression (87).

Many diagnostic tools are available for evaluating the functional and structural aspects of nerve roots. MRI offers the best noninvasive view of the nerve roots and surrounding structures. Computerized tomography has some value when bone details are needed. Invasive myelography, with the instillation of intrathecal contrast, continues to have a role diagnostically, especially when combined with post-myelogram computerized tomography. Sometimes it is important to evaluate the cerebrospinal fluid for signs of infection, inflammation, neoplasia, or hemorrhage by determining the cell count along with protein, glucose, and microbiologic studies (88–90).

The functional status of nerve roots can be tested with nerve conduction studies that include antegrade and retrograde response to stimulus (F responses and the H reflexes). Nerve conduction studies and electromyography can reveal the presence of radiculopathy, but the abnormalities detected are a function of the chronicity of the lesion. Electrophysiologic testing of the nerve roots can also be done with somatosensory evoked potentials (91–93).

The physical findings in myelopathy classically reveal a sensory level. Spinothalamic-mediated pain and temperature, and dorsal column-mediated touch, vibration, and position sense are disturbed below the level of spinal cord disturbance. Typically, this affects pain and temperature beginning several segments below the actual level of the lesion. Usually both sides are affected. Because primarily upper motor neurons are involved, the motor examination reveals a spastic increase in tone and an increase in the muscle stretch reflexes below the level of the lesion. Weakness is diffuse and can be mild or severe. The distribution of weakness reflects the pathologic condition in the anterior horn cells or corticospinal tracts. Depending on the level of the lesion, the patient can have positive Babinski signs and ankle clonus in the lower extremities and positive Hoffman signs in the upper extremities. Sphincter tone can be increased. Gait can be disturbed by spasticity, weakness, or sensory ataxia. Patients with dorsal column sensory loss lose their balance and fall when asked to stand unaided with their eyes closed (Romberg sign). If the patient's neck is flexed, he or she could experience an electric sensation traveling the spinal cord and the extremities (Lhermitte sign), which is the result of stretching the long dorsal column fibers (87).

When specific disease of the spinal column is identified, institute appropriate treatment. When there is structural weakness, supportive bracing can be used. Physical therapies are often valuable. Therapeutic exercise regimens are an essential component to all comprehensive treatment plans. Consider nutritional assessment and supplementation when necessary. Use medications with analgesic, antiinflammatory, and bone supportive properties. Anesthetic blocks of locally irritable structures (or facets) can be effective (94).

OMT is useful in a wide range of vertebral column disorders, including those of somatic dysfunction (95–100). MacDonald (101) demonstrated responses to osteopathic manipulation for low back pain of 14 to 28 days' duration on the basis of outcome studies. In 1995 the Agency for Health Care Policy and Research (AHCPR) concluded manipulation to be safe and effective for patients in the first month of acute low back pain symptoms without radiculopathy (102). Osteopathic treatment is derived from the more comprehensive nature of the osteopathic neurologic evaluation. The examination can yield information local to the area of chief complaint, as well as more general information on the effects of interrelated problems. For example, a person with mechanical low back pain could have an associated visceral disease (such as endometriosis) that can contribute viscerosomatically to the physical findings that the patient presents. Likewise, a similar low back pain could be related to a problem with the foot or leg. By identifying contributing elements, a more complete diagnostic understanding can be reached and a more comprehensive treatment undertaken.

Standard treatment of radiculopathy is appropriately directed to the specific pathologic condition involved. For example, antiviral agents are used for herpes zoster infection, or antineoplastic agents for carcinomatous radiculopathy. For degenerative spine conditions causing radiculopathy, physical measures to reduce compression and deformation with traction, physical therapy, and therapeutic exercise are beneficial. Attempt to decrease inflammation with oral corticosteroids or nonsteroidal antiinflammatory medication. Sometimes the corticosteroids, along with anesthetic agents, are introduced into the epidural space, usually lumbar but occasionally thoracic or cervical (103,104). Patients are given extensive education about provocative aspects of their lifestyle, work, and habits with a goal of minimizing aggravating factors. If persistent radiculopathy causes progressing sensory or motor findings or pain that cannot be controlled, surgical decompression is advisable. When the cauda equina is affected, a particular urgency exists to diagnose and decompress. In these cases, a delay in treatment can be associated with a marked increase in morbidity and with lingering bladder, bowel, sexual, and lower extremity dysfunction.

Specific intervention with OMT has to be undertaken cautiously, if at all, for patients with radiculopathy. Any manipulative procedures that increase nerve root compression or deformation can be potentially injurious. Nonetheless, in careful hands, the use of knowledgeably applied gentle manipulative forces might improve conditions for the nerve root and could potentially affect arterial, venous, and lymphatic circulation, as well as improve local biomechanical factors. At the least, OMT can be useful in alleviating some of the secondary musculoskeletal reaction that develops in the face of nerve root pathologic conditions.

PERSONAL APPROACH TO NEUROLOGIC DIAGNOSIS

When patients present with variable complaints of pain, sensory disturbance, or weakness, it is the neurologist's job to answer three questions. These are:

i. Is there a neurologic abnormality?
ii. Can the neurologic abnormality be localized?
iii. Can a differential diagnosis be generated for the abnormality in question?

For example, if a patient presents with neck or back pain, the physician attempts to localize the symptom by history. An effort is made to differentiate spinal cord disorders, nerve root syndromes, or vertebral disorders.

In the general history, it is necessary to know the patient's past personal history of illness, trauma, and surgery. Knowing the family history is valuable as a potential source of hereditary or constitutional susceptibility. The general history includes a search into the history for abuse (substance, physical, sexual, and emotional). At the same time, explore the psychosocial background of the patient and his or her family. Inquire into the patient's nutrition, work, and exercise habits, sleep patterns, and potential risk exposures. A mental status examination to evaluate the higher cortical functions and arousal system should be followed by a complete neurologic examination. This examination includes evaluation of the cranial nerves and the motor and sensory system. Test coordination and gait. Motor examination includes an assessment of

muscle tone, muscle strength, muscle bulk, and the activity of the associated myotendinous reflexes. Sensory examination includes tests of light touch, pain, temperature, vibration, and proprioception. In addition to a routine neurologic examination, perform a musculoskeletal structural examination for patients with spinal complaints, including (105):

i. Inspection of the patient walking and standing, from an anterior, posterior, and lateral view, looking for static and kinetic structural asymmetries.
ii. Performance of the standing flexion test.
iii. Performance of the standing lateral flexion test.
iv. Performance of the seated flexion test.
v. Assessment of seated trunk rotation.
vi. Assessment of seated lateral flexion.
vii. Seated cervical assessment for flexion, extension, lateral flexion, and rotation.
viii. Supine rib testing.
ix. Supine upper extremity testing.
x. Supine and prone lower extremity testing.

The musculoskeletal structural examination provides structural signs of asymmetry (e.g., scoliosis, an increase in kyphosis or lordosis, or significant deviation from balanced gravitational centering). In addition, the limbs and vertebral complex can be assessed for characteristics of motion by adding a palpatory examination of the soft tissue (muscles, ligaments, tendons, deep and superficial fascia, and the subcutaneous structures). The site of the primary musculoskeletal problem can often be determined. It is possible to know what biomechanical problems are helping to create, maintain, and aggravate the primary problem. In the areas of clinical interest, make the soft tissue examination, the motion testing, and the static structural examination precise to identify the local elements of dysfunction.

The musculoskeletal findings are often secondary to another disease of the musculoskeletal system, a reaction to internal disease, or a compensatory response to the presence of pain. Assessing the patient more thoroughly allows a more inclusive diagnosis with the possibility of a more extensive treatment program, increasing the potential for success. The ability to exclude the more unusual and potentially morbid conditions can only result from such an osteopathic evaluation. Additionally, this approach offers the ability to choose among multiple and costly diagnostic possibilities.

ENTRAPMENT NEUROPATHIES

Entrapment neuropathies represent a localized injury or irritation to one of the peripheral nerves. They are caused by the mechanical effects of the impinging adjacent tissues. The typical anatomic causes include entrapment within the osseofibrous tunnels where the nerve changes course against fibrous and muscular bands. Entrapment can be precipitated by trauma; once the trauma occurs, the local anatomic configuration often causes a repetition of a mechanical injury. This local anatomic configuration can result in local compressive injury to the neural elements. The neural elements at risk include both the axon and the associated myelin. It can compromise local circulation, including arterial, venous,

TABLE 30.3. SITES OF NERVE ENTRAPMENT AND TREATMENTS

Nerve	Site of Entrapment	Treatment
Median	Carpal tunnel, pronator teres, anterior interosseous syndrome	OMT, splint, exercise, surgery
Ulnar	Elbow, cubital tunnel, canal of Guyon, thoracic outlet	OMT, exercise, surgery
Radial	Supinator muscle	OMT, exercise, surgery
Brachial	Thoracic outlet scalenes, pectoralis minor, cervical rib	OMT, exercise, surgery
Sciatic	Pelvic outlet piriformis muscle	OMT, exercise, surgery
Posterior tibial	Tarsal tunnel	OMT, exercise, surgery
Common peroneal	Fibular head	OMT, exercise, surgery
Obturator	Obturator foramen	OMT, exercise, surgery
Femoral	Pelvic brim inguinal ligament	OMT, exercise, surgery
Ilioinguinal	Abdominal wall	OMT, exercise, surgery
Intercostal	Rib cage	OMT, exercise, surgery
Trigeminal	Foramen ovale, foramen totundum, petrosphenoid ligament, Meckel's cave	OMT, surgery
Cranial nerves II, III, IV, V, VI	Orbital apex, exit foramina, reciprocal tension membrane, cavernous sinus	OMT, surgery
Cranial nerves VIII, IX, X, XI, XII	Basisphenoid, basiocciput, jugular formina, hypoglossal canal	OMT, surgery
Cranial nerves VII, VIII	Temporal bone, internal auditory meatus	OMT, surgery
Cranial nerve I	Ethmoid, cribriform plate, sphenoid, lesser wing	OMT, surgery

OMT, osteopathic manipulative treatment.

and lymphatic influences. Table 30.3 represents specific sites of nerve entrapment (106,107).

Carpal Tunnel Syndrome

Carpal tunnel syndrome is the result of entrapment of the distal branches of the median nerve as it passes through the carpal tunnel. The tunnel is formed by the carpal bones and the carpal ligaments. The contents of the tunnel are flexor tendons and the median nerve. Either strong flexion or extension of the wrist can impact the median nerve. There can be acute compression with mechanical deformation and ischemic change. Chronic progressive compression can result in vascular compromise. The first effect of increased compression is an obstruction of venous return from the nerve, which leads to increased capillary distension and further increases in intratunnel pressure. This continues to self-amplify in a cyclic fashion, impairing nutrition to the nerve. The large, myelinated fibers are most vulnerable. At this stage, symptoms appear with pain, and paresthesia is usually transient and reversed by restoring proper circulation. As things get worse, the capillary circulation is sufficiently slowed to create endoneurial edema, epineural edema, and intratunnel edema. This edema can still be reversed if adequate decompression is obtained. In the final stages, there is arterial insufficiency and increasing mechanical deformation, resulting in nerve fiber destruction and ultimate fibrous replacement.

Carpal tunnel can be caused by trauma to the wrist, hypertrophic arthritides, or thickening of the flexor retinaculum. Hypertrophic neuropathy, local edema, ganglion cysts, and tenosynovitis can all compromise the carpal tunnel. Some systemic diseases are predisposing, such as:

Hypothyroidism
Diabetes mellitus
Pregnancy
Leukemia
Paraproteinemia
Gout

The diagnosis depends on a careful history to differentiate local disease from systemic disease. With systemic disease, the symptoms are frequently bilateral. The history is important in understanding predisposing biomechanical factors. These factors are often related to work, hobbies, or chronic behaviors. The patient complains of pain and paresthesias in the thumb, index, and long finger. Aching can spread proximally to the arm and forearm. Early, the pain is transient; later, it becomes permanent. Commonly, it is worse at night or during provocative activities. In the earliest stages, a shake of the hand can restore circulation and relieve symptoms. Later, immobilization with a splint can be relieving. Vague weakness, often described as dropping things, is common.

Physical examination reveals a sharply demarcated median nerve sensory deficit, confined to the palm, often splitting along the long finger or ring finger. Motor examination reveals a weakness of the thumb abductor, thumb opposer, and distal thumb flexor. In the more advanced stages, atrophy of the thenar eminence is evident. Tinel sign is often positive, with percussion of the nerve at the wrist producing a tingling into the hand. Phalen test, forced wrist flexion, can reproduce the pain and paresthesias. Even a reversed Phalen test, forced wrist extension, can be provocative.

Electrodiagnostic tests are helpful in corroborating the diagnosis and quantifying the degree of abnormality. The finding of prolongation of the distal motor and/or sensory latencies is an early sign of demyelination. Axonal involvement and degeneration are demonstrated by the appearance of neurogenic atrophy on electromyography. The electromyogram can be useful to rule out more proximal lesions, such as a radiculopathy. The carpal tunnel itself may be demonstrated on plain radiogram, computed tomogram, and even better with MRI, which can reveal the structural consequences of an anatomic compression.

The standard treatment has consisted of immobilization with wrist splints and avoidance of the provocative activities related to the carpal tunnel syndrome. Paraneural infiltration with local anesthetics and corticosteroids is sometimes used. When conservative measures fail, surgical decompression is the appropriate treatment (108).

The osteopathic neurologist begins with a more thorough evaluation. Not only is the biomechanical function of the wrist examined but the biomechanics of the fingers, hand, forearm, elbow, arm, shoulder, cervical and thoracic spine, and rib cage are also assessed. This assessment is performed in the context of a complete osteopathic structural examination. Restrictive lesions along the upper extremity and shoulder girdle can influence circulation (venous, lymphatic, and arterial) and mechanical deformation of the median nerve that begins at the nerve root, runs through the brachial plexus, and terminates in the median nerve that runs through the arm and forearm before passing through the carpal tunnel. Whole body mechanical issues, like slumped posture, can influence the local conditions at the carpal tunnel. The veins and lymphatics drain proximally into the superior vena cava and thoracic duct. Mechanical dysfunction in the rib cage and cervicothoracic region are as relevant as the mechanics of the arm itself. Arterial insufficiency can be affected similarly at multiple levels. The sympathetic component, often understated, can be influenced from the root of the neck, where the sympathetic ganglia are found, through the upper extremity itself.

The treatment, then, is to treat general structural problems with OMT and exercise. Direct manipulation to the functional releasing of biomechanical barriers at the:

Neck
Upper back
Shoulder
Rib cage
Thoracic inlet and outlet
Upper arm
Forearm
Wrist
Hand
Fingers

The techniques can be direct or indirect, and numerous examples of osteopathic treatment approaches have been proposed. These include myofascial release, muscle energy, thrusting, and functional techniques (97,100,109). Sucher (109) has demonstrated a model for clinically, electrophysiologically, and graphically evaluating carpal tunnel syndrome. He has shown the pathologic changes on neurologic examination, through distal nerve latency studies, and by obtaining MRI images of the carpal tunnel to measure its volume. He has then proceeded to treat these patients with OMT. He retests his patients and demonstrates objective changes in neurologic findings, distal nerve latencies, and carpal tunnel volume, as measured by MRI. Sucher (110) presents strong evidence for the therapeutic value of osteopathic management techniques.

Another syndrome of nerve entrapment is thoracic outlet syndrome. This is a syndrome affecting the brachial plexus at the level of the cervicobrachial junction. It is associated with abnormal cervical ribs and most often with disturbed myofascial relations. Thoracic outlet syndrome most typically affects the lower trunk of the brachial plexus. Compression can occur over the slope of the first rib, in the triangle made by the scalenus anterior and medius, along fibrotendinous attachments of any of the scalenes, along fibrosseous cervical rib rudiments, or under the pectoralis minor.

Patients might also complain of pain and numbness of the upper extremity typically extending along the ulnar aspect of the hand. The pain is usually worse with the arm elevated or abducted. Thoracic outlet syndrome can be associated with pain, weakness, and a variety of sensory complaints. Physical findings include sensory loss, particularly in the ulnar distribution. Weakness of intrinsic, ulnar innervated muscles is an unusual late finding in thoracic outlet syndrome. Provocative tests are helpful to diagnose and localize the syndrome. Depending on the site of entrapment, there might be localized tenderness. For example, with symptoms elicited on isometric scalene contraction, the entrapment can be localized to the scalene triangle and is associated with localized tenderness of the brachial plexus at this site. When hyperabduction with extension is the culprit, the site of entrapment is often the tendon of the pectoralis minor and local pectoral hypertonicity; tenderness is typical. Sometimes a bruit of the subclavian artery can be auscultated at the site of its compression (111).

Electrodiagnostic confirmation is frequently difficult. Prolonged nerve conduction velocity across the thoracic outlet can be demonstrated; in more advanced cases, axonal involvement might be encountered on electromyography. Somatosensory evoked potentials of the upper extremity can be localizing (112). Imaging of the region in question is best attempted with MRI; however, MRI findings are frequently inconclusive. Simple cervical spine radiograms might reveal the presence of cervical ribs.

Standard management includes exercises to improve posture, reduce mechanical stress, lengthen shortened muscles, and avoiding symptom-producing circumstances. Analgesics, antiinflammatory agents, muscle relaxants, and physical therapies are used. Progressive stretching exercises are included when indicated. When conservative measures fail, surgical intervention remains.

Osteopathic management of thoracic outlet syndrome includes appropriate structural evaluation with particular attention to the cervical, thoracic, costal, scapular, and brachial mechanical relationships. In comparison with carpal tunnel, the thoracic outlet syndrome involves a more widely affected area. It is therefore more difficult to define the inciting event and to establish targeted therapy. Evaluation of posture reveals a high incidence of posture with head forward and with rounded, upward, and anterior displaced shoulders. Evaluation of the work station and of the habits of the patient can reveal a subset of behaviors that are dysfunctional. OMT consisting of myofascial-releasing maneuvers to the restrictive musculoskeletal structures can be useful. When they are only temporarily useful and symptoms return when the patient resumes his or her unaltered lifestyle, efforts to modify the patient's life circumstances are employed. These efforts include modification and elimination of occupational and avocational mechanical stressors and the promotion of postural awareness with training in postural modification. The most important long-term aspects are the identification of the specific biomechanical restrictors and the prescription and training of the patient in the performance of self-administered stretching exercises (113–116). As a general concept, the temporary beneficial response to manipulative therapies can be understood using this model. When the pathologic process involves chronically acquired, well-learned maladaptive somatic behaviors, it is not surprising that a single manipulation does not eradicate such a process. Multiple strategies are necessary. Patient education, instruction, and performance in a protracted therapeutic exercise program is often most useful. In this way, the neuromusculoskeletal system can be reeducated.

A particularly osteopathic approach to the cranial neuropathies can be based on the writings of Sutherland as outlined by Magoun (107). In this text, the anatomy of the nerves and their relationship to dural investments, nearby vasculature, bony foraminae, and osseoligamentous structures are elaborately described. The naturally mobile aspect of these cranial and intracranial structures was appreciated. Sutherland and Magoun recognized the potential for vulnerability to mechanical distortion and compression with the resultant production of symptoms, often directly localized to individual cranial nerves. Such symptoms can be related to trauma, developmental phenomena, inflammation, or ischemia.

Chronic Pain Syndrome

There is a difference between patients suffering acute pain and those suffering chronic pain (see Chapters 8, 15, and 35). Patients with acute and subacute pain syndromes typically have some degree of tissue injury with nociceptive activation. These can be recurring events, as in rheumatoid arthritis, migraine headache, or trigeminal neuralgia. Ongoing acute pain is usually the result of continued nociceptive input from a destructive type of lesion, such as a malignant neoplasm.

Conversely, chronic benign nonmalignant pain syndromes last for more than 6 months without obvious signs of ongoing tissue damage. These chronic pain syndromes can be associated with adequate or inadequate coping by the patient. When coping is insufficient, the pain becomes the central focus for the patient. Patients with this problem are believed to have continuous low-level nociceptive barrage or alteration of central processing pathways. This nociceptive barrage can be the result of musculoskeletal or other peripheral pathologic processes with nociceptor activation. It can also reflect a pathologic condition of the nociceptors, their axons, and their central connections (117).

Clinical experience demonstrates a high incidence of biomechanical dysfunction in the patient with the chronic pain syndrome. It is not uncommon that patients with this type of pain syndrome are under recognized as having a significant structural pathologic condition. In fact, significant biomechanical dysfunction can be present, representing either a primary or secondary process. This information can go unrecognized by the majority of evaluators who use only standard neurologic and medical evaluation. Patients can begin with one pathologic problem and over time develop secondary somatic dysfunction. Conversely, patients can begin with a primary biomechanical insult that eludes recognition. In either event, the recognition of somatic dysfunction and its appropriate management are helpful in the global management of the patient with chronic pain.

One outcome of a good structural examination is the diagnosis of the common and often overlooked myofascial pain syndrome (see Chapter 66). This syndrome requires the palpatory identification of tender trigger points in muscles that, when palpated, cause pain to be referred to distant sites. These patterns of referral have been meticulously detailed by Travell and Simons (23). The muscles can harbor painful nodules and bands that act as trigger points and are associated with pain, stiffness, limitation of motion, and weakness. Identified appropriately, the muscles are responsive to a variety of different treatments directed at the active trigger point. When these trigger points are deactivated by deep pressure, dry needling, local infiltration, stretching, or OMT, they no longer serve as a source for pain generation (118).

Nonpharmacologic therapies focused on enhancing the self-healing capacities of an individual are particularly important in the overall therapeutic formulation. These nonpharmacologic therapies include:

- Nutritional evaluation and counseling
- Evaluation and education in therapeutic sleep hygiene
- Instruction and prescription of appropriate relaxation
- Stress reduction techniques
- Therapeutic exercise
- Positive visual imagery
- Promotion of a positive attitude through education about the nature of their pain problem
- Formation of realistic objectives of management

All of these techniques involve the patient as an active participant in his or her own therapy.

CONCLUSION

It is clear that assessing the patient more completely generates a more comprehensive diagnosis. This fosters the prescription for a multifaceted treatment program that increases the potential for success. An additional advantage includes an ability to exclude more unusual yet potentially morbid causes of chronic pain. Furthermore, it offers the osteopathic neurologist the tools to rationally choose among the multiple and costly diagnostic and therapeutic possibilities. The osteopathic approach offers a successful model for integrated multidimensional treatment with the patient as the focus and the physician as the facilitator (119).

REFERENCES

1. Still AT. *Autobiography of A. T. Still*. Kirksville, MO: published by the author; 1897.
2. Denslow JS. Neural basis of the somatic component in health and disease and its clinical management. *J Am Osteopath Assoc.* 1972;72:149–156.
3. Brodal A. *Neurological Anatomy In Relation to Clinical Medicine*. New York, NY: Oxford University Press; 1981.
4. Kandel E, Schwartz J, Jessell T. *Principles of Neural Science*. New York, NY: Elsevier Science; 1991:326–380.
5. Denslow JS. An analysis of the variability of spinal reflex thresholds. *J Neurophysiol.* 1944;7:207–216.
6. Denslow JS, Korr IM, Krems AD. Quantitative studies of chronic facilitation in human motoneuron pools. *Am J Physiol.* 1947;150:229–238.
7. Korr IM. Somatic dysfunction, osteopathic manipulative treatment, and the nervous system: a few facts, some theories, many questions. *J Am Osteopath Assoc.* 1986;86:111–114.

8. Patterson MM. A model mechanism for spinal segmental facilitation. *J Am Osteopath Assoc.* 1976;76:62–72.

9. Korr IM. The spinal cord as organizer of disease processes. I. Some preliminary perspectives. *J Am Osteopath Assoc.* 1976;76:35–45.

10. Korr IM. Spinal cord as organizer of disease processes. II. The peripheral autonomic nervous system. *J Am Osteopath Assoc.* 1979;79:82–90.

11. Korr IM. Spinal cord as organizer of disease processes. III. Hyperactivity of sympathetic innervation as a common factor in disease. *J Am Osteopath Assoc.* 1979;79:232–237.

12. Johnson R, Lambie D, Spalding J. The autonomic nervous system. In: Baker AB, Baker LH, eds. *Clinical Neurology.* New York, NY: Harper & Row; 1985:57.

13. Adams T, Steinmetz M, Heisey S, et al. Physiologic basis for skin properties in palpatory physical diagnosis. *J Am Osteopath Assoc.* 1982;81:366–377.

14. Beal MC. Viscerosomatic reflexes: a review. *J Am Osteopath Assoc.* 1985;85:786–800.

15. Johnston W, Hill J, Elkiss M, et al. Identification of stable somatic findings in hypertensive subjects by trained examiners using palpatory examination. *J Am Osteopath Assoc.* 1982;81:830–836.

16. Schwartz J. Synthesis and trafficking of neuronal proteins. In: Kandel E, Schwartz J, Jessell T, eds. *Principles of Neural Science.* New York, NY: Elsevier Science; 1991:57–65.

17. Korr IM. The spinal cord as organizer of disease processes. IV. Axonal transport and neurotrophic function in relation to somatic dysfunction. *J Am Osteopath Assoc.* 1981;80:451–467.

18. Denslow JS. Pathophysiologic evidence for the osteopathic lesion: the known, unknown, and controversial. *J Am Osteopath Assoc.* 1975;74:415–421.

19. International Headache Society. Classification of headaches. *Cephalalgia.* 1988;8(suppl 7).

20. Jessell T, Kelly D. Pain and analgesia. In: Kandel E, Schwartz J, Jessell T, eds. *Principles of Neural Science.* New York, NY: Elsevier Science; 1991:389–392.

21. Magoun H. Trauma: a neglected cause of cephalgia. *J Am Osteopath Assoc.* 1975;74:400–410.

22. Lay E. Osteopathic management of trigeminal neuralgia. *J Am Osteopath Assoc.* 1975;74:373–389.

23. Travell JG, Simons DG. *Myofascial Pain and Dysfunction: The Trigger Point Manual.* Baltimore, MD: Williams & Wilkins; 1983.

24. Rossman M. *Healing Yourself.* New York, NY: Bantam Books; 1987.

25. Welch KMA. Migraine: a biobehavioral disorder. *Arch Neurol.* 1987;44:323–327.

26. Moskowitz MA. The neurobiology of vascular head pain. *Ann Neurol.* 1984;16:157–168.

27. O'Connor T, Vanderkoop D. Pattern of intracranial and extracranial projections of trigeminal ganglion cells. *J Neurosci.* 1986;6:2200–2207.

28. Brodal A. The cranial nerves. In: *Neurological Anatomy in Relation to Clinical Medicine.* New York, NY: Oxford University Press; 1981:508–513.

29. Bowles DB. Visual field effects of classical migraine. *Brain Cogn.* 1993;21:181–183.

30. Pederson DM, et al. Migraine aura without headache. *J Fam Pract.* 1991;32:57.

31. Bickerstaff ER. Basilar artery migraine. *Lancet.* 1961;1:1520.

32. Blend R, Bull J. The radiological investigation of migraine. In: Smith R, ed. *Background to Migraine: First Migraine Symposium.* London, England: Heinemann Medical Books Ltd; 1967:110.

33. Davidoff RA. Treatment of the acute attack. In: *Migraine: Pathogenesis, Manifestations, and Management.* Philadelphia, PA: FA Davis Co; 1995:194–220.

34. Davidoff RA. Trigger factors and non-pharmacologic approaches. In: *Migraine, Manifestations, and Management.* Philadelphia, PA: FA Davis Co; 1995:183–193.

35. Kidd RF, Nelson R. Musculoskeletal dysfunction of the neck in migraine and tension headache. *Headache.* 1993;33(10):566–569.

36. Blau J, Macgregor E. Migraine and the neck. *Headache.* 1993;33(10):88–91.

37. Weiss H, Stern B, Goldberg J. Post-traumatic migraine: chronic migraine precipitated by minor head or neck trauma. *Headache.* 1991;31:451–456.

38. Kudrow L. Cluster headaches new concepts. *Neurol Clin.* 1983;2:369–384.

39. Hardebo J. How cluster headache is explained as an intracavernous inflammatory process lesioning sympathetic fibers. *Headache.* 1994;34:125–126.

40. Gawel M, Krajewski A, Luo Y, et al. The cluster diathesis. *Headache.* 1990;30:652–655.

41. Graham J. Cluster headache: the relation to arousal, relaxation, and autonomic tone. *Headache.* 1990;30:145–148.

42. Sanin L, Matthew N, Ali S. Extratrigeminal cluster headache. *Headache.* 1993;33:369–370.

43. Matthew N, Rueveni V. Cluster-like headache following head trauma. *Headache.* 1988;28:297–299.

44. Hardebo J. Subcutaneous sumatriptan in cluster headache. *Headache.* 1993;33:1819.

45. Langemark M, Olesen J. Pericranial tenderness in tension headache: A blind, controlled study. *Cephalalgia.* 1987;7:249–256.

46. Schoenen J, Jamart B, Gerard P, et al. Exteroceptive suppression of temporalis muscle activity in chronic headache. *Neurology.* 1987;37:1834–1836.

47. Silberstein S. Tension-type headaches. *Headache.* 1994;34:S2–S7.

48. Olesen J. Clinical and pathophysiological observations in migraine and tension-type headache explained by integration of neural, vascular, and myofascial inputs. *Pain.* 1991;46:125–132.

49. Meloche J, Bergeron Y, Bellavance A, et al. Quebec Headache Study Group. Painful intervertebral dysfunction: Robert Maigne's original contribution to headache of cervical origin. *Headache.* 1993;33:328–332.

50. Michler R, Bovim G, Sjaastad O. Disorders in the lower cervical spine: a cause of unilateral headache. *Headache.* 1991;31:550–551.

51. Hack G, Koritzer R, Robinson W, et al. Anatomic relation between the rectus capitis posterior minor muscle and the dura mater. *Spine.* 1995;20:2484–2486.

52. Olesen J, Rasmussen B. Management of acute nonvascular headache: The Danish experience. *Headache.* 1990;30:541–543.

53. Miller H. Head pain. *J Am Osteopath Assoc.* 1972;72:135–143.

54. Upledger J, Vredevoogd J. *Craniosacral Therapy.* Chicago, IL: Eastland Press; 1983:297–299.

55. Vick DA, McKay C, Zengerle CR. The safety of manipulative treatment: Review of the literature from 1925 to 1993. *J Am Osteopath Assoc.* 1996;96:113–115.

56. Raskind R, North CM. Vertebral artery injuries following chiropractic cervical spine manipulation: Case reports. *Angiology.* 1990;41:445–452.

57. 57. Powell F, Hanigan W, Olivero W. A risk/benefit analysis of spinal manipulation therapy for relief of lumbar and cervical pain. *Neurosurgery.* 1993;33:73–79.

58. Hart R, Easton J. Dissections of cervical and cerebral arteries. *Neurol Clin.* 1983;1:155–182.

59. Okawara S, Nibbelink D. Vertebral artery occlusion following hyperextension and rotation of the head. *Stroke.* 1975;5:23.

60. Elkiss M. Chronic headache pain, an osteopathic perspective. Washington, DC: Testimony before the Agency for Health Care Policy and Research; October 31, 1995. Transcript of Open Forum, Duke University, Durham, NC.

61. Lowe R. Aetiology of the anatomical basis for primary angle closure glaucoma. *Br J Ophthalmol.* 1970;54:161–169.

62. Day J, Raskin N. Thunderclap headache: symptom of unruptured cerebral aneurysm. *Lancet.* 1986;11:1247–1248.

63. Buchbinder R, Detsky A. Management of suspected giant cell arteritis. *J Rheumatol.* 1992;19:1120–1122.

64. Herndon R, Rudick R. Multiple sclerosis and related conditions. In: Baker AB, Baker LH, eds. *Clinical Neurology.* New York, NY: Harper & Row; 1987:33, 45–46.

65. Kokkinos J, Levine S. Neurologic complications of drug and alcohol abuse. *Neurol Clin.* 1993;11:577–590.

66. Fisher CM. The headache and pain of spontaneous carotid dissection. *Headache.* 1982;22:60–65.

67. Mokri B, Sundt T, Houser D. Spontaneous internal carotid dissection, hemicrania, and Horner's syndrome. *Arch Neurol.* 1979;36:677–680.

68. Weinberg S, Lapointe H. Cervical extension:flexion injury (whiplash) and internal derangement of the temporomandibular joint. *J Oral Maxillofac Surg.* 1987;45:653–656.

69. Dubner R, Sharov Y, Gracely R, et al. Idiopathic trigeminal neuralgia: Sensory features and pain mechanisms. *Pain.* 1987;31:23–24.

70. Moore J, Patcher M, Waldenmaier N, et al. High field magnetic resonance imaging and perinasal sinus and inflammatory disease. *Laryngoscope.* 1986;96:267–271.

71. Wall M. Idiopathic intracranial hypertension. *Neurol Clin.* 1991;9:73–95.

72. Martin E. Headache during sexual intercourse (coital cephalgia): a report of 6 cases. *Ir J Med Sci.* 1974;148:342–345.

73. Salter RB. Degenerative disorders of joints and related structures. In: *Textbook of Disorders and Injuries of the Musculoskeletal System.* Baltimore, MD: Williams & Wilkins; 1970:200–230.

74. Henson RA, Urich H. Involvement of the vertebral column and spinal cord. In: *Cancer and the Nervous System.* Oxford, England: Blackwell Science; 1982:120–150.

75. Salter RB. Inflammatory disorders of bones and joints. In: *Textbook of Disorders and Injuries of the Musculoskeletal System.* Baltimore, MD: Williams & Wilkins; 1970:165–166.

76. Finneson B. The lower back in the diagnosis of rheumatic diseases. In: *Rheumatic Diseases Diagnosis and Management.* Philadelphia, PA: JB Lippincott Co; 1977:114–135.

77. Salter R. Generalized and disseminated disorders of bone. In: *Textbook of Disorders and Injuries of the Musculoskeletal System.* Baltimore, MD: Williams & Wilkins; 1970:129–149.

78. Davis C. Extradural spinal cord and nerve root compression from benign lesions of the lumbar area. In: *Youmans Neurological Surgery.* Philadelphia, PA: WB Saunders; 1982:2535–2555.

79. Arbit E, Patterson R. Extradural spinal cord and nerve root compression from benign lesions of the dorsal area. In: *Youmans Neurological Surgery.* Philadelphia, PA: WB Saunders; 1982:2562–2568.

80. Ehni G. Extradural spinal cord and nerve root compression from benign lesions of the lumbar area. In: *Youmans Neurological Surgery.* Philadelphia, PA: WB Saunders; 1982:2574–2604.

81. Bradley W. Diseases of the spinal roots. In: Dyck P, Thomas P, Lambert E, et al, eds. *Peripheral Neuropathy.* Philadelphia, PA: WB Saunders; 1984:1368–1382.

82. Mulder D, Dale A. Spinal cord tumor and disks. In: Baker AB, Baker LH, eds. *Clinical Neurology.* New York, NY: Harper & Row; 1975:44, 125.

83. Moossy J. Vascular disease of the spinal cord. In: Baker AB, Baker LH, eds. *Clinical Neurology.* New York, NY: Harper & Row; 1988:46, 114.

84. Doyle W, Cooper P, Wilmot C, et al. Trauma of the spine and spinal cord. In: Baker AB, Baker LH, eds. *Clinical Neurology.* New York, NY: Harper & Row; 1991:47, 144.

85. Kincaid J. Myelitis and myelopathy. In: Baker AB, Baker LH, eds. *Clinical Neurology.* New York, NY: Harper & Row; 1989:48.

86. Jessell T, Kelly D. Pain and analgesia. In: Kandel E, Schwartz J, Jessell T, eds. *Principles of Neural Science.* New York, NY: Elsevier Science; 1991:388–389.

87. DeJong R. *The Neurologic Examination.* Hagerstown, MD: Harper & Row; 1979.

88. Wagle W. Neuroradiology. In: Baker AB, Baker LH, eds. *Clinical Neurology.* New York, NY: Harper & Row; 1990:2, 178–233.

89. Latchaw R, Taylor S, Meyer J, et al. The spine. In: *Computed Tomography of the Head, Neck, and Spine.* Chicago, IL: Year Book Medical Publishers; 1985:595–695.

90. Norman D. The spine. In: Brant-Zawadzki M, Norman D, eds. *Magnetic Resonance Imaging of the Central Nervous System.* New York, NY: Raven Press; 1987:289–328.

91. Aminoff M. Electromyography. In: Aminoff M, ed. *Electrodiagnosis in Clinical Neurology.* New York, NY: Churchill Livingstone; 1980:197–220.

92. Daube J. Nerve conduction studies. In: Aminoff M, ed. *Electrodiagnosis*

93. in *Clinical Neurology.* New York, NY: Churchill Livingstone; 1980:229–260.

Chiappa K, Jayakar J. Evoked potentials in clinical medicine. In: Baker AB, Baker LH, eds. *Clinical Neurology.* New York, NY: Harper & Row; 1989:7, 148.

94. Bonica J, Buckley P. Regional analgesia with local anesthetics. In: *The Management of Pain.* Philadelphia, PA: Lea & Febiger; 1990:1883–1960.

95. Greenman P. Manipulation with the patient under anesthesia. *J Am Osteopath Assoc.* 1992;92:1159–1170.

96. Shepelle P, Adams A, Chassin M, et al. Spinal manipulation for low back pain. *Ann Intern Med.* 1992;117:590.

97. Greenman PE. *Principles of Manual Medicine.* Baltimore, MD: Williams & Wilkins; 1989.

98. Stiles E. An osteopathic approach to low back pain. *Osteopath Ann.* 1976;4:44–48.

99. Stoddard A. *Manual of Osteopathic Technique.* London, England: Hutchison Medical Publications; 1961.

100. Ward R. *Myofascial Release Technique: Tutorials on Level I, II, and III.* East Lansing, MI: Michigan State University College of Osteopathic Medicine; 1992.

101. MacDonald R, Bell C. An open controlled assessment of osteopathic manipulation. *Spine.* 1990;15:364–370.

102. Bigos S, Bowyer O, Braen G, et al. *Acute Low Back Problems in Adults. Clinical Practice Guideline.* Rockville, MD: US Department of Health and Human Services. Public Health Service. Agency for Health Care Policy and Research; 1994.

103. Anderson KH, Mosdal C. Epidural application of corticosteroids in low back pain and sciatica. *Acta Neurochir (Wein).* 1987;87:52–53.

104. Bush K, Hiller SA. Controlled study of caudal epidural injections of triamcinolone plus prosoine for the management of intractable sciatica. *Spine.* 1991;16:72–75.

105. Moran P, Pruzzo N. In: Mitchell Jr FL, ed. *An Evaluation and Treatment Manual of Osteopathic Manipulative Procedure.* Kansas City, MO: Institute for Continuing Education in Osteopathic Principles; 1973:15–17.

106. Sunderland S. *Nerves and Nerve Injuries.* London, England: Churchill Livingstone; 1978:653–1021.

107. Magoun HI. *Osteopathy in the Cranial Field.* Kirksville, MO: The Journal Printing Co; 1966:95, 184, 207, 251, 259, 294.

108. Sunderland S. The carpal tunnel syndrome. In: *Nerves and Nerve Injuries.* London, England: Churchill Livingstone; 1978:711–723.

109. Sucher BM. Palpatory diagnosis and manipulative management of carpal tunnel syndrome. *J Am Osteopath Assoc.* 1994;94:647–663.

110. Sucher BM. Myofascial manipulative release of carpal tunnel syndrome: Documentation with MRI. *J Am Osteopath Assoc.* 1993;93:1273–1278.

111. Sunderland S. Disturbances of brachial plexus origin associated with unusual anatomical arrangements in the cervico-brachial region: The thoracic outlet syndrome. In: *Nerves and Nerve Injures.* London, England: Churchill Livingstone; 1978:901–917.

112. Synek VM. Diagnostic importance of somatosensory evoked potentials in the diagnosis of thoracic outlet syndrome. *Clin Electroencephalogr.* 1986;17:112–116.

113. Sucher BM. Thoracic outlet syndrome: A myofascial variant. I. Pathology and diagnosis. *J Am Osteopath Assoc.* 1990;90:686–704.

114. Sucher BM. Thoracic outlet syndrome: A myofascial variant. II. Treatment. *J Am Osteopath Assoc.* 1990;90:810–823.

115. Sucher BM, Heath DM. Thoracic outlet syndrome: A myofascial variant. III. Structural and postural considerations. *J Am Osteopath Assoc.* 1993;93:334–345.

116. Dobrusin R. Osteopathic approach to conservative management of thoracic outlet syndromes. J Am Osteopath Assoc. 1989;89:1046–1057.

117. Bonica J. General considerations of chronic pain. In: *The Management of Pain.* Philadelphia, PA: Lea & Febiger; 1990:8, 180–195.

118. Sola A, Bonica J. Myofascial pain syndromes. In: *The Management of Pain.* Philadelphia, PA: Lea & Febiger; 1990:21, 352–366.

119. Elkiss M, Jerome J. Chronic back pain syndrome: an analysis of current therapies. *Mich Osteopath J.* 1978:21–28.

31

OBSTETRICS

MELICIEN TETTAMBEL

KEY CONCEPTS

■ Somatic dysfunction in normal pregnancy, including low back pain, other musculoskeletal problems, fluid circulation, and hormonal changes

■ Indications and contraindications for osteopathic manipulative treatment during pregnancy

■ Examination, viscerosomatic reflexes, skeletal changes, and biomechanical changes in each trimester of pregnancy

■ Evaluation of lumbosacral spine and pelvis for labor and birth; possible rupture of pubic ligaments

■ Somatic dysfunction and treatment in the postpartum period

An up-to-date osteopath must have a masterful knowledge of anatomy and physiology. He [sic] must have brains in osteopathic surgery, osteopathic obstetrics, and osteopathic practice. —A.T. Still (1)

Osteopathic management of an obstetric patient requires knowledge of the influence of the maternal structural framework on the pregnancy and the effect of the pregnancy on the patient's structure. Somatic dysfunction, as defined in the American Osteopathic Association's glossary, is "impaired or altered function of related components of the somatic (body framework) system; skeletal, arthrodial, and myofascial structures, and related vascular, lymphatic, and neural elements" (2). Evaluation and treatment of somatic dysfunction enhances homeostasis, facilitates maternal adaptation to structural and hormonal changes, and may alleviate maternal discomfort caused by an enlarging uterus.

During the process of evaluating and treating somatic dysfunction, the osteopathic obstetrician monitors fetal well being and addresses potential stresses in the mother's body that can occur as a result of pregnancy, labor, and birth. Physical changes and stresses in maternal structures, even apart from psychological aspects, are common. More than half of all pregnant women report some kind of musculoskeletal pain during pregnancy (3,4). There are several aspects of the changing maternal–fetal structural relationships that may cause somatic dysfunction at any time from conception to postpartum. These relationships can be organized, like pregnancy, into trimesters. Obstetric conditions

that may respond particularly well to osteopathic manipulative treatment (OMT) or that may be relative contraindications to such treatment are of special interest.

SOMATIC DYSFUNCTION IN NORMAL PREGNANCY

Three broad areas of somatic dysfunction effect changes in both mother and fetus. These include:

■ Changes in maternal structure and biomechanics as a result of the developing fetus
■ Changes in body fluid circulation
■ Hormonal changes

These are listed in descending order of our ability to treat osteopathically. Although most of these changes are reversible, wide variability exists among patients in the time interval after birth before complete reversion to the pregravid condition. The most obvious changes that occur during pregnancy are in the musculoskeletal system. The nongravid pelvis assumes a new angle when filled with a growing fetus, and must be able to support the weight and volume of the enlarging uterus and fetal structures (often up to 6 kg). During fetal growth, the mother's center of gravity shifts forward. In compensation, the lumbar spine assumes an increased lordotic posture, with a resultant increased pelvic tilt. This tilt is defined by the angle between the horizontal and the posterior superior and posterior inferior iliac crests (angle theta in Fig. 31.1) (5). The thoracic spine also increases its kyphotic posture. The changes in body fluid circulation and hormones during pregnancy are generally less obvious, less well studied, and more controversial regarding their origins than are the changes in the musculoskeletal system.

Low Back Pain

One of the most common complaints and complications of pregnancy is low back pain, which has been traditionally accepted as inevitable by women and their physicians (6). The majority of published reports regarding its cause are either anecdotal or reflect data taken from patient questionnaires. Only two studies have employed a traditional detailed physical examination of patients to properly diagnose the source of back pain (7,8). Several

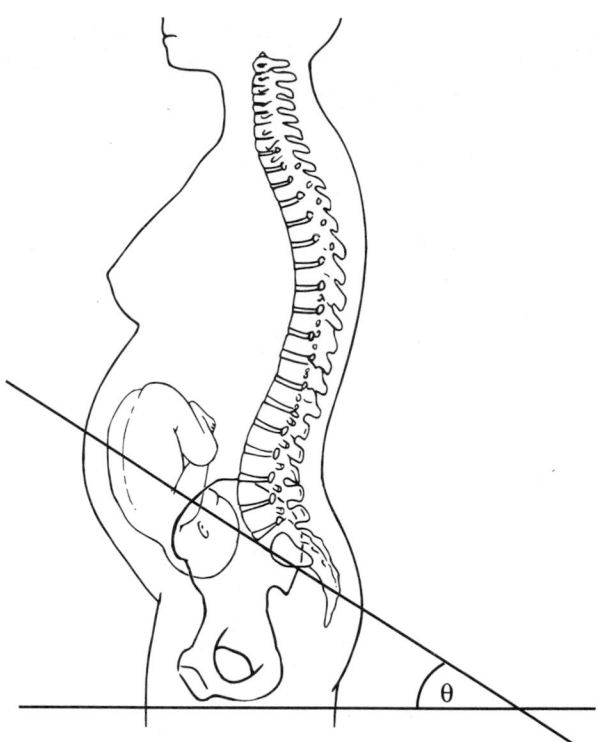

FIGURE 31.1. Spinal and pelvic changes in pregnancy. (Adapted from DiGiovanna EL, Schiowitz S. *An Osteopathic Approach to Diagnosis and Treatment.* Philadelphia, PA: JB Lippincott Co; 1992.)

studies have found that heavy manual labor and smoking are risk factors for the development of low back pain symptoms during pregnancy (7–12). Parity, age, and previous history of low back pain have also been associated with such symptoms in most studies, but other reports have not supported these conclusions, perhaps because of limitations in study design, methods, and/or statistical power. The following have not been found to correlate with the development of low back pain symptoms during pregnancy (4).

- Race
- Occupation
- Fetal weight
- Pre-pregnancy maternal weight
- Weight gain
- Exercise habits
- Sleeping posture
- Mattress type
- Shoe heel heights (13)
- Previous epidural anesthesia
- Previous history of low back pain

The gravid uterus and the compensatory lordosis that it causes create a tremendous mechanical burden on the lower back (14,15). This altered posture increases stress across the vertebral facets of the lumbar spine, and increases shear forces across the intervertebral disc spaces. The paraspinal muscles shorten posteriorly, and are unbalanced by overstretching abdominal muscles anteriorly. Fast and colleagues clinically illustrated the abdominal weakness in pregnancy by comparing the abilities of two groups

(a 36-week pregnant cohort and an age- and weight-matched group of nonpregnant women) to perform a sit-up. Of the pregnant patients, 86% could not perform a single sit-up, compared to just 11% of the nonpregnant controls (16). This major difference in ability to perform a simple exercise involving the abdominal musculature is thought to be indicative of the major change in both normal structure and function during pregnancy.

Hyperlordosis is often implicated in the etiology of low back pain. While radiographic studies have not verified this to date, Bullock and associates used an inclinometer to measure the progression of kyphosis, lordosis, and pelvic tilt in 34 pregnancies (17). In their study, thoracic kyphosis increased an average of 6.6 degrees, lumbar lordosis 7.2 degrees, and pelvic tilt only 1.9 degrees throughout the course of pregnancy. These small degrees of increase and tilt did not correlate with development of low back symptoms in their study group. Snijders and coworkers studied 16 pregnant women, using a combination of reflectometers and mathematical modeling to measure curvature of the spine in the weeks just before and just after delivery (18). Their patients were an average of 10-mm taller before delivery and kyphosis and lordosis were less marked before delivery than after. They postulate that these findings are a result of a relaxation of the psoas muscle, which allows the normally present lordosis to flatten. Östgaard and colleagues have concluded that pregnant women compensate for intrapelvic changes by subtle lumbar lordosis. These investigators postulate this lordosis comes about by extension of the upper trunk and neck and hip joint extension, rather than lumbar spine extension (19).

Pain in the sacroiliac region has been suggested to result from excessive connective tissue stretch and microtrauma, as a consequence of the trunk extensor muscle forces that balance the anterior tilt of the pelvic brim caused by the growing uterus (20). Distention of the pelvis further increases mobility of the sacroiliac joints (Fig. 31.1). The transition between physiologic and pathologic pelvic relaxation, resulting in pain, is indistinct. At first, the main symptoms of pelvic relaxation are spontaneous pain and tenderness of the sacroiliac joints elicited by direct or indirect pressure (21,22). Later, sacroiliac relaxation results in lumbar backache that radiates down the back of the thighs. Occasionally, pain may radiate over the anterior aspects of the lower part of the abdomen and thighs (23,24).

Another type of back pain that commonly affects a large group of pregnant women is located in the posterior part of the pelvis, distal and lateral to the lumbosacral junction. Pain radiates to the posterior part of the thigh, may extend below the knee, and thus may be interpreted as sciatica or posterior joint syndrome. A study of 436 pregnant women by Östgaard and colleagues revealed that this condition, given the name "posterior pelvic pain," is different than sciatica, in that it is less specific than the nerve root syndrome in distribution and does not extend down into the ankle and foot (25). This pain is different from posterior joint syndrome because it does not emerge from the lumbar area. Additionally, it does not include muscle weakness or sensory impairment, and reflexes are unchanged. Therefore, posterior pelvic pain associated with pregnancy should not be treated as low back pain or sciatica because it is not the result of nerve compression. The patient should be evaluated for postural imbalance and possible spinal segment facet problems.

Radicular symptoms often accompany low back discomfort associated with pregnancy (6). Despite increased shear placed across the disc space (which varies among individuals), herniated nucleus pulposus during pregnancy is uncommon, having an incidence of only 1:10,000 (26). It has been postulated that direct pressure on nerve roots/plexi by the gravid uterus is responsible for many of the radicular symptoms (27). "Parietal neuralgia of pregnancy" was first described by Bushnell in 1949 (28). He proposed that mechanical pressure of ligamentous structures of the spine on nerve roots (resulting from increased lordosis of pregnancy) was responsible for radicular pain of pregnancy. The symptoms present primarily as paresthesias in the distribution of the ilioinguinal and iliofemoral nerves. Also occasionally associated with radicular symptoms is "lightening," an event that generally occurs during the final 4 weeks of pregnancy. The presenting part of the fetus settles into the pelvis, thus "lightening" the pressure against the diaphragm and upper abdominal cavity (29). Breathing becomes much easier for the mother, but she may also experience radicular symptoms, which have been attributed to direct pressure of the gravid uterus on components of the lumbosacral plexus that coalesce into the sciatic nerve. A recent study using magnetic resonance imaging demonstrated that bulges or herniations of lumbosacral discs are common in women of childbearing age and that pregnant women do not have an increased prevalence of disc abnormalities (30).

Pregnancy may cause preexisting scoliosis to progress. Berman and co-workers identified an increased progression of the curve in three of eight patients who had idiopathic scoliosis (31). They proposed a link between the effects of the hormone relaxin and the mechanical stress of pregnancy that causes scoliotic curves of more than 25 degrees to progress. In contrast, in a large retrospective review of 355 women who had idiopathic scoliosis (175 of whom had been pregnant and 180 of whom had not), Betz and associates concluded that pregnant scoliotic patients are not at risk for an increase in the progression of spinal curvature (32). Scoliotic curves tend to progress in adulthood, but pregnancy does not seem to aggravate the rate of increase. In addition, mild-to-moderate idiopathic scoliosis does not appear to create problems with pregnancy. The rate of successful pregnancy outcomes in women who had scoliosis did not differ from those without scoliosis (32). However, one review suggests that patients with scoliosis had more premature births than were expected (33). Women with previous posterior spinal fusion for idiopathic scoliosis have also been shown to have no increased risk of development of low back pain during pregnancy (32).

Other Musculoskeletal Problems

Although certain musculoskeletal changes occur during pregnancy, pregnancy itself may affect some preexisting musculoskeletal conditions such as rheumatoid arthritis and ankylosing spondylitis. Pregnancy may have ameliorating effects on most women who have rheumatoid arthritis, usually beginning as soon as they become pregnant and continuing until about 6 weeks after delivery (34). The signs and symptoms of the disease may recur with a flare-up in the postpartum period. Some investigators have speculated that rheumatoid arthritis tends to improve in pregnancy because of increased cortisol secretion (35). Others have proposed that increased α-glycoprotein in the maternal serum decreases inflammation (36,37). Some researchers also assert that substances derived from the fetal tissues alter the severity of this autoimmune disease, perhaps through secretion of cortisol or other substances (38). Whereas rheumatoid arthritis generally improves with pregnancy, ankylosing spondylitis is often aggravated by pregnancy, perhaps because of the increased stresses on the sacroiliac joints during enlargement of the nearby uterus (39). Overall, the course of the disease (over decades) is not affected positively or negatively by one or more pregnancies (39). Even though ankylosing spondylitis often limits motion of the pelvic joints, it is usually not a hindrance to vaginal delivery (40–42).

Changes in Body Fluids and Circulation

Increased circulation to the pelvic organs is necessary to meet the metabolic needs of fetal development. Unfortunately, this increase is sometimes accompanied by insufficient return of fluid into maternal systemic circulation. Either of these can result in congestion or edema of maternal organs and tissues. Fluids increase an average of 6.5 L over the course of pregnancy (43). Hemorrhoids or varicosities of the vulva or lower extremities may occur as a result of sluggish venous return influenced by pressure of the uterus on the venous plexi in the pelvis. Back pain may also be related to development of varicosities (43–45). Some women complain of night back pain 1 to 2 hours after lying down, which may awaken the patient from sleep. Fast and others note that dependent edema accumulates when a pregnant woman is in the upright position during the day (43). When she lies down at night, the changes in osmotic forces allow some of this fluid to return to the intravascular space, resulting in increased venous return. This increased venous return, coupled with venous blockage that occurs by pressure of the fetus on the vena cava, results in decreased blood flow through the pelvis. A delayed, stagnant hypoxia of the neural tissue and the vertebral bodies ensues, producing the delayed low back pain (and, sometimes, radicular symptoms) that awaken the patient (45).

Physical factors of pulse and respiration changing pressure gradients between the abdomen and the thorax alter venous flow dynamics, causing congestion (Fig. 31.2) (46). Because of this flow alteration, a change in volume of abdominal organs (e.g., liver, pancreas) also occurs, which tends to increase abdominal cavity pressure. This reversal of venous flow into vertebral and spinal membranes causes central nervous system congestion, resulting in complaints of headache, nausea, and light-headedness. Because the venous system of the spine is valveless (47), blood from the spinal cord, membranes, and spine passes through communicating veins to the azygous and hemiazygous systems (which do not have individual veins for all thoracic and lumbar spinal levels). Venous blood from these areas usually drains into the heart via the superior vena cava. Decreased efficiency of this closed system may decrease oxygen and cardiac output as arterial blood volume is influenced by cardiac contractions "pushing" venous blood, and as respiration "pulls" venous blood with breathing effort. Nausea, headache, and congestion of the liver and pancreas may result from venous stasis also caused by the gravid uterus on the vena cava, as well as the venous plexi emanating from the spine (48).

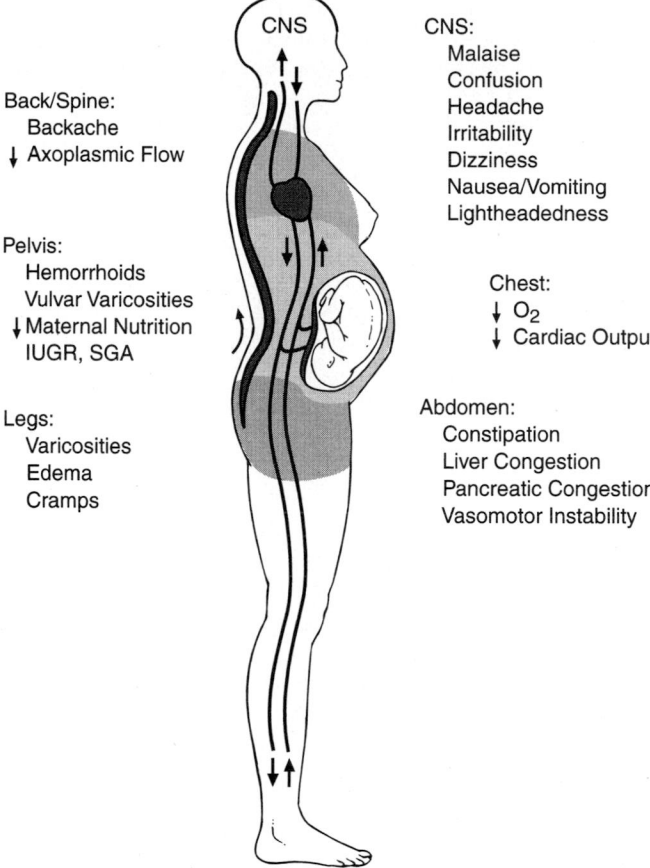

Back/Spine:
  Backache
  ↓ Axoplasmic Flow

Pelvis:
  Hemorrhoids
  Vulvar Varicosities
  ↓ Maternal Nutrition
  IUGR, SGA

Legs:
  Varicosities
  Edema
  Cramps

CNS:
  Malaise
  Confusion
  Headache
  Irritability
  Dizziness
  Nausea/Vomiting
  Lightheadedness

Chest:
  ↓ O₂
  ↓ Cardiac Output

Abdomen:
  Constipation
  Liver Congestion
  Pancreatic Congestion
  Vasomotor Instability

FIGURE 31.2. Diagram of pathophysiology of congestion during pregnancy. (Adapted from Kuchera M, Kuchera W. *Osteopathic Considerations in Systemic Dysfunction*, 2nd ed. Kirksville, MO: KCOM Press; 1992.)

Hormonal Changes

During pregnancy, alterations in hormonal levels cause physical changes in many parameters. One of the most dramatic of these changes is the widening and increased mobility of the sacroiliac joints and the symphysis pubis, which begins at the 10th to 12th week of pregnancy. The increased width of the symphysis pubis can be detected radiographically as early as the first trimester and reaches its maximum near term. The hormone relaxin has been identified as a major contributor to these changes in joint laxity during pregnancy (15). Relaxin is secreted by the ovarian corpus luteum during pregnancy (49,50). Concentrations of relaxin are elevated during the first trimester and then decline early in the second trimester to a level that remains stable throughout the rest of the pregnancy until labor (49). Interestingly, the level of relaxin is not increased with twin gestations. Lower concentrations have been found, however, after 43 weeks of gestation, and in women in premature labor (50). Primary target tissues are the cervix, uterus, and ligamentous structures of the pelvis. In preparation for passage of the fetus during the birthing process, pelvic articulations are relaxed by the hormone relaxin (51). MacLennan and colleagues report that women who have been incapacitated by low back pain during pregnancy have extremely high levels of relaxin (52), suggesting that excessive relaxin is not innocuous.

Another major change during pregnancy related to hormonal alterations occurs in the respiratory system. During pregnancy, there are relatively large changes in the mechanical configuration of the thoracic cage, most of which occur before the uterus enlarges sufficiently to account for such increases. The chest circumference increases 5 to 7 cm, the subcostal angle increases from 68 to 103 degrees, and the diaphragm is pushed superiorly by about 4 cm, but increases in excursion by 1 to 2 cm (53). These changes lead to a 30% to 40% increase in tidal volume, and a similar increase in minute ventilation, since the respiratory rate is essentially constant. These changes are usually attributed to the effects of higher levels of circulating progesterone in pregnancy (based on physiologic studies of progesterone-treated, nonpregnant animals), but relaxin possibly also plays an important role.

Elevations in steroid hormonal levels (especially progesterone) may promote fluid retention, which enhances congestion in both local tissues (e.g., periuterine) and distant sites (e.g., pedal edema, exacerbated by gravity). This congestion may decrease oxygenation and metabolism at the cellular level, leading to accumulation of metabolic waste products in soft tissues, as well as in the gastrointestinal tract (54).

FIRST TRIMESTER

At the initial prenatal visit (usually after the first or second missed menstrual period), the obstetrician obtains a full health inventory and performs a complete physical examination (54). In addition to performing a traditional pelvic examination, the osteopathically trained obstetrician may also perform further palpatory structural examination to identify somatic dysfunction that could affect the outcome of pregnancy. Asymmetry of bony landmarks, joint motion tests, tissue texture changes, and local tenderness are used to confirm areas of somatic dysfunction. Palpatory examination of the paraspinal tissues is performed to identify areas of tissue texture changes that represent viscerosomatic reflex sites (55). Special attention is given to evaluation of any tissue texture change at the costotransverse area because of the belief that autonomic nerve effects on segmental muscles are specific. Spinal segmental sites for somatic dysfunction associated with visceral disease are related to the autonomic nervous system supply for various organs (47,56–62). Hansen and Schliak have identified spinal reflex sites at thoracolumbar levels T10-L2 (Fig. 31.3) (63) affecting:

- Large bowel
- Appendix
- Kidney
- Ureter
- Adrenal medulla
- Testes
- Ovaries
- Urinary bladder
- Uterus

Woods reports that presurgical palpatory findings of a viscerosomatic reflex correlated with the diagnosis in 10 of 13 patients who had acute abdominal disorders (64). Palpatory diagnosis of viscerosomatic reflexes should assist the physician in the

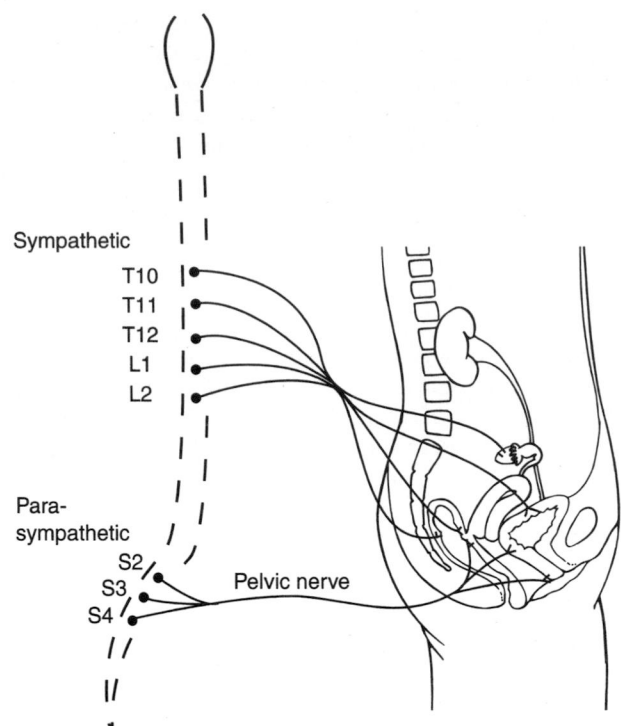

FIGURE 31.3. Sympathetic and parasympathetic innervation of the female pelvis. (From DiGiovanna EL, Schiowitz S. *An Osteopathic Approach to Diagnosis and Treatment.* Philadelphia, PA: JB Lippincott Co; 1992, with permission.)

differential diagnosis of somatic pain. When combined with other historical or physical evidence, a positive reflex may enhance the predictive value of the diagnosis of visceral disease.

OMT of viscerosomatic reflexes has been advocated on the basis that it is designed to reduce residual effects in the somatic structures following a visceral disorder, or to influence the viscus through stimulation of somatovisceral effects (65). Osteopathic physicians have advocated manipulative treatment as a part of the treatment regimen for organic problems, as well as for preoperative and postoperative management of patients with organic disease (66–69).

In the first trimester of pregnancy "morning sickness," or hyperemesis, is a common complaint. The precise cause of the nausea and vomiting remains unclear (54). Viscerosomatic reflexes may be identified on structural examination and often respond to OMT (61). Chapman reflexes (70) are anterior and posterior myofascial tender points related to organ function, which have been "geographically charted" on the body (Fig. 31.4). Evaluation of C2 and T5-9 may identify digestive disturbances (71). Tenderness of a Chapman anterior point can be used for diagnosis, as well as an indicator to evaluate the degree of success in relieving organ dysfunction. Posterior points are less sensitive to palpation and are usually used for treatment. Anterior points should be used for treatment when attempts at a posterior approach are unsuccessful. The indications and contraindications for OMT during pregnancy are summarized in Table 31.1.

Pregnant women often inquire about exercise at the first prenatal visit. Selection of exercises should reflect a consideration of the changes in the patient's weight, body habitus, and balance

to minimize the risk of injury to the patient and fetus (3,23,72). Maintenance of good abdominal tone should be encouraged (73). Current recommendations from the American College of Obstetricians and Gynecologists are that pregnant women exercise for no longer than 15 minutes at a time and that they maintain a pulse rate of less than 140 beats per minute and a core body temperature of less than 38°C (74). It has been shown that the second stage of labor lasts only half as long in athletes as in nonathletes (75). Of course, regimens should be individualized. High-risk patients, such as those who have diabetes, hypertension, defects of the cervix, or a history of miscarriage may not be able to exercise (76). In addition to exercise, weight gain has been advised to be limited to a total of 9.1 to 13.6 kg (approximately 1.4 kg per month) during the course of pregnancy.

SECOND TRIMESTER

In the second trimester of pregnancy, the uterus is emerging from the pelvis into the abdomen. The patient may become aware of fetal motion, as well as stretching pains above the pubic symphysis. If the patient has had abdominal or pelvic surgery, pain may be augmented by stretching of previously formed adhesions. Fascial release (direct or indirect) treatment may provide some relief in this situation. Round ligament pain may correspond to anterior counterstrain points L3-5 (Fig. 31.5).

Structural examination of the pelvis at this time may address restrictions of motion of the sacrum and related ligamentous and muscular structures that could result in backache, sciatica, cramps, or posterior pelvic pain (25). The patient may be treated in the sitting, standing, prone, or supine position—whichever position she can best tolerate. Almost any type of treatment modality (both direct action or indirect method) can be used, depending on operator skill and patient acceptance. Although complaints related to skeletal changes continue in the second trimester, the second most frequent area of musculoskeletal symptoms during pregnancy is pain in the hands and wrists (3). Carpal tunnel syndrome (CTS) occurs most frequently in the second trimester, and is the cause of these symptoms for many women. Symptoms of CTS often include the classic triad of numbness, tingling, and pain at night, usually bilaterally (28,77). CTS probably results from localized edema and swelling in the carpal tunnel. It occurs twice as commonly in pregnant patients who have swelling of the fingers as in those who do not. It also occurs more commonly in those women with preeclampsia and hypertension (78). In one study, CTS occurred in 2% of 2,358 pregnant women (79), and in another study, 25% of 1,000 women had median nerve compression at some time during pregnancy (78). These symptoms are somewhat more common in older primiparous women who have generalized edema (79).

CTS in pregnancy virtually always resolves completely soon after delivery (80). Palliative management is indicated for patients who are sufficiently symptomatic to warrant any treatment. Nighttime splinting of the wrist to support it in neutral or slight dorsiflexion has been reported to be successful (79). Sucher has demonstrated improvement of nerve conduction studies and magnetic resonance changes resulting from osteopathic treatment with myofascial technique (81,82).

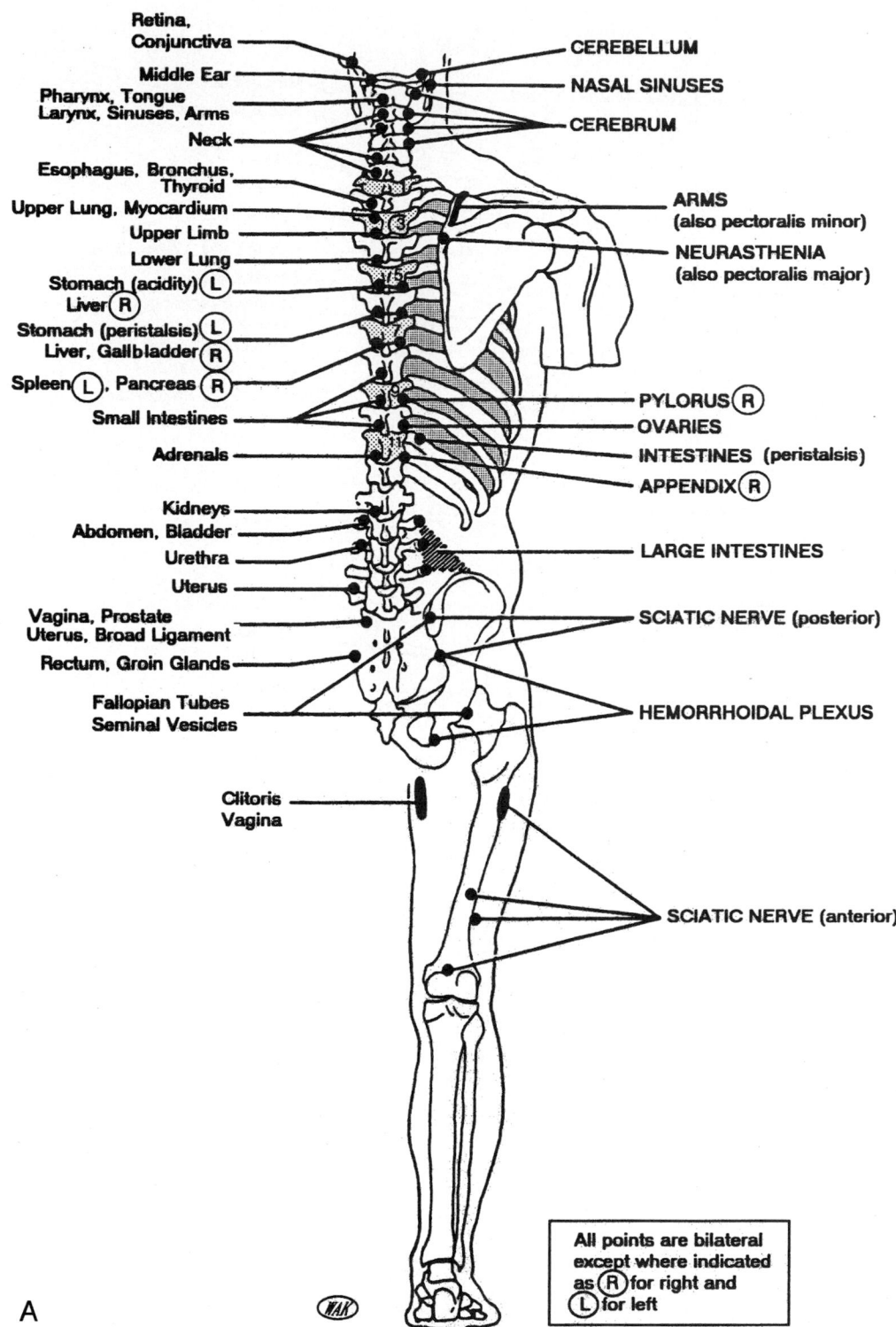

Retina,
Conjunctiva

Middle Ear

Pharynx, Tongue
Larynx, Sinuses, Arms

Neck

Esophagus, Bronchus,
Thyroid

Upper Lung, Myocardium

Upper Limb

Lower Lung

Stomach (acidity) Ⓛ
Liver Ⓡ

Stomach (peristalsis) Ⓛ
Liver, Gallbladder Ⓡ

Spleen Ⓛ, Pancreas Ⓡ

Small Intestines

Adrenals

Kidneys

Abdomen, Bladder

Urethra

Uterus

Vagina, Prostate
Uterus, Broad Ligament

Rectum, Groin Glands

Fallopian Tubes
Seminal Vesicles

Clitoris
Vagina

CEREBELLUM

NASAL SINUSES

CEREBRUM

ARMS
(also pectoralis minor)

NEURASTHENIA
(also pectoralis major)

PYLORUS Ⓡ

OVARIES

INTESTINES (peristalsis)

APPENDIX Ⓡ

LARGE INTESTINES

SCIATIC NERVE (posterior)

HEMORRHOIDAL PLEXUS

SCIATIC NERVE (anterior)

A

All points are bilateral
except where indicated
as Ⓡ for right and
Ⓛ for left

FIGURE 31.4. Diagram of Chapman reflexes.

THIRD TRIMESTER

In the last 3 months of pregnancy, gravitational effects on the uterus and its contents accentuate abdominal fascial drag on inguinal tissues, causing pressure on the venous and lymphatic return flow from the lower extremities, and also on the inferior vena cava. Leg edema and hemorrhoids are common complaints. The pregnant woman may find it difficult to lie in a supine position without experiencing nausea or dizziness from hypotension that results from vena caval compression.

During the third trimester, the mechanical and structural changes in the woman become maximal. As a result of these

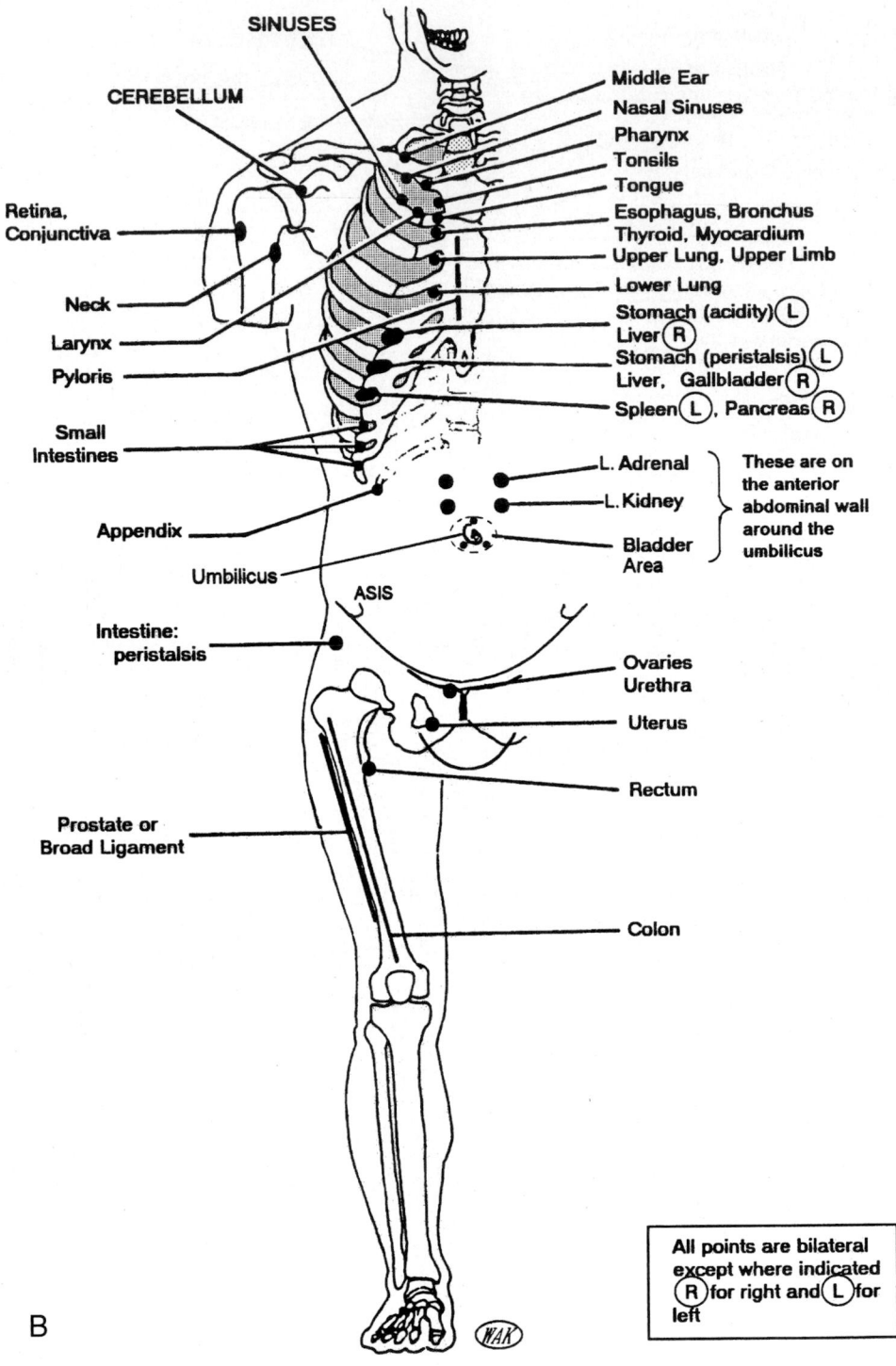

SINUSES

CEREBELLUM

Retina, Conjunctiva

Neck

Larynx

Pyloris

Small Intestines

Appendix

Umbilicus

Intestine: peristalsis

Prostate or Broad Ligament

B

Middle Ear
Nasal Sinuses
Pharynx
Tonsils
Tongue
Esophagus, Bronchus
Thyroid, Myocardium
Upper Lung, Upper Limb
Lower Lung
Stomach (acidity) (L)
Liver (R)
Stomach (peristalsis) (L)
Liver, Gallbladder (R)
Spleen (L), Pancreas (R)

L. Adrenal
L. Kidney
Bladder Area

These are on the anterior abdominal wall around the umbilicus

ASIS

Ovaries
Urethra
Uterus

Rectum

Colon

All points are bilateral except where indicated (R) for right and (L) for left

FIGURE 31.4. *(continued)*

changes in biomechanics, complaints attributable to loss of balance, changes in gait, and especially low back pain are very common. Constipation and reflux esophagitis are also frequent, again due to near-maximal changes in structures, fluids, and/or hormones. Myofascial or soft tissue osteopathic treatment may be utilized to mobilize fluids from extremities to the systemic circulation. Specific palpatory structural examination to identify gastrointestinal viscerosomatic reflexes for treatment may also be

helpful. Treatment of the pelvic diaphragm to lift pelvic contents may relieve constipation. Treatment of somatic dysfunction in the midthoracic spine may relieve gastrointestinal complaints, such as esophagitis or gastroesophageal reflux symptoms.

Osteopathic treatment to relieve somatic dysfunction should focus on spinal segmental levels of T10-L2, the sympathetic nerve supply that influences adrenal and ovarian function, as well as uterine contractility. Gitlin and Wolf (83) have provoked uterine

TABLE 31.1. INDICATIONS AND CONTRAINDICATIONS FOR OSTEOPATHIC MANIPULATIVE TREATMENT DURING PREGNANCY

Indications:
- Somatic dysfunction during pregnancy
- Scoliosis or other structural condition associated with pregnancy
- Edema, congestion, or other pregnancy-associated condition amenable to osteopathic manipulative treatment

Contraindications:
- Undiagnosed vaginal bleeding
- Threatened or incomplete abortion
- Ectopic pregnancy
- Placenta previa
- Placental abruption
- Premature rupture of membranes (preterm)
- Preterm labor (relative contraindication)
- Prolapsed umbilical cord
- Eclampsia and severe preeclampsia
- Surgical or medical emergencies (other than those listed above)

contractions in a small group of women with term pregnancies following use of osteopathic cranial manipulation. Additional case histories pertaining to osteopathic management of pregnancy, with discussion of treatment techniques, may be found in *Osteopathy in the Cranial Field* (84).

LABOR AND DELIVERY

After the 36th or 37th week of gestation, prior to active labor, pelvic examination is performed to evaluate fetal size, presentation, and pelvic outlet accommodation for the fetus. An assessment of the patient's chances for delivering vaginally can be made by interpreting the examination of the "true pelvis" (inlet, midpelvis, and outlet). The pelvic inlet is bounded anteriorly by mentally constructing a line from the iliopectineal lines along the pectineal eminence and pubic crest to the symphysis. Posteriorly, the inlet is bounded by the sacrum at the level of termination of the iliopectineal lines. The sacral base is not included, as it is superior to this territory. The plane of the pelvic inlet is a flat surface bounded similarly, but usually inclined horizontally (with the patient in a standing position) at a 40- to 60-degree angle. The pelvic outlet is bounded by the pubes, ischial tuberosities, and coccyx. The midpelvis contains all structures between the pelvic inlet and outlet.

Caldwell-Moloy classification of pelvic types provides the standard for learning the identifying features of four basic pelvic types (85):

- Gynecoid
- Android
- Anthropoid
- Platypelloid

This classification is based on normal variation in the following pelvic features (Figs. 31.5 to 31.7):

- Shape of inlet
- Splay of pelvic sidewalls
- Prominence of ischial spines

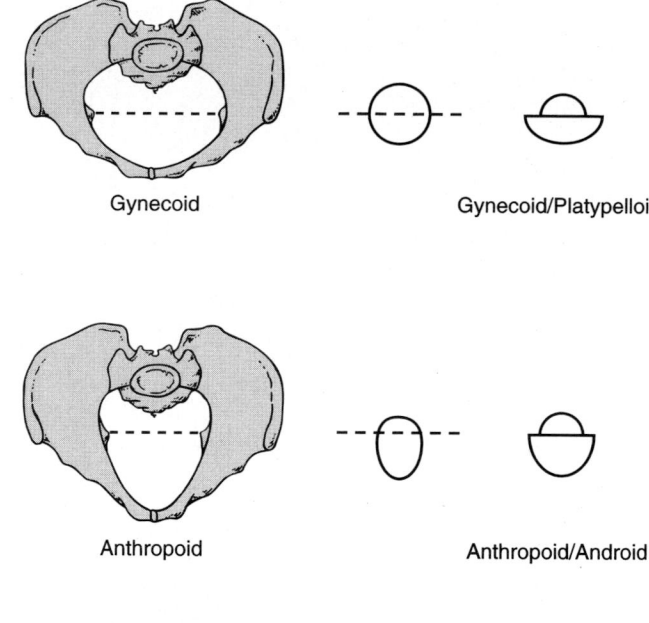

Gynecoid — Gynecoid/Platypelloid

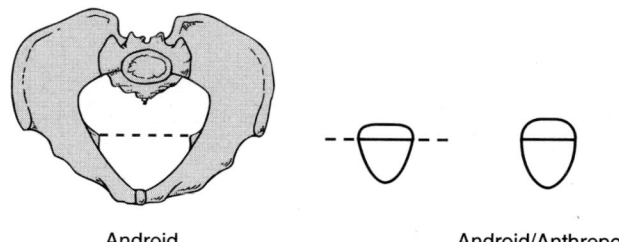

Anthropoid — Anthropoid/Android

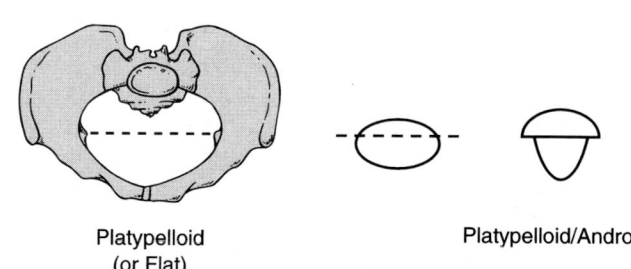

Android — Android/Anthropoid

Platypelloid (or Flat) — Platypelloid/Android

FIGURE 31.5. Pelvic types. The four "classic types," as defined by Caldwell-Moloy classification of pelvic types are shown in the left column. The shapes of the pelvic space for each type are shown in the center column. "Mixed" pelvic types are shown in the third column; these are named by the posterior shape first, followed by the anterior shape.

- Height of pubic symphysis
- Transverse diameter of pelvic outlet
- Width of pubic arch
- Curvature and inclination of the sacrum

Early pelvic typing may become necessary if there is a past history of trauma or fracture, or if the baby's size seems greater than that indicated by menstrual date. Definitive pelvic typing is not clinically helpful prior to 32 weeks of gestation. If delivery occurs before this time, the baby may be so small that bony architecture may not be a major factor in the labor and delivery process. The closer to term the pelvis is evaluated, the less patient

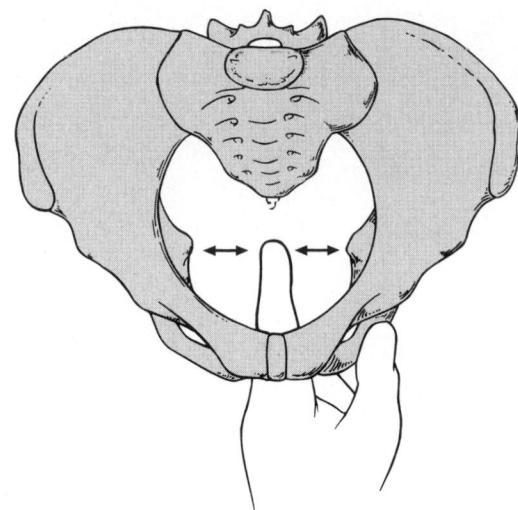

FIGURE 31.6. Evaluation of the transverse diameter. The lateral motion of the gloved finger is limited by the transversely narrowed pelvis (as indicated by the *arrows*). (From Steer CM. Maloy's evaluation of the pelvis. In: Steer CM, ed. *Obstetrics.* Philadelphia, PA: WB Saunders; 1959, with permission.)

discomfort there is likely to be, as pelvic tissues become more softened and relaxed as a result of hormonal and physiologic effects of pregnancy on the musculoskeletal system.

In individuals, "pure" pelvic types are unusual. Despite a great variation in individual features of the bony pelvis, the birth canal is curved anteriorly in nearly all women (Fig. 31.8). To be born,

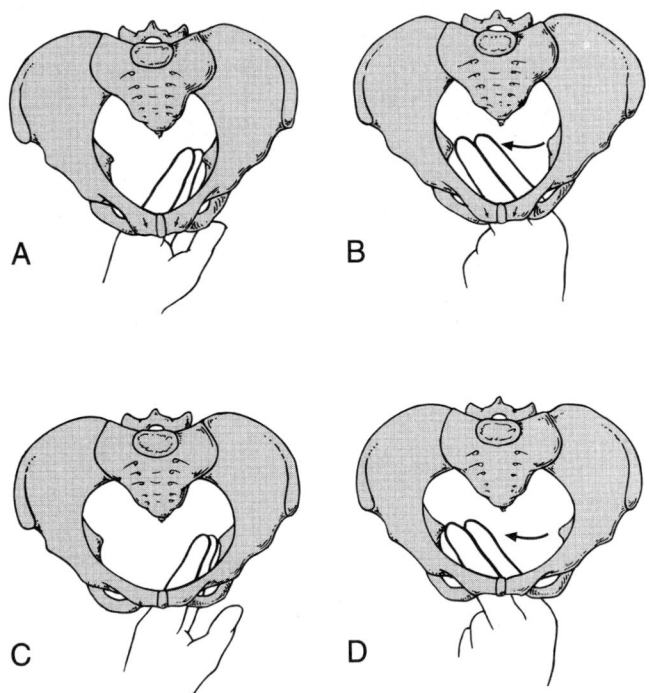

FIGURE 31.7. Estimation of width of subpubic arch. Panels **A** and **B** indicate the method of examination to determine the narrowed diameters in the mid- and lower pelvis. Panels **C** and **D** indicate the estimation of the wide diameters of the mid- and lower pelvis. (From Steer CM. Maloy's evaluation of the pelvis. In: Steer CM, ed. *Obstetrics.* Philadelphia, PA: WB Saunders; 1959, with permission.)

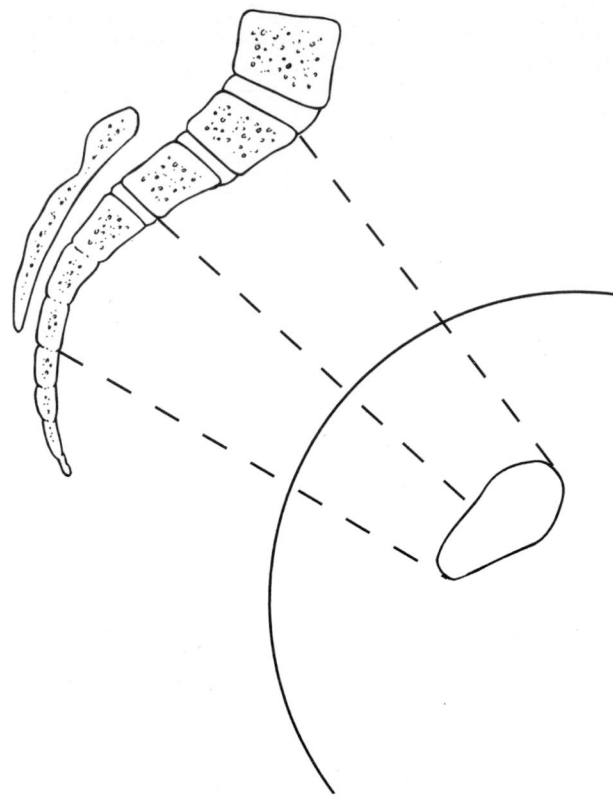

FIGURE 31.8. Axis of the pelvis, seen on sagittal section. Note that the curve is relatively straight throughout the inlet, but curves anteriorly in the midpelvis. The dashed lines indicate planes of the pelvic inlet, midpelvis, and outlet, top to bottom. (From Scott JR, DiSaia P. *Danforth's Obstetrics and Gynecology,* 7th ed. Philadelphia, PA: JB Lippincott; 1994:105–128, with permission.)

the fetal presenting part must negotiate both the pelvic curve and any narrow areas that may be present in the pelvis. Other maternal and fetal variables to contend with during labor are the quality of uterine contractions, head molding ability, and head flexion capability. Most normal labors require minimal intervention.

Osteopathic structural evaluation of the patient in labor should focus on the lumbosacral spine and pelvis, especially on mobility of the sacrum. Manipulative management considerations might include gentle techniques (such as soft tissue or myofascial stretching) that cooperate with natural forces of labor; pregnant patients do not tolerate active or aggressive manual procedures at this time. Treatment of the thoracic spine with soft tissue techniques may regulate uterine contractions via sympathetic influence (86). Treatment of sacral base dysfunction may influence cervical dilation. Osteopathic treatment of the cranium has been shown to influence uterine contractions (83).

A posterior sacral base provides ample space throughout the course of fetal descent; however, the fetal occiput may maintain the posterior position at delivery. If the sacral base is restricted anteriorly in its lower portion, the occiput tends to rotate into the anterior pelvis, usually maintaining the occiput anterior position for delivery. If the entire sacrum persists in an anterior position throughout its long axis (i.e., a flat pelvis), the head descends through the midpelvis in the transverse position. Sometimes a cesarean section becomes necessary for delivery because the head cannot descend any further or cannot rotate for a vaginal delivery. OMT of the maternal pelvis with the objective of addressing sacral motion restrictions may assist the labor and birth process.

Despite the variety of pelvic types and distortions, the fetal head may traverse the pelvis uneventfully, if the pelvis is large enough to accommodate the size of the infant (87). The most deleterious conditions are those encountered when an average-sized head attempts to squeeze through an average-sized android, or "funnel" pelvis in which the spines are prominent, sidewalls convergent, lower sacrum anterior, and subpubic arch narrow. When the subpubic arch is wide, the occiput may position itself with ease. If the arch is narrowed, the occiput remains posterior, in the area of the sacrum. With prolonged maternal pushing, in addition to possibly unsatisfactory placement of the maternal legs in stirrups, iliac dysfunction, sacral base restriction, back and leg pain with resultant neuropathy, and even pubic symphysis separation may occur (88,89).

True rupture of the ligaments supporting the symphysis pubis during labor does occur. Lindsey and Leggon believe that rupture is caused by the wedge effect of the forceful descent of the fetal head against the pelvic ring, usually during delivery, creating a separation of more than 1 cm (90). Normal physiologic separation has been reported not to exceed 10 mm, and this amount of separation causes only slight symptoms or no symptoms at all (91). Characteristically, when the pubis ruptures, there is an often audible "crack" with acute pain in the region that may radiate to the back or thighs. Walking and bending aggravate the pain, and the patient develops a waddling gait. On examination, a distinctive gap may be palpable at the symphysis. There may also be soft tissue swelling and tenderness over the area. Treatment usually consists of conservative measures: bed rest in the lateral decubitus position and a restrictive pelvic binder to reduce the separation and to maintain the reduction (3). Additional osteopathic structural evaluation of the spine and pelvis, and manipulative treatment of additional areas of somatic dysfunction, may help to stabilize the pelvis and to reduce soft tissue swelling. Although subsequent pregnancies are generally unaffected (92,93), some patients may experience pain in the suprapubic region during subsequent pregnancies, especially in the third trimester.

POSTPARTUM

The osteopathic physician can maximize a successful experience for the mother. She may also need treatment of residual somatic dysfunction in the postpartum period. The most obvious challenge is to assist the postpartum patient in returning her pelvis, axial skeleton, and the supporting soft tissues to their pregravid state; this often calls for OMT. King and Hitchcock have demonstrated the benefit of OMT in the reduction of morbidity and mortality due to complications of labor and delivery (94,95).

Although CTS usually occurs in the second or third trimesters, Wand reports its development in 18 patients, not during pregnancy but while they were nursing (80). These symptoms resolved when breast-feeding ceased. Snell and co-workers report similar findings in 5 patients in the puerperium and attribute the problem to fluid retention caused by the hormone prolactin (96).

Another frequently encountered cause of pain in the hand and wrist is de Quervain tenosynovitis, which results from compression and irritation of the extensor pollicis brevis and abductor pollicis longus tendons as they pass through the first dorsal compartment of the wrist near the styloid process of the radius (3). Fluid retention has been suspected as an initiator of this problem, which is intensified by the use of the hand and fingers and by movement of the wrist (97,98). Patients who have persistent symptoms have reported that infant care activities (97), as well as breast-feeding (98,99), aggravate the condition.

Although back pain is the most common complaint of expectant mothers, persistent back pain can also become a problem during the postpartum period. Russell and associates have investigated factors associated with long-term backache after childbirth in 299 patients, especially those factors that may have been associated with epidural anesthesia during labor (100). They concluded that, although new long-term backache was reported by the women given epidural analgesia in labor, the pain tended to be postural and not severe. Also, no differences existed in the nature of the backache between those who did or did not receive epidurals during labor. Although back pain during or after pregnancy may be common, it should not be dismissed on the basis that it is a normal accompaniment of pregnancy. The lumbosacral spine should be evaluated for extended segmental dysfunction. Back pain can also be addressed by normalizing structures passing through the obturator canal.

CONCLUSION

A systematic approach by the osteopathic obstetrician who has been trained to identify and treat somatic dysfunction may reveal underlying sources of discomfort. In this situation, OMT may be used to effect a more comfortable and enjoyable childbearing experience.

REFERENCES

1. Still AT. *The Philosophy and Mechanical Principles of Osteopathy.* Kansas City, MO: Hudson-Kimberly Publishing Co; 1902.
2. D'Alonzo G. *2000–2001 Yearbook and Directory of Osteopathic Physicians,* 91st ed. Chicago, IL: American Osteopathic Association; 2000.
3. Heckman JD, Sassard R. Musculoskeletal considerations in pregnancy. *J Bone Joint Surg Am.* 1994;76:1720–1730.
4. Rungee JL. Low back pain during pregnancy. *Orthopedics.* 1993;16:1339–1344.
5. DiGiovanna EL, Schiowitz S. *An Osteopathic Approach to Diagnosis and Treatment.* Philadelphia, PA: JB Lippincott Co; 1992:459.
6. Mantle MJ, Greenwood RM, Currey HLF. Backache in pregnancy. *Rheumatol Rehabil.* 1977;16:95–101.
7. Berg G, Hammar M, Moller-Nielson J, et al. Low back pain during pregnancy. *Obstet Gynecol.* 1988;71:71–78.
8. Daly JM, Frame PS, Rapoza PA. Sacroiliac subluxation: a common, treatable cause of low back pain during pregnancy. *Fam Pract Res J.* 1991;11:149–159.
9. Nwuga VC. Pregnancy and back pain among upper class Nigerian women. *Aust J Physiother.* 1982;28:8–11.
10. Östgaard HC, Andersson GBJ, Karlsson K. Prevalence of low back pain during pregnancy. *Spine.* 1991;16:549–552.
11. Östgaard HC, Andersson GBJ. Previous back pain and risk of developing back pain in a future pregnancy. *Spine.* 1991;16:432–436.

12. Svensson H-O, Andersson GB, Hagstad A, Jansson P-O. The relationship of low back pain to pregnancy and gynecologic factors. *Spine.* 1990;15:371–375.

13. Bendix T, Sorensen SS, Klausen K. Lumbar curve, trunk muscles, and line of gravity with different heel heights. *Spine.* 1984;9:223–227.

14. Freeman WS. Common complaints during pregnancy. *Res and Staff Physician.* 1979;25:69–73.

15. Laros RK Jr. Physiology of normal pregnancy. In: Willson JR, Carrington ER ed. *Obstetrics and Gynecology.* St. Louis, MO: Mosby-Year Book; 1991:242.

16. Fast A, Weiss L, Duccommun E, et al. Low back pain in pregnancy—abdominal muscles, sit up performance, and back pain. *Spine.* 1990;15:28–30.

17. Bullock J, Juli GA, Bullock M. The relationship of low back pain to postural changes during pregnancy. *Aust J Physiother.* 1987;33:10–17.

18. Snijders CJ, Seroo JM, Snijder JG, Hoedt HT. Change in form of the spine as a consequence of pregnancy. Digest of the 11th International Conference on Medical and Biological Engineering; 1976:670–671.

19. Östgaard HC, Andersson GB, Schultz AB, Miller JA. Influence of some biomechanical factors on low-back pain in pregnancy. *Spine.* 1993;18:61–65.

20. McGill S. A biomechanical perspective of sacro-iliac pain. *Clin Biomech.* 1987;2:145–151.

21. Epstein JA, Benton J, Browder J, et al. Treatment of low back pain and sciatic syndromes during pregnancy. *N Y State J Med.* 1959;59:1757–1768.

22. Hagen R. Pelvic girdle relaxation from an orthopaedic point of view. *Acta Orthop Scand.* 1974;45:550–563.

23. Lotgering FK, Gilbert RD, Longo LD. The interactions of exercise and pregnancy: a review. *Am J Obstet Gynecol.* 1984;149:560–568.

24. Sands RX. Backache of pregnancy: a method of treatment. *Obstet Gynecol.* 1958;12:670–677.

25. Östgaard HC, Zetherstrom G, Roos HE, Svanberg B. Reduction of back and posterior pelvic pain in pregnancy. *Spine.* 1994;19:894–900.

26. LaBan MM, Perrin JCS, Latimer FR. Pregnancy and the herniated lumbar disc. *Arch Phys Med Rehabil.* 1983;64:319–321.

27. Wells J. Osteitis condensans ilii. *AJR.* 1956;76:1141.

28. Bushnell LF. The postural pains of pregnancy, part I: parietal neuralgia of pregnancy. *West J Surg Obstet Gynecol.* 1949;57:123–127.

29. American College of Obstetricians and Gynecologists. Pregnancy and the postnatal period. In: *ACOG Home Exercise Program.* Washington, D.C.: ACOG, 1985:1–5.

30. Weinreb JC, Wolbarsht LB, Cohen JM, et al. Prevalence of lumbosacral intervertebral disk abnormalities on MR images in pregnant and asymptomatic nonpregnant women. *Radiology.* 1989;170:125–128.

31. Berman AT, Cohen DL, Schwentker EP. The effects of pregnancy on idiopathic scoliosis: a preliminary report on eight cases and a review of the literature. *Spine.* 1982;7:76–77.

32. Betz RR, Bunnell WP, Lambrecht-Mulier E, MacEwen GD. Scoliosis and pregnancy. *J Bone Joint Surg.* 1987;69-A:90–96.

33. Visscher W, Lonstein JE, Hoffman DA, et al. Reproductive outcomes in scoliosis patients. *Spine.* 1988;13:1096–1098.

34. Heckman JD. Managing musculoskeletal problems in pregnant patients. *J Musculoskel Med.* 1984;1:35–40.

35. Rhodes P. Orthopaedic conditions associated with childbearing. *Practitioner.* 1958;181:304–312.

36. Kangilaski J. Why does arthritis pain diminish with pregnancy? *JAMA.* 1981;246:317.

37. Kay NR, Park WM, Bark M. The relationship between pregnancy and femoral head necrosis. *Br J Radiol.* 1972;45:828–831.

38. Froelich CJ, Goodwin JS, Bankhurst AD, Williams RC Jr. Pregnancy, a temporary fetal graft of suppressor cells in autoimmune disease? *Am J Med.* 1980;69:329–331.

39. Østensen M, Husby G. Seronegative spondylarthritis and ankylosing spondylitis: biological effects and management. In: Scott JS, Bird HA, eds. *Pregnancy, Autoimmunity, and Connective Tissue Disorders.* New York, NY: Oxford University Press; 1990:163–184.

40. Østensen HC, Romberg Ø, Husby G. Ankylosing spondylitis and motherhood. *Arthritis Rheumat.* 1982;25:140–143.

41. Pregnancy worsens course of ankylosing spondylitis. *Orthoped Rev.* 1980;9:81.

42. Steinberg CL. Ankylosing spondylitis and pregnancy. *Ann Rheumat Dis.* 1948;7:209–215.

43. Fast A, Weiss L, Parich S, Hertz G. Night backache in pregnancy—hypothetical pathophysiological mechanisms. *Am J Phys Med Rehabil.* 1989;68:227–229.

44. Fast A, Shapiro D, Ducommon EJ, et al. Low back pain in pregnancy. *Spine.* 1987;12:368–371.

45. LaBan MM, Wesolowski DP. Night pain associated with diminished cardiopulmonary compliance. A concomitant of lumbar spinal stenosis and degenerative spondylolisthesis. *Am J Phys Med Rehabil.* 1988;67:155–160.

46. Kuchera M, Kuchera W. *Osteopathic Considerations in Systemic Dysfunction.* 2nd ed. Kirksville, MO: KCOM Press; 1992:149.

47. Clemente CD. *Gray's Anatomy,* 30th ed. Philadelphia, PA: Lea & Febiger; 1985.

48. Zink JG, Lawson WG. Pressure gradients in the osteopathic manipulative management of the obstetrical patient. *Osteopath Ann.* 1979;7:208–214.

49. Sherwood OD. Relaxin. In: Knobil E, Neill J, eds. *The Physiology of Reproduction.* New York, NY: Raven Press; 1988:585–658.

50. Szlachter BN, Quagliarello J, Jewelewicz R, et al. Relaxin in normal and pathogenic pregnancies. *Obstet Gynecol.* 1982;59:167–170.

51. Cunningham FG, MacDonald PC, Gant NF. *Williams' Obstetrics,* 18th ed. San Mateo, CA: Appleton & Lange; 1989:134–135.

52. MacLennan AH, Nicolson R, Green RC, Bath M. Serum relaxin and pelvic pain of pregnancy. *Lancet.* 1986;2:243–245.

53. Cugell DW, Frank NR, Gaensler ER, Badger TL. Pulmonary function in pregnancy. I. Serial observations in normal women. *Am Rev Tuberc Pulm Dis.* 1953;67:568–584.

54. Scott JR, DiSaia P. *Danforth's Obstetrics and Gynecology,* 7th ed. Philadelphia, PA: JB Lippincott Co; 1994:105–128.

55. Beal MC. Viscerosomatic reflexes: a review. *JAOA.* 1985;185:786–801.

56. Bonica JJ. Autonomic innervation of the viscera in relation to nerve block. *Anesthesiol.* 1968;29:793–813.

57. Head H. On disturbances of sensation with special reference to the pain of visceral disease. *Brain.* 1893;16:1–133.

58. House EL, Pansky B. *A Functional Approach to Neuroanatomy,* 2nd ed. New York, NY: McGraw-Hill;1967.

59. Crosby EC, Humphry T, Lauer EW. *Correlative Anatomy of the Nervous System.* New York, NY: Macmillan; 1962.

60. Bhagat BD, Young PA, Biggerstaff DE. *Fundamentals of Visceral Innervation.* Springfield, IL: Charles C Thomas Publisher; 1977.

61. Pottenger FM. *Symptoms of Visceral Disease,* 5th ed. St. Louis, MO: CV Mosby; 1938.

62. White JC, Smithwick RH, Simeone FA. *The Autonomic Nervous System,* 3rd ed. New York, NY: Macmillan; 1952.

63. Hansen K, Schliack H. *Segmental Innervation.* Stuttgart, Germany: G. Thieme; 1962.

64. Woods ER. The viscerosomatic reflex in acute abdominal disorders. *JAOA.* 1962;63:239–242.

65. Hix EL. Reflex viscerosomatic reference phenomena. *Osteopath Ann.* 1976;4:496–503.

66. Conley GJ. The role of the spinal joint lesion in gallbladder disease. *JAOA.* 1944;44:121–123.

67. Larson NJ. Manipulative care before and after surgery. *Osteopath Med.* 1977;2:41–49.

68. Young GS. Gently applied manipulation eases post-op convalescence. *Clin Trends Osteopath Med.* 1978;4–7.

69. Drew EG. The role of the secondary lesion from the surgical standpoint. *JAOA.* 1939;38:377–378.

70. Owens C. *An Endocrine Interpretation of Chapman's Reflexes,* 2nd ed. Chattanooga, TN: Chattanooga Printing & Engraving Co; 1937.

71. Taylor G. The osteopathic management of nausea and vomiting of pregnancy. *JAOA.* 1949;48:581–582.

72. Huch R, Erkkola R. Pregnancy and exercise—exercise and pregnancy: a short review. *Br J Obstet Gynecol.* 1990;97:208–214.

73. Wiskstrom J, Haslam ET, Hutchinson RH. Backache during pregnancy—its etiology and management. *J Louisiana State Med Soc.* 1955;107:490–494.

74. Mersy DJ. Health benefits of aerobic exercise. *Postgrad Med.* 1991;90:103–107, 110–112.

75. Women say running helped pregnancy, labor. *Phys Sportsmed.* 1981;9:24–25.

76. Pregnant women advised to consider exercise risks. *Phys Sportsmed.* 1982;10:27.

77. Nygaard IE, Saltzman CL, Whitehouse MB, Hankin FM. Hand problems in pregnancy. *Am Fam Phys.* 1989;39:123–126.

78. Voitk AJ, Mueller JC, Farlinger DE, Jonston RU. Carpal tunnel syndrome in pregnancy. *Can Med Assoc J.* 1983;28:277–281.

79. Eckman-Ordeberg G, Sälgeback S, Ordeberg G. Carpal tunnel syndrome in pregnancy: a prospective study. *Acta Obstet Gynecol Scand.* 1987;66:233–235.

80. Wand JS. Carpal tunnel syndrome in pregnancy and lactation. *J Hand Surg.* 1990;15B:93–95.

81. Sucher BM. Myofascial manipulative release of carpal tunnel syndrome: documentation with magnetic resonance imaging. *JAOA.* 1993;93:1273–1278.

82. Sucher BM. Palpatory diagnosis and manipulative management of carpal tunnel syndrome. *JAOA.* 1994;94:647–663.

83. Gitlin RS, Wolf DL. Uterine contractions following osteopathic cranial manipulation—a pilot study. *JAOA.* 1992;92:1183.

84. Magoun H. *Osteopathy in the Cranial Field.* Kirksville, MO: Journal Printing Company; 1966.

85. Steer CM. Maloy's evaluation of the pelvis. In: Steer CM, ed. *Obstetrics.* Philadelphia, PA: WB Saunders; 1959.

86. Guthrie RA, Martin RH. Effect of pressure applied to the upper thoracic versus lumbar areas for inhibition of lumbar myalgia during labor. *JAOA.* 1982;82:247–251.

87. Frymann V. Relation of disturbances of cranio-sacral mechanisms to symptomatology of the newborn: study of 1250 infants. *JAOA.* 1966;65:1059–1075.

88. Whiting L. Osteopathic prevention of certain complications of labor and the puerperium. *JAOA.* 1945;44:495–498.

89. McCormick J. Some variations can be made in the "obstetrical workshop." *JAOA.* 1944;44:195–197.

90. Lindsey RW, Leggon RE. Separation of the symphysis pubis in association with childbearing: a case report. *J Bone Joint Surg.* 1988;70-A:289–292.

91. Young J. Relaxation of the pelvic joints in pregnancy: pelvic arthropathy of pregnancy. *J Obstet Gynecol Br Empire.* 1940;47:493.

92. Cibils LA. Rupture of the symphysis pubis: a case report. *Obstet Gynecol.* 1971;38:407–410.

93. Dhar S, Anderton JM. Rupture of the symphysis pubis during labor. *Clin Orthopath.* 1992;283:252–257.

94. King HH. Osteopathic manipulative treatment in prenatal care: evidence supporting improved outcomes and health policy implications. *AAOJ.* 2000;10:25–33.

95. Hitchcock ME. Osteopathic care in pregnancy. *Osteopath Ann.* 1976;4:405–411.

96. Snell NJ, Coysh HL, Snell BJ. Carpal tunnel syndrome presenting in the puerperium. *Practitioner.* 1980;224:191–193.

97. Schned ES. De Quervain tenosynovitis in pregnant and post-partum women. *Obstet Gynecol.* 1986;68:411–444.

98. H R Schumacher HR Jr, Dorwart BB, Korzeniowski OM. Occurrence of De Quervain's tendonitis during pregnancy. *Arch Intern Med.* 1985;145:2083–2084.

99. Johnson CA. Occurrence of De Quervain's disease in post-partum women. *J Fam Pract.* 1991;32:325–327.

100. Russell R, Groves P, Taub N, et al. Assessing long term backache after childbirth. *BMJ.* 1993;306:1299–1303.

32

ONCOLOGY

MICHAEL I. OPIPARI
AUGUSTINE L. PERROTTA
DAVID R. ESSIG-BEATTY

KEY CONCEPTS

- Philosophic principles of care of the patient with cancer
- Malignancies that appear as disease involving bone and soft tissue structures, the central nervous system, or the peripheral nervous system, including renal cell cancer, lung carcinoma, and plasma cell neoplasm
- Manifestations of malignancy in musculoskeletal system, including back pain, joints, muscle, and skin
- Manifestations of malignancy in the central nervous system, including cerebral and indirect paraneoplastic malignancies
- Manifestations of malignancy in peripheral nervous system, including remote peripheral manifestations, spinal cord compression, and other causes of peripheral neuropathy
- Viscerosomatic-type oncologic responses
- Presenting diagnostic and treatment options to patients
- Supportive care of patients with cancer including symptom and pain relief, blood and blood products, and general supportive care
- Stress and treatment
- Osteopathic approach, including indications and contraindications for osteopathic manipulative treatment

---

Osteopathic physicians do not treat disease, they treat patients (1). —Philip E. Greenman, DO

Care more particularly for the individual patient than for the special features of the disease (2). —Sir William Osler

INTRODUCTION

Medical oncology is a subspecialty of internal medicine and represents that branch of medicine dealing with the incidence, prevention, diagnosis, and medical management of malignancy. Cancer is the second leading cause of mortality in the United States. The field of study surrounding oncology is constantly changing due to progress of cancer research in diagnosis and treatment over the past 30 years. Medical oncology has grown as a specialty over these years with the advent of subspecialty fellowships since the mid-1960s. This 3-year training program is taken after completion of 3 years of training in general internal medicine.

Primary care physicians or surgeons generally refer patients to oncologists when they either suspect or have diagnosed malignant tumor disease. In most cases, the oncologist will serve as the guide for a patient's care through the maze of cancer diagnosis, surgical and radiation treatment and/or delivery of chemotherapy and, when necessary, through end-of-life and palliative care.

Significant advances leading to cure and long, functional disease-free intervals are now commonplace.

ONCOLOGY

The patient with a cancer diagnosis presents a complex series of events for the primary care physician. The clinical manifestations of this family of diseases are many and may be secondary to altered structure or function at the primary site of tumor involvement or due to involvement of a secondary site with metastatic disease or remote tumor effects such as paraneoplastic syndromes. Often the malignant process may present with signs or symptoms unrelated to the primary site, and without any clinical evidence of metastasis. Metastasis may occasionally be present and subclinical, yet produce symptoms, or indeed metastasis may be totally absent with the primary tumor manifesting itself through a paraneoplastic mechanism. Through this mechanism a malignancy may affect a hormonal cytokine or metabolic process to exert effects at distant sites or within other organ systems without metastasis being present.

Patients with cancer, as in all persons with chronic disease, are still people. They are human beings with families, with thoughts, feelings, hopes, and dreams. They have parents and children, friends and colleagues. These are not cancer patients but people with cancer. They are not interesting cases with great physical findings but are living and breathing people. Therefore, discussion concerning their disease and plans and options for treatment must be carefully individualized. These persons must be offered choices and options that are neither right nor wrong but may be correct for one person while not for another. The oncologist and primary care physician should always care for the person, even if treatment for the disease is unavailable. There must always be optimism. These patients must always be offered the comfort of care even if treatment is unavailable. This care will include prevention of and meeting needs for pain and other symptoms if necessary. This will include supporting the person's fullest level of functioning at home with family and loved ones, or traveling or even working.

In many cases there arrives a time in the course of a disease when no further treatment is available. At that time it is especially important that the treating physician refocus attention from the incurable disease to the person who has to live with the disease. This treatment involves treatment of mind, body, and spirit including the individual's belief system or spirituality. Often, listening is all that is needed. Lack of emotional and physical abandonment is essential in spite of inability to treat disease. Healing a person can occur while losing a battle to disease. This is a significant opportunity for the caregiving physician. Although treatment of the whole person is the foundation of the physician's interactions with the patient, it is especially important to emphasize this aspect of the relationship when you can no longer treat the disease.

THE WHOLE PATIENT: DEFINITION

Throughout this chapter, the reader will see reference several times to the phrase "*whole patient.*" The context in which this is used refers to a person or human being together with a disease, and not only an illness to be diagnosed and managed. That human being presents a constellation of potential issues related or unrelated to the disease. They may be represented as personal, social, financial, or spiritual in nature. The treating oncologist needs to be aware and, at various times, involved in any or all of these aspects, together with the diagnosis and management of the malignancy. This defines the "whole patient," and although a humanistic quality to be strived for by all physicians, is especially linked to the osteopathic, "holistic" philosophy associated with treating a fully integrated/interrelated system.

OSTEOPATHIC PHILOSOPHIC PRINCIPLES OF CARE OF THE PATIENT WITH CANCER

Traditional cancer therapy includes surgery, radiation therapy, and drug therapy. We must continue to use each and all of these modalities. However, we must never forget that we are caring for a person rather than a tumor. Patient decisions and actions are often based on their thoughts, feelings, and perceptions.

To Treat or Not To Treat

Many physicians assume that all cancer must be treated, whether or not there is anything effective to offer. Remember, we must treat every patient, but have no need to treat every cancer. In many cases more benefit can be provided to the patient with careful understanding, supportive therapy, and meeting the needs of the patient than with definitive antineoplastic therapy. Therefore, honesty with the patient is necessary; honesty regarding the availability of effective treatment modalities and regarding cure. A life-threatening disease, such as metastatic renal cell cancer, can be discussed in a positive and optimistic fashion. The patient can be informed regarding the unpredictable natural history of the disease, which can have long-term stable control in some patients. Immunotherapeutics such as interferon and interleukin (IL)-2 can be discussed and offered if the patient is an appropriate candidate. The patient, however, must be reassured that the physician will be available throughout the treatment course. Patients must be reassured that they will not be permitted to remain uncomfortable and that multiple modalities are available for relief of discomfort. They are reassured that the physician will discuss all decisions regarding therapy with them and assist them in decision making. The physician must inform and support the family if the patient wishes. Throughout the discussion, which may become more repetitious and personal as the relationship develops, touching of the patient is important. The patient must leave the physician after each visit confident that a partnership has developed.

Touching as Communication

Some patients complain that the only time a physician has touched them in the past was in the process of physical examination or the placing of a stethoscope on a chest. Patients with cancer feel comforted by an appropriate touch of a hand or even, on occasion, a tear shed with theirs. Touching is a nonverbal communication with the patient that says, I recognize you as a whole person, not only a diseased body or organ or an interesting case. Recognition of the *whole person* encompassing the cancer is to recognize the integration of all of the body systems. This offers the consideration that no system can alone become diseased or healthy without impact or benefit to the whole person or other systems. They must all get well and survive together. The basic osteopathic philosophy emphasizes the need to treat the person as a whole. This approach must consider the patient with the disease as well as the patient's environment. This full embodiment of supportive care can facilitate patient care and provide patient benefit to a greater degree than traditional anticancer therapy.

Osteopathic physicians are known for their respect for the role of the neuromusculoskeletal system in health and disease. Palpatory diagnosis and treatment of neuromusculoskeletal dysfunctions have been hallmarks of this profession from its inception.

Within this chapter, the disease of malignancy as a whole will be discussed with an emphasis on its manifestations/effects on the neuromusculoskeletal system. The relationship of the neurostructural presentation of a patient with malignancy versus a nonneoplastic structural lesion can be interesting and deceiving.

Three separate malignancies are presented as index tumors, and serve as prototypes for the variety of neuromusculoskeletal presentations to be discussed. All three of these malignant diseases have the potential to present as disease involving bone and soft tissue structures, the central nervous system (CNS), or peripheral nervous system.

RENAL CELL CANCER

This disease (hypernephroma, Grawitz tumor) is an elusive, unpredictable one, accounting occasionally for prolonged delays in diagnosis. Renal cell carcinoma makes up only 2% to 3% of all malignant disease (3). The classic triad of presentation including hematuria, flank pain, and abdominal mass is infrequent, occurring in less than 10% of cases (4,5). The presenting symptoms, however, are more commonly associated with distant manifestations, either metastatic or paraneoplastic. As many as 34% of patients have metastasis at the time of diagnosis (6). When present, metastases occur most commonly in lung, bone, liver, and lymph nodes (6,7). This tumor is commonly referred to as the "internist's tumor" due to its presentation with humoral or systemic signs and symptoms of a medical nature rather than a urologic nature. The systemic manifestations may include anemia or erythrocytosis, fever of unknown origin, weight loss and hypercalcemia, all of which may occur in the absence of metastatic disease. The hypercalcemia is often related to elaboration of an ectopic parathyroid hormonelike substance from the tumor (parathyroid hormone-related peptide, or PTHrP). In addition, a hepatic dysfunction syndrome may occur in up to 15% of patients without metastasis manifesting as significantly altered hepatic enzymes (8).

The natural history of renal cell carcinoma is unpredictable. Patients with metastatic disease may remain stable for months to years and suddenly develop progressive metastasis leading to death. Patients with progressive disease may likewise suddenly stabilize for prolonged periods of time. Renal cell carcinoma is one of the most common tumors to be reported to undergo spontaneous regression after removal of the primary site (9). However, the majority of these cases have not been histologically confirmed.

Neuromusculoskeletal metastasis may occur to the spine producing back pain, to soft tissue areas as a mass, a compression of spinal cord, or nerve root producing peripheral neuropathic symptoms, or can produce CNS signs and symptoms due to direct metastasis or paraneoplastic effects (hypercalcemia).

The diagnosis of renal cell cancer is most commonly accomplished by radiologic techniques (computed tomography [CT] scan, magnetic resonance imaging [MRI], intravenous pyelogram, and ultrasonography). Treatment with surgery is most effective when the disease is localized. If metastatic disease is present, the extent and location will dictate whether surgery is appropriate. Radiation and chemotherapy are palliative and of limited benefit. Immune-modulating therapy with IL-2 and/or α-interferon hold some promise.

LUNG CARCINOMA

Lung cancer is the most common cancer and most common cause of cancer death in both men and women. The use of cigarettes and tobacco products accounts for over 30% of cancer deaths and is responsible for 80% to 85% of lung and laryngeal cancers. A rapid rise in lung cancer incidence and death in women is due to an increase in smoking among women. In men, the rate has stabilized and may be showing early evidence of reversal due to smoking discontinuation. At the time of diagnosis, the disease generally has spread to regional lymph nodes or distant sites. Small cell lung cancer (oat cell cancer) is one of the four major cell types of lung cancer arising from the bronchial surface epithelium and originating as a submucosal growth. Epidermoid (squamous cell) cancer, adenocarcinoma, and large cell carcinoma make up the other major varieties. Small cell lung cancer is generally an aggressive, rapidly growing neoplasm making up approximately 20% to 25% of lung cancers. Once, the most common variety of lung cancer, epidermoid carcinoma now has a 25% to 30% incidence, with adenocarcinomas comprising 40%, and large cell cancer 15% of lung tumors (10). Traditionally survival has been believed to be the best in epidermoid cancers. However, with the recent advent of intensive combination chemo/radiation therapy, small cell lung cancer has shown an improvement with up to 20% long-term survivals. Due to its aggressive behavior, small cell lung cancer has approximately a 70% incidence of regional lymph node involvement at the time of surgical resection (11). At autopsy, lung cancer metastasis has been shown to be present in every body organ with small cell cancer having absolute likelihood of extrathoracic metastasis. Common clinical problems relate to distant metastasis including CNS metastasis with neurologic deficits; bone metastasis presenting with bone or back pain and pathologic fracture; liver metastasis; adrenal metastasis; and lymph node and skin metastasis.

Bronchogenic carcinoma may present as a Pancoast syndrome with pain in the neck, axilla, anterior lower ribs, and scapular region, with thoracic paraspinal muscle spasm and paresthesia in the upper extremity (12). Significant relief of pain may be achieved with osteopathic manipulative therapy (OMT) while undergoing definitive radiation therapy and/or chemotherapy.

Paraneoplastic syndromes occur commonly with lung cancer. Some occur more specifically with individual histologic varieties of lung cancer. These may represent presenting symptoms, without metastasis, or even prior to the diagnosis of the primary lung cancer. Paraneoplastic syndromes seen include Cushing syndrome, syndrome of inappropriate antidiuretic hormone (SIADH), nonmetastatic hypercalcemia (PTHrP), subacute cerebellar degeneration, dementia syndromes, peripheral neuropathies, and polymyositis, as well as dermatomyositis. Any of these syndromes may present as altered CNS function and may create difficulty in discussing appropriate treatment options and decisions. A frequent musculoskeletal paraneoplastic manifestation is hypertrophic pulmonary osteoarthropathy. While the previously noted endocrine syndromes, except for PTHrP production, are particularly common with small cell carcinoma, the osteoarthropathy is most commonly seen with adenocarcinoma. Lung cancer should be included as a part of the differential diagnosis in all patients with paraneoplastic syndromes.

A type of paraneoplastic syndrome occurring with lung cancer involves the ectopic production of bombesin, a multiple amino-acid neuropeptide hormone. Since bombesin was first isolated from amphibian skin the mammalian equivalent, gastrin-releasing peptide (GRP) or human bombesin, has been found in tumors of neuroendocrine and some non-neuroendocrine origins (13). Bombesinlike immunoreactivity has been found in human brain, spinal cord, gastrointestinal (GI) mucosa, and pulmonary neuroendocrine cells. High levels of this immunoreactivity are noted in up to 50% of pulmonary carcinoid tumors and in many small cell (oat cell) lung cancers (14). This substance is particularly interesting because of its apparent autocrine growth-enhancing ability imposed on the tumors.

The diagnosis of lung cancer requires tissue confirmation by biopsy, surgical resection, or cytology of sputum or selected bronchial washings. Therapy varies with the specific cell type and stage but commonly involves a combination of surgery, radiotherapy, and/or chemotherapy. Overall survival at 5 years after surgical resection for all resectable stage cell types varies between 30% and 80%, although the previously noted negligible survival rates for small cell cancer are improving due to the use of intensive combination chemotherapy (15).

PLASMA CELL NEOPLASM (MULTIPLE MYELOMA)

This is a neoplasm of B-lymphocytes of monoclonal origin that progresses to a large cellular population. The plasma cells produce immunoglobulins or immunoglobulin fractions that can be distinguished and detected in blood and urine as monoclonal or M protein on a protein electrophoresis pattern. The diagnosis of this neoplasm is made by the demonstration of bone marrow plasmacytosis, monoclonal immunoglobulin detection, anemia, and bone pain (16). This disease is the most common primary tumor to involve medullary bone and may often be overlooked in a patient presenting with back pain. Often the symptoms are vague and nonspecific. Typical lytic "punched out" bone lesions may be absent and a diffuse osteoporosis pattern may be seen on radiograph. The incidence of myeloma is reported to be between two to four per 100,000 population with a higher rate in blacks than whites. Plasma cell tumors may originate in extramedullary sites as well. They have been known to arise in almost any organ with the upper air passages (nasal sinuses, nose, nasopharynx, tonsil) being the most frequent extramedullary sites. These tumors may also arise in skin and subcutaneous tissue, thereby presenting as soft tissue masses. At least two-thirds of patients present with the skeletal symptom of bone pain, especially in the spine and ribs. Pathologic fractures are very common. Spinal cord compression and nerve root compression are common complications of this disease and may produce radicular pain. Peripheral neuropathies may occur as a result of amyloid deposition in nerves or perineural vasculature.

Other clinical problems common in the patient with myeloma include hypercalcemia, which is reported in up to 35% of patients at presentation (17). The progressive confusion and drowsiness in these patients may resemble CNS disease. GI symptoms of nausea, vomiting, and constipation together with polyuria may signal the onset of hypercalcemia. A hyperviscosity syndrome is also a complication of myeloma, especially immunoglobulin A (IgA) myeloma, and is due to a change in concentration, size, and shape of the monoclonal globulin. If the serum viscosity relative to water rises above 4, symptoms occur. These may include cephalalgia, visual disturbance, fatigue, vertigo, nystagmus, paresis, and eventually confusion and coma. This combination of symptoms may closely resemble CNS metastasis. Hyperviscosity is treated by plasmapheresis and specific chemotherapy including steroids and alkylating agents.

Attempts should be made to diagnose myeloma earlier than presentation with pathologic fracture. Anemia, proteinuria, and rouleaux formation on a peripheral smear report, or a report of bone demineralization may be early clues.

Myeloma usually enters a chronic phase that is easily responsive to steroids and alkylating drugs. Pathologic fractures may be surgically treated with pinning for long bone disease. Impending fractures and spinal cord/nerve root compression should be irradiated. Maintaining activity and ambulation is essential in treatment of this disease. Fluid hydration is beneficial for the renal complications and in preventing hyperviscosity. Eventually the patients enter an acute phase characterized by packing of the marrow with plasma cells producing pancytopenia leading to infection. Infection and renal failure are often terminal events.

We have evaluated two relatively common malignant diseases and one extremely common malignant tumor. All three were selected due to their frequent ability to present with signs or involvement of the nervous, muscular, or skeletal system. The impact of these tumors may affect soft tissue and bone simultaneously, sequentially, or not at all. Any physician following or treating a patient with malignancy must be aware of the natural history potential of such presentations.

UNIQUE NEUROMUSCULOSKELETAL MANIFESTATIONS OF MALIGNANCY

The manifestations discussed within this section will be divided into musculoskeletal, central nervous system, and peripheral nervous system. Metastasis can often influence the presentation within these systems. Metastasis is often overlooked because of the site of involvement. The major mechanisms of metastasis involve direct tumor extension and lymphatic and hematogenous dissemination. The specific vasculature invaded in the process of metastasis may determine the site that will be involved in the distribution of the bloodborne metastasis (14,15). This is typified in prostatic carcinoma and other pelvic tumors by metastatic spread to the vertebral spine, or in carcinoma of the breast by spinal metastasis in the absence of pulmonary spread (18,19). This metastatic pattern to vertebral bone may occur as a result of the vertebral venous plexus, a system of valveless vessels extending along the spine and forming anastomoses with veins extending from the brain to the pelvis. Batson, who described the anatomy of this system that now carries his name, demonstrated extensive retrograde-antegrade vascular flow potential in this venous system as related to posture and abdominal pressure (18,19).

Musculoskeletal System

Back Pain

The bony skeleton is the second most common metastatic site of malignancy in terms of frequency (20). Over 80% of the metastatic tumors originate within breast, prostate, lung, kidney, and thyroid gland (21). Microscopically, at autopsy, a much higher rate of metastasis to bone is present than is noted clinically, with in excess of 80% in breast and prostate cancer, 50% in thyroid cancer, and 40% in lung and kidney cancers (21). The spine is involved most often with a reducing order of frequency extending from lumbar to dorsal to cervical areas of the spine (22–24). Back pain is often the first indication of metastatic disease. Metastatic bone disease is much more common than primary bone tumors. Metastatic bone disease in the spine may be lytic (clastic or destructive) or blastic (sclerotic) or a mixture of both, depending on the predominant process of formation or destruction of bone which occurs in metastases. Back pain may be present for varying periods of time before the onset of neurologic signs or symptoms, which usually occur secondary to compression of a nerve root or the spinal cord. The origin of back pain may be difficult to localize in the skeletal system due to the vagaries of diagnostic tests available. Radiographs do not visualize osseous changes as early as radionuclide scans. Scans depend on osteoblastic activity for demonstration of abnormalities (25). Actual loss of bone density of at least 50% is required to demonstrate metastasis by radiograph. Without the osteoblastic process and in purely lytic bone disease, a false-negative bone scan may therefore occur. In the older adult patient, a reactive or inflammatory process such as arthritis or degenerative vertebral disease can mimic the metastatic process and create a false-positive bone scan. Therefore, bone scan abnormalities require radiographic, CT, or MRI confirmation of metastases.

Two procedures are often indicated for comparison prior to a definitive diagnosis and initiation of treatment. CT and MRI, which have a greater degree of resolution, are often helpful in detection of otherwise silent lesions. Often, with a high index of clinical suspicion and without imaging documentation, localization by specific sensory or dermatomal level can focus an area to permit treatment by radiation therapy. In evaluation of the patient with back pain, one must always consider malignancy, especially prostate cancer in a man over 55 years of age. Additional systemic manifestations may include weight loss, pain unrelated to motion or position, and pain unresponsive to analgesic medications. Oftentimes there is an urgency in considering spinal metastasis so that appropriate therapy and maintenance of neurologic function can be maintained in patients with spinal cord compression.

Leptomeningeal carcinomatosis is seen most often in small cell lung cancer, breast cancer, and leukemia. In these patients, a variety of diagnoses may precede the diagnosis of leptomeningeal disease. These include cerebral tumor, meningitis, psychoses, hysteria, and polyneuritis (26). This manifestation of systemic malignancy may occur as a presenting symptom. The presenting symptoms often include low back pain, nonspecific leg pain (radicular), headache, and mental status change in addition to extremity weakness, neck pain, and nuchal rigidity (27). The diagnosis is confirmed by finding malignant cells in the cerebral spinal fluid (CSF) as well as elevated CSF protein and low CSF glucose levels (27). The evaluation of these patients, without knowledge of the presence of a related malignancy, can easily lead to mistaken diagnosis for the back and leg pain resulting from a "musculoskeletal somatic lesion" rather than malignancy.

Joints

The joints may be involved with malignancy by either a primary tumor or metastatic process to the bone or synovium. This presents as a picture of asymmetric arthritis, or diffuse articular changes caused by an indirect, humoral-related process as in hypertrophic osteoarthropathy. Leukemia in children has been reported to present as localized or diffuse bone pain associated with joint swelling and pain (28). Bronchogenic carcinoma has

likewise been reported to present with symmetric painful swelling of the digits resembling early rheumatoid arthritis as a result of metastasis (29). Undiagnosed renal carcinoma has been reported by Ritch and colleagues in three cases to present and be treated as shoulder arthritis, prior to discovery of metastasis to the clavicle or upper humerus (30).

Hypertrophic pulmonary osteoarthropathy (HPOA) is a paraneoplastic syndrome presumed to be due to secretion of estrogen, growth hormone, or neurogenic factors in patients with intrathoracic tumors (31). This syndrome produces a symmetric clubbing of fingers and toes, periostitis of long bones, and polyarthritis resembling rheumatoid arthritis (32). The joints most frequently involved are the knees, ankles, and wrists. The clinical presentation is pain, tenderness, and swelling of the affected joints. Involvement of the metacarpal-phalangeal and proximal interphalangeal joints has been reported. A classic finding is periosteal tenderness and radiographic evidence of periosteal elevation. Lung cancer is the most frequent malignancy associated with HPOA, which occurs in 12% of patients with adenocarcinoma and less often in squamous cell cancers (32). Osteoarthropathy is negligible in small cell cancer of the lung. Upon synovial fluid analysis, generally a noninflammatory fluid finding is noted (33,34). In ruling out rheumatoid involvement, the rheumatoid factor is absent in HPOA. Perhaps the most characteristic finding is the dramatic symptom relief that may occur within hours of primary tumor resection (28).

Muscle and Skin

A wide spectrum of skin, muscle, and connective tissue manifestations are associated with previous, current, or as yet undiagnosed malignancy. These may be secondary to direct or metastatic involvement or due to a paraneoplastic effect. Adenocarcinoma of bronchial origin has been discovered as a mass of the calf (35). Previously undiagnosed renal carcinoma has been reported as a large, growing vascular mass of the biceps muscle (7). Metastatic soft tissue or muscle masses can occur and have been reported in any anatomic area. These may produce pain and affect function due to compression of muscle or to nerve invasion. These masses may occasionally be small, deep-seated, and not readily detectable. Therefore, they may be overlooked and treated inappropriately (36).

A malignancy incidence of up to 50% has been reported with dermatomyositis and polymyositis (32). These conditions may precede the malignancy by days or years. The skin manifestations when present include a purplish erythema. The predominant clinical complaint is a progressive proximal muscular weakness developing over weeks to months. Muscle biopsy, elevated erythrocyte sedimentation rate and muscle enzymes, and abnormal electromyogram (EMG) all play a role in the diagnosis. This syndrome, more common in men, is often labeled carcinomatous myopathy or neuromyopathy due to the diminished to absent deep tendon reflexes. The predominant associated malignancies are lung and gastric cancer.

Acanthosis nigricans, a hyperpigmented, hyperkeratotic skin lesion in intertriginous or flexor areas of axillary, neck, or anogenital areas is often associated with gastric carcinoma or other abdominal malignancies.

Asymmetric shoulder girdle and arm pain may occasionally present as a structural problem simulating cervical nerve root irritation or brachial plexopathy, as in thoracic outlet syndrome. This may be seen in lung cancer with apical involvement and brachial plexus compression by a superior sulcus (Pancoast) tumor.

Occult Malignancy Presenting with Musculoskeletal Symptoms

Children

Cancer in children is more insidious than in adults and may mimic musculoskeletal disease, developmental processes, or childhood psychological problems (37). Occult cancer in children presenting with musculoskeletal symptoms is an especially poignant example of why a high index of suspicion should be triggered when a child presents with disproportionate pain levels or an "atypical" pattern of arthritis that is not characteristic of a specific rheumatic disease. Although underlying neoplasm is found in less than 1% of such patients complaining of musculoskeletal symptoms (39), cancer kills more children than any other disease (37).

In 10 of 1,254 such children, there were 6 acute lymphoblastic leukemia; 2 lymphomas; 1 Ewing sarcoma; and 1 neuroblastoma (38). In a retrospective survey of 29 children ultimately diagnosed with malignancy and referred to a pediatric rheumatology clinic, provisional diagnoses included:

juvenile rheumatoid arthritis (12 children);
nonspecific connective tissue disease (4 children);
discitis (3 children);
spondyloarthropathy (3 children);
systemic lupus erythematosus (2 children);
Kawasaki disease (2 children); and
Lyme disease, mixed connective tissue disease, and dermatomyositis (1 child each) (39).

The final diagnoses were 13 cases of leukemia; 6 neuroblastoma; 3 lymphoma; 3 Ewing sarcoma; and 1 each of ependymoma, thalamic glioma, epithelioma, and sarcoma. The children, between the ages of 1 to 15 years (19 boys and 10 girls), had symptoms or signs of musculoskeletal pain (82%); fever (54%); fatigue (50%); weight loss (42%); hepatomegaly (29%); and arthritis (25%). Features that suggested malignancy included nonarticular "bone" pain (68%); back pain (32%); bone tenderness (29%); severe constitutional symptoms (32%); and features "atypical" of most rheumatic diseases (48%). The "atypical" features were considered to be night sweats (14%); ecchymoses and bruising (14%); abnormal neurologic signs (10%); abnormal masses (7%); and ptosis (3%).

Adults

Malignant neoplasms in the adult are associated with a wide variety of paraneoplastic hematologic syndromes. The most frequently recognized are hypertrophic osteoarthropathy, carcinomatous polyarthritis, dermatomyositis/polymyositis, and paraneoplastic vasculitis (40). Lesser-known associations are fasciitis, panniculitis, erythema nodosum, Raynaud phenomenon, digital gangrene, erythromelalgia, and lupuslike syndromes (40).

Paraneoplastic musculoskeletal manifestations of malignancy may coincide, follow, or antedate the diagnosis of cancer or herald its recurrence. The clinical course parallels that of the primary tumor, and treatment of the underlying malignancy often results in the regression of the rheumatic disorder. Rheumatic manifestations suggesting a hidden cancer include: rapid onset of an unusual inflammatory arthritis; clubbing or diffuse bone pain in a patient 50 years or older; chronic unexplained vasculitis; refractory fasciitis; Raynaud syndrome unresponsive to vasodilator therapy; rapidly progressing digital gangrene; or Lambert-Eaton myasthenic syndrome (40). Management of paraneoplastic rheumatic syndromes consists in control of the underlying cancer; symptomatic treatment of the rheumatic syndrome with a nonsteroidal antiinflammatory disease modifier, cyclo-oxygenase-2 inhibitor, or glucocorticoid; and appropriate osteopathic muscle energy and manipulative techniques.

Central Nervous System

Although the CNS is a composite of both brain and spinal cord, only those manifestations related to the brain will be discussed here. This will include malignant disease involvement of the brain and those manifestations associated with primary malignancy that give rise to CNS symptoms without a direct metastatic relationship.

Direct Cerebral Malignancy

Malignant disease may occur in the brain either as a primary tumor or as metastasis from an extracranial primary site. The symptoms noted are referable to the region of the brain involved. Of the extracranial tumors that often spread to the brain, the most common are lung and breast. Autopsy studies have shown that of all cerebral metastasis, approximately 65% are multiple in occurrence (41), thus the rationale for utilizing whole brain irradiation as therapy rather than surgery. Surgical therapy is limited to selected situations (true solitary lesions) in metastatic brain disease. In most circumstances, adequate control of symptoms, as well as maintenance of CNS function, will be attained with whole brain irradiation until the primary disease progresses.

Indirect Paraneoplastic

Various syndromes have been described that may indirectly affect the CNS. These syndromes affect the CNS less often than the peripheral nervous system (42). One of the most common syndromes is subacute cerebellar degeneration. This manifests as a progressive symmetric disabling cerebellar failure and clinically includes ataxia and dysarthria (43). Other cerebellar features may also occur. Dementia is often associated with the cerebellar degeneration. There is generally progressive clinical deterioration with an occasional report of clinical improvement with removal of the primary tumor (42). The most frequent malignancies associated with subacute cerebellar degeneration are lung, prostate, and colorectal cancer. Other dementia syndromes can also occur and are often associated with hematologic malignancies (progressive multifocal leukoencephalopathy).

A number of endocrinologic manifestations of malignancy occur in which there are indirect CNS signs. These are not a result of metastasis, but due to polypeptide hormonelike substances or cytokines produced by the primary tumor. These hormones are autonomous in their production and not regulated by normal hormonal feedback control. The three most frequent of these syndromes are Cushing syndrome, SIADH, and nonmetastatic hypercalcemia.

The ectopic ACTH syndrome (Cushing syndrome) is most commonly associated with lung cancer, especially small cell (oat cell) lung cancer. In small cell cancer of the lung, 25% of patients have either the clinical syndrome or significant elevations of ectopic-produced ACTH (32). Clinical manifestation is by signs of corticoid excess, which include muscle weakness, hypokalemia, edema, hyperglycemia, hypertension, and neurologic syndromes of altered mental status. The same syndrome may occur in other tumors as well. The most effective therapy is treatment of the primary tumor.

The syndrome of inappropriate antidiuretic hormone also occurs most commonly in lung cancer, especially the small cell variety with 8% to 10% of these patients having the clinically evident syndrome (32). The hormone arginine vasopressin (AVP) is produced in high quantities by the tumor. The major laboratory features are hyponatremia, reduced serum osmolality, and increased urine osmolality relative to serum. The significant clinical symptoms include altered mentation, confusion, lethargy, psychosis, seizures, and coma. This may mimic a primary CNS tumor.

Hypercalcemia is the most frequent metabolic complication associated with malignancy. It occurs commonly with breast, lung, renal carcinomas, head/neck cancers, and multiple myeloma. This entity occurs in approximately 10% of all patients with cancer. Approximately 15% to 20% of this group of patients will not have evidence of bone metastasis (32). Hypercalcemia associated with breast carcinoma and multiple myeloma is usually secondary to bone metastasis with calcium release from bone into the serum. Lung cancer, especially of the epidermoid and large cell varieties, and kidney cancer are most frequently associated with nonmetastatic hypercalcemia. Both of these tumors account for over 50% of the cases of tumor produced PTHrP. It is not unusual for either of these tumors to present clinically with symptoms due to hypercalcemia before a diagnosis of malignancy has been made or suspected. The major clinical signs and symptoms of hypercalcemia occur with serum calcium levels in excess of 14 microfarad (μF) per dL. Serum calcium levels measured as ionized calcium or total calcium must be adjusted by formula based on serum albumin levels. It is only the ionizable (free or unbound) portion that is clinically significant.

The clinical effects of hypercalcemia are predominant on four systems. The GI system effects include nausea, emesis, anorexia, and constipation. The renal manifestations are polyuria, and polydipsia, with a late effect of nephrocalcinosis. Cardiovascular effects include significant echocardiographic alterations, arrhythmias, hypertension, and a marked increase in digitalis sensitivity. The neurologic effects, which not uncommonly resemble metastatic CNS disease, include depression, lethargy, hyporeflexia, progressive stupor and eventual coma, and possibly death. Treatment should begin promptly and include intravenous hydration and avoidance of calcium administration. Selected use of drugs includes osteoclast inhibitors such as mithramycin, calcitonin, and bisphophonates. In addition, definitive treatment of the primary tumor by surgical resection, radiation, or chemotherapy is essential.

Peripheral Nervous System

This section will discuss the direct and remote effects of the malignant process from the standpoint of symptoms related to peripheral motor or sensory nerve involvement in the extremities. Although it is acknowledged that many of these problems have their origin within the CNS, oftentimes the end effects manifest themselves peripherally in the extremities. Therefore, these considerations will occur from the point of signs and symptoms rather than origin.

Remote Peripheral Manifestations

Peripheral neurologic problems are common in many patients with cancer. The most frequent etiology of these problems is direct invasion by primary or metastatic tumor. However, neuropathic symptoms (carcinomatous neuropathy) due to remote effects of the malignancy on the peripheral nervous system can occur but are quite uncommon. Therefore, in addition to the discussion of the myasthenic syndrome and sensory motor polyneuropathy, this section will describe spinal cord disease with nerve root and plexus involvement.

Myasthenic syndrome, also known as Eaton-Lambert syndrome, is especially associated with small cell lung carcinoma. This disorder is characterized by proximal pelvic girdle muscle weakness. Other muscle symptoms may occur and other tumors may be associated. This syndrome is unlike myasthenia gravis in that the EMG muscle potential and clinical strength improve with repeated stimulation or with exercise (44,45). The Tensilon test (diagnostic for myasthenia gravis by instant relief of muscle weakness after Tensilon administration) is not responsive as it is with myasthenia gravis. Treatment of this disorder rests essentially with treatment of the primary malignancy (small cell lung cancer with chemotherapy).

Mixed sensory-motor polyneuropathy is most commonly seen associated with malignancy. This entity is most often seen with lung, breast, and GI malignancy (46). The involvement produces distal extremity muscle weakness and wasting of muscles associated with distal sensory loss and areflexia. EMG studies have shown denervation of muscle and slowed nerve conduction time, while, histologically, axonal degeneration and demyelination are noted (42). Recovery appears to be rare.

Spinal Cord Compression

Epidural metastasis and spinal cord compression occurs in 5% to 10% of patients with cancer (47). The vertebrae are the most common sites of bone metastasis, which may lead to vertebral collapse and compressive involvement of the spinal cord and nerves. This subject is of importance because of the frequency with which it occurs and the devastating effects that result if the signs and symptoms are not recognized in time to intervene. It is common for patients with vertebral metastasis to present to emergency rooms or primary care physicians with low back pain and have this approached as a structural or somatic problem. It is of ultimate importance that spinal cord compression, which is a true oncologic emergency, be considered clinically and evaluated carefully. Of course, certain signs may exist which should direct one's attention to this consideration. These include age over 50 years, recent weight loss, presence of lymphadenopathy, pain nonresponsive to previous treatment measures, and neurologic deficits in a patient with a history of malignancy (47). Constans and colleagues report on a review of 600 cases of spinal metastases with neurologic manifestations and note that 53% had thoracic spine localization, 32% lumbosacral spine localization, and 15% cervical spine localization (48). Therefore, it appears appropriate to recommend radiographic evaluation for patients with thoracic back pain without a known etiology. This recommendation however does not apply to patients with lower back discomfort, the most common back pain complaint seen by primary care physicians. In Constans' review, the most common primary tumor in men was in the lung (19.17%), and in women was in the breast (53.31%) (48).

Tumor metastasis to the vertebrae occurs most commonly due to a system of valveless, small veins known as the Batson plexus. These are richly connected to other venous systems with the pelvic, retroperitoneal, extraabdominal, and thoracic areas allowing freedom of movement of tumor cells to implant and metastasize within the spine. However, blood flow alone does not account for the osteotropism of some tumors—notably prostate and breast cancers.

The primary presenting symptom of spinal cord compression is back pain, which in most cases is localized to the involved area of vertebral damage. In reported series in which radiographic and surgical findings are noted, osteolytic lesions are usually present (71%), with osteoblastic lesions in 21% and mixed lytic-blastic lesions in 8% (48). The back pain may have been present for days to weeks or longer and seldom, by itself, is it a major reason to seek attention. The progression of symptoms to motor weakness, numbness (sensory loss), and finally bladder or rectal dysfunction (autonomic loss) will create concern for the patient. The entire process may have a variable rate of progression. The significant pathophysiologic process is related to spinal cord and nerve infarction due to arterial or venous occlusion by the compression process.

As the progression of neural compression occurs, the symptom focus shifts from that of back pain to localization of neurologic symptoms in the extremities with pain, weakness, or numbness. Radiculopathy, identified by pain referred from the primary spinal site, dermatomal sensory changes, and altered deep tendon reflexes, is common, especially in the lower extremities. This process may be bilateral or unilateral. If bilateral, it is not unusual for one side to progress more rapidly than the other side. Occasionally, an entire nerve plexus (cervical or lumbar plexopathy) may be involved, producing pain or aching in a single extremity only, without a dermatomal pattern.

The anatomic site of the radiculopathy or plexopathy may be determined by the primary tumor. Most cervical spinal cord compression is noted with lung cancer (40%), followed by breast cancer. Brachial plexus involvement occurs most often in association with lung cancer. Apical or superior sulcus tumors of the lung commonly predispose to brachial plexopathy resulting in arm and hand symptoms of pain, swelling, and loss of function.

Lumbar plexopathy is most often associated with pelvic tumors, especially colorectal cancer and sarcomas (49). The symptom complex presented is generally the same as with spinal cord compression, with pain the first and predominant symptom. The pain is radicular in approximately 85% of cases (49). Plexopathy in the lumbar area can also present as unilateral or bilateral lower extremity symptoms. Specific areas of paresis, paresthesia, or pain can help to localize tumor involvement to a specific portion of the plexus.

Diagnostic tests beyond the plain x-ray film are needed to localize the tumor and plan therapy. MRI is the modality of choice in spinal cord compression and can often provide the necessary information for treatment planning. When suspicion exists for spinal cord or plexus compression, diagnostic imaging studies should be done quickly.

Treatment is initiated for suspected spinal cord compression with corticosteroids such as high-dose dexamethasone. It is administered as soon as the diagnosis is suspected and before diagnostic studies are completed. The beneficial effect of steroids may be only short term and may result in pain relief by relieving inflammatory edema. Steroid administration is usually continued through the immediate therapy period and then tapered. Definitive therapy requires surgical laminectomy and/or radiotherapy. Surgery is preferred in radioresistant tumors (renal carcinoma) or in cases of tumor recurrence after previous radiation. Thus far, most radiation results are comparable to surgical results. The responses are variable and must be judged by the degree of symptoms and neurologic deficit with which the patient presents at diagnosis. Most patients with significant paresis or paraplegia at diagnosis will not regain neurologic function. Patients who maintain neurologic function at diagnosis will generally retain function after therapy. Spinal cord compression must be considered in any cancer patient with back pain and/or lower extremity symptoms.

Other Causes of Peripheral Neuropathy

Other phenomena may produce peripheral neuropathy with direct tumor or paraneoplastic involvement. Neurotoxic chemotherapy (Vinca alkaloids, cisplatin, taxanes) may produce paresthesia, muscle weakness, and hyporeflexia. Other neuropathic effects have been reported such as neuronal deposition of amyloid in multiple myeloma, or hemorrhage into nerves in leukemia.

In conclusion, it is not uncommon for malignant tumors to present at onset or through the course of disease progression with neurologic, muscular, or skeletal symptomatology. Often the symptoms may mimic osteopathic musculoskeletal lesions with or without accompanying neurologic components. An overview of many of the most frequently encountered central or peripheral neurologic and musculoskeletal findings has been presented here.

A Possible Viscerosomatic-Type Oncologic Response

Tumor Necrosis Factor (Cachectin)

A variety of cytokines can act as immune system modulators and have been shown *in vitro* and *in vivo* to have antitumor effects.

These include the interleukins, interferons, and tumor necrosis factor (TNF). TNF can serve as an example of a potential viscerosomatic antineoplastic response. TNF is a polypeptide hormone secreted principally by macrophages (50). This substance is produced in the body in response to various stimuli including neoplasms and infection. After attack of an organ or system it is speculated that the body responds in a self-protective manner by signal between cells involved in immunity and inflammation (51). Multiple biologic responses may occur which may be either beneficial or harmful to the body. The responses are dependent on the level of TNF released, the duration of the exposure, and other factors (52). It is believed that excessive production and exposure associated with infection may lead to tissue destruction and endotoxic shock (52). Cachexia, frequently associated with malignancy, infection, and other processes, is believed to be secondary to TNF, hence the name cachectin. Antineoplastic activity of TNF has been noted against a wide variety of tumors (53). The cytolytic effect of TNF is directed toward tumor cells but not on normal cells (50). The mechanism of action may be related to a direct cellular attack as well as an indirect attack through tumor vascular damage (53). In addition to the antitumor effects noted, TNF may also exert mitogenic properties as well as inflammatory properties such as fever induction. TNF appears to be a prime mediator of the immune system interacting with immune responses, such as enhanced cytolysis when combined with interferon, enhanced macrophage and neutrophil function, activation of T cells, and control of some leukocyte precursor differentiation (50). In addition, evidence now exists that TNF has antibacterial and antiviral properties.

Cytokines create potential treatment opportunities. Combinations with immune modulators, or even chemotherapeutic agents, are being attempted for possible enhanced synergistic response (52). Burgess and colleagues report an increased antitumor activity against renal cell carcinoma metastasis in an animal model by combining recombinant human TNF plus VP-16 chemotherapy (53).

TNF represents an excellent model in oncology of a somatic response to stimulation of a viscera or organ system by invasion of tumor or infection. The response provides evidence for the self-regulatory and self-protective healing capacity of the somatic structure.

ETHICS OF PRESENTATION OF DIAGNOSTIC AND TREATMENT OPTIONS TO THE PATIENT

When discussing the finding of malignancy or the effectiveness of treatment, the cardinal rule must always be to tell the truth. A patient must never be deceived. It may not be unusual that protective family members or a spouse will request that the patient not be informed of the presence of malignancy, but it is often themselves that these families are protecting since the patient usually does far better in accepting information. When a patient asks a question they must be answered truthfully. However, additional information need not be offered all at one time unless requested. Patients handle information better when it is given over time, rather than all at one time. Patients and families need truth and honesty and should always be left with optimism.

Optimism may not always relate to effectiveness of treatment or longevity, but must offer assurance of comfort, symptom control, and lack of physician abandonment if no further disease treatment is available. Therefore, the physician must

1. Tell the truth, never lie.
2. Remember that all of the truths are not necessary unless asked specifically.
3. Offer optimism and reassurance.

Relating the diagnosis of cancer to the patient and discussing the disease, prognosis, and diagnostic and treatment options must be done with knowledge and understanding of the perceptions of the patient. This aspect of patient care is extremely significant. As an osteopathic physician, one has a distinct advantage in these discussions because of the osteopathic philosophy of treating the *whole patient* rather than only the disease. Most patients continue to perceive a future with cancer as a short, lonely, painful, and helpless prospect. The initial discussion with the patient may be by the oncologist or the primary care physician. The philosophy used when presenting a cancer diagnosis to the patient and family is based on hope, realistic goal setting, honesty, integrity, and the knowledge that the individual is more than their disease.

It is important to inform the patient and family that the diagnosis is malignancy or cancer. Use of the term tumor should be avoided, as it is often confusing and may be deceiving. The patient should be asked whether or not to include their spouse or family in the initial discussion. In most instances, a strong suspicion already exists and the patient may prefer support from spouse or family. It is important to sit with the patient and discuss the diagnosis in a supportive, unhurried fashion. The understanding and support offered at this time will set the tone and pattern for the remainder of the treatment relationship with the patient. A fully informed, trusting, and cooperative patient will, in most cases, remain cooperative and trusting.

After informing the patient about the diagnosis, a distinction should be made for the patient about cure of disease and control of disease based on realistic expectations of what is possible. Patients and families need an opportunity to think, ask questions, discuss, and express feelings. They may feel abandoned if they are hurried through a brief one-sided discussion, informed they will be referred to an oncologist, and sent on their way before they can ask a question. The physician should ask the patient and their family what they have been told before beginning a discussion. Speak in lay language no matter what the educational level of the patient. Stress that something positive can be done for the patient. The greatest fear of the patient is that they will be told there is nothing that can be done. Even in the case of a medically untreatable cancer, the patient can be given hope of support, comfort, and caring. A supportive attitude is sometimes difficult for the patient to accept from a family member, therefore, this attitude must be conveyed from the physician. If surgery, radiation, or chemotherapy is available and to be offered, the patient is informed, but always with the knowledge that general supportive care will be available at the same time if needed. In the event of metastatic disease that cannot be cured, stress the potential long-term control of the chemotherapy or radiation to be utilized. Indicate that the purpose of the systemic therapy is to at least stabilize the disease at present levels and prevent further growth or spread, if not shrink disease. Throughout the entire interaction, an atmosphere is to be created of concern for the *whole patient* rather than only interest in the disease. The patient is to be cared for while the disease is attacked. Throughout the course of the conversation, do not hesitate to hold the patient's hand, arm, or shoulder or to pat their hand or arm. Patients and families have indicated that this seems to convey even more sincerity in caring about the *whole patient* than any level of discussion.

Often when discussing therapy, especially chemotherapy, a patient may be very resistant to discuss treatment options due to previous unfounded "horror stories." It is appropriate to be aggressive in encouraging chemotherapy when it has a known good outcome in a particular malignancy and the likelihood is high of a beneficial effect. Otherwise, therapy, including investigational or cooperative group protocols, can be offered in an objective manner while informing the patient of all benefit and risk potentials. If the patient is strongly opposed to the uncertain benefit of a treatment program, reassure the patient and allay any guilt. This can be done by informing the patient, and especially the family that, in many malignancies, there is no definite right or wrong therapy. This is the reason investigational treatment protocols are available. The right choice is the choice that leaves the patient and family comfortable with their decision and does not create conflict between patient and family, especially in the later phases of the disease process. The physician must support the patient's choices, unless proven benefit is being deprived by the choice made by the patient. This may not apply at the time of initial discussion and therapy presentation, but later when searching for a subsequent therapy or when choosing to discontinue an ineffective or toxic therapy. The support by the physician of the patient's choices reaffirms the care and importance of the patient in the total treatment of the disease. The patient's needs must be met.

Discussion of prognosis is generally avoided at the initial consultation with the patient. Address this question by a statement indicating the need to wait to observe the response of the planned treatment. The presence or absence of a response and type of response will influence and may change prognosis.

Often during the initial presentation, it is helpful to sit beside or across from the patient, without a desk in the middle, or at the side of the hospital bed. Closeness to the patient, body language, and verbal communication consistent with empathic discussion of support and concern, and the agreement to work as a partner in treating the patient, all help to create an integral relationship between patient and physician. The key element throughout the entire future relationship with a patient must be the treatment of the *whole patient* rather than a diseased organ. The patient must know that throughout the course of the disease and treatment, the less that can be done for the disease, the more will be done for the patient.

At the initial consultation or at subsequent visits after discussion of response or suggested changes in treatment protocol, the patient will often have a desire to take the physician's hand or embrace the physician in gratitude. One may participate in this gesture with the patient.

Patients who have been treated with the holistic philosophy discussed have been observed to have improved longevity and function over comparable patients who have been treated with only an objective, rigid, scientific philosophy of an investigational study without personalization.

SUPPORTIVE CARE OF THE PATIENT WITH CANCER

The supportive care that the patient may require at certain times during their illness carries an equal weight to the specific antineoplastic therapy used. In the event of a patient who declines specific antitumor therapy or who terminates such therapy after a trial, supportive care becomes of paramount importance during the patient's remaining life with the disease.

Supportive care consists predominantly of three categories: symptom control and pain relief, blood and blood products, and general supportive medical care. The latter category includes infection prevention and treatment, nutrition support, and rehabilitative support and may also include psychosocial, legal, and pastoral care support, all of which are components of hospice care.

The discussion on medical management of pain control, use of blood and its products, nutrition, and infection therapy will be limited here. These subjects are well reviewed and documented in the medical literature. Rather, these subjects will be reviewed from the philosophic viewpoint of a medical oncologist with an osteopathic background and experience.

Symptom and Pain Relief

Symptoms other than pain and discomfort are important to address for the cancer patient. Anxiety and apprehension may be addressed by spending time in discussion with the physician, social worker, nurse, psychiatrist, or psychologist. Simple treatment program adjustments may be made to correct the symptom. Pain should always be treated. This seems the least a physician can do for a patient, especially if cure of disease is not possible. The patient must not be forsaken in favor of the disease process. A large number of traditional modalities are available to treat pain including analgesics and various delivery methods to improve effectiveness (intrathecal or intraventricular injections, continuous infusion pumps, self-delivery pumps, etc.). In addition, neurosurgical procedures such as cordotomy and rhizotomy are available as well as anesthetic blocks. However, although no scientific data are yet available, another modality is also useful in selected patients to alleviate anxiety and pain symptoms. Simple, gentle, soft tissue manipulation without any pressure or thrust can be effective, especially in late stage, inactive, and bed-bound patients. The procedure permits the physician to touch the patient and commit time to care for the patient in addition to the disease.

Blood and Blood Products

Red blood cell transfusions to correct anemia, granulocyte transfusions during prolonged suppression in sepsis, and platelet transfusions to prevent bleeding during bone marrow suppression, are all supportive measures that are occasionally needed. These may be needed during periods of disease complications or during toxicity from systemic therapy. This support is often lifesaving. However, continued support with expensive or scarce blood products must be balanced with the benefit to be attained in end-stage patients in the terminal phase of the disease process.

General Supportive Care

Nutritional support of the patient with malignancy is essential whether the patient is actively being treated or not. Malnutrition is part of a general failure-to-thrive syndrome commonly associated with cancer. The patient may need other supportive care such as antibiotics, blood products, and psychosocial support in order to assist with nutrition. In addition, nutritional counseling with a dietician may be helpful as well as nutritional supplements, which are available as commercial products for high-protein enteral support. Total parenteral nutrition administered through percutaneous or surgically placed venous access may also be used for hospitalized patients for whom the enteral approach is not possible due to small intestinal or other specific circumstances.

Anti-infective therapy may be lifesaving during periods of increased risk, such as granulocytopenia after chemotherapy. It may also be provided as combination antibiotic therapy to treat documented infection, sepsis, or fever during granulocytopenia. Specific antimicrobial therapy is guided by culture and sensitivity results.

Mobility and bowel or bladder functions are areas of general supportive care not only for the patient with cancer but also for any geriatric patient or patient who is critically ill. All patients can be encouraged to be mobilized out of bed as much as possible. A positive attitude on the part of the patient can be maintained to a greater degree with increased mobility. This may lessen stress and anxiety and even support the immune system in its attack on the disease. In addition, mobilization enhances venous blood return and reduces the risk of venous thrombosis, decubitus ulceration, edema, and constipation. Many patients with cancer have prolonged periods of bed rest due to bone pain, pathologic fracture, or paraplegia due to spinal cord compressive disease. In these patients, mobilization is essential to maintain even minimal functional ability. If assisted ambulation is possible, it should be encouraged. If ambulation is impossible due to pain, fracture, weakness, or neurologic deficit, sitting in a chair may be possible. For the totally bed-bound patient, side-to-side moving with mild soft tissue manipulation can be offered.

Bowel function can be maintained with appropriate hydration, nutrition, and activity. Stool softeners and other medications or maneuvers such as manual (suppository or digital) stimulation can be used. Constipation can provide significant discomfort to an immobile patient especially one with bone pain or fracture.

Bladder function and control is also essential for patients confined to bed. If incontinence is present, an indwelling catheter can be useful. However, every attempt should be made to remove the catheter and resume normal function if possible. If it is not necessary, a catheter will only keep patients in bed and inactive for prolonged periods and impair the benefits of physical activity.

Rehabilitative care is often an essential element in symptomatic and supportive management of the patient with cancer. Rehabilitation may include physical, occupational, and speech therapy. This may be indicated after management of spinal cord compression syndrome, cerebral metastasis, and head and neck malignancies. Often rehabilitative care assists with functional palliation in patients who may have 6 or more months of life expectancy.

Hospice care is becoming widely recognized and used as an effective modality in the care of terminally ill persons. Hospice focuses on meeting the needs of the patient and the family after effective therapy for the disease is no longer available. The hospice philosophy is focused on effective pain and symptom management while also meeting other physical, social, emotional, and spiritual needs with the aid of a multidisciplinary team of specialists in each area. The patient is maintained in an environment of warmth and caring with family, in the home, except when this is not possible or is unavailable. Dealing with pain and preparation for death is very difficult or impossible for some physicians and represents a deficiency in medical training. Hospice meets this need, so death can be accepted as a natural phase of life.

STRESS OF DISEASE AND TREATMENT OF THE PATIENT AS MODULATORS OF BIOLOGIC RESPONSE

Psychoneurobiology refers to the interrelationship between emotions, the CNS, and somatic cellular biologic responses. There is little argument that the immune system plays a significant role in the initiation and course of malignant disease. The role of T- and B-cell lymphocytes and helper, suppressor, and natural killer (NK) cells together with interferons have all been extensively reviewed in the literature. It appears that the connection between the CNS and the systemic response to illness is often mediated by the endocrine system with the assistance of cortisol, the endogenous opiates (endorphins and enkephalins), and other steroids and hormones that can regulate some aspects of cellular biologic response (54). Nerve endings have been demonstrated within lymphoid organs (nodes and spleen). In addition, receptors have been demonstrated on the surface of lymphocytes for hormones such as ACTH (54). Thus, it is conceivable to believe that certain stresses on the human body can alter the biologic response in terms of enhanced or suppressed output or function of substances including interferon, NK cells, and so forth (55,56). One can then speculate on the effect of the cancer process, which can produce further suppression of an already suppressed immune system.

Although interesting to speculate, the concept of immunologic surveillance has not been able to be confirmed in clinical or human research definitively, particularly as applied to the effect of stressors. Stress and anxiety may lead to increased output of cortisol and catecholamines through pituitary ACTH. The cortisol then may initiate an immune suppressive response (54,57). Glaser and colleagues have demonstrated depressed interferon production by leukocytes concomitant with a reduced interferon regulation of NK activity at times of increased stress (58). The endogenous opiate polypeptides, B-endorphin, and the enkephalins have been demonstrated to enhance NK cell production and activity as well as inhibit metastasis in laboratory animals (59,60).

Although no definitive scientific evidence yet exists, it appears possible that alterations in the emotional state and spirit of the patient with cancer, assisted by the physician through optimism, support, and empathy, can result in an enhanced biologic response. Recognition and treatment of the *whole person* can produce this alteration in the patient's emotional status. The oncologist often encounters a patient with advanced metastatic disease who, without specific antitumor therapy, is able to continue to live and function while waiting for important life event to occur (i.e., a child to graduate, a marriage, the birth of a grandchild). The emotional state and the will to live seem to have the ability to affect the biologic behavior of the disease and the well being of the patient.

OSTEOPATHIC MANIPULATIVE TREATMENT FOR THE PATIENT WITH CANCER

Many osteopathic physicians have mistakenly believed that manipulative treatment is contraindicated for the patient with cancer. While this may be true for some techniques or for some patients, other techniques can be helpful for relieving pain, improving visceral function, reducing tension and stress, and improving the doctor–patient relationship through touch. This section will review the contraindications, indications, and specific techniques for OMT in the patient with cancer.

Contraindications for Osteopathic Manipulative Treatment

While OMT in general is not contraindicated (Table 32.1), treatment of the area immediately surrounding a cancer is contraindicated because of the risk of hematogenous spread. This is particularly true for the vertebral column where the Batson venous plexus, a system of valveless vessels anastomosing with brain and pelvic veins, provides a two-way route of metastasis. Therefore, OMT for the entire vertebral column is contraindicated when there is known or suspected vertebral tumor. A primary or metastatic vertebral cancer should be suspected when there is acute back pain associated with systemic symptoms such as fever, chills, night sweats, fatigue, and weight loss. Persistent back pain despite adequate treatment also raises a possibility of vertebral tumor. And, of course, back pain in a patient with another known cancer or a suspected cancer at a site that commonly metastasizes to the spinal column should raise the index of suspicion (Table 32.2).

Two types of manipulative techniques do pose some risk when used for the patient with cancer. High velocity low amplitude (HVLA) techniques have been reported to cause pathologic rib fractures in patients with osteoporosis. Presumably, these thrust

TABLE 32.1. MANIPULATIVE TECHNIQUES BEARING CONSIDERATION AND POTENTIAL CAUTION

Thrust near bone/joint cancer
Lymphatic pumps
Effleurage
Any technique in immediate vicinity of cancer

TABLE 32.2. PRIMARY MALIGNANCIES WHICH COMMONLY METASTASIZE TO THE VERTEBRAL COLUMN AND SPINAL CORD, LISTED IN DESCENDING ORDER OF FREQUENCY

Vertebrae	Spinal Cord
Breast	Lung
Prostate	Breast
Lung	Colon
Kidney	Sarcoma
Thyroid	

techniques could result in fracture of a rib or other bone weakened by primary or metastatic tumor. Therefore, HVLA technique is contraindicated for joints associated with bones that have known or possible cancer (61). Thrust technique can be safely applied to the oncology patient as long as metastasis to the area being considered for treatment has been ruled out by MRI, CT scan, or bone scan. Other techniques, such as muscle energy or indirect techniques, can be safely applied for joint somatic dysfunction even when there is documented bony involvement, as long as there is no direct extension of tumor into the area being treated.

Other potentially risky techniques for patients with known or suspected cancer are lymphatic pumps and effleurage. Since one route of metastasis is lymphogenous spread, these techniques could contribute to spread of cancer. Factors known to contribute to lymphogenous spread include passive limb exercise, prior cortisone therapy, extent of local disease, and lymphatic invasion and obstruction (62–64). This potential for lymphatic metastasis appears to be due to normal lymphatic transport of cells and lymph node efficiency at filtering and disseminating such cells (65–67). While lymphatic pumps have never been demonstrated to increase lymphatic transport, their purported mechanism suggests a potential contribution to lymphogenous spread of cancer cells. Tissue massage has been demonstrated to stimulate lymph transport and to reduce lymphedema (68,69).

Conversely, there is increasing evidence that physical exercise can reduce risk for breast and colon cancers (70–75). While the mechanism for this decrease in cancer risk with exercise is uncertain, there is some support for a hypothesis that moderate exercise improves immune function (76). A short-term enhancement of antibody response has also been demonstrated for lymphatic pumps (77–80). Soft tissue massage has been shown to increase NK cell number in human immunodeficiency virus (HIV)-positive patients (81,82). Massage has also been shown to reduce pain and anxiety in cancer patients (83–87).

The balance of evidence cited here suggests that lymphatic pumps and effleurage should be applied with caution in patients with cancer. Passive lymphatic treatment can be substituted for active lymphatic pumps and effleurage when lymphatic metastasis is a concern. Myofascial techniques for the thoracic inlet and abdominal diaphragm as well as pectoral traction can be safely applied in patients with cancer with pneumonia, lymphedema, or other problems for which a lymphatic pump or effleurage might have otherwise been considered (88,89). Soft tissue techniques other than effleurage (see Chapter 56) may be helpful in reducing pain and anxiety in patients with cancer when not applied in proximity to tumor sites.

INDICATIONS FOR OSTEOPATHIC MANIPULATIVE TREATMENT IN THE ONCOLOGY PATIENT

OMT, if judiciously applied, can be a very valuable tool for the care of oncology patients, who have the same potential for noncancerous somatic dysfunction and pain as anyone else but with more psychosocial stress (Table 32.3). In addition, the patient with cancer may be saddled with postsurgical pain as well as cancer pain. Furthermore, the terminally ill patient may have immobility-related visceral dysfunction amenable to OMT.

For patients with known cancer, the primary indication for OMT is musculoskeletal pain associated with somatic dysfunction but not directly related to the tumor. The somatic dysfunction can be unrelated to or secondary to the cancer or its treatment. For instance, a patient who underwent median sternotomy and resection of a lung cancer may develop thoracic and intercostal pain from a preexisting somatic dysfunction made worse by the surgery, a viscerosomatic reflex from the lung to the thoracic spine, or surgical trauma to the costovertebral or costochondral joints. The choice of techniques for treating somatic dysfunction in the patient with cancer and musculoskeletal pain is highly individualized and depends on age, severity of illness, previous injuries, other diseases, and time since surgery. In general, indirect methods, such as myofascial release and counterstrain techniques, are more applicable when there is acute or severe illness, and with advancing age. Direct methods such as thrust and muscle energy should be reserved for the stable patient and when metastasis to the area being treated has been definitively ruled out.

OMT is also indicated for prevention or treatment of immobility-related complications in the bedridden patient who is terminally ill with cancer. Prolonged immobility can cause atelectasis predisposing to pneumonia or constipation, which may already be present as a side effect of narcotic analgesics. To prevent and treat atelectasis or constipation, thoracolumbar soft tissue and rib-raising treatment can be applied daily, in many cases by family members instructed to do these techniques at home. The initiation of rib raising should be preceded by treatment of significant vertebral and rib somatic dysfunction to prevent exacerbation of visceral facilitation.

Extremity lymphedema with swelling and pain, especially common after radical mastectomy for breast cancer, can be helped by OMT. Initially, the fascial diaphragms are treated to reduce tension around proximal lymphatic vessels, thereby facilitating lymph drainage from the extremity. If the cancer is cured or the risk for lymphogenous metastasis is insignificant, effleurage to the involved extremity or a lymphatic pump can be applied immediately following diaphragm treatment. If helpful, effleurage

and lymphatic pumps can be taught to a family member to be applied once or twice a day for lymphedema.

Pain, immobility and its consequences, and postsurgical lymphedema are common problems in patients with cancer that can be readily treated with OMT. An additional benefit of treatment is an improved sense of well being which many patients report. It is entirely possible that this period of well being is due to enhancement of the immune system with elevated output of cellular immune substances, NK cells, or endogenous opiates. It has been demonstrated that prognosis may be predicted in patients with breast cancer by the sustained level of NK cell activity (90). A future study to measure serum and CSF levels of various immune substances in response to OMT would be an invaluable addition to the osteopathic literature.

COMPLEMENTARY AND ALTERNATIVE MEDICINE IN ONCOLOGY

Although little objective research has yet been accomplished in the use of alternatives in cancer treatment a number of modalities have been used anecdotally for discomfort or symptom control and general immune enhancement. These include acupuncture and static magnets for control of discomfort and better rest and reduced need for analgesics. Massage and other relaxation techniques may assist in stress reduction. Herbal products are often considered to enhance the immune system as well as for cancer prevention but must be used with caution, considering potential drug interactions with prescribed pharmaceuticals. Perhaps a more studied technique has been visualization or guided imagery to aid in stimulating immune response to assist with traditional chemotherapy or radiation therapy benefit.

CONCLUSION

The osteopathic physician has a special opportunity and obligation to treat the patient with cancer as a whole patient, not just a disease. Practitioners of the osteopathic approach, with its emphasis on touch and healing, can provide patients with cancer and their families with the information and support they need.

REFERENCES

1. Greenman P. The osteopathic concept in its second century. Is it still germane to specialty practice? *JAOA.* 1976;75:589–595.
2. Bean RB, Bean WB. *Sir William Osler Aphorism.* New York, NY: Henry Schuman, Inc; 1950.
3. Parker SL, Tony T, Bolder S, Wingo PA. Cancer statistics. American Cancer Society *CA-A Cancer J Clin.* 1996;46:1.
4. Cherukuri SV, Johenning PW, Ram MD. Systemic effects of hypernephroma. *Urology.* 1977;10:93–97.
5. Bellinger MF, Koontz WW, Smith MJV. Renal cell carcinoma: twenty years of experience. *VA Mod.* 1979;106:819–824.
6. Paulson DF, Perez CA, Anderson T. Genito-urinary malignancies. In: DeVita VT, Hellman S, Rosenberg SA, eds. *Cancer: Principals and Practice of Oncology.* Philadelphia, PA: JB Lippincott, 1982;23:733.
7. Chandler RW, Schulman I, Moore TM. Renal cell carcinoma presenting

TABLE 32.3. INDICATIONS FOR OSTEOPATHIC MANIPULATIVE TREATMENT IN PATIENTS WITH CANCER

Indications

Pain and somatic dysfunction
Constipation
Atelectasis
Pneumonia
Postsurgical lymphedema

as a skeletal mass: a case report. *Clin Orthop Relat Res.* 1979;145:227–229.

8. Chisolm GD. The systemic effects of malignant renal tumors. *Br J Urol.* 1971;43:687–700.

9. Richie JP, Garneck MB. Primary renal and ureteral cancer. In: Rieselbach RE, Garanick ME, eds. *Cancer and the Kidney.* Philadelphia, PA: Lea & Febiger; 1982:17:665.

10. DeVita VT, Hellman S, Rosenberg SA. *Cancer: Principles and Practice of Oncology.* Philadelphia, PA: JB Lippincott; 1993:23:673

11. DeVita VT, Hellman S, Rosenberg SA. *Cancer: Principles and Practice of Oncology.* Philadelphia, PA: JB Lippincott; 1993:24:731.

12. Downs SE. Bronchogenic carcinoma presenting as neuromusculoskeletal pain. *J Manipulative Physiol Ther.* 1990;13(4):2214.

13. Alexander RW, Upp JR, Poston GJ, et al. Effects of bombesin on growth of human small cell lung carcinoma in vivo. *Cancer Res.* 1988;314(6):375.

14. Sunday ME. Weekly clinicopathological exercises, case 5-1986. *N Engl J Med.* 1986;314(6):375.

15. Holland, JF, Frei E, Bast R, et al. *Cancer Medicine.* Philadelphia, PA: Lea & Febiger; 1993;28:1285.

16. Tula CJ, Berman L, Alexanian R. Connective tissue disease manifested as multiple myeloma. *South Med J.* 1984;77:1580–1581.

17. Hoffaan R, Benz EJ, Shattil SJ, et al. Hematology. In: *Basic Principles and Practice.* New York, NY: Churchill Livingstone; 1991:1026–1031.

18. Batson OV. The function of the vertebral veins and their role in the spread of metastases. *Ann Surg.* 1940;112(1):138–148.

19. Batson OV. The role of the vertebral veins in metastatic processes. *Ann Intern Med.* 1942;16:3845.

20. Hendrickson FR, Sheinkop MB. Management of osseous metastases. *Semin Oncol.* 1975;2:399–404.

21. Cadman E, Bertino JR. Chemotherapy of skeletal metastases. *Int J Radiat Oncol Biol Phys.* 1976;1:1211–1215.

22. Behallia KS. Metastatic disease of the spine. *Clin Orthop.* 1970;73:52–60.

23. Drew M, Dickson RB. Osseous complications of malignancy. In: Lokich JJ, ed. *Clinical Cancer Medicine: Treatment Tactics.* Boston, MA: GK Hall, 1980:97.

24. Berrettoni BA, Carter JR. Mechanisms of cancer metastasis to bone. *J Bone Joint Surg.* 1986;68-A(2):308–312.

25. Swanson DA, Bernardino ME. Silent osseous metastasis in renal cell carcinoma: value of computerized tomography. *Urology.* 1982;20(2):201–212.

26. Willis RA. *The Spread of Tumors in the Human Body,* 3rd ed. London, England: Butterworth; 1973:259–268.

27. Smalley RV. The management of disseminated breast cancer. In: Carter SK, Glatstein E., Livingston RB, eds. *Principles of Cancer Treatment.* New York, NY: McGraw-Hill; 1982:327–341.

28. Schaller J. Arthritis as a presenting manifestation of malignancy in children. *J Pediatr.* 1972;81(4)793–797.

29. Karten I, Bartfeld H. Bronchogenic carcinoma simulating early rheumatoid arthritis. *JAMA.* 1962;162:170–172.

30. Ritch, PJ, Hansen RM, Collier BD. Metastatic renal cell carcinoma presenting as shoulder arthritis. *Cancer.* 1983;51:968–972.

31. Jao JY, Barlow JJ, Krant MJ. Pulmonary hypertrophic osteoarthropathy, spider angiomata and estrogen hyperexcretion in neoplasia. *Ann Intern Med.* 1969;70:581.

32. Minna JD, Higgins GA, Glatstein EJ. Cancer of the lung. In: DeVita VT, Hellman S, Rosenberg SA, eds. *Cancer: Principles and Practice of Oncology.* Philadelphia, PA: JB Lippincott, 1982;14:396–474.

33. Schumacher H Jr. Articular manifestations of hypertrophic pulmonary osteoarthropathy in bronchogenic carcinoma. *Arthritis Rheum.* 1976;18:629–636.

34. Rooney TW. Musculoskeletal manifestations associated with malignancy. *Osteopath Ann.* 1983;11(10):437–442.

35. Alburquerque TL, Ortin A. Cacho J. Metastases in deep calf muscles as first manifestation of bronchus adenocarcinoma. *Ann J Med.* 1987;83:606–607.

36. Damron TA, Heiner J. Distant soft tissue metastases: a series of 30 new patients and 91 cases from the literature. *Ann Surg Oncol.* 2000;7(7):526–534.

37. Starling KSA, Shepherd DA. Symptoms and signs of cancer in the school age child. *J Sch Health.* 1977;47(3):144–146.

38. Trapani S, Grisolia F, Simonini G, et al. Incidence of occult cancer in children presenting with musculoskeletal symptoms: a 10-year survey in a pediatric rheumatology unit. *Semin Arthr Rheum.* 2000;29(6):348–359.

39. Cabral DA, Tucker LB. Malignancies in children who initially present with rheumatic complaints. *J Pediatr.* 1999;134(1):53–57.

40. Fam AG. Paraneoplastic rheumatic syndrome. *Best Pract Res Clin Rheumatol.* 2000;14(3):515–533.

41. Sugarbaker PH, Dunnick NR, Sugarbaker E. Diagnosis and staging. In DeVita VT, Hellman S, Rosenberg SA, eds. *Cancer: Principals and Practice of Oncology.* Philadelphia, PA: JB Lippincott, 1982;11:232.

42. Riddoch D. Neurological manifestations of cancer. *Practitioner* 1981;225:819–826.

43. Brain WR, Wilkinson M. Subacute cerebellar degeneration associated with neoplasms. *Brain.* 1965;88:465.

44. Lambert EH, Eaton LM, Rooke ED. Defect of neuromuscular condition associated with malignant neoplasms. *Am J Physiol.* 1956;187:612.

45. Lambert EH, Rooke ED. Myasthenic state and lung cancer. In: Brain WR, Norris FH Jr. eds. *The Remote Effects of Cancer on the Nervous System.* New York, NY: Grune & Stratton; 1965:67–80.

46. Croft PB, Urich H, Wilkinson M. Peripheral neuropathy of sensorimotor type associated with malignant disease. *Brain.* 1967;90:31–66.

47. Bates DW, Reuler JB. Back pain and epidural spinal cord compression. *J Gen Intern Med.* 1988;3:191–197.

48. Contans JP, de Divitiis E, Donzelli R, et al. Spinal metastasis with neurological manifestations. *J Neurosurg.* 1983;59:111–118.

49. Jaeckle KA, Young DF, Foley, KM. The natural history of lumbosacral plexopathy in cancer. *Neurology.* 1985;35:815.

50. Van Der Merwe PA. Tumor necrosis factor. *S Afr Med J.* 1988;74:411–417.

51. Abraham E. Tumor necrosis factor. *Crit Care Med.* 1989;17:590–591.

52. Tracey KJ, Vlassara H, Cerami A. Cachectin/tumor necrosis factor. *Lancet.* 1989;1:1122–1126.

53. Burgess JK, Marshall FF, Isaacs JT. Enhanced anti-tumor effects of recombinant human tumor necrosis factor plus VP-16 on metastatic renal cell carcinoma in a xenograft model. *J Urol.* 1989;142:160–164.

54. Glaser R, Kiecolt-Glaser J. Stress-associated immune suppression and acquired immune deficiency syndrome (AIDS). *Adv Biochem Psychopharmacol.* 1988;44:203–215.

55. Glaser R, Kiecolt-Glaser JF, Stout K, et al. Stress-related impairments in cellular immunity. *Psychiatry Res.* 1985;16(3):233–239.

56. Glaser R, Kiecolt-Glaser JK. Stress and immune function. *Clin Neuropharmacol.* 1986;9[Suppl 4]:485–487.

57. Southam CM. Emotions, immunology and cancer: how might the psyche influence neoplasia? *Ann NY Acad Sci.* 1969;164(2):473–475.

58. Glaser R, Rice J, Stout JC, Kiecolt-Glaser JK. Stress depresses interferon production by leukocytes concomitant with a decrease in natural killer cell activity. *Behav Neurosci.* 1986;100(5):675–678.

59. Faith RE. Inhibition of pulmonary metastasis and enhancement of natural killer cell activity by methionine-enkephalin. *Brain Behav Immun.* 1988;2:114–122.

60. Williamson SA, Knight RA, Lightman SL, Hobbs JR. Differential effects of B-endorphin fragments on human natural killing. *Brain Behav Immun.* 1987;1:329–335.

61. Kuchera WA, Kuchera ML. *Osteopathic Principles in Practice,* 2nd ed. Kirksville, MO: KCOM Press; 1992:295.

62. Schmidt JD, McLaughlin AP, Saltzstein SL, Garcia-Reyes R. Risk factors for the development of distant metastases in patients undergoing pelvic lymphadenectomy for prostatic cancer. *Am J Surg.* 1982;144(1):131–135.

63. Stoker TA. The effect of cortisone therapy and limb exercise on the dissemination of cancer via the lymphatic system. *Br J Cancer.* 1969;23(1):132–135.

64. Yamagata K, Kumagai K. Experimental study of lymphogenous peritoneal cancer dissemination: migration of fluorescent-labelled tumor cells in a rat model of mesenteric lymph vessel obstruction. *J Exp Clin Cancer Re.* 2000;19(2):211–217.

65. Gendreau KM, Whalen GF. What can we learn from the phenomenon of preferential lymph node metastasis in carcinoma? *J Surg Oncol.* 1999;70(3):199–204.

66. Sleeman JP. The lymph node as bridgehead in the metastatic dissemination of tumors. *Recent Results Cancer Res.* 2000;157:55–81.

67. Verhoeven D, Buyssens N. Macrophages and carcinoma cells migrate at the same pace to the lymph nodes. *Lymphology.* 1989;22:141–143.

68. Potapov IA, Abisheva TM. The action of massage on lymph formation and transport. *Vopr Kurortol Fizioter Lech Fiz Kult.* 1989;5:44–47.

69. Wozniewski M. Value of intermittent pneumatic massage in the treatment of upper extremity lymphedema. *Pol Tyg Lek.* 1991;46(30–31):550–552.

70. Batty D, Thune I. Does physical activity prevent cancer? *Br Med J.* 2000;321:1424–1425.

71. Carpenter CL, Ross RK, Paganini-Hill A, Bernstein L. Lifetime exercise activity and breast cancer risk among post-menopausal women. *Br J Cancer.* 1999;80(11):1852–1858.

72. Gerhardsson M, Floderus B, Norell SE. Physical activity and colon cancer risk. *Int J Epidemiol.*1988;17(4):743–746.

73. Longnecker MP, Gerhardsson M, Frumkin H, Carpenter C. A case-control study of physical activity in relation to risk of cancer of the right colon and rectum in men. *Int J Epidemiol.* 1995;24(1):42–50.

74. Marti B. Exercise and cancer: an epidemiologic short review of the effects of physical activity on carcinoma risk. *Schwiez Med Wochenschr.* 1992;122(27–28):1048–1056.

75. Thompson HJ. Effect of exercise intensity and duration on the induction of mammary carcinogenesis. *Cancer Res.* 1994;54[7 Suppl]:1960s–1963s.

76. Lee IM. Exercise and physical health: cancer and immune function. *Res Q Exercise Sport.* 1995;66(4):286–291.

77. Breithaupt T, Harris K, Ellis J, et al. Thoracic lymphatic pumping and the efficacy of influenza vaccination in healthy young and elderly populations. *JAOA.* 2001;101(1):21–25.

78. Jackson KM, Steele TF, Dugan EP, et al. Effect of lymphatic and splenic pump techniques on the antibody response to hepatitis B vaccine: a pilot study. *JAOA.* 1998;98(3):155–160.

79. Measel JW. The effect of the lymphatic pump on the immune response: I. Preliminary studies on the antibody response to pneumococcal polysaccharide assayed by bacterial agglutination and passive hemagglutination. *JAOA.* 1982;82:59–62.

80. Mesina J, Hampton D, Evans R, et al. Transient basophilia following the application of lymphatic pump techniques: a pilot study. *JAOA.* 1998;98(2):91–94.

81. Diego MA, Field T, Hernandez-Rief M, et al. HIV adolescents show improved immune function following massage therapy. *Int J Neurosci.* 2001;106(1–2):35–45.

82. Ironson G, Field T, Scafidi F, et al. Massage therapy is associated with enhancement of the immune system's cytotoxic capacity. *Int J Neurosci.* 1996;84(1–4):205–217.

83. Ferrell-Torry AT, Glick OJ. The use of therapeutic massage as a nursing intervention to modify anxiety and the perception of cancer pain. *Cancer Nurs.* 1993;16(2):93–101.

84. Grealish L, Lomasney A, Whiteman B. Foot massage: a nursing intervention to modify the distressing symptoms of pain and nausea in patients hospitalized with cancer. *Cancer Nurs.* 2000;23(3):237–243.

85. Stephenson NL, Weinrich SP, Tavakoli AS. The effects of foot reflexology on anxiety and pain in patients with breast and lung cancer. *Oncol Nurs Forum.* 2000;27(1):67–72.

86. Weinrich SP, Weinrich MC. The effect of massage on pain in cancer patients. *Appl Nurs Res.* 1990;3(4):140–145.

87. Wilkinson S, Aldridge J, Salmon I, et al. An evaluation of aromatherapy massage in palliative care. *Palliative Med.* 1999;13(5):409–417.

88. Kuchera ML, Kuchera WA. *Osteopathic Considerations in Systemic Dysfunction,* 2nd ed. Kirksville, MO: KCOM Press; 1992:28.

89. Essig-Beatty DR, Steele KM, Mann J. *Myofascial Release & Systemic Dysfunction Manual.* Lewisburg, WV: WVSOM; 2001:105.

90. Levy S, Herberman R, Lippman M, d'Angelo T. Correlation of stress factors with sustained depression of natural killer cell activity and predicted prognosis in patients with breast cancer. *J Clin Oncol.* 1987;5(3):348–353.

33

ORTHOPEDICS

RICHARD A. SCOTT
MICHAEL L. KUCHERA
JEFF J. PATTERSON

KEY CONCEPTS

- Value of orthopedic training to osteopathic physicians
- Elements of an osteopathic orthopedic examination
- Osteopathic orthopedic approach to developmental dysplasia of the hip, hip fracture in the geriatric population, osteoarthritis of the knee, low back pain, and shoulder instability
- Osteopathic approaches to ligamentous laxity and tendonosis
- Specifics of history and physical examination, pathophysiology, differential diagnosis, and management

The study of orthopedics is an integral part of osteopathic education. After residency, osteopathic orthopedic surgeons make up one of the specialty colleges in the osteopathic profession. Orthopedics is the specialty of medicine concerned with the preservation of the health and restoration of function of the skeletal system and its associated structures (i.e., spinal and other bones, joints, and muscles) (1). Orthopedic training is essential to the osteopathic physician; orthopedic knowledge extends the ramifications of somatic dysfunction into the structural and anatomic-pathologic arena. Orthopedic knowledge is vital in the differential diagnosis of patients presenting with musculoskeletal complaints; it offers unique insights into the diagnosis and treatment of traumatic and nontraumatic diseases of the musculoskeletal system. Many osteopathic orthopedic physicians specialize in sports medicine or devote a portion of their practice to this field. They have skills and a special perspective in treating the structural and functional problems arising from sports injuries. Through prevention and rehabilitation, they want to encourage maximum function within the athlete's structure.

The emblem of the orthopedic society is based on an 18th century drawing by Nicholas Andry (Fig. 33.1) that depicts a tree curved and twisted by the winds and weather, held upright by a series of ropes and splints (2). This image continues to influence the orthopedic community. By molding the growing skeleton, orthopedic physicians help a child grow into a straighter

and more functional adult. The etymology of the term orthopedics reflects this perspective as well: *ortho* means to straighten, and *pedic* refers to the pediatric population. The osteopathic orthopedic physician, with their emphasis on structure-function interrelationships, understands and respects this perspective.

The field of orthopedics has subsequently been divided into orthopedic medicine and orthopedic surgery. Beginning in the 1930s, James Cyriax, MD, a British orthopedist, applied the concept of interrelated structure and function and developed a diagnostic and treatment system that is now known as orthopedic medicine, in contradistinction to orthopedic surgery. He authored a series of original papers and the definitive text, *Textbook of Orthopedic Medicine*, which describes the importance of making a precise anatomic diagnosis based on:

- Joint range of motion patterns and their end-feel
- Referred pain patterns
- Differentiation of contractile and inert structures
- Understanding of selective tension

He also created his own system of manual techniques to be incorporated into treatment.

Until his death in 1989, Cyriax believed that the intervertebral disc was the source of almost all spinal pain. While alive, his influence and his dogmatic teaching did not allow alternative ideas to compete (3). Since his death, however, orthopedic medicine in the United States has expanded its paradigm to embrace an understanding of myofascial and ligamentous pain. The American Association of Orthopedic Medicine (AAOM) consists of MDs and DOs who find value in Cyriax's commitment to make a specific anatomic diagnosis using standardized physical examination of the somatic system and who wish to emphasize conservative management of orthopedic cases. This organization embraces the diagnosis of somatic dysfunction and uses manipulative techniques in their treatment regimens; it is also the North American representative of the international organization of fully licensed physicians interested in manual medicine. AAOM has officially adopted the Glossary of Osteopathic Terminology to maintain consistency in their discussions of diagnoses amenable to manipulation. Treatment tools in orthopedic medicine include:

- Manipulation
- Prolotherapy

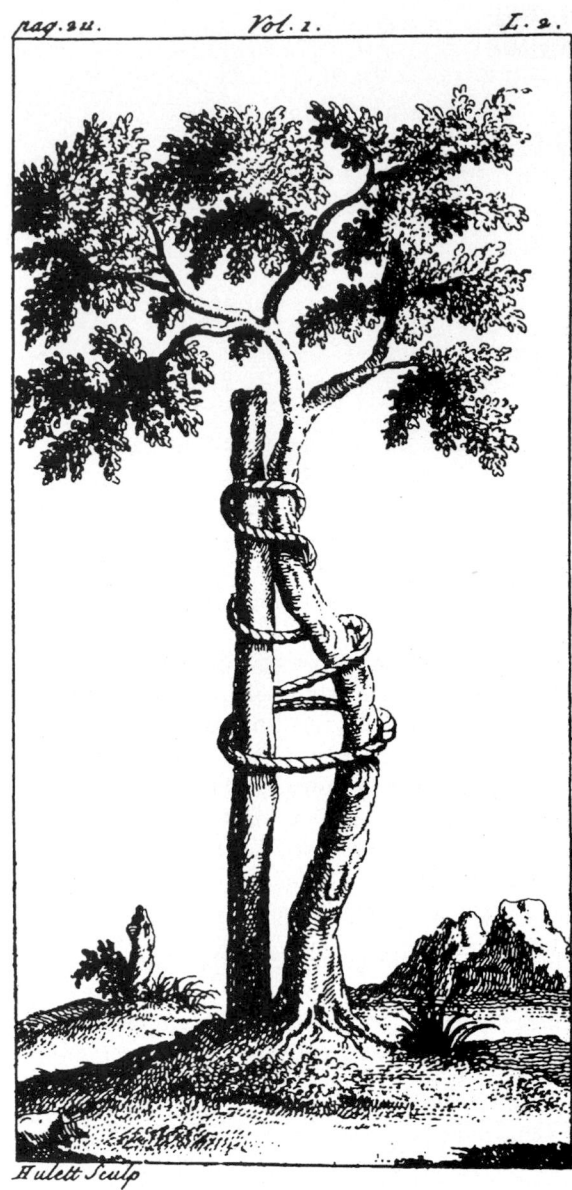

FIGURE 33.1. An important basic orthopedic principle is embodied in the figure of the tree. The bone is not an inert, calcified, fibrous material. It is a growing, plastic, dynamic structure with an active metabolism that responds to a wide variety of stimuli, and is as truly alive as any other structure in our bodies. "Just as the twig is bent, the tree's inclined," wrote Alexander Pope. (From Peltier LF. *Orthopedics: A History and Iconography.* San Francisco, CA: Norman Publishing; 1993. Art from Andry N. L'Orthopedie. Paris: La veuve Alix, 1741, with permission.)

- Trigger point therapy
- Orthotics
- Exercise prescription
- Commitment to an orthopedic perspective

Orthopedic surgery in the osteopathic profession is almost as old as the profession itself. At the American School of Osteopathy (ASO) in Kirksville, Missouri, at the beginning of the 20th century, George Laughlin, DO, was gaining acclaim as an orthopedic surgeon by applying European techniques to perform bloodless surgery on congenital hip dislocations and in other orthopedic cases. The surgical team at the ASO at this time also included Andrew Taylor Still, MD, DO, who is credited with revolutionizing the practice of surgery by osteopathy by employing osteopathic manipulative treatment (OMT) in preoperative and postoperative care (4). Research on the efficacy of the osteopathic approach for reducing postoperative surgical complications with OMT was carried out many years later by another Kirksville orthopedic surgeon, Edward Herrmann, DO (5).

The osteopathic orthopedic specialist has been influenced by adherence to the principles of osteopathic medicine. Even if most of the time in orthopedics is spent in busy mechanical pursuits, equally important moments are spent practicing as an osteopathic physician. In this sense, the orthopedist approaches patient care with a keen awareness that the orthopedic problem is but one part of an entire medical and social paradigm. It is in these moments of interaction with internists, family practitioners, and patients' family members that the orthopedist brings into play much of their osteopathic orientation. One of the goals in osteopathic orthopedics is to inculcate this attitude of wholeness in treatment, lest the specialist in training take the easy route and forget that their area of expertise is only part of the whole.

An osteopathic physician treating an orthopedic problem adjusts or modifies their approach in a manner different from that of a nonosteopathic physician. Osteopathic orthopedic surgeons are in the subsection of orthopedic surgeons who have been trained osteopathically, but they are essentially surgeons. The thought processes of surgeons, different from that of nonsurgeons and internists, involve an approach to problem solving that has an immediacy based on the need for urgent decision making. Farmer has studied the educational process and methodology used in training physicians to become surgeons and has noted differences in affect and approaches from that of general internal medicine, where the educational process has been studied more thoroughly (J.A. Farmer, unpublished work, 1992).

One of the aspects that may make orthopedics alluring today is the tremendous advance in the ability of physicians to diagnose and surgically treat and thus modify diseases and problems that, in the past, could only be watched as they progressed. What differentiates the orthopedist from other physicians and surgeons includes often lengthy technical procedures using saws, drills, and metallic implants, as well as the activities associated with fracture reduction and casting, juxtaposed to delicate repairs of tendons and nerves under magnification. Before a surgical procedure, the orthopedic surgeon performs appropriate diagnostic examinations and tests and formulates a treatment protocol. After surgery, prevention of complications, education about postoperative nutrition, and rehabilitation necessitate a wide range of physician knowledge and skill.

One aspect of orthopedics, both surgical and nonsurgical, deals with the diagnosis and treatment of traumatic and nontraumatic diseases of the musculoskeletal system. Many health professionals address these issues today. Who should examine and who should treat the injured or aching skeleton? Among the many who offer health care are:

- Physician's assistants
- Nurse practitioners
- Specialty-trained registered nurses

- Chiropractic doctors
- Physical therapists
- Massage therapists

In the hospital, the surgeon faces a bewildering, ever-changing number of possible procedures and implants with differing materials and engineering designs. The surgeon must also work closely with the medical managers and hospital administrators who control the expenditures for this technology. Ultimately, these procedures and tests are done for and on people who are not growing properly, have suffered traumatic injury, have developed arthritis, or have intractable pain.

INTEGRATED OSTEOPATHIC ORTHOPEDIC EXAMINATION

The integrated osteopathic examination is detailed in other chapters, but certain principles bear summary here. Recognition of referred pain patterns from nerve roots, peripheral nerves, myofascial trigger points, and ligamentous structures is a prerequisite for the integrated osteopathic orthopedic examination. A neurologic screening examination is also important for differential diagnosis and prognosis in patients referred for orthopedic evaluation.

Use of selective tension in the examination relies on the observation that normal structures are painless and/or strong when stressed; inflamed or strained structures are painful or weak. Orthopedic examination employs selective tension to evaluate muscle, meniscal, tendinous, and ligamentous structures and functions, looking for evidence of inflammation or strain. The physician isolates somatic structures and gently but specifically stresses them, looking for pain, weakness, and crepitus. The McMurray meniscal test and Yergason test are examples of this form of examination.

The orthopedic physical examination of the somatic system evaluates specific joint characteristics, including range-of-motion and the end-feel associated with major and minor joint motions. Often the same test of joint motion allows for structural and dysfunctional interpretations: excessive motion and/or a sloppy end-point to the motion may suggest a ligamentous laxity, while a restrictive barrier at the end of motion testing may suggest a somatic dysfunction. It is important to recall that, in somatic dysfunction, the restrictive barrier appears in one combination of directions and is absent in the opposite combination of directions; the barrier is also reversible with manipulation. Restriction in all directions is characteristic of a capsular pattern seen in pathologic conditions such as arthritis or the fibrotic reaction to trauma or overwhelming stress. In such structural diagnoses, somatic dysfunction is also often secondarily present and can be appropriately treated to the patient's benefit. After the secondary somatic dysfunction is treated, the primary structural barrier characteristics remain.

This chapter is intended for generalists and primary care physicians and reviews a few types of orthopedic diseases while discussing how the orthopedist sees these problems biologically, mechanically, and socially. The chapter discusses what may be distinctive aspects of an osteopathic practitioner's approach to six commonly seen orthopedic problems:

- Developmental dysplasia of the hip
- Geriatric hip fractures
- Osteoarthritis of the knee
- Acute low back pain
- Instability of the shoulder
- Ligamentous laxity and tendonosis

DEVELOPMENTAL DYSPLASIA OF THE HIP

The osteopathic physician, in examining the child at the time of birth and afterwards, first evaluates the whole child. In so doing, the physician looks for dysmorphic features that may be associated with multiple anomalies: the child who has cardiac or gastrointestinal abnormalities, failure to thrive, supernumerary digits, or the inability to bend limbs after delivery (6). A child with multiple congenital anomalies may have abnormalities of the musculoskeletal system that occurred at the same moment in embryogenesis.

Instability of the hip is one of the more common problems in newborn children (7). To evaluate hip stability, the physician observes any abnormalities in skin creases or gluteal folds, leg lengths, and inequalities, and watches for spontaneous motion and activities. The physician evaluates the hip while passing it through a range of motion, checks to see if there is easy and full abduction, and feels the placement and fluidity of motion of the femoral head in the acetabulum (the ball in the socket). An abnormality discovered in any of these observations or tests points to a problem.

Most physicians know the Ortolani sign, which is a palpable sensation of a rapid motion of the femoral head or a "clunk" felt as the dislocated head is reduced into the hip socket from its dislocated position. Here, as Figure 33.2 shows, the femoral head is gently lifted over the labrum and into the socket. In the case of a reduced hip that is unstable, the Barlow test dislocates the hip as the femur is gently adducted with the hip flexed. The physician gently applies pressure over the medial proximal femur and, while doing so, can feel the femoral head slip out of the socket. As the hip is dislocated, gentle pressure on the thigh or knees gives the feeling that the head is not articulating with the socket but that there is a soft end point as the pressure is applied. Moreover, the thigh appears shorter. A positive result in any of these tests, performed routinely in the neonatal examination, suggests further studies or treatment. These tests are performed easily and simply by the osteopathic physician and are examples of the preeminence of a physical examination and the significance of palpatory findings in the evaluation. In the early period of neonatal development, these physical examination tests are more significant than are most imaging modalities, although the recent use of diagnostic ultrasonography has increased the accuracy and sensitivity of the diagnosis of the dysplastic hip. Ultrasonography is especially useful with abnormalities in the development of the soft tissues of the acetabular region, which are not visualized on x-ray films (8). During treatment, various images such as x-ray studies and computed tomography (CT) scans can be used to assess the accuracy and adequacy of the treatment as the child grows or to confirm the physical diagnosis.

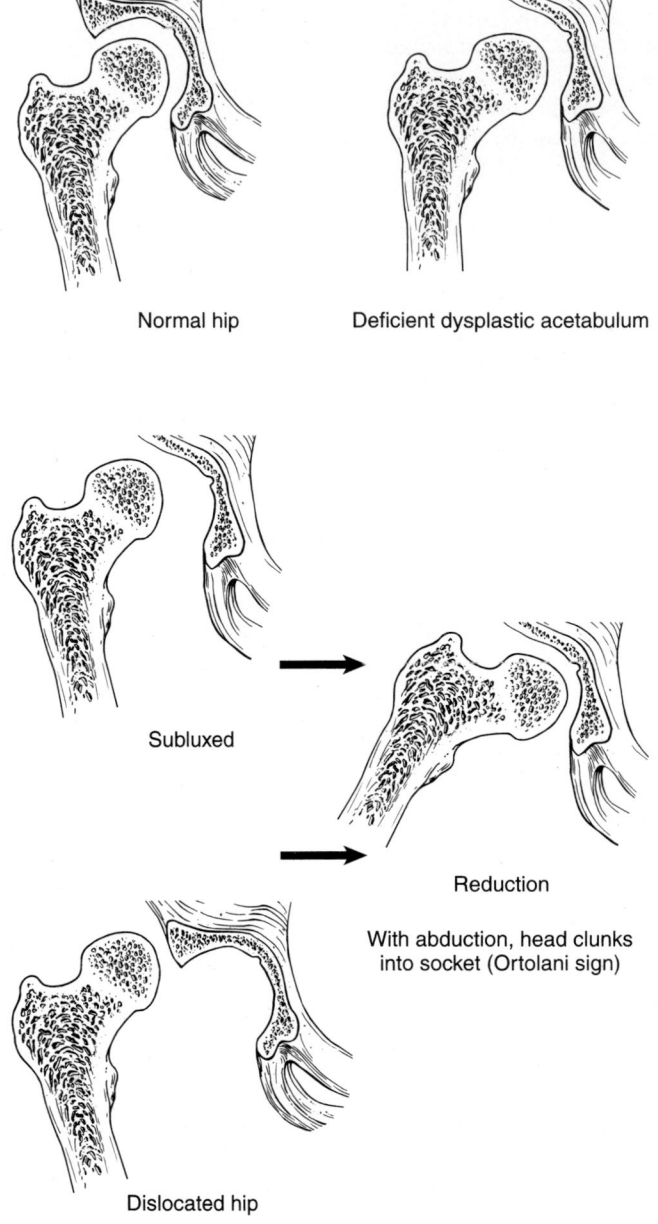

Normal hip   Deficient dysplastic acetabulum

Subluxed

Reduction

With abduction, head clunks
into socket (Ortolani sign)

Dislocated hip

FIGURE 33.2. Ortolani sign.

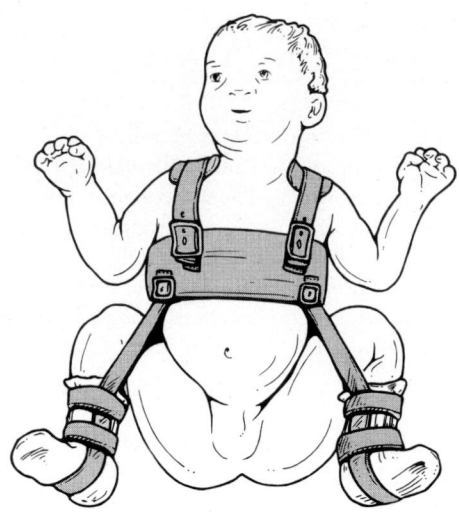

FIGURE 33.3. Pavlik harness.

Treatment of developmentally dysplastic and dislocated hips involves the application of a fundamental osteopathic precept: that growth and maturation of the skeleton follows function. A properly positioned joint with good, easy motion and adequate blood supply and muscle balance grows and develops normally. The orthopedist's goal in the treatment of the dysplastic hip is to place that hip in a position whereby normal stimulation for growth of the acetabulum and proximal femur occurs. One can use external position devices such as casts or braces, internal fixation devices, or structural changes operationally to change the alignment of the bones so that they are allowed to grow and mature in an improved position.

In most cases, a dislocated or dislocatable hip can be either reduced shortly after birth or, if not reducible, held in a position

in which the proximal femur is heading or pointing toward and centered over the triradiate cartilage, the middle portion of the acetabulum. Many orthopedists today use the Pavlik harness to hold such a hip in a position of flexion and abduction while allowing the child to flex the hip and kick at will (Fig. 33.3). The position utilizes a safe zone whereby the femoral head is securely placed and at low risk of dislocation while the patient is harnessed. The pressures on the shaft are such that there is less risk for avascular necrosis of the femoral head than in those patients fixed in a rigid cast, which was the older method of treatment. The position in which the hips are placed is termed the human position, in contradistinction to older forms of immobilization in which the neonate's hip might be held in a position more akin to an amphibian or a frog. The principle is of essential importance: placing the hip within the socket in a stable position allows the body to continue to nourish the hip socket and allows its normal growth over a period of time. Pavlik himself stated, "with the help of stirrups, we want to achieve suitable flexion of the hips, and non-violent unforced abduction of the hips with simultaneous facilitation of movement in the hip joints. Centralization of the femoral heads in the acetabulum results spontaneously." While this has proven successful in most cases, there is still controversy regarding when to apply and how to define if the treatment is successful. One may use ultrasonography or magnetic resonance imaging (MRI) as well as CT scans to help determine adequacy of reduction and position. The risk of complications such as femoral palsy from tight straps over the femoral nerve above the knee or of avascular necrosis from constriction of the epiphyseal blood supply are rare (9–11).

The second form of treatment of the growing child involves the realignment of the proximal femur and acetabulum to center the growing femoral head within the acetabulum. A typical case of a late, unrecognized dislocation presents in a child of early walking age, at approximately 1 year. Such a toddler presents with a shortened leg or a waddling gait. As the child has grown with the hip in a dislocated position, the femur has progressed into a more valgus position at the femoral neck shaft angle (Fig. 33.4). The acetabulum is deformed and shallow, and the cartilaginous

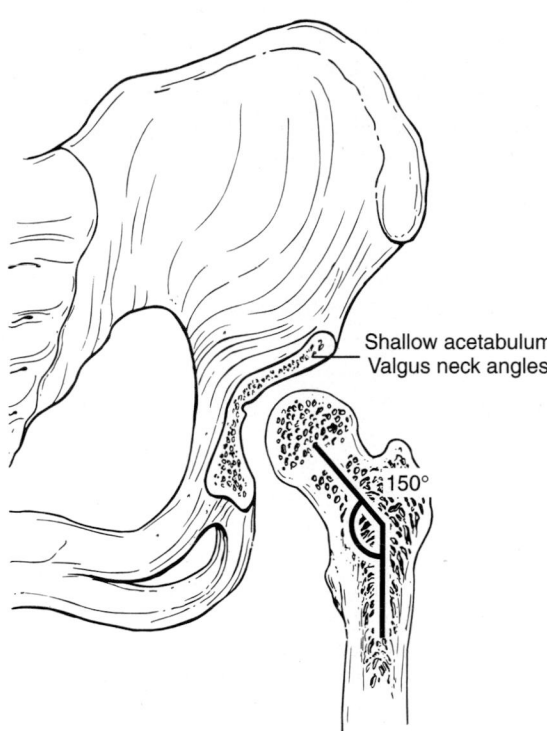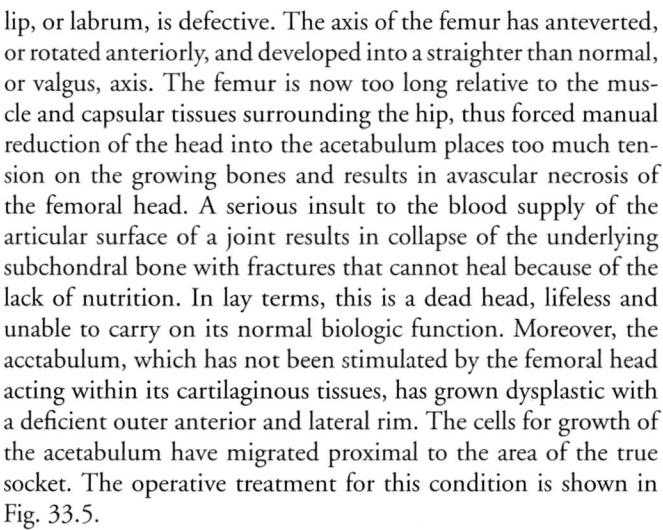

FIGURE 33.4. Long-standing hip dislocation.

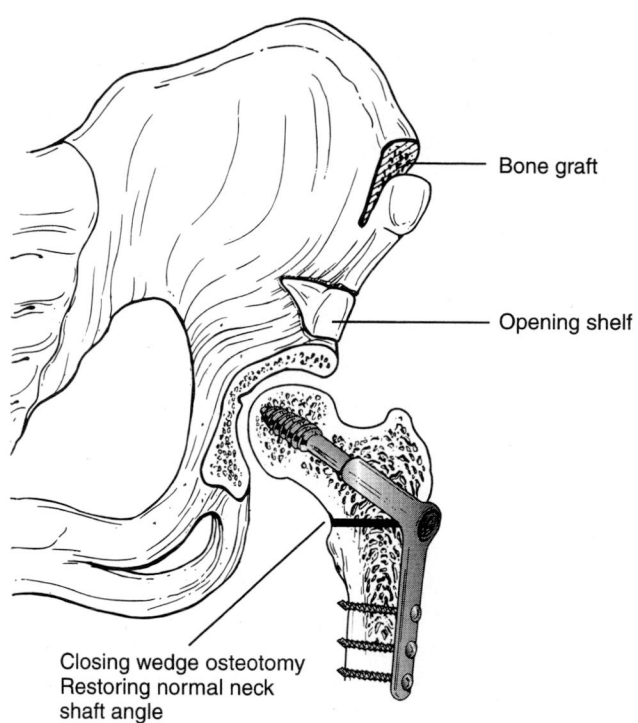

FIGURE 33.5. Open correction of late deformity.

lip, or labrum, is defective. The axis of the femur has anteverted, or rotated anteriorly, and developed into a straighter than normal, or valgus, axis. The femur is now too long relative to the muscle and capsular tissues surrounding the hip, thus forced manual reduction of the head into the acetabulum places too much tension on the growing bones and results in avascular necrosis of the femoral head. A serious insult to the blood supply of the articular surface of a joint results in collapse of the underlying subchondral bone with fractures that cannot heal because of the lack of nutrition. In lay terms, this is a dead head, lifeless and unable to carry on its normal biologic function. Moreover, the acctabulum, which has not been stimulated by the femoral head acting within its cartilaginous tissues, has grown dysplastic with a deficient outer anterior and lateral rim. The cells for growth of the acetabulum have migrated proximal to the area of the true socket. The operative treatment for this condition is shown in Fig. 33.5.

This operation requires that the superior and inferior sides of the hip joint, the femur and the acetabulum, be addressed simultaneously. In the femur, a shortening, varus osteotomy allows the femoral head to be reduced without undue pressure and changes the neck-shaft angle to a more normal degree from its valgus position. In the acetabulum, a more horizontal socket is formed by either placing a bone graft at the rim or performing an osteotomy above the rim and bending the growing cartilage. If the femoral head is kept reduced into the acetabulum and held there while the tissues heal, it stimulates joint growth and encourages continued normal development over time.

Bones and joints are plastic and develop as a result of the forces that are applied to them. One of the joys of treating young people is to watch the growing child mature over time. The physician

can guide this development in many ways. The old saying, "As the twig is bent, so grows the tree," implies a molding of the whole person. This image continues to influence the orthopedic community: by molding the growing skeleton, orthopedists help children grow into straighter, more functional adults.

The term dysplastic hip is used for the abnormality in appearance and congruity of the child's hip. The proper terminology is developmental dysplasia of the hip, which implies that dysplasia may occur not only at birth but also after birth. Congenital dysplasia implies that all dysplastic hips are present at birth. If that were the case, then all should be recognizable at birth. Some hips, however, are normal at birth but become dysplastic in the extrauterine environment. It is important that the physician routinely examine the well baby's hips at regular office visits. The physician should check the child's hips for symmetry, leg length, and equality of abduction at the first postpartum office visit, at 6 weeks of age, and at 6 months of age. The final examination is at 2 years of age, when standing ability and balance are included (7).

The physician who treats the child with a dysplastic hip is treating not only a mechanical problem in a child but also a child in a family, a small member of a complicated social structure. For the young child, nutritional, educational, and emotional support are paramount. The physician needs to encourage the parents to provide the child with sufficient protein, minerals, and vitamins for growth. The physician also needs to encourage the parents to continue to supply intellectual stimuli or the school system to provide homebound instruction, since these children will have difficulty attending classes. Ensure that parents, siblings, and other nurturing family members provide emotional support to the child in a cast or in bed. A family with a child with hip dysplasia worries that the child will not walk and be active in life.

They need encouragement that the child will probably be able to enjoy a lifestyle not unlike that of his or her friends.

HIP FRACTURE IN THE GERIATRIC POPULATION

One of the drawbacks of aging is the progressive loss of bone mineral universally noted in men and women after they enter their mid-70s. Weight-bearing bones develop osteopenia and have a resultant structural weakness, particularly in the hip, which must withstand heavy forces. When the structural inadequacy of the hip bone is joined with diminished visual acuity, balance, and coordination, falls and fractures are common. In treating an aging population, the physician will encounter geriatric fracture problems.

The patient with a hip fracture presents with not only a mechanical problem to solve but also a personal and social problem. The personal upheaval in lifestyle and abilities as well as the severe economic hardships to the injured person and their family profoundly influences all caregivers, illustrating a major problem for public health providers. The number of aging persons with hip fractures is huge, and the costs of treatment for the fracture and its associated morbidity are staggering. It is estimated that 280,000 Americans suffered hip fractures in 1994. The cost in 1994 was nearly $10 billion. If a disease becomes a public health problem when it affects a significant portion of the population, it is incumbent on the public and on physicians to attempt to prevent or control the disease rather than simply treat the disease as it occurs.

In the aging population, fractures of the hip are of multiple types and are somewhat dependent on the forces that act through the hip. These fractures are described according to their location. There are subtrochanteric and intertrochanteric fractures and subcapital fractures. Each particular type of fracture has its own treatment approach. Those fractures that are within the cancellous bone of the intertrochanteric region, if not comminuted or broken into many fragments, generally heal rapidly with stable internal fixation. Fractures in the subcapital region have multiple treatment protocols, and the approach is more difficult. The younger the patient, the more the physician should attempt to bring the bones to a physiologic healing.

The blood supply to the femoral head is precarious. Simply aligning the bones and holding them together does not necessarily ensure healing. Just as in the growth of the immature skeleton, healing of fractures requires adequate oxygenation, nutrition, and blood supply. For any patient with a subcapital fracture, the risk of avascular necrosis is high; nevertheless, with adequate protection and limited weightbearing, union can occur. The surgeon may try to reestablish circulation to the femoral head through a revascularization procedure in which a pedicle of bone attached to a blood supply is rotated into the proximal femur. One method one of the authors (RAS) has used with success is the transfer of a pedicle of bone from the trochanteric region attached to the quadratus muscle along with its large artery. This pedicle is implanted into the femoral head and neck. For younger patients, the surgeon tries to avoid prosthetic hip joint replacement, which is the alternative to internal fixation of the fracture. The younger the patient, the more likely it is that a prosthesis will fail before

the patient has completed their active weightbearing life. To recapitulate, fractures in the subcapital region should be treated with internal fixation in the hope that healing will occur. However, if the fracture is severely displaced or if there appears to be a high risk of diminished blood supply to the femoral head, a prosthetic replacement is indicated.

As a person ages and the bone becomes more porotic, subcapital fractures become more impacted or displaced, and the treatment protocol separates those that are stable or minimally displaced from those that are displaced. For the first group, internal fixation with cannulated screws is recommended; in the latter group, prostheses are recommended. As a person ages more and the ability to ambulate or even get out of bed disappears, the protocol again becomes more complex because the physician needs to weigh the costs of hospital and surgical treatment and the high mortality rates against the possible alleviation of the acute fracture pain. A period of immobilization with traction may be sufficient for a fibrous healing in very old or cognitively impaired patients because it allows turning and protection from bed sores. For others, a replacement with an endoprosthesis may allow an earlier discharge from the acute care hospital to the extended care facility with a lessened incidence of contractures, decubitus ulcers, heart failure, and pneumonia. In the treatment of the older adult patient with hip fracture, the osteopathic physician needs to address the respiratory, cardiac, and alimentary systems, as well as take steps to decrease the incidence of thrombophlebitis. The physician must realize that after a trauma, such as a fracture and fracture surgery, derangements occur in all of the body systems. The physician must be vigilant and treat these derangements as they occur rather than simply pay attention to the hip alone. Mobilization of the thoracic spine often increases cardiorespiratory function and stimulates activity.

Osteopathic physicians need to use their skills and knowledge to help society as a whole in its efforts to increase the quality and quantity of life. Hip fractures occur partly because of biochemical changes associated with aging. The physician should understand how they can help older adults maintain their bony structure and integrity. The basic substrates needed for bone production include protein and calcium. Physicians understand that the absorption of calcium through the gastrointestinal tract partly depends on the interaction of vitamin D and its various active hydroxylated forms with circulating hormones such as calcitonin and estrogen. In nonsmokers, 5 years of estrogen use may reduce annual hip fracture rate by more than 50%.

Bone mineral production also is influenced by the basic principle that if an organ or structure is not used, it wastes away. If bone is not used or stressed, calcium is not deposited. A limb at rest or not stressed by gravity, as in a space station astronaut or in a person on bed rest, quickly becomes osteopenic. A physician can help patients maintain bone production by ensuring dietary and supplemental control of essential vitamins, minerals, and hormones. Patients should be encouraged to exercise, particularly in a weightbearing or an antigravity mode. Regular loading of the appendicular and axial skeleton is the best way to enhance sustained mineral production. To decrease the incidence of hip fractures in older adults, the orthopedic osteopathic physician should begin by encouraging middle-aged female patients to monitor their estrogen levels, replacing the estrogen particularly in those who are prematurely estrogen-depleted or who have prematurely estrogen-depleted or who have proven accelerated bone loss. All bone will not be maintained strong enough not to fracture, despite these measures. The home and workplace must be made safer. Obstacles that may cause one to trip and fall should be removed. Finally, the balance and agility of the older adult should be evaluated regularly and appropriate steps taken to control seizures or to prevent vision loss.

The incidence of hip fractures is increasing as the population is aging. This is a population that is nutritionally and hormonally depleted. Moreover, it is a population that has forgotten to walk. Regulation of these factors as well as decreasing the extrinsic risk factors in the environment helps decrease the numbers of hip fractures. One of the ways in which the physician can decrease the risk of fractures is to decrease the amount of sedatives and drugs that can impair balance. A novel method for increasing stamina and balance has been proposed by Wolf. Based on a study performed by the National Institute of Aging, Wolf recommends that older adults practice the ancient Chinese exercise, tai chi (12).

The osteopathic physician has a major role in helping the individual patient as well as the population at risk for these fractures. In the treatment of a patient with a hip fracture, the goal is to control pain and return the patient to a nonhospital environment. How the physician treats or recommends treatment depends on the anatomic type of fracture as well as on the physiologic status of the patient.

Figure 33.6 represents the types of fracture and the treatment options. Fractures of the proximal femur are generally classified as intracapsular (occurring within the joint) or extracapsular (which are usually intertrochanteric), in which the fracture line goes between or through the greater and lesser trochanters. When possible, intracapsular fractures are treated with reduction and pin fixation. When this is not possible, prosthetic replacement is necessary. Intertrochanteric fractures are usually held in a reduced position with the use of a sliding compression screw.

OSTEOARTHRITIS OF THE KNEE

To examine and treat the arthritic knee requires that one understand how arthritis affects the whole body. The term arthritis is used with little specificity and can refer to different types and causes of joint pain. Arthritis is joint inflammation. An arthritic problem can be the result of a systemic disorder that may be immunologically based, the effect of infection, or a metabolic disorder such as rickets. It can be a late effect of trauma such as a fall, a vehicular accident, or a sports-related ligamentous injury. Before evaluating the joint for which a patient presents to the office because of pain or swelling, the physician must first ascertain if there is a systemic cause for arthritis. Often the types and presentations of the common arthritides are recognizable with a thorough history and physical examination. A careful history allows the physician to recognize that a young woman who presents with morning stiffness and symmetric polyarticular disease might have rheumatoid arthritis. It allows for the assumption that a middle-aged man with a history of recurrent great toe pain associated with dietary indiscretions, who presents with a hot, inflamed knee joint, probably has gout. Examination of the

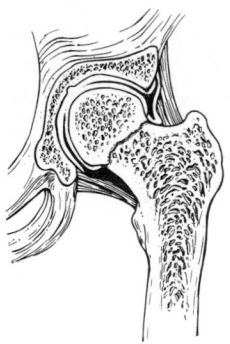

Intracapsular fracture

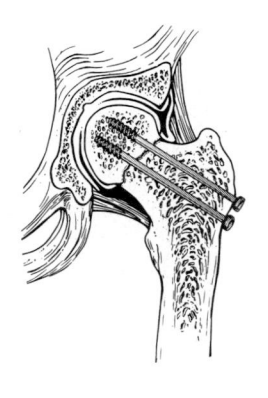

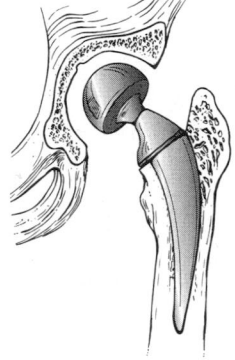

Screw fixation   Prosthetic replacement

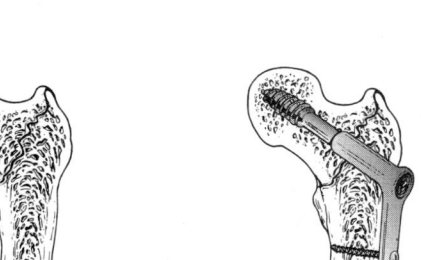

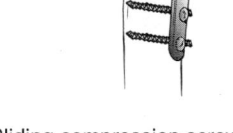

Intertrochanteric fracture   Sliding compression screw

FIGURE 33.6. Fractures of proximal femur.

gowned patient forces even the most casual examiner to recognize advanced psoriatic skin changes in an arthritic patient. To paraphrase one of the tenets of osteopathic medicine, a patient's disease affects their entire body system. It is appropriate and necessary that the osteopathic physician understand the relationship of an arthritic joint to the whole patient.

The most common kind of knee arthritis that presents to the orthopedist is that of a wearing out or erosion of the articular surface of the medial compartment of the knee, called osteoarthritis. This is usually the result of repeated major and minor trauma or

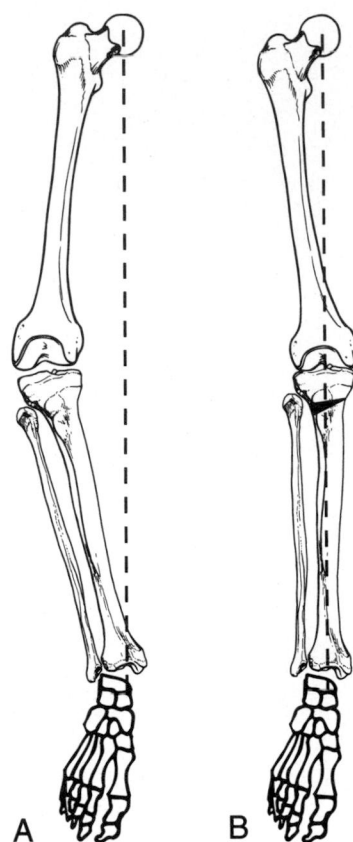

FIGURE 33.7. Genu varum. **A:** A lower extremity with extreme genu varum in which the weightbearing line from the hip to the foot passes medial to the knee joint. **B:** A limb after a high tibial osteotomy in which the weightbearing line passes through a point lateral to the center of the knee joint.

wear. Oftentimes, this is coupled with a normal varus or mild bowlegged body habitus. As shown in Fig. 33.7A, in this presentation, a line of weightbearing from the center of the axis of the femur passing to the center of the ankle joint passes inside of or medial to the center of the knee. In this case, the vast amount of forces and stresses that pass through the knee pass entirely through the medial compartment or through the medial femoral condyle and tibial plateau. If there has been an injury to the ligaments or cartilage of the knee, with time and the increase of stresses, there is increasing wear and debris in the joint. To optimize treatment requires some understanding of how articular cartilage is nourished, what steps can be taken to decrease the wear debris or particulate gravel in the knee, and how to diminish stresses in the medial joint.

The articular surface, or the cartilaginous weightbearing element of a joint, is made up of a matrix of water-heavy proteins with few living chondrocytes present. This anatomic area has no direct blood flow. The metabolites necessary for the nutrition and repair of the cartilage pass into the structure through the spongelike cartilage. With pressure from weightbearing or muscle contracture, the cartilage surfaces collapse, pushing the fluid into the joint. As the pressure is relieved, the joint fluid seeps back into the cartilaginous matrix, bringing the necessary metabolites and oxygen required for cell life. Therefore, it is important to

maintain the motion and normal stresses to the knee. As part of the treatment of the arthritic patient, the osteopathic physician needs to encourage motion and activity. Some of the kinds of activities that are helpful in the maintenance of joint structure include low-impact aerobics, water exercises, and repetitive low-stress activities such as treadmills, cross-country skiing, and bicycling. Eccentrically loaded high-stress activities such as jumping are not recommended because the stresses across the joint are too great. Twisting or torquing motions, especially in a joint with weak ligaments, increase the forces and shear that occur across the cartilaginous area. If, as a result of previous trauma or the ravages of aging, the cartilage of the joint is damaged, then the irregularly shaped edges of this normally smooth articular cartilage may be easily ripped or torn with compression and shear. Judicious exercise is important to maintain the metabolic nutrition of the cartilaginous matrix, but overuse may cause serious problems. Assisting the patient to obtain and maintain a body weight within normal limits also helps to diminish the stresses in the joint.

Disabling unilateral medial knee arthritis has other effects as well. The patient with a painful joint has an antalgic gait: he or she limps. Limping causes a twisting motion to the joints above and below the painful joint. A common problem with limping is an imbalance in the sacroiliac articulation with a resultant somatic dysfunction in this joint. Often, as the knee bows medially, an effective leg length difference occurs that may need to be addressed with a lift. Patients with pronated feet increase the stresses over the medial knee joint. The use of a custom orthosis in the shoe often changes the dynamics, relieves pain, and allows the patella to track more normally in the patella-femoral trochlear groove. With pain, the patient fails to exercise and becomes deconditioned; their entire cardiopulmonary status may deteriorate if left unattended. Many patients with pain cannot work as hard at their jobs and their hobbies as they would like and become depressed. Counseling and the use of antidepressant medications may be helpful.

At the present time in the development of orthopedic implants, laboratory designed and manufactured biomaterials do not have the same degree of biologic function as do normal tissues. They are not self-reparative. They have different moduli of elasticity than the human tissues; they do not bend the same amount with forces as do human bones. The result of this is increased stress at the interface between the implant and the biologic tissue. Recently, researchers and clinicians have discovered that particles of wear debris that occur normally with time, particularly those of the high-density polyethylene that serves as the bearing surface in most prostheses, are read by the host cells as foreign. This causes an intense foreign body reaction in some patients. A side effect of this foreign body reaction is a release of biologically active mediators from the tissue macrophages and other immunologically competent cells of osteoclast-stimulating factors. These in turn cause the body, sometimes quickly, to resorb the bone surrounding the implant, weakening the junction between the prosthesis and the bone and allowing loosening, pain, and fracture to occur.

The options for the physician treating osteoarthritis are limited because no surgical implant can guarantee a relief of pain. As in the case of the younger patient with a hip fracture, replacement arthroplasty should be avoided for as long as possible. The following paragraphs and the accompanying diagrams describe the various braces used and surgical procedures done to alleviate discomfort. A physician recommends one modality for a particular patient with knee arthritis based on the understanding of that patient's physiology, age, life requirements, and goals, as well as on their knowledge of the types of treatment available.

One of the simplest treatments is the application of a knee brace that applies pressure to the tibia below and the femur above, thereby increasing the forces applied over the lateral joint line. This brace is similar to those worn by athletes with torn ligaments; in fact, it was developed for use in arthritic patients through an offshoot of the sports medicine designs. For many the brace is successful for pain relief, although it may be cumbersome to apply and bulky under clothes.

For those who have an angular deformity that is severe and painful, osteotomy may realign the mechanical problems associated with genu varum. As depicted in Fig. 33.7B, a simple form of osteotomy removes a wedge of bone from the lateral proximal tibia. If this wedge is properly calculated, when the osteotomy heals, the center of gravity or the forces acting through the knee pass through the lateral joint, thus diminishing the forces through the arthritic medial joint.

For many, as an adjunct to or substitute for osteotomy or bracing, arthroscopy may afford relief. If there is a degree of effusion and torn tissues with multiple loose particles floating inside the knee joint, a debridement or vacuuming of the knee can wash out the offending particles. While this is not curative, for many it affords a long period of pain relief.

For those whose knee joint is not a candidate for osteotomy and whose lifestyle and physiologic age are appropriate, joint replacement arthroplasty is indicated. Joint replacement arthroplasty requires adherence to a host of mechanical constraints. The joint must be in a normal and mechanically sound position, and the components need to be securely fixated to the bones of the knee joint. There are many options, ranging from the unicompartmental hemiarthroplasties that simply replace the damaged medial compartment to constrained systems in which the design attempts to substitute for damaged ligaments.

The osteopathic physician needs to understand some of the features of the implants and the physiologic changes that occur with implant arthroplasty. The risks of thrombophlebitis are high. Precautions are necessary, ranging from early activity and external compression devices to therapeutic anticoagulation with warfarin, heparin, or dextran derivatives. The risk of infection, both early and late, although not great is disastrous when it occurs. The risks are diminished through good surgical technique, by decreasing the number of bacteria that can come into contact with the wound, and with the use of appropriate antibiotics. Finally, the physician must recognize that a joint implant is a foreign body. With any systemic infection, circulating bacteria may adhere to the implant and cause a late infection. The judicious use of antibiotics in the face of systemic infections or bacteremia may decrease the incidence of infection. Many physicians recommend the prophylactic use of antibiotics with oral surgical procedures or at other times of predictable risk for bacteremia.

The osteopathic physician who evaluates the patient for a total joint arthroplasty must address the variety of problems that are involved in knee arthritis. Weight control, physical conditioning, exercise, and proper nutrition are helpful to encourage healing and to maximize the gains from the procedure. Ongoing research into the efficacy of osteopathic manipulative procedures in the preoperative period should encourage the physician to maintain a normalized spine. A study of the adjunctive use of OMT in the early postoperative period following joint arthroplasty showed that those who underwent OMT reported less pain, used fewer analgesic medications, and walked farther than those patients who were not manipulated (13).

LOW BACK PAIN

The most frequently seen problem for general orthopedists today is low back pain. Back pain is ubiquitous in the population. The costs of treatment, the expenses of failed work, and the problems frequently associated with blame and the legal system make these the treatment of low back pain one of urgency. The patient and family need to have a return-to-work schedule and sense of normalcy restored; society needs some surcease from the huge costs necessitated by the disability structure. Every physician sees the patient with acute disabling back pain who is unable to walk and unrelieved of discomfort. From the orthopedist's point of view, the urgency to relieve pain and disability quickly makes a dispassionate evaluation and treatment plan impossible. The new technological advances in imaging and in surgical technique have led many patients to believe that a rapid, easy, risk-free anodyne is available by surgery. Everyone has known someone who, following a back surgery, did not get better but may have gotten worse. The litigants would have us believe it is because of faulty technique or poor technology or inadequate screws. Spine surgeons are still evolving techniques, materials, and methods to find out which patients with low back pain can benefit from which procedure. Other surgeons often do not want to examine, evaluate, or treat the patient with acute or chronic back pain because such patients are often difficult and demanding.

The osteopathic orthopedic surgeon approaches the patient with low back pain with a systematic protocol. The primary objective for all physicians and surgeons is to define a distinct diagnosis: a diagnosis that has an accurate anatomic and pathologic basis. The great problem for surgeons in general and for orthopedists in particular is to identify appropriate surgical pathologic conditions. Most back pain does not need to be treated surgically. In a great percentage of patients with low back pain, the final diagnosis is idiopathic. This means essentially that nobody knows what is the cause of the disease. Some estimates indicate that more than 50% of all patients with low back pain do not have a firm, accurate, anatomically defined reason for their pain. To operate is problematic if the diagnosis is uncertain.

Just because a surgeon may be predisposed to seek a surgical solution to a problem does not mean that the spine surgeon looks to operate first. Spine surgeons realize that for people with the same pathologic diagnosis, the long-term result of surgical and nonsurgical treatment may be the same. The outcome in equivalent groups of patients with low back pain and myelographically proven herniated discs is the same as for those who have undergone surgery and those treated nonsurgically. This does not mean that the patient with a frank neurologic deficit, weakness, numbness, and intractable pain over the ipsilateral dermatome should not be operated on. The immediate results of pain relief usually outweigh the fact that later, after the settling down of the disc space and the degenerative changes that occur in the surrounding structures, the postsurgical patient may subsequently have episodes of severe back and buttock pain. The spine surgeon approaches each patient who has been referred as having problematic back pain, pain that the referring physician thinks is severe enough to warrant consideration for operative treatment.

The orthopedic spinal surgeon who evaluates the patient referred by the family practitioner, emergency room physician, internist, or family members first has to understand the reasons for referral. Back pain that is severe enough to make the bearer nauseous, that has defied the palliative or curative modalities that often prove successful, and that is unrelieved by narcotic medications, rest, and antiinflammatory shots, pills, and emollients must be a surgical disease. If pain is the anathema of life or, as Herkowitz has stated, "Life is the avoidance of pain" (Annual Spine Session, 1993), then those who suffer and complain have an urgent imperative to seek the services of the surgeon. Patients and physicians are eager believers in the curative possibilities of the newer technologies. If MRI shows a bulging disc and a person has back pain, it follows that the excision of the disc will relieve the pain. This does not always prove true. The fact that the patient may not improve following a surgical experience does not necessarily mean that the surgeon was inept. The imaging diagnostics may not have been as precise or as helpful as we would want, or the acute episode is but one point in time of an ongoing process.

Asymptomatic herniations in the lumbar spine are common (14). It is impossible for the person suffering severe intractable back pain to think rationally about the nature of their pain. As compassionate as the physician-surgeon may be, it is their job to review the possible causes of back pain (Table 33.1) to be able to outline the appropriate steps to best understand and treat the acute episode.

Low back pain is so ubiquitous that its definition is elusive. In the context of this chapter, low back pain is that symptom complex in which the person experiencing pain describes it as encompassing the area of the lumbar spine and the associated musculature of the lumbar spine, as well as the sacrum and buttocks. Pain in the lumbar spine may be of local origin or may be referred. Disorders causing low back pain may, in turn, cause radiculopathy, which is a pain radiating through the peripheral nervous system, usually into a defined dermatome or somatome. There are large lists of entities that can be associated with back pain. Lists in medicine are useful if only to refresh our memories of possibilities in diagnosis not readily at hand. Too often, however, they serve as diagnostic maps in which the observer-physician finds an easy way to choose tests for diagnostic possibilities. For instance, most people with back pain do not have myeloma. To run a gamut of blood and urine tests on an otherwise healthy 30-year-old to rule out myeloma is not reasonable until the more common and statistically significant clinical entities have been differentiated.

Tests should be chosen with a degree of scientific aplomb, using the test to help firm up a diagnosis only after a careful history has been elicited and a physical examination has explored abdominal, pelvic, and spinal structures. In *Acute Low Back Problems in Adults* (15), a clinical practice guideline published by the U.S. Department of Health and Human Services, the authors have included a series of red flags that help alert the examiner to responses or findings that merit detailed evaluation. Their algorithm (Fig. 33.8) outlines an approach to assessing low back pain symptoms. Throughout the patient evaluation, as the physician is considering the diagnostic tests and therapeutic regimens, they should be continually asking if there is some reason for this pain outside of or beyond the spinal area. The red flags that can suggest to the examiner that a serious underlying condition, such as cancer, is present include:

Age of 50 years or older
Previous history of cancer
Unexplained weight loss
Failure to improve with 1 month of therapy
No relief with bed rest

For a patient suffering from a known trauma or with a history of corticosteroid use, fracture is suspected. Intravenous drug abuse, urinary tract infection (UTI), or skin infection in a patient with back pain suggests osteomyelitis or discitis. Sciatica suggests disc herniation and pseudoclaudication; the symptom of increasing leg pain or weakness that is eased with forward flexion or rest suggests spinal stenosis (15).

History and Physical Examination

As in most areas of medical care, the history is of primary importance. A quiet listening attitude on the part of the physician may encourage the patient to be more open and frank. The algorithm for the evaluation of back pain is so large that one item or another from the history given by the patient leads the physician interviewer to follow one pathway in his or her continued questioning and in test ordering. Examples of questions that can help guide

TABLE 33.1. CAUSES OF BACK PAIN

Mechanical	Tumor
Spinal arthritis	Primary
Degenerative disk disease	myeloma
Facet arthritis	sarcoma
Fracture	neural tumor
Spondylolysis	Secondary (metastatic)
Spondylolisthesis	prostate
Congenital	lung
genetic malformations	breast
achondroplasia	kidney
Nonmechanical	Rheumatologic
Viscerogenic	Seronegative spondyloarthropathy
renal colic	ankylosing spondylitis
inflammatory bowel disease	psoriatic arthritis
endometriosis	Reiter syndrome
Vasculogenic	Behçet syndrome
aortic aneurysm	fibromyalgia
ischemic spinal claudication	polymyalgia rheumatica
epidural venous anomalies	Rheumatoid arthritis
Infection	Metabolic
Discitis	Osteoporosis
Herpes zoster	Paget disease
Osteomyelitis	

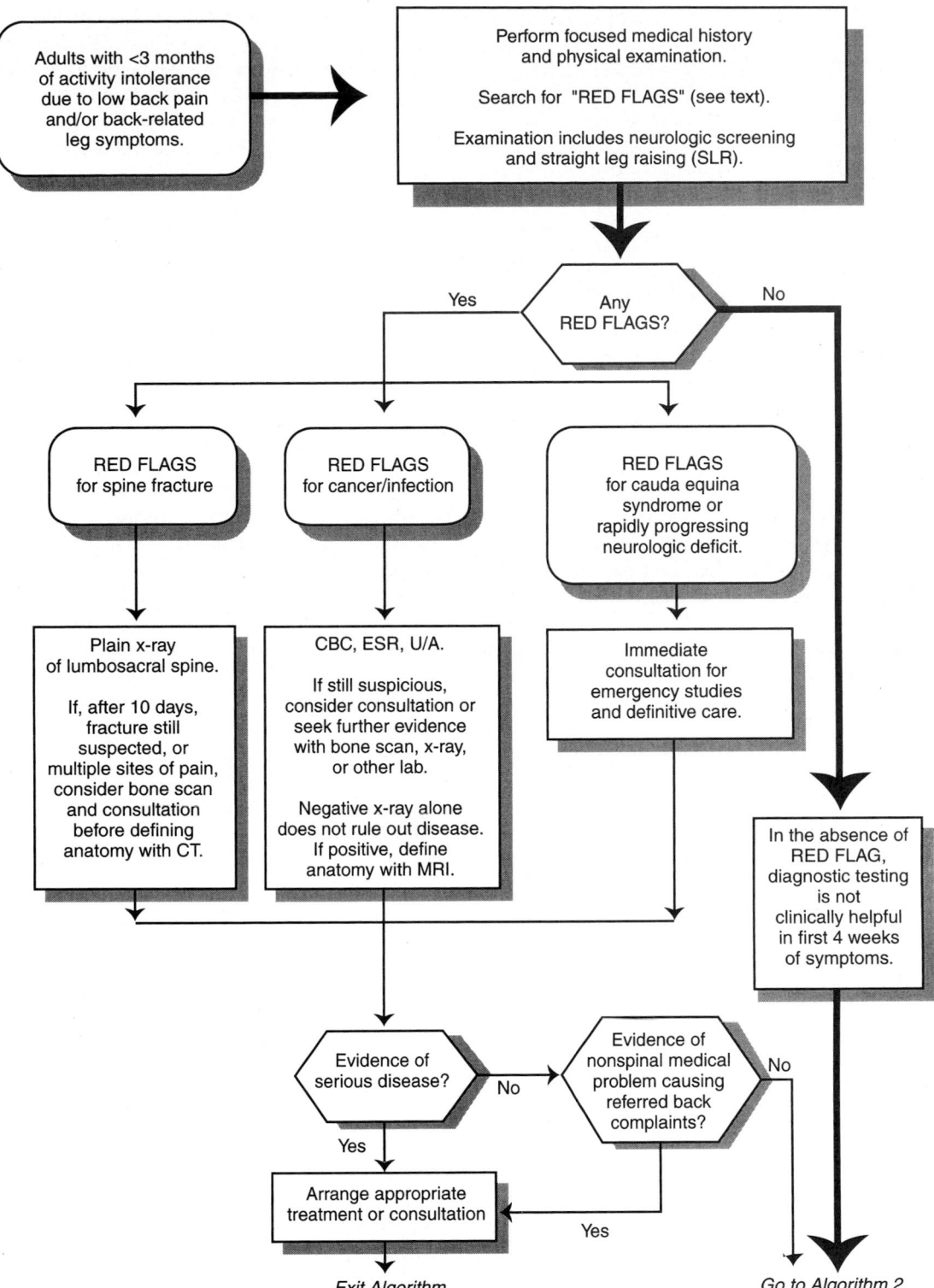

FIGURE 33.8. Initial assessment of acute low back pain symptoms. *CT*, computed tomography; *CBC*, complete blood count; *ESR*, erythrocyte sedimentation rate; *U/A*, urine analysis. (From Bigos S, Bowyer O, Braen G, et al. *Acute Low Back Problems in Adults*. Clinical Practice Guideline, No 14. Rockville, MD: US Department of Health and Human Services; December 1994. Public Health Service, Agency for Health Care Policy and Research AHCPR publication 95-0642, with permission.)

the examiner include:

When did the pain begin?
When is it worse?
What aggravates the pain?
What relieves the pain?
Have other family members had similar problems?
Was the onset associated with a traumatic episode?
Is litigation pending?

Although many of the tests are essential to confirm a diagnosis, the physical examination is crucial. Physical examination includes:

Observation
Palpation and manual motion testing
Neuromuscular examination
Vascular assessment

Although additional tests may later be employed, these four aspects of examination are essential. Many can be performed quickly and concurrently while distracting the patient. All require that the patient be gowned so that their back and legs can be observed and palpated. Examination of a fully clothed patient is inadequate.

Observation requires a keen eye. Watch the patient while they move from chair to examining table and note their ability to get off and on the examining table with or without assistance. Note the gait to ascertain if limp, foot drag or drop, or lurch exists. Note the use of an assistive device, cane, or walker, as well as any alteration of muscle mass, tone, or atrophy, and the presence of any scars.

Palpation of the back and limbs can be performed in multiple positions. Note the tone of the muscles and the turgor of the skin in the extremities. Examine the spine in standing and supine positions, noting areas of discomfort, pain provocation, asymmetries, or muscle spasm. As the spine is placed through ranges of motion, note individual segments with abnormal findings and make measurements of the ranges of rotation, side bending, and flexion. Perform percussion of the spinous process and palpation of contiguous areas such as ischial tuberosity, greater trochanter, and groin.

The neuromuscular examination tests motor power, particularly the strength of the ankle and toe flexors and extensors, hip flexors, gluteal muscles, and rectal tone. The ability to stand on toes or heels unassisted is a sensitive evaluator of leg strength and the presence of intact S1 or L5 nerve roots. Test for absent, present, or hyperesthetic sensation in legs, thighs, back, and perineum. Check deep tendon reflexes as well as the presence of clonus or a Babinski reflex. Assess the presence or absence of pressure on the nerve roots in the lumbar spine through the use of the straight leg-raising maneuver, which can be performed with the patient sitting and supine. This maneuver is performed as the patient flaxes the hip while keeping the knee extended. Record symptom provocation in the form of back or ipsilateral or contralateral thigh and leg pain. Vascular assessment includes palpation of peripheral pulses and auscultation of abdominal, iliac, and femoral vessels.

Multiple tests and signs can elicit symptoms and help in the diagnosis. Examination of contiguous joints, such as the hip, may elicit a cause of referred pain. Frequently, the examiner finds patients with exaggerated complaints. Sometimes the patient may appear hysterical, to magnify the symptoms or to be a malingerer. Careful recording of these findings will help the examiner arrive at a meaningful conclusion. Waddell and colleagues have listed tests and suggested evaluation for those with atypical findings (16).

Pathophysiology

The study of low back pain begins with an anatomic and pathologic consideration of the basis for pain. The basic structural element of the spine is the functional spinal unit (FSU). The FSU is the motion segment and is the smallest segment of the spine that exhibits biomechanical characteristics similar to those of the entire spine. It consists of two adjacent vertebrae and the connecting ligamentous tissues (17). How an FSU behaves depends on the structure of each of the elements and its characteristics, strength, flexibility, and responses to stress. Each FSU is part of the entire axial skeleton from the inion to the coccyx, and each has a mechanical role to support the mass of the body as it moves in space and time.

The anatomic basis for disease encourages our understanding of the FSU. Disease can emanate from the bony structure, the synovial joints, and the ligaments constraining the adjacent vertebra. Moreover, disease can be caused by problems of the intervertebral disc. Figure 33.9 shows the anatomic basis of the FSU. The FSU contains the elements to contiguous spinal vertebrae, their connecting discs, and the associated ligaments and muscles. The posterior elements consist of the spinous processes, ligaments, muscles, and facet joints. The middle segment contains the bony spinal canal and its contents, the neural elements, fat, and vasculature. The anterior elements include the vertebral bodies and the disc. In thinking about the spine as a source of pain, remember this anatomic image. Figure 33.10 describes the type of motions the FSU undergoes in response to applied forces. This is a three-dimensional image. Over the last century, most physicians have relied on two-dimensional imaging such as radiograph and other modalities. Newer technology, such as real time three-dimensional computerized technology scans, allows us to better define the normal ranges for each of the motions. At present, definitions of measured abnormalities or segmental instability are unclear. The American Academy of Orthopedic Surgeons offers this definition: "Segmental instability is an abnormal response to applied loads, characterized by movement in motion segments beyond normal constraints" (18). Concrete numbers based on an x-ray study or on goniometric measurement to define a pathologic instability and prove that it is associated with a painful problem are lacking, except in cases of gross luxation or angular change as seen in fractures. Palpatory diagnosis, in which the end point of vertebral motion is ill defined and either restricted from normalcy or lacking uniformity, offers meaningful data to the examining physician.

The stability of the osseous spine depends on three zones, consisting of the anterior, middle, and posterior elements. This model, devised after a retrospective analysis of spinal fractures in the thoracic and thoracolumbar spine, has been widely adapted for use by spinal surgeons to arrange the thought processes in a more logical manner (19). This discussion centers on the

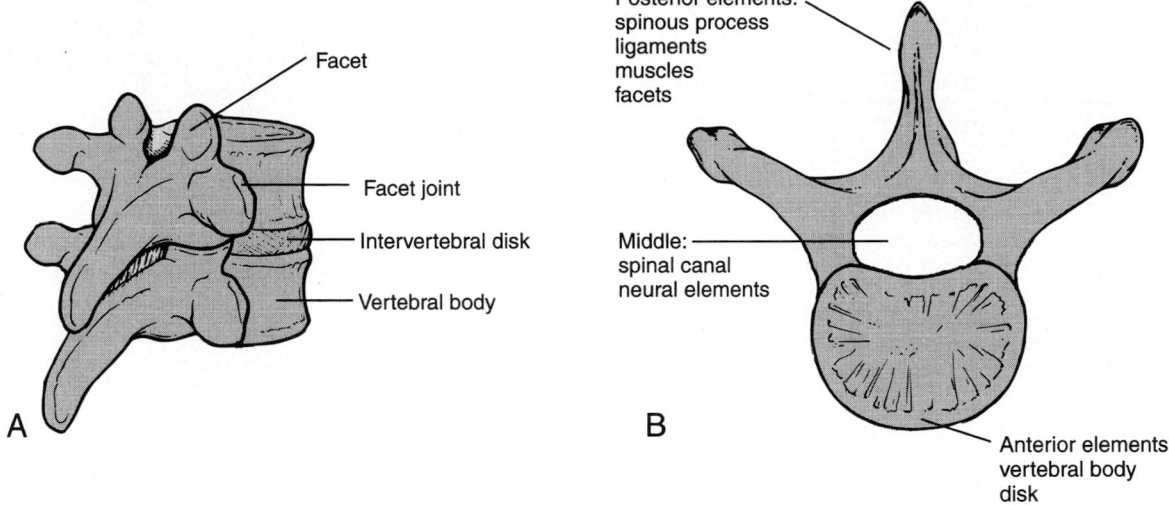

FIGURE 33.9. Functional spinal unit (FSU) seen from oblique projection (**A**) and end-on projection (**B**).

problems of the bony and soft tissue structures. The three columns as described by Denis include the posterior column formed by the posterior bony complex alternating with the posterior ligamentous complex (supraspinous ligament, interspinous ligament, capsule, and ligamentum flavum). The posterior longi-

tudinal ligament, the posterior annulus fibrosus, and the posterior wall of the vertebral body form the middle column. The longitudinal ligament, the anterior annulus fibrosus, and the anterior part of the vertebral body form the anterior column (19).

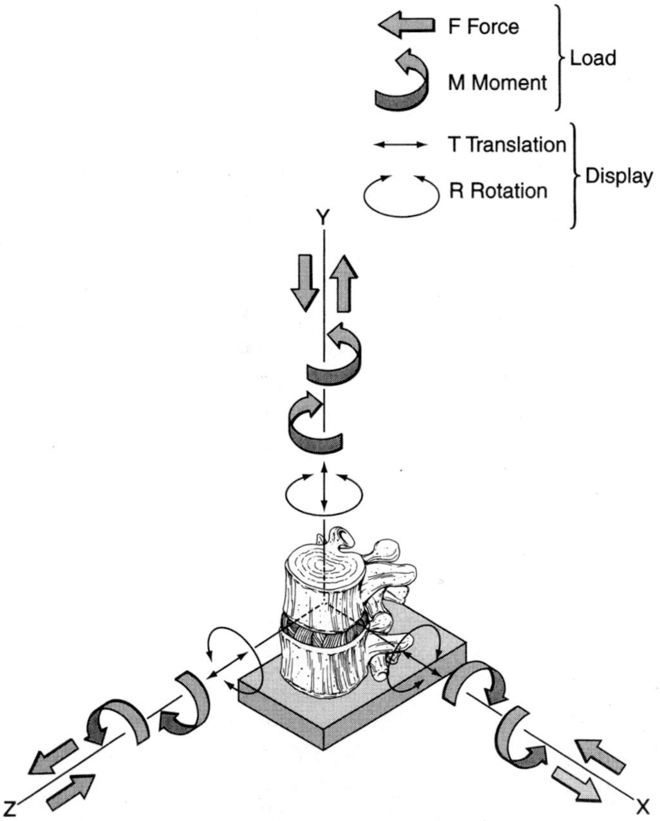

Denis designed his classification in an attempt to better understand the biomechanical changes found in the common and often devastating thoracic and thoracolumbar fractures. In his retrospective study, he described fractures at risk for neurologic compromise based on injury of the middle column. Although fractures of the low back or lumbar and lumbosacral spine are uncommon, the risk of damage to neural elements from middle column disruption in the lumbar spine is less because the cord usually stops above this area. The bony spinal canal is larger, and the cauda equina can be remarkably resistant to compressive damage from fracture fragments. For the anatomic basis of low back pain, the arbitrary separation of the spine into three segments is helpful. It allows the physician to focus on the anatomic element that is the pain generator.

Gunnar Andersson has divided the spine into anterior and posterior segments for ease in isolating causes of disease (20). This author has labeled the central spinal canal as the middle column to isolate those entities that can cause back pain and may be present in the spinal canal alone (Fig. 33.9B).

Entities that may cause acute back pain in the anterior spine include fractures and invasive diseases of the vertebral body and disc, which include tumor, infection, and traumatic disc disruption. The Schmorl node or herniation of the disc through the vertebral end plate often characterizes traumatic disc disruption. The disc has often been implicated as the major source of spinal pain. Certainly, as the disc ages, undue stresses may be placed on the facet joints and arthritic spurs may compress into the spinal canal. However, in the normal spine, the disc under load bulges as a viscoelastic shock absorber (Fig. 33.11). The normal disc behaves in a viscoelastic manner under pressure. During bending (flexion, extension, lateral bending), one side of the annulus is subjected to compression while the other side is put under tensile load. Although it is normal for the disc to bulge in a degenerated state or with a deficient annulus, the disc can herniate or

FIGURE 33.10. Three-dimensional coordinate system fixed in space. Twelve-load components (forces or torques) are depicted. Application of any one of load's components produces displacement of upper vertebra with respect to lower vertebra, consisting of translation and rotation, further divisible with respect to coordinate axes.

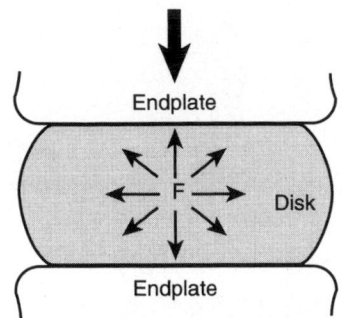

Disk under compressive force-normal.
Disk pushes, "bulges" annulus outward and
compresses end plates.

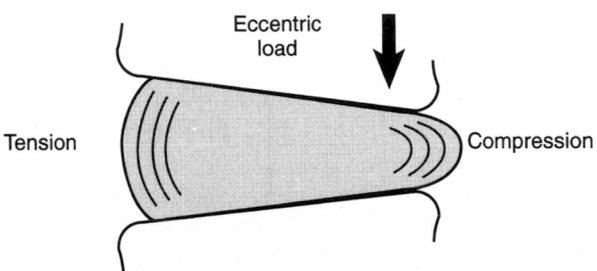

With bending, eccentric loads cause tensile forces
or unloading on one side and higher compressive
loads on the flexion side.

FIGURE 33.11. Disc stresses. *F*, force.

protrude through the ligament and irritate, compress, or damage the neural structures.

Diseases of the middle column include those that compress the contents of the spinal canal; these can be either intrinsic or extrinsic to the canal. Examples of the latter are fragments of bone or disc that are herniated into or compress the thecal sac and neurofibromas or metastatic tumor masses that have entered the canal through the neural foramina and caused compression of the canal. Intradural tumors, meningeal infections, or the sequestered disc when free within the spinal canal can cause intrinsic compression of the spinal cord, as can extradural benign tumors or fibromas. Any narrowing of the spinal canal causes stenosis, a constricting and narrowing of the space available for the spinal nerves and the cauda equina (21). Most often, spinal stenosis is a problem caused by bony changes, which are usually developmental and associated with aging and degenerative changes. These changes of stenosis rarely occur because of genetic problems, as in the case of the achondroplastic dwarf whose ossification has prevented the development of a large enough spinal canal. The cauda equina syndrome is a syndrome of low back pain, characterized by involvement of the sacral nerves causing numbness around the perineum and loss of bladder and bowel function (20).

Changes in the posterior column are common and often related to age or activity. The posterior elements contain the major motion segments of the spinal column including the apophyseal joints and the spinous processes. Fractures of the posterior elements may be associated with severe trauma; most often, severe sprains of the posterior elements are associated with rotatory and translational forces. Fractures, sprain, and somatic dysfunction are part of a spectrum of derangements of the FSU. Mechanical means such as manipulation or traction provide proper realignment of the FSU in these conditions.

The patient with acute low back pain often has a combination of preexisting problems associated with aging (22). Such changes involve desiccation of the disc with loss of disc height and elasticity, the development of spurs at areas of excessive traction, and inflammation of the apophyseal joint with the production of synovial hypertrophy. For many patients, combinations of factors work together to summate the pain load at each of the areas that generate low back pain. Often, bearable, yet constant, low back pain caused by the inevitable aging process may be increased by a mechanically minor twisting in the posterior elements. When the threshold is reached, the resulting pain drives the patient to see the physician. More often than not, attention to the posterior elements with the use of manipulative techniques spares the expense of multiple diagnostic procedures and surgeries.

Spondylolysis is the most common structural problem found in the pediatric population; it often is not diagnosed until radiologic examination is performed on the adult patient. Spondylolysis is a defect in the pars intraarticularis, the bony bridge between the two facet joints; it is most often developmental or caused by a structural weakness. It may also be caused by an acute fracture, as in the case of the gymnast who repetitively stresses the area in hyperextension activities or in the contact athlete who acutely loads the spine in lordosis. Although the radiologic findings in the oblique, lumbar spinal x-ray view might suggest a more serious problem, most patients with acute low back pain and spondylolysis do get better. With progressive motion, a vertebra can move or slip on the inferior vertebra; this is called spondylolisthesis. In the vertebra above the lumbosacral segment and most often in the aging spine, this is called pseudospondylolisthesis because it is not associated with a traumatic, developmental, or congenital weakness of the pars intraarticularis.

Differential Diagnosis

The thought processes involved in diagnosis require separating into definable groups the different known entities with which acute and chronic back pain are associated. One of the ways to separate the different types of back pain is to ask a few elementary questions:

1. Is the pain intrinsic or extrinsic to the spine?
2. Does the pain emanate from some deranged structure in the spine or is it directed to the spine from a distant or contiguous area?
3. Is the nature of the pain related to an injury, an inflammatory condition, an infection, a congenital anomaly, or compression of a neurologic structure?

The extrinsic causes of back pain are associated with viscerogenic and vasculogenic causes. Any visceral disease can manifest as back pain. The pain associated with pancreatitis is classic for irresolvable, unrelenting paroxysms of back discomfort. Prostatitis, renal colic from infection or an obstructed ureter, colitis, or perforated viscus and metastasis of cancer from the colon, ovary, or other contiguous organs may all present as back pain. Most often a quick but deliberate palpatory examination of the abdomen and rectum differentiate these entities.

Vasculogenic causes of back pain are associated with claudication. Usually claudication presents with leg pain after or during exertion. It is uncommon but not rare for the ischemic spine to present with pain. The vasculogenic cause of low back pain that is the most urgent is that of the abdominal aortic aneurysm. Remembering that this is not an uncommon entity in the elderly population prone to atherosclerosis leads the physician to palpate and auscultate the abdomen.

Of the myriad other causes of back pain, those that are systemic in origin tend to act directly on the spine rather than from a distant focus. There are systemic diseases of inflammation, infection, and metastasis that cause back pain. Of the inflammatory diseases, the arthritides are most important; that which presents most insidiously is ankylosing spondylitis, one of the spondyloarthropathies. The diagnosis is difficult in the patient who has not developed the classic, late radiologic changes but who presents with severe episodic nontraumatic low back pain and stiffness in bending. For this patient, the appropriate blood studies may help confirm the diagnosis. The other seronegative spondyloarthropathies and the inflammatory bowel diseases present with back pain for which the treatment is nonsurgical.

Infections of the spine have been rare, but they may become more prevalent in the near future as viral diseases increase in a population with primary and secondary immunosuppression. In the proper host, any organism, if unchecked, is able to invade the paravertebral tissues, disc, or vertebral body. The paravertebral plexus of veins of Batson, for example, drains the organs of the pelvis and has been implicated as the conduit down which clusters of tumor cells or aggregates of bacterial organisms pass. These cells may then grow as a metastatic site in a vertebral body or in the epidural space. An awareness of the problem leads to appropriate differential diagnosis followed by controlled biopsy, aspiration, and culture.

Multiple myeloma is an example of a tumor that spreads to bone, particularly the marrow-rich vertebral body. Myeloma and all the myeloproliferative diseases are systemic diseases that tend to grow in the vertebral body, rendering it structurally weak and ready to fracture even with minimally applied force. The more common tumors to spread to bone are:

Breast
Prostate
Kidney
Thyroid
Lung

If faced with a middle-aged patient with low back pain and radiographic suggestions of a metastatic bone tumor, first ascertain whether the more common tumors have become metastatic. There are multiple tumors, benign and malignant, primary and metastatic, that can cause back pain. Figure 33.12 is an algorithm for diagnosis of spine tumors as proposed by James Weinstein, DO, a tertiary spine specialist (23).

The physician and orthopedist evaluating the patient with low back pain must include tumor as a possible cause of the pain, realizing that it is an uncommon cause. All of the following should alert the physician that there may be a remote source of the low back pain:

Malaise
Fevers
Weight loss
Increased incidence of infections
Change in stool character
Blood in urine, sputum, or feces

A history of night or rest pain greater than pain with activity also is suggestive of tumor spread to bone. Of the various tests performed in physical examination, the most important is that of percussion. In tumor and infection of the spine, percussion of the spinous process of the affected vertebra causes severe pain out of proportion to that which might be expected.

The physician who meets a patient whose low back pain is a sign of metastatic disease may not find the diagnosis unexpected, although such a diagnosis usually startles the patient and the family. The patient with a somatoform disorder or psychogenic pain is not rare. Sometimes there are clues indicating a hysterical or hypochondriac pain pattern, such as frequent trips to the hospital or multiple operations, which may suggest some nonorganic cause of back pain. Hysterical paralysis, reputed to be common in Freud's time, is rarely encountered today. Nevertheless, we all see patients for "executive back pain" or back pain caused or amplified by the stresses of life. The terminology used by people to describe their symptoms is often suggestive of nonorganic pain. "My fellow worker gives me a headache," "My job is a pain in the buttocks," or "I feel like I'm carrying the weight of the world on my shoulders" are all examples of the kind of metaphors used by patients in describing their somatic complaints. These may suggest there are additional factors in back pain not associated with structural lesions. It is helpful to include in the patient history form a pain drawing in which the patient pencils in the anatomic site of their pain (Fig. 33.13). For those who are hysterical, characteristic patterns of nonanatomic pain radiation are present (24). Just as it is important for the examining orthopedist to remember that metastatic disease is an omnipresent possibility and that a careful history and physical examination directs them to that possibility, it is equally important to remember that the sick patient can have disease. Patients with psychoses and neuroses also have infections, tumors, fractures, and discogenic disease (25).

Management

Most often, the orthopedist is encouraged to believe that the referring generalist has evaluated the possibility of nonlocalized origin of back pain. Although the orthopedist runs through a checklist of nonlocalized possibilities during the interview and examination of the patient, the thoughts center on the kinds of problems that are mechanical or structural and might require some form of operative intervention. Most acute low back pain improves over a period of rest or over time. Many patients can be assisted by manipulative treatment. Certainly many of the acute episodes of low back myositis and fibromyalgia are amenable to fascial massage and mobilization, counseling, and antidepressants.

Over the last 15 years, there have been major efforts to understand the nature of back pain. What are the sites or pain generators

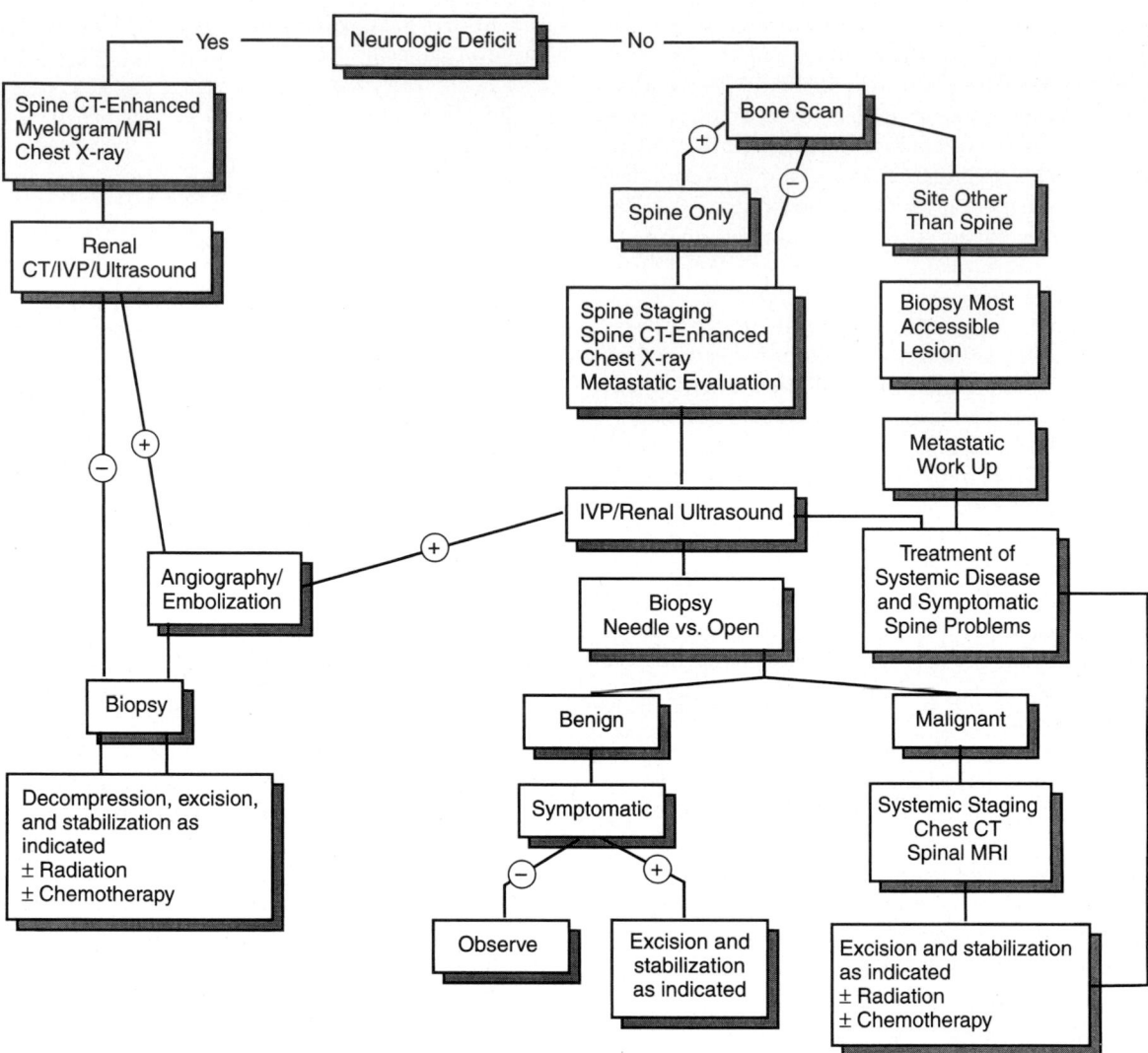

FIGURE 33.12. Algorithm of approach to spine tumors. (From Weinstein J. Differential diagnosis and surgical treatment of primary benign and malignant neoplasms. In: Frymoyer JW, ed. *The Adult Spine.* New York, NY: Raven Press; 1991;41:851, with permission.)

that transmit nociceptive impulses (26). Operating orthopedists are attempting to develop surgical designs to stabilize the unstable spine, as well as to define what stability is (27). They have also been refining approaches and tools to decompress the stenotic spine or entrapped nerve root.

New technologies and materials are expanding the physician's ability to manage back pain and spinal conditions both surgically and nonsurgically. For patients with chronic low back pain without spinal nerve impingement, the pain generator is thought to be pain receptors innervating the disrupted annular fibers of the intervertebral disc. This "discogenic" back pain, confirmed by a provocative diagnostic injection into the disc itself, has eluded a surgical therapy short of removing the functioning but painful disc or fusing the functional spinal unit to obliterate irritant motion. Nevertheless, there are ongoing biologic and biomechanical studies to design and build appropriate implants, which might enable the maintenance of stability and normal spinal unit motion. Long-term studies on human implants, in which the implants reproduce stability and the normal viscoelastic behavior of the human intervertebral disc, are lacking. A recent therapy has developed where a catheter, similar to that used in discography, is placed into the disc percutaneously allowing heat to be delivered to the disc by a radiofrequency probe. The mechanism of how heating the disc reduces pain is elusive, though neurolysis of the free nerve endings has been suggested. The IDET procedure (Intra Discal Electrothermal Therapy) is now being performed by thousands of orthopedists, neurosurgeons, and pain management physicians. The long-term effects of the procedure, especially how IDET affects the stiffness of the disc and its implications for disc functional integrity are unknown at this time (28–30).

Disc herniations resulting in sciatica that do not respond to conservative measures often drive a patient who is suffering to seek a surgical alternative. Removal of the offending disc material that is compressing nerves concordant with the patient's symptoms is generally accepted to bring short-term pain relief to 90% of properly selected patients (31). A variety of surgical techniques for open discectomy, microdiscectomy, percutaneous, and endoscopic techniques exist. With current technology, success rates

Mark the area on your body where you feel the described sensations. Use the appropriate symbol. Mark areas of radiation. Include all affected areas.

| Numbness | — | Increased Sensitivity | 0000 |
| Constant, throbbing Ache | xxx | Sharp Twinge | /////// |

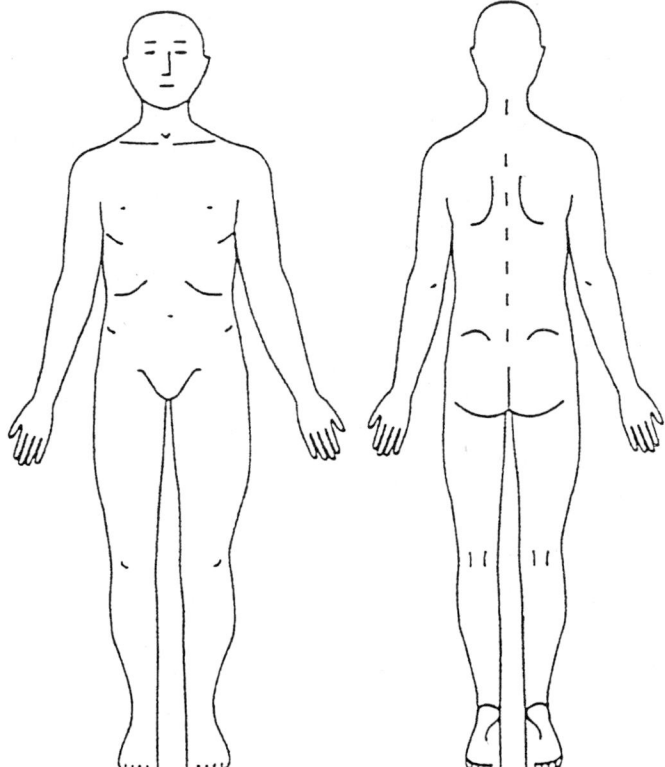

FIGURE 33.13. Pain drawing used by patient to depict severity, type, and location of pain. (From Bigos SJ. *Acute Low Back Problems in Adults*. Clinical Practice Guideline, No 14. Rockville, MD: US Department of Health and Human Services; December 1994. Public Health Service, Agency for Health Care Policy and Research AHCPR publication 95-0642, with permission.)

The bisphophonates (like alendronate) increase bone mass by inhibiting the normal bone resorptive process. It has been proven that alendronate can reduce the risk of a new vertebral fracture by 50% in postmenopausal women with osteoporosis. At least one study has shown that alendronate therapy is effective in reducing back pain and improving functional status in patients with already existing vertebral fractures (35).

Surgical treatment of intractable back pain from vertebral compression fractures has previously necessitated major open procedures. Anterior surgical approaches to the spine are necessary to attempt to restore height to the vertebral body thus restoring the normal contour to the spinal column. The morbidity associated with this type of invasive procedure, especially in the patient age group associated with osteoporotic fractures, has limited it as a feasible option for treating pain alone.

Kyphoplasty has developed as a reasonable treatment for intractable pain secondary to osteoporotic vertebral compression fractures. Considered to be a minimally invasive surgery, the operation is performed percutaneously under fluoroscopic guidance. Catheters placed through the back into the crushed vertebra allow the passage of balloons into the vertebral body. The balloons are inflated under pressure, restoring height to the fractured vertebra. The vertebra is then injected with cement, stabilizing its height. Many centers allow patients to return home the same day. Previous techniques (vertebroplasty) have not provided restoration of vertebral height, only stabilization with cement. Initial studies indicate pain relief to be significant and long lasting in these types of vertebral fractures (36).

A variety of degenerative spinal conditions causing pain and neural compromise (i.e., degenerative disc disease, spinal arthritis, degenerative scoliosis, spinal stenosis, degenerative spondylolisthesis) are often refractory to other therapies and are amenable only to surgery to relieve pain and improve function. Most procedures involve fusion of the involved functional spinal units as the common final step. Similar to other procedures to cease motion across a joint, spine surgeons have tried a variety of methods to achieve a bony fusion and remove pain by obliterating motion.

Basics of spinal fusion necessitate removing cartilage from the opposing facet joint surfaces, holding the segments in a relatively motionless position by external bracing or internal hardware, and waiting months for transplanted bone to complete the osseous bridge across the motion segments, achieving fusion. The difficulty of obtaining a solid fusion in the best of circumstances is best appreciated in light of confounding factors. These include patient compliance with an uncomfortable brace, preexisting medical conditions that hamper bone graft incorporation, corticosteroid use, and smoking (a proven detriment to the local environment necessary for fusion to occur).

The intervertebral surfaces have become another potential site for fusion. Traditionally the posterolateral bony surfaces of the vertebra (transverse process, pars, lamina) have been exposed and bone graft applied over successive levels to create the fusion mass. By removing a portion or all of the already degenerated disc and applying bone graft into that potential space, a greater surface area for fusion is available, increasing the likelihood of achieving the arthrodesis. Recently developed prosthetic devices, known collectively as "cages," are applied into the disc space in place of the degenerated disc, maintaining or even restoring the disc

decline and recurrence increases with the invasiveness of the procedure. Currently open discectomy or microdiscectomy is considered the standard, with microdiscectomy edging out open discectomy in randomized trials for shorter hospital stay and return to work. In the foreseeable future, image-guided stereotactic percutaneous surgical procedures will be the accepted mode for removing small offending tissues from the offended nerve root (32,33).

The vertebral bodies are among the most common sites of osteoporotic fractures and, hence, back pain in older adults, particularly in postmenopausal women of European descent. Rates of vertebral fracture approaching 25% in women over 80 have been reported (34). Increased back pain and the resulting functional limitations are a significant cause of medical visits. Two therapies have emerged in the prevention and treatment of these causes of back pain.

space height, while awaiting bony growth to bridge the space. The largest multicenter trial of one type of cage device reported fusion rates in 196 patents with 4-year follow-up to be 95% (37). These procedures most often involve supplemental internal hardware to stabilize the spine, which may have reduced the necessity of bulky braces to reduce unwanted motion during healing.

Strides are being taken to establish objective data regarding the efficacy of manipulative medicine. The osteopathic profession is challenged to perform objective studies carried out in a blinded prospective scientific manner. Accurate and reproducible data are difficult to obtain. More information that exemplifies current research in manipulative medicine, the majority of which supports a beneficial effect of manipulative treatment in the management of low back pain, is available from various sources (38–56).

Spinal surgeons who deal with complex curves in major adolescent and adult scoliosis must approach the skeleton as a whole as they plan their surgery to balance the weight of the body over the sacrum with an instrumented spinal fusion. The geometric designs require four-dimensional analyses using the x, y, and z axes as well as vector and torsional forces over time (57). The approach to an 11-year-old with a paralytic curve and hydrocephalus is different from that of a 40-year-old with a 60% thoracic scoliosis resulting from Scheuermann disease, a developmental disorder with progressive localized kyphosis. Most osteopathic physicians have been well trained in the palpatory diagnoses of the small curves, rotations, and compensatory changes found remote from the primary lesion of somatic dysfunction. Osteopathic physicians should find the three-dimensional aspects of scoliosis easy to conceptualize.

Summary

Despite the exciting approaches and materials now available, surgery is only useful to try to stabilize or decompress the spine. Most of the time, surgery is unnecessary. Just as treatment for disorders of the growing skeleton is directed toward helping the patient's body mature under guidance, in most cases of acute low back pain, restoration of nutrition, strength, and normal intersegmental motion alleviates pain. The use of algorithms or flow charts, although not foolproof, offer the clinician and the patient the greatest opportunity not to miss causes of back pain that are dangerous and life-threatening, such as fractures or tumors, or are unusual, such as aneurysm or spondylitis. Most often, based on the history and presentation, these life-threatening diseases that can be associated with back pain are ruled out. Nonoperative treatment consists of encouragement that the body will heal, medications to accelerate the healing, and manipulation and exercise to restore segmental normalcy and strength.

INSTABILITY OF THE SHOULDER

Injuries to the ligamentous structures of the major joints are common. The average layperson and general practitioner understand that a sprained ligament is painful and causes swelling and edema. All respect the need for ice, compression, and elevation (ICE) and protection of the injured joint until healing has occurred. This section of the chapter discusses injuries of the shoulder joint as

a model for sprains, or ligamentous injuries, the biomechanical changes that occur with sprains, and recognition of laxity of ligaments with instability or tightness of joint structures causing adhesions. The spectrum flows from those joints unable to be maintained within normal physiologic ranges and those unable to have normal physiologic motion. The goal of this section is to introduce the student to the osteopathic approach to the joint, to understand the biomechanical aspects of joint stability, and to review possible mechanisms of treatment.

The osteopathic physician needs to be able to recognize the unstable and the dislocated shoulder. Many physicians see patients with shoulder problems soon after a traumatic episode, such as an auto accident or sports-related injury. Other times, weeks may pass after an injurious event before the patient presents to the physician with pain and instability. Physicians also need to be able to recognize the unusual dislocation that occurs after seizure or electric shock.

Sprains are either acute or chronic. The acute injury is associated with tearing of structures; the chronic with stretched or inadequate structures. Instability is also characterized by degree: complete dislocation versus subluxation or subtle instability, such as is found in the "dead shoulder" of baseball pitchers who have pain associated with the overhead pitching motion. Instabilities are also diagnosed by direction: anterior, posterior, inferior, and multidirectional. A most interesting case of fracture-dislocation was recently reported in which the humeral head was not seen on radiograph and was found in the retroperitoneum. This was a case of intrathoracic dislocation following massive trauma. While this incomplete list of classification may seem daunting it should not, as the physician should cover these aspects in the history and physical examination of the patient (58).

As in other areas of the orthopedic structural examination, the physician should *listen, look,* and *feel.* One can often learn more about the structure from finding out how and when the initial injury occurred, how often it has happened, and what the shoulder or joint looks or looked like when it was injured than from sophisticated images. Imaging, such as MRI and ultrasonography, is helpful to confirm a clinical diagnosis. In our society a corroborative image may be necessary prior to invasive treatment. Imaging, however, often lacks in specificity and sensitivity. Sometimes the readily obtained radiographs are not helpful.

As a case example, a common presentation to the emergency room is of a middle-aged, cachectic alcoholic man with seizure history and multiple co-morbidities. He presents postictally complaining of pain over the front of his shoulder and holds his arm protectively. Radiographic examination is negative. The physical examination is diagnostic. If the shoulder is posteriorly dislocated there is a palpable hollowness anteriorly, and as the elbow is brought posterior to the midaxillary line with gentle pressure on the humeral head, the examiner can feel the shoulder return to its normal position. Often the reverse examination in the shoulder that has spontaneously reduced will allow the physician to feel the head slide out of the joint. The patient examined long after the original injury will often have symptoms when the arm is circumducted.

Posterior dislocations account for 5% of all acute dislocations. Nearly half are missed at initial presentation. We mention them because the examination is diagnostic just as in the

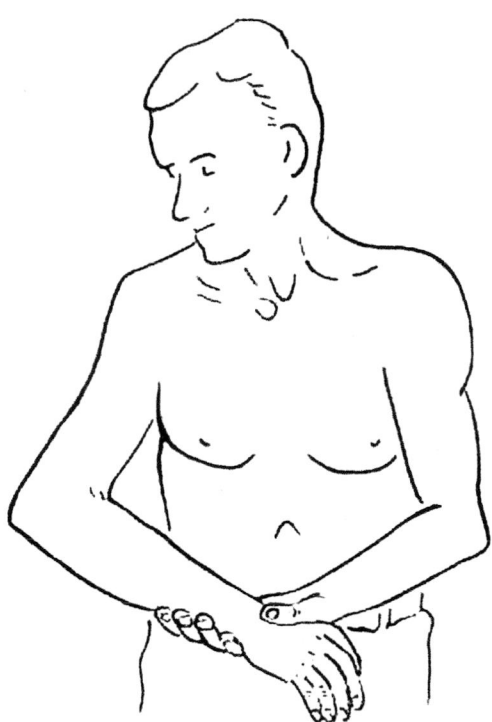

FIGURE 33.14. Typical appearance of a dislocated shoulder.

other directions of instability. The interested reader can read more about these problems in a textbook that details shoulder problems (59) (Fig. 33.14).

Many factors are associated with joint stability. Problems with the osseous structures are common static factors. These include abnormal version of either glenoid or humerus, crushed glenoid, in which the defect in the structure allows the humeral head to slide out of the joint, and the Hill-Sachs lesion, wherein a defect or grooved fracture in the humeral articular surface induces recurrent instability. The ligaments are thickenings of the capsular structure, which provide stability in the multiple positions in which the shoulder can be moved. The ligaments are mostly type I collagen. The strength, aging characteristics and repair mechanisms of torn ligaments are important factors in the healing process.

Thickening of the capsule on the periphery of the joint results in the formation of the labrum, or lip. The labrum has an essential stabilizing force for the shoulder in increasing its depth, as the joint is inherently unstable. Arthroscopic visualizations, anatomic dissections, and MRI imaging have helped us understand the anatomy and function of the ligamentous structures. The small amount of fluid within the joint acts as a fluid membrane allowing sliding or slipping, but inhibiting separation. This force is analogous to that of two wet glass plates that will slide on each other easily but are difficult to separate (60).

The study of what makes the shoulder stable continues but the answers are elusive. The interested reader is referred to the studies of Soslowsky and colleagues on contact areas of the glenohumeral joint, and to the recent analysis of the role of the labrum in centralization of the humeral head by Halder and others (61,62).

The many muscles around the shoulder are essential to stability and important in dysfunction. The biceps, the rotator cuff, and

the scapulothoracic musculature are secondary stabilizers. If torn the shoulder may displace. If healed and tightened too much they can cause adhesions. The osteopathic examiner should palpate and test the function of the various muscles of the shoulder girdle. Treatment then can be directed toward stretching the fibrosed muscle and exercising the weak or lax muscle. Electromyographic studies may help to ascertain if there is a neuromuscular etiology to dysfunctional shoulder girdle. In a high-performance, throwing athlete these can be augmented with video of the throwing motion that can help in planning treatment.

The goal of treatment of the unstable shoulder is to bring the patient to a painless, stable state in which they can carry out normal life functions. Most people who have dislocated their shoulder have learned how to protect themselves from recurrent dislocations. Strengthening of weakened secondary stabilizers will often assist this. Older people have fewer recurrent dislocations than younger people. In the noncompetitive athlete it is often prudent to assist the body in healing itself.

Practitioners should beware of the voluntary recurrent dislocator who can show you how they can actively, Houdini-like, dislocate the shoulder. Treatment for these individuals may not be rewarding. Abnormal collagen structure or a neuromuscular abnormality may be the cause.

If the acute dislocation is a result of a tearing of fibers, the goal of treatment is to hold the joint in a position of protection. Keeping the torn fibers approximated allows them to heal with the least amount of scar or laxity. Apply the principle to our case of seizure with posterior dislocation by holding the arm in a thoracobrachial cast or brace in which the elbow is posterior to the chest wall and the arm is externally rotated. It is intuitive to maintain the shoulder in this unusual position. Practice moving the arm around and reduplicate the position of dislocation; a posterior dislocation occurs often when the arm is extended forward and a large force directs the humeral head out the back of the joint. It is then obvious that reversing these positions would tend to keep the shoulder in a "reduced" position. Recent information has demonstrated that the position that approximates the torn fibers of the joint capsule in an "anterior" dislocation (the most common type of dislocation seen) is not what we most commonly use. Normally a "reduced" anterior dislocation is kept in an arm sling with the arm internally rotated. Itoi and coresearchers found, with the use of MRI, that the torn anterior capsule was most closely approximated with the arm held at 90 degrees of external rotation (63). This can be a difficult position to hold the patient in. Protection while healing is the precaution to take to allow the body to heal its injured tissues in the best way. Athletes can be protected from reinjury with braces. Hockey players may benefit from straps that inhibit the checking opponent from lifting their arm overhead, which may be the unstable position.

A tear of the labrum may not heal. A tear of the labrum at the anterior portion of the glenoid is called a Bankart lesion. If this is found in a recurrent dislocator or in a young athlete with an acute dislocation then surgical repair may be necessary. Surgery of the shoulder to repair instability is either open, through incisions, or endoscopic. More tools for minimally invasive repairs are becoming available. The results of acute repair of Bankart lesions are promising. In recurrent instability the goal of treatment is improvement (88,89). A double-blinded study on prolotherapy in knee osteoarthritis revealed statistically significant improvement in joint pain, subjective joint swelling, flexion range of motion, and knee buckling. There was also anterior cruciate ligament tightening by objective measures in the prolotherapy group (90).

Further information on this approach to soft tissue problems can be found in "Prolotherapy in the Lumbar Spine and Pelvis" (91). Internet resources can be located easily by logging onto the American Osteopathic Association website (*www.aoanet.org*) and following the links to the American Academy of Sclerotherapy, which contains multiple links that provide more information.

CONCLUSION

This chapter is not meant to discuss in any detail the surgical aspects of orthopedic treatment, even though these are the more exciting avenues for the surgeon. Acknowledgment and respect for the whole person and their inherent healing capacity, the interdependent relationship of structure and function and the need for rational therapeutic approaches form the foundation of the osteopathic approach to orthopedic medical and surgical problems. And so the reader is led back to the first illustration in this chapter, in which Andry likened the orthopedic surgeon to the gardener who nurtured his fruit trees so that, by gentle, steady guidance, they grew strong and straight. Andry espoused principles of orthopedic medicine that will always stay in favor (92).

John Spears, D.O., helped update the section on low back pain.

REFERENCES

1. Micropedia. *The New Encyclopaedia Britannica.* Vol VIII. Chicago, IL: Encyclopedia Britannica, Inc; 1987:1017.
2. Andry N. *L'Orthopedie.* Paris: La veuve Alix, 1741, as referenced in Peltier L. *Orthopedics: A History and Iconography.* San Francisco, CA: Norman Publishing; 1993:22.
3. Gracer R. Educational Committee Report. American Association of Orthopedic Medicine (AAOM). Board of Directors Meeting, June 5–6, 1993.
4. Walter GW. *The First School of Osteopathic Medicine.* Kirksville, MO: Thomas Jefferson University Press; 1992:63.
5. Herrmann E. Precepts and practice. *The DO.* October 1965:163–164.
6. Goldberg MJ. *The Dysmorphic Child: An Orthopedic Perspective.* New York, NY: Raven Press; 1987.
7. Staheli LT. *Fundamentals of Pediatric Orthopedics.* New York, NY: Raven Press; 1992.
8. Hensinger R. The changing role of ultrasound in the management of developmental dysplasia of the hip (DDH) [Editorial]. *J Pediatr Orthop.* 1995;15(6):723–724 . [This issue is a symposium discussing the complexities of DDH.]
9. Pavlik A. Stirrups as an aid in the treatment of congenital dysplasia of the hip in children. *J Pediatr Orthop.* 1989;9:157–159.
10. Mostert A, Pulp N, Castelein R. Results of Pavlik harness treatment for neonatal hip dislocation as related to Graf's sonographic classification. *J Pediatr Orthop.* 2000; 20:306–310.
11. Laor T, Roy DR, Mehlman CT. Limited magnetic resonance imaging examination after surgical reduction of developmental dysplasia of the hip. *J Pediatr Orthop.* 20(5):572–574.
12. Wolf S. In: Apple DF Jr, Hayes WC, eds. *Prevention of Falls and Hip Fractures in the Elderly.* Rosemont, IL: American Academy of Orthopedic Surgeons; 1994:120.
13. Loniewski EG, Williams JL, Jarski R, et al. The effectiveness of osteopathic manipulative treatment after hip or knee arthroplasty: a prospective, controlled, randomized, single-blinded outcome study. *JAOA.* 1995;95:492(abst).
14. Herzog RJ. Magnetic resonance imaging of the spine. In: Frymoyer J, ed. *The Adult Spine.* New York, NY: Raven Press; 1991:475.
15. Bigos S, Bowyer O, Braen G, et al. *Acute Low Back Problems in Adults.* Clinical Practice Guideline, No. 14. Rockville, MD.: US Department of Health and Human Services; December 1994. Public Health Service, Agency for Health Care Policy and Research. AHCPR publication 95-0642.
16. Waddell G, McCulloch JA, Kummel E, et al. Non-organic physical signs of low back pain. *Spine.* 1980;5:117–125.
17. White AA, Panjabi MM. *Clinical Biomechanics of the Spine,* 2nd ed. Philadelphia, PA: J.B. Lippincott Co; 1990:45.
18. American Academy of Orthopedic Surgeons. A glossary on spinal terminology. Quoted in: Frymoyer J, Pope MH. Segmental instability. *Semin Spine Surg.* 1991;3(2):109.
19. Denis F. The three-column spine and its significance in the classification of acute thoracolumbar spine injuries. *Spine.* 1983;8:817–831.
20. Andersson GB, McNeil T. *Lumbar Spine Syndromes, Evaluation and Treatment.* New York, NY: Springer-Verlag, 1989.
21. Mirkovic S, Garfin SR. Spinal stenosis: history and physical examination. In: Schafer M, ed. *Instructional Course Lectures.* Vol 43. Taunton, MA: American Academy of Orthopedic Surgeons; 1994:435–439.
22. Frymoyer JW, Gordon SL. *New Perspectives on Low Back Pain.* Park Ridge, IL: American Academy of Orthopedic Surgeons; 1989:217–241.
23. Weinstein J. Differential diagnosis and surgical treatment of primary benign and malignant neoplasms. In: Frymoyer JW, ed. *The Adult Spine.* New York, NY: Raven Press; 1991:41:851.
24. Ransford AO, Cairns D, Mooney V. The pain drawing as an aid to the psychological evaluation of patients with low-back pain. *Spine.* 1976;1(2):127–134.
25. Stein D, Floman Y. Psychologic approaches to the management and treatment of chronic low back pain. In: Weinstein JN, Wiesel SW, eds. *The Lumbar Spine.* Philadelphia, PA: WB Saunders; 1990:811–827.
26. King AI, Cavanaugh J, Fairbank J, et al. Diagnosis and neuromechanisms. In: Weinstein JN, Wiesel SW, Eds. *The Lumbar Spine.* Philadelphia, PA: WB Saunders; 1990:74–162.
27. Weinstein J, LaMotte R, Rudevile B. Nerve. In: Frymoyer JW, Gordon SL, eds. *Perspectives on Low Back Pain.* Park Ridge, IL: American Academy of Orthopedic Surgeons; 1989;4:35–110.
28. Barendse GA, Kessels AH, van den Berg S, et al. Randomized controlled trial of percutaneous intradiscal radiofrequency thermocoagulation for chronic discogenic back pain. *Spine.* 2001;3:287–292.
29. Saal JS, Saal JA. Management of chronic discogenic low back pain with a thermal intradiscal catheter. *Spine.* 2000;3:382–388.
30. Karasek M, Bogduk N. Twelve-month follow-up of a controlled trial of intradiscal thermal annuloplasty for back pain due to internal disc disruption. *Spine.* 2000;20:2601–2607.
31. McCulloch JA. Focus issue on lumbar disc herniation: Macro- and microdiscectomy. *Spine.* 1996;21[Suppl 24]:45S–56S.
32. Kahanovitz N, Viola K, McCulloch J. Limited surgical discectomy and microdiscectomy: a clinical comparison. *Spine.* 1989; 14:79–81.
33. Andrew DW, Lavyne MN. Retrospective analysis of microsurgical and standard lumbar discectomy. *Spine.* 1990;15:329–335.
34. Melton LJ, Kan SH, Frye MA, et al. Epidemiology of vertebral fractures in women. *Am J Epidemiol.* 1989;129:1000–1011.
35. Nevitt MC, Thompson DE, Black DM, et al. Effect of alendronate on limited-activity days and bed-disability days caused by back pain in postmenopausal women with existing vertebral fractures. *Arch Intern Med.* 2000;160:77–85.
36. Lieberman IH, Dudeney S, Reinhardt MK, Bell G. Initial outcome and efficacy of "kyphoplasty" in the treatment of painful osteoporotic vertebral compression fractures. *Spine.* 2001;26:1631–1638.
37. Kuslich SD, Danielson G, Dowdle JD, et al. Four-year results of lumbar spine arthrodesis using the Bagby and Kuslich lumbar fusion cage. *Spine.* 2000;20:2656–2662.
38. Anderson R, Meeker WC, Wirick BE, et al. A meta-analysis of clinical trials of spinal manipulation. *J Manipulative Physiol Ther.* 1992;15:181–194.

39. Andersson GB, Lucente T, Davis AM, et al. A comparison of osteopathic spinal manipulation with standard care for patients with low back pain. *N Engl J Med.* 1999;341 (19):1426–1431.

40. Atchison JW. Manipulation for the treatment of occupational low back pain. *Occup Med.* 1998;13(1):185–197.

41. Brodin H. Inhibition facilitation technique for lumbar pain treatment. *Manual Med.* 1987;3:24–25.

42. Bronfort G. Spinal manipulation. Current state of research and its indications. *Neurolog Clin North Am.* 1999;17(1):91–111.

43. Carey TS, Garrett J, Jackman A, et al and the North Carolina Back Pain Project. The outcomes and costs of care for acute low back pain among patients seen by primary care practitioners, chiropractors, and orthopedic surgeons. *N Engl J Med.* 1995;333:913–917.

44. Chrisman OD, Mittnacht A, Snook GA. A study of the results following rotatory manipulation in the lumbar intervertebral disc syndrome. *J Bone Joint Surg.* 1964;46:517–524.

45. Deyo RA. Non-operative treatment of low back disorders: differentiating useful from useless therapy. In: Frymoyer JW, ed. *The Adult Spine: Principles and Practice.* New York, NY: Raven Press; 1991:1567–1579.

46. Greenman PE. Syndromes of the L-spine, pelvis and sacrum. In: Stanton D, ed. *Manual Medicine. Physical Med Rehabil Clin North Am.* New York, NY: WB Saunders; 1996;7(4):733.

47. Haldeman S, Phillips RB. Spinal manipulative therapy in the management of low back pain. In: Frymoyer JW, ed. *Adult Spine: Principles and Practice.* New York, NY: Raven Press; 1991:1581–1605.

48. Koes BW, Assendelft WJ, van der Heijden GJ, Bouter L M. Spinal manipulation for low back pain. An updated systematic review of randomized clinical trials. *Spine* 1996;21(24):2860–2873.

49. MacDonald R, Bell CMJ. An open controlled assessment of osteopathic manipulation in nonspecific low back pain. *Spine.* 1990;15:364–370.

50. Mannion AF, Muntener M, Taimela S, Dvorak J. A randomized clinical trial of three active therapies for chronic low back pain. *Spine.* 1999;23:2435–2448.

51. Mein E. Low back pain and manual medicine. A look at the literature. In: Stanton D, ed. *Manual Medicine. Physical Med Rehabil Clin North Am.* New York, NY: WB Saunders; 1996;7(4):715–729.

52. Pope MH, Phillips RB, Haugh LD, et al. A prospective randomized three-week trial of spinal manipulation, transcutaneous muscle stimulation, massage and corset in the treatment of subacute low back pain. *Spine.* 1994;19(22):2571–2577.

53. Powell FC, Hanigan WC, Olivero WC. A risk/benefit analysis of spinal manipulation therapy for relief of lumbar or cervical pain. *Neurosurgery.* 1993; 33(1):73–78 (commentary: 78–79).

54. Seferlis T, Nemeth G, Carlsson AM, Gillstrom P. Conservative treatment in patients sick-listed for acute low-back pain: a prospective randomised study with 12 months' follow-up. *Eur Spine J.* 1998;7(6):461–470.

55. Shekelle P, Adams A, Chassin M, et al. Spinal manipulation for low back pain. *Ann Intern Med.* 1992;117:590–598.

56. Van Tulder MW, Koes BW, Bouter LM. Conservative treatment of acute and chronic nonspecific low back pain. A systematic review of randomized controlled trials of the most common interventions. *Spine* 1997; 22(18):2128–2156.

57. Asher MA, Strippgen W, Heinig C, Carson W. Isola instrumentation. In: Weinstein SL, ed. *The Pediatric Spine.* New York, NY: Raven Press; 1994:1619–1657.

58. Andrews JR, Zarins B, Wilk KE. *Injuries in Baseball.* Philadelphia, PA: Lippincott-Raven, 1998.

59. Norris T, ed. *Orthopedic Knowledge Update: Shoulder and Elbow.* Rosemont, IL: American Academy of Orthopedic Surgeons, 1997.

60. Cole BJ, Warner JJP. Anatomy, biomechanics, and pathophysiology of glenohumeral instability. In: Ianotti JP, Williams GR, eds. *Disorders of the Shoulder: Diagnosis and Management.* Philadelphia, PA: Lippincott, Williams & Wilkins,1999:207–232.

61. Soslowsky LJ, Flatow EL, Bigliani LU, et al. Quantitation of in situ contact areas at the glenohumeral joint. *J Shoulder Elbow Surg.* 1998;74: 46–52.

62. Halder AM, Kuhl SG, Zobitz ME, et al. Effects of the glenoid labrum and glenohumeral abduction on stability of the shoulder joint through concavity compression. *J Bone Joint Surg.* 2001;83-A(7):1062–1068.

63. Itoi E, Sashi R, Minagawa H, et al. Positions of immobilization after dislocation of the glenohumeral joint. A study with use of magnetic resonance imaging. *J Bone Joint Surg.* 2001;83-A(5):661.

64. Chester JB. Whiplash, postural control, and the inner ear. *Spine.* 1991;16(7):247.

65. Astrom M, Rausing A. Chronic Achilles tendinopathy: a survey of surgical and histopathologic findings. *Clin Orthop.* 1995;316:151–164.

66. Khan KM, Bonar F, et al. Patellar tendinosis (jumper's knee): findings at histopathologic examination. US and MR imaging. *Radiology.* 1996;200(3):821–827.

67. Nirschl RP, Pettrone FA. Tennis elbow: the surgical treatment of lateral epicondylitis. *J Bone Joint Surg (Am).* 1979;80(5):832–839.

68. Kraushaar BS, Nirschl RP. Tendinosis of the elbow (tennis elbow): clinical features and findings of histological, immunohistochemical, and electron microscopy studies. *J Bone Joint Surg (Am).* 1999; 81(2):269–278.

69. Ollivierre CO, Nirschl RP, et al. Resection and repair for medial tennis elbow: a prospective analysis. *Am J Sports Med.* 1999;23(2):214–221.

70. Khan KM, Cook JL, et al. Overuse tendinosis, not tendinitis. *Physician Sports Med.* 2000;28(5):38–48.

71. Puddu G, Ippolito E, et al. A classification of Achilles tendon disease. *Am J Sports Med.* 1976;4(4):145–150.

72. Kapetanos G. The effect of the local corticosteroids on the healing and biomechanical properties of the partially injured tendon. *Clin Orthop.* l982;163:170–179.

73. Ketchum LD. Effects of triamcinalone on tendon healing and function. Plast Reconstr Surg 1971;47:471.

74. Speed CA. Corticosteroid injections in tendon lesions. *BMJ.* 2001;1: 532–536.

75. Astrom M. Partial rupture in chronic Achilles tendinopathy: a retrospective analysis of 342 cases. *Acta Orthop Scand.* 1998;69(4):404–407.

76. Hay EM, Paterson SM, et al. Pragmatic randomised controlled trial of local corticosteroid injection and naproxen for treatment of lateral epicondylitis of elbow in primary care. *BMJ.* 1999;319:964–968.

77. Banks, AR. A rationale for prolotherapy. *J Orthop Med.* 1991;12(3): 54–59.

78. Oates JA, Fitzgerald GA, et al. Clinical implications of prostaglandin and thromboxane A2 formation. *N Engl J Med.* 1988;319(11):689–698.

79. Fuller RB. *Synergetics.* New York. NY: Macmillan; 1975.

80. Nelson KD. Continuous tension, discontinuous compression structures. 1965.

81. Levin SM. The icosahedron as the three-dimensional finite element in bio-mechanical support. In: *Proceedings of the Society of General Systems Research Symposium on Mental Images, Values, and Reality.* St. Louis, MO: Society of General Systems Research; 1986.

82. Levin SM. The importance of soft tissues for structural support of the body. In: Dorman T, ed. *Spine: State of the Art Reviews.* Philadelphia, PA: Hanley & Belfus, Inc. 1995;9:357–363.

83. Kroto H. Space, stars, C60, and soot. *Science.* 1988;242:1139–1145.

84. Ingber DE. The architecture of life. *Scientific American.* January 1998;48–57.

85. Chen CI. Tensegrity and mechanoregulation: from skeleton to cytoskeleton. *Osteoarthritis and Cartilage.* 1999;7(1):81–94.

86. Still AT. *The Philosophy and Mechanical Principles of Osteopathy.* Kansas City, MO: Hudson-Kimberly Publishing Co; 1902.

87. Liu YK, Tipton CM, et al. An in situ study of the influence of a sclerosing solution in rabbit medial collateral ligaments and its junction strength. *Connect Tissue Res.* 1983;11:95–102.

88. Ongley MJ, Klein RG, et al. A new approach to the treatment of chronic low back pain. *Lancet.* 1989;143–146.

89. Klein RG, Eek BC, et al. A randomized double-blind trial of dextrose-glycerine-phenol injections for chronic low back pain. *J Spinal Disord.* 1993;6:23–33.

90. Reeves KD, Hassanein K. Randomized prospective double-blind placebo-controlled study of dextrose prolotherapy for knee osteoarthritis with or without ACL laxity. *Alter Ther Health Med.* 2000;6(1): 68–80.

91. Dorman TA, ed. Prolotherapy in the lumbar spine and pelvis. *Spine, State of the Art Reviews.* Philadelphia, PA: Hanley and Belfus, Inc; 1995;9(2) (ISSN 00887-9869).

92. Peltier LF. *Orthopedics: A History and Iconography.* San Francisco, CA: Norman Publishing; 1993:21.

34

PULMONOLOGY

GILBERT E. D'ALONZO, JR.
SAMUEL L. KRACHMAN

KEY CONCEPTS

- Tight interaction between respiratory structure and function
- Viscerosomatic and somatovisceral reflexes and lung disease
- Thoracic lymphatic drainage
- Osteopathic manipulatory effects on pulmonary function and lymphatic drainage
- Prevention and treatment of lung disease, including pneumonia, chronic obstructive pulmonary diseases, respiratory distress syndrome, and postoperative pulmonary complications

Pulmonology is the study of lung diseases and it is a subspecialty of internal medicine. Having its beginnings in the diagnosis and treatment of tuberculosis, pulmonary medicine accelerated with the use of spirometry, flexible bronchoscopy, and the use of the mechanical ventilator outside of the operating room. Advances in cardiology and cardiothoracic surgery further supported the need for pulmonologists who have, for the most part, dominated the area of critical care medicine. Most recently, pulmonologists have become intimately involved in sleep medicine.

Osteopathic pulmonologists have been involved in the entire evolutionary process of pulmonary medicine. Osteopathic physicians who practice pulmonary, critical care, and sleep medicine are growing in number. The respiratory system is an absolutely ideal model to learn and explore osteopathic medicine and its practice and principles. Furthermore, the practice of both critical care and sleep medicine requires a keen knowledge of the body as a whole, with all of its integrative and communicative mechanisms. Osteopathic physicians are conceptually well prepared for these areas. The lungs are totally dependent on the thoracic pump, which is influenced by the entire musculoskeletal system and controlled by a large variety of neural and humoral signals. This makes the respiratory system, in both health and disease, a prime target for osteopathic research.

The respiratory system includes all of the components of the upper airway; the tracheobronchial tree, lungs, and pulmonary circulation which are enclosed in the thoracic cage and diaphragm; and the central nervous system with its peripheral connections. The central nervous system performs as a system controller, regulating the activity of the respiratory muscles and the thoracic cage, which functions as a pump. The pumping action of this organ system is essential for the lung's mechanism to exchange oxygen for CO_2 but it also assists in the return of venous and lymphatic fluids to the chest. This system provides adequate oxygenation, which is vital to end-organ function, releases at least one major end product of metabolism, CO_2, and participates in the homeostasis of acid-base metabolic balance on a moment-to-moment basis. The lungs are also involved in the elimination of various toxins and drugs, vocalization, and with pressurization of the abdomen, defecation, urination, parturition, and physical work. Malfunction of an individual component of the respiratory system or alterations of the relationships among various components can lead to disturbances in end-organ function and, eventually, in total body performance. The respiratory system is completely dependent on the musculoskeletal system for optimal performance.

The respiratory system, like other body components, is constructed to preserve function and maintain health. It depends on the proper function of other systems, and, of course, other systems depend on the process of respiration. Additionally, the lungs are organs that interface with the environment through the exchange of air that occurs with each breath. Each day, the lungs are exposed to more than 10,000 L of ambient air that may contain microorganisms, dusts, and chemicals. The exposure to these noxious substances is likely responsible in part for a wide variety of diseases, including infections, inflammatory conditions, and malignancies. However, the lungs possess certain defenses that reduce the likelihood that injury and disease will develop. The lungs and the entire breathing process participate in the body's self-regulatory, self-healing, and health maintenance processes.

Proper respiratory function depends on a delicate harmony with other systems, notably, but not exclusively, the cardiovascular, neuromuscular, and skeletal systems. Disease cannot occur in one system without affecting other body systems. The eventual extent generally depends on the severity of the initial disruption. In essence, the body attempts to function as a unit with a cadre of purposeful interrelationships and interdependencies between structure and function. Its goal is to enhance optimal function, ensure health, and prolong survival.

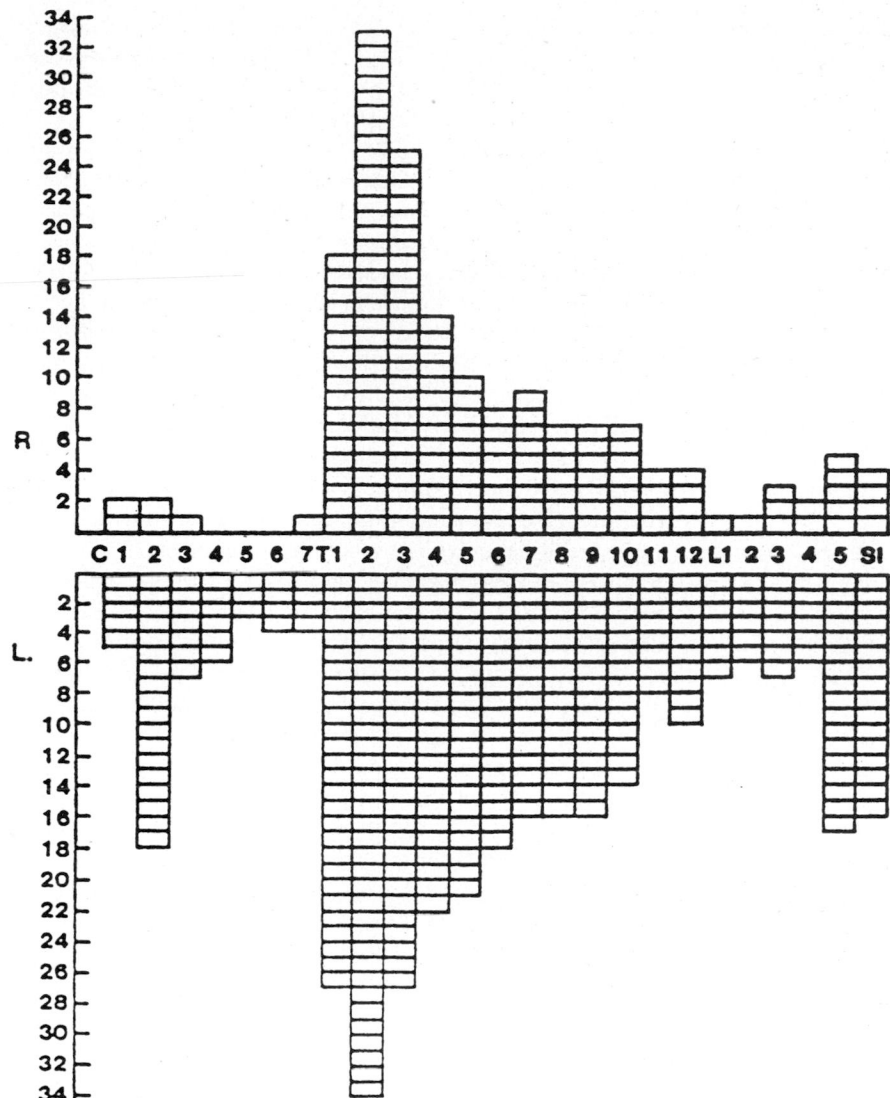

FIGURE 34.6. Location of somatic dysfunction in 40 patients with pulmonary disease.

thoracic excursion. OMT should not only improve breathing and respiration but also enhance the healing process for patients with inflammatory and infectious diseases involving the lung. Additionally, if manipulative treatment can enhance thoracic lymphatic drainage, then this process can also be associated with accelerated healing. Prophylactic rib elevation and thoracic pump techniques are likely useful in the prevention of venous stasis. They should play a role in prophylaxis of deep venous thrombotic disease and pulmonary embolism for patients at bed rest.

OMT may do more than improve motion and enhance blood and lymphatic flow related to the thoracic cage. Improving thoracic motion may have a positive influence in maintaining proper lung function and enhancing healing. Manipulation potentially has direct effects on the lung parenchyma itself. OMT likely affects the neurohumoral system in a way that benefits the lungs. Osteopathic research can make a major contribution to the health care of patients suffering from respiratory disease. Through the use of manipulative treatment, patients with respiratory disease could have improved functional performance during the daytime.

They could also enjoy enhanced sleep at night, with or without the concomitant use of standard medical therapy.

PULMONARY FUNCTION

Attempts have been made to determine how OMT alters physiologic function. Eggleston (16) and Detwiler (17) have observed the immediate favorable effects of OMT on vital signs, including respiratory rate. The design of these studies lacked proper controls, however, making it difficult to draw conclusions from their data.

A more carefully controlled study by Ortley and associates (18) designed experiments to determine, in healthy subjects, if measurable physiologic changes resulted from manipulation. Healthy male medical students were selected and participated in five interventional sessions, which included two control periods. There was an emphasis on observing the effects of OMT on respiration. High-velocity, short-amplitude manipulation was used as osteopathic intervention. A decrease in heart rate in a number of subjects and a decrease in skin resistance and respiratory rate in four of six subjects was found. In the four subjects who showed a drop in respiratory rate, three had a compensatory increase in tidal volume (V_T). The increase in V_T appeared to be the result of a greater abdominal diaphragmatic movement component. Manipulation had no effect on expiratory or inspiratory reserve volumes, VC, forced expiratory volumes, and maximal midexpiratory flow rate as determined by pulmonary function testing. Obvious problems with the study were that the subjects were healthy and only a few were studied.

A series of experiments observing the effects of OMT on pulmonary function was conducted by Murphy (19–21). Restricted breathing, including a loss in lung compliance, has been associated with altered lung gas exchange and the eventual development of hypoxemia. Improving restricted breathing improves gas exchange.

Murphy attempted to examine the influence of thoracic mobilization on selected pulmonary functions (19). Pulmonary function tests were performed before and after each thoracic mobilization or restriction procedure. Her early findings indicated that thoracic mobilization techniques in healthy subjects tend to decrease the FRC and RV, while increasing the total thoracic compliance. Restriction techniques tend to decrease the FRC and total compliance. RV appears to be increased, and it may be that air-trapping or uneven lung ventilation distribution is responsible for this change. In further studies, Murphy found that there is an increase in V_T and respiratory rate after thoracic mobilization, which results in an increase in alveolar ventilation (20).

In a technique that restricts breathing and thoracic mobilization, a decrease in V_T and an increase in respiratory rate are noted. At times there are minute ventilation increases, but overall alveolar ventilation remains decreased. Looking at the effect of nitrogen clearance from the lungs, thoracic mobilization clears nitrogen from the lungs faster. Any procedure that restricts breathing, creating a rapid shallow breathing pattern, reduces the clearance rate of this gas.

Murphy used a subsequent mathematical model to analyze the various factors that may have influenced the clearance of nitrogen from the lung. She concluded that, for nitrogen clearance to be enhanced, it is important to increase V_T and improve the distribution of gas in a homogeneous fashion throughout both lungs. This means that manipulation likely not only improves movement but also may improve ventilation homogeneity. In other words, OMT not only may improve movement factors of the thorax increasing bulk airflow with each breath but also may, with each breath taken, distribute air more evenly through the lungs, improving ventilation-perfusion relationships.

Finally, in her effort to further study this observation, Murphy used I-131-labeled human albumin to study the effect of thoracic mobilization on pulmonary capillary circulation (21). The method was used to look at the distribution of blood flow throughout the lungs. In healthy subjects, blood flow distribution may reflect the distribution of ventilation, since perfusion usually matches ventilation in lung disease and in healthy subjects. Murphy reported that thoracic mobilization increases the density of radioactivity throughout the lungs. This finding suggests that enhanced movement of the chest improves ventilation as suggested by these changes in lung perfusion. This process leads to improved lung oxygenation since ventilation-perfusion relationships within the lungs are enhanced.

Doran and colleagues (22) studied the role of spinal curvature on respiratory mechanics. They hypothesized that an alteration in lumbar lordosis induces changes in respiration. Their experience had been that many patients in the initial physical examination have an increased lumbar lordosis that manipulation can decrease. Experiments were performed to establish the reproducibility and variability of a table that they constructed to quantify the degree of lumbar lordosis. Once the reliability of their measurement table was determined, they recruited young adult volunteers. They assessed how OMT would affect respiratory function.

The test was administered using high velocity, low amplitude (HVLA) techniques with emphasis placed on treatment of the transitional areas of the spine. Respiratory function was measured for 15 minutes using both a pneumotachograph and a respiratory plethysmography, which assessed thoracoabdominal motion and timing. Following manipulative treatment, which often successfully decreased the lumbar lordotic curvature, there was a corresponding decrease in respiratory rate and an increase in V_T. A larger abdominal component to each breath, as compared with the thoracic component, was noted.

The Doran group concluded that one of the significant factors that correlates with impairment of respiration is the lordotic curve, and that OMT can alter this curve and favorably affect the mechanics of respiration.

These investigations, reported in abstract form, are hard to interpret. Most of the conclusions are based on minimal published data. A need exists for extensive controlled studies exploring the effect of OMT on pulmonary mechanics and gas exchange.

THORACIC PUMP

The thoracic pump has been investigated for its effect on respiratory function and its immunomodulating effect by a variety of techniques. Since the early reports of Miller in the 1920s (23,24), the thoracic lymphatic pump technique has been used as a research and treatment tool. More recently, Allen has been responsible for readdressing the potential value of the thoracic pump technique. He proposed a study to investigate the effects of this intervention on respiratory function in healthy subjects (25). The results of this study have yet to be published, but they have been obtained for some patients with respiratory disease who have received thoracic pump intervention. These patients have shown an improvement in VC, improved mobilization of the thoracic cage and spine, and more rapid clearing of airway secretions (26).

In a subsequent editorial, Allen and Kelso stated that patients who have been treated with the thoracic pump and mobilization of the thoracic cage and spine nearly uniformly experience a sense of well being and relief from pulmonary congestion, dyspnea, and the milder forms of air hunger (27). They claim that physicians have also observed improved sputum expectoration. In this same editorial, the authors provoke the osteopathic profession's interests in establishing a national clinical trial to explore not only the physiologic changes that occur with this form of manipulative intervention but also how these changes improve the quality of care of our patients.

Additional proposed mechanisms for the effectiveness of thoracic pump therapy center on an enhancement of immune function. In a preliminary investigation, Measel studied the effect of the thoracic pump on the immune response of healthy male medical students by measuring how two serologic tests changed in response to a subcutaneous administration of pneumococcal polysaccharide antigen, administered subcutaneously (28). The students, once treated by the thoracic pump technique, had an increased immune response on the basis of testing for polysaccharides 1, 3, 4, 6, 8, 14, 23, 25, and 56 by passive hemagglutination. This study suggests that the thoracic pump had a significant effect on the humoral or B-cell component of the immune system.

On follow-up Measel, in a double-blind study, evaluated the effect of the thoracic pump technique on peripheral blood, bone marrow, and thymic-derived cells, again in medical students (29). Preliminary results indicate that white cell counts rose and lymphocyte numbers decreased following lymphatic pump intervention. Additionally, the percentage of circulating T cells and B cells increased following therapy.

It appears, therefore, that thoracic pump therapy significantly changes the peripheral leukocyte blood picture in healthy individuals. In a pilot study, Paul and co-workers (30) attempted to determine whether interferon, an antiviral and antibacterial chemical, could be released or induced by thoracic pump manipulation. Twelve healthy adults were studied in a controlled fashion. Serum samples were drawn immediately before and at different times during the 24-hour period after manipulative intervention. Interferon levels were determined by a tissue culture technique that used a reduction of cytopathic effect as the endpoint variable. Mean pretreatment serum interferon levels were no different than the posttreatment levels in this acute study. This study does not discount the effectiveness of the thoracic pump maneuver in the treatment of infectious lung disease. It is possible that the classic agents necessary for interferon production may be required to initiate stimulation of interferon production and that the thoracic pump served to augment or enhance the response. Further research is necessary to clarify the usefulness of the thoracic pump technique for the augmentation of body interferon production.

A more recent study used a guinea pig model to explore the effect of thoracic pump technique on macrophage activity during lung infection with *Streptococcus pneumoniae* (31). This study may or may not relate to humans, but the sequence of experiments performed indicate that the thoracic pump technique has an effect on macrophage enzyme activity that could be important for the control of pneumonia with this organism in humans. Again, further controlled studies are necessary.

PREVENTION AND TREATMENT OF LUNG DISEASE

Osteopathic physicians typically treat respiratory disease by conventional means, but their options expand to a new level and

intensity with the appropriate use of OMT. As discussed earlier, a variety of manipulative techniques are useful in relieving thoracic cage discomfort, in facilitating inhalation and exhalation, and in improving overall ventilation and perfusion of the lungs. In addition to techniques that concentrate on paravertebral muscle disease, other techniques concentrate on improving rib motion and enhancing the performance of the secondary muscles of respiration, such as the cervical strap muscles and the superficial muscles of the thorax.

Thoracic pump techniques have been used to enhance the elimination of airway secretions and perhaps even increase the movement of fluids from lung parenchyma and pleural space. The thoracic pump techniques are often employed with rib elevation techniques. This combination of techniques has been proposed to prevent venous stasis throughout the body and to enhance fluid movement from the parenchyma of the lung.

Most osteopathic physicians do not treat specifically for the thoracic problem that is present but expand their therapy to treat the entire body. Although special attention might be directed at the cervical and higher thoracic area, for patients with respiratory disease it is not unusual to also treat somatic dysfunctions found in the lower thoracic, lumbar, and sacral areas. Treating the lower thoracic and lumbar areas can favorably influence abdominal muscle performance, which, at times, is essential in respiration. The patient's condition and response to manipulation should govern the frequency and intensity of each osteopathic manipulative intervention. Optimal timing has not been established.

Clinical studies of the effectiveness of the use of OMT in visceral diseases have been anecdotal, with small numbers of patients. The use of manipulation has been explored for patients with a variety of infectious diseases of the airways and lungs and with COPD, including asthma and emphysema. Limited information is available on using manipulative techniques in the management of respiratory distress syndrome and for the prevention of postoperative pulmonary complications.

RESPIRATORY INFECTION

The early osteopathic literature is full of anecdotal case reports and information discussing the use of OMT in the treatment of acute and chronic pneumonia. From the beginning of the 19th century to the middle of the 20th century, pulmonary tuberculosis was often treated adjunctively with manipulative intervention (32–38).

The older literature also has many articles focusing on using manipulative treatment in the management of patients who had bacterial pneumoniae other than tuberculosis (39–61). Most notably, several articles taught the effectiveness of osteopathic manipulative support for patients suffering from influenza pneumonia during the great flu epidemic of 1918 (48–53). These older studies are primarily anecdotal; no data are presented but there are eloquent descriptions of the benefits of OMT. Nonetheless, osteopathic physicians at that time and even today are convinced that manipulative treatment improves the course and outcome of patients with both acute and chronic infections of the chest. The literature cited in this chapter contains excellent descriptions of the techniques of manipulation used in treating pneumonia.

OSTEOPATHIC PHYSICAL MEDICINE AND REHABILITATION

J. MICHAEL WIETING
JAMES A. LIPTON

KEY CONCEPTS

- Definition of the specialty of Physical Medicine and Rehabilitation (PM&R)
- History of osteopathic PM&R
- Patient evaluation by the osteopathic PM&R specialist
- Use of osteopathic manipulation by PM&R physicians
- Research concepts and status
- Illustrative cases in osteopathic PM&R practice

DEFINITION OF THE SPECIALTY OF PHYSICAL MEDICINE AND REHABILITATION

Physical methods of healing have been practiced since prehistoric time; however, the specialty of physical medicine and rehabilitation (otherwise known as physiatry) did not become a recognized medical specialty until 1947. Most widely known as physical medicine and rehabilitation, this specialty is also known as rehabilitation medicine, physical and rehabilitation medicine, and as physiatry. The specialty today comprises the disciplines of physical medicine, rehabilitation medicine, and electrodiagnostic medicine.

Osteopathic physicians (DO) and allopathic physicians (MD) who specialize in physical medicine and rehabilitation (colloquially known as "PM&R") are called physiatrists. Physiatrists are specialists in the diagnosis and treatment of patients of all ages in three major subspecialty realms:

i. Physical medicine: diagnosis and treatment of musculoskeletal injuries and pain syndromes, including acute and chronic musculoskeletal diseases, sports and occupational injuries, and degenerative diseases including low back pain.
ii. Rehabilitation medicine: comprehensive rehabilitation of neurologic and musculoskeletal conditions, such as stroke, brain injury, spinal cord injury, amputations, burns, sports injuries, and others. The physiatrist often practices rehabilitation medicine while directing a team of medical rehabilitation professionals including, but not limited to, physical and occupational therapists, rehabilitation nurses, rehabilitation psychologists, speech-language pathologists, social workers/discharge planners, recreation therapists, vocational rehabilitation counselors, case managers, and others.
iii. Electrodiagnostic medicine: physical medicine and rehabilitation is the only specialty in medicine in which training in electrodiagnosis (nerve conduction studies, electromyography, and evoked potentials) is required.

Physiatrists are physicians who use physical agents and other medical therapeutic methods to assist in the healing and rehabilitation of patients. Treatment involves the entire person and addresses the physical, social, psychological, and emotional needs of the patient to achieve optimal restoration of quality of life so that potential for recovery is reached. Osteopathic physiatrists incorporate fundamental concepts of the body as a unit, the body's capability of self-healing/health maintenance, the interrelationship of structure and function, and the basis of treatment on understanding of body unity, self-regulation, and structure-function interdependence. Additionally, osteopathic physiatrists incorporate the use of osteopathic manipulative medicine (including structural diagnosis and osteopathic manipulative treatment) in their approach to treating patients.

After graduation from medical school, a minimum of 4 years of postdoctoral graduate medical education is needed for training as a specialist in physical medicine and rehabilitation. One year of this training, the internship, is devoted to the development of fundamental clinical skills; this year includes experiences in family practice, internal medicine, pediatrics, and general surgery or other critical care medicine. The remainder of the year may include any combination of a multitude of specialty experiences, including, but not limited to, neurology, orthopedic surgery, psychiatry, radiology, rheumatology, sports medicine, urology, or subspecialties of internal medicine (such as cardiology, pulmonology, nephrology, or oncology). On completion of the internship, an additional 3 years of residency training are needed in PM&R, which includes training regarding electrodiagnostic medicine, and the diagnosis, etiology, treatment, prevention, and rehabilitation of neuromusculoskeletal, cardiovascular, pulmonary, and other system disorders in patients of all ages.

Board certification may be awarded to physicians who complete a comprehensive written examination at the end of (or after completing) residency training and a rigorous oral examination after at least 1 year of full-time clinical practice, fellowship training, or an acceptable combination of these experiences.

HISTORY OF PHYSICAL MEDICINE AND REHABILITATION

It is well established that the use of manual procedures and manipulation dates back several centuries. Evidence exists to place the use of manipulation and manual procedures in Thailand over 4,000 years ago. The use of the hands to treat injuries and diseases was practiced by the ancient Egyptians, and the writings of Galen, Oribasius, and Celisies refer to manual procedures in medical practice. The 18th and 19th centuries saw renewed interest in the use of manual procedures. Dr. Edward Harrison, a 1794 graduate of the University of Edinburgh, developed a reputation in London for using manual procedures. Bonesetters became popular in England and the United States in the 19th century. Skilled bonesetting practitioners, such as Hutton, led the renowned Drs. James Paget and Wharton Hood to report in *The Lancet* and the *British Medical Journal* that medicine of the day should pay attention to the successes of contemporary bonesetting practitioners. The disenchantment of A. T. Still with the medical practice of his day led to the formulation of his new medical philosophy, which was called osteopathic medicine (1).

Physical medicine also dates back to ancient times. Hippocrates used traction and leverage to treat spinal deformities. Heliotherapy and hydrotherapy were recognized and used in Roman times. There was a void in the reported use of manual procedures that seems to correspond to the time of the split between physicians and barber surgeons. The role of manual techniques in patient care declined as physicians became less involved in patient contact and hands-on care was allocated to barber surgeons. This was also at the time of the bubonic plague, and it is possible that physicians were reluctant to have close personal contact with patients.

In the late 18th and early 19th centuries, applications of galvanic and faradic currents were prescribed as valuable therapeutic procedures for a variety of diseases and conditions. Around 1890, high-frequency currents from spark-gap diathermy machines were introduced to medical practice by d'Arsonval in France. In the early 1900s, the profession of physical therapy was developing along with new increased interest on the part of allopathic physicians who began to see the value of the approach to patient care that had been promulgated by the osteopathic profession for over a quarter of a century by then. The early 1900s was also a time of increased empirical trials, which provided evidence that physical medicine and manipulation were effective methods of intervention in musculoskeletal and other disease and injuries. The osteopathic profession was the source of many of these efforts, including the pioneering work of Dr. Louisa Burns and others. Osteopathic physicians, for example, were noted to apply the principles of hyperemia (stimulating blood flow to the spinal cord) in the treatment of infantile paralysis (2). During World War I, diathermy, electrical stimulation, heat, massage, and exercise were increasingly used as therapeutic tools in the U.S. (3). The early 20th century also saw proponents of electromagnetic therapy for musculoskeletal conditions. Allopathic physicians of that time began to join osteopathic physicians in the practice of "physiotherapy," using techniques gleaned from literature and from demonstrations in the U.S. and Europe. Col. Harry Mock of the U.S. Army medical corps referred to the importance of the use of physical and occupational therapies in the rehabilitation of wounded and other disabled persons in World War I (4). This was echoed after World War II by Dr. John Coulter, also of the Army medical corps (5). After World War I, empirical trials provided evidence that physical methods were useful to augment traditional medical care (6). Additionally, physicians were pioneering new medical applications of radiographs and other therapeutic methods. Investigations were initiated regarding the effectiveness of using functional activities to provide exercise and retrain coordination.

In the early 1920s, medical organizations, such as the American Medical Association Council on Physical Therapy and the American Society of Physical Therapy Physicians, were formed (6). These organizations (whose names were later changed numerous times) included physicians who practiced in the areas of physical medicine, physical therapy, radiology, and rehabilitation. The major organizations for physicians in the field of physical medicine and rehabilitation today include the American Osteopathic College of Physical Medicine and Rehabilitation, the American Academy of Physical Medicine and Rehabilitation, the Association of Academic Physiatrists, the International Society of Physical and Rehabilitation Medicine, and the American Congress of Rehabilitation Medicine. These organizations collectively represent approximately 75 years of development of the field of physical medicine and rehabilitation. Additionally, two major American medical journals have been developed to publish research in the specialty, the *Archives of Physical Medicine and Rehabilitation* and the *American Journal of Physical Medicine and Rehabilitation*. Journals are also published in Europe, the Middle East, and Asia.

Formal education for allopathic specialists in physical medicine and rehabilitation began in 1926 with short courses, 3 to 6 months in duration, in physical medicine at Northwestern University Medical School; these were later extended to 1 year. Before those courses, training in physical medicine was accomplished by preceptorships with experienced practitioners. Formalized training programs for physicians subsequently began to develop, initially under the auspices of the American Registry of Physical Therapists. In 1936, Dr. Frank Krusen established the first 3-year physical medicine residency program at the Mayo Clinic (6). Dr. Krusen, who coined the word "physiatry" to describe physicians who were dedicated to adding physical medicine to traditional medical therapeutics to treat neuromusculoskeletal disorders, is considered the "Father of physical medicine" (6). After World War II, with the advent of antibiotics and the addition of new medical technology, the awareness of American society of the need for more advanced treatment and rehabilitation care for disabled persons became heightened due to large numbers of soldiers returning from war with injuries and disabilities that had previously proved fatal. Additionally, the poliomyelitis epidemic received extensive publicity in the media of the day. These events created an increased demand for physicians who were trained in comprehensive medical and physical rehabilitation.

An interesting parallel event added to the demand for the specialty of physical medicine and rehabilitation. After World War II, Dr. Howard Rusk, a traditionally trained internist and military physician, noted that inactive, non-physically involved rehabilitation in convalescence resulted in functional deterioration in soldiers who were recovering from trauma or disease. As a result, the military had unprecedented numbers of soldiers who were not allowed to return to active duty. Dr. Rusk carried out a controlled experiment that demonstrated a dramatically improved return of strength, endurance, and overall function with an aggressive, patient-centered approach to rehabilitation. Subsequent to his military career, Dr. Rusk began private medical practice and made initial efforts to train physicians in the specialty of physical medicine and rehabilitation.

As the specialty of physiatry grew, the need for ongoing research and training programs became evident. Bernard Baruch, a noted philanthropist, chaired a committee that awarded grants to hospitals and medical schools to establish physical medicine and rehabilitation teaching and research programs. By the mid-1940s, numerous postdoctoral training programs in physical medicine and rehabilitation were established through this funding. In January of 1947, the advisory board of medical specialties (the precursor of the current American Board of Medical Specialists) formally recognized the American Board of Physical Medicine as a credentialing organization (6). In 1949, the name was changed to include rehabilitation to recognize that phase of the specialty. Early after the specialty was organized under one governing body, electrodiagnosis was introduced to the field for the purpose of evaluating neuromusculoskeletal pathology. It became evident that electrodiagnosis allowed physicians to more efficiently evaluate, from a qualitative, as well as a quantitative standpoint, pathology of the neuromusculoskeletal system.

After the 1950s, the specialty of physical medicine and rehabilitation grew rapidly. Increased research showed throughout the latter part of the 20th century that comprehensive rehabilitation decreased dependency and increased functional independence and quality of life for disabled persons. This created new demand for physiatrists and pointed to a need for additional training programs. Physical medicine and rehabilitation became a "shortage specialty" and remains so at this time. The specialty grew at unprecedented rates in the 1980s and the 1990s, and has continued to grow; however, as with other numerous other medical specialties, an inconsistent distribution of physiatrists from a geographic standpoint has developed. Today, the specialty of physical medicine and rehabilitation is a vibrant, thriving, exciting group of physicians who practice physiatric medicine in a variety of settings with a wide scope of interests and practice styles. There are currently over 80 accredited residency programs graduating over 300 physicians annually. The sole osteopathic program is at Michigan State University College of Osteopathic Medicine (and is dually/allopathically accredited as well). It is anticipated that the future will see additional osteopathically accredited residency programs in physical medicine and rehabilitation.

The 21st century brings many new challenges to physical medicine and rehabilitation. Much research is ongoing and many medical advances are anticipated. With these advances come new issues that bring technology to bear on medical ethics and the appropriate use of technology.

In the osteopathic profession, the specialty of rehabilitation medicine began in the late 1940s in response to osteopathic physicians who were interested in structural diagnosis and manipulation and the rehabilitation process. It became evident that an additional level of care was needed, and the osteopathic profession developed the practice affiliate, the American Osteopathic College of Rehabilitation Medicine, in 1954. The American Osteopathic Association added physiatry as a specialty in 1954. The prevailing attitude within the osteopathic profession at that time was that specifying "physical medicine" was a redundancy, as osteopathic training at that point emphasized physical medicine-oriented treatment, as opposed to allopathic medical schools, which neglected it. Thus, the osteopathic profession elected to designate the specialty as rehabilitation medicine. (This organization was renamed the American Osteopathic College of Physical Medicine and Rehabilitation in 2001.) The American Osteopathic Board of Rehabilitation Medicine (also recently renamed the American Osteopathic Board of Physical Medicine and Rehabilitation) was organized in 1954 to provide a credentialing mechanism for osteopathic physicians in the specialty of physiatry.

The specialty of physical medicine and rehabilitation is very compatible with the basic tenets of osteopathic medicine, which place emphasis on the concept based on the linkage of the science and art of medicine. Osteopathic physiatrists naturally embrace the concept of the body as a unit of the person—the body, mind, and spirit, the body's capability of self-regulation, healing, and health maintenance, the inter-relationship of structure and function, and the basis of treatment on these concepts.

An essential activity of the physiatrist is to establish lines of communication among members of the comprehensive rehabilitation team, which includes the patient, family and significant others, employer, and third-party payers, as applicable. Physiatrists evaluate disability using the concept of structure/function relationship, as patients must be actively involved in their own rehabilitation program.

PATIENT EVALUATION BY THE OSTEOPATHIC PHYSIATRIST

The osteopathic physiatrist practices from the perspective of the osteopathic philosophy of health enhancement and preventive health care with the belief that structure and function are integrated in healthy and diseased states. The osteopathic physiatrist makes use of the physical and biologic sciences related to health maintenance and disease prevention, and typically looks beyond the patient's presenting complaint in specific diagnosis and treatment. Biologic, psychological, behavioral, sociocultural, occupational, and environmental factors related to the patient's life are explored (7). These factors may have significant effect on the patient's illness and disability and may preclude maximal physical and psychological recovery. This broad-based approach to treatment addresses the body as an entire unit and from a functional point of view. As osteopathic physicians use manipulative procedures in the context of total patient care along with other accepted modalities, a systematic approach to medical problems has developed, which is properly designated as "manual medicine" (7).

The physiatric history and physical examination is the basis for all subsequent therapeutic decisions. The osteopathic physiatrist may encounter patients through referral from primary care, via secondary or tertiary specialists, or, as in many military and civilian settings, directly via an initial patient-physician contact. The patient's needs are variable—a simple, new diagnosis, a rehabilitation program for a well-established diagnosis, or perhaps an additional structural evaluation. Although any physiatrist can prescribe medications, modalities, or other therapies, the osteopathic physiatrist can provide a distinctive evaluation that is well-grounded in manual medicine. There are some diagnoses that are particularly amenable to such care. A good example would be the common condition of interscapular rib restriction. Although antiinflammatory medications can be used, expertly applied osteopathic manipulative medicine can immediately and safely address the root cause of the pain in a cost-effective manner. In addition to the conventional history and physical examination, the physiatric evaluation is somewhat different. The physiatric evaluation is based on a conventional history and physical examination; however, the physiatrist tailors the procedures of the conventional process to further clarify the functional problems of the patient. The physiatrist emphasizes functional capacity in the home and community throughout the evaluation. The osteopathic physiatrist determines not only physical deficits but also the functional impact of those deficits, because identification of functional problems allows determination of functional goals that become the basis for developing a therapeutic management strategy.

Evaluation by the osteopathic physiatrist identifies patient impairments (losses or abnormality of psychological, physiologic, or anatomical structure or function), disability (a restriction resulting from an impairment of the ability to perform an activity in the manner that is considered "normal"), and handicap (disadvantage resulting from the fulfillment of a societal role that is considered "normal" for an individual). Though patients may have multiple impairments, these might not cause disabilities or handicaps unless they affect the patient's ability to function in the home or community.

The physiatric history generally includes chief complaint, history of present functional problem, and functional history. The functional history typically will include assessment of mobility activities, activities of daily living (dressing, bathing, and hygiene activities), household and community activities, assessment of cognition, communication, vocational and avocational status, and the need for assistive devices. Psychosocial history will usually include assessment for substance abuse, psychiatric, or sexual history, and an evaluation of the patient's current living situation, vocational, and financial status. Medications, allergies, diet, past medical and surgical history, family history, and review of systems will also be included. In addition to the traditional examination, physiatric physical examination will focus on assessing function in the areas of mobility, activities of daily living, household activities, and driving. The examination will be focused on the neuromusculoskeletal system using inspection, palpation, evaluation of range of motion and contractures, assessment of joint stability, and manual muscle testing. Neurologic examination will evaluate the patient's overall cognitive status (including level of consciousness, mental status, and communication) and will also include assessment of sensation, cerebellar function, cranial nerves, muscle stretch reflexes, manual muscle testing, and speech and language function. The osteopathic physiatrist is trained to make unswerving use of a comprehensive history, physical examination, and diagnostic evaluation for even the most routine-sounding complaint. As an example, assessment of how the forces of gravity and impaired coping skills can affect a patient's overall function may need to be considered in developing a risk-benefit ratio associated with a proposed treatment regimen. A patient with low back pain may not achieve symptom relief unless both somatic dysfunction and concomitant gait dysfunction are addressed; if the patient also smokes as a reaction to stress, this may affect the number, types, and locations of other somatic dysfunctions (as in the rib cage) that can interfere with the primary complaint of interest. After collection of data and physical examination, the osteopathic physiatrist will formulate a problem-oriented summary that identifies the patient's major problems, which will include pertinent impairments, functional deficits, and medical and surgical issues. From this, the osteopathic physiatrist formulates a problem list with recommendations regarding rehabilitation issues along with a subsequent management plan noting treatment options for rehabilitation, as well as medical and surgical problems. The physiatric management plan is typically interdisciplinary and addresses functional deficits, physical impairments, psychosocial, medical, and surgical issues. Therapeutic precautions and appropriate treatment settings are also identified. Treatment goals are determined based on a realistic appraisal of rehabilitation and medical status and what is attainable after completion of the proposed treatment plan. Potential obstacles to achieving functional goals and the estimated time to achieve goals are also determined.

THE USE OF MANIPULATION IN PHYSIATRIC PRACTICE

The physiatrist is usually able to identify, through focused musculoskeletal examination, patients who are most likely to benefit from manipulative care. Although some manipulation techniques have applicability to hospitalized patients, most patients in physiatric practice who are appropriate for manipulation are encountered in the outpatient setting. This constituency includes patients with structural problems, such as vertebral rotations, pelvic asymmetry, sacral torsion, or other entities in which diagnosis relies on palpatory skills.

After performing a general physiatric examination, the osteopathic physiatrist will identify and treat any underlying pathology, including fractures, herniated discs, sprains, strains, hematomas, joint injuries, and peripheral and central neurologic injuries. Additional diagnostic studies will be employed as necessary. The physiatrist contemplating manipulative intervention performs a focused detailed history and structural examination in the area suggested by the symptoms or by the general examination. This typically involves observation, active gross and fine motion assessment, and general palpatory/motion examination. The structural and functional evaluation should begin from the moment the physician's senses contact the patient. Listening to and observing ambulation patterns, measuring symmetry of paired structures (such as malleoli, anterior and posterior superior iliac spines, inferior lateral sacral angles, and sacral-sulci), and observing transfers, dressing, and so on, may provide indispensable insights into the cause and treatment of multifaceted clinical presentations. Success of manipulative therapy in physiatric practice, as in other specialties, often depends on accurate palpatory diagnosis. Palpatory and segmental autonomic changes may be significant components of structural diagnosis.

Bony structure asymmetry, restrictive vertebral motion relative to adjacent vertebrae in flexion, extension, side bending and rotation, tissue texture changes, local tolerance to palpation or induced motion, and tenderness elicited over vertebral processes or by induced motion are generally included in evaluation of vertebral or segmental levels. Evaluation of passive motion for range, symmetry and amount of force needed to achieve full range is assessed in terms of quality or "end-feel" motion (1). Evaluation of combinations of vertebral motions are also included.

The osteopathic physiatrist will often "spring" vertebrae and examine for areas of tenderness or local pressure on interspinous ligaments; these techniques are useful in determining musculoskeletal function and loss of joint mobility (8). Subcutaneous tissue texture changes, such as edema or fibrosis, may also be noted on palpation and may indicate musculoskeletal pathology with associated segmental autonomic changes (8). Examination of the ribs, occiput, and pelvis in the structural examination is often included. The osteopathic physiatrist may determine that hypermobile musculoskeletal segments may not be amenable to manipulative intervention, but may indicate the presence of hypomobile segments in other locations and, if nontender, may be amenable to manipulation to resolve distant hypermobility (1). Thorough structural examinations, as noted, may add 5 to 10 minutes to an initial visit and less than 5 minutes to subsequent examinations. The osteopathic physiatrist choosing manipulation is advised that they should possess a relatively high degree of basic palpatory skills so that referral to another physician or a nonphysician manipulative practitioner can include specific identification of structural dysfunction. In addition, palpatory examination allows the osteopathic physiatrist to determine areas needing manipulative treatment and to establish a potential end point of manual care. The osteopathic physiatrist who possesses expertise in manipulative care has the ability to provide the patient (or referral source) a "one stop shop," at which a comprehensive evaluation, diagnosis, and nonsurgical treatment regimen can be provided. Osteopathic physiatrists who use manipulation have a variety of approaches available to them for manual treatment. Their individual armamentarium of treatment techniques depends on their training, their study with mentors, and the integration of and comfort level with particular techniques. Choice of technique may also depend on the patient being served. Many different treatment approaches are available; the interested reader is referred to numerous selected references for further inquiry in this particular area.

The availability of manipulative care depends significantly on geographic location and regional practice patterns. Osteopathic physiatrists who wish to use manipulation but do not provide it themselves generally refer patients to either a physician or licensed nonphysician provider. Referral to another physician practitioner generally works well, but potential problems exist, especially regarding referral of that patient. This issue can be satisfactorily addressed through a specific referral that states the exact nature and scope of evaluation and treatment requested, encouragement of discussion with the referring physician, and a statement that makes clear the intent of the physiatrist to resume the remainder of the patient's care. When referring to another physician (physiatrist or otherwise) for manual care, consideration should be given to how to recognize appropriate skill and training. Possible avenues to obtain skill in manipulation include certification by an osteopathic specialty board (which requires evaluation of capability in osteopathic principles and practice), attendance at postdoctoral courses offered by numerous osteopathic and allopathic sponsors, and certification of proficiency for competence in a particular manipulative approach (such as cranial osteopathy). The American Osteopathic Board of Neuromusculoskeletal Medicine (NMM) provides full board certification in osteopathic manipulative medicine and the American Academy of Osteopathy confers Fellowship on physicians certified in NMM who have undergone further testing in manipulative medicine and who have contributed in a significant way to the body of knowledge related to manipulation. If referral is to a licensed nonphysician practitioner, the problem to be treated must first be accurately diagnosed and a specific prescription must be written for manipulative care. Manipulative care can also be provided as part of a comprehensive therapy program; however, the physician should write a detailed prescription for the specific area to be treated and identify the diminished motion to be restored, as well as frequency and length of treatment. This enables the physician to monitor patient progress objectively and determine the end point and benefit of manipulative treatment.

Three main obstacles have been identified for physiatrists interested in performing manipulation: skill acquisition, skill maintenance, and economic considerations. Manipulative techniques are best learned on colleagues and fellow learners under close supervision. Studies suggest that the minimum learning time required may vary from 3 to 12 months depending on the modality (9,10). This extended period has significant ramifications for the practitioner. Because of enhanced safety and small potential for harm, sufficient skill can be acquired by most practitioners in 1 to 2 weeks of formal training in each of the types of manipulation, including isometric/muscle energy, counterstrain, myofascial release, and articulatory techniques. Training time for these approaches is shorter because inappropriate or nonindicated indirect technique, unless repeated frequently or over a prolonged period of time, rarely causes detrimental effects. These time frames are predicated on the osteopathic physiatrist having achieved basic skill proficiency in manipulative care during their initial medical training.

RESEARCH REGARDING MANIPULATION IN PHYSIATRIC PRACTICE

In recent years, scientific evidence for the efficacy of manipulation has been mounting in the treatment of numerous clinical entities that are commonly addressed by physician specialists in physical medicine and rehabilitation. Most inquiry has been aimed at acute musculoskeletal conditions and pain syndromes (11). The process has been somewhat slower in the area of chronic pain; however, objective evidence is becoming more apparent. The efficacy of manipulation for low back pain, for example, has been addressed in many previous studies and reviews. Manipulation was one of the recommended treatments for acute low back pain in the 1994 Agency for Health Care Policy and Research (now the Agency for Health Care Research and Quality) guidelines. Koes et al. (12) reported a randomized, prospective clinical trial of manipulative therapy for persistent, nonspecific back and neck pain. In this study, one group of patients with nonspecific back and neck pain complaints of at least 6 weeks duration received chiropractic spinal manipulative therapy and a second group received only exercise. Improvement in pain complaint was greater in the group receiving manipulative therapy than the other group after 12 months of follow-up. Vernon et al. (13) reported that manipulation was able to increase local paraspinal pain threshold levels in patients with chronic mechanical neck pain syndromes. Hurwitz (14) did an extensive review of randomized clinical trials of manipulation for persons with neck pain and headaches. Many high-quality studies demonstrated at least short-term benefits of manipulation. Gross and Fiechtner (15,16) demonstrated that the effectiveness of manipulation is enhanced when used with other concurrent treatment approaches, such as exercise and ergonometric adjustments. Winters showed that manipulation was very efficacious in treating shoulder disorders based on complaint, duration, and rate of treatment success (17).

Few studies have been reported that evaluate the efficacy of manipulation of sports injuries in controlled interventional trials. Cibulka and Delitto (18) have reported a statistically significant difference between hip mobilization versus sacroiliac manipulation in 20 runners with hip pain and sacroiliac dysfunction. Several studies have attempted to clarify the relationship between lower extremity function, lumbopelvic mobility, and sacroiliac and low back pain. Although these studies are primarily descriptive, they do have clinical relevance. Muscle imbalances, with resultant pain and dysfunction, have been described by Janda (19) and others (20). The collaborative efforts of Greenman, Janda, and Bookhout have provided a working clinical paradigm that, when used diagnostically and as a basis for exercise prescription, enhances manual medicine treatment (1). The exact physiologic reasons for the efficacy of manual treatments are not often well understood. There are theoretical constructs that address, among other things, a bony alignment, muscle link, muscle and spindle tone, neurologic and nociceptive input, central nervous system processing, psychological factors, and others (21). The actual act of human touch undoubtedly contributes to the patient's experience (21). This is a complicated issue that incorporates many aspects of the human experience, including pain, function, philosophy, psychology, and social milieu (21). It is hypothesized that if these issues are more rigorously researched, it is likely that the efficacy of manual therapy (as is true in many other aspects of medicine) will be multifactorial in nature.

In the area of chronic pain, Greenman and associates (1) found that manipulation can be quite effective in not only relieving acute musculoskeletal pain caused by manipulable somatic dysfunction, but also may occasionally help in reducing reported pain levels in the chronic pain population (7). Manual medicine has recently been shown to be useful for chronic neck and low back pain (22,23). The most valuable purpose of manipulation in the chronic pain population is to assist in increasing physical activity to productive levels. These researchers have two hypotheses regarding the relationship between chronic pain and somatic dysfunction:

i. The somatic dysfunction may have been a primary pain generator during the acute stage (which had not yet completely resolved), and this unresolved dysfunction had been an ongoing source of nociception responsible for causing changes in the central nervous system (functional pathology), which perpetuates pain perception. The somatic dysfunction may have continued or recurred as a pain responder and may have developed into a secondary pain generator. Had this dysfunction been treated in a timely fashion (during the acute phase), central changes may not have occurred and the chronic pain syndrome would not have developed.

ii. The somatic dysfunction may primarily be a response to an already altered central nervous system output (pain responder) caused by a nonrelated source of nociception, such as degenerative disc disease.

Because of the vicious cycle that is established in both of these hypotheses, treatment could result in improved motion, but pain relief may not occur, or be short-lived, even if the somatic dysfunction can be corrected. Dependency on manipulation (as with any other passive modality) could quite easily occur because of temporary pain relief. In their chronic pain population, Greenman, Stanton, and Wieting found that maximal benefit was usually obtained with eight to ten sessions of manipulation over a 2 to 3 month period (7). The judicious, periodic use of manipulation to maintain achieved levels of musculoskeletal function is often necessary over longer periods of time. Exercises prescribed specifically for persistent or recurrent somatic dysfunction have been found to be effective by Bourdillon et al. (24). These exercises can be easily learned and performed independently by the patient. Regular daily physical activity (e.g., work) has also been shown to be effective in maintaining restored musculoskeletal function. Numerous studies have shown that rest and sedentary activities are counter-productive.

An additional benefit is obtained by body contact through the application of hands directly on the areas of complaint. Symptoms can often be reproduced during the palpatory structural examination. This evaluation facilitates trust in the physician by demonstrating attention to those specific areas that have been perceived by the patient as being a causative factor of pain. This is consistent with the patient's expectations for evaluation and treatment. Further, the manipulative process by the astute physiatrist may, on occasion, facilitate an emotional response on the part of the patient that is manifested by voluntary disclosure of personal information, and which allows the physician and patient to gain insight into the stressors and suffering that often are a significant part of a chronic pain syndrome. Healing is facilitated by creating an effective connection between mind and body, thus rejecting the Cartesian theory of mind/body separation (7). It is felt that this connection must be augmented through a cooperative effort between the physician, the patient, and other members of the treatment team. The chronic pain patient is best served by assisting with restoration of normal physiologic movement patterns and with the development of health-promoting thought patterns and beliefs. The patient regains physical and psychological "normalcy," and the central nervous system "resets" and readapts to a more physiologic mode. To achieve desired total outcome, functional restoration must also include social and vocational integration within the family and community.

Physiatrists see a preponderance of individuals with "failed low back pain syndrome." The goal of rehabilitation is to achieve functional restoration with return to full activity, including work, on a long-term basis. Greenman (25) reported the incidence of sacroiliac dysfunction, for example, in a population of 183 such low back pain patients. An increase in the incidence of restricted motion in the sacroiliac joint and symphysis pubis was noted. These dysfunctions (lesions of skeletal, arthrodial, myofascial, or related structures) included pelvic obliquity and sacral base unleveling (short leg/pelvic tilt syndrome), pubic dysfunction, anterior nutational restriction of the sacrum, innominate sheer dysfunction, nonneutral lumbar dysfunction, and muscle imbalance of the lower extremities and trunk. Two or more of these aforementioned dysfunctions were found in 86.3% of patients, and only five patients had none (25). Diagnosis was made with a thorough history and physical, including palpatory structural examination. Indicated imaging and laboratory studies were also recommended to rule out other causes. The patient's usual presentation was with a history of low back pain, usually unilateral, overlying the sacroiliac region and radiating to the buttock and lower extremity, usually involving the posterior and posterior-lateral thigh. Seventy-five percent of patients were able to return to full premorbid activity, including work for those who were employed, after completing a manual medicine and functional restoration rehabilitation program lasting approximately 7.8 months (with the majority completing this program in less than 6 months) (25).

It would seem that the vast majority of persons with chronic pain adapt, compensate, and continue to function well without incapacitating distress. There are, however, many who, for whatever reason, have extreme distress, suffer significantly, and are unable to maintain their usual roles within the family and community. A clear distinction should be made between the physical impairment, the suffering, and the disability. It generally makes no difference whether or not there is demonstrable evidence of injury (i.e., verifiable anatomic change); the net effect is the same. Those who become dysfunctional are dependent on their families, the health care system, and the social welfare system (including worker's compensation) in varying degrees. Successful treatment approaches must address this dependency. Psychological variables have been shown to be related to both chronic pain and the transition from acute to chronic pain (26). Ten percent of chronic back pain individuals in the worker's compensation system, for example, account for 80% of the cost to that system (27). Much of the dependency seen in the chronic pain population is iatrogenic with all specialties and treatment approaches implicated. Manipulation is no exception. Any treatment approach must help patients understand their situation, promote a healthy functional belief system, encourage physical activity, promote social and vocational reintegration, restore self-esteem and confidence, and teach strategies to allow patients to control their pain rather than the pain controlling them. The job of the osteopathic physiatrist in this case is to help patients conquer the chronic pain syndrome, not to blame them for it.

The successful outcome of any procedure depends on the expectation for it. The osteopathic physiatrist, in approaching chronic pain patients, acts consistently as if the persistent pain is caused by functional pathology within the central nervous system, which cannot be objectively identified by currently available methods. Regardless of proven or suspected initial etiologic nociceptive sources, the objective is to treat with the hope of pain relief but not to expect it. As Wall (28) eloquently stated, "Our task is not so much to cure pain as to aid recovery."

RETURN TO WORK/DUTY ISSUES

The cost-avoidance and potential savings experienced through a fiscally responsible evaluation and treatment program is of interest to both allopathic and osteopathic physicians. The osteopathic physiatrist can, and often does, diagnose, treat, and resolve many simple and complex issues through effective use of osteopathic principles and manipulative care. This is particularly valuable in the instance of patients in military and critical nonmilitary functions. In these cases, the return to full duty of a person with work restrictions results in significant recovery of lost productive time and cost savings. Maximal operational efficiency of military personnel may, in fact, be essential to national security. There are many specific diagnoses where osteopathic care (including manipulation) may offer the fastest, safest, most specific treatment course possible. In a nation faced with staggering losses of productivity and associated cost from musculoskeletal conditions, specific, effective care using osteopathic principles offers an especially attractive option to improve health and work force effectiveness.

ILLUSTRATIVE CASES OF OSTEOPATHIC PHYSIATRIC PATIENT CARE

Low Back Pain

Low back pain is second only to headache as a cause of pain in the industrialized world, and it is the leading cause of financial expenditure for worker's compensation (29). In the U.S., the annual cost of low back pain is approximately 16 billion dollars per year (30). Studies have suggested that 25 million Americans have lost one or more days of work annually because of low back pain, and approximately 2% of workers each year submit disability claims attributed to low back pain (31).

It is estimated that 50% to 80% of adults will have low back pain in their lifetime (32). A 1985 telephone survey of 1,254 Americans revealed that 56% of the adult population of the United States had some low back pain in the year preceding the survey, and that 3% of those had low back pain for more than 1 month (31). Studies have suggested a lifetime low back pain rate of about 60% to 90%, and an annual rate of about 5% (33,34). Low back pain is commonly addressed in physiatric practice. To evaluate low back pain, the osteopathic physiatrist must understand pertinent risk factors (which include occupational, patient-related (such as age, gender, postural, mobility, strength and fitness considerations), and the anatomy and kinesiology of the lumbosacral spine. The evaluation of the patient with low back pain begins with history but also includes physical examination (via inspection, palpation and percussion, and assessment of range of motion) a neurologic evaluation (including gait, station, coordination, muscle stretch reflexes, muscle bulk and strength, and sensation), and appropriate diagnostic studies (including, but not limited to, imaging studies and electrodiagnosis) as appropriate.

Structural and manual medicine evaluation should include motion testing (of the thoracolumbar region) with emphasis on forward and backward bending, side-bending, and rotation. Intrasegmental motion testing should be accomplished in positions of rotation, flexion, extension, and side-bending. Additionally, evaluation for scoliosis is also indicated. Both direct and indirect manipulative techniques can be brought to bear on low back pain. Muscle energy techniques can address both type I neutral (group) curves and type II somatic dysfunctions (involving single segments). Counterstrain can be employed to treat anterior tender points, (especially in the supine position) and posterior tender points (with the patient prone). Common tender points include L1, L2, abdominal L2, L3, L4, and L5 anteriorly, and L1 and the posterior points of L1-5, L3-5 upper pole, and L5 lower pole. High velocity/low amplitude thrust can also be used effectively to treat somatic dysfunctions of the lumbar spine.

An apparently healthy aviator in his early 40s presented with a complaint of lumbar pain that prevented him from flying, presumably from the forces encountered during take off. None of his fellow aviators had complained of back pain, although they experienced the same schedule of flight operations. The patient was reluctant to complain of pain and would rather have deferred seeking medical attention. He did his best to downplay his pain, yet his seeking medical care was significant. The patient's medical history was completely unremarkable except for awaking at night to note low back pain. Nonstructural physical examination was unremarkable until structural components were examined. The patient was noted to have a physiologic short right leg, elevated right anterior superior iliac spine, and a right-on-right (forward) sacral torsion. Although diagnosis of gait dysfunction and sacral somatic dysfunction was considered and addressed, it is important to also consider other etiologies of this musculoskeletal presentation. Additional diagnostic studies were ordered, including complete blood count, erythrocyte sedimentation rate, blood chemistry, urine analysis, and plane films of the lumbosacral spine. The patient was noted to have markedly elevated urine protein. An orthosis and manipulation reduced the patient's back pain by two-thirds within 3 days and completely eliminated it within 1 week. On repeat testing, urine protein continued to be markedly elevated. After referral to a nephrologist, the patient eventually underwent renal biopsy confirming the additional diagnosis of focal glomerular nephrosis. The patient was subsequently placed under treatment with an angiotensin-converting enzyme inhibitor and scheduled to receive appropriate physiatric and nephrologic follow-up. After additional care, the patient ceased to have nocturnal awakening, his back pain did not return, and he resumed normal flight status.

In addition to manipulative care, a comprehensive approach also includes therapeutic exercise that is designed to establish and maintain musculoskeletal structural integrity. Evaluation of lumbar lordosis and the muscles that act to attain and maintain it is indicated. Strengthening of the upper and lower abdominal muscles, stretching of low back and gluteal muscles, as well as pelvic tilt to decrease lumbar lordosis and exercise to increase lumbar

flexibility are also appropriate. Stretching of back extensors and anterior pelvic muscles, as well as hip flexors and hamstrings is a part of manual care. Maximizing the patient's involvement in a therapeutic exercise program is needed to optimize functional outcome.

Carpal Tunnel Syndrome

Carpal tunnel syndrome is one of the most common forms of repetitive stress injury. It is a condition that can be caused by repetitive motion, often in the workplace or during leisure activities. This painful condition is caused by swelling of the flexor tendons of the hand. The flexor tendons, median nerve, and deep radial artery and vein pass from the forearm to the hand through the narrow carpal tunnel, which is composed of bones and ligaments in the wrist. When these tendons and surrounding membranes swell, pressure is exerted on the median nerve, causing pain, numbness, or tingling. Repetitive stress injuries, such as carpal tunnel syndrome, are some of the fastest growing workplace injuries. Carpal tunnel syndrome is one of the leading causes of lost work days, with employees averaging 30 days away from work. Repetitive stress injuries often top the list of lost time injuries and illnesses reported by American employers. Treatment of carpal tunnel syndrome by the osteopathic physiatrist can be simple or complex depending on the severity and frequency of symptoms. Treatments can include physical therapy, stretching, special braces or splints, ice, strengthening exercises, and antiinflammatory medications or steroid injections. Surgery is usually a last resort for patients who do not respond to conservative treatment. Early diagnosis and treatment improves the chances for successful functional recovery.

Sucher (35) demonstrated that physician-applied, three-phase soft tissue myofascial release, in combination with self-stretch of the carpal canal, is very effective in the treatment of mild to moderately severe cases. This manipulative approach involves:

i. "Opening" the carpal canal with stretching and release of the transverse carpal ligament to increase space within the canal, thereby decreasing pressure on the median nerve. This procedure reverses the natural tendency toward flexion of the carpal canal and subsequent narrowing of the carpal space.
ii. Release of the true myofascial component of the carpal canal, the attachment of the abductor pollicis brevis muscle.
iii. Indirect stretch of the distal carpal canal with internal distention/dilation of the canal.

Through magnetic resonance imaging analysis of the cross-sectional area of the carpal tunnel and electrodiagnostic study, this technique has been shown to produce clinical improvements in the form of reduced distal latencies and increased motor response amplitudes (36). Additionally, the antero-posterior and transverse dimensions of the carpal canal were shown to significantly increase after this treatment (36). Further studies by Sucher and Hinrichs (37) have shown that osteopathic manipulative techniques show promise for nonsurgical relief of pressure on the median nerve in patients with carpal tunnel syndrome through lengthening the distal transverse carpal ligament.

Cervical Sprain/Strain

Perhaps the most commonly encountered cervical disorders in physiatric practice involve sprain and strain trauma to the cervical spine. A sprain is a tearing or stretching of ligament or tendon structures due to joint trauma; a strain is a muscular injury. The most frequent cause of cervical sprain/strain in the U.S. is "whiplash," with greater than one million cases reported per year (38). The classical mechanism of injury involves cervical spine hyperextension as the result of a motor vehicle collision from the rear, or if the patient is in a moving vehicle that strikes a nonmoving object. Although such injuries may involve ligaments, tendons, and muscles, the osteopathic physiatrist must also consider potential injury to the nerve root, cranial nerves, or associated joints (such as the temporomandibular joint).

A diagnosis includes history of neck and headache pain and possibly associated stiffness and fatigue. Physical examination frequently reveals diminished range of motion of the neck, tenderness to palpation (both anteriorly and posteriorly), and facet joint tenderness. Special attention should also be given to structural abnormalities and somatic dysfunctions involving cervical and other areas of the spine, as well as assessment of areas of sympathetic hyperactivity. Treatment should be individualized for the patient and may include medications (such as nonsteroidal antiinflammatory drugs and other analgesics) for pain or sleep disturbance and physical therapy modalities (such as massage, ultrasound, electrical stimulation, and any therapeutic exercise program that focuses on appropriate neck muscle position and posture).

Manipulative treatment should be used to decrease edema and acute tissue reaction. Generally, gentle indirect approaches using myofascial or facilitated positional release or counterstrain are most helpful in acute injury to the cervical and upper thoracic region. Passive range of motion exercises and lymphatic drainage can also be used. Subsequently, muscle energy and/or myofascial release can be used to restore respiratory motion in the cranium and sacrum and to restore motion in the pelvis and sacrum. Patients with more long-term symptoms may require manipulation of other areas of the body in addition to the cervical region. Beginning with soft tissue techniques, the osteopathic physiatrist can then employ direct or indirect techniques along with a vigorous active range of motion program.

Manipulation in Sports Rehabilitation Medicine

The purpose of using manipulation in the practice of sports rehabilitation medicine is to provide an adjunct in the treatment of many nonsurgical musculoskeletal mobility impairments resulting from injury or, occasionally, to provide primary treatment to decrease pain and speed return to activity. The global objective is to restore normal pain-free motion with the highest level of motor control and coordination in a state of postural balance that allows the athlete to perform at the highest level of his or her ability.

Manipulation is an appropriate adjunct to the rehabilitation of sports-related injuries. Timing, however, should be appropriate. Treating an acutely inflamed area with direct techniques may aggravate inflammation and increase pain. Indirect techniques (such as counterstrain and myofascial release) may help to decrease inflammation. A manual medicine approach should be considered an integral part of comprehensive sports rehabilitation. In addition to the PRICE (protection, rest, ice, compression, elevation) protocol, nonsteroidal and other antiinflammatory medications, muscle relaxants, analgesic medications, as well as physical and occupational therapy and physiatric-directed therapeutic exercise can also be employed. Because of the benefits of manipulation and pain relief resulting from muscle relaxation, the use of medications can often be minimized. This is helpful to athletes in sanctioned sports, as well as recreational athletes, who avoid medication because of the side effects and disallowance of competition. Many medications (including narcotics, analgesics, and some muscle relaxants) are banned by athletic organizations.

As an example, the knee is the most frequently injured joint in sport activity (39). Diagnosis and management of knee injuries requires a detailed knowledge of functional knee anatomy, mechanism of injury, the pertinent sport, and the most common sport-related knee injuries. Structural examination of the knee must certainly include evaluation of patellar tracking, tibial head motion, assessment of any effusion, edema, pain, popping, locking, or "giveaway," as well as range of motion and leg length symmetry. Evaluation of a knee injury should also include assessment of the hip, ankles, feet, and lumbar spine, as well as the function of pertinent muscles in other structures of the knee joint. Patellofemoral dysfunction, iliotibial band syndrome, patellofemoral dislocation, tendonitis, and anterior cruciate ligament trauma should also be evaluated.

In an osteopathic manual medicine approach to knee injury, evaluation and treatment of acute fractures and other serious injuries is accomplished first, with soft tissue and other structural problems being treated secondarily. Knowledge of the pertinent sport, as well as its associated equipment, will give the osteopathic physiatrist insight into the effect that these factors may have on injury to the knee. Classically, shoe spikes, playing surface, and other factors may affect the likelihood of injury. Manipulative treatment may be used to regain or maintain range of motion while the knee is healing and to correct or prevent contractures associated with the healing process. In the initial manipulative approach to restoring motion of the knee and its associated components, a passive indirect technique, such as myofascial release, counterstrain, and soft tissue, may be employed. These can be later followed with more direct approaches, such as muscle energy and high velocity/low amplitude thrust. As in previous examples, manipulative treatment should also have, as an adjunct, an appropriately directed therapeutic exercise program that will generally involve stretching and strengthening of knee flexors and extensors, paying special attention to the medial quadriceps. Prokop and Wieting (40) describe stretching and articulatory technique approaches to increase joint play in patellar restriction. These techniques are often helpful for treating knee injuries to football players, runners, and athletes participating in other sports.

Many patient complaints to osteopathic physicians in all specialties are musculoskeletal in nature and may be ideally treated by physical rather than pharmacologic or surgical approaches. The osteopathic approach involves a comprehensive, patient-centered system of health care with manipulation as a useful adjunct. Manipulation and manual medicine are natural compliments to other methods of musculoskeletal care. Palpatory skills are an essential aspect of patient examination and evaluation, and manipulation is very useful in improving range of motion and decreasing pain, thereby increasing functional benefits to the patient. Manual medicine, and more specifically manipulation, have benefited from the rehabilitative concepts of functional reactivation and transitioning from patient-passive to patient-active care, as promulgated by Stanton and Mein (41). Although the use of manipulation is not intended as an all-inclusive treatment approach, it is a valuable system of patient care when used in the context of total care integrated with other appropriate procedures. It is our hope that this chapter will stimulate the interest of the reader in the valuable role of manual medicine and manipulative procedures in physiatric practice, and that the reader's appetite to learn more about manual medicine and the specialty of physical medicine and rehabilitation will be stimulated.

ACKNOWLEDGMENTS

The authors appreciate and acknowledge the assistance of Debra Summers, Curatorial Assistant at the Still National Osteopathic Museum, and the National Center for Osteopathic History in Kirksville, Missouri, in researching the early history of osteopathic physical medicine.

REFERENCES

1. Greenman PE. *Principles of Manual Medicine.* Philadelphia, PA: Williams & Wilkins; 1989:1–2.
2. Millard FP, ed. *Poliomyelitis.* Kirksville, MO: Journal Printing Co; 1918.
3. Krusen FH. *Physical Medicine: The Employment of Physical Agents for Diagnosis and Therapy.* Philadelphia, PA: WB Saunders; 1941:9–143.
4. Mock HE. Rehabilitation. *Arch Phys Med Rehabil.* 1943;24:676–78.
5. Coulter JS. History and development of physical medicine. *Arch Phys Med Rehabil.* 1947;28:600–602.
6. The History of Physiatry. Association of Academic Physiatrists website. Available at: http://www.physiatry.org. Accessed , May 14, 2002.
7. Stanton DF, Wieting JM. Osteopathic Medicine and the Role of Manipulation in the Treatment of Chronic Pain. In: Anchor KN, Felicetti TC, eds. *Disability Analysis in Practice.* Dubuque, IA: Kendall Hunt; 1999:112–113.
8. Rechtien JJ, Andary MT, Holmes TG, et al. Manipulation, Massage, and Traction. In: DeLisa JA, ed. *Rehabilitation Medicine: Principles and Practice,* 3rd ed. Philadelphia, PA: Lippincott-Raven Publishers; 1998:523.
9. Lewitt K. *Manipulation Therapy in the Rehabilitation of the Motor System.* London, England: Butterworth-Heineman; 1985.
10. Maigne R. *Diagnosis and Treatment of Pain of Vertebral Origin.* Baltimore, MD: Williams & Wilkins; 1996.
11. U.S. Department of Health and Human Services. Acute Low Back Problems in Adults (AHCPR Publication No. 95-0642). Washington, DC: U.S. Government Printing Office; 1994.
12. Koes BW, Bouter LM, Van Mamereu H, et al. Randomized clinical trial of manipulative therapy for persistent back and neck complaints: Results of one year follow-up. *BMJ.* 1992;304:601–605.
13. Vernon HT, Aker P, Burns S, et al. Pressure pain threshold evaluation of the effect of spinal manipulation in the treatment of chronic neck pain: A pilot study. *J Manipulative Physiol Ther.* 1990;13(1):13–16.
14. Hurwitz EL, Aker PD, Adams AH, et al. Manipulation and mobilization of the cervical spine: A systematic review of the literature. *Spine.* 1996;21(15):1746–1759.
15. Gross AR, Aker P, Quartly C, et al. Musculoskeletal medicine: Manual therapy in the treatment of neck pain. *Rheum Dis Clin North Am.* 1996;22(3):579–598.
16. Fiechtner JJ, Brodeur RR. Manual and manipulation techniques for rheumatic disease. *Rheum Dis Clin North Am.* 2000;26(1):83–96.
17. Winters JC, Sobel JS, Groenier KH, et al. Comparison of physiotherapy, manipulation, and corticosteroid injection for treating shoulder complaints in general practice: Randomized single blind study. *BMJ.* 1997;314:1320–1325.
18. Cibulka MD, Delitto A. A comparison of two different methods to treat hip pain in runners. *J Orthop Sports Phys Ther.* 1993;17:172.
19. Janda V. *Muscle Function Testing.* London, England: Butterworth-Heineman; 1983.
20. Geraci MC. Rehabilitation of pelvis, hip, and thigh injuries in sports. *Phys Med Rehabil Clin N Am.* 1994;5:157.
21. Schlinger M, Andary MT. Massage and Manual Medicine. In: O'Connor FG, Wilder RP, eds. *Textbook of Running Medicine.* New York, NY: McGraw-Hill; 2001:561.
22. Rogers RG. The effects of spinal manipulation on cervical kinesthesia in patients with chronic neck pain: A pilot study. *J Manipulative Physiol Ther.* 1997;20:80–85.
23. Triano JJ, McGregor M, Hondras MA, et al. Manipulative therapy versus education programs for chronic low back pain. *Spine.* 1995;20:948–953.
24. Bourdillon JF, Day EA, Bookhout MR. *Spinal Manipulation,* 5th ed. Oxford, UK: Butterworth-Heineman; 1992.
25. Greenman PE. Sacroiliac Dysfunction in the Failed Low Back Pain Syndrome. In: Vleeming V, Mooney C, et al, eds. Conference Proceedings of the First Interdisciplinary World Congress In Low Back Pain and Its Relation to the Sacroiliac Joint. Netherlands: European Conference Organizers; 1992.
26. Linton SJ. A review of the psychological risk factors in back and neck pain. *Spine.* 2000;25(9):1148–1156.
27. Battie ML, Bigos SJ. Industrial Back Pain Complaints: A Broader Perspective. In: Brown MD, Rydevik BL, eds. *The Orthopedic Clinics of North America,* 22. Philadelphia, PA: WB Saunders; 1991:273–282.
28. Wall PD. Introduction. In: Wall PD, Melzack R, eds. *Textbook of Pain,* 2nd ed. New York, NY: Churchill Livingstone; 1989:1–18.
29. Sinaki M, Mokr B. Low Back Pain and Disorders of the Lumbar Spine. In: Braddom RL, ed. *Physical Medicine and Rehabilitation.* Philadelphia, PA: WB Saunders; 2001:853.
30. Grazier KL, Holbrook TL, Kelsey JL, et al, eds. *The Frequency of Occurrence, Impact and Cost of Selected Musculoskeletal Conditions in the United States.* Chicago, IL: American Academy of Orthopedic Surgeons; 1984.
31. Taylor H, Curran NM. *The Nuprin Pain Report.* New York, NY: Louis Harris and Associates; 1985.
32. Biering-Sorensen F. A prospective study of low back pain in a general population. I. Occurrence, recurrence, and etiology. *Scand J Rehabil Med.* 1983;15:71.
33. Biering-Sorensen F. Physical measurements as risk indicators for low back trouble over a one year period. *Spine.* 1984;9:106.
34. Frymoyer JW, Pope MH, Clements JH, et al. Risk factors in low back pain: An epidemiological survey. *J Bone Joint Surg Am.* 1983;65:213.
35. Sucher BM. Myofascial release of carpal tunnel syndrome. *J Am Osteopath Assoc.* 1993;93(1):92–101.
36. Sucher BM. Myofascial manipulative release of carpal tunnel syndrome: Documentation with magnetic resonance imaging. *J Am Osteopath Assoc.* 1993;93(12):1273–1278.
37. Sucher BM, Hinrichs RN. Manipulative treatment of carpal tunnel syndrome: Biomechanical and osteopathic intervention to increase the length of the transverse carpal ligament. *J Am Osteopath Assoc.* 1998;98:(12):679–686.
38. Evans RW. Some observations on whiplash injuries. *Neurol Clin.* 1992;10:975–997.
39. Mellion MB. *Sports Medicine Secrets.* Philadelphia, PA: Henley and Belfus; 1994.
40. Prokop LL, Wieting JM. The Use of Manipulation in Sports Medicine Practice. In: Kruft GH, ed. *Physical Medicine and Rehabilitation Clinics of North America.* Philadelphia, PA: WB Saunders; 1996:926.
41. Stanton DF, Mein EA. Preface. In: Kraft GH, ed. *Physical Medicine and Rehabilitation Clinics of North America.* Philadelphia, PA: WB Saunders; 1996:XV.

RHEUMATOLOGY

J. MICHAEL FINLEY

KEY CONCEPTS

- Frequency, impact, and costs of rheumatic diseases
- Inflammatory arthritides
- Osteoarthritis
- Soft tissue injury and fibromyalgia
- History
- Physical examination
- Specific rheumatologic examination
- Differential diagnosis
- Inflammatory arthritides
- Degenerative arthritis
- Nonarticular rheumatism
- Management
- Osteopathic Principles

Rheumatology is defined as the subspecialty of internal medicine that deals with the medical evaluation and treatment of the musculoskeletal system. Rheumatologists are specialists who devote themselves to the diagnosis and management of the both rheumatic and non-rheumatic soft tissue and joint-related medical problems. Musculoskeletal complaints affect approximately 33% of the North American population, and are frequently cited as among the most common reasons for patient visits to physicians. The social and economic impact of these conditions is enormous. The Arthritis Foundation reports that there are more than 100 different forms of arthritic diseases (1). Clinically, they account for more impairment and functional limitation among middle-age and older adults than any other disease category (2).

Prevalence is highest among older adults, but all age groups are affected. Impairment, disability, and job loss are frequent. In a North American study of patients over age 65, musculoskeletal symptoms, including knee trouble, back trouble, and unspecified joint pain, were more common in this population than in any other group (3). Prevalence rates increase with age, and are rare under age 18 (4). Among those over age 65, arthritic diseases are among the leading causes of physician visits. Patient surveys document that a majority of individuals aged 75 and over report having arthritis (5).

Self-reported arthritis is more common in women than men. Among racial and ethnic groups, it is more prevalent in American Indians, and slightly more so in blacks. It is less prevalent in Hispanics than whites. In general, arthritis is more likely to cause activity limitation in older persons, women, and nonwhites.

In 1992, the last year available, total expenditures for musculoskeletal-related problems were $118.5 billion per year, excluding fractures and acute injuries.

Costs continue to increase due to both population aging and better overall survival rates. In the 1960s and 1970s, overall costs accounted for approximately 0.7% of the gross domestic product. By the late 1980s, they had increased to 2.5%, and even more during the 1990s. Work loss and rehabilitation costs add to indirect costs, accounting for anywhere from 50% to 76.5% of all medical costs. Studies of costs incurred by patients with the most common rheumatic diseases, rheumatoid arthritis (RA), osteoarthritis (OA), and fibromyalgia (FM) have documented that these diseases have much higher than expected direct medical costs when compared with patients of similar ages without arthritis. Not surprisingly, those with the most severe and disabling diseases incur the highest costs (6). This review of rheumatology is in no way exhaustive. Drawing from Bernard Rubin's material in the first edition of this text (7), this chapter highlights the integration of osteopathic principles with management of rheumatic and non-rheumatic problems.

PATIENT EVALUATION AND PROBLEM-SOLVING (SEE CHAPTER 19)

Because of their ability to use palpatory skills, osteopathic physicians are uniquely qualified to evaluate patients presenting with musculoskeletal complaints. Along with empathetically sensitive interview and other examination methods, this particular skill is useful for establishing trusting relationships. More precisely defined and described patient problems are often identified with these special skills.

Younger patients often assume that rheumatic diseases are afflictions of older patient. They are also apt to assume that their problems are self-limited or curable when they are not. On the other hand, even today, many physicians either miss or delay a diagnosis of rheumatologic disease, sometimes with devastating long-term consequences.

Establishing a precise history is vital for a correct diagnosis. In general, patients seek help for pain, pain equivalents, depression, and anxiety. Painful sensations have many elements. Some are physiologic, but many are perceptually driven, i.e., they are learned behaviors. Feelings of helplessness and hopelessness are common in this population, particularly among those who make frequent physician visits. (See Chapters 6, 8, 15, 17, and 19.) Pain equivalents include unpleasant (not necessarily painful) sensations, such as itching, aching, stiffness, and nausea. The history should include detailed inquiry about the patient's motivation for coming to the doctor, especially in the absence of pain or pain equivalent (8). As a consequence, successful treatment depends on pain relief and its interpretations. Clearly stated and understandable explanations are the keys for long-term success.

History Taking (8) (See Also, Chapter 19)

In general, do the symptoms raise the possibility of systemic disease(s), or local conditions? A localized condition may affect multiple sites. What joints or other structures are involved? What is the pattern of involvement? In what order does joint involvement occur? How fast does it occur? At what time of the day does it start? If joint involvement is painful, severity is estimated by whether it interferes with function of the affected extremity, or with sleep and work. Is involvement self-limited, migratory, or progressive? If limited, how long do episodes last? Are they migratory or progressive?

Migratory means that the process subsides completely before moving to another apparently normal joint. *Progressive* means that the first joint stays afflicted as the pathologic process moves on to additional joints. Has this problem been treated previously? What was done and for how long? Was disease progress affected? What was its effect on the disease? Were there any drug side effects?

The *duration of morning stiffness* serves as a convenient, nonspecific index of inflammatory activity. Typically, it is directly proportional to the severity of the inflammatory process. Variations in duration are readily used to evaluate inflammation and responses to treatment. For example, the duration of morning stiffness is a more precise assessment than the erythrocyte sedimentation rate for rheumatoid inflammation.

If a structure is severely inflamed, motion usually causes pain unless there are neurologic problems that interfere with nociception. In general, pain arises from stimulation of synovial, capsular, periosteal, ligamentous, or tendinous free, unmyelinated nerve endings. Mechanical irritation and inflammation are common causes. Both pain and numbness occur in association with nerve entrapments in the carpal tunnel, for example. Other common sites are the suprascapular nerve in the shoulder and radicular syndromes arising from arthritic and degenerative changes in the neck. Intermittent muscle spasm and chronically increased muscle tone are common in this group of patients.

As joint involvement advances, disuse muscle atrophy occurs rapidly in affected muscles, often within in a few days. Diffuse systemic rheumatic diseases may also demonstrate characteristic muscle pathology. For example, upper-limb involvement commonly causes clumsiness of varying types, with loss of hand strength as a common complaint. Difficulty in rising from a chair or climbing and descending stairs signals both hip girdle and lower limb involvement (9).

Depression is common in individuals with chronic arthritis. Two types are common, primary and reactive. Primary depression

occurs particularly frequently in fibromyalgia patients, over 95% of whom are women. Living alone, having maladaptive thoughts, and expressing more functional limitations are particularly common in about half of these patients (10). Some (11) believe this common, ambiguous diagnostic category has a significant limbic nervous system and neuroendocrine component that affects specific aspects of brain, brainstem, and spinal cord functioning. "Some scientists believe . . . the syndrome may result from a trauma affecting the central nervous system . . . Others believe the syndrome may be triggered by an infection, such as a virus." No one knows for sure (11).

Rheumatic diseases, on the other hand, tend to create long-term problems as a consequence of mounting frustration with loss of personal autonomy. Reactive depression is common in this group (See Chapters 15 and 17). The problem frequently arises or is aggravated with the onset of pathologic fatigue. Emotional lability, including crying, morbid thoughts, temperamental outbursts, and withdrawal are common under these circumstances. These symptoms often disappear as the disease remits (8).

A number of questionnaires are available for long-term evaluation: the Stanford Health Assessment Questionnaire, Functional Disability Index, and Arthritis Impact Measurement Scales. These instruments document the patient's functional status with results comparable to traditional measures of disease-related joint activity, such as tender point count, radiographic joint erosion score, and erythrocyte sedimentation rate (12).

Other historic cues, such as chorea or "growing pains" in childhood may aid in differentiating rheumatic fever or juvenile rheumatoid arthritis (JRA) in an adult patient. A history of recent exposure to ticks or viral illness may clarify an otherwise obscure arthritis.

Even more important is a sexual history in a patient suspected of having gonorrheal arthritis or reactive arthritis, such as Reiter syndrome. Diabetes is often associated with adhesive capsulitis of the shoulders, Dupuytren contracture, and OA.

A family history of arthritis may or may not be helpful. The stability of family life and the stability and type of job are important points to establish (11).

Avocations should also be recorded because these, too, must often be dealt with in designing a treatment program. Current drug intake should be listed here, including alcohol and tobacco.

A mental status examination is important to establish the patient's level of emotional maturity and reality testing. Organic brain disease, including the late effects of brain injuries, dementia, and Alzheimer disease, is particularly important when assessing treatment compliance issues (8).

PHYSICAL EXAMINATION

Palpation

A standard, disciplined routine examination of the musculoskeletal system is essential. A number of excellent monographs are available to provide more detailed descriptions (13,14).

The physician's hands and fingers are important physical examination tools. Although various mechanical devices are useful for quantifying tenderness, joint swelling, and skin temperature, none are as useful as the fingers. A typical peripheral joint and spinal screening examination should take 5 or 6 minutes, on average.

Osteopathic physicians, with their special backgrounds using palpatory diagnosis, are particularly suited for this work. A working knowledge of both topographic and functional anatomy is essential to know which structures lie under the palpating hand.

Joint and muscle tenderness are nonspecific, but very sensitive signs of trouble. Some experts use a great deal of force, although other clinicians are gentler. In general, inexperienced practitioners tend to use too little force when evaluating superficial structures. On the other hand, some experts, such as McCarty (15,16), recommend force sufficient to blanch the thumbnail to rule out active disease (when examining areas that are not obviously inflamed). If tenderness is present, then either a low pain threshold or pathologic change may be responsible. Fortunately, most tenderness due to an organic cause is accompanied by more specific findings, such as swelling, crepitus, and increased local heat. Classic fibromyalgia tender point sites should be routinely evaluated on every patient (17).

Areas of tenderness can be "controlled" by applying similar pressure over nearby areas. A neurotic patient may be tender everywhere on the body.

Tender bones should be distinguished from aching soft tissues. For example, the anterior tibia is often tender in older subjects for unknown reasons. Bone tenderness may also present in severe osteoporosis and other forms of systemic bone disease.

Range of Motion

Passive joint motion testing embraces a set of common and familiar osteopathic palpatory procedures. It is used to evaluate all peripheral, spinal pelvic mechanics for altered tissue tension, asymmetry, restricted motion capability, and tenderness (TART). (See Glossary and Section VII, Chapters 38 through 73.) It is also a *method* for eliciting pain and joint contractures.

Swelling

Swelling of joints, bursae, and tendons is always abnormal. Unlike tenderness, swelling specifically indicates organic disease. Swelling is most often due to underlying inflammation and can be due to synovial thickening, increased volume of joint fluid, or local edema. If thickened tissue is felt, particularly in multiple areas, synovium is probably thickened, owing either to inflammatory proliferation or to storage of abnormal material, such as amyloid. Synovial thickening in a tendon sheath, common in Reiter syndrome or psoriatic arthritis, produces a "sausage finger" or "sausage toe" appearance. In general, synovial swelling is most pronounced on extensor surfaces of joints, where the capsule is more distensible.

Effusions are particularly common in large weight-bearing joints. Thus, fluid is often found in the knee, and is less common in the hip. It is even less common in ankles, upper limbs, hands, and wrists because of their tighter capsules. Nodular swellings over peripheral joints commonly signal osteophytes and osteoarthritis. Less frequently, they mark the presence of rheumatoid nodules. A number of less common conditions also occur.

Clinically, a pathologic nodule cannot be accurately identified without a biopsy. Most turn out to be synovium herniated through defects in the joint capsule, and are most commonly associated with RA, or systemic lupus erythematosus.

Other Clinical Findings

Increased skin temperature is a common and usually nonspecific finding. See TART, above. Sometimes crepitus (joint noises) occurs during passive range of motion testing. Generally, the finer the crepitus, the more clinically significant it is. Sometimes tendons will snap over joint surfaces and bony prominences. Typically, the noise is due to tendons snapping over bony prominences.

DIFFERENTIAL DIAGNOSIS AND USE OF DIAGNOSTIC TOOLS

The general category in which a problem falls is usually obvious from the history and physical examination. To pinpoint the diagnosis, however, laboratory examination, including gross and microscopic joint fluid analysis, radiologic study, specialized tests, and occasionally, biopsy for ordinary or special microscopy, are often indicated (18).

Routine laboratory tests include complete blood count, chemistry panel, and urinalysis. Synovial fluid examination in selected individuals commonly provides useful diagnostic information. Autoantibody and immune complex assays are indicated when specific inflammatory rheumatic diseases are suspected.

One must be alert to a number of diagnostic pitfalls. Patients with rheumatoid arthritis can have a positive antinuclear antibody titer. Persons over 60 years old can have rheumatoid factor in the absence of rheumatoid arthritis. An elevated sedimentation rate indicates the presence of any type of inflammation or infection, even unrelated to a rheumatic disease, and an abnormal creatine phosphokinase (CPK) value is not necessarily diagnostic of polymyositis (7).

Radiographic examination is important for differentiating inflammatory from non-inflammatory disorders. X-ray imaging is often used to stage disease progression and to follow progress once therapy has been instituted. In general, joint inflammation, whether from long-term infection or an autoimmune process, leads to osteopenia and joint erosions. On the other hand, non-inflammatory rheumatic diseases frequently cause an increase in bone as a result of subchondral sclerosis, osteophyte formation, and bridging of joint spaces. The latter are commonly seen on plain spinal films.

Local ultrasound (US), magnetic resonance imaging (MRI), and computerized tomography (CT) are also helpful.

INFLAMMATORY ARTHRITIDES
Rheumatoid Arthritis

Rheumatoid arthritis (RA) is a systemic inflammatory disease with its primary manifestation in the synovium that results in substantial morbidity and premature death (19–21). The diagnosis of RA should be considered in any patient with polyarticular inflammatory arthritis of greater than 6 weeks duration, especially if the hands and feet are involved (22).

The hallmark of the disease is a chronic, symmetric polyarthritis (synovitis) that typically affects the hands, wrists, and feet initially, and later may involve any joint lined by a synovial membrane, most frequently the knees, ankles, hips, elbows, and shoulders (22). Although RA primarily involves the synovium, features of systemic disease are also present in almost all patients, ranging in severity from fatigue, low-grade fevers, and mild to moderate anemia, to serositis (pleural or pericardial effusions) and severe multisystemic vasculitis. Fortunately, recent pharmacologic advances with disease-modifying antirheumatic drugs (DMARDs), slow-acting antirheumatic drugs (SAARDs), and TNF-α inhibitor therapy is significantly improving treatment outcomes (23).

Four of seven distinct criteria establish the diagnosis of RA (24). They include at least 6 weeks of:

i. Morning joint stiffness for at least one hour.
ii. Simultaneous soft tissue swelling in three or more joint groups.
iii. Hand involvement for the previous.
iv. Symmetric involvement, i.e., same joints on the right and left.
v. Rheumatoid nodules.
vi. Serum rheumatoid factor (RF).
vii. Radiographic evidence of typical RA bone erosions of the hands and wrists.

The 6 week requirement for diagnosis is necessary, because there are many other causes of symmetric polyarthritis (viral and others) that often mimic RA but are of shorter duration (22).

During both acute and chronic phases of the RA process, osteopathic physicians can offer patients range-of-motion exercises. The use of any of several indirect osteopathic manipulative procedures is also helpful.

Seronegative Spondyloarthropathies

A patient presenting with an asymmetrically distributed inflammatory arthritis, with or without spinal joint involvement, a diagnosis of seronegative spondyloarthropathy.

The *seronegative spondyloarthropathies* are characterized by sacroiliitis, peripheral inflammatory arthritis, and the absence of serum rheumatoid factor (RF) (5). There is an association with the HLA-B27 allele in many cases, although, the presence of this genetic marker is neither diagnostic nor predictive of spondyloarthropathies. Examples of seronegative spondyloarthropathies include juvenile and adult ankylosing spondylitis (AS), Reiter syndrome, spondylitis associated with chronic inflammatory bowel disease, or psoriatic arthritis.

Some forms of reactive arthritis follow enteric infection, with such organisms as *Yersinia, Shigella, Salmonella,* and *Campylobacter.* All share similar clinical manifestations. The prevalence of sacroiliitis is high, along with extraarticular manifestations, including uveitis and, occasionally, oral ulcers (5).

Chronic low back pain and stiffness are typically the first symptoms of AS (25–27). Onset is usually insidious rather than abrupt, and patients often cannot date when symptoms first began or precisely localize the areas affected (28). Complaints of alternating pain, first in one buttock and then the other, occasionally with radiation down the posterior thigh, can be elicited from some

patients and probably represent sacroiliac involvement. Often these symptoms are incorrectly ascribed to hip disease or sciatica.

Because low back discomfort is such a common malady in the population at large, much attention has been directed at attempting to differentiate inflammatory from non-inflammatory back pain (25). Characteristically, inflammatory back symptoms are suggested by prominent stiffness and pain in the morning or after other periods of rest (gel phenomenon) that improve with exercise. Such symptoms are most likely to reflect AS in a person younger than 40 years. Additional historic data suggesting AS include back pain that forces the individual out of bed at night or is not relieved by lying down, as well as concomitant chest-wall pain (26). Enthesitis, especially involving Achilles or plantar tendon insertions and causing heel pain, may appear alone or with arthritis (29,30).

Juvenile Rheumatoid Arthritis

Juvenile rheumatoid arthritis (JRA), known outside of North America as Juvenile Chronic Arthritis, occurs in patients younger than 18 years of age. Approximately 250,000 children in the United States have JRA (31). JRA takes many forms, including systemic-onset JRA, also known as Still disease. Still disease is associated with negative rheumatoid factor, negative antinuclear antibody, high fevers, and a rash. A small percentage goes on to have chronic destructive arthritis. Pauci-articular JRA occurs in half of all patients with juvenile rheumatoid arthritis, with four or fewer joints affected; pauci means few. Young girls with positive antinuclear antibody and pauci-articular JRA are at risk for iridocyclitis, which can cause potentially serious eye inflammation. Regular ophthalmologic visits with thorough slit lamp examinations are necessary until they reach adulthood. Older boys with pauci-articular JRA who are HLA-B27 positive might also have a form of juvenile ankylosing spondylitis manifested by sacroiliitis and asymmetric lower extremity arthritis (7).

Crystal-Induced Arthritis

Crystal-induced arthritis primarily includes gout and pseudogout. The latter is classified as calcium pyrophosphate deposition disease. Gout, itself, is probably the second most common inflammatory arthritis in the United States. Both are monoarticular, and polarized microscopy of synovial fluid identifies the crystals (7,32,33).

Gouty arthritis, recognized since antiquity, remains common. It mainly affects middle-aged and older men, in contrast to RA, OA, and most other connective tissue diseases that seem to occur more often in women (5).

DEGENERATIVE ARTHRITIS
Osteoarthritis

Osteoarthritis (OA) is a slowly evolving articular disease characterized by the gradual development of joint pain, stiffness, and limitation of motion (34). At present, the terms OA, osteoarthrosis, and degenerative joint disease are used interchangeably. It is the most common of all joint diseases. Its importance derives from its economic impact, in terms of both productivity (single greatest cause of days lost from work) and cost of treatment (chronic use of analgesics and antiinflammatory drugs) (35).

Degeneration of cartilage is the most prominent pathologic change. Both experimental (36) and clinical (37) studies have shown mild-to-moderate synovitis, although inflammatory changes may be absent early (38). Although OA is often benign, severe degenerative changes often cause serious disability.

Although the etiology of the disorder is still not clearly understood, osteoarthritis has been shown to be a family of disorders with cartilage as a target organ. Biomechanical factors play a central role, with risk factors, such as age, weight, and occupation acting as major variables. With more severe disease, pain may be persistent and interfere with normal activities of daily living. A chronic loss of restorative sleep with attendant increases in pain reports is common in this group.

Pain is the predominant symptom and initially often involves only one joint. Others tend to occur as time passes. The pain is most often described as a deep ache that is frequently accompanied by joint stiffness after periods of inactivity, such as on rising in the morning and after sitting. Pain is aggravated by using the involved joints, and may radiate or be referred to surrounding structures. In the early stages it is commonly relieved by rest.

Because no treatment can currently prevent or ameliorate the basic disease process, medical treatment is aimed at relieving pain, with orthopedic intervention largely reserved for situations that cannot be controlled with more conservative therapy (35). Newer concepts of pathogenesis suggest that OA is not an inevitable sequence of aging itself and raise the possibility of rational preventive and therapeutic approaches in the future (34).

The most effective symptomatic therapy combines several approaches and is often more effective if a multidisciplinary approach is followed. Typical participants are the primary care physician, rheumatologist, physiatrist, orthopedist, physical therapist, occupational therapist, psychologist, psychiatrist, nurse/nurse coordinator, dietitian, and social worker.

NONARTICULAR RHEUMATISM

Fibromyalgia

Primary fibromyalgia (FM) has been defined as chronic, widespread musculoskeletal pain and tenderness at 11 of 18 specified sites established by the American College of Rheumatology (39). Qualitatively, the FM tender point count has been referred to as a "sedimentation rate" for distress (40).

The absence of signs of connective tissue or other musculoskeletal disease is implicit in this definition. Because of its subjective nature and its frequent association with disturbed sleep, chronic fatigue, headaches, and irritable bowel syndrome, the validity of classifying FM as a (rheumatic) disease rather than a "syndrome of being out of sorts" has been challenged (41–48).

Patients often appear anxious and depressed, and studies have shown that they may feel dissatisfied with all aspects of their lives. Strong evidence has been given for an association between FM and major depressive disorder. Nevertheless, the specific charac-

teristics of anxiety and depression have not been identified consistently on psychological testing. On the other hand, it has been suggested that chronic pain and fatigue of any cause regularly engenders anxiety and depression (49,50).

Despite their subjectivity, symptoms of FM tend to be constant over many years. Decreased threshold to pain on pressure over certain sites and increased skin fold tenderness have led to numerous attempts to demonstrate localized peripheral abnormalities and to speculation that FM is a disorder of pain modulation (40).

There are no irrefutable biochemical, immunologic, or anatomic abnormalities detected in FM. However, studies of biopsied muscle samples have found decreased levels of adenosine triphosphate and phosphocreatine both at rest and after exercise (51). These findings have been confirmed by magnetic resonance spectroscopy in a small number of patients (52). Other findings, such as decreased regional cerebral blood flow with low cerebrospinal fluid metabolite levels, have been cited as evidence for functional dysregulation of central pain pathways (53–55).

RHEUMATIC DISEASE MANAGEMENT

Management of rheumatic diseases is predicated on an accurate diagnosis. Once a diagnosis is established, interventions and recommendations should be based on evolving evidence that most rheumatic diseases are neither benign nor inevitably disabling. As with many other chronic conditions, such as diabetes mellitus and hypertension, treatment focuses on quality-of-life issues with strategies designed to prevent adverse outcomes to the extent possible. Fortunately, both medical personnel and the public-at-large have a much better understanding of these situations than they did only a few years ago. The good news is that, with proper care, most can function at quite high levels with only minor impact on their daily lives.

Nonpharmacologic Treatments (7)

Nonpharmacologic therapies for rheumatic diseases are often rewarding, generally providing an assistive role. Along with improving general physical fitness, both physical therapy and occupational therapy are fundamental components of treatment for both rheumatic and nonrheumatoid disorders. (Also see Chapter 35, Osteopathic Physical Medicine and Rehabilitation.)

No single modality has proven to be most successful. However, treatment of the somatic component of any arthritic process by administration of appropriately chosen manipulative treatment is often helpful in relieving both pain and emotional distress (56,57). Manipulative techniques also supplement other adjunctive measures. Indirect approaches are particularly useful, using strain and counterstrain, myofascial release, and functional techniques. (See Chapters 58–66.) Exercise, muscle strengthening, weight and nutrition management, along with general home and workplace considerations, are also factored in, including appropriate ergonomic advice.

Both OA and FM have proven to be particularly responsive to osteopathic manipulative methods. Medical management generally focuses on symptom management because, until recently, no single intervention has been proven to cure the primary disease processes, including DMARDs and SAAMARDs. Nonsteroidal antiinflammatory drugs (NSAIDs) are particularly useful, and their generic forms are inexpensive.

A carefully graded, incremental exercise program is essential. If the regimen advances too quickly, symptoms may worsen, threatening compliance. Importantly, the patient should be advised that worsening pain is a warning sign that exercise tolerance has been reached (58). Symptomatic relief commonly also occurs using both heat and cold.

MEDICATIONS

Pharmacologic therapies are generally nonspecific, although recent research has focused on underlying cellular physiology and targeting specific parts of the immune response.

Antiinflammatory Drugs (59)

NSAIDs are fundamental to the treatment of most rheumatic diseases. They are useful as both analgesic and antiinflammatory agents, and are generally inexpensive when generics are prescribed.

Salicylates are also inexpensive and generally well tolerated. In general, larger doses are required than those used for primary analgesia. A constant blood level of 20 to 30 mg/dL is needed, which for most patients, requires between 3 and 6 grams of aspirin daily. All patients should be monitored for toxic blood levels and side-effects, including tinnitus, deafness, and gastrointestinal intolerance. Recent evidence suggests that the latter occurs more often when *Helicobacter pylori* infection is present. Eradication of the *H. pylori* then allows for safer use of these products (60).

Overt gastrointestinal tract hemorrhage or ulceration is infrequent, but when it occurs, it dictates discontinuation of the drug and exploration for *H. pylori* infection (60). In most cases, concomitant administration of proton pump inhibitors significantly reduces NSAID-induced gastrointestinal toxicity (59).

Corticosteroids

Local injection of corticosteroids into affected joints and myofascial trigger points often produces dramatic symptomatic and functional improvements. Unfortunately, long-term side effects make them unrealistic choices except for the unresponsive patient with aggressive joint disease that threatens loss of functional abilities. Oral prednisone, given every other day, is commonly helpful in this group of patients. Higher doses are necessary for patients with neuropathy, vasculitis, pleuritis, pericarditis, scleritis, and related conditions (59).

DISEASE-MODIFYING THERAPIES

Disease-modifying antirheumatic drugs (DMARDS) (59), the more slowly acting drugs, include antimalarials, methotrexate, gold salts, penicillamine, sulfasalazine, and minocycline. Antimalarials are usually given as hydroxychloroquine (Plaquenil), 200 mg once or twice daily. This drug may cause retinal lesions and loss of vision, making regular annual ophalmologic evaluations a necessity.

Currently, the most widely used and effective form of long-term therapy for RA appears to be methotrexate. An oral dosage of 7.5 to 25 mg one time per week is usually effective. A therapeutic response usually occurs within several weeks. Side effects include hepatotoxicity with a possibility of cirrhosis, bone marrow suppression, oral ulcers, and potentially life-threatening pneumonitis. Methotrexate may also cause a leukocytoclastic vasculitis that promotes formation of more rheumatoid nodules. This condition is called systemic nodulosis. Simultaneous treatment with folic acid 1 mg per day reduces methotrexate toxicity without impairing efficacy.

Leflunomide (Arava), a pyrimidine antagonist that selectively inhibits activated T lymphocytes, has been recently introduced for long-term treatment of RA.

Sulfasalazine in large doses is effective in some patients. Minocycline has also been found to be effective in RA (61).

Gold salts, rarely used, are given in weekly intramuscular injections. It produces remission in many cases. Common side effects include pruritic skin rashes and painful mouth ulcers. Severe manifestations include bone marrow suppression (usually leukopenia or thrombocytopenia), renal damage with proteinuria, and rarely, nephrotic syndrome. Frequent urinalyses and blood counts must be performed, especially during the early phases of treatment. In general, gold salts have fallen out of favor as more effective and better tolerated treatments have become available.

Penicillamine is also effective. Like gold salts however, its effects begin slowly. Bone marrow and kidney toxicity are more common side effects. It also has the potential for inducing other autoimmune diseases, such as myasthenia gravis, Goodpasture syndrome, and lupus erythematosus. As a result, both gold salts and penicillamine are rarely used today.

Immunosuppressive agents, such as azathioprine, cyclophosphamide, chlorambucil, and cyclosporine have been used to treat especially severe, unremitting RA.

Etanercept (Enbrel), a soluble recombinant TNF-α receptor inhibitor, has recently been introduced for severe RA management. To date, it has proven to be highly effective at controlling symptoms and, seemingly, disease progression, in many patients. Toxicity appears to be low, but concerns about potential cancer induction and infectious complications resulting from TNF-α blockade remain to be determined. High cost is a particular disadvantage along with the need for twice weekly injections.

Infliximab (Remicade), a chimeric TNF-α receptor antagonist is also available via intravenous infusion every 6 to 8 weeks. Concerns also exist about potential long-term side effects.

Surgery

Surgical joint replacement has been a major benefit for thousands of disabled arthritis sufferers. Prosthetic devices for hip and knee joints generally give excellent results, and devices for ankle, elbow, and shoulder replacement are improving.

OSTEOPATHIC MANIPULATIVE TREATMENT: EFFICACY AND RESEARCH

Arthritis patients appear to experience improved quality of life when offered OMT, as opposed to more traditional pharmacologic therapy.

Research studies involving large numbers of patients followed for months or years have not yet been done. The long-term benefits of OMT are unknown in these conditions. A study examining the use of OMT as an adjunct in the management of systemic lupus erythematosus has begun (62), but results are not yet available.

Tucker (63) examined the treatment of osteoarthritis using manual therapy. His work, published almost 30 years ago, has conclusions that are valid today regarding the early use of physical measures for the treatment of osteoarthritis followed by more traditional pharmacologic therapy (7). He believed that the early use of manipulative treatment might be beneficial, but if symptoms persisted after 6 months, more aggressive traditional therapy should be considered.

CONCLUSION

Osteopathic principles and concepts are particularly useful when working with arthritic patients of all types. Palpatory diagnosis and manipulative treatment are particularly applicable for this population.

With the possible exception of infectious arthritis, no rheumatic disease can truly be cured. By combining appropriate neuromusculoskeletal and laboratory diagnoses with carefully selected pharmacologic therapy and manipulative treatment, the patient can experience both symptomatic and functional improvements, including an improved sense of well-being.

Clinical research will answer lingering questions regarding the benefits of osteopathic manipulative treatment in this population. Recent studies dealing with fibromyalgia and systemic lupus erythematosus are among the first efforts to examine osteopathic manipulative treatment in a defined population (64,65). More controlled studies of this nature are planned for the future.

ACKNOWLEDGMENTS

This chapter is dedicated to my wife, Michelle Miller, and sons Richard and Casey. Their support and indulgence allowed me to complete this project. The intellectual support and patience of my co-workers, who helped me find the time in an overworked schedule to complete this project is appreciated. Not to be forgotten are the other members of the Western University College of Osteopathic Medicine of the Pacific staff, Drs. Michael Seffinger and Ehab Tuppo, and Christine Jacobson, MA, who offered important suggestions. I thank each of you for your support in helping to bring forth this chapter.

REFERENCES

1. Decker JL, Glossary Subcommittee of the ARA Committee on rheumatologic practice. American Rheumatism Association nomenclature and classification of arthritis and rheumatism. *Arthritis Rheum.* 1983;26:1029–1032.
2. Haber LD. Disabling effects of chronic disease and impairment. II. Functional capacity limitations. *J Chronic Dis.* 1973;26(3):127–151.
3. Verbrugge LM. From sneezes to adieux: stages of health for American men and women. *Soc Sci Med.* 1986;22(11):1195–1212.
4. Lawrence RC, Helmick CG, Arnett FC, et al. Estimates of the prevalence of arthritis and selected musculoskeletal disorders in the United States. *Arthritis Rheum.* 1998;41(5):778–799.
5. Felson D. Epidemiology of the Rheumatic Diseases. In: Koopman WJ, ed. *Arthritis and Allied Conditions,* 14th ed. Philadelphia, PA: Lippincott Williams & Wilkins; 2001.
6. Yelin E, Callahan LF. The economic cost and social and psychological impact of musculoskeletal conditions. National Arthritis Data Work Groups. *Arthritis Rheum.* 1996;39(11):1931.
7. Rubin B. Osteopathic Considerations in the Clinical Specialties—Rheumatology. In: Ward R, ed. *Foundations of Osteopathic Medicine,* 1st ed. Philadelphia, PA: Lippincott Williams & Wilkins; 1995.
8. McCarty DJ. Differential Diagnosis of Rheumatic Disease: Analysis of Signs and Symptoms. In: Koopman WJ, ed. *Arthritis and Allied Conditions,* 14th ed. Philadelphia, PA: Lippincott Williams & Wilkins; 2001.
9. Csuka ME, McCarty DJ. A rapid method for measurement of lower extremity muscle strength. *Am J Med.* 1985;78:77–81.
10. Okifuji A, Turk DC, Sherman JJ, et al. Evaluation of the relationship between depression and fibromyalgia syndrome: Why aren't all patients depressed? *J Rheumatol.* 2000;1:212–219.
11. NIAMS/NIH Website. Fibromyalgia Research: Challenges and Opportunities. http://www.niams.nih.gov/hi/topics/fibromyalgia/fibromya.htm. Accessed May 15, 2002.
12. Gordon DA. Approach to the Patient with Musculoskeletal Disease. In: Goldman L, Bennett JC, eds. *Cecil Textbook of Internal Medicine,* 21st ed. Philadelphia, PA: WB Saunders; 2000.
13. Polley HF, Hunder GG. *Rheumatologic interviewing and physical examination of the joints,* 2nd ed. Philadelphia, PA: WB Saunders; 1978.
14. Doherty M, Doherty J. *Clinical Examination in Rheumatology.* London, England: Wolfe; 1992.
15. McCarty DJ, Gatter RA, Phelps P. A dolorimeter for quantification of articular tenderness. *Arthritis Rheum.* 1965;8:551–559.
16. McCarty DJ, Gatter RA, Steele AD. A twenty-pound dolorimeter for quantification of articular tenderness. *Arthritis Rheum.* 1968;11:696–698.
17. Wolfe F, Smythe HA, Yunus MB, et al. The American College of Rheumatology 1990 criteria for the classification of fibromyalgia. Report of the multicenter criteria committee. *Arthritis Rheum.* 1990;33:160–172.
18. Shmerling RH, Liang MH. Laboratory Evaluation of Rheumatic Diseases. In: *Primer on the Rheumatic Diseases,* 10th ed. Atlanta, GA: Arthritis Foundation; 1993:64–66.
19. Scott DL, Symmons DPM, Coulton BL, et al. Long-term outcome of treating rheumatoid arthritis: Results after 20 years. *Lancet.* 1987;1:1108–1111.
20. Pincus T, Brooks RH, Callahan LF. Prediction of long-term mortality in patients with rheumatoid arthritis according to simple questionnaire and joint count measures. *Ann Intern Med.* 1994;120(1):26–34.
21. Wolfe F, Mitchell DM, Sibley JT, et al. The mortality of rheumatoid arthritis. *Arthritis Rheum.* 1994;37(4):481–494.
22. O'Dell JR. Rheumatoid Arthritis: The Clinical Picture. In: Koopman WJ, ed. *Arthritis and Allied Conditions,* 14th ed. Lippincott Williams & Wilkins; 2001.
23. American College of Rheumatology Ad Hoc Committee on Clinical Guidelines. Guidelines for the management of rheumatoid arthritis. *Arthritis Rheum.* 1996;39(5):713–722.
24. Arnett FC, Edworthy SM, Bloch DA, et al. The American Rheumatism

Association 1987 revised criteria for the classification of rheumatoid arthritis. *Arthritis Rheum.* 1988;31(3):315–324.

25. Calin A, Porta J, Fries JF, et al. Clinical history as a screening test for ankylosing spondylitis. *JAMA.* 1977;237(24):2613–2614.

26. Blackburn Jr WD, Alarcon GS, Ball GV. Evaluation of patients with back pain of suspected inflammatory nature. *Am J Med.* 1988;85(6):766–770.

27. Gran JT. An epidemiologic survey of the signs and symptoms of ankylosing spondylitis. *Clin Rheum Dis.* 1985;4:161–169.

28. Arnett FC. Ankylosing Spondylitis. In: Koopman WJ, ed. *Arthritis and Allied Conditions,* 14th ed. Lippincott Williams & Wilkins; 2001.

29. Ball J. The enthesopathy of ankylosing spondylitis. *Br J Rheumatol.* 1983;22(suppl):25–28.

30. Olivieri I, Barozzi L, Padula A. Enthesopathy: clinical manifestations, imaging and treatment. *Baillieres Best Pract Res Clin Rheumatol.* 1998;12:665–681.

31. Singsen BH. Epidemiology of the rheumatic diseases of childhood. *Rheum Dis Clin North Am.* 1990;16:581–599.

32. McCarty DJ. Coexistent gout and rheumatoid arthritis. *J Rheumatol.* 1981;8:253–254.

33. Lawrence RC, Hochberg MC, Kelsey JL, et al. Estimates of the prevalence of selected arthritic and musculoskeletal diseases in the United States. *J Rheumatol.* 1989;16:427–441.

34. Moskowitz RW, Holderbaum D. Clinical and Laboratory Findings in Osteoarthritis. In: Koopman WJ, ed. *Arthritis and Allied Conditions,* 14th ed. Lippincott Williams & Wilkins; 2001.

35. Schnitzer TJ. Osteoarthritis (Degenerative Joint Disease). In: Goldman L, Bennett JC, eds. *Cecil Textbook of Internal Medicine,* 21st ed. Philadelphia, PA: WB Saunders; 2000.

36. Moskowitz RW, Goldberg VM, Berman L. Synovitis as a manifestation of degenerative joint disease: an experimental study. *Arthritis Rheum.* 1976;19:813(abst).

37. Goldenberg DL, Egan MS, Cohen AS. Inflammatory synovitis in degenerative joint disease. *J Rheumatol.* 1982;9:204–209.

38. Myers SL, Brandt KD, Ehrlich JW, et al. Synovial inflammation in patients with early osteoarthritis of the knee. *J Rheumatol.* 1990;17:1662–1669.

39. Wolfe F, Smythe HA, Yunus MB, et al. The American College of Rheumatology 1990 criteria for the classification of fibromyalgia. Report of the multicenter criteria committee. *Arthritis Rheum.* 1990;33:160–172.

40. Ball EV. Non-articular Rheumatism. In: Goldman L, Bennett JC, eds. *Cecil Textbook of Internal Medicine,* 21st ed. Philadelphia, PA: WB Saunders; 2000.

41. Bennett RM. Fibromyalgia and the facts. Sense or nonsense. *Rheum Dis Clin North Am.* 1993;19:45–59.

42. Granges G, Littlejohn GO. A comparative study of clinical signs in fibromyalgia/fibrositis syndrome, healthy and exercising subjects. *J Rheumatol.* 1993;20:344–351.

43. Powers R. Fibromyalgia: an age-old malady begging for respect. *J Gen Intern Med.* 1993;8:93–105.

44. Waylonis GW, Heck W. Fibromyalgia syndrome. New associations. *Am J Phys Med Rehabil.* 1992;71:343–348.

45. Veale D, Kavanagh G, Fielding JF, et al. Primary fibromyalgia and the irritable bowel syndrome: different expressions of a common pathogenetic process. *BMJ.* 1991;30:220–222.

46. Littlejohn GO. A database for fibromyalgia. *Rheum Dis Clin North Am.* 1995;21:527–557.

47. Jacobsen S, Petersen IS, Danneskiold-Samsøe B. Clinical features in patients with chronic muscle pain with special reference to fibromyalgia. *Scand J Rheumatol.* 1993;22:69–76.

48. Yunus MB, Masi AT, Aldag JC. A controlled study of primary fibromyalgia syndrome: clinical features and association with other functional syndromes. *J Rheumatol.* 1989;16:62–71.

49. Hudson JI, The relationship between fibromyalgia and major depressive disorder. *Rheum Dis Clin North Am.* 1996;22(2):285–303.

50. Goldenberg D. A randomized, double-blind crossover trial of fluoxetine and amitriptyline in the treatment of fibromyalgia. *Arthritis Rheum.* 1996;39(11):1852–1859.

51. Jacobsen S, Bartels EM, Danneskiold-Samsoe B. Single cell morphology of muscle in patients with chronic muscle pain. *Scand J Rheumatol.* 1995;20(5):336–343.

52. Van-Denderen JC, Boersma JW, Zeinstra P, et al. Physiological effects of exhaustive physical exercise in primary fibromyalgia syndrome (PFS): Is PFS a disorder of neuroendocrine activity? *Scand J Rheumatol.* 1995;21(1):35–37.

53. Jacobsen S, Jensen KE, Thomsen C, et al. Phosphorus 31 magnetic resonance spectroscopy of skeletal muscle in patients with fibromyalgia. *J Rheumatol.* 1994;19(10):1600–1603.

54. Russell IJ, Vaeroy H, Javors M, et al. Cerebrospinal fluid biogenic amine metabolites in fibromyalgia/fibrositis syndrome and rheumatoid arthritis. *Arthritis Rheum.* 1995;35(5):550–556.

55. Russell IJ, Michalek JE, Vipraio GA, et al. Platelet tritiated imipramine uptake receptor density and serum serotonin levels in patients with fibromyalgia-fibrositis syndrome. *J Rheumatol.* 1994;19(1):104–109.

56. Fiechtner JJ, Brodeur RR. Manual and manipulation techniques for rheumatic disease. *Rheum Dis Clin North Am.* 2000;26:83–96.

57. Tettambel MA. Osteopathic treatment considerations for rheumatic diseases. *J Am Osteopath Assoc.* 2001;101(4)(Part 2 Suppl):S18–S20.

58. Lozada CJ, Altman RD. Management of Osteoarthritis. In: Koopman WJ, ed. *Arthritis and Allied Conditions,* 14th ed. Lippincott Williams & Wilkins; 2001.

59. Arnett FC. Rheumatoid Arthritis. In: Goldman L, Bennett JC, eds. *Cecil Textbook of Internal Medicine,* 21st ed. Philadelphia, PA: WB Saunders; 2000.

60. Huang J-Q, Sridhar S, Hunt RH. Role of Helicobacter pylori and nonsteroidal anti-inflammatory drugs in peptic ulcer disease: a meta-analysis. *Lancet.* 2002;359:14–22.

61. Tilley BC, Alarcon GS, Heysc SP, et al. Minocycline in rheumatoid arthritis. A 48 weeks, double blind, placebo controlled trial. MIRA Trial Group. *Ann Intern Med.* 1995;122(2):81–89.

62. Pertusi RM, Rubin BR, Davis GC. Instruments to assess quality of life in SLE. *J Am Osteopath Assoc.* 1993;93(9).

63. Tucker WE. Treatment of osteoarthritis by manual therapy. *Br J Clin Pract.* 1969;23(1):38.

64. Rubin BR, Cortez CA, Gamber R, et al. Treatment options in fibromyalgia syndrome. *J Am Osteopath Assoc.* 1990;90(9):844.

65. Rubin BR, Gamber R, Shores J, et al. The effect of treatment options on perceived pain in fibromyalgia syndrome. *Arthritis Rheum.* 1991;34(5):R33.

AN OSTEOPATHIC APPROACH TO SPORTS MEDICINE

P. GUNNAR BROLINSON
KURT HEINKING
ALBERT J. KOZAR

KEY CONCEPTS

- Appreciate the unique role of osteopathic medicine in sports medicine
- Understand the roles and responsibilities of the sports medicine team
- Understand the pathomechanics of sport and exercise-related disease and dysfunction
- Describe the relationship between somatic dysfunction and common sports-related injuries and how osteopathic manipulative treatment is integrated in the treatment of the injured athlete
- Understand the unique challenges associated with sideline coverage and event management medical issues
- Understand the rational behind treatment and what factors need to be considered prior to returning the athlete to play

Sports medicine is the branch of the healing arts profession that uses a holistic, comprehensive approach to the prevention, diagnosis, and management of sports and exercise-related injuries. Osteopathic sports physicians apply their medical and scientific knowledge with a philosophy that the athlete's structure and function are interrelated. Osteopathic physicians must look at the entire scope of an athlete's problem, including the mechanism of injury, environmental influences, inherent postural and muscle imbalances, the psychological effects of injury and rehabilitation, and finally, to the athlete's safe return to play. The osteopathic primary care physician can also play a key role in sports medicine.

Although only 20% of the American population regularly participates in an exercise program, our population is becoming more active, health conscious, and physically fit (1). This increase in athletic participation does not only include the younger athletic male. Participation in sports by children and adolescents has dramatically increased over the last few years. The number of adolescent athletes involved in formal sports participation continues to increase yearly in the United States and now totals more than

12 million. Due to the affects of Title IX, and the Amateur Sports Act of 1978, there has also been a major impact on the field of sports medicine for young women. Now more than 55 million women participate in recreational sports annually (2). Growing numbers of senior athletes are exercising routinely and participating in competitive sports. By the year 2030, 20% of our population will be over the age of sixty-five. It is also encouraging to see that 2 to 3 million people with disabilities participate in sports each year in the United States (3). It is this diversity that makes the field of sports medicine so exciting and challenging.

However, this rise in physical activity has been accompanied by an increase in the number of sports-related injuries. It is estimated that over 17 million Americans seek medical care each year because of athletic and recreation-related problems (4). Due to the enormous volume of participants and numbers of injuries, medical practitioners of all fields need to be educated on the diagnosis and treatment of athletic injuries.

WHY IS THERE SUCH AN "EXERCISE BOOM?"

Over the last 2 to 3 decades, hundreds of studies delineating the beneficial effects of exercise have emerged. National recommendations advocating the development and maintenance of lifelong patterns of physical activity have been published. Many serious health problems can be controlled, improved, or eliminated through moderate, consistent physical activity. Considerable evidence suggests that regular exercise in conjunction with other risk-reducing behaviors, will protect against an initial cardiac episode (primary prevention); will aid in the recovery of patients with myocardial infarction, coronary bypass surgery, or angioplasty; and will reduce the risk of recurrent cardiac events (secondary prevention). Due to the beneficial effects of exercise and dietary modification, coronary artery disease has decreased 30% in the United States since 1960. Aerobic exercise and endurance training can also lead to numerous favorable metabolic effects. These include but are not limited to: a more favorable lipid profile, control of obesity, decreased blood pressure, improved glucose tolerance, higher bone density, and improved self-image (3,5).

Improving physical health also improves emotional health. It has been known for many years that chronic psychological and emotional distress is associated with a deterioration of health. When comparing exercise programs with relaxation techniques and psychotherapy, exercise was proven to be more effective at decreasing depression than relaxation techniques and was equally as effective as psychotherapy. There is a high correlation between regular exercise and intellectual function, memory, and improved self-concept (6). Regular exercise and appropriate training in older adults increases physical safety, reduces susceptibility to acute and chronic disease, and improves psychological outlook (7).

PRACTITIONERS

Ideally, the field of sports medicine consists of health care providers who work in synchrony to provide a "team approach" to achieve better health for the patient. At the head of this team of professionals is the physician who diagnoses the condition and directs the treatment plan. The team physician must have an unrestricted medical license and be responsible for treating and coordinating the medical care of athletic team members. The primary responsibility of the team physician is to provide for the well being of the individual. The team physician should possess special proficiency in the care of musculoskeletal injuries and medical conditions encountered in sports. The team physician also must actively integrate medical expertise with other health care providers, including medical specialists, athletic trainers, and allied health professionals. The relationship of the physician and athletic trainer is critical, as is the link between the coach, physician, athlete, and family members. This "team approach" helps to motivate the discouraged player, evaluate the injured player, and eliminate risks to the player who is coming back from an injury. The athletic trainer not only carries out the physician's treatment plan, but is a highly skilled practitioner. The team physician must ultimately assume responsibility within the team structure for making medical decisions that affect the athlete's safe participation. The team physician is the "final authority" to determine the mental and physical readiness of athletes in organized programs (8).

The osteopathic physician has a unique role in the total care of the athlete or active patient. Our philosophic approach is patient, not disease, oriented. This philosophic approach lends itself to this population, because athletic patients are generally healthy and motivated to return to better health. Palpatory skills provide osteopathic physicians with a distinct advantage over other health care practitioners in determining the location, extent, and associated manifestations of athletic injury. Finally, osteopathic physicians who effectively use OMT have another "tool in the toolbox" with which to treat an important component of athletic injury—somatic dysfunction.

TRAINING

Sports medicine physicians can enter this field of medicine through numerous pathways. The physician must decide early on if he/she wants to practice surgically oriented medicine. If this is the case, a common approach is to do a sports medicine fellowship after an orthopedic surgical residency. Some neurosurgeons also practice sports medicine.

If a primary care emphasis is sought, then a sports medicine fellowship can be completed after a family practice, pediatrics, emergency medicine, or internal medicine residency. For those interested in a purely manipulative practice, a sports medicine fellowship can follow a residency in osteopathic manipulation. Not all practitioners of sports medicine have postgraduate or fellowship training. However, it adds exposure, extra training, and confidence, and is now a requirement to sit for the certification examination of added qualification in sports medicine offered by the American Osteopathic Association (AOA). The American Osteopathic Academy of Sports Medicine (AOASM) is the professional organization of the AOA in which osteopathic sports medicine professionals meet, exchange ideas, and develop new knowledge.

HISTORY OF SPORTS MEDICINE AND OSTEOPATHIC SPORTS MEDICINE

Physicians have been caring for athletes since ancient times. Herodicus, the teacher of Hippocrates, was the most well known Greek physician around 400 B.C. In those days, they supervised the training and care of Olympic athletes. In the second century A.D., Galen, the first to be called team physician, served as the physician to Roman gladiators. His knowledge of exercise physiology greatly influenced the practice of medicine for the next millennium.

A. T. Still's teachings on the importance of structure and function and the significance of the musculoskeletal system in the maintenance of health were keys to his philosophy. It should surprise no one, that Still and the administration of American School of Osteopathy (ASO) encouraged new students, both men and women, to join the Athletic Association (9). Professional and collegiate sports were just becoming popular at the turn of the 19th century. As Still's reputation grew as a highly skilled practitioner in providing relief of sprains, strains, and dislocations, many injured athletes came to him to be treated. Accordingly, Still became known as a pioneer in sports medicine (10). In 1901, the first athletic director was named at the American School of Osteopathy while both intramural and intercollegiate sports, including football, baseball, and basketball, prevailed in Kirksville. The ASO teams were charter members of the Missouri Intercollegiate Athletic Association. The Osteopaths, as they were known, took on major universities including Notre Dame and Nebraska. ASO teams were often very good and gained so much reputation for the school that many famous athletes later came back to attend. Forrest "Phog" Allen, an illustrious coach whose teams won 771 basketball games during his long career at the University of Kansas, was probably the best known sports figure to attend ASO.

PRE-PARTICIPATION PHYSICAL

One of the most important functions of a sports medicine professional is to perform a thorough pre-participation physical examination (PPE). The pre-participation history and physical examination has numerous functions, with the screening for life-threatening conditions at the top of the list. This examination may be the only time the athlete will have contact with a medical professional during the teen years. The PPE was originally designed to clear those athletes who were eligible for competition and hold out those who were not. In 1992, the American Academy of Pediatrics (AAP), the American Academy of Family Practice (AAFP), the American Medical Society of Sports Medicine (AMSSM), the American Orthopedic Society for Sports Medicine (AOSSM) and the AOASM, published *Pre-participation Physical Evaluation* (11), in an effort to provide a common format for practitioners to use. In 1996, the American Heart Association produced a document entitled *Cardiovascular Preparation Screening of Competitive Athletes* at the 26th Bethesda Conference on Cardiovascular Health (12,13).

In the challenge to decrease the risk of sudden cardiac death, they determined the following:

- A complete medical history, physical examination, and brachial artery blood pressure should be performed before participation in organized high school (grades 9 through 12) and college sports.
- Screening should be repeated every 2 years; in intervening years, a history should be taken.
- A national standard for pre-participation examinations should be developed.
- A health care worker with the training, skills, and background necessary to reliably obtain a detailed cardiovascular history, perform a physical examination, and recognize heart disease should perform athlete screening.

Although these guidelines are clinically useful, there is no nationally accepted form for completing the pre-participation physical examination. However, the following are goals and objectives that should be considered during the pre-participation examination:

- Screen for life-threatening conditions
- Decide eligibility or restriction of play (based on classification of sport: contact, limited contact, non-contact)
- Determine disqualifying medical conditions for sport participation
- Evaluate the function of the musculoskeletal system and prior injuries
- Record a baseline mini-mental status examination
- Check for communicable diseases
- Counsel/educate on athletic injury prevention and cancer screening examinations based on the population
- Establish rapport with athletes
- Evaluate for the potential of injury and areas of performance enhancement
- Educate the athlete on closed head injury, used of ergogenic aids, and proper protective equipment
- *Osteopathic physicians should perform a screening musculoskeletal examination with emphasis on evaluation for the presence of somatic dysfunction*

The pre-participation physicals should take place at least 6 to 8 weeks prior to the sports season. The history is the primary focus for all athletes. An athlete who reports syncope or chest pain during exertion is waving a "red flag" during the examination. It is also crucial to inquire about any alterations in consciousness or concussions during sports, asthma, recent history of mononucleosis, and menstrual history. All athletes should be asked if they are using any medications, OTC preparations, or performance-enhancing drugs. Family history should elicit if there has been a cardiac-related death in a first-degree relative under the age of 50, and any known congenital heart disease.

The physical examination is a screening examination only, but should include a thorough cardiac evaluation in at least two positions carried out with maneuvers. The musculoskeletal screening should include not only evaluation of symptomatic joints, but also a general screening examination, a focused palpatory examination, and motion testing of body areas that contain significant tissue texture abnormality.

Osteopathic physicians have unique palpatory skills. These skills can be very useful in determining if there is a somatic component to a patient's medical condition or somatic dysfunction that may lead to overuse injury. Consider an asthmatic patient with upper thoracic and rib dysfunction. Palpating for these viscerosomatic reflexes gives the clinician useful information regarding management and sports participation. This approach allows the osteopathic physician additional structural and functional information.

The following clinical examples highlight the importance of an osteopathic examination during the pre-participation physical:

i. A baseball pitcher with significant thoracolumbar motion restriction may not transfer the ground reactive force through his legs and trunk to the upper extremity. Because of this, he tries to throw harder with his arm, producing an overuse syndrome of the upper extremity.

ii. A female tennis player with a history of dysmenorrhea develops central low back pain during her season. This may be treated symptomatically or prevented if related somatic dysfunction is diagnosed and/or addressed during the PPE.

iii. Consider a patient with posterior and lateral knee pain, yet a normal orthopedic examination. It is not uncommon to find somatic dysfunction of the ilium and fibular head. Treatment of the ilium, hamstring, and fibula prior to the season may decrease the incidence of a hamstring strain while competing.

Osteopathic physicians have unique skills to offer our competitive young athletes. It is important to use these skills right from the beginning of care—integrated into the PPE.

THE OSTEOPATHIC APPROACH TO THE INJURED ATHLETE

History

An osteopathic approach to the injured athlete is a unique approach that is important because many musculoskeletal injuries or athletic-based illnesses have a somatic component. History taking in the athletic population should include all of the components of the routine history, yet also cover questions regarding the athlete's level of play, type of sport(s), positions, and prior injury or illness. These questions will help the physician determine the mechanism of injury, whether the injury is an exacerbation of a pre-existing illness, or if it is perhaps a new, undiagnosed medical condition. One must not settle on the obvious diagnosis based on the chief complaint; the history must be focused to probe for factors contributing to the *cause* of the obvious diagnosis. Many times, an athlete will see a physician not because they are in pain but because of a decline in their athletic ability or performance. It is important to find out if the symptoms are progressing, staying the same, or improving. If progressive symptoms are present, how has the athlete changed their activity or lifestyle to cope with this? What is the athlete's emotional state?

Young athletes may not give a reliable history. Obtaining the history from family members can sometimes be beneficial. Parents of athletic children may have a different viewpoint of the events surrounding the injury or illness. Parents or family members are a more reliable source of how the patient is psychologically responding to the situation. Obtaining this information will allow you to also make return-to-play recommendations and, if indicated, what type of restriction is necessary. From the history, a differential diagnosis is produced; the physical examination and diagnostic tests help narrow the focus.

Physical Examination

The appreciation of tissue texture abnormality is fundamental to the evaluation of the patient. The experienced osteopathic physician uses palpation and a detailed functional biomechanical evaluation to make an assessment that is not limited to the patient's subjective complaint.

Osteopathic physicians also examine not only the injured region but also distant, potentially related sites. Often, there is a direct anatomic correlation. The body is interconnected through various complex fascial, neurologic, reflexive, and metabolic relationships. Athletes especially rely on the transfer of energy between these different regions of the body. Osteopathic manipulative therapy can correct these segmental and regional dysfunctions and thereby improve the transfer of energy that is required for various athletic demands.

Osteopathic sports physicians develop both their hands and minds and are trained to evaluate injuries differently. Consider a common sports medicine "itis," such as tendonitis, periostitis, or bursitis. It is commonplace to quickly diagnose an "itis" in an athlete. An osteopathic physician can use palpatory skills to determine where the "itis" is located, its severity, and chronicity. They also look for the "why" behind the injury. Was there a predisposing structural or functional imbalance between the muscles, joints, or connective tissues? Was it just a situation of too much, too soon, or too fast? If so, what are the psychological or social factors motivating the patient?

Lastly osteopathic doctors (DOs) do not have to rely solely on the prescription pad to relieve pain, decrease edema, or improve performance. Many athletic injuries can be treated effectively using osteopathic techniques.

Standing Screening/Scanning Examination

The standing screening examination in the athlete is performed in the same fashion as for the general population; however, it is not uncommon to find some differences. Consider the evaluation of spinal A-P curves. Athletes may develop unique postural characteristics associated with their particular sport, which must be taken into account.

On forward bending, asymmetry of muscle mass in the paraspinal muscles is not uncommon. This paravertebral muscle "humping" or prominence may be related to spinal idiopathic scoliosis, functional group curve mechanics, or as a developmental response on the dominant hand side. This is especially true in athletes who predominately use one extremity (quarterback or place kicker). Athletes who perform repetitive motions (like golfers) can have lateral spinal curves due to muscle tightness from the patterned repetitive movement.

Volleyball and basketball players (especially tall, thin females) are commonly found to have general ligamentous laxity and recurvatum at the elbows and knees. Arm span longer than height, arachnodactyly (long, thin fingers), and kyphoscoliosis may tip off the doctor to Marfan syndrome. Because of potential aortic and cardiac structural abnormalities, these patients need a thorough cardiovascular workup prior to competition.

Runners may have a variety of foot problems, including asymmetric pes planus, which can present as a short leg on structural examination. In this situation, the iliac crest and greater trochanter may be low on the same side. Pelvic side shift will be away from the short leg side. A lumbar spinal convexity is commonly palpated on the short leg side.

Asymmetric hamstring tension can affect posture and the standing flexion test. A tight hamstring muscle may hold the innominate inferiorly, giving a false negative test on the same side. A tight iliopsoas muscle may produce pelvic side shift away from the psoas spasm. A tight iliopsoas affects the standing examination. The patient may appear bent over forward and to the side of the spasm. Their belt line may appear low on one side.

In weight lifters, protracted shoulders may lead to rotator cuff impingement syndromes. This is usually attributed to poor posture, over-development of the pectorals, inhibited rhomboids and lower trapezius muscles. These areas are prone to extended segmental dysfunctions that are painful and persistent. Treating these dysfunctions throughout the rehabilitation is crucial for restoration of a functional thoracic kyphosis (Fig. 37.1). Evaluating and treating these types of muscle imbalances is a key to preventing or treating shoulder complaints.

Palpatory Examination

Athletic patients have an overall tone to their muscles and tissues that is not found in the general population. Healthy muscle feels smooth and homogeneous, with taught fascia and less subcutaneous findings. The palpatory examination can determine the presence and severity of tissue texture abnormality, as well as the size, shape, and tone of the muscles. The extent and location of muscle splinting (which is a common finding in athletic injury) needs to be determined with palpation. For example, muscle splinting of the hamstrings can give a false negative anterior drawer test at the knee.

Palpation can be used as part of the neurologic examination, because flaccid or atrophic muscles may be related to a lower motor neuron lesion. Athletes with a herniated lumbar disc and radiculopathy may have palpable findings in the affected leg.

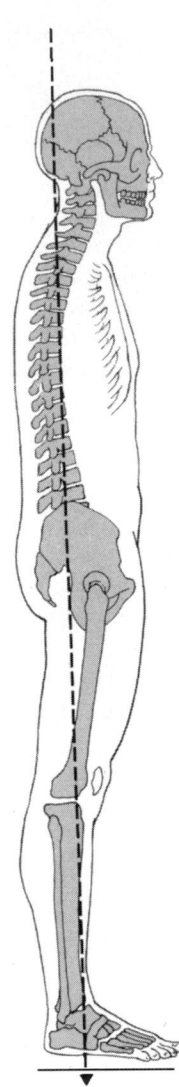

FIGURE 37.1. Flat Back Posture. (From Kendall FP, McCreary EK, Provance PG. *Muscles Testing and Function with Posture and Pain,* 4th ed. Baltimore: Williams & Wilkins; 1993:76, with permission.)

Palpation may also reveal injury to ligamentous structures, such as in the acute ankle sprain. Torn ligaments are locally tender and may have a palpable defect. Rents (tears) in the fascia with or without muscle herniation can also be palpated. In children, a frequent area of injury is the apophysis (where the tendon inserts on bone), which can be palpated. In compartment syndromes of the extremities, increased tissue tension, muscle firmness, fullness, and pain to applied pressure are common palpatory findings.

It is important to palpate the injured area (and sometimes distant areas) when the athlete is performing a particular motion, such as performing a sit-up. Tenderness, muscular findings, or even a hernia may be accentuated at this time. Tenderness of muscle during a concentric or eccentric contraction may indicate a muscular strain. Scar tissue does not actively contract and may be locally tender during this examination.

Observation and/or palpation of muscle firing patterns can also provide useful information. Palpation at this time also allows the physician to determine if a particular muscle is "turning on" or if it is inhibited. Consider the vastus medialis muscle. It

commonly becomes flaccid and atrophic after knee arthroscopy or injury. This is a neurologic inhibition, not a true weakness. This factor is important to determine and treat prior to prescribing more advanced therapeutic exercises.

There are particular patterns of muscular contraction seen in various movements. Patients who have significant muscular imbalances, somatic dysfunction, or injury are prone to having these abnormalities. Consider the low back pain patient who fires their lumbar paraspinals instead of their gluteus with each hip extension. This pattern becomes learned and will persist and lead to further injury or incomplete recovery if not corrected by appropriate neuromuscular retraining.

Motion Testing

Motion testing should include joints, soft tissues, fascia, and cranial motion. It is performed in areas that contain significant tissue texture abnormality. Prior to motion testing, it is important to understand that athletes may have very different qualities of motion, yet these are still "normal" findings. For example, motion testing in an athlete's innominates may reveal a symmetric yet firm compliance. A sedentary patient is typically found to have a soft compliant pelvis.

Some athletes have significant flexibility of their ligaments and joints, yet this is not appreciated readily because of the generalized tone of the muscles. Clinically, it is more difficult to palpate areas of articular hypermobility than hypomobility. Adolescent females are commonly found to have ligamentous laxity or hypermobility. This is commonly seen at the knees and shoulders. Sports that accentuate this laxity include gymnastics and swimming. Other athletes appear to be stiffer. These differences in flexibility may be genetically related. Symmetric range of motion and an appropriate range of motion for a given activity are important factors in motion testing and later on during rehabilitation.

Articular Motion Testing

Motion testing includes an evaluation of *the quantity and quality of motion.* Articular somatic dysfunction typically occurs in the joint's minor motions. A significant variable during motion testing is the concept of "end-feel." End-feel is a qualitative finding of reluctance or resistance to further motion. It is a qualitative descriptor of the restrictive barrier. Microtraumatic injuries (repetitive overuse) may have a firm end-feel due to muscle tightness. Macrotraumatic injuries evaluated within the "golden hour" may produce a loose or sloppy end-feel, especially if ligamentous disruption occurred. After this, muscle splinting of the injured area occurs, and the end-feel may become firm. Viscerosomatic reflexes may produce a rubbery end-feel to the tissues. The type of restriction found during motion testing helps guide the selection of manipulative treatment.

The Functional Biomechanical Examination

Sport performance is primarily a function of the musculoskeletal system. The body economy (including the cardiovascular and pulmonary systems) is constantly tuned to the high and variable demands of the musculoskeletal system. The athlete is subject to the biomechanical strength and flexibility demands of his or her particular sport, as well as the gravitational challenges producing the ground reaction forces of the associated sports performance. When approaching the injured athlete, it is important to think of functional anatomy, understanding the joints are both mechanical and sensory organs that produce both proprioceptive and nociceptive information. The processing of this altered information may change motor patterns and produce dysfunction and/or injury. The most important symptom of disturbed motor function is usually pain. As sports medicine clinicians, we want to avoid falling into the trap of treating symptoms. We must learn to identify dysfunctional patterns and seek to guide our athletic patients in neuromusculoskeletal behavioral patterns that are less costly biomechanically and more favorable to health and efficient function.

To treat dysfunction, we must first understand function. We often recognize athletes by characteristic movements, such as running gait, golf swing, pitching motion, or other particular sport-related movements. Every individual acquires highly characteristic motor patterns during growth and development. There are no norms to movement patterns. As sports medicine clinicians, we sometimes identify "functional pathology," recognizing that characteristic motor patterns have been altered under the influence of injury, fatigue, and/or abnormal compensations. We must therefore develop the ability to be accurate in reproducing a functional profile of the injured segments, as well as the relationships of the segments to the whole. Compensations that can occur to the neuromusculoskeletal system allow us to adapt to both internal and external stressors. Some compensation can be normal, whereas others are abnormal and can be indicative of or create functional pathology. Part of the difficulty in determining which compensations are normal and which are not demonstrates one of the central challenges of sports medicine. Gravity, ground reaction, and momentum are the primary drivers for functional compensations that can be influenced by extrinsic environments, as well as intrinsic causes, such as structural malalignment, strength, endurance, and flexibility of the connective tissue. It is important to remember that all motion at all joints involves three planes: sagittal, frontal, and transverse, *with appropriate neuromuscular control.* Generally, each joint will have a dominant plane of motion for a given activity; however, injury can occur in a non-dominant plane. A typical example is the knee joint, which is primarily a sagittal plane dominant joint, but is often injured in the transverse or frontal plane.

To evaluate and rehabilitate athletic injuries with intelligence, we must think in terms of a functional kinetic chain. The injured tissue response needs to be predicted and evaluated with reference to ability to decelerate, stabilize, and accelerate specific functional athletic motions. A non-functional approach may try to initially isolate the injured tissue with inappropriate stretching techniques, exercises, and non-physiologic application of stress in an artificially designed, non-functional environment. This may ultimately inhibit the ability of the involved tissue to heal successfully. As a result, this allows us to understand the integrated ground reaction force, center of body weight, muscle movements, and other complementary forces. We can then successfully integrate the involved tissue into the entire kinetic chain system.

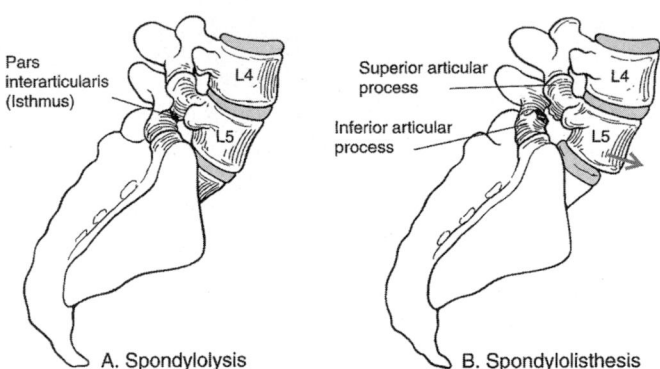

FIGURE 37.2. A fatigue fracture to the pars interarticularis is called **(A)** spondylolysis. When the fracture occurs laterally, **(B)** spondylolisthesis develops. (From Hamill J, Knutzen KM. *Biomechanical Basis of Human Movement.* Baltimore: Williams & Wilkins; 1995:310 [Figure 7-22], with permission.)

Somatic Dysfunction and Sports-Related Injuries

The following clinical examples demonstrate the importance of diagnosing and treating somatic dysfunction that accompanies four common sports injuries.

Back Pain and Spondylolysis

Back pain is commonly seen in adolescent athletes. A spondylolysis is a stress fracture of the pars-interarticularis of the posterior elements of the vertebrae (Fig. 37.2). It is most commonly seen at the L5 level and produces localized pain, especially with extension of the spine. The mechanism of injury is typically one of repetitive hyperextension stress; however, macrotrauma can also produce this injury. Patients typically present with central low back pain, which does not typically radiate into their legs. Pain may be reproduced with the patient bearing weight on a single leg and backward bending. Initial radiographs may show the classic "collar around the Scotty dog's neck" on oblique views, or they may be initially negative. A SPECT bone scan helps to confirm the diagnosis.

It is common to find significant somatic dysfunction along with this injury. Common areas of somatic dysfunction in this injury include:

■ Iliopsoas spasm
■ Flexed upper lumbar dysfunction
■ Sacroiliac/sacral torsion dysfunction
■ Innominate dysfunction

Iliopsoas Spasm

During the evaluation of gait, if the patient walks in a forward bent position, they may have an iliopsoas spasm (Fig. 37.3). The following specific findings on physical examination may indicate this somatic dysfunction. A beltline that is low on one side may indicate the presence of a psoas spasm or short leg. A tight psoas may be associated with a flexed dysfunction in the upper lumbar spine (L1). Pelvic side shift frequently occurs toward the side

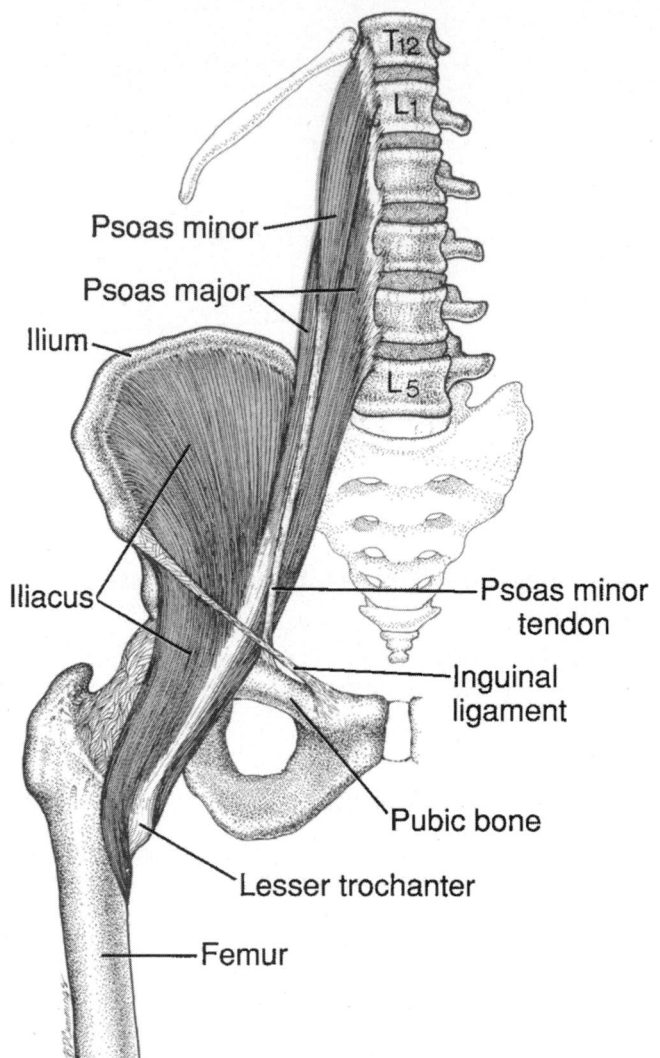

FIGURE 37.3. Attachments of the right psoas major, psoas minor, and iliacus muscles. The psoas major crosses many articulations, including those of the lumbar spine and the lumbosacral, sacroiliac, and hip joints. The psoas minor does the same, except that it does not cross the hip joint. The iliacus, on the other hand, crosses only the hip joint. Psoas. (From Greenman PE. *Principles of Manual Medicine.* Baltimore: Williams & Wilkins; 1996:462 [Figure 20.15b], with permission.)

of the longer leg or opposite to the side of the tighter psoas muscle. A tight iliopsoas resists hip extension. In a patient with spondylolysis, decreasing psoas hypertonicity is a priority. Many times, a flexed Fryette type II dysfunction is commonly found in the upper lumbar region. Treating the flexed lumbar component followed by stretching the tight psoas muscle accomplishes this. Care must be taken as not to apply excessive forces through the area of spondylolysis in accomplishing this.

Sacroiliac/Sacral Torsion Dysfunction

Sacroiliac dysfunction is also commonly present. The type of sacroiliac dysfunction is variable. A sacrum that freely extends is typically more painful and harder to treat. It may be related to flexed lumbar dysfunction or A-P curve problems. A bilaterally flexed sacrum is seen with an increased lumbar lordosis. Treat-

ment of the psoas hypertonicity typically helps sacroiliac dysfunction. If significant sacral dysfunction is still present after treating the psoas, muscle energy, myofascial, or indirect techniques for the sacrum are useful. Dysfunction of the innominates or pubes may maintain sacroiliac dysfunction. Do not forget that the ilium is the other half of the sacroiliac joint!

Treatment

The first goal of manipulative treatment in the acute spondylolysis is to do no harm. *Do not forget that this is a fracture and fractures are treated with immobilization not manipulation!* However, it is of paramount importance to relieve as much of the *associated* somatic dysfunction as possible. Gentle indirect techniques or muscle energy techniques may be appropriate. Tenderness at L5 and the iliolumbar ligament responds well to counterstrain techniques. Myofascial release of the lumbosacral area can decrease pain and improve motion.

Orthopedic treatment may include the use of a custom neutral lumbar orthosis. This brace is typically worn around the clock initially, and then tapered as the patient improves over the next 6 to 8 weeks. Some athletes may still be able to practice or compete in the brace. Each case needs to be treated individually. Repeat x-ray imaging or a thin-cut computerized tomography (CT) scan can help determine healing; however, the patient's symptoms typically guide the treatment. Watkins (14) describes the orthopedic management of spondylolysis in a variety of sports.

Consider the osteopathic approach to the patient with spondylolysis and psoas spasm. Achieving appropriate muscle firing during hip extension prior to strengthening is crucial. According to Janda's research (described by Dr. Philip Greenman) (15), the muscle-firing pattern for hip extension is: hamstrings, gluteus maximus, contralateral lower lumbar erector spinae, and their ipsilateral lower erector spinae (Fig. 37.4). "The most common alteration of this pattern is failure of activation and weakness of the gluteus maximus, with substitution by the hamstrings and erector spinae musculature, particularly in the upper lumbar and lower thoracic regions." OMT is a crucial component as the athlete retrains weakened abdominal and paraspinal muscles. Treatment of the thoracic, lumbar, and pelvic regions with OMT improves the activation of these patterns and sets the stage for appropriate rehabilitation.

Hip Joint Extension

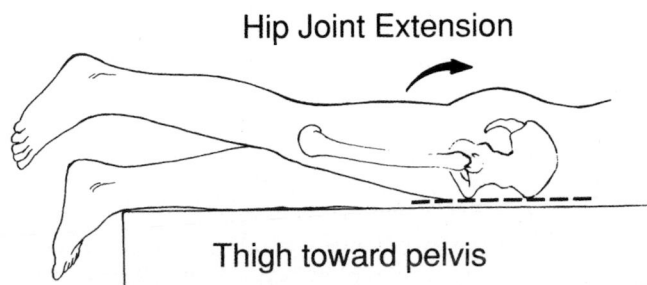

FIGURE 37.4. Hip joint extension. (From Kendall FP, McCreary EK, Provance PG. *Muscles Testing and Function with Posture and Pain,* 4th ed. Baltimore: Williams & Wilkins; 1993:20, with permission.)

Anterior Knee Pain

Anterior knee pain is a common finding in the athletic population. There are many entities that are grouped in this category. These include: patellofemoral pain syndrome, chondromalacia of the patella, miserable malalignment syndrome, and patellar tracking abnormality, to name a few. This painful condition is a spectrum of overuse; however, occasionally there may be a traumatic insult that starts the process. Overuse may result from training errors or underlying malalignment. Overload is characterized by abnormal tensions across the patellofemoral joint with resultant inflammation and microinjury. As the process continues, the cartilage on the under surface of the patella becomes softened and somewhat eroded away. Patients complain of anterior pain around the patella with a variable amount of local swelling. A common complaint is that the knee is painful with activity, especially negotiating stairs or hills. The knee will lock temporarily if the patient was sitting for a while and then stands up. This is called the "theatre sign," and it is pathognomonic (16).

During examination of the patellofemoral joint, it is common to palpate crepitation when motion is introduced to the patella. The traditional orthopedic examination of the patella looks for ballotment (effusion), lateral laxity, and the "patellofemoral grind test." This test is performed by having the supine patient contact their quadriceps while an inferior pressure is applied on the patella. This test generally hurts the patient. Skilled hands can palpate subtle amounts of crepitation, excessive motion, and tracking abnormalities throughout flexion and extension.

The osteopathic palpatory examination not only palpates for restrictions of patellar motion and crepitation but also for the ability of the vastus medialis oblique muscle to "turn on." Atrophy, flaccidity, or inhibition of this muscle is common in this condition. The muscle may become neurologically inhibited from axial somatic dysfunction or inhibited due to pain or disuse. Whatever the cause, the first step in rehabilitating these patients is to gain the ability of this muscle to fire.

Associated physical findings of this condition also include increased hamstring tension, fibular motion restriction, and interosseous membrane tension. Increased tension of the hamstrings will increase pressure between the patella and femoral condyles (Fig. 37.5). This can aggravate inflammation and cartilage damage at the undersurface of the patella. Increased tension in the biceps femoris, iliotibial band (ITB), and lateral fascia of the thigh can cause motion restriction of the fibula and interosseous membrane. This constellation of findings is commonly seen in patellar tracking abnormalities. Subtle restrictions of fibular motion can be appreciated by translating the proximal fibula or lateral malleolus anteriorly or posteriorly. Interosseous membrane tension can also be assessed through internal and external rotation of the tibia and fibula. OMT can be applied to these dysfunctions with retraining of the vastus medialis muscle, thus improving hamstring and ITB tension.

Rotator Cuff Tendonitis/Impingement Syndromes

Rotator cuff tendonitis and subacromial bursitis are common sports medicine diagnoses. The history can help pinpoint the

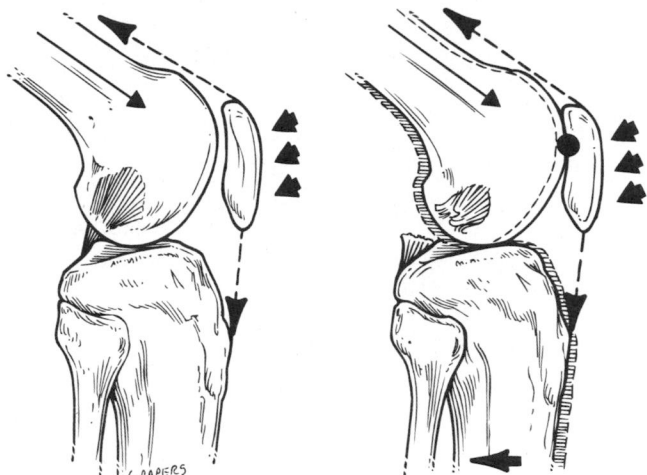

FIGURE 37.5. Patellofemoral compression. A functioning quadriceps mechanism is necessary for proprioceptive control of the knee. The static stability provided by the cruciate ligament protects the patellofemoral mechanism and the menisci, and stops the femur from being driven into the tibia in deceleration and descending movements. (From Baker CL. *The Hughston Clinic Sports Medicine Field Manual.* Baltimore: Williams & Wilkins; 1996:228 [Figure 20-9], with permission.)

diagnosis in upper extremity complaints. For example, pain into the deltoid insertion at night may indicate a rotator cuff tear. A clicking or snapping deep in the shoulder may indicate a labrum tear. Apprehension with external rotation may indicate instability.

It is important to realize that although these are common conditions, not all shoulder pain is due to rotator cuff problems. Somatic dysfunction plays a major role in the pathogenesis of shoulder pain. In young healthy patients, most shoulder complaints are due to abnormal muscular tensions or forces across the pectoral girdle. Occasionally, bony abnormalities, fracture, arthritis, infections, or tumors are diagnosed. Injuries to the glenohumeral joint almost always lead to a restriction of motion. Consider the entire pectoral girdle and axial spine when assessing these injuries and conditions.

Impingement syndromes can occur due to multiple factors. The space between the undersurface of the acromion and humeral head is called the impingement interval. This space narrows with arm abduction (Fig. 37.6). Any condition that further narrows this space can cause impingement. Several classification systems have been described. Neer (17) described three stages of injury based on patient age and pathologic changes in the rotator cuff. Impingement syndromes can also be divided into external and internal impingement. In external impingement, there is not enough room under the acromion for the supraspinatus tendon to glide freely. An example of this is outlet obstruction, where an arthritic spur or anatomic variant at the acromion may narrow the space. This usually occurs in patients older than 35 years of age. Another factor may be postural, where protracted (rolled forward) shoulders, weak cuff muscles, and poor humeral head depression cause a limited subacromial space.

A common internal factor that causes impingement includes instability of the glenohumeral joint. This usually occurs in patients less than 35 years old, and may be associated with a superior glenoid labrum tear (SLAP lesion), a fracture (Bankart lesion), or a depression-type fracture of the humeral head

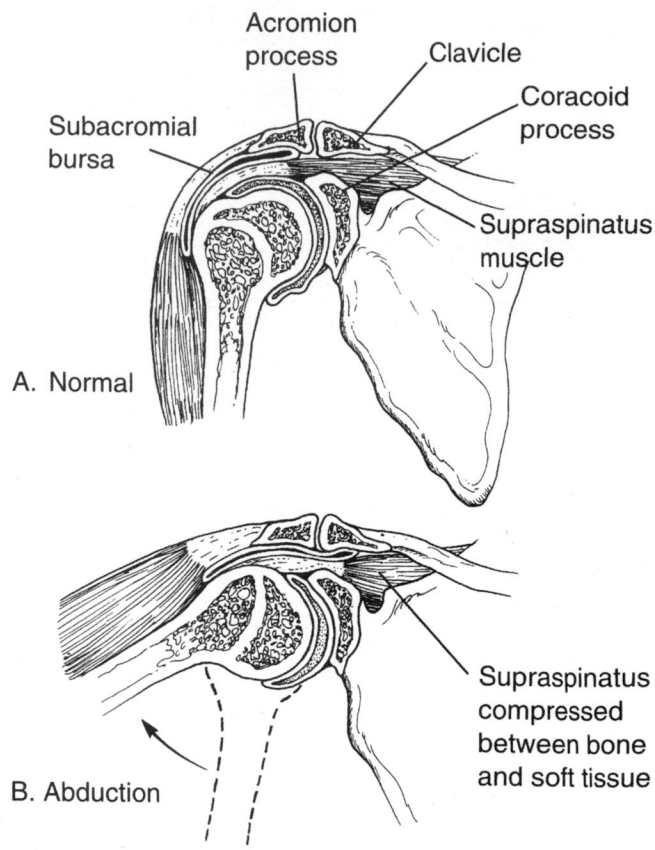

FIGURE 37.6. Supraspinatus/Impingement. (From Anderson MK, Hall SJ. *Fundamentals of Sports Injury Management.* Baltimore: Williams & Wilkins; 1997:405 [Figure 11.16], with permission.)

(Hill-Sachs deformity). This impingement occurs more distal to the acromioclavicular joint. Overuse, instability, and microtrauma contribute to this condition. The most common form of instability is anterior and inferior. The deficiency is in the anterior inferior glenohumeral ligament complex. Posterior, inferior, and multidirectional instabilities also occur. There are specific tests for each of these.

Diagnosis of the Somatic Component

Whether or not there is an axial (spine and torso) component to the patient's complaint, it is prudent to include evaluation of the upper thoracic and cervical spine, the costal cage, and internal organs of the chest and abdomen in each patient with an upper extremity problem. The patient's history will occasionally steer the physician to the workup of visceral disease referring pain to the upper extremity. The physical examination, including palpation of the upper extremity for evidence of somatic dysfunction, will elucidate the diagnosis. Occasionally, cardiopulmonary disease may be the cause of the somatic findings and pain in the upper thoracic spine and upper extremity. It is not uncommon to find somatic dysfunction between T5-9 due to a viscerosomatic reflex from stomach or duodenal inflammation secondary to the prolonged consumption of nonsteroidal antiinflammatory medications that are often used to relieve the pain in the upper extremity. Even after resolution of upper extremity pathophysiology, persistence of upper extremity pain may be due to referred visceral

pain or upper and/or mid-thoracic viscerosomatic dysfunction. This, of course, requires further evaluation and treatment of the visceral component of the problem.

In addition to the upper extremities, the upper thoracic and cervical spine are important areas to palpate and evaluate for somatic dysfunction. The upper thoracic cord, especially at levels T1-4, supplies sympathetic efferents to the head, neck, and upper extremities. These efferents are involved in the regulation of blood flow and also innervate the musculature, modulating muscle tone (18). Additionally, afferent fibers from the cervical spine and paraspinal soft tissues synapse in the upper thoracic spinal cord (intermediolateral cell column). Somatic dysfunction in the cervical region causes increased afferent input into the upper thoracic spinal cord. This can, in turn, facilitate upper thoracic sympathetic hyperactivity and contribute to upper extremity dysfunction. Most mechanical neck problems are accompanied by identifiable upper thoracic and upper extremity somatic dysfunctions that are partly through this mechanism. Upper thoracic sympathetic hyperactivity (often from levels T2 and T3) can refer pain, tingling, or abnormal temperature sensations to the arm.

Whenever there is a dysfunction in any one part of the neuromusculoskeletal system, it is imperative to evaluate the entire kinetic chain as a dynamic unit of function in posture and motion. Investigating along these lines would lead the osteopathic physician to ask:

i. Are there abnormal neurologic reflexes or asymmetric muscle strength, tone or size?
ii. Is there evidence of joint dysfunction?
iii. Is postural imbalance contributing to the problem or complaint?
iv. Is the painful extremity on the concave or convex side of a spinal dysfunction?
v. Is there evidence of compensation contributing to spinal or extremity dysfunction?

Dysfunction in the upper extremity will also affect scapular position and motion (Fig. 37.7). Somatic dysfunction of the upper thoracic spine and ribs can also affect scapulohumeral rhythm and scapular position. Smooth, efficient movement of the scapula and coordinated strength of the scapular stabilizing muscles are necessary to prevent upper quarter dysfunction (including rotator cuff problems).

Cervical spine diseases (i.e., herniated disc, osteoarthritis, stenosis) may refer pain to the upper thoracic region, shoulder, arm, and hand. Somatic dysfunction of the lower cervical and cervical-thoracic junction can produce arm symptoms through three mechanisms:

- Direct irritation of cervical spinal nerves
- Neurovascular compression (thoracic outlet syndromes)
- Myofascial restrictions resulting in lymphatic obstruction

OMT directed at somatic dysfunction of the upper thoracic spine and ribs, cervical spine, and then to the myofascial structures of the pectoral girdle and arm is an important component of treatment in patients with rotator cuff disease.

MOVEMENTS OF THE SCAPULA

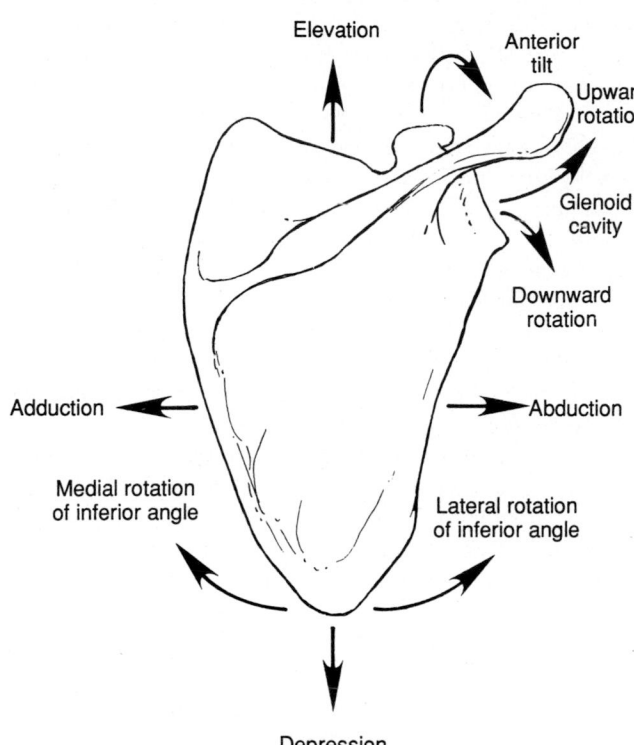

FIGURE 37.7. Scapular Motion. (From Kendall FP, McCreary EK, Provance PG. *Muscles Testing and Function with Posture and Pain,* 4th ed. Baltimore: Williams & Wilkins; 1993:16, with permission.)

Inversion Ankle Sprain

Ankle sprains are the most common athletic injury. They make up 45% of all injuries in basketball, 31% in soccer, and 25% in volleyball. Inversion-type ankle sprains make up 85% of all ankle sprains (19).

The ankle is a hinge type of synovial joint. The distal ends of the tibia and fibula form a "mortise" into which the superior aspect of the talus fits. The talus is wider anteriorly than posteriorly (wedge-shaped). Plantar flexion decreases the stability of the ankle because the anterior aspect of the talus is no longer wedged between the malleoli. Because of this anatomy, most ankle injuries occur in the plantar flexed position. Ankle injuries should be assessed as soon as possible after the injury before swelling commences. Because less than 15% of ankle injuries are found to result in significant fracture, the Ottawa ankle rules were developed to guide clinicians as to when to obtain a radiograph (20).

Supination (inversion) stresses the lateral ankle ligaments (Fig. 37.8). Most inversion sprains occur with the ankle in the plantar-flexed position. Various physical tests are used for assessing the ankle ligaments. Palpable tissue texture changes are usually found over the injured ligament(s). Palpation for tissue texture changes is very valuable, especially when the patient is experiencing too much pain to tolerate stress testing for ligament integrity. Tears of the anterior talofibular ligament are very common and are likely if the talus may be moved forward (and into slight internal rotation) 4 mm or more on physical testing. This test is called

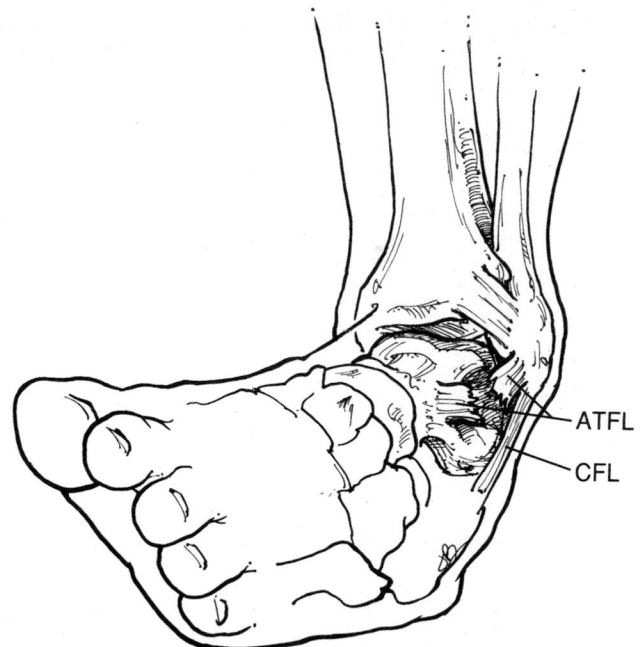

FIGURE 37.8. Inversion Ankle Sprain. (From Baker CL. *The Hughston Clinic Sports Medicine Field Manual.* Baltimore: Williams & Wilkins; 1996:240 [Figure 22-1], with permission.)

the anterior drawer test. The ability to tilt the ankle or invert it more than 25 to 30 degrees implies rupture of the lateral ligaments. Grading ankle sprains is based on clinically determining if a minor incomplete, moderate incomplete, or total rupture of the lateral ligaments has occurred. The medial deltoid ligament is strong and thick; injury to it usually results in a bony avulsion. Always palpate for bony pain, crepitation, or point tenderness when considering a potential fracture.

Most ankle sprains will be associated with dysfunction of the lateral malleolus and, frequently, with restrictions at the fibular head. Restriction at either the proximal (head) or distal (lateral malleolus) end of the fibula can alter normal ankle motion and produce pain and dysfunction in both the ankle and the knee, increasing the amount of time to recovery. A key mobilization to help restore full range of motion is the "Talar Tug," where the talus is distracted from the calcaneus, allowing a resetting of the articular facets.

The venous and lymphatic drainage must travel through myofascial structures associated with the ankle, knee, and hip on their way back to the heart. Dysfunction in any of these structures can disrupt both lymphatic and venous drainage and interfere with healing. Prolonged swelling alters the proprioceptive ability of the ankle and may predispose this area to further injury. Addressing somatic dysfunction may assist in the removal of swelling from the area and may ultimately speed the recovery from such injuries.

Consider the individual's gait biomechanics in their ankle rehabilitation. When the heel first strikes the ground, the foot is in the supinated (inverted) position. As the body's weight is transferred anteriorly, the foot pronates (everts). A flat foot is frequently associated with over pronation (foot eversion). This will place excessive stress on the ligaments of the medial ankle and may lead to pain in this area. An excessive range or rate of pronation may also be associated with shin splints. A high arch is frequently associated with excessive supination (foot inversion). This will place excessive strain on the ligaments of the lateral ankle and may lead to lateral foot pain.

A useful manipulative approach in the acute ankle sprain uses myofascial and indirect techniques. As the swelling subsides, muscle energy, articulatory, or other direct techniques can be used. For persistent ankle pain after an inversion injury, a direct myofascial release of the medial deltoid ligament and fascial structures seems to work well. OMT is useful to decrease edema and pain, allowing the patient to begin a functional ankle rehabilitation program sooner. It is also useful to treat secondary symptoms (such as low back pain) that can occur from a change in gait after an ankle injury.

PRINCIPLE CENTERED REHABILITATION

Principles are natural laws that, for the most part, are intuitively obvious. We hope that by introducing you to principles rather than practices and describing the principles behind some of the practices, you will be better prepared to handle the current challenges of sports medicine rehabilitation, as well as the unknown challenges of the future (21). We hope to be able to prepare you to handle each patient and the situations unique to each patient. This approach tends to orient you away from a particular treatment protocol and will provide you with a philosophic approach that will hopefully allow your patients to have outstanding functional outcomes.

Inherent in this process is differentiating between "treatment" thinking versus "preventive" thinking. Sports medicine clinicians need to avoid falling into the trap of "treating symptoms" and initiate a reevaluation and reprogramming process that prevents the injury from recurring. Identify the *root cause* of the injury and orient the rehabilitative process to attack the root cause rather than simply treating the symptom of the injury.

Be cognizant of the natural laws taught in the disciplines of anatomy and physiology, which includes biochemistry and the biomechanics that govern successful (or unsuccessful) function of the neuromusculoskeletal system in the performance of the sport being played. These natural laws usually cannot be violated with impunity, or dysfunction and/or injury will occur. The more physiologically aligned our athletes are with these basic principles, the less the opportunity for injury and the greater the chance for success.

Albert Einstein once said, "The significant problems we face cannot be solved by the same level of thinking that created them." We must be able to transform our patients to a new level of function to successfully reintegrate them into sports-related activities and prevent reinjury.

Functional Approach

As we begin to approach the strategy for the design of a functional rehabilitative process for our injured athletes, it is useful to think of the locomotor system as a "kinetic chain." Some things that are part of this chain include, but are not limited to, the joints, muscles, bones, and proprioceptors that help to guide our patients in successful athletic activities. As such, we must begin to appreciate that there is a strange relationship between the cause and the cure of injuries. The ultimate goal of rehabilitation of an injured athlete is to return the injured individual back safely to the activity that directly contributed to the injury! In general, athletes enjoy having the opportunity to return to the activity that originally caused their pain in a successful and pain-free manner.

Therefore, a vital component of the functional rehabilitative environment will actually be the causative activity. Therein lies the challenge of rehabilitation . . . to transform the cause into the cure. This transformation is the rehabilitation. Through rehabilitation, we must transform the injured tissue into tissue that successfully deals with the loads and motions of the causative activity. We must reintegrate the injured tissue into a more effective and efficient functional chain reaction system.

For this transformation and reintegration to occur and be successful, a logical progression of clinically controlled techniques that are symptom and performance directed must be accomplished. Intelligent management of these techniques requires and is based on a strong biomechanical understanding of the kinetic chain and the pathophysiology of injury.

Central to the understanding of kinetic chain muscle function in the locomotor system is understanding the concept of an oxymoron—a unique combination of two incongruent qualities juxtaposed to form a more meaningful concept. To wit, the integrated use of opposite words provides an understanding synergistically greater than the combined understanding of each word used in an isolated manner. "Functional oxymorons" provide us with the necessary foundation to design and manage biomechanically reactive rehabilitative environments (i.e., "causative cure").

The isolation of a soft tissue in an integrated system begins to describe the concept of "integrated isolation" (another functional oxymoron). Initially, one must isolate the involved tissue to fully understand the site of injury, the extent of injury, and the effect of injury. Concurrently, one must appreciate the actual function of the involved tissue and how its integration into the functional compensation system allowed for the excessive mechanical loading of the tissue and the resultant injury.

To determine the integrated isolated function of this tissue in the kinetic chain, what this tissue does in real life must be comprehended in a practical sense. The following questions need to be addressed and answered to appreciate the causes and compensations resulting in tissue failure:

i. To what forces does the tissue react?
ii. What joints and motions does the tissue decelerate, stabilize, and accelerate?
iii. In what planes and with what other tissues does it function?
iv. How does the tissue dynamically integrate its isolated function?

Answering these inquiries will lead to the successful design of the appropriate functional environment for rehabilitation, helping to transform the injured tissue into healthy tissue, and then reintegrate it into the functional system.

Therefore, the rehabilitative strategy is to design the environment to facilitate the appropriate reaction of the target tissue with functional, progressive exercises and appropriate therapeutic modalities. This is controlled clinically by modulating the stress and strain of the activity, controlling the joints that dominate the activity, and determining in what plane the reaction/action predominantly takes place.

Compensations

Compensation occurs in the neuromusculoskeletal system that allows us to adapt to both internal and external stressors. Some compensation can be normal; however, others are abnormal and can be indicative of or create functional pathology. Part of the difficulty in determining which compensations are normal and which are abnormal demonstrates the cause and effect relationship between functional activity and the resultant compensations. Gravity, ground reaction, and momentum are the primary drivers for functional compensations. Footwear and various orthotic interfaces are examples of extrinsic environments that a functional system can react with and compensate for. Compensations can be caused by interacting with various forms of equipment, therapeutic or otherwise, as well as types of terrain (playing fields, etc.).

Structural malalignment abnormalities are examples of intrinsic causes of compensations. Intuitively, the strength, endurance, and flexibility of the connective tissue have a direct effect on the compensation of the linkage system. Additionally, balance and other neuromuscular considerations, such as proprioceptive ability and muscle tone, have a dramatic effect on function and functional compensation. Determining the actual cause or causes of the compensation and what relationship the compensation has to the contribution of excessive mechanical loads to the involved tissue is the major task of the biomechanical evaluation. Understanding the potential causes and resultant compensation is based on the biomechanics of function and the timing of function. This understanding allows for more effective treatment of the causes of the injury and the resultant compensations, as well as the symptoms (pain).

Real World Muscle Function

Clinicians typically describe muscle function in three ways: concentric, eccentric, and isometric. We think of a concentric muscular contraction as a functional shortening of the muscle while it contracts. Eccentric contraction is a functional lengthening of the muscle while it contracts. Isometric contraction is a stabilizing force during which neither shortening nor lengthening of the muscle occurs.

As we begin to understand the real world function of muscles and groups of muscles, we begin to understand that muscles may function concentrically at one joint, eccentrically or isometrically at another joint, or in another plane at the same joint at the same time. This occurs within the kinetic chain, reacting with and against gravity, ground reaction, and momentum, in multiple planes of motion. This concept of chain reaction muscle function is best summed up in the phrase "econcentric." This concept of econcentric muscle function allows clinicians to understand the causes and compensations of both acute and overuse injuries and gives us an enhanced ability to determine the appropriate

econcentric reaction of the injured tissue to facilitate healing and enhance function.

To intelligently rehabilitate injuries, we must know not only what the affected tissue is doing during the activity that contributed to its breakdown, but also what it does, when it does, and why it does. As previously noted, we must also know how the involved tissue is integrated into the entire kinetic chain system.

Pronation and Supination

Understanding pronation and supination gives us a head start in our thought process to determine potential causes of dysfunction and the resultant symptoms. Understanding functional chain reaction pronation and supination gives us the ability to begin to determine which dynamic compensations are normal and which are abnormal. This also allows us to understand the integrated isolated function of the involved tissue with the other tissues that synergistically work in the kinetic chain with the symptomatic tissue. This understanding also allows us to begin to take advantage of the concept of econcentric muscle function.

Pronation is a collapsing of the chain, while supination is a regirding of the chain. Pronation is shock absorption, while supination is propulsion. Pronation is a reaction caused by the effects of gravity and ground reaction forces. Supination is a reaction resulting from pronation. Pronation succumbs to gravity, while supination overcomes gravity. The transformation of pronation into supination is the key to the success of the locomotor system in sport movement. Pronation and supination occur at all joints and in all planes of motion of the locomotor system.

Remember that pronation and supination many times have more to do with the timing of motions at certain joints and in certain planes than with the actual amount of motion of the joint. Pronation is dominated by eccentric (deceleration) muscle function. Supination is dominated by concentric (acceleration) muscle function. Therefore, the transformation of pronation into supination is dominated by isometric (stabilizing) and econcentric muscle function—deceleration of motion at one joint and acceleration of motion at another joint or in another plane, all at the same time.

Osteopathic Manipulative Therapy and Rehabilitation

Somatic dysfunction frequently develops in the human neuromusculoskeletal system in the course of adapting to the relentless force of gravity. The athlete's ability to adapt is additionally challenged by the particular demands of his or her sport. OMT is a vital step to restore balanced structure and function. Once structure and function have been improved, comprehensive neuromuscular retraining as previously described can be undertaken.

The Success Imperative

Successful rehabilitation depends on the ability to take advantage of just the right amount of motion, at just the right joint, in just the right plane, in just the right direction, at just the right time. A basic principle of functional rehabilitation is to allow the patient to be successful and to allow this success to ultimately transform into the ultimate goal of returning the athlete to his or her sport. However, we must remember that the health and safety of the athlete is our primary concern. Our ability to successfully return athletes to the environment of sport is based on the integrative findings of the comprehensive biomechanical examination and an in-depth understanding of the pathophysiology of injury, as well as the loads and motions of the particular sport.

We must be always mindful that the examination, diagnosis, and treatment of an athletic injury include a dialogue between two human beings, involving physical, physiologic, and psychological linkages. This is a complex transaction that, when skillfully performed, can result in a profound and long-lasting effect. The clinician interested in neuromusculoskeletal medicine quite literally has at his or her fingertips an extensive document of the patient's history, including indications of general health and the extent of structural adaptation to the environment, as well as challenges produced in the pursuit of sport.

CONCUSSIONS, HEADACHES, AND NEUROLOGIC DEFICITS IN ATHLETES

Headache is the most common neurologic disease. Hippocrates was the first physician to describe a sports headache. The international headache society describes 13 categories of headaches and about 150 headache syndromes. In the young athletic population, there is about a 35% incidence of headache. A slightly greater incidence of headache (46%) is described in young athletic males. This is likely secondary to higher numbers of males participating in contact sports. When evaluating an athletic headache, it is important to rule out other forms of headache, which may be secondary to medication, intracranial mass, sinusitis, or other medical ailments.

The most common sports headache is the effort headache. There is an equal incidence in both males and females. This is felt to be secondary to increased intracranial pressure associated with athletic effort. It typically has a rapid onset and is described as a frontal or bi-frontal type of headache. Duration can be from several minutes to up to 24 hours.

Another common sports-related headache is the cervicogenic headache, or headache related to cervical sprain. This is felt to be secondary to stretching of cervical ligaments and tendons, which results in a reflex muscle contraction, or spasm, of the paracervical musculature. This headache is probably more common in males, and is frequently associated with combative sports, such as football, boxing, wrestling, or martial arts. Because of the tremendous forces generated in luge and bobsled, this headache is also frequently described in these athletes as well. Typically, patients will complain of pain in the upper cervical, occipital, and/or parietal regions, and the pain may last for several days or weeks.

Acute effort migraine may also occur in athletes. This typically follows short, intense activity. Mechanism for this is unclear, but is felt to be related to decreased cerebral CO_2 secondary to hyperventilation, which results in vasoconstriction. Contributing factors may also include caffeine use or discontinuance, poor nutrition, dehydration, head load, hypoglycemia, and alcohol use. Interestingly, similar to the refractory period that can be induced

in exercise asthma, a gradual warm-up may help in prevention by inducing this "refractory period" with respect to migraine. A trauma-triggered migraine is initiated by head trauma and is found to be more common in athletes with a prior history of migraine headache. This is seen more commonly in contact or collision sports, and usually responds to the patient's typical treatment for migraine.

Posttraumatic headache may also occur in athletes and is more common in males that are involved in contact and combative sports. It is important to note that the intensity of headache may not be related to the severity of trauma, and that this is a headache that is also often associated with concussion. Duration of this headache may be from hours to weeks.

One of the biggest issues facing the sports medicine clinician is concussion. Sports that are at highest risk for concussion include football, gymnastics, ice hockey, and wrestling. In U.S. football alone, 250,000 head injuries are estimated per year. Unfortunately, there is no universal agreement on the definition of concussion or the various grades or severity of concussion. As a result, multiple different evaluation systems have developed (Table 37.1). Some athletes may develop post-concussive syndrome, which can include on-going headache, headache with exertion, dizziness, fatigue, irritability, impaired memory, and decreased concentration. This is felt to be most likely secondary to altered neurotransmitter function posttraumatically.

Decisions governing return to sports after head injury most often lies with the primary care physician (22). There are a number of clinical guidelines in the literature that are intended to help physicians. The guidelines (Table 37.1) most widely accepted are those proposed by Cantu (23, 24), by the Colorado Medical Society (25), and by the American Academy of Neurology (26). None of these guidelines are based on prospective studies. Currently, there is no consensus in the sports medicine community as to which guidelines are most appropriate. Further leading to confusion, a recent study by Lovell (27) questions the validity of guidelines that use loss of consciousness as a marker of concussion severity in return-to-play decisions.

The long-term health and the prevention of secondary neurologic injury to the athlete should be the only concern that guides return-to-play timing and permission from the team physician. The restriction from play of any athlete with persistent symptoms is generally accepted (22). To avoid second-impact syndrome, return to contact sports should only be allowed after the athlete is asymptomatic both at rest and with exertion. Further, repeat concussions generally require a longer period of asymptomatic rest, although the exact amount is unclear. A number of studies have demonstrated that neuropsychiatric testing, through a battery of tests, can detect cognitive impairment after mild traumatic brain injury (28–32). Any athlete with repeat concussions should probably undergo multidisciplinary evaluation, including neuropsychiatric testing prior to return to play.

In general, athletic headache management strategies include both an acute management component and a prophylactic component. The pathophysiology is felt to be secondary to a number of factors, including the so-called neuroinflammatory model, with vascular involvement, as well as stimulation of nociceptive nerve fibers. Management strategies include both non-drug

TABLE 37.1. GUIDELINES FOR RETURN TO PLAY AFTER CONCUSSION

Concussion Grade	Features	Management	Return to Play
Cantu (23, 24)			
1 (mild)	No loss of consciousness; posttraumatic amnesia <30 min.	Remove from contest; observe on sidelines.	May return if asymptomatic[a]; second grade-1: May return in 2 weeks if asymptomatic for 1 week; third grade-1: terminate season, may return next year if asymptomatic.
2 (moderate)	Loss of consciousness <5 min OR posttraumatic amnesia >30 min.	Remove from contest and disallow return that day; athlete should be evaluated by a neurologist at a medical facility; cervical spine precautions as indicated.	Return after asymptomatic for 1 week; second grade-2: wait at least 1 month, may return then if asymptomatic for 1 week, consider terminating season; third grade-2: terminate season, may return next year if asymptomatic.
3 (severe)	Loss of consciousness >5 min OR posttraumatic amnesia >24 hrs.	Transport athlete to nearest hospital with neurosurgical facilities with head and neck immobilization; admit to hospital and check for intracranial bleeding.	Wait at least 1 month, may return if asymptomatic for 1 week; second grade-3: terminate season, may return next season if asymptomatic.
Colorado Medical Society (25)			
1 (mild)	No loss of consciousness; confusion without amnesia.	Remove from contest; examine immediately and at 5 min intervals for development of mental status changes or postconcussive symptoms at rest with exertion.	May return if asymptomatic at least 20 minutes; second grade-1 in same contest: disqualify athlete for that day; third grade-1: terminate season.
2 (moderate)	No loss of consciousness; confusion with amnesia.	Remove from contest and disallow return that day; examine on site frequently for signs of evolving intracranial pathology.	May return after 1 full asymptomatic week; second grade-2: return to play after 1 month symptom, consider termination of season; third grade-2: terminate season.
3 (severe)	Any loss of consciousness.	Transport athlete to nearest ER by ambulance with cervical spine precautions; CT scan or MR imaging if symptoms worsen or persist > than 1 week.	May return after 1 month if asymptomatic for at least 2 weeks; second grade-3: terminate season, return to any contact sport seriously discouraged.
American Academy Neurology (26)			
1 (mild)	No loss of consciousness; transient confusion; concussion symptoms <15 min.	Remove from contest; examine immediately and at 5 min intervals for development of mental status changes or postconcussive symptoms at rest and with exertion.	May return if symptoms clear <15 min; second grade-1 in same contest: disqualify athlete, return in 1 week if asymptomatic.
2 (moderate)	No loss of consciousness; transient confusion; concussion symptoms >15 min.	Remove from contest and disallow return that day; examine on site frequently for signs of evolving intracranial pathology.	May return after 1 fully asymptomatic week; second grade-2: return to play after 2 weeks symptom free.
3 (severe)	Any loss of consciousness, either brief (seconds) or prolonged (minutes).	Transport athlete to nearest ER by ambulance with cervical spine precautions; CT scan or MR imaging if symptoms worsen or persist >1 week.	Brief (seconds) grade-3 concussion: no play until asymptomatic for 2 wks; second grade-3: withold from play for a minimum of 1 asymptomatic month.

[a]All asymptomatic periods mean asymptomatic both at rest and with exertion. Asymptomatic means no headache, dizziness, or impaired concentration plus the ability to fully recall the events occurring before injury.

treatments, such as appropriate conditioning and warm-up, avoidance of triggers, osteopathic manipulation, and physical therapy, as well as drug treatment which might include antiserotonergic and nonsteroidal antiinflammatory medications, beta blockers, calcium channel blockers, and judicious use of narcotics as rescue medication. The sports medicine clinician must always be aware of special considerations regarding drug therapy when treating athletes and being aware of banned substances, as well as the ergolytic effects of certain medicines on athletic performance. Convenience and ease of use of medication is also a consideration when they are to be used at or around the time of athletic competition.

RETURN-TO-PLAY CONSIDERATIONS

There is not a simple algorithm that determines return to play after sport injury. Medical factors are paramount, although a variety of non-medical factors (e.g., age of the athlete, level of competition, psychosocial issues) can influence return-to-play decisions. Although the decision to return to play can be complex, some medical sequelae of sports injuries do represent absolute contraindications to return to contact sports.

Some specific examples would include neck injuries resulting in permanent central nervous system (i.e., spinal cord) dysfunction, permanent and significant peripheral nerve (i.e., nerve root) dysfunction, and certain infectious diseases in the active stages. Some other conditions, for example concussions and some heart conditions, represent relative contraindications to return to play, even in the setting of full recovery. Community physicians are asked to make return-to-play decisions regarding a wide variety of musculoskeletal conditions. Carefully designed symptom-directed functional testing can be invaluable in assisting the clinician in making these sometimes challenging decisions. A typical example would be returning an athlete with an ankle sprain to his/her sport. One can design a series of progressive functional tests that simulate the loads and motions of the sport and evaluate the athlete's performance. Physical therapists and athletic trainers can provide assistance in this regard.

Long-term health and prevention of secondary injury to the athlete should be the only concerns that guide return-to-play timing and permission from the team physician. A licensed, well-trained sports medicine physician who is then responsible for making the final return-to-play decision should evaluate each case individually and completely.

PERFORMANCE ENHANCEMENT

Today's athletes are bigger, stronger, and faster than ever before. This is accomplished by aggressive off-season training through physical, nutritional, and psychological means. As a team physician, it is important to evaluate those athletes with injuries during the season to be sure they have been maximally rehabilitated during the off-season.

Today's athletes improve performance by working specifically on flexibility, speed, strength, and endurance. Integral components to improved performance that are often overlooked are balance and functional strength. As discussed earlier in various sections, training the body in various neuromuscular patterns that are sport specific is the key to performance enhancement. Improved neuromuscular coordination is achieved through removal of somatic dysfunction and postural and muscle imbalances while repetitively training to improve balance, energy transfer, and functional strength throughout sport-specific joint motions. Static pure strength is unimportant without balance and provides minimal advantage to the athlete. An athlete's ability is enhanced through a combination of improved flexibility, proprioception, strength, and practiced movement patterns, which all aim to build better neuromuscular coordination.

The Use of Performance-Enhancing (Ergogenic) Drugs

The term ergogenic means any method to enhance athletic performance. Its Greek root "Ergon" means "to work." Historically, the ancient Greek Olympic athletes are believed to have used both herbs and mushrooms to enhance their performance. Drug abuse in the modern era of athletics became a recognized problem in the 1950s when the use of stimulants was reported during the 1952 winter Olympics in Oslo, Norway. Philosophically, athletes will always look to gain an edge. Genes, nutrition, training techniques, and mental discipline best predict athletic success.

Categories of ergogenic aids include pharmacologic, nutritional, and physiologic, such as blood boosting. Recently, there has been increased emphasis on the psychological aspect of sports performance, with many elite athletes using mental imagery and a number of other relaxation techniques to enhance performance. We must also not forget about the various technological and mechanical aids that are available, including such things as oversized tennis racquets, titanium materials used in golf clubs, lightweight racing shoes, and a host of other developments specifically related to each specific sport.

In general, here in the United States, there seems to be a cultural bias toward the use of medication to "solve" problems. The American public is inundated with television and print ads encouraging the public to solicit prescription medications from their physicians to treat medical problems and enhance their quality of life. Superimposed on these issues are the use and abuse of alcohol and recreational drugs that are defined as nonprescription drugs used for mood altering purposes.

With respect to pharmacologic aides, the most commonly used substances include creatine, anabolic steroids, and human growth hormone. Regarding anabolic steroids, the mechanism of action is felt to be related to increased protein synthesis, increased red blood cell production, and central nervous system effects that include increased aggressiveness. Incidence of use has been variously reported in the 3% to 12% range. Anabolic steroids are considered a controlled substance (class III) with a multitude of potential side effects on the cardiovascular system, the reproductive system, and the endocrine system. Research is limited and difficult to carry out due to the fact that these are banned substances; it is difficult to get athletes to participate in these types of studies.

Human growth hormone is another commonly used ergogenic aid that cannot be detected using current drug testing methodology. It is produced using recombinant DNA technology, and its high cost does in some ways limit its abuse. Proposed mechanisms of action include increased transport of amino acids into tissue, as well as stimulation of mobilization of fat as an energy source. Potential side effects include those mentioned for anabolic steroids, as well as possible acromegaly, diabetes mellitus, heart failure, and osteoporosis. As with any injectable drug, the risk of infectious disease secondary to needle sharing must also be taken into consideration.

Amphetamines have been used for over 50 years. They were initially used in World War II to prevent "battle fatigue." Mechanism of action includes central nervous system stimulation, speeding of reaction time, and masking of symptoms of fatigue. Potential of serious side effects include cardiovascular collapse, hypertension, hallucinations, irritability, and restlessness. All are currently banned substances. Caffeine is a special subclass of stimulant that may enhance performance in endurance athletic events. A mechanism of action is not clearly understood, but may be related to central nervous system stimulation and enhanced energy utilization. Caffeine is widely considered to be one of the safest, most effective, and extensively studied ergogenic aids. Incidence of use is estimated at approximately 60%, and it is legal for use in low doses (5 to 10 mg per kilogram). This dose represents about three to four cups of strongly brewed coffee (about a 300 mg dose). Potential side effects can include GI intolerance, dehydration, cardiac arrhythmia, tremor, and headaches.

Blood doping is also employed by endurance athletes. Initially, the technique was to donate two units of autologous blood approximately 8 to 12 weeks prior to the athletic event and then reinfuse this blood about 1 week prior to competition. The mechanism of action was to increase oxygen-carrying capacity. More recently, athletes have used erythropoietin, which is an injectable medication that stimulates red blood cell production by bone marrow. Potential side effects of these techniques include stroke, blood clots, sudden death, transfusion reaction, headache, and hypertension.

Proper nutrition is one of the most important contributing factors to enhancing athletic performance. Deficiency of key nutrients will impair performance; however, in a non-deficiency state, the effect of supplementation is often unclear and over stated. Several reports suggest that the two factors leading to improvement in athletic records over the last few years are improved diet and enhanced training techniques. A comprehensive discussion of nutrition is beyond the scope of this chapter, but the consumption of a diet balanced in carbohydrate, protein, and fat is extremely important. Probably the most often overlooked nutrient is water, and athletes must consume more water than the general population to replace sweat losses. There are a number of "sports drinks" that are commercially available that do an excellent job of replacing fluid electrolytes and carbohydrates. Several studies have indicated enhanced performance in endurance athletics. It is important when using sports drinks to make sure to use them in practice prior to using them in competition, as they may cause gastrointestinal distress.

With regard to technological aids, great strides have been made in many sports to enhance an athlete's mechanical advantage. The use of oversize tennis racquets and titanium woods and graphite shaft golf clubs are just a few of the more commonly used technological aids. Lightweight and aerodynamic bicycles and components can result in significant time savings during racing. Regarding running shoes, a 200 gram reduction in shoe weight improves running efficiency by about 1%. For an elite marathon runner, this can result in as much as a minute and a half in time savings over the course of a marathon race.

In summary, genetic endowment is the key to high performance. There is no substitute for hard work and good nutrition. Technology may be of benefit. Mental imagery and relaxation techniques are an emerging area. Nutritional technology has advanced, and research, although limited, does support the ergogenicity of some nutrients, but more work in this area is needed. The International Olympic Committee doping legislation states that any physiologic substance taken in an abnormal quantity with the intention of artificially and unfairly increasing performance should be construed as doping and is illegal. One must always understand and appreciate the ethics of sports performance when considering the above issues.

SIDELINE AND EVENT MEDICAL MANAGEMENT ISSUES

A physician with an interest in sports medicine is often called on to provide medical services or coverage for an athletic event. This involvement may be limited to providing medical coverage or services as part of a medical team or a more comprehensive role with a commitment to assisting in planning, organizing, and administering the event medical team. The primary responsibility remains the health and safety of the athlete. The event physician may also have an implied role to protect the event organization from medical liability.

Acute injury management during a mass participation event is often more complex, because the athlete will often present without an available medical database to the physician. As a result, appropriate medical management may require interaction with coaches, athletic trainers, and parents. The event physician should evaluate the athlete, treat if required, and make recommendations regarding return to play or further evaluation in the emergency room or with the athlete's primary care physician.

The event physician must not only be knowledgeable in musculoskeletal medicine, but must be prepared to deal with environmental concerns, as well as injuries specific to the event being covered. This is especially true of mass participation endurance events, such as marathons and triathlons. Specific recommendations for event equipment and protocols can be found in the *ACMC Handbook for the Team Physician* (33). In general, the physician at every event should initially and periodically assess the environment when appropriate, introduce all medical personnel to one another, and review an emergency response plan, including the chain of command. At least one physician and four medical personnel per 250 participants and one physician and two medical personnel per 10,000 spectators should be present and planned for. Available equipment, including communication equipment, should be evaluated prior to the event. The closest emergency room should be notified ahead of time of potential injuries that might be anticipated.

CONCLUSIONS

From its beginnings, osteopathic medicine has taken an active role in promoting participation in athletics as a means to a healthy lifestyle and providing specialized treatment of athletes. Osteopathic principles and practice, including the use of manual medicine, have a large role in the treatment of the athlete. Each athlete should be evaluated and treated on an individual basis, including a comprehensive evaluation of both structure and function when appropriate. Because of the wide variety of potential injuries and medical maladies that can affect the athlete, the sports medicine physician must be comprehensively trained. Finally, physicians must always keep the health of the athlete as their primary goal when considering return-to-play decisions.

REFERENCES

1. Patrick K, Sallis JF, Long B, et al. A new tool for encouraging activity: Project PACE. *Physician Sports Med.* 1994;22:45–52.
2. Lopiano DA. Modern history of women in sports. *Clinics in Sports Medicine.* 2000;19(2):163–173.
3. Strauss RH. Cardiovascular benefits and risks of exercise: The scientific evidence. In: Wickland Jr EH, ed. *Sports Medicine,* 2nd ed. Philadelphia, PA: WB Saunders; 1991:72–80.
4. Scuderi GR, McCann PD, Bruno PJ, et al, eds. *Sports Medicine Principles of Primary Care,* 1st ed. St. Louis, MO: Mosby–Year Book; 1997.
5. Dailey SM, Oberman A. The athletic heart. *Heart Disease and Stroke.* 1993;2:53–58.
6. Anthony J. Psychologic aspects of exercise. *Clinics in Sports Medicine: The Exercise Prescription.* 1991;10(1):171–179.
7. Elia EA. Exercise and the elderly. *Clinics in Sports Medicine: The Exercise Prescription.* 1991;10(1):141.
8. Anderson MK, Hall SJ. *Fundamentals of Sports Injury Management.* Baltimore, MD: Williams & Wilkins; 1997.
9. Walter GW. *The First School of Osteopathic Medicine.* Kirksville, MO: The Thomas Jefferson University Press; 1924 (Reprinted 1992):39–45.
10. Still Jr CE. *Frontier Doctor—Medical Pioneer: The Life and Times of A. T. Still and His Family.* Kirksville, MO: The Thomas Jefferson University Press; 1907 (Reprinted 1991):205–216.
11. AAFP, AAP, AMSSM, AOASM, AOSSM. *Pre-Participation Physical Evaluation,* 2nd ed. Minneapolis, MN: McGraw-Hill; 1997.
12. Herbert DL. Pre-participation cardiovascular screening: Toward a national standard. *Physician Sports Med.* 1997;25(3):112–117.
13. Maron BJ, Thompson PD, Puffer JC, et al. Cardiovascular pre-participation screening of competitive athletes. A statement for health professionals from the Sudden Death Committee (clinical cardiology) and Congenital Cardiac Defects Committee (cardiovascular disease in the young), American Heart Association. *Circulation.* 1996;94:850–856.
14. Watkins RG. *The Spine in Sports.* St. Louis, MO: Mosby–Year Book; 1996.
15. Greenman PE. *Principles of Manual Medicine,* 2nd ed. Baltimore, MD: Williams & Wilkins; 1996:452–456.
16. Post WR. Patellofemoral pain: Let the physical exam define treatment. *Physician Sports Med.* 1998;26(1):68–78.
17. Neer CS, 2nd. Impingement lesions. *Clin Orthop* 1983;3:70–77.
18. Kuchera ML, Kuchera WA. *Osteopathic Considerations in Systemic Dysfunction,* 2nd ed. Columbus, OH: Greyden Press; 1994.
19. Trojian TH, McKeag DB. Ankle sprains. *Physician Sports Med.* 1998;26(10):29–40.
20. Tandetter HB, Shvartzman P. Acute ankle injuries: Clinical decision rules for radiographs. *Am Fam Physician.* 1997;55(8):2721–2727.
21. Brolinson PG. Principle Centered Rehabilitation. In: Garrett WE, Kirkendall DT, Squire DL, eds. *Principles and Practice of Primary Care Sports Medicine.* Philadelphia, PA: Lippincott Williams & Wilkins; 2000:645–652.
22. Amann CM. Office management of trauma. *Clin Fam Pract.* 2000;2(3):599–611.
23. Cantu RC. Guidelines for return to contact sports after a cerebral concussion. *Physician Sports Med.* 1986;14:75–76, 79, 83.
24. Cantu RC. *Neurologic Athletic Head and Spine Injuries.* Philadelphia, PA: WB Saunders; 2000.
25. Colorado Medical Society Sports Medicine Committee. Guidelines for the management of concussions in sports. Denver, CO: Medical Society; 1991.
26. Kelly JP, Rosenberg JH. Practice parameters: The management of concussion in sports. Report of the Quality Standards Committee. *Neurology.* 1997;48:581–585.
27. Lovell MR, Iverson GI, Collins MW, et al. Does loss of consciousness predict neuropsychological decrements after concussion? *Clin J Sport Med.* 1999;9:193–198.
28. Collins MW, Grindel SH, Lovell MR, et al. Relationship between concussion and neuropsychological performance in college football players. *JAMA.* 1999;282:964–970.
29. Echemendia RJ, Putukian M, Mackin RS, et al. Neuropsychological test performance prior to and following sports-related mild traumatic brain injury. *Clin J Sport Med.* 2001;11(1):23–31.
30. Jones RD. Neuropsychological Assessment of Patients with Traumatic Brain Injury: The Iowa-Benton Approach. In: Rizzo M, Tranel D, eds. *Head Injury and Postconcussive Syndrome.* New York, NY: Churchill Livingstone; 1996.
31. King NS. Emotional, neuropsychological, and organic factors: Their use in the prediction of persisting postconcussion symptoms after moderate and mild traumatic injuries. *J Neurol Neurosurg Psychiatry.* 1996;61:75–81.
32. Maddocks D, Saling M. Neuropsychological deficits following concussion. *Brain Inj.* 1996;10:99–103.
33. American College of Sports Medicine. *ASCM Handbook for the Team Physician.* Baltimore, MD: Williams & Wilkins; 1996.

OSTEOPATHIC CONSIDERATIONS IN PALPATORY DIAGNOSIS AND MANIPULATIVE TREATMENT

INTRODUCTION

JOHN M. JONES, III
ROBERT E. KAPPLER

The following chapters contain detailed descriptions of musculoskeletal examination and various treatment techniques commonly taught at osteopathic medical colleges in the United States. We would like to gratefully acknowledge the contributions made by the faculties of those colleges. Andrew Taylor Still never taught what he called techniques and explicitly recommended against teaching osteopathy in that fashion. He felt that if the physician knew anatomy, it was unnecessary to teach techniques, because the method to be used for a particular patient's problems should be obvious. So why do we teach techniques at our colleges today?

In 1892, when Still founded the American School of Osteopathy, he established a curriculum dominated by anatomy. This was partly because he discarded much of the standard medical curriculum; it was of little use to the physician and largely harmful to the patient. There has been an explosion of knowledge in both the basic and clinical sciences since that time. To the medical student, it often seems that all the knowledge accumulated in the last century has been retained in the curriculum, without the deletion of a single element of medical minutiae. This may be true to an extent. Currently, only about 10% of the curriculum in the first 2 years of osteopathic education is reserved for teaching the philosophy, principles, and mechanics of osteopathic manipulative diagnosis and treatment.

FORMS OF TREATMENT

There are many forms of osteopathic manipulation. Only the basic types taught during the first 2 years at United States colleges of osteopathic medicine are presented in the following chapters. Other forms of osteopathic manipulation, such as visceral manipulation, are left for later work. Also, not every possible form of a particular technique is included. For example, there are at least six ways to do high-velocity/low-amplitude (HVLA) thrust technique on a typical cervical vertebra. Only representative samples of the techniques are included.

These samples of treatment can be classified as soft tissue techniques, articulatory techniques, or direct and indirect methods of treatment. Techniques named according to the activating forces used are muscle energy, springing, or high-velocity/low-amplitude thrust. Those referring to a concept of treatment are called strain/counterstrain, myofascial release, or osteopathy in the cranial field. Related topics of release by positioning are discussed, as well as Simon and Travell's system of trigger points. Though trigger point diagnosis and treatment is not classified as osteopathic, it fits well into the practice of musculoskeletal medicine and is used by many osteopathic physicians.

MODELS

In each of these classifications of treatment techniques, the diagnosis and treatment are based on a mental model, a cognitive system of reference that is workable when applied to patients with somatic dysfunctions. Models have limitations. They cannot explain everything; that is not their purpose. They are designed to correlate certain gathered information with a diagnosis and to relate this diagnosis to a successful treatment. The muscle energy model of sacral torsion does not delineate the exact biomechanics of the sacrum or which specific muscle(s) are involved in the treatment. However, if the physician collects data, arrives at a diagnosis, and treats the disorder as indicated, the somatic dysfunction should resolve. The muscle energy model relates to the body in terms of simplified biomechanics. Many physicians use the muscle energy model not because it is perfect but because it works and they are pragmatic.

Models that survive the test of time and propagate are those that have empirically proven themselves by benefiting the patients. The models in the following chapters are examples of ways to accomplish biomechanical changes and achieve treatment goals. They are not the only way. If you understand anatomy, you can use a variety of ways to achieve the same objective. If you do not understand anatomy, following a protocol may do the patient no good; the patient's physique may not conform to the 5' 10", 170-pound model on which the protocol was based. Knowing anatomy, however, is not enough by itself.

You may, for instance, adapt a technique by using muscle energy activation on a position normally followed by HVLA. You base this on what you palpate and sense happening with the patient and on the patient's unique response to past or current treatment. You may use treatment in two planes rather than three, because of positional limitations imposed on the patient because of surgery, trauma, or the formation of osteophytes in osteoarthritis. You might more appropriately make a completely different choice of treatment technique because of the positional limitation. For example, the muscle energy model requires flexion to confront an extension lesion. If the surgeon wants the head to remain flat, you may elect to use indirect myofascial release at the cervical segment level, requiring only a few degrees of motion, which would not raise the head off the pillow.

PHYSICIAN KNOWLEDGE AND EXPERIENCE

The choice of technique depends on the knowledge and experience of the physician, as well as the limitations of the patient.

When a patient has a diagnosable somatic dysfunction in the cervical region, you have many treatment options. Some may be contraindicated, as illustrated by the case of a male septuagenarian who was in the hospital for cardiac electrophysiologic studies. He lost consciousness several times before admission—when he turned his head. During provocative testing, his heart stopped beating for 6 seconds, until defibrillation was used to restart cardiac performance. Normally, one would think that use of strain/counterstrain techniques would be much easier on a patient than most other treatments. However, in this case, treatment by strain/ counterstrain is contraindicated. Muscle energy, HVLA, or articulatory treatment would also be inadvisable. Osteopathic diagnosis and treatment provide the alternatives of indirect segmental treatment or osteopathy in the cranial field (with caution in this case). Carefully consider your patient's limitations, along with your own skill level, when choosing which technique to use. Clinical judgment about "when to use what" is often difficult until one acquires a certain body of clinical experience. This is accomplished largely by observing decisions made by other physicians.

TECHNIQUE VERSUS TREATMENT

Another problem is making the jump between performing a technique and doing an osteopathic treatment. Osteopathic manipulation can be reduced in scope to the point where it appears to be a series of specific treatments for specific problems. If it is carried out in this fashion, however, it loses its identity as osteopathic manipulation and becomes merely manual medicine. The term manual medicine implies a form of treatment applied by the hands. The term osteopathic manipulation indicates more than that; it indicates that the physician is applying the four basic principles of osteopathic philosophy. One of these principles is that the body is a unit. The true osteopathic approach cannot be broken down into isolated procedures specific for particular complaints; the osteopathic approach treats the patient as a whole.

It is often said that when you see an osteopathic physician for treatment of a low back problem, the doctor might check your feet, your knees, and your neck. The goal of osteopathic treatment includes consideration of the entire person, not a specific dysfunctional muscle. Though its success helps the patient overcome the dysfunction or disease, the osteopathic treatment is performed to support the patient, in whatever way is indicated.

That is the osteopathic ideal. Realistically, there are many times in medical practice where the dictates of time, resources, and energy direct you to apply this ideal in limited form. The effects of applying specific procedures to a specific dysfunction have far less profound effects than a total treatment. The degree to which you apply osteopathic philosophy is determined by the degree to which you are practicing osteopathy. To offer an analogy, an engine sometimes needs an overhaul but sometimes only a minor adjustment or a single part. In the same way, time constraints may indicate that a specific procedure should be provided today, with a more thorough treatment in the scheduled follow-up visit. A single procedure that treats the body's needs may be preferable to no treatment at all, or to merely writing a prescription to treat the disease. At no time should you lose sight

of the impact of that procedure on the total body. The body is constantly trying to maintain optimal homeostasis, using its self-healing ability and self-regulatory mechanisms. By directing the osteopathic manipulation to a prime site, the body may be able to continue improvement. At the next visit, you can reevaluate body needs and administer further treatment as necessary.

Beginning physicians often hesitate to use manipulation on hospital patients. There is the fear of treating an already debilitated patient. Always bear in mind that a physician is expected not to use techniques that could hurt the hospital patient but to use common sense and clinical judgment as to what the patient needs and is able to tolerate. Particularly if you are working in a non-osteopathic institution or with preceptors who learned only direct methods of treatment, there is the supposition on the part of the preceptor that you would use HVLA without proper consideration. There may be many osteopathic techniques; always discuss which techniques are best for the particular patient with the best risk:benefit ratio for treatment.

The verbalization of osteopathic manipulative treatment is always limited in scope. We attempt to put into words an experience that includes:

> Palpatory assessment
> Other tactile and proprioceptive input
> Integration of those data on a nonverbal level
> Kinesthetic response through our hands and/or other parts of the anatomy

We do all of this based on cognitive knowledge. We do it to change the motion characteristics, fluid flow patterns, and sensorimotor responses of our patients. It is not always possible to verbalize everything we do, partially because so many things happen simultaneously. This makes it difficult to adequately describe each factor. Proprioception is difficult to describe, because the feeling of where one is in space is unique to each individual. Because language is linear and sequential, the description of two synchronous events might be perceived in a sequenced linear fashion. Because most mental processing is on a nonverbal level, it is often difficult to describe portions of it at all. Korr (1) described the experience of diagnosis and treatment as a nonverbal dialogue between the osteopathic physician and the patient.

ART OF OSTEOPATHIC MEDICINE

Osteopathic manipulative diagnosis and treatment are part of a complex process involving three domains:

> Affective
> Cognitive
> Psychomotor

The physician must have enough interaction with the patient to achieve relaxation and trust. The physician's brain must receive proper palpatory, visual, and auditory input, which is processed through previously gained cognitive knowledge. Reacting to this input, the physician's processing and kinesthetic output take place in a real-time, ongoing fashion. This all occurs simultaneously, in many forms of treatment, without stopping.

The art of medicine is not strictly fact-oriented. From initial observation and facts, a diagnosis may appear accurate, but further observation can show otherwise. A diagnosis may be accurate for a limited time, after which different characteristics prevail. Patience and persistence help you adapt, accepting art in medicine, as well as science. Learning manual medicine skills is not like learning facts of biochemistry. Only a small portion of the data can be grasped by memorization of facts. As with any psychomotor skill, seeing or doing something once is only a beginning. Repeated practice of the technique is necessary to gain skill.

Different patients also respond in different ways to the same technique. An individual also has a unique response to different technique types. Each practitioner becomes part of this human equation and is also unique. The way you are taught a skill during training may be different than the way you finally employ that skill. As you practice, you master the skill. An old story is told about an education professor who was approached by a teacher. "I've taught second grade for 20 years," she told the professor, who replied, "Have you really taught second grade 20 years? Or have you taught 1 year 20 times?" Attention to variations in input from patients, as well as following the results of research, leads to constant refinement in skills. Merely learning treatment protocols and applying them in the same fashion never produces improvement. The human being who is your patient is both your school and one of your teachers.

In a simplistic way, each osteopathic technique system could probably be assigned to deal better with certain types of physical ailments. However, this analogy ignores the complex human factor. Physicians who use one type for all problems may have selected it because it is the one with which they are most comfortable or at which they are most adept. Their practices may be self-selecting for patients who benefit from what they do, with others leaving to find help elsewhere. A physician practicing the highest form of osteopathy is one who uses the approach, method, techniques, or plan that best matches the patient asking for help. If the indicated osteopathic manipulative treatment is HVLA, that becomes the highest form of treatment for that patient. If it is osteopathy in the cranial field, then that is the one that is most appropriate.

Some may feel that OMT is singularly effective for a wide range of clinical problems. Others are somewhat skeptical, often because they have not seen a patient who presented to a physician with a clinical problem.

Some patients, often those with problems associated with motion loss from a non-recurring physical force or trauma, respond immediately and dramatically. Some resolutions take longer, as the body requires time to respond; healing takes time. Observe the effects of watering a brown lawn. Immediately after watering, the lawn is still brown, but it turns green with time.

Sometimes somatic dysfunction is secondary to postural, mechanical, or visceral disorders. In these cases, OMT provides temporary relief, but the somatic dysfunction tends to return because the cause is still present. A psychic or emotional component is sometimes the major cause. These patients do not get better until the emotional component is resolved.

In some cases, OMT is used to provide maintenance treatment. The term maintenance is prejudicial, because insurance companies will not pay for maintenance, even though this treatment enables better function and quality of life. The treatment is indicated and is proper.

On occasion, patients just do not get better despite the best efforts of the physician. The physician must constantly reexamine such cases, analyzing the data to see if a different approach or type of treatment would be more effective. The only way to know what OMT does is to try it and gain clinical experience by following the patients. Remember as you use this approach that you are promoting the efficiency of natural function in your patients, enabling the human organism to function at its individual optimal level.

ANATOMY

To diagnose and treat a patient efficiently and effectively, you must know anatomy. There are several ways to know anatomy. One way is by being able to locate and name every structure. Another is by being able to successfully palpate and mentally interpret the response of tissues from the proprioceptive input from your hands. All osteopathic techniques produce functional and physiologic changes in tissue, in the following ways:

Lengthening
Shortening
Increase in tone in some muscles
Corresponding decrease in tone of their antagonists
Increase in motion in one or more directions
Decrease in other directions

The effects of osteopathic manipulation go beyond their obvious impact on the neuromusculoskeletal system, such as a decrease in pain or an increase in motion. Profound changes are seen in:

Blood and lymphatic fluid flow
Neural system
Endocrine system
Respiration
Autonomic balance

Improvement of homeostatic mechanisms increases functional efficiency of the tissues, enhances quality of life, and increases resistance to illness and injury.

ASPECTS OF LEARNING

When learning and practicing, remove as many distractions from the situation as possible. Ensure that neither your own needs nor the environment distracts you. If you are training the sense of touch, remove the distraction of sight and sound by closing your eyes and focusing on palpation in a quiet environment. If you are focusing on the need to go to the lavatory, you are not able to concentrate on sensory input related to the patient, because your brain is directing attention to your own internal sensations. Hunger or thirst can be tremendously distracting. An emotional upset may make it temporarily impossible for you to effectively receive input unless you can put the distraction out of your mind.

Thinking about how much time you are taking or how much you have to do may block immediate proprioceptive interpretations.

You may be learning a new field in an area totally different from the cognitive skills at which you have excelled. Be patient with yourself and realize that your learning may not proceed at the same pace as the learning of others. Sometimes it may be rapid; other times, slow. Continuous progress should be your goal, but be patient with yourself as you learn this challenging integrative process.

Is any one method or type of activation the most profound form of manipulative treatment in osteopathy? Which one gets the best results from the body? Is direct treatment superior to indirect treatment? At times, listening to one physician or a special interest group of physicians makes it seem as if this were so. However, the original question makes as much sense as asking if the knife, fork, or spoon is the superior instrument for dining. Each has its place. Each has its function, to which the others are less well adapted. Can you use a knife to pick up peas? Certainly.

However, most of us prefer one of the other instruments, because they are better adapted to that function.

CONCLUSION

An osteopathic physician looks at the study of osteopathic diagnosis and treatment as a lifelong discovery process that combines art and science. Your understanding and application of these principles will, because of your commitment and receptivity to new input, continue to develop and refine over your professional life.

REFERENCES

1. Korr IM. Somatic dysfunction, osteopathic manipulative treatment and the nervous system: a few facts, theories, many questions. *J Am Osteopath Assoc.* 1986;86:109–114.

PALPATORY SKILLS AND EXERCISES FOR DEVELOPING THE SENSE OF TOUCH

ROBERT E. KAPPLER

KEY CONCEPTS

- Art of palpation, including practice using hands and fingers
- Identification of dominant eye and hand in palpatory technique
- Present progressive exercises for developing palpatory skills to refine and improve beginning practitioners' sense of touch
- Perception of tactile differences in tissue texture and motion
- Perception on palpation of layers and structures of the body
- Palpation of thoracic and lumbar areas with passive flexion
- Palpation for somatic dysfunction in cervical, thoracic, lumbar, and sacroiliac areas
- Development of finely tuned sensory perception and mental filters in palpatory skill
- Motion perception
- Palpation of acute and chronic somatic dysfunction
- Perception of tactile differences in tissue texture and motion
- Perception on palpation of layers and structures of the body
- Palpation of thoracic and lumbar areas with passive flexion
- Palpation for somatic dysfunction in cervical, thoracic, lumbar and sacroiliac areas

This chapter introduces the art of palpation. Being efficient and accurate with palpation is an asset for any physician regardless of specialization. Palpation is especially important to osteopathic manipulative diagnosis and treatment because it is fundamental to functional and structural evaluation. Two of the essentials of effective practice are palpatory skill in locating and defining somatic dysfunctions and manipulative skill to appropriately treat them. The *Glossary of Osteopathic Terminology* (1) defines palpation as the application of variable manual pressure to the surface of the body for the purpose of determining the shape, size, con-

sistency, position, inherent motility, and health of the tissues beneath. Another definition (DiGiovanna E. New York College of Osteopathic Medicine. OPP course syllabus, 1992) puts it another way: Palpation consists of lightly placing the hands or fingers on the patient's body to discover changes in the normal condition of soft tissues, bones, or organs beneath the surface of the skin, as well as the skin itself. Still another definition includes the descriptive words "gentle handling," an important point to remember when applying this skill. Skill in recognizing normal tissue movements along with changes that signal dysfunction or disease can be acquired with continued practice.

ART OF PALPATION

The art of palpation requires discipline, time, patience, and practice. To be most effective and productive, palpatory findings must be correlated with knowledge of functional anatomy, physiology, and pathophysiology. It is much easier to identify frank pathologic states (a tumor, for example) than it is to describe signs, symptoms, and palpatory findings that lead to or identify pathologic mechanisms (2). This is analogous to learning to read an electrocardiogram or a sonogram: it takes time to develop the vocabulary of sight that allows a person to distinguish and describe true pathologic patterns. Through repetitive palpatory experiences, physicians realize ranges of normal and correlate significant findings with:

Past and present history
Tissue texture changes
Restriction of motion
Asymmetry
Subjective tenderness
Related symptomatology

Considering these factors together strengthens the differential diagnostic decision (Frymann V. College of Osteopathic Medicine of the Pacific. Syllabus for workshop on palpation, 1990). Treatment then follows.

PALPATION WITH FINGERS AND HANDS

Palpation with the fingers and hands provides sensory information (Frymann V. Syllabus for workshop on palpation, 1990) that the brain interprets as:

Temperature
Texture
Surface humidity
Elasticity
Turgor
Tissue tension
Thickness
Shape
Irritability
Motion

LEARNING PALPATORY TECHNIQUE

To accomplish this task, it is necessary to teach the fingers to feel, think, see, and know. One feels through the palpating fingers on the patient; one sees the structures under the palpating fingers through a visual image based on knowledge of anatomy; one thinks what is normal or abnormal; and one knows with a confidence acquired by practice that what is felt is real and accurate.

Through complex peripheral and central processing, the smallest sensory perception can be amplified to the point of conscious recognition and analysis.

Exercise 1: Palpating Inanimate Objects
Goal

To perceive slight tactile differences of tissue texture and motion. Exercises on inanimate objects serve to sharpen tactile concentration and attention. Concentration is essential. Close the eyes to eliminate extraneous stimuli. Pay attention to kinesthetic sensations received through the fingers.

Procedure

i. Put a mixture of coins in a pocket or purse. By touch, distinguish between heads and tails, and between pennies, dimes, nickels, and quarters. Identify date lines on the coins.
ii. Locate a hair that has been placed under a sheet of paper; attempt to estimate its length. Add sheets of paper until you can no longer palpate the hair.
iii. Palpate several types of human bones. Identify the bones and their component parts, envisioning the tissue that normally surrounds them.
iv. Palpate a human bone and a solid plastic imitation of the same bone. Identify the characteristics of the human bone that distinguish it from the replica.

Mitchell (2) calls palpation a two-way communication system in which the patient's tissues react to the presence of the palpator's hand. This is more likely to occur when palpation has been practiced over a period of time.

Three steps define the process. The first is detection, the second is internal amplification or magnification, and the third is analysis and interpretation. This last step translates palpatory findings into meaningful anatomic, physiologic, or pathologic states (Frymann V. Syllabus for workshop on palpation, 1990). Familiarity with osteopathic terminology permits description of palpatory findings in consistent terms.

Effective palpatory technique cannot be learned by observation. Watching another physician palpate a patient indicates where the hands are placed but gives little or no indication of the feel of tissues being palpated.

Many individuals have a dominant hand with which they prefer to palpate or motion test. This may or may not be the hand with which they write. Recognition of a dominant hand will allow the individual to develop a compensatory mechanism to obtain accurate information when using both hands.

Exercise 2: The Dominant Hand
Purpose

The purpose of this exercise is to determine the dominant hand. It is believed that when a person does not consciously think about it, he or she will put his or her dominant hand on top when the hands are clasped.

Position

This exercise can be done in a standing or sitting position.

Procedure

Without consciously thinking about it, clasp your hand together in front of you, with one hand on top of the other.

Results

The hand that *is* on top will most likely be your dominant hand. It is also believed that palpatory results are more consistent if the examiner has the dominant eye over the area that is being palpated.

For example, if one hand is stronger than the other, practice in applying equal pressure over equivalent structures can result in accurate interpretation of such manual information.

Interpretation of dominant and nondominant proprioceptive feedback from each hand is also a response that the individual can adjust.

Exercise 3: The Dominant Eye
Purpose

The purpose of this exercise is to determine the dominant eye. Some believe that palpation and the interpretation of palpatory findings are more accurate if palpation is performed with the dominant eye over the area being palpated.

Position

This exercise can be performed standing or sitting with a distant clock or visible object to look at.

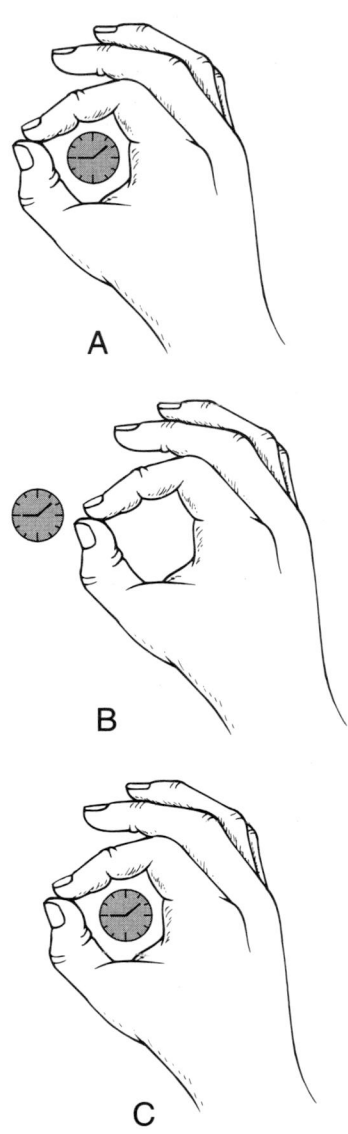

FIGURE 38.1. Right eye dominance. **A:** Both eyes open. **B:** Right eye closed; left eye open. **C:** Left eye closed; right eye open. (Modified from WA Kuchera, with permission.)

Procedure

   i. Look at the distant object with both eyes open (Fig. 38.1).
  ii. Extend your dominant hand and make a circle with your thumb and index finger that encircles your view of the distant object.
 iii. Now, close one eye, then open it and close the other eye.

Result

The eye that saw the object encircled with the fingers of your dominant hand is generally your dominant eye (2). Recognition of dominance, if it exists, and development of a compensatory mechanism is the main issue here; in time, apparent palpatory ambidexterity may result.

There are more touch (kinesthetic) nerve endings in the pads of the fingers than elsewhere in the hand. It is generally agreed that the thumb and/or the first two finger pads, rather than the fingertips, are the most sensitive part of the hand to train and use for palpation (Frymann V. Syllabus for workshop on palpation, 1990).

Some physicians find that variations in skin temperature are best perceived by the dorsum of the hand, especially the dorsum of the middle phalanges of fingers two, three, and four; others use the palmar surface. Try both and see which is more effective for you. The coordinated use of the palms and the fingers around an object is best suited for obtaining a stereognostic sense of contour (3).

Flexibility of the joints of the elbows, wrists, hands, and fingers is important. Relaxation is also important to eliminate any muscle tension that would block perception. Strength of hands and fingers can be increased by using a finger exerciser, squeezing a ball, or playing a musical instrument that requires fingering. Because the hands are so important to a physician, they should be carefully protected and cared for. They are sensitive diagnostic instruments.

Light touch is thought by many persons experienced in palpation to be the most useful and easy to use. Very light touch, or light touch, consists of laying the hands passively on the skin or moving the hands lightly over the skin. Such light touch can be used to determine skin temperature, texture, moistness, oiliness, resistance, tone, and elasticity. It may be possible to determine skin temperature sensation by passing the hand just above the skin. Firmer pressure communicates with the deeper cutaneous layers and fascial sheaths. It explores superficial muscles to determine their tone and mobility. Firm pressure and compression explore deeper muscle, fascia, and bony relationships.

Exercise 4: Layer Palpation

Goal

The goal of this exercise is to palpate your own tissues and concentrate and perceive various layers and structures of the body by varying the pressure of palpation.

Position

The position for this exercise is seated comfortably beside a table with your nondominant arm resting on the table.

Procedure

   i. Close your eyes and relax. Concentrate your attention through the palpating fingers of your dominant hand.
  ii. Lightly palpate the dorsum of the nondominant hand using the fingers of your dominant hand. Scarcely touching the surface, feel the contour of the hand.
 iii. Test palpation with the dorsal and palmar aspects of the palpating fingers to determine which is most sensitive to temperature.
  iv. Using very light touch, palpate and describe skin texture, moisture, and thickness.
   v. Gently pinch the skin on the back of the hand. Elevate it and release it. How long did it take for the skin to resume its normal configuration?
  vi. Evaluate skin drag on both the palm and dorsum of the hand. Skin drag is the estimation of the amount of resistance experienced when the pads of the fingers are lightly applied and moved (dragged) over the skin surface. On which aspect of the hand do the palpating fingers move

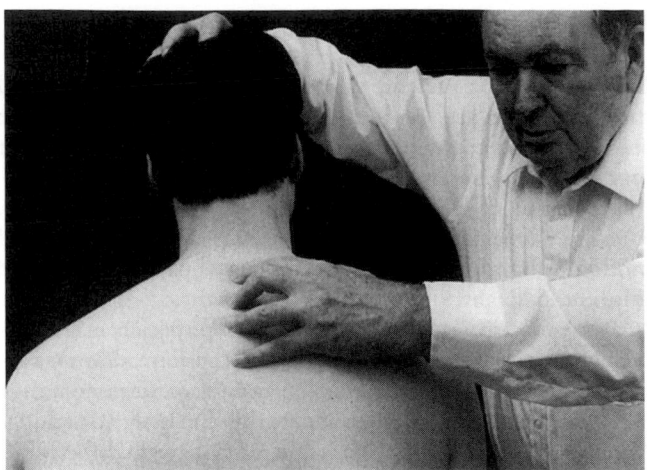

FIGURE 38.2. Palpating upper thoracic flexion-extension.

ii. Locate the spinous processes and interspinous ligaments, noting how they feel. Compare differences between the feel of the bone and the feel of the ligament.

iii. Passively flex the head and neck while sensing for increasing tension of the interspinous ligaments. Note: One spinous process may move more easily than another (Fig. 38.2).

iv. Using the fingers of both hands, palpate for temperature differences along the paravertebral thoracic and lumbar spine. Use either the palmar or dorsal surface of your fingers, depending on which you find to be more sensitive.

v. Using both hands simultaneously, stroke the back from C7 to L5. Which areas are warmer? Try to find a segment within the thoracic area that is either warmer or cooler than another segment. Compare left with right sides, and superior with inferior. Stroking of this type is useful in identifying changes in contour, as well as identifying areas of edema and increased tissue tension.

vi. Palpate for moisture differences, noting stickiness, dryness, wetness, waxiness, and slipperiness.

vii. Proceeding from T2 to L5, lightly compress the paravertebral soft tissues. Then use deeper pressure, but less pressure than that required to palpate bone. You may notice that in some areas, tissues compress more easily while in others, there is more resistance. Significant resistance indicates an area of tissue texture abnormality (TTA) (1), which bears further investigation.

viii. Lightly palpate the skin and subcutaneous tissue over the resistant site. This helps you identify the outer limits of tissue texture involved.

SOMATIC DYSFUNCTION PALPATION

The osteopathic physician uses all palpatory skills to diagnose somatic dysfunction. The definition of somatic dysfunction is impaired or altered function of related components of the somatic (body framework) system: skeletal, arthrodial, and myofascial structures, and related vascular, lymphatic, and neural elements (1).

The osteopathic diagnostic criteria for somatic dysfunction are discerned through palpation and can be conveniently recalled through the mnemonic TART. These letters stand for:

T: Tissue texture abnormalities
A: Asymmetry (static, motion, tonicity, turgor, color, temperature)
R: Restriction of motion
T: Tenderness (in the area of the abnormality)

By grouping these palpatory findings according to the characteristics of acute and chronic inflammation, somatic dysfunction can be further classified, as shown in Table 38.1.

ACUTE SOMATIC DYSFUNCTION

Palpate with light to somewhat firmer touch. Several types of change may be present; biochemically mediated tissue texture changes often predominate. First, the skin over the somatic dysfunction may feel warmer. The skin and deeper tissues directly

TABLE 38.1. CLASSIFICATION OF SOMATIC DYSFUNCTION

Acute	Chronic
History: recent; often an injury	History: long-standing
Pain: acute pain, severe, cutting, sharp	Pain: dull, achy; paresthesias (crawling, itching, burning, gnawing)
Vascular: vessels injured, release of endogenous peptides = chemical vasodilation, inflammation	Vacular: vessels constricted because of sympathetic tone
Skin: warm, moist, red, inflamed (via vascular and chemical changes)	Skin: cool, pale (via chronic sympathetic vascular tone increase)
Sympathetics: systemically increased sympathetic activity but local effect overpowered by bradykinins so there is local vasodilation due to chemical effect	Sympathetics: has vasoconstriction due to hypersympathetic tone; regional sympathetic hyperactivity; systemic sympathetic tone may be reduced toward normal
Musculature: local increase in muscle tone, muscle contraction, spasm, increased tone of the muscle spindle	Musculature: decreased muscle tone, flaccid, mushy, limited range of motion because of contracture
Mobility: range often normal, quality is sluggish	Mobility: limited range, with normal quality in the motion that remains
Tissues: boggy edema, acute congestion, fluids from vessels and from chemical reactions in tissues	Tissues: chronic congestion, doughy, stringy, fibrotic, ropy, thickened, increased resistance, contracted, contractures
Adnexa: moist skin, no trophic changes	Adnexa: pimples, scaly, dry, folliculitis, pigmentation (trophic changes)
Visceral: minimal somatovisceral effects	Visceral: somatovisceral effects are common

(From Kuchera WA, Kuchera ML. *Osteopathic Principles in Practice*, 2nd ed. Columbus, OH Greyden Press; 1994:25, with permission.)

over the area of somatic dysfunction may be tender. The skin and subcutaneous tissues may also feel tense and less mobile. Superficial muscle tension may be detected through a slight increase in palpatory pressure. Finally, there may be fullness caused by edema.

Deep palpation, defined as pressure sufficient to contact the periaxial soft tissues of the spinal column, can also identify several types of change. Pain or tenderness over acute areas of dysfunction is common. It is also common to find swelling in the deep periarticular tissues, giving the area a soggy, swollen texture. Muscles directly concerned with the affected vertebral segment demonstrate a doughy tightness or hypertonicity. Finally, there are perceptible changes in interosseous relations that are best evaluated by motion testing a vertebral unit. This reveals restricted motion in one direction and a preference or freedom of movement in the other direction.

CHRONIC SOMATIC DYSFUNCTION

Palpation with light to slightly more firm touch may elicit evidence of several types of chronic tissue changes. The skin may be somewhat immobile and tense in the presence of chronic fibrotic changes beneath the skin. These changes reduce the skin's elasticity. Temperature changes in the skin may be present or absent. Usually the skin is cool to touch. The muscles have a hard, ropy, and nonresilient texture as a result of fibrotic changes. When the dysfunction is chronic, it may actually have lost its tone and not feel fibrotic. The amount of tenderness is less than that found in acute dysfunction, often described as a dull, uncomfortable, or burning pain. In the absence of irritation, inflammation may subside and there may be little or no tenderness.

Deeper palpation reveals additional changes. Most notably, there is a decreased range of motion between the vertebral segments. As stated before, often there is little or no tenderness. It is helpful to evaluate mobility changes and interosseous changes together, using each to check the other. At this level, too, fibrotic changes replace edema. When a chronic somatic dysfunction has reached an advanced stage, fibrotic changes result in dysfunction of the surrounding fascias, musculature, and ligaments, sometimes to a point of producing contractures and joint ankylosis.

Exercise 8: Palpation for Somatic Dysfunction

Goal

(Review the types of tissue changes that are encountered in patients with vertebral somatic dysfunction before undertaking the final exercises in this section.) The goal of this exercise is to be able to palpate each area of the spine and detect tissue changes that may be perceived in areas of somatic dysfunction. These exercises assume a classroom situation, in which partners take turns acting as the patient.

Cervical Region

Position

Stand or sit at the head of the table behind your supine patient.

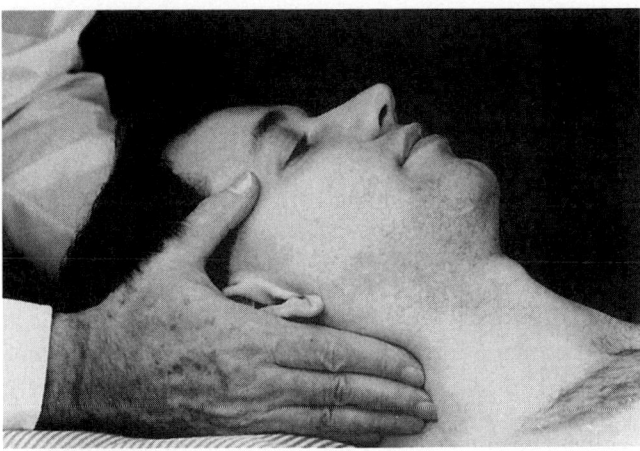

FIGURE 38.3. Assessing cervical spine side-bending translation.

Procedure

i. Cradle the patient's occiput in your palms. This position frees the fingers for checking cervical soft tissue and vertebral mechanics.
ii. Lightly palpate the posterior cervical skin. If you identify an area of localized tissue tension, palpate for swelling, deep muscle tension, and interosseous mobility.
iii. Straighten the cervical curve by passively flexing the neck. Place the pads of the fingers of one hand between the spinous processes and check for separation of the spinous processes.
iv. Reverse the procedure with passive backward bending of the head and neck. What happens to the spinous processes?
v. Assess side-bending and translational movements (1). With the pads of the fingers on either side of the articular column and directly across from each other, assess side-bending by translating to the right, then left (Fig. 38.3).
vi. Using deep pressure over the posterolateral margin of the articular column, translate anteriorly (both right and left sides), checking for spontaneous vertebral rotation capability.

Thoracic Region

Position

Stand behind your seated patient. The pads of the thumbs are most effective for palpation in this exercise.

Procedure

i. Lightly stroke the skin over the thoracic area, noting any temperature difference. For this part of the exercise, you may find that the dorsal surfaces of the middle phalanges are more sensitive to temperature change (Fig. 38.4).
ii. With a slightly deeper touch, palpate the subcutaneous and myofascial structures, noting soft tissue changes, such as muscle tension and swelling.
iii. Increase the depth of touch until you can feel the periarticular tissue changes; note the deeper tissue characteristics.
iv. Examine the facets and transverse processes, one side at a time and together, along with the spaces between spinous processes.

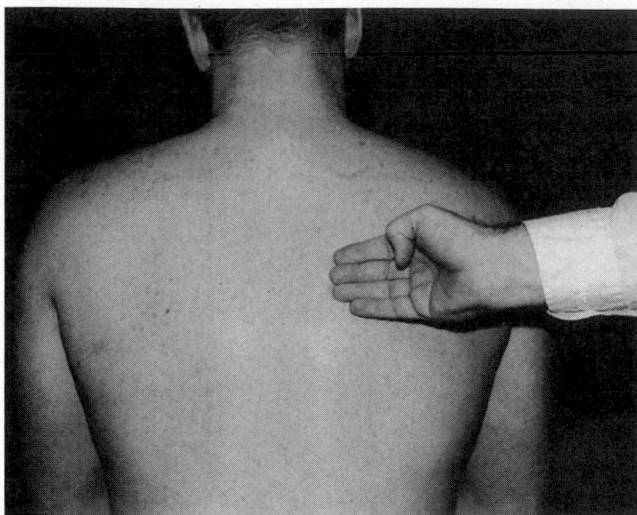

FIGURE 38.4. Checking temperature using back of hand and fingers.

v. Check motion response during passive flexion, extension, rotation, and side-bending of the thoracic area.

Lumbar Region

Position

Stand to the side of your prone patient, at the level of the patient's hips.

Procedure

i. Using light touch, palpate bilaterally for lumbar contour and any tissue texture abnormalities. Systematically compress the tissues over the transverse processes until you feel bony resistance.

ii. Test passive and active motion capability of individual vertebrae. Induce rotation by direct anterior pressure over one transverse process while no pressure is on the contralateral side. Then test rotation to the opposite side (Fig. 38.5).

iii. Induce side-bending to one side by applying lateral trans-

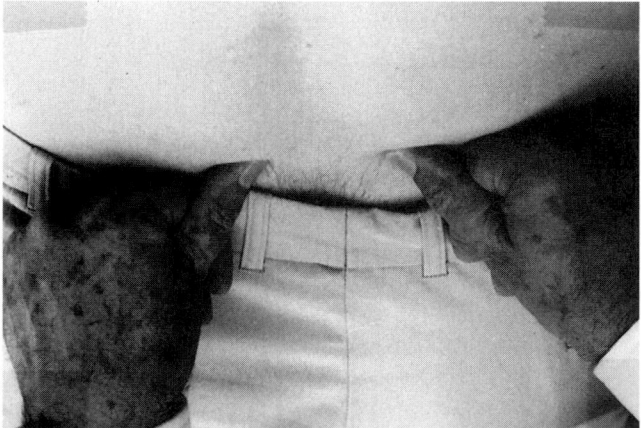

FIGURE 38.5. Testing lumbar spine rotation.

lational force to one transverse process, then test the other direction.

iv. Note differences in the mechanical response when the patient is seated and prone. Maximum spinal loads occur when seated; they are the least when supine.

Sacroiliac Region

Position

Stand to the side of your prone patient, at the level of the hips.

Procedure

i. Palpate the entire gluteal area. The palm of the hand is useful for palpating gross muscle changes. Ask the patient to extend the opposite hip as you palpate the contraction of the gluteus maximus muscle. Compare the right and left sides.

ii. Now assess the superficial tissues overlying and lateral to the superior and inferior poles of the sacroiliac joint, noting any tension in the gluteal muscles. Adjust your depth of touch as needed to assess various tissue layers. The pads of the thumbs are best used for this deep palpation, although other methods may be used (Fig. 38.6).

iii. Bilaterally check the posterior superior iliac spines for asymmetry. Use the pads of each thumb, placed directly caudad to the posterior superior iliac spines (PSIS) and note their levels. The PSIS are called pure landmarks, because they can be affected only by the position of the innominates. The level of the PSIS is a clue to possible innominate rotation. Is one more cephalad or more caudad (Fig. 38.7)?

iv. Check depth of the sulcus between the posterior surface of the PSIS of the ilium and the posterior surface of the sacrum. This sulcus depth is called a mixed landmark, because its depth can be affected by the innominate or the sacrum.

v. To determine rotation of the sacrum, palpate deeply in the sulci using the tips of the thumbs. Is the sacral base level, or is

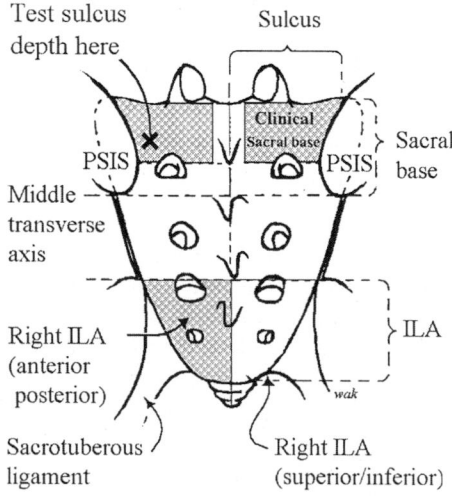

FIGURE 38.6. Posterior pelvic landmarks. (Illustration by WA Kuchera, with permission.)

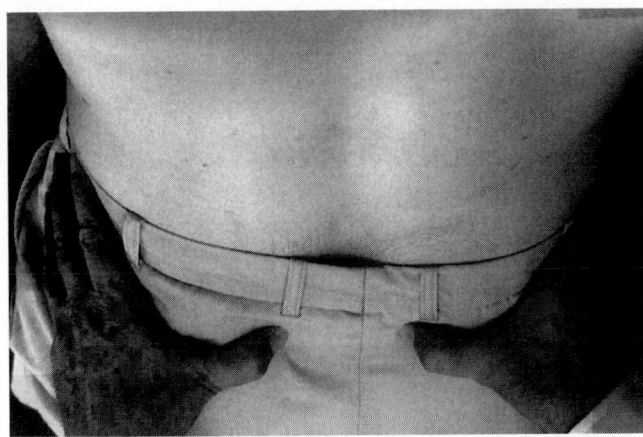

FIGURE 38.7. Checking level of the posterior superior iliac spine (PSIS) with the patient prone.

one side more anterior or posterior than the other side? This is a pure landmark that indicates sacral base rotation. Check for rotation of the innominates by evaluating the anteroposterior levels of the PSIS on both right and left.

CONCLUSION

Position your dominant eye over the structure being palpated. Place thumbs or finger pads over the area to be palpated. To ensure greater accuracy, mentally transfer your thoughts to the interface of your hand with the patient's body. Realize that resiliency or resistance to motion can be sensed in the initial movement during motion testing. You can miss these subtle findings and get hung up on gross motion restrictions, for example, how far a vertebral joint or tissue moves rather than the quality of the movement. Avoid these common errors in palpation:

Lack of concentration
Too much pressure
Excessive movement

These palpatory skills provide a method of obtaining practical experience in developing the art of palpation. There are many other exercises. Initially, palpation is practiced on a partner in the skills laboratory. During clinical clerkships, one gains additional experience by examining attending physicians' patients. Ultimately, palpatory experience is gained from palpatory examination of the physician's own patients. The physician continues to learn and never stops gaining experience. The preceding section shows how to get started in the process of obtaining palpatory data from the patient.

Remember that development of a high level of palpatory skill is an ongoing process, requiring patience and practice.

ACKNOWLEDGMENTS

Barbara Peterson collected the materials and Judith McPherson organized and assisted with the writing of this chapter.

REFERENCES

1. The Glossary Review Committee of the Educational Council on Osteopathic Principles. Glossary of Osteopathic Terminology. In: D'Alonzo Jr GE, ed. *AOA Yearbook and Directory of Osteopathic Physicians.* Chicago, IL: American Osteopathic Association; 2000.
2. Mitchell Jr F. The training and measurement of sensory literacy in relation to osteopathic structural and palpatory diagnosis. *J Am Osteopath Assoc.* 1976;75:881.
3. Kuchera WA, Kuchera ML. Palpation of soft tissue. In: *Osteopathic Principles in Practice,* 2nd ed. Columbus, OH: Greyden Press; 1994: 112.
4. Kappler RE, Larson NJ, Kelso AF. A comparison of osteopathic findings on hospitalized patients obtained by trained student examiners and experienced osteopathic physicians. *J Am Osteopath Assoc.* 1971;70(10):1091–1092.
5. Van Allen P, Stinson J. The development of palpation. *J Am Osteopath Assoc.* 1941;40(5):207, 208.
6. Greenman PE. *Principles of Manual Medicine,* 2nd ed. Baltimore, MD: Williams & Wilkins; 1996.

EXAMINATION AND DIAGNOSIS: AN INTRODUCTION

MICHAEL L. KUCHERA

KEY CONCEPTS

An integrated osteopathic neuromusculoskeletal regional examination that links structure and function:

- Specifically identifies somatic dysfunction
- Provides somatic clues to internal or systemic disease
- Expands the database for diagnosis and treatment

Recognition of patterns of somatic dysfunction:

- Facilitates diagnosis of impending or underlying problems before there is subjective evidence of that primary diagnosis or disease process
- Permits implementation of preventive education or action

Information from an integrated osteopathic examination used in a management program:

- Directs specific treatment of neuromusculoskeletal dysfunction, primary musculoskeletal overuse syndromes, trauma, strains, and sprains
- Supports homeostatic mechanisms
- Aids the patient's own body defenses in the fight against a systemic disorder

An osteopathic perspective provides unique insights into physical examination and the formulation of a differential diagnosis. This orientation begins on the first day of anatomy class and continues throughout a lifetime of osteopathic practice. Osteopathy emphasizes the interrelationship between structure (anatomy) and function (physiology), and this leads to physical examination skills that many consider to be second to none [1,2]. Without specific knowledge of pertinent anatomy and physiology, the osteopathic approach could be very time-consuming. With focused knowledge, however, it is not only time efficient but also cost effective [3–5]. A strong case can be made that the true diagnosis is reached more quickly, with fewer unnecessary expensive tests and that disorders are identified at the earliest dysfunctional state, when prognosis is good and treatment costs are relatively minimal.

THE OSTEOPATHIC EXAMINATION

Emphasis on the neuromusculoskeletal system, supported by an in-depth knowledge of functional anatomy and physiology, provides osteopathic practitioners the opportunity to consider and incorporate additional viscerosomatic and somatovisceral reflex clues that are largely unavailable in many other health care systems. This is one reason that the complete history and physical of each patient admitted by an osteopathic physician to an American Osteopathic Association (AOA) accredited hospital is to include an osteopathic structural examination [6]. A professional standardized osteopathic structural examination for hospitalized patients is discussed in Chapter 71.

Integration of these physical findings is further enhanced by the profession's emphasis on understanding body unity as completely as possible. A survey of patient stressors and the individualized response to those stressors is necessary, along with information on the following:

Symptoms and pain patterns
Activities and ergonomics of daily living
Past accidents, surgeries, and significant illness
Medications, supplements, and toxins
Nutritional, lifestyle, and environmental data

These can all be translated or interpreted with an understanding of their anatomic and/or physiologic impact on the patient's body unity, and provides insight into the unique individual who is placing his or her trust in the physician's skill and judgment. A hands-on approach and willingness to listen to the patient (often cited by patients as a characteristic of an osteopathic physician) initiate within the patient subtle therapeutic mechanisms, even as data are being gathered to make a diagnosis. Patients are highly satisfied with this type of attention, examination, and synthesis.

An osteopathic physician examines the homeostatic reserve of each patient and seeks optimum function within each structure. *"To find health is the object of the physician; anyone can find disease"* [7]. This portion of the examination is essential for determining prognosis and treatment design when host mechanisms are compromised. It is also helpful in the examination of noncompromised or compensated hosts, in designing preventive strategies, or in directing a patient toward optimum health levels. It is central in the sports medicine approach. In an osteopathic approach to examination and diagnosis, it is not enough to study the disease and its by-products; an intimate and thorough knowledge of the individual is essential.

Analyzing an individual's homeostatic reserve considers the impact on the whole body but screening may focus on historic, observational, or manual testing factors in a singular region. For example, in the respiratory-circulatory model (8), observation of passive respiration extending motion down to the pubic symphysis provides the osteopathic physician with a screening assessment of the homeostatic capabilities of that patient to move venous and lymphatic fluids. The degree to which a patient is able to mount a fever in response to an infection provides information about that individual's immune status. A synopsis of general reactions to emotional or job-related stress provides insights into the reactivity of the sympathetic nervous system. Even postural alignment provides information on the compensatory capabilities of the neuromusculoskeletal system. Each speaks to homeostatic mechanisms inherent to maintaining the health of the patient.

An osteopathic examination strives to provide all pertinent information needed for diagnosis. The osteopathic physician practicing osteopathic medicine must diagnose beyond the disease; osteopathic diagnosis strives to know all about the whole person. A whole person approach is one that encompasses structure-function interactions, self-healing mechanisms, and unique responses to stressors, all within the context of that individual patient's internal and external environments. The osteopathic examination is not just a standard history and physical examination with a palpatory diagnosis of somatic dysfunction added to it.

CHAPTER SCOPE AND DESIGN

This chapter provides a framework for applying the basic skills discussed in the previous chapter and provides an introduction for the "Overview: Evaluation and Management" chapters that follow (Chapters 40 through 44). Other portions of this text will elaborate on the general perspectives that this chapter introduces.

The regional chapters of this text (Chapters 45 through 53) emphasize functional anatomy and diagnostic tests that are central to an osteopathic examination of each body region. Information in these chapters is selected to examine representative structural and functional considerations that may produce symptoms or compromise homeostasis. The process of arriving at a differential diagnosis using the osteopathic approach is enhanced through more thorough discussions of a select number of common clinical conditions. (Also see Chapter 19, Clinical Problem-Solving.)

This text does not attempt to replace standardized texts on physical examination or medical and surgical differential diagnosis, nor does it attempt to replace exhaustive anatomy, physiology, or physical examination texts. Instead, chapters are designed to augment and focus the osteopathic physician's synthesis of skills needed to perform an osteopathic medical examination. They are designed to raise awareness and recognition of functional disturbances that influence a patient's progress (therefore requiring additional attention) and to make a presumptive diagnosis and transition from examination to treatment.

The "Palpatory Diagnosis and Manipulative Treatment" chapters of this text (Chapters 54 through 73) discuss specific options and outcomes of various treatment techniques or approaches.

These chapters rely on applying "evaluation and management principles" to improve the function of the body and to manage somatic dysfunction identified in the overall examination and diagnosis.

The importance of synthesizing individual tests and historic information into a working knowledge of a complete individual is the overall perspective that this chapter emphasizes. To recognize individual (host) strengths and weaknesses in such fashion permits a patient-physician interaction that promotes health and reduces dysfunction and disease.

FUNCTIONAL ANATOMY

A fundamental understanding of anatomy is the basis of the osteopathic examination. Knowledge of the body framework—of pertinent skeletal, arthrodial, and myofascial structures—is essential. Emphasis is placed on how these anatomic structures relate to their intended functions—alone and in interrelated units. Functional relationships of somatic structures extend to anatomically and physiologically related neural, lymphatic, and other vascular elements.

In an osteopathic examination, viscera are examined individually, in relationship to their respective organ system, and as they are structurally and functionally related to the body framework.

A complete understanding of function and its interrelationship with structure leads to the ability of the physician to recognize dysfunction, often before the dysfunction progresses to the classic signs, symptoms, and anatomic alterations that can be diagnosed as disease. The definition of somatic dysfunction (9) requires an assessment of the functional and physiologic interrelationships between certain anatomic structures, including:

Skeletal tissues
Arthrodial tissues
Myofascial tissues
Nerves (including the autonomic system)
Arteries and veins
Lymphatics

It also warrants assessment of these factors of possible interrelationships between somatic and visceral structures.

The physical examination for somatic dysfunction, rarely covered in other medical texts, is a central component (but not the only component) in the osteopathic medical examination. Therefore, the chapters in this and other sections of *Foundations of Osteopathic Medicine* therefore center on the anatomic and physiologic information that is provided by discovering somatic dysfunction. Most employ one or more representative clinical conditions to enhance understanding of the application of the osteopathic examination in arriving at a presumptive diagnosis and/or in initiating treatment.

ANATOMY AND SOMATIC DYSFUNCTION
Structures Predisposing to Somatic Dysfunction

Identification of structure predisposing to somatic dysfunction is important in differential diagnosis, in selecting diagnostic tests or denotes that T5 on T6 is extended, rotated right, and side-bent right with freedom of motion in that direction and restriction in attempting to flex, rotate, and side-bend left.

Through discussions coordinated by the Educational Council on Osteopathic Principles (ECOP), the nomenclature for describing spinal motion has evolved to where the profession uses the terms neutral (N) and nonneutral (NN) as adjectives to describe specific types of mechanics, positions, and tests. The "neutral" and "nonneutral" adjectives may also be employed to name and record the diagnosis of specific somatic dysfunctions derived from synthesizing the motion characteristics palpated using passive or active motion testing in neutral and/or nonneutral positions (Fig. 39.1).

- Example 1: A person's lumbar spine would have been moved into a "nonneutral position" if that sagittal plane position would typically induce "nonneutral mechanics."
- Example 2: Palpation of motion characteristics consistent with coupled motion in one neutral mechanical pattern that simultaneously resists motion in the diametrically opposed opposite neutral mechanical pattern is diagnosed as a "neutral somatic dysfunction."
- Example 3: A specific "neutral somatic dysfunction" at the fifth thoracic vertebral unit could be recorded as "T5 N S_RR_L" if there was no preference ascertained for flexion or extension at that vertebral unit; as "T5 F S_RR_L" if flexion was also free and extension was restricted.

For those wishing more background, complicated combinations of interacting neutral and nonneutral mechanics are described by Hoover in a 1950 paper (20).

A third principle, described by Beckwith (21) and Hoover and Nelson (22) came later. It suggests that initiation of vertebral segment motion in any one plane modifies and reduces movement in all other planes. As mentioned previously, coupled motions change in response to the anteroposterior curves of the vertebrae.

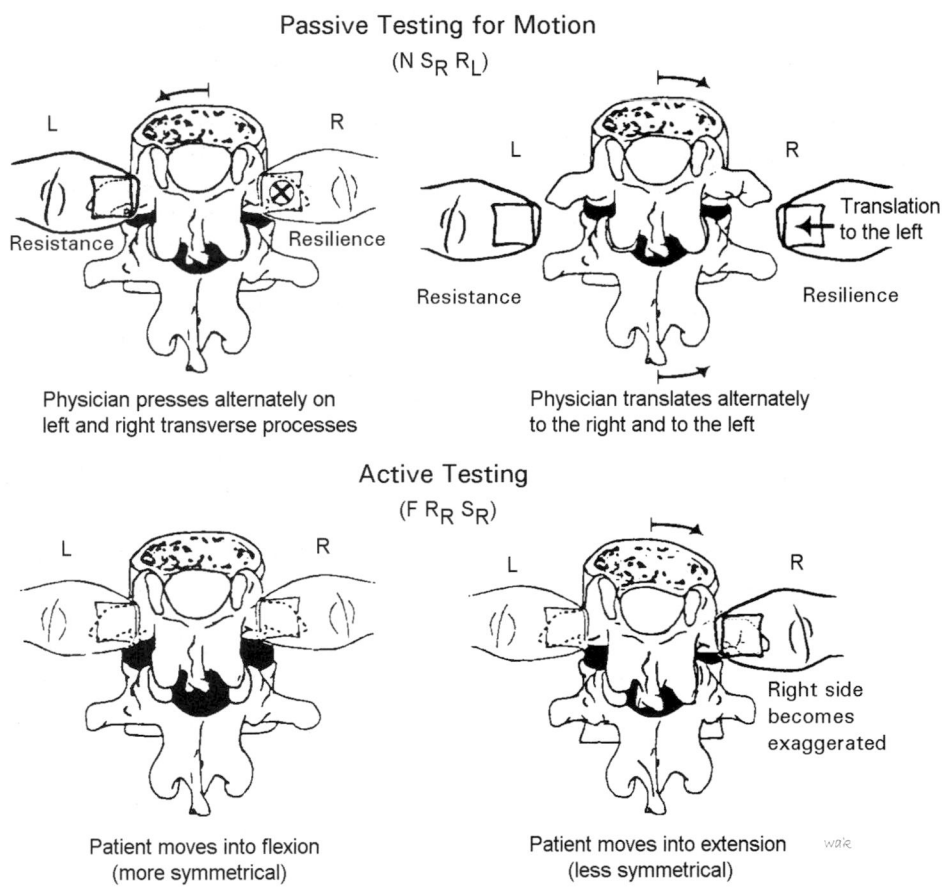

Passive Testing for Motion
(N S_R R_L)

Physician presses alternately on left and right transverse processes

Physician translates alternately to the right and to the left

Active Testing
(F R_R S_R)

Patient moves into flexion (more symmetrical)

Patient moves into extension (less symmetrical)

FIGURE 39.1. Motion Testing. *Passive motion testing (top)* involves the physician pressing alternatively over each transverse process and translating between spinal segments to assess the quality of the barrier at the end of motion. In the diagram, the left thumb meets sudden resistance in both side-bending and rotation while the end-feel for both is springy under motion initiated by the right thumb. The somatic dysfunction is a spinal segment that is side-bent right and rotated left (NS$_R$R$_L$). In *active motion testing (bottom),* the patient flexes and extends while the physician palpates the motion over the transverse processes. In the diagram, both thumbs move forward equally with flexion. With extension, the right facet closes but the left does not. At the end of extension, the right transverse process is more posterior that the left. Here, the dysfunction is flexed, rotated, and side-bent right (FR$_R$S$_R$). (From Kuchera ML. Gravitational stress, musculoskeletal strain, and postural alignment. *Spine: State of the Art Reviews.* 1995;9(2):463–490, with permission.)

Furthermore, a common application of this principle is observed in the setup of manipulative techniques. For example, side-bending and/or sagittal plane motion is often introduced to limit the amount of rotation needed to engage a barrier.

Active and Passive Motion Testing

According to the *Glossary of Osteopathic Terminology* (9), "active motion" refers to patient-initiated voluntary motion. Conversely, "passive motion" is induced in a subject by the physician with the subject remaining passive or relaxed. These terms may also be applied to palpatory tests used to diagnose somatic dysfunction.

Passive motion testing of a vertebral unit assesses the direction, quantity, and end-feel of each motion individually in each of the three cardinal planes of motion. It is usually assessed with that region of the patient's spine in an anatomically neutral position. Passive motion testing components may be used as a screening examination or to specifically identify and name somatic dysfunction.

Active motion testing assesses the vertebral unit's combined motion by palpating over the transverse process area as the patient bends forward and backward outside the "easy and free" neutral range. The changes in position of the palpated site, found at the extremes of flexion and extension and as the vertebral unit moves from the neutral position to these nonneutral sagittal plane positions, provide significant information (see Chapter 52, Fig. 52.16). Active testing may be used to palpate normal spinal mechanics or to identify somatic dysfunction.

Each motion testing system provides valuable information about different aspects of vertebral unit motion. Each can be used to identify impaired or altered function. Each provides sufficient information to "name" somatic dysfunction and to formulate a treatment plan to reestablish motion. Some practitioners incorporate only one system of palpation; others combine or integrate systems of diagnosis.

Neutral (Type I) Mechanics

Neutral (type I) mechanics typically occur in the thoracic and lumbar spine in the presence of free and easy articular and soft tissue motion (9,18). Side-bending movements are accompanied by vertebral segments rotating away from formed concavities and toward the convexities. Clinically, the transverse processes rotate posteriorly on the side of the formed convexity. For example, in the neutral position, right lumbar side-bending creates left rotation of one or more vertebral segments. A typical neutral, type I, response involves three or more segments.

Nonneutral (Type II) Mechanics

Nonneutral (type II) ERS/FRS segmental motions occur in the thoracic and lumbar regions when vertebral facets, soft tissues, and costovertebral attachments are asymmetrically engaged during compound movements. This is especially likely to occur outside of the easy neutral range described previously (see Chapter 52, Fig. 52.16). The sooner facets and soft tissues asymmetrically engage, the earlier the nonneutral, type II, responses

TABLE 39.1. PHYSIOLOGIC SPINAL MOTIONS

Segmental Region	Physiologic Motion(s)
C0–1 (occipitoatlantal joint)	F or E; SxRy only; combinations
C1–2 (atlantoaxial joint)	Rx or Ry only
C2–7 (typical cervicals)	F or E; SxRx; combinations
T1–12 (typical thoracics)	F or E; type I (SxRy) or type II (RxSx); combinations
L1–5 (typical lumbars)	F or E; type I (SxRy) or type II (RxSx); combinations

begin. Under these conditions, the involved segments and unit (or units) rotate into the intended concavity.

Mechanics in Other Anatomic Regions

The spinal mechanics outlined above for the thoracic and lumbar regions are normal physiologic motions for these regions. The specific motions that normally occur, however, depend on the anatomy of the structure being examined. Different normal physiologic mechanics are found for varying structures in different regions (e.g., cervical, sacral, rib, sternal, pelvic, and extremity regions).

In the cervical region, for example, the anatomy of the most superior two vertebral segments of the superior cervical division are very different from each other and from the other vertebral segments in the inferior cervical division (C2-7). This variation in structure results in three different sets of motion mechanics in this one region of the spine alone. Refer to specific regional chapters (Chapters 45 through 53) to understand the normal physiologic motions that exist in the various regions of the body from head to toe. See Table 39.1 for a summary of physiologic spinal motions.

Physiologic Mechanics and Somatic Dysfunction

Somatic dysfunction demonstrates impaired or altered function of somatic structures, and altered motion characteristics are one objective finding in the osteopathic examination that defines it. It may be initiated by a variety of causes, and a number of postulated mechanisms have been advanced for its continued presence (16).

Somatic dysfunction commonly occurs while engaged in common daily activities. Osteopathic examination reveals that a significant amount of somatic dysfunctions demonstrate the arrested physiologic motion specific to the region and activity involved. Motion findings in this type of somatic dysfunction typically reveal one combination of permitted physiologic motion with simultaneous restrictions in each of the opposing directions. The pattern of motion permitted is typically consistent with the physiologic motion that was occurring at the time the dysfunction was initiated.

Traumatic causes are another story, due to the uncontrolled forces that impacted the body region. Traumatically induced somatic dysfunction may or may not result in patterns associated with the patient's position or activity; it may not even follow the physiologic motion pattern of the region traumatized.

DIAGNOSIS AND PLAN FOR MANUAL TREATMENT: A PRESCRIPTION

ROBERT E. KAPPLER
WILLIAM A. KUCHERA

KEY CONCEPTS

- Definition of somatic dysfunction, and possible causes
- Essential elements of diagnosing somatic dysfunction, including observation, screening tests, palpation, and motion testing
- Effects of somatic dysfunction on range of motion and end-feel
- Decisions physician must make after diagnosis of somatic dysfunction
- Answers to: When is it important to use manipulative treatment?
- Considerations when developing a treatment plan, including sequence in which somatic dysfunctions should be treated, dose and frequency of treatments, and choice of techniques

Many treatment procedures follow the principles of osteopathic philosophy. The use of manual intervention to remove impairment of normal body function was emphasized by A. T. Still. This intervention, osteopathic manipulative treatment (OMT), requires a careful evaluation and diagnosis of the patient before, during, and after treatment. The evaluation of the patient leads to a precise and individual plan for treatment.

The plan is the guide for the patient's treatment developed from observations and findings about him or her at that moment. The plan is written in the record for later reference. A note is recorded stating whether the procedure was effective or ineffective.

Osteopathic examination methods and procedures have been categorized. Dinnar (1,2) listed four categories:

General impressions
Regional motion testing
Superficial and deep tissue evaluation
Local characteristics of motion

DIAGNOSIS

Somatic dysfunction is an impaired or altered function of related components of the somatic (body framework) system, such as these elements:

Skeletal
Arthrodial
Myofascial
Vascular
Lymphatic
Neural

Four criteria are used for diagnosis of somatic dysfunction:

i. Tissue texture abnormalities (T)
ii. Asymmetry of bony landmarks (A)
iii. Restriction of motion (R)
iv. Tenderness or soreness to examiner pressure (T)

These form the acronym TART.

The following is a plan for conducting an osteopathic evaluation for diagnosis of somatic dysfunction. The physician first looks at the whole person, noting characteristics of gait and evidence of asymmetries. Screening tests are performed. Abnormal findings on general impression tests, such as asymmetrical bony landmarks or regional motion, suggest regions that require further palpatory evaluation for tissue texture changes and asymmetry of segmental motion characteristics.

Palpation reveals localized areas that stand out from surrounding areas by exhibiting temperature differences, swelling, hyperesthesia, or firmness, which can be identified as tissue texture changes (TTC). Palpation of these areas is almost always tender.

The segmental areas of TTC and tenderness are then tested for motion characteristics. Motion testing may be active or passive. The characteristics of motion of a joint and its tissues can be described in various ways (Fig. 40.1). It may involve rotation around one of three axes (vertical, transverse, anteroposterior) or translation in one of the three planes of the body, or it may be a shearing of myofascial tissue layers.

For the spine, forward and backward bending indicates motion in the sagittal plane about a transverse axis. Pressure on the transverse process initiates rotation in a horizontal plane

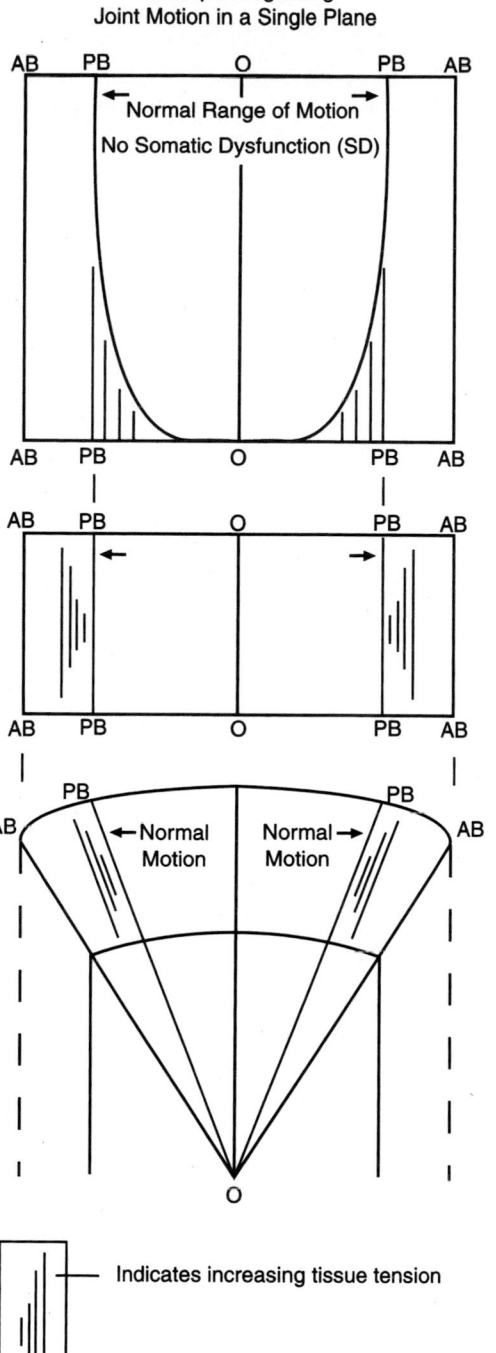

FIGURE 40.1. Normal motion in a single plane: three methods of illustration. AB, anatomic barrier; PB, physiologic barrier; RB, restrictive barrier.

about a vertical axis; side-to-side translation of the vertebral body produces side-bending. Regardless of how the segments of a region are tested, the questions that must be answered are:

Does it move?
Does it move appropriately? (Is it restricted in motion?)

What is the quality of motion?
What does the end range of motion feel like?

Motion has direction, range, and quality. Visual observation measures the range of motion; palpation reveals the quality of motion. The quality of motion is described as:

Smooth
Ratcheting
Restricted
Exhibiting resistance to the motion introduced

The presence of normal passive motion in one direction of one plane of motion and resistance in the other is presumptive evidence of somatic dysfunction.

The range of motion with somatic dysfunction is decreased. This decrease of motion occurs within the normal range of motion for the joint. The quality of motion can be shown in a graph (Fig. 40.2). The joint will move farther in the direction in which the somatic dysfunction occurred; its movement is restricted in the opposite direction. There is a restriction to motion in one direction, called a restrictive barrier. As the joint is moved in the direction of the restrictive barrier, the curved line of resistance rises at a much more rapid rate than the resistance encountered when moving toward the physiologic barrier in the opposite direction. The restrictive barrier of the joint occurs before motion reaches the physiologic barrier on that side.

Kappler (3) describes the resistance near the limits of motion as end-feel. The end-feel of motion in a direction toward the somatic dysfunction (restrictive barrier) is different from the end-feel away from the direction of the somatic dysfunction. The end-feel in a normal joint should be the same in either direction. End-feel characteristics may be used to differentiate which of the many manipulative procedures to use.

TREATMENT

Approach

Somatic dysfunction is identified with the following diagnostic findings:

Asymmetry of tissue texture
Range of motion
Perception of tenderness
Characteristics of the end-feel

The physician makes further decisions based on the answers to these questions:

i. Are the findings significant and related to the patient's problem(s)?
ii. Should the findings be altered by manipulation?
iii. If so, which of the many techniques are indicated and likely to be effective for this patient?

Additional questions relate to the areas of restricted motion. Are they:

i. A primary somatic dysfunction related to the musculoskeletal system?

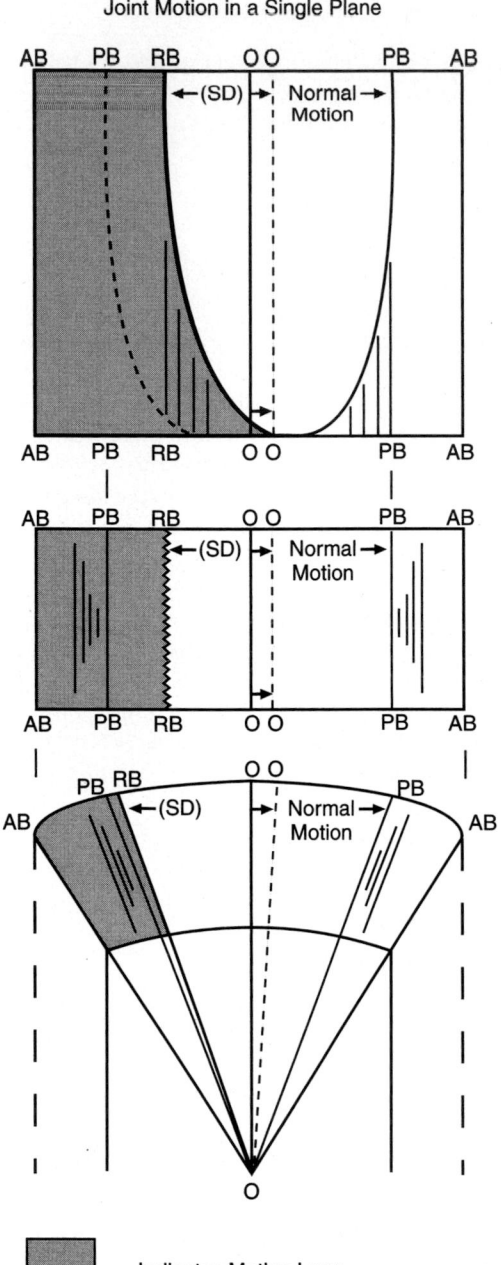

Concepts Regarding
Joint Motion in a Single Plane

Indicates Motion Loss

FIGURE 40.2. Somatic dysfunction in a single plane: three methods of illustrating the restrictive barrier (the restrainer). AB, anatomic barrier; PB, physiologic barrier; RB, restrictive barrier; SD, somatic dysfunction.

ii. A somatosomatic reflex related to some other musculoskeletal problem?

iii. A viscerosomatic reflex from a dysfunctional or diseased organ? Clinical investigations (4) have found the presence of somatic components related to visceral disturbances.

iv. A mechanism protecting some damaged tissue or weakened structure? Treatment of the somatic dysfunction in this situation is not indicated at this time; strengthening of the weakened area is indicated (5).

The positional and motion aspects of somatic dysfunction can be described using two parameters:

i. The position of a body part, as determined by palpation and referenced to its adjacent defined structure (the upper segment is named in relation to the lower).

ii. The directions in which motion is more free and the directions in which motion is restricted (6).

The goal of treatment is to enhance movement to resolve somatic dysfunction.

Hoag (5) asked, "When is it important to use manipulative treatment?" He answered the question as follows:

■ When the challenge is not overly severe, but the body is not responding adequately to the appropriate treatment regimen, or when appropriate (manipulative) treatment may aid the body's response or may accelerate the healing process.

■ When the body is critically ill, and life's continuance is in the balance, a more optimal musculoskeletal reaction to illness may be the factor that tips the balance of recovery in favor of the patient.

■ Zink and Lawson (7) answered, "The findings are significant to treat until a physiologic state existed that included eupnea in the supine position. The osteopathic physician focuses on the whole person. While the person's symptom may be localized, the major influence can be elsewhere."

Methods

i. The dose of treatment is limited by the patient's ability to respond to the treatment. The physician may want to do more and go faster; however, the patient's body must make the necessary changes toward health and recovery.

ii. The physician's ability to execute a technique effectively is a major factor in determining which techniques to use. There are many different technique approaches. The physician must choose from the various techniques that are effective in his or her hands.

iii. There must be an objective to be accomplished by the treatment. Treatment should be outcome-oriented, meaning that the intended objective is accomplished. Do not allow OMT to become oriented only to the process, meaning that once you have given the OMT, the process is viewed as completed. Examples of objectives are: mobilize the sacrum, decrease rib tenderness, improve motion at T5, or relax cervical muscles.

iv. The objective is the constant; the method is the variable.

v. The technique chosen must be safe and potentially effective. Risk/benefit relationships must always be considered.

vi. The physician must be able to execute the technique effectively. The technique must be modified to meet the needs of the patient and the physician.

Sequence

There are different opinions regarding what should be treated first. Absolute rules for sequencing do not exist. Patient problems vary and may require deviation from the physician's usual approach. One school of thought suggests that the initial approach is to balance the pelvis. Another opinion suggests that the sacrum should be treated first because the sacrum is the base of support. A sample sequence is as follows:

i. For low back pain, especially with psoas involvement, treat the lumbar spine first.
ii. Treat the upper thoracic spine and ribs before treating the cervical spine.
iii. Treat the thoracic spine before treating specific rib dysfunctions.
iv. For very acute somatic dysfunctions, treat secondary or peripheral areas to allow access to the acute area.
v. Cranial treatment can produce relaxation and allow OMT to work in other areas.
vi. For extremity problems, treat the axial skeletal components first (spine, ribs, sacrum).

These guidelines on sequencing are not absolute rules. Each physician, after gaining experience, develops his or her own approach.

Dose and Frequency

A quotation frequently repeated in osteopathic circles is attributed to A. T. Still: Find it, fix it, and leave it alone. The statement addresses dosage, with the admonition to resist continuing treatment but give the patient time to respond. The ability of patients to respond is variable. Pediatric patients respond quickly, while geriatric patients respond more slowly. Patients who are very ill and debilitated respond slowly; they cannot respond appropriately to a treatment dose that is appropriate for an ambulatory patient. Some forms of osteopathic manipulative treatment, such as thoracic pump, may be performed several times a day. Soft tissue stretching may be performed frequently. Specific joint mobilization is an example of a treatment approach that requires a longer interval between treatments.

The frequency of visits for ambulatory patients has several guidelines, as well as some confounding factors. The availability of time in the physician's appointment schedule is a practical factor in the scheduling of the next visit. The physician may work at more than one site and not be available at a particular location every day. Patient availability must be considered, as well as factors such as travel distance, work, and prior commitments. Apart from physician or patient availability, the acuteness of the patient's problem is a major consideration in the scheduling of the next visit. The ambulatory patient disabled with an acute low back problem would be reevaluated in 24 to 48 hours. A patient with chronic low back discomfort might be seen every 2 weeks. Consider response to treatment in a decision for timing the next visit. A favorable response suggests lengthening the interval. A poor response might suggest that the patient is not yet able to respond appropriately and should be seen again when the ability to respond improves.

At times, the patient may exhibit more dysfunctions than can be appropriately handled in one visit. A plan of treatment involves immediate objectives along with longer-term objectives. Provide palliative treatment with the understanding that the real task is yet to be addressed.

DOSE GUIDELINES

i. The sicker the patient, the less the dose.
ii. Caring, compassionate novices often err on the side of overdose.
iii. Allow time for the patient to respond to the treatment.
iv. Do not waste the dose on insignificant areas. Concentrate on key areas needing treatment.
v. Chronic disease requires chronic treatment.
vi. Pediatric patients can be treated more frequently; geriatric patients need a longer interval to respond to the treatment.
vii. Acute cases should have a shorter interval between treatments; as they respond, the interval is increased.

Direct or Indirect Method

Two major factors determine choice of technique:

The ability of the patient to respond to the treatment
The ability of the physician to execute the technique

We lack precise answers for when to choose one technique instead of another. There are only general guidelines. Sometimes certain techniques are inappropriate to achieve the intended objective. There are times when the risk/benefit relationship is such that certain techniques should be avoided. The use of forceful high-velocity technique in a patient with advanced osteoporosis might lead to pathologic fracture. This text contains chapters on a number of technique types and their use.

The ability of the physician to execute the technique is probably the greatest factor in determining choice of technique. For many years, direct action thrust techniques were taught and were used very successfully by osteopathic physicians in the treatment of their patients. Those physicians did not face the challenge of trying to decide which type of technique to use. They knew thrust techniques and learned how to modify the techniques to make them work.

Some osteopathic physicians tended to use one type of technique approach other than high-velocity/low-amplitude force (HVLA) direct action thrust. Some physicians used only muscle energy. Others used only functional or indirect techniques. Many of these physicians were considered experts in their field. This illustrates the reality that there is more than one method to achieve the objective. Precise answers to choice of technique do not exist. Indirect technique is of no value to a physician who lacks skills in using indirect technique. HVLA is of no value to a physician who lacks skills to use that technique.

The model for today's osteopathic physician is eclectic, with knowledge and skill in a broad spectrum of techniques. The more methods available, the greater the chance is of success in treating a wide range of patients and patient problems.

Techniques are classified as direct and indirect. Direct technique means that the initial positioning of the patient's somatic dysfunction is in the direction of the restrictive barrier, and then a final activating force is applied. Indirect technique involves positioning away from the restrictive barrier.

Indirect technique is usually comfortable for the patient because the physician is moving the tissues in a direction that is freer, in a direction the tissues want to go. Most of these procedures involve holding in the proper position; release is by inherent forces rather than physician forces. Examples of the indirect method are the Sutherland ligamentous release technique (8), functional technique, and counterstrain technique.

Direct technique usually involves a greater amount of force. Procedures of this type are soft tissue, articulation, myofascial, muscle energy, and thrust techniques. Descriptions of these techniques are found in other chapters in this text.

A muscle energy procedure for the treatment of a patient with an acute, stiff neck is clinically effective, but the initial positioning is not toward or away from the restrictive barrier. The neck is positioned in a neutral, pain-free position and held while the physician instructs the patient to turn the neck in a direction in which it will not move. The muscles that are contracting are not the shortened, painful muscles, but the antagonist, non-painful group. After the patient completely relaxes this contraction, the physician rotates the neck a few degrees toward the new barrier, being careful to avoid a painful position. This procedure is repeated several times and usually results in significant improvement of the patient's condition.

An osteopathic manipulative treatment has been described as a transaction between two unique persons (9). The amount of HVLA used for one patient may be inappropriate for another. The presence of osteoporosis suggests a lesser force. Thus, thrust or impulse must be titrated. How much force should be used in a HVLA thrust? Kimberly (10) states " ...enough to affect a physiologic response (increased joint mobility, produce a vasomotor flush, produce palpable circulatory changes in periarticular tissues, and/or provide pain relief) but not enough to overwhelm the patient."

Plan of Intervention

A plan of intervention requires a specific diagnosis. Decisions must be made based on the answers to these questions:

What doesn't move?
What direction will it move?
In which direction doesn't it move?

The plan includes the decision to use a direct or indirect method of treatment to improve the movement. It considers in what direction the treatment can most effectively be applied. It includes choosing the best technique for the patient from the variety of therapeutic procedures available.

The plan of treatment and the patient's response to the treatment should be recorded in the chart's progress note. A review of the record at a follow-up visit can change the plan for the next visit. The record also is used for purposes of research, reimbursement, or legal documentation. One example of the subjective, objective, assessment, plan note (SOAP) method of recording an osteopathic office call follows:

SOAP

S: Subjective

A 28-year-old woman complains of a cold with coughing, difficulty getting a deep breath, fatigue, and low back pain. The symptoms have been present for 5 days. She complains of nasal discharge and postnasal drip. She has had a mild fever. She has no known allergies, has otherwise been very healthy, and has had OMT in the past with no complications. There has been no change in bowel or bladder activity.

O: Objective

The patient's heart rate is 88 and regular, blood pressure is regular at 130/72, temperature is 99° F orally, and respirations are 16 and not labored but shallow. There is anterior and posterior tender lymphadenopathy, the pharynx is hyperemic, and the nasal passages are congested and contain thick creamy mucus. The umbo of the tympanic membranes is congested and hyperemic, but no fluid is seen, and there is a normal cone of light. The chest is clear to auscultation over all lobes, and auscultation of the heart revealed no murmurs or adventitious sounds. There is decreased diaphragmatic breathing with best motion on the left side; C2-4 is $R_R S_R$, the thoracic inlet is side-bent and rotated left; T12 is N RL S_R. The anterior superior iliac spines (ASIS) are inferior and the PSIS are superior on the left.

A: Assessment

i. Acute upper respiratory infection
ii. Somatic dysfunction of the cervical, cervicothoracic, thoracolumbar, and pelvic regions

P: Plan

i. Cervical soft tissue
ii. Direct action side-bending thrust to C3
iii. Indirect action myofascial unwinding to thoracic inlet
iv. Effleurage of face and neck provided. Soft tissue to thoracolumbar region and direct action muscle energy to T12 SD. Diaphragm re-domed with indirect method. Classic lymphatic pump soft tissue given
v. Counterstrain treatment of anterior innominate
vi. Prescribe amoxicillin 250 mg, 30 tabs, 2 tabs four times a day

Manipulation was successful and the patient left the clinic improved with this note: *Take all of the prescription and expect to be improved in 24 hours and know you are better in 48 hours. If this is not the case, or you have any problem with medications, call me or come to clinic for recheck.*
(Personal Signature, DO)

CONCLUSION

There are several parts to a treatment plan, including the sequence in which somatic dysfunctions should be treated, the dose and frequency of treatments, and the choice of techniques. Such intervention requires a careful evaluation and diagnosis of the patient before, during, and after treatment. The evaluation of the patient leads to a precise and individual plan for his or her treatment.

REFERENCES

1. Dinnar U. Classification of diagnostic tests used with osteopathic manipulation. *J Am Osteopath Assoc.* 1980;79:451–455.
2. Dinnar U. Description of fifty diagnostic tests used with osteopathic manipulation. *J Am Osteopath Assoc.* 1982;81:314–321.
3. Kappler RE. Direct action techniques. *J Am Osteopath Assoc.* 1981; 81(4):239–243.
4. Beal MC. Viscerosomatic reflexes: a review. *J Am Osteopath Assoc.* 1985; 85:786–801.
5. Hoag JM. The musculoskeletal system: a major factor in maintaining homeostasis. *1977 American Academy of Osteopathy Yearbook.* Newark, OH: American Academy of Osteopathy; 1979: 516.
6. The Glossary Review Committee of the Educational Council on Osteopathic Principles. Glossary of Osteopathic Terminology. In: Allen TW, ed. *AOA Yearbook and Directory of Osteopathic Physicians.* Chicago, IL: American Osteopathic Association; 1990:675.
7. Zink JG, Lawson WB. An osteopathic structural examination and functional interpretation of the soma. *Osteopath Ann.* 1979;7:12.
8. Lippincott H. The osteopathic techniques of Wm. G. Sutherland, D.O. In: Northup TL, ed. *AOA Yearbook.* Indianapolis, IN: American Academy of Osteopathy; 1949:124.
9. Korr IM. Somatic dysfunction, osteopathic manipulative treatment and the nervous system: a few facts, some theories, many questions. *J Am Osteopath Assoc.* 1986;86:109–114.
10. Kimberly P. Forming a prescription for osteopathic manipulative treatment. *JAOA.* 1980;79:512.

41

CONSIDERATIONS OF POSTURE AND GROUP CURVES

MICHAEL L. KUCHERA
ROBERT E. KAPPLER

KEY CONCEPTS

- What constitutes optimal posture
- Factors that produce postural decompensation
- Mechanisms of compensation and spinal patterning
- Mechanics of group curves
- Physical findings that occur with group curves and their clinical significance
- Role of central nervous system in maintaining posture
- Possible treatments for postural decompensation
- Direct osteopathic manipulation treatment techniques for group curves

"If we regard posture as the result of the dynamic interaction of two groups of forces—the environmental force of gravity on one hand, and the strength of the individual on the other—then posture is but the formal expression of the balance of power existing at any time between these two groups of forces. Thus, any deterioration of posture indicates that the individual is losing ground in his contest with the environmental force of gravity" (1).

Analysis of a patient's posture provides an enormous amount of information about the body. The endurance of antigravity (postural) muscles, the capability of the musculoskeletal system to adjust homeostatically to physical stressors, the presence and type of group spinal curves, and the locations of postural spinal crossovers all offer insight into structure-function relationships on a physical level. Observation of posture may also offer the clinician the first clues to the emotional, spiritual, and psychological elements of a patient's health.

Treatment of posture has wide implications in the general health status of each patient. It especially involves reduction or elimination of a constant precipitating and perpetuating factor of group curves and recurrent somatic dysfunction. Postural treatment can also play a significant role in the treatment of certain specific spinal conditions associated with postural decompensation, such as scoliosis and spondylolisthesis. Finally, postural treatment can be effective in improving symptoms associated

with a tremendous number of neuromusculoskeletal conditions, including myofascial pain syndromes, trigger points, segmental facilitation, and recurrent somatic dysfunction.

According to *Osteopathic Research: Growth and Development,* "Biomechanics from the osteopathic perspective has evolved into a dual study of the adaptive responses of the body to gravitational force and the effects of alterations in joint mechanics that result from injury or impaired function" (2).

ASPECTS OF POSTURE

Base of Support

Posture is the distribution of body mass in relation to gravity over a base of support. The base of support includes all structures from the feet to the base of the skull. The effect of the lower extremities, (3) pelvis, (4) and base of the skull (5) are especially important. Distribution of weight over the base of support depends on the following:

- Energy requirements for homeostasis
- Integrity of musculoligamentous structures
- Compensation that structures at or below the base of the skull have on the visual and/or balance functions of the body

Optimal Posture

Optimal posture is a balanced configuration of the body with respect to gravity. It depends on normal arches of the feet, vertical alignment of the ankles, and horizontal orientation (in the coronal plane) of the sacral base. The presence of an optimum posture suggests that there is a perfect distribution of the body mass around the center of gravity. The compressive force on spinal discs is balanced by ligamentous tension; there is minimal energy expenditure from postural muscles (6,7). Structural or functional stressors on the body, however, may prevent achievement of optimum posture. In this case, homeostatic mechanisms provide for compensation in an effort to provide maximum postural function within the existing structure of the individual. Compensation is the counterbalancing of any defect of structure or function (8).

Compensated Posture

A compensated posture is considered to be the result of the patient's homeostatic mechanisms working through the entire body unit to maximize function. Postural compensation in the musculoskeletal system occurs in all three planes of body motion to keep the body balanced and the eyes level. The central nervous system (CNS) places a high priority on visual and vestibular (balance) functions. Spinal compensation involves CNS correlation of proprioceptive information from tendons and muscles as well as vestibular information from the semicircular canals. The CNS also integrates this proprioceptive information with information received from the eyes (9).

Postural homeostatic lessons are learned gradually by the CNS from visual and proprioceptive input as the individual grows and develops. The process has implications for treatment protocols that include postural reeducation; this should be progressive and consistent if it is to succeed. Structural compensation allows a person to function despite musculoskeletal imbalances. Because of an accumulated history of genetic, traumatic, and habitual processes requiring compensation, few patients have ideal posture.

Posture is both static (structural) and dynamic (functional). It is static in its alignment of body mass with respect to gravity. It is dynamic because this alignment constantly adjusts to the individual's changing postural demands.

Over time, individual static postural alignment conforms to inherent connective tissue structure. It also responds to the cumulative functional demand placed upon it by static and dynamic postural conditions. Both static and dynamic postures are influenced by and influence soft tissue functions. Examination includes analysis of static postural alignment in the upright weight-bearing position. It also includes osteopathic examination of the selective tensions of the soft tissues. Palpatory examination of dynamic posture and segmental motion testing is vital to understanding structure-function interrelationships. This combination of examinations provides clinical clues about the inherent capability of the patient's neuromusculoskeletal system to balance and maintain biomechanical alignment. Radiographic analysis of bony postural relationships can further add to this understanding (see Chapter 42).

Group Curves

A group curve is a spinal curve that involves several segments. The motion pattern in these curves follows the first principle of physiologic motion of the spine. When the spine is in neutral position, that is, with an absence of marked flexion or extension, and side bending is introduced, the vertebrae rotate into the produced convexity (10). In these curves, rotation is to the opposite side of side bending.

Compensatory changes of the spine are often named according to the group curve with the most prominent postural feature (Fig. 41.1). Lateral group curves that exceed 5 degrees as measured by the Cobb method are called scoliosis. Group curves in the sagittal plane are called kyphotic or lordotic curves. Scoliotic curves are sometimes referred to as rotoscoliotic curves because rotation and side bending are inseparable. A curve may be called a kyphorotoscoliotic curve if all three planes are significantly involved.

MECHANICS OF GROUP CURVES

Spinal joints are designed to provide motion; spinal motion is necessary in most of our ordinary activity. Most spinal motion involves a group of vertebral segments. This motion follows the first principle of physiologic motion of the spine and is necessary to allow for positional changes of the body. Every time a person bends to the side, a lateral curve is produced. This sometimes leads to restriction of motion. Lateral curves become a problem when restriction occurs and the spine no longer straightens.

Spinal curves may be produced by unilateral muscle contraction. This muscle pull creates a concavity, resulting in a curve. The vertebrae rotate into the convexity. This type of lateral curve disappears when the muscle hypertonicity is gone.

Another type of lateral curve involves long-term anatomic adaptation associated with positional change. Examples would include the spine that is initially in a curved position to compensate for an anatomic short leg or certain structural deformities, postural balance adaptation, or even long-term positional change (such as may be required for a certain occupation) that becomes a pattern. Over time, the tissues associated with this curve change. Tissues on the convex side become lengthened. Tissues on the concave side become shortened. Deformity of a vertebral body with lateral wedging results in a spinal curve. Long-standing curves with anatomic adaptation resist change. Over time, the curved position becomes the neutral position.

DIAGNOSIS OF GROUP CURVES

A patient presents with humping of a paravertebral region on the convex side of a coronal plane curve as a result of stretched muscles or deformation of ribs brought about by rotation of the vertebrae in the curve. Stretched muscles may be tender to palpation. Side bending is toward the concavity, and rotation occurs into the convexity with maximal rotation occurring at the apex of the curve.

The physician should consider a diagnosis of kyphoscoliosis. Anteroposterior (AP) curves may be increased at the apex. AP curves flatten at the crossover. The crossover is a point where an S curve crosses the midline to the other side. By international convention, scoliotic curves are named for their convex side. For example, rotoscoliosis right means a curve that is convex to the right by being side bent to the left.

POSTURAL DECOMPENSATION

Gravitational force acts universally to affect upright posture. Decompensation occurs when an individual's homeostatic mechanisms are overwhelmed (11). Several conditions can overwhelm host factors.

Traumatic decompensation occurs when macrotrauma or recurrent microtrauma disrupts ligamentous stability of the spine. Fractures of the spine, pelvis, or lower extremity may produce sacral base unleveling or the need for other compensatory changes above the area of the trauma.

Congenital or acquired structural changes may create chronic postural strain and decompensation. Conversely, chronic postural

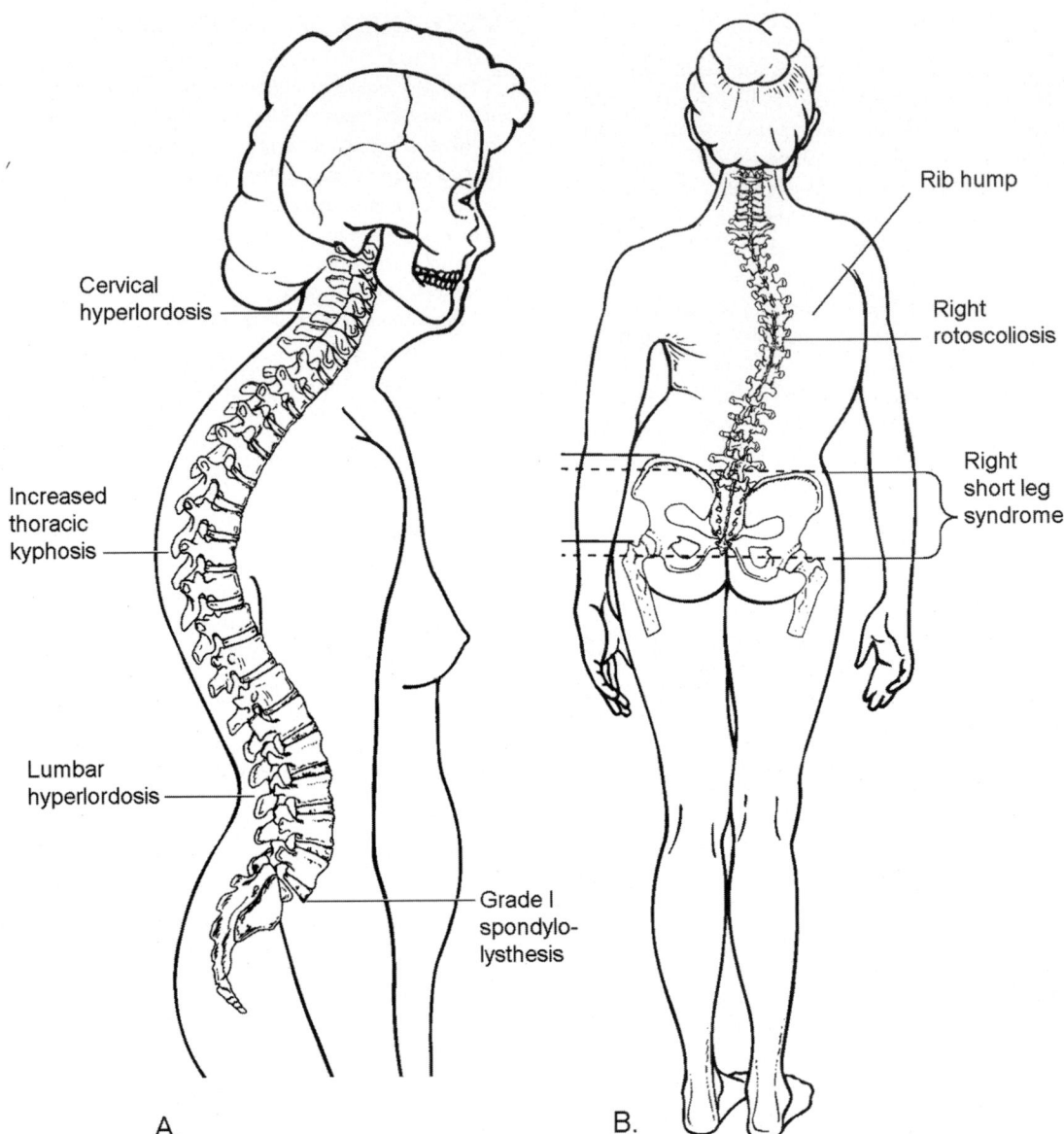

Cervical
hyperlordosis

Increased
thoracic
kyphosis

Lumbar
hyperlordosis

Grade I
spondylo-
lysthesis

A.

Rib hump

Right
rotoscoliosis

Right
short leg
syndrome

B.

FIGURE 41.1. A: Disorders in the coronal and horizontal plane: short leg syndrome and rotoscoliosis. **B:** Disorders in the sagittal plane: lumbar and cervical hyperlordosis, thoracic kyphosis, and L5-S1 isthmic spondylolisthesis. (From Kuchera WA, Kuchera ML. *Osteopathic Principles in Practice*, 2nd ed rev. Columbus, OH: Greyden Press; 1994:47, with permission.)

stress can initiate structural change. This is a classic example of the reciprocity of structure-function interrelationships. Unleveling of the sacral base or a deformed vertebra due to fracture or congenital deformation leads to compensatory curvatures of the spine. Occasionally an unlevel sacral base is observed in an x-ray image with a straight spine above it. This requires muscular effort, resulting in spinal musculoligamentous strain that may manifest as back pain or even as headache. As the person grows older and the muscular compensation becomes inadequate, functional scoliosis manifests and structural scoliosis eventually develops (12). Likewise, isthmic L5-S1 spondylolisthesis is a bony structural change often initiated by stress occurring predominantly in the sagittal plane (13). This leads to decompensation, spondylo*lysis*, and finally spondylo*listhesis*. These acquired bony structural changes often necessitate functional demand on

musculoligamentous structures to resist postural stresses in the region.

Personal conditions, inactivity, and aging potentially predispose people to decompensation of the spine. Changes of body habitus that accompany pregnancy, obesity, muscular weakness related to aging, and poor sitting or standing habits produce postural stress and can initiate decompensation. Work environments or recreational activities requiring strenuous posturing may also result in postural decompensation.

Abnormal gait may initiate the need for compensation or precipitate decompensation. Examples include the gait produced from unilateral pes planus (flat foot), wearing shoes with high or worn heels, and dysfunctional gait following ankle sprains or strains. These conditions affect the base of support and therefore stimulate compensatory changes in posture. If continued

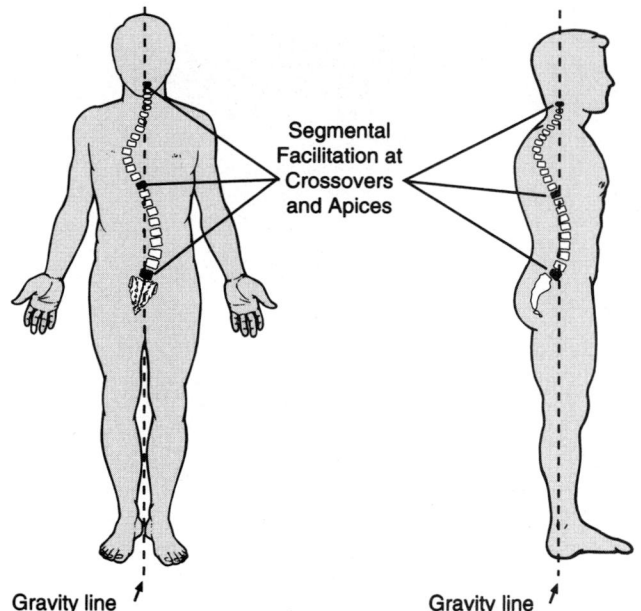

FIGURE 41.2. Gravitational strain pathophysiology. Crossover sites are found where the center of gravity line crosses bony posture. These sites have a high incidence of segmental facilitation. (From Kuchera WA, Kuchera ML. *Osteopathic Principles in Practice*, 2nd ed rev. Columbus, OH: Greyden Press; 1994:47, with permission.)

indefinitely, these changes could progress to decompensation with rotation, scoliosis, lordosis, and/or kyphosis.

Postural progression from a healthy state to a dysfunctional state leads to symptoms and a structural pathologic state. The body first tries to compensate for imbalance by altering motion characteristics and tissues in its spinal structure. The result is a functional scoliosis in the coronal plane. If this remains too long, it develops a fixed component and becomes a structural scoliosis (12).

Other symptoms occur in a person with spinal decompensation. These usually originate at the areas of crossover where the spinal curve crosses from side to side or anterior to posterior across the weightbearing line (Fig. 41.2). These crossover points may be the site of local subjective joint and tissue symptoms. They could also result in facilitated segments (14,15) and somatovisceral reflexes, producing inappropriate increases in sympathetic activity and related organ dysfunction.

PATTERNING

Spinal Patterning

The nature of postural compensation is to react to a disturbance of posture with change throughout the remaining somatic tissues. These changes tend to overcorrect slightly for postural disturbances. They alternate from one body region to the next and tend to occur in regions above and below the initial change. Most commonly these changes occur at the so-called transition zones, areas where anatomic structure changes create the potential for the greatest functional change (Fig. 41.3). Describing these regional changes in a patient can lead to recognition of patterns (16–18). Patterning provides a convenient way of summarizing common

prototypes of compensation. Postural patterns or patterning refer to classifiable combinations of regional compensatory change.

Compensation involves all three cardinal planes because spinal motions are biomechanically linked (10). Scoliotic, rotational, lordotic, or kyphotic group curves can therefore develop as compensation for postural stressors. The curve in a given plane often occurs in one direction in one region and in the opposite direction in the next spinal region so that the body can maintain some type of postural balance.

Postural patterns can be classified by whether they can be reduced by specific functional maneuvers. If some spinal motion such as side bending can reduce a lateral curve, it is known as a functional or secondary scoliotic curve. If it is unable to be reduced, it is known as a structural, fixed, or primary scoliosis. Functional scoliosis is reversible. Structural scoliosis is fixed. Because structure and function are interrelated, many scoliotic curves are a mixture of these two classifications. This phenomenon is also seen with postural patterns in the other planes.

Clinical Significance of Group Curves

Lateral curves contribute to postural imbalance by producing positional asymmetry that may lead to back pain or predispose a patient to recurrent somatic dysfunctions. They may involve a loss of energy because of the increased active muscle contraction (19) needed to counteract gravity or need to ambulate. Not all anatomic asymmetries can be corrected. In searching for an answer to the significance of a lateral curve in a patient, consider both structure and function. Although the physician often tries to improve the structure, reducing asymmetry does not necessarily improve the function of the patient. The objective of treatment is to maintain or improve function of the patient within their existing structure.

Group curves (type I, neutral) typically involve multiple segments. Often the longer outer muscles are involved rather than the short, deep segmental muscles. Multiple segments lack segmental specificity in terms of altered neural activity. By contrast, type II nonneutral dysfunction typically involves single segments. Segmental dysfunction is more likely to be associated with changes in spinal cord function, which osteopathic physicians associate with somatic dysfunction.

Osteopathic physicians differ regarding the significance of group curves. Some physicians focus on nonneutral type II single segmental dysfunction, while others emphasize treating group curves as well. The approach should depend on the individual patient: what is the functional significance of a group curve for the patient? If the group curve contributes to dysfunction of the patient, it should be treated.

Clinical Significance of Fascial Patterns

Postural patterning influences and is influenced by the fascias and related structures. J. Gordon Zink described patterns (18) that are clinically relevant to the diagnosis and treatment of fascial compensation and decompensation. Based on the palpatory fascial preference to motion (see Chapter 68), these fascial patterns may be classified as ideal, compensated, or uncompensated (Fig. 41.4). The postural influence on fascial patterning is important

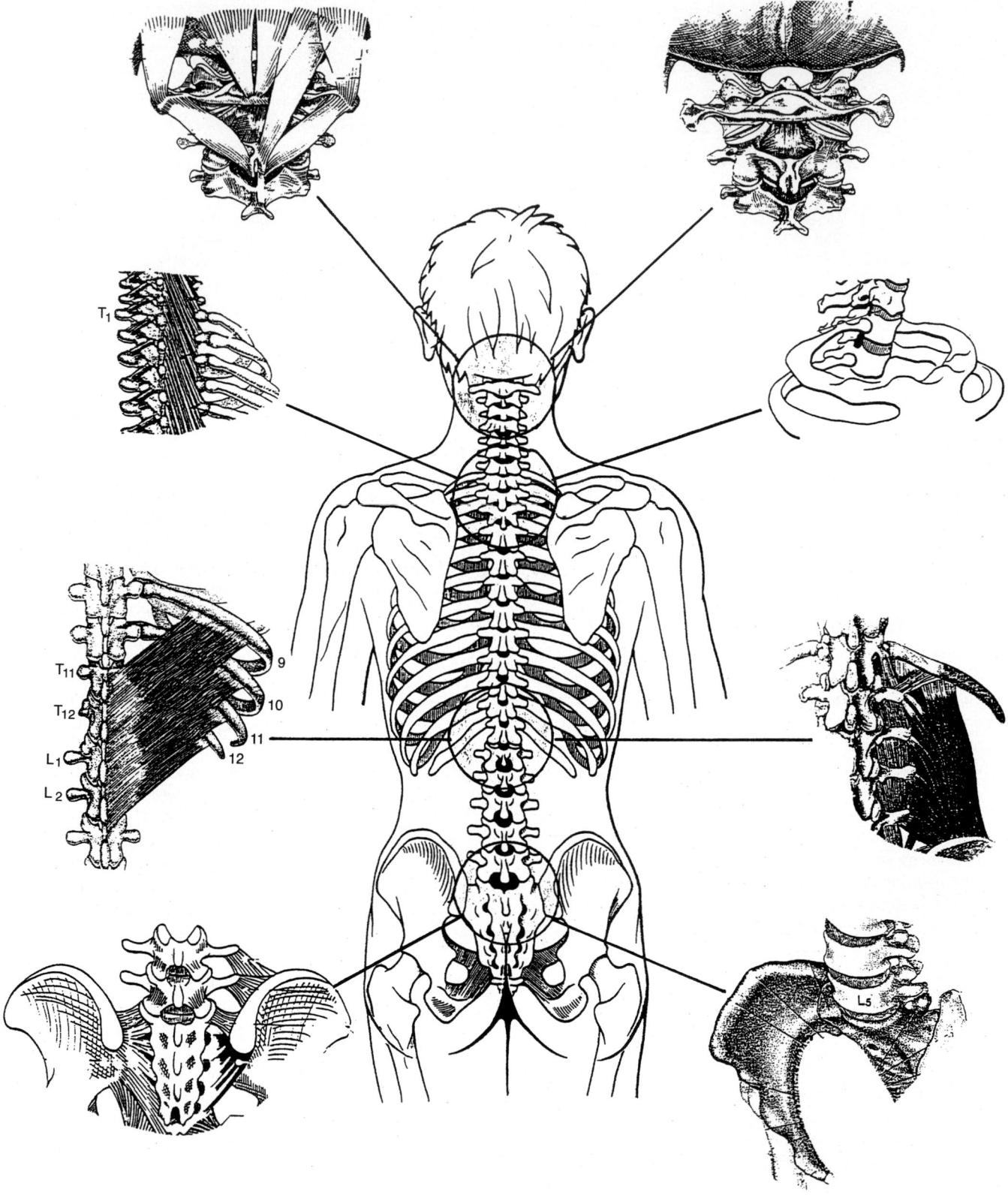

FIGURE 41.3. Transition zones are anatomically defined and their function is affected by skeletal, arthrodial, and myofascial anatomy. Transition zones occur at occipitocervical junction, cervicothoracic junction, thoracolumbar junction, and lumbosacral junction. Between each transition zone lies a definable region of spine. (From Kuchera WA, Kuchera ML. *Osteopathic Principles in Practice*, 2nd ed rev. Columbus, OH: Greyden Press; 1994:47, with permission.)

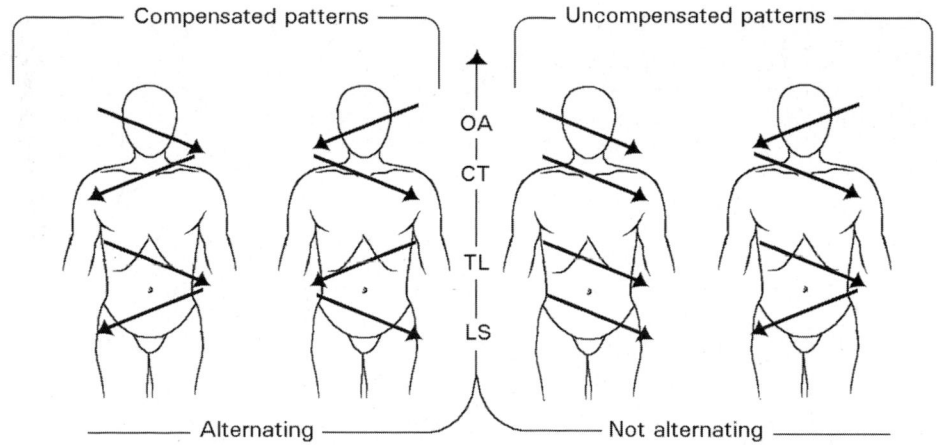

FIGURE 41.4. Fascial patterns that alternate in direction from region to region are typically compensated patterns. Those that do not are uncompensated and usually traumatically induced. *OA*, occipitoatlantal; *CT*, cervicothoracic; *TL*, thoracolumbar; *LS*, lumbosacral. (From Kuchera WA, Kuchera ML. *Osteopathic Principles in Practice*, 2nd ed rev. Columbus, OH: Greyden Press; 1994:47, with permission.)

for understanding the effect that postural management has in improving the respiratory-circulatory model (20). Conversely, fascial preference influences tissues and skeletal structures of each region producing the dynamic postural characteristics of that body region. Tensegrity is an additional model in which fascial patterning and musculoligamentous tensions take on primary importance. Described by Buckminster Fuller in 1929, tensegrity modeling explains a number of low-energy integrated structure-function arrangements. A number of clinical models cite tensegrity principles (21,22,33) with respect to orthopedic medicine, osteopathic medicine, and postural balance.

Clinical Significance of Musculoligamentous Patterning

Musculoligamentous structure and function are also significantly influenced by, and responsible for, static and dynamic postural alignment. Gravitational stress placed on these structures to maintain a patient's posture is a constant and greatly underestimated stressor. In a patient with less than ideal postural alignment, gravitational stresses are amplified. When the viscoelastic deformation properties of muscle are unable to resist the stress imposed, predictable pathophysiologic changes occur (23). These changes are both functional and structural. The elastic component represents the transient functional change in connective tissue length occurring in response to stress. The viscous component, on the other hand, is responsible for the more permanent deformation of connective tissue that occurs with static postural change.

Musculoligamentous structures are affected early in patients with gravitational strain and can be easily recognized. The symptoms arising from the resultant pathophysiologic condition have certain associated palpable characteristics, including the following:

- Muscle spasm in postural (antigravity) muscles
- Subtle weakness to muscle testing in postural antagonist (phasic) muscles
- Tenderness over ligamentous and osseotendonous attachments involved in postural stability

- Myofascial trigger points
- Edema or bogginess

Not missing such palpable changes or postural pattern clues is important. Myofascial structures undergo sustained changes in length; studies (24) suggest that deleterious change is most pronounced in shortened muscles. New collagen, with a half-life of 10 to 12 months, realigns the connective tissues in response to vectors of stress, perpetuating postural problems and maintaining the biomechanical amplification of gravitational stress. Postural patterns that are compensated can decompensate.

The structure of the muscle and its function are related. Structure and function play a major role in the muscle patterns commonly seen in posture-initiated pain and dysfunction. Postural stress on muscles leads to chronic, recurrent trigger points (25), consistent myotomal and sclerotomal pain patterns (26), and predictable functional changes. Postural muscles are structurally adapted to resist fatigue and function in the presence of prolonged gravitational exposure. When their capacity to resist stress is overwhelmed, these postural muscles become irritable, tight, and shortened (27). Many muscles, antagonists to these postural muscles (27), react when stressed by becoming weak or pseudoparetic. Therefore, gravitational strain patterns reveal a dysfunctional pattern of tight and weak muscles in a postural pattern (Fig. 41.5) (13,27). Patterned involvement of a number of the muscles shown in Tables 41.1 and 41.2 should alert the osteopathic physician to this underlying cause. In these patients, treatment of the dysfunctional postural alignment yields more lasting results than treatment of the recurrent myofascial trigger points or muscle imbalances in isolation.

TREATMENT

Treating a patient with postural decompensation requires appropriate diagnosis of the functional capabilities of that individual's structure. The treatment goals may depend on how long the imbalance has been present and how much decompensation has already occurred. Structural treatment goals are directed at

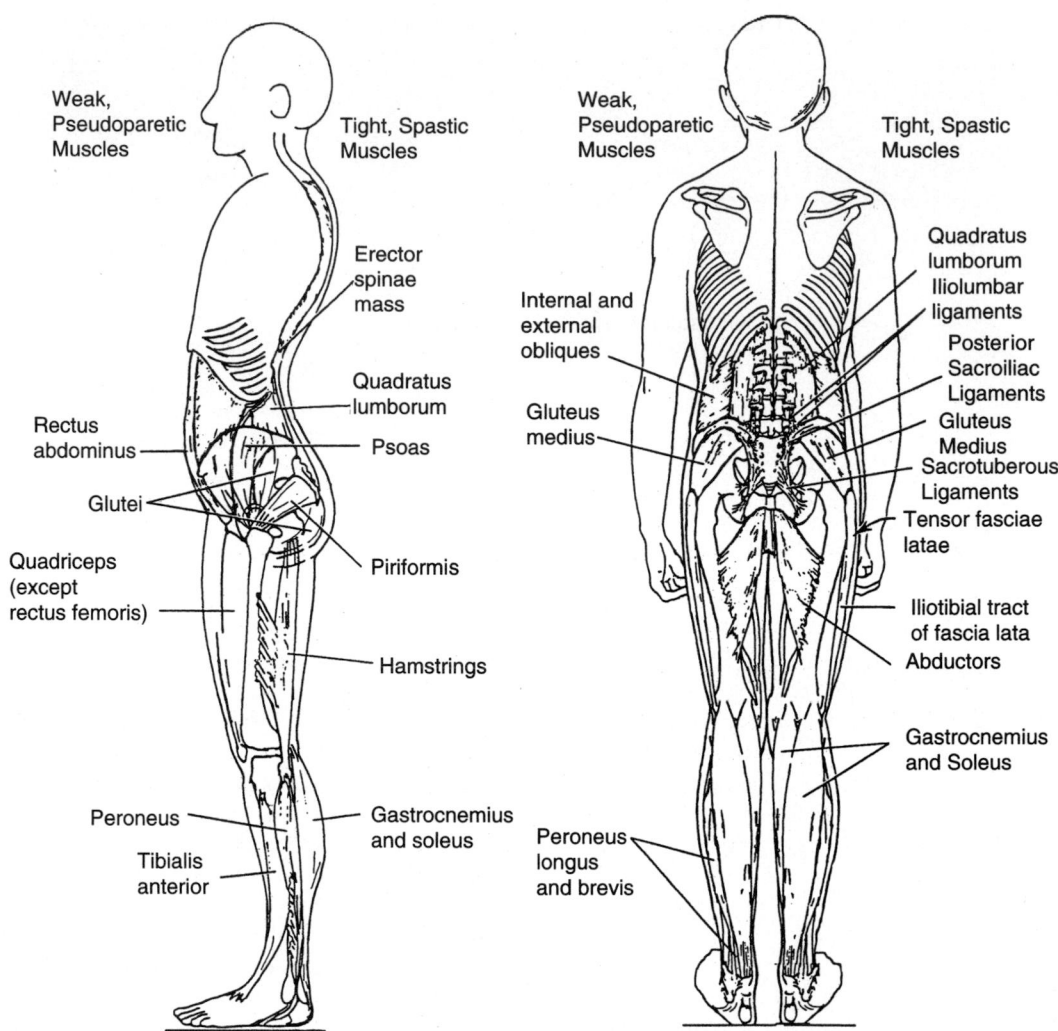

FIGURE 41.5. Coronal and horizontal postural patterns usually alternate from side to side in adjacent regions with stressed muscle groups typically on the convex side of each postural curve. Sagittal plane postural patterns involve postural muscles and their antagonists as listed in Tables 41.1 and 41.2. (From Kuchera WA, Kuchera ML. *Osteopathic Principles in Practice*, 2nd ed rev. Columbus, OH: Greyden Press; 1994:47, with permission.)

establishing the optimal function their existing structure is capable of achieving. Functional treatment goals promote free motion within an optimally balanced posture.

Treatment of postural problems emphasizes compliance, especially in the initial phases of the reeducation program. Compliance by the patient is essential and can be enhanced if the patient understands the rationale behind the treatment procedures and requirements.

The choice of treatment modalities to achieve these goals also depends on the degree of decompensation present in the patient and an estimate of the patient's homeostatic reserves. The physician may choose a combination of the modalities discussed in the following sections of this chapter and discussed more fully in Chapter 43.

Osteopathic Manipulative Treatment

Manipulation plays an intimate role in the formulation of any postural treatment protocol. Manipulation is defined as the use of the hands in a patient management process using instructions and maneuvers to achieve maximum painless movement of the musculoskeletal (motor) system in postural balance.

Osteopathic manipulative treatment (OMT) helps prepare muscles, joints, ligaments, and other supportive soft tissue to better accept positive postural change. Tension that is not addressed in these structures often prevents an optimal compensatory response. Additionally, hypomobility often creates pain or ache in the sites seeking to compensate or change under the forces of homeostasis.

Manipulative Treatment of Group Curves

Several principles govern the management of group curves.

First, the physician needs to identify and treat the cause of the curve. If a patient has an anatomic short leg with sacral base unleveling, the short leg is treated to level the sacral base and decrease the curve. As a patient adjusts to treatment for postural rebalancing, the spine must remain mobile to compensate for

reeducation. Promotion of flexibility for realignment and selective strengthening for stability in hypomobile areas are goals for postural exercise.

Postural Bracing

Static structural bracing has both positive and negative aspects. Although such devices support the structure and initially reduce ligamentous and muscular stress, the muscles soon become dependent on the support provided. The longer the brace is worn, the weaker the patient's own muscles become. It is therefore imperative that the physician links the patient's brace treatment with an ongoing exercise program. Static braces are better for providing rest in an acute condition than for treating a chronic one. Ideally a physician should not introduce a static brace without having a plan to replace it (31).

Postural Orthotics

Functional orthotics serve to direct, guide, and/or reeducate the body, as opposed to directly taking over support. They are capable of influencing physiologic parameters and reducing associated low back pain. With respect to postural realignment, this class of treatment modalities includes several specific orthotics (see Chapter 43). The Levitor® pelvic orthotic, which was biomechanically designed specifically to reduce gravity-induced musculoligamentous stress, has its greatest effect within the sagittal plane. Foot orthotics incorporating heel lifts have their effect primarily within the coronal plane. Anterior sole lifts maximally affect the horizontal plane. All three of these examples, however, affect posture in all cardinal planes simultaneously (32), and each ultimately has systemic effects. Functional orthotics in conjunction with an osteopathic approach have been documented (13) to reduce or reverse lordosis, kyphosis, and scoliosis, decrease low back pain and other musculoskeletal symptoms, improve respiratory-circulatory functions, decrease energy demands, and decrease segmental facilitation. Flexible foot orthoses and the Levitor® pelvic orthotic do not replace normal muscular function. Therefore, their use does not weaken associated muscles.

Electrical Stimulation and Posture

Electrical stimulation of paraspinal muscles has been used in some centers. Electrodes are placed in the muscles on the side of the spinal convexity. The electrodes are connected to a direct current from a control box. An electrical current causes contraction of the muscles on the side of the convexity and is postulated to help reduce scoliotic curvature. Research suggests, that used alone, this modality is not effective in reversing scoliotic curves but is recommended by some centers as part of a unified treatment regimen to assist in muscle strengthening or pain relief.

Prolotherapy

Prolotherapy (sclerotherapy) is injection of a proliferant solution into a ligament (26). When postural strain biomechanically overwhelms structural integrity, ligamentous laxity can result. Injection of a proliferant solution into the ligament at its fibro-osseous insertion can increase stability. Combined with exercise, OMT,

and postural realignment to prevent return of musculoligamentous strain, this protocol can be an effective conservative approach to hypermobility and ligamentous laxity (33).

Surgery in Postural Decompensation

When an insurmountable problem is primarily structural, its treatment is primarily structural. In unstable situations, or in situations that have not responded to conservative care, surgery may be performed. In the case of severe scoliosis or highly symptomatic spondylolisthesis, this could consist of fusing vertebrae. Surgical implantation of orthopedic rods or other stabilizing apparatuses may also be required. Surgical techniques have even been successfully used to lengthen anatomically short legs.

CONCLUSION

Postural diagnosis and treatment are perfectly consistent with the tenets of the osteopathic philosophy. Careful exploration of the homeostatic response of the body unit as reflected in the structure and function of that individual's posture permits specific treatment design for total patient management.

Posture is not just a stack of spinal curves with musculoligamentous connectors. Posture is influenced by the patient's emotional-spiritual-psychological self. It has been astutely observed that posture, to a large degree, is also a somatic depiction of the inner emotions. In this fashion there is no doubt that posture can be considered a "somatization of the psyche" (34). Postural realignment requires reintegration of peripheral and central factors that are physiologically, psychologically, and biomechanically linked.

Several conservative modalities are available to the osteopathic physician to aid in the realignment process. These include OMT, functional orthotics and orthopedic braces, exercise protocols, and patient education. There is an intimate relationship between OMT and postural balance. The osteopathic physician seeks to achieve maximum function of the neuromusculoskeletal system in postural balance and to prepare the patient's neuromusculoskeletal system to respond to postural realignment. Postural treatment generally supports the patient's homeostasis.

Postural gravitational stress should be considered a factor in the general health status of each and every patient. It should not be reserved only for consideration in cases of recurrent somatic dysfunction, myofascial trigger point syndromes, scoliosis, or spondylolisthesis. Rather, consider postural treatment strategies (Chapter 43) whenever postural patterning of group spinal curves or recurrent skeletal, arthrodial, or myofascial dysfunction is diagnosed.

REFERENCES

1. Jungmann M, McClure CW. Backaches, postural decline, aging and gravity-strain. Abstract delivered at the New York Academy of General Practice; October 17, 1963; New York, NY.
2. Beal MC. Biomechanics: A foundation for osteopathic theory and practice. In: Northup GW, ed. *Osteopathic Research: Growth and Development.* Chicago IL: American Osteopathic Association; 1987:37–58.

3. Hiss JM. A classification of feet. *JAOA*. 1931;30:260–261.

4. Vleeming A, Mooney V, Dorman T, et al, eds. *Movement, Stability and Low Back Pain: The Essential Role of the Pelvis*. New York, NY: Churchill Livingstone; 1997.

5. Lewit K. Disturbed balance due to lesions of the craniocervical junction. *J Orthop Med*. 1988;(3):58–59.

6. Kappler RE. Postural balance and motion patterns. In: Peterson B, ed. *Postural Balance and Imbalance (1983 AAO Yearbook)*. Newark, OH: American Academy of Osteopathy; 1983:612.

7. Kuchera ML, Kuchera WA. Postural decompensation. In: *Osteopathic Principles in Practice*, 2nd ed rev. Columbus, OH: Greyden Press; 1994.

8. *Dorland's Medical Dictionary*. Philadelphia, PA: WB Saunders; 1989.

9. Cohen LA. Role of eye and neck proprioceptive mechanisms in body orientation and motor coordination. *J Neurophysiol* 1961;24:1–11.

10. Fryette HH. Physiologic movements of the spine. *JAOA*. 1917 (Sep):18:1–2.

11. Denslow JS, Chase JA. Mechanical stresses in the human lumbar spine and pelvis. In: Peterson B, ed. *Postural Balance and Imbalance (1983 AAO Yearbook)*. Newark, OH: American Academy of Osteopathy; 1983:76–82.

12. Giles GF, Taylor JR. Lumbar spine structural changes associated with leg length inequality. *Spine*. 1981;6:510–521.

13. Kuchera ML. Treatment of gravitational strain patholophysiology. In Vleeming A, Mooney V, Dorman T, et al, eds. *Movement, Stability and Low Back Pain: The Essential Role of the Pelvis*. New York NY: Churchill Livingstone; 1997:477–499.

14. Thomas PE, Korr IM, Wright HM. A mobile instrument for reading electrical skin resistance patterns of the human trunk. *Acta Neuroveg*. 1958;VVII (1–2):97–100.

15. Thomas PE, Korr IM. Relationship between sweat glands and electrical resistance of the skin. *J Appl Physiol*. 1957;10:505–510.

16. Dunnington WP. A musculoskeletal stress pattern: observations from over 50 years' clinical experience. *JAOA*. 1964;64:366–371.

17. Heilig D. *Patterns of Still Lesions and an Evaluation of Some Diagnostic Criteria in Altered Vertebral Postural Patterns* [master's thesis]. Philadelphia, PA: Philadelphia College of Osteopathy; 1957.

18. Zink JG, Lawson WB. An osteopathic structural examination and functional interpretation of the soma. *Osteopath Ann*. 1979;7:12–19.

19. Zink JG. Respiratory and circulatory care: the conceptual model. *Osteopath Ann*. 1977;5(3):108–112.

20. Strong R, Thomas AE, Earl WD. Patterns of muscle activity in leg, hip, and torso during quiet standing. *JAOA*. 1967;66:1035–1038.

21. Levin SM. A different approach to the mechanics of the human pelvis: tensegrity. In: Vleeming A, Mooney V, Dorman T, et al, eds. *Movement, Stability and Low Back Pain: The Essential Role of the Pelvis*. New York NY: Churchill Livingstone; 1997:157–167.

22. Cummings CH. A tensegrity model for osteopathy in the cranial field. *AAOJ*. 1994;4:2(Summer):9–13, 24–27.

23. Kuchera ML. Gravitational stress, musculoskeletal strain, and postural alignment. *Spine. State of the Art Reviews*. 1995;9(2):463–490.

24. Gossman MR, Sahrmann SA, Rose SJ. Review of length-associated changes in muscle. *Phys Ther*. 1982;62(12):1799–1807.

25. Travell JG, Simons DG. *Myofascial Pain and Dysfunction: A Trigger Point Manual*. Vol II. Baltimore, MD: Williams & Wilkins, 1992:547.

26. Hackett GS. *Ligament and Tendon Relaxation Treated by Prolotherapy*, 3rd ed. Springfield, IL: Charles C Thomas; 1958.

27. Janda V. Muscle weakness and inhibition (pseudoparesis) in back pain syndromes. In: Grieve GP, ed. *Modern Medicine Therapy of the Vertebral Column*. Edinburgh, Scotland: Churchill Livingstone; 1986:197–200.

28. Kimberly PE, Funk SL. *Outline of Osteopathic Manipulative Procedures: The Kimberly Manual Millennium Edition*. Marceline, MO: Walsworth Publishing Company; 2000.

29. Travell JG, Simons DG. *Myofascial Pain and Dysfunction: The Trigger Point Manual*. Vol I. Baltimore, MD: Williams & Wilkins; 1983:680.

30. Kuchera WA, Kuchera ML. *Osteopathic Principles in Practice*, 2nd ed rev. Columbus, OH: Greyden Press; 1994:385–389.

31. Grieve GP. Lumbar instability. *Physiotherapy*. 1982;68(1):29.

32. Kuchera ML, Irvin RE. Biomechanical considerations in postural realignment. *JAOA*. 1987;87(11):781–782.

33. Dorman T. Pelvic mechanics and prolotherapy. In: Vleeming A, Mooney V, Dorman T, eds. *Movement, Stability and Low Back Pain: The Essential Role of the Pelvis*. New York NY: Churchill Livingstone; 1997:501–522.

34. Calliet R. *Low Back Syndrome*. 3rd ed. Philadelphia, PA: FA Davis; 1981:24.

RADIOGRAPHIC ASPECTS OF THE POSTURAL STUDY

MICHAEL L. KUCHERA
WILLIAM A. KUCHERA

KEY CONCEPTS

- Use of postural study x-ray series
- Importance of standardization of postural x-ray series
- Equipment used in performing a postural study
- Essential views for complete postural x-ray series
- Methods for obtaining postural x-ray series and reasons for following standardized procedures
- Explanations of concepts related to radiographic image analysis:
  —Vertebral rotation and side bending
  —Cobb angles
  —Sacral base unleveling
  —Pelvic rotation
  —Angle of sacral base
  —L3 weightbearing line
  —Pelvic index
  —Lumbosacral and lumbo-lumbar lordotic angles
  —Evidence-based reliability and validity

Osteopathic physicians have used radiographs for many years to better understand and study structure and function. The roentgen ray was discovered in 1895; by 1898 the American School of Osteopathy in Kirksville, Missouri had acquired the second machine west of the Mississippi. In 1898, this equipment provided the earliest roentgenologic studies of circulation (1). Hoskins and Schwab introduced the standing postural x-ray series in 1921, opening the field for clinical interpretation and integration. Martin Beilke in 1936 acknowledged the value of the technique by observing: "The osteopathic profession can lay claim to these contributions as being strictly original and especially applicable to our approach in finding etiological factors in a given pathological process and in applying corrective measures" (2).

For many years, lack of standardization for a postural x-ray procedure prevented the profession from combining important multicenter data. It also prevented universal clinical interpretation of postural studies. J. Stedman Denslow and his co-workers called for standardization in 1955 (3), although even today, outside of the osteopathic profession, relatively few academic medical institutions have adopted that recommendation. Standard protocols provide measurable, accurate, reproducible data to correlate with the osteopathic palpatory structural examination.

Standardized postural x-ray views document "repeatable findings when the state of the patient is unchanged and provide valid information concerning improvements or regressions in skeletal structure which are associated with changes in the patient's condition." (3). Postural x-ray views taken according to a standardized protocol can be accurately and consistently measured for postural information by radiologists or attending nonradiologist physicians (4).

Many radiologists are not trained to do postural studies specifically for osteopathic analysis but will conduct them for referring physicians if given an appropriate protocol. This chapter provides a method (5) for evaluating the pelvis and spine. This method has the following advantages:

- Standardized
- Accurate
- Reproducible
- Practical
- Inexpensive

The measurements obtained through the use of this protocol can be interpreted clinically in the context described in other chapters of this text, including postural diagnosis and treatment (see Chapters 41 and 43).

MATERIALS

The following equipment is needed to employ this standardized protocol:

1. Vertical Bucky diaphragm
2. Adjustable holder for plumbed wire
3. Piano wire or metal core fishing line
4. Plumb bob
5. Level metal base plate or level floor

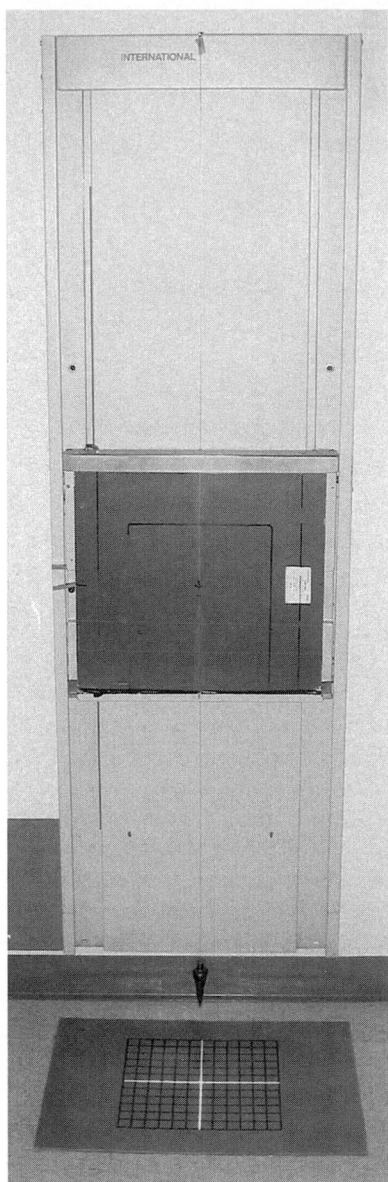

FIGURE 42.1. Vertical Bucky diaphragm and piano wire reference.

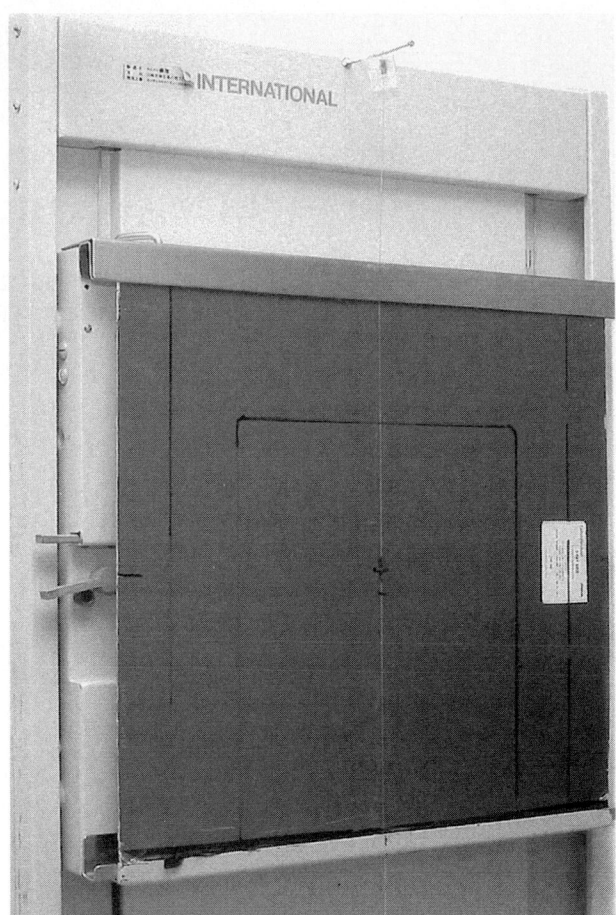

FIGURE 42.2. Adjustable film cassette holder.

The vertical Bucky diaphragm is mounted on the wall for best results (Fig. 42.1). The adjustable holder (Fig. 42.2) is designed to move the plumbed wire exactly over the desired point on the base plate. Piano wire, 0.020 inches in diameter, is ideal for this system. It is pliable and durable for adjusting to the desired shape, and it is readily identified on the exposed film because of its density. Alternatively, metallic core fishing line has been used and is reported to kink less over time. A plumb bob (Fig. 42.3) of any size or configuration is attached to the wire. These items are relatively inexpensive and available from hardware stores.

A level, rectangular metal base plate (Fig. 42.4) is made from $1/4$-inch gauge steel and measures 70×50 cm. It is leveled and cemented or fixed to the floor. This insures a level plane for the patient to stand on (unlevel floors may accentuate or hide an unlevel sacral base). The floor may be used instead of the metal plate if it is absolutely level in two planes. A modified

cross-hatched grid is permanently marked on the surface of the plate or on the floor to ensure accurate alignment of the patient's feet.

The metallic wire is attached to the adjustable holder. If possible, it is passed behind the protective covering on the Bucky diaphragm (Fig. 42.1). The plumb bob is attached to the wire to establish a vertical reference line. It is adjusted to lie directly over two main cross-sectional base lines that are perpendicular to each other (Fig. 42.4). The posterior line (Fig. 42.4, *1*) lies in a plane parallel to the film and the coronal plane of the body. The midheel line (Fig. 42.4, *2*) and the plumbed wire lie in the sagittal plane of the body, perpendicular to the posterior line. This plane is equidistant from both heels when exposing the anteroposterior (AP) view. It is just anterior to the lateral malleolus for exposure of the lateral view.

The reference line in the AP radiograph is also known as the midheel line. In the lateral radiograph, the reference line is referred to as the postural or weightbearing line (WBL).

PROCEDURE

In patients with suspected postural disorders, a palpatory examination and osteopathic manipulative treatment of somatic dysfunction followed by reevaluation ideally precedes referral for

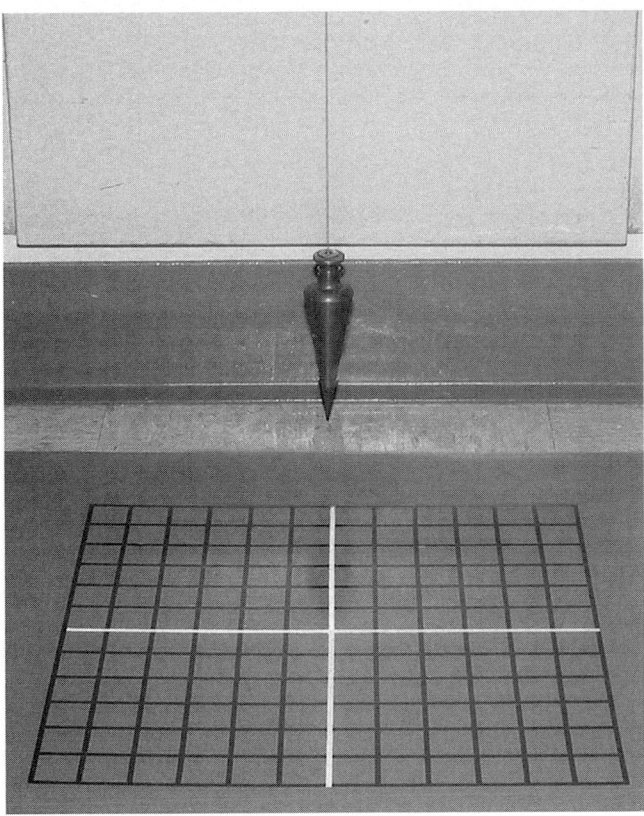

FIGURE 42.3. Plumb bob and piano wire.

a postural radiograph. The somatic dysfunctions most likely to create significant transient postural asymmetry are:

- Sacral shear (unilateral sacral flexion)
- Innominate shear (upslipped innominate)
- Psoas muscle spasm
- Quadratus lumborum spasm
- Innominate rotation

Prior to referral for a postural x-ray series and again immediately prior to this procedure, it should be ascertained that the patient is not pregnant.

The patient prepares for postural x-ray views by removing all clothing and putting on a gown. He or she stands on the adjustable metal base plate with the back facing, but not touching, the Bucky diaphragm (Fig. 42.5). Postural films of the pelvis or any section of the spine are then exposed at a consistent film-tube distance of 40 to 44 inches (72 inches is used by some centers). Information, including radiographic factors and the position of the feet, is recorded on a separate form that is filed with the patient's radiographic records so that positioning of the patient is consistent when a postural x-ray is repeated at a future date (see example in Table 42.1). Future examinations are then performed using the same technical factors. This ensures a uniform, acceptable, and reproducible method.

The metallic piano wire, located behind the patient but in front of the Bucky diaphragm and film, will be recorded in an undistorted fashion on the film. It becomes a relevant reference line for assessing deviation from ideal weightbearing in AP and

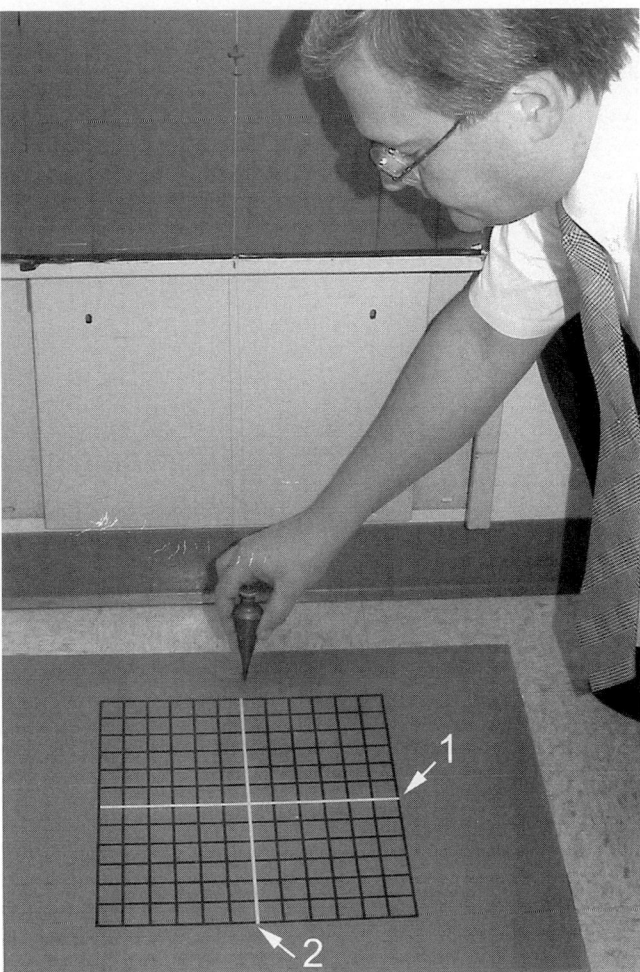

FIGURE 42.4. Rectangular metal base plate with reference lines. *1*, posterior line; *2*, midheel line.

lateral films. Radiographic measurements can then be obtained using this reproducible gravitational reference line.

Anteroposterior Postural Radiographs

To obtain radiographic information relative to coronal or horizontal plane posture, AP standing postural views are exposed.

The patient is asked to stand on the level floor plate with the head facing forward, eyes looking straight ahead, arms relaxed to the sides, and knees extended in a locked but comfortable position (Fig. 42.5). The feet are positioned equidistant from and parallel to the midheel base line (Fig. 42.6), far enough apart so that they are directly under the femoral heads. This distance is recorded by noting the distance from the midheel line to the medial aspect of the heels, as indicated by the markings on the base plate. The heels are placed equidistant from the posterior line (Fig. 42.4, *1*), with the patient standing as close to the film as possible, in a relaxed posture. This method ensures a reproducible, standard position for the feet (the base for support of posture).

The Bucky diaphragm is adjusted to the desired height so that the AP lumbopelvic film includes the femoral heads, the pubic symphysis, and most of the lumbar vertebrae. The lower part of the Bucky will be slightly lower than the femoral greater

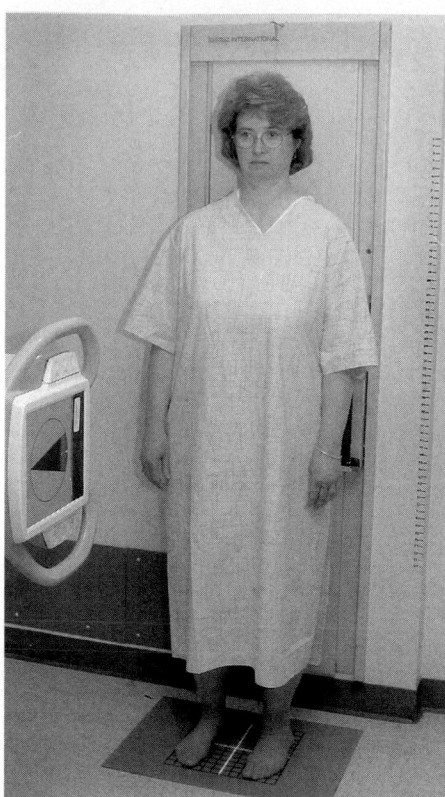

FIGURE 42.5. Patient positioned for anteroposterior postural x-ray view.

TABLE 42.1. SAMPLE ANALYSIS REPORT ON WEIGHT BEARING POSTURAL X-RAY SERIES

Subject _____ Examiner _____ Date _____

Other Examiners: _____

Height of Femur Heads:
(Indicate side of shortness by R or L; measure in millimeters.)

Height of Iliac Crests:
(Repeat process used above.)

Sacral Base:
(Is it level or is it depressed? How many millimeters on R or L side? How does this finding relate to the plane of the femoral heads?)

Lumbar Rotation:
(Indicate R or L and which ones.)

Lumbar Lateral Flexion:
(Indicate side-bending, right or left, and vertebrae involved.)

Pelvic Rotation:
(R or L; measure millimeter difference.)

Pelvic Tilt:
(R or L)

Lateral Disalignment of Trunk:
(At L5; R or L)

Lumbosacral Angle:
(Degrees)

Relation of L3 to the Sacral Base:
(Where is the weight-bearing line in relation to the sacrum?)

Lordosis:
(Qualitative: Normal, decreased, or increased? Quantitative: Measurement of lumbosacral or lumbolumbar lordotic angle.)

Pelvic Index:
$X =$ _____ mm
$Y =$ _____ mm
$PI = X/Y =$

Anomalies:
(Bat-wing, sacralization, lumbarization, facet asymmetry, spina bifida, etc.)

Summary:
(Comment concerning disalignment and related disturbances. This includes changes in the density of both osseous and soft tissues such as muscles and ligaments.)

trochanters in order to include the entire pelvis including the pubic symphysis. For a lumbopelvic x-ray exposure, the central ray should be at the level of the iliac crest.

When taking an AP postural study of the thoracic spine, the Bucky height is adjusted and the central beam is aimed at the xiphoid process, which corresponds to approximately the T9 level.

Lateral Postural Radiograph

To obtain radiographic information relative to sagittal plane posture, a lateral standing postural view is exposed.

The lateral view is obtained by having the standing patient turn to the lateral position so that the ankle closest to the wire is in a position where it lies just anterior to the ankle's lateral malleolus (Fig. 42.7). This positioning is very important, because the metallic wire will then identify the plane of the patient's lateral WBL. In a patient with an ideal posture, the lateral WBL (gravitational line) should pass through a point just anterior to the lateral malleolus, and through the greater trochanter, the center of the L3 vertebral body, and the external auditory canal. (6) The other foot is positioned parallel to the contralateral foot and the same distance apart as was determined when the AP x-ray view was exposed.

The patient's arms are crossed in front of the body to obtain an unobstructed view of the spine. The knees are locked and the normal posture maintained as for the AP view (Fig. 42.8). The Bucky diaphragm and the central ray are adjusted as described in

the AP view to insure inclusion of lumbar vertebrae, lumbosacral junction, sacrum, and pubic bones.

General Considerations

The x-ray method described is amenable to rapid adjustment and placement, making it useful in a busy department. It also positions the patient in a weightbearing posture that is reproducible and records an independent vertical reference line on the film (see Fig. 42.11, *RL*) that can be used to obtain accurate measurements. The reference line is unrelated to the position of the cassette, yet it is perpendicular to the line of the horizon. Measurements taken from the edge of the film may be inaccurate because of the variable position of the film within the cassette and therefore would produce misleading or nonreproducible results (7).

AP and lateral postural films are typically performed with the patient's shoes off to determine postural discrepancies. At times, films may also be obtained with the patient wearing their shoes, with a therapeutic lift in place, to determine the amount of sacral base unleveling that still remains to be corrected. Both views are exposed immediately after positioning the patient to eliminate movement from fatigue.

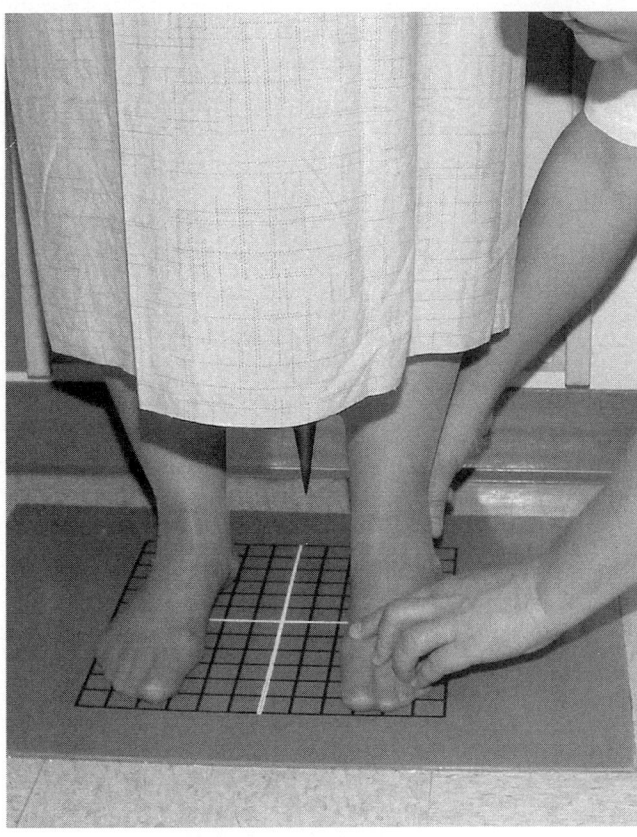

FIGURE 42.6. Midheel positioning.

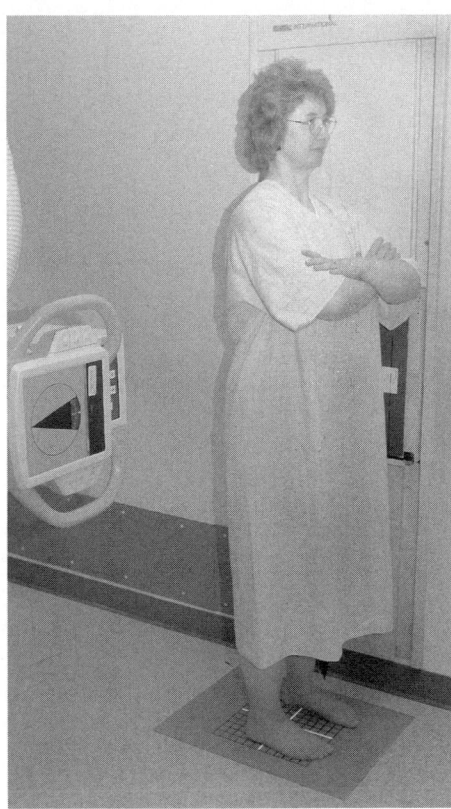

FIGURE 42.8. Patient positioned for lateral postural x-ray view.

Sometimes both right and left oblique x-ray views are necessary to evaluate the neural arches, the intervertebral foramina, and a patient with suspected spondylolysis. Such oblique views may be obtained with the patient standing, although this has not proved helpful in evaluating a patient's posture.

The exposure of the patient to ionizing radiation in this study is minimal. For example, this protocol is calculated to expose the patient to 0.12 rad for the AP postural view but could be reduced even further with only 0.011 rad to the gonads, using a lead gonadal shield (7).

RESULTS

Admittedly, clinical correlation with radiographic findings of lumbosacral anomalies is not as straightforward as many would like. Static findings from postural radiographs should be correlated with various dynamic aspects of the clinical examination, including palpation. In this manner, relevant structure-function and postural-biomechanical insights may be uncovered. In 1934 Ferguson noted, "Our spines were developed for the four-footed position and are not yet adapted to the erect, so mechanical weakness at the lumbosacral area is usual rather than exceptional. We must consider the lumbosacral area, not as normal or abnormal, but as mechanically sound or mechanically unsound (8)."

In judging whether the lumbopelvic region is mechanically sound, a standard postural x-ray series may reveal a number of findings that may or may not be clinically relevant, including:

- Facet tropism
- Sacralization
- Lumbarization
- Scoliosis
- Spondylolisthesis
- Spondylosis
- Facet arthritis
- Small hemipelvis
- Fracture

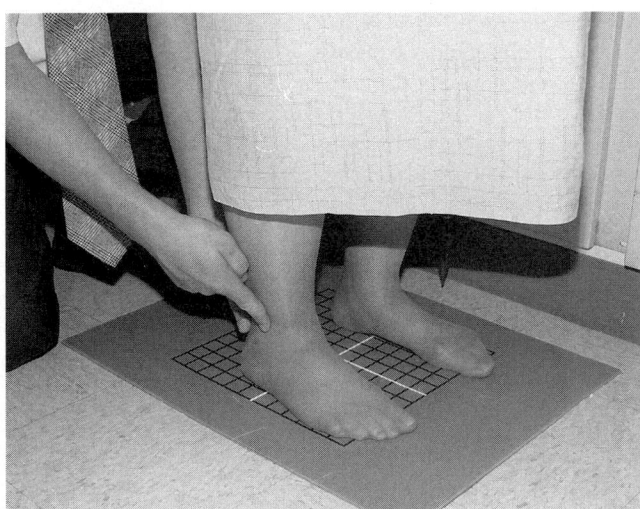

FIGURE 42.7. Patient's feet positioned for lateral postural x-ray view.

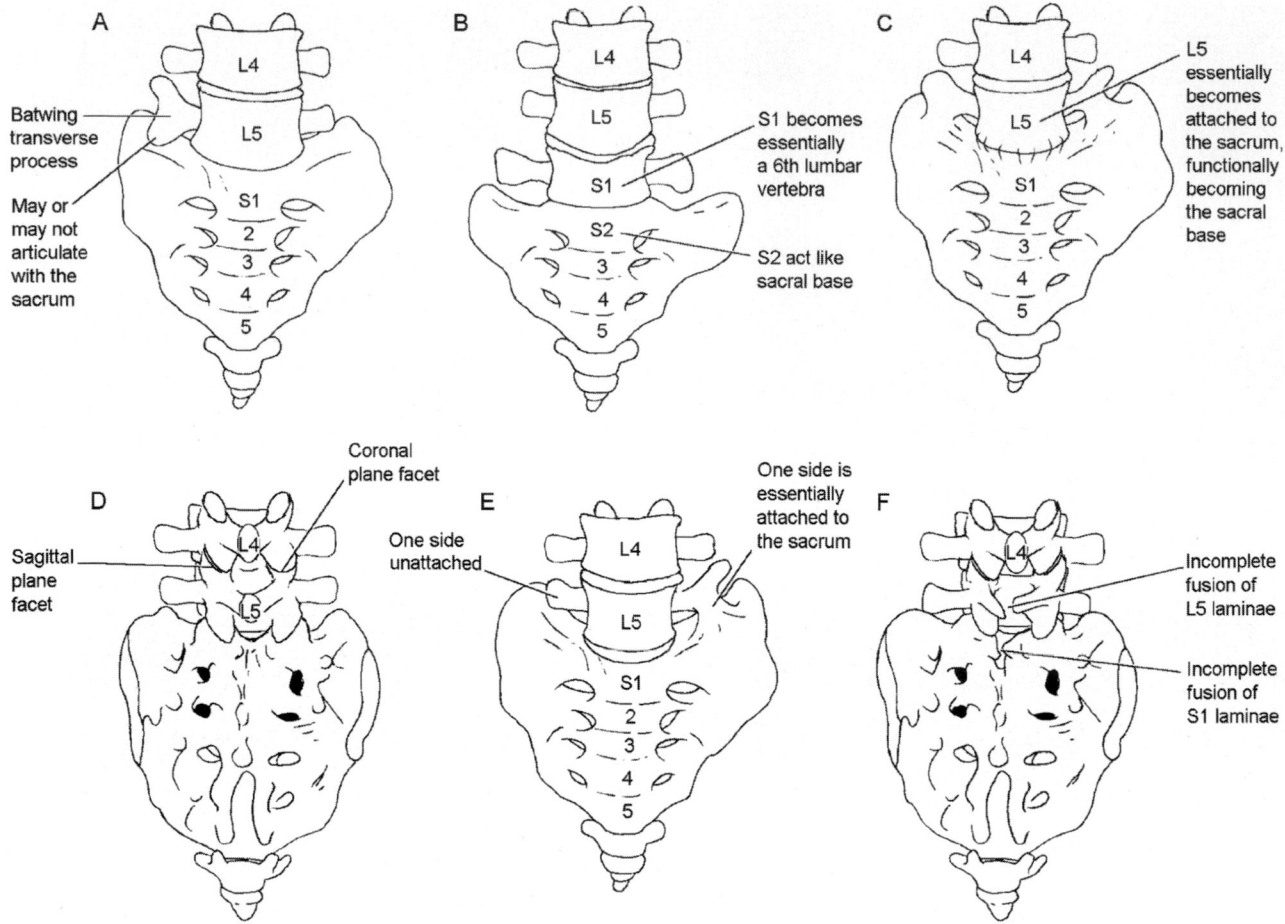

FIGURE 42.9. Common lumbosacral anomalies: **A:** Batwing transverse processes of L5. **B:** Lumbarization of S1. **C:** Sacralization of L5. **D:** Facet asymmetry (zygopophyseal tropism) of L4. **E:** Partial sacralization of L5 (Bertolotti). **F:** Spina bifida occulta of both L5 and of S.

Common lumbosacral anomalies appearing radiographically are depicted in Fig. 42.9. Several of these anomalies complicate selection of landmarks used in postural measurements or interpretation of postural radiographic data. A few are recognized to cause low back pain or instability in a percentage of patients; others are widely believed to be incidental insignificant anomalies. Some may be viewed as "risk factors;" others are potentially complicating findings in those patients diagnosed to have regional instability.

Interpreting Anteroposterior Thoracic and Lumbar Postural Radiographs

The standing AP film of the thoracic and lumbar regions contains both qualitative and quantitative information about posture in the coronal and horizontal planes.

By noting the relative positions of the two pedicles and the spinous process, vertebral rotation can be qualitatively assessed (Fig. 42.10B). In the absence of vertebral rotation, the spinous process is located equidistant from each pedicle. With right vertebral rotation (named in relation to the direction of movement of a reference point on the anterior portion of the vertebral body),

the spinous process visualized on the x-ray film appears closer to the left pedicle. With left vertebral rotation, the spinous process appears closer to the right pedicle on the x-ray film.

Vertebral side bending is also easily observed on this radiographic view and can be qualitatively reported. Quantitative measurement of group curves is often more formally reported using scoliosis nomenclature. Scoliosis, by convention, is reported in reference to the convexity of the curve. A right scoliosis is side-bent left (convex right). The Cobb method is commonly used to measure scoliotic curves (Fig. 42.10A). Lines are constructed across the top of the superior vertebral segment and across the bottom of the inferior vertebral segment of a spinal scoliotic curve. Perpendicular lines are then constructed from these lines. These perpendicular lines intersect to form an angle, the Cobb angle measurement. (Scoliosis, its diagnosis and treatment, is more fully discussed in Chapter 43.)

Interpreting Anteroposterior Postural Radiographs of the Pelvis

The standing AP film of the pelvis contains coronal and horizontal plane postural data. This film is especially important in

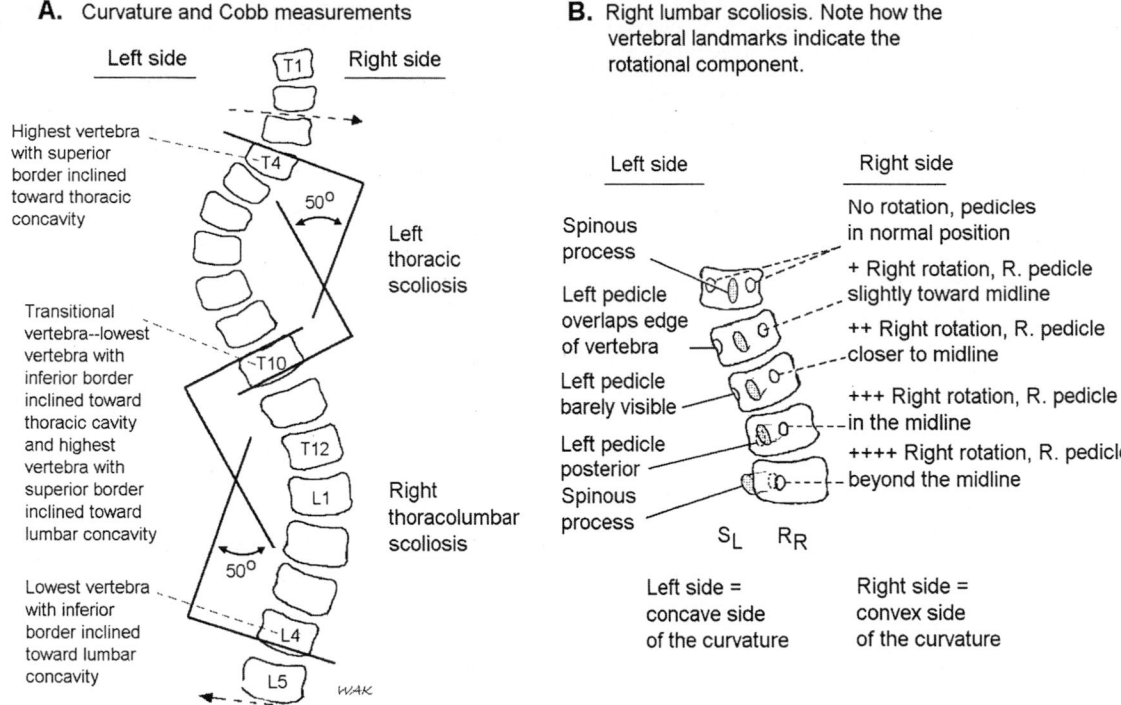

A. Curvature and Cobb measurements

Left side | Right side

Highest vertebra with superior border inclined toward thoracic concavity

Left thoracic scoliosis

50°

Transitional vertebra--lowest vertebra with inferior border inclined toward thoracic cavity and highest vertebra with superior border inclined toward lumbar concavity

Right thoracolumbar scoliosis

50°

Lowest vertebra with inferior border inclined toward lumbar concavity

B. Right lumbar scoliosis. Note how the vertebral landmarks indicate the rotational component.

Left side | Right side

Spinous process — No rotation, pedicles in normal position

Left pedicle overlaps edge of vertebra — + Right rotation, R. pedicle slightly toward midline

Left pedicle barely visible — ++ Right rotation, R. pedicle closer to midline

Left pedicle posterior — +++ Right rotation, R. pedicle in the midline

Spinous process — ++++ Right rotation, R. pedicle beyond the midline

S_L R_R

Left side = concave side of the curvature

Right side = convex side of the curvature

FIGURE 42.10. Measurement of curvature and rotation by Cobb method. (Illustration by W.A. Kuchera.)

evaluating the degree of sacral base unleveling as well as determining structural leg lengths and pelvic rotation with the patient in a weightbearing position. Refer to Fig. 42.11 when reading the following description of measuring postural radiographs.

Lines are drawn from the most superior aspect of the femoral heads (*D*), perpendicular to the reference line, and discrepancies are measured in millimeters. Similar lines are drawn from the superior margins of the iliac crests (*E*), perpendicular to the reference line, to determine the relative iliac crest heights.

A sacral base line (*7*) is constructed either from the junction of the articular pillars and the sacral ala (*a–a'*), the sites where the sacral ala and the iliac crests cross each other on the x-ray film (*b–b'*), or, alternatively, along the line of eburnation across the top of the sacrum (*c–c'*, as shown in Fig. 42.11B). The alternative selected should be the one that has the least ambiguity or in which the set of reference points are most easily and accurately identified (9,10). For clinically relevant reasons, this line is extended to the vertical lines extending from the femoral heads (*3,4*). The amount of sacral base unleveling is reported as the measured height differential of the sacral base as extrapolated by the sacral base line intersecting the femoral head lines (points *C* and *C'*).

The margin of error in measuring sacral base unleveling, using this radiographic protocol, has been reported to be ±0.75 mm (7). Measurements using the different choices of landmarks for identifying the sacral base are reported to have a variability of up to 2 mm (4,7).

The osteopathic physician is more interested in leveling the sacral base than making the leg lengths equal, that is, the sacral base unleveling is usually of more clinical significance than comparison of anatomic leg lengths. In the presence of sacral base un-

leveling, the direction of the lumbar side-bending component is also clinically relevant. Roughening of the iliac crest where the iliolumbar ligament attaches or calcification of the iliolumbar ligament (11) should be noted, as these are markers for postural stress.

Pelvic rotation is recognized qualitatively by observing asymmetry of the obturator foramina. It can be quantified by measuring the distance between the pubic symphysis and either the dark line representing the air in the gluteal crease or the median sacral crest (*F* to *G*). (12) The pelvis is said to rotate in the direction in which the anterior portion of the pelvis (pubic symphysis) moves. In Fig. 42.11A the pelvis is rotated to the left.

Interpreting Lateral Postural Radiographs of the Pelvis

The standing lateral film of the pelvis provides a means for determining a number of sagittal plane postural measurements. These include the angle of the sacral base, the WBL from L3 relative to the sacral base, lumbar lordotic angles, and the pelvic index (PI) (Fig. 42.11C) (see Chapter 43).

The angle of the sacral base, also known as the Ferguson angle, or the lumbosacral angle (LSA), is calculated by drawing a line (*A*) across the sacral base. Another line (*B*) is constructed to cross line *A* and to be perpendicular to the reference line (Fig. 42.11C, lines *A* and *B*).

The ideal line of weightbearing, previously described as running just anterior to the lateral malleolus, is represented by the lucent line produced by the image of the metallic reference wire on the x-ray film. This reference line (*RL*) can also be used to evaluate the position of the center of gravity (normally located

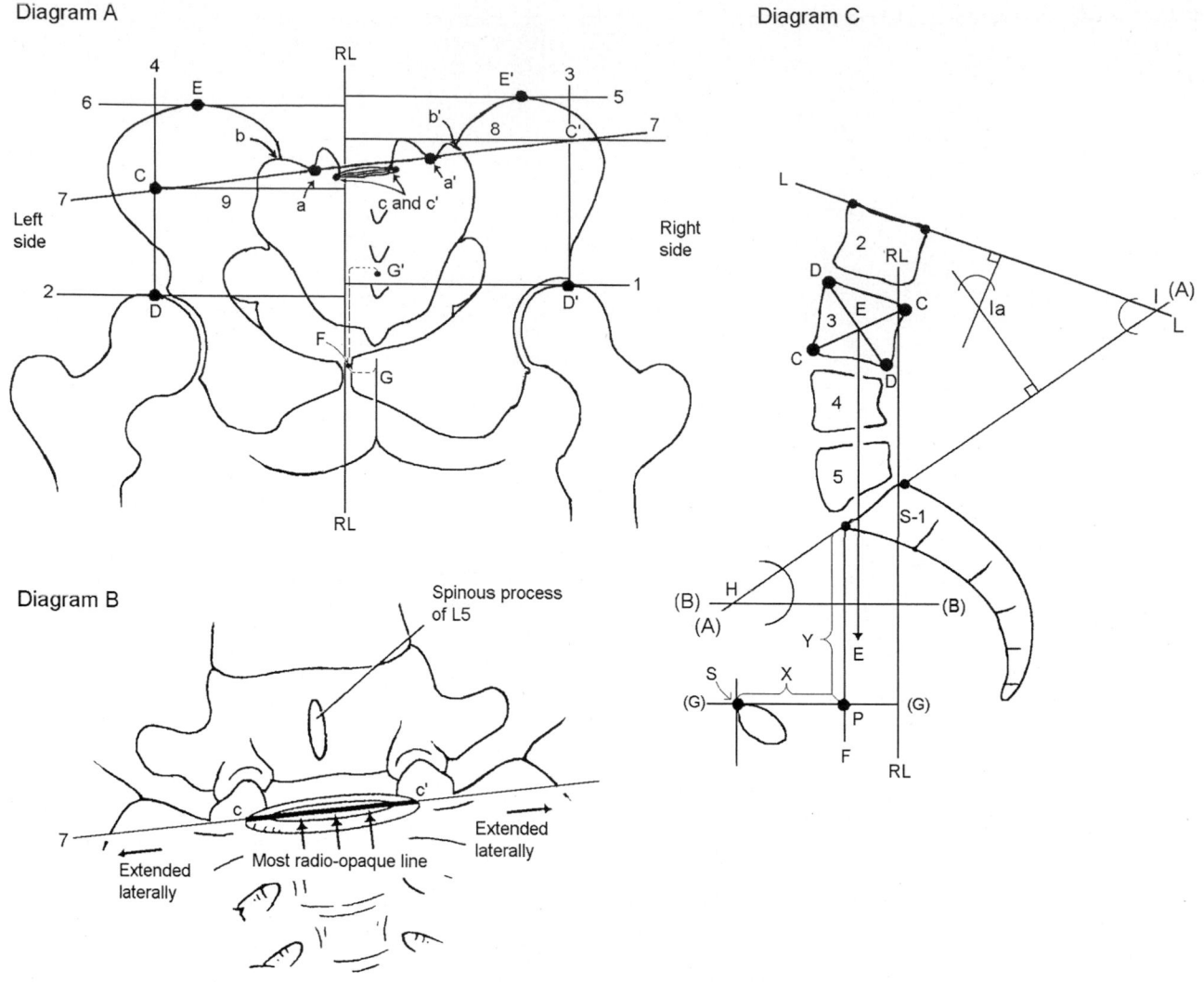

FIGURE 42.11. Measurements for postural x-ray view. **A:** Anteroposterior postural measurements. **B:** Landmark options for measuring sacral base unleveling. **C:** Lateral postural measurements. (Figs. 42.11A and C adapted from Kuchera WA, Kuchera ML. *Osteopathic Principles in Practice*, 2nd ed rev. Columbus, OH: Greyden Press; 1994:63. Fig. 42.11B adapted from Irvin RE. Suboptimal posture: the origin of the majority of idiopathic pain of the musculoskeletal system. In Vleeming A, Mooney V, Dorman T, et al, eds. *Movement, Stability and Low Back Pain: The Essential Role of the Pelvis*. New York, NY: Churchill-Livingstone; 1997:133–155.)

in the center of L3) relative to the lateral malleolus of the ankle, the sacral base, and the femoral heads. The measured L3 WBL is created by constructing a line parallel to the gravitational reference line through the center of the third lumbar vertebra (line *E* in Fig. 42.11C). This L3 WBL should ideally fall through the anterior one-third of the sacral base. If this line falls posterior to the sacral base, the lumbar facets are subject to increased load. Especially in the case of long-standing, significant stress, the involved facets on the radiograph will exhibit arthritic change, seen as eburnation (increased density) of these articulations.

The PI is calculated from measurements obtained from the lateral postural x-ray view (Fig. 42.11C). The PI is a calculation of the ratio of measurements, in millimeters, of x/y (Fig. 42.11C, *letters F, G, x,* and *y*). PI quantitatively reflects the relative position of the innominates to the sacrum. Normal PI values are age-related (13) and are typically less than 1.00. As the patient ages, this pos-

tural intrapelvic ratio approaches (or, in the same conditions, may exceed) the value of 1.00. PI has been documented to be increased in some patient populations (Fig. 42.12), including those with chronic low back pain and those with L5-S1 isthmic spondylolisthesis (14). In this latter group, patients with an extremely high PI for their age should be examined for spondylolysis or spondylolisthesis. Conversely, PI has been shown to decrease in patient populations with L4-5 degenerative spondylolisthesis (15).

Lumbar lordosis can be qualitatively assessed as normal, increased, or decreased. It can be quantified by measuring the angle created by lines along the top of L2 and S1 (Fig. 42.13—*lumbosacral lordotic angle*), or the top of L2 and the bottom of L5 (Fig. 42.14—*lumbo-lumbar lordotic angle*) (16). These angles average 60 and 43 degrees, respectively (17). A synopsis of normative values for measurements reflecting postural relationships in the sagittal plane are found in Fig. 42.15.

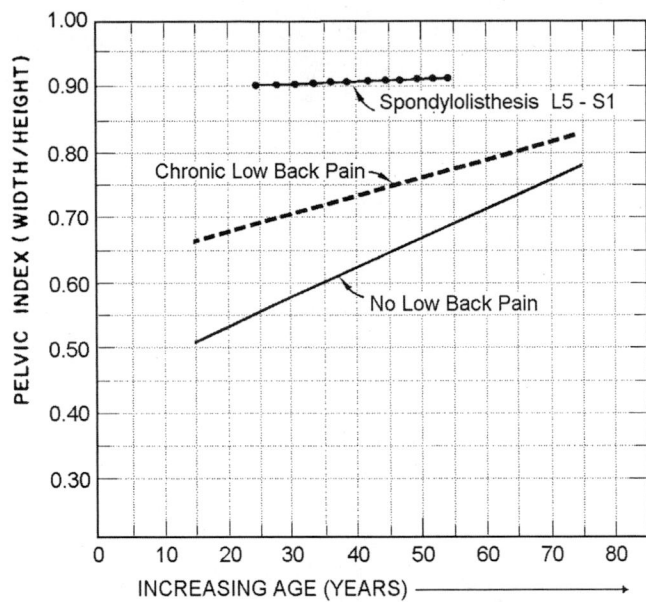

FIGURE 42.12. Pelvic index. (Illustration by W.A. Kuchera.)

EXERCISE IN MEASUREMENT OF POSTURAL RADIOGRAPHS

Two exercises follow. One is for measurement of the AP postural radiograph and the other is for measurement of the lateral postural radiograph (see Figs. 42.11A, B, C). These exercises provide step-by-step practice in measuring postural x-ray films taken with the method described in this chapter.

Exercise One: Anteroposterior Postural X-Ray View of Pelvis (Fig. 42.11A, B)

Initial Markings and Measurements

1. Using a fine tip marker, make a dot at the most superior margin of each iliac crest (E and E').
2. Place a dot at the most superior margin of each femoral head (D and D').
3. Also make a dot at any one of these pairs of sites, whichever are the most easily and accurately identified (any one of these

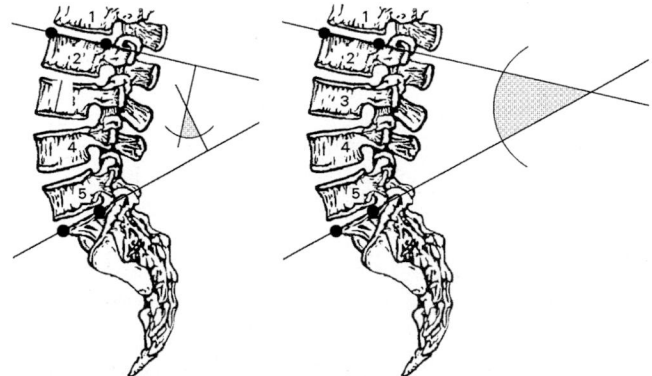

FIGURE 42.13. Lumbosacral lordotic angle using L2 and S1 (average 60 degrees). (Illustration by W.A. Kuchera.)

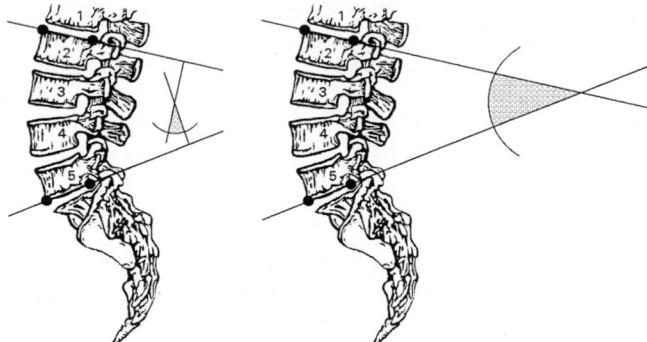

FIGURE 42.14. Lumbo-lumbar lordotic angle using L2 and the bottom of L5 (average 43 degrees). (Illustration by W.A. Kuchera.)

pairs determine a line parallel to the sacral base):
   a. Where the superior articular processes of the sacrum intersect the sacral ala (a-a'), *or*
   b. Where the sacral ala and the iliac crest intersect (b-b'), *or*
   c. At the right and left margins of the line of eburnation (i.e., the "most prominent radio-opaque line" (c-c') running along the top of the S1 segment (Fig. 42.11B).

4. To measure femoral head height discrepancies ("short leg"):
   a. Draw lines *1* and *2* perpendicular to the reference line (RL). One line passes through D and the other through D'.
   b. Measure the difference, in millimeters, between the points where lines *1* and *2* intersect the reference line (RL).

5. To measure iliac crest height discrepancies:
   a. Draw lines *5* and *6* perpendicular to the reference line (RL). One passes through E and the other passes through E'.
   b. Measure the difference, in millimeters, between the points where lines *5* and *6* intersect the reference line (RL).

6. To measure sacral base height discrepancies (the unlevel sacral base):
   a. Draw lines *3* and *4* parallel to the reference line (RL). One passes through D and the other passes through D'. These lines indicate the WBLs of each femoral head.
   b. Using your choice of a-a', b-b', or c-c' in step 3 above, draw line *7* to pass through this selected pair. The sacral base line, *7*, must be long enough to intersect at points C and C' on lines *4* and *3*, respectively (constructed in step 6a above).
   c. Draw lines *8* and *9* perpendicular to the reference line (RL). One passes through C and the other through C'.
   d. Measure the difference, in millimeters, between the points where lines *8* and *9* intersect the reference line (RL).

7. To measure the amount of pelvic rotation present:
   a. Make a dot with a fine tipped marker on the middle of the pubic symphysis (F).
   b. Identify the gluteal crease (G) which appears as a dark line in the region of the lower pelvis, *or* identify and place a dot on the median sacral crest (G).
   c. Measure the difference, in millimeters, for one of the following:
      i. Distance between the pubic symphyseal dot (F) and the gluteal crease (G), *or*
      ii. Distance between the pubic symphyseal dot, F, and point G on the median sacral crest.

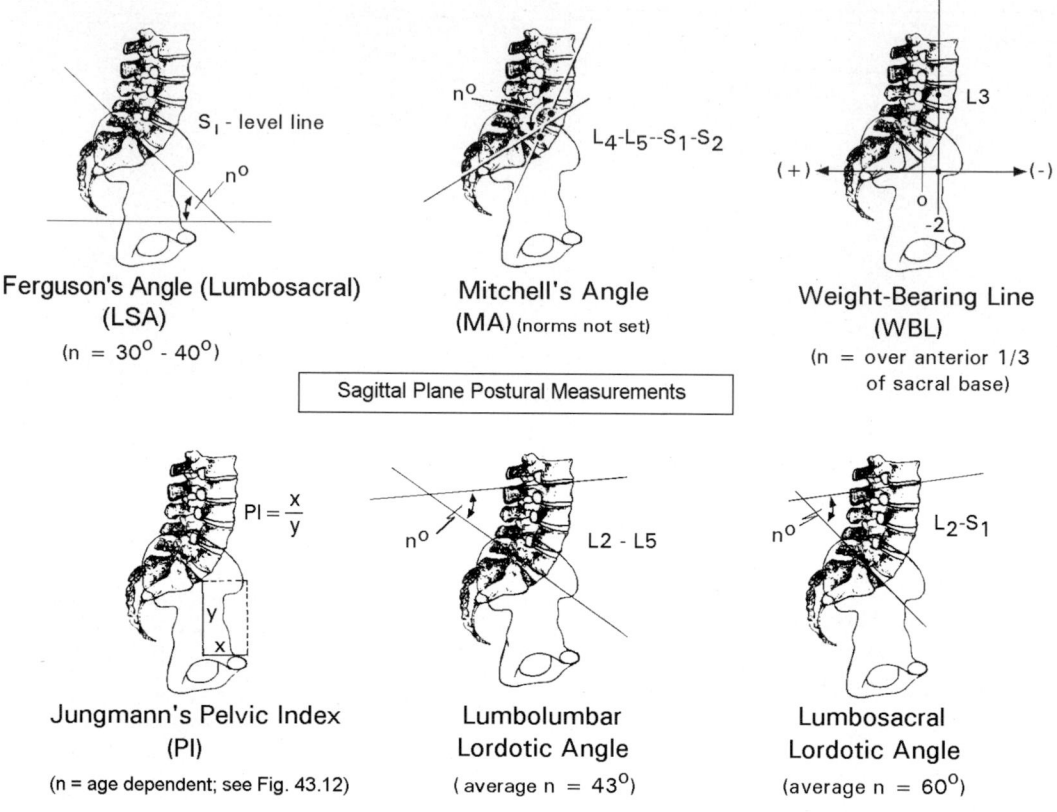

FIGURE 42.15. Sagittal plane standing postural radiographic measurements and their normal ranges.

Exercise Two: Lateral Postural X-Ray View of the Lumbopelvic Region (Fig. 42.11C)

Initial Markings and Measurements

1. Identify the center of the L3 vertebral body.
   a. Place a dot with a fine tipped marker at each of the four corners of the L3 vertebral body.
   b. Construct diagonal lines from the dots on the corners of L3 so that they intersect at a midpoint.
2. Identify the superior surface of the L2 vertebral body.
   a. Put a dot at the anterior and posterior corners of the superior surface of the L2 vertebral body.
   b. Draw a line, *L*, that passes through these two dots on L2 and extends some distance posteriorly.
3. Identify the sacral base.
   a. Place a dot at the sacral promontory and another dot at the posterior-superior extent of the vertebral body of S1.
4. To assess the center-of-gravity L3 WBL:
   a. From the midpoint in the body of L3 (step 1 above), construct line *E* parallel to the reference line (*RL*) of gravity.
   b. Line *E*, the L3 WBL, should ideally pass through the anterior third of the sacral base.
5. To measure the LSA (also known as the Ferguson angle, or sacral base angle):
   a. Draw line *A* that passes through two points marking the sacral base.
   b. Draw line *B* that crosses line *A* (point *H*) and is perpendicular to the reference line (*RL*).

c. Measure the angle formed between lines *A* and *B*. This is the LSA, alternatively referred to in the literature as the Ferguson angle or sometimes as a sacral angle.
6. To measure lordosis (lumbosacral lordotic angle and lumbolumbar lordotic angle; Fig. 42.13):
   a. If lines *L* and *A* intersect posterior to the lumbar spine (point *I*), measure the angle they form. This is the lumbosacral lordotic angle (Fig. 42.13).
   b. If lines *L* and *A* will run off before they intersect on the radiograph posterior to the lumbar spine, construct lines that are perpendicular to lines *A* and *L* so that these perpendicular lines cross (point *1a*). Measure the angle superior or inferior to point *1a*. Mathematically, this also measures the lumbosacral lordotic angle and should be identical to that measured by the method used in 6a above.
   c. The lumbo-lumbar lordotic angle (Fig. 42.14) is measured by drawing an alternative line (*A*) across the inferior margin of the body of L5 rather than through the top of the body of S1. Using the line, *L* and the "alternate line *A*," steps 6a or 6b can be employed to determine the lumbo-lumbar angle.
7. To measure PI (Fig. 42.11C):
   a. Put a dot on the most anterosuperior point of the pubic symphysis (*S*).
   b. Draw a line (*G*) through point *S* that is perpendicular to the reference line (*RL*).
   c. Now construct a line *F* that passes caudally from the sacral

promontory and is parallel to the reference line (*RL*). This line must cross line G (point *P*).

d. The distance, in millimeters, from the most anterosuperior point of the pubic symphysis (*S*) to this intersection point (*P*) is the measurement "*x*."

e. The distance, in millimeters, from the sacral promontory to this intersection point (*P*) is the measurement "*y*."

f. The PI is a calculated ratio determined by dividing measurement *x* by measurement *y*. (PI = *x/y*; see Fig. 42.12 for age-dependent values.)

Clinical interpretation of all measurements obtained using the exercises outlined here are dependent upon observing standard osteopathic postural protocols before and during the radiographic studies described.

THE EVIDENCE BASE

Reproducibility and Validity

Lack of a standard osteopathic postural radiographic protocol renders many measurements meaningless for the purposes of postural diagnosis, patient follow-up, or research. In the context of standard protocols however, many postural measurements have been studied extensively for reproducibility, validity, and clinical relevance (21,29).

Greenman notes the importance of first removing somatic dysfunction and normalizing lumbopelvic mechanics (9) before obtaining a postural x-ray series. Others point out that muscle imbalance involving the quadratus lumborum (7) or iliopsoas (14), for example, distorts postural interpretations. Interexaminer standard measurements of error are acceptably small and are remarkably consistent in multiple studies (18–20) using the standard protocols. These might best be summarized as a mean error of less than 1.0 mm and a maximum error of 2.0 mm for linear measures and 2 degrees for angular measures. These were also the conclusions obtained when manual and computer-assisted measurements by different practitioners (radiologist, primary care physicians, and osteopathic medical students) (4) were compared.

For decades, osteopathic literature has documented the natural history of postural changes and also the consistency of radiographic postural findings (21,22). Repeat studies on leg length inequality of 108 subjects found 85% with less than a 1.5-mm difference in measurement and 10% with less than a 3-mm difference; in only 3 subjects did the repeat study differ as much as 5 mm (23).

The incidence of low back pain symptomatology and coronal plane postural asymmetry is more completely discussed in Chapter 43, however, prevalence data and radiographic measurements definitely correlate much better than either of the following clinical estimates of postural asymmetry:

Comparison of malleolar levels (24)
Mechanical assessment of leg length with a tape measure (7,25)

Postural radiographic measurements in the coronal plane have also been correlated with degenerative osteoarthritis of the hip, (23) lumbar osteophytes, (26,27) lumbar vertebral wedging, (26) and a variety of somatovisceral symptoms (10,28).

CONCLUSION

The postural x-ray protocol described in this chapter provides a simple and inexpensive way to obtain accurate, reproducible structural measurements for either research or clinical interpretation (Table 42.1). In those sites without a standardized protocol, the radiographic technical requirements are easily shared with and implemented by a consultant DO or MD radiologist.

Application of a standardized protocol results in consistent AP standing (postural) views of the lumbopelvic and thoracic regions as well as lateral standing views of the lumbopelvic region. A reliable gravitational reference line is produced on each radiograph—essential for proper evaluation of the patient when various postural treatment strategies are being considered or applied (see Chapter 43). These protocols and measurement methods provide a means of comparing a patient's present posture with established standards of other patients of the same age. It also provides a means of gathering data from which, at some future date, a patient's weightbearing posture can be reliably and accurately calibrated and compared, determining if there has been continued decompensation with age or an improvement in posture, following some form of corrective treatment.

Just as important, these static (structural) findings can be effectively correlated with dynamic (functional) physical findings for a more complete assessment and follow-up of patients with suspected postural problems.

REFERENCES

1. Smith W. Skiagraphy and the circulation. *J Osteopath.* 1899;3:356–378.
2. Beilke M. Roentgenological spinal analysis and the technic for taking standing x-ray plates. *JAOA.* 1936;35:414–418.
3. Denslow JS, Chace JA, Gutensohn OR, Kumm MG. Methods in taking and interpreting weight-bearing films. *JAOA.* 1955;54:663–670.
4. Kuchera ML, Bemben MG, Kuchera WA, Willman MK. Comparison of manual and computerized methods of assessing postural radiographs. *JAOA.* 1990;90(8):714–715.
5. Willman MK. Radiographic technical aspects of the postural study. *JAOA.* 1977;76:739–744.
6. The Glossary Review Committee of the Educational Council on Osteopathic Principles. Glossary of osteopathic terminology. In: D'Alonzo GE Jr, ed. *AOA Yearbook and Directory of Osteopathic Physicians.* Chicago IL: American Osteopathic Association; 2000:860.
7. Travell JG, Simon DG. *Myofascial Pain and Dysfunction: The Trigger Point Manual.* Vol II. Baltimore MD: Williams & Wilkins; 1992: 22–88.
8. Ferguson AB. The clinical and recent roentgenographic interpretation of lumbosacral anomalies. *Radiology.* 1934;22:548–588.
9. Greenman PE. Lift therapy: use and abuse. *JAOA.* 1979;79:238–250.
10. Irvin RE. Suboptimal posture: the origin of the majority of idiopathic pain of the musculoskeletal system. In Vleeming A, Mooney V, Dorman T, et al, eds. *Movement, Stability and Low Back Pain: The Essential Role of the Pelvis.* New York, NY: Churchill-Livingstone; 1997:133–155.
11. Lapadula G, Covelli M, Numo R, Pipitone V. Iliolumbar ligament ossification as a radiologic feature of reactive arthritis. *J Rheumatol.* 1991;18:1760–1762.
12. Denslow JS, Chace JA. Mechanical stresses in the human lumbar spine and pelvis. Postural balance and imbalance. In: Peterson B, ed. *1983 AAO Yearbook.* Newark, OH: American Academy of Osteopathy; 1983:76–82.
13. Kuchera ML. Aging, postural decompensation and low back pain. *JAOA.* 1986;886(10):74.

14. Kuchera ML. Treatment of gravitational strain pathophysiology: In Vleeming A, Mooney V, Dorman T, et al, eds. *Movement, Stability and Low Back Pain: The Essential Role of the Pelvis.* New York, NY: Churchill-Livingstone; 1997:477–499.

15. Kuchera ML, Miller K. Postural measurements in L4 degenerative spondylolisthesis. *JAOA.* 1995;95(8):496.

16. Fernand R, Fox DE. Evaluation of lumbar lordosis: a prospective and retrospective study. *Spine.* 1985;10(9):799–803.

17. Kuchera ML, Gitlin R, Frey-Gitlin K. Aging, lumbar lordosis and low back pain. *JAOA.* 1992;92(9):1182.

18. Friberg O. Clinical symptoms and biomechanics of lumbar spine and hip joint in leg length inequality. *Spine.* 1983;8:643–651.

19. Friberg O. The statics of postural pelvic tilt scoliosis: a radiographic study on 288 consecutive chronic LB patients. *Clin Biomech.* 1987;2:211–219.

20. Henrad J-Cl, Bismuth V, deMolmont C, Gaux J-C. Unequal length of the lower limbs: measurement by a simple radiographic method: application to epidemiological studies. *Rev Rheum Mal Osteoartic.* 1974;41:773–779.

21. Peterson B, ed. *Postural Balance and Imbalance (1983 AAO Yearbook).* Newark, OH: American Academy of Osteopathy; 1983.

22. Hagen DP. A continuing roentgenographic study of rural school children over a 15 year period. *JAOA* 1964;63:546–557.

23. Gofton JP, Trueman GE. Studies in osteoarthritis of the hips, Part II. Osteoarthritis of the hip and leg length disparity. *Can Med Assoc J.* 1971;104:791–799.

24. Friberg O, Nurminen M, Korhonen K, et al. Accuracy and precision of clinical estimating of leg length inequality and lumbar scoliosis and comparison of clinical and radiological measurements. *International Disability Study.* 1988;10:49–53.

25. Beal MC. A review of the short-leg problem. *JAOA.* 1950;50:109–121.

26. Giles LGF, Taylor JR. Lumbar spine structural changes associated with leg length inequality. *Spine.* 1981;6:510–521.

27. Morscher E. Etiology and pathophysiology of leg length discrepancies. *Prog Orthop Surg.* 1977:9–19.

28. Kuchera ML, Kuchera WA. *Osteopathic Considerations in Systemic Dysfunction,* 2nd ed rev. Columbus, OH: Greyden Press; 1994.

29. Mense S, Simons DG. *Muscle Pain: Understanding Its Nature, Diagnosis, and Treatment.* Philadelphia, PA: Lippincott, Williams & Wilkins; 2001.

43

POSTURAL CONSIDERATIONS IN CORONAL, HORIZONTAL, AND SAGITTAL PLANES

MICHAEL L. KUCHERA

KEY CONCEPTS

General Principles

- Anatomic landmarks associated with the ideal postural weightbearing line
- Implications of faulty postural alignment
- General somatic patterns in primary postural dysfunction
- Specific effects of gravity on postural muscles and ligaments
- Clinical relevance of gravitational strain pathophysiology
- Observation, palpation, and radiology in evaluating postural decompensation and instability
- Osteopathic manipulative treatment used in postural problems
- Orthotics and types of devices in treating postural insufficiencies

Coronal and Horizontal Plane Posture

- Short leg syndrome as a misnomer
- Biomechanical changes contributing to short leg syndrome
- Biomechanical principles and osteopathic manipulative treatment in treatment of short leg syndrome
- Treatment modalities for pelvic rotation
- Major classification criteria for scoliosis
- Treatment goals for scoliosis, and implications of each treatment modality as it relates to the patient's lifestyle and activities

Sagittal Plane Posture

- Modalities useful in treating hyperlordosis and spondylolisthesis
- Classification and general structural condition of spondylolisthesis
- Radiographic grading severity of spondylolisthesis

- Clinical presentation of spondylolisthesis and different age-related manifestations
- Two basic rules of exercise and importance of patient compliance

Be sure the foundation is level and all will be well.

—A.T. Still

GRAVITATIONAL STRAIN AND POSTURAL DECOMPENSATION

Gravity is one of the major disrupters of postural homeostasis (1,2). Although it exerts a constant force on all structures, some individuals appear to be less capable of resisting gravitational stress than others. These individuals often have weakened support mechanisms, increased functional demand on postural structures, and/or biomechanical risk factors that augment the gravitational stress challenging their homeostatic resources (1–5). A postural treatment approach to these patients is often effective in ameliorating their recurrent, predictable patterns of pain and dysfunction as well as relieving a wide range of secondary complaints (6).

A homeostatic response to gravity begins as soon as the individual assumes an upright position (Fig. 43.1) and continues throughout life. Two secondary lordotic curves normally develop in the cervical and lumbar regions to counterbalance the primary thoracic curve present at birth. These three spinal curves together will resist gravity much better than one single sagittal plane curve. They allow a person to function in an upright position; however they also result in some uniquely human problems affecting both structure and function. These problems are characterized by coordinated compensation occurring in multiple regions and planes.

The presence of a number of anatomic and/or congenital conditions can create significant homeostatic stress on postural mechanisms or can aggravate existing postural decompensation. These

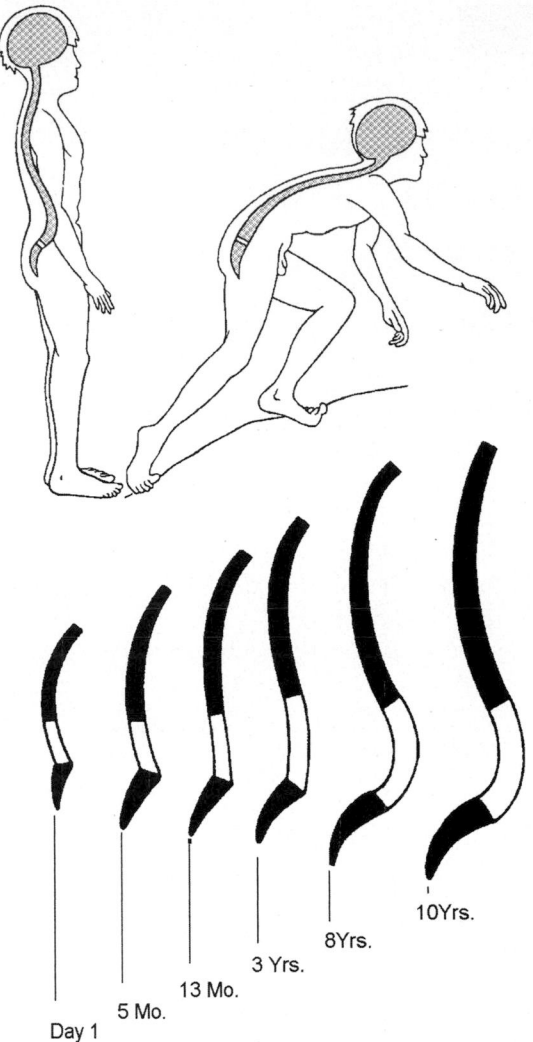

FIGURE 43.1. Changes in sagittal plane spinal curves from day 1 through age 10 years. (From Kapandji IA. *The Physiology of the Joints.* Vol 3. New York, NY: Churchill- Livingstone; 1974:17, with permission.)

include:

- Anatomic short leg
- Scoliosis
- Small hemipelvis
- Spondylolisthesis
- Wedge vertebrae

Diagnosis of any one or a combination of these disrupts symmetry and requires the body to compensate in order to maintain postural balance.

Ideal postural alignment depends, in part, on balancing the cervical, lumbar, and thoracic curves against the effects of gravity. Failure to do so in the sagittal plane results in lordosis or kyphosis and numerous symptoms associated with postural decompensation. Lordosis has been implicated as a destabilizing factor in the development and progression of scoliosis (7).

Ideal standing postural alignment in the coronal plane will place the center of gravity line midway between the feet, extend superiorly up the midline of the spine, and divide the body into

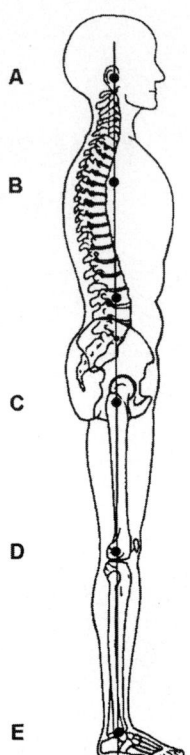

FIGURE 43.2. Ideal postural alignment of body in relation to gravitational line. **A:** External auditory meatus. **B:** Shoulders. **C:** Center of the body of L3. **D:** Through the knee. **E:** Just anterior to the lateral malleolus.

two equal parts. Ideally, there would be no rotation in the horizontal plane of any body region and no coronal plane side-bending asymmetry.

Ideal postural alignment in the sagittal plane (Fig. 43.2) has a center of gravity or weightbearing line that passes through the following anatomic landmarks:

- Just anterior to the lateral malleolus
- Just behind the mid-knee
- Femoral head
- Anterior third of the sacral base (x-ray landmark)
- Middle of the body of the L3 vertebra (x-ray landmark)
- Humeral head
- External auditory meatus

Failure of the body to align with respect to its center of gravity functionally stresses the soft tissues and joint facets. These structures are not designed for weightbearing. Structural change and pain is the result of postural decompensation (1).

Postural Homeostasis and Strain

Each person with asymmetric postural stress will progressively compensate in a different way depending, in part, on his or her unique biomechanical risk factors. Nonetheless, certain guiding postural principles apply. Postural changes will take place throughout the musculoskeletal system in an attempt to coordinate visual, vestibular, and kinesthetic input and to distribute stress. Typically, the changes occur more predictably in the lumbopelvic region because of its proximity to the center of gravity.

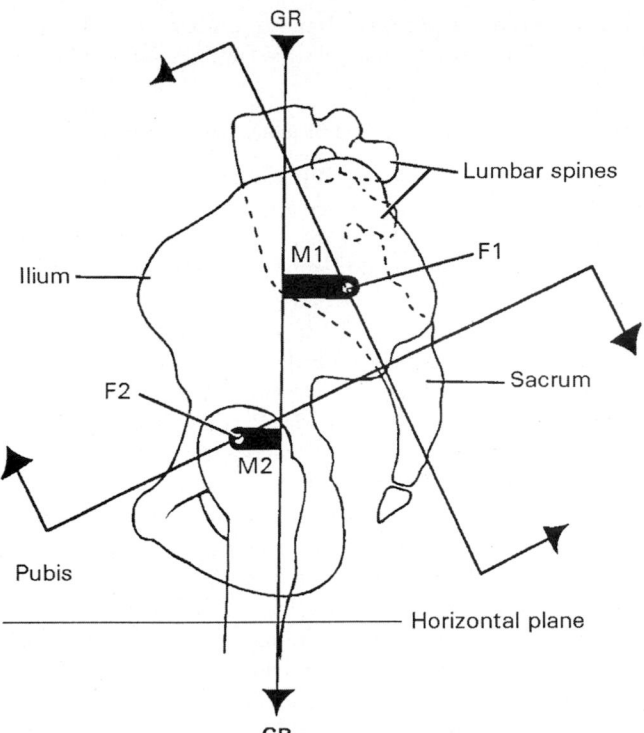

FIGURE 43.3. Pelvic mechanics. Intrapelvic rotations occur biomechanically about their axes of rotation in relation to gravitational line *(GR)*. The sacrum rotates anteriorly because weightbearing falls anterior to its S2 axis *(F1)*. Innominates rotate posteriorly because weightbearing is posterior to femoral axes *(F2)*. (From Jungmann M. *The Jungmann Concept and Technique of Antigravity Leverage.* Rangely, ME: Institute for Gravitational Strain Pathology, Inc; 1982, with permission.)

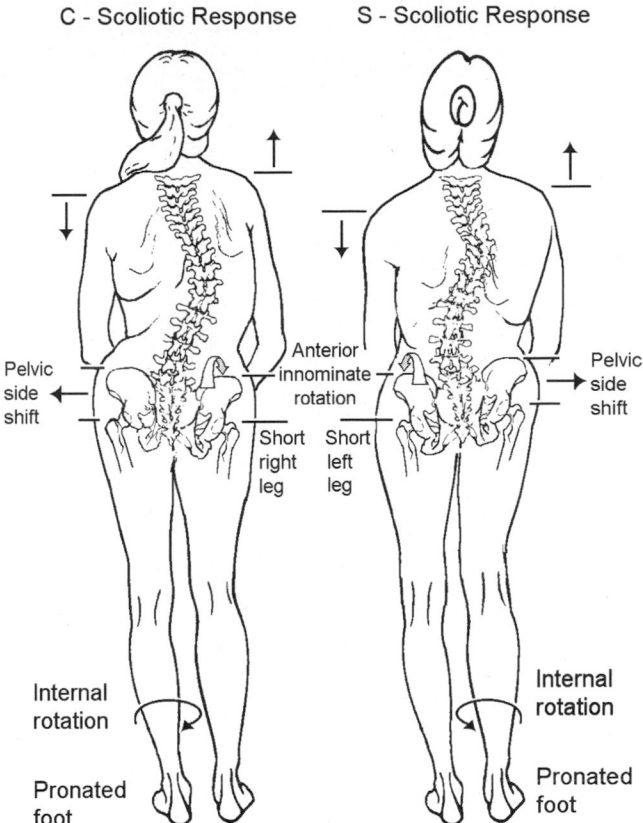

FIGURE 43.4. Typical postural compensation for short leg syndrome.

Biomechanics

The biomechanical principles that govern gravity's effect on the lumbopelvic region are specific. In the sagittal plane, gravity encourages the sacral base to rotate anteriorly and encourages innominates to rotate posteriorly (Fig. 43.3) (8,9). This occurs because the L3 weightbearing gravitational line falls anterior to the middle transverse sacral axis and behind the femoral axis. Homeostatic mechanisms to resist this counter-rotation are provided by muscular tone as well by as pelvic and lumbosacral ligaments (10).

The body's response to sacral base unleveling in the coronal plane also follows homeostatic biomechanical principles. The lumbar spine side bends away from and rotates toward the low sacral base. The biomechanics of the typical spinopelvic response to sacral base unleveling is shown in Fig. 43.4. As a curve forms in one spinal region there is a change in the curvature of all other spinal regions. Early compensation is associated with the development of a single, long scoliotic curve in the lumbar or lumbothoracic spine. In this C-shaped curve, the horizontal cephalad planes are typically depressed on the side opposite the depressed pelvic horizontal plane. Later, the compensatory mechanisms redistribute postural responsibilities resulting in the formation of several lateral curves. In an S-shaped scoliotic curve, the shoulders and the greater trochanteric planes are typically depressed on the same side as the depressed sacral base.

Compensatory changes associated with leg length inequality can also be generalized. The pelvis as a unit typically side shifts and rotates toward the long leg side. The innominate may attempt to compensate for the "short leg" by rotating anteriorly on the short leg side. This functionally lengthens that extremity. The innominate on the side of the apparent long leg may rotate posteriorly to functionally shorten that extremity. Often, on the long leg side, the foot assumes a pronated position, and the lower extremity internally rotates. The lumbosacral angle (LSA) (see Chapter 42) increases 2 to 3 degrees. The increased LSA and pelvic rotation often mask the presence of an unlevel sacral base (11). The vertebrae of the most caudal scoliotic curve usually side bend away from and rotate toward the side of the apparent short leg.

Pelvic rotation in the horizontal plane occurs concomitantly with biomechanical stresses in the coronal plane (such as the short leg syndrome) (12). This can present a therapeutic challenge when prescribing foot orthotics in an attempt to treat leg length and/or to level the sacral base. Alternating directional patterns of the transitional regions of the body occur in compensation (61) to the rotation of one or more of these regions (Fig. 43.5).

Somatic Structures Stressed: Muscles

Gravity stresses a number of somatic structures involved in homeostasis. Each of these structures responds predictably when stressed. For example, postural muscles that are structurally adapted for prolonged stress typically respond by becoming tight

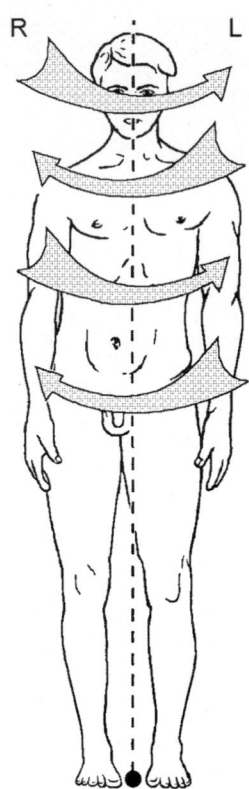

FIGURE 43.5. Compensation in the horizontal planes: Alternating pattern of rotation at transition zones.

when overstressed. Postural antagonists (phasic muscles) typically become pseudoparetic and are somewhat weak when tested (Table 43.1) (13). Patients with postural stress will also often have trigger points in a number of the muscles listed in Table 43.1. In combination, the responses of the many individual structures create a recognizable pattern of postural decompensation (1,14). Such patterns of involvement should alert the osteopathic clin-

TABLE 43.1. POSTURAL ANTAGONISTS

Postural Muscles	Phasic Muscles
Cervical and upper thoracic muscles	
Upper trapezius muscle	Latissimus dorsi muscle
Levator scapulae muscle	Mid/lower trapezius muscles
Pectoralis major (upper part)	Rhomboid muscles
Pectoralis minor muscle	Anterior cervical muscles
Cervical erector spinae muscles	
Scalenus muscles	
Lumbar and lumbopelvic muscles	
Tensor fasciae latae muscle	Quadriceps muscles
Hamstring muscles	Dorsiflexor muscles
Hip adductor muscles	Abdominalis muscles
(short adductors)	
Gastrocnemius/soleus muscles	Gluteus maximus muscle
Piriformis muscle	
Iliopsoas muscles	

Reprinted with permission from Kuchera M. Gravitational stress, musculoligamentous strain and postural alignment. In: Dorman T, ed. *Spine: State of the Art Reviews on Prolotherapy.* Philadelphia, PA: Hanley and Belfus; 1995:463–490.

ician to consider a postural diagnosis and can often be traced biomechanically to gravitational stress on these muscles.

Somatic Structures Stressed: Ligaments

Gravity's effect on individuals with postural imbalance or diminished homeostatic abilities to resist gravity functionally stresses a number of stabilizing ligaments. These ligaments include the iliolumbar, sacrotuberous, and long dorsal (posterior) sacroiliac ligaments.

The iliolumbar ligaments (ILL) are critical structures for stabilizing the lumbar vertebrae on the sacral base (10). They are usually the first structures to be involved with postural decompensation and are affected by both sacral and innominate rotations (Fig. 43.6). When stressed, the attachments of these ligaments become bilaterally tender to palpation. Unilateral stress and tenderness are very common in coronal plane postural strain; bilateral tenderness is more common in sagittal plane strain conditions. ILL calcification may be seen when there has been long-standing postural strain because calcium is laid down along lines of stress (Wolff's law) (15). Functional changes include tenderness, edema, and pain referred to the lower extremity (Fig. 43.7); these findings disappear with treatment.

The sacrotuberous ligament (STL) and long dorsal sacroiliac (LDSI) ligament respectively resist anterior and posterior rotation of the sacrum (Fig. 43.8) (16). The LDSI ligament connects the sacrum and the posterior superior iliac spine (PSIS) whereas the main part of the STL connects the sacrum and ischial tuberosity with fibers connecting to the iliac bone as well.

Postural stress involves a more complex biomechanical interaction than is depicted in Figs. 43.6 and 43.8. It involves interaction between these ligaments, the sacroiliac joint, the thoracolumbar fascia, and a variety of muscles including the multifidi, biceps femoris, and glutei (16). The pelvic girdle as a foundation for function and support must therefore be interpreted in its relationship to other areas of the spine and all four extremities.

Somatic Structures Stressed: Skeletal—Arthrodial

Bone remodels over time in response to the stress placed upon it (15). Over time, the vertebrae of patients with exaggerated or lateral postural curves will develop wedging of the vertebral body and exostoses (spurs). Posterior weightbearing mechanics transfer weight onto the spinal facets resulting in modified function, increased calcium deposition that may appear on radiographs, and pain.

Degenerative structural change in joints is also common when there is accentuated functional demand and asymmetry. This affects both spinal joints and other weight bearing structures, such as the hip joint. Degenerative arthritis of the hip joint often develops on the long leg side, (17) and is accompanied by tenderness over that greater trochanter.

Long-term radiographic postural studies (see Chapter 42) have shown chronic, progressive postural decline. The resultant postural pattern of spinal curvature continued to evolve with age in one-third of the population studied (18). The likelihood that several lateral curves will evolve is higher when the leg length

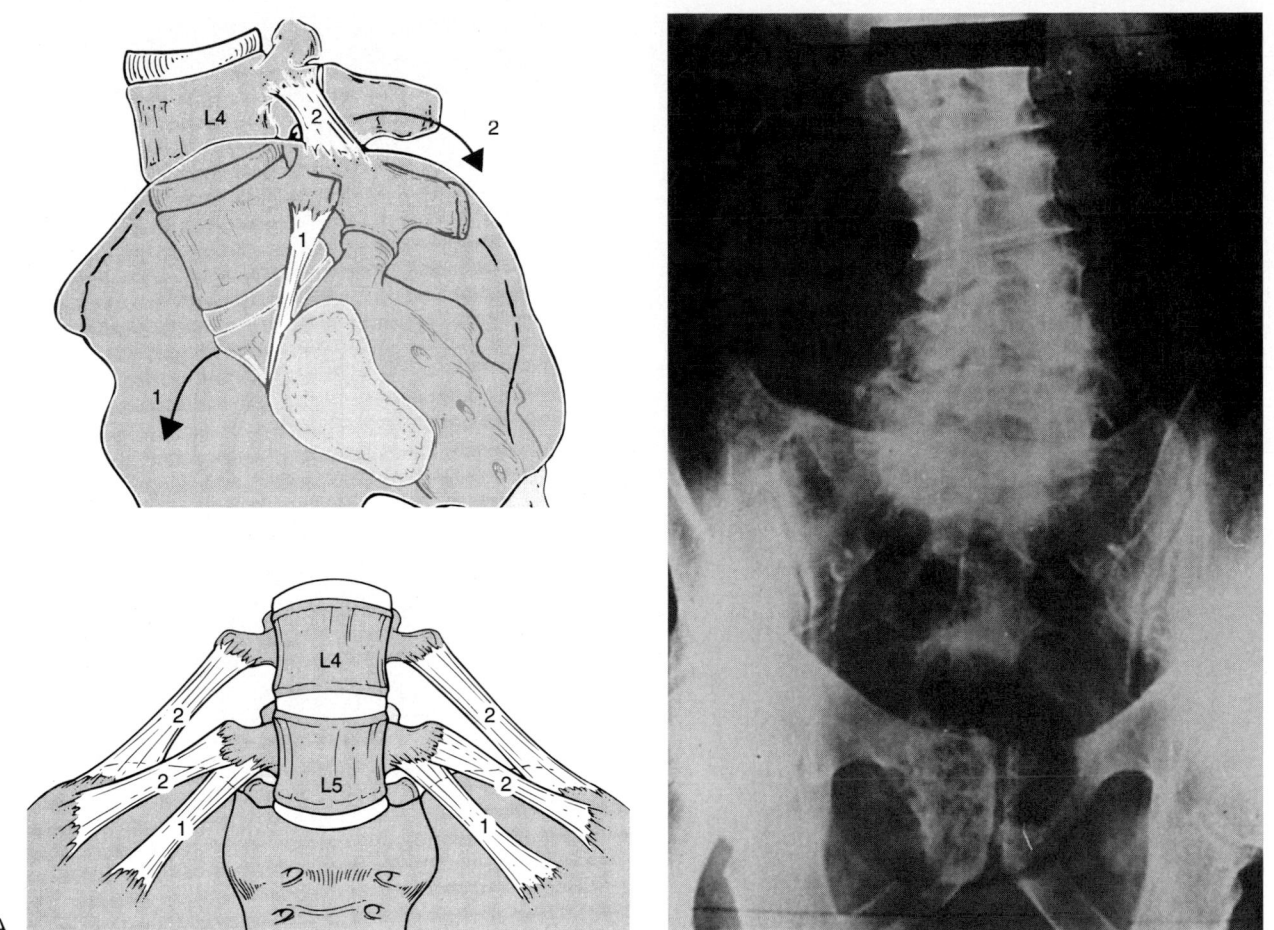

FIGURE 43.6. A: Anterior rotation of sacrum bilaterally stresses fibers labeled 1. Posterior rotation of innominates bilaterally stress fibers labeled 2. **B:** Calcification of iliolumbar ligament is an excellent example of structural change resulting from excessive functional demand. (Radiograph from the Institute for Gravitational Strain Pathology, Inc., with permission.)

inequality is greater than 10 mm (19). The stereotypic posture of the geriatric patient depicts a decrease in total height as their kyphotic and lordotic curves accentuate and the radiographic measurements show a height diminution (an increased pelvic index ratio) within the pelvis (see Chapter 42) (2,20).

POSTURAL DIAGNOSIS

Accurate postural diagnosis requires an understanding of both static and dynamic components of postural stress. Important postural information is gained from independent and interactive examination of each of these components. These components must then be interpreted with respect to their relative contributions to the stress upon the person as a whole functional being.

Correlation of static-dynamic information within the structural-functional continuum of a given postural diagnosis plays a significant role in postural treatment regimens and in providing patient education concerning prognosis. Observation and palpation form the cornerstones of postural evaluation. Radiographic and computerized range-of-motion analyses provide additional or supportive information.

Initial observation of asymmetry provides the initial clue to variance from the "ideal." Looking at the space around the body in addition to spinal alignment is also very insightful. Is the space between one arm and the body greater on one side than the other? Look for the presence of group curves (Chapter 41). Screen for rotoscoliosis by comparing symmetry in levelness of key paired landmarks with the patient in the static anatomic position and then when the patient bends forward (see the "Screening and Symptoms" section under " Scoliosis" later in this chapter).

Palpation identifies key landmarks for structural symmetry and gathers information about the functional characteristics of the body unit. It is also the best tool for uncovering patterns of somatic dysfunction, pain and strain, or adaptations characteristic of postural disorders. Palpation of the postural response to certain movements helps to differentiate the degree to which a given postural curve is structural (fixed) or functional (flexible) (i.e., does it stay the same or increase or does it reduce or disappear?).

Radiographic analysis (see Chapter 42) is used to quantify static postural distortion from the ideal. It may also be used to objectively monitor progress of a postural treatment regimen. Furthermore, it can indicate congenital or acquired abnormalities

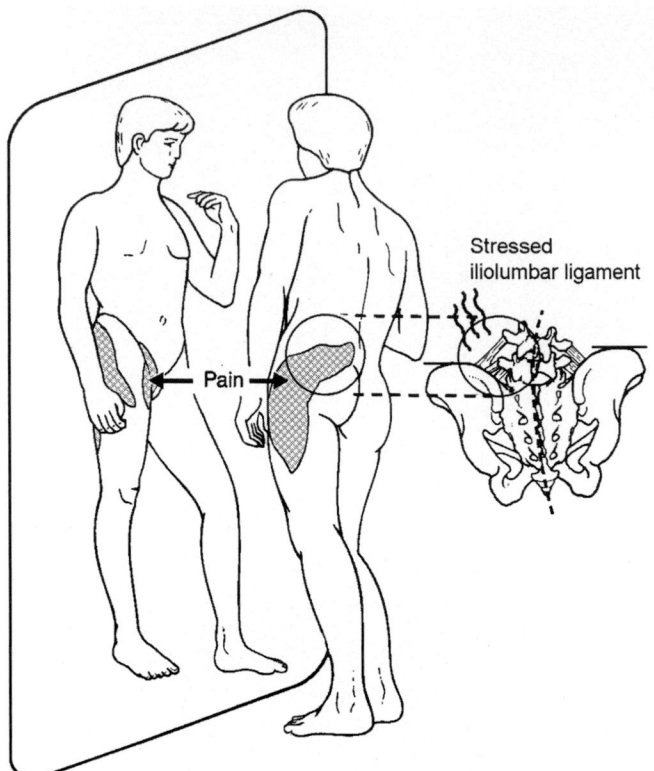

FIGURE 43.7. Iliolumbar ligament pain pattern from postural imbalance.

that predispose the patient to postural decline or that will compromise the results of a treatment program.

Observation and Palpation

Observation and palpation of the spine and pelvis are essential when evaluating the dynamic or functional component of posture.

Observation and palpation of postural muscles, their antagonists, and regional or group spinal curves should be performed with the patient in an upright, weightbearing position. With the patient in this upright position, they are asked to move into various positions to determine whether any observed thoracic or lumbar rotoscoliotic group curve asymmetry can be functionally reduced or eliminated. The structural component in these planes is represented by the spinal asymmetry that is not modified by active or passive motion.

With the patient supine, the physician determines whether the lumbar curve can relax and be flat against the table. In functional lumbar lordosis, bending the knees as shown (Fig. 43.9) should permit the lumbar region to flatten onto the table (or floor). Inability to flatten this curve actively or passively represents a sagittal plane structural component. Be sure to palpate the lumbar spine when evaluating this element, as hypertrophy of soft tissues in the adjacent flanks may mask the lordotic curve.

Alternatively, or additionally, objective measurements can be ascertained using varying computerized measuring instruments. Some of these instruments can measure intersegmental as well as regional motions and are used to reinforce the palpatory

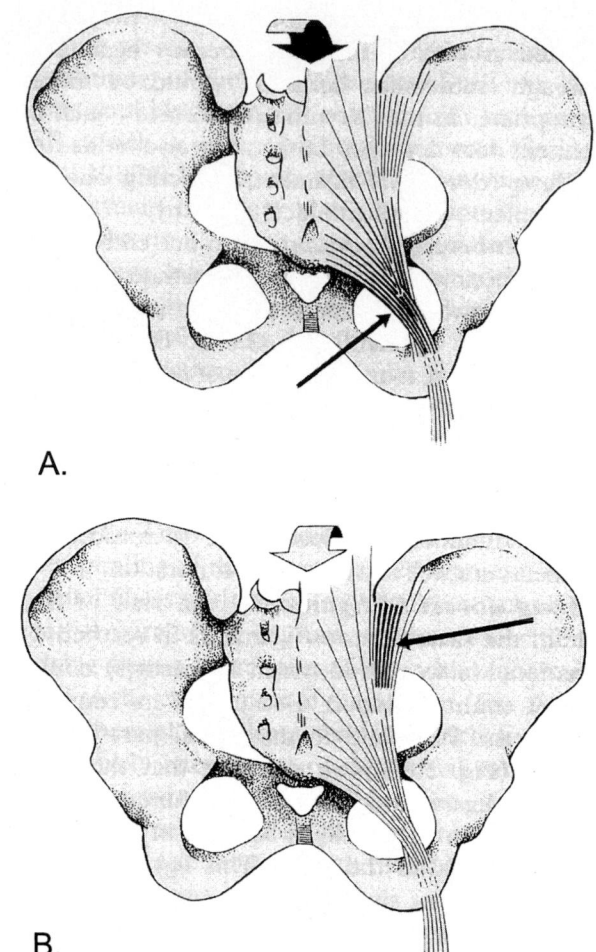

A.

B.

FIGURE 43.8. A: Sacrum rotating anteriorly winds up sacrotuberous ligament. **B:** Sacrum rotating posteriorly winds up the long dorsal sacroiliac ligament. (From Vleeming A, Snijders CJ, Stoeckart R, Mens JMA. The role of the sacroiliac joints in coupling between spine, pelvis, legs and arms. In: Vleeming A, Mooney V, Dorman T, et al., eds. *Movement, Stability and Low Back Pain: The Essential Role of the Pelvis.* New York, NY: Churchill-Livingston, 1997, with permission.).

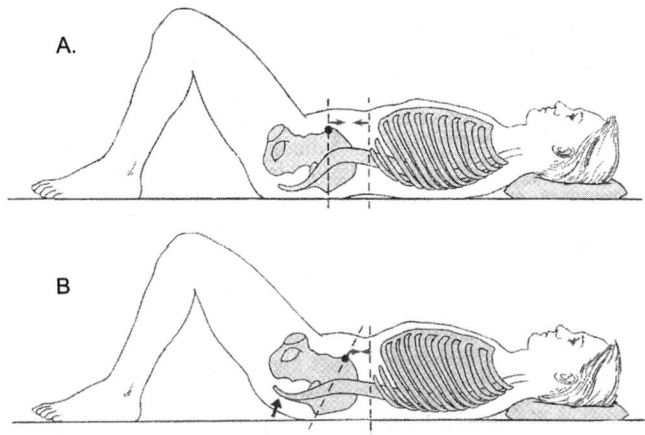

FIGURE 43.9. Lumbar lordosis, with patient actively attempting to flatten spine to table. **A:** Structural component (no reduction of lordotic curve). **B:** Flattening indicative of functional lordotic curve. (From Simon DG, Travell JG, Simons LS. *Myofascial Pain and Dysfunction: The Trigger Point Manual.* Vol I. Baltimore, MD: Williams & Wilkins; 1999, with permission.)

determination of areas requiring manipulative treatment (hypomobile areas) and those that need strengthening exercise, prolotherapy, or extrinsic stabilization (hypermobile areas).

Coronal plane decompensation is suspected with certain constellations of asymmetry, recurrent somatic dysfunction, and tissue texture change. When this diagnosis is the result of leg length inequality, the standing trochanteric plane, the plane of the PSIS, and the iliac crests are usually depressed on the side of the depressed sacral base. Usually the more horizontal cephalad planes (shoulders, occipital) are also depressed to compensate for the unlevelness of the sacral base (19). The number of curvatures between the pelvis and the upper body will determine on which side the more horizontal cephalad planes are depressed in relation to the sacral base. The following horizontal planes (Fig. 43.10) are assessed by standing behind the patient and palpating these key anatomic landmarks:

- Mastoid processes
- Acromioclavicular joints
- Inferior scapula
- Iliac crests

- PSIS
- Greater trochanters
- Knee creases

These static landmarks are helpful in predicting underlying spinal response to coronal plane postural asymmetry.

Sagittal plane decompensation is associated with alteration of the anteroposterior regional curves of the body and specific palpable somatic patterns. In addition to myofascial and ligamentous clues, anterior sacral base and lumbar hyperlordosis, craniosacral extension mechanics often accompanies this condition. The extension phase of the craniosacral mechanism is often accompanied by fatigue, loss of energy, and/or psychological depression. It is clinically important to recognize that these patients may have problems in many activities of daily living as well as poor compliance, even with an apparently appropriate postural treatment program.

Radiographic Findings

As mentioned, posture and postural diagnoses involve the understanding of both static (structural) and dynamic (functional) characteristics. X-ray images primarily visualize the static or structural aspect of posture. They also aid in identifying congenital anomalies and other structural deficiencies that enable gravitational and other functional strain to overcome the body's homeostatic mechanisms. Finally, postural radiographs may be used to quantify spinal decompensation in the coronal and horizontal planes using the Cobb method (Fig. 43.11) for rotoscoliosis and the Meyerding or Taillard classification systems (Fig. 43.12) for spondylolisthesis in the saggital plane.

Abnormal static postural measurements can be viewed as being biomechanical (or functional) risk factors for a patient. Using a standard protocol (21), radiographic measurements outside the normative range suggest a biomechanical disadvantage that increases functional demand. As the number of biomechanical risk factors increases, homeostatic maintenance of posture is more likely to fail. These factors not only strain musculoligamentous structures but also predispose the patient to the development of scoliosis, spondylolysis or spondylolisthesis (22), or other postural diagnoses.

A number of coronal plane radiographic studies (23) indicate that sacral base unleveling and leg length inequality are fairly common. About 50% of an unselected population had radiographic leg length inequality of more than $^3/_{16}$ of an inch. Approximately equal declination of femoral head, sacral base (extrapolated laterally to the femoral head line), and iliac crest were often present. Other radiographic studies have also documented the distribution of lumbopelvic positional relationships with respect to providing a foundation for the lower extremity. Yet other studies have monitored scoliotic patterns with regard to natural history or in response to treatment.

Radiographic series are also extremely valuable in measuring sagittal plane posture. Key radiographic measurements (Fig. 43.13) used to evaluate a patient for postural management of sagittal plane problems are the weightbearing line from L3 (*n* = anterior one-third to one-half of the sacral base) and the modified LSA of Ferguson (*n* = 30 to 40 degrees).

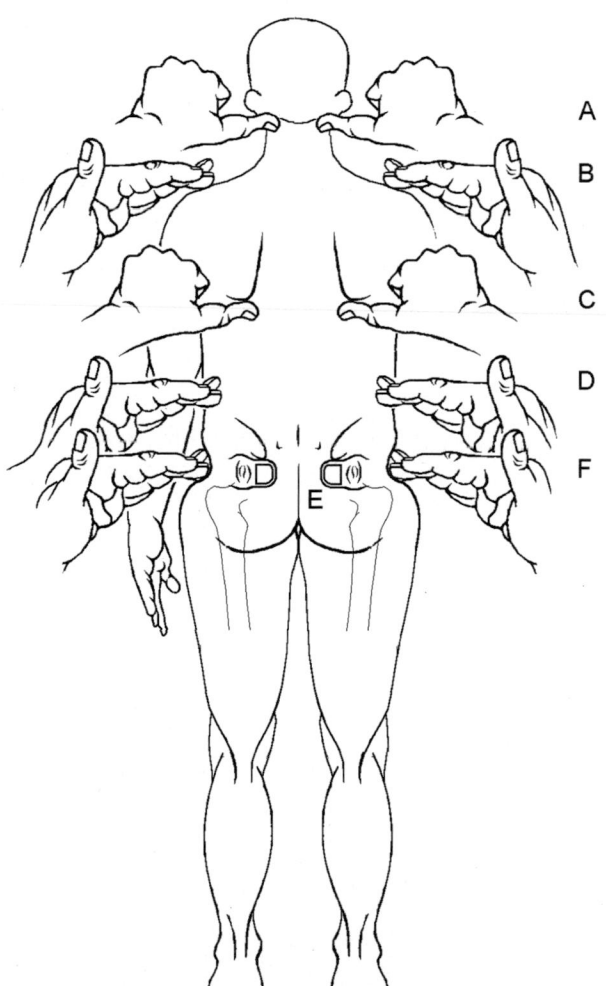

FIGURE 43.10. Levelness of horizontal planes. **A:** Occipital plane. **B:** Shoulder plane. **C:** Scapular plane (inferior). **D:** Iliac crest plane. **E:** Posterior superior iliac spine plane. **F:** Greater trochanteric plane.

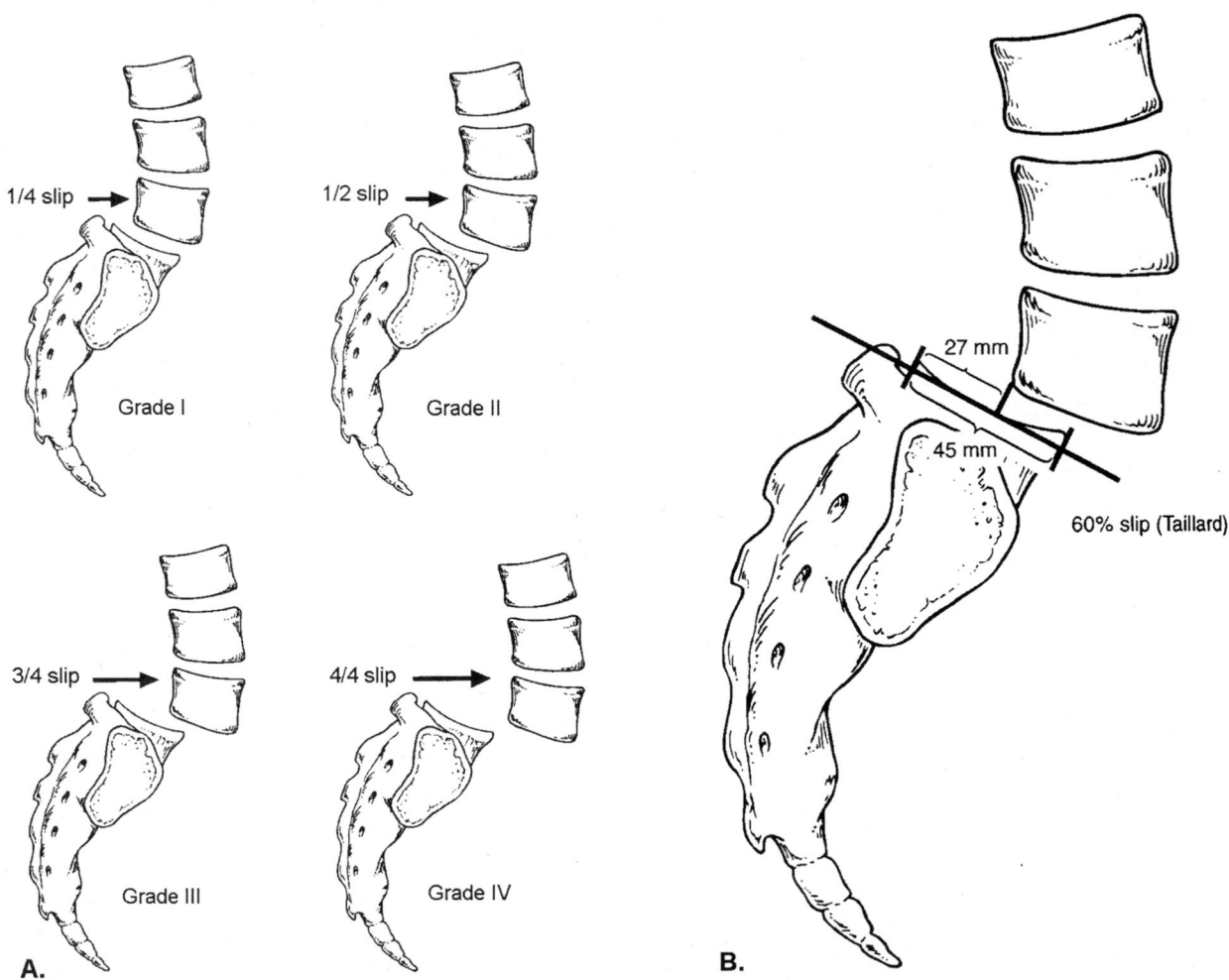

A. Curvature and Cobb measurements

Left side   T1   Right side

Highest vertebra with superior border inclined toward thoracic concavity — T4

50°

Left thoracic scoliosis

Transitional vertebra--lowest vertebra with inferior border inclined toward thoracic cavity and highest vertebra with superior border inclined toward lumbar concavity — T10

T12

L1

Right thoracolumbar scoliosis

50°

Lowest vertebra with inferior border inclined toward lumbar concavity — L4

L5

WAK

B. Right lumbar scoliosis. Note how the vertebral landmarks indicate the rotational component.

Left side   Right side

No rotation, pedicles in normal position

Spinous process

Left pedicle overlaps edge of vertebra — + Right rotation, R. pedicle slightly toward midline

Left pedicle barely visible — ++ Right rotation, R. pedicle closer to midline

Left pedicle posterior — +++ Right rotation, R. pedicle in the midline

Spinous process — ++++ Right rotation, R. pedicle beyond the midline

S_L R_R

Left side = concave side of the curvature

Right side = convex side of the curvature

FIGURE 43.11. Measurement of curvature and rotation using the Cobb method. In the Cobb method, identification of the top and bottom of each curve is most important.

1/4 slip ➡   Grade I

1/2 slip ➡   Grade II

3/4 slip ➡   Grade III

4/4 slip ➡   Grade IV

A.

27 mm

45 mm

60% slip (Taillard)

B.

FIGURE 43.12. A: Classification of spondylolisthesis using the Meyerding system. **B:** Taillard method of classifying spondylolisthesis.

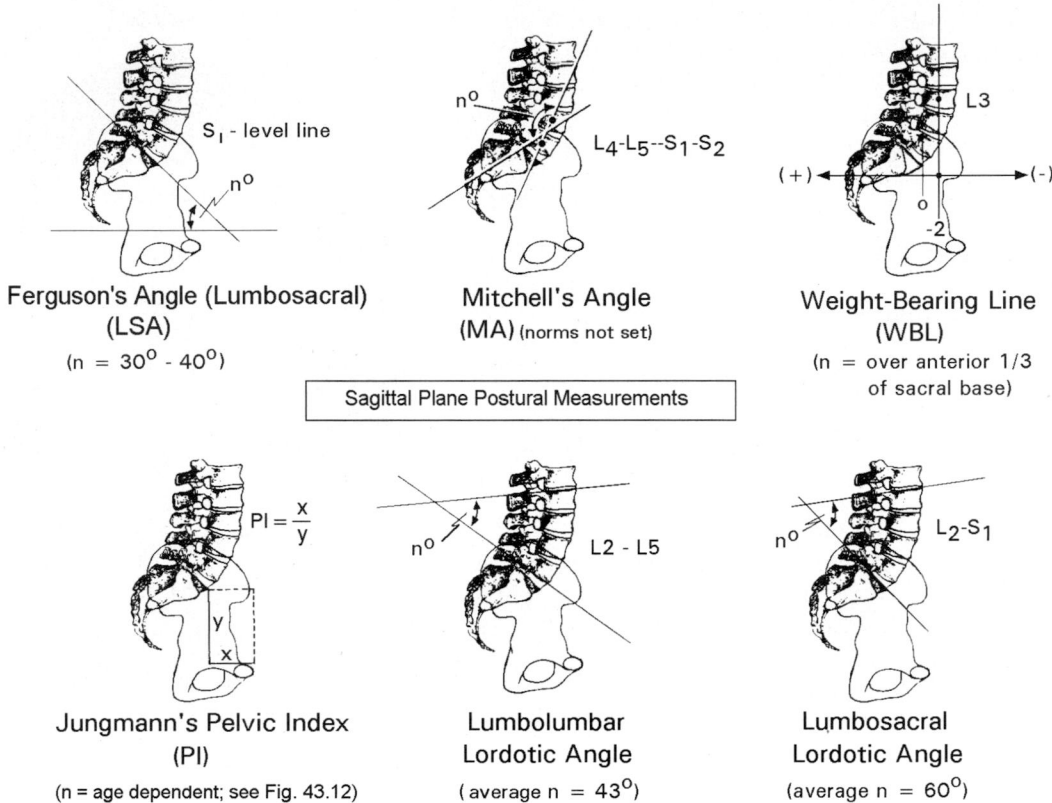

Ferguson's Angle (Lumbosacral)
(LSA)
$(n = 30^\circ - 40^\circ)$

Mitchell's Angle
(MA) (norms not set)

Weight-Bearing Line
(WBL)
$(n = $ over anterior 1/3
of sacral base)

Sagittal Plane Postural Measurements

Jungmann's Pelvic Index
(PI)
$(n = $ age dependent; see Fig. 43.12)

Lumbolumbar
Lordotic Angle
(average $n = 43^\circ$)

Lumbosacral
Lordotic Angle
(average $n = 60^\circ$)

FIGURE 43.13. Sagittal plane postural (standing) radiographic measurements and their normal ranges.

Another clinically relevant sagittal plane radiographic measurement is the Jungmann pelvic index (age-dependent normative values). This pelvic index (PI) is the ratio of measurements representing the position of the sacrum relative to the innominates. The index appears to rise as gravity overcomes the individual's homeostatic ability to resist it. The index is higher for patients with chronic low back pain (20) and for those with other elevated sagittal plane postural measurements (24). It is also elevated for athletes with high functional demand in the sagittal plane (5). The highest PI measurements are seen in people with isthmic (L5-SI) spondylolisthesis (64). For this reason, if the PI is very high and spondylolisthesis is not visualized on routine lumbopelvic x-ray views, the clinician may elect to order oblique films of the lumbosacral area to detect a spondylolytic defect at the pars interarticularis (Fig. 43.14).

Lumbo-lumbar or lumbosacral lordotic angles are objective measurements of lumbar lordosis (25). The observation of hyperlordosis is significant in the evaluation of patients with sagittal

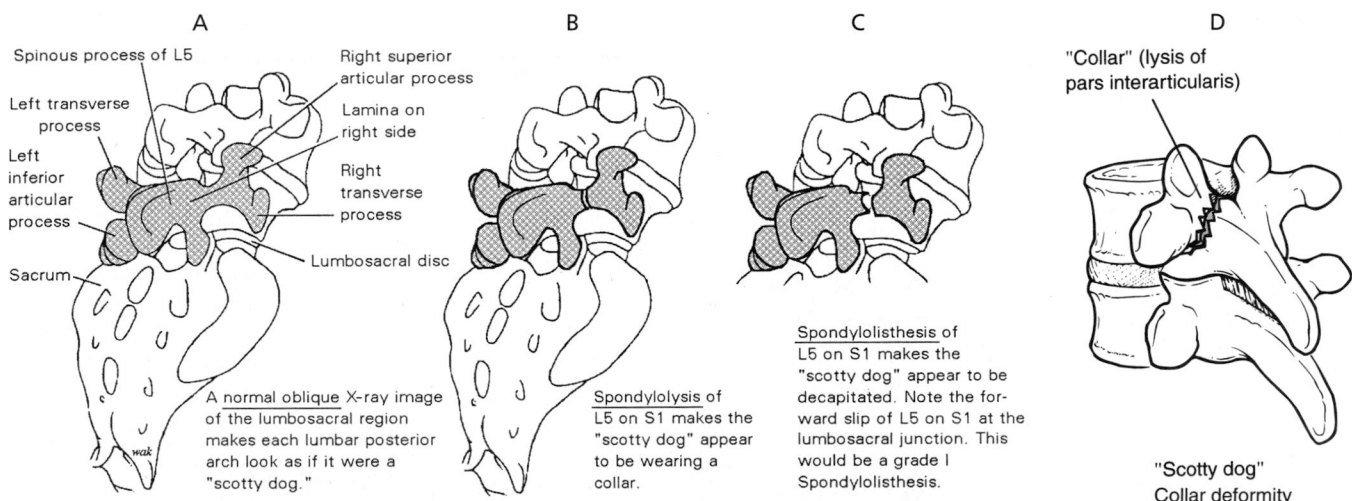

FIGURE 43.14. A: Normal 45-degree oblique radiographic view best visualizes pars interarticularis. **B:** Spondylolysis. **C:** Spondylolisthesis. **D:** Lysis pars interarticularis appearance as a collar. (From Roy S, Irvin R. *Sports Medicine: Prevention, Evaluation, Management, and Rehabilitation.* Englewood Cliffs, NJ: Prentice-Hall; 1983:280, with permission.)

plane postural problems. Some of these measurements may eventually prove to be relevant, whereas others may never add any clinical relevance. Current research by the Institute for Gravitational Strain Pathophysiology at the Kirksville College of Osteopathic Medicine is delineating these and other postural measurements that may add to the understanding of postural decompensation.

POSTURAL TREATMENT: OVERVIEW

Regardless of the planes involved, the principles used to prescribe individualized treatment plans for patients with postural decompensation do not vary significantly. Rational treatment depends on an accurate diagnosis, recognition that every postural curve has both a structural and a functional component, and the consideration of the homeostatic, structure-function characteristics of the specific patient that is being treated. Identification of dysfunctional factors, such as muscle imbalance and joint somatic dysfunction, focuses strategies for treatments designed to reduce postural stress and reverse the process of postural decompensation. Identification of structural involvement also provides insight into the patient's prognosis.

If compensatory mechanisms are overwhelmed, treatment of postural decompensation should include some combination of the following:

1. Sound *biomechanical and ergonomic education.* This includes emphasizing appropriate footwear including the reduction of high heels, promotion of functional arches, and correction of pronation. Other useful education includes proper lifting technique and dietary counseling when necessary for appropriate weight distribution.

2. Functional *orthotics* such as a heel lift, a sole lift, or a Levitor to biomechanically reverse the mechanics involved in decompensation.

3. Specific *exercise* designed first to rest and then to functionally enhance ineffective soft tissue structures.

4. *Osteopathic manipulative treatment* (OMT) addresses the somatic dysfunction that consistently and recurrently accompanies postural problems and facilitates postural compensation that will be associated with treatment intervention.

5. Injection techniques using proliferative medication (*prolotherapy*) for ligamentous laxity if other conservative modalities alone fail to restore stability.

Compliance is a must, especially in the initial phases of the program of reeducation or in the wearing of an orthotic. It can be enhanced if the patient understands the rationale behind the treatment procedures and requirements. The amount of compliance that can be expected from a person can be estimated by evaluating body unity factors including vanity, dedication, self-image, energy levels, and a number of biopsychosocial factors.

Exercise

Exercise is an often misunderstood and misused activity. Clinically, the patient needs a precise and realistic prescription for the goal, the dose, the frequency, and the duration of physical activities. In this manner, an exercise prescription can help the patient

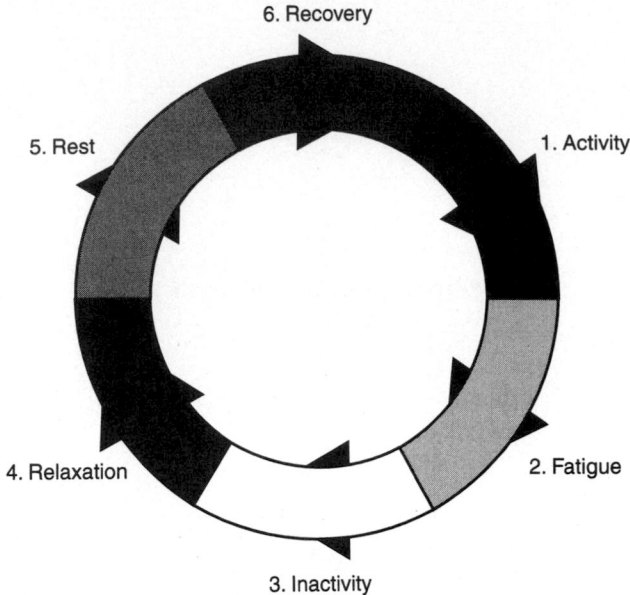

FIGURE 43.15. Bioenergetic model. (Modified from Jungmann M. *The Jungmann Concept and Technique of Antigravity Leverage.* Rangely, ME: Institute for Gravitational Strain Pathology, Inc; 1982.)

achieve rest, flexibility, strength, and endurance, depending on the desired goal. Further tissue damage may also be prevented.

Exercise prescriptions should always consider the present status of the muscles and their ability to respond to a desired goal. In general, a person with decompensated posture requires a period of rest before exercise and compensation are effective; overly stressed or strained muscles cannot effectively be exercised until they have first recovered (26). Thus, rest, medication, indirect OMT, and certain physical modalities may be necessary before beginning an individually designed exercise program; the appropriate exercise prescription for a patient with postural decompensation may be to *decrease* activities of daily living.

The bioenergetic cycle (Fig. 43.15) espoused by Jungmann (27) describes the requirement of resting the body until it is physiologically capable of resuming its postural fight against gravity. Energy expenditure throughout each day is cyclic; sequencing is important for the efficacy of the process. Postural strain increases the load in the early stages of the cycle and delays or even subverts later stages. When a person whose homeostatic reserves have been exceeded first lies down at night, it may take 30 minutes (or more) before the erector spinae and quadratus lumborum muscles relax and allow comfort in the supine position. These muscles, therefore, need to be monitored. The reduction in iliolumbar ligament tenderness and edema are indicators of when active postural exercises may be introduced to achieve strength, stability, and proprioceptive reeducation.

The exercise prescription should promote healing of strained and injured tissues before striving to accomplish any other postural goal. Two basic rules of exercise are advocated for these patients (28):

1. Avoid exercising to the point of fatigue.
2. Discontinue any exercise that causes pain until a reason for the pain is discovered.

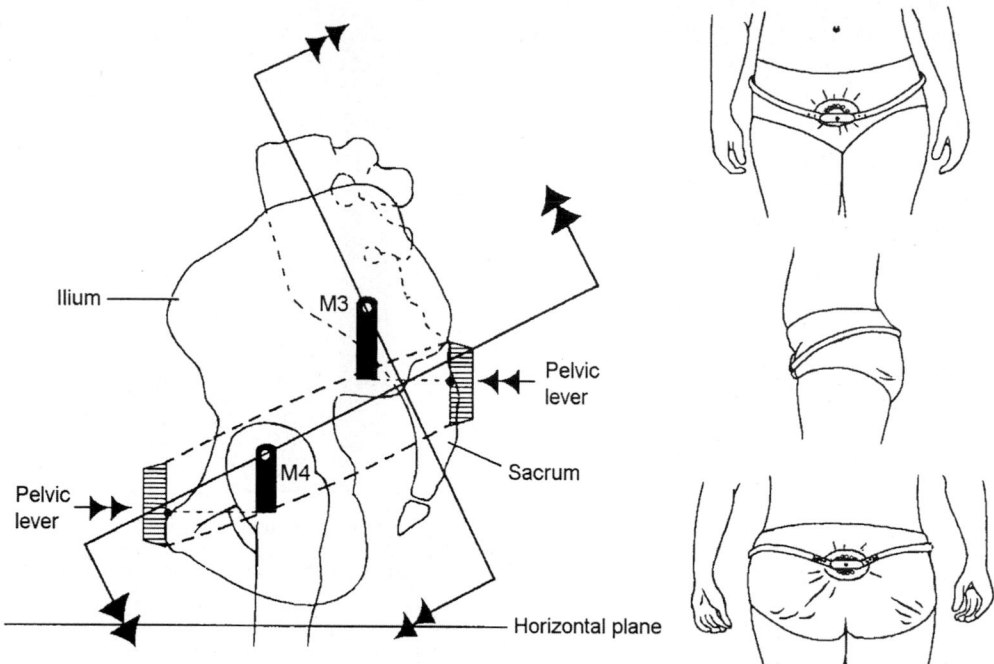

FIGURE 43.16. Pelvic lever action and Levitor®. (From Jungmann M. *The Jungmann Concept and Technique of Antigravity Leverage.* Rangely, ME: Institute for Gravitational Strain Pathology, Inc; 1982, with permission.)

Osteopathic Manipulative Treatment

OMT should be selected to improve structure-function relationships with a minimum of side effects for patients with posture-induced pathophysiologic change. Indirect method OMT is particularly useful for treating somatic dysfunction in hypermobile areas. It should be recognized that hypermobile areas may represent either primary traumatized tissue or regions of secondary compensation for other regions of restricted motion. Direct methods, physical modalities, and stretching exercises are particularly useful in regions of hypomobility. The percussion hammer technique, as was taught by Robert Fulford, DO, is clinically helpful in treatment of some chronic postural problems.

Orthotics, Braces, and Other Adjunctive Treatment

Adjunctive therapy is often necessary. Static braces are often helpful by promoting rest and healing in a region of acute strain. Chronic postural strain, however, is a situation in which the use of functional orthotics or elimination of biomechanical risk factors is required to support homeostasis. Its chronicity precludes replacing function and mandates that functions be modified. Use of static bracing in chronic situations requires careful and continuous exercise as well as care designed to prevent muscle atrophy and the patient's dependence on the static brace.

A functional orthosis, such as the Levitor®, is a more appropriate choice than a static brace for patients with chronic postural decompensation. This pelvic orthosis has been used in the United States since 1939 and is a prescription, custom-fitted device. It weighs 6 ounces and is made of a high-test aluminum alloy that transfers pressure to cushioned pads, one over the superior portion of the pubic symphysis and the other on the posterior part of the sacral apex below the S2 middle transverse axis. This orthosis was specifically designed to resist the counter-rotation of the sacrum and innominates (Fig. 43.16) that occur under the influence of the strain of gravity. It aids but does not replace the function of postural muscles, thus avoiding the dependency side effects of static bracing.

A functional orthosis is added to a patient's treatment regimen to enhance homeostatic postural mechanisms and increase efficacy. A functional orthosis is indicated in those chronic or recurrent conditions resulting from, or aggravated by, postural strain or decompensation. Its use can realistically be expected to improve the body's ability to resist strain and decompensation by altering biomechanical alignment or assisting soft tissue structures. Concomitant symptoms such as back pain, headache, fatigue, muscle imbalance, and functional visceral complaints may be relieved in a program that incorporates a functional postural orthosis, OMT, and patient education. These symptoms alone in the absence of the underlying postural cause are not a sufficient indication for the use of orthoses.

Functional orthotics may be especially indicated for patients who have had failed back surgery for chronic back pain or patients with chronic disc disease, spondylolisthesis, or who have had failed medical treatment for low back arthritic conditions. All of these structural conditions make it more difficult for the patient to functionally resist gravity.

A functional orthosis should not to be used alone. It requires systemic OMT and carefully prescribed exercise to be maximally effective. Conversely, the effects of OMT and exercise for patients with chronic postural decompensation may be greatly benefited by the addition of an orthotic device. Adjunctive use of the Levitor®, for example, has been demonstrated to improve measurable sagittal plane risk factors and to reduce posture-related low back pain (29,30). In a 1985 study involving 109 patients with recalcitrant chronic low back pain 30% of patients were found to improve with manipulation and postural exercise alone. When a functional orthosis (Levitor®) was added to this program, 76% improved. The likelihood of improved results is achieved by decreasing functional demand on postural structures, modifying biomechanical risk factors, and allowing postural homeostatic mechanisms to operate under more optimal conditions.

In summary, numerous modalities are used to assist the body's postural response to gravity. An individually designed program includes a carefully selected combination of patient education, OMT, exercise, and functional orthotics. All of these are aimed at modifying the structure-function relationship and enhancing the body's ability to self-heal. Postural balancing therefore requires an understanding of the biomechanical nature and functional anatomy of each patient and a full understanding of osteopathic philosophy.

CORONAL AND HORIZONTAL POSTURAL CONDITIONS

Scoliosis and rotoscoliosis are postural diagnoses with origins dating back to ancient Greece. References to the existence of leg length inequality in 90% of the population have appeared in the medical literature since the latter half of the 1800s (31–33). John Hilton specifically mentioned lift therapy as a treatment for this problem in 1863:

> Thus I have seen many patients wearing spinal supports, in order to correct a lateral curvature when the deformity might have and has been subsequently, corrected by placing within the shoe or boot a piece of cork thick enough to compensate for the shortness of the less well developed limb (34).

The osteopathic profession began studies on the diagnosis and treatment of coronal plane asymmetry in 1921, when Hoskins and Schwab introduced the standing postural x-ray view (35,36). A compilation of many of the classic osteopathic articles discussing diagnosis, clinical impact, and treatment of this and other postural subjects can be found in the *1983 Yearbook of the American Academy of Osteopathy, Postural Balance and Imbalance* (23).

SHORT LEG SYNDROME

Within the profession, the term "short leg syndrome" is recognized as a misnomer. This text, however, will continue to refer to short leg syndrome because of historical precedence. Regardless of the name, the actual cause of the condition may not be related to the actual length of the legs at all. It is called a syndrome because it is associated with a variety of biomechanical findings and symptoms.

An unlevel sacral base is the clinically relevant element in this so-called short leg syndrome. Because a short lower extremity

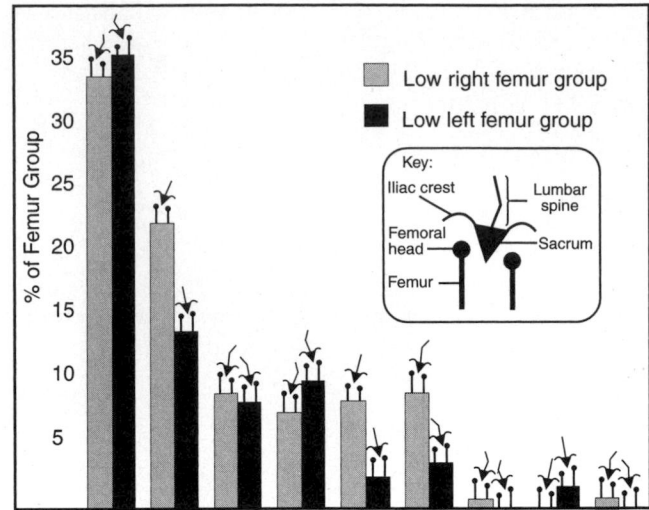

FIGURE 43.17. Frequency distribution of lumbosacral relationships to unlevel femoral head heights. *N* = 738. (From Kirksville College of Osteopathic Medicine, Kirksville, MO, with permission.)

usually results in an unlevel sacral base, the spine compensates by changing its spinal curvatures. Subsequently, the person often must stand and walk differently. If the sacral base is unlevel for any reason, the innominates often rotate to compensate. This creates the appearance of a functionally short lower extremity. In either case, the most common spinal response is development of a rotoscoliosis with side bending of the most caudal curve toward the side that is opposite the low sacral base, or short leg. Atypical patterns do occur, however, and provide clinically challenging cases (Fig.43.17).

Diagnosis

Compensatory measures are sometimes so good that any single landmark measurement may fail to provide a true and accurate diagnosis. Neither alignment of spinous processes nor level of iliac crests is a good single indicator of sacral base unleveling or short leg syndrome. Anterior superior iliac spine (ASIS) or hip-to-ankle measurements using a tape measure are also inaccurate (37,38). Comparison of the levels of the medial malleoli in the supine position is similarly inaccurate or misleading (39). The greater trochanters in the standing position are somewhat more helpful clinically but can be in error when unilateral coxa varus or coxa valgus is present (40). Therefore, it is difficult and not always accurate to make a diagnosis based on clinical findings alone. In one study of standing patients with known radiographic leg length inequality, the wrong extremity was identified as being short in 13% of the clinical observations; more than half of the 196 clinical estimates of leg length were incorrect by more than $^3/_{16}$ of an inch (41).

Recurrent somatic dysfunction of the pelvis, spine, cranium, or myofascial structures may also be a clue that the sacral base is unlevel or that a short leg is present. Soft tissue involvement with respect to the compensation occurring in the short leg syndrome is particularly common and a cause of many patient complaints. Tissues on the concavity shorten and demonstrate increased electromyographic activity (42,43). Tissues on the convex side lengthen. Patients with coronal plane postural imbalance develop tight abductors on one side and tight thigh adductors on the contralateral side. Associated horizontal plane imbalance often results in tight hamstrings on one side and tight rectus femoris on the other thigh.

The iliolumbar ligament on the side of the convexity of the lumbopelvic curve is often the first structure to react to added stress in the lumbosacral area. The iliolumbar ligament is pain-sensitive. The point of maximal tenderness to palpation is typically located over the attachments of the iliolumbar ligament at the iliac or L4 or L5 transverse processes. When stressed, it often refers pain around the ipsilateral side to the groin, and sometimes into the testicle or the labia and the upper medial thigh (Fig. 43.7) (44). The pain may be mistaken for arthritis of the hip, greater trochanteric bursitis, or even an inguinal hernia.

The sacroiliac ligaments on the side of the convexity may also become stressed and tender to palpation and may refer pain down the lateral side of the leg. Unilateral sciatica and hip pain, as well as pain over the greater trochanter however, are more often expressed on the long leg side. Numerous postural muscles are strained, and significant physiologic changes related to segmental facilitation have been documented. Subsequently, there may be visceral dysfunction related to increased sympathetic hyperactivity coming from spinal crossover areas located between T1 and L2.

Before definitive diagnosis of a patient's posture, a thorough OMT should be directed to all somatic dysfunction. It is extremely important not to overlook sacral or innominate shear somatic dysfunctions. After OMT, the presence of a positive standing flexion test coexisting with a negative seated flexion test should raise the suspicion that lower extremity influences, such as a short lower extremity, are affecting the function of the sacroiliac joint and the patient's posture (45).

When the spine is as mobile as possible and any nonphysiologic (shear) somatic dysfunctions have been removed, it is a good idea to obtain a standard standing postural x-ray series (see Chapter 42). After first removing the patient's somatic dysfunction, this x-ray series primarily portrays structural data associated with the best homeostatic compensation possible by the patient at the time. These standardized standing postural x-ray images can then be used to measure coronal plane values accurately, including the following:

- Iliac crest heights
- Femoral head heights
- Sacral base unleveling
- Degree, location, and type of scoliotic compensatory curvatures

When reading the x-ray image (Fig. 43.18) obtained by standard methods, remember that there is still potentially a 2-mm human error in measurement. This can occur even with flawless technique by the radiologic technician and perfect patient cooperation. There can also be up to a 25% bony magnification (distortion) (46,101).

Compensatory changes such as innominate rotations, pelvic rotation, and changes in the LSA may alter the x-ray appearance.

This can misrepresent the extent of the patient's actual problem. For these reasons, a leg length difference of less than 5 mm may not be treated unless the patient has other clinically relevant complaints and risk factors. Conversely, the desire to attain "peak physical performance" may be an indication for treating a patient in this case. Patterns of imbalance recorded along the spine may be caused by as little as a $1/16$ of an inch (1.5 mm) difference in leg length. Clinical symptoms can occur in these cases, including low back pain (19,47).

Lift Therapy

Typically, treatment of the short leg syndrome involves lifting the heel of the leg on the side of the depressed sacral base. This is especially true if there is a compensatory curvature that side bends to the side opposite the short leg. In the less common situation where the curve has its concavity toward the side of the short leg, it may be necessary to lift the side of the long leg. This first effects a change in the lumbar scoliosis and also relieves some of the pelvic and lumbar strain (48). The lift on the long leg side is later reduced to begin lifting the depressed side of the unlevel sacral base.

Heel lift treatment within the osteopathic profession is always combined with OMT and is usually not attempted until after an appropriate trial of OMT. The rationale for both was clearly implied by Harrison Fryette:

> In the average case I do not attempt a correction until I have mobilized the lumbar joints and established rotation in them; furthermore, if this region cannot be rotated toward the midline, the lift will not do what it is intended of it, for the correction will not take place in the lumbar region—the spine higher up will compensate by increasing its curve and only more trouble will result (49).

OMT may alleviate a functional condition that presents as an apparent short leg syndrome. In the situation in which lift therapy is indicated, OMT prepares the somatic tissues to accept the realignment needed in response to the newly established sacral base level.

Whenever lift therapy is initiated, osteopathic physicians consider the implications of postural realignment and reeducation, which must take place throughout the entire body. For many reasons, the initial amount of lift selected is rarely the full amount needed. In most cases, compensation and decompensation have occurred over a period of time, leading to shortening and fibrosis of soft tissues, bony remodeling, and regional somatic dysfunction. The easiest but least sensitive guideline used by clinicians is to select an initial lift that is one-third to one-half of the measured sacral base difference.

Attempts to formulate specific guidelines to better quantify the amount of lift are best appreciated by studying the writings of David Heilig (50). Heilig found that one-third to one-half the measured sacral base unleveling was too much initial lift in selected clinical situations. He developed a formula (50) (Table 43.2) that considered the amount of lift to be directly proportional to the measured sacral base unleveling and inversely proportional to host factors such as the age, duration of the condition, and amount of compensation or adaptation acquired by the body.

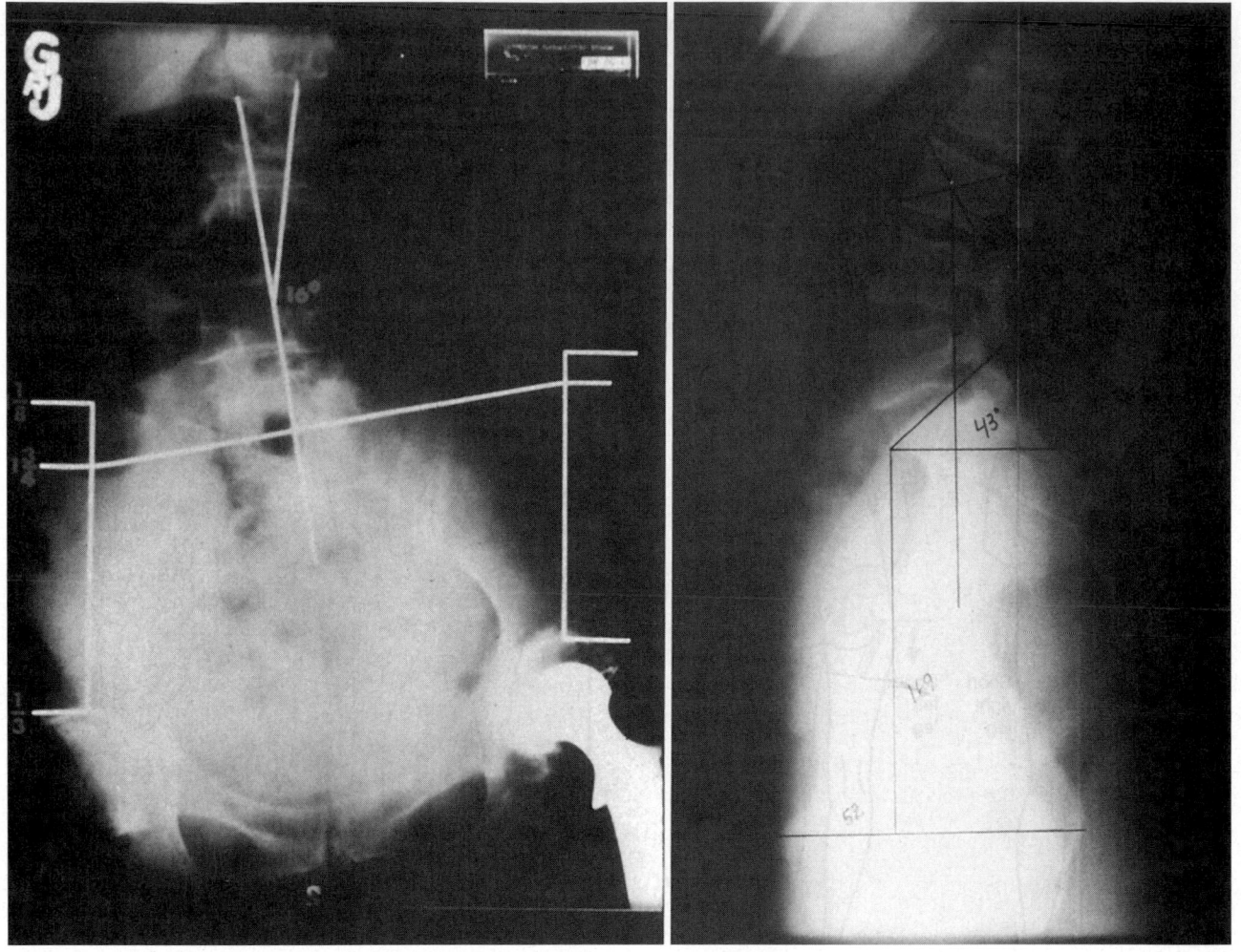

FIGURE 43.18. X-ray image marked for coronal **(A)** and horizontal **(B)** plane measurements. Ideal values would be no side-to-side unleveling of any of these landmarks and no pelvic rotation.

Heilig offered examples of patients who all had a $1/2$-inch sacral base unleveling but who, based on the formula, would receive different initial lifts (Table 43.3).

One of the safest protocols taught at many of the colleges of osteopathic medicine is less complicated than the Heilig formula yet sensitive to individual host factors. It employs conservative rules of thumb that can later be modified by the physician's clinical experience and judgment. This protocol is designed to avoid any unexpected flare-ups of pain or somatic dysfunction that can occur if lift therapy is introduced too rapidly or if it exceeds the capability of the body to realign in response to the changes being made in the sacral base level.

TABLE 43.2. THE HEILIG FORMULA

The Heilig formula suggests that the initial lift can be calculated as follows:

L < [SBU]/[D + C]

L, lift required; SBU, sacral base unleveling; D, duration; C, compensation. Duration allotted as: (D = 1), 0–10 years; (D = 2), 10–30 years; (D = 3), 30+ years. Compensation allotted as: (C = 0), none observed; (C = 1), rotation of lumbar vertebrae into convexity of compensatory side-bending; (C = 2), wedging of the vertebrae, altered size of facets, horizontal osseous developments from endplates, and/or spurring.

The following are only guidelines for the application of conservative lift treatment and must be adapted to each patient according to their individual evaluation and response (51).

- If lift therapy is required and if the patient is considered to be a fragile patient (arthritic, osteoporotic, elderly, having significant acute pain, etc.), begin with a $1/16$-inch lift and lift no faster than $1/16$ of an inch every 2 weeks.
- If the spine is flexible and no more than mild-to-moderate strain is noted in the myofascial system, begin with a $1/8$-inch

TABLE 43.3. PATIENTS WITH SAME SACRAL BASE LEVELING BUT RECEIVING DIFFERENT LIFTS

Case 1: Following fracture, minimal duration, no compensatory changes
  L = [SBU]/[D + C] = $1/2''$/[0 + 1] = $1/2''$
Case 2: Patient age 35, injured in early youth, minimal compensation
  L = [SBU]/[D + C] = $1/2''$/[2 + 1] = $1/2''$/3 = $1/6''$
Case 3: Patient age 75, injured in youth, spurring, horizontal endplate development, rotation is marked
  L = [SBU]/[D + C] = $1/2''$/[3 + 2] = $1/2''$/5 = $1/10''$
Case 4: Patient age 26, polio affecting right leg in youth, minimal compensatory change
  L = [SBU]/[D + C] = $1/2''$/[2 + 0] = $1/2''$/2 = $1/4''$

lift and lift at a rate no faster than $^1/_{16}$ of an inch per week, or $^1/_8$ of an inch every 2 weeks.

■ If there was a recent sudden loss of leg length on one side, as might occur following fracture or a recent hip prosthesis, and the patient had a level sacral base before the fracture or surgery, lift the full fractional amount that was lost.

Regardless of the method used to select the amount of the initial lift, certain other guidelines should be followed for optimum clinical results.

■ Because of magnification, measurement error, and compensatory changes, the final lift height in a chronic short leg syndrome may only be one-half to three-fourths of the shortness in that leg measured by the standard standing x-ray method.
■ When a proper lift has eventually been reached and there are no pelvic or lower extremity somatic dysfunctions, the standing flexion test should become negative. If a repeat x-ray image is desired, it should be taken using the same radiographic protocol and parameters that were used in the initial x-ray series, but with the shoes on and the lift in place.

Guidelines used in lift treatment are not absolute rules. One aspect of the art of medicine is an appreciation of the concerns that patients have about cost, cosmetic appearance, and convenience. Ideally, the shoe is rebuilt with every increment of lift to prevent alteration of foot mechanics and introduction of unwanted pelvic rotation. Few patients, however, would agree with this approach. The following guidelines emphasizing clinical tolerances can be pragmatically used in lift treatment. If problems arise, reducing the tolerances or insisting on the ideal may be necessary.

■ The true height of a lift is measured from the bottom of the lift to a point where the calcaneal bone strikes the lift; it is not measured at the posterior edge of the lift.
■ Up to and including $^1/_4$-inch of replaceable lift can be used inside of the shoe before the shoe no longer fits well.
■ Up to and including a total of a $^1/_2$-inch lift can be placed between the heel of the patient's foot and the floor before foot mechanics are significantly disturbed.
■ As a heel is progressively lifted, there is an increased tendency toward pelvic rotation, muscle imbalance, and alteration of foot mechanics.

Application of these principles to change the relative leg length by $^1/_2$ inch may result in:

■ a $^1/_4$-inch lift being placed inside the shoe and $^1/_4$ inch added to the heel of that shoe
■ $^1/_2$ inch added to the heel of one shoe
■ $^1/_4$ inch added to one sole and $^1/_4$ inch removed from the opposite sole (50–52).

Many other combinations exist within these general guidelines, permitting the osteopathic practitioner the latitude to balance nonphysical factors (such as vanity and cost) with those related to posture.

Any increase in height beyond the $^1/_2$-inch heel lift must be added to the heel and also to the anterior half-sole of the shoe (Fig. 43.19). This principle preserves the relationship of the heel to the forefoot by maintaining a certain normal angle.

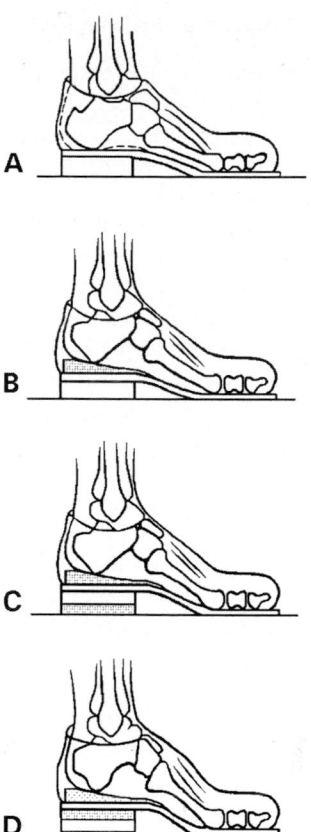

FIGURE 43.19. Principles of lift therapy. Heel lift measurements made at midcalcaneal line. **A:** Foot in a typical shoe. **B:** Heel lift in place. Maximum left in shoe is $^1/_4$ inch. **C:** If more lift is needed, add to outside heel. **D:** If more than $^1/_2$ inch is required, or to create minimal disturbance of foot mechanics, the entire sole can be lifted.

Studies (4,47) indicate that an 80% reduction in subjective pain and other posture-related symptoms could be expected as a result of properly balancing the sacral base with lift therapy to within 1 mm of levelness.

The physician must try to balance the weight of both shoes, especially if large lifts are required. If a big lift is needed, cork material between the shoe and the heel may be necessary to reduce the weight being added to one side. In some cases, small lead weights may be added to the other shoe to maintain balance.

OMT helps the patient's spine to compensate better for the new posture that results from lift therapy for a short leg.

Compressive force makes bone grow faster. A lift under a growing child's short leg may be expected to stimulate faster growth in that leg. The physician must therefore closely monitor leg lengths when using lift therapy for a child. The height of the lift must be adjusted according to clinical responses and the results observed on follow-up x-ray studies. In growing athletes, alternating lower extremity growth parameters have been reported (50). This has prompted the clinical recommendation to check the pelvic and extremity levels at regular intervals. Fryette even remarked: "In the last 15 years I have added lifts to the short side in many cases under the age of fourteen and in every case that I have kept under my observation for some time I have been astonished to find that the legs grew to the same length" (53).

Anterior Lift Therapy: Pelvic Rotation

The clinical use of anterior sole lifts (in distinction from heel lifts) or the combination of an anterior lift in one shoe and/or a heel lift in the opposite shoe to affect posture in the horizontal plane has largely been explored by Ross Pope and James Carlson (54). An increase in the sole height of a shoe encourages rotation of the pelvis toward that same side. A unilateral heel lift rotates the pelvis to a lesser degree and rotates it away from the lifted side (51). Because this method is new, few clinical trials have been performed. The predominance of clinical experience, however, suggests the following guidelines, which are adapted to each individual patient's evaluation and response.

Anterior lift therapy rotates the pelvis toward the same side; heel lifts may rotate the pelvis away from the lift side. Treatment of both planes simultaneously is often warranted, as side bending and rotation are biomechanically linked motions. A heel lift pushes that side of the pelvis anteriorly in the horizontal plane because the lift is behind the axis of motion (i.e., rotates the pelvis away from the side of the heel lift). Anterior sole lifts are in front of the axis and so they rotate that side of the pelvis posteriorly in a horizontal plane (i.e., rotate the pelvis toward the side of the sole lift) (Fig. 43.20).

In the treatment of pelvic rotation assuming coexistent sacral base unleveling, follow these principles:

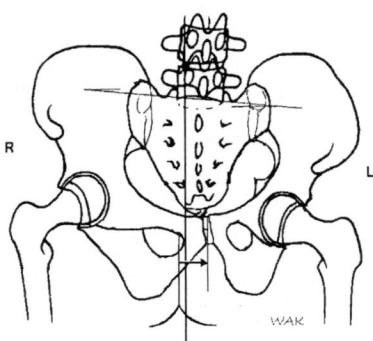

With lifts in the heel or in the opposite half sole, the pelvis can be derotated.

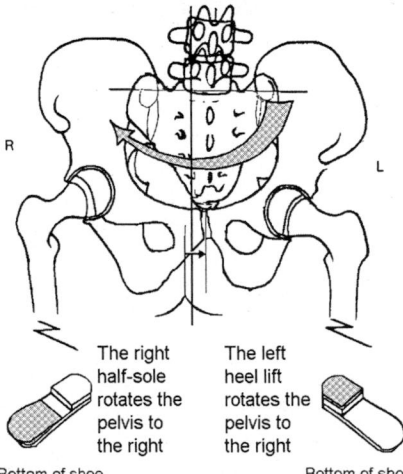

The right half-sole rotates the pelvis to the right   The left heel lift rotates the pelvis to the right

Bottom of shoe   Bottom of shoe

FIGURE 43.20. Right anterior half-sole lift and/or left heel lift rotating pelvis to the right.

For pelvic rotation less than 5 mm: Usually it is not necessary to treat a pelvic rotation less than 5 mm. However, if the sacral base unleveling is treated with heel lifts, this should be done according to the principles outlined for coronal plane postural balancing. Recheck to determine if any unwanted pelvic rotation occurs secondary to the heel lift therapy.

For pelvic rotation of 5 to 10 mm: For pelvic rotation of 5 to 10 mm, both sacral base (coronal plane) and rotational (horizontal plane) components are treated simultaneously. Begin with appropriate $1/8$-inch anterior and heel lifts, progressively increasing in $1/8$-inch increments every 2 weeks.

For pelvic rotation greater than 10 mm: Pelvic rotations more than 10 mm should first be treated with an anterior (sole) lift of $1/4$ inch, and the postural study then rechecked before attempting heel lifts. Thereafter, sacral base unleveling and pelvic rotation are treated simultaneously with 1/8-inch incremental changes in anterior (sole) and heel lifts every 2 weeks.

Lift Summary

Lift therapy is initiated to help the body return to better structural alignment and function. Properly managed, the patient's postural mechanisms are reeducated toward the ideal posture. Balancing mechanisms have been shown to become more precise as evidenced by graphic center-of-gravity plots before and after appropriate lift therapy. Paraspinal muscle tension and various spinal physiologic parameters become more symmetrically normalized, and patient symptoms throughout the body are dramatically reduced.

SCOLIOSIS (ROTOSCOLIOSIS)

Ten in every 200 children (10:200) develop scoliosis by the age of 10 to 15 years; 1 in every 200 (1:200) has clinical symptoms related to the curvatures. Boys and girls are equally affected, but the curvatures in girls are 3 to 5 times more likely to progress and produce subjective symptoms.

Curvatures are more likely to progress during times of rapid bone growth. Most cases (75% to 90%) of scoliosis in children are discovered between the ages of 10 and 15 because of widespread screening programs and because this is the time when rapid bone growth occurs.

Diagnosis

Scoliosis primarily affects the coronal plane. It is officially named according to the direction of the convexity of the curve. A curve that is side bent to the left is called a right scoliosis because the convexity of the curve is toward the right.

Scoliosis may be classified by its reversibility, severity, cause, or location.

Classification: Reversibility

Scoliosis can be functional or structural. A simple physical examination technique to assess the proportion of functional to structural scoliosis can be accomplished by standing behind a

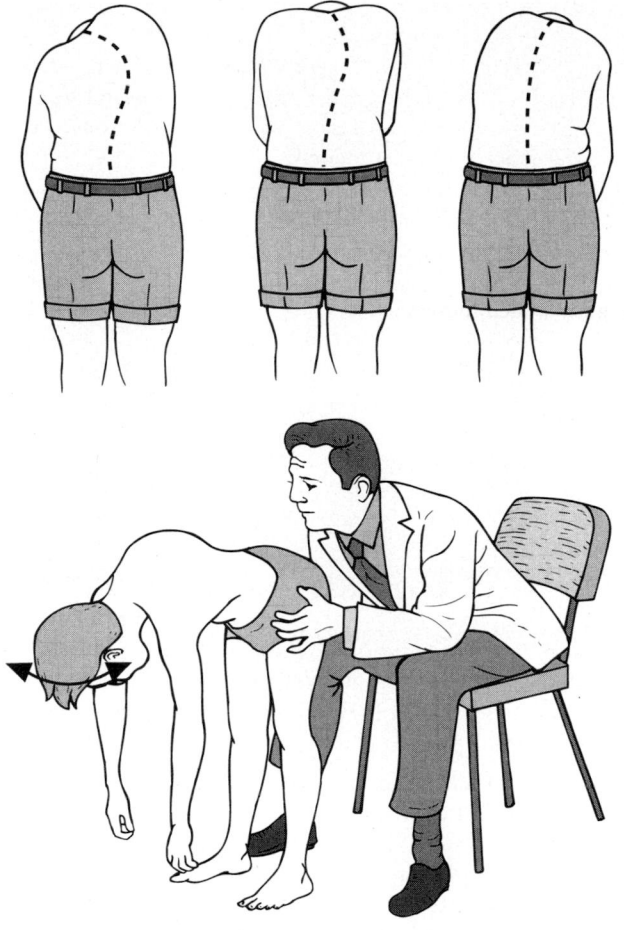

FIGURE 43.21. Assessment of structural or functional scoliosis.

patient (Fig. 43.21). The patient bends forward until maximal rib hump appears on horizon. With that much of the body forward bending, the patient swings the upper body first left, then right, while the clinician observes the functional ability of rib hump to reduce. The amount of rib hump remaining during this maneuver indicates the associated structural scoliotic component. Functional scoliotic curves go away with side bending, rotation, or forward bending. If they remain in the body too long, they may become structural (55). Structural scoliotic curves are fixed curves that do not reduce with side bending, rotation, or lift therapy.

Classification: Severity

There are four degrees of severity. The normal case shows no scoliosis. A curve of 5 to 15 degrees is classified as mild (Fig. 43.22). Moderate scoliosis curves measure 20 to 45 degrees. Severe scoliosis has a curve of more than 50 degrees. Severe scoliosis affects structure and systemic function. A thoracic curve of more than 50 degrees compromises respiratory function. A thoracic curve of more than 75 degrees compromises cardiovascular function.

Classification: Cause

The following causes are listed according to decreasing frequency.

Idiopathic

This diagnosis accounts for 70% to 90% of scoliotic curves. By definition, the term "idiopathic" implies that there is no known reason for this type of scoliosis to occur. Osteopathic physicians believe that some of these may be explained as compensatory curves occurring because of an unlevel sacral (47) or cranial base (56). In those cases where such a biomechanical basis exists for the development of scoliosis, a diagnosis of an idiopathic scoliosis is inappropriate. Other clinicians have implicated sagittal plane biomechanics in the genesis and progression of different types of idiopathic scoliotic patterns (7). Better understanding of scoliosis may further reduce the number of cases classified as idiopathic.

Congenital

Of congenital cases, 75% are progressive. This classification is the second most common type according to cause of scoliosis.

Acquired

Acquired scoliosis may result from the following conditions:

- Osteomalacia
- Response to inflammation or irradiation
- Sciatic irritability
- Psoas syndrome
- Healed leg fracture
- Following a hip prosthesis

Obviously, if a short leg syndrome is documented as the reason for the patient's scoliosis, this should be reclassified as an acquired scoliosis.

Classification: Location

Various locations of scoliosis are given here according to decreasing frequency (Fig. 43.23). Regions involved in scoliosis may be balanced or unbalanced. Unbalanced curves are more likely to decompensate, while balanced curves are subject to degeneration at crossovers.

Double Major Scoliosis

These are balanced curves but they are subject to degeneration at the crossover regions of the spine (see Glossary at the end of the textbook). This is the most common scoliosis, with a thoracic and lumbar combination being the most frequent.

Single Thoracic Scoliosis

Cosmetically, this curve is rather noticeable. It is usually side-bent right and rotated left, producing a left paraspinal rib hump. If this type of curve should progress, it could compromise the function of the heart or lungs. It is the second most common scoliosis.

Single Lumbar Scoliosis

This curve is associated with arthritic change. It is the third most common scoliosis.

Junctional Thoracolumbar Scoliosis

This single curve scoliosis often results in structural (arthritic) change because it tends to be a longer curve that functionally overstresses the spine. It is not a common scoliosis.

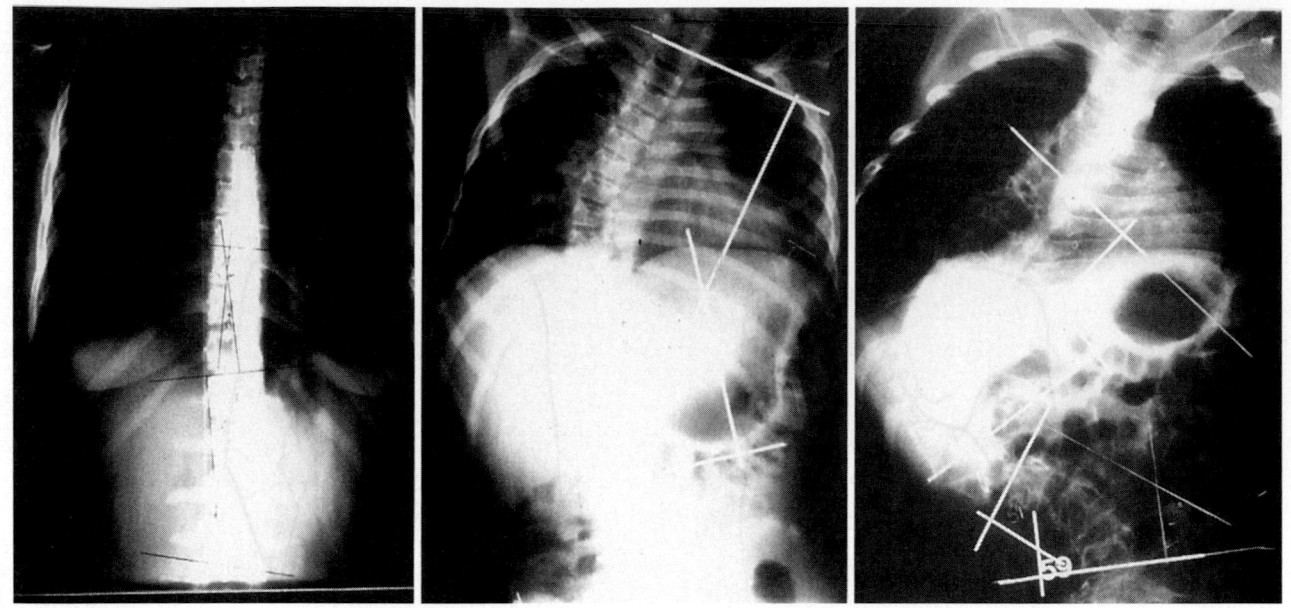

A,B   C

FIGURE 43.22. Curve patterns in idiopathic scoliosis. **A:** Mild (14 degrees and 15 degrees). **B:** Moderate (38 degrees). **C:** Severe (59 degrees and 85 degrees). Assessment of scoliotic severity defined by Cobb angle measurements (see Fig. 43.11) for each portion of coronal plane curve. Classification system quoted allows a 5-degree gray zone between severity classes.

Junctional Cervicothoracic Scoliosis

This scoliosis is very uncommon.

Symptoms and Screening

Children with scoliosis are usually asymptomatic, yet by checking them between the ages of 10 to 15 years when they are experiencing rapid bone growth, the scoliosis can be found. For this reason, school children should be routinely screened for scoliosis.

An adolescent with scoliosis is also often asymptomatic and therefore would be overlooked unless a spinal screening examination was performed. The patient may have only noticed that clothing does not fit properly.

As the person gets older, several symptoms bring the scoliotic patient to the physician. These include:

■ Arthritic symptoms
■ Backaches
■ Chest pains
■ Neck aches
■ Headaches
■ Symptoms of organ dysfunction

Physicians casually looking for scoliosis may miss a curve of up to 35 degrees. Careful screening with physical examination alone should pick up all types of scoliosis more than 10 degrees.

In the standing position, the space around the patient's body is analyzed, especially in the arm and waist area. Observe whether one hand hangs by the side and the other hand lays on or over the thigh. Look at the levelness of the occipital, shoulder, iliac crest, PSIS, and trochanteric planes (Fig. 43.10). Run your fingers along the spinous processes from top to bottom. Have the patient forward bend and observe for an asymmetric "hump" along the horizon of vision. Its presence would indicate rotoscoliotic

deformity with rotation to that side and side bending of the spine to the side opposite the hump.

If spinal curvature is found, have the patient bend over to that area of the spine and determine if the asymmetry goes away with side bending toward the side of the rib hump (Fig. 43.21). Check the patient for conditions that could give the appearance of a short leg, such as sacral shear somatic dysfunction on that side. If you find somatic dysfunction, it can be corrected with manipulation. Recheck following OMT for a lower extremity induced postural problems.

Radiographic Measurement

If there is continued recurrence of a scoliotic curve, provide OMT until there is good mobilization of the spine and then obtain a standardized standing postural x-ray image (see Chapter 42). The x-ray image provides the quantitative data to determine:

■ Bony pathology
■ Type and severity of spinal curvatures
■ Amount of sacral base unleveling
■ Femoral head and iliac crest levelness

Scoliotic curvatures are measured from the radiographs by the Cobb method (Fig. 43.11). The same vertebrae used to define the top and the bottom of the curve are used for future Cobb measurements to see if the curve is progressing. Scoliosis often increases rapidly during the growth spurt of adolescence. Take an x-ray image of the hands and epiphyses and obtain a bone age for those patients who have significant scoliotic progression. For females, the scoliosis is more likely to undergo a rapid progression. Significant progression of the curve is considered to be occurring if, on a second standardized postural x-ray taken within

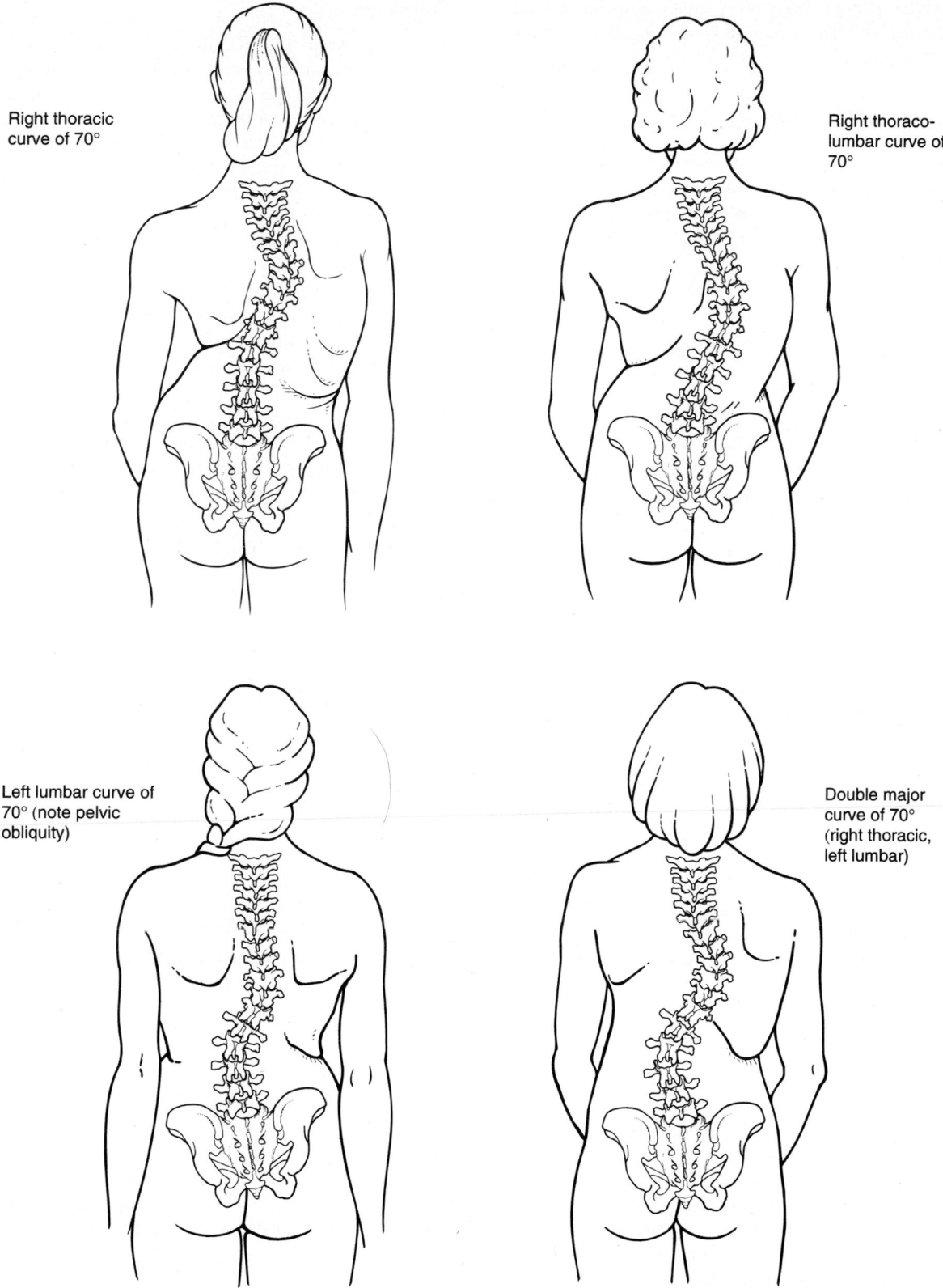

Right thoracic
curve of 70°

Right thoraco-
lumbar curve of
70°

Left lumbar curve of
70° (note pelvic
obliquity)

Double major
curve of 70°
(right thoracic,
left lumbar)

FIGURE 43.23. Curve patterns in idiopathic types of scoliosis classified by location.

5 months of the first one, there is a 5-degree or greater increase in the curvature. The Cobb method is used to classify scoliosis by severity (Fig. 43.22).

Treatment of Rotoscoliosis

Appropriate treatment protocols are based on classification of the scoliosis, taking into consideration factors affecting potential compliance. The treatment for scoliosis according to its severity follows these general guidelines (51).

For mild scoliosis, use:

- OMT
- Konstantin exercises
- Functional orthotics
- Patient and family education

For moderate scoliosis, use:

- OMT
- Konstantin exercises
- Patient and family education
- Bracing
- (Electrical stimulation—debatable efficacy)

For severe scoliosis, consider surgery and adjunctive measures, including those listed for moderate scoliosis.

Anyone with scoliosis of more than 15 to 20 degrees, with progression of curvature, or with intractable low back pain in spite of adequate conservative treatment measures, should be referred to a physician who specializes in the treatment of this condition.

The goals of treatment are to obtain flexibility and improved balance of the spine. Decide what can be improved and then correct the primary cause or at least prevent the scoliosis from progressing. Postpone fusions as long as possible without endangering function or the patient's life. Osteopathic manipulation is a definite part of the management of a patient with scoliosis. The person with scoliosis must be able to compensate for the new posture that is introduced by the treatment methods used to prevent progression or reduce the severity of the curvatures.

Osteopathic Manipulative Treatment

When structural scoliosis is present, the goal of direct manipulation is to optimize the function of the existing structure. It is not primarily intended to straighten the curvatures. Treatment should remove joint somatic dysfunction but should also include improvement of the general range of body motion through soft tissue, fascial releases, and indirect treatments. Stretch the lumbosacral tissues and institute exercises to reduce the LSA and strengthen the psoas and abdominal muscles. After structural strains are allowed to heal, introduce Konstantin exercises.

Orthopedic appliances, orthotics, braces, and electrical stimulation may also be used in the management program. These adjunctive modalities were conceived to support, align, or prevent deformity and may stabilize function of a hypermobile part of the body. Braces are more effective if the scoliosis is moderate, if the spine is mobile, and if the spine still has not fully matured.

Braces

The Milwaukee brace (Fig. 43.24) was introduced in 1945 and has been the standard for scoliotic bracing for many years. It is individually fitted and easy to prescribe, but it is also hard to wear and is costly. It is worn 23 hours a day with only 1 hour allowed out of the brace for applying skin care. This brace is used in a growing patient with 20- to 40-degree curves. It works to control the scoliotic (lateral) curves until the spine matures, which is generally around age 21.

It is necessary to exercise the muscles that are supported by static braces or appliances. Studies suggest that even for patients with a good reduction in the Cobb measurements, after a few years their curves return to approximately the extent present at the time that the brace was introduced.

An alternative brace for some patients with scoliosis is the Boston brace (Fig. 43.25). This brace is made of plastic and is designed to work on deformities such as lordosis and rotation as well as scoliosis. The Boston brace can be used only if the apex of the curve is below T10. In these particular patients, it is helpful in addressing postural curves in all three cardinal planes.

Electrical Stimulation

Electrical stimulation was introduced in the 1970s. It was applied to the convexity of the curve and may be considered when the curve is in the thoracic region, it measures 10 to 40 degrees, and the spine is flexible. This concept enjoyed some degree of popularity but is not often used today. Its efficacy is debatable. If electrical stimulation is applied to a patient's lumbar curve, it increases the lumbar lordosis.

Surgery

Surgical fusion is performed only in 1 of every 1,000 cases of scoliosis. It is usually considered for patients with progressing scoliotic curves at 45 to 50 degrees to prevent the heart and lung complications that accompany curvatures over 50 degrees. The placement of stainless steel Harrington rods (Fig. 43.26) and spinal fusion is an extensive surgery. The mechanical power of the body is dramatically demonstrated by the propensity of the rods to become stressed and break, requiring another extensive surgery to replace them.

SAGITTAL PLANE DISORDERS

Posture-related disorders in the sagittal plane include those defined by their lordotic and kyphotic curves; those defined by their distinctive pattern of somatic dysfunctions including muscle imbalance and trigger points; and those with related structural change such as isthmic L5-S1 spondylolisthesis. As with any spectrum ranging from functional to structural disorders, there can be a great deal of overlap in diagnostic findings and treatment strategies. Each relies upon the biomechanical principles discussed in the earlier sections of this chapter. Often treatment focuses on modifying the underlying functional disorders that aggravated or precipitated the eventual structural changes that define the structural, codable diagnosis.

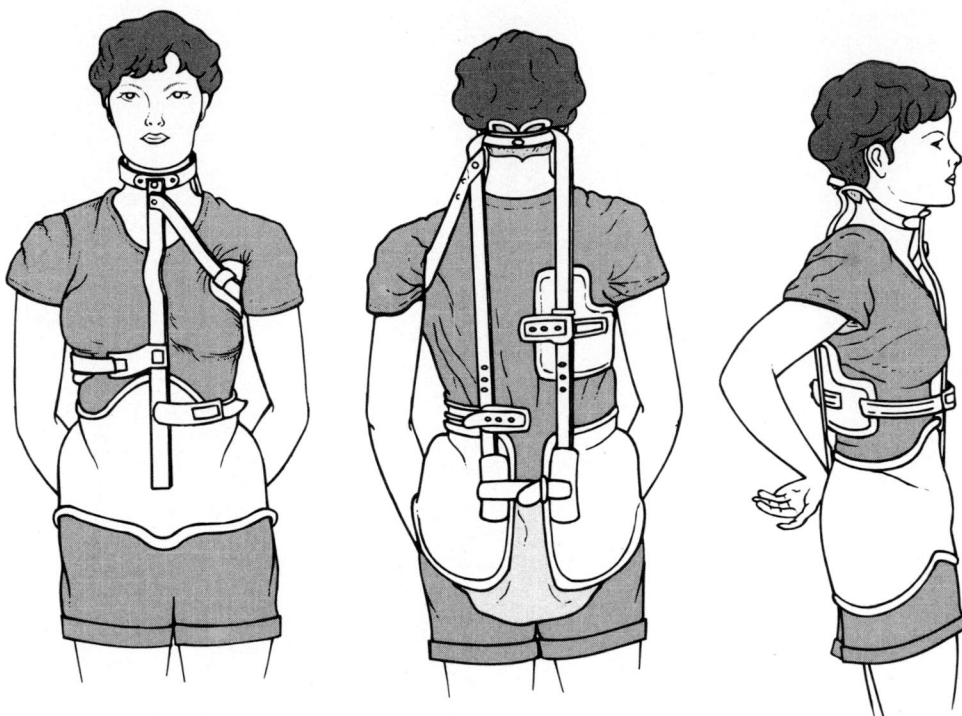

FIGURE 43.24. Milwaukee brace.

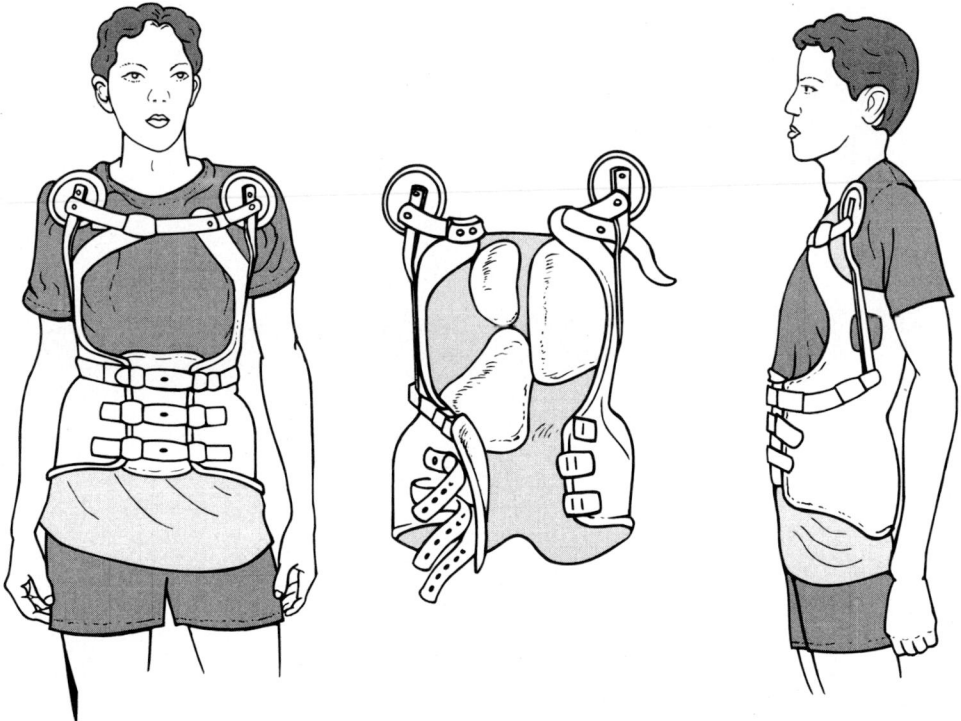

FIGURE 43.25. Boston brace.

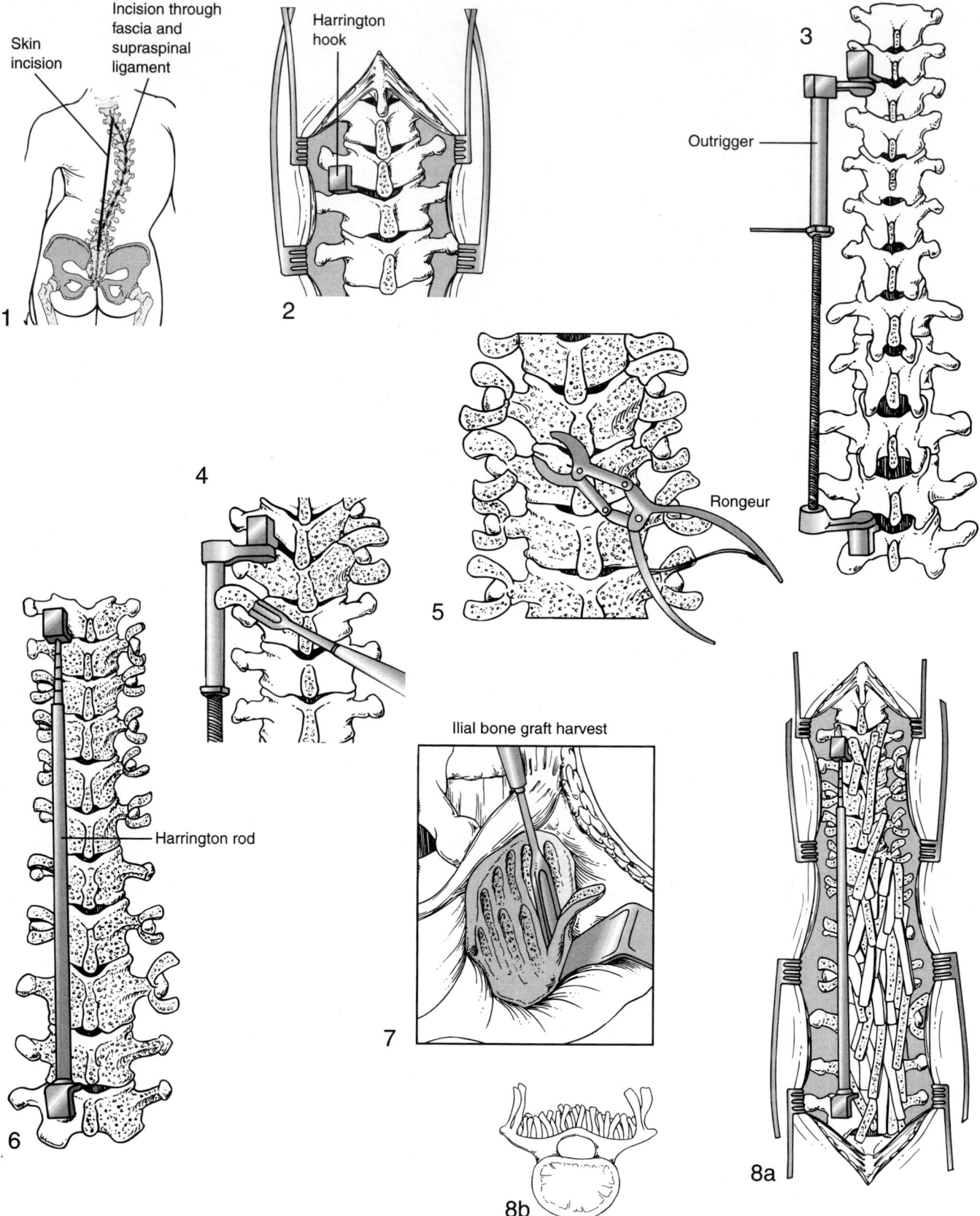

FIGURE 43.26. Surgical fusion with Harrington rod implantation. This extensive surgery is reserved for patients with curves greater than 45 degrees. A major clinical goal is to stop structural progression of a curve before it seriously compromises cardiopulmonary function.

SPONDYLOLISTHESIS

The biomechanical principles of diagnosis and treatment of patients with sagittal plane postural problems can be directly applied to the management of patients with spondylolisthesis. The generic term spondylolisthesis is derived from Greek roots roughly meaning "vertebra sliding down a slippery path." It describes the common finding of a group of spinal disorders in which there is a forward displacement of one vertebra over another, usually the fifth lumbar over the body of the first sacral segment.

Classification

With the advent of modern radiology, the study of spondylolisthesis began, including its true incidence, location, classification, and significance. The classification of spondylolisthesis subsequently evolved into the currently accepted causal categories delineated by Wiltse, Newman, and MacNab (57) shown in Table 43.4.

Causes

Regardless of specific hereditary and developmental factors, spondylolisthesis refers to a group of disorders having a particular common mechanical consequence. Applying the mechanical perspective permits better understanding of the general symptom complex. Applying mechanical treatment protocols provides the rational basis for osteopathic conservative management of patients diagnosed as having spondylolisthesis.

Hereditary Predisposition

Two observations argue against a person having a direct inheritance of spondylolisthesis. First, although there is an increased incidence of spondylolisthesis within family groups (58,59), a significant number of these family members exhibit different types of spondylolisthesis. Second, infants are rarely reported to have spondylolysis, or prespondylolisthesis. The incidence increases after children assume an active upright position and continues up until age 20, when it matches the 5% incidence of the general population (60).

The genetic link appears more likely to involve those factors that predispose the region to instability. Posterior defects such as spina bifida occulta and open sacrum are almost invariably inherited in dysplastic spondylolisthesis and in a third of patients with the isthmic type (60). This lack of posterior support may concentrate postural weightbearing forces in the area, resulting in forward subluxation of the entire L5 unit in dysplastic spondylolisthesis. In this fashion and under certain biomechanical stressors, genetics could predispose a patient to stress fracture of the pars interarticularis and then sliding of the anterior elements of L5 on S1 in isthmic spondylolisthesis (59).

Conversely, degenerative spondylolisthesis (formally called pseudospondylolisthesis), occurs two to three times more frequently in African Americans, who are also known to have greater L5-S1 stability (62). In general, patients with degenerative spondylolisthesis have a low PI for age (63) and higher incidences of sacralization of L5 and/or block-shaped L5 vertebrae. They also have a much lower incidence of posterior defects (62) than seen in the general population. The increased stability at L5 encourages instability higher in the lumbar spine.

Developmental Factors

Certain developmental factors have been statistically and/or logically implicated in spondylolisthesis. Foremost among these factors are posture and microtrauma (64–69).

Posture is strongly implicated in the development of spondylolisthesis and spondylolysis (prespondylolisthesis). Spondylolysis does not develop prior to the assumption of the standing posture. In one study of 125 institutionalized patients who had never assumed a standing position, none demonstrated a pars defect (65). No other primate has fully adopted human upright posture, nor does any other primate develop a lytic type of spondylolisthesis.

Postural decompensation as measured by the Jungmann PI is substantially higher in patients with L5-S1 spondylolisthesis (64) than in the general population. Increasing PI and increasing lumbosacral instability may, in part, address Wiltse's observation (57) that many patients develop lesions in the pars at approximately age 6 and then have no problems with it until their mid-30s.

Hyperlordosis, in particular, has been the postural fault most implicated in isthmic spondylolysis and spondylolisthesis (67,69,70). Increased lordosis transfers weightbearing from the vertebral bodies onto the articular facets in joint capsules (28). These structures are ill-designed to carry the body's weight continuously. An anterior weightbearing line is also known to create similar mechanics and should be looked for and evaluated. Certain activities such as gymnastics further increase backward bending demands in the lumbar spine. Subsequently, many young gymnasts permanently adopt an exaggerated lordotic posture. Not surprisingly, many female gymnasts demonstrate spondylolysis, having an incidence four times that of the general female population (71).

Other groups are specifically subject to increased stress in the lumbopelvic area and each has been shown to have an increased incidence of spondylolysis. These included weight lifters, soldiers carrying backpacks, and college football linemen. Repetitive lumbosacral motion is a common characteristic in all types of spondylolisthesis except that due to trauma. Therefore, frequent stress in posturally or congenitally unstable areas is implicated, especially during the adolescent growth spurt, in the development of fatigue fracture, the proposed basic lesion in isthmic spondylolisthesis (59).

Diagnosis

Of the estimated 5% of the population with spondylolisthesis, approximately half are asymptomatic (72). Those who become symptomatic do so commonly after the age of 20. Preventive care depends on early and accurate diagnosis.

Diagnostic testing should include the following:

- Radiography
- PI measurement
- History
- Physical examination

TABLE 43.4. CLASSIFICATION OF SPONDYLOLISTHESIS

Diagnosis	Type	Percent	Criteria	Comments
Type I Dysplastic spondylolisthesis 	Dysplastic	21	Congenital deficiency of neural arch of L5 or upper sacrum. Insufficiency of superior sacral facets.	2 girls: 1 boy is the ratio; almost exclusively L5; lumbosacral facets also approach horizontal
Type IIA Isthmic spondylolisthesis Type IIB 	Isthmic Subtype A Subtype B Subtype C	51	Pars interarticularis defect A. Lytic-fatigue fracture of pars B. Elongated but intact pars C. Acutely fractured pars	Almost exclusively L5 A. Most common type below age 50 years B. Probably due to repeated microfractures healing elongated fashion as slippage occurs C. History of severe trauma may heal with immobilization
Type III Degenerative spondylolisthesis 	Degenerative	25	Degenerative changes at apophyseal joints due to long-standing intersegmental instability	4 female: 1 male; 3 black: 1 white; 6–9 times more common at L4; sacralization 4× general population; not seen before age 40; rare between 40–50; slippage 30% maximum
Type IV Traumatic spondylolisthesis 	Traumatic	1	Due to fractures in other areas of the bony hook than the pars	Heals with immobilization
Type V	Pathologic	2	Generalized or localized bone disease	Neoplasm, osteogenesis imperfecta, Paget's disease, arthrogryposis, iatrogenic postlumbar fusion; Kuskokwim disease

Reprinted with permission from Kuchera WQ, Kuchera ML. *Osteopathic Principles in Practice*. Columbus, Ohio: Greyden Press; 1994.

- Spinal palpation
- Neurologic testing

Radiographic Analysis

Radiology has greatly enhanced our ability to diagnose spondylolisthesis even in totally asymptomatic patients; it is a modality that provides prognostic data (64,73). It must be realized that there are significant differences between the measurements obtained from weightbearing and non-weightbearing x-ray films (73,74). From a pragmatic point of view, the standardized postural standing film series offers reproducible, functional, postural data and is preferred.

Radiographically, gross spondylolisthesis can be seen and quantified on a lateral x-ray view. However, 45-degree oblique films may be necessary to see a subtle or unilateral spondylolysis (Fig. 43.14). In this view, the pars interarticularis in isthmic type II-B spondylolisthesis has been described as the Greyhound of

Hensinger because of the "long neck" rather than the "collar" on the "Scotty dog" (75).

Meyerding (76) provided the simplest system of grading (Fig. 43.12). Spondylolisthesis is assigned the classification of I, II, III, or IV, respectively, for each one fourth of the vertebral body that the upper vertebra is displaced forward on the vertebra below. The more precise displacement measurement of Taillard (77) can detect minor progression but it is rarely needed clinically. The Meyerding system is more commonly used, more quickly applied, and is clinically relevant.

The fastest progression of isthmic spondylolisthesis is seen between ages 9 and 15. Rarely is there progression in the Meyerding grading over the age of 20, especially in patients having a sclerotic buttress on the anterior lip of the sacrum (65,78).

Other signs of instability or its effects in the area can be seen with radiographic analysis (9,20,24,70,79), including:

- Angle of slip
- Osteophytes
- Calcified ligaments (especially iliolumbar)
- Increased PI
- Anterior weightbearing mechanics
- Increased lordosis or LSA
- Disc narrowing

Whenever possible, radiographic typing of the spondylolisthesis should be performed because it may affect treatment or prognosis.

Clinical

The age of the symptomatic patient determines the clinical presentation. While spondylolisthesis is perhaps the most common cause of persistent low back pain and sciatica in children and adolescents (80), most children with spondylolisthesis in this age group do not have pain. These individuals are often identified when a school official or parent notes a change in gait or posture (80). If any pain is expressed, it is usually described as a dull ache in the buttock or posterior thigh. Symptoms are rarely expressed below the knee (75).

Tight hamstrings (73,81) are found in 80% of young people with symptomatic spondylolysis or spondylolisthesis and to a lesser extent in asymptomatic patients. This finding probably results from postural stress and an attempt to stabilize the unstable lumbosacral junction (and is not from root impingement). Inability to bend over to touch one's toes reveals this deficit. It can also be used to uncover the nonfixed scoliosis (65,82) that exists in approximately 30% of these patients secondary to lumbar irritation and paraspinal spasm. Furthermore, as a result of having tight hamstrings, those patients having spondylolisthesis rated greater than grade II have a pathognomonic stiff-legged, short stride, waddling gait (81,83) in which the pelvis rotates with each step.

Distortion of the pelvis and trunk appears in patients having a Meyerding grade II or III (81,83). They have a flared ilia in the back and an abdomen that is thrust forward. These young people have a short waist, a transverse abdominal crease at the level of the umbilicus, and flattened heart-shaped buttocks. Only 2% of young people demonstrate any objective neurologic change (28) requiring extensive electromyographic or myelographic workup.

One of the most consistent physical findings associated with patients younger than 30 years of age and with dysplastic or isthmic spondylolisthesis is tight hamstrings that restrict forward flexion of the trunk. In contrast, the most constant physical finding in patients older than 50 years of age with degenerative spondylolisthesis is the ease with which they are able to touch their toes without bending their knees or obliterating their lumbar lordosis.

The flexibility of a patient with degenerative spondylolisthesis is thought to result from laxity of the pelvicotrochanteric and hamstring muscle groups. The unstable spondylolisthetic joint at the L4-5 level predisposes the patient to manifest L5 root neurologic symptoms. The patient is more likely to have somatovisceral complaints of a hypersympathetic nature including constipation or irregular menses (2). Symptoms of pelvic congestion and vague complaints in the lower extremity are also common in adults with spondylolisthesis. These result from the hyperlordosis, visceroptosis, and poor thoracic abdominal diaphragmatic function that accompanies spondylolisthesis (2,61,84,85).

Adult patients are more likely to complain of pain. Their pain is usually aggravated by moderate activity or prolonged standing and relieved by rest or limited activity. Because of chronic overt instability of the lumbosacral region, these patients have poorly responsive soft tissues (86), somatic dysfunction, and multiple myofascial points that, when stressed, react out of proportion to the initiating event and produce palpable spasm and low back pain. Pain can thus be caused by several structures in the area other than the spondylolisthetic segment. These structures are also subject to the instability of the region and the mechanical disadvantage that is localized there. It is, therefore, difficult to sort out when the pain is caused by spondylolisthesis, when it is the result of somatic dysfunction of muscular, ligamentous, or joint structures, or when it is of discogenic origin.

In patients older than 20 years of age with spondylolisthesis of less than 33%, pain is probably caused by one of three mechanisms (65):

- Disc degeneration at the level of the defect
- Root impingement by fibrocartilaginous build-up
- Referral from stressed posterior ligaments and soft tissues

In our clinical experience, pain in these patients is most commonly referred from trigger points in the quadratus lumborum, glutei, and piriformis muscles, and from iliolumbar and posterior sacroiliac ligaments. This best supports the third mechanism above.

The cauda equina becomes physically involved in isthmic spondylolisthesis patients with more than a 50% slip (more than a grade II) (65). In these patients, low back pain is attributed directly to the spondylolisthesis itself. Because the dysplastic type carries the posterior arch forward, no more than 25% slippage is necessary to manifest a cauda equina syndrome (59). Degenerative spondylolisthesis, by nature of its mechanism, does not progress beyond a 30% slip (59,65,70). The instability of this joint (usually L4-5), coupled with physical continuity with the posterior arch, usually results in L5 root impingement. Myelograms performed on these patients generally show hourglass constriction (70) at that level. Therefore, the differential and accurate diagnosis of the primary cause of back pain in a patient with spondylolisthesis requires careful palpatory and neurologic physical examination and diagnosis in addition to the radiographic and historical findings just outlined.

Palpatory

Increased intersegmental motion in the lumbosacral region is usually a sign of instability and severe degeneration. This increased motion is grossly apparent even on x-ray films. However, palpatory evidence (86) by those trained to palpate segmental motion is generally considered to have twice the diagnostic yield for instability (28.6%) when compared to diagnosis by x-ray studies (15%).

Palpatory findings in patients with spondylolisthesis reveal an anteriorly located spinous process (Fig. 43.27) or drop-off sign. The anterior spinous process is associated with the vertebra that has slipped forward in dysplastic and degenerative spondylolisthesis. It is the adjacent vertebra, above the slipped segment, in isthmic spondylolisthesis.

Sacral base motion is excessively lax when it is rocked anteriorly around the middle transverse axis; this may also result in associated subjective buttock or posterior thigh discomfort. If testing sacral base motion causes neurologic symptoms, particular care should be taken in designing a treatment protocol that does not produce neurologic symptoms.

Paraspinal tissues vary in palpatory quality depending on the degree of symptoms present. Often they display multiple myofascial tender points. Even in the asymptomatic state, they are slow to relax and are somewhat boggy (congested) to palpation. Muscle strength testing of the low back muscles demonstrates nearly full flexibility but decreased strength and endurance.

The iliolumbar ligament should be palpated bilaterally in every patient with symptomatic spondylolisthesis. Attached to the transverse processes of L5, the anterior sacroiliac joint, and the iliac crest, the iliolumbar ligament is anatomically positioned to resist any forward slip of L5 on the sacrum (10). Bilateral palpatory tension and subjective tenderness are often noted over its attachments. The patient may experience lateral thigh and/or groin referral (Fig. 43.7). Palpation of the iliolumbar ligament is a valuable and sensitive indicator of the success of conservative management programs designed to reduce mechanical stress in patients with symptomatic spondylolisthesis.

Neurologic

The physical examination of each patient should include a neurologic evaluation including deep tendon reflexes, muscle strength testing, and straight leg raising. Electromyographic testing and/or myelography are indicated if radicular symptoms are present. It is especially important to assess the condition of the L4 disc (65) if surgical fusion is contemplated.

Treatment

Conservative management is 85% to 90% successful in degenerative spondylolisthesis (65,70). In the minority of children who are symptomatic, only 50% are successfully managed with conservative care (65,75). For immature patients with Meyerding grade

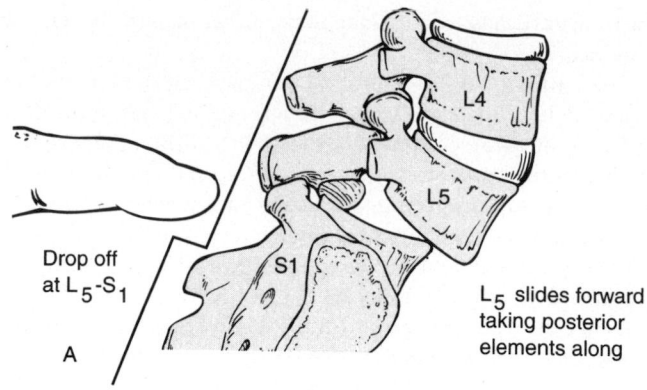

A — Drop off at L₅-S₁ — L_5 slides forward taking posterior elements along

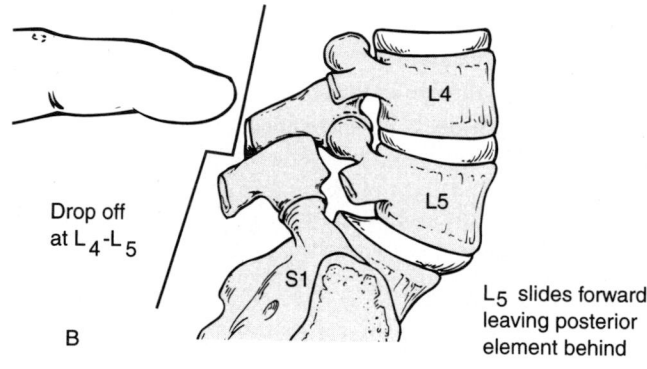

B — Drop off at L₄-L₅ — L_5 slides forward leaving posterior element behind

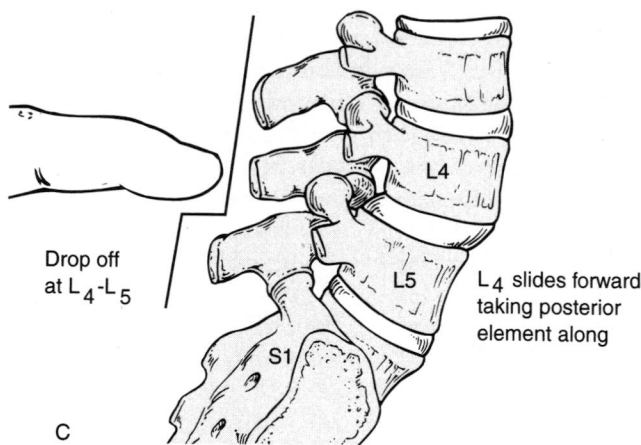

C — Drop off at L₄-L₅ — L_4 slides forward taking posterior element along

FIGURE 43.27. Location of anteriorly located spinous process (drop-off sign) depends on underlying mechanism of spondylolisthesis. **A:** In dysplastic spondylolisthesis, L5-S1 horizontal facets allow entire spine to glide forward creating drop-off between L5 and S1. **B:** In isthmic spondylolisthesis, pars defect between L5 and S1 allows anterior elements of L5 to slide forward along with the rest of the spine. Posterior elements of L5 remain behind with the sacrum creating drop-off between L4 and L5. **C:** Degenerative spondylolisthesis at L4-5 does not affect anterior and posterior elements of the vertebral unit and therefore the drop-off sign is located between L4 and L5.

III or IV spondylolisthesis, those with progressive subluxation, or those with spondylolisthesis secondary to acute fractures, conservative management is probably not indicated without extensive bracing or surgical fusion. The acute fracture group responds best to immediate immobilization (65).

For those patients requiring surgery (or bracing), conservative management should be added afterward because the conditions that led to the instability preoperatively are still present postoperatively. In all cases, conservative management should attempt to maximize structure-function relationships.

Patient Education

Education is a key element in conservative management (72,87,88) of the patient with either asymptomatic or symptomatic spondylolisthesis. Goals center on decreasing stress in the unstable lumbosacral region through application of back mechanics, proper exercise and nutrition, and improvement of posture. Back schools, offering 36 hours of instruction in teaching back mechanics and appropriate choices for optimum back care, are effective (87). These approaches immensely increase patient compliance. In the absence of a back school, the individual practitioner should use a minimum of one patient visit (more if necessary) to explain lumbosacral mechanics. Patients are taught to lift properly and to avoid improper lifting, especially over the head, as this increases lumbar lordosis.

The osteopathic physician should advocate proper footwear; high heels in particular increase lumbar lordosis (28). Patients should be advised on correct sleeping, sitting, and standing postures; they should also be counseled on weight loss, if necessary. This minimal investment of time reduces the frequency of reinjury or the failure of an otherwise well-conceived conservative program.

Pregnancy significantly affects posture by shifting the weight-bearing line anteriorly and accentuating the lumbar lordotic curve. Unfortunately, this postural stress occurs at a time when the hormonal changes of pregnancy also reduce soft tissue stabilization. Women with spondylolisthesis contemplating pregnancy should prepare their posture and muscle tone in advance, if possible. They should also strictly adhere to their obstetrician's weight gain limits. Often the addition of a Levitor® is extremely beneficial, even if it is only for the duration of the pregnancy.

For asymptomatic young people with less than a Meyerding grade I spondylolisthesis, avoid creating a back cripple with excessive restrictions. It is wise to direct these individuals toward a vocation not requiring heavy lifting or strenuous activity (89). In asymptomatic young people with more than grade I spondylolisthesis, the same vocational goals are upheld but these individuals should also avoid contact sports. Inform young patients and their parents of the concerns and uncertainties involved; stress the need for close follow-up.

Exercise

The response to exercise does not depend on the type of spondylolisthesis (I, II, or III) (88). The goals of exercise are to eventually stabilize the lumbosacral region and diminish the lumbar lordosis (84,88). Weight loss for an overweight patient can also be facilitated by exercise.

Exercise should be of a flexion-type only, rather than flexion-extension combination programs (82). Gramse has reported excellent results with the flexion program (88). The variables examined included relief of pain, need for back supports, return to work status, and recovery. Combination flexion-extension exercise significantly reduced the effectiveness in all of these variables. Pelvic narrow and coil exercise (90–92,98) with the knees bent in the supine position is extremely effective (Fig. 43.9), although flattening the back against the wall while standing or bringing the chest to the thigh while sitting in a chair can also be beneficial.

The patient must be able to demonstrate their ability to maintain a reduced lordosis before abdominal strengthening exercises such as bent-knee sit-ups are considered. Good abdominal strength adjunctively supports weightbearing and unloads the spine. Gymnastics, diving, and contact sports are not encouraged. Swimming, however, is considered an excellent activity to cultivate.

Manipulation

Several authors report a benefit (2,6,9,28,93) from the manipulative management of patients with spondylolisthesis. Manipulative treatment of the patient with spondylolisthesis is extremely helpful in attempting to redress some of the postural decompensation that has occurred over time and to alleviate segmental limitation of motion known to upset the forces resisting spondylolisthesis (70).

The goals (2,6,9,93,94) are reduction of lumbar lordosis and somatic dysfunction. This transfers weightbearing from the posterior elements and tissues back to the vertebral bodies. It specifically relaxes strained, irritable lumbar paraspinal tissues, permitting them to better resist stresses of the activities of daily living. It also reduces the patient's somatic pain and somatovisceral symptomatology. These goals seek gradual reestablishment of fascial and muscular balance to promote maximal functional weightbearing posture.

The manipulative program is not just directed to the lordosis and specific somatic dysfunctions, but to all support structures as well. Because of the instability and injury in the lumbosacral junction, high-velocity techniques should be avoided in that area.

In correcting lordosis and recurrent lumbopelvic clinical conditions, the first concern is often balancing the pelvis horizontally (11,28,95). An undiagnosed or uncorrected unilateral, sacral shear somatic dysfunction thwarts the most expert manipulator in achieving this goal and renders functional orthoses such as the Levitor ineffective. This and other nonphysiologic somatic dysfunctions can be treated promptly and effectively with OMT.

An unlevel sacral base needs gradual heel lift orthotics before instability and recurrent somatic dysfunction can be effectively addressed. A minimal heel lift, when indicated, can reduce the LSA by 2 to 4 degrees (11) and may move an anterior weightbearing line as much as an inch posterior (96). Correction of a short leg is also extremely helpful in reducing long-term strain on the iliolumbar ligament. It eliminates somato-somatic referral of groin pain from this structure as well as reduces low back pain and instability in the lumbosacral junction (94,97). A heel lift may also be helpful to the one-third of spondylolisthetic young people who have concomitant scoliotic change and the long-term somatovisceral changes resulting from it.

Any intrapelvic somatic dysfunction should be removed; the sacroiliac articulations should be freely mobile. Tight hamstring muscles are gently stretched with isometric muscle energy technique. The use of a vapocoolant spray and stretch over the hamstrings to achieve this goal is often helpful (see Chapter 66). Fascial unwinding of the lower extremities is well received by patients and eliminates many of the vague congestive complaints in this area (J.G. Zink, personal communication, 1978).

The thoracic spine and thoracolumbar junction are addressed next. Schwab (93) reported improvement of compensatory lumbar lordotic stresses with mobilization of increased thoracic kyphosis. Fryette (28) emphasized that somatic dysfunction in this area must be corrected before any effective changes could be maintained in the lower lumbosacral junction. Additional consideration of the diaphragm and quadratus lumborum has proven particularly successful in helping to promote lymphatic drainage (61). The quadratus lumborum and the iliolumbar ligament are functionally and structurally related (97) and both should be treated.

Lastly, the lower lumbar region should be approached in a general manner with soft tissue, counterstrain, myofascial release, and fascial unwinding techniques. Address any specific somatic dysfunction with indirect technique. A clinically useful end point is achieved when the intrinsic rhythm of the craniosacral mechanism is easily palpated between hands that are monitoring both the thoracolumbar junction and sacrum.

Orthotics, Braces, and Casts

Orthotics play a significant role in the conservative management of patients with spondylolisthesis. The benefits of a heel lift orthotic in helping to lend stability to the lumbosacral region have already been discussed, and the heel lift orthotic is potentially a permanent part of the patient's treatment program. A corsetlike lumbosacral support, conversely, should only be considered for short-term stability (72,86). Grieve (86), however, writes that a support should never be supplied without a plan to eliminate it. Most lumbosacral supports worn for prolonged periods weaken the patient's own supportive mechanisms (72), thereby increasing long-range instability and promoting dependence on the support. For short-term management of lumbar strain, however, these supports can be invaluable in reducing pain and preparing the tissues for a subsequent exercise program.

Types of immobilization, ranging from knee to nipple casting to ordinary body casts and corsets, have been studied for use by patients with spondylolisthesis resulting from an acute fracture (75). The latter two types of immobilization suppress the extremes of bending but do a poor job of diminishing lumbosacral motion with walking (78).

The Levitor® functional pelvic orthotic has proven extremely effective as an adjunct in the long-term management of symptomatic isthmic spondylolisthesis (2,9,22). Exerting pressure between the pubic symphysis and the base of the sacrum, the Levitor® effectively (30) aids in decreasing postural decompensation as measured by PI, in reducing the LSA, and in transferring weightbearing off the posterior tissues and forward to the ver-

tebral bodies. By reducing the chronic strain on these tissues, symptomatic relief from low back pain is accomplished in days to weeks, and implementation of an exercise program can begin shortly thereafter.

Medication

Antiinflammatory medication, analgesics, muscle relaxants, and bowel softeners all have a limited role in the symptomatic relief of various common symptoms experienced by patients with spondylolisthesis. Because spondylolisthesis is a chronic problem, narcotics have no place in symptom management of these patients. Vapocoolant spray-and-stretch technique (98) and trigger point injection with local anesthetics (98) may be helpful in relieving the secondary myofascial points that occur (see Chapter 66). Injections of proliferative agents are also useful for cases of ligamentous laxity uncorrected by conservative means (99).

CONCLUSION

Patients' philosophies toward illness, their way of life, and the environment in which they function may affect their compliance, in turn affecting the outcome of the treatment program. Conservative protocols, including individually adapted combinations of OMT, orthotics, exercise, patient education, and other modalities, help the patient's spine compensate better for the new posture that results from treatment for functional disorders. These disorders range from short leg syndrome to hyperlordotic conditions as well as structural component disorders such as scoliosis or spondylolisthesis.

Rational, conservative management of a patient with orthopedic and structural disorders with postural components presupposes early and accurate diagnosis and a thorough understanding of the biomechanics involved. While the cause is important for prognosis, treatment addressing the underlying instability, spinal mechanics, and patient homeostasis provides optimum benefit. Postural decompensation in the sagittal plane is particularly prominent in patients with isthmic spondylolisthesis and in the coronal and horizontal planes of patients with rotoscoliosis. These patients must be treated to maximize both patient homeostasis and body mechanics.

Finally, physicians' changing perspectives on posture mechanisms as a dynamic process affecting interrelated structures throughout the body (9,100) have allowed postural treatment approaches to evolve and improve. As stated by Hippocrates nearly 2,500 years ago: "The regimen I adopt will be for the benefit of my patients according to my abilities and judgment." The guidelines in this chapter provide principles to enhance your ability to design an individualized treatment regimen for patients with postural components. They will benefit from your continued study and total body application of postural homeostatic mechanisms and structure-function interrelationships.

REFERENCES

1. Kuchera ML. Gravitational stress, musculoskeletal strain, and postural alignment. *Spine.* State of the Art Reviews. 1995;9(2):463–490.

2. Kuchera ML. Diagnosis and treatment of gravitational strain patho-physiology: research and clinical correlates (parts I & II). Vleeming A, ed. *Low Back Pain: The Integrated Function of the Lumbar Spine and Sacroiliac Joints.* Proceedings of the 2nd Interdisciplinary World Congress; November 9–11, 1995:659–693; University of California (San Diego).

3. Cathie AG. The applied anatomy of some postural changes. In: Peterson B, ed. *Postural Balance and Imbalance (1983 AAO Yearbook).* Newark, OH: American Academy of Osteopathy; 1983:44–46.

4. Irvin RE. Suboptimal posture: the origin of the majority of idiopathic pain of the musculoskeletal system. In: Vleeming A, Mooney V, Dorman T, et al, eds. *Movement, Stability & Low Back Pain: The Essential Role of the Pelvis.* New York, NY: Churchill-Livingstone; 1997:133–155.

5. Kuchera ML, Bemben MG, Kuchera WA, Piper F. Athletic functional demand and posture. *JAOA.* 1990;90(9):843–844.

6. Kuchera ML. Treatment of gravitational strain pathophysiology. In: Vleeming A, Mooney V, Dorman T, et al, eds. *Movement, Stability & Low Back Pain: The Essential Role of the Pelvis.* New York, NY: Churchill-Livingstone; 1997:477–499.

7. Cruickshank JL, Koike M, Dickson RA. Curve patterns in idiopathic scoliosis: a clinical and radiographic study. *J Bone Joint Surg.* 1989;71B(2):259–263.

8. Beal MC. The sacroiliac problem: review of anatomy, mechanics, and diagnosis. *JAOA.* 1982;81(10):667–679.

9. Jungmann M. *The Jungmann Concept and Technique of Antigravity Leverage.* Rangeley, ME: Institute for Gravitational Strain Pathology, Inc; 1982.

10. Willard FH. The muscular, ligamentous and neural structure of the low back and its relation to back pain. In: Vleeming A, Mooney V, Dorman T, et al, eds. *Movement, Stability & Low Back Pain: The Essential Role of the Pelvis.* New York, NY: Churchill-Livingstone; 1997:3–35.

11. Kuchera ML, Irvin RE. Biomechanical considerations in postural re-alignment. *JAOA.* 1987;87(11):781–782.

12. Denslow JS, Chase JA, Gardner DL, Banner KB. Mechanical stresses in the human lumbar spine and pelvis. *JAOA.* 1962;61:705–712.

13. Janda V. Muscle weakness and inhibition (pseudoparesis) in back pain syndromes. In: Grieve GP, ed. *Modern Manual Therapy of the Vertebral Column.* Edinburgh, Scotland: Churchill-Livingstone; 1986:197–210.

14. Kuchera ML. Gravitational strain pathophysiology and "Unterkreuz" syndrome. *Manuelle Med.* 1995;33(2):56.

15. Wolff J. Die innere Architekur der Knochen. *Arch Anat Phys* 1870;50.

16. Vleeming A, Snijders CJ, Stoeckart R, Mens JMA. The role of the sacroiliac joints in coupling between spine, pelvis, legs and arms. In Vleeming A, Mooney V, Dorman T, et al, eds. *Movement, Stability and Low Back Pain: The Central Role of the Pelvis.* New York, NY: Churchill-Livingstone; 1997:53–71.

17. Gofton JP, Trueman GE. Studies in osteoarthritis of the hip: part II. Osteoarthritis of the hip and leg-length disparity. *Can Med Assoc J.* 1971;104:791–799.

18. Hagen DP. A continuing roentgenographic study of rural school children over a 15-year period. *JAOA.* 1964;63:546–557.

19. Travell JG, Simons DG. *Myofascial Pain and Dysfunction: A Trigger Point Manual.* Vol II. Baltimore, MD: Williams & Wilkins; 1992:47.

20. Kuchera ML. Aging, postural decompensation and low back pain. *JAOA.* 1986;86(10):74.

21. Willman MK. Radiographic technical aspects of the postural study. *JAOA.* 1977;76:739–744.

22. Kuchera ML. *Conservative Management of Symptomatic Spondylolisthesis.* On file with the American Academy of Osteopathy (Newark, OH) in partial fulfillment of FAAO; 1987.

23. Peterson B, ed. *Postural Balance and Imbalance. (1983 AAO Yearbook).* Newark, OH: American Academy of Osteopathy; 1983.

24. Kuchera ML, Barton J. Sagittal plane postural measurements. *JAOA.* 1990;90(10):932.

25. Fernand R, Fox DE. Evaluation of lumbar lordosis: a prospective and retrospective study. *Spine.* 1985;10(9):799–803.

26. Semon RL, Spengler D. Significance of lumbar spondylolysis in college football players. *Spine.* 1981;6(2):172–174.

27. Gallant R, ed. *The Jungmann Concept and Technique of Anti-Gravity Leverage: A Clinical Handbook,* rev 2nd ed. Rangeley, ME: Institute for Gravitational Strain Pathology, Inc; 1992:46.

28. Luibel GJ. Lordosis. *JAOA.* 1954;54(3):126–130.

29. Kuchera ML. Alteration of intrapelvic spatial relationships utilizing an external pelvic orthosis in patients with low back pain. Originally published in *Proceedings of the International Society for Prosthetics and Orthotics.* June 1992:291. Also see *JAOA.* 1992;92(9):1182.

30. Kuchera ML, Jungmann M. Inclusion of Levitor Orthotic Device in the management of refractive low back pain patients. *JAOA.* 1986;86(10):673.

31. Hunt W. Inequality to length of the lower limbs, with a report of an important suit for malpractice; and also a claim for priority. *Am J Med Sci.* 1879;77:102–107.

32. Cox WC. On the want of symmetry in the length of opposite sides of persons who have never been the subject of disease or injury to their lower extremities. *Am J Med Sci.* 1875;69:438–439.

33. Garson JG. Inequality in length of lower limbs. *J Anat Physiol.* 1879;13:502–507.

34. Hilton J. *Rest and Pain,* 6th ed. Philadelphia, A: JB Lippincott Co; 1950:404.

35. Schwab WA. Principles of manipulative treatment: II. Low back problem. *JAOA.* 1932;31:216–220.

36. Beilke MC. Roentgenological spinal analysis and the technic for taking standing x-ray plates. *JAOA.* 1936;35:414–418.

37. Nichols PJR, Bailey NTJ. The accuracy of measuring leg-length differences. *Br Med J.* 1955;2:1247–1248.

38. Clarke GR. Unequal leg length: an accurate method of detection and some clinical results. *Rheum Phys Med.* 1972;11:385–390.

39. Beal MC. The short-leg problem. *JAOA.* 1950;50:109–121.

40. Hoskins ER. The development of posture and its importance: III. Short leg. *JAOA.* 1934;34:125–126.

41. Friberg O, Nurminen M, Korhonen K, et al. Accuracy and precision of clinical estimation of leg length inequality and lumbar scoliosis: comparison of clinical and radiological measurements. *International Disability Studies.* 1988;10:49–53.

42. Strong R, Thomas PE. Patterns of muscle activity in the leg, hip, and torso associated with anomalous fifth lumbar conditions. *JAOA.* 1968;67:1039–1041.

43. Strong R, Thomas PE, Earl WD. Patterns of muscle activity in the leg, hip, and torso during quiet standing. *JAOA.* 1967;66:1035–1038.

44. Hackett GS. *Ligament and Tendon Relaxation Treated by Prolotherapy,* 3rd ed. Springfield, IL: Charles C Thomas; 1958:27.

45. Sutton SE. Postural imbalance: Examination and treatment utilizing flexion tests. In: Peterson B, ed. *Postural Balance and Imbalance (1983 AAO Yearbook).* Newark, OH: American Academy of Osteopathy; 1983:102–112.

46. Denslow JS, Chace JA, Gutensohn OR, Kumm MG. Methods in taking and interpreting weight-bearing x-ray films. In: Beal MC, ed. *Selected Papers of John Stedmen Denslow (1993 AAO Yearbook).* Indianapolis, IN: American Academy of Osteopathy; 1993:109–120.

47. Irvin RE. Reduction of lumbar scoliosis by use of a heel lift to level the sacral base. *JAOA.* 1991;91(1):34–44.

48. Beal MC. A review of the short-leg problem. In Peterson B (ed). *Postural Balance and Imbalance (1983 AAO Yearbook).* Newark OH: American Academy of Osteopathy; 1983:26–38.

49. Fryette HH. Some reasons why sacroiliac lesions recur. *JAOA.* 1936;36:119–122.

50. Heilig D. Principles of lift therapy. In: Peterson B, ed. *Postural Balance and Imbalance (1983 AAO Yearbook).* Newark, OH: American Academy of Osteopathy; 1983:113–118.

51. Kuchera WA, Kuchera ML. Postural decompensation. In: *Osteopathic Principles in Practice,* rev. 2nd ed. Columbus, OH: Greyden Press; 1994:343–356.

52. Greenman PE. Lift therapy: use and abuse. In: Peterson B, ed. *Postural Balance and Imbalance (1983 AAO Yearbook).* Newark, OH: American Academy of Osteopathy; 1983:123–134.

53. Patriquin DA. Lift therapy: a study of results. In: Peterson B, ed. *Postural Balance and Imbalance (1983 AAO Yearbook).* Newark, OH: American Academy of Osteopathy; 1983:119–122.

54. Carlson JA, Carlson JM, Earl DT. Three-dimensional counter-strain lifts (3-DCL)–theoretical concept and applications. *AAOJ.* 1995;5(2):23–27.

55. Giles LGF, Taylor JR. Lumbar spine structural changes associated with leg length inequality. *Spine.* 1982;7:159–162.

56. Magoun HI. Idiopathic adolescent spinal scoliosis: a reasonable etiology. In: Peterson B, ed. *Postural Balance and Imbalance (1983 AAO Yearbook).* Newark, OH: American Academy of Osteopathy; 1983:94–100.

57. Wiltse LL, Newman PH, MacNab I. Classification of spondylolysis and spondylolisthesis. *Clin Orthop.* 1976;117:23–29.

58. Friberg S. Studies on spondylolisthesis. *Acta Chir Scand.* 1939;82[Suppl 55]:1440.

59. Wiltse LL, Widell EH, Jackson DW. Fatigue fracture: the basic lesion in isthmic spondylolisthesis. *J Bone Joint Surg.* 1975;57A:1722.

60. Wiltse LL. Spondylolisthesis in children. *Clin Orthop.* 1961;21:156–163.

61. Zink JG, Lawson WB. An osteopathic structural examination and functional interpretation. *Osteopath Ann.* 1987;7(12):12–19.

62. Rosenberg NJ. Degenerative spondylolisthesis–predisposing factors. *J Bone Joint Surg (Am).* 1975;57(4):467–474.

63. Kuchera ML, Miller K. Postural measurements in L4 degenerative spondylolisthesis. *JAOA.* 1995;95(8):496.

64. Kuchera ML. Postural decompensation in isthmic spondylolisthesis. *JAOA.* 1987;87(1l):781.

65. Finneson BE. *Low Back Pain.* Philadelphia, PA: JB Lippincott Co; 1973:276–288.

66. Krauss H. Effect of lordosis on the stress in the lumbar spine. *Clin Orthop.* 1976;117:56–58.

67. Newman PH. The etiology of spondylolisthesis. *J Bone Joint Surg.* 1963;45B:39–59.

68. Wynne-Davies R, Scott JHS. Inheritance and spondylolisthesis: a radiographic family survey. *J Bone Joint Surg.* 1979;61B:301–305.

69. Troup DG. Mechanical factors in spondylolisthesis and spondylolysis. *Clin Orthop.* 1976;117:59–67.

70. Farfan HF, Osteria V, Lamy C. The mechanical etiology of spondylolysis and spondylolisthesis. *Clin Orthop.* 1976;177:40–55.

71. Jackson DW, Wiltse LL, Cirincione RJ. Spondylolysis in the female gymnast. *Clin Orthop.* 1976;117:68–73.

72. Magora A. Conservative treatment in spondylolisthesis. *Clin Orthop.* 1976;117:74–79.

73. Boxall D, Bradford DS, Winter RB, Moe JH. Management of severe spondylolisthesis in children and adolescents. *J Bone Joint Surg.* 1979;61A:479–495.

74. Lowe RW, Hayes TD, Kaye J, et al. Standing roentgenograms in spondylolisthesis. *Clin Orthop.* 1976;117:80–91.

75. Hensinger RN, Lang JR, MacEwen GD. Surgical management of spondylolisthesis in children and adolescents. *Spine.* 1976;1:207–216.

76. Meyerding HW. Spondylolisthesis. *Surg Gynecol Obstet.* 1932;54:371–377.

77. Taillard WF. Le spondylolisthesis chez l'enfant et l'adolescent. *Acta Orthop Scand.* 1955;24:115–144.

78. Eisenstein S. Spondylolysis: a skeletal investigation of two population groups. *J Bone Joint Surg (Br)* 1978;60:488–494.

79. Hoyt H, Bard D, Shaffer F. Experience with an antigravity leverage device for chronic low back pain: a clinical study. *JAOA.* 1981;80(7):474–479.

80. Laurent LE, Oskman K. Operative treatment of spondylolisthesis in young patients. *Clin Orthop.* 1976;117:85–91.

81. Phalen GS, Dickenson JA. Spondylolisthesis and tight hamstrings. *J Bone Joint Surg.* 1961;43A:505–512.

82. Fisk JR, Noe JH, Winter RB. Scoliosis, spondylolysis, and spondylolisthesis. *Spine.* 1978;3(3):234–245.

83. Newman PH. A clinical syndrome associated with severe lumbosacral subluxation. *J Bone Joint Surg.* 1965;47B(3):472–481.

84. Freeman JT. Posture in the aging and aged body. *JAMA.* 1957;165(7):843–846.

85. Kimberly P. Visceroptosis: an osteopathic explanation of cause and symptoms. *JAOA.* 1944;43(6):270–273.

86. Grieve G. Lumbar instability. *Physiotherapy.* 1982;68(1):29.

87. Fisk JR, DiMonte P, Courington SM. Back schools—past, present and future. *Clin Orthop.* 1983;179:18–21.

88. Gramse RR, Sinaki M, Ilstrup DM. Lumbar spondylolisthesis—a rational approach to conservative treatment. *Mayo Clin Prac.* 1980;55:681–686.

89. Wiltse LL. The etiology of spondylolisthesis. *J Bone Joint Surg.* 1962;44A:536–569.

90. Cochran A. Useful exercises for pelvis and spine. Derived from "Physio-synthesis." Handout distributed at Kirksville College of Osteopathic Medicine, Kirksville, MO: 1983.

91. Lay EM. Personal communication. Lectures delivered annually while teaching at Kirksville College of Osteopathic Medicine, Kirksville, MO: 1976–1982.

92. Pheasant HC. Practical posture building. *Clin Orthop.* 1962;25:83–91.

93. Schwab WA. Principles of manipulative treatment—low back problem. In: Barnes MK, ed. *1965 AAO Yearbook.* Carmel, CA: Applied Academy of Osteopathy; 1965:90–94.

94. Cathie AG. Structural mechanics of the lumbar spine and pelvis. In: Barnes MW, ed. *1965 AAO Yearbook.* Carmel, CA: Applied Academy of Osteopathy; 1965:14–20.

95. Friberg O. Clinical symptoms and biomechanics of lumbar spine and hip joint in leg length inequality. *Spine.* 1983;8(6):643–651.

96. Magoun HI Sr. Mechanics of chronic spinal lesion. *JAOA.* 1943;42:489–500.

97. Luk KDK. The iliolumbar ligament. *J Bone Joint Surg.* 1986;68B:197–200.

98. Simons DG, Travell JG, Simons LS. *Travell & Simons' Myofascial Pain and Dysfunction: The Trigger Point Manual.* Vol I. Baltimore, MD: Williams & Wilkins; 1999.

99. Dorman T, Ravin T. *Diagnosis and Injection Techniques in Orthopedic Medicine.* Baltimore, MD: Williams & Wilkins; 1991:34–35.

100. Levin SM. A different approach to the mechanics of the human pelvis: tensegrity. In: Vleeming A, Mooney V, Dorman T, et al, eds. *Movement, Stability & Low Back Pain: The Essential Role of the Pelvis.* New York, NY: Churchill-Livingstone; 1997:157–167.

101. Kuchera ML, Bemben MG. Comparison of manual and computerized methods of assessing postural radiographs. *JAOA* 1990;90(8):714–715(abst).

MUSCULOSKELETAL EXAMINATION FOR SOMATIC DYSFUNCTION

WILLIAM A. KUCHERA
ROBERT E. KAPPLER

KEY CONCEPTS

- Elements, procedure, and interpretation of initial osteopathic musculoskeletal screening examination
- Additional, more focused, screening examination
- Musculoskeletal examination of hospitalized patients and outpatients.
- Examination of ambulatory patients
- Recording of examination findings

INTRODUCTION

An osteopathic musculoskeletal examination is preceded by taking and recording the patient's history. Its significance includes:

- Indication of the patient's mental, physical, and physiologic concerns
- Directing the physician's physical examination by indicating the significance of certain body regions
- Indicating regions of the body related to the patient's complaints and/or concerns
- Uncovering significant history that the patient may not have thought was significant to his or her complaints
- Helping the physician decide on the method, type, activating force, duration, and frequency of manipulative treatment when indicated.

Evaluation of the musculoskeletal portion of an osteopathic physical examination helps the physician in many ways. Clues obtained from a musculoskeletal examination relate to:

- Information about the present efficiency of the musculoskeletal system
- Musculoskeletal indications to dysfunction of other systems
- The general health status of the patient
- Musculoskeletal problems
- Somatic response to systemic problems
- Information about the primary etiology of a dysfunction

- Areas in which somatic structures are in need of help and support
- Areas where manipulative treatment can help relieve a somatic component of disease
- Areas in which manipulative treatment can improve the body's natural support and defense mechanisms

Sometimes musculoskeletal examinations may be conducted for the purpose of collecting osteopathic research data to be analyzed at a later date in accordance with the research protocol.

IDENTIFICATION OF SOMATIC DYSFUNCTION

An osteopathic examination is unique in that palpation, integrated with motion testing, is the major component of the musculoskeletal portion of the physical examination. Discovery of musculoskeletal dysfunction often provides additional physical clues that direct, focus, and/or expand the physical examination. Interpretation of the data gathered from a musculoskeletal dysfunction or diagnosis expands the logical conclusions that can be drawn from the physical examination. Several researchers have discussed aspects of the musculoskeletal examination (1–8).

A physician uses trained, skilled hands as primary tools for this portion of the physical; they gather information necessary to evaluate and assess tissue texture change, quality or motion, and quantity of motion. Tenderness is a relatively objective response of the patient elicited by the physician's palpation. Tenderness alone can not be an indication of somatic dysfunction.

Osteopathic diagnostic criteria for identifying somatic dysfunction can be recalled with the mnemonic TART:

T: Tissue texture abnormalities. This is a palpatory assessment of quality of tissues, usually paraspinal. Tissue changes accompany somatic dysfunction. Skilled osteopathic physicians recognize immediately the palpatory quality of tissue texture abnormality. Tissue texture abnormality could be described as palpable evidence of disturbed physiology in the tissues. Tissue texture change is evaluated in layers, from superficial or skin to deep, such as deep muscle. Tissue texture changes are described as acute or chronic.

A: Asymmetry of position of bony (or other) landmarks. Findings are discovered by inspection. Though the key element in determining the presence or absence of asymmetry is observation, or visual inspection, palpatory asymmetry is also evident.

R: Restriction of motion. Active motion testing involves instructing the patient to move, with the physician observing and recording range of motion. Passive motion testing involves the physician slowly introducing motion (with the patient inactive or passive). The quantity of motion is assessed by taking the joint to the end point of motion in both directions, or in all directions if multiple planes of motion are being assessed. Quality of motion is assessed by palpation, that is, the physician introduces motion and assesses compliance or resistance to the motion being introduced. The motion quality of somatic dysfunction is asymmetric, with relative freedom in one direction and relative restriction in the other direction. Motion restriction occurs within the limits of normal physiologic motion of a joint.

T: Tenderness. Tenderness is said to be present when the physician applies a stimulus, usually palpatory pressure, and the patient reports discomfort, flinches, has a facial change, or otherwise indicates discomfort. The test is objective in that the physician applies a measured force to the patient. Patient response involves a degree of subjectivity, depending on the individual's sensitivity or threshold for pain. Tenderness differs from pain. Pain is a totally subjective cerebral (cortical) perception of nociceptive input reported by the patient in the absence of palpatory stimulus.

A MUSCULOSKELETAL EXAMINATION

A musculoskeletal examination for somatic dysfunction is best performed in stages, progressing from overview or screening examinations to a more detailed segmental definition of TART at specific joints, facets, myofascial tissues, or vertebral units and their related vascular, lymphatic, and neural elements. This progressive approach, from a screening examination to a more detailed examination, is applicable in most situations. The patient may be outpatient and ambulatory. They may be a hospitalized patient or a patient with a specific musculoskeletal problem who is referred to the physician who has a special proficiency in osteopathic manipulative medicine.

The following is an example of a multistep musculoskeletal examination. For the purpose of simplicity, the components of this examination are identified as stage I (general or screening) or stage II (more focused or segmental) tests. We realize that there are many tests that could be performed. Basic screening and segmental examples are presented here. The physician does not do all of these tests. Those that best fit the investigative needs as indicated by the patient's history and the physician's knowledge and experience in working through a differential diagnosis are chosen. The medical student needs practice and should preform a complete regional physical examination on each patient. After this is completed the student usually looks at the results and then tries to make a working diagnosis. With this repetition during medical school and in the early practice years as a physician, the physician becomes able to perform any combination of these and other regional physical examinations and tests with ease and efficiency. During the history and routine physical, an experienced physician mentally formulates the most likely regions and/or systems that are directly or indirectly and/or anatomically or physiologically related to the patient's complaints. The physical examination may focus more on some systems than others. This chapter presents a simple musculoskeletal examination that can be performed by a medical student or a beginning practitioner. A method of recording results of this examination is also presented. Following these presentations, examples of applying a simple musculoskeletal screening examination for an ambulatory patient and a patient that is bedfast at home or in the hospital are presented.

An osteopathic musculoskeletal examination is a prerequisite for manipulative treatment and determines where to treat and how to treat. Rarely, if ever, will a physician include all of these test procedures in a single examination. If a problem is suspected in a specific region, as many tests as indicated are performed to gather as much information as is needed with the patient in a specific position. The goal is to develop a time-efficient examination sequence and a method that will gather enough information from each patient to allow the student or physician to make a working diagnosis. How much information? What tests? This is based upon the experience of the physician and his or her preference using treatment procedures.

For efficiency, it is important that the examination sequence be organized and responsive to the patient's chief complaint requires minimal changes of a patient's position and is responsive to the physician's preferred treatment procedures. The structural examination portion must identify obvious significant musculoskeletal changes (false-negative results must be minimized). Its database of findings must be sufficient to begin development of a treatment plan. Again, with experience, one better understands how the various findings are interrelated within the whole body.

Some musculoskeletal examinations may not lead to an immediate musculoskeletal treatment plan following the examination. A musculoskeletal screening examination, as is often performed on the hospitalized patient, may be used to identify potential problem areas that will be further evaluated and treated later, maybe in the physician's office after the patient has been released.

An organized total body musculoskeletal screening examination includes inspection, palpation, and motion testing to identify a problem or problems in one or more of the body's regions:

Regions Examined	Somatic Dysfunction (SD) Severity of Examined Regions
Cranial Cervical Thoracic Costal Lumbar Abdomen Pelvis Appendages	0 No somatic dysfunction (SD) or background (BG) levels 1 Obvious TART findings (especially restriction of motion and Tissue texture changes, with or without patient symptoms 2 More than BG levels and minor TART findings present 3 A key lesion (inciting SD), symptomatic patient, and restriction of motion and tissue texture changes stand out.

The physician considers these questions and relationships while examining the patient:

1. Is a problem (dysfunction) present?
2. Is there a problem with the base of support or is it a weight-bearing problem?

3. Is the problem in one or more regions of the body, and if so, which ones?

4. Is there tissue texture abnormality (temperature, turgor, tension, or discomfort with compression)?

5. Is there asymmetry?

6. Is there a restriction of active, passive, or inherent motion?

7. Is there tenderness?

8. How do the findings correlate with known medical, personal, and social histories?

9. How do these areas correlate with the areas of sympathetic or parasympathetic innervation to the viscera, that is, can they be attributed to or result from a visceral dysfunction or disease?

10. Are there other objective findings associated with the same segmental level?

11. How do the findings correlate with a common or known pattern, such as the common compensatory pattern of the fasciae of the body? (9)

12. What are the identified problems and can they be listed clearly?

The brief initial screening examination is a scan of all areas of the body, while focusing attention on the area involved in the patient's history of the chief complaint and/or the viscerosomatic region or regions related to it. Remember that the optimal functions of the thoracic inlet, the abdominal diaphragm, the thoracic and upper lumbars, and the craniosacral mechanism, within the capacity of the patient to respond, are important to the health of every individual. Also remember that a "hyperactive sympathetic nervous system" is detrimental to the healing process and to the maintenance of health.

Record the result of the examination on the patient's chart, documenting all areas that were examined and the basic elements of somatic dysfunction that were or were not diagnosed in a given region. It is very helpful to include a specific segmental diagnosis in the report to support the somatic dysfunction in the region, especially if osteopathic manipulative treatment (OMT) will be performed that day as part of the patient's treatment program. This last statement is meant to emphasize that a musculoskeletal segmental examination must be performed in the region or regions to be treated before an OMT is performed. This is repeated previous to each OMT as it directs the goal, method, and activating force that is needed. It is then rechecked after treatment to assess the results.

AN OVERALL EXAMPLE OF A MUSCULOSKELETAL EXAMINATION (TABLE 44.1)

Specific Tests for the Musculoskeletal Examination

The following are examples of some of the screening tests used in an organized, multistep musculoskeletal screening (scanning) examination.

General appearance: Look for asymmetry of the body; is the body type typical? Estimate the nutritional status; does the weight and height look proportional? Observe posteriorly, lat-

erally, and anteriorly (Figs. 44.1 through 44.3). Observe head carriage (rotation or side bending in relation to shoulders), shoulder and scapular levels, rib cage configuration, sternal deformities (pectus carinatum, pectus excavatum), clavicular deformities or elevation, supraclavicular fossae for fullness and depth, carrying angle of elbows, linea alba hair patterns, or scars.

Record the body type, muscle development, weight, and nutritional status. *Palpate for more segmental asymmetry* of paraspinal muscles. Palpate relative thickness and tension of the Achilles tendons (unilateral fullness is indicative of congestion, tension is indicative of increased weightbearing on that side); and relative tension of the right and left muscle groups, such as the trapezius, erector spinae, gluteus maximus, hamstrings, and gastrocnemius. *Palpate for hypertonicity* (tight) or hypotonicity (loose) of left and right trapezius, erector spinae, iliolumbar ligament attachments, gluteus maximus, iliotibial bands, hamstring, and gastrocnemius. *Palpate arches of feet for height* and tension.

Note: Was there change in these results when the patient performed active motion while in the sitting position? If so, record these changes.

Observe gait: Describe the gait in medical terms, if possible, or be brief but as descriptive as possible. Is weight transferred in a continuous manner from heel to toe for push off? Is there a limp? Is there toeing in, toeing out, or excessive pronation or supination? Is either leg internally or externally rotated? Is there symmetric motion through the pelvis and lumbar area, through the thoracic area, the shoulders? Is arm swing present and equal bilaterally?

Observe symmetry of the body and the space around it (Figs. 44.1 through 44.3): This includes observation of the patient from the front, side, and back, describing the resting position of one upper extremity in relation to the other, and the anterior, posterior, lateral, and paraspinal symmetry of the body. It also includes any obvious rotational positions of one body region in relation to the next. The rotation of body regions is best observed when the physician is looking down on the patient from a cephalad vantage point (Fig. 44.4).

Spinal curvatures (Figs. 44.1 through 44.3): Examine the patient, especially from the front and side. (Findings may include visual evidence of scoliosis, kyphosis, or lordosis.) This part of the screen is done while observing the general appearance.

Again observe symmetry and curvatures

Posterior screen for evidence of lateral spinal curvatures (scoliosis). Sometimes this is expected by having the patient bend forward at the waist as the physician observes the horizon of the patient's back. A rib hump or paraspinal asymmetry in thoracic or lumbar regions may indicate presence of rotoscoliosis (Fig. 44.5).

Anterior screen of the body (see Fig. 44.3).

Lateral screen for anterior/posterior asymmetry and for increased lordosis or kyphosis in cervical, thoracic, and lumbar areas (Fig. 44.2). Observe to determine if the weightbearing line passes through the external auditory meatus, acromioclavicular joint, greater trochanter, or lateral malleolus. The patient's knees should be partially flexed or hyperextended.

Horizontal plane levelness: Posterior and anterior evaluations take place here.

TABLE 44.1. A PROGRESSIVE MUSCULOSKELETAL EXAMINATION: AN EXAMPLE

Stage I Examination (Screening)	Stage II: Examination of Regions Failing Stage I Screens
STANDING	
General appearance, body type, estimate nutritional status, weight and height	*Record:* appearance and body type; weigh the patient and check his/her height.
Observe gait	*Record:* the gait
Observe symmetry of the body and space around it	Consider postural decompensation, unleveled sacral base, congenital deformities
Spinal curvatures—AP and lateral (scoliosis, kyphosis, lordosis)	*Record:* region, extent, apex. *Observe*—with forward bending and *Record*—degree of functional or structural scoliosis.
Horizontal plane levelness	Consider spinal curvatures, muscular imbalances
Standing flexion test	Consider dysfunction in structure or muscles of lower extremity or of the sacroiliac joint on the positive side
Active screening motion tests (cervical), thoracic, upper extremities, and lumbar spinal regions	Segmentally test the regions involved
Hip drop test	Consider lumbar and thoracolumbar junction dysfunctions
Pelvic side-shift test	Consider postural problem
SEATED	
Observe symmetry—did it change?	*Record*
Observe curvatures—did they change?	General appearance—describe spinal curvatures
	AP curves—identify range and apex
	Lateral curves—classify as mild, moderate, or Severe (see Chapter 43, "Osteopathic Considerations in Coronal, Horizontal, and Sagittal Planes")
Palpate for apparent elevated first rib (elevated rib or thoracic inlet dysfunction?)	*Seated:* Thoracic inlet—depth of infraclavicular space; inhalation test the first rib. Segmentally test upper thoracic region. *Supine:* coracoclavicular angle and spring upper rib region.
Active motion testing of cervical spine (and upper extremities)	*Supine:* segmental cervical motion testing
Passive motion testing of upper and lower cervical divisions	Segmentally test regions involved
Palpation for rib angle tenderness	Segmentally test atypical and typical rib motion (Figs. 44.13 and 44.18)
or	
Six-quadrant rib cage screen (see Fig. 44.16)	
Alternate straight leg raising test	Consider lumbar and pelvic region dysfunctions
Trunk sidebending test (acromion drop test)	Consider upper thoracic somatic dysfunction
Seated flexion test	Consider sacroiliac dysfunctions on the positive side
Palpation of thoracic and lumbar paraspinal regions for tissue texture changes and tenderness—fairly easy in this position	Passive or active segmental motion tests for thoracic and lumbar spine (See Chapter 39, Fig.39.1, and Chapters 48 and 50)
SUPINE POSITION *(properly position the patient)*	
Palpate CRI and sphenobasilar symphyseal motion—added experience necessary	*Supine:* Basic Diagnostics: sphenobasilar motion pattern and synchrony of the temporal bones.
	Complete Diagnosis: for somatic dysfunction of cranium—special training required
Observe symmetry of rib cage, pelvis, and lower extremities	Specific segmental tests for region with asymmetry
Abdominal palpation	Correlate findings with paraspinal thoracic and upper lumbar paraspinal tissue texture changes
Anterior pelvic landmark levelness	Correlate with posterior landmarks. *Prone:* segmental diagnosis of sacrum and innominates
Palpate cervical region for tissue texture changes and tenderness (see also Chapter 46)	*Supine:* segmental cervical motion testing
Rib compression tests	*Seated or Supine:* segmentally test atypical and typical rib motion (Figs. 44.13 and 44.18; see also Chapter 49)
Palpate thoracic and lumbar paraspinal regions for tissue texture changes and tenderness—more difficult in this position	Segmental diagnosis of thoracic and lumbar regions—more difficult (see Chapters 48 and 50)
Passive flexion screen of lower extremities (see also Chapter 53)	Segmentally test the joints failing the flexion screen (see Chapter 53)
ASIS compression test (See Chapter 52, Fig. 52.8)	*Record:* segmental pelvic palpatory data for the side of the positive compression test
PRONE POSITION	
Posterior pelvic landmark levelness	*Prone:* complete segmental testing of sacrum and innominates including motion testing
Spinal compression test or spinal spring test (thoracic and lumbar spinal regions)	*Prone:* Segmentally test for rotation; then test asymmetric regions for sidebending preference
Palpate thoracic and lumbar paraspinal regions for tissue texture changes and tenderness—easiest in this position	Segmental diagnosis of thoracic and lumbar regions (See Chapters 48 and 50)
Test rotation of each lumbar vertebral unit	*Prone:* segmentally test sidebending of lumbar spine, if R and S to same side, also test preference of F or E

AP, anteroposterior; ASIS, anterior posterior iliac spines; CRI, cranial rhythmic impulse
Note: Finding any abnormalities during stage I screen warrants a more detailed evaluation and segmental diagnosis of the region as suggested in stage II. Some of the more detailed tests are explained. In order to make these findings clinically helpful in the treatment of the patient, it is necessary to postulate on how those findings affect the total patient.

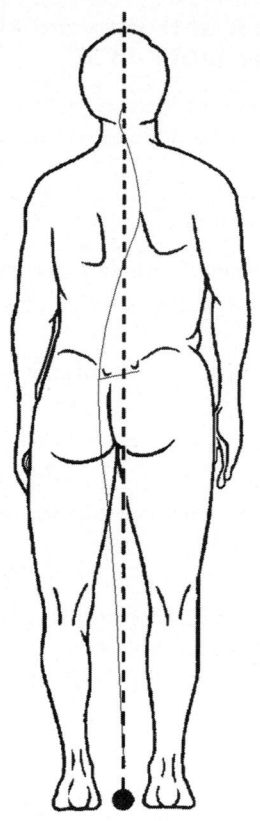

FIGURE 44.1. Observe posterior body alignment.

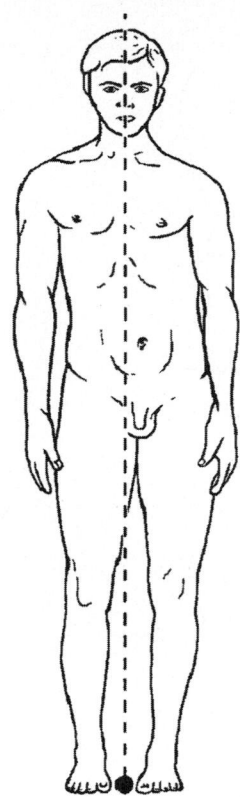

FIGURE 44.3. Observe anterior body alignment.

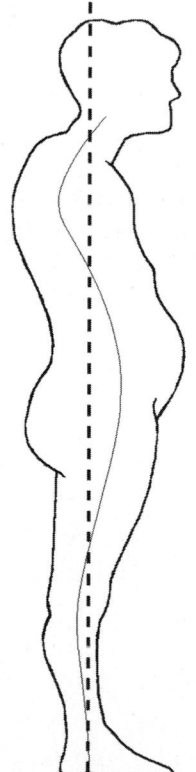

FIGURE 44.2. Observe lateral body for anteroposterior and weight-bearing alignment.

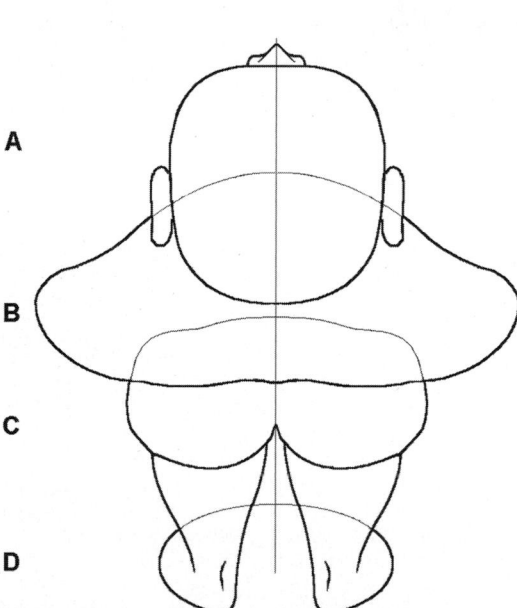

FIGURE 44.4. Observe cephalad/caudad for horizontal plane body alignment.

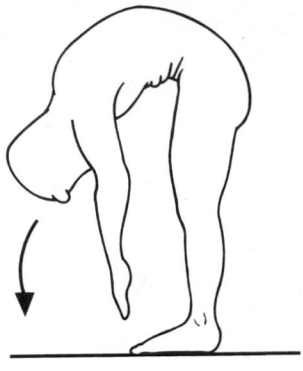

Forward bend

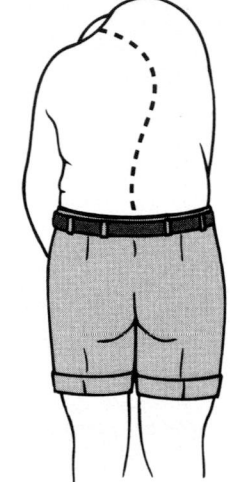

Side-bending left

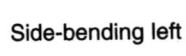

Forward bending

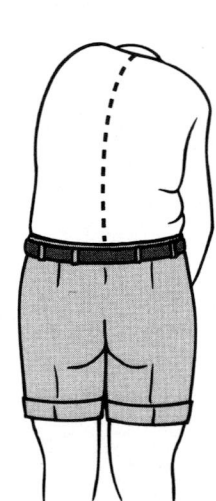

Side-bending right

FIGURE 44.5. Standing forward bending test.

Posterior Screen of Horizontal Planes (Fig. 44.6 or see Table 44.3).

This screen determines the levelness of bilateral structures.

Position: Patient standing and physician stands behind the patient

Procedure:

1. Assess mastoid processes with the transverse plane (Fig. 44.6A)
2. Assess acromion processes with the transverse plane (Fig. 44.6B)
3. Assess inferior angle of scapulae with transverse plane (Fig. 44.6C)
4. Assess iliac crests with the transverse plane (Fig. 44.6D)
5. Assess PSISs with the transverse plane (Fig. 44.6E)
6. Assess superior aspect of the greater trochanters with the transverse plane (Fig. 46.6F)

Interpretation: If a plane or planes are not level consider lower extremity abnormalities, an unlevel sacral base, spinal scoliosis, and/or congenital vertebral abnormalities.

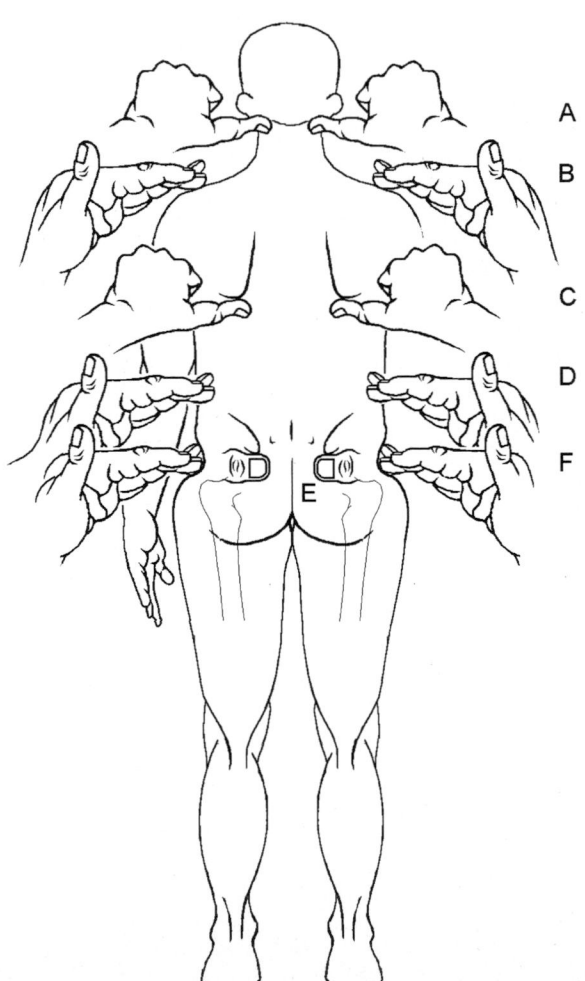

FIGURE 44.6. Posterior examination of bony landmarks (horizontal planes) of the body.

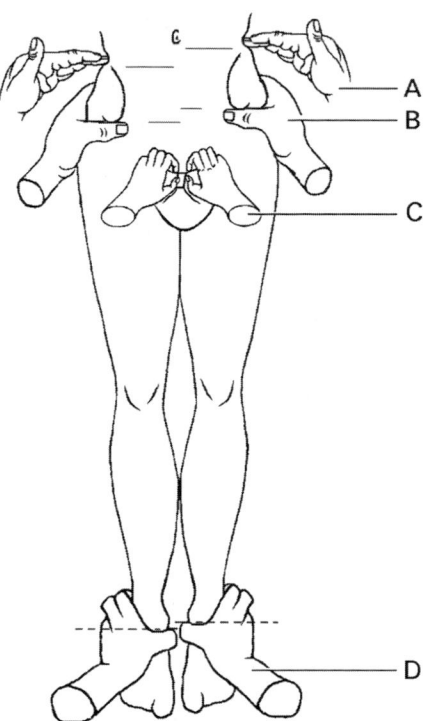

FIGURE 44.7. Anterior examination of bony landmarks (horizontal planes) of the body.

Anterior Screen of Horizontal Planes (Fig. 44.7)

Position: Patient supine and physician stands behind the patient

Procedure:

1. Hip flop test is done to align the patient on the table.
2. Assess iliac crests with transverse plane (Fig. 44.7A).
3. Assess anterior superior iliac spine (ASIS) levels with transverse plane (Fig. 44.7B).
4. Assess pubic tubercles with transverse plane (Fig. 44.7C).
5. Assess medial malleoli levels with transverse plane (Fig. 44.7D).

Interpretation: If a plane or planes are not level consider lower extremity abnormalities, an unlevel sacral base, spinal scoliosis, and/or congenital vertebral abnormalities.

Test for Clue to Early Postural Decompensation (Iliolumbar Ligament Palpation)

After screening for posterior superior iliac spine (PSIS) levels, move the palpating thumbs 1 inch lateral and 1 inch cephalad from their position on the PSISs. This will place them approximately over the iliac attachment of the iliolumbar ligaments to the ilium (see Chapter 50, Fig. 50.8). Press toward the iliac crests, testing for tissue texture changes and tenderness of these attachments.

Positive test: Tenderness of these attachments to the ilia.

Interpretation: These are normally not tender but become tender if there is postural decompensation and may be tender if there is innominate or lumbosacral somatic dysfunction. Early postural decompensation may be asymptomatic to the patient but can be indicated if these ligaments are tender to palpation. With a positive test, question the patient further about back fatigue or backache when they first lie down at night. Test for a short leg with an unlevel sacral base and for scoliosis.

Upper Extremity Screen for Joint Dysfunction: Extend Arms over Head, Active (or Passive) (Fig. 44.8)

Position: Patient is standing or seated and the physician stands in front or behind the patient. If the patient is supine, the physician stands beside the table or bed.

Procedure: The patient actively and fully abducts both arms in the coronal plane over their head, first with the backs of the hands together and then with the palms together.

Interpretation:

Negative test: With the head and neck in a neutral position, the medial surface of the upper arms should touch the ears. The elbows should be straight, the arms touching the ears, the forearms pronated and the hands equally approximated with the backs of the hands together over the head. This is repeated with the patient putting the palms together over his or her head. If all this can be accomplished, the joints of the shoulder, elbow, radioulnar, and wrist are probably normal.

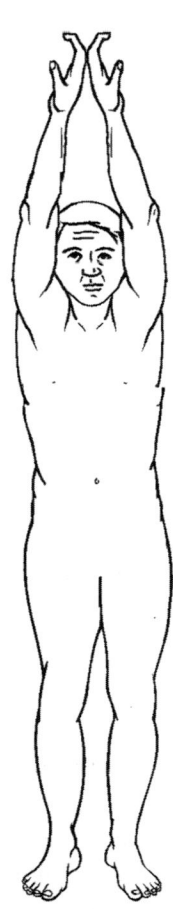

FIGURE 44.8. Upper extremity screen for joint dysfunction.

Negative test: The AC horizontal plane depresses 20 to 25 degrees on both sides.

Passive Motion Tests of Thoracolumbar Side Bending and Rotation

Procedure (Table 44.3): An additional method for passive testing of any of the gross motions of the upper thoracic spine is to place one hand on the patient's head and introduce flexion down to the cervicothoracic junction. The other hand contacts the upper thoracic area and monitors further motion flexion, side bending and rotation being introduced through the head and neck. The upper thoracics can be tested in neutral, flexed, or extended position by producing these motions beyond the cervicothoracic junction.

Hip Drop Test (Fig. 44.11)

The hip drop test is an active test. It screens for the ability of the lumbar and lumbothoracic region (especially the lumbosacral region) to side bend away from the side of the hip drop.

Position: The patient is standing and the physician kneels or sits behind the patient.

Procedure:

1. The physician's fingers are placed on the superior and most lateral surface of the patient's iliac crests, palms facing downward (parallel to the floor), and a mental note is made of the observed horizontal plane passing through these two contact points.

2. The patient is instructed to bend one knee without lifting the heel from the floor and let the hip drop downward. The patient must do this in a manner that does not rotate the pelvis in the transverse plane, nor translate the pelvis in a coronal plane.

3. The physician again observes the levelness of the horizontal

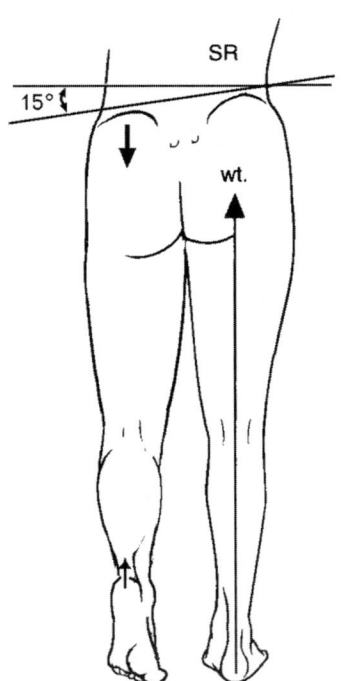

FIGURE 44.11. Positive left hip drop test.

plane through the contact points on the patient's iliac crests. These findings are compared with those observed in step 1.

4. Steps 2 and 3 are repeated with the patient's other lower extremity.

Interpretation:

Negative test: Indicates normal side-bending ability of the lumbar and thoracolumbar regions of the spine to the contralateral side of the hip drop test. Normal is a hip drop of 20 to 25 degrees and a smooth curve away from the side of the hip drop test (its convexity is on the same side as the hip drop).

Positive test: The plane of the iliac crests drops less than 20 degrees and/or the lumbar and thoracolumbar spine does not side bend with a smooth lateral curve, or is flat, or is angled at one unit in its attempt to side bend away from the side being tested. The test is called positive on the side that was being tested. A positive hip drop test indicates that there is some somatic dysfunction or pathology in the lumbars or thoracolumbar junction that prevents the region of the spine from side bending normally to the side opposite the hip drop.

Example of a Positive Hip Drop Test (Fig. 44.11): With weight being supported on the right leg, the left hip drops only 15 degrees and there will also be an angled curvature observed in the lumbar region. This indicates that lumbar and the thoracolumbar spine should be segmentally examined to determine the site of the side-bending dysfunction.

Note: In all cases, as the hip drops the lumbar spine and thoracolumbar junction side bends away from the test side. Under normal conditions the side that drops the most has the greatest convexity of lumbar/thoracolumbar curve on the side of the test. The hip drop test can also be used to estimate the type of scoliosis present in a patient. If you observe a left scoliosis (thoracic region side bent to the right) in a patient and the left hip drop test is negative, a C curve (side-bent right) is most likely present. If the right hip drop test is negative in that person, an S-type spinal curvature is most likely present. The area of flattened or angled spinal curvature seen in this patient is probably where the contralateral curves meet and is often called a crossover point. Somatic dysfunction at a crossover has expanded significance because it is more likely to be associated with visceral dysfunction in organs receiving sympathetic innervation from that level of the spinal cord.

Pelvic Side-Shift Test (Passive) (Fig. 44.12)

With perfect posture, viewed from the back, the midline of the sacrum should be in the midheel line (the anteroposterior vertical gravitational line) and should not deviate to the right or left. This test determines whether the sacrum, as the center of the pelvis, is in the midline.

Position: The patient is standing and the physician stands behind the patient.

Procedure:

1. The physician's left hand is placed on the lateral side of the left pelvis of the patient.

2. The physician's right hand is placed on the patient's right shoulder to stabilize the thoracic spinal segments.

3. The physician translates the patient's pelvis to the right side (while stabilizing the shoulder with his or her right hand).

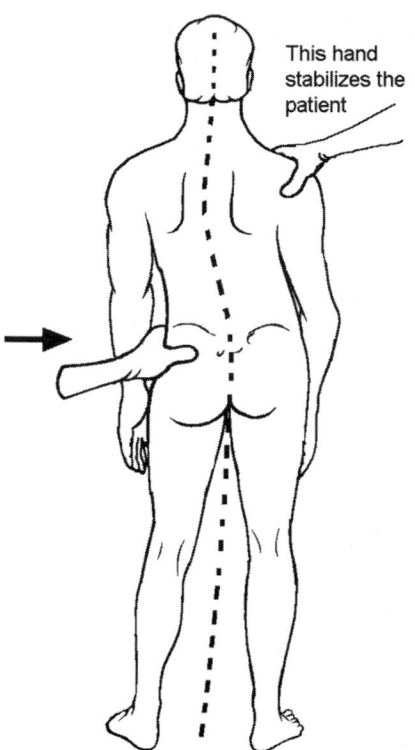

FIGURE 44.12. Right pelvic side-shift test.

4. The physician switches hand placements and translates the patient's pelvis to the left side.

Interpretation: The physician is aware of amount of movement, resistance to movement, and the end-feel at the barrier.

Positive test: A positive test reveals freer translation to the side of side shift. This means that the sacrum (base of support) is positioned on the side of the freer motion. If the deviation to one side is obvious with gross observation, pelvic shift is confirmed and this test need not be performed.

Palpate for Elevated First Rib (Fig. 44.13A)(See also Chapter 49.)

The most posterior part of the first rib in located in the fleshy part of the cervicothoracic junction just below and ¹/₂-inch lateral to the end of the articular column of the cervical spine. Each is palpated with the index and middle finger of each hand and the horizontal plane through these contact points is estimated.

Position: Patient can be seated or supine. Seated examination seems to be easier to evaluate.

Positive test: The rib head and posterior end of the first rib is elevated in comparison with the opposite side.

Note: This is only a presumptive sign and must be supported with first rib motion testing. This is because an apparent elevation of the first rib is present on the side opposite the side-bending

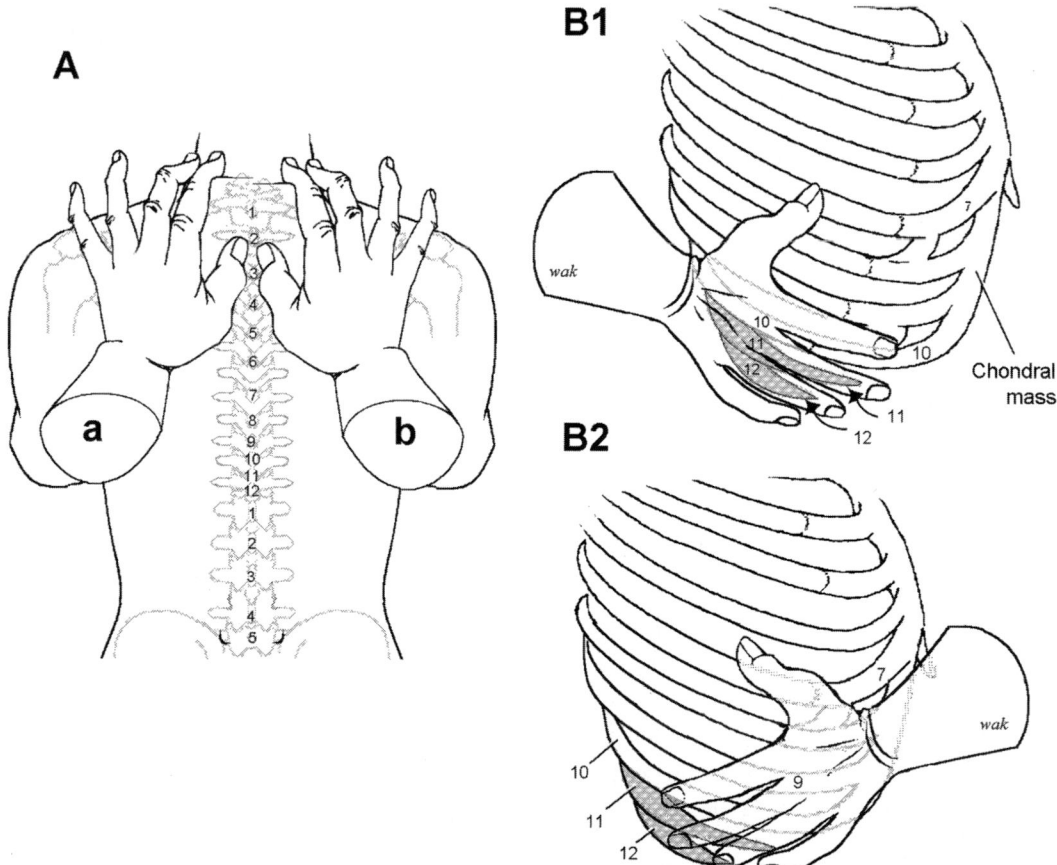

FIGURE 44.13. A, B1, B2. Segmental diagnosis of atypical ribs.

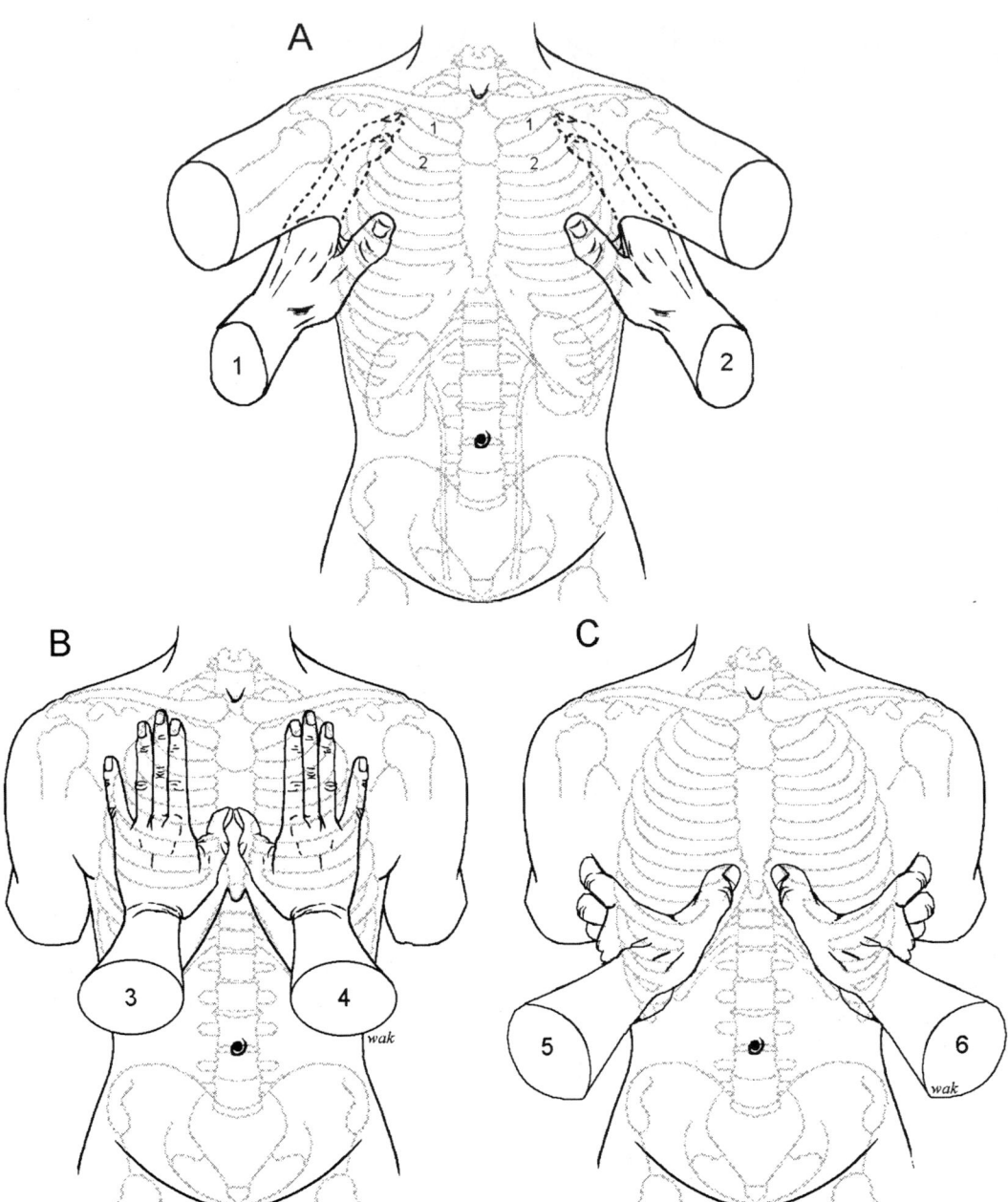

FIGURE 44.16. Six-quadrant rib screen.

Optimal Patient Position for Segmental Musculoskeletal Examination of Body Regions (Table 44.2)

Paraspinal palpation is an art perfected with time and practice. It is usually accomplished using the index and middle fingers of each hand to sense the superficial and then deep fasciae and muscular layers of the paraspinal regions. It can be performed in any position. Various characteristics are noted and expressed (Fig. 44.17).

Segmental Motion Testing

For spinal complaints and dysfunction, record findings on the side of the positive seated flexion test. If a lower extremity dysfunction is possible but not evident, record the lower extremity findings on the side of the standing flexion test (Table 44.3).

Passive Cervical Segmental Motion Testing

See Chapter 46 for supine cervical segmental motion testing. For rotation and side bending, contact the articular column on both sides. Anterior pressure tests for rotation to the opposite side. Lateral translation tests for side bending to the side opposite the direction of translation. (For flexion and extension, monitor the spinous process–interspinous area.)

Passive Segmental Testing for Joints of the Upper Extremity

This is discussed in Chapter 47.

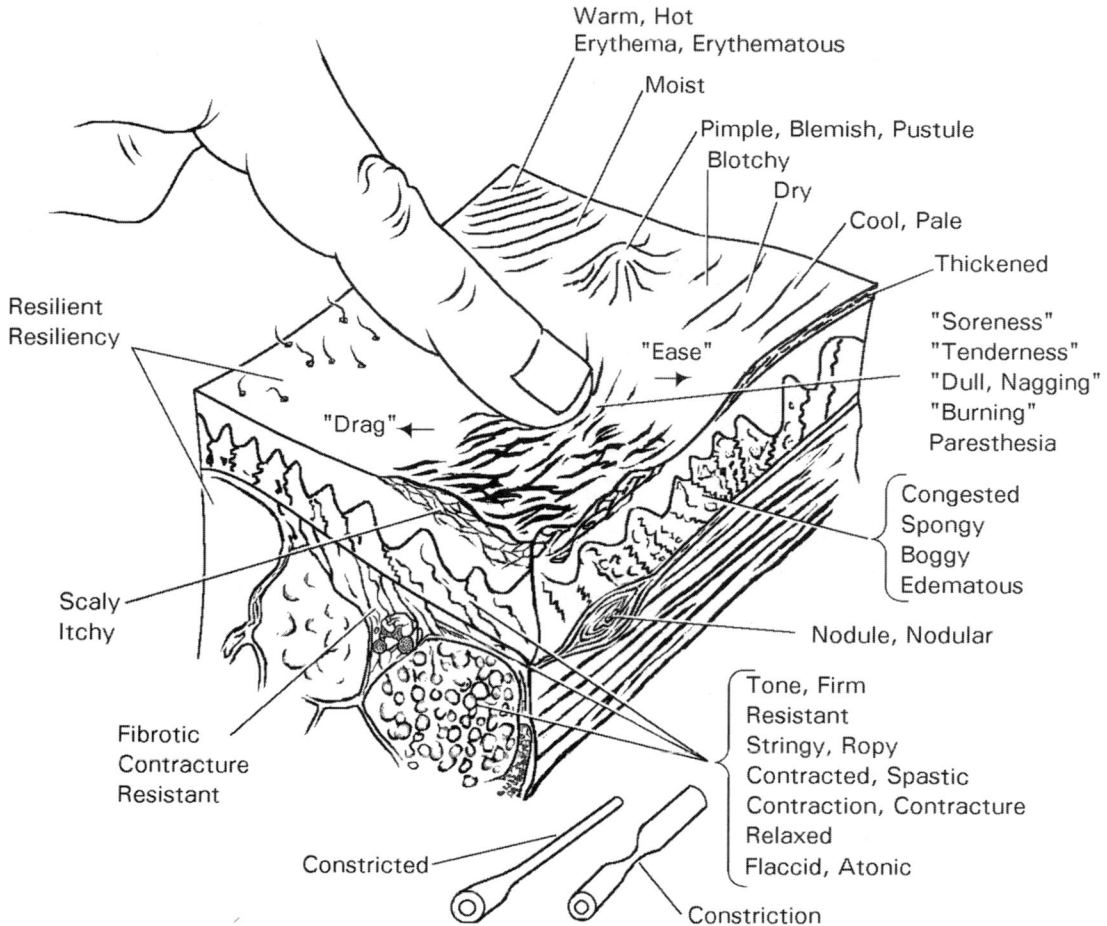

FIGURE 44.17. Palpation of tissue properties and abnormalities. (Reprinted with permission from Kuchera W, Kuchera M, *Osteopathic Principles in Practice*. 2nd ed rev. Greyden Press: Columbus, OH; 1994:20.)

Active Typical Rib Segmental Motion Testing (Figs. 44.18A and B)

Position: Patient is seated or supine and physician stands behind or at the side of the table.

Procedure:

1. The physician uses the index and middle fingerpads of one hand to straddle the rib angle and the index and middle finger of the other hand to straddle the same rib at its midclavicular line. The thumbs can be placed on the rib shaft at the midaxillary line to evaluate bucket handle motion of the rib.

TABLE 44.2. BEST POSITION FOR A PATIENT'S EXAMINATION

Region	Position
Cervical	Supine
Thoracic	Seated or prone
Ribs	Seated or supine
Lumbar	Seated or prone
Sacrum	Prone
Pelvis	Supine
Upper Extremities	Seated or supine
Lower extremities	Seated or supine

2. The patient is instructed to take a deep breath in and out, with the mouth open.

Positive test: The rib will move freely throughout one of these phases but not move completely throughout the other phase of the respiratory cycle. The rib somatic dysfunction is named for the motion and axis in which it moves. Example: Rib 5, exhalation, pump handle rib (about a transverse axis).

Active Atypical Rib Segmental Motion Testing

First rib segmental testing (see Fig. 44.13 A)

Rib 11 or 12 segmental testing (see Figs. 44.13B1 and B2)

Passive Lumbar Segmental Motion Testing

This screen is done by paraspinal thumb pressure over the transverse processes, looking for rotation preference.

Position: Patient is prone and the physician stands to the side of the patient.

Procedure:

Assess rotation:

1. The physician places the pads of their thumbs over the transverse processes of a single vertebral segment with the rest of the hand wrapped around the lumbar paraspinal area.

2. The physician "grabs some torso" (i.e., hold the torso), and

TABLE 44.3. SCREENING MUSCULOSKELETAL EXAMINATION FOR THE AMBULATORY PATIENT

Tests	Test Results		Explanation
	Neg.	Pos.	
Body Planes			Estimate levelness of horizontal planes under the mastoid bones, shoulders, inferior scapular angles, iliac crests, posterior superior iliac spines (PSIS), and the cephalad margins of the greater trochanters. Positive = unleveled horizontal planes. This indicates postural change that could be related to compensatory mechanisms, visceral dysfunction, and/or scoliosis.
Arms	Neg.	Pos.	The patient raises his/her arms above the head; upper arms touch ears, back of hands are together. Repeat the test having patient put palms together over the head. Positive = unable to fully extend the extremity with upper arms alongside of the ears and hands together. Indicates dysfunction in any one or combination of the joints of the upper extremity and also includes the upper back and upper thoracic region. Individual joints listed above are specifically examined according to the patient's history and concerns.
Legs	Neg.	Pos.	The patient squats down and returns to upright position. This tests hips, knees, ankles, and strength of the legs. Positive = inability to flex legs while weightbearing to a point where the thighs are at least level with the ground or patient is unable to return to the upright position without help. Individual joints listed above are specifically examined *according to the patient's history and concerns.*

(continued)

TABLE 44.3. (continued)

Tests	Test Results		Explanation
Standing Flexion Test	Neg.	Pos.	The physician monitors the inferior notches of the PSISs as the patient bends forward with arms hanging toward the floor. This localizes pelvic and/or leg somatic dysfunction to one side. (A rib hump can also be visualized at this time if there is thoracic rotoscoliosis.) Positive = the PSISs rise asymmetrically. It is the PSIS that rises farthest and last with forward bending: and/or there is a "rib hump" visualized. Because the patient is weightbearing this test indicates dysfunction *in the leg and/or in the pelvis on the "positive" side*. (A rib hump indicates rotoscoliosis with rotation toward the side of the hump and side bending away; often due to scoliosis resulting from an unleveled sacral base.)
Seated Flexion Test	Neg.	Pos.	The physician monitors the inferior notches of both PSISs while the patient bends forward with arms hanging toward the floor. The test localizes somatic dysfunction to one side of the pelvis. (A rib hump can also be visualized at this time if there is thoracic rotoscoliosis.) Positive = the PSISs rises asymmetrically. It is the PSIS that rises farthest and last with forward bending: and/or there is a "rib hump" visualized. Because the patient is *not weightbearing* the positive side indicates some problem with the innominate or sacral joints on the positive side. (A rib hump indicates rotoscoliosis.)
Trunk Rotation Screen	Neg.	Pos.	Passive rotation of the trunk is produced to the right and to the left. Normal = 90°. Positive = rotation restricted in one direction. Indicates restriction to rotation somewhere in the thoracolumbar spine. If there is a problem in rotation there is a problem in side bending. If screen fails, follow with segmental examination for somatic dysfunction and correlate findings with neurologic examination.
Upper Trunk Side Bending and Rotation Test (Acromion Drop Test)	Neg.	Pos.	The physician depresses the shoulder on one side and then the other. This action tests side bending and rotation of the upper thoracic spine. Normal = acromion drops 25°. Positive = acromion does not drop as far on one side as on the other (i.e., drops less than 25°). Indicates restriction of the upper thoracic area to side bend toward the side of the positive test. With neutral dysfunctions those units rotate to the opposite side of side bending. With non-neutral dysfunction the vertebral unit rotates to the same side as the side bending.

(continued)

Outpatient Osteopathic Assessment and Plan Form

wak SOAP version B 5:021402

Office of:	
For office use only:	

A Patient's Name _____   Date _____

Dx No.	ICD Code	Written Diagnosis	Dx No.	ICD Code	Written Diagnosis
	739.0	Somatic Dysfunction of Head and Face		739.4	Somatic Dysfunction of Sacrum
	739.1	Somatic Dysfunction of Neck		739.5	Somatic Dysfunction of Pelvis
	739.2	Somatic Dysfunction of Thoracic		739.9	Somatic Dysfunction of Abd / Other
	739.8	Somatic Dysfunction of Ribs		739.6	Somatic Dysfunction of Upper Extremity
	739.3	Somatic Dysfunction of Lumbar		739.7	Somatic Dysfunction of Lower Extremity

Physician's evaluation of patient prior to treatment: First visit ☐   Resolved ☐   Improved ☐   Unchanged ☐   Worse ☐

P ☐ All not done

Region	OMT Y	OMT N	ART	BLT	CR	CS	DIR	FPR	HVLA	IND	INR	LAS	ME	MFR	ST	VIS	OTH	R	I	U	W
Head and Face	☐	☐	☐	☐	☐	☐	☐	☐	☐	☐	☐	☐	☐	☐	☐	☐	☐	☐	☐	☐	☐
Neck	☐	☐	☐	☐	☐	☐	☐	☐	☐	☐	☐	☐	☐	☐	☐	☐	☐	☐	☐	☐	☐
Thoracic T1-4	☐	☐	☐	☐	☐	☐	☐	☐	☐	☐	☐	☐	☐	☐	☐	☐	☐	☐	☐	☐	☐
T5-9	☐	☐	☐	☐	☐	☐	☐	☐	☐	☐	☐	☐	☐	☐	☐	☐	☐	☐	☐	☐	☐
T10-12	☐	☐	☐	☐	☐	☐	☐	☐	☐	☐	☐	☐	☐	☐	☐	☐	☐	☐	☐	☐	☐
Ribs	☐	☐	☐	☐	☐	☐	☐	☐	☐	☐	☐	☐	☐	☐	☐	☐	☐	☐	☐	☐	☐
Lumbar	☐	☐	☐	☐	☐	☐	☐	☐	☐	☐	☐	☐	☐	☐	☐	☐	☐	☐	☐	☐	☐
Sacrum	☐	☐	☐	☐	☐	☐	☐	☐	☐	☐	☐	☐	☐	☐	☐	☐	☐	☐	☐	☐	☐
Pelvis	☐	☐	☐	☐	☐	☐	☐	☐	☐	☐	☐	☐	☐	☐	☐	☐	☐	☐	☐	☐	☐
Abdomen/Other	☐	☐	☐	☐	☐	☐	☐	☐	☐	☐	☐	☐	☐	☐	☐	☐	☐	☐	☐	☐	☐
Upper Extremity	☐	☐	☐	☐	☐	☐	☐	☐	☐	☐	☐	☐	☐	☐	☐	☐	☐	☐	☐	☐	☐
Lower Extremity	☐	☐	☐	☐	☐	☐	☐	☐	☐	☐	☐	☐	☐	☐	☐	☐	☐	☐	☐	☐	☐

(Treatment Method columns; Response columns R I U W)

Meds: _____   PT: _____

Exercise: _____   Other _____

Nutrition: _____

Complexity / Assessment / Plan (Scoring) *Default to level 2—same criteria

Problems		Risk: (presenting problem(s), diagnostic procedure(s) and management options)		Data	Maximum Points
Self	1 (2 max.)	Minimal = Min.		Lab	1
Established problem improved / stable	1	Low		Radiology	1
Established—worsening.	2	Moderate = Mod.		Medicine	1
New—no workup	3 (1 max.)	High		Discuss with performing physician	1
New—additional workup	4			Obtain records or Hx from others	1
				Review records, discuss with physician	2
				Visualization of tracing, specimen	2

Level I	Level II	Level III	Level IV	Level V	Level I	Level II	Level III	Level IV	Level V	Level I	Level II	Level III	Level IV	Level V
	≤1 pt.	2 pt.	3 pt.	≥4 pt.		Min.	Low	Mod.	High		≤1 pt.	2 pt.	3 pt.	≥4 pt.
	☐	☐	☐	☐		☐	☐	☐	☐		☐	☐	☐	☐

Requires only 2 above 3 (problems, risk and data).   Level of complexity = average of included areas.

Traditional Method—Coding by Components

History	I	II	III	IV	V
Examination	I	II	III	IV	V
Complexity / Assessment Plan		II	III	IV	V
Final level of service	☐	☐	☐	☐	☐

All these areas required. Average of three levels of service.

Optional Method—Coding by Time

When the majority of the encounter is counseling / coordinating, the level is determined by total time.

	I	II	III	IV	V
New patients (minutes)	10	20	30	45	60
Established patients (minutes)		10	15	25	40
Final level of service	☐	☐	☐	☐	☐

Dictate total time and counseling / coordinating time plus a brief description of topics discussed

Minutes spent with the patient:	☐ 10	☐ 15	☐ 25	☐ 40	☐ 60	☐ >60	Follow-up:	☐ 1	☐ 2	☐ 3	☐ 4	☐ 5	☐ 6	☐ 7	☐ 8	☐ 9	☐ 10	☐ 11	☐ 12	Units:	☐ D	☐ W	☐ M	☐ Y	☐ PRN

OMT performed as Above: 0 areas ☐   1-2 areas ☐   3-4 areas ☐   5-6 areas ☐   7-8 areas ☐   9-10 areas ☐

Other Procedures Performed:	CPT Codes:							
	Written Dx:							

E/M Code:	New	☐ 02	☐ 03	☐ 04	☐ 05	EST ...	☐ 11	☐ 12	☐ 13	☐ 14	☐ 15	Consults ...	☐ 41	☐ 42	☐ 43	☐ 44	☐ 45
Write 992 plus ...																	

Signature of transcriber: _____   Signature of examiner: _____

Funded by a grant from the Bureau of Research. © 2002 American Academy of Osteopathy.
Designed to coordinate with Outpatient Osteopathic SOAP Note Form. Recommended by American Association of Colleges of Osteopathic Medicine.

D

FIGURE 44.19. *(continued)*

SAMPLE HISTORY AND OSTEOPATHIC MUSCULOSKELETAL EXAMINATION

A 38-year-old woman presents with low back pain of insidious onset and of 3 months duration. She is examined in standing, seated, prone, and supine positions. Review of systems is not relevant (NR). The back pain is worse at the left lumbosacral area. Neurologic examination is NR.

The patient failed screening examination for body planes, standing and seated flexion tests, collateral ganglia, and fascial planes.

Standing: right iliac crest, trochanter, and PSIS planes ↓. (+) right standing and seated flexion tests. Right lumbar paravertebral hump, apex at L2. Anteroposterior curves appear normal.

Supine: abdominal tenderness in subxiphoid and right epigastric regions; celiac ganglion tender; right ASIS ↓, left ASIS ↓. Cranial screen and cervical spine negative.

Prone: Right PSIS ↓ and left PSIS ↑; right sacral sulcus deep; tenderness TTA present. Right ILA posterior and ↓. Ischial tuberosities are level. Right lumbar paravertebral muscle mass; tenderness and TTA right paravertebral lumbar musculature. Lumbars S_LR_R; TTA at right T6-9 region, T8 is ES_RR_R. Patient denies food intolerances.

Segmental Musculoskeletal Findings

T8 ES_RR_R, standing and seated FT +R, R PSIS ↓, R ASIS ↑, R sulcus deep, R ILA post. and ↓, ischial tuberosities are level; inlet fascia R_LS_L; TL fascias R_L.

Working Diagnosis

1. Somatic dysfunction (SD) of pelvis: right sacral shear and posterior right innominate
2. SD of thoracic region: nonneutral T8 SD
3. Probable subacute dysfunction of gallbladder
4. Myofascial SD

Rx

1. Lateral recumbent pull for shear
2. ME for posterior right innominate
3. Rib raising, midthoracic
4. Paraspinal soft tissue
5. Myofascial direct method treatment to dome diaphragm
6. ME to inlet fasciae
7. High velocity/low amplitude technique to thoracic SD (pillow localization)
8. Avoid concentrated fatty foods
9. Recheck in 1 week, (consider possible gallbladder dysfunction)

Note: Although this example does not follow the proposed new recording forms, the Louisa Burns Research Committee has produced, and the American Academy of Osteopathy has recently adopted, standardized subjective, objective assessment plan (SOAP) note forms to simplify the physician's recording of "essential" history, examination, and treatment documentation concerning patients seen in the office (Fig. 44.19A through D). Actual preliminary clinical trials using these forms have revealed improved completeness and recording accuracy. Up to a 33% increase in collections has been reported. These and a SOAP Note Form Usage Guide, instructing the physician on how to use these forms, are available from the American Academy of Osteopathy, 3500 DePauw Blvd, Suite 1080, Indianapolis, IN 46268-1136; phone (317) 879-1881; *www.academyofosteopathy.org.*

CONCLUSION

The osteopathic musculoskeletal evaluation provides information about the musculoskeletal system and musculoskeletal clues to dysfunction of other systems or of the general health status of the patient. It is unique in that palpation integrated with motion testing is the major component of that portion of the examination. Discovery of musculoskeletal dysfunction often provides additional clues that direct, focus, or expand the examination; the musculoskeletal diagnosis also expands the logical conclusions that can be drawn from that examination.

REFERENCES

1. Dinnar U. Classification of diagnostic tests used with osteopathic manipulation. *JAOA.* 1980;79:451–455.
2. Dinnar U, et al. Description of fifty diagnostic tests used with osteopathic manipulation. *JAOA.* 1982;81:314–321.
3. Johnston WE. Hip shift: testing a basic postural dysfunction. *JAOA.* 1964;63:923–930. Reprinted in Peterson B, ed. *Postural Balance and Imbalance.* Newark, OH: American Academy of Osteopathy; 1983:109–112.
4. Kappler RE. Postural balance and motion patterns. *JAOA.* 1982;81:598–606. Reprinted in Peterson B, ed. *Postural Balance and Imbalance.* Newark, OH: American Academy of Osteopathy; 1983:612.
5. Mitchell FL Jr, Moran PT, Pruzzo NA. *An Evaluation and Treatment Manual of Osteopathic Muscle Energy Procedures.* Published by the authors, Valley Park, MO; 1979.
6. Sutton SE. Postural imbalance: examination and treatment utilizing flexion tests. *JAOA.* 1978;77:456–465. Reprinted in Peterson B, ed. *Postural Balance and Imbalance.* Newark, Ohio: American Academy of Osteopathy; 1983:102–108.
7. Sutton SE. An osteopathic method of history taking and physical examination, part I. *JAOA.* 1978;77:780–788.
8. Sutton SE. An osteopathic method of history taking and physical examination, part II. *JAOA.* 1978;77:845–858.
9. Zink JG, Lawson WA. An osteopathic structural examination and functional interpretation of the soma. *Osteopath Ann.* 1979;7(5):208–214.
10. Glossary Review Committee of the Educational Council on Osteopathic Principles. Glossary of osteopathic terminology. In: Allen TW, ed. *AOA Yearbook and Directory of Osteopathic Physicians.* Chicago, IL: American Osteopathic Association; 1994.
11. Kuchera ML, Kuchera WA. *Osteopathic Considerations in Systemic Dysfunction,* 2nd ed rev. Columbus, OH: Greyden Press; 1994.

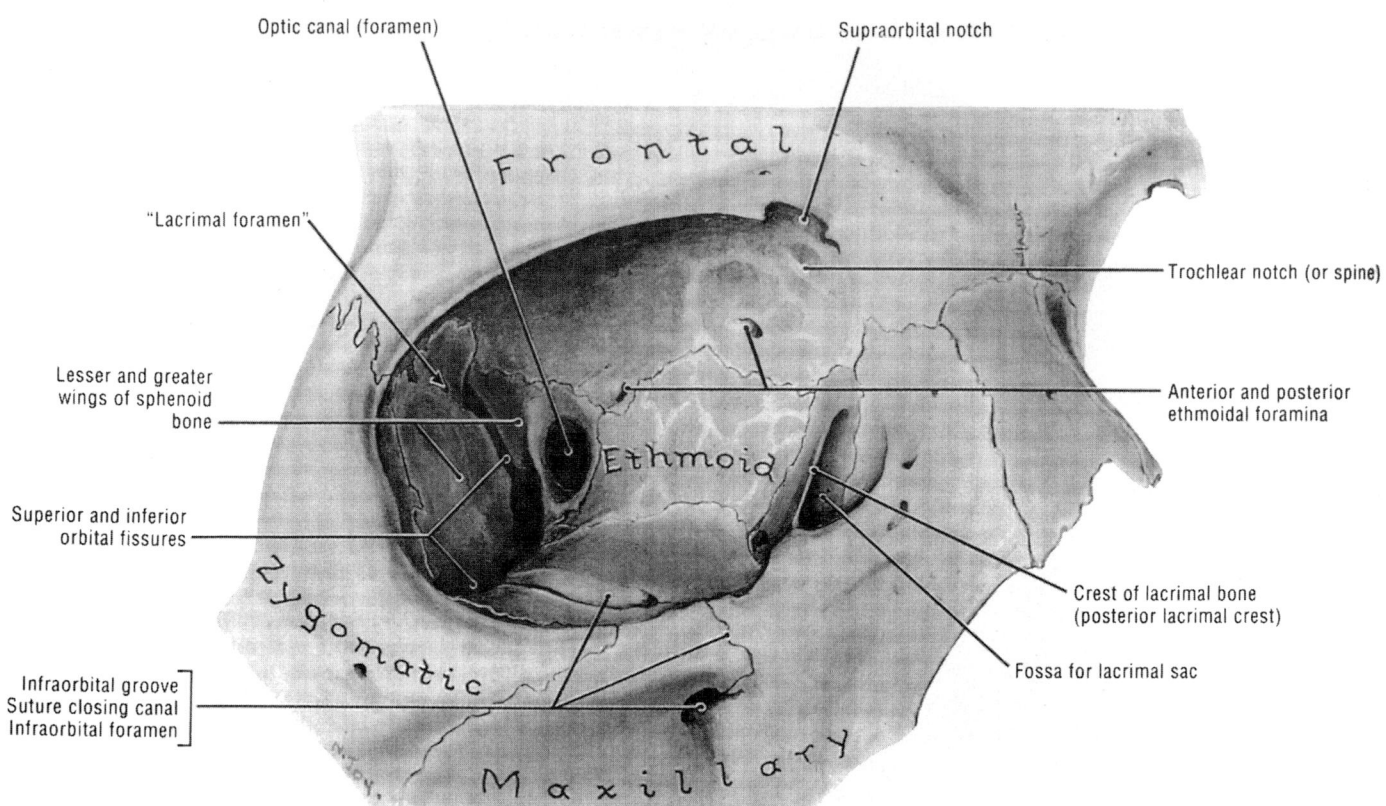

FIGURE 45.2. Orbital view of skull. (From Agur AMR. *Grant's Atlas of Anatomy*, 9th ed. Baltimore, MD: Williams & Wilkins; 1991:482.)

ARTERIAL SUPPLY

The face and scalp are supplied by branches of the external carotid artery (primarily the facial artery) (3). The internal structures of the head are primarily supplied by the internal carotid and vertebral arteries (Fig. 45.12). The internal carotid artery passes through the carotid canal in the petrous portion of the temporal bone. It supplies the anterior portions of the cerebrum (3). Cranial dysfunction in the articulations between the temporal bones, occiput, and sphenoid can alter the normal function of these arteries (3). This can produce symptoms including weakness and altered sensation on the opposite side of the body. The vertebral arteries arise from the subclavian artery and ascend through the transverse foramen of C6-C3. At C2 they make several right angle turns before piercing the dura to angle anteriorly and enter the skull through the foramen magnum (3). The vertebral arteries supply the visual area of the cerebrum (occipital lobe), brainstem, and cerebellum. Dysfunctions affecting this artery can be associated with visual abnormalities and dizziness (3).

VENOUS DRAINAGE

Approximately 85% of the venous drainage from the head occurs via the internal jugular veins (Fig. 45.13). These veins pass through the jugular foramen which is formed by both the occiput and temporal bones and is located along the occipitomastoid

suture. An occipitomastoid compression can compromise venous flow through the jugular foramen, leading to congestion of the large valveless venous sinuses within the head. Sacral, upper thoracic, cervical, and associated regional connective tissue dysfunction can also contribute to congestion and impaired venous flow from the head (2).

LYMPHATIC DRAINAGE

A knowledge of lymphatic drainage patterns assists the physician in localizing pathologic conditions in the head (Fig. 45.14). Lymphatic vessels in the forehead and anterior part of the face drain into the submandibular lymph nodes. Lymph vessels from the lateral face and eyelids drain inferiorly toward the parotid lymph nodes and ultimately drain into the deep cervical lymph nodes (3). The superficial lymph nodes of the head include the submandibular, occipital, retroauricular, and superficial parotid lymph nodes.

Lymph from the occipital region of the scalp drains into the occipital lymph nodes. The temporoparietal region drains into the retroauricular lymph nodes. The frontoparietal region drains into the superficial parotid lymph nodes. Lymph from the superficial lymph nodes eventually drains into the cervical lymph nodes. The deep cervical lymph nodes are located along the internal jugular vein. Lymph from the deep cervical structures passes through the jugular trunk into the left (thoracic duct) and right lymphatic trunks (Fig. 45.15) (3).

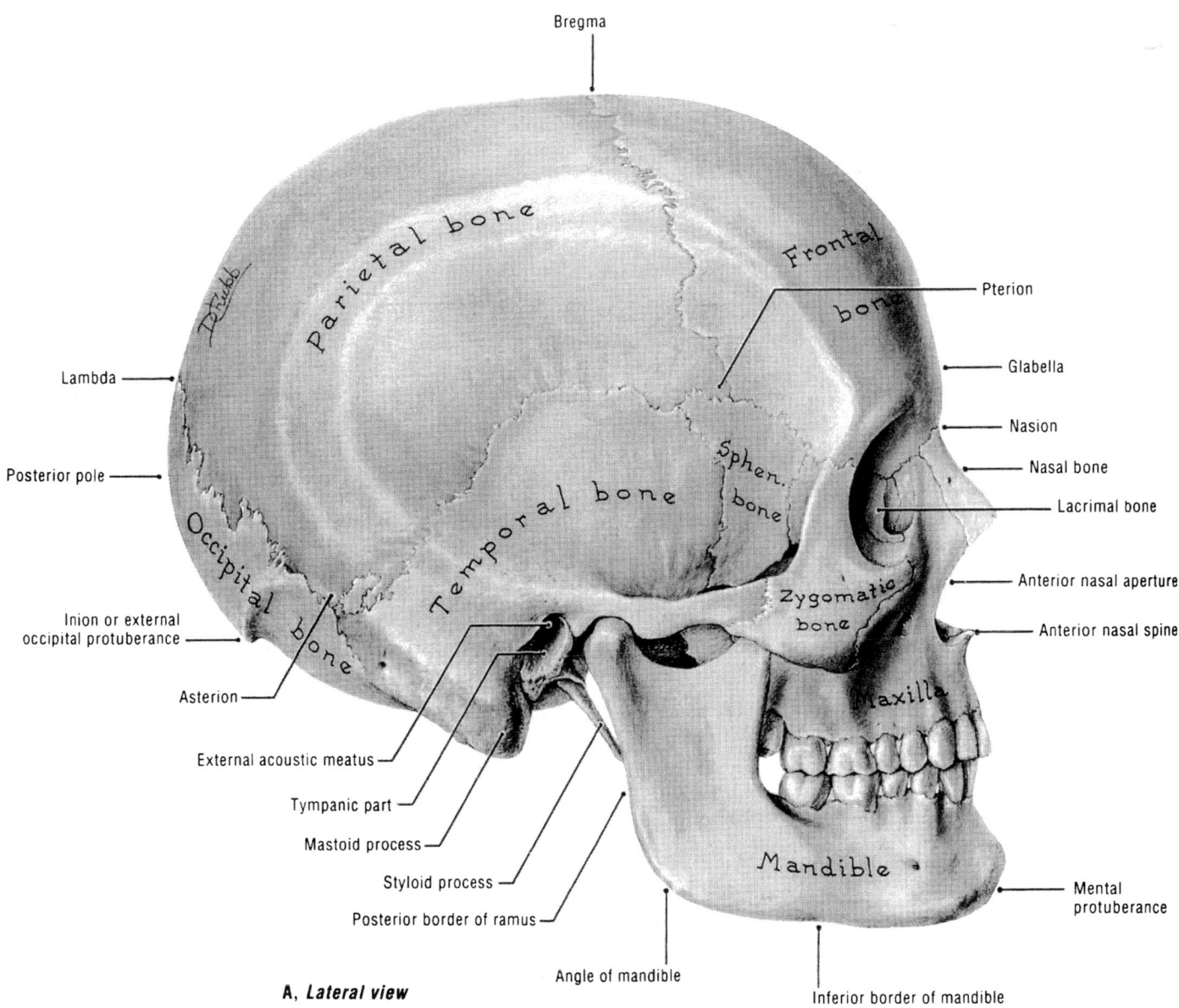

Bregma

Parietal bone

Frontal bone

Pterion

Glabella

Nasion

Nasal bone

Sphen. bone

Lacrimal bone

Temporal bone

Lambda

Posterior pole

Occipital bone

Zygomatic bone

Anterior nasal aperture

Anterior nasal spine

Maxilla

Inion or external occipital protuberance

Asterion

External acoustic meatus

Tympanic part

Mastoid process

Styloid process

Posterior border of ramus

Mandible

Mental protuberance

Angle of mandible

Inferior border of mandible

A, *Lateral view*

FIGURE 45.3. Lateral view of skull. (From Agur AMR. *Grant's Atlas of Anatomy*, 9th ed. Baltimore, MD: Williams & Wilkins; 1991:454.)

All drainage from the head passes through the neck, cervical fasciae, and thoracic inlet to return to the general circulation. Dysfunction in any of these structures can hinder the pathways and lead to lymphatic congestion. Increased sympathetic stimulation constricts the smooth muscle of the larger lymphatic vessels of the head and neck (associated with upper thoracic and cervical dysfunction), leading to decreased lymphatic drainage (2).

PARASYMPATHETICS

Parasympathetic nerve fibers to the pupil are supplied by cranial nerve (CN) III (oculomotor nerve) (Fig. 45.16). They innervate the ciliary muscle and cause constriction of the pupil. Parasympathetic activity shortens the focal length of the lens and is associated with visual disturbance. Parasympathetic fibers to

the lacrimal gland and nasopharyngeal mucosa originate in CN VII (facial nerve). They synapse in the sphenopalatine ganglion (Fig. 45.17). The postganglionic fibers then travel in the maxillary branch of CN V to the lacrimal gland. Parasympathetic hyperactivity resulting from sphenoid, maxilla, and palatine dysfunction results in excessive tear production and profuse, clear, thin secretions from the mucosa of the nasopharynx and sinuses. Parasympathetic nerves to the thyroid gland arise from the superior and inferior laryngeal nerves, a branch of the main vagus nerve (CN X) (2).

SYMPATHETICS

The structures of the head and neck obtain their sympathetic innervation from cell bodies located at spinal cord levels T1-4

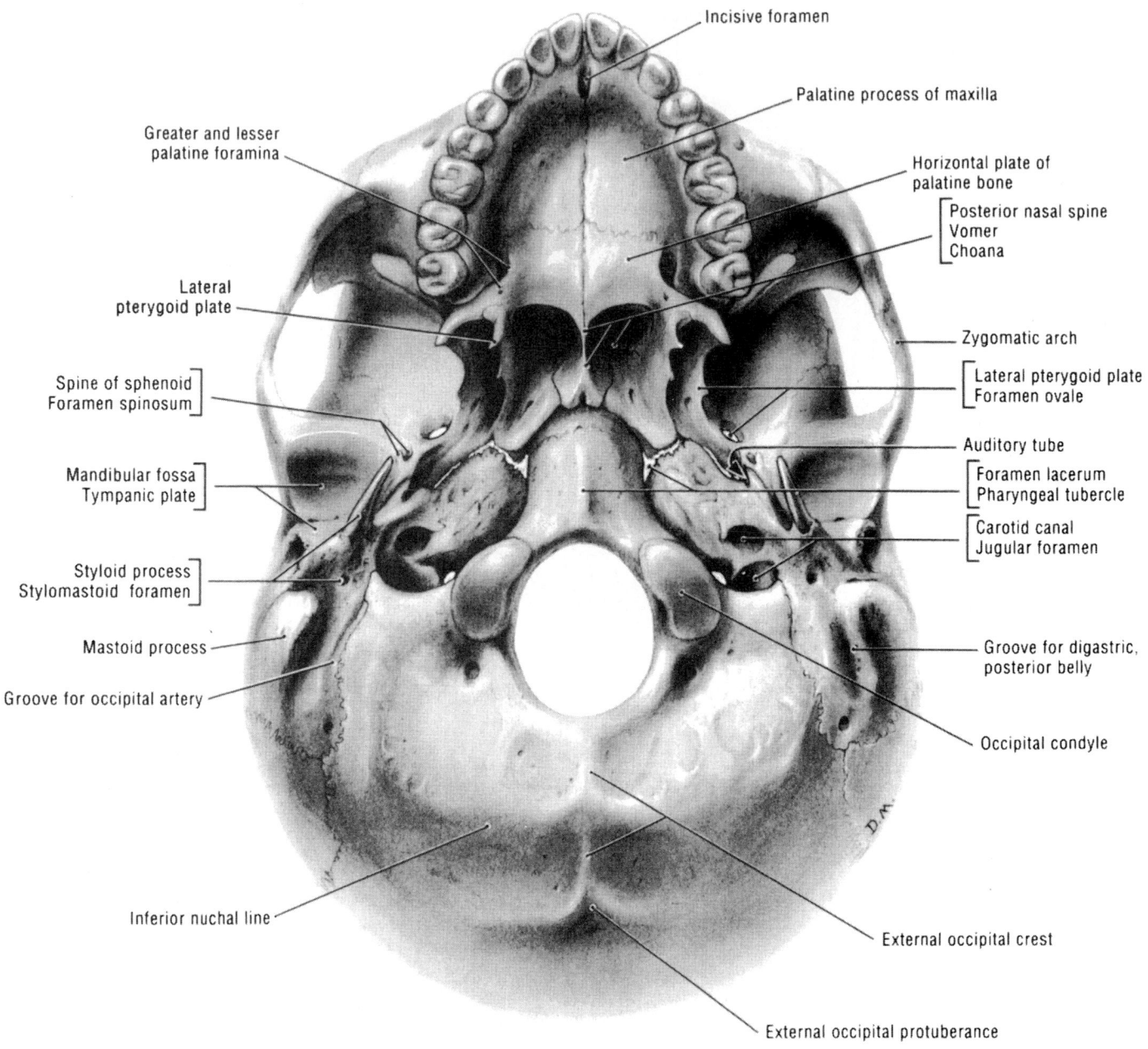

FIGURE 45.7. Inferior view of skull. (From Agur AMR. *Grant's Atlas of Anatomy*, 9th ed. Baltimore, MD: Williams & Wilkins; 1991:582.)

mount an immune response and obtain effective concentrations of medications is reduced in areas of vasoconstriction and tissue congestion (2).

Prolonged sympathetic stimulation changes the composition of the cells of the respiratory epithelium resulting in nasal and pharyngeal secretions that are thick and sticky, thereby reducing effective cleaning and clearing by the pseudostratified ciliated epithelium of the mucosa. Epithelial hyperplasia is present, with a relative increase in the activity and number of goblet cells, constriction of arterioles, decreased vascular and lymphatic drainage of the tissues, and the mechanical difficulty in moving the mucus. Sympathetic stimulation also produces vasoconstriction and inhibits secretion, leading to dryness of the nasopharyngeal mucosa. Dryness and cracking of the mucosa breaks down the normal

TABLE 45.1. BONES OF THE ADULT SKULL

Cranial Group (8)	Facial Group (14)	Miscellaneous (7)
Occiput	Vomer	Six middle ear ossicles
Sphenoid	Mandible	Hyoid bone
Ethmoid	Paired maxillae	
Frontal	Paired palatine	
Paired temporals	Paired zygoma	
Paired parietals	Paired lacrimal	
	Paired nasal	
	Paired inferior conchae	

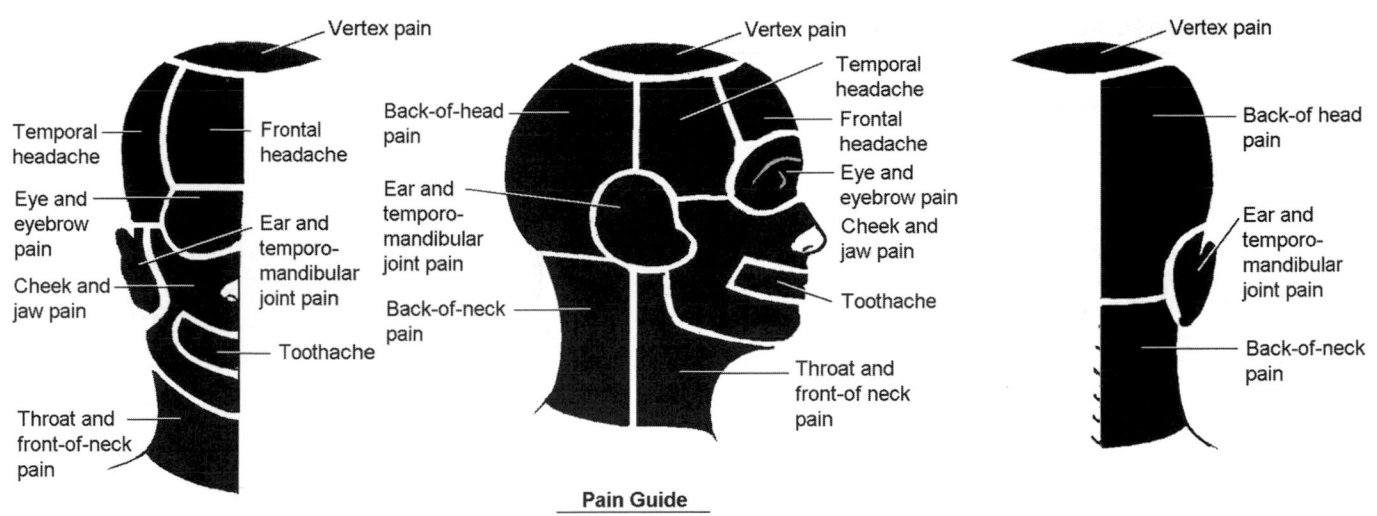

Pain Guide

Vertex pain

Sternocleidomastoid (sternal)
Splenius capitis

Back-of-Head Pain

Trapezius (TP1)
Sternocleidomastoid (sternal)
Sternocleidomastoid (clavicular)
Semispinalis cervicis
Splenius cervicis
Suboccipital group
occipitalis
Digastric
Temporalis (TP4)

Temporal Headache

Sternocleidomastoid (clavicular)
Sternocleidomastoid (sternal)
Semispinalis capitis
Frontalis
Sygomaticus major
Zygomaticus major

Frontal Headache

Sternocleidomastoid (clavicular)

Sternocleidomastoid (sternal)
Semispinalis capitis
Frontalis
Zygomaticus major

Ear and Temporomandibular pain

Lateral pterygoid
Masseter (deep)
Sternocleidomastoid (clavicular)
Medial pterygoid

Eye and Eyebrow Pain

Sternocleidomastoid (sternal)
Temporalis (TP1)
Splenius cericis
Masseter (superficial)
Suboccipital group
Occipitalis
Orbicularis oculi
Trapezius (TP1)

Trapezius (TP1)
Trapezius (TP2)

Trapezius (TP3)
Multifidi

Levator scapulae
Splenius cervicis
Infraspinatus

Throat and front-of-neck pain
Cheek and jaw pain

Sternocleidomastoid (sternal)
Masseter (superficial)
Lateral pterygoid
Trapezius TP1)
Masseter (deep)
Digastric
Medial pterygoid
Platysma
Orbicularis oculi
Zygomaticus major

Toothache

Temporalis (TPs1,2,3)
Masseter (deep)
Digastric (anterior)

Back-of-Neck Pain

Sternocleidomastoid (sternal)
Digastric
Medial pterygoid

FIGURE 45.8. Muscle trigger points pain guide **(left)** and areas of referred pain **(right)** in the head and neck. (From Travell JG, Simons DG. *Myofascial Pain and Dysfunction: The Trigger Point Manual. The Upper Extremities.* Vol 1. Baltimore, MD: Williams & Wilkins; 1983:166–167.)

mucosal defenses, thereby permitting secondary bacterial infection (2).

Dilation of the pupil (mydriasis) also occurs with increased sympathetic activity to the eye. This elevates intraocular pressures in patients with narrow angle glaucoma. Prolonged upper thoracic and cervical dysfunctions have been associated with the development cloudiness of the lens (2). The Barr-Lieou syndrome (vertigo, ataxia, vasodilation, and eye pain) results from hypersympathetic activity and proprioceptive dysfunction that often follows whiplash injuries.

The sympathetics innervate blood vessels that supply the thyroid and innervate the cells that produce thyroid secretions. Increased sympathetic stimulation may alter thyroid gland secretion (2).

CRANIAL NERVES

There are 12 sets of cranial nerves (Fig. 45.19). The actions, associated symptoms, and somatic dysfunction considerations are summarized in Appendix I. The reader is referred to *The Netter Atlas of Human Anatomy*, plate 7, published by Ciba-Geigy Corp. (Summit, NJ), which correlates the cranial nerves with associated foramina.

Olfactory Nerve (I)

The nerve of smell has olfactory neurosensory cells located in the olfactory neuroepithelium covering the superior conchae of the nasal cavity and the superior portion of the nasal septum.

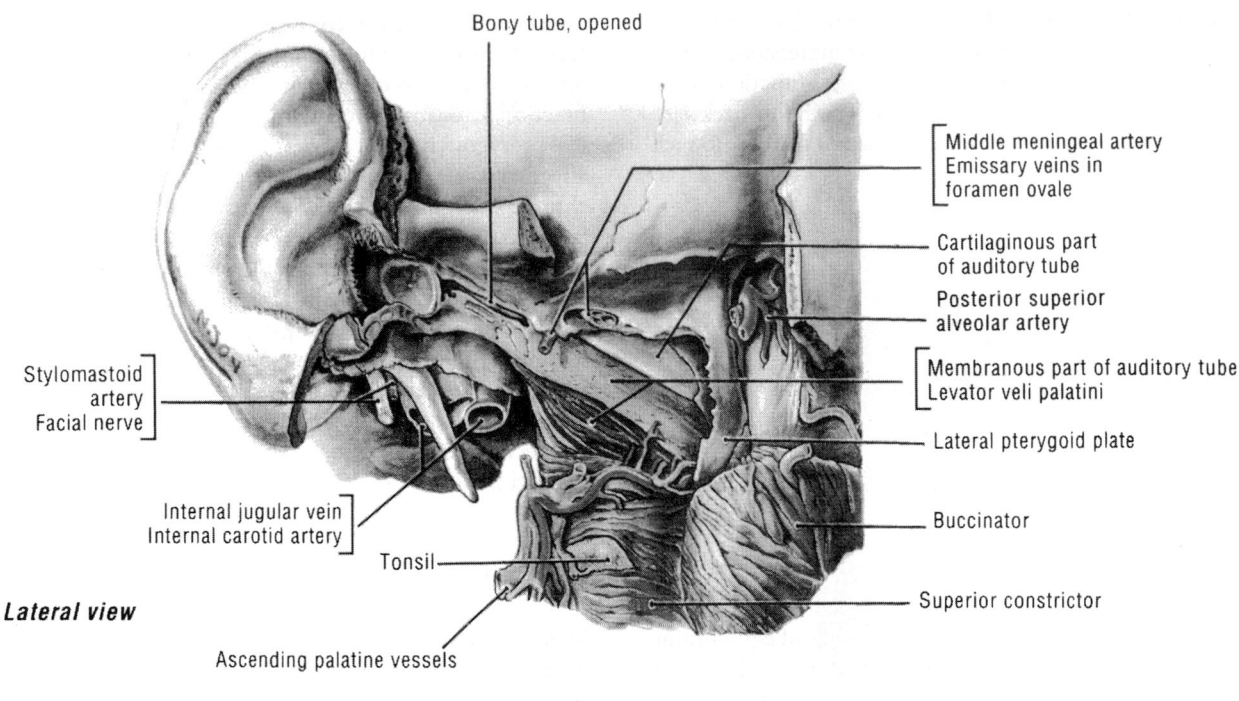

FIGURE 45.24. Connection of middle ear to nasopharynx. Lateral view. (From Agur AMR. *Grant's Atlas of Anatomy*, 9th ed. Baltimore, MD: Williams & Wilkins; 1991:541.)

tubes. Osteopathic treatment:

1. Improves the blood supply
2. Increases venous and lymphatic drainage from the affected area
3. Relieves muscle spasm, thereby improving breathing
4. Relieves pain
5. Reduces reflex disturbances
6. Improves circulation to and from the reticuloendothelial system and thereby improves immune function

Treatment of cranial dysfunction assists in managing a patient with sinus congestion. Circular pressure applied to the supraorbital and infraorbital nerves eases sinus pain. Treatment of the upper thoracic spine (rib raising) and cervical spine reduces excessive sympathetic outflow to the nose, sinuses, and bronchial tubes and aids the body in producing thin, saliva-like secretions. Treatment of cervical myofascial and articular dysfunctions and fascial torsions at the thoracic inlet improves lymphatic and venous drainage (2). Facial effleurage and lymphatic pump procedures augment drainage. These manipulative treatment measures assist in cleansing the structures of the head and upper airways.

HEADACHE

Headache is one of the most common conditions seen in a primary care practice. Every year, 40 to 50 million Americans seek treatment for headaches (5). This condition can be caused by a number of intracranial and extracranial abnormalities. The underlying cause of many headaches is often described as "un-

known" or "idiopathic." A thorough knowledge of anatomy and physiology and ability to diagnose structural abnormalities of the cranium, neck, upper thoraces, and sacrum often allows a physician to logically explain and treat previously unknown causes of headache. The implementation of a rational treatment plan significantly reduces suffering of the patient and improves overall functioning.

The head and scalp contain many pain-sensitive structures. These include:

- Skin and its blood supply
- Muscles of the head and neck
- Great venous sinuses and their tributaries
- Portions of the dura mater at the base of the brain
- Dural arteries
- Intracranial arteries
- Cervical nerves
- Trigeminal (V), abducens (VI), and facial (VII) nerves

The brain parenchyma itself is not sensitive to pain. Pain from structures above the tentorium cerebelli travel via the trigeminal nerve, so pain referred from structures above the tentorium cerebelli is perceived in the frontal, temporal, and parietal regions of the head. Pain fibers from structures below the tentorium cerebelli travel via the glossopharyngeal (IX) and vagus (X) nerves and the upper cervical spinal nerve roots. Therefore, pain referred from structures below the tentorium cerebelli is perceived in the occipital region (5).

Structural abnormalities, usually acting via the fasciae, place tension on pain-sensitive structures and cause discomfort. Example: parietal bone dysfunction produces strain on the superior sagittal sinus, producing discomfort in the parietal region. Upper cervical dysfunction leads to discomfort in the occipital region. Gastrointestinal abnormalities result in headache in the occipital region via vagal transmission.

A detailed history is vital to the diagnosis and treatment of headache, especially if they are recurrent or chronic in nature. Information regarding the patient's birth history (length of mother's pregnancy, maternal complications, length of labor, method of delivery, use of forceps, pitocin or vacuum extraction, neonatal complications) and childhood growth and development may shed light on the precipitating factors for headache. A history of trauma is often important. Clinical experience has revealed that a forgotten fall or head injury that has resulted in a sacral shear has often been overlooked and is the key to providing effective treatment of a chronic headache. Family history should be obtained (5), including information about:

- Headache: onset, frequency, location, duration, and severity
- Associated symptoms
- Trigger factors
- Previous medical, surgical, and dental history
- Prior headache therapy

A complete physical examination is performed, including a neurologic evaluation, in addition to the structural examination. Carefully document your findings. Always rule out serious organic causes of headache, such as brain tumor, aneurysm, arteriovenous malformation, hemorrhage, and temporal arteritis. Neuroradiologic studies such as computed tomography (CT), magnetic resonance imaging (MRI), and/or magnetic resonance angiography (MRA) are needed if any of the aforementioned are suspected (5).

There are four major classifications of headache (5):

1. Vascular (migraine and cluster)
2. Tension (muscle contraction)
3. Traction and inflammatory type (brain tumor, infection, cerebrovascular disease)
4. Cranial neuralgias (trigeminal neuralgia, TMJ)

Migraine

Migraine headaches are recurrent and vary widely in intensity, frequency, and duration. The pain is often described as a unilateral throbbing, pounding pain. It may later radiate to the opposite side. Migraine headaches can be associated with:

- Nausea
- Vomiting
- Diarrhea
- Vertigo
- Tremors
- Photophobia
- Phonophobia
- Sweating
- Chills

They are often preceded by:

- Aura
- Scotomas (blind spots)
- Photopsia (flashing lights)
- Paresthesias
- Visual, olfactory, and auditory hallucinations
- Vertigo
- Syncope

The initial episode most often occurs during puberty but can occur at any age between 5 and 40 years. Migraine headaches may be triggered by (5):

- Head injury or other trauma
- Stress
- Hormone fluctuations
- Fasting
- Oversleeping and undersleeping
- Vasoactive substances in foods (wine and cheese, cold foods)
- Changes in weather and temperature (bright light, poor ventilation)
- Physical stimuli (smoking)

The production of migraine symptoms involves two major events: vasoconstriction and vasodilation. The cerebral blood vessels can be divided into two major systems: the innervated adrenergic system and the noninnervated arterial system. The large innervated vascular system consists of the arteries at the base of the brain and the pial arteries. These have a rich adrenergic nerve supply and respond to catecholamines. The noninnervated vascular system consists of the parenchymal arteries and the terminal high-resistance arteries. They respond to local metabolic factors.

Trigger factors (listed above) produce unilateral cerebral vasoconstriction via the adrenergic nervous system. Platelets systemically aggregate and release serotonin, which augments vasoconstriction of these adrenergically innervated blood vessels. The overall result is vasoconstriction with a reduction in cerebral blood flow. When blood flow is sufficiently reduced, an aura develops with symptoms occurring as a consequence of which brain region is affected by the constriction. The vasoconstriction phase causes local anoxia and acidosis and a systemic drop in serotonin. Serotonin sensitizes the pain receptors in the blood vessels. In response to local metabolic factors (anoxia and acidosis), the vessels of the noninnervated arterial system dilate, increasing cerebral blood flow and promoting local vasomotor changes resulting in a combined dilation of the innervated extracranial and intracranial arteries on the same side. This vasodilation, along with the sensitization of pain fibers, produces the pain of migraine (5).

A trigeminal vascular reflex may also explain some of the events seen in the production of migraines. Afferent pain fibers from the cortex, thalamus, hypothalamus, and cervical roots C1-3 communicate with the spinal nucleus of the trigeminal nerve. These impulses can then travel via the facial nerve (CN VII) to produce parasympathetic dilation of the internal and external carotid arteries. Pain perception is increased when the effects of this dilation feed back into the spinal nucleus of the trigeminal nerve. Stimulation of the trigeminal ganglion, through vasodilation, can also produce edema in the dura (5).

How might somatic dysfunction play a role in the genesis of migraines? Somatic dysfunction in the upper thoracic spine increases the level of sympathetic tone to the innervated blood vessels of the head. Increased sympathetic tone produces

DIAGNOSIS

Inspection

Observe the skin for color changes. Look for asymmetry of position, including:

Flexion or extension
Side-bending to the right or left
Rotation to the right or left
Anterior posterior curves
Relationship of the head to the lateral weight-bearing line

Active Motion Testing

With the patient seated, ask him or her to:

Rotate to the right and to the left
Side-bend right and left (attempt to touch the ear to the shoulder)
Flex or touch the chin to the chest
Extend or backward bend

Occasionally, extension may produce lightheadedness. Record these motions in degrees. Measure the range with a goniometer. Osteopathic physicians may elect to bypass active motion testing and proceed directly to passive motion testing. If the patient has neck complaints or has sustained trauma, first determine the amount the patient can move.

Palpation

The cervical spine may be palpated in the seated position or in the supine position. Tissues on the anterior and lateral portions of the neck can be comfortably assessed with the patient seated and the physician standing behind the patient. Palpate muscle tension, tenderness, and tissue texture abnormality (scalenes, sternocleidomastoid, and trapezius). Examination of the neck with the patient seated and examination of the upper thoracic spine are often integrated. Passive motion testing to evaluate the ability of muscles to lengthen is sometimes performed (for example, side bend the cervical spine to evaluate scalene tension).

Palpation of the cervical spine with the patient supine allows for a detailed evaluation of tissue texture abnormality and tenderness surrounding the cervical spine. The suboccipital region contains muscles that are more lateral than the mid and lower cervical region, so paraspinal palpation must involve a more lateral placement of the fingers. Significant suboccipital tissue texture abnormality is usually associated with changes in the ipsilateral upper thoracic and rib angle area; look for them. Palpation over the posterior portion of the articular pillars reveals local muscle hypertonicity, tenderness, and tissue texture abnormality associated with segmental dysfunction. These changes are usually apparent with rotational restriction.

Palpate the lateral margins of the articular pillars (locate fingers laterally and direct the palpatory force medially) to reveal tenderness and tissue texture abnormality over the convex (anterior component) side of segmental dysfunction. For example, given C4 rotated and side-bent right with restriction of left rotation and side-bending, the posterior portion of the articular pillar is tender on the right side; the lateral margin of the articular pillar is tender on the left side.

The terms open facet and closed facet are sometimes applied as positional descriptors of cervical spine somatic dysfunction. Flexion motion (in a normal spine without motion restriction) causes the facets to open, and extension motion closes the facets. Side-bending motion with coupled rotation to the same side produces a concave side and a convex side. The facets on the concave side are closed while the facets on the convex side are open. Given a condition of C5 extended, rotated, and side-bent right (restriction of flexion, rotation, and side-bending left), the right side is the concave side and the left side is the convex side. In motion testing, extension is free so both facets close. During flexion motion testing, the facet on the right side is closed and resists opening. This produces palpable asymmetry in which the right transverse process (technically, the articular pillar) is more posterior, and the paraspinal muscle over C5 right is tight and palpable. This concept can be applied to C2-7 segmental motion testing. If a segment is extended (flexion restriction), rotated, and side-bent right (restriction of rotation and side-bending left), flexing this segment, which is engaging the barrier, intensifies the palpable posterior transverse process on the right, as well as the palpable muscle change. From this position of flexion, motion testing reveals a dominant restriction of left rotation and side-bending. If this segment is extended, the motion restriction is significantly less. Engaging the barrier in flexion or extension intensifies the rotation and side-bending restriction.

Passive Motion Testing

Regional Motion

Test the range of regional cervical rotation, side-bending, flexion, and extension with the patient in the supine position. Evaluate these motions by contacting the head bilaterally and introducing the motions through the head. The range of extension may be difficult to evaluate with the patient supine because the table gets in the way.

Segmental Motion

A novice may test every segment. The experienced clinician tests those segments in which palpation and screening motion tests suggest a problem.

The suboccipital area can be confusing. Neurologically, C1 and C2 are considered a common neurologic segment. Hyperactivity of the C1-2 segment potentially involves three joints: the occipito-atlantal (O-A) joint, the atlanto-axial (A-A) joint, and C2/C3. Therefore, positive palpatory findings in the suboccipital region demand testing of these three joints. Each joint is different in its motion, so they must be individually tested.

Occipital Motion Testing of C0-1

Lateral Translation Test

The physician stands or sits at the head of the supine patient. Grasp the head with both hands, with the fingertips of the index and middle fingers over the occipital articulation (Fig. 46.1).

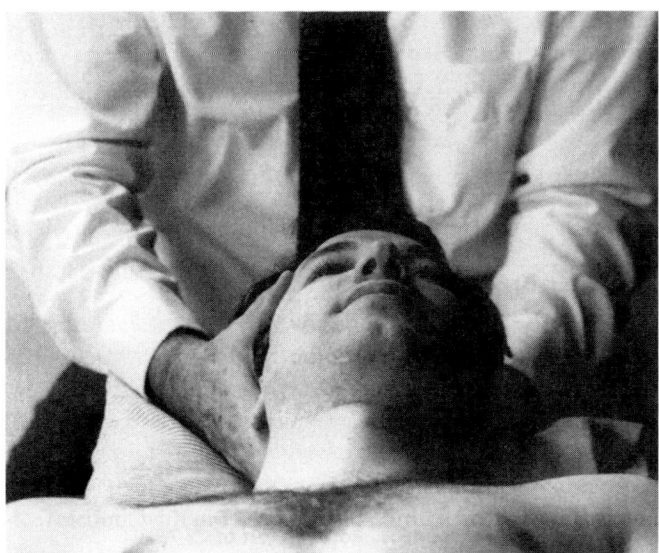

FIGURE 46.1. Lateral translation test for occipital motion.

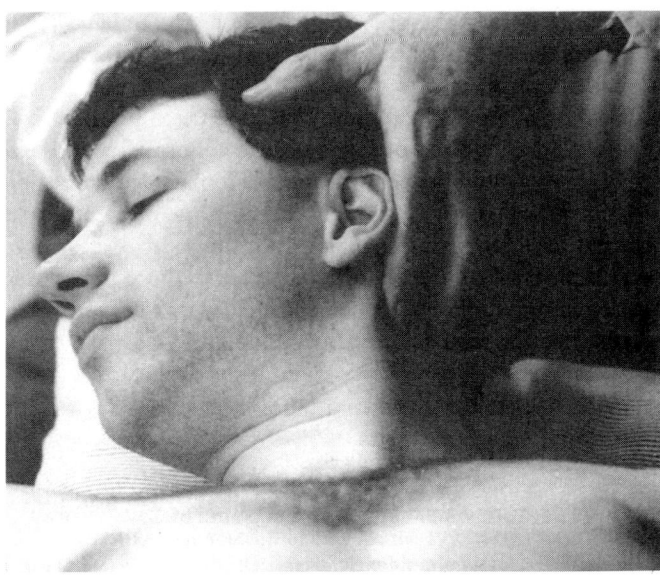

FIGURE 46.2. Rotation test for atlas motion.

Translate the head to the right and to the left, evaluating freedom or resistance. A more precise method is to perform the lateral translation test in flexion and in extension. Flex the occiput (O-A), and then translate to the right and to the left. Then extend the occiput and translate to the right and to the left. Restriction of right translation with freedom of left translation suggests an occiput rotated left and side-bent right (occiput posterior left). If translation is done in flexion and extension, restriction is encountered when the barrier is engaged. Restriction of right translation in the flexed position suggests an occiput that is extended, rotated left, and side-bent right with restriction of flexion, rotation right, and side-bending left.

There are two O-A joints, one on each side. Given a condition of occiput rotated right and side-bent left, the dominant restriction, tenderness, and tissue texture abnormality may be on the right side or it may be on the left side. In treating this dysfunction with high-velocity technique, it may be appropriate to localize force precisely to one side or the other. The terminology that has been used by the osteopathic profession for years is positional terminology. This in no way implies that positional diagnosis is preferred; identification of motion restriction is imperative. In the above example of the occiput rotated right and side-bent left, the right side is called posterior occiput and the left side is called anterior occiput. A posterior occiput right exhibits motion restriction, tissue texture abnormality, and tenderness on the right side. An anterior occiput left exhibits motion restriction, tissue texture abnormality, and tenderness left. Do confirmatory motion tests. Focusing on one side at a time, assess freedom of flexion and extension. The posterior occiput side exhibits restriction of extension. The anterior occiput side exhibits restriction of flexion.

Atlas Motion Test

The atlas rotates in relation to the axis and becomes restricted in rotation. The motion test of atlas function is a rotation test. It is convenient to isolate cervical rotation to the atlas by flexing the cervical spine prior to rotation. This produces physiologic locking of C2-7. This is an example of the third principle of physiologic motion of the spine. Flexion of C2-7 effectively eliminates rotation in this area.

Stand or sit at the head of your supine patient. Grasp the head with fingertips contacting the lateral mass of the atlas. Flex the cervical spine. Rotate to the right and to the left, assessing the range of motion and freedom or resistance (Fig. 46.2).

A right-rotated atlas exhibits restriction of left rotation. Osteopathic positional terminology for this dysfunction is posterior atlas right. Flexion, extension, and side-bending motions are not tested.

Some osteopathic physicians refer to an anterior atlas. The anterior side is opposite the posterior atlas. Given an example of atlas rotated right with restriction of left rotation, the right side would be the posterior atlas side. If the left side exhibited tenderness and tissue texture abnormality, it would be referred to as an anterior atlas left. These are not common, but when present, they are very symptomatic and tender. Retro-orbital pain is often associated with an anterior atlas.

C2-7 Motion Testing

Flexion and Extension Test

At a segmental level, C2-7 motion is difficult to assess by directly flexing and extending, although this has been the method used by many osteopathic physicians in the past. The lateral translation test, which was used extensively by the muscle energy tutorial committee (15), provides a more precise method of evaluating flexion and extension while evaluating side-bending.

Lateral Translation Test

The lateral translation test is similar to the occiput lateral translation test, except that the hand placement is on the cervical region with the fingertips over the lateral portion of the articular pillars. Stand or sit at the head of the supine patient. Support the patient's

Sympathetics

The sympathetic innervation to the upper extremities arises from the upper thoracic spinal cord. The sympathetic ganglia lie anterior to the rib head, in the fascia common to both structures. Dysfunction in the upper thoracic spine and ribs may increase sympathetic tone to the upper extremity and produce altered motion, nerve dysfunction, and lymphatic and venous congestion. Increased sympathetic tone is accompanied by palpatory findings in the upper thoracic/rib area and increased sensitivity to painful stimulus. It also prevents arterial blood from getting to the structures of the arm and reduces the amount of lymphatic fluid returning from the arm via the lymphatic vessels. The cause of these musculoskeletal findings may be viscerosomatic; they may be primary somatic in the area, or they may be reflex from the cervical spine. Nociceptive afferents from the cervical spine travel in the sympathetic chain and synapse in the intermediolateral cell columns of the upper thoracic cord. This produces an irritable focus in the cord, with resulting somatic and sympathetic hyperactivity.

Brachial Plexus

Nerve roots C5-8 and T1 form the brachial plexus. These nerve roots pass through the intervertebral foramen of the cervical vertebrae and pass between the anterior and middle scalene muscles. The roots unite to form successive trunks, divisions, cords, and branches. The nerve trunks extend from the scalene triangle (formed by the anterior and middle scalenes and the clavicle) to the clavicle. Nerve divisions extend from a position posterior to the clavicle to the axilla. Nerve cords are found in the axilla. Nerve cords divide into branches that innervate various structures in the upper extremity. The neurovascular bundle of the arm contains the subclavian artery, subclavian vein, brachial plexus, and the sympathetic nerve plexus.

DIAGNOSIS

History

When is arm pain something more? Upper extremity discomfort cannot always be attributed to dysfunction in this area. A good clinician must determine whether the discomfort is primarily caused by dysfunction in the extremity or referred from another area.

If the cause lies in the upper extremity itself, there is generally restricted motion. Pain is usually localized to specific dermatomes and may be described as acute, sharp, and severe. Discomfort is usually improved by rest, is frequently reproduced by motion, and may lead to the perception of strength loss.

If the discomfort is referred from another area (e.g., the lungs, diaphragm, stomach, intestines, heart, or cervical spine), passive motion does not appear to be restricted. Pain is diffuse, poorly localized, and may be described as nagging, achy, or dull. Discomfort is usually worse at night. Discomfort is frequently related to symptoms in other areas (difficulty breathing, chest pain, cough, gastrointestinal upset) and may not be reproduced by motion. Motion is generally good, but decreased strength or muscle atrophy is possible (e.g., disc herniation).

Observation

Observation begins the moment the patient walks into the room. Observe overall posture and motion. Is there any abnormality? Observe the patient in the standing position. Look at the height of the shoulders. A low shoulder may be the result of a short leg or a lateral curve. Look at the spine from the side. Is the thoracic kyphotic curve normal, increased, or decreased? An area of thoracic spine flattening may indicate the presence of an extended somatic dysfunction. Dysfunction in the upper thoracic spine may alter sympathetic tone and produce dysfunction in the upper extremity. Begin at the shoulder and examine the skin of the upper extremity. Is there any asymmetry? Areas that appear reddened or have pigment changes may have somatic dysfunction. Observe the various muscle groups bilaterally. Is there evidence of hypertrophy or atrophy? Look for the presence of fasciculation (small tremors) in the muscle.

Palpation

Begin by palpating the superficial tissue of the shoulders. Palpate into the deeper tissues. Look for signs of acute or chronic tissue texture change. Remember to compare the right side with the left side and areas located superiorly with areas located inferiorly. Compare muscle groups bilaterally for size and tone.

Pulses

Thorough examination of the upper extremities necessitates an examination of the brachial and radial pulses. The brachial pulse is found on the medial surface of the arm just medial to the biceps tendon. The radial pulse is best palpated over the lateral and ventral side of the wrist. Examine the arterial pulses with the distal pads of the second, third, and fourth fingers. Palpate firmly but not so hard that the artery is occluded. Arterial pulses can be examined for:

> Heart rate and rhythm
> Pulse contour (wave form)
> Amplitude (strength)
> Symmetry

Lack of symmetry between the left and right extremities suggests impaired circulation. The amplitude of the pulse can be described on the scale shown in Table 47.8 (4).

Reflexes

The three basic reflexes that evaluate the integrity of the nerve supply to the upper extremity are the biceps reflex, the brachioradialis reflex, and the triceps reflex. Each of these is a deep tendon

TABLE 47.8. STANDARD METHOD FOR RECORDING AMPLITUDE OF THE PULSE

4/4	Bounding
3/4	*Full, Increased*
2/4	Expected
1/4	*Diminished, barely palpable*
0	Absent, not palpable

TABLE 47.9. STANDARD METHOD FOR RECORDING AMPLITUDE OF A REFLEX

0	Absent
1/4	*Decreased but present*
2/4	Normal
3/4	*Brisk with unsustained clonus*
4/4	Brisk with sustained clonus

reflex (lower motor neuron reflex) transmitted to the cord as far as the anterior horn cells and returning to the muscle via the peripheral nerves. Reflexes may be increased in the presence of an upper motor neuron lesion or may be decreased in the presence of a lower motor neuron lesion (bulging disc).

Biceps Reflex

This primarily tests the integrity of neurologic level C5. Place the patient's arm over your opposite arm so that it rests on your forearm. With your elbow supporting the patient's arm under the elbow's medial side, place your thumb on the tendon of the biceps in the cubital fossa. Instruct the patient to rest the arm on your forearm and relax. Tap your thumbnail with a neurologic hammer. The biceps should jerk slightly. You should be able to see or feel its movement.

Brachioradialis Reflex

This tests neurologic level C6. Support the patient's arm in the same manner used to test the biceps reflex. Tap the brachioradialis tendon at the distal end of the radius with the neurologic hammer.

Triceps Reflex

This reflex tests neurologic level C7. Use the same position as above. Tap the triceps tendon where it crosses the olecranon fossa (2). Remember to use bilateral comparison. Reflexes may be graded as shown in Table 47.9.

Motor Strength

The strength of various muscle groups can be evaluated by applying force in a manner that loads the muscle as the patient resists. Remember to test the uninjured side first. Table 47.10 shows a standard method of recording motor strength.

Differences in muscle strength may be subtle. Compare the strength of various groups in different positions to get the full

TABLE 47.10. STANDARD METHOD FOR RECORDING MOTOR STRENGTH

5/5	Normal	Complete range of motion against gravity with full resistance
4/5	Good	Complete range of motion against gravity with some resistance
3/5	*Fair*	*Complete range of motion against gravity*
2/5	Poor	Complete range of motion with gravity eliminated
1/5	*Trace*	*Evidence of slight contractility; no joint motion*
0	Zero	No evidence of contractility

clinical picture. There are some simple screening procedures that are useful. Although not a test of strength, palpation for flaccidity may reveal muscles that should be tested. For cervical root or brachial plexus problems, perform a grip strength test by asking the patient to squeeze two of your fingers. Another simple test is to ask the patient to squeeze the thumb and index finger together while you try to pull them apart. If normal strength is present, it is difficult to pull them apart.

Sensation

This can be tested by light touch, pinprick, or two-point discrimination. Compare both sides and areas located superiorly with areas located inferiorly. Look for areas of either decreased or increased sensation. Sensation around the upper extremity is controlled by five different nerve supplies:

1. C5 controls the lateral arm
2. C6 controls the lateral forearm
3. C7 controls the index finger
4. C8 controls the medial forearm
5. T1 controls the medial arm

Motion Testing
Shoulder Motion

Shoulder motions can be screened by using gross motion analysis or by the seven motions of Spencer. Gross motions can be screened by asking the patient to:

Abduct the arms to put the palms together overhead
Abduct the arms to put the backs of the hands together overhead
Reach across the chest to touch the opposite shoulder
Reach behind the body to scratch the opposite shoulder (Apley scratch test)

Internal and external rotation may be tested as follows: (5)

1. With the arm at the side, the forearm is flexed 90 degrees at the elbow and the elbow is supported. The forearm is turned medially to test internal rotation and laterally to test external rotation.
2. With the arm abducted 90 degrees at the shoulder, the forearm is flexed 90 degrees at the elbow and the elbow is supported. An anterior arc of the forearm produces internal rotation, and a posterior arc produces external rotation.

Testing of the shoulder can be localized to the glenohumeral joint by stabilizing the scapula with one hand as the arm is moved with the other. A gross test of stability of the glenohumeral joint is to stabilize the scapula and translate the head of the humerus anteriorly and posteriorly. Compare both sides. An unstable joint moves too freely; with adhesive capsulitis, there is no motion. Motion of the entire shoulder girdle is evaluated without stabilizing the scapula to isolate glenohumeral motion. In evaluating total shoulder girdle motion, observe the amount of scapulothoracic motion as the shoulder girdle moves. Most shoulder problems involve dysfunction of muscles. Malposition of the scapula alters the working length of a shoulder girdle muscle. Treatment of

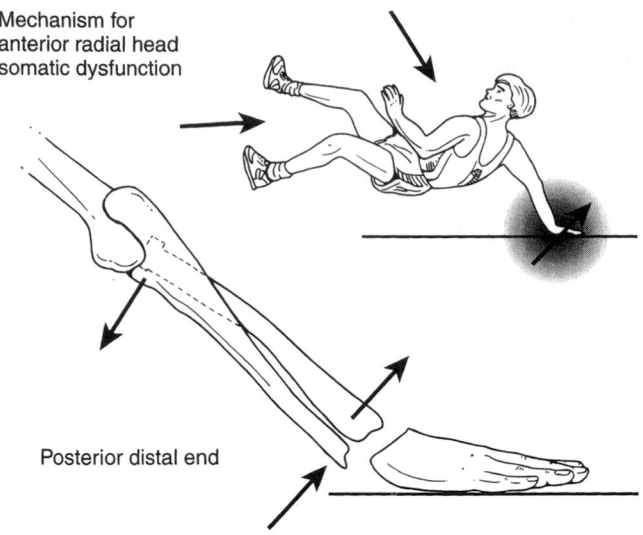

FIGURE 47.10. Fall backward on extended arm. (Illustration by W. A. Kuchera.)

axis and can abduct 20 degrees and adduct 50 degrees about its anteroposterior axis. Combined motion about both of these axes permits a motion called circumduction. Figures 47.11 and 47.12 illustrate normal motion of flexion and extension.

Somatic Dysfunction of the Wrist

Somatic dysfunction is not related to the gross motions of the wrist but to dysfunction of the slight gliding motions of the carpal bones on the radius as the wrist is moved. In Figures 46.10 and 46.11, notice the direction of glide of the carpal bone during each of these wrist motions.

Somatic dysfunction of the wrist is named according to the direction of motion preference. If a wrist extends and is re-

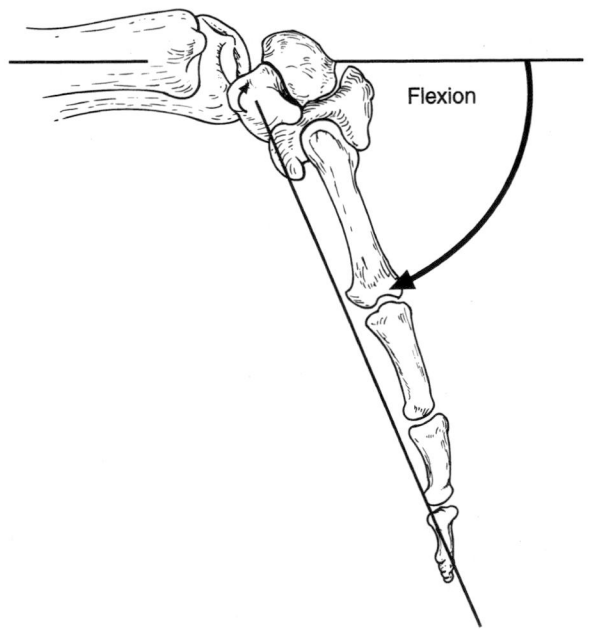

FIGURE 47.11. Wrist flexion: dorsal glide of proximal carpal bones. (Illustration by W. A. Kuchera.)

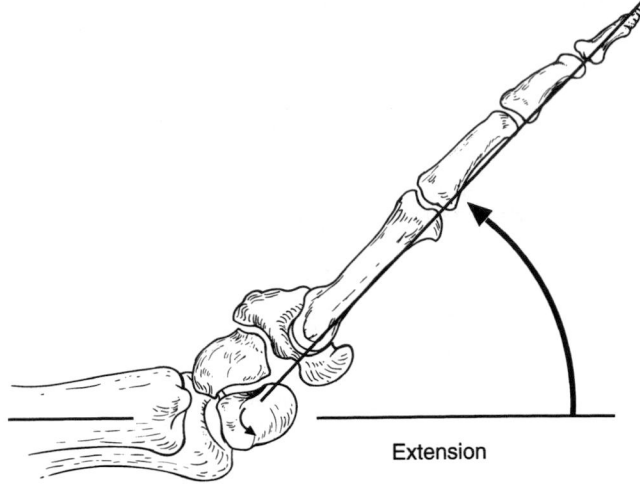

FIGURE 47.12. Wrist extension: anterior (ventral) glide of proximal carpal bones. (Illustration by W. A. Kuchera.)

stricted in its full flexion, it is an extension somatic dysfunction (Fig. 47.13), with the wrist restricted in flexion. In this extension somatic dysfunction, the three carpal bones glide ventrally and are restricted in gliding dorsally. The opposite is true for a flexion somatic dysfunction of the wrist; similar relationships occur for the other wrist motions.

Several principles describe somatic dysfunction of the wrist:

1. Observation is not very helpful when looking for somatic dysfunction; swelling of the wrist is an inconsistent sign.
2. Painful compression means dysfunction is present, but this test does not diagnose the specific problem that is present.
3. Radial glide and limited parallelogram motions are not obvious until the opposite motion is attempted. If there is an adduction somatic dysfunction at the wrist with a proximal shift of the radius, the problem may not be evident until abduction of the wrist is tested and the results are compared with the opposite side.
4. Flexion extension somatic dysfunction of the wrist is usually caused by a trauma that overcomes the ligamentous restraints and opposing muscle pull. This can often result if a strain or sprain exceeds the extent of a somatic dysfunction. Restricted extension of the wrist is its most common major motion loss caused by dysfunction.

Somatic Dysfunction of the Hand

Intercarpal Joints

Intercarpal somatic dysfunction often occurs from a fall on an outstretched hand. For this reason, somatic dysfunction in these areas is very likely to have a compression component. If the wrist joint is swollen, the physician must rule out fracture of the navicular bone (scaphoid). This is also true if there is pain on pressure over the snuffbox, or if there is persistent pain and dysfunction after proper conservative care, even if the initial post-trauma radiographs showed no evidence of fracture. Sometimes the scaphoid does not reveal evidence of fracture until the disruption in its blood supply slowly produces degeneration of the bone.

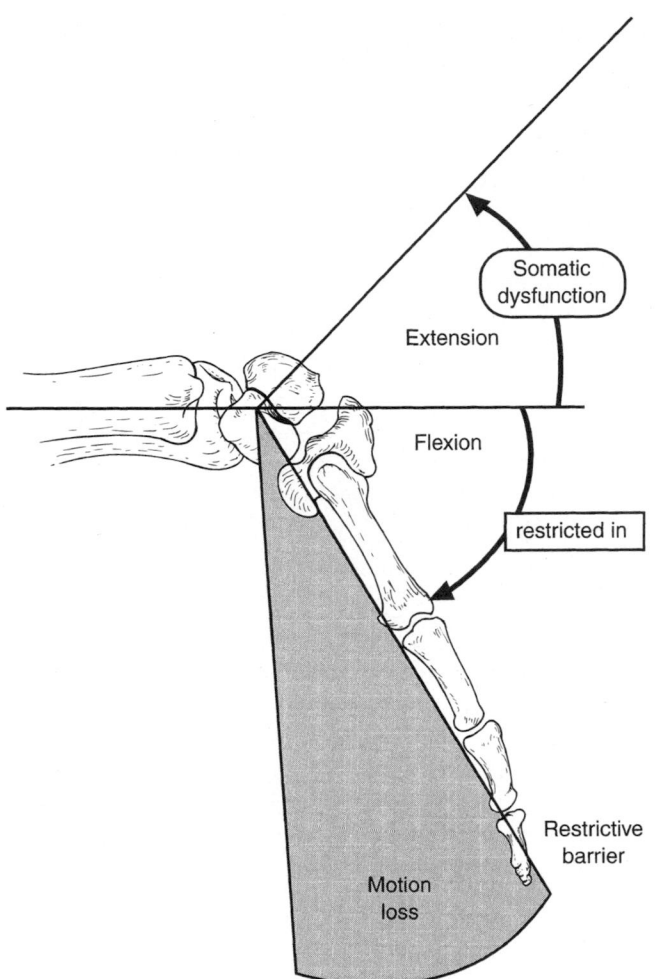

FIGURE 47.13. Wrist extension: somatic dysfunction. (Illustration by W. A. Kuchera.)

Carpometacarpal Joints

All of these joints, except the thumb, are classified as plane synovial joints, which share a common joint cavity with the intercarpal joints. Their main type of somatic dysfunction is a dorsal glide with restriction in ventral glide.

The carpometacarpal joint of the thumb is different; it is a separate saddle-type joint, having both a concave and a convex articular surface. This configuration permits angular movements in almost any plane with the exception of limited axial rotation. Only a ball and socket joint has more motion than the carpometacarpal joint of the thumb. Because it has very good motion, it is more likely to have compression strain or sprain of the ligaments than to have somatic dysfunction.

Metacarpophalangeal and Interphalangeal Joints

The metacarpophalangeal (MP) joints and all the interphalangeal (IP) joints of the hand are gliding joints. The fifth MP joint has the most motion; there is less motion in the fourth MP joint, and the third and second MP joints have the least motion. The MP and IP joints may develop somatic dysfunction in any one of a combination of six gliding motions:

Anteroposterior glide
Mediolateral glide
Internal-external rotational glide

All of these motions are minor and cannot be initiated directly by muscle action.

Diagnosis

Compression is always part of MP and IP somatic dysfunctions, as when a ring on a finger gets caught as a person jumps over a wire fence. Intermetacarpal cramps and pain may be a sign of MP or IP somatic dysfunction. Pain in the metacarpal joints may be referred from an ulnohumeral joint somatic dysfunction.

SPECIAL TESTS FOR THE UPPER EXTREMITY

Adson Test

The Adson test is used to determine the state of the subclavian artery, which may be compressed by an extra cervical rib or by tightened anterior and middle scalene muscles. To perform Adson test, take the patient's radial pulse at the wrist. Continue to feel the pulse while abducting, extending, and externally rotating the arm. Then instruct the patient to take a deep breath and turn the head toward the side being tested. Marked diminution or absence of the radial pulse indicates compression of the subclavian artery (2).

Yergason Test

The Yergason test determines whether the biceps tendon is stable in the bicipital groove. Instruct the patient to fully flex the elbow. Grasp the flexed elbow in one hand while holding the wrist with your other hand. To test the stability of the biceps tendon, externally rotate the patient's arm as he or she resists, and at the same time, pull downward on the elbow. If the biceps tendon is unstable in the bicipital groove, it pops out of the groove and the patient experiences pain. If the tendon is stable, it remains secure and the patient experiences no discomfort. This procedure may also be performed using one hand to palpate the tendon and the other hand to introduce motion (2).

Drop Arm Test

The drop arm test detects whether or not there are any tears in the rotator cuff. First, instruct the patient to fully abduct the arm. Then instruct the patient to slowly lower the arm to the side. If there are any tears in the rotator cuff (especially in the supraspinatus muscle), the arm drops to the side from a position of about 90 degrees abduction. The patient is not able to lower the arm smoothly and slowly no matter how many times they try. If the patient is able to hold the arm in abduction, a gentle tap of the forearm causes the arm to fall to the side (2).

Apprehension Test

The apprehension test detects chronic shoulder dislocation. Abduct and externally rotate the patient's arm to a position where it might easily dislocate. If the shoulder is ready to dislocate, the patient has a noticeable look of apprehension or alarm on his or her face and resists further motion (2).

Bicipital Tendonitis

The long head of the biceps muscle extends intraarticularly under the acromion through the rotator cuff to insert at the top of the glenoid. Impingement may result in inflammation of the tendon. This condition may also result from subluxation of the tendon out of the bicipital groove. Pain is usually localized to the proximal humerus and the shoulder. Resistive supination of the forearm aggravates pain. The distal portion of the biceps tendon is palpated in the cubital fossa medial to the tendon of the brachioradialis muscle. If the tendon is inflamed, the area may feel puffy and may be sensitive to touch. Also examine the coracoid process of the scapula, as the tendon of the short head of the biceps attaches there.

Apley Scratch Test

The Apley scratch test is used to evaluate the range of shoulder motion. First, to test abduction and external rotation, ask the patient to reach behind his or her head and touch the superior medial angle of the opposite scapula. To test the range of internal rotation and adduction, instruct the patient to reach in front of the head and touch the opposite acromion. To further test internal rotation and adduction, instruct the patient to reach behind the back and touch the inferior angle of the opposite scapula. Observe the patient's movement during all phases of testing for any limitation of motion or for any break of normal rhythm or symmetry.

Alternatively, instruct the patient to abduct the arms to 90 degrees, keeping the elbows straight. Then instruct the patient to turn the palms up in supination and continue abduction until the hands touch overhead. This tests full bilateral abduction and provides instant bilateral comparison. Next, instruct the patient to place the hands behind the neck and push the elbows out posteriorly to test abduction and external rotation. Finally, test adduction and internal rotation by instructing the patient to place the hands behind the back as high as they will go to scratch the inferior angle of the scapula (2).

Tinel Sign

Tinel sign is used in the diagnosis of carpal tunnel syndrome. Attempt to elicit or reproduce pain or tingling in the distribution of the median nerve by tapping over the transverse carpal ligament (2).

Phalen Test

The Phalen test is also used in the diagnosis of carpal tunnel syndrome. Attempt to elicit or reproduce symptoms by flexing the patient's wrist to its maximum degree and holding it in that position for at least 1 minute (2).

Allen Test

The Allen test determines whether or not the radial and ulnar arteries are supplying the hand to their full capacity. Instruct the patient to open and close the fist several times and then squeeze the fist tightly so that the venous blood is forced out of the palm. Place your thumb over the radial artery and your index and middle fingers over the ulnar artery. Press both arteries against the underlying bones to occlude them. Instruct the patient to open the hand. The palm of the hand should be pale. Release one of the arteries at the wrist while maintaining pressure on the other one. Normally, the hand flushes immediately. If it does not react or flushes very slowly, the released artery is partially or completely occluded. Test both arteries (2).

Tennis Elbow

Tennis elbow is also known as lateral epicondylitis. This condition is an inflammatory response to overuse of the extensor muscle group attached to the lateral epicondyle of the humerus. It is usually caused by repeated overload of the musculotendinous units. This condition produces pain that may be localized to the lateral epicondyle or may radiate down the forearm extensor group or up into the brachioradialis muscle. The pain is intensified by resistive extension of the wrist and fingers, or by shaking hands. Pressure over the lateral epicondyle is painful (7,8).

TREATMENT

Carpal Tunnel Syndrome

This condition is most commonly described as an entrapment neuropathy of the median nerve at the wrist producing paresthesia and weakness of the hands (9). Carpal tunnel syndrome is frequently associated with repeated or sustained activity of the fingers and hands. Incidence rates are reported as high as 25.6 cases per 200,000 work hours (10) and involving 10% of workers. Medical cost estimates vary from $3,500 to $60,000 per case (11).

Patients experience numbness or paresthesia on the palmar surface of the thumb, index, and middle fingers, and radial half of the ring finger. Numbness and paresthesia of the whole hand may also occur. Pain may be referred to the forearm and, less commonly, to the neck and forearm regions. Pain or tingling of the fingers often occurs at night and is relieved by shaking or exercising the hand. Weakness and atrophy of the thenar muscles usually appear late and can occur without significant sensory symptoms. On examination, symptoms may be reproduced by percussion over the volar surface of the wrist (Tinel sign) or by full flexion of the wrist for one minute (Phalen maneuver). Decreased touch may be demonstrated over the fingers supplied by the median nerve. Nerve conduction studies are considered to be the gold standard for the diagnosis of this condition (9).

The syndrome is traditionally described as resulting from pressure on the median nerve where it passes with the flexor tendons of the fingers through the tunnel formed by the carpal bones and the transverse carpal ligament (9). Additional explanations exist.

Single compressions of dog sciatic nerves have failed to produce significant conduction loss. Both proximal and distal compressions have produced conduction blocks in 50% of test animals (12).

In 1973, Upton and McComas (13) proposed the existence of the "double crush syndrome." This syndrome hypothesizes that neural function is impaired when single axons that are compressed on one region become especially susceptible to damage in another area. The authors report that a slight compression may cause a reduction in axoplasmic flow that is too small to result in denervation changes; but when coupled with the onset of a slowed lesion, might further reduce axoplasmic flow below the safety margin for prevention of denervation at a distal lesion, and clinical symptoms ensue (13). Abramson demonstrated that decreased blood supply to a nerve alters conduction (14). Larson suggested that upper thoracic dysfunction alters upper extremity vasomotion (15). Hurst demonstrated a relationship between cervical arthritis and bilateral carpal tunnel syndrome (16). Sunderland has suggested that lymphatic and venous congestion contribute to this disorder (17).

The treatment of carpal tunnel syndrome has traditionally involved the use of wrist splints, antiinflammatory drugs, and local injection of steroids. Surgical decompression of the carpal tunnel with release of the transverse carpal tunnel ligament is used if symptoms persist or if motor abnormalities are present (9,18). Evidence in the preceding paragraph suggests that the hand symptoms may be related to dysfunctions in the upper extremity, and the cervical and thoracic spine. Osteopathic treatment incorporates the modalities described above and should also include:

1. Reducing sympathetic tone to the upper extremity by correcting upper thoracic and upper rib dysfunctions. This directly affects nerve function by improving blood flow and reducing congestion through improved lymphatic and venous drainage. An internally rotated temporal bone may be associated with increased sympathetic tone in the upper thoracic spine and, if it is diagnosed, should also be treated.
2. Removing cervical somatic dysfunction to improve brachial plexus function.
3. Removing myofascial restrictions in the upper extremity, thereby removing potential sites of additional compression.
4. Increasing space within the carpal tunnel using direct release techniques.

Reflex Sympathetic Dystrophy

Reflex sympathetic dystrophy (RSD) is characterized by pain and tenderness (usually in the distal extremity) that is accompanied by vasomotor instability, trophic skin changes, and rapid development of bone demineralization. A precipitating event can be identified in two-thirds of the cases. These include:

Trauma
Myocardial infarction
Stroke
Peripheral nerve injuries

RSD is observed most often in individuals over the age of 50. An entire hand or foot is usually affected. The pathogenesis of RSD is poorly understood. The vasomotor manifestations are thought to be caused by abnormal stimulation of the sympathetic nervous system (9). Larson (15) implicates the upper thoracic spinal segments with facilitating a vasomotor response in the upper extremity.

RSD evolves through three clinical phases. The clinical manifestations of the first phase are pain and swelling that develop weeks to months after the precipitating event. The pain has an intense, burning quality. The involved extremity is warm, edematous, and tender, especially around the joints. Increased sweating and hair growth occur. In 36 months, the skin gradually becomes thin, shiny, and cool (second phase). Clinical features of the first two phases overlap. In another 36 months, the skin and subcutaneous tissues become atrophic, and irreversible flexion contractures of the hand or foot develop (third phase). Motion of the shoulder on the affected side is frequently painful and greatly restricted, a condition referred to as the shoulder-hand syndrome (9).

Early recognition and treatment are important to prevent permanent disability. RSD may be reversible in its early phases. Appropriate mobilization of the patient after a myocardial infarction, stroke, or injury may help prevent this condition. Pain should be properly controlled. Exercises are helpful. Sympathetic nerve blocks may be initially effective, but the response may not be sustained. High-dose prednisone has benefited some patients (9). Osteopathic treatment should focus on reducing sympathetic tone to the extremity. This includes correcting cervical, upper thoracic, and upper rib dysfunctions. Apply gentle articulation and mobilization techniques. Always treat the whole patient.

Adhesive Capsulitis

Also known as "frozen shoulder," this condition is characterized by pain and restricted movement of the shoulder, usually in the absence of intrinsic shoulder disease. Adhesive capsulitis may follow bursitis or tendonitis of the shoulder or may be associated with systemic disorders, such as chronic pulmonary disease, myocardial infarction, and diabetes mellitus. Prolonged arm immobility contributes to the development of this condition. Reflex sympathetic dystrophy is thought to be a pathogenic factor. The capsule of the shoulder is thickened, and a mild, chronic, inflammatory infiltrate and fibrosis may be present.

Pain and stiffness usually develop gradually over several months to a year, but may progress rapidly in some patients. Pain may interfere with sleep. The shoulder is tender to palpation, and active and passive motions are restricted (9).

Early mobilization after an injury to the arm or shoulder may help prevent the development of this condition. Local injection of corticosteroids and administration of nonsteroidal antiinflammatory drugs and physical therapy may help (9). Osteopathic manipulation should be directed to the upper thoracics, upper ribs, and entire shoulder complex. The objective is to improve motion. Avoid taking the patient into the "crampy" pain zone. This only slows progress. Only progress as fast as the patient can respond. Indirect techniques may be especially effective in the initial treatment phases.

Myofascial Triggers

See Chapter 66, "Travell and Simons' Myofascial Trigger Points."

Chapman Points

See Chapter 67, "Chapman Reflexes."

Thoracic Outlet Syndrome

This condition results from compression of the neurovascular bundle (subclavian artery, subclavian vein, and brachial plexus) as it courses through the neck and shoulder. Several dysfunctions may compress the neurovascular bundle as it passes from the thorax to the arm, including:

Cervical ribs
Excessive tension in the anterior and middle scalene muscles
Dysfunction of the clavicle, upper ribs, or upper thoracics
Abnormal insertion of the pectoralis minor muscle

Patients may develop:

Shoulder and arm pain
Weakness
Paresthesia
Claudication
Raynaud phenomenon
Ischemic tissue loss
Gangrene

Examination is often normal unless provocative maneuvers are performed. Occasionally, distal pulses are decreased or absent and digital cyanosis and ischemia may be evident. Tenderness may be present in the supraclavicular fossa (9). Some forms of thoracic outlet syndrome are associated with sympathetic autonomic dysfunction, which produces upper extremity symptoms. Sympathetic dysfunction has accompanying palpatory findings in the upper thoracic or rib area. Most patients can be conservatively managed. Patients should avoid positions that aggravate symptoms. Osteopathic treatment should be directed toward improving mechanics in the:

Cervical region
Upper thoracics
Upper ribs
Clavicles
Scalene muscles
Muscles of the shoulder and pectoral girdle

Surgical intervention is a last resort.

CONCLUSION

Understanding the structure and function of the upper extremities leads to effective diagnosis and treatment of disabilities in this area, and therefore improves the overall function of the patient.

REFERENCES

1. Truhlar RE. *Doctor A. T. Still in the Living.* Published by the author; 1950.
2. Hoppenfeld S. *Physical Examination of the Spine and Extremities.* Norwalk, CT: Appleton & Lange; 1976:25.
3. Moore KL. *Clinically Oriented Anatomy,* 3rd ed. Baltimore, MD: Williams & Wilkins; 1992:528.
4. Seidel HM, Ball JW, Dains JE, et al. *Mosby's Guide to Physical Examination.* St. Louis, MO: Mosby; 1987:309–311.
5. Kuchera WA, Kuchera ML. *Osteopathic Principles in Practice,* 2nd ed. rev. Columbus, OH: Greyden Press; 1994:539.
6. Kuchera WA, Kuchera ML. *Osteopathic Principles in Practice.* 2nd ed. rev. Columbus, OH: Greyden Press; 1994:615–629.
7. Roy S, Irvin R. Throwing and tennis injuries to the shoulder and elbow. In: *Sports Medicine: Prevention, Evaluation, Management, and Rehabilitation.* Salt Lake City: Prentice Hall, 1983:221–222.
8. Gunter-Griffin, Letha Y. *Athletic Training and Sports Medicine,* 2nd ed. Rosemont, IL: The American Academy of Orthopedic Surgeons; 1991:274.
9. Wilson JD, et al. *Harrison's Principles of Internal Medicine,* 12th ed. New York, NY: McGraw-Hill; 1991:1487.
10. Armstrong TJ. *An Ergonomics Guide to Carpal Tunnel Syndrome. Ergonomics Guide Series.* Akron, OH: American Industrial Hygiene Association; 1983.
11. Hiltz R. Fighting work-related injuries. *Natl Underwriter.* 1985;89:15.
12. Nemoto K. Experimental study on the vulnerability of the peripheral nerve. *Nippon Sea Gakkai Zasshi.* 1983;57:1773–1786.
13. Upton A, McComas AJ. The double crush in nerve entrapment syndromes. *Lancet.*1973;2:359.
14. Abramson DI, Rickert BL, Alexis JT, et al. Effects of repeated periods of ischemia on motor nerve conduction. *J Appl Physiol.* 1971;30:636–642.
15. Larson NJ. Osteopathic manipulation for syndromes of the brachial plexus. *J Am Osteopath Assoc.* 1972;72:94–100.
16. Hurst LC, et al. The relationship of double crush syndrome to carpal tunnel syndrome (an analysis of 1000 cases of carpal tunnel syndrome). *J Hand Surg.* 1985;10:202.
17. Sunderland S. The nerve lesion in the carpal tunnel syndrome. *J Neurol Neurosurg Psychiatry.* 1976;39:615.
18. Anonymous. Carpal tunnel syndrome: getting a handle on hand trauma. *Occup Hazards.* 1987;42:45–47.

48

THORACIC REGION

RAYMOND J. HRUBY

KEY CONCEPTS

- Importance of the thoracic region for normal function
- Structure and function of the thoracic area, including lymphatics, connective tissues, neural connections, and motion
- Clinical characteristics of thoracic movements
- History and physical examination, including observation, palpation, and motion testing
- Assessment, diagnosis, and treatment of structural dysfunction

Because the heart and lungs are contained in the thorax, this region's unique significance in life has long been recognized. The inability to draw breath or the perception of pain in the thorax often constitutes real or imagined immediate and life-threatening problems. Movement of the thorax is necessary for normal function in both obvious and not-so-obvious ways. Because much of the regulatory outflow of the sympathetic nervous system originates in the thoracic spinal cord, disturbances in the muscles and joints of the thoracic region often mimic life-threatening problems. Injury to thoracic vertebrae can cause long-term sequelae for health and survival. The complexities of the thoracic region and the vital importance of its organ systems underscore the necessity for the osteopathic physician to understand its many functions, diagnoses, and potential treatment approaches.

The thoracic region is bounded by the cervical region above and the lumbar region below. In diagnosis and treatment, it cannot be considered as separate from the other body regions, because dysfunction in it or other regions is always interdependent.

ANATOMY AND PHYSIOLOGY

Thoracic Region

The thoracic cage includes 12 thoracic spinal vertebrae, 12 pair of ribs, and the sternum (Fig. 48.1). (See also Chapter 51, Figure 51.1.) Although the scapula overlies the posterior portion of the rib cage, is connected to the sternum through the clavicle, and is often involved in thoracic injuries and pain syndromes, this structure is more properly considered a part of the upper extremity (see Chapter 47).

White and Panjabi (1) divide the thoracic spine into three anatomical regions:

Upper (T1-4)
Middle (T4-8)
Lower (T8-L1)

It is also helpful to divide the thoracic and upper lumbar spine into four functional divisions that roughly correspond to the thoracolumbar outflow of the sympathetic system:

T1-4: Sympathetics to head and neck, with T1-6 to the heart and lungs.
T5-9: All upper abdominal viscera: stomach, duodenum, liver, gall bladder, pancreas, and spleen.
T10-11: Remainder of the small intestines, kidneys, ureters, gonads, and right colon.
T12-L2: Left colon and pelvic organs.

This functional division is often very useful to the osteopathic physician, because visceral, afferent (generally nociceptive; see Chapter 7) neurons usually follow the same pathway as the sympathetic outflow. Visceral disturbances often cause increased musculoskeletal tension in the somatic structures that are innervated from the corresponding spinal level through the viscerosomatic reflexes (see Chapter 9). Manipulative treatment at that spinal level is used to reduce somatic afferent input from the associated facilitated segments, which, in turn, reduces somatosympathetic activity to the affected viscus (2).

Generally, the thoracic spine has a mildly kyphotic, forward-bending curve that varies from person to person. In the osteoporotic or older patients, the angle of this curve can become more acute, causing biomechanical problems and necessitating compensatory adaptation in other regions of the spine and in general posture. Individual thoracic vertebrae are parts of a continuum with the cervical and lumbar vertebrae; size increases from cervical to lumbar to account for increased weight bearing. The spinous processes of the thoracic vertebrae are particularly large and easily palpated, pointing increasingly caudad from T1 through T9 and back to an almost anteroposterior orientation from T10-12.

Thoracic vertebral facet joints are plane-type synovial joints. The interarticular surfaces of these joints are smooth, shiny,

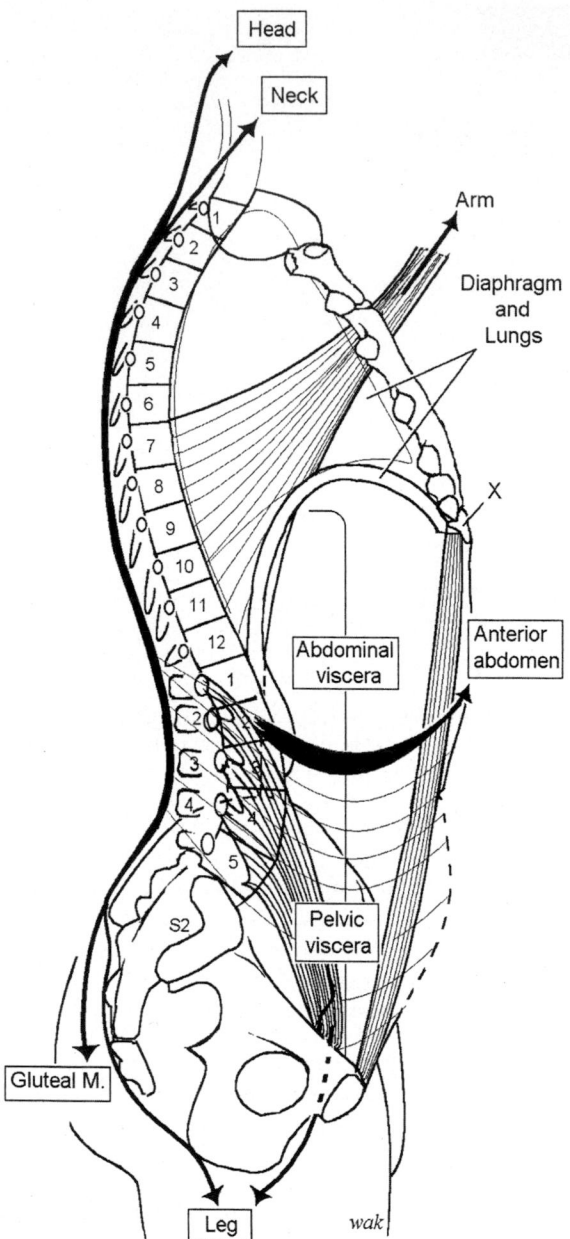

FIGURE 48.1. The thoracic region and its relationships.

a functional transition to the lumbar spine. The inferior facet of each thoracic vertebra faces in the opposite direction from the superior and has a slightly concave surface.

The thoracic vertebrae are separated by discs, as are the cervical and lumbar vertebrae. The discs act as shock absorbers and permit flexibility between the vertebrae. Each disc is composed of an outer anulus fibrosus and an inner nucleus pulposus, a gel at the center of the disc that acts like a semifluid hydrophilic ball bearing that becomes less hydrated and broader under sustained compression. The anulus fibrosus is composed of concentric lamellae of fibrocartilage, running at right angles to the fibers of adjacent layers. Its structural arrangement is more vulnerable to tears posteriorly, where the lamellae are thinner and less numerous. However, the restricted motion of the thoracic spine due to the attachments of the rib cage and the fairly broad posterior longitudinal ligament make ruptured thoracic discs relatively uncommon. On the other hand, discopathy from trauma, aging, and degenerative disease is relatively common in the thoracic area.

Muscles of the Thoracic Area

The muscles of the thoracic area are involved in:

Actions of the ribs and vertebrae
Posture
Head and neck control
Breathing
Locomotion
Stabilization of the extremities
Visceral function

Table 48.1 lists the major muscles of the thoracic area, with the action, proximal and medial attachments, distal and lateral attachments, and innervation of each. It is especially important to note the action of each muscle, because altered tone in these muscles can affect the function of not only the bones to which the muscles are attached but other body areas as well. In addition, increased or decreased tone has the capacity to alter both general and microcirculation in a myriad of ways, such as altered homeostatic regulation and cellular immunity.

As with all muscles, the thoracic muscles are fed not only by circulatory elements but also by physiologically active trophic substances delivered directly by nerves (3). In addition, there is evidence that the sympathetic nerve supply to striated and smooth muscles alters muscle tone and contractile forces. Therefore, attention to the palpatory cues associated with altered muscle tone implies the presence of many differential diagnostic factors that are discussed throughout this text.

The larger muscles of the head, neck, shoulder girdle, and thorax control much of the activity of the thoracic cage and help stabilize the cervical and cranial areas, as well as the arms and shoulder girdle. For example, the splenius capitus and cervicis muscles originate on the lower cranial and upper cervical areas and attach distally along the middle thoracic spine, as low as T6-8 in some cases. Vertebral dysfunction in the upper thoracic areas can affect the action of these muscles, causing problems with motion outside the thoracic area in the head and neck. Lower down, the internal and external oblique muscles are generally viewed as trunk rotators, but they also attach to the lower ribs along with the diaphragm. Altered tone in these muscles can alter diaphragmatic

compact bone that is covered with hyaline cartilage. The joints are surrounded by a thin, loose articular capsule that is lined with synovial membrane. The facet joints guide and limit gross, segmental, and coupled movements. The superior facets of each thoracic vertebra are slightly convex and face posteriorly (backward), somewhat superiorly (up), and laterally. Their angle of declination averages 60 degrees relative to the transverse plane and 20 degrees relative to the coronal plane. A tool to remember the facet facing is the mnemonic BUL (backward, upward, and lateral). This is in contrast to the cervical and lumbar regions, where the superior facets face backward, upward, and medial (BUM). Thus, the superior facets are BUM, BUL, BUM from cervical to thoracic to lumbar. In the lower portion of the thoracic spine, the superior facet surface begins to face more posteriorly than laterally, and at T12, it may even face medially, as part of

TABLE 48.1. REGIONAL THORACIC MUSCLES

Muscle	Action	Proximal/Medial Attachments	Distal/Lateral Attachments	Innervation
Pectoralis major	1. *Clavicular head:* flexion, adduction, horizontal flexion, and medial rotation of the humerus at the shoulder. 2. *Sternocostal head:* flexion, adduction, medial rotation, and horizontal flexion of the humerus at the shoulder. Also extends flexed humerus. Through its action on the humerus, it depresses, protracts, and rotates downward.	1. *Clavicular division:* anterior surface of the medial $\frac{1}{2}$ of the clavicle. 2. *Sternocostal head:* sternum to 7th rib, cartilages of true ribs and aponeurosis of external abdominal oblique muscle.	1. *Clavicular division:* lateral lip of the intertubercular groove of the humerus. 2. *Sternal division:* lateral lip of the intertubercular groove of the humerus.	1. *Clavicular head:* lateral pectoral, C5, C6. 2. *Sternocostal head:* pectoral, C7, C8, T1.
Pectoralis minor	Depresses scapula and rotates scapula inferiorly. Important anterior shoulder stabilizer.	Anterior surfaces of 3rd, 4th, and 5th ribs near the costal cartilages.	Coracoid process of the scapula.	Medial pectoral, C6, C7, C8.
Teres major	Adducts and medially rotates humerus at the shoulder. Extends the shoulder joint.	Dorsal surface of inferior angle of the scapula.	Medial lip of intertubercular groove of humerus. Medial to latissimus dorsi tendor.	Lower subscapular, C6, C7.
Teres minor	Lateral rotation of humerus at the shoulder. Stabilization of head or humerus.	Superior $\frac{2}{3}$ of dorsal surface of lateral border of scapula.	Inferior aspect of greater tubercle of the humerus, capsule of the shoulder joint.	Axillary, C5, C6.
Trapezius	1. *Lower fibers:* depress the scapula. Retract the scapula. Rotate the scapula upward so the glenoid cavity faces superiorly. Give inferior stabilization of scapula. Help maintain spine in extension. 2. *Middle fibers:* retract and aid in elevation of scapula. 3. *Upper fibers:* elevate the scapula as in shrugging the shoulders. Rotate the scapula upward so the glenoid cavity faces superiorly. When acting with the other sections of the trapezius, it retracts the scapula.	1. *Lower fibers:* spinous processes of 6th–12th thoracic vertebrae. 2. *Middle fibers:* spinous processes of 1st–5th thoracic vertebrae. 3. *Upper fiber:* external occipital protuberance, medial $\frac{1}{3}$ of superior muchal line, ligamentum nuchae, and spinous process of the 7th cervical vertebra.	1. *Lower fibers:* medial $\frac{1}{3}$ of spine of the scapula. 2. *Middle fibers:* superior border of spine of scapula. 3. *Upper fibers:* lateral $\frac{1}{3}$ of clavicle and acromion process.	1. *Lower division:* spinal root of accessory and anterior primary rami C3, C4. 2. *Middle division:* spinal root of accessory and anterior primary rami C3, C4. 3. *Upper division:* spinal root accessory and anterior primary rami C3, C4.
Latissimus dorsi	Extends, retracts, and medially rotates the humerus at the shoulder. Through its action on the humerus, it depresses, retracts, and rotates the scapula downward. Assists in forced expiration.	Flat tendon that twists on itself to insert into the intertubercular groove of the humerus, just anterior to and parallel with tendon of pectoralis major.	Broad aponeurosis that originates on the spinous processes of lower 6 thoracic and all lumbar vertebrae; posterior crest of ilium, posterior surface of sacrum, lower 3 or 4 ribs, and an attachment to the inferior angle of the scapula.	Thoracodorsal C6, C7, C8.
Levator scapulae	Elevates the scapula and rotates the scapula downward so the glenoid cavity faces inferiorly. Working with the upper fibers of the trapezius, it elevates and retracts the scapula. *Reversed action:* when the scapula is fixed, it laterally flexes and slightly rotates the cervical spine to the side.	Transverse processes of first four cervical vertebrae.	Vertebral border of scapula between superior angle and scapular spine.	Dorsal scapular C5 and anterior primary rami C3, C4.
Rhomboid	1. *Minor:* retracts and elevates the scapula. Assists in rotating the scapula downward. 2. *Major:* retracts and elevates the scapula. Inferior fibers aid in rotating the glenoid cavity inferiorly.	1. *Minor:* lower part of ligamentum nuchae, spinous processes of C7 and T1. 2. *Major:* spinous processes of T2–5.	1. *Minor:* medial border of scapula at the root of the spine of the scapula. 2. *Major:* medial border of scapula from spine to inferior angle.	1. *Minor:* dorsal scapular, C4, C5. 2. *Major:* dorsal scapular, C4, C5.

(continued)

TABLE 48.1. (*continued*)

Muscle	Action	Proximal/Medial Attachments	Distal/Lateral Attachments	Innervation
Quadratus lumborum	Lateral flexion of lumbar vertebral column; helps the diaphragm in inspiration.	Iliolumbar ligament, posterior part of the iliac crest.	Inferior border of the 12th rib and transverse processes of the upper four lumbar vertebrae.	Anterior primary rami T12, L1, L2, L3.
Serratus anterior	1. Accessory muscle of respiration. 2. Protraction of the scapula.	Superior lateral surfaces of upper 8 ribs at the side of the chest.	Costal surface of the medial border of scapula.	Long thoracic, C5, C6, C7.
Serratus posterior (superior/ inferior)	Accessory muscles of inspiration. Superior elevates superior ribs; inferior depresses inferior ribs.	1. *Superior:* lower portion of ligamentum nuchae and spinous processes of the 7th cervical and 1st, 2nd, and 3rd thoracic vertebrae. 2. *Inferior:* spinous processes of 11th and 12th thoracic and 1st, 2nd, and 3rd lumbar vertebrae, and the thoracolumbar fascia.	1. *Superior:* superior borders of 2nd–5th ribs distal to the angles. 2. *Inferior:* inferior borders of lower 4 ribs just beyond their angles.	1. *Superior:* anterior primary rami T2–5. 2. *Inferior:* anterior primary rami T9–12.
Intercostals	1. Keep the intercostal spaces from bulging and retracting with respiration. 2. Elevate the ribs anteriorly with inspiration.			
External intercostals Internal intercostals Innermost intercostals				
Subcostals	Depress the ribs.			
Transversus thoracis	Depress the second to sixth ribs.			
Levatores costarum	Elevate the ribs.	Transverse processes of the 7th cervical and upper 11 thoracic vertebrae.	The outer surface of the rib immediately below the vertebrae from which it takes origin, between the tubercle and the angle.	Anterior primary rami of the corresponding intercostal nerves.
Splenius	1. *Capitis:* acting bilaterally, extends the head and neck. Acting unilaterally, laterally flexes and rotates the head and neck to the same side. 2. *Cervicis:* laterally bends and rotates the neck.	1. *Capitis:* spinous processes of C7–T3, inferior half of ligamentum nuchae. 2. *Cervicis:* spinous processes of 3rd–6th thoracic vertebrae.	1. *Capitis:* mastoid process and lateral third of the superior nuchal line. 2. *Cervicis:* transverse processes of 1st, 2nd, 3rd, and 4th cervical vertebrae on the posterior aspect.	1. *Capitis:* posterior primary rami of the middle cervical spinal nerves. 2. *Cervicis:* posterior primary rami of the lower cervical spinal nerves.
Spinalis	1. *Cervicis:* laterally bends and rotates the neck. 2. *Thoracis:* acting unilaterally, lateral flexion of the spine. Acting bilaterally, extension of the spine.	1. *Cervicis:* lower portion of ligamentum nuchae, spinous processes of the 7th cervical and 1st and 2nd thoracic vertebrae. 2. *Thoracis:* spinous processes of the 1st and 2nd lumbar vertebrae, thoracic vertebrae 11 and 12.	1. *Cervicis:* spinous process of the axis and the 3rd and 4th cervical spinous processes. 2. *Thoracis:* spinous processes of upper thoracic, vertebrae T4–T8.	1. *Cervicis:* posterior primary rami of the spinal nerves. 2. *Thoracis:* posterior primary rami of the spinal nerves.
Semispinalis	Extends the thoracic and cervical region and rotates it toward the opposite side.	1. *Capitis:* between superior and inferior nuchal lines of the occipital bone. 2. *Cervicis:* spinous processes of 2nd–5th cervical vertebrae. 3. *Thoracis:* spinous processes of the 1st–4th thoracic vertebrae and 6th and 7th cervical vertebrae.	1. *Capitis:* 7th cervical and 1st–6th thoracic transverse processes, and articular processes of 4th, 5th, and 6th cervical vertebrae. 2. *Cervicis:* transverse processes of the 1st–6th thoracic vertebrae. 3. *Thoracis:* transverse processes of 6th–10th thoracic vertebrae.	1. *Capitis:* posterior primary rami of cervical spinal nerves. 2. *Cervicis:* posterior primary rami of cervical spinal nerves. 3. *Thoracis:* posterior primary rami of thoracic spinal nerves, T1–6.

(*continued*)

TABLE 48.1. (continued)

Muscle	Action	Proximal/Medial Attachments	Distal/Lateral Attachments	Innervation
Longissimus	1. *Capitis:* acting bilaterally, extends the head; acting unilaterally, laterally flexes and rotates the head to the same side. 2. *Cervicis:* acting unilaterally, laterally flexes the neck. Acting bilaterally, laterally flexes the vertebral column. Acting bilaterally, extension of vertebral column; draws ribs down.	1. *Capitis:* transverse processes of the 1st–5th thoracic vertebrae and the articular processes of the 4th–7th cervical vertebrae. 2. *Cervicis:* transverse processes of the 1st–5th thoracic vertebrae. 3. *Thoracis:* the common broad thick tendon with the iliocostalis lumborum, fibers from the transverse and accessory processes of the lumbar vertebrae and thoracolumbar fascia.	1. *Capitis:* the posterior margin of the mastoid process. 2. *Cervicis:* transverse processes of the 2nd–6th cervical vertebrae and transverse process of the atlas. 3. *Thoracis:* the tips of transverse process of all thoracic vertebrae and the lower 9 or 10 ribs between the tubercles and angles.	1. *Capitis:* posterior primary rami of spinal nerves. 2. *Cervicis:* posterior primary rami of spinal nerves. 3. *Thoracis:* posterior primary rami of spinal nerves.
Iliocostalis	1. *Cervicis:* acting bilaterally, extension of the spine; acting unilaterally, laterally flexes the vertebral column. 2. *Thoracis:* acting bilaterally, extension of the spine; acting unilaterally, laterally flexes the spine. 3. *Lumborum:* acting bilaterally, extension of the spine; acting unilaterally, laterally flexes the spine.	1. *Cervicis:* the posterior tubercles of the transverse processes of the 4th, 5th, and 6th cervical vertebrae. 2. *Thoracis:* into the angles of the upper 6 or 7 ribs and into the transverse process of the 7th cervical vertebra. 3. *Lumborum:* inferior borders of the angles of the lower 6 or 7 ribs.	1. *Cervicis:* superior borders of the angles of the 3rd–6th ribs. 2. *Thoracis:* superior borders of the angles of lower 6 ribs medial to the tendons of insertion of the iliocostalis lumborum. 3. *Lumborum:* anterior surface of a broad and thick tendon, which originates from the sacrum, spinous processes of the lumbar and 11th and 12th thoracic vertebrae, and from the medial lip of the iliac crest.	1. *Cervicis:* posterior primary rami of spinal nerves, C6, C7, C8. 2. *Thoracis:* posterior primary rami of spinal nerves. 3. *Lumborum:* posterior primary rami of spinal nerves.
Rotatores	Rotate the vertebral column	1. *Brevis:* bases of the spinous processes (lamina) of the 1st vertebra above. 2. *Longus:* bases of the spinous processes (lamina) of the 2nd vertebra above.	1. *Brevis:* transverse processes of the vertebrae. 2. *Longus:* transverse processes of the vertebrae.	1. *Brevis:* posterior primary rami of spinal nerves. 2. *Longus:* posterior primary rami of spinal nerves.
Multifidus	1. Rotate the vertebral column toward the opposite side. 2. Stabilize the vertebral column.	Spinous processes of all the vertebrae except the atlas.	Posterior surface of the sacrum, the dorsal end of the iliac crest, the mammary and transverse processes of lumbar and thoracic vertebrae, and the articular processes of the 4th–7th cervical vertebrae.	Posterior primary rami of spinal nerves.
Interspinales	1. Unite the spinous processes. 2. Produce slight extension of the vertebral column.	Pairs of small muscles joining the spinous processes of adjacent vertebrae, one on each side of the interspinous ligament. Continuous in the cervical region extending from the axis to the 2nd thoracic vertebra and in the lumbar region from the 1st lumbar vertebra to the sacrum.	*See proximal/medial attachment.*	Posterior primary rami of spinal nerves.
Intertransversarii	1. Unite the transverse processes. 2. Produce lateral bending of the vertebral column.	Unite transverse processes of consecutive vertebrae. Well developed in the cervical region.	*See proximal/medial attachment.*	Anterior and posterior primary rami of spinal nerves.

(continued)

TABLE 48.1. (continued)

Muscle	Action	Proximal/Medial Attachments	Distal/Lateral Attachments	Innervation
Diaphragm	Contracts into the abdomen with inhalation and relaxes into the thorax with exhalation.	The central tendon, which is an oblong sheet forming the summit of the dome.	An approximately circular line passing entirely around the inner surface of the body wall: 1. *Sternal portion:* two slips from the back of the xiphoid process. 2. *Costal portion:* the inner surfaces of the cartilages and adjacent portions of the lower 6 ribs on either side, interdigitating with the transversus abdominis. 3. *Lumbar portion:* medial and lateral arcuate ligaments and right and left crura from the anterolateral surfaces of the bodies and discs of the upper three lumbar vertebrae.	Phrenic nerve, C3, C4, C5.
Obliquus capitis inferior	Rotates the atlas, turning the face toward the same side.	Apex of the spinous process of the axis.	The inferior and dorsal part of the transverse process of the atlas.	Posterior primary rami of C1.
Subclavius	Depresses clavicle, draws it medially.	1st rib at junction with costal cartilage.	Groove on the inferior surface of the clavicle, between the costoclavicular and conoid ligaments.	Subclavius, C5, C6.

and respiratory function and vice versa. Experienced palpation readily identifies these relationships.

Of special note are the erector spinae groups (Fig. 48.2), which extend and side-bend the vertebral column, and allow smooth flexion by gradually decreasing resistance to forward bending. These muscles are often involved in group or multiple movement dysfunction (i.e., altered coupling or non-neutral vertebral unit dysfunction), and are vulnerable to insult with unplanned movements or trauma. The deep back muscles, especially the rotatores and multifidus, are also implicated in this type of problem. These small muscles are richly innervated with muscle spindles, which provide proprioception. In fact, one of their primary tasks is to signal position and speed of motion of the vertebral column. (This task makes them important in the maintenance of posture and in directing movement.) They are also very vulnerable to sudden stretch and unplanned movement, which appears to alter the sensory input to the spinal cord and brain, with resultant development of altered motion and pain typical of vertebral somatic dysfunction (4–6).

Lymphatics

As blood moves through the capillaries, fluid filters into the interstitial tissues. The return of interstitial fluid through the lymphatic system is necessary for health and proper function, and is even more important when the patient has disease. Lymphatic drainage from the lower half of the body is supplied by the thoracic duct (or left lymphatic duct). Smaller lymphatic vessels drain into the cisterna chyli in the abdomen. Trunks from the left side of the head, the left arm, and the thoracic viscera also empty into the thoracic duct before it drains into the junction of the left internal jugular and left subclavian veins (Fig. 48.3). In approximately 20% of the population, three trunks, the right jugular, the right subclavian, and the right transverse cervical join to form the right lymphatic duct. The remainder of the population varies in the way the three trunks empty into the jugulosubclavian junction in the anterior neck. The right lymphatic duct enters the junction of the right internal jugular and right subclavian veins (7).

Connective Tissue and Fascia

Connective tissue unites and surrounds all other tissues. It is found between the cells of organs, as tendons of muscles, and as ligaments joining skeletal parts. Of special importance to the osteopathic physician are the fasciae of the body. These connective tissues surround virtually all organs, muscles, and vessels (8). Fascial elements called the pericardium and pleura even surround the heart and lungs, respectively. Fascia is a fibrous tissue that is effectively wound around the invested organs at various angles.

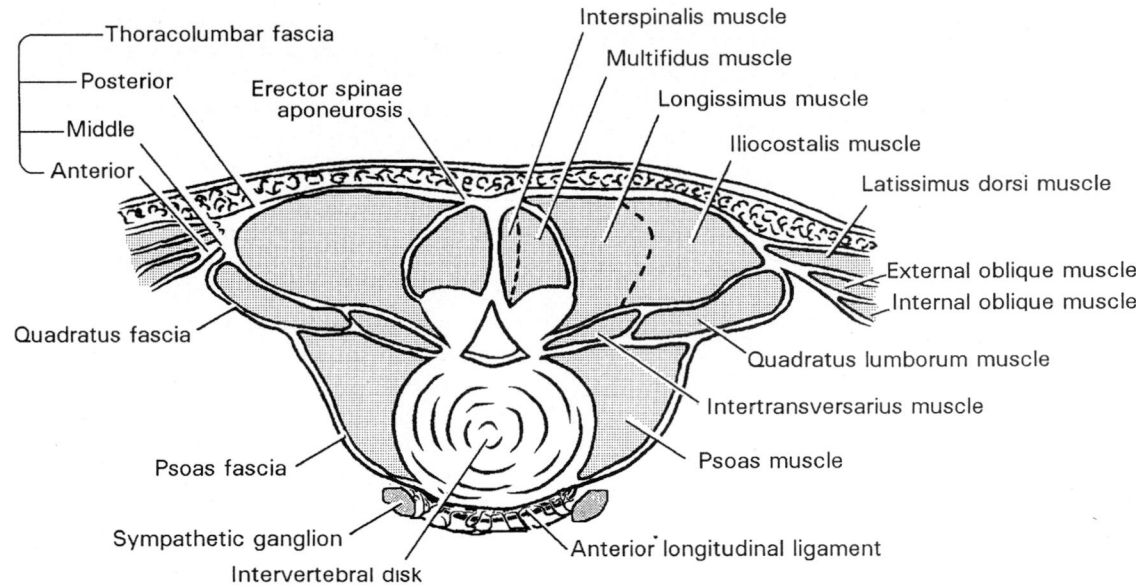

FIGURE 48.2. The erector spinae muscle groups of the thoracic region.

Trauma, chemical alterations of the bathing fluids (immune changes), and other pathologic agents alter the angles of the fascial bands and change cross-linkages between the bands, causing altered tensions of the fasciae throughout the body. An increase in tension in the fascial sheets leads to altered interstitial fluid (lymph) flows, decreased blood flow, and decreased efficiency of organ function. Normalization of the fascial tensions returns the body to more efficient function, thereby using less energy.

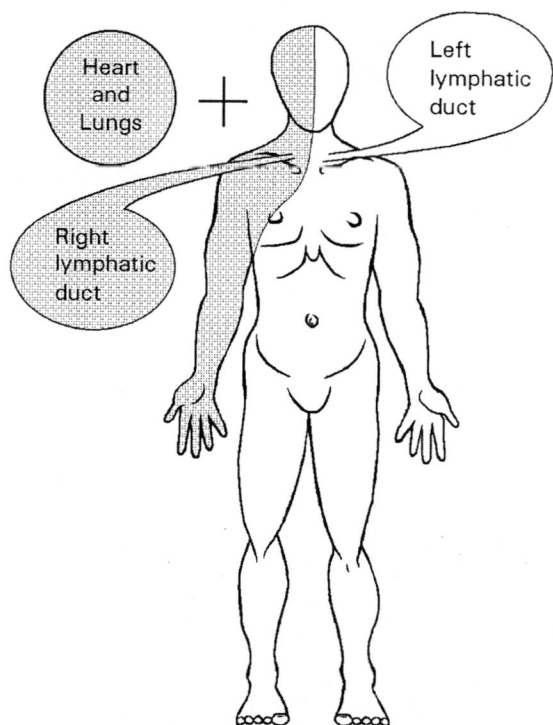

FIGURE 48.3. The lymphatic system of the body.

Osteopathic manipulative techniques, including direct and indirect myofascial release, have been developed to address these problems in ways not generally found to be effective with most other manipulative techniques. The thoracic fasciae are often involved in dysfunction due to thoracic trauma.

Neural Connections of the Thoracic Area

The neural connections of the thoracic area are of vital importance to all body functions. Not only do the usual connections to the musculoskeletal system exit the spinal cord in the thoracic region, but a large part of the sympathetic nervous system also originates in the thoracic region (Fig. 48.4). The composite autonomic innervation of the body is shown in Chapter 73. An understanding of the relationships between the thoracic nerves, as well as their relationships to the bony landmarks is vital to understanding neurologic problems associated with the thoracic region.

The spinal cord, which runs from the brainstem to about the level of L3, is a continuous structure with no segmentation. During embryologic development, the spinal nerve bundles are gathered into spinal nerve roots that course between the encircling bones through the intervertebral foramina. This imposes what appears to be a dermatomal segmentation effect. Inherently, however, the function of the spinal cord is not segmented.

The spinal nerves exit through the intervertebral foramina, which identify their vertebral level. Each spinal nerve is numbered at the level at which it exits, except in the cervical region, because there are eight cervical nerve roots and seven cervical vertebra. Spinal nerve C1 exits above the atlas, and the eighth root exits below C7. All other roots exit below their corresponding vertebrae. Because the intervertebral foramen is a bounded space and the nerve roots share that space with other tissues, the roots are especially vulnerable to pressure from herniated nucleus pulposus and even edema. Somatic dysfunction in a thoracic area

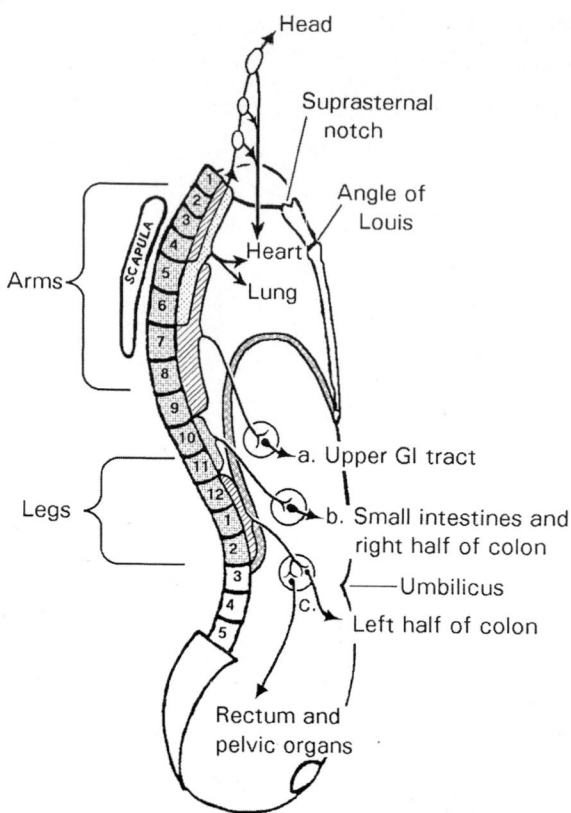

FIGURE 48.4. The sympathetic innervation of the body.

may cause local edema and tissue tightening, which can exert pressure on the nerve root and, importantly, can alter blood and fluid flows to and from the nerve sheaths. Such pressure can alter neural conductivity in the affected roots, although the lack of proper blood and fluid flow to the sheaths can cause irritability in the nociceptors of the sheath, causing pain along the nerve distribution (9). Local disturbances can often be relieved with proper manipulative treatment that is designed to restore proper motion and fluid flow to the region. As stated previously, radiculopathy is somewhat rare in the thoracic region, although discopathy is less rare. These problems in the thoracic area are not easy to diagnose because of overlapping dermatomes and a lack of readily testable deep tendon reflexes (see Chapter 30).

The abdominal diaphragm receives its motor innervation through the phrenic nerves coming from C3-5. Perhaps more importantly, sensory nerves of the diaphragm innervate the mediastinal pleura, the fibrous pericardium, and the parietal layer of the serous pericardium (10). This relationship helps explain the very common palpatory findings of cervical tension and somatic dysfunction associated with pericardial or diaphragmatic irritation that are mediated via the viscerosomatic reflexes (see Chapter 9). Manipulative treatment of the involved cervical segments is designed to ameliorate thoracic and diaphragmatic dysfunction through somatovisceral reflex pathways.

Parasympathetic innervation to the thoracic viscera and many of the abdominal viscera comes through the vagus nerve (cranial nerve X). These relationships are shown in Chapter 73 and are also discussed in Chapter 6. Treatment of problems encountered

in the function of the thoracic viscera must include assessment and treatment of cranial and cervical areas to normalize vagal function.

The majority of the outflow of the sympathetic system originates in the thoracic region (see Chapters 6 and 73). The distribution of the sympathetic system to almost every tissue and area of the body makes this system a very important one for all body functions. It is even becoming evident that the sympathetic system is vitally important in regulating immune function (11) (see Chapter 8). The importance of the sympathetic nervous system for all body functions suggests that disturbances within the thoracic vertebra and their associated musculature that affect the function of the sympathetic system can have widespread consequences. Identification and treatment of somatic dysfunction in the thoracic region is especially important in treating problems ranging from infectious processes to functional abnormalities.

Visceral dysfunction that alters input to the spinal cord not only increases the sympathetic outflow back to the visceral areas through viscerovisceral reflex pathways but also alters somatic outflow in often unexpected patterns. Understanding this phenomenon provides insight on how to treat many painful and/or functional problems. Due to the overlap of visceral afferents onto spinal pathways that also receive somatic afferents, the sensory experience of visceral irritation is often one of referred pain to a somatic structure, with concomitant increased somatic muscle tone. One of the most common of these patterns is the shoulder pain and muscle tension associated with acute myocardial infarction. The nociceptive input from the compromised myocardium is experienced as shoulder or chest pain. Often, a vicious circle of increased somatic involvement results, as increased somatic activity also increases sympathetic outflow to the heart, further exacerbating the pathologic process. Although obviously not the only course of treatment, treating the somatic component of the process can be beneficial. Recognition of the visceral origin of referred pain patterns can save the osteopathic physician much time and missed diagnoses. Likewise, recognizing that osteopathic treatment of the involved somatic structures can also help the course of the problem. Understanding the somatic areas likely to show effects of underlying visceral pathologic conditions through viscerosomatic reflexes (2) provides the osteopathic physician with another important diagnostic and treatment tool.

VARIATION AND DYSFUNCTION

Vertebral and Costal Cage Motion

Thoracic spinal movement is an integral part of total body movement and includes intimately detailed, interdependent functions with both the craniocervical and lumbopelvic systems. Both bony and general configuration anomalies are common; Wolff's law is always at work. Wolff's law states that bones and soft tissues deform (are strained) according to the stresses (forces applied over an area) that are placed on them. Examples of general configuration alterations affecting both shape and movement characteristics are seen with scoliosis, kyphosis, the arthritides, and leg length inequalities.

General body shapes and movement characteristics are also affected by growth, aging, and lifestyle factors. For example, experienced tennis players tend to develop thoracic alterations in association with repetitive twisting and stressing from the dominant hand side. So do automobile assembly line workers as they bend, twist, and turn in the same direction hundreds of times a day. On the other hand, age-induced osteoporosis and arthritic changes also affect these same characteristics. Interdependent spinal movements are always changing as life processes unfold.

Thoracic Spinal Motion

Available thoracic spinal motion is generally less than in the cervical or lumbar areas. This is because all planes of motion are affected by costal cage mechanics and their complicated relationships with head, neck, shoulder girdle, and lumbopelvic anatomy. Thoracic spinal motion is further complicated by a number of other factors that go beyond basic costovertebral configuration and mechanics. A few of the elements include configuration characteristics of the anteroposterior curves in the sagittal plane, such as:

Kyphosis
Costal cage asymmetries, such as pectus excavatum and pectus carinatum
Osteoporosis/osteoarthritis effects
Increased chest wall diameter associated with a variety of cardiopulmonary problems
Cervical, shoulder girdle, rotator cuff influences (i.e., anterior muscles are generally tighter than posterior groups); under these circumstances, anteroposterior curves tend to become more kyphotic
Effects of lifestyle and affective states, such as slumping with depression

Characteristics of primary and secondary lateral deviations include:

Scoliosis with and without kyphosis
Effects of upper and lower motor neuron lesions
Effects of repetitive motion activities
General thoracic spinal motion characteristics

Because of configuration changes in size and shape, thoracic spinal motion characteristics vary markedly from the cervicothoracic to thoracolumbar junctions. The upper and middle portions demonstrate greater rotation than elsewhere in the spine, with the exception of the atlanto-axial (A-A) joint. Generally, flexion capability is greater than extension. Side-bending capability is even less, because of rib cage constraints. In the lower portions, flexion and extension capacities are greatest, although side-bending abilities exceed those of rotation (i.e., they are more like lumbar spine mechanics).

In general, thoracic spinal motion occurs according to the mechanical principles formulated by Fryette. Thus, both neutral (type I) and non-neutral (type II) vertebral unit dysfunction is common in the thoracic spine. Neutral/type I asymmetries typically involve three or more segments that are neither flexed nor extended; they are mildly scoliotic. Non-neutral/type II vertebral unit dysfunction generally involves a single vertebral unit with both proximal and distal neutral/type I responses.

However, there are times when variations from Fryette principles occur in thoracic vertebral motion. Upper thoracic vertebrae may exhibit neutral/type II motion, which may occur as low as T4, and movements are similar to normal cervical spine behavior. Some suggest that these motions are associated with the interdependent combination of asymmetrical vertebral and upper rib shapes and attachments and their interactions with cervical muscle extensors and side-benders that attach as low as T5 and T6 (splenius mechanics).

Middle thoracic vertebral motion is commonly a mix of neutral/type I and non-neutral/type II movements, which may produce rotation to either the formed convexity or to the formed concavity.

Lower thoracic vertebral motion is more apt to be similar to lumbar neutral/type I mechanics.

Clinical Characteristics of Thoracic Movement

Clinically, there is a constant tendency for spinal flexion because of the effects of gravity and the tendency for the back extensors to become inhibited while flexors tend toward contraction. Clinically, it seems that the rotatores, intertransversarii, and multifidi are often involved in postural stress, somato-somatic, and viscero-somatic reflexes (see Chapters 7 and 30). When these muscles are reflexively affected by facilitation, they are often responsible for maintaining non-neutral somatic dysfunction of the vertebral units that are innervated by the involved muscle, neural network, or viscera. Some refer to this phenomenon as the somatic component of impairment, illness, or disease (see also Chapter 73).

Neurologic pathologic conditions, trauma, visceral disease, and intrinsic mechanical asymmetries are common sources of spinal dysfunction. Trauma, for example, often flexes, extends, and/or twists the spine simultaneously in such a way that the accumulated forces localize around a vertebral unit, thereby disturbing the mechanics of both the single vertebral segment and the vertebral units. Deforming injuries of this type often alter physical shapes; that is, they cause plastic deformations with permanent stretching of ligaments and distortions in facet joints and osseous-ligamentous relationships. Not surprisingly, recurring non-neutral/type II vertebral unit dysfunction is common under these circumstances. This type of vertebral unit change is sometimes associated with altered visceral functions; for example, somatic dysfunction is superimposed on vertebral segment and vertebral unit changes with resulting facilitated peripheral, autonomic, and centrally mediated reflex activities (see Chapters 7 and 30). Patients report many clinical symptoms when these processes occur.

HISTORY AND PHYSICAL EXAMINATION

The evaluation of the thoracic region includes:

Elements of history taking
Observation
Auscultation
Percussion

Palpation
Motion testing

The following sections focus on aspects of the history and physical examination that are uniquely osteopathic in nature.

History

Ask standard questions of the patient as part of the total evaluation of the thoracic region. Do a history of the systems most closely associated with this region, including the cardiac, pulmonary, and gastrointestinal systems. Ask if there has been any history of trauma. This information is particularly important to the osteopathic physician, as trauma to the thoracic region may have produced disturbances in structural relationships that have resulted in disturbances in visceral function. Historic information should also include when the complaint first appeared, whether a similar complaint has occurred in the past, and whether there are any underlying predisposing conditions. If there is pain, ask:

About its location
About its duration
Whether it is constant or intermittent
Whether anything has ameliorated or exacerbated it
The quality (stabbing, aching, burning, or like an electrical shock)
Whether it radiates to any other location
How much stress the patient has recently been experiencing

Information gathered during history taking helps in formulating hypotheses as to the nature of the problem. Combined with the physical examination findings, the history allows development of a working diagnosis and an appropriate comprehensive treatment approach that includes osteopathic manipulative treatment.

Observation

Observe certain aspects of the thoracic region with the patient standing, seated, supine, and prone. These observations help determine whether more detailed examination is warranted. Observations include:

1. The skin, noting such characteristics as color, skin rashes or eruptions, and hair distribution.
2. The relationship of the neck to midline. This gives information about rotation and side-bending abilities of both the neck and upper thoracic regions.
3. The sternum, observing for pectus excavatum (hollow chest, depressed sternum) or pectus carinatum (pigeon chest, protruding sternum).
4. The levelness of the clavicular heads.
5. The shoulders for excessive rounding.
6. The nipple heights.

In the standing position, observe the patient from the front, noting shoulder heights and the general shape and contour of the thoracic region. Also observe the patient from the back, taking note of shoulder heights, scapulae position, the contour and shape of the thoracic region, and any observable evidence of lateral spinal curvature, such as scoliosis. Observing the patient from each side, note the shape and contour of the thoracic region, including observable evidence of changes in the sagittal spinal curves, such as lordosis and/or kyphosis. Make the same observations with the patient seated.

Evaluate the patient for trunk side-bending abilities. With the patient standing, observe right and left side-bending from the back without forward bending. Observe for symmetry of motion of the induced spinal curve. A normal curve should be a smooth C-shaped curve with paravertebral muscle fullness on the side of the convexity. Lack of a C-shape to the induced spinal curve suggests the presence of vertebral motion segment dysfunction in the region.

Also from the back, observe forward bending as the patient attempts to touch the floor. Follow the formed contour of the spine and thoracic cage. Asymmetrical changes anywhere along the spine and rib cage raise the suspicion of vertebral motion restriction and possible somatic dysfunction in the area. Observe lateral posture using an imaginary vertical line that lies along a path drawn from the external auditory meatus to the tip of the acromion, through the middle of the femoral trochanter, ending just anterior to the lateral malleolus (see postural line in Glossary). Thoracic kyphosis and lordosis suggest the need for more detailed evaluation. Prone and supine observations assess general thoracic shape, symmetry, and contour.

Examination

When the history and screening examination indicate thoracic region dysfunction, look for more specific signs of vertebral motion segment or soft tissue myofascial dysfunction. The following points are helpful in learning to identify and describe pertinent thoracic anatomic landmarks.

Thoracic vertebral motion segments are identified by the letter T followed by a number from 1 to 12, for example, T1, T2, and so on.

It is important to distinguish C7 from T1 when evaluating the thoracic region. This can easily be done using the following method. Ask the patient to try to touch his or her chest with the chin. With the head in this position, the seventh cervical vertebra (C7) usually has the most prominent spinous process in the cervicothoracic region. Place a finger on the tip of this spinous process and ask the patient to look up toward the ceiling. In this position, the spinous process of C7 translates anteriorly. The spinous process of the vertebra just below this one is then identified as T1.

The sternal notch is located at the superior border of the manubrium between the two sternoclavicular joints. This structure is anterior to and at the same horizontal level as the second thoracic vertebra.

The sternal angle is the point at which the body of the sternum and manubrium unite. It is located anterior to and in the same horizontal plane as the fourth thoracic vertebral segment. The costal cartilage of the second rib inserts at the sternal angle. This is a clinical guide to the numbering of the ribs. The sternal angle lies anterior and in the same horizontal plane as the fourth thoracic vertebra. The xiphisternal angle is located at the inferior end of the sternum and is also anterior to and in the same horizontal plane as the ninth thoracic vertebra.

The spine of each scapula is usually at the level of the spinous process of T3. The inferior angle of each scapula is usually at the level of the spinous process of T7.

A useful way of identifying the thoracic vertebrae involves the rule of threes. This rule is a generalization that is only approximate but positions the palpating fingers in a position for locating individual thoracic vertebrae:

1. The spinous processes of T1, T2, and T3 project directly posteriorly so that the tip of each spinous process is in the same plane as the transverse processes of its associated vertebra.
2. The spinous processes of T4, T5, and T6 project in a slightly caudal direction so that the tip of each spinous process is in a plane that is approximately half way between the transverse processes of its associated vertebra and those of the vertebra immediately below.
3. The spinous processes of T7, T8, and T9 project caudally at a sharper angle so that the tip of each spinous process is in the same plane as the transverse processes of the vertebra immediately below it.
4. For the T10, T11, and T12 vertebrae, the spinous processes are placed as follows. The spinous process of T10 is similar to those of T7-9. The spinous process of T11 is similar to those of T4-6. T12 is similar to those of T1-3.

Palpation

Observation and the screening examination provide information about body regions that may have significant somatic dysfunction. Palpation is used to further investigate these areas and to further localize and identify the somatic dysfunction that may be present. Somatic dysfunction may be representative of musculoskeletal dysfunction, viscerosomatic reflex changes, or both.

Palpation of the thoracic spine can find tissue texture abnormalities and restricted motion. When either is found, more palpation may be used to identify somatic dysfunction in specific vertebral segments.

Palpate for tissue texture changes by lightly stroking the paravertebral soft tissues in a cephalocaudal direction, either bilaterally or unilaterally. The search is for changes in tissue texture defined as:

Increased tone or tension (hypertonicity)
Spasm
Fasciculation
Ropiness
Bogginess (indicative of edema)
Increased or decreased temperature
Moisture

Warm, moist, and boggy tissue usually suggests acute somatic dysfunction, although cold, dry, ropy tissue suggests chronic somatic dysfunction. If an area has abnormal tissue texture, asymmetry, restricted motion, or tenderness, perform a more detailed assessment.

Perform the red reflex test by firmly (but with slight pressure) stroking two fingers on the skin over the paraspinal tissues in a cephalad to a caudad direction. The stroked areas briefly become erythematous and then almost immediately return to their usual color. If the skin remains erythematous longer than a few seconds, it may indicate acute somatic dysfunction in the area. As the dysfunction acquires chronic tissue changes, the tissues blanch rapidly after stroking and are dry and cool to palpation.

In addition to palpating the paravertebral tissues, assess the tips of the spinous processes and the interspinous ligaments for evidence of gross asymmetry, edema, or tenderness. Palpation also extends laterally to the transverse processes, the costotransverse articulations, and the rib angles; look for tissue texture changes and tenderness.

MOTION TESTING

Thoracic region motion testing further identifies areas of altered movement of the vertebrae, ribs, and soft tissues. Use more detailed palpation of vertebral motion segments and soft tissues to assess areas where gross motion restrictions are located.

Motion restriction evaluation involves both active and passive motion testing. Active motion testing assesses voluntary motions produced by the patient. Passive motion testing is induced while the patient remains as passive and relaxed as possible.

Active Motion Testing of the Thoracic Spine

Flexion/Extension: Sagittal Plane Bending

The patient sits on the examination table or on a stool with the feet on the floor. The physician palpates for asymmetries and vertebral motion segment restrictions while the patient bends forward and backward.

Side-Bending

The patient side bends right and left as the physician palpates for restriction in spinal curves and for neutral and non-neutral dysfunction in vertebral motion segments. Identify the level of the apex of any curve where limitation is found.

Rotation

The patient rotates right and left as the physician notes restriction in spinal and vertebral unit motion segments, both unilaterally and bilaterally, to identify the spinal segmental level where limitation occurs.

Active Motion Testing of the Vertebral Motion Segment

The physician places his/her thumbs on the posterior surfaces of the left and right thoracic transverse processes at the level to be evaluated. Then the patient is asked to slightly flex, extend, side bend right, side bend left, rotate right, and rotate left as the physician palpates to determine the site(s) of greatest restriction in comparison with vertebral segments above and below.

Passive Motion Testing

Regional Examination of the Upper Thoracic Spine

Flexion and Extension

1. Place one hand posteriorly on the patient's upper thorax and the other on top of the patient's head.
2. Bend the head and neck forward until flexion creates movement in the upper thorax (T1-4). Note flexion restrictions as the process proceeds.
3. Bend the head backward until extension creates movement in the upper thorax, again noting any movement restrictions.

Side-Bending

1. With a hand on the patient's upper thorax, bend the head and neck to one side and then the other side.
2. Note any side-bending restrictions.

Rotation

1. With one hand on the patient's upper thorax, use the other hand to rotate the head and neck right and left.
2. Palpate for upper thoracic rotation restrictions.

Regional Examination of the Lower Thoracic Spine

Flexion/Extension

1. Place the palmar surface of one hand on the patient's lower thorax.
2. Place the other hand on the opposite shoulder.
3. Bend the torso forward and backward, noting any flexion and extension restrictions with the hand palpating the lower thorax.

Rotation

1. Place the palmar surface of one hand on the patient's lower thorax.
2. Place the other hand on the opposite shoulder.
3. Rotate the torso to the left and to the right, noting any rotation restrictions with the hand palpating the lower thorax.

Side-Bending

1. Place the palmar surface of one hand on the patient's lower thorax.
2. Place the other hand on the opposite shoulder.
3. Side bend the torso to the left and to the right, noting any side-bending restrictions with the hand palpating the lower thorax.

Segmental Examination of the Upper Thoracic Spine

Segmental motion tests are most commonly done with the patient seated.

Flexion/Extension

1. Place the fingertips of one hand between the spinous processes of the first four thoracic vertebrae.

2. Use the other hand to move the head and neck passively into flexion and extension.
3. Assess each vertebral motion segment as the process unfolds.
4. Typically, the spinous process of the superior vertebra moves anteriorly and superiorly before those that are more distal. If a vertebral motion segment does not move freely into flexion, it is defined as being in an extended position, such as an extended–rotated–side-bent vertebral unit dysfunction that is restricted during flexion movements.
5. Examine extension in a similar manner, using passively induced backward bending.
6. If a vertebral motion segment does not extend well, it is in a flexed position, such as a flexed–side-bent–rotated vertebral unit dysfunction that is restricted during extension movements.

Side-Bending

1. Place the fingertips of one hand between the transverse processes of the first four thoracic vertebrae.
2. Use the other hand to move the head and neck passively into left and right side-bending.
3. Assess each vertebral motion segment as the process unfolds.
4. If the transverse process of one segment does not approximate the transverse process of the segment below, it is restricted in side-bending right or left in accordance with the restriction.

Rotation

1. Place the index and long fingers over the transverse processes of the upper thoracic segment to be examined.
2. Rotate the head and neck passively right or left until the segment begins to rotate in the same direction.
3. Restricted right rotation restriction suggests that the segment is positionally rotated left.

Segmental Examination of the Lower Thoracic Spine

Motion testing is performed with the same maneuvers used on the upper thoracic segments. However, instead of using the head and neck as a lever, do the following:

1. For example, to examine the patient from the patient's right side, the physician stands on the patient's right side.
2. The physician places the index and long fingers of his/her left hand on the transverse processes of the lower thoracic segment to be examined, in the same manner as described for the upper thoracic segments.
3. The physician places his/her right axilla over the top of the patient's right shoulder, then reaches across the patient's chest and places his/her right hand on the patient's left shoulder.
4. The physician then uses the patient's upper trunk as a lever to move T5-12.

Diagnosis

Use active and passive motion testing to formulate a specific positional diagnosis for a given spinal segment. For example, if

T2 moves more easily into flexion than into extension, it is in a flexed position. If it rotates more easily to the right than to the left, it is rotated right. If it side bends more easily to the right than to the left, it is side-bent right.

Examine all the lower thoracic segments for flexion/extension, right and left side-bending, and right and left rotation movements.

The principles of physiologic motion of the spine are used to identify any specific segmental motion restrictions. For example, if the examination reveals that a vertebral segment moves more easily into extension, left rotation, and left side-bending, this indicates that the vertebra is positionally extended, and rotated and side-bent to the left (ER_LS_L).

If the motion restriction is most noticeable with the patient in the neutral position (that is, motion improves in flexion and extension), then the motion restriction is described as a neutral vertebral motion segment dysfunction. For example, if the vertebrae are rotated to the left and side-bent to the right in the neutral position, the segmental dysfunction is recorded as NR_LS_R.

CONCLUSION

The thoracic cage is a complex region of the body, containing and protecting many vital organs. Osteopathic physicians must understand the proper function, diagnosis, and treatment of the thoracic area.

REFERENCES

1. White AA, Panjabi MM. *Clinical Biomechanics of the Spine.* Philadelphia, PA: JB Lippincott Co; 1978:44–56.
2. Patterson MM, Howell JN, eds. *The Central Connection: Somatovisceral/Viscerosomatic Interaction.* Indianapolis, IN: American Academy of Osteopathy; 1992.
3. Korr IM. The spinal cord as organizer of disease processes. IV. Axonal transport and neurotrophic function in relation to somatic dysfunction. *J Am Osteopath Assoc.* 1981;80(7):451–459.
4. Korr IM. Proprioceptors and somatic dysfunction. *J Am Osteopath Assoc.* 1975;74(7);638–650.
5. Patterson MM, Steinmetz JE. Long-lasting alterations of spinal reflexes: A basis for somatic dysfunction. *Man Med.* 1986;2:38–42.
6. Van Buskirk RL. Nociceptive reflexes and the somatic dysfunction: a model. *J Am Osteopath Assoc.* 1990;90(9):792–804.
7. Gallaudet BB. *A Description of the Planes of Fascia of the Human Body.* New York, NY: Columbia Press; 1931.
8. Budgell B, Sato A. Somatoautonomic reflex regulation of sciatic nerve blood flow. *J Neuromusculoskeletal Sys.* 1994;2:170–177.
9. Moore KL. *Clinically Oriented Anatomy,* 2nd ed. Baltimore, MD: Williams & Wilkins; 1985.
10. Warwick R, Williams P, eds. *Gray's Anatomy,* 35th ed. Edinburgh, Scotland: Churchill Livingstone; 1973.
11. Willard FH, Patterson MM, eds. *Nociception and the Neuroendocrine-Immune Connection.* Indianapolis, IN: American Academy of Osteopathy; 1994.

49

THE RIB CAGE

RAYMOND J. HRUBY

KEY CONCEPTS

- Importance of the rib cage for normal function
- Structure and function of the rib cage, including lymphatics, connective tissues, neural connections, and motion
- Clinical characteristics of rib movements
- History and physical examination, including observation, palpation, and motion testing
- Assessment, diagnosis, and treatment of structural dysfunction

Respiration is a process involving the participation of several systems of the body, none the least of which is the musculoskeletal system. As Cathie (1) noted, "Respiratory activity requires motion in a greater number of articulations and with a greater frequency than any other musculoskeletal function." This not only includes the intervertebral joints of the thoracic spine but also the costovertebral and costotransverse joints at the posterior aspects of the ribs. In addition to the articular motion, optimal respiration also requires a degree of elasticity of the ribs and costal cartilages. The biomechanical architecture among the vertebrae and ribs may be thought of as a complex system of levers; anything that alters the normal movement of this system of levers may impair respiration.

ANATOMY AND PHYSIOLOGY

The Costal Skeleton

The 12 sets of ribs correspond with the 12 thoracic vertebrae. All ribs are composed of a bony segment and a costal cartilage. Each rib has a cup-shaped depression in its bony segment where the costal cartilage fits into the costochondral joint and where the periosteum of the rib joins the perichondrium of the rib cartilage. The rib heads join with the thoracic vertebrae at the costovertebral articulations. The heads of ribs 2 through 9 articulate with a demifacet on the vertebra above and below. For example, rib 2 articulates by demifacets with T1 and T2. The heads of ribs 1 and 10–12 articulate with unifacets on their corresponding ver-

tebrae. The transverse processes of vertebrae T1-10 also have synovial costotransverse joints with the tubercle of the corresponding rib.

Ribs 1, 2, 11, and 12 are called atypical ribs. Rib 1 is the flattest, shortest, broadest, strongest, and most curved. The subclavian artery and the cervical plexus are vulnerable to muscular compression where they pass over the first rib between the tubercles and attachments of the anterior and the middle scalene muscles (the so-called scalenus anticus syndrome). The latter is one of several conditions clinically labeled as thoracic outlet syndrome (see Chapter 30). The subclavian vein may also be compressed between the first rib and the clavicle. Rib 2 is considered anatomically atypical because of its tuberosity that attaches to the proximal portion of the serratus anterior muscle. Ribs 11 and 12 are anatomically atypical because they do not have tubercles, do not attach to the sternum or other costal cartilages, and have tapered ends. These two ribs are also called floating or vertebral ribs. Rib 10 is sometimes considered atypical because of its single articulation between the rib head and T10.

The anatomy of the rib cage is shown in Figure 49.1. Anatomically typical ribs (3–9, and in most respects 10) have heads, necks, tubercles, angles, and shafts that connect directly or via chondral masses to the sternum. Rib 1 and ribs 2–7 connect directly with the sternum by their own individual cartilaginous synovial joints (rib 1 with a stable synchondrosis); therefore, they are often called the true ribs. Ribs 8–10 merge into a single cartilaginous mass that attaches to the sternum; therefore, these are called vertebral chondral ribs. Ribs 11 and 12 do not connect with the sternum and are hence called floating ribs. Because ribs 8–12 do not connect directly to the sternum, they are often called the false ribs.

The costovertebral joints between the heads of the ribs and the vertebral bodies allow gliding or sliding costal motions. The costotransverse joints at the tubercle of the typical ribs, with the facets at the tip of the transverse processes of their own vertebra, a synovial membrane, and a thin articular capsule, allow gliding and slight rotational motions. When these motions are restricted, respiratory movements are commonly impeded.

The sternum has three parts:

Head or manubrium
Body or gladiolus
Tail or xiphoid process

The superior portion of the manubrium cradles the clavicles at the sternoclavicular joints, forming the sternal notch or

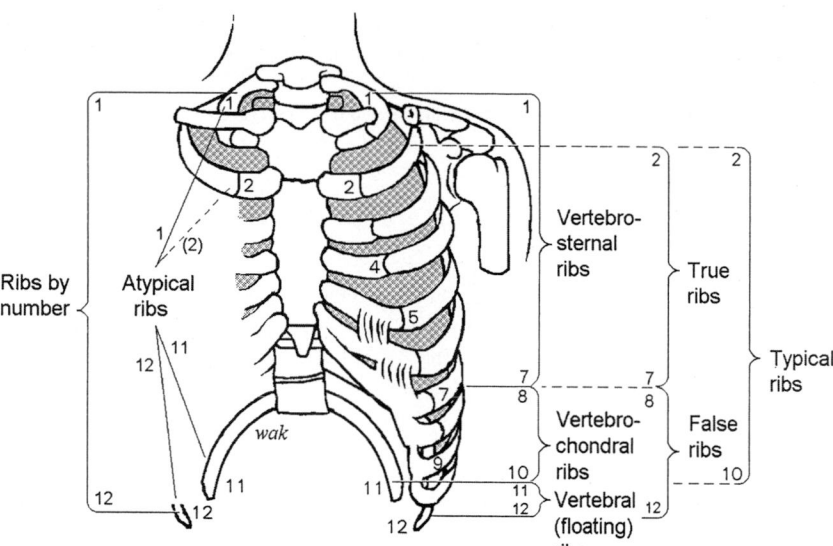

FIGURE 49.1. The bony anatomy of the rib cage and the naming of rib types.

jugular notch, which is a landmark for several anterior thoracic strain/counterstrain tender points. The sternal notch lies almost directly anterior to the T2 vertebral body. The manubrium joins the sternal body via a fibrocartilaginous symphysis, or secondary cartilaginous joint, called the sternal angle or angle of Louis. This joint lies anterior to the fourth thoracic vertebra. Because the second rib attaches to the manubrium and sternal body with a synovial joint, the sternal angle is an anterior landmark for counting the ribs. The xiphisternal joint is located anterior to the ninth thoracic vertebra. It is also a hyaline cartilage symphysis that fuses into a synostosis in the fifth decade.

Muscles of the Costal Area

The muscles of the thoracic area are involved in:

Actions of the ribs and vertebrae
Head and neck control
Breathing

For specific information regarding individual muscles of the rib cage, see Table 50.1 in Chapter 50. As with all muscles, the rib cage muscles are fed not only by circulatory elements but by physiologically active trophic substances delivered directly by nerves themselves (3). In addition, there is evidence that the sympathetic nerve supply to striated and smooth muscles alters muscle tone and contractile forces. Attention to the palpatory cues associated with altered muscle tone therefore implies the presence of many differential diagnostic factors that are discussed throughout this text.

The abdominal diaphragm is the primary muscle of respiration. It forms the floor of the thorax and attaches to the xiphoid process, the internal surface of the inferior six ribs, the upper two (left) or three (right) lumbar vertebrae, and their intervertebral discs. Its fibers converge into a common central tendon that has no bony attachment. When the diaphragm contracts with inhalation, it descends into the abdomen; when it relaxes during exhalation, it moves upward into the thorax. This up and down movement produces pressure gradients between the thoracic and abdominal cavities, and is important for both efficient respiration and circulation. Because there are one-way valves in the larger lymphatic vessels, the pressure gradients also enhance the movement of lymph and venous blood toward the heart. When the dome of the diaphragm is flattened because of asymmetric load and/or tonus, respiration and lymphatic drainage from anywhere in the body becomes less efficient.

Three apertures occur in the diaphragm: one for the vena cava at about the level of T8, another for the esophageal hiatus at T10, and the third for the aorta at the level of T12 (Fig. 49.2). Diaphragmatic muscle fibers are arranged so that when it contracts in inspiration, the vena caval opening dilates, permitting

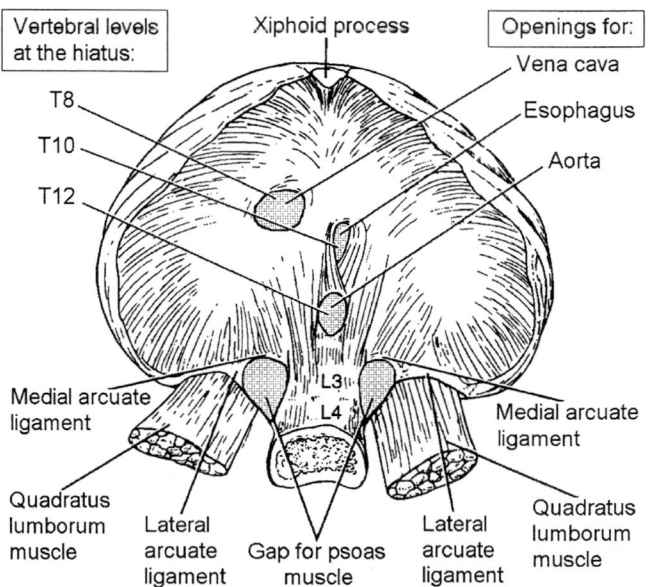

FIGURE 49.2. Apertures of the abdominal diaphragm.

more venous blood to pass from the abdomen to the thorax; at the same time, the esophageal hiatus constricts to prevent gastric contents from rising in the esophagus. Its contraction has no influence on the aortic hiatus, which lies posterior to the diaphragm and does not truly pierce the diaphragm.

The diaphragm does most of the work of breathing under normal conditions and during moderately forced inspiration. With increased respiratory demands, accessory muscles of respiration become involved to move the ribs even more. The scalene muscles, attached to the upper two ribs, assist inhalation. Hypertonicity or hypotonicity of segmental intercostal muscles alters rib behavior, making breathing less efficient. Actual spasm in these muscles can result in pain at rest or especially with each deep breath or cough. Quiet exhalation creates passive recoil of the lung as the diaphragm relaxes. Forced exhalation also involves the inferior internal intercostal and abdominal muscles, including the trunk rotators and erector spinae.

Osteopathic manipulative treatments can often restore or partially rehabilitate altered diaphragmatic function. These treatments are designed to increase motion of the lower costal cage by freeing the diaphragm for better excursion. This, in turn, helps improve breathing mechanics and assists in venous blood return and lymphatic flow. This approach can be especially helpful for individuals with asthma, respiratory infections, loss of general lung compliance, and associated disorders.

Lymphatics

In general, the superficial lymph vessels of the thoracic wall ramify subcutaneously and converge on the axillary nodes (2). The lymph nodes from the deeper tissues of the thoracic wall drain into three groups of nodes:

1. The parasternal (internal thoracic) lymph nodes. These are four or five pairs of nodes located at the anterior ends of the intercostal spaces.
2. The intercostal lymph nodes, located in the posterior parts of the intercostal spaces in relation to the heads and necks of the ribs.
3. The diaphragmatic (phrenic) lymph nodes, located on the thoracic surface of the diaphragm.

Connective Tissue and Fascia

Like all other muscles of the body, the muscles of the thoracic cage are invested with fascia. The internal thoracic wall is covered by a parietal layer of fascia called the endothoracic fascia. This deep fascia invests the internal intercostal, subcostal, and transversus thoracis muscles (3). This fascia blends with the periosteum of the ribs and sternum and with the perichondrial tissue of the costal cartilages. The endothoracic fascia also covers the superior surface of the diaphragm, thus becoming the superior diaphragmatic fascia. The endothoracic fascia is also continuous with the prevertebral layer of the cervical fascia and with the scalene fascia (also called Sibson fascia), where it attaches along the inner border of the first rib. Behind the sternum, it is also continuous with the fascia of the infrahyoid muscles. This

parietal thoracic fascia proceeds through the openings of the diaphragm to become continuous with the transversalis fascia of the abdomen.

In addition, there are specialized fascial elements that comprise the pericardium, pleura, and mediastinum.

Neural Connections of the Thoracic Cage

A detailed description of the nerve supply to the thoracic area is given in Chapter 50. The ventral rami of the first 11 thoracic nerves are called *intercostal nerves* (4). They are located between the ribs, although the 12th thoracic nerve lies below the last rib and is thus called the *subcostal nerve*. Each of these nerves is connected to the sympathetic chain ganglia via the *white and gray rami communicantes*. The intercostal nerves provide innervation chiefly to the thoracic and abdominal walls. The first six nerves provide innervation to the thoracic wall, with the first two nerves also providing fibers to the upper extremity. The lower five nerves are distributed to the thoracic and abdominal walls, and the subcostal nerve innervates the abdominal wall and the skin of the gluteal area.

The abdominal diaphragm receives its motor innervation through the phrenic nerves coming from C3-5. Perhaps more importantly, sensory nerves of the diaphragm innervate the mediastinal pleura, the fibrous pericardium, and the parietal layer of the serous pericardium (2). This relationship helps explain the very common palpatory findings of cervical tension and somatic dysfunction associated with pericardial or diaphragmatic irritation that are mediated via viscerosomatic reflexes (see Chapter 9). Manipulative treatment of the involved cervical segments is designed to ameliorate thoracic and diaphragmatic dysfunction through somatovisceral reflex pathways.

RIB MECHANICS

During inhalation, the thoracic cage widens its vertical, transverse, and anteroposterior dimensions as the diaphragm contracts. With deep inhalation, the anterior ends of the superior ribs move more anteriorly and superiorly along with the sternum (Fig. 49.3).

Typical ribs are attached to the sternum by the costal cartilage, and their pump-handle movements displace the anterior component of the costosternal system upward and anteriorly. (See Glossary for more detailed definition.) The rib shaft is the handle of the bucket and the vertebral column is the pivot point (Figs. 49.3 and 49.4).

Even though the first ribs are described as being elevated or depressed when they have somatic dysfunction, the vertebrosternal ribs (1 and 2) and vertebrochondral ribs (8–10) move in a bucket-handle manner (Figs. 49.5 and 49.6). They are described as moving about functional pivots posteriorly and anteriorly. Functionally, their shafts move laterally and superiorly during inhalation, increasing the transverse diameter of the costal cage. The anterior/posterior (AP) diameter of the chest is increased as the anterior ends of ribs 8–10 are elevated by the contraction of the diaphragm. Ribs 11 and 12 are called vertebral ribs, because they do not attach to the sternum or the chondral mass.

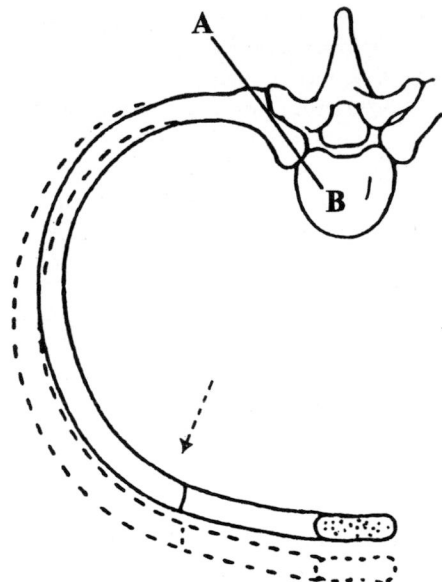

FIGURE 49.3. Functional transverse rib axis. (From *Gray's Anatomy*, 35th ed. Edinburgh, Scotland: Churchill Livingstone; 1973:421, with permission.)

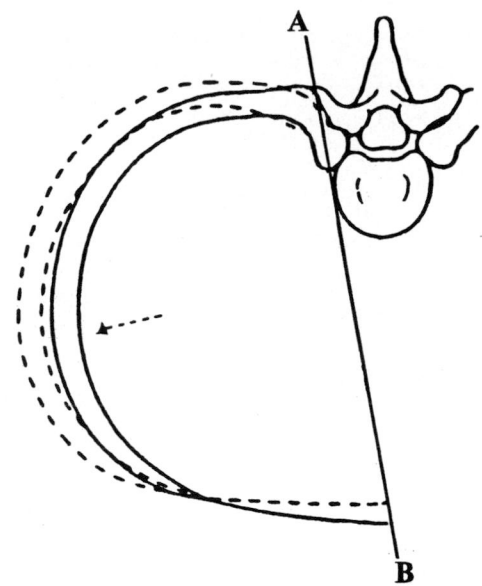

FIGURE 49.5. Functional anteroposterior rib axis. (From *Gray's Anatomy*, 35th ed. Edinburgh, Scotland: Churchill Livingstone; 1973:421, with permission.)

These two atypical ribs have a pincer-type motion. The types of rib motion described clinically are depicted in Figure 49.7.

HISTORY AND PHYSICAL EXAMINATION

The evaluation of the rib cage includes:

Elements of history taking
Observation
Auscultation
Percussion
Palpation
Motion testing

The following sections focus on the aspects of the history and physical examination that are uniquely osteopathic in nature.

History

Ask standard questions of the patient as part of the total evaluation of the rib cage. Do a history of the systems most closely associated with the rib cage. This includes the cardiac, pulmonary, and gastrointestinal systems. Ask if there has been any history of trauma. This information is particularly important to the osteopathic physician, as trauma to the ribs may have produced disturbances in structural relationships that have resulted in the presenting symptoms. Historic information should also include when the complaint first appeared, whether a similar complaint has occurred in the past, and whether there are any underlying predisposing conditions. If there is pain, ask:

About its location
About its duration
Whether it is constant or intermittent
Whether anything has ameliorated or exacerbated it

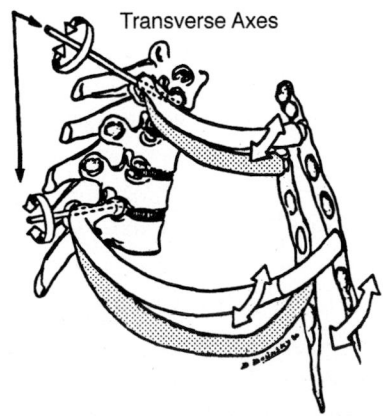

Transverse Axes

FIGURE 49.4. Pump-handle rib motion.

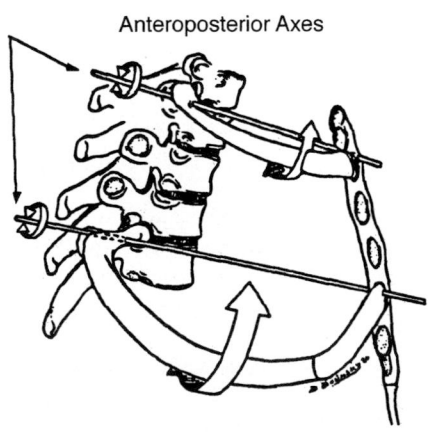

Anteroposterior Axes

FIGURE 49.6. Bucket-handle rib motion.

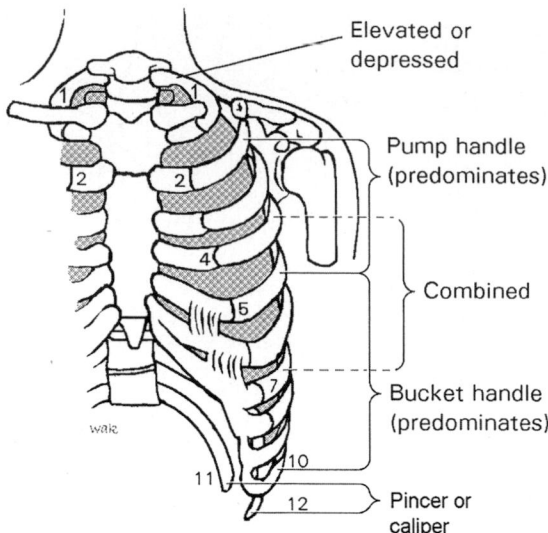

FIGURE 49.7. Clinical rib movement.

The quality (stabbing, aching, burning, or like an electrical shock)

Whether it radiates to any other location

How much stress the patient has recently been experiencing

Information gathered during history taking helps formulate hypotheses as to the nature of the problem. Combined with the physical examination findings, the history allows development of a working diagnosis and an appropriate comprehensive treatment approach that includes osteopathic manipulative treatment.

Observation

Observe certain aspects of the rib cage with the patient standing, seated, supine, and prone. These observations help determine whether a more detailed examination is warranted. Observations include:

1. The skin, noting such characteristics as color, skin rashes or eruptions, and hair distribution.
2. The tissue textures of the muscles, fasciae, and ligaments associated with the rib cage.
3. The sternum, observing for pectus excavatum (hollow chest, depressed sternum) or pectus carinatum (pigeon chest, protruding sternum).
4. Any asymmetry of the bony components of the rib cage.
5. Tenderness or pain of the ribs and associated structures.

In the standing position, observe the patient from the front, noting shoulder heights and the general shape and contour of the thoracic cage. Also observe the patient from the back, taking note of shoulder heights, position of the scapulae, the contour and shape of the thoracic cage, and any observable evidence of lateral spinal curvature, such as scoliosis. Observing the patient from each side, note the shape and contour of the thoracic cage, including observable evidence of changes in the sagittal spinal curves, such as lordosis and/or kyphosis. Make the same observations with the patient seated.

With the patient standing, observe for symmetry of rib cage motion as the patient side bends right and left without bending forward. Observe forward bending as the patient attempts to touch the floor. Follow the formed contour of the rib cage. Asymmetrical changes anywhere along the rib cage raise the suspicion of motion restriction and possible somatic dysfunction in the area.

Prone and supine observations assess general costal shape, symmetry, and contour. Respiration is best observed with the patient supine. Is respiratory effort mostly thoracic or abdominal, or a combination of each? Altered patterns often indicate somatic, visceral, or neurosensory problems reflected partially as somatic dysfunction in the ribcage.

Examination

When the history and screening examination indicate rib cage dysfunction, look for more specific signs of somatic dysfunction of the ribs. Motion dysfunction of the ribs is designated as either structural or respiratory. Specific structural dysfunction includes:

Superior subluxation of the first rib
Anterior or posterior subluxations
External rib torsions
Anteroposterior compression
Lateral compressions
Laterally flexed ribs

Respiratory dysfunction is classified as either inhalation or exhalation dysfunction, and may involve either single ribs or groups of ribs.

Evaluation for Structural Rib Dysfunction

Evaluation of First Rib for Superior Subluxation

The first rib is evaluated for superior subluxation as follows:

1. The patient is seated on the examination table.
2. The physician stands behind the patient.
3. The physician grasps the anterior and superior aspect of the trapezius muscle on both sides and retracts the tissues posteriorly.
4. The physician then directs the long fingers caudally to make bilateral contact with the posterior shafts of the first ribs.
5. A positive finding is unleveling of the first ribs.
6. The patient is instructed to inhale and exhale deeply.
7. The inability of one or the other first rib to descend into the exhalation position confirms the diagnosis of superior subluxation of that rib.

Evaluation of Ribs 2–10 for Structural Rib Restrictions

Evaluate for structural rib restrictions in this region as follows:

1. The patient is seated on the examination table.
2. The physician first stands behind the patient and assesses the posterior contour of the rib cage by palpating over the area of the rib angles. The physician assesses whether one rib angle is more or less prominent than another.

3. The physician then assesses whether there is a normal posterior convexity with the inferior border of each rib being more easily palpated than the superior border.
4. The posterior rib cage is also assessed for muscle hypertonicity and tenderness.
5. The width of the intercostal spaces is assessed for symmetry, intercostal muscle hypertonicity, and tenderness. Each intercostal space should be symmetrical with the one on the opposite side and with the one immediately above and below.
6. The physician next stands in front of the patient and examines the anterior contour of the rib cage. Palpation is done at the costochondral junctions, assessing the rib contours and intercostal spaces in a manner similar to that described in step 5 above.
7. The physician then similarly evaluates the lateral rib cage, palpating in the mid-axillary line.

The diagnostic criteria for structural rib dysfunction are described as follows:

1. Anterior subluxation.
   A. Posteriorly, the rib angle is less prominent.
   B. Anteriorly, the rib shaft is more prominent.
   C. There is associated tenderness and muscle hypertonicity.
2. Posterior subluxation.
   A. Posteriorly, the rib angle is more prominent.
   B. Anteriorly, the rib angle is less prominent.
   C. There is associated tenderness and muscle hypertonicity.
3. External rib torsion.
   A. The superior border of the involved rib is more prominent.
   B. The inferior border of the involved rib is less prominent.
   C. There is a wider intercostal space above and a more narrow intercostal space below the involved rib, with associated muscle hypertonicity and tenderness.
4. Anteroposterior rib compression.
   A. There is less prominence of the involved rib both anteriorly and posteriorly.
   B. There is increased prominence of the involved rib in the midaxillary line.
   C. The intercostal space above and below the involved rib reveals tenderness and increased muscle tension.
5. Lateral rib compression.
   A. There is more prominence of the involved rib in the anterior and posterior rib cage.
   B. There is less prominence of the involved rib in the midaxillary line.
   C. The intercostal space above and below the involved rib reveals tenderness and increased muscle tension.
6. Laterally flexed rib.
   A. There is prominence of the involved rib in the midaxillary line.
   B. There is a narrow intercostal space above and a wider intercostal space below the involved rib.
   C. There is marked tenderness, usually in the intercostal space above the involved rib.
   D. This restriction is most commonly seen in the second rib.

Evaluation of the First Rib for Respiratory Rib Restriction

The first rib is evaluated for respiratory restriction as follows:

1. The patient is seated or supine on the examination table.
2. The physician stands behind the seated patient or sits at the head of the examination table if the patient is supine.
3. The physician grasps the anterior and superior aspect of the trapezius muscle on each side and retracts the tissues posteriorly.
4. The physician then directs the long fingers caudally to make bilateral contact with the posterior shafts of the first ribs.
5. The patient is instructed to inhale and exhale deeply.
6. The inability of one or the other first rib to descend into the exhalation position indicates inhalation restriction of that rib. The inability of one or the other first rib to ascend into the inhalation position indicates exhalation restriction of that rib.

Evaluation of Ribs 2–10 for Respiratory Rib Restrictions

This can be done in the following manner:

1. The patient lies supine on the examination table.
2. The physician stands at the side of the table so that his or her dominant eye is over the patient's midline.
3. The physician places his or her hands over the patient's upper anterior thoracic cage so that the tips of the middle fingers contact the inferior borders of the clavicles.
4. The patient is asked to inhale deeply and then exhale fully; assess pump-handle motion of the upper ribs, looking for asymmetry of motion between the left and right sides of the upper rib cage (see Glossary).
5. Evaluate the upper rib cage in the same manner, but along the midaxillary line. This maneuver assesses bucket-handle motion of the upper rib cage (see Glossary).
6. This process is repeated for the middle and lower rib cage regions.

Asymmetry of motion in any of the rib cage areas indicates the presence of respiratory rib dysfunction in that region. Respiratory rib dysfunction has either inhalation or exhalation restriction. There is usually one rib within a group of ribs that is responsible for maintaining the inhalation or exhalation restriction. This rib is referred to as the key rib and is the rib that must be identified and treated to remove the group restriction.

To identify the key rib within a group of ribs, examine each rib in the group individually. This is done by doing the following:

1. Place a finger on each pair of ribs in the group, first at the parasternal area (for pump-handle restriction) and then in the midaxillary line (for bucket-handle restriction).
2. For each placement, ask the patient to inhale and exhale. Palpate successive pairs of ribs within the group until symmetry of motion on respiration is noted.
3. With inhalation restriction, the key rib is found at the top of the group, but it is located at the bottom of the rib group with exhalation restrictions.

In summary, inhalation restrictions involve a rib or group of ribs that first stops moving during inhalation. The key rib is the top rib in the group. Exhalation restrictions involve a rib or group of ribs that stops moving first during exhalation. The key rib is the bottom rib in the group.

Evaluation of Ribs 11 and 12

Ribs 11 and 12 have no anterior cartilaginous attachment and therefore do not exhibit pump-handle or bucket-handle movement. Instead, they move posteriorly and laterally with inhalation, and anteriorly and medially during exhalation. This motion is sometimes described as caliper motion.

Assessment for respiratory dysfunction of ribs 11 and 12 is as follows:

1. The patient lies prone on the examination table.
2. The physician stands at the side of the patient, with his or her dominant eye over the patient's midline.
3. The physician places his or her hands over the 11th and 12th ribs, contacting the rib shafts with the thumbs and thenar eminences.
4. Ask the patient to inhale and exhale fully; note any asymmetry of motion in the ribs.
5. If either of the ribs does not move posteriorly with inhalation, it has an inhalation restriction. Conversely, if the ribs do not move anteriorly with exhalation, exhalation restriction is present.

Diaphragm Evaluation

One method of examining the diaphragm for motion restriction is as follows:

1. The patient is seated on the examination table.

2. The physician stands behind the patient.
3. The physician passes his or her hands around the thoracic cage under the arms of the patient.
4. Assess diaphragmatic motions by gently but firmly introducing the finger pads upward and medially under the costal margins.
5. Testing is easier when the patient leans slightly backward against the physician's chest in a slightly slumped position. This position lessens tension of the muscular attachments on and around the costal margins, making palpation easier.
6. Assess motion restriction and asymmetry by passively rotating the diaphragm gently right and left.

Sternum Evaluation

Compression and decompression of the sternum can be a valuable diagnostic test, for many reasons. Two common examples are sternocostal problems associated with seat belt injuries in car accidents and mechanical chest wall problems secondary to coronary artery bypass surgery.

Sternal Compression

Testing the sternum involves gentle compression and release with particular attention to respiratory, mechanical, and pain-related responses arising both locally and from points distant. Functional and myofascial approaches are particularly useful (see Chapters 61 and 62).

To test the motion of the sternum:

1. Place one hand longitudinally on the manubrium and the body of the sternum, and place the fingers of the other hand on top of the first hand (Fig. 49.8).
2. Compress slightly, noting any indication that the tissue moves more easily in one or more directions as the patient goes through the respiratory cycle.

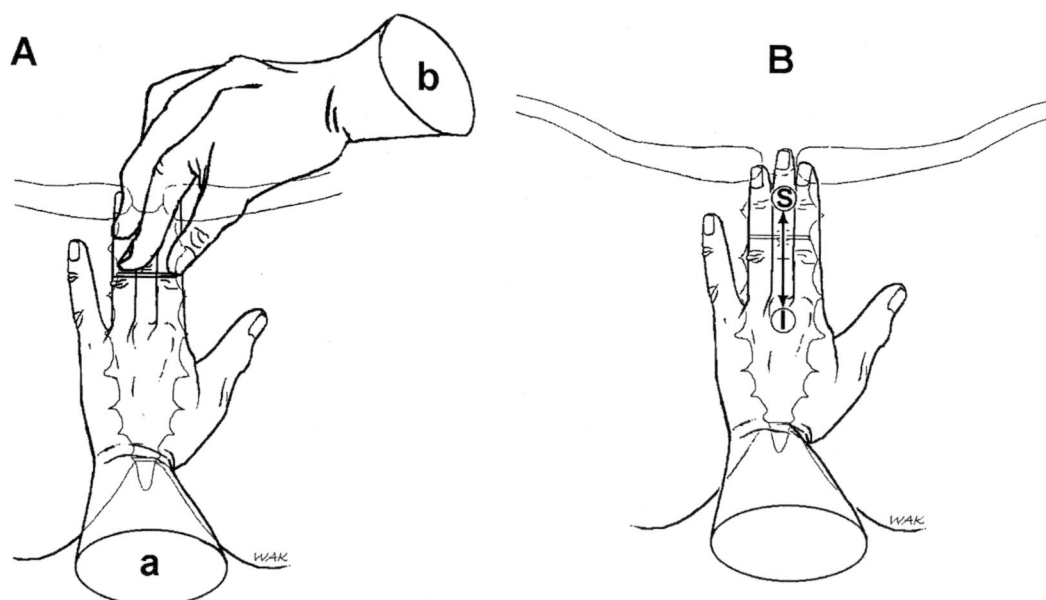

FIGURE 49.8. Evaluation of the sternum. **A:** By Compression. **B:** By superior and inferior gliding motion.

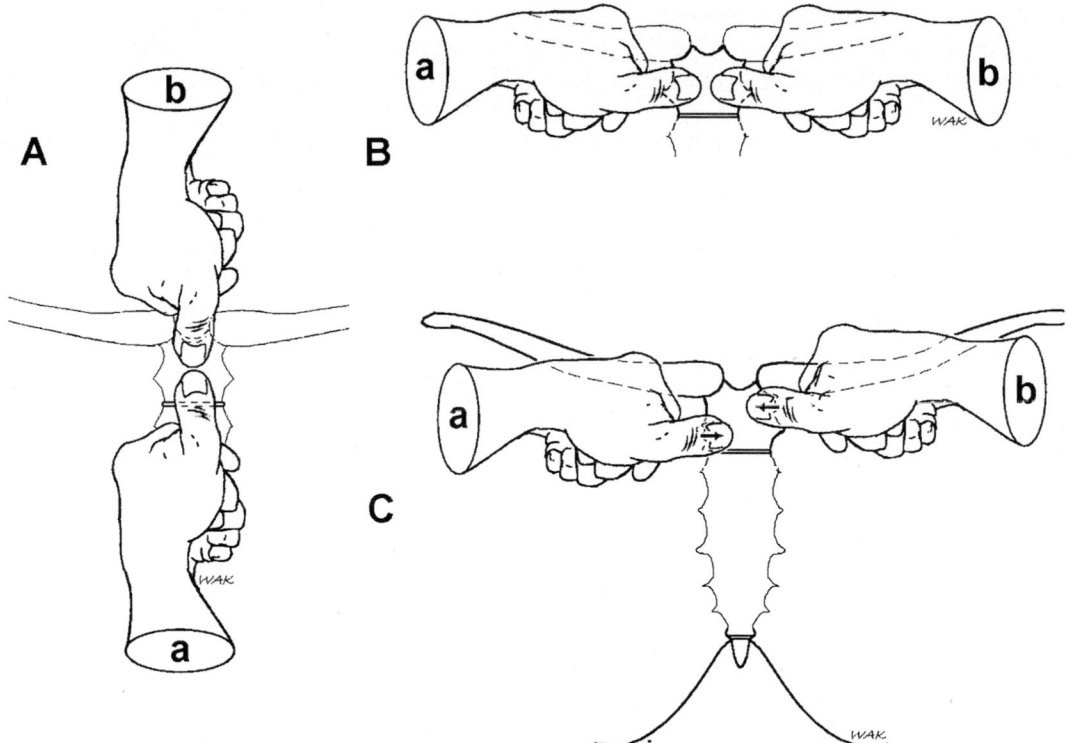

FIGURE 49.9. Segmental evaluation of the manubrium of the sternum.

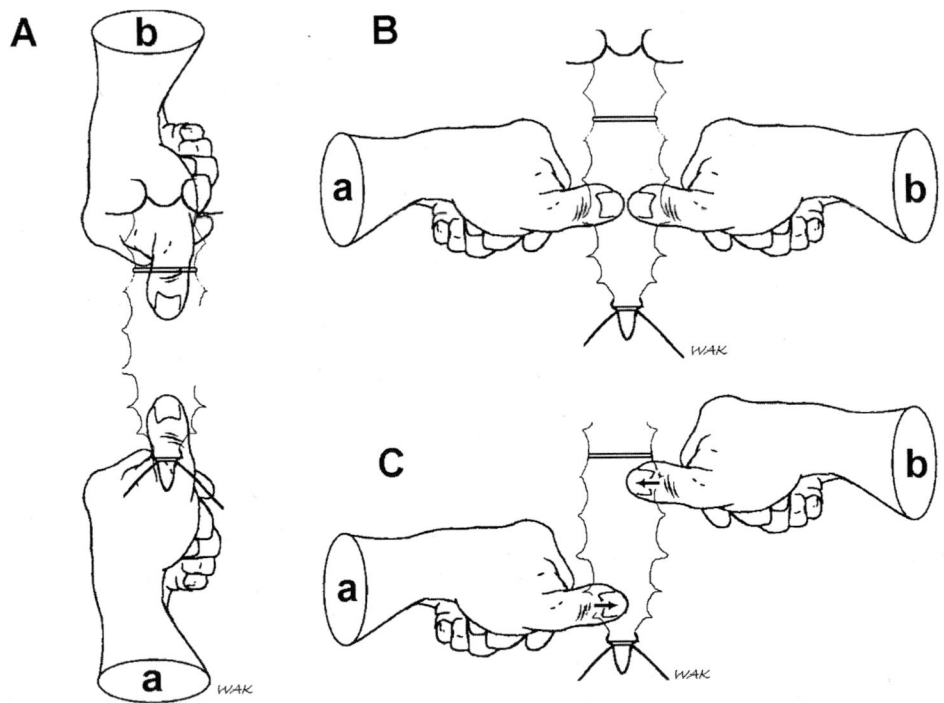

FIGURE 49.10. Segmental evaluation of the body of the sternum (gladiolus).

3. Place one hand longitudinally on the manubrium and body of the sternum and apply a superior and inferior gliding motion, noting whether motion is restricted in one direction or the other (Fig. 49.8).

The sternum may also be examined segmentally as follows:

1. The manubrium may be tested by placing the thumbs first on the upper and lower portions of the manubrium in the midline (Fig. 49.9), then on the anterolateral aspects of the middle portion of the manubrium, and finally on the upper and lower opposite corners of the manubrium. Motion of the manubrium can be tested around transverse, longitudinal, and oblique axes, respectively.

2. A similar approach may be used to test the motion of the body of the sternum (Fig. 49.10).

3. Perform a motion test at the xiphisternal joint using one thenar eminence on the sternum and a single finger (or the thumb and a finger) on the inferior border of the xiphoid. Maintain slight pressure on the sternum while depressing and then lifting the xiphoid with slight anterosuperior pressure, and note any tendency for the tissues to move toward a position of ease.

OTHER DIAGNOSTIC INDICATORS

Palpation that elicits tenderness, complaints of pain, wincing, grunting, or grimacing provides valuable assessment information. For example, point tenderness over a bone may be an indication of a fracture, sprain, infection, or even cancer. Pain in muscle and connective tissue in the absence of trauma is more indicative of musculoskeletal dysfunction or connective tissue disorder. Palpating for tender spots and trigger points is often helpful (Chapters 66 and 67).

CONCLUSION

The rib cage is a complex region of the body, containing and protecting many vital organs. Osteopathic physicians must understand the proper function, diagnosis, and treatment of the thoracic area. Osteopathic manipulation is used to improve sympathetic and parasympathetic factors, diaphragm excursion, spinal and rib mechanics, and vascular and lymphatic flow (which improves breathing). The goal is to decrease sympathicotonia and energy wasted on inefficient breathing by decreasing abnormal mechanoreceptor and nociceptive input to the central nervous system (decreasing pain) and assisting the body in mobilizing the immune system.

REFERENCES

1. Cathie AG. Physiological motions of the spine as related to respiratory activity. *AAO Yearbook.* Colorado Springs: American Academy of Osteopathy 1974:59.
2. Warwick R, Williams P, eds. *Gray's Anatomy,* 36th ed. Edinburgh, Scotland: Churchill Livingstone; 1985.
3. Moore KL. *Clinically Oriented Anatomy,* 2nd ed. Baltimore, MD: Williams & Wilkins; 1985.
4. Gardner E, Gray DJ, O'Rahilly R. *Anatomy,* 4th ed. Philadelphia, PA: WB Saunders; 1975.

LUMBAR REGION

WILLIAM A. KUCHERA

KEY CONCEPTS

- Functional anatomy of the lumbar region, including skeleton, ligaments, muscles, fascia, vasculature, lymphatics, and nerves
- Normal motion and somatic dysfunction of the lumbar region
- Aids to diagnosis, including patient history, physical examination, observation, palpation, reflexes, muscle strength, and motion testing
- Treatment examples, including abdominal aneurysm, cauda equina syndrome, psoas syndrome, radiculopathy, iliolumbar ligament syndrome, meralgia paresthetica, "the dirty half-dozen," hypermobility, and radiculopathy

The lumbar spine normally consists of five vertebrae and forms a smooth lordotic curve just above the pelvis. Lumbosacral anomalies are fairly common (see Radiologic Aspects of the Postural Study, Fig. 42.9) Sometimes during embryologic development, a sixth vertebra forms. Although this alters muscular attachments, it usually does not hinder stability during activity. The lumbar region normally has a lumbo-lumbar lordotic angle extending from L2-5 that averages 43 degrees (see Radiologic Aspects of the Postural Study, Fig. 42.14). The normal lordotic curve of the lumbar spine functionally permits more extension than flexion before the sagittal plane reaches a position where non-neutral multiple plane mechanics occur with motion.

The lumbar spine occupies half to two-thirds of the posterior skeletal and myofascial wall of the true abdomen (Fig. 50.1). It is directly linked to the thoracic and pelvic regions. Because of its functional anatomic connections, it can influence the head and neck, the upper extremities, the lower extremities, and even the viscera (Fig. 50.1). This means that the location of symptoms does not necessarily indicate the region of their etiology. Problems in the pelvis, abdomen, leg, arm, head and thoracic regions, as well as the lumbar region, need to be considered.

Although the lumbar facets are relatively aligned in the sagittal plane, analysis reveals that the lumbar and thoracolumbar regions provide most of the motion of the trunk. The facets of the thoracic region, oriented in a coronal plane, would seem to allow more motion around all three axes. However, the rib cage hinders the ability of the thoracic region to rotate, side-bend, flex, or extend.

The lumbar region is a frequent site for strain, pain, and disability. Back pain afflicts up to 85% of all people at some time in life (1,2). It is the most common reason for limited activity in people younger than 45 years, the second most frequent reason for visits to the physician, the fifth-ranking cause of admission to the hospital, and the third most common site for surgical procedures (3,4). Low back dysfunction constitutes a large percentage of compensation claims and is often the reason for a worker's absence from work, an employer's need to complete an insurance claim, and for insurance companies sending out disability payments. Successful and long-lasting treatment must be directed toward the primary cause and not only toward the symptom of "a backache" or "a back problem." To do this effectively and efficiently, the physician must have functional anatomic knowledge of the lumbar region and its neurophysiologic connections with the rest of the body (Fig. 50.1).

FUNCTIONAL ANATOMY

The Anterior Element

Vertebral Body

A lumbar vertebra is larger than other spinal vertebrae. It is distinguished by the absence of costal facets (like the thoracic vertebrae) and transverse foramina (like the cervical vertebrae). The vertebral body is wider transversely and deeper anteroposteriorly than any other vertebrae (5). This large, cross-sectional area and its longitudinal and vertical trabecular arrangement (Fig. 50.2) increase its strength and stability. Lumbar vertebrae are capable of sustaining the heavy, functional, longitudinal loads that will surely be acting on them. The vertebral bodies also act as accessory organs for hematopoiesis.

Despite their apparent strength, the lumbar spine is the most common site for compression fracture. This is because there is a weak spot located in the anterior portion, where the trabecular arrangement and density is reduced (Fig. 50.2). Sufficient flexion with anterior stress can result in a compression fracture of the vertebral body. This anterior area fractures at 75% of the force needed to fracture the posterior portion of the vertebral body. With or without lifting, compression fractures occur most frequently in persons who have reduced calcium and/or frank

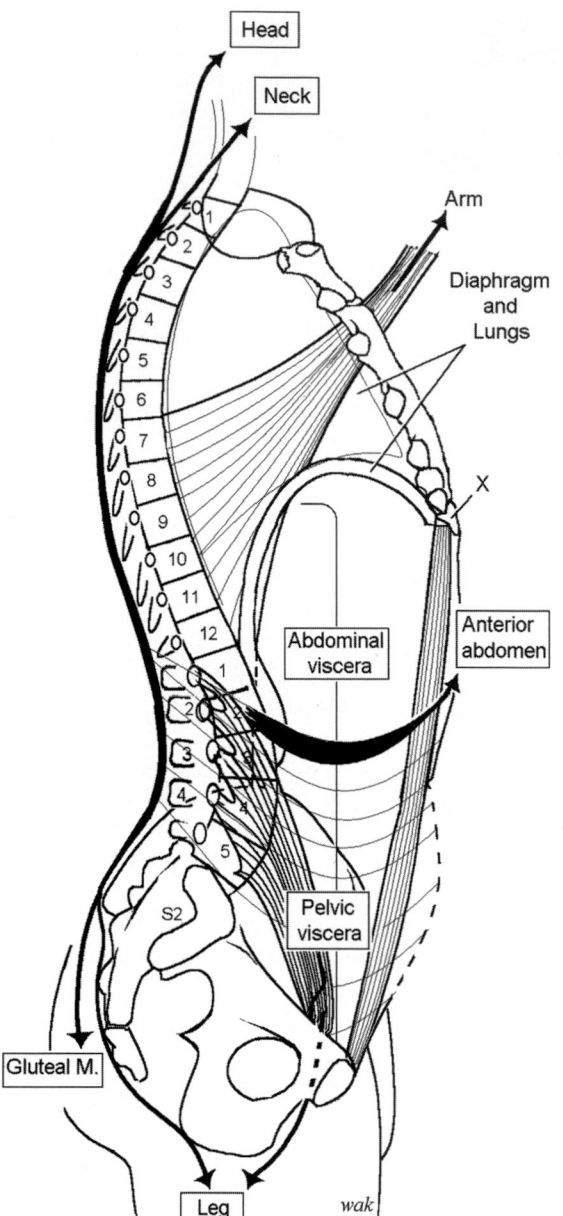

FIGURE 50.1. The lumbar region and its functional anatomic relationships with the rest of the body.

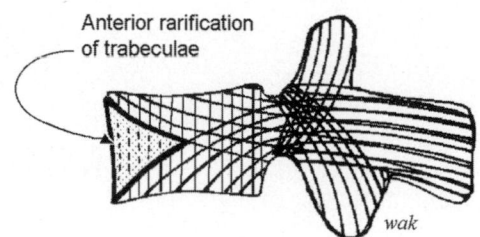

FIGURE 50.2. Trabeculae of a lumbar vertebra, illustrating the weak anterior region of the vertebral body.

The physical examination will reveal discomfort, even with light palpation, percussion, or vibration over the spinous process of the involved vertebra. Palpatory discomfort and a history of discomfort with certain spinal motions will be out of proportion to the physical signs of injury. Pain is usually increased by leaning on the patient's shoulders, causing compression of the spinal column, and is eased by pulling cephalad from under the patient's arms, or by holding a gentle extension to the patient's spine. The physician who mistakenly believes the problem is a strain and begins manipulative treatment or who only prescribes medications with physical therapy soon finds out that this management is ineffective and not pleasing to the patient.

Although pain in the low back is usually immediate, it will be several days after the accident before a routine lateral lumbar radiograph will show a compression deformity of the vertebral body. Apparently, initial compression of the bone is followed by a rebound of its tissue matrix. Decalcification and anterior vertebral compression then occur, finally revealing the tell-tail sign: a wedged vertebral body. The spine then angulates at the site of the compression fracture, and the spinous process at that vertebral unit becomes more prominent than normal. If both the anterosuperior and anteroinferior aspects of a vertebra are clearly wedged on an early radiograph, and especially if there is eburnation of the bone, the defect is old and due to osteochondritis rather than fracture.

For treatment, the patient is given instructions and exercises that encourage gradual extension of the lumbar region, and/or a brace that is specifically ordered for the patient and is applied to prevent active flexion and maintain slight extension. Adequate pain relief medication is provided, taking care not to induce dependency or habituation. The use of codeine in lumbar fractures may be counter productive, as both the pharmacologic properties of the medication and the nociceptive thoracolumbar reflex facilitation from the injury tend to constipate the patient. Most types of direct osteopathic manipulative treatment over the site of a compression are contraindicated, although classic direct and indirect myofascial treatment may be used to improve lymphatic flow, to reduce segmental facilitation, and to comfort the patient. Pain and nociception are also reduced by myofascial treatment directed toward relief of sympathicotonia and general improvement of lymphatic drainage. Secondary sites of somatic dysfunction that develop as a result of the injury are treated to reduce their secondary facilitation of related cord segments. Only methods and activations that are comfortable for the patient and that do not stimulate the site of injury are used to reduce discomfort and promote normal healing.

osteoporosis. Risk factors include: poor diet, prolonged inactivity, or hypoparathyroid disease. It may also be a consequence of a malignancy. Even in the absence of risk factors, a compression fracture may be produced in anyone by forceful flexion, for example, in automobile accidents, pratfalls, and jumping off or falling from a considerable height. Sometimes the precipitating event is unknown to the person; they only know that they began to have a deep nagging back discomfort that did not go away.

Early clues to a vertebral compression fracture are provided by the history and physical examination—not radiographs. The history will most likely reveal activities or risk factors like the ones described. If a compression fracture is suspected, do not ask the patient to perform flexion or side-bending. Instead, place the person in a lateral recumbent position for an examination.

Intervertebral Disc

An intervertebral disc is located between each lumbar vertebra. Though gross anatomists do not consider the intervertebral disc a part of the anterior vertebral element, it is certainly associated with it when functional anatomy is considered. If all the intervertebral discs were stacked up one on another, they would normally account for one-fourth of the length of the spine. Lumbar discs are large and built to tolerate and dissipate heavy loads. They are composed of:

Glycosaminoglycans
Mucopolysaccharides
Proteoglycans
Collagen

Intervertebral discs are named according to their region (lumbar in this case) and numbered according to the vertebral unit of which they are a part (i.e., the number corresponds to the first vertebra of the vertebral unit). Example: The intervertebral disc for the L2 vertebral unit would be the second lumbar disc. Each disc is joined to the inferior plate of the vertebra above it and the superior plate of the vertebra below it.

There is a compressible nucleus pulposus located at its center, and this is surrounded by layers of the anulus consisting of concentric lamellae of collagenous fibers. These anular fibers are oriented 65 degrees from vertical, and the layers alternate in a right/left direction as they encircle and contain the nucleus pulposus. Clinically, it is important to note that the anulus of a lumbar disc is fairly thick anteriorly but is noticeably thinner posteriorly. Historically, L4 and L5 intervertebral discs are at the greatest risk for rupture.

The nucleus pulposus is composed of 70% to 90% water, and is semifluid and hydrophilic. It is deformable but not compressible. With postural weight bearing, the nucleus expands laterally against the anulus, and these two parts work together mechanically to act as a shock absorber between each vertebral body of the spine. When load is applied and the nucleus is compressed, it loses water. This results in a 1.5 mm creep in the first 2 to 10 minutes of compressive stress. Resting supine with the lower extremities flexed and raised is the optimal position for rehydrating the discs. With this rest, discs normally return to their full or optimal height. With aging, however, the hydrophilic properties of a disc are reduced, just as is its ability to reform after being stressed by prolonged pressure or a sudden and severe stress.

The Posterior Elements

Pedicles

Pedicles connect the posterior elements to the vertebral body and mark the site where the posterior vertebral elements begin. In the lumbar region, pedicles are located on the superior third of the posterior surface of the vertebral body. This protects the nerve root of a vertebral unit from being injured by a significantly herniated intervertebral disc of that same unit (Fig. 50.3). The nerve winds around the pedicle and exits its intervertebral foramen before it crosses the intervertebral disc.

Anatomically and radiographically, all of the posterior elements of a vertebra can be accurately identified if the pedi-

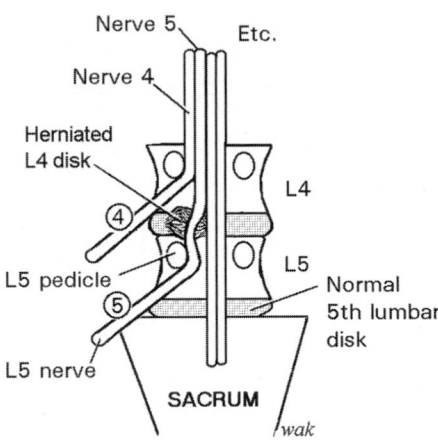

FIGURE 50.3. Pedicles located on the superior third of the posterior side of a lumbar vertebra protect the nerve from being injured by a herniated disc at its own level. It is more likely that a lumbar nerve would be affected by a herniated disc of the previous vertebral unit. That is why an S1 nerve root is usually affected by a herniated L5 intervertebral disc.

cles of that vertebra are first identified. On an anteroposterior (AP) radiograph, the pedicles appear as two longitudinal rows of opaque ovals on the lateral, superior third of the vertebral bodies (Fig. 50.4). These are used as landmarks for finding the other posterior elements.

Transverse Processes

A transverse process projects laterally from the region of each pedicle. In the lumbar region, these processes are anatomically located directly lateral (in the same horizontal plane) to the spinous process of the vertebra of their origin. This fact helps in locating and palpating the pair of associated lumbar transverse processes after palpating and identifying a specific lumbar spinous process. This also permits accurate testing of the proper vertebra for rotational motion of a specific lumbar vertebral unit. However, when looking at an AP radiograph of the lumbar region, the transverse processes will not be located directly lateral to the spinous process of their parent vertebra. In the exposure required to obtain a standard AP lumbar radiograph, the central x-ray beam is not placed directly over the lumbar vertebral bodies. With this positioning of the central ray, the surrounding angled, paracentral x-ray beams project, distort, and magnify the images of the bony structures they pass through.

Superior and Inferior Articular Processes

An inferior articular process projects in a caudad direction from the region of the pedicle, and its articular facet faces laterally. A superior articular process projects cephalad from the same pedicle, and its facet faces medially.

The joint space of an intervertebral synovial joint is formed by the facet of an inferior articular process of one vertebra and the facet of a superior articular process of the next vertebra. A lumbar joint space generally has a sagittal plane orientation, so it is best viewed on an AP radiograph of the lumbar region, where it appears as a gray or dark line between two articular processes.

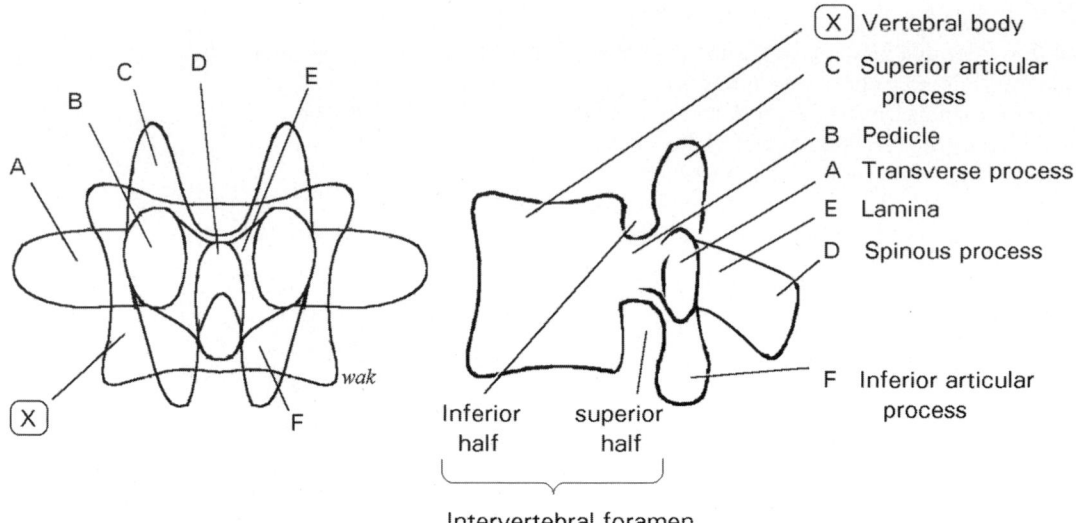

FIGURE 50.4. Illustration of an x-ray view of a lumbar vertebra. The pedicle acts as a landmark for identification of the other parts of the posterior elements of a vertebra.

Zygapophyseal tropism is the most common lumbar congenital abnormality, and is found in 30% of patients (see Radiologic Aspects of the Postural Study, Fig. 42.9D). This term describes a composite arrangement where the articular pillars on one side of a vertebral unit are twisted so that the plane of the resulting synovial intervertebral joint on that side does not match the orientation of the synovial joint on the other side. Asymmetry of lumbar facets (just as finding six lumbar vertebrae) should not keep an employer from hiring that person for a job. However, asymmetric joints at the same level may be associated with asymmetric muscle tensions and altered spinal motions.

Lamina

A lamina projects medially and caudad from each pedicle, and normally meets its partner in the posterior midline to form a typical rectangular lumbar spinous process. In some instances, the laminae will not completely meet in the midline, and a spina bifida is produced (Fig. 50.5). The most common congenital anomaly of this type is the "hidden" spina bifida, called spina bifida occulta. Spina bifida occulta is frequently found at the L5-S1 level of the spine (see also Fig. 42.9F). The only physical clue to its presence may be a midline patch of coarse hair on a patient's skin over its site. In this type of spina bifida, the skin is intact and

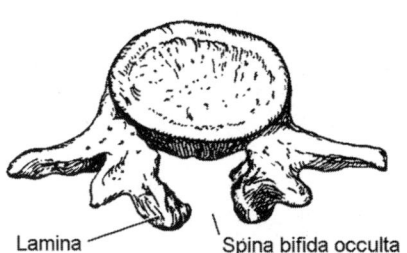

FIGURE 50.5. A spina bifida deformity. The laminae do not completely meet to form a spinous process. Spina bifida occulta is relatively benign, but a spina bifida that contains meningeal or neural elements is very serious and disabling.

there are no meningeal components. An employer should not use this type of spinal bifida as a reason to refuse hiring a person. It may modify muscle attachments, however, and can be associated with a higher incidence of other posterior vertebral anomalies, including congenital or acquired spondylolisthesis (see Chapter 43, Postural Considerations in the Sagittal, Coronal, and Horizontal Planes). In the more serious forms of spina bifida, meningocele and meningomyelocele, the spinal membranes protrude, with or without cord tissue. These are disabling.

Spinous Processes

Clinically, the spinous process of a lumbar vertebra is located in the same horizontal plane as its associated transverse processes. Lumbar spinous processes are distinguished by their palpable, thick, quadrangular, "spade-like" distal ends. This is in contrast to the fingertip-shaped palpatory characteristic of the thoracic spinous processes. Their distinguishing shape provides palpatory evidence of where the lumbar region begins and where the thoracic spine ends. This also aids in counting lumbar or thoracic vertebrae. There is one exception; the spinous process of the fifth lumbar vertebra is smaller, lies in a hollow just above the sacral base, and its distal end is about one-third smaller than the rest of the lumbar spines. It feels more like a thoracic than a lumbar spinous process (Fig. 50.4). This L5 spinous process characteristic helps to identify it as the last lumbar vertebra and not the first spinous process of the sacrum. Another, less accurate way of counting lumbar vertebrae is to find the most superior portion of the iliac crests and then follow a horizontal plane from there to the midline. This should cross the spinous process of L4, and counting can begin from there.

Spinal Canal

The spinal canal is actually an anatomic space between the posterior margin of a vertebral body and parts of its posterior elements (i.e., its two pedicles, and the laminae). It contains the dural tube, spinal cord, and origins of the spinal nerves down to approximately the L2-3 level, where the spinal cord ends. From that level on, the dural tube contains the cauda equina and the filum terminalis interna (Fig. 50.12). The entire spinal canal is wider transversely than it is anteroposteriorly. In the lumbar spine, it is also triangular. The spinal cord usually terminates at the L2 level as the conus medullaris. Each of the remaining dorsal and ventral roots of the lumbar, sacral, and coccygeal nerves hang in the dural tube and spinal canal, forming the cauda equina (horse's tail); they exit the conus medullaris or the dural tube as they approach their appropriate intervertebral foramen.

The Intervertebral Foramen

Intervertebral foramen (one on the right and one on the left) are formed by two adjacent vertebrae of a vertebral unit. They are defined by:

Two adjacent vertebral bodies and the intervertebral disc between them
Two adjacent pedicles
The inferior articular process of one vertebra and the superior articular process of the next, including the synovial joint between them

A spinal nerve and a recurrent meningeal nerve, each carrying the same identification number as the vertebral unit, pass through a lumbar foramen. The recurrent meningeal nerve then re-enters the foramina (Fig. 50.6L). These nerves only occupy 35% to 40% of the foramina area. A lumbar intervertebral foramen is normally two to three times larger than the area taken up by the lumbar nerves, so it seems that compression of the nerve would be difficult. With flexion, the facets and pedicles glide away from one another, and the size of the intervertebral foramen increases. With extension, the pedicles glide toward one another, and the foramen is reduced in size. Reduction of the foramen size also results from arthritis or spurs, hypertrophy of the posterior longitudinal ligament, extrusion of the nucleus pulposus, tissue congestion or edema, inflammation, and perineural edema. Removal or reduction of the effect produced by any of these factors may be enough to allow a symptomatic patient to become asymptomatic—pain free and able to work. This is important to remember when considering management of patients with back pain etiologies, paresthesias, or radiculopathies.

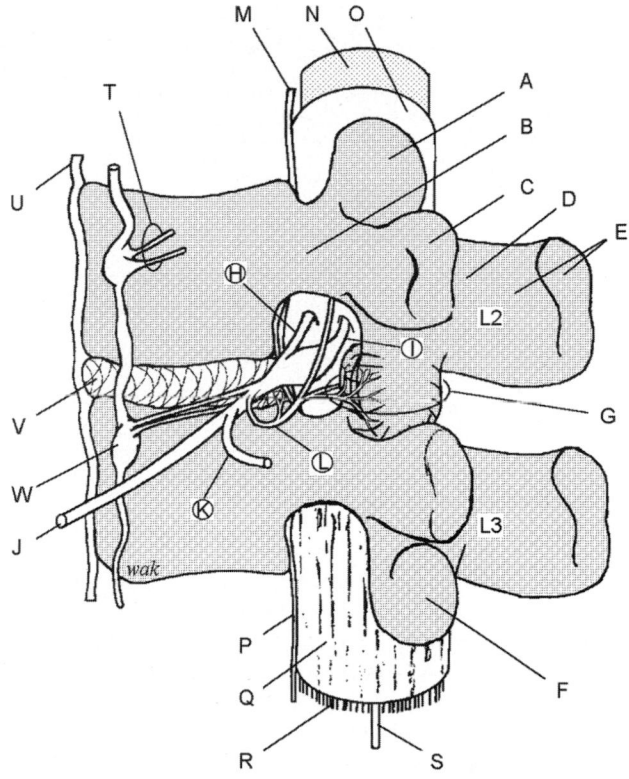

FIGURE 50.6. Diagrammatic representation of the L2 intervertebral foramen. **(A)** superior articular process, **(B)** pedicle, **(C)** transverse process, **(D)** lamina, **(E)** spinous process, **(F)** inferior articular process, **(G)** L2 synovial joint and capsule, **(H)** L2 ventral root, **(I)** L2 dorsal root, **(J)** ventral ramus of L2 nerve, **(K)** dorsal ramus of L2 nerve, **(L)** recurrent meningeal nerve, **(M)** posterior longitudinal ligament, **(N)** spinal cord, **(O)** dural tube containing spinal cord and approaching conus medullaris at L2 region, **(P)** posterior longitudinal ligament, **(Q)** dural tube containing cauda equina, **(R)** ventral and dorsal roots of the cauda equina, **(S)** filum terminalis internus, **(T)** gray and white rami, **(U)** anterior longitudinal ligament, **(V)** intervertebral disc, and **(W)** L2 chain ganglion.

Ligaments (Table 50.1)

The Posterior Longitudinal Ligament

The posterior longitudinal ligament is broad in the cervical region, and begins to narrow when it reaches the first lumbar vertebra. It takes on a scalloped appearance, and is only one-half

TABLE 50.1. LUMBAR LIGAMENTS

Ligament	Comment
Of the Posterior Elements:	
Supraspinous ligament	Degenerated in the adult lumbar spine and possibly ruptured.
Interspinous ligament	Between the lumbar spinous processes (weak and often absent).
Ligamentum flava	Between one lamina and the next. They are punctured when the patient is given an epidural or spinal anesthetic.
Capsular ligament	Supplied by nociceptive fibers that report somatic dysfunction.
Of the Anterior Element:	
Anterior longitudinal ligament	Wide and strong.
Posterior longitudinal ligament	Narrowed and scolloped in the lumbar spine producing a posterolateral deficiency over the intervertebral disk.
Other Ligaments:	
Iliolumbar ligament	Joins the lumbar spine to the ilium of the pelvic region. Can produce symptoms that mimic an inguinal hernia.

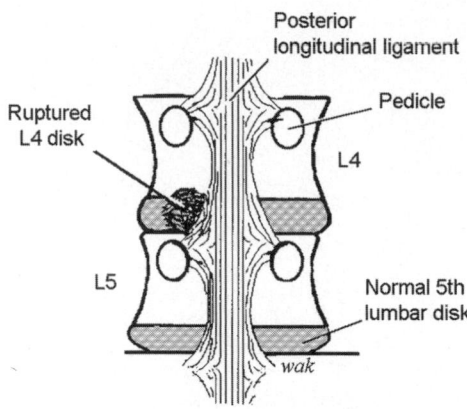

FIGURE 50.7. A left-sided L4 intervertebral disc herniation. The posterior longitudinal ligament is normally narrowed, thinned, and scalloped in the lumbar region. This leaves the lateral margins of a lumbar intervertebral disc vulnerable to herniation.

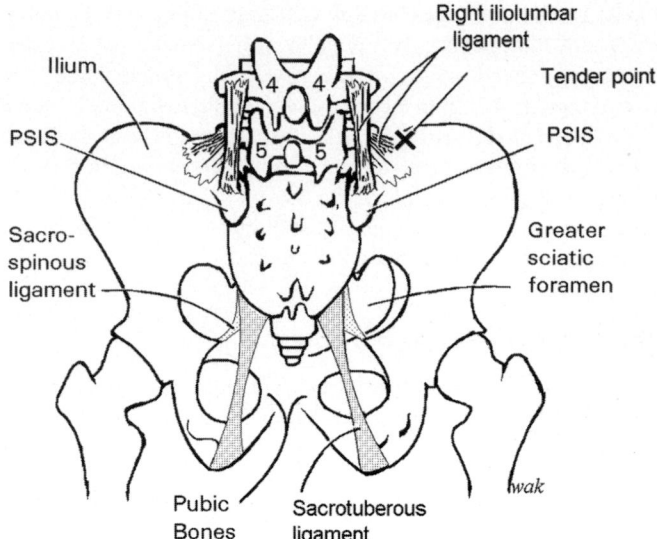

FIGURE 50.8. The iliolumbar ligaments and the location of the right iliolumbar ligament tender point. The iliolumbar ligament is the first to become tender to palpation when there is postural decompensation. Radiation of pain into the groin/testicle may incorrectly suggest an inguinal hernia on that side.

its original width when it reaches L5. The scallops produce a deficiency in the posterior longitudinal ligament that is located over the posterolateral portions of each lumbar intervertebral disc (Fig. 50.7). The posterior portion of the intervertebral disc is also the thinnest portion of the anulus. Therefore, this is the region of a lumbar disc that is most likely to rupture; if it does, it is most likely to be associated with nerve root pressure.

The Iliolumbar Ligament

This ligament is located in the lumbosacral region. It is attached to the transverse processes of L4 and L5, and extends to the iliac crest and the anterior and posterior regions of the sacroiliac joint (Fig. 50.8). It has been reported that this "ligament" may consist of muscle fibers in neonates and children and gradually becomes ligamentous over the next thirty years, but this has recently been disputed by some anatomists.

Remember that the iliolumbar ligament is typically the first ligament to become tender to palpation when there is lumbosacral postural stress and decomposition. A tender point on the iliac crest, located 1 inch superior and lateral from the inferior margin of the PSIS and in the iliolumbar ligament, becomes acutely tender to palpation (Fig. 50.8). Patients with early postural decompensation may not realize that the iliac attachment of this lig-

ament is tender until it is palpated. Its tenderness is a physical clue that should prompt the physician to ask questions about posture and to carefully examine the spine, lower lumbar, and sacroiliac joints for somatic dysfunction, scoliosis, and/or evidence of sacral base unleveling. An example would be an adult who has, for years, been successfully compensating for continuous low back strain secondary to a congenital sacral base unleveling or an acquired short leg. As a result of decompensation in the lumbosacral region, this patient finally becomes symptomatic with back pain. The first complaint of a patient with irritation of the iliolumbar ligament may be, "I think I have a hernia." (See Iliolumbar Ligament Syndrome in the Treatment of Non-Medical/Non-Surgical Etiologies section below.)

Muscles and Fascia (Tables 50.2 and 50.3)

The first few lumbar vertebrae provide posterior attachments for the abdominal diaphragm. The left crura of the diaphragm attaches to the first two, and the right crura attaches to the first three

TABLE 50.2. EXTRINSIC LUMBAR MUSCLES FOR MOVEMENT OF RESPIRATION, THE SPINE, AND THE LIMBS

Muscle	Origin	Insertion	Comments
Abdominal diaphragm	Bodies of L1–3	Lower 6 ribs and xiphoid process	(See Chapter 51, Abdominal Region.)
Quadratus lumborum	Iliolumbar ligament and iliac crest	Tips of the L1–4 transverse processes and the anterior surface of the 12th rib	Functionally considered a posterior inferior extension of the abdominal diaphragm.
Serratus posterior inferior	Last two thoracic and first two lumbar spinous processes	Inferior border of the lower 3 or 4 ribs	Functionally connects the thoracolumbar region with the lower ribs.
Latissimus dorsi	Thoracolumbar fascia, iliac crest and spinous processes of lower 6 thoracic vertebrae	Intertubercular groove of the humerus	Functionally connects the lumbar, thoracic, and pelvic regions to the upper extremity.
Erector spinae mass (spinalis, longissimus, and iliocostalis)	Iliac crest and sacrum	Lumbars, thoracic, ribs, cervicals, and occiput	Connects to the entire spine and to the lower extremity through the lumbo-thoracic fascia.

TABLE 50.3. INTRINSIC LUMBAR MUSCLES FOR MOVEMENT OF THE VERTEBRAL COLUMN

Muscle	Origin and Insertion	Comments
Erector spinae mass (ESM)	Iliac crest and sacrum to lumbars, thoracics, ribs, cervicals and occiput.	Connect to entire spine and through the lumbo-thoracic fascia, to the lower extremity.
Spinalis dorsi	Spinous processes of L1 and L2 to upper 8 thoracic spines.	
Interspinalis portion of the medial spinalis group (part of the ESM)	One spinous process to the next.	From lumbar region to second cervical vertebra.
Longissimus dorsi (part of the ESM)	Transverse processes and lumbo-dorsal fascia to lower 10 thoracic transverse processes and their ribs, medial to the rib angles.	
Iliocostalis lumborum (part of the ESM)	Iliac crest and sacrum.	These attach to the posterior angles of the lower 6 to 7 ribs and mark the most lateral extent of the ESM muscle group.
Intertransversarii	One transverse process to the next.	Most developed in lumbar and cervical regions.
Multifidus[a]	One mammary process to the next.	Only in lumbar region.

[a]Multifidi muscles in the L1 and L2 region are usually the first to become involved by viscerosomatic reflexes from irritation of the left colon and/or pelvic organs. Their involvement usually results in non-neutral (type II) somatic dysfunctions of those vertebral units that are usually rotated toward the side of the involved organ. (See lumbar motion and Chapter 51, Abdominal Region.)
ESM, erector spinae mass.

lumbar vertebral bodies. The diaphragm then arches cephalad past these and the lower thoracic vertebrae, with its apex sometimes as high as the fifth intercostal space. It then curves caudad to attach to the xiphoid process (Figure 50.1 and Chapter 51, Abdominal Region). For this reason, somatic dysfunction of the first three lumbar vertebrae can be associated with a flattened, ineffective, dysfunctional, resting abdominal diaphragm. A flattened diaphragm is often associated with a lumbar lordosis and/or psoas and quadratus muscle spasms. In this flattened resting condition, the diaphragmatic dome is unable to develop efficient, appropriate pressure gradients between the thorax and abdomen during contraction and relaxation, and this results in decreased lymphatic flow and venous return from anywhere in the body. The physician should also remember that the innervation to the diaphragm is the phrenic nerve, which originates from nerve roots C3-5 of the spinal cord. Therefore, cervical somatic dysfunction can be involved in diaphragmatic dysfunction.

The lumbar spine also supplies partial origin for the erector spinae mass of muscles that extend from the pelvis all the way to the occiput. Unilateral contraction of extrinsic or intrinsic muscles of the back will side bend or rotate the spine. When working together, these muscles extend the spine. Through the lumbosacral aponeurosis and fascial divisions, the lumbar region is functionally attached to the gluteal muscles, the hamstrings, and via the iliotibial band, to the lower extremity. Through the lumbodorsal fasciae, with its continuity surrounding the external and internal oblique muscles and the rectus abdominus muscle, the posterior lumbar region is functionally related to the lateral and anterior abdominal wall (Fig. 50.1).

Thoracolumbar Aponeurosis

The thoracolumbar deep fascia surrounds, compartmentalizes, and protects all of the lumbar muscles and bones (Fig. 50.9). This fascia gives attachment to the latissimus dorsi muscle, which extends to the proximal end of the humerus. Next to the spine, it compartmentalizes the interspinalis, multifidi, and rotatores muscles. More laterally, but still near the midline, it encloses the

longissimus muscle. Even more laterally, it encloses the iliocostalis muscle group that inserts on and provides a landmark for locating the angles of the ribs. The angle of the ribs marks the most lateral extent of the erector spinae mass. Deeper layers of the deep fascia form compartments for the intertransversarii. Anterior to the transverse processes, the deep fascia surrounds the psoas and quadratus lumborum muscles. The quadratus lumborum muscle can clinically and functionally be thought of as the posteroinferior extension of the abdominal diaphragm.

Mesenteries

Approximately 30 feet of small intestines and portions of the ascending and descending colon are located anterior to the lumbar region. The abdominal mesenteries are formed by reflections of the parietal peritoneum from the posterior abdominal wall (Fig. 50.10). These mesenteries carry arteries and efferent autonomic nerve fibers to the viscera. They also carry veins, lymphatic vessels, and visceral afferent nerves away from the viscera. In this way, somatic dysfunction of the myofascial tissues of the lumbar region can functionally influence the local environment of the abdominal viscera.

Myofascial trigger points in the gluteus medius, rotatores, multifidi, iliopsoas, quadratus lumborum, and the piriformis muscles produce pain patterns in the lumbar region and sometimes into the sacral region and lower extremities (6,7) (Fig. 50.11).

Spinal Cord and Lumbar Nerves

Spinal Cord

In an adult, the spinal cord usually terminates at the L2 level as the conus medullaris (terminal range T12-L2, and some say to T3). The dural sac and a string of fibrous tissue and pia, known as the filum terminalis internus, continue on. The dural sac terminates by attaching to the spinal canal at the S2 level. Fibrous tissue and cells from the dura continue on as the filum terminalis externa, which attaches to the first coccygeal segment (Fig. 50.12). Remember that the posterior longitudinal ligament is anterior

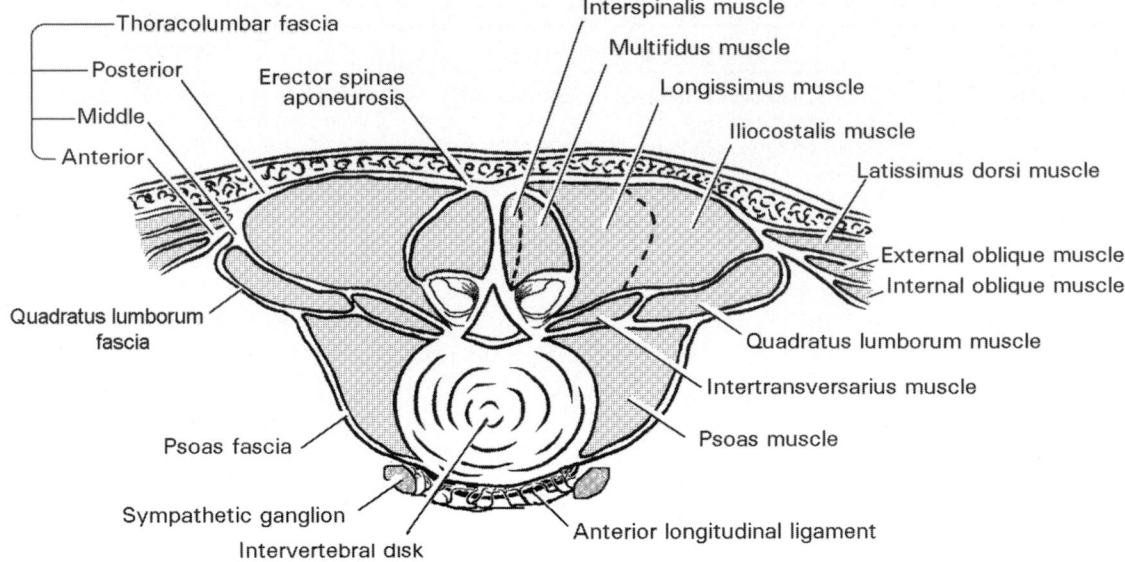

FIGURE 50.9. The deep fascia and thoracolumbar aponeurosis of the low back. It compartmentalizes, protects, and gives attachments for the erector spinae mass and lumbar muscles.

to the spinal cord and has lateral deficiencies in the areas of the lumbar discs (Fig. 50.7). The dural sac of the spinal canal, below the conus medullaris, contains the filum terminalis internus and lower lumbar, sacral, and coccygeal dorsal and ventral rootlets of the cauda equina (see Posterior Elements: Spinal Canal, above).

The lumbar spinal canal takes on a triangular configuration and normally decreases in its anteroposterior dimension as it progresses from L1 to L5. As a person ages, the diameter of the lumbar spinal canal or intervertebral canal may be further compromised by factors that include:

Hypertrophy of the posterior longitudinal ligament
Thickening of the ligamentum flava on its anterior wall
Osteoarthritis
Exostoses
Osteophytes
Tumors
Ruptured lumbar intervertebral discs

Tissue congestion, frank edema, and perineural edema can also compromise the nerves in the spinal canal or an intervertebral foramen, especially if the region already has somatic dysfunction and/or an anatomic/pathologic deformity. If there is enough pressure on the spinal cord or the nerves in the cauda equina, there will be loss of reflexes, weakness of muscles, and paralysis of the lower extremities and sphincters of the bladder and rectum. This symptom complex describes a severe form of spinal stenosis called cauda equina syndrome (see Treatment of Non-Medical/Non-Surgical Etiologies: Cauda Equina Syndrome below).

Lumbar Plexus

The lumbar plexus (Table 50.4) is composed of nerve roots L1-4 and a branch from T12. Lumbar nerve roots enter directly into the psoas muscle, where the lumbar plexus is formed. Lumbar nerves emerge from the borders and surfaces of the psoas muscle (5).

Dermatomes, Myotomes, and Sclerotomes

Lumbar dermatomes are located on the posterior lumbar paraspinal region and the anterior part of the thigh, leg, and foot (Fig. 50.13). Pain or paresthesia in these areas of skin provides clues to the level of nerve root involvement and nerve dysfunction and/or irritation. Hoppenfeld (8) has provided the easiest pattern to remember (Fig. 50.13). He advises that the physician mentally construct three oblique lines, from superolateral to inferomedial, on the anterior thigh, dividing it into three equal sections. The inferior of these three oblique lines must go through the patella. From superior to inferior, these lines delineate

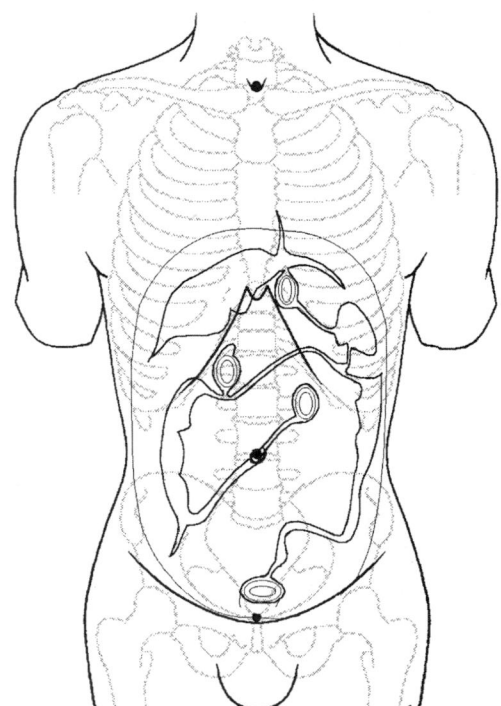

FIGURE 50.10. The location of the posterior abdominal roots of the abdominal visceral mesenteries.

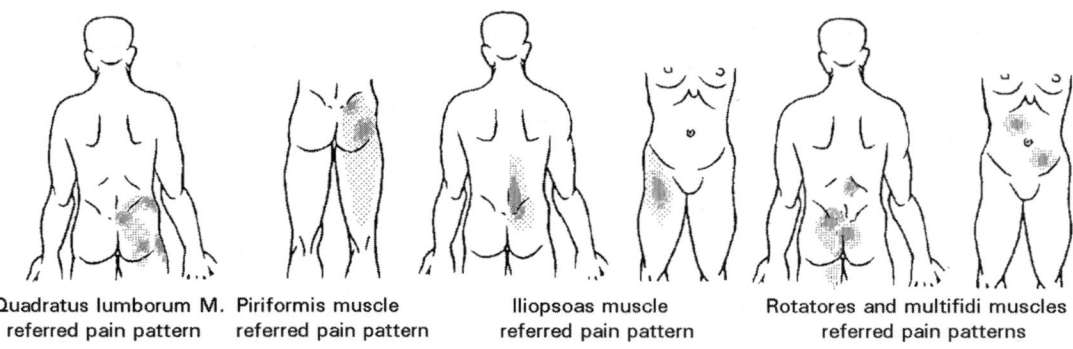

Quadratus lumborum M.   Piriformis muscle   Iliopsoas muscle   Rotatores and multifidi muscles
referred pain pattern   referred pain pattern   referred pain pattern   referred pain patterns

FIGURE 50.11. Pain patterns produced by myofascial trigger points in the quadratus lumborum, piriformis, iliopsoas, rotatores, and multifidi muscles of the back.

dermatomes L1, L2, and L3. A line visualized from the patella to the big toe delineates the medial L4 dermatome from the lateral L5 dermatome. A small section on the lateral side of the foot is the first sacral dermatome. This schematic approximates the location of lumbar dermatomes of any patient. Note that different books illustrate dermatomal patterns of various complexities. However, remembering that these divisions will vary slightly from person to person, the Hoppenfeld diagram provides an easy to recall, good general clinical pattern from which to work.

Myotomal pain is associated with cramps, weakness, and myofascial trigger points in the muscles that share innervation from the same irritated nerve roots.

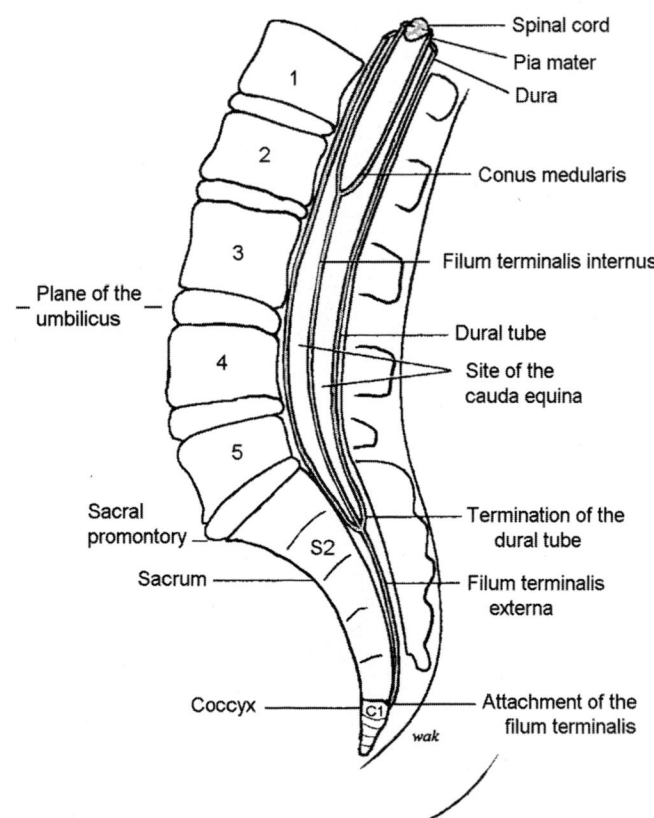

FIGURE 50.12. The relationships of the spinal cord, dural tube, conus medullaris, filum terminalis internus, cauda equina, and filum terminalis externa to the lumbar and sacral regions.

Sclerotomal pain is described as vague, deep, toothache-like pain (see Chapter 53, Lower Extremity, Fig. 53.30). It arises from ligaments, bones, or joints that share innervation from the same irritated nerve root. Knee pain, for example, can be the result of irritation of the L3 vertebra, ligaments in the L3 region, the pubic symphysis, the hip, or the knee. All of these sites have the same L3 sclerotomal origin.

Vasculature and Lymphatics

Blood Vessels

The lumbar spinal cord receives its arterial blood supply from segmental radicular arteries. In the lumbosacral region, one of these radicular arteries, the arteria radicularis magna, is larger than the rest, and is the source of blood for the inferior two-thirds of the spinal cord (9). The rest of the cord receives blood from associated segmental arteries. Arteries supplying a lumbar vertebra enter around the circumference of the vertebral body, especially near its transverse processes.

Venous blood drains the spinal cord via a profuse plexus of thin-walled veins that communicate with the profuse, valveless venous plexus in the vertebrae and the anterior and posterior longitudinal veins of the dura. Venous blood from the profuse vertebral plexus of valveless veins drains into a large basivertebral vein (10), which exits from a foramen located in the posterior surface of each vertebral body. *All of these veins are valveless.* Venous blood from the spinal cord can drain into radicular veins or can drain cephalad into the large, valveless venous sinuses of the dura.

The profuse, valveless venous plexus of the spinal cord, vertebrae, communicating veins, and large, intracranial venous sinuses are of great clinical importance. An increase in intraabdominal or intrathoracic pressures, as occurs with coughing, Valsalva maneuvers, or fascial tensions, can reverse the flow of venous blood and become a factor in the metastasis of primary abdominal and pelvic malignancies to the spine and brain (11) (Fig. 50.14). This mechanism also explains headaches and other central nervous system symptoms from increased venous pressure associated with visceral, spinal cord, or vertebral dysfunction.

The blood from the muscles of the lumbar region drains into the inferior vena cava. It does not drain into mesenteric veins or pass through the portal system of the liver, as the venous blood from the abdominal and pelvic viscera does.

TABLE 50.4. NERVES OF THE LUMBAR PLEXUS

Nerve	Roots	Comments
Femoral	L2, 3, 4	Exits femoral canal to innervate the quadriceps muscles of thigh and provides sensory fibers to skin of anterior thigh.
Obturator	L2, 3, 4	Exits obturator foramen to innervate the adductor muscles of thigh and provide sensory fibers from medial portion of the thigh.
Lumbar muscular branches	—	Innervate the psoas major, psoas minor, iliacus, and quadratus lumborum muscles.
Iliohypogastric Ilioinguinal Genitofemoral	L1 L1 L1, 2	The iliohypogastric, ilioinguinal, and genitofemoral nerves carry sensory fibers from lateral skin of the gluteal region, root of the penis or mons, and upper part of scrotum and labia, inguinal and femoral triangle, and cremasteric muscle, respectively.
Lateral femoral cutaneous	L2, 3	Emerges from psoas just superior to iliac crest, runs over iliacus muscle, passes through or under the inguinal ligament just medial to ASIS. Provides sensory fibers for a large oval area on the anterolateral thigh.

ASIS, anterior superior iliac spine.

Lymphatics

Lymphatic fluid from all abdominal and pelvic viscera drains into the thoracic duct, which is also called the left lymphatic duct (LLD). All somatic lymphatic vessels at and inferior to a horizontal plane through the umbilicus drain into the inguinal nodes, the deep pelvic external and common iliac nodes, the preaortic and lateral aortic nodes, and then into the LLD (Fig. 50.15). Note that lymphatic vessels from the gonads or the viscera *do not* drain into the inguinal region, but drain into the deep lymphatic vessels of the pelvis and then into the cisterna chyli. Therefore, gonadal and prostate inflammation or malignancy is not associated with enlarged, palpable inguinal nodes. (See Chapter 71). The LLD

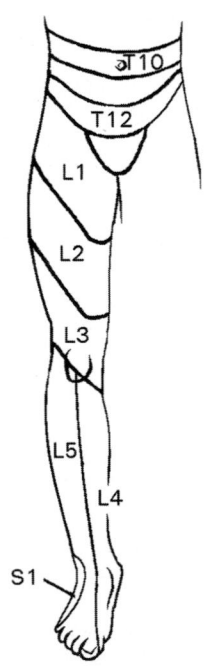

FIGURE 50.13. Dermatomes of the lumbar nerves.

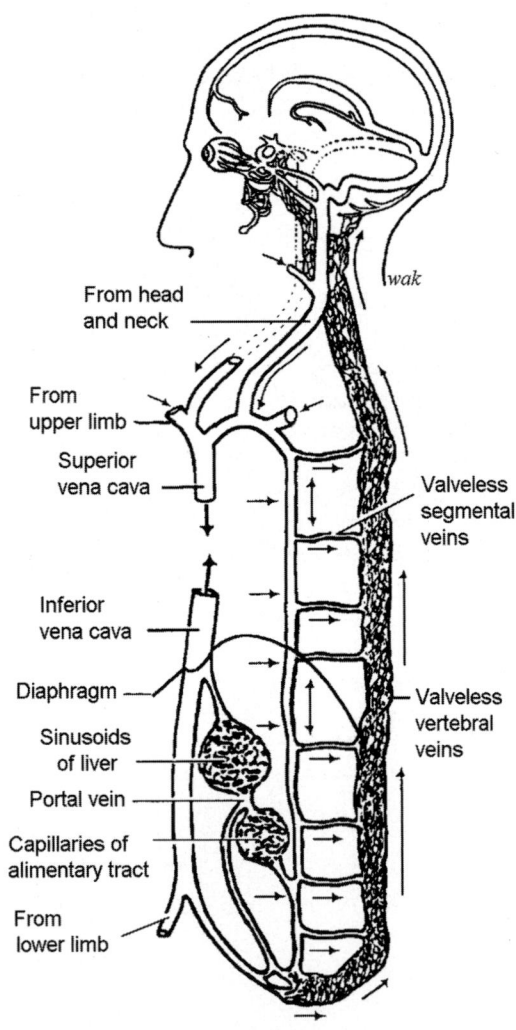

FIGURE 50.14. The profuse valveless venous system of the spinal cord, spinal vertebrae, and the brain. (Modified from Millard FP.)

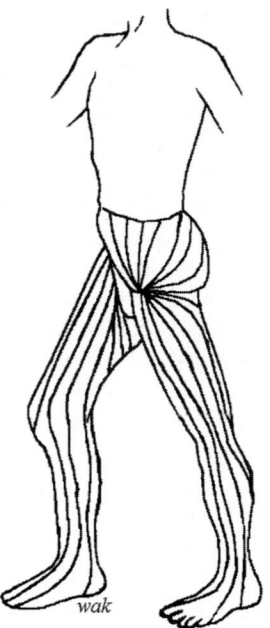

FIGURE 50.15. Lymphatic drainage from somatic tissues below the level of the umbilicus will drain into the inguinal lymph nodes, into the deep lymphatic vessels of the pelvis, and then into the cisterna chyli and thoracic duct (the left lymphatic duct).

passes through the fasciae of the left side of the thoracic inlet twice before emptying into the left brachiocephalic vein. All lymphatic fluid (from anywhere in the body) must pass through the fasciae of the thoracic inlet on its way to the venous circulation and the heart.

Motion

The Vertebral Unit

From a functional anatomic or osteopathic perspective, a vertebral unit "is composed of two adjacent vertebrae with their associated disc, arthrodial, ligamentous, muscular, vascular, lymphatic, and neural elements" (12). In "Clinical Biomechanics of the Spine," White and Panjabi label a vertebral unit as a functional spinal unit (FSU) (13). They define FSU as "two adjacent vertebrae and the connecting ligamentous tissues." Therefore, the vertebral unit is different and more comprehensive than the FSU of the orthopedic specialist; the two should not be confused when communicating or when reading the literature. With stress, a vertebral unit behaves according to its structure, strength, flexibility, and the functional ability of its ligaments, muscular, neural, vascular, and lymphatic connections. Both the vertebral unit and the FSU are given the same number as the cephalad vertebra of the unit. For example, the third lumbar unit is named L3. According to the vertebral unit definition, however, it not only indicates L3 moving on L4, but also includes their associated disc, arthrodial, ligamentous, muscular, vascular, lymphatic, and neural elements.

Normal Motion

Moore (9) sites that the cervical and lumbar regions of the vertebral column are the most mobile and the most common sites of aches and pains. Lumbar motion is especially visible when the

vertebrae of the lumbar spinal region move together as a group. The major motions are:

> Flexion
> Extension
> Side-bending
> Rotation

Note that side-bending and rotation are coupled motions. Their direction of motion may be opposite (type I motion) or in the same direction (type II motion), but side-bending and rotation occur together in the lumbar spine; one cannot occur without the other.

There are also minor translatory motions occurring in opposite directions on each of the three planes of motion. A vertebral unit normally has 12 possible movements available to it and, therefore, 12 movements that can be restricted in a somatic dysfunction of a joint. Somatic dysfunction usually involves these minor motions, and that dysfunction then affects the major motions that are possible for that joint. The pattern for multiple plane motion of a vertebral unit depends on the position of the sagittal plane of the spine when a vector of rotation or side-bending is introduced.

When the spine is in its neutral positional range (Fig. 50.16), side-bending and rotation normally occur to opposite sides in multiple units, and this is called type I motion or type I mechanics. Type I motion occurs when it is predominately the vertebral bodies and discs that influence spinal action.

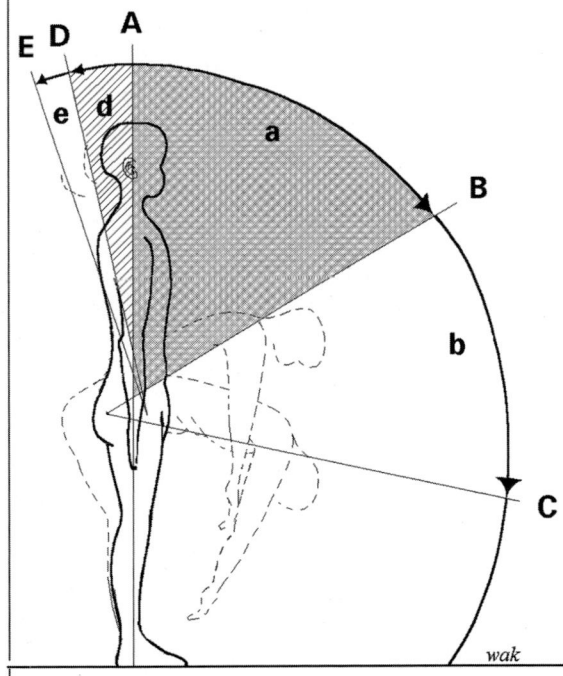

FIGURE 50.16. The position of the body in neutral or non-neutral sagittal plane ranges determines multiple-plane spinal motion mechanics. Flexion and extension within ranges A–B or A–D are within the sagittal plane range where multiple-plane motion results in neutral mechanics. Flexion or extension within ranges B–C + or D–E are within the sagittal plane ranges where multiple-plane motion typically results in non-neutral (type II) mechanics.

When the lumbar spine is flexed far enough or extended far enough that it is out of the neutral sagittal plane range and into the non-neutral sagittal plane range (Fig. 50.16), rotation and side-bending normally occur to the same side, usually in the vertebral unit where the forces are localized. This is called type II motion or type II mechanics. Type II motion occurs when the facets exert the major influence on spinal motion.

There is another way of stating these two normal motion principles. In the neutral mechanical range for the sagittal plane (where multiple plane motion is predominately directed by the vertebral bodies and discs), side-bending and then rotation occur to opposite sides in a group of vertebrae, or rotation occurs toward the convexity of the curve. This is type I motion and is expected to occur in a group of vertebral units because of the joint facings, as well as the construction and ligamentous attachments of the lumbar vertebrae. In the lumbar region, this type of multiple plane motion occurs through a greater arc of extension than flexion.

If the lumbar sagittal plane is in a mechanical range where flexion or extension is sufficient to engage the facets as the prime movers of the spine, multiple plane motion will result in rotation and then side-bending occurring to the same side. This can also be stated as rotation into the concavity of the intended side-bending, and is type II motion or type II mechanics. Positioning in the sagittal plane that is sufficient to induce type II mechanics with multiple plane motion is usually localized in a single vertebral unit. After type II motion occurs in that one vertebral unit, the other vertebral units involved in the group side-bending curve normally move according to type I mechanics.

Neutral, type I, and non-neutral, type II, motions are a usual and normal biomechanical occurrence during the performance of daily activities. When an activity is over, the spinal units that are free of somatic dysfunction will return to their neutral, resting positions. If motion is tested, they will exhibit ease of motion in all of their usual planes of motion.

Although the lumbar spine can normally flex about 40 degrees and extend about 30 degrees, non-neutral, type II motion is more likely to occur in the lumbar and thoracic spine when the spine is in a straightened configuration. Therefore, non-neutral mechanics with type II motion for the lumbar spinal region are more likely to occur when the lumbar spine is flexed. However, it is possible to produce type II motion with extreme lumbar hyperextension, as might occur when a high diver enters the water, when a gymnast does a back walkover, or when a painter stands on a ladder and reaches up to paint a high ceiling.

Somatic Dysfunction

Somatic dysfunction occurs when, for some reason, the spine does not return to its usual resting, neutral position after an activity is completed. This restriction is found to be within the joint's normal range of motion. Most somatic dysfunction involves restrictions of the minor gliding motions of a joint, which then restricts the major range of motion in one direction around an axis. The restriction usually occurs during the routine activities of daily living when, for some reason, the biomechanical or physiologic spinal motions do not return to their normal resting position. It is especially likely when muscles have been previously fatigued or stressed by thermal, biophysiologic, or biomechanical stress, such as overuse, chilling, postural strain, psychological stress, or excessive load.

Therefore, neutral or non-neutral somatic dysfunction of the lumbar spine can develop depending on the position of the sagittal plane when the joint motion became restricted. Somatic dysfunction is found by identifying *t*enderness, *a*symmetry, *r*ange of motion differences, and *t*issue texture changes (TART characteristics) (12) during motion testing of a spinal region or its vertebral units. When the patient is tested, the lumbar units with somatic dysfunction will exhibit the motion preference that was maintained when the dysfunction occurred (even if the patient is prone, sitting, or supine and in a "neutral" position). The patient will also simultaneously exhibit motion restriction in the opposite direction of the motion permitted. For this reason, when a physician finds a somatic dysfunction, he or she can reasonably conclude what motion the person was performing at the time the somatic dysfunction was initiated.

Anatomic variations, physiologic conditions, trauma, and so on may alter the "usual" motion patterns described above. Therefore, the specific diagnosis for indicated treatment depends on testing the site of the dysfunction, as it may not always follow the expected patterns of motion.

Note that the typical vertebral units of the spine can also have a somatic dysfunction that only involves a single plane (flexion or extension). Also, if motion is found to be restricted in both directions and in multiple planes, the patient's joint may be demonstrating a "capsular pattern" of barriers. Capsular patterns are seen in pathologic conditions, such as arthritis, and warrant further diagnosis and treatment beyond the manipulative treatment of simple somatic dysfunction (see also Chapter 53, Lower Extremity). In capsular patterns, the restrictive barriers of joint motion have less resilience and a definite, firm end-feel.

For the initial musculoskeletal examination on a hospitalized patient, the physician need only look for and document regional tissue texture change, and/or asymmetry of tissues, and/or restriction of motion, and/or tenderness (TART), and the name of the spinal region in which any of these were palpated. (See Chapter 71, Treatment of the Acutely Ill Hospital Patient, Fig. 71.1.) Specific segmental diagnosis is not necessary in this initial hospital patient encounter unless a specific manipulative treatment is to be given right at that time. However, segmental diagnosis of a spinal region or other regions of somatic dysfunction must be performed, each time, before a manipulative treatment for the somatic dysfunction is administered.

Writing a somatic dysfunction formula without an additional qualifier assumes that the formula is a statement of the preference for motion of the vertebral unit(s). To indicate that the formula describes the restrictions of motion, the physician must precede the written formula using the word, "restricted." Examples:

L1-4 S_L R_R (also L1-4 N S_L R_R) or L1-4 restricted S_R R_L (motion present and then motion restricted)

L5 F R_R S_R or L5 restricted E R_L S_L (motion present and then motion restricted)[1]

---

[1] When the somatic dysfunction is type I, the sagittal plane does not have to be determined, but if the somatic dysfunction is type II, the sagittal plane preference for flexion or extension must be determined and indicated.

These formulae are not appropriate for recording capsular patterns. The above formulas should be reserved for describing somatic dysfunction.

EXAMINATION

History

Consideration of the onset, duration, and progression of a complaint is essential. An inventory by systems is taken, especially those systems that could be related to the lumbar complaints. Although the history is discussed as an entity that precedes the physical examination, further questioning (history) may take place as positive clues obtained from the history are combined with functional anatomic knowledge and considerations. This approach to history will prompt the physician to ask questions about areas that the patient does not consider important enough to mention initially, and it yields an organized, total etiologic list of conditions to be considered by the physician in his or her differential diagnosis of the complaints. For example, if a patient complains of lumbar dysfunction, questions about bowel and bladder function, whether the urinary stream is full and forceful, and whether there is any pain or burning on urination are all functionally relevant questions to ask. During the physical examination, if the patient complains of acute tenderness when the iliotibial bands are palpated, questions about bowel habits and function are relevant. In women, these findings should also initiate questions about menses and pelvic discomfort; in men, questions about prostate or penile discomfort, or deep, uncomfortable pressure in the perineal region are indicated. Asking if chilling or muscle-stressing activities increase the symptom might alert the physician to consider and examine for select myofascial trigger points related to the symptomatology.

When planning total management of patients with lumbar complaints, it is also important to ask the patient about past "pratfalls" or accidents that could have produced a unilateral sacral flexion or an up-slipped innominate (shears), upset spinal mechanics, or affected the craniosacral mechanism. Most patients forget about these types of accidents because they think, "I didn't break anything when I fell, I recovered, and therefore, it is not important and could not be related to my problems." Or they think, "I almost fell but I caught myself, so that couldn't have stressed my body—it was not an accident."

Ask the patient about choking feelings (thyroid) and breast changes or masses (breast tumors). These questions explore the possibility of cancer of the organs that usually metastasize to bone and can produce pain in the back. Other positive answers during a history provide clues requiring a differential diagnosis: chilling (myofascial triggers?), frequency and burning (infection of the genitourinary tract?), blood in the stool and/or changes in bowel habit or function (colon dysfunction or cancer?), pratfalls (non-physiologic shear somatic dysfunction and/or somatic dysfunction in the cranial field?), and so on.

Physical Examination

A complete physical examination is performed, with special emphasis on regions that are spotlighted by the history or that have functional association with the symptomatic region. In this chapter, only the more common points related to a patient with lumbar complaints are described.

If the patient has leg pain or paresthesia, ask the patient to show exactly where it is located, and then decide if this could represent a dermatomal, myotomal, sclerotomal or radicular pain pattern. Sclerotomes and myotomes have been documented and mapped. They are important and are often overlooked pain patterns (see Dermatomes, Myotomes, and Sclerotomes in this chapter and Chapter 53, Lower Extremity, Fig. 53.30). A radicular pattern would indicate that there may be nerve root pressure, perhaps related to a herniated intervertebral disc or a tumor in the cauda equina. In this particular case, traditional orthopedic and neurologic testing, which includes deep tendon reflex assessment, assessment of muscle strength/weakness, and testing key dermatomes for sensation and/or pain are important. The physical examination is extremely important in formulating a differential diagnosis.

Observation

What is the patient's appearance? Observation of posture and activity often provide the first clue to dysfunction. Posture mimics a patient's inner self more than their complaints or responses to direct questioning. An example would be the slumped posture of a depressed patient.

Is there asymmetry of a region of the body when the whole body is observed? Clues to lumbar dysfunction may be indicated by observing the spacing difference between the arms and the hip/waist on each side of the body (Fig. 50.17). This sign may indicate the presence of scoliosis, strain from sacral base

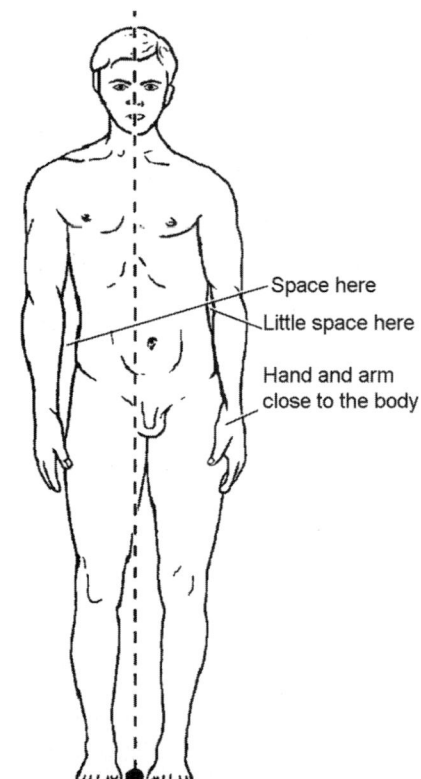

Space here
Little space here

Hand and arm
close to the body

FIGURE 50.17. The space around the patient provides clues to postural imbalances, such as scoliosis, unlevel sacral base, and so on.

unleveling, or a unilateral muscle spasm. Could there be sacral base unleveling? If the patient likes to stand in a forward-bent position, consider bilateral psoas muscle spasm of mechanical or visceral etiology, or a condition that is putting pressure on lumbar nerves in the intervertebral foramen. If the patient is leaning forward, to one side, and has the ipsilateral foot everted when standing or walking, consider a unilateral psoas spasm. If this develops into a full psoas syndrome on one side, the patient may also complain of pain in the contralateral hip and leg, rarely past the knee (see Clinical Examples: Psoas Syndrome and Fig. 50.25). When a patient stands very erect and dislikes bending forward, he or she may be protecting a herniated disc or be suffering the effects of spinal stenosis, especially if there are other symptoms, such as muscular weakness, reflex changes, or muscle atrophy.

Auscultation

Auscultate the four quadrants of the abdomen to determine the presence, location, frequency, and pitch of peristaltic waves. An intermittent, low, occasional slow gurgle is normal. Conversely, high-pitched tinkling sounds may denote a developing bowel obstruction. Absence of bowel sounds may indicate a paralytic ileus. A bruit in the midline of the abdomen between the xiphoid process and the umbilicus could indicate renal stenosis or abdominal aortic aneurysm (especially when associated with a pulsating abdominal mass). A bruit at the junction between the middle and outer two-thirds of the inguinal region could indicate a significant atherosclerosis of the common iliac or femoral artery. A bruit over the umbilical region could indicate a saddle thrombosis or severe atherosclerosis at the bifurcation of the abdominal aorta. Other physical examination tests for the abdomen of a patient are covered in other chapters (see Chapter 51 and Chapter 71).

Palpation and Motion Testing

Anterior Chapman points related to organs associated with symptoms in the lumbar region (Fig. 50.18) are located around the umbilicus, the pelvis, and in the iliotibial bands. Tender points in these locations may be associated with hypersympathetic activity resulting from viscerosomatic reflexes initiated in an irritated colon or pelvic organ, and the physician should question the patient regarding dysfunction of the organ most likely to be associated with that particular tender point (see Chapters 51, 66, and 67). A positive response to specific questioning helps position a somatic clue according to its significance and rank when considering a differential diagnosis.

The abdomen is also palpated for masses. Palpation is aided by mental visualization of the liver, kidneys, stomach, small intestines, bifurcation of the aorta at the level of the umbilicus, and the colon (Fig. 50.19).

The midline region between the xiphoid and umbilicus should be palpated for any pulsating tumor (abdominal aneurysm). Anteriorly occurring pulsations are normal, but lateral pulsations of the aorta suggest an aneurysm, especially if it is widened greater than 1 inch (a normal adult abdominal aorta should not be wider than 1 inch). Palpate the inguinal area, evaluating and comparing the right and left femoral pulses. If a decreased pulse is found on one or both sides, ask the patient about claudication. Palpate the

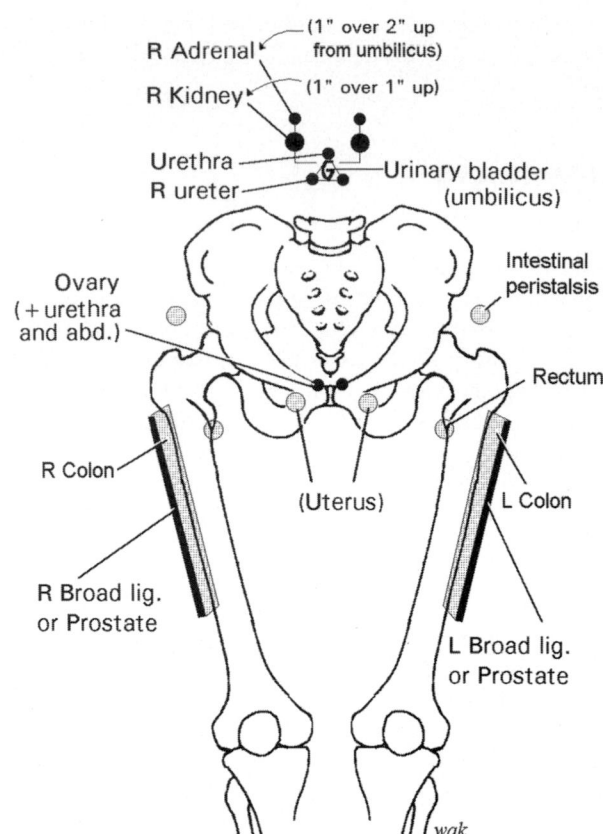

FIGURE 50.18. These Chapman points in the anterior abdominal wall around the umbilicus, around the pelvis, and/or in the iliotibial bands may provide non-invasive clues to visceral irritation or dysfunction that can produce symptoms in the lumbar region of the body.

pulse of the popliteal, posterior tibial, and dorsal pedis arteries in that leg and compare them with the pulses of the opposite leg.

Neurologic Testing and Muscle Strength

For an excellent summary on neurologic testing and muscle strength, see Table 50.5 and Table 50.6. For the standard method of recording reflexes, see Chapter 47, Table 47.9. For the standard method of recording muscular strength, see Chapter 47, Table 47.10.

Specific Tests

Testing the Abdominal Diaphragm

For additional information on testing the abdominal diaphragm, see Chapter 68, The Lymphatic System: Lymphatic Manipulative Techniques. This test is for the diagnosis of abdominal diaphragmatic dysfunction, or testing for evidence of flattening of the dome of the diaphragm.

Position: The patient is supine, and the physician stands beside the patient's hips with his or her dominant hand nearest the patient's feet.

1. The physician grasps the lateral sides of the patient's lower rib cage and tests for right and left rotational preference of the deep fasciae. Freedom of rotation in both directions is a negative test (i.e., no somatic dysfunction is present).

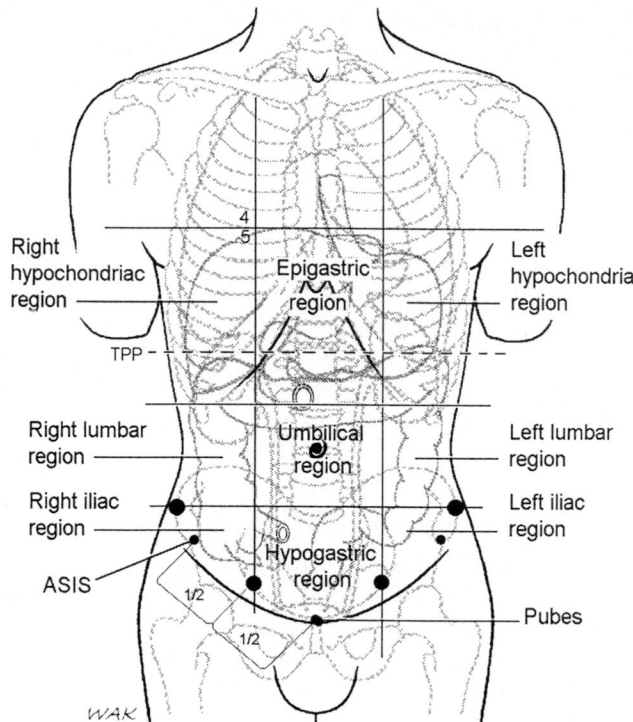

FIGURE 50.19. The approximate location of major abdominal viscera. Knowing the approximate locations helps a physician better interpret abdominal palpatory findings.

2. If rotational preference is present, side-bending preference will also be present and usually to the same side. Side-bending and rotational preference at the thoracolumbar junction indicates that diaphragmatic function is compromised, and its "dome" is probably flattened, in the resting position, on one or both sides.

Abdominal Diaphragmatic Re-doming

For more information on re-doming techniques, see Chapter 68, The Lymphatic System: Lymphatic Manipulative Techniques. Direct or indirect methods of manipulative treatment may be used. Direct myofascial, muscle energy treatment to re-dome the abdominal diaphragm:

Position: The patient is supine and the physician stands beside the patient's hips with his or her dominant hand nearest to the patient's feet.

1. The physician holds the patient's myofascial tissues of the thoracolumbar region in the direction of its restriction for rotation.

TABLE 50.5. REFLEXES FOR EVALUATING THE LUMBAR REGION

Reflexes	Comments
Patellar	L4 nerve root.
Achilles	S1 nerve root.
Cremasteric	L1 and L2. Usually tested only if specific history or physical findings indicate possible involvement.

TABLE 50.6. TESTS FOR EVALUATING LUMBAR INNERVATION USING MUSCULAR STRENGTH

Muscle Innervations and Strength	Comments
Quadriceps and anterior tibialis	Innervation predominately L4
Extensor digitorum longus, brevis, and hallucis longus	Innervation predominately L5
"Walk on your heels."	Tests strength of L5
Gastrocnemius/soleus and intrinsic foot muscles	Innervation predominately S1
"Walk on your toes."	Tests strength of S1

2. The patient is instructed to, "Take a deep breath in and out." At this point, if the patient has a flattened diaphragm, movement can be detected on only one side of the thoracoabdominal region. The physician adds thoracolumbar side-bending toward himself or herself, carrying it to its restrictive barrier by pulling his or her caudad hand contact toward, and his or her cephalad contact away. At the same time, the physician continues to adjust rotation to its restrictive barrier. At that point, it will be sensed that both sides of the thoracolumbar region begin to move with inhalation.

3. The physician holds the thoracolumbar region in that position as the patient is instructed to take three or four deep inhalations and exhalations. With this positioning and the patient's respiratory efforts, the diaphragm re-domes itself.

4. The physician returns the thoracolumbar region to a neutral position and rechecks movement of that region as the patient takes a deep breath in and out (also see Chapter 68, The Lymphatic System: Lymphatic Manipulative Techniques).

Hip Drop Test

For additional information on the hip drop test, see Figure 50.20 and Chapter 44, Musculoskeletal Examination, Figure 44.11.

Negative test: The iliac crest on the unsupported side drops 20 to 25 degrees, and there is a smooth lumbar curvature toward the weight bearing side of the body.

Positive test: The iliac crest *does not* drop 20 to 25 degrees on the non-weight-bearing side, and there is an angled, uneven, or poor lumbar spinal curve toward the weight-bearing side. A positive test indicates that the lumbar and/or thoracolumbar spine has difficulty side-bending toward the weight-bearing side of the body (i.e., the side *opposite* the positive test).

Because rotation and side-bending are linked motions, the physician may elect to screen the lumbar spine using only the segmental rotational test or the hip drop test. Neither test is as sensitive as segmental palpation, but when properly performed, a positive finding on either test identifies a need for segmental diagnosis of the lumbar spine.

Thoracolumbar Rotation Screen

See Chapter 44, Musculoskeletal Examination, and Table 44.3, to read about the trunk rotation test.

Negative test: Normal rotation is equal motion in both directions—about 90 degrees in both directions.

Positive test: Failure to rotate as far in one direction as in the other *or* a qualitatively different end-feel to each barrier. This

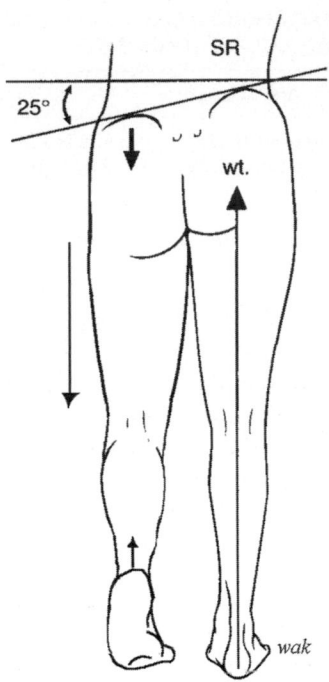

FIGURE 50.20. A negative left hip drop test.

suggests a problem that is restricting rotation somewhere in the lumbar spine, especially at the thoracolumbar junction.

Anterior Spinal Compression (Spring) Test

Table 44.1, Compression Test, in Chapter 44, Musculoskeletal Examination, provides further information about this test. It is a screening examination to determine the ability of the thoracic or lumbar spine to extend.

Position: The patient is prone and the physician stands beside the table near the patient's hips.

Procedure: The physician intermittently applies anterior pressure over the spine of the thoracic and lumbar regions of the body.

Positive test: Compression is resisted (end-feel is abrupt). This means that the thoracic or lumbar spine will not extend and is flexed. Note that the lumbar spine can normally extend through more degrees than it can flex and still be in the neutral sagittal plane range of multiple-plane lumbar motion (Fig. 50.16). If the anterior compression test is positive, the vertebral unit resists extension and probably prefers to flex. Multiple-plane lumbar somatic dysfunction of a vertebral unit with a preference for flexion is more likely to be symptomatic and to be associated with type II somatic dysfunction in a single vertebral unit. Therefore, if a lumbar compression test is positive, the vertebral unit(s) must be segmentally tested for rotation and side-bending. If a type II somatic dysfunction involves the L1 or L2 vertebral unit, there is also the probability that it may be associated with visceral dysfunction of the descending colon or a pelvic organ; alternately, it may be associated with a psoas syndrome. Testing for the rotational preference of each vertebra is a more efficient way of screening the lumbar spine, because it identifies asymmetry in rotation, which can then be correlated with segmental side-bending to provide a specific diagnosis of somatic dysfunction.

In the thoracic region, a positive compression test is more often associated with finding type I somatic dysfunction in a group of vertebral units, because the thoracic spine can flex more easily than it can extend. A group of thoracic, type I somatic dysfunction that resists extension and is flexed will have a positive anterior compression test.

Negative test: If the thoracic or lumbar spine does not resist anterior compression, the test is considered to be a negative compression test. Yet this lumbar spine could still have type I somatic dysfunction. Now if there were a type II, lumbar non-neutral dysfunction, the physician may not catch the resistance of this one vertebral unit in five and report a false negative compression test. For this reason, testing for rotational preference of each lumbar vertebra is more time-efficient and will help clarify this possible confusion (see Lumbar Rotation Screen, below).

Spinal Lumbosacral Spring Test

This test is a part of some physicians' tests for segmental sacral diagnosis. It is easily confused with the anterior spinal compression test, because some physicians (and instructors) say that they "spring" the vertebral column anteriorly when referring to the anterior compression test. Results are used to help diagnose sacral somatic dysfunction and are interpreted in relationship to findings from segmental testing of the sacrum.

Position: The patient is prone, sometimes resting on his or her elbows, and the physician stands to one side near the patient's pelvis.

Procedure:

1. The physician places his or her caudad hand over the lumbosacral region and reinforces it with the palm of the cephalad hand.
2. Repeated anterior and slightly cephalad pressure is applied to this region of the spine.

Positive test: If no spring to this region of the lumbar spine is found, it is believed to be due to posterior motion of the sacral base, which locks the lumbar spine.

Negative test: This is believed to be normal for the lumbar spine or associated with somatic dysfunction of the sacrum, where segmental tests indicate the base has moved anteriorly.

Lumbar Rotation Screen

Additional information on this topic can be found in Chapter 44, Musculoskeletal Examination, Segmental Motion Testing, Passive Lumbar Segmental Motion Testing.

Note that if rotational preference of a lumbar vertebra is found in one direction with restriction in rotation in the opposite direction, side-bending preference will also be present and must be tested. If preferences for side-bending and rotation occur to the same side, then flexion or extension must also be tested to determined preference for sagittal plane motion in those segments. Rotation testing of each of the five lumbar vertebrae is the most accurate and time-efficient method of screening for lumbar somatic dysfunction, because the transverse processes are directly lateral to the spinous process of the lumbar vertebra being tested. The rotational screen also begins segmental lumbar testing.

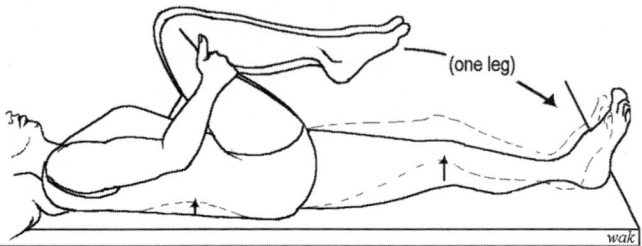

FIGURE 50.21. The Thomas test for finding iliopsoas spasm or contracture.

Paraspinal Palpation for Tissue Texture Changes

See Chapter 44, Musculoskeletal Examination, Palpation for Tissue Texture Abnormalities and Tenderness and Figures 44.17.

Positive test: Tissue texture asymmetry is palpated. Vertebral units with palpable tissue texture abnormality have segmental somatic dysfunction. If found at the L1 or L2 level, then viscerosomatic reflexes from irritation of a kidney, the descending colon, or pelvic organs (T10-L2) must also be considered.

Thomas Test for Psoas Shortening

Figure 50.21 shows this test. Psoas shortening can be acute, chronic, or subacute. (See also Chapter 53, Lower Extremities.) Patients are tested in the supine position.

Positive test: If the iliopsoas muscle is shortened, the lower extremity on that side will be unable to fully extend at the hip (i.e., the thigh and popliteal region do not lie flat on the table).

Psoas Test Variations

The patient may also be tested in the prone or lateral recumbent position. Though a patient with chronic or subacute shortening of the psoas muscle can usually lie prone, the patient with acute psoas spasm or shortening cannot usually lie prone flat on the table. In this case, the physician can have the patient turn to the lateral recumbent position and attempt to extend the leg at the hip.

Positive test: It is not comfortable for the leg to be in the fully extended position. When the psoas is involved, the patient becomes especially uncomfortable when anterior thigh extension is attempted. If the extension of the thigh produces pain in the posterior sacroiliac joint, also consider dysfunction of the hip or sacroiliac joint on that side.

Tender Points and Trigger Points Relating to the Lumbar Region

The multifidi next to the spines, the quadratus lumborum muscle, and/or the gluteus medius attachments to the lateral iliac crest may contain Travell tender points (Fig. 50.11), which can refer pain to the lumbar region. Tender points for the iliopsoas muscle are located approximately 1 inch medial to each anterior superior iliac spine (ASIS) on the anterior side of the body. An iliopsoas tender point is deep in the abdomen, not on the posterior wall and not in the superficial abdominal wall.

If Chapman myofascial tender points for the lumbar region are evaluated (Fig. 50.18), palpate for them at the beginning of the physical examination, because motion and repeated palpation or stretching of the myofascial tissues in their location will decrease their sensitivity and diagnostic value; their tenderness to palpation will disappear, at least for a period of time. Chapman points found around the umbilicus may be related to the bladder, kidney, or adrenal glands. Those over the pubic symphysis may be related to gonadal tissue. Posterior Chapman points to the large intestine lie in a triangular area on either side of the lower lumbar spine. If large bowel problems are suspected, do not give lumbar soft tissue treatment until you have palpated the anterior points related to the colon (found in the iliotibial bands) to secure data that would help confirm this suspicion. Chapman points should be carefully correlated with history, palpation, tenderness of the collateral abdominal ganglia, and spinal somatic dysfunction, as well as with the palpation of the suspected organ system to determine the ranking, significance, and value of the tender point in the differential diagnosis (see Chapter 51, Abdominal Region). Chapman reflexes are one of the early diagnostic clues to irritation and dysfunction of viscera.

TREATMENT: LUMBAR SOMATIC DYSFUNCTION

Specific manipulative treatment methods and activating forces used to treat somatic dysfunction in any region of the body are found in the different palpatory diagnosis and treatment chapters of this book. The indications and goals of osteopathic manipulative treatment of the total patient include:

Treat the patient according to that patient's physiologic needs.
Reduce or remove symptoms and spinal cord facilitation due to primary somatic dysfunction.
Reduce or remove facilitated spinal cord segments due to secondary somatic dysfunction.
Support the body's homeostatic mechanisms during natural stresses (e.g., pregnancy) and illness, preoperatively, and after postoperative complications.
Support the body's immune system.
Provide comprehensive and efficient total body treatment.
Comfort the patient and help alleviate anxiety during the workup for conditions that may primarily require medical/surgical treatment.
Enhance other medical or surgical treatments.
Prevent the likelihood of reoccurrence of the dysfunction.

Clinical Examples: Treatment for "Back Pain"
Treatment for Medical/Surgical Etiologies

Any physician who is adept at finding and treating somatic dysfunction should remember that approximately 10% of patients complaining of back pain will primary have a medical or surgical etiology for their complaint. Medical/surgical conditions that refer pain to the lumbar region include:

Two surgical emergencies: dissecting abdominal aneurysm and cauda equina syndrome (14)

Secondary (medical) somatic dysfunction: kidney dysfunction, ureteral obstruction, irritation of the left colon, and prostate or bladder irritation

Primary cancers that metastasize to bone (most common in patients over 50 years of age): thyroid, breast, lung, kidney and prostate

Abdominal Aneurysm

Both anatomic relationships and a good history help more accurately determine the cause of a patient's complaints. For example, an older, hypertensive patient complaining of severe back pain, numbness of the lower extremities, and a bruit over the abdominal aorta (with or without a palpable abdominal mass) could have either an abdominal aneurysm or renal artery stenosis. The abdominal aorta divides into the common iliac arteries at the level of the umbilicus. The umbilicus is located anterior to and in a horizontal plane running through the L3-4 disc space. Bruits from an abdominal aortic aneurysm are often identified by auscultation near or anterior to the umbilicus. The sudden onset of severe, tearing abdominal pain that radiates through to the back and is associated with palpation of an abdominal mass and the auscultation of a bruit most likely indicates a dissecting abdominal aneurysm. A dissecting abdominal aneurysm is a surgical emergency; surgical consultation should be immediately obtained. A bruit from renal artery stenosis is also auscultated at the midline but higher in the epigastric region, and the abdominal aorta is not enlarged.

Any ventral abdominal osteopathic techniques or thrust activations for manipulative treatment of the thoracic, lumbar, or sacral regions should be avoided in these patients. If somatic dysfunction is present and located in the midcervical region, thoracic inlet, or the abdominal diaphragm, it should be treated using gentle, indirect methods (if necessary). Gentle paraspinal inhibition with the patient in the supine position is indicated (or may be tolerated) in nonemergent cases to prepare the patient for surgery.

Cauda Equina Syndrome

The typical patient with this problem complains of backache and paralysis that begins in the feet and progresses upward. If asked, he or she will usually give a history of bladder and/or anal sphincter weakness, because the sphincters are often involved early. Paralysis may develop slowly or occur very rapidly (progressing to complete paralysis of the lower extremities within an hour). Therefore, immediate surgical consultation and timely emergency surgical decompression of the nerves is mandatory if full use of the lower extremities is to be achieved. Although surgery is able to completely decompress the nerves, if surgery is delayed too long, motor function of the lower extremities and/or sphincters may never return.

Osteopathic manipulative treatment is definitely secondary to immediate surgical care for patients with surgical emergencies, but it is definitely indicated in the postoperative period, where it supports abdominal diaphragmatic function, improvement of lymphatic drainage, and the reduction of postoperative sympathicotonia of the GI tract (which could progress to paralytic ileus).

Others

These include uterine spasm or irritation, renal calculi, and orthopedic problems (see Chapter 51, Abdominal Region, and Chapter 52, Pelvis and Sacrum). When examining a patient with low back pain, orthopedic problems must be ruled out. Orthopedists divide the vertebra into three parts to help with the differential diagnosis and treatment considerations—a posterior element, a middle element, and an anterior element (Fig. 50.22). Scott states that Gunnar Anderson does not consider the intervertebral disc with the middle elements, instead placing it with the anterior elements. In this classification, only the spinal cord and spinal canal remain with the middle elements. In his Orthopedics chapter in the first edition of *Foundations for Osteopathic Medicine*, Scott mentions the etiologies for back pain (Table 28.1).

Somatic dysfunction of the first two lumbar vertebral units may also be related to viscerosomatic reflexes from left colon or pelvic organ irritation, especially if they are diagnosed as exhibiting a non-neutral mechanical preference. L1 and L2 are the only lumbar nerves with white rami that carry sympathetic efferent neurons, the neurons that carry outgoing sympathetic messages. It is possible that somatic dysfunction of either, or both, of these two vertebral units is a secondary result of viscerosomatic reflexes from primary dysfunction irritating the left colon, pelvic splanchnic nerves, or pelvic organs. In these conditions, nociceptive impulses are transmitted up through the paraspinal sympathetic chain ganglia to the T12-L2 spinal cord levels. Here, they facilitate the T12-L2 cord segments. Then, through "cross-talk" in the spinal cord with somatic motor nerves in the dorsal horn of the T12-L2 segments, secondary somatic dysfunction develops in the joints and tissues associated with T12-L2 somatic innervation. The upper lumbar region may also be painful and exhibit somatic dysfunction as a result of primary problems in an organ innervated by parasympathetic sacral nerves, S2-4. For example, although pain fibers from the cervix of the uterus refer to the pelvic splanchnic nerve centers (S2, S3, and S4), pain fibers from an irritation of the fundus of the uterus refer to the upper lumbar region (see Chapter 51, Abdominal Region).

Treatment of Non-Medical/Non-Surgical Etiologies

The same caution that was given to the physician "specializing" in osteopathic manipulative medicine must be given to an internist or surgeon, but worded differently: "Not all back pain is due to medical or surgical problems." In fact, most are not. Ninety percent of patients with back pain have conditions that do not require surgery or primary medical care. Most conditions are due to mechanical dysfunction of the posterior elements of a vertebra (Fig. 50.22) or other distant and/or nonarticular somatic structures functionally related to the lumbar spine, including shoulder dysfunction from lumbosacral somatic dysfunction via the latissimus dorsi muscle, and dermatome, myotome, or sclerotome pain referred to the lower extremity (see Chapter 53, Lower Extremities, Fig. 53.30). It also includes patients with primary somatic dysfunction, strains, sprains, postural decompensation, or overuse syndromes, and patients with hypermobility. Most will have a primary diagnosis of somatic dysfunction and/or postural decompensation. Sometimes the decompensation is due to

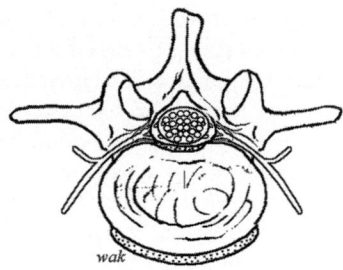

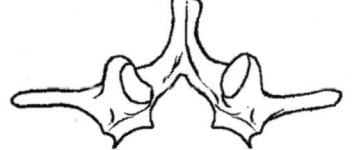
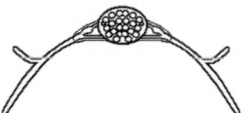
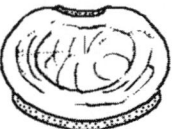

FIGURE 50.22. Vertebral divisions that help a physician consider possible etiologies for back pain. The vertebra is divided into the posterior bony elements, the middle meningeal and neurologic elements, and the vertebral body and disc (Table 50.7).

TABLE 50.7. POSTERIOR, MIDDLE, AND ANTERIOR SPINAL ELEMENTS RELATED TO BACK PAIN

Elements	Possible Etiologies
Posterior Elements—most common	
Spinous process, transverse processes, lamina, pedicles, ligaments and joint capsule, intervertebral joints	Somatic dysfunction–TART[a] Especially the "half-dirty dozen" (15) Age-related and activity-related strains–arthritis, overuse Severe or chronic twists Strains and sprains Spondylosis, overuse, or chronic trauma Spondylolisthesis Severe trauma and twists Fractures of pedicle, transverse process, or spinous process[b]
Middle Elements	
Central spinal canal, meninges, spinal cord and nerves	Compression of the spinal canal or nerve root Cauda equina syndrome[b] Intrinsic Intradural tumors Meningeal infections Extrinsic pressure through foramen and/or the thecal sac Metastatic tumors Ruptured disc with contents free in spinal canal Neurofibromas Spurs or other symptoms, of aging or degenerative conditions (osteoarthritis) Benign tumors or fibromas Reflex etiologies–visceral dysfunctions and disease
Anterior Elements	
Posterior longitudinal ligament, vertebral body, anterior longitudinal ligament, and intervertebral disk	Compression fractures of the vertebral body Vascular causes–abdominal aneurysm[b] Traumatic disc disruption with pressure on nerve root or thecal sac Infection

[a]Glossary of osteopathic terminology. *AOA Yearbook and Directory*, 91st ed, Chicago, IL: American Osteopathic Association; 2000:869.
[b] Surgical emergency.

chronic, untreated somatic dysfunction. Sometimes the primary etiology arises from an unlevel sacral base, which is usually asymptomatic unless left undiagnosed and untreated for a significant length of time (perhaps years). Over time, the patient usually begins to complain of localized discomfort or pain brought about by compensatory changes that are actually located cephalad from the unlevel sacral base (see Chapter 44, Postural Consideration in the Sagittal, Coronal, and Horizontal Planes).

Dirty Half-Dozen
This designation was coined by Phil Greenman (15) for a cluster of somatic findings that often underlie the complaints of patients who have been diagnosed with "failed low back syndrome" (Fig. 50.23). This dysfunction includes:

Non-neutral lumbar somatic dysfunction.
Dysfunction of the symphysis pubis (pubic shear).
Restriction of the anterior movement of the sacral base. This could be either a posterior sacral base or a posterior backward torsion (non-neutral sacral rotation on an oblique sacral axis).
Innominate shear dysfunction.
A short leg and pelvic tilt syndrome.
Muscular imbalance of the trunk and lower extremity (including psoas syndrome).

Over years of practice, many patients that were referred to me for "failed low back syndrome" were often found to have a unilateral sacral flexion (sacral shear) that had been overlooked. Innominate shears or sacral shears may be asymptomatic at their site, but eventually result in secondary subjective symptoms in the patient's lumbar, upper rib, cervical, suboccipital, or cranial regions. These are regions of increased stress brought about by the body's attempt to compensate for the persistent dysfunction and the pelvic base. Because shears are non-physiologic, the body is often unable to remove them without outside specific treat-

ment; so it tries to compensate for their presence. A pelvic shear may even prevent successful manipulative treatment of other somatic dysfunction. The presence of a shear is also associated with the continuance or return of symptoms shortly after other diagnosed somatic dysfunction has been successfully treated and removed. When a patient complains of pelvic symptoms with persistent and/or recurrent "usual" sacroiliac somatic dysfunction (regardless of receiving "effective" manipulative treatment), look for other dysfunction that refers pain to the lumbosacral region, including mechanical, surgical, and/or medical.

Iliolumbar Ligament Syndrome
The back pain experienced by a patient with iliolumbar ligament syndrome is located in the sacroiliac, posterior thigh, and/or inguinal regions (Fig. 50.24). In fact, the presenting complaint is often, "I think I have a hernia," and then the patient points to the inguinal region. Check for an inguinal hernia, but regardless of the actual presence or absence of a hernia, palpate the attachment of the iliolumbar ligaments to the ilia for a tender point. If the iliolumbar ligament is stressed and irritated, its tender point will be on the iliac crest, located on the ipsilateral side of the complaint 1 inch superior and lateral to the undersling of the posterior superior iliac spine (Fig. 50.8). This tender point in the iliolumbar ligament may or may not refer pain to the inguinal region. If the patient has a hernia *and* a tender point in the iliolumbar ligament, even successful surgical repair of the hernia, without treating the etiology for the iliolumbar ligament syndrome, may leave the patient with continued symptoms of "the inguinal hernia."

Also remember that the iliolumbar ligament is the first ligament stressed when there is postural decompensation. So, if a patient's iliolumbar ligament is tender to palpation, also check for an unlevel sacral base, scoliosis, short leg, and so on, and provide corrective treatment as indicated by your diagnostic findings. Injection of a local anesthetic into the tender point located at

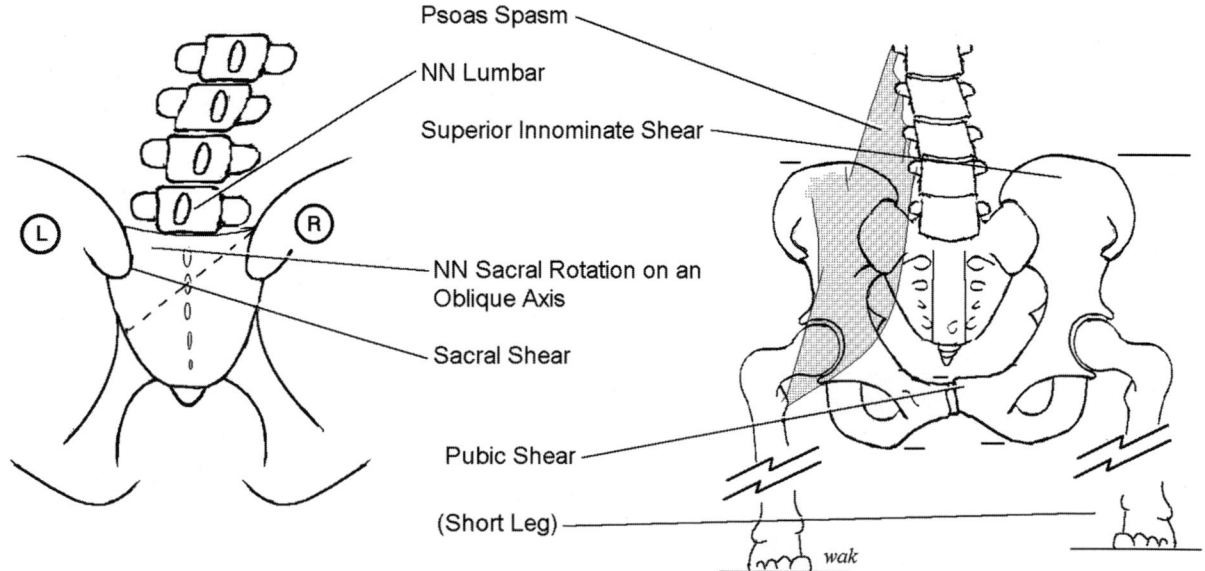

FIGURE 50.23. The "Dirty Half-Dozen." This term, popularized by Phil Greenman, lists the common mechanical etiologies for somatic dysfunction in patients with "failed low back syndrome."

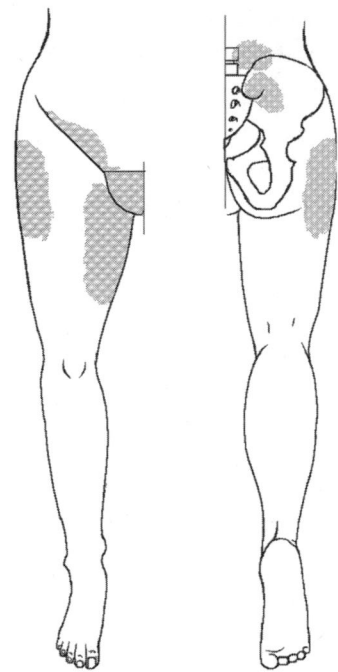

FIGURE 50.24. Referral pain pattern of a patient with an irritated right iliolumbar ligament syndrome (see also Fig. 50.8).

the attachment of the ligament to the ilium will often relieve or reduce the pain while definitive diagnosis and specific treatment for the primary problem is instituted.

Meralgia Paresthetica

This condition may or may not be associated with back pain, but it does involve the lumbar region. The patient complains of numbness, paresthesia, or hypoesthesia in a fairly large oval region on the lateral side of the thigh, which can cover any portion of the area from the lateral buttock to the knee. History usually supplies no apparent clue for its occurrence. Examination of gait, weight-bearing posture, and a radiograph of the back may all be normal. This condition is due to pressure somewhere along the course of the lateral femoral cutaneous nerve (formed from the L2 and L3 nerve roots). This nerve passes through the psoas major muscle, runs inferolateral on the iliacus muscle, *under* (and sometimes through) the inguinal ligament just medial to the ASIS, and then passes into the thigh. Somatic dysfunction may involve the L2 or L3 vertebral units, the psoas muscle, the innominate, or the fasciae of the thigh or innominate. Manipulative treatment of any of this somatic dysfunction is indicated, if present. Sometimes, very constrictive clothing (jeans) or some other external mechanical force will have initiated this condition.

Hypermobility

In some symptomatic "back pain" patients, motion of the lumbar region seems unusually free and easy. This can be especially true with extension motion at the L5 level, and this finding suggests hypermobility from relaxed ligaments and contributes to instability of the involved vertebral unit. Patients with stressed low back ligaments often complain of severe back discomfort that lasts for minutes to an hour or more when they first lie down to relax or sleep. They are also unable to sit or stand in one place for any length of time, and are continually shifting to find a comfortable position when they have to sit for a period of time. The patient presentation of the latter has been called "theater cocktail syndrome."

Hypermobility may be a relative contraindication for the use of thrust-type activation in the treatment of somatic dysfunction in that region. Patients with this problem usually respond better to indirect or gentle and specific muscle energy procedures, because these activations produce less stress on structures that are already over-stretched. A region of *hyper* mobility may need to be strengthened with graded exercises or treated with a regimen that includes sclerotherapy. Interestingly, areas of hypermobility often resolve when adjacent areas of *hypo* mobile somatic dysfunction are treated. In those cases, the hypermobility was apparently compensatory for the adjacent hypomobile region. In any case, primary causes of hypermobility, including postural-gravitational strain, overuse phenomena, and so on should be sought and treated.

Psoas Syndrome

"The iliopsoas muscle is the hidden prankster in the sense that it serves many critically important functions, often causes pain, and is relatively inaccessible" (6). The psoas muscles are attached to the vertebral bodies and the anterior surface of the transverse processes of the lumbar vertebra. They pass along the superior border of the true pelvis, are joined by the iliacus muscles, pass over the superior ramus of the pubes, and then turn posteriorly to insert on the lesser trochanter of each femur via common tendons (Fig. 50.25).

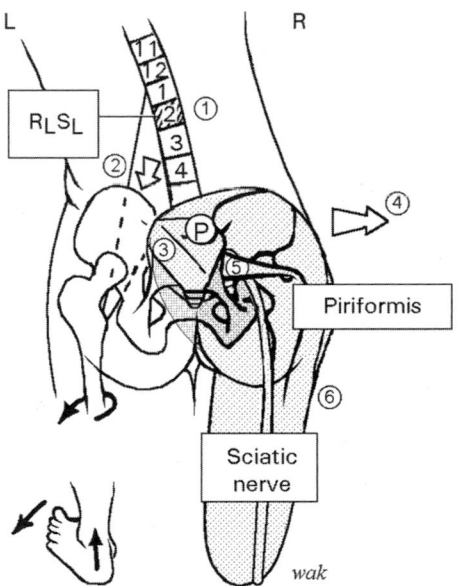

FIGURE 50.25. Full-blown left psoas syndrome. The patient is forward bent, leans to the left side, and the left foot is everted. Signs and symptoms include: (1) the key, non-neutral somatic dysfunction at L1 or L2 that is side-bent left, (2) marked left psoas muscle spasm, (3) rotation of the sacrum on a left oblique axis (often of the non-neutral type), (4) right pelvic side shift, (5) right piriformis spasm and myofascial tender point, and (6) pain in the right hip, down the back side of the right leg, but not usually past the knee.

Psoas syndrome is usually initiated when a person assumes any number of positions that shorten the origin and insertion of the psoas muscle for a significant length of time and then gets up quickly, suddenly lengthening the origin and insertion, and attempts to assume normal upright activity. The initial positions that might bring about this syndrome include sitting in a soft easy chair or recliner, bending over from the waist for a long period of time, working at a desk, or weeding in the garden. Psoas syndrome can also be precipitated by overuse, such as doing sit-ups with the lower extremities fully extended. Apparently, each of these situations creates a neuromuscular imbalance that results in psoas muscle hypertonicity. The subsequent formation of somatic dysfunction then affects the psoas muscle and the lumbar spine. Once a patient realizes that he or she has been in one of these positions, the possibility of initiating a psoas syndrome can usually be avoided if he or she *slowly* returns to a neutral postural position.

The physician must be aware that there are organic causes for psoas tension or spasm, and if suspected, these must be ruled out by history and/or physical examination and special tests. These include:

Femoral bursitis
Arthritis of the hip
Diverticulosis of the colon
Ureteral calculi
Prostatitis
Cancer of the descending or sigmoid colon
Salpingitis

The key somatic dysfunction initiating or perpetuating psoas syndrome is believed to be a type II (non-neutral) somatic dysfunction (F Rx Sx) usually occurring in the L1 or L2 vertebral unit, where "x" is the side of side-bending of the somatic dysfunction. If this key somatic dysfunction remains, the patient's symptoms may progress to full-blown psoas syndrome (Fig. 50.25). Symptoms of this syndrome include:

The key, non-neutral (type II) somatic dysfunction at L1 or L2
Sacral somatic dysfunction on an oblique axis, usually to the side of lumbar side-bending
Pelvic shift to the opposite side of the greatest psoas spasm
Hypertonicity of the piriformis muscle that is opposite the side of greatest psoas spasm
Sciatic nerve irritation on the side of the piriformis spasm
Gluteal muscular and posterior thigh pain that does not go past the knee, on the side of the piriformis muscle spasm

Manipulative treatment is preceded by ruling out psoas involvement caused by one of the organic etiologies previously listed. Effective treatment of the "key" somatic dysfunction (usually found at L1 or L2) is essential for the patient's comfort and for effective, long-lasting effects of manipulative treatment, regardless of the administration of other indicated medicines, chemotherapy, radiation, or surgery. Removing somatic dysfunction, wherever it occurs in the body, reduces afferent load to the spinal cord from secondary somatic sources and lessens the segmental activity of the primary facilitated spinal cord segments.

This makes the patient more comfortable and supports the body's homeostatic and defense mechanisms, thus hastening recovery.

Radiculopathy

Radiculopathy is a general diagnosis that involves several etiologic conditions affecting a nerve root. "Radicular" pain describes pain that follows the distribution of an involved nerve root. Common mechanisms include conditions that produce pressure (pressure radiculopathy) or inflammation (radiculitis) of the nerve root. The lumbar region is a common site for radiculopathies.

Multiple, specific etiologies exist for this condition, and diagnosis can be difficult. Etiologies include a ruptured disc with material from the nucleus pulposus pressing on the nerve root or cord, and pressure exerted by bone tumors, exostoses, spinal stenosis, or irritation from an infection. Radiculopathy is often precipitated or aggravated by acute somatic dysfunction, especially if the intervertebral foramen and/or the spinal cord had already been compromised by some chronic process.

A ruptured and protruding disc producing pressure on the nerve root is often the first condition that the physician considers when a patient presents with pain referred into the lower extremity. As mentioned in the functional anatomy section of this chapter, the L4 and L5 discs are at greatest risk for rupture, as they undergo the most lumbar motion and experience significant functional and/or postural stress. Also, the width of the posterior longitudinal ligament at L4 and L5 is only one-half the width it was at L1, producing a posterolateral weakness over the intervertebral disc at each of these sites (Fig. 50.7).

Because the pedicles of a lumbar vertebra are located on the superolateral one-third of the lumbar vertebral body, a lumbar nerve winds around a pedicle and passes through its foramen, before it passes over the disc of that vertebral unit (Fig. 50.3). It is therefore more common to see the L5 nerve irritated by pressure from a ruptured L4 herniated disc, and the S1 nerve root irritated by pressure from a ruptured L5 herniated disc. Remember that it is not a reported "bulging disc" that produces symptoms. It is the significant pressure of a bulging or ruptured disc on a nerve root that is responsible for the patient's complaints, and it is helpful if magnetic resonance imaging indicates this connection at the site of the pressure.

Lumbar radiculopathy produces paresthesia in a dermatomal pattern. These are located on the anterior portion of the thigh, leg, and/or foot (Fig. 50.13). Myotomal distribution also results in decreased or absent deep tendon reflexes, muscle weakness, and atrophy of the muscles associated with the level of the ruptured disc (Figs. 50.26 and 50.27). Sclerotomal pain associated with discogenic disease is referred to the pelvis and over the lower extremity, as seen in Chapter 53, Lower Extremities, Figure 53.30. It also predisposes to trigger points in the involved musculature.

If any one of these three effects is seen (paresthesias, reflex changes, and muscle atrophy) and involve the same nerve root or roots, conservative care with adequate follow-up is indicated. A poor response to conservative treatment indicates that more aggressive care is indicated to prevent permanent weakness or loss of leg function; a consultation is recommended for these patients.

Surgical consultation (orthopedic and/or neurologic) and special tests are indicated if certain conditions are present. These

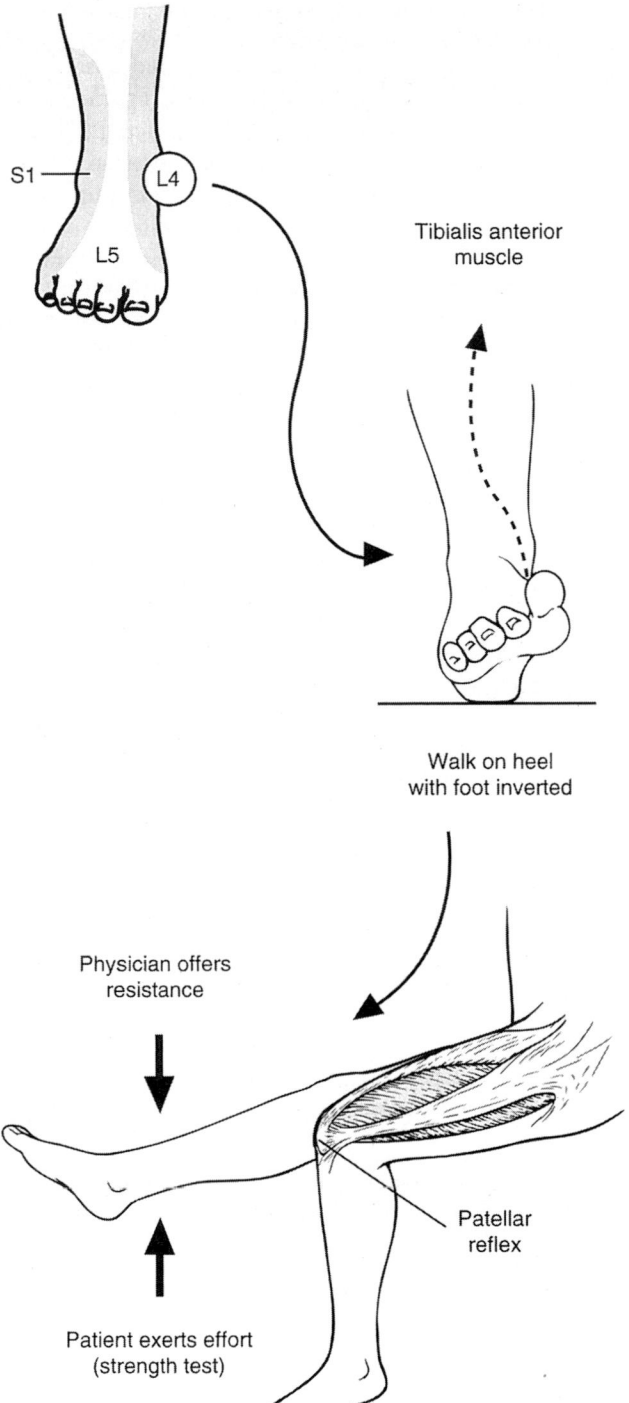

FIGURE 50.26. Tests for L4 nerve dysfunction.

Conservative care includes reduction of as many of the possible contributing factors as is practical. This may include specific treatment of postural imbalance and somatic dysfunction, adequate relief of pain, treatment of contributing or primary medical factors, and reduction of any other mechanical, structural, or psychological stresses.

Anatomically, the contents of the intervertebral foramen fill only one-third of the cross-section of the foramen, so it seems that the nerve roots should have plenty of room. Remember, 90% of low back pain is due to mechanical causes (11). Studies have shown that probably only 5% of patients that actually have ruptured discs require surgery (14). Osteopathic manipulation is effective in improving biomechanical function and is a primary treatment for radiculopathy due to functional causes. Removal of somatic dysfunction may be just enough to make a patient with a ruptured disc comfortable or asymptomatic. Furthermore, removal of adjacent *hypo* mobile somatic dysfunction may eliminate lumbar vertebral units that are exhibiting *hyper* mobility stress.

include:

- 6 to 8 weeks of conservative care that has not been accompanied by steady progress toward reversal of and/or resolution of the symptoms and signs
- Poor clinical response associated with any two or all three of the following: paresthesia, reflex changes, and muscle atrophy
- If the symptoms increase in intensity despite good ongoing conservative care

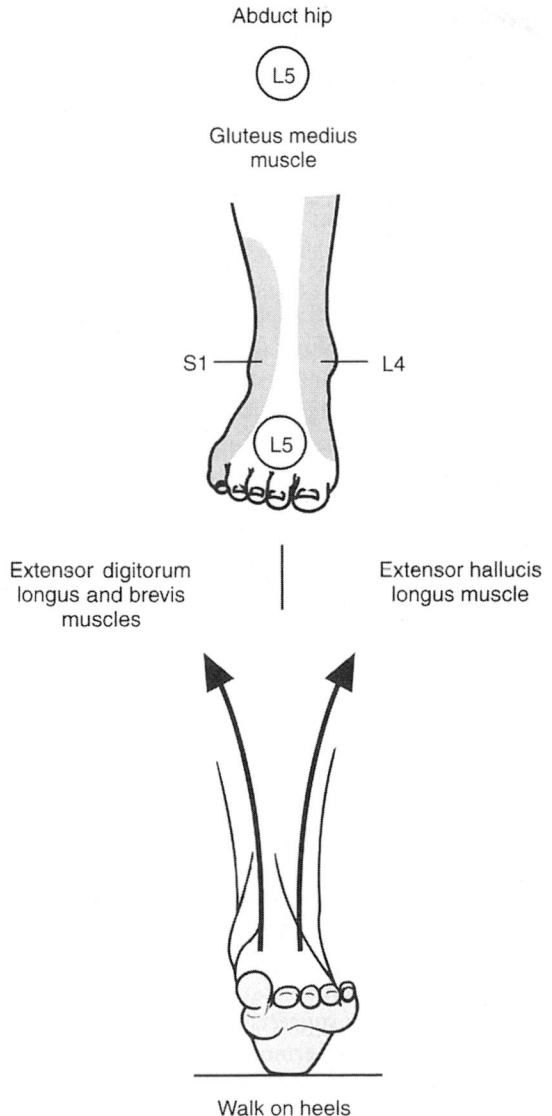

FIGURE 50.27. Tests for L5 nerve dysfunction.

As a patient gets older, several infirmities commonly compromise an intervertebral foramen and disc:

Arthritis
Ligament hypertrophy
Disuse atrophy
Disc degeneration
Muscle imbalance
Inherent tissue qualities
Somatic dysfunction

Manipulation is also indicated in the 10% of patients with medical or surgical problems. It makes the patient more comfortable and normalizes local biophysiologic responses while the specific primary care is being administered. Removal of somatic dysfunction supports the body's self-healing mechanisms during recovery from primary medical or surgical conditions. Sympathetic tone can be reduced, the thoracic inlet fascia normalized, and the diaphragm domed, preparing the patient's own systems and defenses for a surgery and/or aiding in postsurgical or medical recovery. Realize that mere "physician frustration" from poor results while using some combination of conservative treatment on a patient with back pain is not, by itself, an indication for recommending surgery.

Adequate pain relief is necessary to prevent reflex muscle spasm and guarding. Failure to adequately control pain usually leads to increased disability and morbidity, but care must be taken not to produce dependency or addiction. Muscle relaxants and physical therapy can be helpful to the patient's conservative care.

The physician should expect that effective conservative treatment of a patient will be accompanied by progressive reduction of subjective and objective signs and symptoms, and will be associated with obvious improvement in the patient. The key to good results with conservative treatment is to provide specific forms of acceptable treatment that are indicated by the pathophysiology and functional status of the patient, to monitor progress, to expect steady improvement, and to modify diagnostic procedures and treatment and/or get a consultation as it becomes clinically indicated. It is unreasonable to expect a patient who has been receiving your best conservative care for a long time and who has failed to make any significant objective and subjective change to suddenly get better with administration of "more of the same."

CONCLUSIONS

This chapter presents some of the unique thought processes used to evaluate the lumbar region and how these thought processes can be used to diagnose and treat patients with lumbar complaints. The physician should consider not only the lumbar site of the complaint but also the functional and reciprocal relationships within the rest of the body as they relate to the lumbar region. This chapter is not meant to provide comprehensive treatment of all lumbar complaints, but to present representative, common examples obtained through clinical experience that illustrate how osteopathic thinking is used in the care of patients with lumbar pain.

Despite the fact that mechanical problems (including somatic dysfunction) are responsible for most complaints of back pain, the physician must always consider and be ready to treat dysfunction in regions that have functional connections to the back. The attending physician should treat or find an internist or surgeon consultant who will treat the patient for any primary medical or surgical problems and emergencies. Do not feel inferior for asking for consultations that are needed.

The lumbar region is a frequent site of strain, pain, and disability. There are many myofascial and neural interconnections between the lumbar region and other regions of the body. For the best results, treatment offered must be directed toward the primary cause and not merely at the symptom of a backache or a back problem.

REFERENCES

1. Deyo RA. Low-back pain. *Sci Am.* 1998;279:48–53.
2. Anderson GBJ. Epidemiological features of chronic low-back pain (review). *Lancet.* 1999;354:581–585.
3. Taylor VM, Deyo RA, Cherkin DC, et al. Low-back pain hospitalization: Recent United States trends and regional variations. *Spine* 1994;19:1207–1212.
4. Hart LG, Deyo RA, Cherkin DC. Physician office visits for low back pain. *Spine.* 1995;20:11–19.
5. Williams PL, Warwick RW, Dyson M, et al. *Gray's Anatomy,* 37th ed. Edinburgh, Scotland: Churchill Livingstone; 1989.
6. Travell JG, Simon DG. *Myofascial Pain and Dysfunction: The Trigger Point Manual The Lower Extremities,* vol. II. Baltimore, MD: Williams & Wilkins; 1992.
7. Travell JG, Simon DG. *Myofascial Pain and Dysfunction: The Trigger Point Manual,* vol. 1. Baltimore, MD: Williams & Wilkins; 1999.
8. Hoppenfeld S, Hutton R. *Orthopaedic Neurology, A Diagnostic Guide to Neurologic Levels.* Philadelphia, PA: JB Lippincott Co; 1977.
9. Moore KL. *Clinical Oriented Anatomy,* 2nd ed. Baltimore, MD: Williams & Wilkins; 1985.
10. Warwick R, Peter WL. *Gray's Anatomy,* 35th British ed. Philadelphia, PA: WB Saunders; 1973:222.
11. Borenstein DJ, Wiesel SW. *Low Back Pain.* Philadelphia, PA: WB Saunders; 1989.
12. Glossary of osteopathic terminology. *AOA Yearbook and Directory,* 91st ed. Chicago, IL: American Osteopathic Association; 2000:869.
13. White AA, Panjabi MM. *Clinical Biomechanics of the Spine,* 2nd ed. Philadelphia, PA: JB Lippincott, 1990:45.
14. Borenstein DG, Wiesel SW. *Low Back Pain: Medical Diagnosis and Comprehensive Management.* Philadelphia, PA: WB Saunders; 1989.
15. Greenman PE. *Principles of Manual Medicine,* 2nd ed. Baltimore, MD: Williams & Wilkins; 1996.

THE ABDOMINAL REGION

RAYMOND J. HRUBY

KEY CONCEPTS

- Osteopathic historical perspective on the abdomen
- The abdominal region defined
- Functional anatomy
- Supportive evidence for the use of osteopathic manipulation in the treatment plan for abdominal disorders
- Osteopathic evaluation of the abdomen
- Osteopathic manipulative approaches and example techniques for the abdomen

HISTORICAL PERSPECTIVE AND SUPPORTIVE EVIDENCE

Osteopathic manipulative techniques can be used as part of a complete treatment approach to abdominal visceral problems. Such techniques have been part of osteopathic practice since the time of Andrew Taylor Still, the founder of osteopathic medicine. One early description of abdominal visceral treatment by Still is that of his first case of "flux," or dysentery, in a 4-year-old boy. He describes his examination of the child, noting that the child's back was hot while the abdomen was cold to the touch. In writing about his treatment, he states:

> I began at the base of the brain, and thought by pressures and rubbings I could push some of the hot to the cold places, and in so doing I found rigid and loose places on the muscles and ligaments of the whole spine, while the lumbar was in a very congested condition. I worked for a few minutes on that philosophy, and told the mother to report next day, and if I could do anything more for her boy I would cheerfully do so. She came early next morning with the news that her child was well (1).

Still described having treated many other similar cases with a high degree of success. His knowledge of the structure-function relationships involved with abdominal conditions was extensive enough to warrant an entire chapter of one of his books being devoted to this topic (2).

Other osteopathic physicians since the time of Still have promoted the use of osteopathic manipulative techniques directed toward the abdominal viscera. Hazzard described how to examine the abdomen, and discussed treatment approaches for various abdominal visceral diseases (3). Conrad (4) devoted a section of his book to diseases of the abdomen, specifically diseases of the stomach, intestines, liver, kidneys, and spleen. He described and illustrated specific osteopathic manual techniques for these organs. In a rather extensive treatise on the abdomen, McConnell (5) talked about the osteopathic approach from the ventral plane of the body, and described "ventral technique." Tender points, described as "gangliform contractions," were noted by Frank Chapman, DO, and came to be known as "Chapman's reflexes." The only known reference text on this topic was published by Owens (6).

In later years other osteopathic researchers published studies illustrating the use of osteopathic manipulative techniques for abdominal conditions. For example, Hermann (7) demonstrated that osteopathic manipulative treatment (OMT) prior to abdominal surgery greatly reduced the incidence of postoperative ileus. He also demonstrated that OMT could be successfully used to treat postoperative ileus when it did occur. In a recent study, Radjieski (8) demonstrated the use of OMT could significantly reduce the length of hospital stay in patients with acute pancreatitis.

Researchers in other health care professions have also noted the clinical relationship between the soma and the viscera. As an example, Pikalov (9) found using spinal manipulative techniques as part of the treatment plan for duodenal ulcer disease resulted in pain relief and clinical remission much sooner than conventional medical treatment alone. Travell and Simons (10) have noted that abdominal myofascial trigger points may produce visceral symptoms such as diarrhea, vomiting, belching, food intolerance, and infantile colic. Barral has published extensively on the use of manual techniques for treatment of the abdominal viscera (11,12). Other authors in this area include Finet (13) and Lossing (see Chapter 69).

Thus it becomes apparent that optimum treatment of abdominal visceral conditions requires an understanding of the underlying structure-function relationships and of the segmental viscerosomatic reflex phenomena that are involved. An understanding of osteopathic philosophy and principles, and the ability to use OMT as part of a complete treatment approach to abdominal disease, is one of the most unique characteristics of the osteopathic physician.

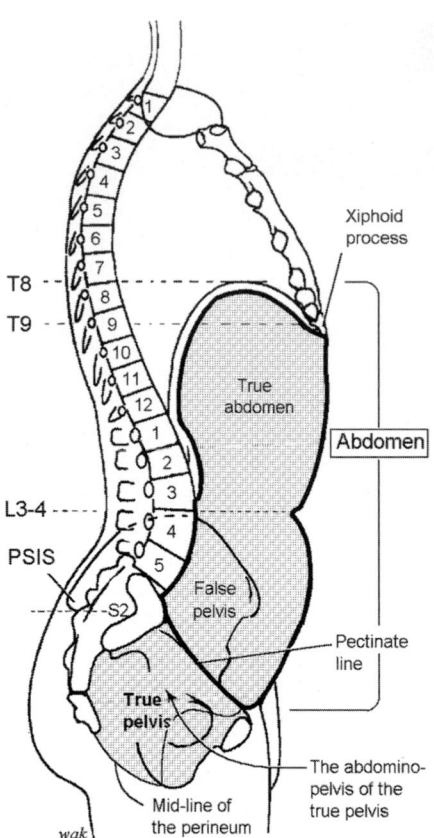

FIGURE 51.1. Boundaries and skeletal elements of the abdomen.

DEFINITION

The abdomen may be defined simply as the region of the trunk below the thoracic diaphragm. This area (Fig. 51.1) consists of two parts: an upper part, the *abdomen proper,* and a lower part, the *lesser pelvis* (14). These two areas are continuous at the plane of the inlet of the lesser pelvis. This inlet is bounded by the sacral promontory, the arcuate lines of the innominate bones, the pubic crests, and the upper border of the symphysis pubis.

FUNCTIONAL ANATOMY

The *abdomen proper* is bounded *superiorly* by the thoracolumbar diaphragm; *inferiorly* it becomes continuous with the pelvis or, as some anatomists describe it, the abdominopelvic portion of the abdominal cavity (15), by way of the superior aperture of the lesser or true pelvis. *Anteriorly* the abdomen is bounded by the abdominal muscles, which include the rectus abdominis, the pyramidales, the external obliques, the internal obliques, and the transversus abdominis. *Posteriorly* the abdomen is bounded by the lower thoracic and the lumbar vertebrae, the crura of the diaphragm, the psoas and quadratus lumborum muscles, and the posterior parts of the iliac bones.

The *lesser pelvis* or abdominopelvic portion of the abdomen is shaped somewhat like an inverted cone. Its *anterolateral* boundary consists of those parts of the hip bones below the arcuate lines and the pubic crests, and the obturator internus muscles; its

superior and dorsal boundary includes the sacrum, coccyx, and the piriformis and coccygeus muscles; and its *inferior* boundary includes the levator ani muscles and fascial coverings (which together form the pelvic diaphragm). For further information regarding the functional anatomy (skeletal, muscles and ligaments, vasculature and lymphatics, nerves) of the thoracic region, ribs, lumbar region, true pelvis, and the perineal region as related to the abdominal region see Chapters 48, 49, 50, and 52.

The abdominal structures of interest in this chapter are the stomach, small intestine, large intestine, liver, gallbladder, spleen, pancreas, kidney, parts of the ureters, suprarenal glands and numerous blood and lymph vessels, lymph nodes, and nerves. The lower ureters, the urinary bladder, and internal genitalia are not covered in this chapter. See Chapter 28 for discussion of these particular organs.

Skeletal

The skeletal elements of the abdomen are the lumbar vertebrae, the sacrum, coccyx, and the innominate bones (Fig. 51.1). Detailed descriptions of these skeletal elements are given in Chapters 48, 50, and 52.

Ligaments, Muscles, and Fasciae

As noted earlier, the muscles of the abdominal cavity include the rectus abdominis, the pyramidales, the external obliques, the internal obliques, and the transversus abdominis, along with the diaphragm, the psoas, and quadratus lumborum muscles.

The muscles of the abdominal region have associated fascial sheaths. The deep fascial layers have names associated with the various abdominal regions. Table 51.1 shows these fascial layers and their associated abdominal regions.

The *peritoneum* is a large serous membrane that consists of two layers: the *parietal* layer, which lines the abdominal wall, and a *visceral* layer, which is reflected over the abdominal viscera. The parietal peritoneum angles from the posterior wall of the abdomen to form very defined mesenteric connections to the abdominal viscera. These mesenteries carry the sympathetic and parasympathetic fibers and arteries to the viscera. They also carry visceral afferent fibers, veins, and lymphatic vessels away from the viscera. The visceral peritoneum is sensitive to stretch. It produces visceral pain only when the distention of the viscus exceeds the length of the visceral peritoneum on the outside of the mesentery.

The root of the mesentery for approximately 30 feet of small intestines is only 6 inches long and is located on the posterior wall

TABLE 51.1. ABDOMINAL REGIONS AND THEIR ASSOCIATED DEEP FASCIAL LAYERS

Region	Fascial Layer
Internal surface of the transversus abdominis	Transversalis fascia
Inferior surface of thoracolumbar diaphragm	Diaphragmatic fascia
Psoas and iliac areas	Iliac fascia
Anterior surface of the quadratus lumborum muscles	Anterior layer of the thoracolumbar fascia
Muscles of the pelvis	Pelvis fascia

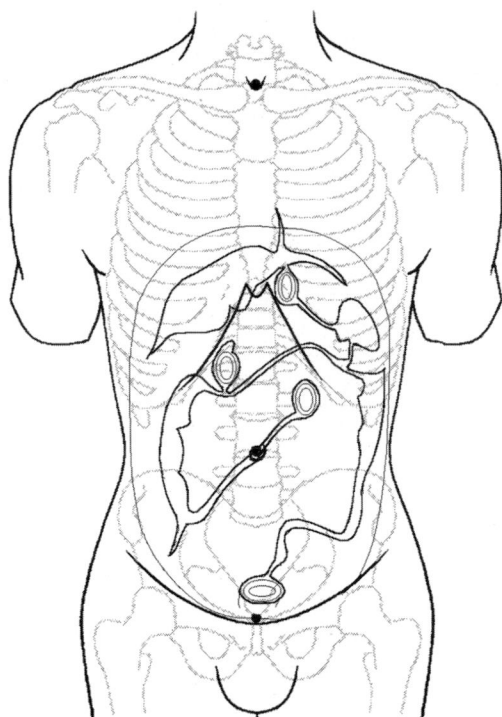

FIGURE 51.2. Roots of the abdominal mesenteries.

of the abdominal cavity, posterior to a point about 1 inch to the left of and 1 inch above the umbilicus (Fig. 51.2). The root of the mesentery runs inferolaterally to a second point just anterior to the right sacroiliac joint. Mental visualization of these mesenteries allows a physician to determine more accurately the origin of palpable masses and the origin of auscultated abnormal sounds. It is also important when performing visceral manipulation to free fascial pathways and improve visceral function.

Vasculature and Lymphatics

The thoracic aorta lies along the anterior and left anterolateral side of the thoracic vertebrae. It enters the abdominal cavity through the aortic hiatus in the abdominal diaphragm at the level anterior to the 12th thoracic vertebra. Here it becomes the abdominal aorta. Its main abdominal branches are the celiac, superior mesenteric, renal, and inferior mesenteric arteries.

Various small veins and plexuses in the pelvis eventually flow into the external and internal iliac veins. The two pairs of external and internal iliac veins unite to form the left and right common iliac veins, and these in turn unite to form the inferior vena cava, which conveys blood to the right atrium of the heart (Fig. 51.3). The veins that collect blood from the digestive tract, spleen, pancreas, and gallbladder join to form the portal vein. The portal vein carries blood to the liver, where this vein branches out into a series of very small vessels called sinusoids. From here, hepatic veins convey the blood to the inferior vena cava.

The left lymphatic duct (the thoracic duct) drains interstitial fluids from the lower extremities, the pelvic and abdominal viscera, the left arm, and the left side of the head (Fig. 51.4). It begins as the cisterna chyli, a 2-inch, yellowish, cylindrical struc-

ture that lies just to the left of the thoracolumbar junction at about the level of the first lumbar vertebra. It receives lymphatic vessels that drain interstitial fluids from all the abdominal organs, the pelvic organs, the lower extremities, and all of the superficial lymphatic vessels located below a horizontal plane of the body running through the umbilicus. The superficial lymphatic vessels drain lymph into superficial inguinal nodes. Lymph then travels into the deep nodes, the deep trunks along the common iliac arteries and the aorta, and finally into the cisterna chyli. It should be noted that lymph from the ovary, testicles, and prostate does not drain into the inguinal nodes but drains into the deep pelvic nodes.

Nerves

Primary sympathetic fibers for innervation of all organs below the diaphragm, except the descending colon and pelvic organs, pass from the intermediolateral cells in the thoracic spinal cord through the thoracoabdominal diaphragm. In the abdomen these primary fibers enter the celiac, superior mesenteric, and the inferior mesenteric collateral ganglia where they synapse (Fig. 51.5). Secondary or postganglionic fibers continue on to innervate specific groups of organs in the abdomen and pelvis. Parasympathetic innervation is supplied from the craniosacral outflow. All abdominal organs down to the midtransverse colon are supplied by the vagus nerve (cranial nerve X); the rest of the abdominal organs and all of the pelvic viscera receive their parasympathetic innervation from the pelvic splanchnic nerves (S2-4).

Visceral Pain

Visceral afferent impulses travel back to the cord using the same course used by the sympathetic efferent nerves to that organ (Fig. 51.6). This pain tends to be vague and gnawing, deep, poorly localized, and midabdominal.

Viscerosomatic Pain

Visceral afferent fibers from the root of the mesentery report to the somatic cord segment of that organ's sympathetic innervation. This type of sensory input produces the paraspinal tissue changes that help the physician to locate the viscus that is most likely dysfunctional. The tissue changes are *t*enderness, *a*symmetry, *r*ange of motion differences, and *t*issue texture changes (TART). The pain and tissue texture changes are primarily localized at the paraspinal level consistent with the organ's sympathetic innervation (Figs. 51.7 and 51.8).

Somatic Pain Caused by the Percutaneous Reflex of Morley

This type of somatic pain is usually located directly over the inflamed organ and is produced by direct contiguous irritation of the parietal peritoneum and the abdominal wall (Fig. 51.9). It is responsible for rebound tenderness and abdominal guarding associated with more severe abdominal pain.

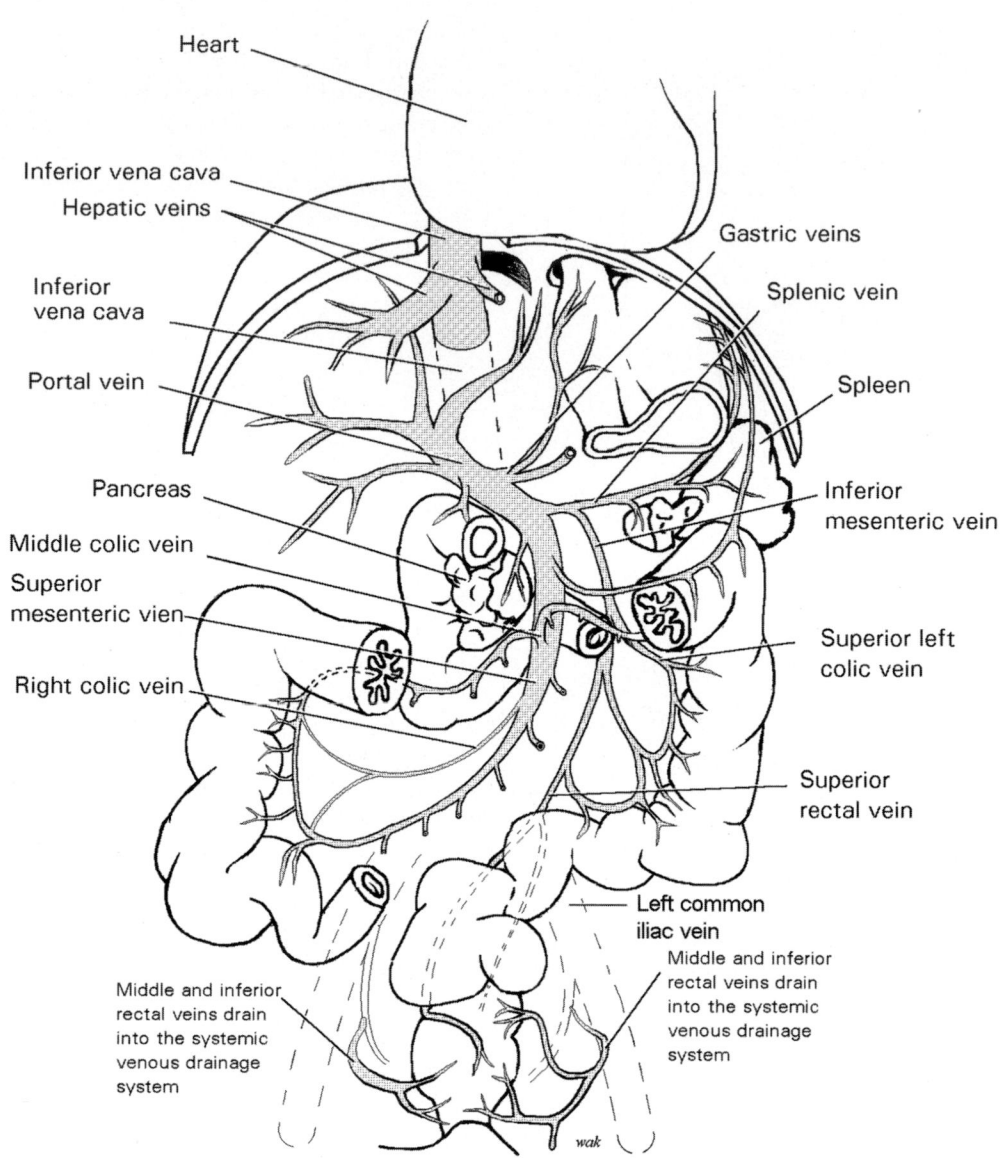

FIGURE 51.3. Venous drainage: portal venous system for the viscera.

TOPOGRAPHIC ANATOMY

There are certain surface landmarks of the abdomen that are palpable (16). These landmarks (Fig. 51.10) include the:

- Costal margins
- Xiphoid process
- Iliac crests
- Anterior superior iliac spines
- Pubic crests and tubercles
- Inguinal ligaments
- Umbilicus
- Linea alba

For purposes of locating abdominal structures and describing abnormalities, the abdomen is conventionally divided into four quadrants (Fig. 51.11). Another method divides the regions of the abdomen into nine sections (Fig. 51.12A). Either method may be used, although division into quadrants is most commonly seen.

The organs with which we are concerned in the abdomen are the following (Fig. 51.12B):

- Stomach
- Liver
- Gallbladder
- Pancreas
- Spleen
- Kidneys
- Urinary bladder
- Small intestine
- Colon
- Aorta and common iliac arteries

The adrenal glands are not palpable. The internal reproductive organs are considered in Chapters 28 and 31.

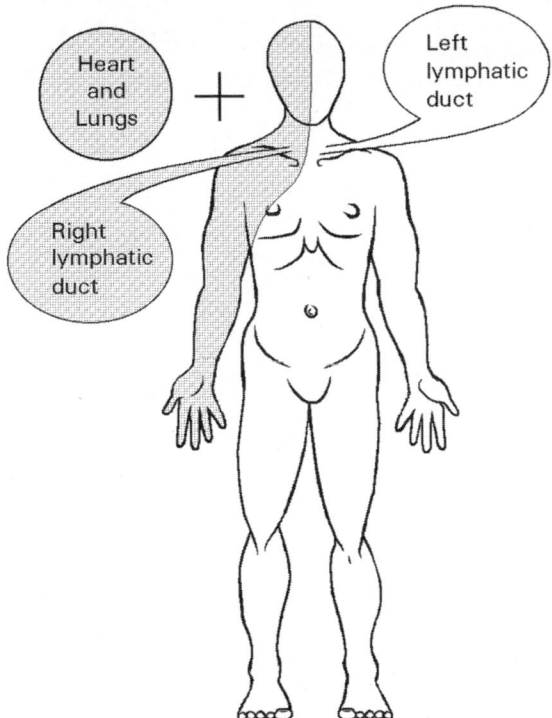

FIGURE 51.4. Main lymphatic ducts of the body.

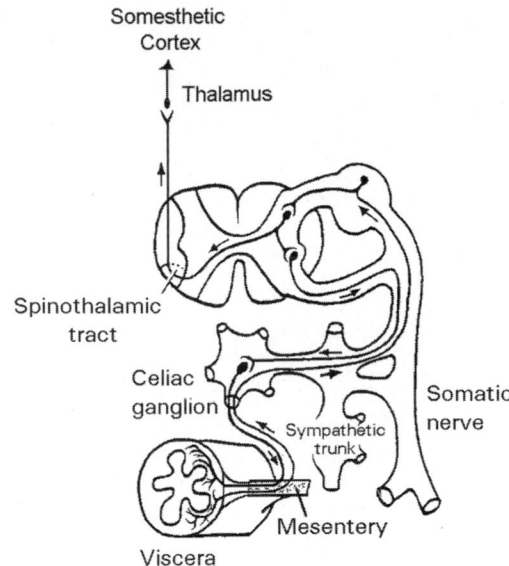

FIGURE 51.6. Neurologic pathway of visceral pain (afferent fibers).

DIAGNOSIS

Patient History

While beyond the scope of this chapter, it must be emphasized that a thorough history is a critical element in making a correct diagnosis of a patient's abdominal problem. The history should include at least the following information:

1. Chief complaint
2. History of the chief complaint
3. Past medical history
4. Past surgical history
5. Current medications
6. Nutritional history
7. Allergies
8. Family and social history
9. Review of systems

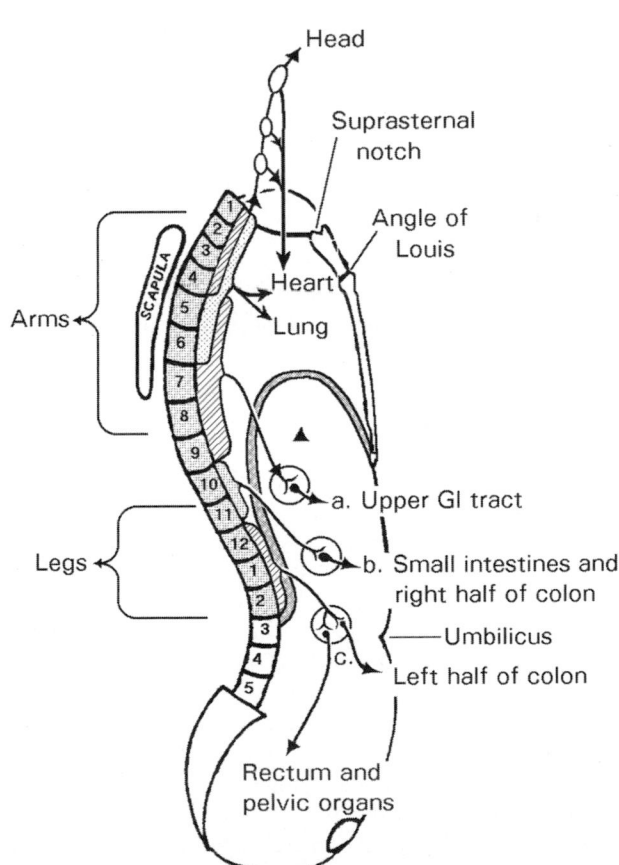

FIGURE 51.5. Primary sympathetic (efferent) nerves of the body.

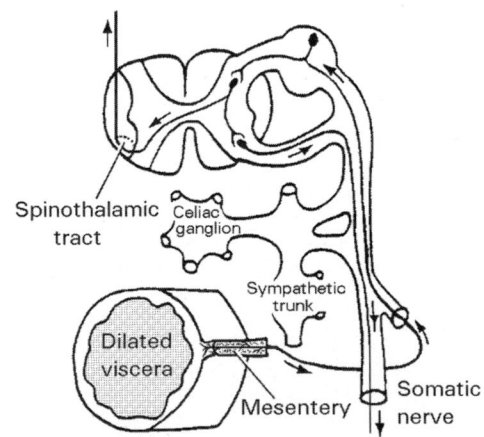

FIGURE 51.7. Neurologic pathway of viscerosomatic pain.

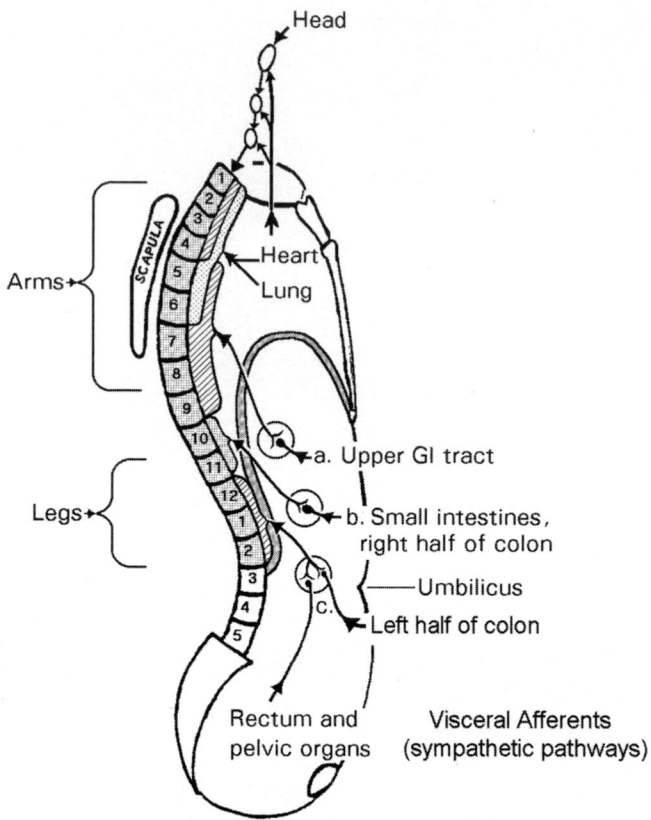

FIGURE 51.8. Visceral afferent fibers.

The reader is referred to standard textbooks on patient interviewing for more information on this topic.

Physical Examination

A complete physical examination is performed with special emphasis on regions that are spotlighted by the history or that might have functional association with the symptoms expressed by the patient. In this chapter, only the more important points as related to a patient with abdominal symptoms are considered.

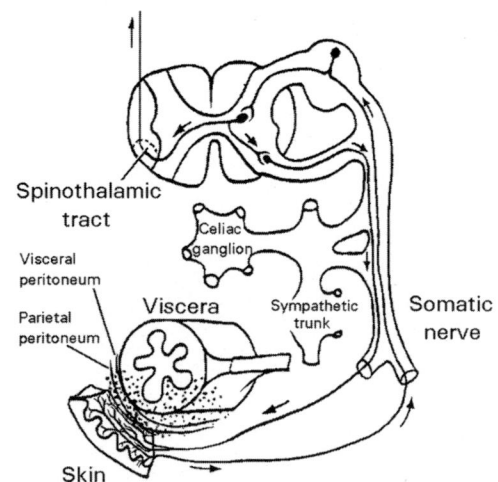

FIGURE 51.9. Neurologic pathway of pain from the percutaneous reflex of Morley.

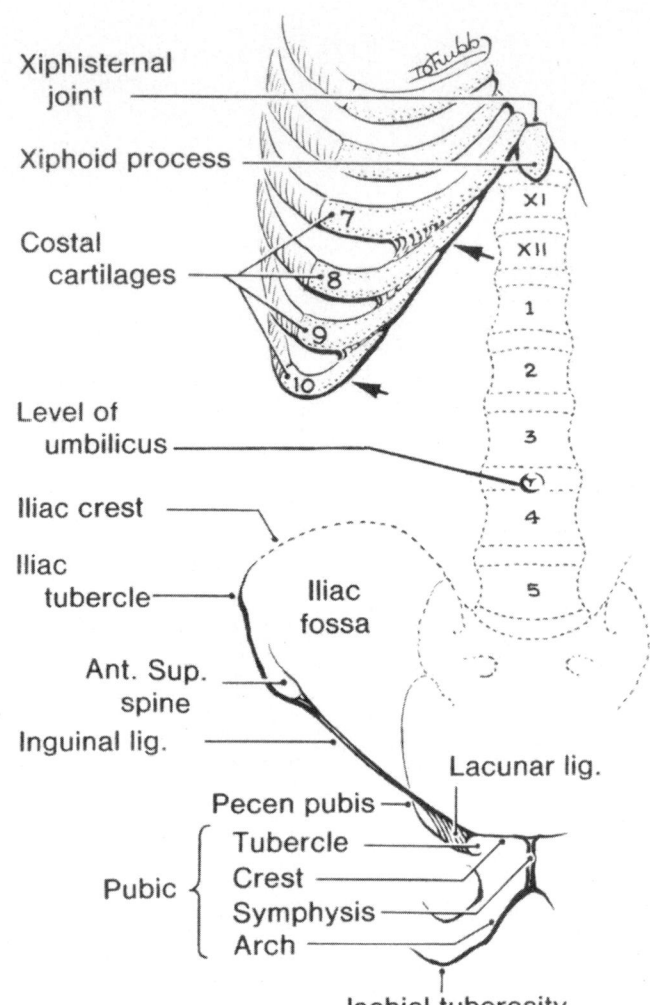

FIGURE 51.10. The abdominal landmarks.

General

Before beginning the abdominal examination, care must be taken to ensure that the patient is as relaxed as possible and in a comfortable position. The examination of the abdomen is commonly done with the patient in the supine position, resting comfortably on an examination table or bed. A pillow supports the patient's head; a patient with increased thoracic kyphosis may require more than one pillow for support of the head and shoulders. A pillow may be placed under the patient's knees for additional comfort. If orthopnea is present, raise and support the trunk with a back rest to relax the abdominal muscles (17). The patient should be draped in a manner that allows the abdomen to be exposed from the xiphoid region to the pubes. The examining room temperature should be adjusted for the patient's comfort, and the room should be adequately illuminated for the performance of the examination. The physician may stand on either side of the patient for the examination. The only instruments required for performing the abdominal examination are the physician's warm hands and warm stethoscope head. The examination should employ the methods of physical examination in the following sequence: observation, auscultation, palpation, and percussion.

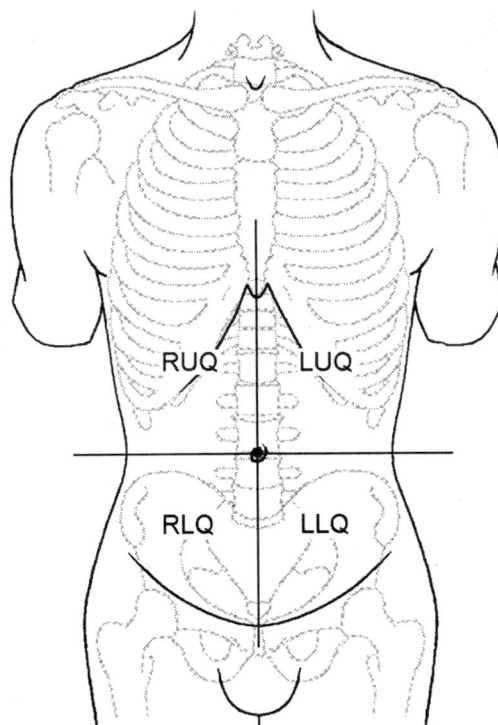

FIGURE 51.11. The four-quadrant abdomen.

The osteopathic physician includes examination for the elements of somatic dysfunction commonly noted by the TART acronym.

Observation

For this part of the examination, the examiner should be seated in a chair at the side of the patient so that the examiner's head is only slightly higher than the abdomen. Ideally, there should be a single source of light that shines across the patient's abdomen toward the examiner, or lengthwise over the patient (17). The abdomen is observed for the following:

1. Symmetry
2. Contour
3. Scars
4. Pulsations
5. Visible masses
6. Engorged veins
7. Visible peristalsis
8. Unusual pigmentation
9. Hair distribution
10. Distention

Auscultation

Auscultate the four quadrants of the abdomen to determine the presence, location, frequency, and pitch of peristaltic waves. This could reveal the intermittent, low-pitched, occasional slow gurgle that is normal, or the high-pitched, tinkling sounds of developing obstruction. Bowel sounds may be absent, indicating possible paralytic ileus. The midline of the abdomen between the xiphoid process and the umbilicus is auscultated for bruits. These could indicate an aneurysm and/or renal artery stenosis. The periumbilical region and the junction between the middle and outer two-thirds of the inguinal region are auscultated for a bruit that could be associated with a significant atherosclerosis of the common iliac or femoral artery.

Palpation

Palpation of the abdomen begins with a touch that is light yet firm, using the palmar surfaces of the approximated fingers to contact the abdominal wall. The physician lightly palpates each quadrant, checking for tenderness, any cutaneous or subcutaneous masses, and any unusual sensitivity. If the patient is apprehensive or is unable to relax during palpation of the abdomen, it is useful to ask the patient to flex his or her hips and knees in order to facilitate relaxation of the abdominal muscles.

During light palpation the physician can assess the abdominal wall for somatic dysfunction. Each quadrant of the abdomen can be palpated for abnormal myofascial tension, and the presence of tender points such as counterstrain points (see Chapter 63), Chapman reflex points (Fig. 51.13; also see Chapter 67), or Travell trigger points (see Chapter 66). One should note that Chapman reflex points related to abdominal visceral pathology are located next to the sternum in the intercostal spaces of ribs 5 through 11 and at the tip of rib 12.

After performing light palpation, the osteopathic physician proceeds to deep palpation of the abdomen. Each quadrant is examined for tenderness, masses, or enlarged organs. At this time the physician also assesses the deep fasciae and soft tissues of the abdomen, looking for abnormal tissue tensions that might indicate disturbance related to the collateral ganglia or mesenteries. The mobility and motility of the various abdominal organs may be assessed according to the theory and techniques described by Sutherland (18), Barral (11), and others (see Chapter 69).

Percussion

Percussion of the abdomen is more commonly performed in the asymptomatic patient, since, in the interest of patient comfort, painful conditions of the abdomen may preclude the use of percussion. Ordinarily percussion is used to outline the borders and help to determine the approximate size and position of solid organs, such as the liver, and hollow fluid-filled organs such as the urinary bladder. In general, the hollow viscera that occupy most of the abdomen contain gas and are usually resonant to percussion.

TREATMENT GOALS

As with OMT to any other body region, OMT should be applied to the abdominal region with specific goals in mind. The goals of treatment will vary with each individual patient. Some of these goals include:

- Addressing asymmetries, motion restrictions, and tissue texture abnormalities that are viscerosomatic reflections of homeostatic disturbances

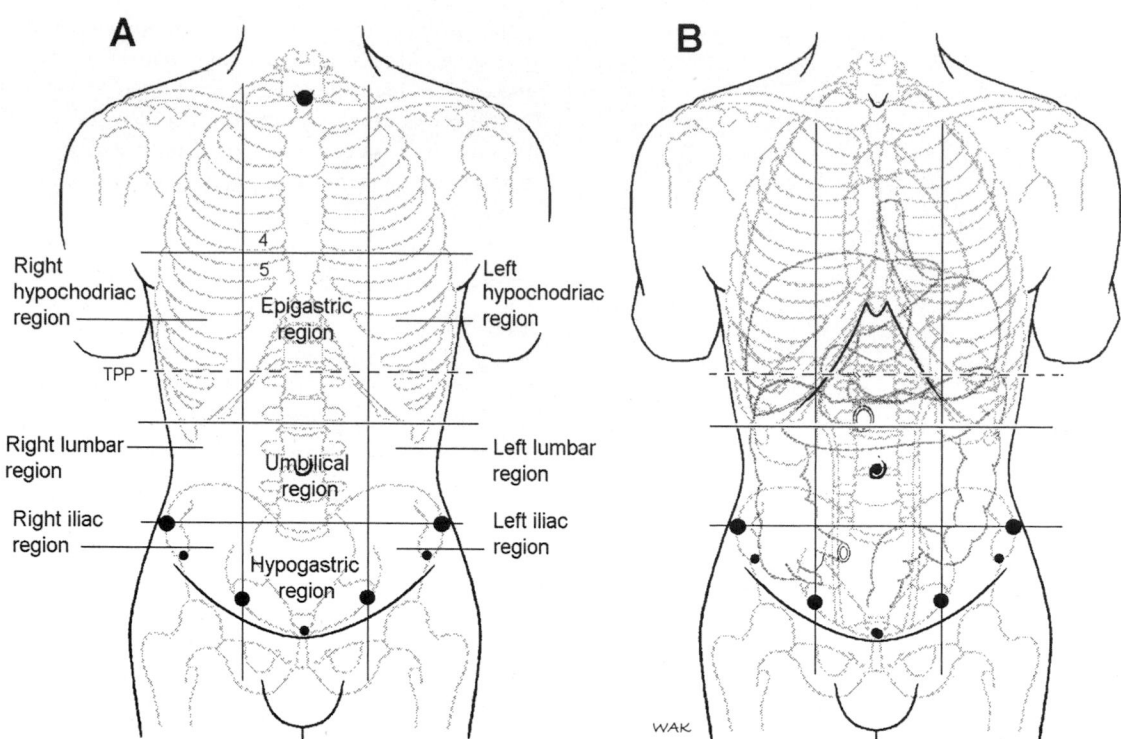

FIGURE 51.12. **A:** The nine-quadrant abdomen. **B:** Approximate location of visceral organs.

- Decreasing or eliminating pain
- Removing segmental motion restrictions
- Improving altered skeletal vertebral unit and myofascial motion arising from aberrant visceral and autonomic activity
- Decreasing or eliminating segmental facilitation
- Decreasing or eliminating trigger point and tender point activity
- Decreasing pathophysiologic musculoskeletal and neuroreflexive factors influencing circulation
- Enhancing musculoskeletal and neuroreflexive-mediated circulatory functions
- Improving organ function
- Altering any or all of the previously mentioned situations as either contributing to, or predictive of, future health problems

APPROACHES TO THE OSTEOPATHIC TREATMENT OF THE ABDOMEN

We may consider three ways to approach the abdomen in order to address structure-function relationships:

1. *From the back.* Any spinal somatic dysfunctions that may relate to an abdominal problem should be treated in order to improve spinal motion and therefore restore normal nerve function in segmentally related areas. This approach includes typical manipulative methods such as high velocity/low amplitude (HVLA), muscle energy, counterstrain, and others. Paraspinal rib raising and paraspinal inhibition are used effectively for treatment of sympathicotonia.

2. *From the periphery.* This approach includes such techniques as thoracic and pedal lymphatic pumps, diaphragmatic redoming, and thoracic inlet and pelvic diaphragm releases. These techniques are used to improve the ability to move fluids throughout the abdominal region, thus improving the delivery of oxygen, nutrients, and arterial blood to affected areas, and facilitating venous and lymphatic drainage for the removal of the waste products of cellular metabolism. This approach also includes the use of diagnostic Chapman reflexes and their soft tissue treatment, such as treatment of Chapman points for the large bowel that are located on the lateral thigh areas.

3. *Direct techniques to the abdomen.* These techniques are applied through the abdominal wall directly to collateral ganglia or the organs to be treated. These techniques are described in the following section.

It should be noted that, as in the approach to other structure-function relationships, these approaches are often used in combination with each other.

Paraspinal Inhibition

Follow the steps below for ileus prevention and treatment of sympathicotonia.

1. The patient is supine.
2. The physician is seated on either side of the patient.
3. The physician's hands are placed under the patient's thoracolumbar spine with the fingertips over the opposite side erector spinae tissues and the thenar and hypothenar eminences over the ipsilateral erector spinae tissues.

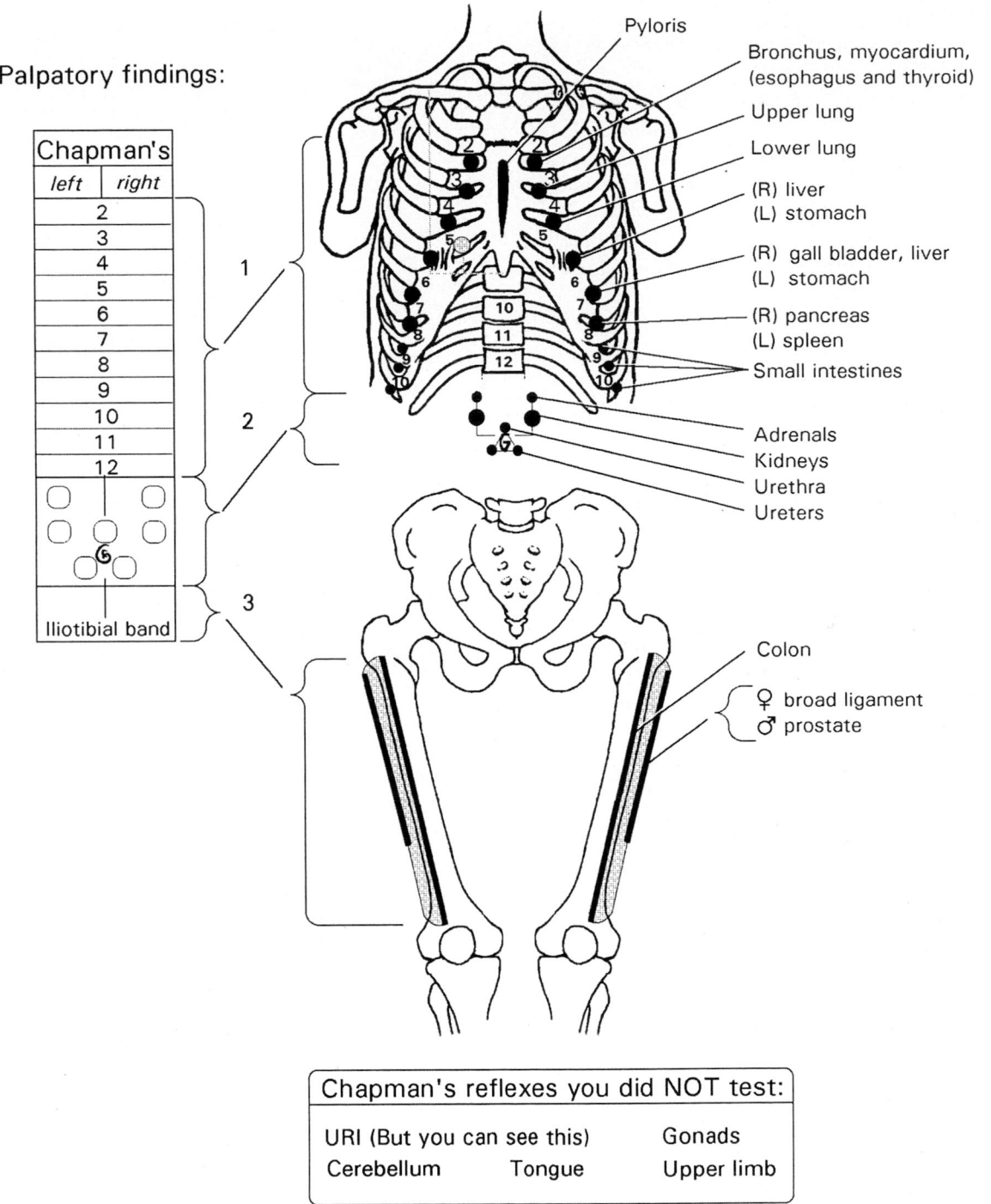

Palpatory findings:

Pyloris

Bronchus, myocardium, (esophagus and thyroid)

Upper lung

Lower lung

(R) liver
(L) stomach

(R) gall bladder, liver
(L) stomach

(R) pancreas
(L) spleen

Small intestines

Adrenals
Kidneys
Urethra
Ureters

Colon

♀ broad ligament
♂ prostate

Chapman's	
left	*right*
2	
3	
4	
5	
6	
7	
8	
9	
10	
11	
12	
Iliotibial band	

Chapman's reflexes you did NOT test:

URI (But you can see this)		Gonads
Cerebellum	Tongue	Upper limb

FIGURE 51.13. Thirty-second screening examination for Chapman reflex points.

4. The physician's fingers are flexed toward the base of the palms and the erector spinae masses are thus gently squeezed, approximating them, and effectively moving the thoracolumbar spine into extension.

5. The point of tissue tension balance or equalization is obtained by adjusting the pressure between the two hands to match the tension in the erector spinae tissues; the forearms can be moved closer to or farther away from the patient's body, if necessary, to equalize tissue tension.

6. Erector spinae tension is maintained until these muscles relax (usually 60 to 90 seconds).

7. The tension in the erector spinae tissues is reassessed.

8. Steps 2 through 5 are repeated until tissue tension is greatly reduced or eliminated.

Collateral Ganglia Inhibition

Follow the steps below for treatment of sympathicotonia.

1. The patient is supine.
2. The physician stands on either side of the patient, facing the patient's abdomen.
3. The length of the examining fingers are standardized by bending the longer fingers.
4. The skin over the celiac (then superior, then inferior) ganglion is contacted with the fingerpads and assessed for tenderness and tension in the soft subcutaneous tissues.
5. When an area of increased tissue tension is noted, the physician instructs the patient to inhale partially and hold their breath as long as possible.
6. When the patient exhales, the physician gently increases the pressure on the tissues as they relax, until the next restrictive barrier is met.
7. Repeat steps 5 and 6 until the tissue tension is greatly reduced or eliminated.

Falciform Ligament (Linea Alba) Release

To relieve fascial tension on the liver and relieve general mental tension, follow these steps:

1. The patient is supine.
2. The physician stands at the left side of the patient.
3. The physician places the fingerpads of both hands on the midline of the patient's abdomen. The physician's right fifth fingerpad is just below the xiphisternal joint.
4. The fingerpads are aligned so they are even in contact with the skin, each fingerpad with the same pressure.
5. The pressure of contact is gently increased, matching the tension of the soft tissues under the fingerpads along the linea alba or falciform ligament as the patient takes long, slow, deep breaths.
6. The pressure of contact is increased as the tissues permit and adjustments are made according to the patient's comfort level.
7. The technique is completed when there is no resistance felt in the soft tissues under the fingerpads.

Mesenteric Releases

To relieve mesenteric tension and thereby improve lymphatic drainage from and innervation and circulation to and from the viscera, follow these steps:

1. The patient is supine.
2. The physician stands at the patient's right side.
3. The physician contacts the mesentery to be treated (ascending colon, descending colon, sigmoid colon, root of the mesentery) with the ulnar edges of their fingers (not the fingerpads).
4. The intestine is gently moved at right angles to the attachment of its mesentery (ascending colon and descending colon are moved medially toward the umbilicus; the sigmoid colon and the root of the mesentery are moved in a diagonal line from the lower left abdominal quadrant toward the upper right abdominal quadrant (Fig. 51.14).

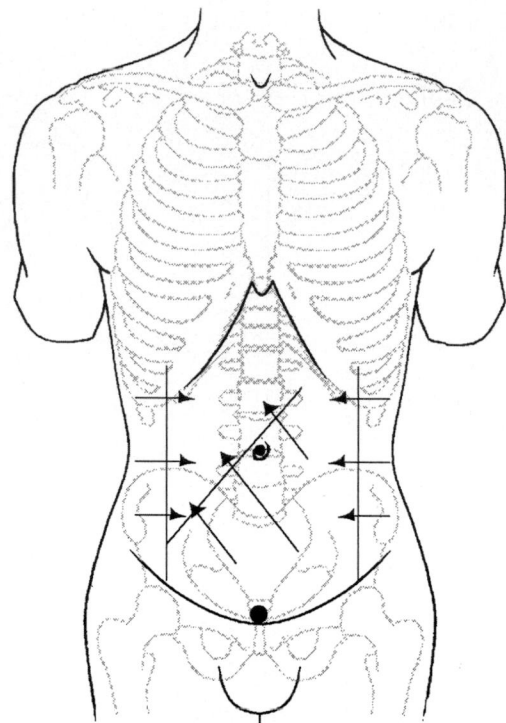

FIGURE 51.14. Direction of hand movement for treatment of abdominal mesenteries.

5. The mesentery to be treated is moved gently until resistance to motion is felt.
6. The patient takes a partial breath in and holds it as long as possible.
7. As the patient exhales, the physician increases the pressure on the tissues until the next restrictive barrier is met.
8. Steps 2 through 5 are repeated until the colon feels compliant to mobility testing.

A variation on this technique is as follows:

9. The tissues are moved only a few centimeters until resistance is felt, then the colon is allowed to recede (recoil).
10. This process is repeated three to four times until the colon feels compliant to mobility testing.

CONCLUSION

One should not forget that somatic dysfunction may be present with abdominal visceral conditions. Optimum treatment of these conditions should be based on osteopathic philosophy and principles, and should include appropriate OMT. Using osteopathic manipulation as part of a complete treatment approach to the patient with an abdominal visceral disorder serves several purposes. It provides a more holistic, total body approach to the treatment of a patient's medical problems, it addresses important structure-function relationships, and it helps to optimize the patient's self-healing and self-regulatory mechanisms.

REFERENCES

1. Still AT. *Autobiography of A. T. Still.* Published by the author, Kirksville, MO; 1897.

2. Still AT. *The Philosophy and Mechanical Principles of Osteopathy.* Kansas City, MO: Hudson-Kimberly Publishing Company; 1902.

3. Hazzard C. *The Practice and Applied Therapeutics of Osteopathy.* Kirksville, MO: The Journal Printing Company; 1901.

4. Conrad CF. *A Manual of Osteopathy,* 4th ed. New York, NY: The University Book Company; 1919.

5. McConnell CP. *Ventral Technique.* Indianapolis, IN: The American Academy of Osteopathy; Yearbook; 1951.

6. Owens C. *An Endocrine Interpretation of Chapman's Reflexes.* Carmel, CA: Reprinted by the American Academy of Osteopathy; 1932.

7. Hermann E. *The DO.* 1965(Oct):163–164.

8. Radjieski JM, Lumley MA, Canteri MS. Effect of osteopathic manipulative treatment on length of stay for pancreatitis: a randomized pilot study. *JAOA.* 1998;98:15.

9. Pikalov AA, Kharin VV. Use of spinal manipulative therapy in the treatment of duodenal ulcer: a pilot study. *JMPT.* 1994;17:5.

10. Travell JG, Simons DG. *Myofascial Pain and Dysfunction: The Trigger Point Manual.* Baltimore: Williams & Wilkins; 1983.

11. Barral JP, Mercier P. *Visceral Manipulation.* Seattle, WA: Eastland Press; 1988.

12. Barral JP. *Visceral Manipulation II.* Seattle, WA: Eastland Press; 1989.

13. Finet G. Wiallame C. *Treating Visceral Dysfunction.* Portland, OR: Stillness Press; 2000.

14. Williams PL, Warwick R, eds. *Gray's Anatomy.* Philadelphia, PA: WB Saunders; 1980:1319.

15. Spraycar M, ed. *Stedman's Medical Dictionary,* 26th ed. Baltimore, MD: Williams & Wilkins; 1999:1.

16. Willms JL, Schneiderman H, Algranati PS. *Physical Diagnosis.* Baltimore. MD: Williams & Wilkins; 1994:347.

17. DeGowin EL, DeGowin RL. *Bedside Diagnostic Examination.* New York, NY: Macmillan; 1969:452.

18. Sutherland WG. In: Wales AL, ed. *Teachings in the Science of Osteopathy.* Fort Worth, TX: The Sutherland Cranial Teaching Foundation; 1990.

PELVIS AND SACRUM

KURT P. HEINKING
ROBERT E. KAPPLER

KEY CONCEPTS

- Functional anatomy of the pelvic girdle
- Motion and dysfunction of innominates, pubes, and sacrum
- Diagnosis and history of pelvic region
- Motion testing of pelvic region, including special tests
- Pelvic diagnoses and causes of sacroiliac dysfunction

Accurate and efficient diagnosis of the pelvic girdle is of great importance to practitioners of manual medicine. The pelvis holds a central role in coupling the mechanical forces of the lower extremities with the axial skeleton above, as it is the foundation for body support and locomotion. Alterations and restrictions of motions in the pelvic girdle may have a profound effect on vertebral function, the thoracoabdominal diaphragm, and the urogenital diaphragm. Alterations in the biomechanical function of the pelvic girdle can also influence the craniosacral mechanism and vice versa. The pelvis functions in reproduction and elimination of wastes and is the site of parasympathetic innervation to the left colon and pelvic organs. Somatic dysfunction of the pelvic girdle may be causative, contributory, or diagnostic for a wide range of patient complaints. Such complaints may be somatic, visceral, or emotional in nature. The role of manual medicine in the management of the pelvic girdle is the restoration of functional symmetry between the arthrodial, neural, vascular, lymphatic, and connective tissue elements.

FUNCTIONAL ANATOMY

Skeletal/Ligamentous Anatomy

The pelvis consists of three bones and three joints forming an open ring shape. The false pelvis is a part of the lower abdomen and is walled laterally by ilia. The true pelvis is located inferior and posterior to the abdomen. It begins at the level of the sacral promontory, arcuate line, pectinate line, and pubic bones, ending with the inferior fascia of the pelvic diaphragm.

In the past the hip bones were referred to as the innominate bones because each was composed of three bones joined together at the acetabular notch. Initially there is a single cartilaginous model for the entire element, and the ischium, ilium, and pubis are the primary ossification centers before birth. Epiphyseal centers form in the cartilaginous iliac crest, anterior superior iliac spine, and ischial tuberosity (at puberty) and eventually fuse in the late teens or early 20s. The only remnants of the original cartilaginous model are the bilateral sacroiliac joints.

The three joints of the pelvis include the symphysis pubis and the two sacroiliac joints. The sacrum is attached to the lumbar vertebra by a lumbosacral disc, two lumbosacral synovial joints, and ligaments. Anomalous development commonly results in asymmetric lumbosacral facets (facet tropism) and, less commonly, incomplete separation and differentiation of the fifth lumbar vertebrae (sacralization). When the transverse processes of the fifth lumbar vertebra are atypically large, a pseudoarthrosis may occur with the sacrum or ilia(um). When this occurs bilaterally, it is termed a bat-wing deformity.

The acetabulum occupies the lateral aspect of the ilium and articulates with the head of the femur to create the hip joint. The two innominates are joined anteriorly by the symphysis pubis and cephalically with the sacrum via the bilateral sacroiliac joints. The female pelvis is less robust than the male pelvis, with smaller weightbearing areas and less height. The female pelvis grows more rapidly in transverse dimensions during adolescence. This growth leads to a larger, more rounded pelvic inlet and outlet, a larger infrapubic angle, and a greater distance between the ischial tuberosities and the coccyx. Functionally, each innominate can be viewed as a lower extremity bone; and the sacrum, as a component part of the vertebral axis.

The pubic symphysis is a fibrocartilaginous joint that has motion determined by its anatomic shape, ligaments, and muscular attachments. Muscular forces acting on each pubic ramus can cause rotation upon each other at the symphysis, about a transverse axis.

The sacrum is shaped like an inverted triangle with the superior aspect being the base and the inferior aspect being the apex. The most anterior and superior portion of the first sacral vertebral body is called the sacral promontory. The anterior surface is concave, and the posterior surface is convex with palpable spinous tubercles. The medial row of tubercles is formed by fusion of the sacral articular processes. The lateral row is formed by the fusion of sacral transverse processes and inferiorly ends in a curve of

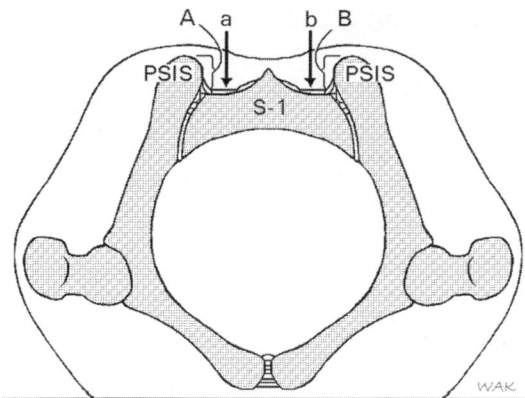

FIGURE 52.1. Cross-section of pelvis. Differential static landmarks for determining sacral sulcus depth *(A and B)* versus sacral base anterior or posterior *(a and b)*. (Illustration by W.A. Kuchera.)

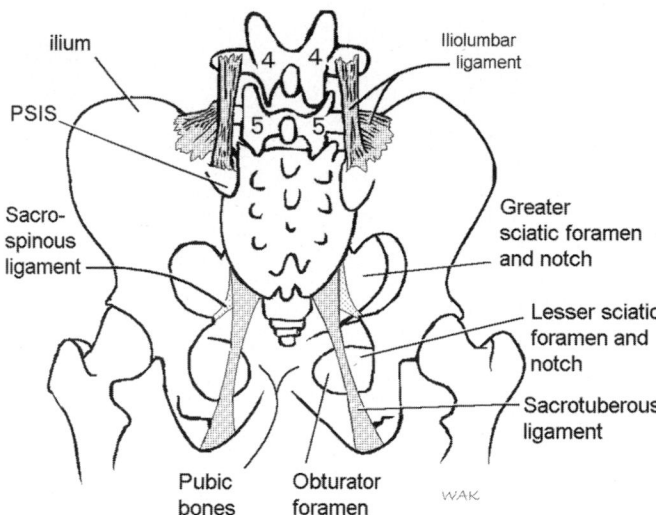

FIGURE 52.2. Pelvic ligaments and foramen. (Modified from Kuchera WA, Kuchera ML. *Osteopathic Principles in Practice*, 2nd ed. rev. Columbus, OH: Greyden Press; 1994.)

the bone called the inferolateral angle. The sacrum contains the sacral canal and four bilateral sacral foramina for the passage of the ventral and dorsal rami of the first four sacral spinal nerves. The sacral hiatus is a defect near the apex, formed by a failure of laminal closure of the fifth sacral vertebra. It is at this location that sacral epidural nerve blocks are performed. The coccyx attaches to the sacral apex via the sacrococcygeal joint. The ganglion impar (where the right and left sympathetic chains join) rests on the anterior surface of the coccyx.

The sacroiliac joints have been described as L- or C-shaped and are contoured with a shorter upper arm and longer lower arm, with the junction occurring approximately at S2. The apex, or junction of the two arms of the sacroiliac joint, points anteriorly. The sacroiliac articulation is typically convex at the upper arm and concave at the lower arm. The sacroiliac joints converge inferiorly and posteriorly. The lumbosacral facets are predominantly coronal with the surface of the inferior lumbar facet slanting posteriorly. The sacral sulcus (Fig. 52.1) is a palpable groove just medial to the posterior superior iliac spine. Much variation exists between anatomic description and an individual patient's anatomy. Weisl's work (1) demonstrates the varying contours of the articular surfaces of the sacrum and the ilia at their articulation with each other.

The sacrum is suspended between the innominate bones by three true and three accessory ligaments. The true pelvic ligaments include the anterior sacroiliac ligaments, interosseous sacroiliac ligaments, and posterior sacroiliac ligaments. The accessory pelvic ligaments include the sacrotuberous, sacrospinous, and iliolumbar ligaments. The iliolumbar ligaments attach from the anterior surface of the iliac crest and the anterior surface of the sacral base to the transverse processes of L4 and L5 (Fig. 52.2).

The lower fibers blend in with the anterior sacroiliac ligament, thus integrating sacroiliac mechanics with the lumbar spine. There are anterior and posterior portions to the sacroiliac ligaments. The anterior ligaments are flat bands, while the posterior ligaments are thicker with multiple layers (2). The bilateral sacrotuberous ligaments run from the inferior medial border of the sacrum and insert on the ischial tuberosities and the posterior margins of the sciatic notches. The bilateral sacrospinous

ligaments lie anterior to the sacrotuberous ligaments and attach to the ischial spines, dividing this space into a greater and a lesser sciatic foramen (Fig. 52.2).

The sacrospinous and sacrotuberous ligaments restrain the anterior movement of the sacrum within the pelvic bones. The anterior, posterior, and interosseous ligaments restrain the posterior, lateral, and axial rotation movements. No muscles are specific for the movement of the sacroiliac joints. Motion at the sacroiliac joints results from actions of muscles that function to move the back or legs (3).

In the weightbearing position, without strong pelvic ligaments, the sacral base tends to rock anteriorly. The downward effects of gravity, combined with environmental and genetic factors, can stress the tensile strength of these ligaments. These ligamentous stresses can create lumbosacral imbalance, chronic back pain, and joint degeneration. The iliolumbar ligament is prone to irritation by lumbosacral instability. When an iliolumbar ligament becomes irritated, its attachments to the crest and transverse processes of L4-5 become tender to palpation. Pain may be referred to the groin via the ilioinguinal nerve, mimicking the pain felt in an inguinal hernia. Palpatory diagnosis should therefore always include ligamentous attachments (Fig. 52.3).

Muscles and Connective Tissue

Muscles and connective tissue of the thoracoabdominal wall aid in coordinating movements and pressures between the thoracic cage and the pelvic girdle. Muscles acting on or through the pelvis can be classified as primary (intrinsic muscles of the pelvic diaphragm) and secondary (muscles considered to have partial attachment to the true pelvis).

PRIMARY MUSCLES

Primary muscles and connective tissue intrinsic to the pelvic girdle include the pelvic and urogenital diaphragms. The pelvic

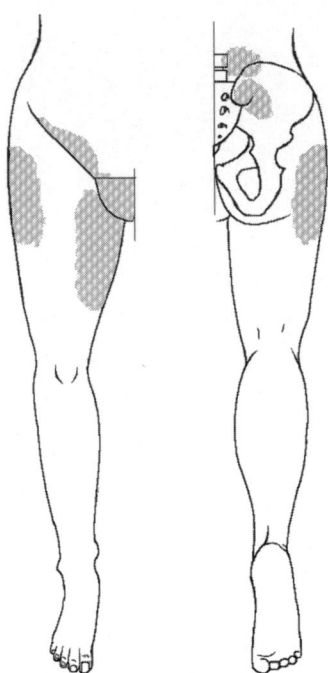

FIGURE 52.3. Pain referral pattern from iliolumbar ligament. (Modified from George S. Hackett, MD.)

diaphragm consists of the levator ani and coccygeus muscles, which form a basin, supporting the pelvic viscera and closing the pelvic outlet. The urogenital diaphragm spans the area between the ischiopubic rami and is formed by the deep transverse perineal and sphincter urethrae muscles and their fasciae. The pelvic diaphragm slants downward from the lateral wall to the midline perineal structures while the urogenital diaphragm is rather level. This creates a small potential fingerlike space (ischiorectal fossa) on either side superior to the urogenital diaphragm and inferior to the pelvic diaphragm, which may provide an anterior avenue for the spread of perineal infections.

SECONDARY MUSCLES

Secondary muscles include:

- Rectus abdominis
- Transverse abdominis
- Internal and external oblique
- Quadratus lumborum

The external abdominal oblique muscle forms the inguinal ligament as it courses between the anterior superior iliac spine and the pubic tubercle.

The lower extremity may influence the pelvic girdle through its musculature and connective tissue. The anterior and medial compartments of the thigh may affect iliac and pubic motion and contain the following muscles:

- Quadriceps femoris
- Sartorius
- Gracilis
- Adductor group

The iliopsoas may also be considered with this group. The deep fascia of the thigh (fascia lata) is continuous with the superficial thoracolumbar fascia of the thorax and splits to form the compartments of the lower extremity. Dysfunction of muscles or fascia of the posterior compartment or gluteal region may affect function of the pelvic girdle. These muscles include:

- Glutei maximus, medius, and minimus
- Piriformis
- Obturator externus
- Superior and inferior gemelli
- Biceps femoris
- Semimembranosus
- Semitendinosus

Collectively, the muscles of the gluteal region, the quadratus femoris and the iliopsoas, comprise the rotator cuff of the hip (Fig. 52.4).

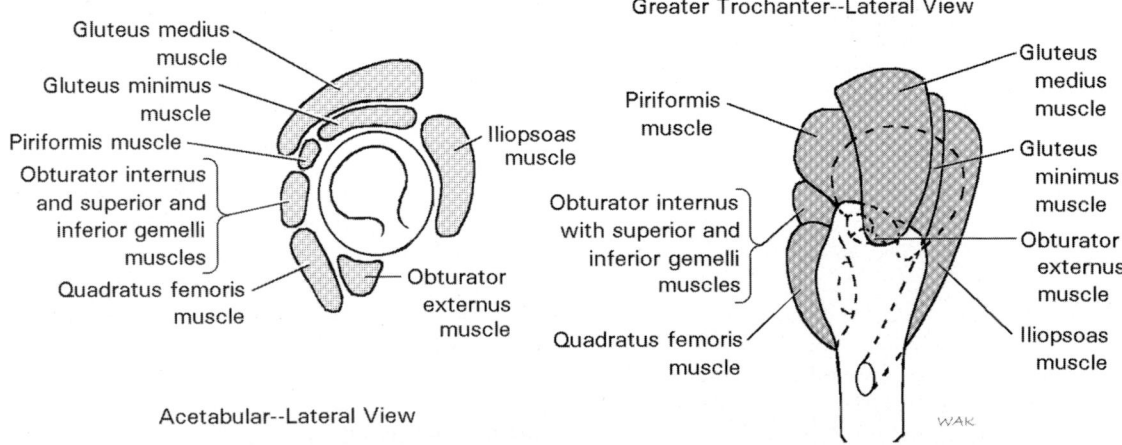

FIGURE 52.4. Rotator cuff muscles of right hip. (Modified from Kuchera WA, Kuchera ML. *Osteopathic Principles in Practice.* 2nd ed. rev. Columbus, OH: Greyden Press; 1994.)

The structure of the pelvic girdle and its function are intimately interrelated. The true pelvis is situated like a cul-de-sac or diverticulum off from the false pelvis and is not in the main stream of lymphatic flow from the legs to the abdomen. The pelvic diaphragm does not rhythmically contract, but when relaxed, it works synchronously with the abdominal diaphragm. This synchronous movement with the abdominal diaphragm preserves interstitial fluid homeostasis in the true pelvic region. A relaxed pelvic diaphragm is absolutely necessary for the efficient movement of lymphatic fluids away from the pelvis and perineal tissues.

Somatic dysfunction of the symphysis pubis or disturbed ilioilial mechanics (asymmetry of the relationship between the two innominates) can place asymmetric tensions on the pelvic and urogenital diaphragms. These tensions may result in tension myalgia of the pelvic floor, low back pain, dyspareunia, and painful defecation with associated constipation (4). Appropriate pelvic musculoskeletal performance is essential for adequate bladder functioning. Tension on the pubovesicular and puboprostatic fascia from innominate dysfunction (especially pubic shears and compressions) may produce urinary tract symptoms such as burning, frequency, fullness, and a weak stream. Such tensions on the inguinal ligament from disturbed ilioiliac mechanics can affect the lateral femoral cutaneous nerve, resulting in anterior thigh pain.

Dysfunction of any of the abdominal muscles or their fasciae may disturb respiratory excursion, compromising the intraabdominal pressure changes that promote lymphatic and venous return. The thoracolumbar and lumbosacral fasciae contribute to the origin of the internal abdominal oblique and the transverse abdominis muscles. Fascial restrictions in these areas can restrict both thoracolumbar and sacral motion. The inner membranous layer of the superficial thoracolumbar fascia (Scarpa) attaches to the iliac crest and pubic symphysis. It is continuous with the fascia of the thigh inferior to the inguinal ligament (fascia lata), the posterior perineal membrane, and the tunica dartos scrota. Fascial restrictions along its course may affect the thigh, perineum, or abdomen, as fluid collections can traverse along these planes.

Dysfunction of the rectus femoris and the ipsilateral adductor group may cause an anterior rotation of the innominate and inferior shear at the pubes. Adductor dysfunction may be related to reflex changes at the ipsilateral iliolumbar ligament, while a pubic shear may affect the pelvic and urogenital diaphragms. Gait may be affected by lumbosacral somatic dysfunction, affecting the superior gluteal nerve (L4-5, S1) and the gluteus medius and minimus. Piriformis hypertonicity related to sacral somatic dysfunction may produce benign sciatica. Hamstring tension may cause a posterior rotation of the innominate and affect pelvic mechanics. Female patients under the influence of hormonal and structural changes during pregnancy, which shifts the center of gravity, are prone to pelvic somatic dysfunction.

Vascular/Lymphatic Anatomy

Following the bifurcation of the abdominal aorta at the approximate level of the umbilicus, the right and left common iliac arteries diverge and descend to the lumbosacral junction. Here they divide into the internal and external iliac arteries. The internal iliac arteries have two trunks that supply the pelvic viscera, perineum, and gluteal region. The proximal anterior trunk supplies the urinary bladder, uterus, vagina, and rectum. Distally the artery branches into the internal pudendal artery, supplying the genitalia and perineum, and the inferior gluteal artery, supplying the gluteal region. The posterior trunk contains the iliolumbar, lateral sacral, and superior gluteal arteries collectively supplying the intrinsic muscles of the pelvis, the sacrum, and the superior gluteal region.

Veins of the pelvic girdle form venous plexi encircling the pelvic organs and the sacrum and generally following the arterial distribution. The rectal venous plexus communicates with the portal system via the superior rectal vein, which is valveless (Fig. 52.5).

Lymphatic drainage from the pelvic girdle generally follows the corresponding arteries. Lymphatic flow from the lower extremities and pelvic viscera (apart from the gut) passes through the pelvic girdle, terminating ultimately in the lateral aortic groups.

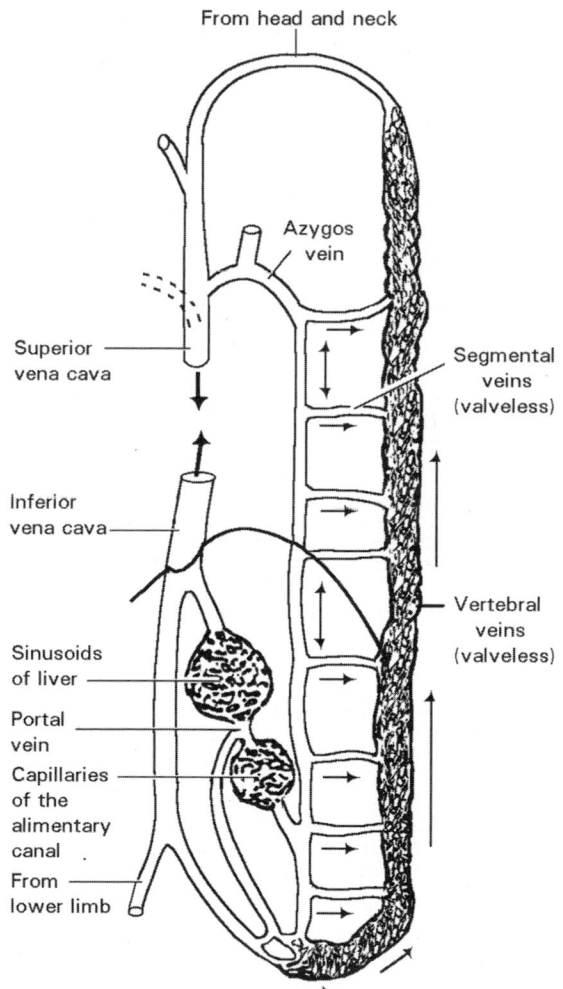

FIGURE 52.5. Valveless vertebral venous plexus. (Illustration by W.A. Kuchera; adapted from G. Zink.)

Organs and tissues drained by these groups include:

- Testes
- Ovaries
- Fallopian tubes
- Uterus
- Kidneys
- Ureters
- Posterior abdominal, pelvic, and perineal walls

Lymph from the remaining viscera (bladder) and gluteal region passes initially to regional nodes along the internal iliac arteries. The external genitalia drain to the inguinal nodes and then deeper into the external iliac and the intermediary lumbar groups.

Lymphatic drainage of the rectum and anal canal is unique in that, above the pectinate line, lymph follows a deep course to the internal iliac nodes and preaortic nodes. Below the pectinate line, the lymph drains superficially to the inguinal nodes. As lymph flows through a number of intermediary groups in the lumbar region, on up to the cisterna chyli and thoracic duct, the diameter of the thoracic duct and lymphatic channels is under sympathetic control similar to blood vessels. Hypersympathetic activity can reduce lymphatic flow capacity. Accumulation of pelvic lymph may occur in the preaortic, lateral aortic, or retroaortic lymph node groups. Peripherally compromised lymphatic drainage has been linked to the pathogenesis of atherosclerosis and to the development of hypertension (5). Correction of pelvic girdle dysfunction may allow improved lymphaticovenous return, blood flow, and gait for a patient whose activities of daily living are already compromised by a cardiovascular condition.

Nerves

The nervous system may influence the pelvic girdle through one of four areas. These are the:

- Lumbar plexus
- Sacral plexus
- Coccygeal plexus
- Autonomic nerves of the pelvis

The lumbar plexus lies between the anterior and posterior masses of the psoas major, anterior to the transverse processes of the lumbar vertebrae. The plexus is formed by the contributions of the ventral rami from T12 to L4 with only partial contributions from T12. The lumbar plexus gives motor supply to muscles in the abdomen and thigh, which act on the pelvic girdle. These muscles include the:

- Psoas major and minor
- Iliacus
- Pectineus
- Internal abdominal oblique
- Transverse abdominis
- Quadriceps group
- Adductor group
- Sartorius
- Gracilis

The lumbar plexus also supplies sensation to the thigh, buttocks, lower abdomen, and pubic area.

The sacrum contains sacral foramen for passage of the sacral nerve roots, which exit anteriorly and posteriorly. The lumbosacral trunk (ventral rami of L4 and L5), the first three sacral ventral rami, and a portion of the fourth form the sacral plexus. The ventral rami divide into anterior and posterior branches. The anterior branch forms anterior nerves that innervate the flexors and adductors; the posterior branch forms posterior nerves that innervate the extensors and abductors. The sacral plexus also has motor and sensory innervations in the pelvis and lower extremities and contains parasympathetic fibers (S2, S3, S4) for innervation of the left colon and pelvic organs. The muscular branches include the:

- Sciatic
- Pudendal
- Superior gluteal
- Inferior gluteal
- Smaller muscular branches

The cutaneous innervation is through the posterior femoral cutaneous nerve.

The sciatic nerve is a muscular branch of the sacral plexus composed of fibers from the ventral rami of L4-S3. Pathology at the L4-5 or L5-S1 level is the usual cause of nerve root compression, as it is uncommon within the sacrum. The sciatic nerve is closely associated with the piriformis muscle. Eighty-five percent of the time the sciatic nerve passes through the greater sciatic notch just inferior to the piriformis; it passes through the muscle in less than 1% of the population. Since injections are sometimes given in myofascial trigger points when the muscle is spastic, it is important to realize that more than 10% of the time the peroneal portion of the sciatic nerve passes through the muscle, and in 2% to 3% of instances it exits above the piriformis and passes posterior to the piriformis muscle (6) (Fig. 52.6). Piriformis hypertonicity can cause sciatica. Evidence indicates that this may not be due to pressure but to a chemical reaction that irritates peroneal fibers of the sciatic nerve. For this reason there is referred pain down the posterior thigh but not past the knee.

The coccygeal plexus is located on the pelvic surface of the coccygeus muscle and formed by the coccygeal nerve with contributions from S4 and S5. This plexus gives rise to the anococcygeal nerve that pierces the sacrotuberous ligament to supply the skin over the coccyx. The autonomic nerves of the pelvis include the sacral sympathetic trunks, the parasympathetic nerves of the pelvic splanchnics, and the inferior hypogastric plexus. The right and left sacral sympathetic trunks are extensions of the lumbar sympathetic chain ganglia and are located on the ventral surface of the sacrum medial to the sacral foramina. They contain four or five ganglia and eventually fuse over the coccyx to form the single ganglion impar. The sacral sympathetic trunks have gray rami communicantes that follow the sacral and coccygeal nerves for innervation of blood vessels and sweat glands in the body wall and extremities. Because the sacral and coccygeal nerves do not have white rami, visceral afferent impulses returning from sites of sympathetic innervation by the sacrum and coccyx refer viscerosomatic symptoms to the thoracolumbar region of the body.

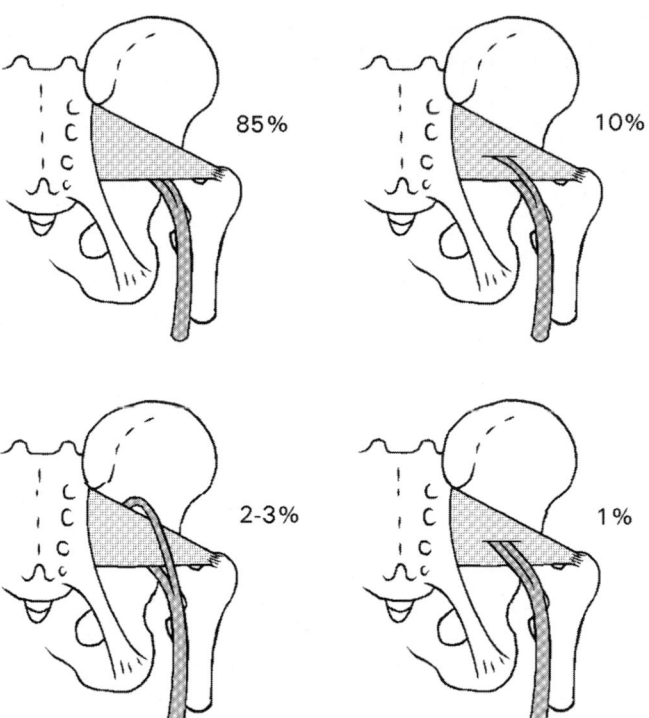

FIGURE 52.6. Position of sciatic nerve in relationship to the piriformis muscle. (Adapted from Beaton LE, Anson BJ. The sciatic nerve and the piriformis muscles: their interrelation as a possible cause of coccygodynia. *J Bone Joint Surg (Br)*. 1938;20:686–688.)

Examples include anterior lower thoracic or sacral exostoses and anterior disc protrusions or ruptures. Contractions of the uterus refer pain to the thoracolumbar region, as the visceral afferent nerves travel to this level from the uterine body.

Sacral splanchnics come off the chain and contribute to the formation of the inferior hypogastric plexus. The pelvic splanchnics arise directly off the ventral rami of S2-4 and supply parasympathetic innervation to the left colon and inferior hypogastric plexus for pelvic viscera. Visceral afferent nerves following parasympathetic nerve pathways produce viscerosomatic symptoms in the sacrum. An example is sacral pain and pressure from uterine contractions.

The inferior hypogastric plexus contains both sympathetic and parasympathetic fibers; it gives rise to smaller plexi to the rectum, bladder, prostate, uterus, and vagina.

Somatic dysfunction of the lumbar spine may affect the lumbar plexus and produce symptoms in both the pelvis and lower extremity. Dysfunction of the quadratus lumborum may produce symptoms similar to a groin pull or hernia, by irritating the ilioinguinal and iliohypogastric nerves (L1) as they pass just anterior to this muscle. Dysfunction of the piriformis, or sacrum, can affect the sciatic nerve and cause signs and symptoms of sciatica.

Many visceral complaints are related to an imbalance in the autonomic control of the pelvic viscera. When irritable bowel syndrome is dominated by parasympathetic hyperactivity (headache, nausea, diarrhea, and cramps), relaxation of the pelvic diaphragm through ischiorectal fossa techniques relieves the congestion and pain by influencing the pelvic parasympathetic (S2, S3, S4). Normalizing parasympathetic tone and encouraging venous and lym-

phatic return with firm continuous pressure over the sacral base treats primary dysmenorrhea.

MOTION AND DYSFUNCTION

The pelvic girdle holds a central role in coupling the mechanical forces from the lower extremities to the axial skeleton. An analysis of the mechanics and motions occurring in the lumbar spine and pelvis during walking demonstrates physiologic motions occurring around various axes of the pelvic girdle. Somatic dysfunction affecting any of these axes hinders gait, requires compensatory changes, and increases energy expenditure. Somatic dysfunction of the pelvis occurs when there are motion preferences during activity that become restricted when activity is completed and the joint has returned to a resting position. Shears are somatic dysfunctions that do not follow an axis.

Individual axes of the pelvic bones are described in the following paragraphs, as well as the motion about or around those axes. This is followed by a discussion of the integration of coupled movements during the motion cycle of walking.

Innominates

The innominates rotate anteriorly and posteriorly about the inferior transverse axis of the sacrum. The innominates may also be considered to rotate posturally around an axis passing through the greater trochanters of the femur. By virtue of their construction, a lower extremity, including the attached innominates, is likely to shear superiorly or inferiorly rather than have true pelvic rotation around an anteroposterior axis.

Reynolds (7) demonstrated that there were multiple varying instantaneous axes of rotation of the ilium about the sacrum when the thigh was used to introduce motion at the sacroiliac joint.

Pubes

The pubic bones may rotate about a transverse axis. Pubic somatic dysfunctions may occur where iliac movement is maximal and pubic shear is minimal. They may also be sheared (subluxed) superiorly or inferiorly along with the rest of the respective innominate. Anterior and posterior shears can also occur. These are rare and usually result from a significant traumatic event.

Sacrum

Ordinarily, sacroiliac motion is a result of mechanical forces acting on the sacrum. These forces can come from above, associated with changes of position or center of gravity within the torso, or from below, as in walking. While muscles are attached to the sacrum, sacral motion is not caused by sacral flexors, extensors, lateral flexors, or rotators (3). Describing motion of the sacrum about certain axes is a model by which we explain how the sacrum seems to work as a result of the forces acting upon it. We are also able to gather palpatory information, use this model, and describe the motion present and motion restricted. This becomes objective evidence of sacroiliac motion disturbances. We can then design methods of manipulative treatment to remove the dysfunctions.

By palpating landmarks and motion testing after manipulation we are able to evaluate the effectiveness of treatment.

AXES OF MOTION

Mitchell (3) describes three transverse axes. The superior transverse axis is at the level of the second sacral segment, posterior to the sacroiliac joint, in the spinous process area. This is the respiratory axis where flexion and extension associated with respiration occur, as well as nutation and counternutation in craniosacral mechanics. The middle transverse axis is located at the anterior convexity of the upper and lower limbs of the sacroiliac joint. Sacral postural flexion and extension occur about this axis. The inferior transverse axis is located at the posteroinferior part of the inferior limb of the sacroiliac joint and is the axis about which innominate (ilial) rotation occurs.

There are two oblique axes of the sacrum, named according to the side of the body toward which the superior end of the oblique axis is located. Motion about an oblique axis may actually result through motions occurring about a vertical and transverse sacral axis (combination of rotation and side bending). Sacral movement can occur around an individual axis or simultaneously around multiple axes. Cadaveric studies of sacral/pelvic motion document movement of the sacroiliac joint and movement of the ilia in relation to the sacrum (8).

TYPES OF SACRAL MOTION

Considering these principles, four types of sacral motion can be described. These include:

- Postural
- Respiratory
- Inherent
- Dynamic

Postural Motion

In the standing or seated patient, postural motion of sacral flexion or extension occurs about a middle transverse axis. Flexion and extension of the sacrum correspond to anatomic nomenclature, with a reference point at the anterior portion of the sacral base. Flexion (forward bending) occurs when the sacral base is moving forward or anteriorly. Extension is backward bending of the sacral base. Terminology for sacral motion uses the same reference point as terminology for spinal motion, the most anterior superior part of the body (in the case of the sacrum, the sacral base). Postural flexion/extension of the sacrum is sometimes referred to as sacral base anterior (for flexion) or posterior (for extension). This prevents confusion of understanding sacral motion that occurs during flexion and extension of the sphenobasilar joint during craniosacral motion (see "Inherent Motion"). When a person is seated and the torso is forward bent, the sacral base moves anteriorly. When a person is standing and begins forward bending, the sacral base begins to move anteriorly, tightening the sacrotuberous ligaments. As forward bending

continues, the pelvis moves posteriorly in relation to the feet. This shift in the base of support causes the sacral base to move posteriorly.

Respiratory Motion

Respiratory motion also affects the sacrum, partially because the diaphragm is attached to the top three lumbar vertebrae (L1-2 on the left and L1-3 on the right). Mitchell and Pruzzo (9) showed that the sacrum moves in response to respiration along a transverse axis. As inhalation occurs, the lumbar lordotic curve decreases, and therefore the sacral base moves posteriorly. As we exhale, the lumbar lordosis increases and the base of the sacrum moves slightly forward.

Inherent Motion

Inherent motion of the sacrum is considered in Chapter 62. Older osteopathic literature regarding the craniosacral mechanism reversed the terms flexion and extension in relating sacral inherent motion to palpated motion of the cranium about the sphenobasilar synchondrosis. However, when the sphenobasilar synchondrosis is in (craniosacral) flexion, the sacrum extends (by postural and respiratory terminology). Because of this confusion, the Educational Council on Osteopathic Principles has encouraged the use of the terms nutation and counternutation to describe sacral movement in the cranial cycle of flexion/extension. Nutation means nodding forward, referring to anterior motion at the sacral base. During the flexion phase of craniosacral inherent motion, the sacrum counternutates. During the extension phase, the sacrum nutates.

Dynamic Motion

Dynamic motion of the sacrum and pelvis occurs during walking. As weightbearing shifts to one leg, unilateral lumbar side bending engages the ipsilateral oblique axis by shifting weight to that sacroiliac joint. The sacrum now rotates forward on the opposite side, creating a deep sacral sulcus. With the next step, this process reverses as weightbearing changes to the other leg. The sacral base is constantly moving forward on one side, then the other, about oblique axes. As this occurs, the two innominates are rotating in opposite directions to each other about the inferior transverse sacral axis. One side rotates anteriorly as the other side rotates posteriorly. With the next step, this process reverses as the anteriorly rotated hip bone moves into posterior rotation.

Interacting with the bony and ligamentous structure during this motion are the viscera, the weight of the upper body, the muscles of locomotion and balance, and the pelvic diaphragm, all revolving around the constantly changing axes at the pelvis.

NORMAL MOTION OF WALK CYCLE

In the following passage from his paper, "Structural Pelvic Function", Mitchell (3) described the interplay of locomotion and balance as being the walking cycle:

> The cycle of movement of the pelvis in walking will be described in sequence as though the patient were starting to walk forward by moving the right foot out first.
>
> To permit the body to move forward on the right, trunk rotation in the thoracic area occurs to the left accompanied by lateral flexion to the left in the lumbar with movement of the lumbar vertebrae into the forming convexity to the right. There is a torsional locking at the lumbosacral junction as the body of the sacrum is moving to the left, thus shifting the weight to the left foot to allow lifting of the right foot. The shifting vertical center of gravity moves to the superior pole of the left sacroiliac, locking the mechanism into mechanical position to establish movement of the sacrum on the left oblique axis. This sets the pattern so the sacrum can torsionally turn to the left, thereby the sacral base moves down on the right to conform to the lumbar C curve that is formed to the right.
>
> When the right foot moves forward there is a tensing of the quadriceps group of muscles and accumulating tension at the inferior pole of the right sacroiliac at the junction of the left oblique axis and the inferior transverse axis, which eventually locks as the weight swings forward allowing slight anterior movement of the innominate on the inferior transverse axis. The movement is increased by the backward thrust of the restraining ground, tension on the hamstrings begins; as the weight swings upward to the crest of the femoral support, there is a slight posterior movement of the right innominate on the inferior transverse axis. The movement is also increased by the forward thrust of the propelling leg action. This iliac movement is also being influenced, directed and stabilized by the torsional movement on the transverse axis at the symphysis. From the standpoint of total pelvic movement one might consider the symphyseal axis as the postural axis of rotation for the entire pelvis.
>
> As the right heel strikes the ground and trunk torsion and accommodation begin to reverse themselves, and as the left foot passes the right foot and weight passes over the crest of the femoral support, and the accumulating force from above moves to the right, the sacrum changes its axis to the right oblique axis and the sacral base moves forward on the left and torsionally turns to the right.
>
> The cycle on the left is repeated identically to the right half movements. The shifting vertical center of gravity moves to the superior pole of the left sacroiliac locking the mechanism into mechanical position to establish movement of the sacrum on the left oblique axis.

Somatic dysfunctions may accentuate and retain portions of the motion described above. These are called physiologic somatic dysfunctions, because the muscles, connective tissue, and joints remain in positions that are normally a part of physiologic motion but are dysfunctional when the body should have returned to a neutral position but did not do so. Nonphysiologic somatic dysfunction is generally induced by trauma. It is evidenced by the joint, muscle, and connective tissue elements being in positions and/or relationships that are not part of the physiologic range of motion and do not involve the physiologic axes of motion. Examples include sacral, innominate, and pubic shears.

HISTORY AND PHYSICAL EXAMINATION

Motion restriction is palpated as part of the osteopathic screening examination. Motion testing is active, passive, regional, and segmental. Active motion testing is part of the observation or inspection. The physician asks the patient to move in a directed fashion. This is often done in cases of trauma before the physician tests for passive motion, allowing the physician to see whether there is a significant problem prior to inducing motion to potentially damaged structures.

A patient may have compensatory motion patterns that cover dysfunction but are revealed by careful inspection of focal areas in an overall pattern of satisfactory motion. Passive motion testing allows the physician to assess the quality and quantity of motion. Motion may be limited by pain rather than by the tightness of muscles. Left and right sides are compared for asymmetry, restriction in motion, and changes in tissue texture. Tenderness is assessed.

The sacral and pelvic regions are examined as part of the screening examination. If the screen is positive, the regions are examined joint by joint, as well as by muscle groups. If indicated, individual muscles, fascial restrictions, and pulses are assessed.

Diagnosis by History and Physical Examination

History

In the diagnosis of pelvic girdle dysfunction, the importance of taking a complete history and performing an in-depth physical examination cannot be overemphasized. The osteopathic examination is not a traditional history and physical with a palpatory examination added to it. An osteopathic examination strives to provide a time- and cost-effective diagnosis while encompassing the interrelationship between structure and function. Integration of the physical findings with the emotional, environmental, and genetic factors allows the osteopathic physician to understand their impact on body unity. In this fashion an osteopathic physician examines the homeostatic reserve of each patient, an area crucial in determining prognosis, treatment design, and prevention. To find health is the object of the physician, anyone can find disease (10).

A history is not just the complaint, the symptoms, and the history of the disease, but it is the history of the patient who has the disease. If the physician listens carefully, the patient's history usually reveals the diagnosis (11).

In patients with pelvic girdle complaints, physicians should always be aware of their expressions, remarks, and gestures. A diseased organ does not walk into the physician's office, but an anxious and fearful patient does, who may misinterpret or be sensitive to the issues at hand.

A physician should never assume that a patient's low back or pelvic pain has a solely muscular cause. The history should always clarify if a visceral or an emotional cause exists.

Because the pelvic region includes the sexual organs, the patient's sexual history needs to be obtained when the patient presents with a complaint in the pelvic region. Considerations of the chief complaint should include several questions (12). Tables 52.1 and 52.2 show the two mnemonics that are widely used. In addition, ask the following questions:

■ Are there any associated symptoms?
■ Is there a relationship to bodily functions and activities?
■ Have there been any changes in bowel or bladder habits?

TABLE 52.1. PQRST MNEMONIC FOR INVESTIGATING PAIN

Position, Palliation	Is it related to a particular position?
	Does anything make it better or worse?
Quality	What is it like? Sharp, stabbing, dull ache, burning, or electric?
Radiation	Where is the pain? Does it go anywhere else?
Severity	On a scale of 1–10, with 10 being worst, how bad is it?
Time	When did it start? How long does it last?

TABLE 52.2. COLDER MNEMONIC FOR INVESTIGATING PAIN

Condition, Character	What does it feel like (character or quality)?
Onset	When did it start? What were the circumstances?
Location	Where is it located? Does it radiate anywhere else?
Duration	How long does it last?
Exacerbation	Does anything make it worse?
Remission	Does anything make it better?

- Was there any previous medical care for a similar condition?
- What was the treatment outcome?
- Is the patient currently on any medications, including over-the-counter medications?
- Are there any allergies?

Even when pain is the primary complaint and clinical suspicion centers on musculoskeletal causes, the physician remembers that pain is a liar and should address the contributory topics listed in Table 52.3.

Physical Examination

The physical examination of the pelvic girdle begins the moment the patient enters the room. Observe the patient's gait, structure, body habitus, and nutritional status. Ask permission to perform a genital or rectal examination. For female patients, a male physician may require a female health care provider to be in the same room during the examination.

Along with general observation, the osteopathic structural examination includes analysis of:

- Gait
- Structural asymmetry
- Curvature of the spine
- Postural balance

A screening structural examination is done to indicate whether a region has problems requiring a more in-depth or segmental ex-

amination. A palpatory examination is essential; the two forms of examination, observation and palpation, focus on the four criteria for identifying somatic dysfunction. The mnemonic TART—*t*enderness, *a*symmetry, *r*ange of motion differences, *t*issue texture changes—(Table 52.4) helps to recall these.

PALPATORY EXAMINATION

The palpatory examination begins with the structural examination as bony anatomic landmarks are found. In the pelvic region, these should include:

- Anterior superior iliac spines (ASISs)
- Pubic symphysis
- Posterior superior iliac spines (PSISs)
- Sacral sulci
- Sacral base
- Inferior lateral angles of the sacrum
- Ischial tuberosities
- Iliac crests
- Greater trochanters

Ligamentous structures to be palpated include the iliolumbar, posterior sacroiliac, and sacrotuberous ligaments. Soft tissue palpation should include:

- Rotator cuff muscles of the hip
- Thoracolumbar and lumbosacral fasciae
- Lumbar paraspinal muscles

TABLE 52.3. CONSIDERATIONS FOR COMPLAINTS OF PAIN

In Male and Female Patients	In the Female Patient	In the Male Patient (16)
Employment risks	Menstrual history	Difficulty maintaining or achieving erection
Exercise risks/contact sports	Obstetric history	Difficulty with ejaculation
Hernia	Cleansing routines	Discharge or penile lesion
Past genitourinary surgeries	Douching history	Infertility
Cancer of the genitourinary tract	Abnormal vaginal bleeding	Urinary symptomatology
Chronic illness	Vaginal discharge	Urinary stream, good or poor
Family history	Date of last pelvic examination	Enlargement of the inguinal area
Psychiatric history	Date of last Pap smear and results	Testicular pain or mass
Medications, including contraceptive use	Past gynecologic procedures or surgery	Testicular self-examination practices
Sexual activity history		
Sexual orientation		
Sexually transmitted diseases		
Cancer of the reproductive organs		
Infertility		
Significant and related medical history (e.g., diabetes)		
Urinary tract symptoms		

TABLE 52.4. TART CRITERIA FOR IDENTIFYING SOMATIC DYSFUNCTION

Tissue texture abnormalities	How the tissue feels to the palpating hand	Classify as acute or chronic
Asymmetry	Apparent relationship of landmarks and tissues	Made by observation, not palpation; is generally static positional asymmetry
Restriction of motion	How the tissue moves	Arthrodial, muscular, or fascial elements
Tenderness	Pain elicited by palpation	Generalized as in traumatic tissue damage, such as contusion, or specific for individual muscles or sclerotomal levels, as in tender point diagnosis

- Trochanteric bursa
- Piriformis and location of the sciatic nerve
- Abdominal wall
- Pelvic diaphragm

Palpation of the lower extremity may be indicated, if the hamstrings or iliopsoas are of unequal length when motion tested.

In addition to generalized changes in the pelvic girdle tissues, the physician may detect small myofascial tender points. Such areas may be characterized by a small, palpable, circumscribed thickening of tissue that is tender with moderate to deep palpation. These tender points may be associated with autonomic dysfunction or refer pain to a neurologic distribution. Muscles containing tender points reveal pain with active or passive range of motion. There may be areas of patchy weakness in the range of motion of muscles containing painful tender points. Joints controlled by muscles with tender points may have a diminished range of motion. The pelvic girdle contains many of these myofascial tender points because myofascial structures are constantly working to maintain postural balance. Numerous authors (13,14) have indicated continuous postural strain as the cause of precipitating and/or perpetuating myofascial tender points.

Osteopathic physicians may discover paraspinal tissue texture changes that have characteristic palpatory qualities and conclude that these changes are due to visceral disturbances. These tissue texture changes are caused more by changes of the spine, subcutaneous tissue, and superficial and deep fascia rather than pinpoint tissues and muscle. The maximum intensity is at the costotransverse area in the thoracic spine and the region of the transverse processes in the lumbar spine. The quality of motion is a reluctance to move rather than an absolute restriction with loss of range. The skin and subcutaneous tissue findings exceed the muscle-bone-joint findings. In chronic viscerosomatic problems, they take on the characteristics of any chronic somatic dysfunction. Sometimes they present as an acute exacerbation of a chronic problem with the superficial puffiness of acute change and the motion restriction of chronic somatic dysfunction.

Skilled osteopathic physicians are able to palpate inherent motion of the human body. This motion has been described as a cyclic, rhythmic wave of motion; Sutherland referred to it as the primary respiratory mechanism (15). This motion has been demonstrated in numerous studies, and there are various theories as to its origin. This motion continues even when the patient holds their breath. Physicians trained in craniosacral diagnosis can palpate this motion in the sacrum as the craniosacral mechanism moves the sacrum between the two ilia. Clinical significance of this motion is discussed in Chapter 64.

The palpatory examination should include an assessment of the patient's cardiovascular status. Pulses should be palpated and auscultated for bruits bilaterally. An abdominal pulse should be identified, classified, and auscultated. Peripheral edema, sacral edema, and trophic changes in the skin should be evaluated.

In addition to the auscultation over arteries in the periphery, auscultation of the heart, lungs, and abdomen should accompany any patient evaluation. If atheromatous disease is suspected, auscultation over the carotid and femoral arteries is imperative, and the diameter of the abdominal aorta is evaluated carefully.

For evaluation of the pelvic girdle, a complete examination of the abdomen is required. Following inspection, auscultation, and palpation, the physician can percuss the liver, spleen, and stomach, and palpate for any pelvic masses. Diaphragmatic excursion can be percussed posteriorly to evaluate respiratory dysfunction. A rectal examination, a pelvic examination in the female, and a prostate examination in the male should be a part of a complete examination of the pelvic/sacral region.

Neurologic Examination of Pelvic Region

Muscle testing and sensation are the focus of the neurologic examination of the pelvis and hip (3).

Muscle Testing

Muscles of the lower extremity and buttocks require assessment when evaluating the pelvis and hip. Descriptions of the innervation, functional anatomy, and dysfunction are discussed in Chapter 57. Primary intrinsic muscles of the pelvis, although not tested for strength, may be palpated for tension, tissue texture changes, and tender points. Lumbar and pelvic muscles that may have trigger points referring pain to the pelvis should also be investigated.

Sensation Testing

The dermatomal distribution of sensory nerves to the pelvic girdle ranges from T10 to S5, involving nerve roots from the thoracic, lumbar, and sacral regions (Fig. 52.7). Dermatomes of the anterior abdominal wall run in transverse and oblique bands. These dermatomes begin at the umbilicus with the T10 strip followed inferiorly by the T11 strip. The T12 strip lies just superior to the inguinal ligament, while L1 lies just inferior to it. Inferior to the L1 dermatome lie the L2 and L3 strips covering the anterior thigh and ending at the patella. The buttocks, posterior superior iliac spines, and iliac crest are supplied by the cluneal nerves (16) (posterior primary divisions of L1, L2, L3). The posterior femoral cutaneous nerve (S2) supplies sensation to a longitudinal band traversing the posterior thigh. The lateral femoral

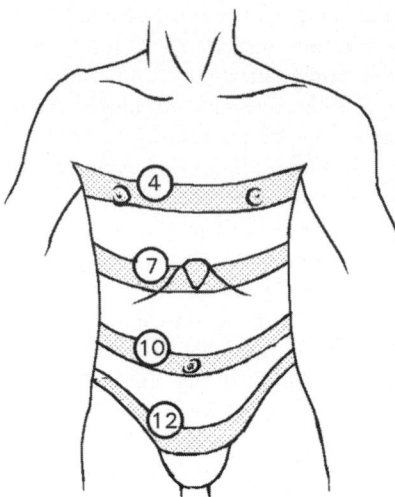

FIGURE 52.7. Anterior thoracic dermatomes. (Reprinted with permission from Kuchera WA, Kuchera ML. *Osteopathic Principles in Practice*, 2nd ed. rev. Columbus, OH: Greyden Press; 1994.)

cutaneous nerve (S3) supplies sensation to the lateral thigh. The cutaneous innervation of the perineum is arranged in concentric rings around the anus: the outermost (S2), middle (S3, S4), and innermost (S5).

MOTION TESTING OF THE PELVIC REGION

Multiple methods are available for motion testing, which is customarily done in an integrated fashion with examination of the anatomic landmarks. The immediate objective of manipulative treatment is to improve motion. An initial diagnosis is made and treatment is begun; repeated integral motion testing and treatment follow. Movement of tissues is continuously assessed, determining freedom of, or resistance, to motion testing.

Anatomic Landmarks Used to Assess Pelvis

To assess static positional relationships and perform motion testing, the physician should be able to correctly locate (in the following positions) several landmarks:

Patient standing

- Level of iliac crests
- PSISs
- Greater trochanters of the femurs

Patient supine

- ASISs
- Pubic symphysis
- Pubic tubercles
- Medial malleoli
- Sacrum

Patient prone

- PSISs
- Sacral sulcus

- Sacral base
- Inferior lateral angle (ILA)
- Sacrotuberous ligament
- Ischial tuberosity
- Iliac crest
- Piriformis muscle
- Iliolumbar ligament insertion on ilium

Motion Testing Sequence

An example of a motion testing sequence follows:

Patient standing

- Trendelenburg test
- Iliac crests
- PSISs
- Standing flexion test
- Pelvic side-shift

Patient seated

- Seated flexion test
- Lateral translation sacroiliac motion test
- Upper lumbar for flexed somatic dysfunction and psoas

Patient supine

- ASISs
- Pubes
- Medial malleoli
- Hamstrings
- Sacrum (for cranial rhythmic impulse)

Patient prone

- PSISs
- Sacral sulci
- Sacral base
- ILA
- Sacrotuberous ligaments
- Spring test
- Backward bending test
- Prone sacral motion tests
- Hamstring palpation for tension

Special Tests of Pelvis

Trendelenburg Test

This test determines the strength of the gluteus medius muscle. During gait, the gluteus medius acts as a stabilizer, preventing the unsupported hip from dropping during the swing phase.

1. Stand behind the patient and observe the sacral dimples. With equal weight distribution over both legs, these dimples should be level.
2. Now have the patient stand on one leg. The opposing gluteus medius should contract, elevating the pelvis on the unsupported side and indicating a negative test. If the muscle is weak, the pelvis on the unsupported side stays level or drops, indicating a positive test.

Conditions that could cause a weakening or paralysis of the gluteus medius include:

- Fractures of the greater trochanter
- Slipped capital femoral epiphysis
- Coxa vera
- Poliomyelitis
- Meningomyelocele
- Nerve root lesions
- Lumbar somatic dysfunction
- Disturbed ilioiliac mechanics

Iliac Crest Levelness

Place your index fingers over the iliac crests, and maintain a position so that your eyes are level with the crests. Inspect to see whether the crests are at equal heights.

Posterior Superior Iliac Spine Levelness

Place your thumbs on the inferior slopes of the PSISs and note whether they are level. If one is more cephalad or caudad at the beginning of the standing flexion test, be sure that you include the difference in your end-point estimate before calling the test positive.

Standing Flexion Test

The standing flexion test identifies the side of iliosacral dysfunction. It does not identify the specific type of dysfunction, only which side to treat. Mechanical forces from the lower extremity may influence this test.

A positive standing flexion test indicates three possibilities:

1. Iliosacral dysfunction
2. Contralateral tight hamstrings
3. Carryover from the seated flexion test

False-positive and false-negative test results do exist. A false-negative standing flexion test may be caused by ipsilateral hamstring shortness, but since hamstring tension can cause a false-negative result on the ipsilateral side, or a false-positive result on the contralateral side, testing for hamstring length identifies a hamstring cause for false-negative or false-positive standing flexion tests. If there are unilaterally tight hamstrings, the dysfunctional side should be treated so that both sides are equal, and the standing flexion test repeated. When the sacroiliac dysfunction is treated, the standing flexion test may become negative.

Some physicians believe that if a patient has unequal iliac crest heights, a false-negative test result may exist unless shimming is done to level the iliac crests prior to performing the test.

Patient Position
Standing with shoes removed, heels on a line and feet under the hips.

Physician Position
Kneeling or standing behind the patient, eyes level with the PSISs.

Procedure
1. Place your thumbs on the inferior slopes of the PSISs, and your fingers on the superolateral surface of the iliac crests. Obtain firm pressure on the PSISs to follow bony landmark motion rather than skin motion.
2. Ask the patient to bend forward, touching the floor if possible, but stopping short of pain.
3. Let your thumbs follow the motion of the PSISs. As the patient bends forward, allow the pelvis to come back toward you. If you do not, the patient will fall forward.
4. Your eyes should be level with the PSISs at all times, so that as the patient bends forward, you rise from a kneeling position to one where you are standing over the PSISs.
5. If one PSIS moves more cephalad at the end range of motion, the test is positive on that side. (Do not count the side that moves superior first as the positive side. Fascial drag can cause the positive side to end up inferior to the negative side at the completion of the test. If both sides are equal, the test is usually interpreted as negative.)

Seated Flexion Test (Seated Forward Bending Test)

A positive seated flexion test indicates sacroiliac dysfunction. In the seated position, mechanics of the lower extremity are not influencing the pelvis. A positive test indicates the dysfunctional side but not the specific type of dysfunction.

Patient Position
Seated, with both feet flat on the floor, or on the rung of a bench, shoulder width apart, and with the popliteal fossa against the edge of the table.

Physician Position
Kneeling or standing behind the patient, with eyes level with the PSISs.

Procedure
1. Place your thumbs on the inferior slopes of the PSISs.
2. Have the patient cross the arms in front of the chest.
3. Ask the patient to bend forward, as far as possible without pain.
4. Note the movement of the PSIS. If one side has moved cephalad at the end point of forward bending, the seated flexion test is positive for that side. If the PSISs remain equal, the test is negative.

Interpretation of Standing/Seated Test Results

If both tests are negative, there is no problem in the sacrum/pelvis. A true positive standing or seated test indicates a problem on that side. If positive, the tests should become negative after proper treatment.

Supine

Align Pelvis on Table

This is sometimes called a hip flop. The purpose of this maneuver is to reset the pelvis so that the least effect of postural muscles is present. This should also be a comfortable position for the patient.

Procedure

1. Ask your supine patient to raise the knees while keeping the feet on the table.
2. Ask the patient to raise the buttocks slightly, so they are off the table.
3. Now have the patient drop the buttocks to the table and then lower the knees.
4. Continue your assessment with the following tests.

Medial Malleoli Levelness

The levelness of the medial malleoli used to be correlated with the findings of the standing structural examination, innominate rotations, and pelvic shears. Medial malleoli levelness is not very reliable for making a diagnosis of innominate dysfunction, as it may not fit the result expected. This is because the ankle, the knee, the hip, and all the fasciae and muscles between the malleoli and the pelvis can affect the levelness of the malleoli. However, when the planes between the malleoli are unlevel, the physician is alerted to leg, hip, and ankle stress; this increases general body stress.

A patient with a short leg is similar to a building with the foundation slightly lower on one side. The body must adapt by seeking a new balance, and this produces tensions in all of the postural muscles. A short leg also places additional stress on the joints of the longer lower extremity. As the body seeks a new level of balance, there is generally a slight scoliotic curve in the lumbar region with the convexity on the short leg side and side-bent toward the long leg side. This is usually then compensated for with additional curve(s) in the superior portions of the spine. The cause of a short leg may be anatomic (e.g., the patient had a fractured tibia as a child and growth was slightly shortened) or functional (e.g., the patient has a posteriorly rotated ilium, sacral torsion, or lumbar curve, causing one leg apparently to be shortened by its displacement in three planes).

Procedure

1. With the patient supine, place your thumbs on the inferior surfaces of the medial malleoli, with your fingers curved around the anterolateral aspect of the ankles.
2. Put slight traction, equal on both sides, on the legs.
3. Note whether one malleolus is more cephalad than the other, and if so, record the difference in length of the short leg.

Hamstring Test

Patient Position
Supine.

Physician Position
Standing at the side of the table, facing the patient.

Procedure

1. Place your cephalad hand on the patient's opposite ASIS.
2. Place your other hand under the ankle of the leg on your side of the table.
3. Slowly lift the leg until you feel slight motion at the opposite ASIS. This occurs after the hamstrings on your side are tight enough to begin rotating the whole pelvis, which is when you feel the motion in your monitoring hand.
4. Note the angle at which this occurs.
5. Perform the same test on the opposite leg (from the opposite side of the table).
6. Mentally compare the angles at which you felt motion at the ASIS. If the leg angles are equal and about 85 to 90 degrees, the test is considered negative. If you felt the motion sooner on one side, that side has restricted (tight) hamstrings.

Note: The hamstrings can be palpated directly for tension with the patient in the prone position. This is a good screening test but does not directly measure hamstring shortness.

Anterior Superior Iliac Spine Levelness

Procedure

1. Place your thumbs on the inferior surface of the ASISs.
2. Note whether one side is more inferior or superior.
3. Note whether one side or the other is more medial or lateral. Integrate this information with the rest of your diagnostics to make an iliosacral diagnosis.

Note: The innominates may be motion tested at this time. Normally, motion is freer in the direction of positional change. With a left posterior innominate, a posterior and superior direction motion to the supine patient's left ASIS is freer. With a left anterior innominate, a posterior- and superior-directed motion to the supine patient's left ASIS is restricted.

Pubic Symphyseal Levelness

Procedure

1. Inform the patient that you will need to palpate the pubic symphysis and ask the patient's permission to do so.
2. Place the heel of your hand at about the level of the umbilicus. With slight pressure, slide it down the patient's abdomen until you reach the pubic symphysis.
3. Place your thumbs or fingers at the superior aspect of the pubic symphysis and move them slightly medial, slightly lateral.
4. Note whether one side is more caudad, the other more cephalad. Note also any tenderness or tissue texture abnormalities. Integrate this information with that from the rest of your diagnostic tests to make an iliosacral diagnosis.

Sacrum: Indirect Diagnosis

This assessment is often made after gross level motion dysfunctions have been treated with muscle energy, high velocity/low amplitude (HVLA), strain/counterstrain, or other techniques.

Patient Position
Supine.

Physician Position
Sitting at the side of the table facing the patient.

Procedure
1. Ask the patient to raise the opposite knee, with the foot on the table, and to roll the opposite hip toward you.
2. Start with hand lateral to the raised hip and place it between the patient's sacrum and the table.
3. Have the patient roll the hip back to regain the supine position, and lower the knee.
4. Assess sacral motion for both respiratory effects and the cranial rhythmic impulse.

Posterior Superior Iliac Spines

Procedure
1. Place your thumbs on the inferior surface of the PSIS.
2. Note whether one side is more inferior or superior than the other.
3. Integrate this information with the results of the rest of your diagnostic tests to make an iliosacral diagnosis.

Note: The innominates may be motion tested at this time. Normally, motion is freer in the direction of positional change.

Sacral Base

Patient Position
Prone.

Physician Position
Standing at the side of the table, dominant eye centered.

Procedure
1. Place your thumb pads about one-half inch above where you tested levelness of the PSISs and curl your thumbs from the iliac crest into the sacral sulcus at the base of the sacrum (Fig. 52.1).
2. Evaluate depth of the sacral sulci as an indication of sacral base position. Are both sides the same? Is the sacral sulcus depth normal? Is one side deep? Is one side shallow?
3. Push forward on one side of the sacral base, then the other. Note which side moves more easily. Motion should be freer on the deep side.
4. Mentally record the position of the sacral base and continue the examination.

Note: At this time, palpation of the sacral sulci for tissue texture abnormality is appropriate.

Sacral Inferolateral Angles

Patient Position
Prone.

Physician Position
Standing at the side of the table, dominant eye centered.

Procedure
1. Place your thumb pads on the inferolateral angles of the sacrum.
2. By inspection, note which side appears (a) anterior/posterior and (b) superior/inferior.
3. Mentally record which side is anterior/posterior and which is superior/inferior from your motion testing and continue the examination.

Notes:

■ The ILA may be equal anteriorly/posteriorly; equal superiorly/inferiorly.
■ One side may be anterior or posterior but level superiorly/inferiorly.
■ One side is anterior and superior; or one side is posterior and inferior.

Motion Test about Transverse Axis

Patient Position
Prone.

Physician Position
Standing at side of table at hip level with palpating hand over sacrum, fingers pointing cephalad.

Procedure
Place your hand over the sacrum with your fingers pointing cephalad. Alternatively apply pressure with the tips of your fingers, then with the heel of your hand in a gentle, slow, rocking motion. This introduces anatomic flexion and extension about a transverse axis. Assess the quality and quantity of motion and note which movement is freer.

Motion Test about Oblique Axis

Patient Position
Prone.

Physician Position
Standing at the side of the patient at hip level.

Procedure
Place the pads of the index and middle fingers of your monitoring hand so that one finger contacts the PSIS and the other finger rests in the sacral base. Place the heel of your active hand in contact with the inferior lateral angle on the contralateral side. With your active hand, apply downward (anterior) pressure on the ILA of the sacrum about an oblique axis. Note freedom or restriction of motion. With your monitoring hand appreciate anterior or posterior motion of the sacral base. Assess both quality and quantity of movement as the forces are slowly introduced. Evaluate motion on both left and right oblique axes. If the sacral base has rotated forward and become restricted, posterior motion

of the sacral base at the sulcus is restricted. Palpatory examination typically finds the restriction; however, somatic dysfunction is named for the freedom of motion.

Test for Posterior Sacrum

This tests for restriction of lower limbs of L (C).

Patient Position
Prone.

Physician Position
Standing at the side of the patient at hip level.

Procedure
Bilaterally contact the inferior portion of sacrum somewhere between the caudal border of the inferolateral angle and where you tested for levelness of the PSIS. Apply a cephalad, downward force. The inferior arms of the sacroiliac joints run anterior and superior, and their posterior borders are about 1 inch inferior to the caudal border of the PSIS. If there is restriction of the lower limb of the sacroiliac joints, this downward, cephalic pressure meets with resistance.

Lumbosacral Spring Test

This test may determine if an increased or decreased lumbar lordosis is present, as well as whether or not the sacrum is tilted forward at the base. If there is increased lumbar lordosis and/or the sacral base is forward, there is increased mechanical stress at the lumbosacral joint and in the articular structures of the lumbosacral region. This comes about because of changes in the postural line of the body. If the sacral base is able to move anteriorly, there is good spring (a negative spring test). If the sacral base is posterior, spring provides poor or nonexistent motion at the sacral base (a positive test).

Patient Position
Prone.

Physician Position
Standing at the side of the table.

Procedure
1. Place the heel of one hand over the lumbosacral junction, and the heel of the other hand on top of it.
2. Apply a gentle but rapid downward pressure on the lumbosacral junction, in a repeated fashion, two or three times.
3. If there is good springing motion, it is a negative test. If there is poor spring or no spring, it is a positive spring test.

Backward Bending Test

This test helps evaluate sacral somatic dysfunction at the upper arm of the sacroiliac joint. If the sacral base is anterior on one side, it continues to move anteriorly with the patient propped up on the elbows. The opposite side of the sacral base also moves anteriorly; the sacral base moves anteriorly (sacral flexion) on both sides, reducing asymmetry at the sacral base. The sacral sulci and ILAs are more equal in position if the lumbar spine is backward bent. If the sacral base is posterior on one side with a shallow sulcus (as with backward torsions), and the lumbar spine is backward bent with the patient propped up on their elbows, the sacral base posterior side (shallow sulcus side) resists anterior movement of the sacral base. The other side of the sacral base will move anteriorly. This increases the asymmetry, making the sacral base, sacral sulci, and ILAs less equal in position.

Patient Position
Prone.

Physician Position
Standing at the side of the table, dominant eye centered.

Procedure
1. Place your thumbs in the sacral sulci or on the ILAs.
2. Ask the patient to take a position propped up on elbows, and then to relax the low back.
3. Examine the sacral sulci and ILAs. Note with each whether one side is deeper or shallower than the other. Test with motion (anterior pressure) on one side, then on the other, to see in which direction the sulcus or ILA moves most easily.
4. Mentally record whether the patient's condition improved (position and motion were more symmetric and appropriate) or became worse in this position.

On a forward torsion, the asymmetry of the sacral base, sacral sulci, and ILAs decreases. On backward torsions, the asymmetry increases.

Anterior Superior Iliac Spine Compression Test

This is a test for lateralization of somatic dysfunction of the sacrum, innominate, or pubic symphysis (Fig. 52.8). It can be used to confirm the findings of the seated flexion test or to help localize to one side or another or both sides when the standing or seated flexion test results are equivocal.

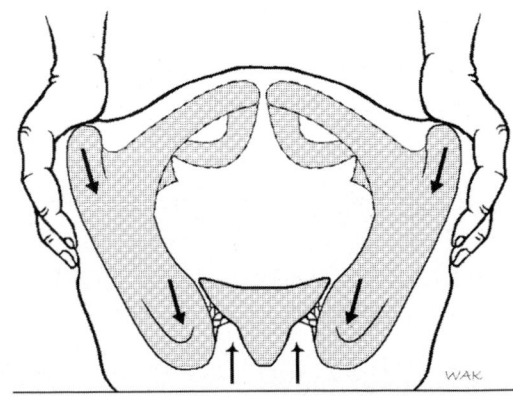

FIGURE 52.8. Anterior superior iliac spine compression test. (Modified from Kuchera WA, Kuchera ML. *Osteopathic Principles in Practice*, 2nd ed. rev. Columbus, OH: Greyden Press; 1994.)

Patient Position

Supine.

Physician Position

Standing at side of the patient, facing the head.

Procedure

Contact the ASISs; apply a posterior compression on one ASIS while stabilizing the other. Test both sides. A posterior compression normally produces a palpatory sense of give or resilience as the innominate glides slightly posterior at the sacroiliac joint on that side. Somatic dysfunction of the pelvis on the side of compression produces resistance to the test. This is interpreted as a positive ASIS compression test.

Bilateral pelvic somatic dysfunction would produce similar findings on both sides and may be interpreted as negative. However, none of the normal resiliency would be found on either side.

Fascial Restrictions of Pelvis

The physician should be able to determine the direction of freer or restricted motion of a fascial plane through palpatory assessment. The direction of the fascia, determined by this palpation, often is a vector in three planes. Fascial assessment is more than an active, doing process. The hands must listen to the tissues and detect change. This is a sensorimotor skill, one in which the physician must "read" or "listen" to the tissues and respond to the palpatory messages received.

A common fascial restriction of the pelvis exists between the two innominates. Positional asymmetry and motion disturbance between the two innominates may be related to fascia as well as to disturbance within the sacroiliac joints.

Patient Position

Supine.

Physician Position

Standing at the side of the table, facing the head, with the dominant eye centered.

Procedure

1. Place your hands on the ASISs and adjoining crests.
2. Apply downward pressure in a posterior superior direction alternatively to each side, monitoring for resistance or freedom of motion.

Freer motion is in the direction of positional change and is how somatic dysfunction is ordinarily named. This dysfunction can be treated using fascial release technique.

PELVIC DIAGNOSES

Mitchell divided pelvic and sacral diagnoses into iliosacral dysfunctions (including innominate and pubic dysfunctions) and sacroiliac dysfunctions (sacral diagnoses). The sacroiliac joint is composed of two bones with a joint separating them. One bone is the sacrum, and the other is the ilium. A disturbance in one will always affect the other. Innominate disturbances may sometimes be a primarily disturbed relationship between the two sides, maintained by muscle and fascial alterations. Within the ten regions of somatic dysfunction (*International Classification of Diseases, Ninth Revision*), iliosacral diagnoses are listed as pelvic diagnoses. In the Mitchell muscle energy model of diagnosis, two assumptions are made when determining an iliosacral diagnosis. The first is that the dysfunction is due to neuromuscular imbalance, with the muscle(s) on one side being hypertonic and their opposites being hypotonic. The second is that the side of dysfunction is the side of the positive standing flexion test.

Iliosacral Somatic Dysfunctions

Iliosacral somatic dysfunctions include:

- Innominate rotations, anterior and posterior
- Innominate subluxations (shears), superior and inferior
- Innominate flares (inflares and outflares)
- Pubic shears (subluxations), superior and inferior
- Unequal hamstring length
- Unequal iliopsoas length

Anterior Innominate Rotation

This exists when the dysfunctional side has the following characteristics:

- Entire innominate appears to be rotated in a direction anterior to the other hip bone
- ASIS is more inferior (caudad)
- PSIS is more superior (cephalad)

Subjective complaints may include ipsilateral hamstring tightness and spasm and sciatica (secondary to piriformis dysfunction). Palpatory findings may include tissue texture changes at the ipsilateral ILA of the sacrum, as well as iliolumbar ligament tenderness. Motion characteristics should indicate freedom of anterior rotation, about a low transverse axis, on supine motion testing, and resistance to posterior rotation.

Posterior Innominate Rotation

This exists when the dysfunctional side has the following characteristics:

- Entire innominate appears to be rotated in a direction posterior to the other hip bone
- ASIS is more superior (cephalad)
- PSIS is more inferior (caudad)

Subjective complaints may include inguinal/groin pain (secondary to rectus femoris dysfunction) and/or medial knee pain (secondary to sartorius dysfunction). Palpatory findings may include inguinal tenderness as well as tissue texture change at the ipsilateral sacral sulcus. Motion characteristics include freedom of posterior rotation about a low transverse axis on supine motion testing and resistance to anterior rotation.

Superior Innominate Shear (Subluxation)

This exists when the dysfunctional side has the following characteristics:

- ASIS is more superior (cephalad)
- PSIS is more superior (cephalad)
- Pubic ramus may be more superior (cephalad)

Note: The reciprocal positioning of the ASIS and PSIS exists only if there is a pure superior shear without any rotation of the innominate.

The two innominates appear to be sheared so that the one hip bone is subluxed superiorly to the other.

Subjective complaints may include pelvic pain. Palpatory findings may include tissue texture changes at the ipsilateral sacroiliac joint and ipsilateral pubes. Motion characteristics include freedom of superior translation.

Inferior Innominate Shear (Subluxation)

This condition exists when the dysfunctional side has the following characteristics:

- ASIS is more inferior (caudad)
- PSIS is more inferior (caudad)
- Pubic ramus may be more inferior

The two innominates appear to be sheared so that the one hip bone is subluxed inferiorly to the other. This condition is rare, and walking tends to reduce it.

Subjective complaints may include pelvic pain. Palpatory findings may include tissue texture changes at the ipsilateral sacroiliac joint and ipsilateral pubes. Motion characteristics include freedom of inferior translation.

Innominate Flares

This condition is a positional change of an innominate in which the ASIS is medial or lateral to its usual position. This may be thought of as rotation of an innominate in relation to a vertical axis.

Flares are determined by imagining a transverse line going through the ASIS. Visually connect this line between the ASIS. Then connect a line from each ASIS to the umbilicus, forming a triangle. Bisect this triangle by visually connecting a line from the umbilicus to the pubic symphysis, dividing the triangle into two triangles. Examine the length of the bisected transverse line between the two ASISs, and determine which ASIS is more medial or lateral. If the ASIS is more lateral on the dysfunctional side, the patient has an innominate outflare. If the ASIS is more medial on the dysfunctional side, the patient has an innominate inflare.

Subjective complaints may include pelvic or sacroiliac pain. Palpatory findings may indicate greater laxity in the muscles on the side that is more lateral and more tautness on the side that is more medial.

Vertical Pubic Shears

Vertical pubic shears (subluxations) may or may not actually exist. There may be evidence of a rotation or subluxation that is difficult to diagnose. However, there are times when the ASISs appear to be equal, the PSISs appear to be equal, and yet the pubes are definitely displaced so that one is detectably superior and the other inferior. Since the ASISs and PSISs are equal, it does not appear that the hip bone is rotated or sheared. When the dysfunctional side is superior, it is said to be a superior pubic shear; if the dysfunctional side is inferior, it is an inferior pubic shear. Anterior pubic shears are uncommon but possible and are usually associated with trauma. In these cases, one side of the symphysis is anterior to the other.

Pubic Symphysis Compressions

Pubic symphysis compressions occur, evidenced by bilateral tenderness. Using the adductor muscles of the thigh in a muscle energy technique can reduce these compressions.

The L5 anterior counterstrain point is also located on the pubes. Treatment of this tender point with counterstrain technique may be appropriate and necessary in treating pubic symphysis symptoms because what appears to be a pubic dysfunction may actually be reflexive evidence of L5 dysfunction.

Unequal Hamstring Length

Unequal hamstring length can be considered either a pelvic or a lower extremity somatic dysfunction because the hamstrings are attached to both the pelvis and the lower extremity.

If the hamstrings are of unequal length, standing flexion test results may be either falsely positive or negative. Therefore, it is imperative to treat the hamstrings and retest. If the standing flexion test and pelvic landmark positions normalize, the dysfunctional hamstrings were the problem. Otherwise, treat as indicated by the second diagnosis.

Unequal Iliopsoas Length

Unequal psoas length may be suspected when pelvic side shift is present, when the upper lumbar lordotic curve is flattened, or when seated or prone evaluation suggests upper lumbar flexed somatic dysfunction.

To test the ability of the psoas muscle to lengthen, place the patient in a prone position. Stand at the side of the table. Grasp the thigh just above the knee and extend the hip until the ASISs begin to rise off the table. Note the ease and degrees (quality and quantity) of hip extension on both sides. Also, on the tighter side the leg appears heavier. Compare the two sides.

DIAGNOSIS OF SACROILIAC DYSFUNCTION

The most common and standard diagnoses of sacroiliac somatic dysfunction include (but are not limited to):

- Sacrum anterior
- Sacrum posterior
- Forward torsions (rotation of the sacrum on the same oblique axis):
  —Left rotation on left oblique axis
  —Right rotation on right oblique axis

- Backward torsions (rotation of the sacrum on the opposite oblique axis):
  —Right rotation on left oblique axis
  —Left rotation on right oblique axis
- Bilateral sacral flexion
- Bilateral sacral extension
- Unilateral sacral flexion (sacral shear)
- Unilateral sacral extension (sacral shear)

In the osteopathic profession, several models of sacroiliac dysfunction have been described. Two systems of nomenclature currently used to define sacropelvic mechanics are those described by Strachan (HVLA) and Mitchell (muscle energy). The HVLA system is described in Walton's text, *Osteopathic Diagnosis and Technique, Sacroiliac Diagnosis* (17). Both models describe similar events, but from differing points of reference. Both systems are based on physiologic motion of the sacrum, pelvis, and lumbar spine. However, the Strachan model does not describe or identify what the Mitchell system refers to as backward sacral torsions, just as the Mitchell system has no equivalent for Strachan's posterior sacrum.

Sacroiliac dysfunction is described in this chapter using the most consistent criteria of both systems. To integrate the following information into the clinical arena, the physician must consider three questions:

1. Is the sacrum in trouble?
2. Why is the sacrum restricted?
3. What are we going to do for the patient?

The information in Table 52.5 can be used clinically in a four-step process using four patient positions. This step-by-step approach can lead to the diagnosis of any somatic dysfunction of the sacroiliac articulation.

Collectively, these four steps integrate information in a logical and time-efficient way of approaching sacroiliac problems. Diagnosing these syndromes is complex, because they may occur in combination, jointly producing symptoms. For this reason, many experienced osteopathic physicians repetitively diagnose during treatment to evaluate the efficacy of their therapeutic decision.

Positional terminology, such as Strachan's, was historically used in naming most somatic dysfunctions, although this did not imply that diagnosis was based on positional observation alone. The glossary of osteopathic terminology states that somatic dysfunction can be named in three ways:

1. Position of body part
2. Direction of freer motion
3. Direction of restriction

Strachan's model describes sacral dysfunction in relation to the ilium rather than to L5. Historically, prior to Mitchell's paper in 1958 on structural pelvic function (3), sacroiliac problems were described as the sacrum in relation to the ilium, or the ilium in relation to the sacrum. Dysfunctions include anterior sacrum and posterior sacrum. Sacral movement is around an oblique axis: motion may be restricted at either the upper or lower arm of the L- (C-) shaped sacroiliac joint. Note that the ILA is not the lower arm of the joint, but a portion of the sacrum used for

TABLE 52.5. EXAMINATION FOR SOMATIC DYSFUNCTION OF SACROILIAC ARTICULATION

Position	Examination	Results
Step 1. Patient standing	Evaluate anatomic landmarks, standing flexion test	A positive standing flexion test means dysfunction in the leg and/or pelvis on that side.
Step 2. Patient seated	Perform seated flexion test	Will specifically determine whether there is a sacroiliac dysfunction, and if so, which side (but not which arm) of the sacroiliac joint is dysfunctional.
Step 3. Patient supine	Positional assessment of ASISs, pubic tubercles, and medial malleoli	Helps determine the etiology of the problem and whether it is purely sacral or a "mixed" problem, incorporating iliac and pubic dysfunction.
Step 4. Patient prone	Palpate for tissue texture changes, motion testing of the sacrum, motion testing of L5, ligamentous tension testing	Helps the physician discover which axis is involved, find what portion of the sacroiliac joint is restricted, determine L5 motion and position, and evaluate pelvic ligamentous tensions.

ASISs, anterior superior iliac spines.

palpation and positional reference. The sacrum is diagnosed as either anterior or posterior to the ipsilateral ilium.

Anterior Sacrum

An anterior sacrum is a positional term describing a somatic dysfunction in which the sacral base has rotated forward and side bent to the side opposite the rotation. The upper limb of the sacroiliac joint has restricted motion, and the dysfunction is named for the side on which forward rotation occurs. An anterior sacrum is probably one type of Mitchell's forward torsion. For example, anterior sacrum left describes a condition in which the sacrum is rotated right and side bent to the left, the directions of ease of motion. (This could also be considered right rotation about a right oblique axis.) There is restriction of left rotation and right side bending. The sacral sulcus is deep on the left, with tenderness and tissue texture abnormality in the left sulcus. When downward pressure is applied over the right ILA, attempting to rotate the sacrum about the right oblique axis, the left superior portion of the sacrum resists moving posteriorly, toward the ilium.

Posterior Sacrum

A posterior sacrum is diagnosed when the sacrum has rotated backward and is side bent to the side opposite of rotation. It is named for the side of the backward or posterior rotation. This rotation side bending to the opposite side could be considered rotation about an oblique axis. The posterior sacrum is on the side opposite the deep sulcus at the inferior pole of the joint. The patient experiences discomfort at the inferior arm of the sacroiliac joint and possibly sciatic pain. There is a pelvic side shift to the side of dysfunction, spinal asymmetry, and postural imbalance. There is a positive seated flexion test on the side of dysfunction, as well as ipsilateral piriformis tension, and the ipsilateral ILA is posterior and inferior. There may be contralateral psoas tension, and there is generally a contralateral short leg. For example, a posterior sacrum right has rotated right and side-bent left, the directions of ease of motion; rotation left and side-bending right are restricted. A posterior sacrum involves restriction of motion at the lower limb of the sacroiliac articulation. Tissue texture abnormality and tenderness are located over the inferior portion of the dysfunctional sacroiliac joint; in this example, the tenderness is on the right. The rotation, in this case, is in relation to the right oblique axis. A posterior sacrum is probably a form of forward torsion in which the major joint motion restriction is on the side opposite the deep sulcus. A motion test for lower pole (lower limb of the L) restriction (e.g., posterior sacrum right) is to contact the inferior borders of the sacrum with both thumbs and apply a cephalad/anterior force, attempting to glide the sacrum in the direction of the lower limb of the joint. Restriction is felt on the posterior sacral side. Although there are similarities between the posterior sacrum and the forward torsion, there is no true Mitchell equivalent to Strachan's posterior sacrum. A posterior sacrum should not be confused with a backward torsion, a posterior sacral base, or an extension of the sacrum.

The Mitchell system, based on the cycle of walking (as previously detailed), describes sacral motion relative to L5. The sacrum can move forward or backward about left and right oblique axes depending on the individual's center of gravity and gait, can flex or extend around a transverse axis, or can shift in the L- (C-) shaped articulation, causing a shear. Mitchell's dysfunctions include sacral torsions, shears, flexion, and extension.

Sacral Torsions

Sacral torsions refer to motion at the lumbosacral junction where the sacrum and L5 are rotating in opposite directions. Rotation of the sacrum is movement about an oblique axis or diagonal axis. Sacral torsion does not describe a relationship between the sacrum and the ilium.

Forward Torsions

Forward torsions occur when the lumbar spine is in neutral. In this example, side bending of the lumbar spine to the left (during the motion cycle of walking) engages the left oblique axis. The lumbar spine, in neutral, rotates right with left side bending. Since the left oblique axis is engaged, the sacrum rotates left about the left oblique axis, producing a deep sacral sulcus on the right. Torsion implies that the sacrum has rotated left, while the lumbar spine has rotated right. (Note that, with neutral lumbar mechanics, left side bending produces rotation right.) The term forward torsion is derived from the observation that, in the erect

TABLE 52.6. POSITION FINDINGS FOR TWO FORWARD TORSIONS

Sacral Rotation on Same Oblique Axis	Left Rotation on Left Oblique Axis	Right Rotation on Right Oblique Axis
Sacral base anterior, deep sacral sulcus	Right	Left
Posterior, inferior lateral angle	Left	Right
Lumbar curve convex to	Right	Left
L5 rotated to	Right	Left

posture, the sacrum is in a flexed forward position (45 to 55 degrees from the vertical, or 35 to 45 degrees from the horizontal). The Ferguson lumbosacral angle is measured from the horizontal. There are two forward torsions: left rotation on a left oblique axis (left on left), and right rotation about the right oblique axis (right on right). Positional findings with each of the two forward torsions include those shown in Table 52.6.

In the normal motion cycle of walking, the sacrum rotates from side to side. Dysfunction in the form of a forward torsion occurs when the sacral base rotates forward, becomes restricted, and does not rotate back as far as it should. The forward sacral torsion and anterior sacrum have several findings in common. Subjective complaints include sacroiliac, inguinal, or groin discomfort and low back pain. Objective findings include freedom of rotation anteriorly about an oblique axis, with sacral side bending and rotation in opposite directions. There is an increased lordotic curve. Spinal asymmetry and postural imbalance are noted: The sacrum has rotated in a direction opposite to the supported lumbars. There is an ipsilateral positive seated flexion test, deep sacral sulcus with tissue texture abnormality, possible psoas tension, and short leg. Neutral mechanics apply to L5, with side bending and rotation to the opposite side. However, rotation of L5 is also in a direction opposite to that of the sacrum.

Backward Torsions

Backward torsions (nonneutral) occur when the lumbar spine is in nonneutral (flexion or, where the curve exceeds normal lordosis, extension) and the sacral base rotates posteriorly about the opposite oblique axis. While they do not occur within the cycle of walking, they are associated with physiologic motion when a person forward bends and then side bends. Consider a patient in the standing position who bends forward. The sacrum actually extends or backward bends at this time. The lumbar spine is flexed to a point where any multiple plane motion results in nonneutral multiple plane motion. The patient reaches sideways to pick up an object. The lumbar spine side bends to the right from the nonneutral sagittal plane position. The right oblique axis is engaged as a result of the right side bending. L5 rotates right according to nonneutral lumbar mechanics. The sacral base moves posteriorly at the left base as the sacrum rotates to the left according to sacral nonneutral mechanics. This example is called left on right (left rotation about the right oblique axis). There are two types of backward sacral torsions: right rotation on a left oblique axis (right on left), and left rotation on a right oblique axis (left on

TABLE 52.7. POSITIONAL FINDINGS FOR TWO BACKWARD TORSIONS

	Sacral Rotation on Opposite Oblique Axis	Right Rotation on Left Oblique Axis	Left Rotation on Right Oblique Axis
Sacral base anterior, deep sacral sulcus	Left (tender right)	Right (tender left)	
Posterior, inferior lateral angle	Right	Left	
Lumbar curve convex to	Right	Left	
L5 rotated to	Left	Right	

right). Positional findings with each of the two backward torsions include those shown in Table 52.7.

A backward torsion is not the same as a posterior sacrum. A posterior sacrum is a type of forward torsion in which the inferior portion of the sacrum is posterior. In a backward torsion, the posterior portion is at the sacral base (the shallow sulcus).

Subjective complaints include low back pain or sacroiliac discomfort that gets worse when bending forward or walking. Objective findings include those listed above, plus a decreased lordotic curve. Palpatory findings include tissue texture abnormality and a shallow sacral sulcus on the side of the dysfunction, with tissue texture abnormality at L5. Nonneutral mechanics apply to L5, with rotation and side bending occurring to the same side and opposite the side of the sacrum's rotation.

Bilateral Sacral Flexion

If the sacrum is flexed forward, with the sacral base anterior, the lumbar lordosis appears to be increased, the seated flexion test is negative, the sacral sulci are bilaterally deep, and the ILAs are posterior. It is postulated that this motion occurs about a middle transverse axis of the sacrum. This is called a bilateral sacral flexion. When the lumbosacral spring test is performed, there is good spring (a negative test) because the sacral base, already anterior, moves forward easily. If the backward bending test is done, the sacral sulci is still deep (if not deeper), and the ILAs are still posterior (or more posterior) because the base of the sacrum normally moves forward and the apex moves posteriorly during backward bending of the lumbar region.

This is an extremely common dysfunction in the postpartum female because of birth mechanics (see Chapter 31). Subjectively, the patient complains of low back pain that becomes worse when bending backward. Objective findings include:

- Increased lumbar curve
- Deep bilateral sacral sulci with tissue texture changes
- Bilateral ILAs posterior
- Negative lumbar spring test
- No change with the hyperextension test

Motion characteristics include resistance to posterior rotation of the base of the sacrum if pressure is placed on the apex.

Bilateral Sacral Extension

In some cases, the patient does not have a positive seated flexion test, yet complains of low back pain, and the sacrum seems to be at the center of the problem. At that time, the sacral sulci should be examined, the ILAs checked, the spring test and backward bending test performed, and a careful analysis made of the relationship of the sacrum to the lumbar spine. The lordotic curve may be increased or decreased. With postural flexion at the lumbar spine (forward bending), the sacrum extends (the base moves posterior), and there is a decrease in the lumbar lordotic curve. If the lordotic curve seems to be decreased, it may be that there is a posterior sacral base. In a bilateral extension, the sacrum is held in a backward bent position and does not easily bend forward. The lumbosacral spring test is therefore positive, which means there is either poor spring or no spring. Sacral sulci and ILAs should appear symmetric in either prone or backward bending positions, and, if there is any difference on the backward bending test, the sulci look more shallow, and the ILAs more anterior.

Subjectively, the patient complains of low back pain or fatigue that becomes worse with forward bending. Objective findings include:

- Decreased lumbar curve
- ILAs equal and perhaps anterior
- Positive lumbar spring test
- ILAs stay equal during hyperextension test (superior/inferior)
- Sacral sulci are bilaterally shallow, with tissue texture changes
- Sacrum resists posteroanterior pressure at base, but yields to posteroanterior pressure on apex

Sacral Shears

The sacrum can appear as if it has slipped anteriorly or posteriorly around a transverse axis that allows it to shift within the L- (C-) shaped sacroiliac joint. If it slips forward, it produces a finding called a sacral shear or unilateral sacral flexions and extensions.

Unilateral Sacral Flexion

If there is a positive seated flexion test, with the base of the sacrum anterior on the dysfunctional side (sacral sulcus deep on that side) and the ipsilateral ILA is posterior, the patient has a unilateral sacral flexion. The ipsilateral medial malleolus is more inferior, and the transverse process of L5 is more posterior on the dysfunctional side. Both sides of the sacral base move anteriorly with exhalation but do not move easily in a posterior direction with inhalation. The spring test should be negative, since the base of the sacrum moves anteriorly easily when it is flexed. The backward bending test should show improvement because, while the one side is flexed forward, making the sacral sulcus deep, when the patient bends backward the other side of the sacral base should be pulled forward, increasing symmetry.

Unilateral Sacral Extension

If there is a positive seated flexion test, with the base of the sacrum posterior on the dysfunctional side (sacral sulcus shallow), and the ipsilateral ILA is anterior, the patient has a unilateral sacral extension. To confirm this, test the patient with the spring test and the backward bending test. The spring test should be positive, since the base of the sacrum does not move anteriorly easily when the sacrum is held in an extension position. On the backward bending test, the sulci and ILAs should look even less symmetric because, while the one side is held backward, making the sacral sulcus shallow, when the patient bends backward, the other side of the sacral base should be pulled forward, making the results look worse.

CAUSES OF SACROILIAC DYSFUNCTION

Psoas

Psoas muscle hyperactivity compresses the lumbosacral area. To test for psoas muscle tension with the patient prone, extend the thigh (hip). Psoas problems also have a flexed upper lumbar somatic dysfunction with restriction of extension. Ordinarily, L1 or L2 is flexed, rotated, and side bent to the side of the shorter psoas.

Short Leg Syndrome

The first symptoms of short leg syndrome are usually sacroiliac discomfort or pain. Symptoms are worse with excessive walking or running. Examination of the sacrum usually reveals a deep sacral sulcus on the short leg side with significant tissue texture abnormality and tenderness.

Postural Imbalance

Spinal asymmetry, lateral curves, and repetitive asymmetric activity can produce sacroiliac dysfunction.

Pelvic Side Shift

When the sacral base is to one side of the midline (e.g., pelvic side-shift right), the compensatory change is for body mass to be moved to the opposite side (e.g., pelvic side-shift right, lumbar curve convex left). In this example, the sacrum has to side bend left to accommodate the lumbar curve. When the sacrum side bends left, it rotates right, producing sacroiliac dysfunction. This is the mechanism of sacroiliac dysfunction associated with a short leg problem.

L5 Problems

L5 problems such as spondylolysis, spondylolisthesis, and congenital anomalies predispose to sacroiliac dysfunction.

Lumbar Somatic Dysfunction

Lumbar somatic dysfunction, particularly type II flexed dysfunctions, may contribute to sacroiliac dysfunction. Effective treatment of the lumbar somatic dysfunction will often release the sacroiliac restriction.

Disc

Disc problems at L4 or L5, in the early stages, radiate pain into the buttock region that is interpreted as sacroiliac pain. Often the sacrum is restricted from secondary muscle hypertonicity. In these cases, treating the sacroiliac restriction is not associated with the relief of pain.

Simple Traumatic Sacral Somatic Dysfunction

These patients usually limp in, leap out, and are forever grateful for the one-treatment cure.

Reflex Causes

Reflex causes such as viscerosomatic reflexes from pelvis or unilateral sympathetic nervous system dysfunction are causes of sacroiliac pain. Viscerosomatic reflexes are associated with tissue texture abnormality along the sacroiliac joint, which is puffy and warm. This is similar to acute tissue texture abnormality found in the thoracic area from abdominal or thoracic visceral problems.

Clinical Pearls on Low Back Pain

1. L5 is a frequent site of pain and may be unstable as well as painful. *Plan:* Mobilize adjacent segments that are restricted. Avoid excessive HVLA to unstable joints.
2. Treat short hypertonic psoas.
3. Sacroiliac pain may be caused by L5 problems. In these cases, mobilization of the sacroiliac joint does not relieve the pain.
4. Iliolumbar ligament insertion on the ilium may be very tender. Causes include ipsilateral lumbothoracic irritability, anterior rotation of L5, and pelvic side shift to that side. This may be the first ligament to be strained with postural decompensation.
5. Nociceptive activity at the lumbosacral junction causes lumbothoracic irritability with increased sympathetic tone.
6. Active exercises are essential to strengthen and stabilize a back. OMT can create an environment that allows exercises to work and compensations to occur. The primary rule for exercise is to stop short of pain.

CONCLUSION

Manual medicine can restore functional symmetry between the arthrodial, vascular, lymphatic, and connective tissue elements of the pelvic girdle. It can relieve a wide range of somatic, visceral, and emotional patient complaints and contribute to the health of vertebral function, the thoracoabdominal diaphragm, and the urogenital area.

REFERENCES

1. Weisl H. The articular surfaces of the sacroiliac joint and their relationship to the movements of the sacrum. *Acta Anat.* 1954;22:1;14.
2. Greenman PE. *Principles of Manual Medicine.* Baltimore, MD: Williams & Wilkins; 1989:226–227.
3. Mitchell FL. Structural pelvic function. In: *American Academy of Osteopathy Yearbook.* Indianapolis, IN: American Academy of Osteopathy; 1958:71–90.
4. Thiele GH. Coccygodynia: cause and treatment. *Dis Colon Rectum.* 1963;6:422–436.
5. Korr IM. Sustained sympathicotonia as a factor in disease. In: *The*

Collected Papers of Irvin M. Korr. Newark, OH: American Academy of Osteopathy; 1979:77–89.

6. Beaton LE, Anson BJ. The sciatic nerve and the piriformis muscle: their interrelationship as a possible cause of coccygodynia. *J Bone Joint Surg (Br).* 1938;20:686–688.

7. Reynolds HM. Three dimensional kinematics in the pelvic girdle. *JAOA.* 1980;80:277–280.

8. Strachan WF, et al. A study of the mechanics of the sacroiliac joint. *JAOA.* 1938;43(12):576–578.

9. Mitchell FL, Pruzzo NA. Investigation of voluntary and primary respiratory mechanism. *JAOA.* 1971;70:1109–1112.

10. Truhlar RE. *Doctor A.T. Still in the Living.* Privately published, Cleveland, OH; 1950. Distributed, Indianapolis, IN: American Academy of Osteopathy; p. 62.

11. Kuchera WA, Kuchera ML. *Osteopathic Principles in Practice.* 2nd ed. rev. Columbus, OH: Greyden Press; 1994.

12. Seidel HM, Ball JW, Dains JE, Benedict GW. *Mosby's Guide to Physical Examination.* St. Louis, MO: CV Mosby Co; 1987.

13. Travell JG, Simons DG. *Myofascial Pain and Dysfunction: The Trigger Point Manual.* Vol 1. Baltimore, MD: Williams & Wilkins; 1983.

14. Kuchera WA, Kuchera ML. *The Kuchera Manual: Osteopathic Principles in Practice.* Kirksville, MO: KCOM Press; 1991.

15. Sutherland AS, Wales AL. *Collected Writings of William Garner Sutherland, D.O., D.Sc. (Hon.).* Produced under auspices of the Sutherland Cranial Teaching Foundation, 1967.

16. Hoppenfeld S. *Physical Examination of the Spine and Extremities.* Norwalk, CT: Appleton & Lange; 1976:151–152, 164.

17. Walton WJ. *Osteopathic Diagnosis and Technique, Sacroiliac Diagnosis,* 1st ed. St. Louis, MO: Matthews Book Co; 1966:187–197. Distributed, Colorado Springs, CO: American Academy of Osteopathy; reprinted, 1970.

53

LOWER EXTREMITIES

MICHAEL L. KUCHERA

KEY CONCEPTS

■ Structure, functional anatomy, and somatic dysfunction of the lower extremities
■ Differential palpatory end-feel characteristics associated with dysfunction, inflammation, and trauma
■ Recognition of each distinctive "capsular pattern" for hip, knee, and ankle
■ Classification of ligamentous sprains
■ Structures and biomechanical factors influencing major and minor motions of lower extremity joint regions
■ Meaning and biomechanical impact of coxa varus, genu valgus, and/or pes planus
■ Motions of fibular head and how motions of ankle affect fibular head motion
■ Most common ankle sprains, how they occur, and related somatic dysfunction
■ Relationship of related neuromuscular, vascular, and lymphatic elements to lower extremity dysfunction and clinical symptoms
■ Neuromuscular imbalance in the lower extremities and myofascial trigger points

The lower extremities provide for support and locomotion with strong bones and powerful muscles. Functionally, the lower extremities extend to the iliosacral joint (covered in Chapter 52); anatomically, most texts begin at the hip. While many clinicians consider the pelvis to be the foundation on which the spine balances, the lower extremities form the final common platform for postural alignment (1). Somatic dysfunction in the lower extremities has local, postural, and systemic implications.

The lower extremities are often the site of referred pain from somatic structures in the lumbar and pelvic regions and/or from certain abdominopelvic viscera. While these relationships are mentioned in this chapter, refer also to those chapters in this text associated with the primary problem. Examples of lower extremity clinical considerations discussed in this chapter include:

■ Ankle sprains
■ Bursitis and arthritis

■ Compartment syndromes
■ Myofascial trigger points
■ Patellar tracking problems

Neuromusculoskeletal system evaluation of the lower extremities typically includes a screening evaluation of the region during walking, standing, and squatting as well as evaluation of a standing flexion test; one-legged stork (also known as Gillet or modified Trendelenburg) test; and straight-leg raising test. These are integrated with standard screening functional tests for neural, lymphatic, and vascular disorders. A positive finding in any of these screening examinations, or an indication in the history of a need for closer scanning of the region, requires palpation; assessment of range of motion of each joint; and assessment of muscle strength, stability, and flexibility. This chapter reviews the functional anatomy and basic examination of the lower extremities in three sections:

1. Skeletal, arthrodial, and ligamentous structure and function
2. Neuromuscular structure and function
3. Vascular and lymphatic structure and function

SKELETAL, ARTHRODIAL, AND LIGAMENTOUS STRUCTURES AND FUNCTION

The bony skeleton of each lower limb (Fig. 53.1) includes the:

■ Innominate (pelvic bone)
■ Femur
■ Tibia
■ Fibula
■ 7 tarsal bones (including the talus, calcaneus, navicular, cuboid, and 3 cuneiforms)
■ 5 metatarsal bones
■ 14 phalanges

Functionally, the joints of the lower extremities include:

■ Hip (femoroacetabular joint)
■ Knee (femorotibial, proximal tibiofibular, and patellar joints)
■ Distal tibiofibular joint
■ Ankle (tibiotalar joint)
■ Subtalar (talocalcaneal joint)

Femoroacetabular Joint

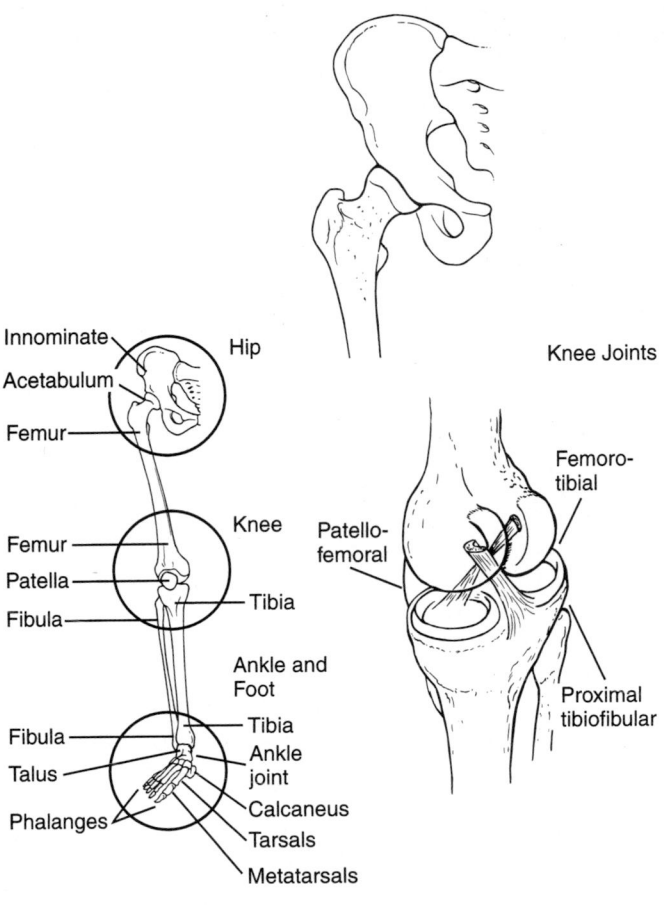

Knee Joints

Ankle and Foot Joints

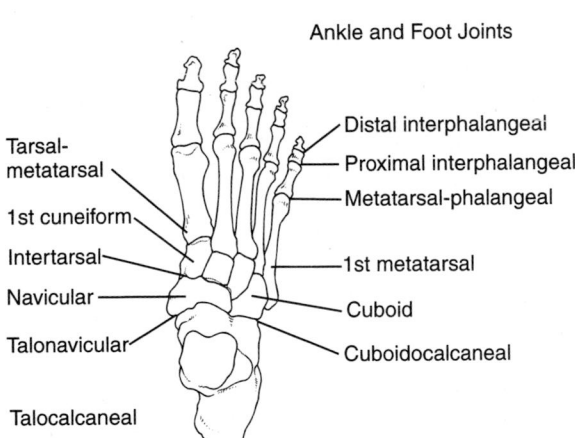

FIGURE 53.1. Bones and joints of the lower extremity.

- Several intertarsal joints (including the talonavicular, the cuboidocalcaneal, and two small talocalcaneal joints) collectively called the Chopart joint
- Numerous tarsometatarsal, metatarsophalangeal, and interphalangeal joints in the foot

The bones making up these joints are covered in articular cartilage. The majority are synovial joints with a capsule and synovial membrane while the distal tibiofibular joint is a fibrous syndesmosis with an interosseous membrane. Each of these joints is stabilized by ligaments, which limit joint motions and are a part of the normal end-feel sensed when palpating joint motion.

Joint capsules are subject to pathologic and inflammatory processes. Such processes result in "capsular patterns" of restricted motion in which all or most passive movements of the joint prove painful and limited. A capsular pattern due to inflammation or pathology is palpably different from the patterns of tenderness and restricted motion assessed in somatic dysfunction (2) (Table 53.1). Palpation of the capsular pattern is also dramatically different from the laxity appreciated in ligamentous sprains. Thus palpation of the end-feel provides significant information about the differential diagnosis of a painful or improperly functioning joint.

In the diagnosis of ligamentous sprains, the joint line and stabilizing ligaments should be palpated directly for tenderness followed by end-feel assessment for arthrodial motion or laxity. The greater the structural damage due to ligamentous spraining, the greater the laxity with resultant loss of normal end-feel and stability. Palpation of joint play end-feel is therefore useful in classification of traumatic and orthopedic conditions including sprains.

Ligamentous Sprain Classification

Ligamentous sprains are generally classified by degree. A first-degree sprain assumes that the integrity of the ligament is undisturbed, resulting in generally intact tensile strength. (Some label this degree of injury a "strain," while others reserve the term, strains, for muscle injuries.) A first-degree sprain, while tender to specific palpation and painful when stressed, is generally stable to most orthopedic ligamentous tests. A first-degree sprain responds well to conservative osteopathic care and recovers with normal function and no ligamentous laxity.

A third-degree sprain (also known as a grade III sprain) indicates complete disruption of the ligament with no remaining tensile strength. Orthopedic testing indicates the sloppy end-feel of complete instability. Good splinting and early surgery may offer the best prognosis when dealing with third-degree ligamentous sprains around the structurally unstable knee; with ligaments of the inherently more stable ankle joint, surgery may be delayed or unnecessary to reestablish stability.

Second-degree sprains make up the ligamentous injuries in between these two diagnoses. Second-degree sprains may be divided into grade I (partial tearing with slight laxity) and grade II (more complete tearing and moderate laxity) sprains. Second-degree sprains, even grade II, do not usually require surgical repair if they are appropriately immobilized for a time appropriate to the amount of structural damage. Prolotherapy (3) and/or

TABLE 53.1. THE CAPSULAR PATTERNS

Region Involving Capsular Pattern (Common Diagnoses)	Capsular Pattern of Motion Specific to Joint (Contrast with Somatic Dysfunction Patterning)	End-Feel and Other Comments
"Sign of the Buttock" Indicates major lesion such as osteomyelitis, ischiorectal abscess, iliac neoplasm, etc.	Passive hip flexion more limited and more painful than straight leg raise	A prematurely empty end-feel on passive hip flexion accompanies the sign of the buttock
Hip Rheumatoid, traumatic, or spondylitic arthritis; osteoarthrosis	Marked limitation of internal rotation and flexion, some limitation of abduction, little or no limitation of adduction and external rotation	Hard end-feel palpated especially at the end of internal rotation (advanced cases: patient may walk with foot turned outward)
Knee Traumatic arthritis, rheumatoid arthritis, osteoarthritis, Baker cyst	Gross limitation of flexion, slight limitation of extension	In arthritis, the palpated end-feel on passive flexion is usually hard. Most common primary capsular conditions signaled by warmth, fluid, and synovial thickening
Ankle Osteoarthrosis, reactive arthritis	More limitation of plantar flexion than of dorisflexion	Capsular patterns unusual
Talocalcaneal Joint Osteoarthrosis, rheumatoid or subacute traumatic arthritis, Sudeck atrophy	Increasing limitation of varus until fixation in valgus position	
Mid tarsal Joint Osteoarthrosis, monarticular or subacute rheumatoid arthritis	Limitation of adduction and internal rotation, other movements full	Peroneal spasm involved
Big Toe Rheumatoid arthritis, osteoarthrosis, gout	Gross limitation of extension, slight limitation of flexion	Advanced pattern demonstrates fixation in neutral position (hallux rigidus)

(From Cyriax JH, Cyriax PJ. *Cyriax's Illustrated Manual of Orthopaedic Medicine,* 2nd ed. Oxford, England: Butterworth-Heinemann Ltd; 1993:6–8, with permission.)

certain rehabilitative procedures may be employed to restore a component of the laxity and lost joint stability.

HIP

The hip, or coxa, is a term used loosely to indicate the articulation of the head of the femur with the acetabular socket of the innominate bone. (Recognize that the term, hip, may also be commonly used to refer to any part of the region between the waist and the thigh.) Throughout this chapter the term, hip, will be interchangeable with the structural and functional elements associated with the femoroacetabular joint itself.

The hip is a ball-and-socket synovial joint with a socket deeper than the glenoid fossa of the shoulder, reflecting the stability characteristic of the joint. In the newborn with a congenitally shallow acetabulum, this lack of stability can be evaluated using the Ortolani test for dislocation (Fig. 53.2) and the Barlow test for reduction (Fig. 53.3). Early discovery permits satisfactory results with triple diapering or conservative brace management. Failure to perform a satisfactory examination risks a late diagnosis and the necessity for surgical correction.

FEMUR

The femur is the longest and heaviest bone in the body, attaining a length about one-fourth the height of an adult (4).

This fact allows the forensic pathologist or archaeologist to estimate an individual's height from the femur alone. The angle formed by the intersection of the anatomic axis of the shaft of the femur and the longitudinal axis of the neck of the femur is called the angle of inclination. This angle normally measures 120 to 135 degrees. If the angle of inclination is larger than 135 degrees, the condition is referred to as coxa valgus. If it measures less than 120 degrees, the condition is called coxa varus (Fig. 53.4). The femoral shaft is twisted so that the condyles of the distal femur are in a transverse plane even though the femoral neck angles forward 12 to 15 degrees. This is called the angle of anteversion.

Longitudinal Axis

The anatomic longitudinal axis running down the shaft of the femur is not its functional axis. The functional longitudinal axis of the femur runs from the femoral head distally to a point midway between the condyles. With internal rotation at the hip on this functional axis, the femoral head glides posteriorly. With external rotation, the femoral head glides anteriorly. Internal rotation with posterior glide and external rotation with anterior glide are minor motions of the femoroacetabular joint.

Since arthritic change modifies gliding motions and occurs early in the minor motions of the joint, (5) screening for arthritic changes in the hip should combine the standard Patrick screening test (Fig. 53.5) with evaluation for a hip capsular pattern. The acronym FABERE is often used to describe the order in which

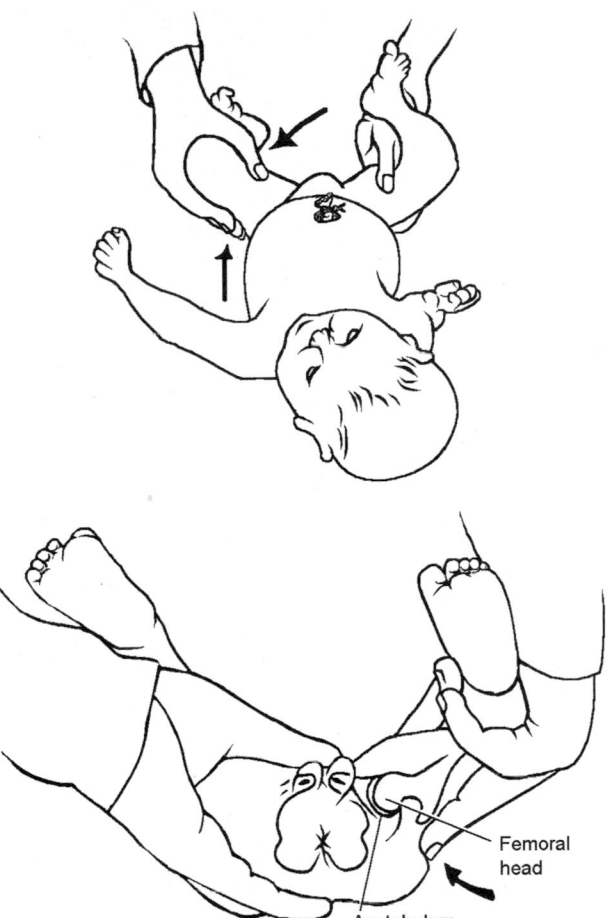

FIGURE 53.2. Ortolani test. Ortolani test for hip dislocation can be used in the first few weeks of life. In a subluxated hip, this maneuver creates resistance felt at 45 to 60 degrees. A positive sign is a palpable click (not heard) when resistance is overcome and the femoral head reduces. (**Top:** From Kuchera ML, Kuchera WA. *Osteopathic Principles in Practice*, 2nd ed. rev. Columbus, OH: Greyden Press; 1994:636, illustration by W.A. Kuchera. **Bottom:** Modified from Burnside JW. *Physical Diagnosis: An Introduction to Clinical Medicine*, 16th ed. Baltimore, MD: Williams & Wilkins; 1981:246.)

the "Patrick FABERE" test is performed:

*F*lexion
*Ab*duction
*E*xternal *R*otation
*E*xtension

Positive without a hip capsular pattern, the Patrick test is more likely to reflect pain from the sacroiliac joint or anterior sacroiliac ligament than hip pathology.

Arthritic change progresses from functional demand accentuated by biomechanical stress to pathophysiologic response to structural change. For example, the biomechanical stress placed on the hip joint by a short lower extremity results in a higher incidence of greater trochanteric bursitis and of osteoarthritis (6,7), both on the long leg side. Somatic dysfunction and arthritic pathology often coexist within this structure-function spectrum. Each should be addressed with appropriate therapeutic tools integrated into a regimen for total patient treatment (8).

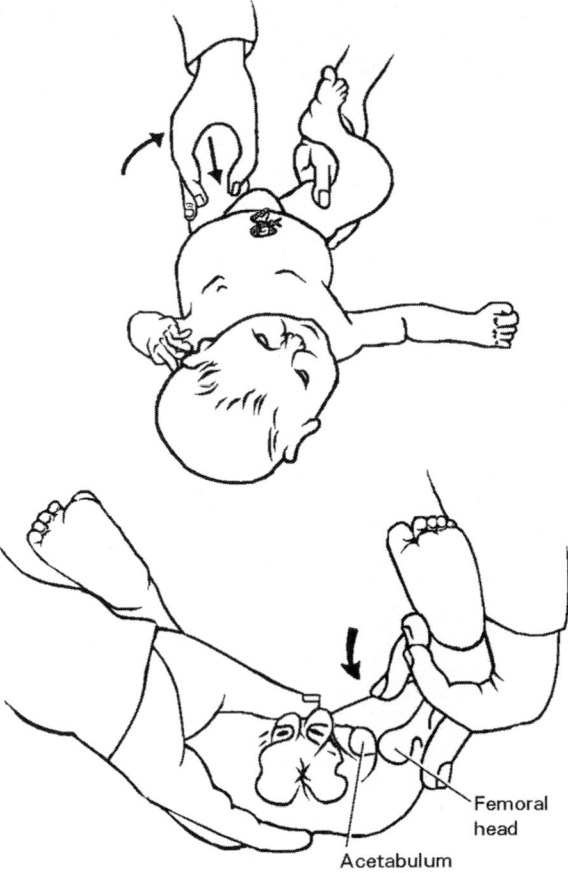

FIGURE 53.3. Barlow test. Barlow test for hip reduction is a modification of the Ortolani test used to identify an unstable hip in infants up to 6 months of age. To perform the Barlow test, the Ortolani test is first performed followed by a posterolateral pressure over the inner thigh. If the femoral head slips out over the posterior lip of the acetabulum and reduces spontaneously when the pressure is released, then the joint is not dislocated but is unstable. (**Top:** From Kuchera ML, Kuchera WA. *Osteopathic Principles in Practice*, 2nd ed. rev. Columbus, OH: Greyden Press; 1994:636, illustration by W.A. Kuchera. **Bottom:** Modified from Burnside JW. *Physical Diagnosis: An Introduction to Clinical Medicine*, 16th ed. Baltimore, MD: Williams & Wilkins; 1981:246.)

Ligaments

The iliofemoral ligament on the anterior aspect of the hip joint is the strongest ligament in the body. Because it is shaped like the letter Y, it is also called the Y-ligament of Bigelow. This ligament tenses with full hip extension. It helps to maintain posture in the military at-ease position with minimal muscle activity. On the posterior side, the ischiofemoral ligament attaches to the ischial portion of the acetabular rim and wraps over the posterior and superior part of the hip joint to attach just medially to the base of the greater trochanter of the femur. This important anatomic configuration tends to screw the femoral head into the acetabulum with extension, thereby preventing hyperextension. Normal extension is limited to about 35 degrees (Fig. 53.6).

Motion

The motions of the hip (femoroacetabular) joint that are grossly tested are:

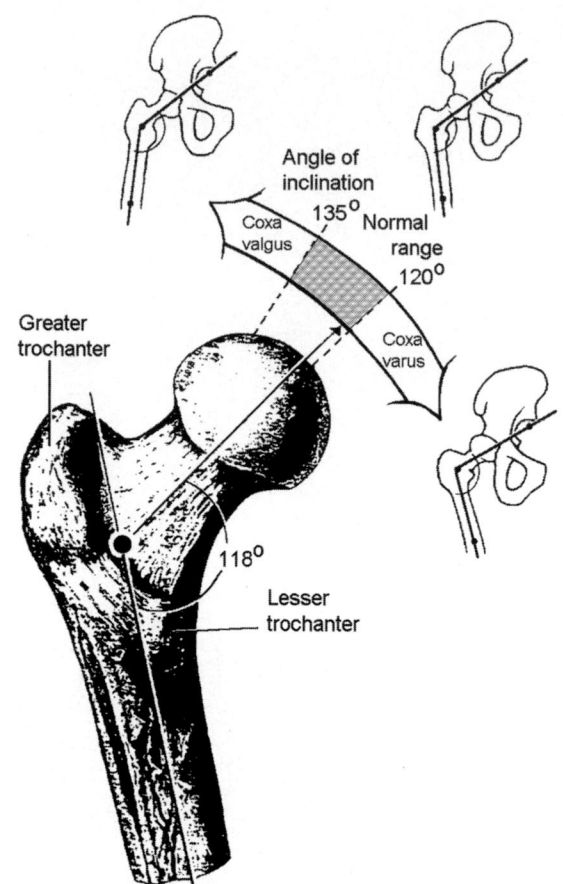

FIGURE 53.4. Angle of inclination in coxa varus (120 degrees) and coxa valgus (135 degrees). (Illustration by W.A. Kuchera.)

■ Flexion–extension
■ Abduction–adduction
■ External rotation–internal rotation

Minor motions of the joint are glides that are assessed with end-feel palpation. For example:

■ Anterior glide occurring with external rotation
■ Posterior glide occurring with internal rotation

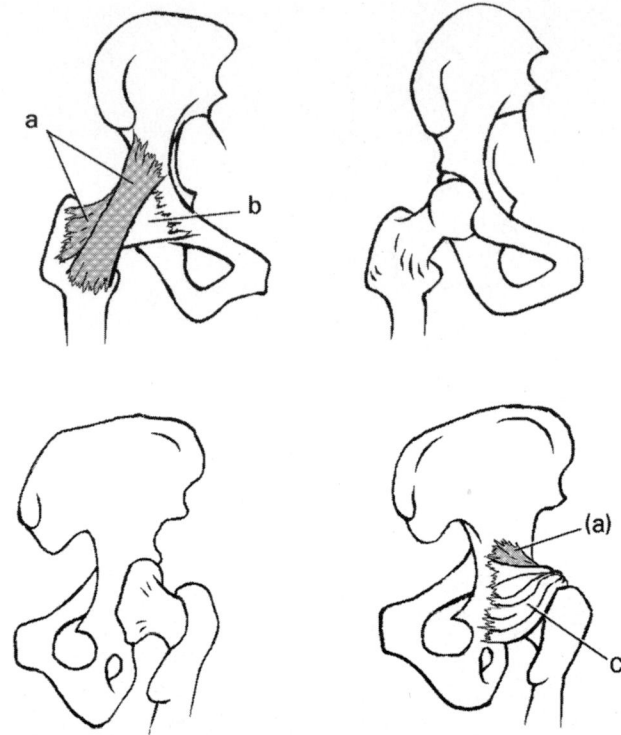

FIGURE 53.6. Top: Bones and ligaments of the right hip (anterior view). **a:** Iliofemoral ligament (Y-ligament of Bigelow). **b:** Pubofemoral ligament. The iliofemoral ligament on the anterior aspect of the joint is the strongest ligament in the body. **Bottom:** Bones and ligaments of the right hip (posterior view). The ischiofemoral ligament on the posterior side of the joint limits extension to 35 degrees. (Illustration by W.A. Kuchera.)

Gross hip ranges of motion and passive assessments of end-feel are usually tested with the patient supine and the pelvis stabilized. Ranges of motion vary from individual to individual and differ in different populations tested. (For example, expect different averages for male high school football players than for teenage female gymnasts.) More important than the absolute number of degrees measured is side-to-side symmetry and the quality of the barrier at the end of motion. This holds true for all lower extremity joints assessed as well. In the presence

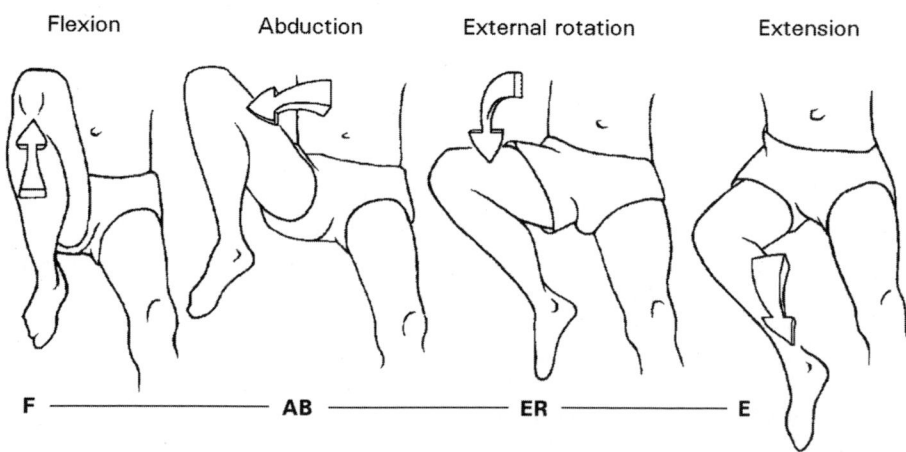

FIGURE 53.5. Patrick FABERE test of the hip. (Illustration by W.A. Kuchera.)

of asymmetric motion, also differentiate hypomobility from hypermobility.

The character and pattern of the end-feel of each hip motion may be springy (physiologic) or it may suggest a capsular, traumatic, or dysfunctional pattern. Subtle differences in somatic dysfunction of myofascial rather than articular origin may also be appreciated by evaluating the end-feel of the hip joint.

The muscles and soft tissues of the hip typically limit flexion more than the ligaments. Straight leg raising at the hip around a transverse axis is limited by the hamstring muscles to 85 to 90 degrees. If the knee is bent to remove the hamstring influence, the thigh can normally be flexed up to 135 degrees at the hip. If significant improvement in range-of-motion is not seen after bending the thigh, the situation is not consistent with a biomechanical cause. Thus when more pain and limitation of motion (with an empty end-feel) occurs with bent-knee hip flexion than with straight-leg raising, a serious condition, such as septic bursitis, ischiorectal fossa abscess, osteomyelitis or neoplasm of the upper femur, or other significant pathology of the ilium, must be ruled out (9) (see Table 53.1.).

Extension with the subject prone and legs extended may measure as much as 35 degrees; bending the hip and knee of the opposite lower extremity relaxes some of the muscular restriction to hip extension and should increase this measurement.

Around an anteroposterior (AP) axis through the femoral head the hip may abduct and adduct as much as 55 degrees and 35 degrees, respectively. To test adduction in a supine patient with the knee locked, the leg must be lifted to cross anterior to the opposite leg.

Around a functional longitudinal axis, hip external rotation may measure up to 55 degrees; internal rotation to 45 degrees.

In summary, the major motions of the hip and the minor motion glides of anterior glide (with external rotation) and posterior glide (with internal rotation) should be assessed and their pattern evaluated. A physiologic end-feel to one motion compared to a barrier in the opposite is consistent with a dysfunctional pattern. A capsular pattern of marked limitation to internal rotation, with limitation to flexion and abduction as well, should raise suspicions of an inflammatory process. If findings do not follow functional biomechanical principles, they warrant further evaluation.

KNEE

While this section also covers the patellofemoral joint, the true knee, genu, or femorotibial joint is a double condylar, complex synovial articulation formed by the femoral condyles and the tibial plateau (Fig. 53.7). This joint contains medial and lateral semilunar cartilages to provide some stability, smoothness, and resilience to pressure.

The medial condyle of the knee is longer than the articular surface of the lateral condyle (Fig. 53.8). This structural configuration affects joint function. With extension of the knee, the lateral condyle reaches its physiologic limit of motion while the medial condyle of the femur continues to track posteriorly on the tibial plateau. This results in posterolateral glide of the

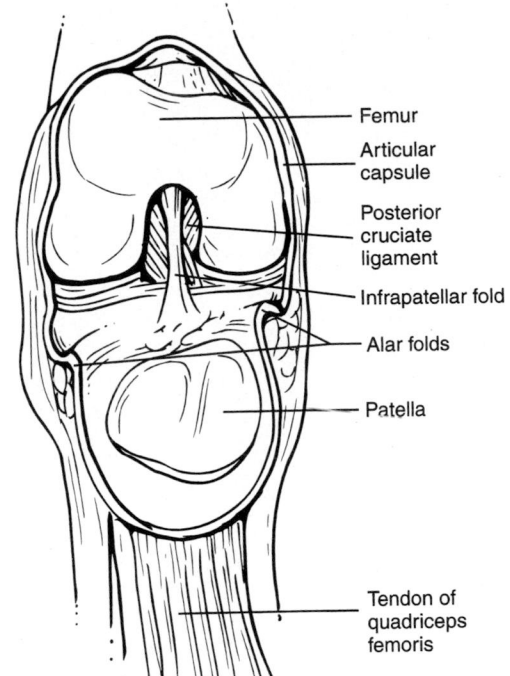

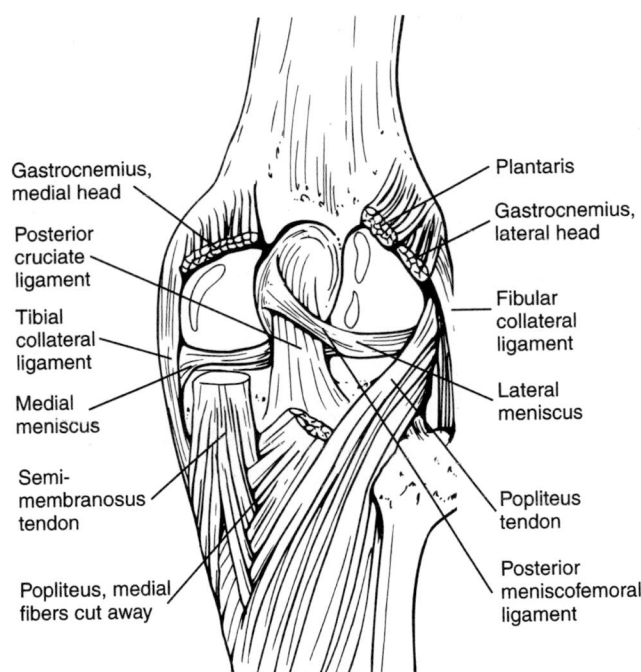

FIGURE 53.7. Knee joint. **Top:** Anterior view. **Bottom:** posterior view.

tibia with full extension of the knee. Full extension locking requires this minor rotational glide. The opposite (anteromedial glide) occurs with full flexion of the knee. These minor motions of the joint should be checked for somatic dysfunction by adding an anteromedial glide while inducing external rotation of the tibial plateau and a posterolateral glide while inducing internal rotation of the tibial plateau (Fig. 53.9).

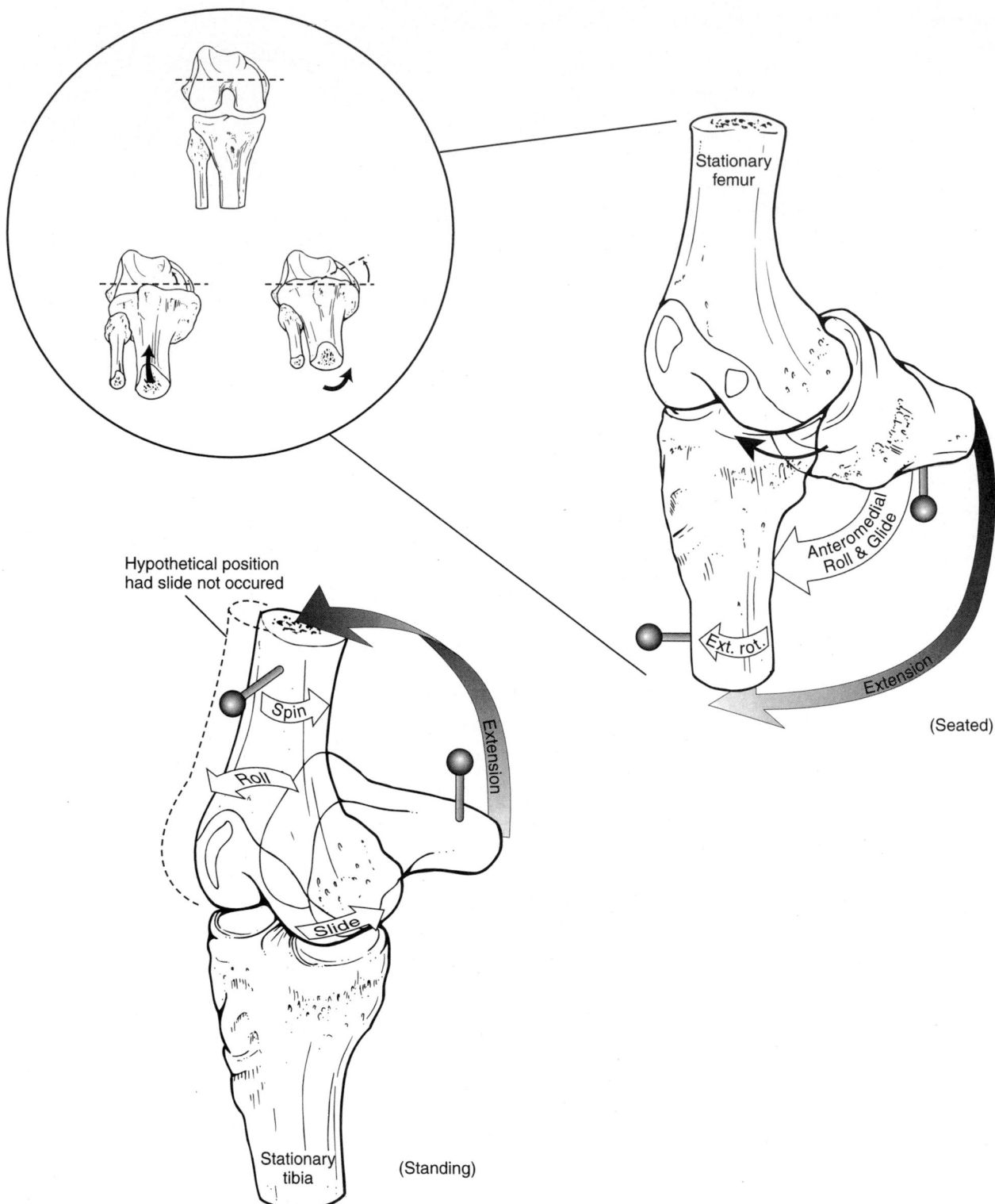

FIGURE 53.8. Structure-function relationship of the medial condyle. In knee extension, the medial, but not the lateral, femoral condyle will continue to track posteriorly, resulting in internal rotation of the femur (if the tibia is stationary) or external rotation (*Ext. rot.*) of the tibia (if the femur is held stationary). The condylar glide occurring with external rotation of the tibia is called the anteromedial glide.

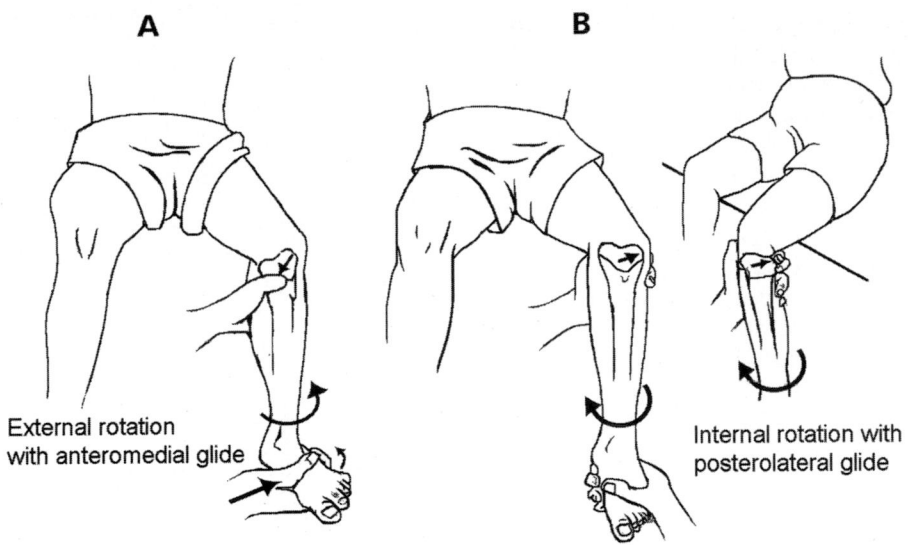

A

B

External rotation
with anteromedial glide

Internal rotation with
posterolateral glide

FIGURE 53.9. Physical examination of anteromedial glide with external rotation **(A)** and posterolateral glide with internal rotation **(B)** of the knee. (Illustration by W.A. Kuchera.)

The osteopathic palpatory examination of the knee incorporates standard knee testing positions and maneuvers while noting the presence and pattern of these findings:

- Gross range of motion
- Restricted gliding minor motions (end-feel)
- Hypermobility and loss of stability (end-feel)

The same testing maneuvers needed to diagnose somatic dysfunction offer orthopedic and rheumatologic information about knee structure. In general during testing, if the end-feel of the test is too loose, there is an orthopedic diagnosis. If generally restricted in both directions of a given paired motion (e.g., flexion–extension), there is often a rheumatologic diagnosis. If a pattern of paired motions are assessed to be physiologically free in one direction but ends too abruptly in the other, the diagnosis is joint somatic dysfunction. Thus, interpreting each test for the available dual structure-function information provides twice the diagnostic information in the same amount of time usually spent in examining the knee structure alone.

Q-Angle and the Patella

The angle formed by the intersection of the functional longitudinal axis of the femur and the tibial longitudinal axis is referred to as the Q- (or *Quadriceps*-) angle. Normally the Q-angle measures 10 to 12 degrees (Fig. 53.10). An angle of 20 degrees or more is definitely abnormal. As the Q-angle increases, the patient appears more knock-kneed, a condition referred to as genu valgus. A bowlegged appearance is known as genu varus. Biomechanically, coxa varus increases the Q-angle, as does a pronated foot. Each enhances the possibility of genu valgus.

The Q-angle has a major effect on the tracking of the patella, a sesamoid bone in the tendon of the quadriceps femoris muscle group. Patellofemoral joint dysfunction and structural change may each arise from abnormal tracking of, or pressure on, the patella.

Accentuated Q-angles may be associated with symptoms of patellar pain due to ligamentous stress at the knee or through

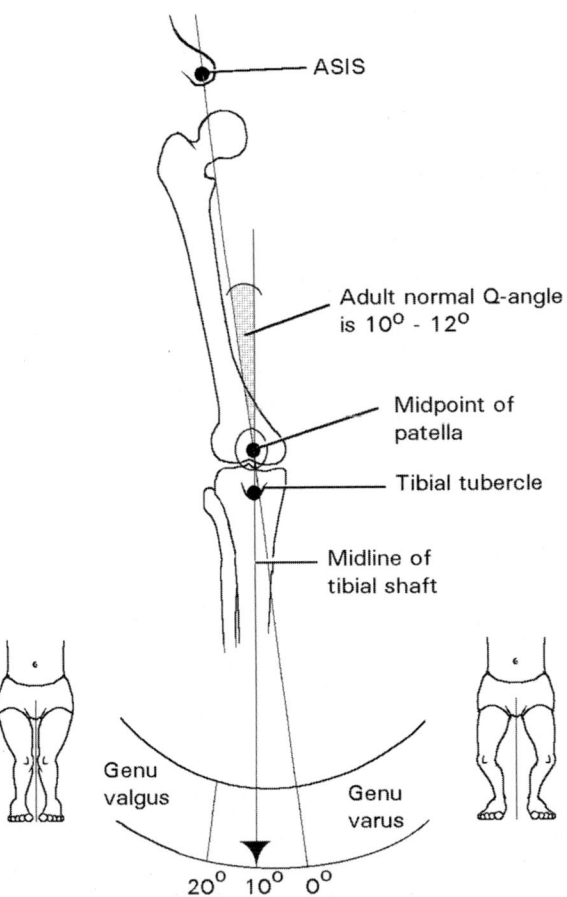

ASIS

Adult normal Q-angle
is 10° - 12°

Midpoint of
patella

Tibial tubercle

Midline of
tibial shaft

Genu
valgus

Genu
varus

20° 10° 0°

FIGURE 53.10. Q-angle (quadriceps angle) normally measures 10 to 12 degrees. Key landmarks for establishing the Q-angle are the anterior superior iliac spine, the patella, and the tibial tuberosity. Note the change in the Q-angle in genu valgus and varus.

secondary development of muscle imbalance and trigger points. The patella may even sublux laterally with these biomechanical forces, especially with dysfunction or weakness of the vastus medialis muscle. Locking of the patella strongly suggests myofascial trigger points in the vastus lateralis muscle. Complete locking of the patella immobilizes the knee joint in slight flexion, while partial locking causes difficulty in straightening the knee after sitting in a chair.

Prolonged patellofemoral dysfunction, due to these biomechanical factors, predisposes to structural change such as irregular or accelerated wearing or roughening of the articular surface on the posterior surface of the patella (chondromalacia patellae). This coexistence of structural and functional disorders must be considered and appropriately diagnosed and treated to encourage optimum healing. Patellar structural problems also arise from:

- Patellar dislocation
- Chronic or direct patellar trauma
- Fracture of the lower extremity

Structural problems of the patella are evaluated, in part, by palpating over and around the patella. Look for subpatellar tenderness, crepitus, grinding, or clicking with compression against the underlying femur (patellar grind test) when gliding the patella medially and laterally as well as superiorly and inferiorly. Effusion within the knee joint also strongly suggests structural change.

As a consequence of secondary bony alignment and muscular imbalance, functional patellar tracking difficulties may also be the presenting symptom of postural disorders (see Chapter 43).

Ligaments and Cartilage

Lateral and medial collateral ligaments, placed to limit lateral glide of the tibia with adduction and medial glide of the tibia with abduction, stabilize the true knee joint. The lateral (fibular) collateral ligament does not attach to the lateral semilunar cartilage (meniscus), while the medial (tibial) collateral ligament does attach to the medial semilunar cartilage (meniscus) (Fig. 53.11).

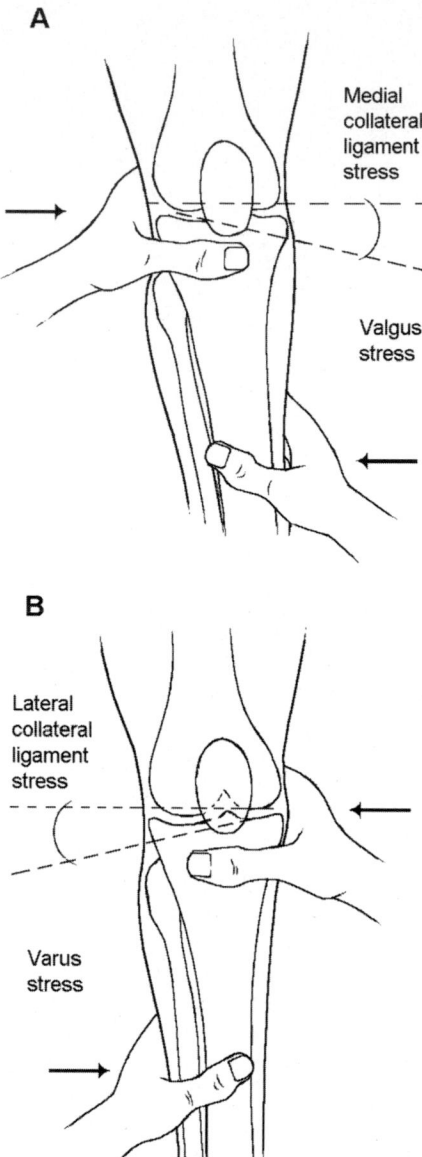

FIGURE 53.12. Tests for collateral ligament injury at the knee. Tibial abduction or genu valgus stress **(A)** tests for medial collateral ligament stability. Tibial adduction or genu varus stress **(B)** tests for lateral collateral ligament stability. (Illustration by W.A. Kuchera.)

This anatomic arrangement makes the medial cartilage more susceptible to injury. It also predisposes to displacement, especially from a blow to the knee that comes through the knee from the lateral to the medial side, or to twisting injuries of the knee.

Valgus stress testing of the knee at 30 degrees (Fig. 50.12A) induces abduction of the tibia with medial glide and provides information on stability of the medial collateral ligament. Varus stress testing at 30 degrees (Fig. 53.12B) induces adduction of the tibia with lateral glide and provides information on stability of the lateral collateral ligament. A palpable click accompanied by pain while performing McMurray meniscal tests (Fig. 53.13) strongly suggests a meniscal tear. In addition to ligamentous evaluation, these positions permit assessment for medial and lateral glide somatic dysfunction.

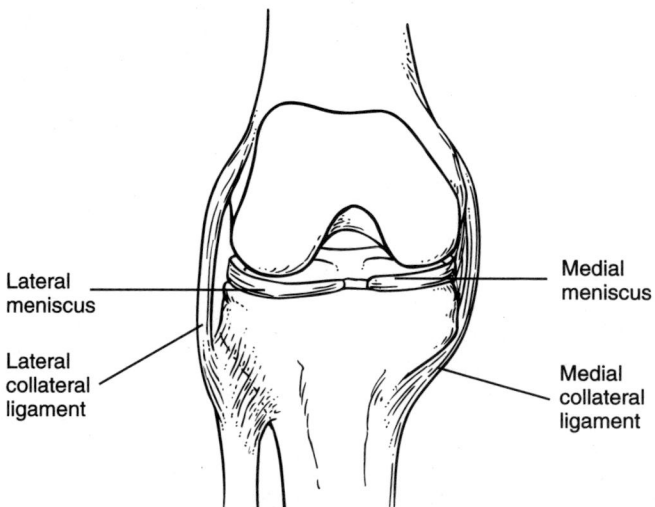

FIGURE 53.11. Relationship of collateral ligaments to knee cartilage (anterior view).

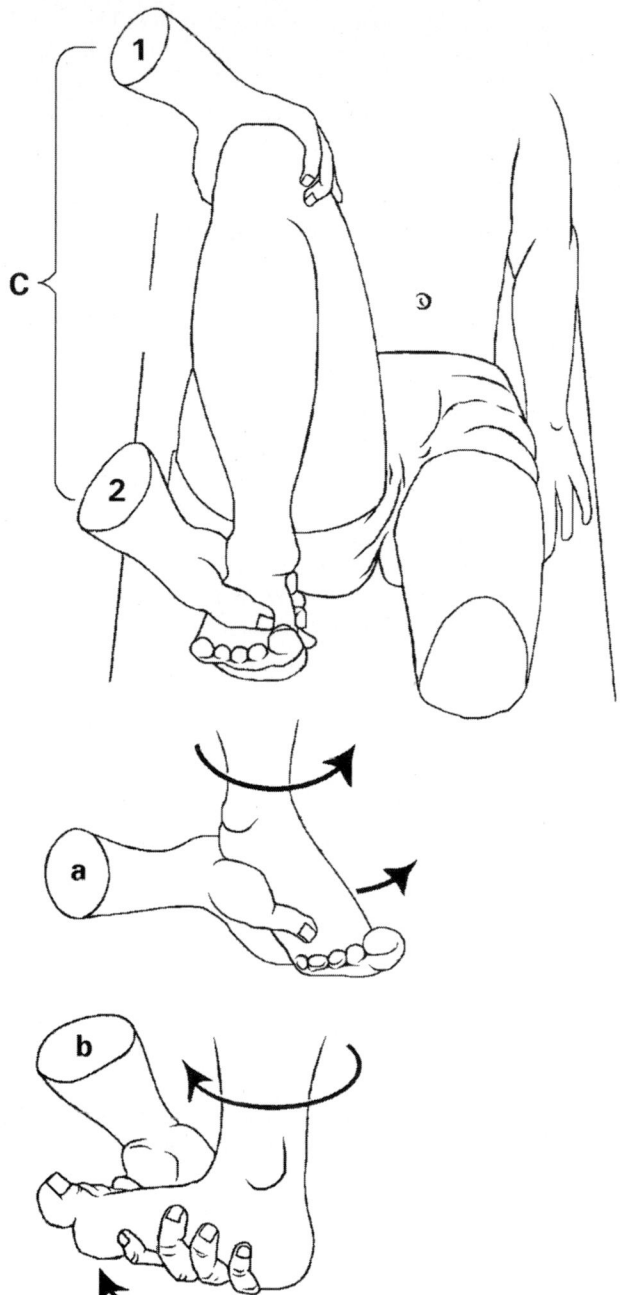

FIGURE 53.13. McMurray test for medial and lateral meniscal injury. The knee is fully flexed. One hand *(1)* palpates the knee at the medial and lateral joint line. The other hand *(2)* holds the foot to control internal *(a)* and external *(b)* rotation of the foot and tibia. A test for lateral meniscus injury: The foot and tibia are internally rotated *(a)*, the two hands *(c)* place the tibia into adduction (genu varus), and while holding this positioning, the leg is extended. A test for medial meniscus injury: The foot and tibia are externally rotated *(b)*, the two hands *(c)* place the tibia into abduction (genu valgus), and while holding this positioning, the leg is extended. (Illustration by W.A. Kuchera.)

The cruciate ligaments run between the tibia and femur and are named according to their tibial attachments. The posterior cruciate ligament attaches to the posterior part of the tibia and prevents excessive posterior glide of the tibia. The anterior cruciate ligament attaches to the anterior part of the tibia and prevents excessive anterior glide of the tibia at the knee joint. Stability of the anterior cruciate ligament (Fig. 53.14A) is checked with an anterior drawer test (knee flexed toward 90 degrees) or, even more specifically, a Lachman test (knee flexed up to 30 degrees). Stability of the posterior cruciate ligament is checked with a posterior drawer test (Fig. 53.14B). These maneuvers also permit assessment of anterior and posterior glide end-feel for dysfunction.

The combination of torn anterior cruciate and medial collateral ligaments along with a torn medial meniscus occurs predictably from certain traumas featuring valgus stress forces (such as a tackle to the outside of the knee with the knee extended fully and the foot fixed). Because this injury causes significant knee instability, historically many clinicians referred to this constellation as the "terrible triad," or "O'Donaghue's triad."

Motion

The major motions of the knee joint are flexion and extension. Because of the irregular shape of the joint surfaces, these two motions are combined with some minor involuntary glides, rolling, and rotational motions. Minor motions of the tibial plateau at the knee include:

- Anterior and posterior glides
- Medial and lateral glides
- Internal rotation with posterolateral glide
- External rotation with anteromedial glide

Complete extension of the knee creates a bony lock. Testing of minor motions of the joint and ligament assessment should therefore be performed with the knee in variable degrees of flexion. Abduction and adduction of the tibia are passive motions of the knee that cannot be voluntarily created by the patient. A varus stress motion applied in an attempt to create adduction of the tibia produces a lateral glide (with slight internal rotation). A valgus stress motion inducing abduction of the tibia produces a medial glide (with slight external rotation) of the tibia. Restriction of glide in one direction suggests somatic dysfunction; laxity in one direction suggests ligamentous sprain or tear.

The knee should move into full extension with locking, freely and without restriction. This is tested by grasping the foot of the supine patient with one hand and raising that lower extremity just off the table. The knee is flexed slightly with the other hand. The slightly flexed knee is then released, allowing it to extend. A normal knee drops freely into extension and bounces off the ligaments. Structural injuries, especially medial meniscal tears, may result in inability to extend fully, or guarding on extension. The hyperextended knee is referred to as genu recurvatum.

A knee with gross limitation of flexion and slight limitation of extension is consistent with a capsular pattern of that joint. This palpatory finding, correlated with history and other physical findings, leads to an appropriate differential diagnosis of varying

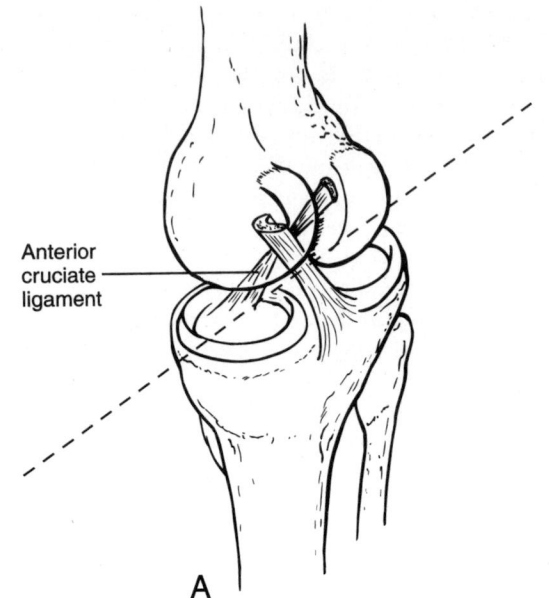

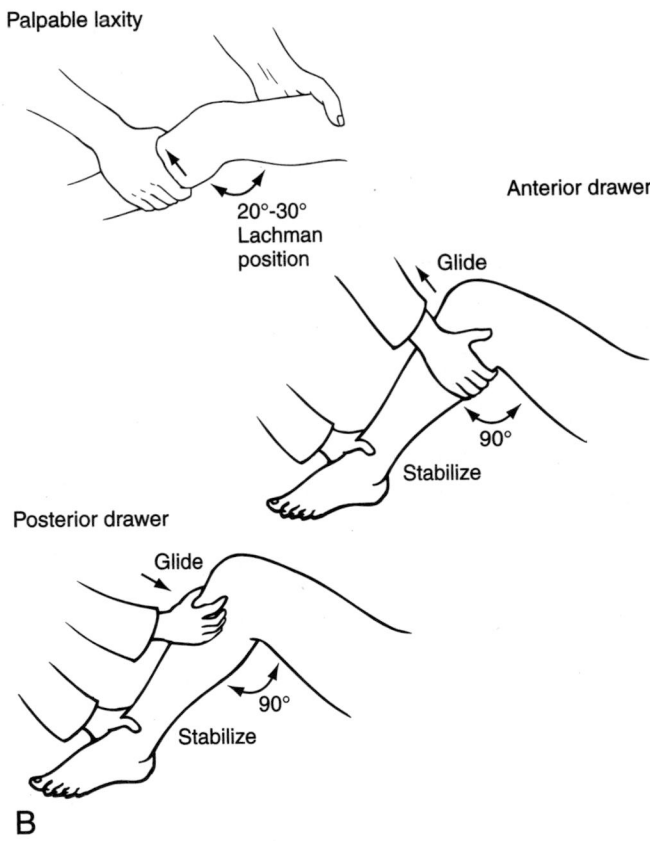

FIGURE 53.14. Structure-function tests of the anterior **(A)** and posterior **(B)** cruciate ligaments using the Lachman and drawer tests.

types of arthritis and synovitis affecting the knee. The capsular pattern of the knee (10) differs significantly from a somatic dysfunction in which minor motions of the joint are restricted in one aspect of each paired motion and free in the opposite direction.

Fibular Motion

The proximal tibiofibular joint is a separate synovial joint at the knee (Fig. 53.15). While the angulation of the articulation actually permits the minor motions of anterolateral and posteromedial glide of the fibular head, clinicians simply report fibular head glide as anterior or posterior. The fibular head lies in the same horizontal plane as the tibial plateau.

The distal tibiofibular articulation is a syndesmosis. This joint allows the fibula to move laterally from the tibia to accommodate the increased width of the talus presented during dorsiflexion. Restricted dorsiflexion of the ankle warrants examination and treatment of this syndesmosis.

When the fibular head glides anteriorly, reciprocal motion is initiated at the distal fibula (lateral malleolus), which glides posteriorly. Posterior fibular head motion is accompanied by anterior motion at the distal fibula. External rotation of the tibia and ankle carry the distal fibula posteriorly and elevate and glide the proximal fibular head anteriorly. The opposite occurs with internal rotation of the tibia and ankle (Fig. 53.16).

With pronation of the foot, ligamentous attachments glide the distal talofibular joint posteriorly with reciprocal glide of the head of the fibula anteriorly. The opposite occurs with supination.

Fibular Head Dysfunction

Fibular head dysfunction is checked by gliding the fibular head posteriorly (and slightly medial) and anteriorly (and slightly lateral). In grasping the fibular head, the physician must take care not to cause undue pressure on the peroneal (fibular) nerve, which lies directly posterior to this structure. Posterior fibular head somatic dysfunction may itself cause symptoms related to entrapment neuropathy or compression of the common peroneal (common fibular) nerve.

Fibular head dysfunction often occurs in recurrent ankle sprains and responds well to manipulative procedures (11). In the more common ankle sprain in which the foot tends to supinate, the distal fibula is often found to be anterior and the fibular head is posterior. In ankle sprains however, the physician must be sure to check both ends of the fibula, because with trauma and ligamentous sprain, the physiologic, reciprocal motion described earlier may not occur.

Palpation and manipulative treatment of tibiofibular interosseous membrane strain may also help in treating patients who have incurred an ankle sprain. This may be achieved with ligamentous balancing techniques between fibula and tibia while palpating at both ends of the fibula.

ANKLE

The ankle has both an upper and lower joint. Together, these joints act as a functional unit (12). The upper joint is the tibiotalar (talocrural) joint and the lower is the subtalar (talocalcaneal)

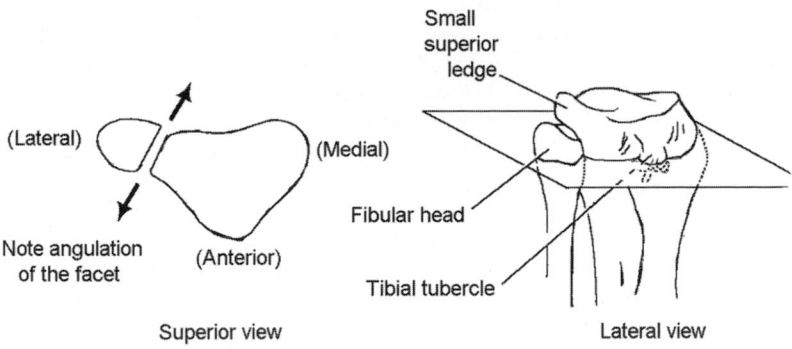

(Lateral) (Medial)

Note angulation
of the facet (Anterior)

Superior view

Small
superior
ledge

Fibular head

Tibial tubercle

Lateral view

FIGURE 53.15. Proximal tibiofibular joint. Note that the fibular head and the tibial tuberosity are on the same horizontal plane.

joint. As the patient walks forward and bears weight on the foot, there is visible medial rotation of the tibia with increasing dorsiflexion at the ankle. The calculated (13) amount of medial rotation of the tibia (13,14) however is greater than can be attributed to movement only at the tibiotalar joint. The increased medial rotation coincides with a relative calcaneal eversion about the subtalar axis. As the stance phase of the walking cycle continues to the toe-off interval, the tibia externally rotates with simultaneous calcaneal inversion about the subtalar axis. Hicks reports that without movement at the subtalar joint it would be difficult for a person to balance their body over one lower limb (15).

Tibiotalar Joint

The tibiotalar (or talocrural joint) involves the talus moving in the ankle mortise. Until the publication of Inman's studies (12,13), the axis of the tibiotalar joint was thought, and described in anatomic textbooks, to be a horizontal axis that corresponded

with the articular surfaces of the joint. Inman demonstrated that a single empirical (functional) axis in 80% of his specimens was not horizontal. He described an oblique axis directed laterally and downward (average 8 degrees) on a coronal plane and laterally and posteriorly (average 6 degrees) on a transverse plane. Despite this knowledge, the major motions of the tibiotalar joint are simply described as dorsiflexion and plantar flexion. Minor motions occur with each, posterior glide with dorsiflexion and anterior glide with plantar flexion. These minor motions are important when setting up manipulative techniques of the fibula.

Adduction, toeing-in, and some supination of the foot accompany plantar flexion. This motion also carries the lateral malleolus anteriorly. Through reciprocal action of the fibula, the proximal fibular head also glides posteriorly and inferiorly. The talus glides anteriorly, placing the narrow portion of the talus in the ankle mortise, a less stable position.

Since the tibiotalar axis passes distally to the tip of each malleolus, its position may be estimated by placing the fingertips at the most distal ends of the malleoli. At this position the fingers are over the transverse axis of the tibiotalar joint.

Abduction, toeing-out, and some pronation of the foot accompany dorsiflexion. This type of motion also carries the lateral malleolus posteriorly, and through reciprocal action glides the fibular head anteriorly and superiorly. With dorsiflexion, the talus glides posteriorly. Because the talus is structurally wider anteriorly, it fits more securely with the posterior glide component in the ankle mortise (Fig. 53.17). Dorsiflexion is therefore functionally a more stable position because of its structure. This stability is the reason taping to treat or prevent ankle sprains usually emphasizes a dorsiflexed position. Ankle sprains, more likely to occur when the tibiotalar joint is plantar flexed, are discussed with foot position (supination and pronation) later in this chapter and were classified by severity earlier in the chapter.

Recurrent somatic dysfunction of the ankle at the tibiotalar joint is more commonly found to prefer plantar flexion with a resistant barrier at the end of dorsiflexion. The tibiotalar capsular pattern however is restricted in both directions, but especially resists plantar flexion.

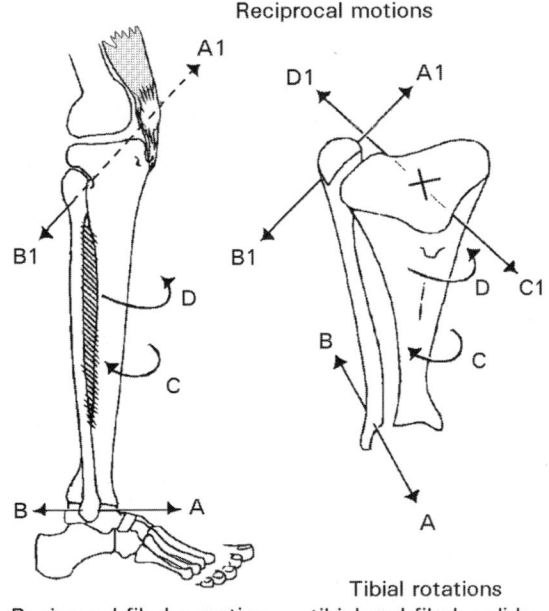

Reciprocal motions

Reciprocal fibular motion

Tibial rotations
tibial and fibular glides

FIGURE 53.16. External rotation of the tibia **(C)** moves the distal fibula posteriorly **(B)** and reciprocally is associated with the fibular head moving anteriorly **(B1)**. The opposite is true **(A, A1)** with internal rotation **(D)** of the lower leg. (Illustration by W.A. Kuchera.)

Subtalar Joint

The subtalar or talocalcaneal joint (Fig. 53.18) has been called the main "shock-absorber" joint (16). It earned this designation

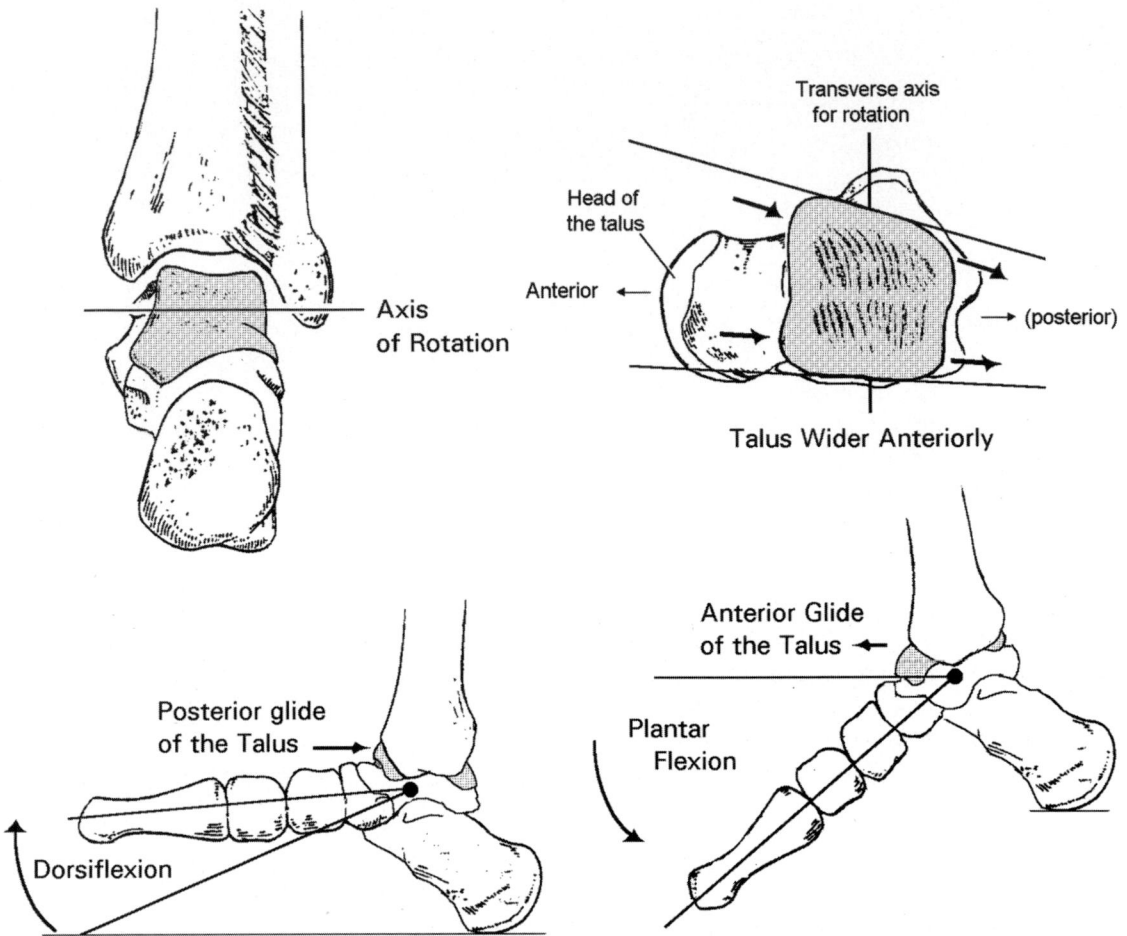

FIGURE 53.17. Ankle major and minor motions. Dorsiflexion with posterior glide is the most stable joint position because the wedge-shaped talus is engaged. (Illustration by W.A. Kuchera.)

because, in coordination with the intertarsal joints, it determines the distribution of forces upon the skeleton and soft tissues of the foot. The strong talocalcaneal ligament stabilizes it. It is a synovial joint with a single oblique axis that declines backward and laterally.

The subtalar joint acts like a mitered hinge so that movement of the calcaneus produces leg rotation. Inversion of the calca-

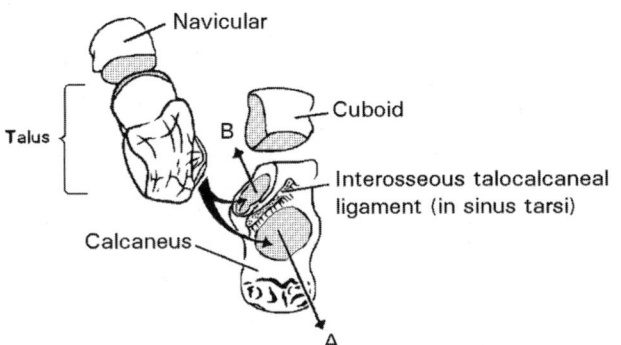

FIGURE 53.18. Subtalar joint. Persons with flat feet have a more horizontal axis and greater foot motion. Those with a more vertical axis have a more rigid, pes cavus foot. **A:** Posterolateral glide. **B:** Anteromedial glide. (Illustration by W.A. Kuchera.)

neus produces external rotation of the tibia, and the talus glides posterolaterally over the calcaneus. Eversion of the calcaneus produces medial rotation of the tibia and anteromedial glide of the talus on the calcaneus. Clinically, these mechanics seem to explain the palpable talocalcaneal motions: posterolateral glide of the talus when the ankle is supinated and the anteromedial glide at the talocalcaneal joint when the ankle is pronated.

Inman (13) found the average inclination of the subtalar axis from the horizontal plane on the sagittal plane to be 42 degrees (ranging from 20 to 68 degrees). If the inclination of the axis is 45 degrees, rotation of the tibia and calcaneus has a one-to-one relationship. The more horizontal the axis, the more the calcaneus rotates and the less the leg rotates. This calcaneal rotation is not very obvious during walking because the metatarsals of the forefoot appear to remain stationary. Inman's studies concluded that approximately half of the population has some linear displacement of the talus along the axis with movement in the subtalar joint.

Pes Planus and Pes Cavus

Persons with pes planus (flat foot) have the more horizontal subtalar axis and greater motion in their feet. This explains why they break down their shoes quickly and prefer to go barefoot. Persons

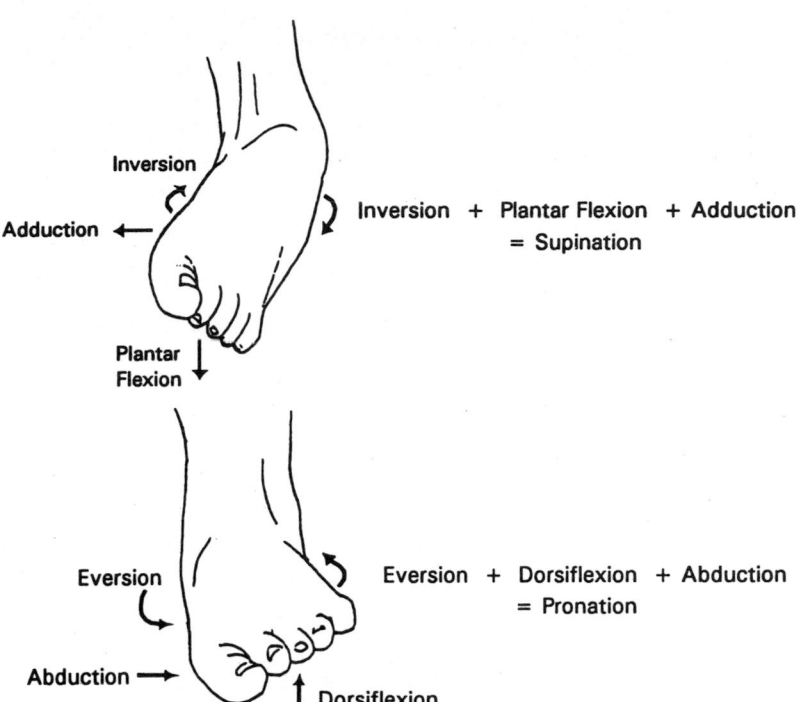

FIGURE 53.19. Inversion, eversion, supination, and pronation of the left foot.

with pes cavus (high arch) have a more vertical subtalar axis angle and a more rigid foot.

FOOT

The movement of the foot (or pes) is a composite movement of the talocalcaneal joint of the hind foot and movement of the forefoot about the talonavicular and calcaneocuboid joints. Inversion is that movement in which the heel (calcaneus) faces medially as the inside edge of the foot is lifted. Eversion occurs when the heel faces laterally as the outside edge of the foot is lifted. In the non-weightbearing foot, inversion and eversion can be applied to the forefoot as it moves more medially or more laterally, respectively (Fig. 53.19).

In the upper extremity, pronation and supination are movements of the forearm and muscles of the forearm produced by supinator and pronator muscles. Supination means that the palm is up, such as when holding the hand out waiting for someone to put something into it. In the foot, however, there are no muscles anatomically labeled as pronators or supinators. An active attempt to supinate the foot results in a combination of adduction, plantar flexion, and inversion of the foot. Likewise, an attempt to pronate the foot results in abduction, dorsiflexion, and eversion.

Gray's Anatomy has described pronation and supination in the foot as movements of the forefoot not including movement of the calcaneus. This is not true with weightbearing and active motion. With weightbearing, supination of the foot is accompanied by eversion of the calcaneus and posterolateral glide of the talus with respect to the navicular at the talocalcaneal joint. While providing less stability at the ankle, supination locks the foot. This allows stabilization at heel strike and propulsion at

toe-off. Pronation during weightbearing stabilizes the ankle and creates eversion of the calcaneus with anterolateral glide of the talocalcaneal joint. Pronation unlocks the foot for surface adaptation and shock absorption during running.

LATERAL STABILIZING LIGAMENTS AND ANKLE SPRAINS

Ankle sprains are very common in a general practice. The supination position, which includes the less stable plantar flexion position, predisposes the ankle to such injuries. Approximately 80% of all sprains are of the supination type (17). These supination sprains traumatize the lateral stabilizing ligaments of the ankle. Additionally, somatic dysfunction occurs during the mechanism of injury, which extends well beyond the local ligamentous stress (Fig. 53.20).

In a supination sprain, eversion of the calcaneus and posterolateral glide at the talocalcaneal joint occurs. Abrupt stretching of the lateral and anterior compartments often initiates peroneus (fibularis) or other myofascial trigger points (Fig. 53.21) (16). The distal fibula may be drawn anteriorly with reciprocal posterior glide of the fibular head. If the anterior talofibular ligament is torn, the distal fibula may move posteriorly with anterior glide of the fibular head. (Because sprains are traumatically induced, somatic dysfunction may therefore not follow simple biomechanical predictions.)

Somatic dysfunction does not stop here. The tibia often externally rotates with an anteromedial glide of the tibial plateau. The femur internally rotates. Myofascial forces (postural forces) then continue upward into the pelvis and spine. Failure to diagnose and treat or rehabilitate beyond the ankle itself increases recurrence rates and prolongs the healing and rehabilitation process.

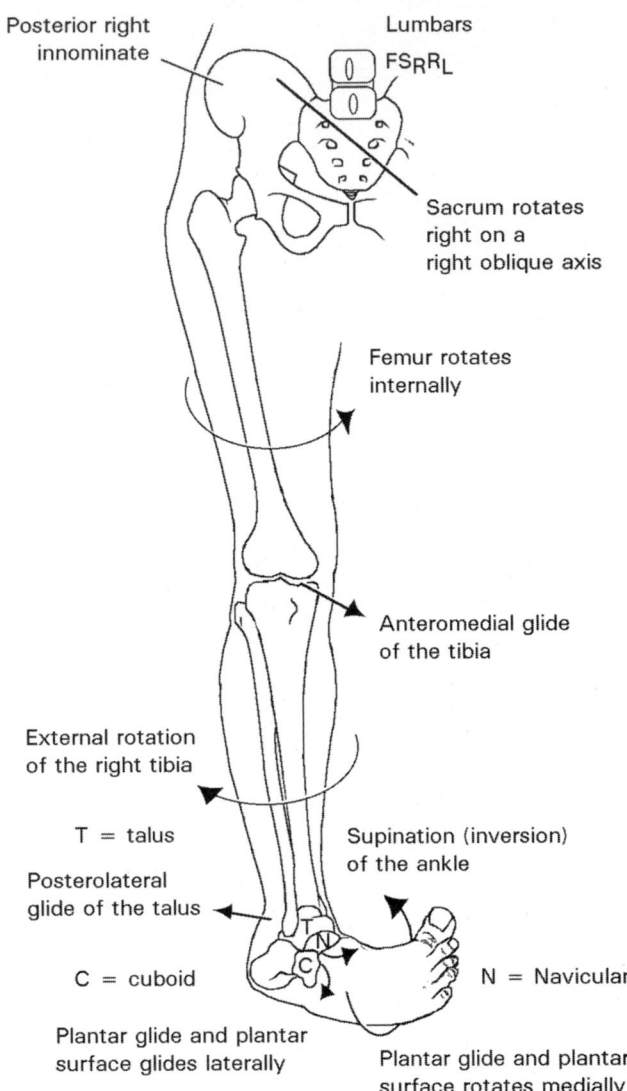

Mechanism of supination (inversion) strain or sprain

Posterior right innominate

Lumbars
FS$_R$R$_L$

Sacrum rotates right on a right oblique axis

Femur rotates internally

Anteromedial glide of the tibia

External rotation of the right tibia

T = talus

Posterolateral glide of the talus

C = cuboid

Supination (inversion) of the ankle

N = Navicular

Plantar glide and plantar surface glides laterally

Plantar glide and plantar surface rotates medially

FIGURE 53.20. Somatic dysfunctions and structural stress occurring in the more common supination ankle sprain.

It also increases complaints in distant sites due to the patient's involuntary attempts to compensate for continued dysfunction.

Three separate ligaments stabilize the lateral side of the ankle (Fig. 53.22). From anterior to posterior, these are the:

- Anterior talofibular ligament
- Calcaneofibular ligament
- Posterior talofibular ligament

Because the biomechanical stresses associated with a supination strain progress from anterior to posterior, ankle sprains are often named by type according to the extent of ligamentous involvement:

Type 1:	Involves anterior talofibular ligament only
Type 2:	Involves the anterior talofibular and calcaneofibular ligaments
Type 3:	Involves all three lateral supporting ligaments.

Classification by severity was discussed earlier in this chapter.

A pure inversion sprain can result in sprain of the calcaneofibular ligament alone. This occurs in basketball players during rebounding when they land directly on the lateral aspect of the foot (without any plantar flexion). An understanding of the biomechanics of the foot and ankle explains why this is an uncommon ankle sprain.

MEDIAL STABILIZING LIGAMENTS

The deltoid ligament (Fig. 53.23) stabilizing the medial side of the ankle is so strong that trauma stressing this structure is more likely to fracture a piece of medial malleolus than tear the ligament. Pronation sprains are uncommon. This is due both to the strength of the deltoid ligament and the stability imparted by gliding the wide portion of the talus into the tibiotalar joint during dorsiflexion.

FUNCTIONAL ARCHES OF THE FOOT

The two main functional arches of the foot are the longitudinal arch (with medial and lateral components) and the transverse arch. They are maintained by:

- Interlocking articular facets of the bones
- Interosseous ligaments
- Special fascial sheaths
- Plantar ligaments
- Muscles and muscle tendons

A so-called "metatarsal arch" is not a functional arch. It refers to the heads of the five metatarsals. Restrictions or altered relationships here are usually secondary to dysfunction of the other arches of the foot (18).

Longitudinal Arch

The longitudinal arch is divided into medial and lateral components. The tibialis posterior muscle supports it. Its tendon attaches to the navicular, first cuneiform, and bases of the second, third, and fourth metatarsals. The bony lateral longitudinal arch is the calcaneus, the cuboid, and the fourth and fifth metatarsals. The bony medial longitudinal arch consists of the talus, navicular, the three cuneiforms, and the first three metatarsals (Fig. 53.24).

Transverse Arch

The transverse arch is composed of the cuboid, the navicular, the three cuneiforms, and the proximal ends of the metatarsals. This arch is supported by the peroneus (fibularis) longus muscle inferiorly and by the tibialis anterior muscle, which attaches to the medial and undersurface of the first cuneiform and proximal first metatarsal (Fig. 53.25).

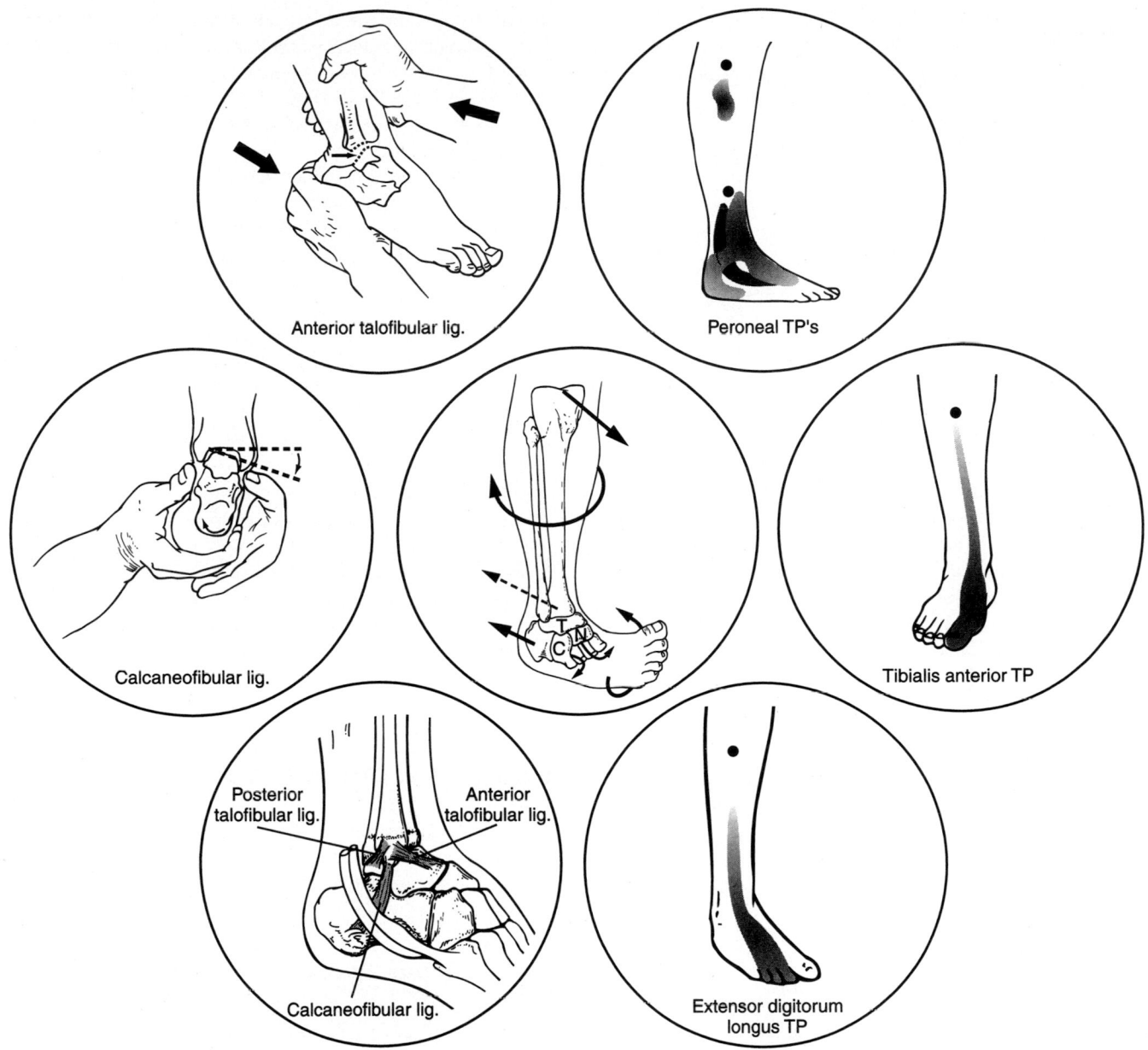

FIGURE 53.21. Trigger points (TPs) and ligamentous strain are somatic sources of pain in the more common supination ankle sprain. Muscles placed on stress are (in order): peroneus, tibialis anterior, and extensor digitorum longus. Ligaments *(lig.)* stressed are (in order): anterior talofibular, calcaneofibular, and anterior tibiotalar. *T*, talus; *N*, navicular; *C*, cuboid.

PLANTAR LIGAMENTS AND FASCIAE

The plantar aponeurosis (Fig. 53.26) extends from the calcaneus to the phalanges and encompasses the sesamoid bones under the great toe. Functional demand causes chronic stress on this structure. Irritation caused by either excessive pronation or a high-arched cavus foot may result in plantar fasciitis. With time, calcium is laid down along lines of stress, leading to formation of a calcaneal heel spur. Correction of the underlying biomechanical dysfunction is the treatment of choice. Surgery is rarely necessary.

The long plantar ligament runs from the calcaneus to the lateral three metatarsals. It forms a tunnel for the passage of the peroneus longus muscle as that tendon passes under the foot to the first cuneiform and first metatarsal. The short plantar ligament is, by definition, short. It lies medial to the lateral longitudinal arch and is attached between the calcaneus and the proximal end of the cuboid.

The spring ligament (calcaneonavicular) runs from the sustentaculum tali of the calcaneus to the navicular. The spring ligament strengthens the medial longitudinal arch.

TRANSVERSE TARSAL JOINT

The transverse tarsal joint contains the talonavicular and calcaneocuboid articulations, which are separate joints that act

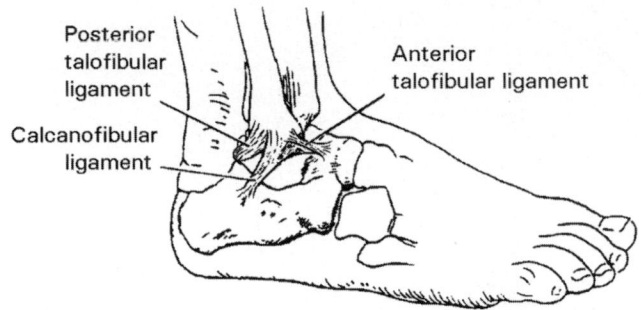

FIGURE 53.22. Ligamentous stability of the lateral ankle.

together as a functional unit. It has its greatest influence during the stance phase of the walking cycle because it responds to eversion or inversion of the heel. The talonavicular and calcaneocuboid joints plus the two small talocalcaneal joints are collectively called the Chopart joint. When amputating a foot, the surgeon follows the articulations of the Chopart joint.

Between the intertarsal joints and the subtalar joint is a groove called the sinus tarsi. Attached along this groove is the very strong interosseous talocalcaneal ligament that provides stability for the subtalar and intertarsal joints.

With internal rotation of the leg and inversion of the heel, the lines of the talonavicular and calcaneocuboid axes coincide. This produces enough freedom in the transverse tarsal joint so that the forefoot can evert or invert to accommodate for an uneven terrain.

When the leg rotates externally and everts the heel on a weight-bearing forefoot, the transverse tarsal joint appears to become more rigid. This is because the two axes do not coincide. The forefoot can no longer accommodate for an uneven terrain in this position.

As the heel rises in plantar flexion, the transverse tarsal joint must follow the movement about the subtalar axis and invert with the heel to assist the toe-off interval.

TARSAL SOMATIC DYSFUNCTION

Somatic dysfunction of the tarsal bones (cuboid, navicular, and/or cuneiforms) is relatively common. In middle- and long-distance runners these bones may even sublux.

Somatic dysfunction of the cuboid involves the edge nearest the middle of the foot. This edge glides toward the plantar sur-

face of the foot and rotates laterally around its AP axis. Somatic dysfunction of the navicular involves the edge nearest the middle of the foot gliding toward the plantar surface and rotating medially around its AP axis (Fig. 53.27). Cuneiform somatic dysfunction is usually manifested by the second cuneiform gliding directly plantarward.

Somatic dysfunction of these tarsal bones can be diagnosed by the combination of tenderness and increased tissue tension over the plantar surface of each of these bones. Osteopathic manipulative treatment (OMT) is effective, although some patients find orthotics to modify predisposing biomechanical factors useful as well.

There are five metatarsophalangeal joints. As the forefoot inverts with plantar flexion, the body weight is transferred to these articulations for push-off. Foot structure provides two functional axes for push-off: an oblique axis that passes through the heads of the second through fifth metatarsals, and a transverse axis that passes through the heads of the first and second metatarsals.

Structurally, a Morton foot is characterized by a short first metatarsal that is not designed to accept the normal weightbearing function involved in the push-off portion of gait. Callus forms under the second and third metatarsal heads as they assume the weightbearing function. Increased functional demand remodels bone. This results in thickening of the second metatarsal; the thickening is evident on x-ray films. Treatment consists of orthotics to modify the structure-function relationships (Fig. 53.28) and OMT to permit realignment.

METATARSAL AND PHALAGEAL FINDINGS

Hallux valgus and bunions have a significant hereditary component. Hammer toes are acquired. Each of these are structural changes with associated biomechanical effects and related somatic dysfunction.

Hallus Valgus, Bunions, and Hammer Toes

Hallux valgus is a structural deformity resulting from contracture of various periarticular structures of the first metatarsophalangeal joint. It is progressive.

Bunion protrusion is accentuated by varus deviation of the first metatarsal. Muscle imbalance aggravates symptoms, but surgical intervention of the structure may be required for symptomatic

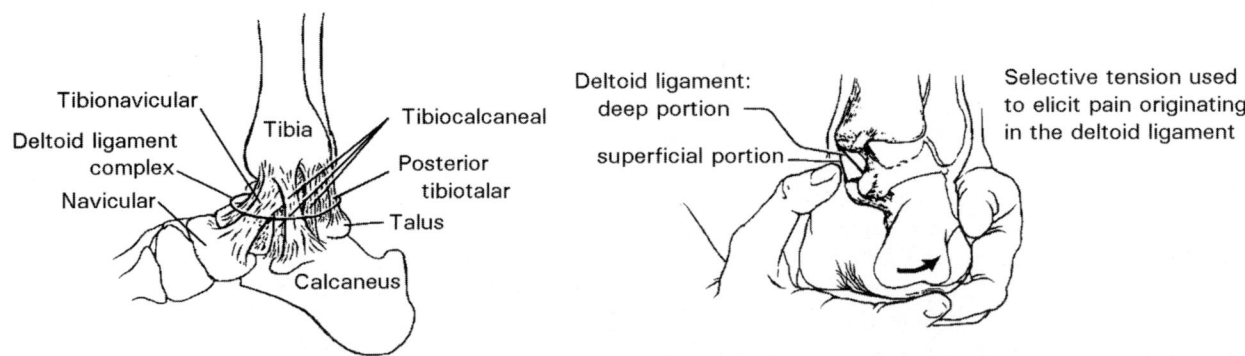

FIGURE 53.23. Deltoid ligament.

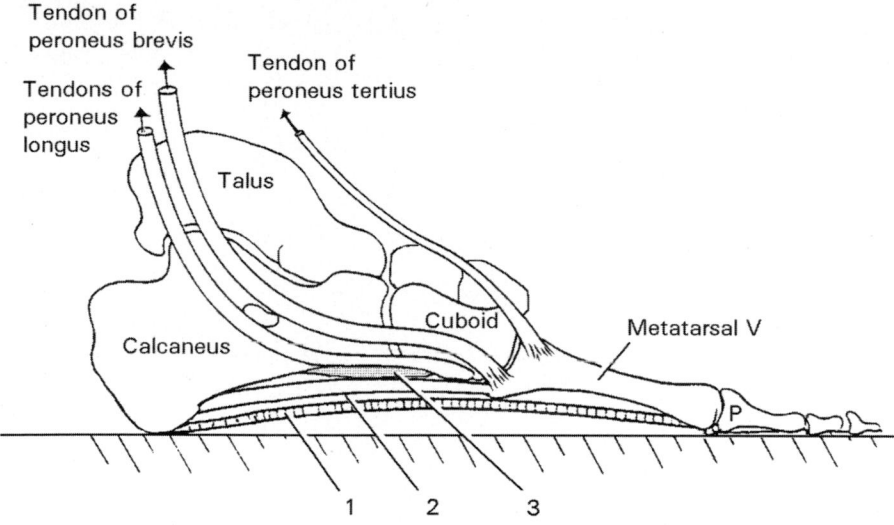

FIGURE 53.24. Supports of the longitudinal arch of the foot. *1*, plantar aponeurosis, abductor digiti minimi, and flexor digitorum brevis IV and V; *2*, long plantar ligament; *3*, short plantar ligament; *P*, phalanges. (From Hamilton JJ, Ziemer LK. Functional anatomy of the human ankle and foot. In: *AAOS Symposium on Foot and Ankle*. St Louis, MO: CV Mosby; 1983:13.)

relief. Counterstrain OMT to a tender point on the medial aspect of the great toe often provides symptomatic relief.

Hammer toes are often functional and may be associated with myofascial trigger points in the dorsal interossei. Deformation may disappear after treatment of this somatic dysfunction (19).

Somatic Dysfunction

Somatic dysfunction of the tarsometatarsal, metatarsophalangeal, and interphalangeal joints involves their minor motions:

- Plantar or dorsal glide
- Internal or external rotation
- Lateral or medial glide

It also involves compression or, less commonly, traction.

Indirect stacking OMTs are especially helpful in jammed toes. A stacking technique is one where the physician moves a joint in the direction of preference in all of its planes, stacking one motion upon the other. Compression or traction is then applied to that combined position. The technique may require holding that position of ease for 90 seconds or until the joint tensions

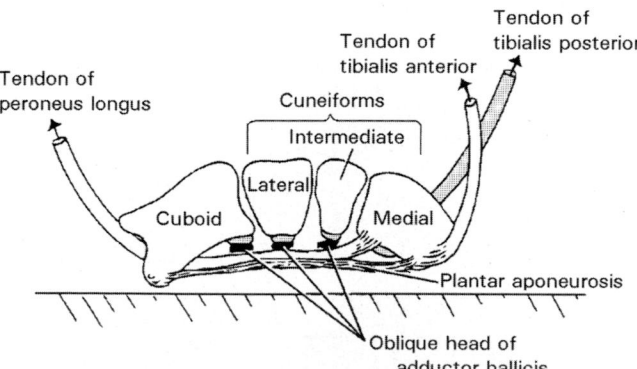

FIGURE 53.25. Supports of the transverse arch of the foot. Stippled tube represents tendon of tibialis posterior; black areas represent oblique head of adductor hallucis. (From Hamilton JJ, Ziemer LK. Functional anatomy of the human ankle and foot. In: *AAOS Symposium on Foot and Ankle*. St Louis, MO: CV Mosby; 1983:13, with permission.)

relax. The joint is then slowly returned to a neutral position and rechecked for motion.

NEUROMUSCULAR STRUCTURES AND FUNCTION

Neurologic Examination

A traditional neurologic examination to rule out associated neurologic disease or a structural problem affecting the nervous system is a part of the lower extremity work-up. This should include Achilles and patellar deep tendon reflexes, assessment for ankle clonus, straight-leg raising assessment, and evaluation of lower extremity muscle tone, strength, flexibility, and coordination. Evaluation of sensation may be indicated as well.

Upper motor neuron disorders are characterized by hyperreflexia, often with pathologic reflexes such as ankle clonus or Babinski upgoing toe reflex. Lower extremity muscles may demonstrate spasticity or rigidity.

Lower motor neuron disorders are generally characterized by hyporeflexia accompanying muscle weakness and/or flaccidity. Dermatomal patterns of pain and/or dysesthesia associated with radicular (nerve root) problems in the lower extremities follow general patterns as depicted in Fig. 53.29. (Depending on the location of the lower motor neuron problem, the pattern may be that of a plexopathy, a neuropathy, or a peripheral neuropathy instead of a radiculopathy.) In any case, review of the lumbar and pelvic regions is necessary to thoroughly understand neuromuscular problems affecting the lower extremities.

Radiculopathy

Radiculopathy may have as its cause, for example, a herniated nucleus pulposus, osteoarthritic spur, advanced spondylolisthesis, or mass lesion. Regardless of the cause, there are relatively predictable structural and functional effects to be evaluated in the lower extremities. History and physical findings will uncover patterns of lower extremity sensory changes, pain, and reflex

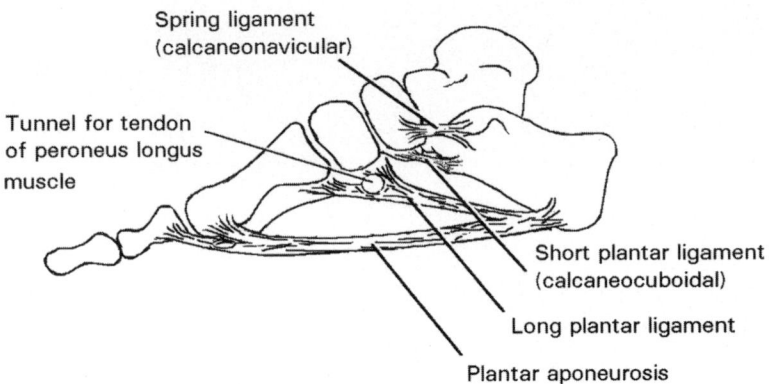

Spring ligament
(calcaneonavicular)

Tunnel for tendon
of peroneus longus
muscle

Short plantar ligament
(calcaneocuboidal)

Long plantar ligament

Plantar aponeurosis

FIGURE 53.26. Plantar ligaments supporting the arches of the foot.

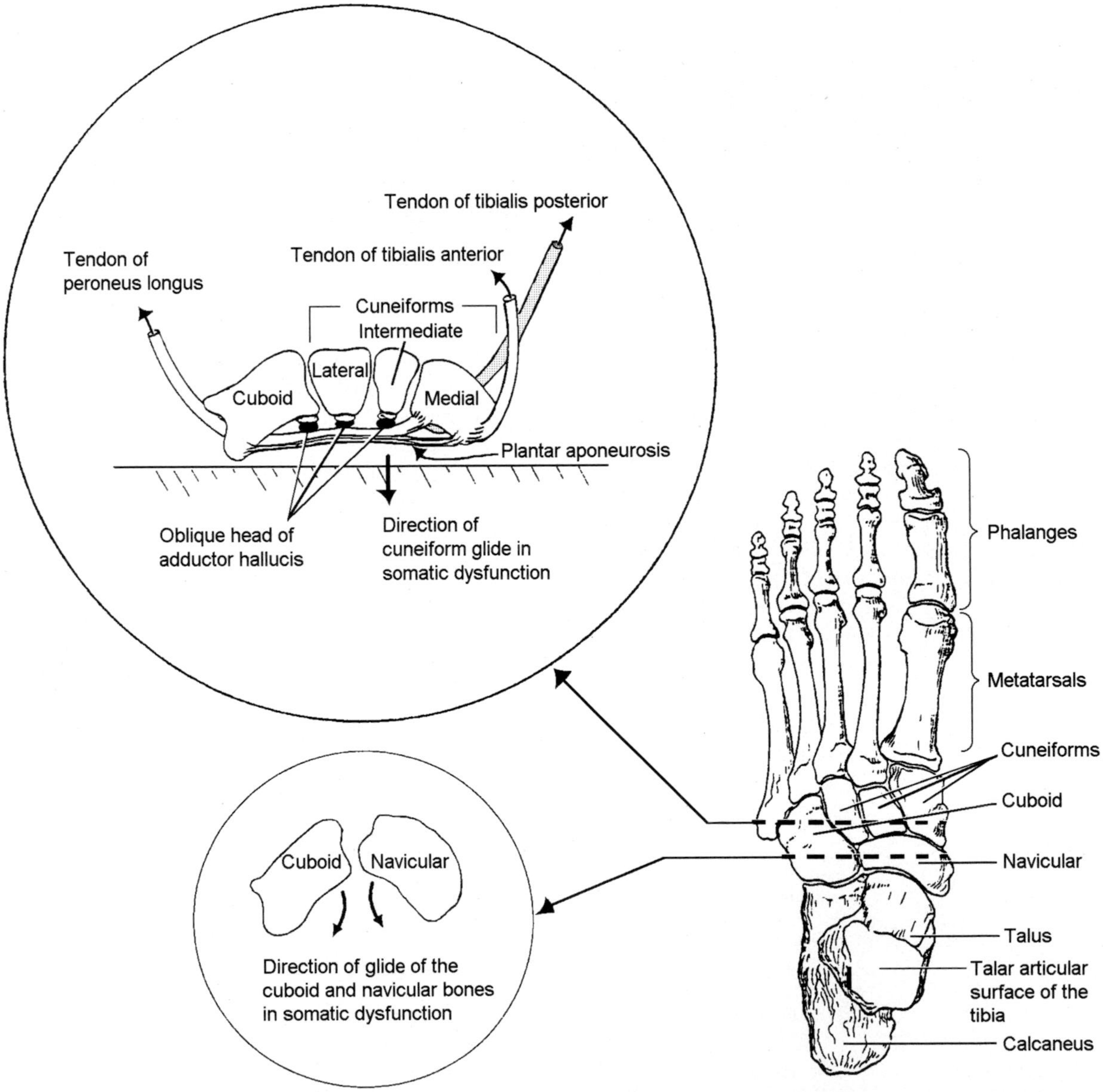

Tendon of tibialis posterior

Tendon of tibialis anterior

Tendon of
peroneus longus

Cuneiforms
Intermediate

Lateral

Cuboid

Medial

Plantar aponeurosis

Oblique head of
adductor hallucis

Direction of
cuneiform glide in
somatic dysfunction

Phalanges

Metatarsals

Cuneiforms

Cuboid

Navicular

Talus

Talar articular
surface of the
tibia

Calcaneus

Cuboid Navicular

Direction of glide of the
cuboid and navicular bones
in somatic dysfunction

FIGURE 53.27. Navicular, cuboid, and cuneiform somatic dysfunction.

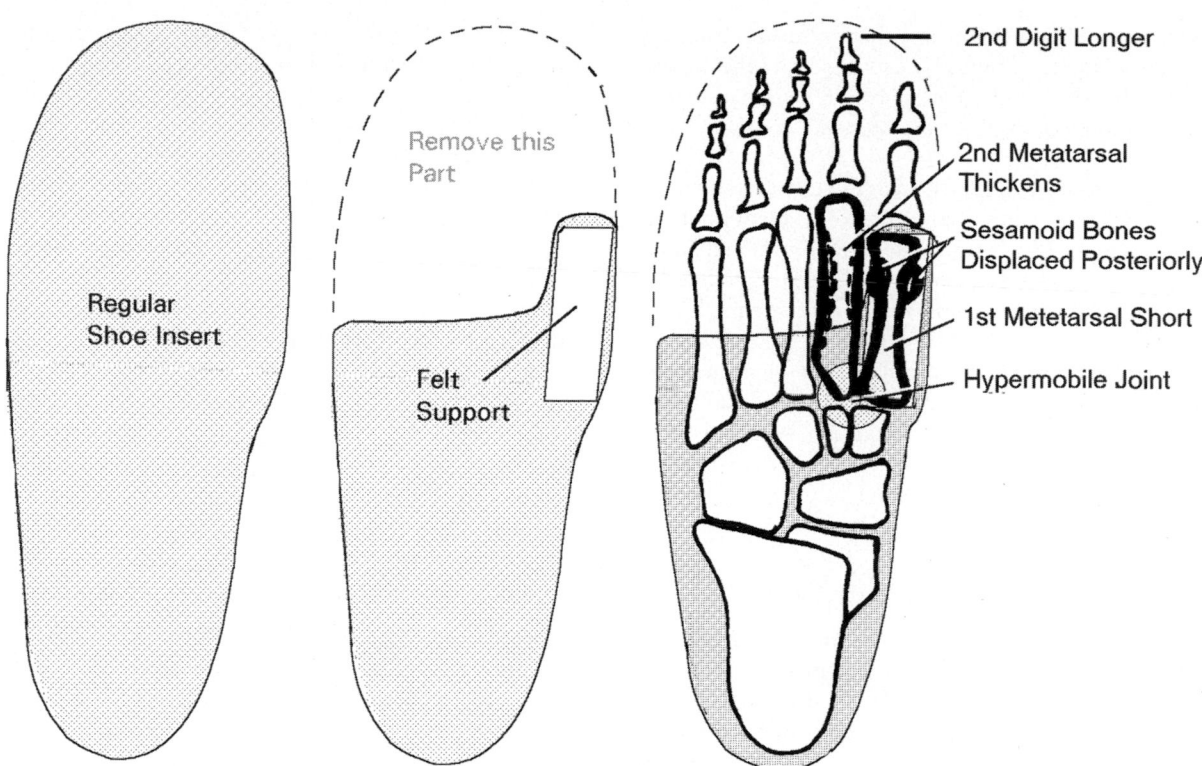

FIGURE 53.28. Orthotic used for Morton foot to modify structure-function relationships. Toe portion of the sole insert is removed so support is under only the first metatarsal head. Lateral side of the support must not extend under second metatarsal head. Insert should reach to the distal end of the first metatarsal.

changes as well as muscle weakness, atrophy, predisposition to trigger points, and imbalance. The diagnosis of lumbar or upper sacral radiculopathies by electromyography focuses on the discovery of fibrillation potentials in patterns of lower extremity muscles sharing a common involved nerve root.

L4 radiculopathy is suspected when there is reduction of the patellar deep tendon reflex, dysesthesia in the L4 distribution, and patterns of weakness, cramping, and/or trigger points in those muscles innervated by the L4 nerve root, such as the quadriceps and tibialis anterior. Often this patient will complain of a knee that gives way or difficulty climbing stairs.

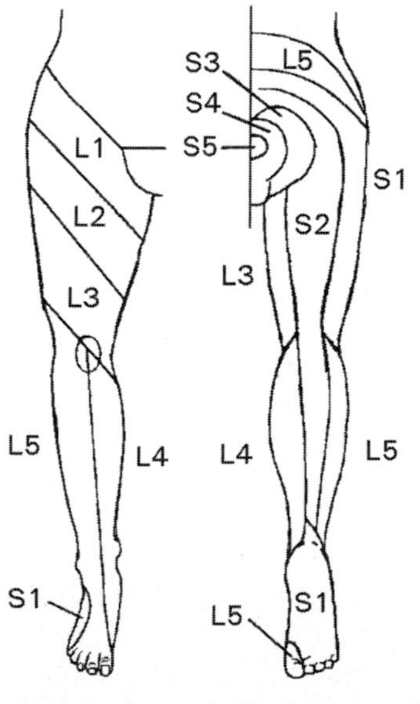

L5 radiculopathy has no abnormal deep tendon reflex; it is suspected when there is dysesthesia in the L5 distribution and patterns of weakness, cramping, and/or trigger points in the gluteus medius and ankle dorsiflexors, such as tibialis anterior, extensor hallucis, and extensor digitorum brevis. This patient may often complain of tripping over carpets or "small cracks in the sidewalk" because of a foot drop.

S1 radiculopathy is suspected with reduction of the Achilles deep tendon reflex, dysesthesia in the S1 distribution, and patterns of weakness, cramping, and/or trigger points of intrinsic foot muscles, the gastrocnemius-soleus complex, and the buttock/gluteal muscles. This is the most common radiculopathy, often resulting from a herniated disc between L5 and S1.

Referred Pain

Pain and dysesthesia are not limited to a nerve root or dermatomal pattern. Pain patterns referred from the facet joints of the lumbar spine overlap myofascial trigger point pain arising from the following muscles (19):

- Multifidi
- Quadratus lumborum
- Glutei
- Piriformis
- Obturator internus

FIGURE 53.29. Dermatomal or radicular (nerve root) patterns. (Illustration by W.A. Kuchera.)

Myotomal referral often results in a charley horse or a crampy sensation. A myotomal distribution is associated with the location of muscles that share the neural (root, plexus, or peripheral nerve) innervation. Muscle innervations are reviewed in Tables 53.2 and 53.3.

Sclerotomal referral is a deep, achy sensation that is toothache-like in quality. Sclerotomal (bony/ligamentous) distribution has also been mapped out (Fig. 53.30) but is often overlooked. Patients may dismiss it as lower extremity arthritic pain. Notice that different aspects of the knee and the hip joints share the L3 and L4 sclerotomes.

Referred pain in general is reproducible. An understanding of the patterns associated with each referral improves patient diagnosis and treatment design. Failure to appreciate nondermatomal patterns may lead a practitioner to incorrectly consider a patient with legitimate symptoms a malingerer.

Referral from Lumbopelvic Structures

In addition to lumbar nerve roots and sclerotomes discussed earlier, a number of other lumbopelvic region myofascial, arthrodial, ligamentous, and visceral structures commonly refer pain to the inguinal area and/or hip. Somatic examples include iliolumbar and posterior sacroiliac ligaments (20), quadratus lumborum muscle (21), and lumbar zygapophysial joints (22). Referral from visceral structures in this region are also often seen, as in a urinary tract stone passing down the ureter radiating into the ipsilateral flank and the inner thigh region (23).

Referral Originating in the Lower Extremities

Structures in the hip region often refer pain to the knee. For example, an adolescent male with knee pain and no sign of knee dysfunction or structural abnormality should have a hip x-ray to rule out a slipped capital epiphysis or other hip joint pathologic conditions. Lower extremity myofascial trigger points create predictable patterns of pain and dysfunction.

Lower Extremity Myofascial Trigger Points

Myofascial trigger points as described by Travell and Simons (19,24) also have predictable referral patterns not associated with dermatomes. See Fig. 66.1 for a synopsis of representative trigger points associated with the lower extremities. By definition, these points are a form of somatic dysfunction (see Chapter 66). They represent impaired or altered function of myofascial tissues with effects also in related neural, vascular, and lymphatic elements.

Asymmetric postural stress creates recurrent predictable patterns of lower extremity muscle somatic dysfunction. Neuromuscular imbalance and/or myofascial trigger points characterize this. In neuromuscular imbalance, stressed postural (antigravity) muscles exhibit increased irritability (short and tight), while their antagonists demonstrate inhibition (weak and atrophic)

(Fig. 53.31) (25). When stressed, the iliopsoas, piriformis, hamstrings, gastrocnemius-soleus complex, adductor magnus, rectus femoris, and tensor fasciae latae all tend to tighten while the vasti (especially the vastus medialis), glutei, peroneus, and tibialis anterior all tend to be inhibited and weak (26). An understanding of the myotatic unit, muscle agonists and antagonists, and patterns of use is necessary for efficient diagnostic and therapeutic approaches in the neuromuscular system.

MUSCLES OF THE HIP

Muscles of the hip are generally large and powerful. They can be grouped according to their functional role (Table 53.2). Dysfunction leads to a number of patient symptoms responding readily to a variety of OMTs, especially soft tissue, muscle energy, and counterstrain activating forces.

Myofascial trigger points in these muscles respond to these techniques as well as adjunctive use of the following:

- Vapocoolant spray and stretch
- Injection of procaine
- Dry needling

Often the joints straddled between muscle origin and insertion need treatment. Alternatively, viscerosomatic referral should be entertained as a primary source of secondary muscle dysfunction, particularly when the historical review of systems is suggestive of the possibility. Because crosstalk between the viscera and the soma tends to take place in the spinal cord, innervation of each muscle becomes clinically relevant for more than just the recognition of nerve root pathophysiology.

NERVE SUPPLY IN THE BUTTOCK AND THIGH

In the buttock and/or thigh, nerve supply may be affected functionally by the piriformis muscle. Biochemical irritation of the sciatic nerve is possible with irritation of the piriformis because of the close anatomic relationship between the two (Fig. 53.32). In approximately 10% of the U.S. population, the peroneal portion of the sciatic nerve actually passes through the piriformis muscle; this occurs in one-third of patients of Asian descent. In the presence of this anatomic variation, peroneal entrapment is likely. Because of this variant anatomy, therapeutic injections (especially those containing a steroid) into the piriformis muscle should be approached with caution to avoid permanent nerve injury.

The sciatic nerve divides into a posterior tibial and common peroneal (common fibular) nerve in the thigh. The obturator and femoral nerves innervate the other thigh muscles. The gluteal nerves innervate the gluteal muscles.

MUSCLES OF THE THIGH AND LEG

Muscles of the thigh and leg include those affecting knee, ankle, and foot function (Table 53.3 and Fig. 53.33). Several thigh

TABLE 53.2. FUNCTIONAL MUSCLE CHART FOR THE HIP

Muscle Innervation	Functional Anatomic Features	Dysfunction
Hip flexors		
Iliopsoas (L2-4)	Strongest flexor of thigh	Psoas posturing and psoas syndrome
	Postural significance: extension of spine while standing (lumbar lordosis); flexion of spine with bending	Activated by sit-ups or bending over a low table
	Psoas attaches to T12-L5 vertebral bodies and associated intervertebral discs	Aggravated by weightbearing; relief recumbent with knees bent
	Psoas crosses lumbar intervertebral, lumbosacral, sacroiliac, and hip joints	Referral back and anterior groin
		Positive Thomas test = iliopsoas contracture
		Usually develops spasm when stressed
Rectus femoris (L2-4; femoral n.)	Crosses both hip and knee	Referral patellar and deep knee pain
	Primarily an extender of the knee; only causes hip flexion when knee extended	Usually develops spasm when stressed
Pectineus	Flexion and adduction of thigh at hip	Referral deep-seated groin ache
	Designed for power not speed	
Also sartorius thigh adductors, t. fascia latae	Contribute to hip flexion	
Hip extensors		
Gluteus maximus (L5-S2; superior gluteal)	Type I (slow twitch) muscle fibers suited for continuous use	Decreases hip flexion
	Location and size unique, providing anatomic basis for upright posture	Restlessness, pain on sitting or walking uphill
	Most powerful extensor	Antalgic gait
		Referral to buttock
		Usually becomes inhibited when stressed
Hamstrings (L5-S2; sciatic n.)	Restrains hip flexion produced by body weight during stance phase of walking; extension during walking	Decreased hip flexion with straight leg raising test
		Pain sitting and walking; disturbs sleep
		Perpetuated by chair pressure under thighs
		Referral posterior thigh
		Usually develops spasm when stressed
Adductor magnus (ischiocondylar portion: L4-S1 sciatic n.)	Only portion of adductor magnus assisting flexion and then only when the femur is flexed more than 70°	Referral to inner thigh
		Usually develops spasm when stressed
Hip abductors		
Gluteus medius (L4-S1; inferior gluteal)	Stabilizes pelvis during single limb stance (prevents nonstance innominate from falling inferior—negative Trendelenburg test)	TPs aggravated by walking, slouching in chair, or lying on back
		Referral to posterior iliac crest, sacroiliac joint, sacrum, and minor to buttock
		Positive Trendelenburg test = weakness in hip abductors
		Usually becomes inhibited when stressed
Gluteus minimus (L4-S1)	Stabilizes pelvis during single limb stance (prevents nonstance innominate from falling inferior—negative Trendelenburg test)	Travell calls TPs in this muscle "pseudosciatica"
		Characteristic pain arising from chair or walking; can be constant and excruciating
		Mistaken for L5 or S1 radiculopathy (but may coexist)
		Antalgic gait
		Referral buttock, lateral and posterior thigh
		Positive Trendelenburg test = weakness in hip abductors
		Usually becomes inhibited when stressed
Piriformis (S1-2)	Acts as abductor when thigh flexed	May entrap peroneal portion of sciatic nerve or cause sciatica
		Perpetuated by sacroiliac somatic dysfunction or irritation (especially sacral shear) and sitting on billfold
		Associated with pelvic floor dysfunction, dyspareunia, prostatodynia
		Usually develops spasm when stressed

(continued)

TABLE 53.2. (*continued*)

Muscle Innervation	Functional Anatomic Features	Dysfunction
Also to lesser extent: sartorius, gluteus maximus, iliopsoas		

Hip adductors
  Adductor longus, brevis and magnus
  (L2-4; obturator n.)
	Early in swing phase, these muscles pull limb toward midline	Referral distal to inguinal ligament, inner thigh, and upper medial knee
		Usually develops spasm when stressed

External rotators of the hip (L5-S2) Obturator internus (L5-S2)	When the thigh is extended, cause external rotation; when flexed, cause abduction	Responsible for pelvic floor symptoms (fullness in rectum) Referral to anococcygeal region (some to posterior thigh)

Internal rotators of the hip
  Gluteus medius and minimus (L4-S1)
  Also from: gemelli and quadratus
  femoris (L4-S1). Less from piriformis
	(See Hip Abductors above)
	Piriformis only involved with external rotation when the femor is extended
		(See Hip Abductors above)

TPs, trigger points.

muscles have already been described in relation to their effect at the hip. These include the:

- Hamstrings
- Rectus femoris
- Tensor fasciae latae

The hamstrings and the short head of the biceps femoris are the chief flexors of the knee. The hamstrings, by definition muscles that attach to the ischial tuberosity, attach to the leg below the knee and are supplied by the tibial division of the sciatic nerve (27). The head of the biceps femoris crosses the knee and is innervated by the peroneal portion of the sciatic nerve. Both heads of the biceps femoris also cause external rotation of the knee while the remaining hamstrings cause internal rotation.

NERVE SUPPLY IN THE THIGH, LEG, AND FOOT

Nerve supply in the thigh, leg, and foot is derived from the posterior tibial and common peroneal (common fibular) nerves (Fig. 53.34). As noted, a vulnerable site for entrapment or trauma exists as the common peroneal nerve passes behind the fibular head. The tibial nerve supplies the posterior compartment of the leg and the muscles of the foot. The deep peroneal nerve supplies the anterior compartment of the leg with sensation to the webbing between the first and second toes. The superficial peroneal nerve supplies the lateral compartment of the leg as well as the skin on the anterolateral side of the leg and the dorsum of the foot.

VASCULAR AND LYMPHATIC STRUCTURES AND FUNCTION

Enhancing homeostasis associated with vascular and lymphatic elements is a significant portion of an integrated osteopathic treatment regimen in the lower extremities. By definition, removal of somatic dysfunction is linked to its influence on related neural, vascular, and lymphatic elements (Fig. 53.35).

Treatment of somatic dysfunction is postulated to improve blood delivery by reducing hypersympathetic activity. This is important for nutrition of the tissues in the lower extremities. It would also benefit delivering medications such as nonsteroidal antiinflammatory drugs to target tissues in the lower extremities where pharmacologic effectiveness is proportionate to tissue or synovial concentration of the drug. Cell bodies for the sympathetic nerve supply of the lower extremities are found at the level of T11-L2.

Opening fascial pathways and eliminating myofascial trigger points can improve venous and lymphatic drainage of the extremities. Drainage can be enhanced using a variety of lymphatic pump techniques. This is especially true of the pedal pump techniques described in other chapters. Lymphaticovenous return is also enhanced by improving the mechanical lymphatic pumping produced by muscular contraction, and maximal pressure gradients between the thorax and abdomen produced by improving respiratory efficacy.

Hip

The inferior margin of the acetabulum is incomplete, forming an acetabular notch through which the hip joint receives its blood vessels (Fig. 53.36). These vessels are easily disrupted by a femoral neck fracture, which creates the possibility of delayed healing or nonunion.

The femoral artery is the major vessel supplying the lower extremities. Easily located in the femoral triangle, this artery is bounded by the sartorius and adductor muscles and the inguinal ligament. The mnemonic NAVEL provides a reminder of the order, from lateral to medial, of the structures in the femoral triangle:

Nerve
Artery

TABLE 53.3. FUNCTIONAL MUSCLE CHART FOR THE THIGH AND LEG

Muscle Innervation	Functional Anatomic Features	Dysfunction
Knee flexors		
Biceps femoris (L5-S2; sciatic n. long head = tibial portion; short head = peroneal portion)	Long head crosses both hip and knee Short head crosses only knee Both heads plus semimembranosus establish a tripartite anchor on the fibular head Short head active in knee flexion for toe clearance during walking Active contraction also induces some external rotation of the knee	Pain referral is distalward from trigger points (TPs) in the posterior thigh to the back of the knee or to the region of the fibular head Often wakes patient at night
Semimembranosus and semitendinosus (L5-S2; sciatic n. tibial portion)	Also hip extensors Hamstrings are not consistently active for knee flexion during walking (passive knee motion when the hip is flexed is more common) Active contraction also induces some internal rotation of the knee	Pain referral proximally to lower buttock; aggravated by walking often causing limp TPs often misdiagnosed as "sciatica" or "osteoarthritis of the knee" or "growing pains"[a] TPs remaining post-op often cause of "postlaminectomy syndrome"[b] Tightness in the hamstrings is associated with inhibition and laxity of the gluteal muscles
Also popliteus and gastrocnemius	Contribute somewhat to knee flexion Popliteus initiates flexion from fully extended position before hamstrings act	
Knee extensors		
Quadriceps (L2-4; femoral n.)	Rectus femoris crosses both hip and knee joints (proximal attachment to anterior posterior iliac spine [ASIS]); also a hip flexor Three vasti cross only knee joint All four tendons unite into patellar tendon with patella anchored to tibial tuberosity by patellar ligament *Q-angle* is the quadriceps angle measured from ASIS to midpatella to tibial tuberosity (Fig. 53.5)	Thigh and knee pain and weakness of knee extension especially going up stairs Anterior knee pain is referred from vastus medialis and rectus femoris; may interrupt sleep Posterior knee pain and pain anywhere along the lateral thigh to the iliac crest are referred from vastus lateralis TPs in v. medialis cause "buckling knee" and may cause patient to fall TPs in v. lateralis may restrict motion of the patella; pain with walking TPs in v. intermedius have difficulty straightening knee after prolonged sitting Imbalance in quadriceps with one another or with the hamstrings predispose to chondromalacia patellae as does an increased Q-angle Direct trauma to the quadriceps should be observed for myositis ossificans Usually becomes inhibited when stressed
Knee external rotator		
Biceps femoris	Also a knee flexor	See description with Knee Flexors above
Knee internal rotators		
Popliteus (L4-S1; tibial n.)	Unlocks knee at the start of weight bearing by "externally rotating the thigh on the fixed tibia"; internally rotates tibia when thigh is fixed Prevents posterior glide of tibia relative to femur while crouching	Pain behind the knee when crouching, walking down stairs, or running downhill Aggravated by braking forward motions during twists (e.g., skiing), high heels by excessive foot pronation,[d] and by training on uneven ground Mimics symptoms of Baker cyst but no associated swelling in the region
Semimembranosus and semitendinosus	Also knee flexors (primary)	See description under Knee Flexors above
Also sartorius (L2-3; femoral nerve) and gracilis (L2-3; obturator n.)	Sartorius is the longest muscle in the body crossing both hip and knee; it is a hip flexor and knee internal rotator Gracilis is the second longest muscle in the body crossing hip and knee	Pain from the sartorius in the anterior thigh is superficial and described as tingling or sharp; may exhibit symptoms of meralgia paresthetica (entrapment of lateral femoral cutaneous nerve)[e] Pain from gracilis is a hot stinging, superficial pain in the medial thigh; it may be relieved by walking

(continued)

TABLE 53.3. (*continued*)

Muscle Innervation	Functional Anatomic Features	Dysfunction
Ankle dorsiflexors		
Tibialis anterior (L4-S1; deep peroneal n.)	An anterior compartment muscle A dorsiflexor at the taloitibial joint Also supinates foot at the talocalcaneal and transverse tarsal joints	Pain and tenderness referred into great toe and anteromedial ankle Weakness leads to varying degrees of foot drop; patients may complain of tripping over carpets, dragging foot, or "foot slap" Weakness in muscle may be caused by L5 radiculopathy, peroneal mononeuropathy, the habit of crossing the legs at the knee, or posterior fibular head somatic dysfunction
Extensor digitorium longus (L4-S1; deep peroneal n.)	Also everts the foot balancing inversion of tibialis anterior Helps prevent posterior postural sway	Pain pattern over dorsum of foot and ankle Dysfunction often results in foot slap after heel strike TPs may entrap fibers of the deep peroneal nerve Muscle imbalance may lead to formation of hammer toes
Peroneus tertitus (L5-S1; deep peroneal n.)	An anterior compartment muscle A dorsiflexor at the talotibial joint Also everts foot Tendon passes in front of lateral malleolus to insert on proximal 5th metatarsal	Pain referred along anterolateral ankle and sometimes to lateral heel; failure to identify and treat TPs post-ankle sprain can prolong rehabilitation process Weakness in ankle dorsiflexion predisposing to ankle instability and repeat sprains May be mistaken for ankle arthritis[f] Weakness in muscle may be caused by L5 radiculopathy, peroneal mononeuropathy, the habit of crossing the legs at the knee, posterior fibular head somatic dysfunction or prolonged immobilization (as in an ankle cast)
Ankle plantar flexors		
Gastrocnemius (L5-S2; posterior tibial n.)	Gastrocnemius-soleus complex referred to as triceps surae; constitutes close functional unit; shares Achilles tendon attachment to calcaneus	Dysfunction often results in nocturnal leg cramps TP pain may be referred to upper posterior calf and/or to instep "Tennis leg" is a partial tearing of the gastrocnemius; symptoms include a sudden intense calf pain, as if kicked, followed by swelling and local tenderness; failure to recognize may lead to a posterior compartment syndrome
Soleus (S1-2; tibial n.)	Gastrocnemius-soleus complex constitutes close functional unit; shares Achilles attachment to calcaneus Soleus function during gait is to add to knee and ankle stability Acts as "second heart"[g] in moving venous and lymphatic fluid from lower extremity (e.g., fainting with military "attention" position) Also aids in inversion of foot and extension of knee	Heel pain with TPs in this muscle and/or may refer proximally to sacroiliac joint or even temporomandibular joint May restrict dorsiflexion at ankle; pain severe walking up hill or stairs May be cause of growing pains in children Soleus TPs easily mistaken for Baker cyst, thrombophlebitis, and/or Achilles tendinitis
Peroneus longus and brevis (L4-S1; superficial peroneal n.)	Lateral compartment muscles Plantar flex and pronate foot p. longus attaches to fibular head and to upper 2/3 of lateral fibula, crosses behind the lateral malleolus over the cuboid, and divides to attach to the 1st cuneiform and the base of the 1st metatarsal p. brevis travels with p. longus but inserts on the lateral aspect of the 5th metatarsal	Pain and tenderness projected to lateral malleolus and some of lateral leg TPs initiated by inversion twisting of ankle or prolonged immobilization in ankle cast Predispose to weak ankles and recurrent sprains May have deep peroneal nerve entrapment with some foot drop p. longus and brevis aggravated by Morton foot structure Pain easily mistaken for arthritis in ankle[h] TPs in p. longus can entrap the common peroneal nerve and weaken both anterior and lateral compartment muscles; numbness often noted in web of great toe

(*continued*)

TABLE 53.3. (*continued*)

Muscle Innervation	Functional Anatomic Features	Dysfunction
Foot supinators Tibialis anterior (L5-S1; deep peroneal n.)	An anterior compartment muscle Supinates foot at talocalcaneal and transverse tarsal joints Also dorsiflexes at the talotibial joint	Pain and tenderness referred into great toe and anteromedial ankle Weakness leads to varying degrees of foot drop; patients may complain of tripping over carpets, dragging foot, or "foot slap" Weakness in muscle may be caused by L5 radiculopathy, peroneal mononeuropathy, the habit of crossing the legs at the knee, or posterior fibular head somatic dysfunction
Foot pronators Peroneal muscles (L5-S1; deep peroneal n.)	Lateral compartment muscles are p. longus and brevis; p. tertius is an anterior compartment muscle Pronate the foot (eversion and abduction) p. tertius also dorsiflexes at the talotibial joint; p. brevis and longus also plantar flex Tendon passes in front of lateral malleolus to insert on proximal 5th metatarsal	Pain referred along lateral ankle and foot; sometimes to lateral heel; failure to identify and treat TPs post-ankle sprain can prolong rehabilitation process Weakness in ankle dorsiflexion predisposing to ankle instability and repeat sprains May be mistaken for ankle arthritis[i] Weakness in muscle may be caused by L5 radiculopathy, peroneal mononeuropathy, the habit of crossing the legs at the knee, posterior fibular head somatic dysfunction, or prolonged immobilization (as in an ankle cast)
Foot and/or toe flexors Flexor digitorum longus (L5-S1; tibial n.) Flexor hallucis longus (L5-S2; tibial n.) Also intrinsic foot muscles		TP pain referred to sole of foot; worse with walking TP perpetuation by Morton foot, running on uneven ground, or barefoot in the sand TP pain referred to plantar surface of great toe and first metatarsal head TP perpetuation by Morton foot, running on uneven ground, or barefoot in the sand Intolerably sore feet, limited walking range, limp
Foot and/or toe extensors Extensor digitorum longus (L4-S1; deep peroneal n.) Extensor hallucis longus (L4-S1; deep peroneal n.) Also intrinsic foot muscles	(See above under Ankle Dorsiflexors)	Dysfunction makes foot less adaptable to the ground while walking TP referred pain to dorsum of foot at the base of the great toe TPs may be perpetuated by L4-5 radiculopathy; often follow anterior compartment syndrome, prolonged jogging, or dorsiflexed ankle position during sleep Intolerably sore feet, limited walking range, limp

[a]Travell JG, Simons DG. *Myofascial Pain and Dysfunction: The Trigger Point Manual,* Vol II. Baltimore, MD: Williams & Wilkins; 1992:324.
[b]Travell JG, Simons DG. *Myofascial Pain and Dysfunction: The Trigger Point Manual,* Vol II. Baltimore, MD: Williams & Wilkins; 1992:324.
[c]Travell JG, Simons DG. *Myofascial Pain and Dysfunction: The Trigger Point Manual,* Vol II. Baltimore, MD: Williams & Wilkins; 1992:250.
[d]Brody DM. Running Injuries. *CIBA Clin Symp.* 1980;32(4):15–16.
[e]Travell JG, Simons DG. *Myofascial Pain and Dysfunction: The Trigger Point Manual,* Vol II. Baltimore, MD: Williams & Wilkins; 1992:229–232.
[f]Travell JG, Simons DG. *Myofascial Pain and Dysfunction: The Trigger Point Manual,* Vol II. Baltimore, MD: Williams & Wilkins; 1992:377.
[g]Travell JG, Simons DG. *Myofascial Pain and Dysfunction: The Trigger Point Manual,* Vol II. Baltimore, MD: Williams & Wilkins; 1992:427.
[h]Reynolds MD, Myofascial trigger point syndromes in the practice of rheumatology. *Arch Phys Med Rehabil.* 1981;62:111–114.
[i]Travell JG, Simons DG. *Myofascial Pain and Dysfunction: The Trigger Point Manual,* Vol II. Baltimore, MD: Williams & Wilkins; 1992:377.

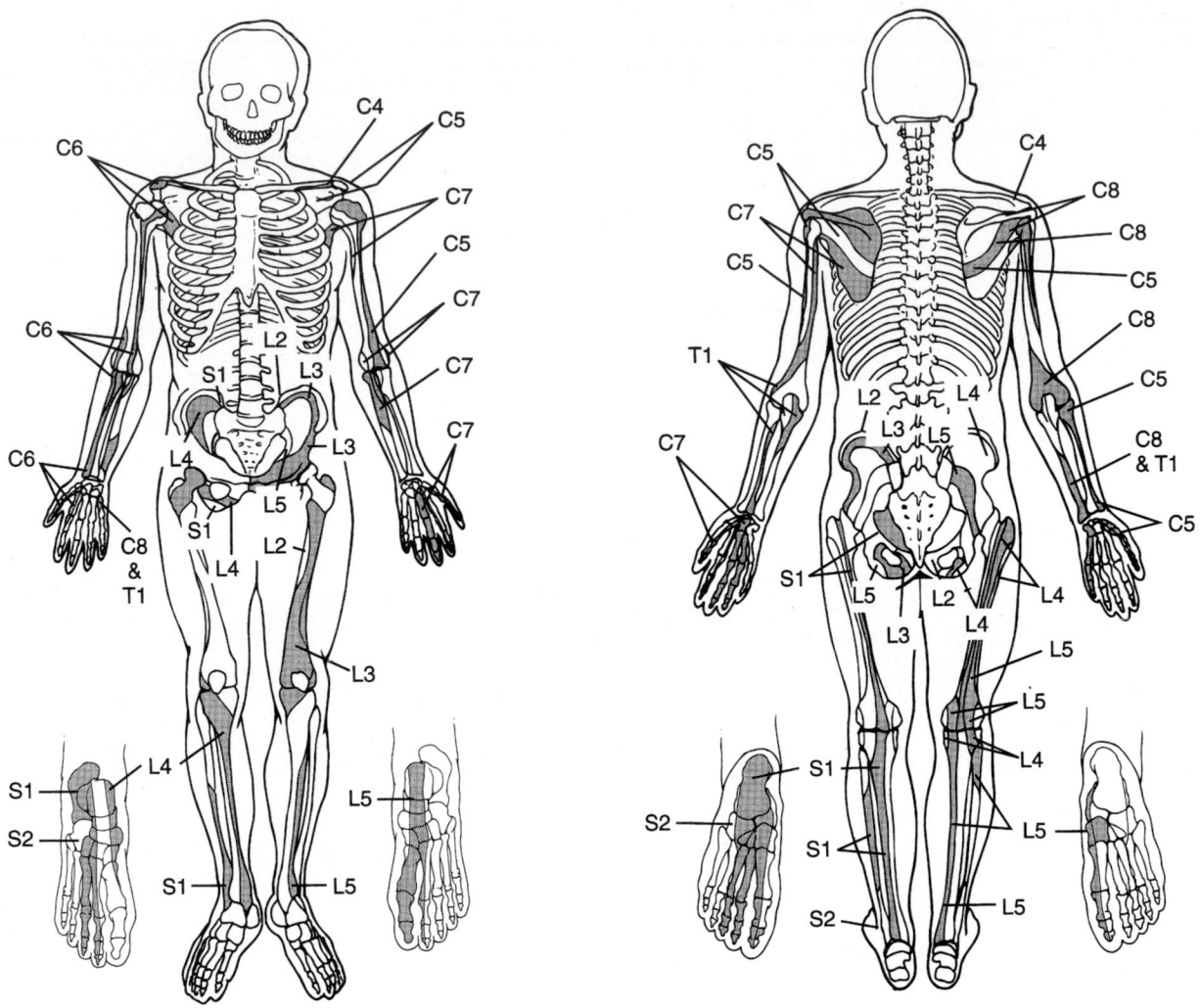

FIGURE 53.30. Sclerotomal pain patterns.

*V*ein
*E*mpty space
*L*ymphatics

Evidence of terminal lymphatic drainage dysfunction for the lower extremities may be palpated just inferior to the inguinal ligament. Dysfunctional drainage results in tissues that are tight, tender, and/or ticklish in this region.

Knee

The vascular supply is very poor to the menisci in the knees (especially the central section) and to synovial joint tissues in general. In large part, nutrition to the joints depends on good blood flow to the region (Fig. 53.35) and then diffusion into the synovial fluids. Metabolic waste products out of the arthrodial tissues likewise diffuse into the synovial fluid.

Intermittent non-weightbearing compression–decompression of the joints (joint pump) provides for fluid movement and may aid in the exchange of nutrients into and waste products out of the arthrodial structures. In rheumatoid arthritis the synovial mem-

brane thickens, and diffusion is impeded while oxygen demands in that joint increase (28).

Lower Leg

The lower leg is divided into three compartments (Fig. 53.37):

- Anterior osseofibrous compartment
- Lateral osseofibrous compartment
- Two posterior osseofibrous compartments—deep and superficial

Clinically, a compartment syndrome can arise from trauma or vigorous overuse, leading to a rise in intracompartmental pressure. This in turn compromises the circulation within that compartment, including venous return.

Recurrent mild compartment symptoms are managed with ice and OMT. Ice decreases pain and metabolic demand after activity. OMT also decreases pain and improves venous and lymphatic return. Management of co-existing trigger points is also helpful but not with injections; they would increase pressure in an

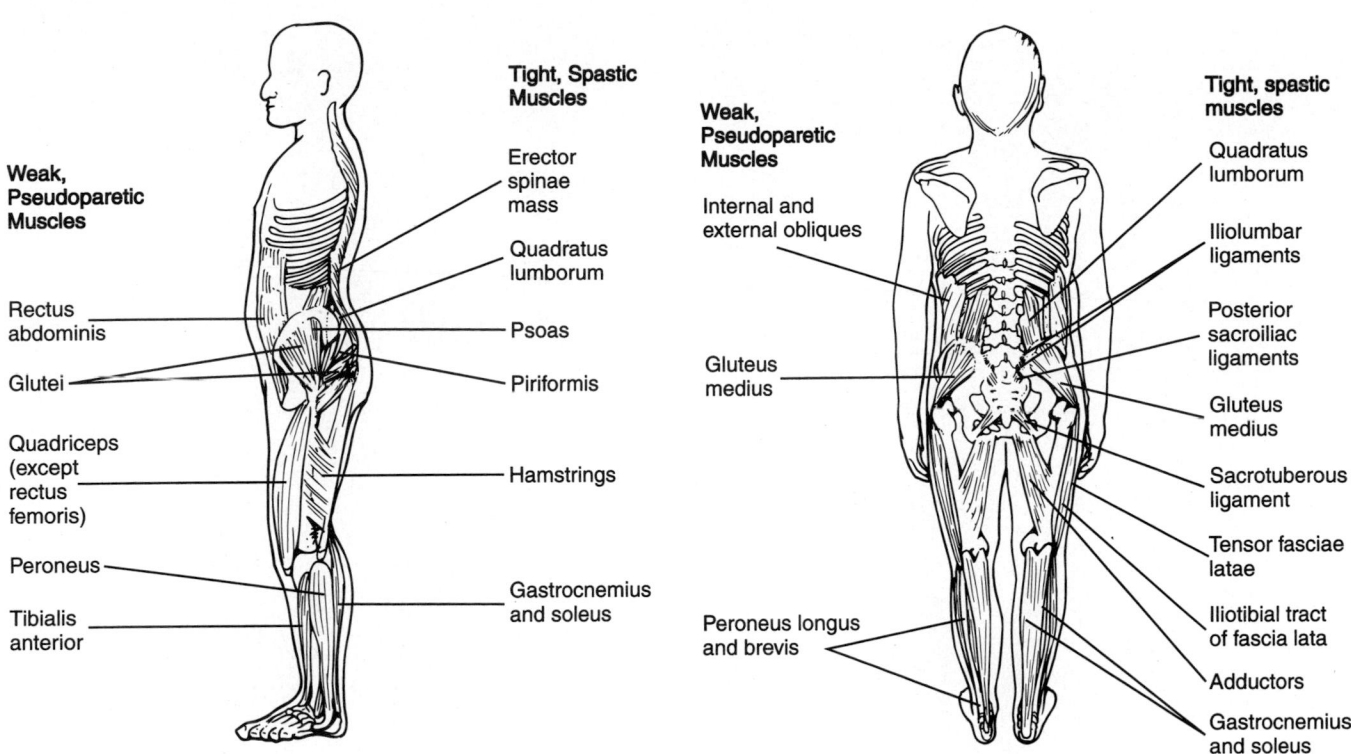

FIGURE 53.31. Muscle imbalance caused by biomechanical stressors.

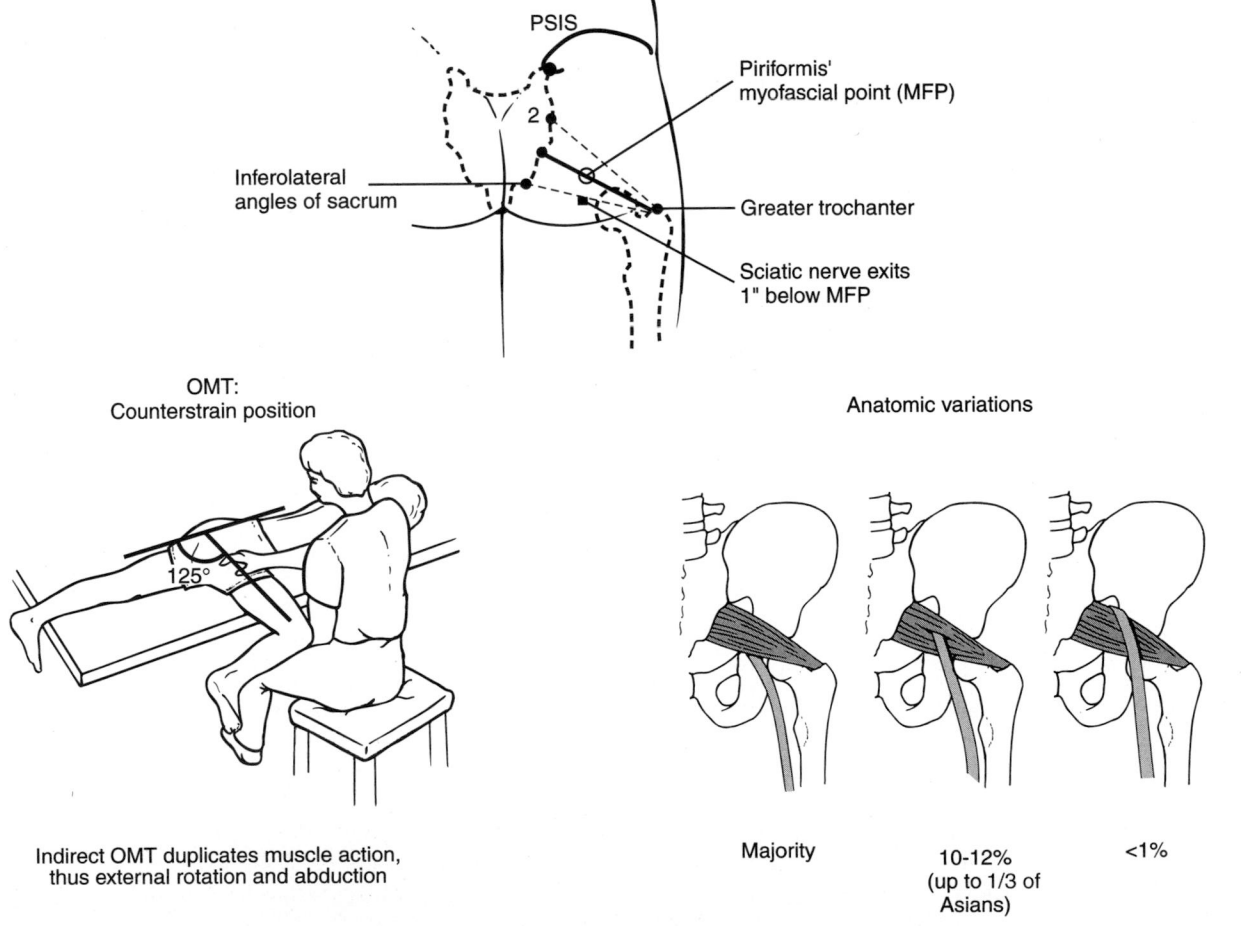

FIGURE 53.32. Piriformis structure-function relationships.

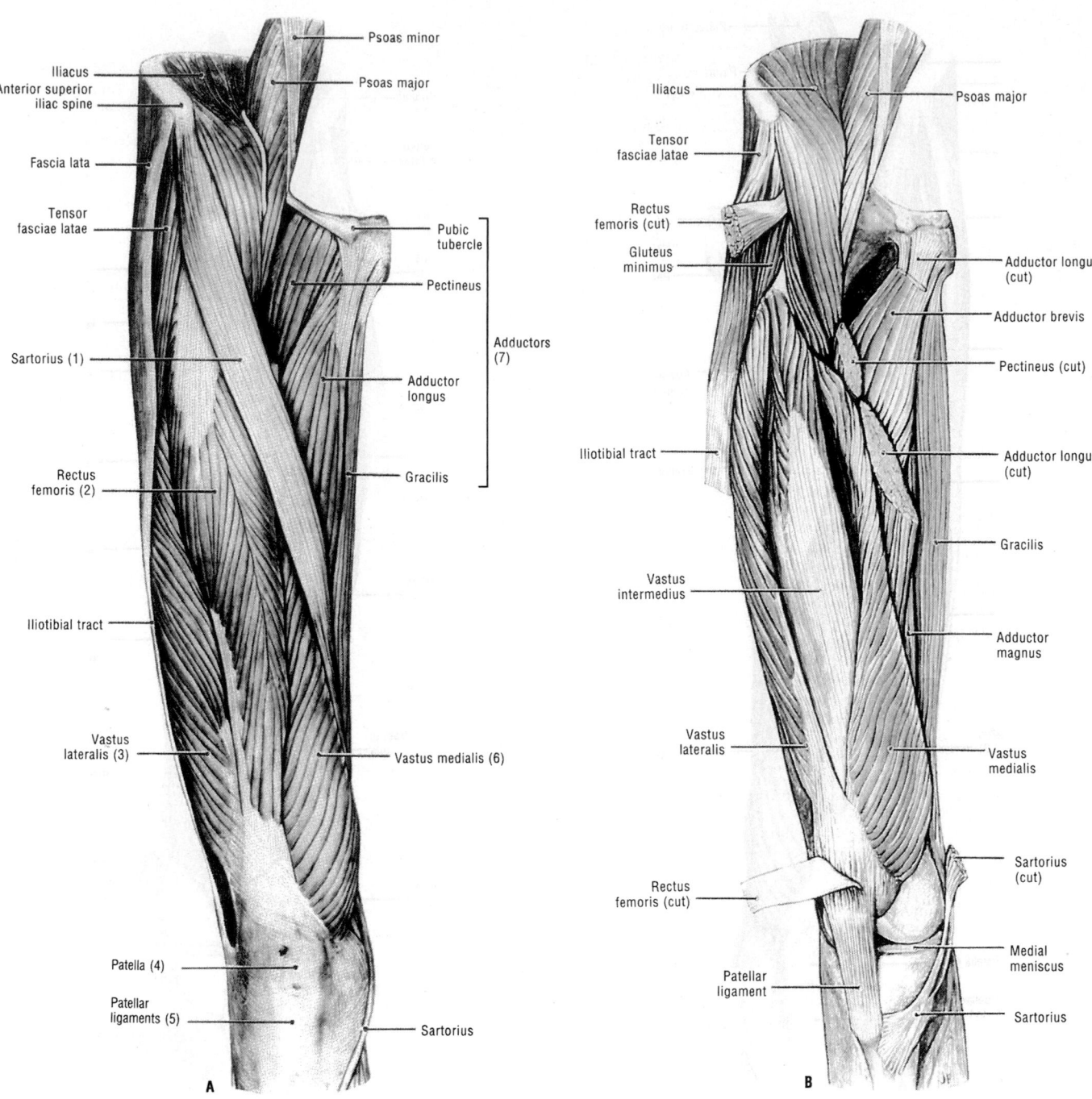

FIGURE 53.33. Muscles of thigh **(A)** and leg **(B)**. (From Moore KL. *Clinically Oriented Anatomy*, 3rd ed. Baltimore, MD: Williams & Wilkins; 1992:394, 395, 442, 453, with permission.)

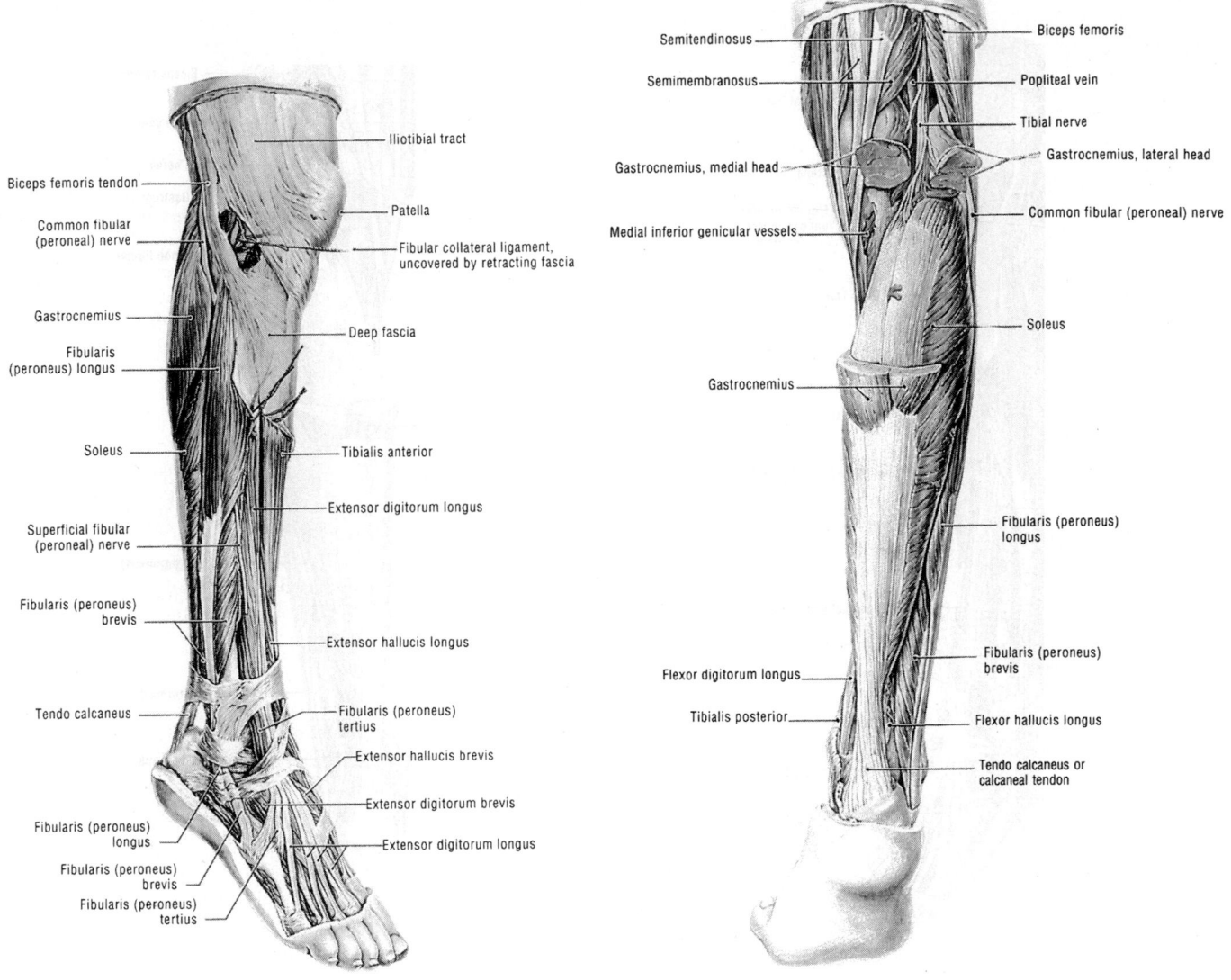

FIGURE 53.33B. (*continued*)

ANTERIOR COMPARTMENT

The anterior compartment is covered anteriorly by a relatively nonexpansile fascia. Structurally, this creates the potential for development of an anterior compartment syndrome. Bleeding into this compartment from a fracture or other trauma creates increased pressure in this enclosed space. For runners, sometimes muscle swelling impairs venous outflow, resulting in a rise in intracompartmental pressure. If intracompartmental pressure becomes great enough, arterial circulation is reduced, and ischemia with potential necrosis of muscle in the compartment can occur. An acute compartment compression is a surgical emergency requiring fasciotomy. Such a situation is more likely to occur in the anterior compartment than in other divisions of the leg. The

already tight compartment. Modification of the running surface or the running shoe may also be required to prevent recurrent compartment syndromes.

acute compartment compression may occur in runners where symptoms of intense pain develop during the run but do not subside afterward.

Palpation reveals the entire tibialis anterior muscle to be hard and tender. Anterior compartment muscles may also exhibit weakness upon testing. Peripheral pulses are usually present. Decreased sensation is often present between the first and second toes as a result of entrapment of the deep peroneal nerve. While primarily a clinical diagnosis, intracompartmental pressure can be measured with a wick catheter (19). Because of the location of the pain on the anterolateral side of the leg, recurrent anterior compartment syndrome is also called anterior shin splints.

LATERAL COMPARTMENT

In the lateral compartment syndrome, pain is located diffusely along the lateral aspect of the lower leg. It recurs in runners with

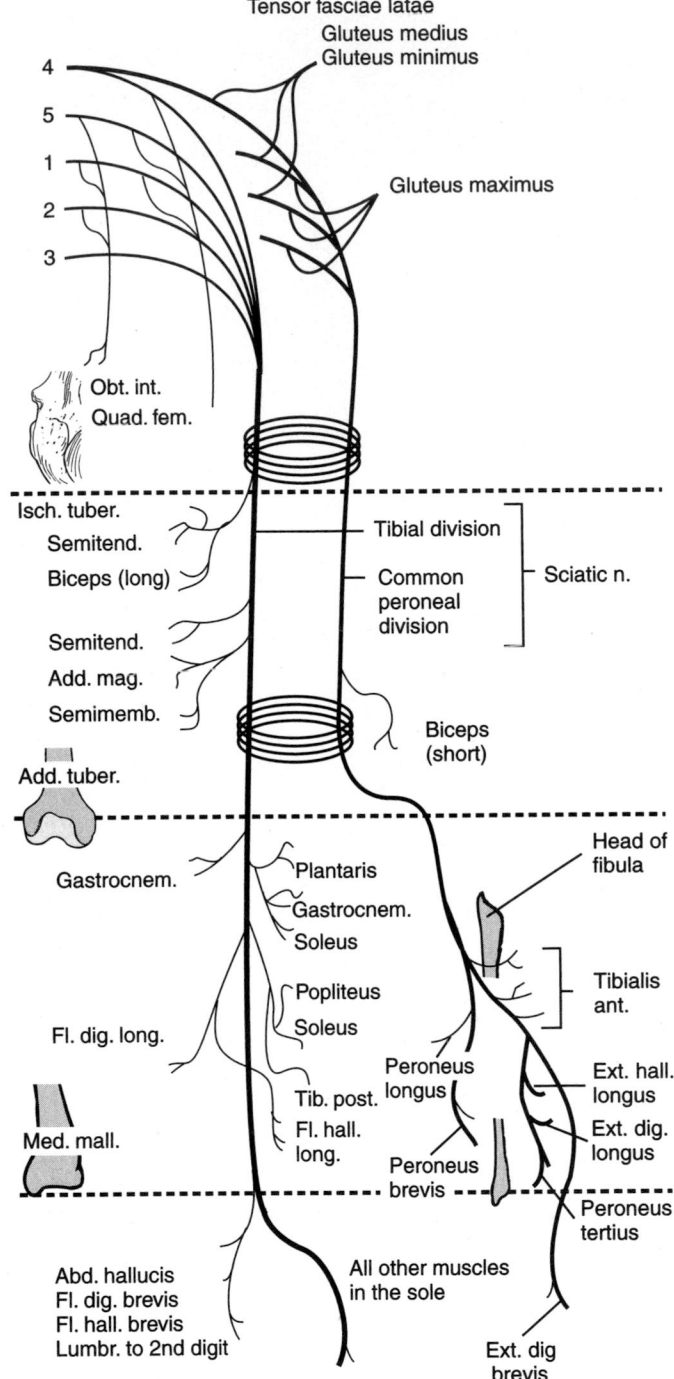

FIGURE 53.34. Nerve supply of the lower extremity arising from the sciatic nerve and its branches.

excessive pronation of the foot or may result from rupture of the peroneus longus muscle.

POSTERIOR COMPARTMENT

The posterior compartment syndromes typically refer pain anteromedially. While some reserve the term shin splints only for periostitis along the line of attachment of a repeatedly overloaded muscle (19), others include posterior compartment syndrome in the differential diagnosis along with stress fractures of the tibia and chronic periostitis (the soleus syndrome). Posterior compartment syndromes are often bilateral and difficult to manage conservatively.

Bursae and Bursitis

A number of bursae are located around the hip, knee, and ankle. They may swell as a response to direct trauma or stresses placed on the joints of the lower extremities (Fig. 53.38). Bursitis is inflammation of a bursa. There is palpable swelling that can be defined and that is sensitive to deep pressure. Pain alone in the region of the bursa often leads to misdiagnosis.

Trochanteric Bursitis

In the hip region, trochanteric bursitis is a common clinical diagnosis or, in many cases, a misdiagnosis. The subgluteus maximus (trochanteric) bursa lies at the root of the iliotibial tract. Here it separates the greater trochanter of the femur from the converging fibers of the gluteus maximus and the tensor fasciae latae. The bursa also separates these fibers from the origin of the vastus lateralis muscle. Trigger points in any of these muscles can refer pain to this site and are commonly misdiagnosed as a trochanteric bursitis. This is also the case in quadratus lumborum trigger points (21) and in the ligamentous pain referral from iliolumbar ligament (20).

True inflammation and swelling of the trochanteric bursa (trochanteric bursitis) causes intense pain over the bursal location with radiation into the lateral thigh. Palpation of the bursa just below the greater trochanter reveals the swelling and heat. Pressure here increases the pain. Walking, hip abduction, and internally rotating the hip can aggravate the pain. Injection of the bursa with a local anesthetic with or without accompanying steroids quickly and significantly reduces pain. A higher incidence of trochanteric bursitis is found on the long leg side of individuals with unequal leg length (7).

Patellar Bursitis

The knee is a common site for trauma to the bursa designed to protect the relatively exposed superficial structures from injury against those underlying them. A large prepatellar bursa separates the patella from the skin anterior to it. Inflammation of this bursa from long-term kneeling or from other trauma results in a condition known as "housemaid's knee."

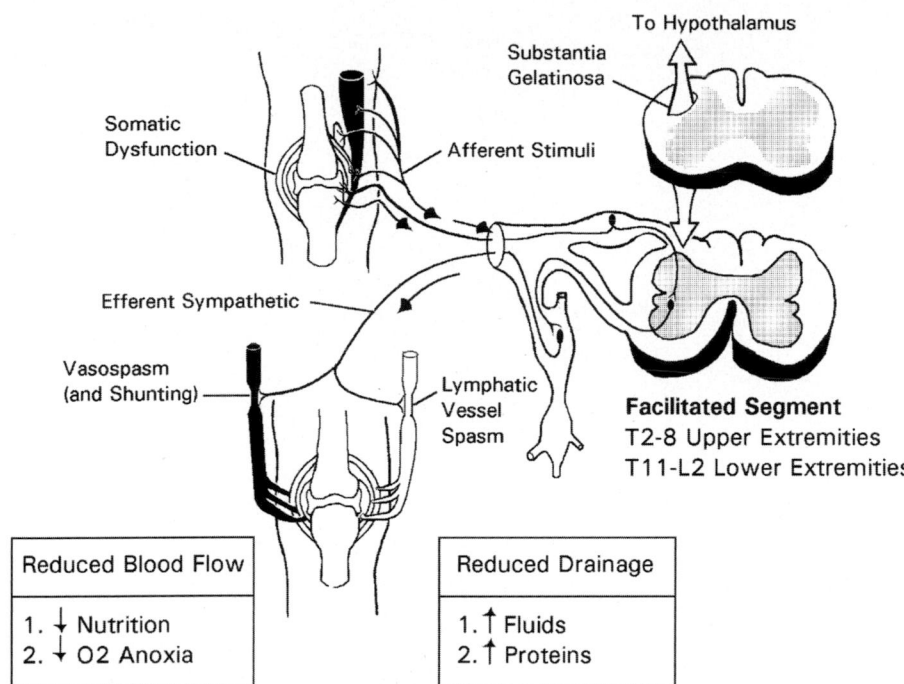

To Hypothalamus
Substantia Gelatinosa
Somatic Dysfunction
Afferent Stimuli
Efferent Sympathetic
Vasospasm (and Shunting)
Lymphatic Vessel Spasm
Facilitated Segment
T2-8 Upper Extremities
T11-L2 Lower Extremities
Reduced Blood Flow
1. ↓ Nutrition
2. ↓ O2 Anoxia
Reduced Drainage
1. ↑ Fluids
2. ↑ Proteins

FIGURE 53.35. Influence of somatic dysfunction on normal vascular and lymphatic elements of the lower extremity. (From Kuchera ML, Kuchera WA. *Osteopathic Considerations in Systemic Dysfunction*, 2nd ed. rev. Columbus, OH: Greyden Press; 1994, with permission.)

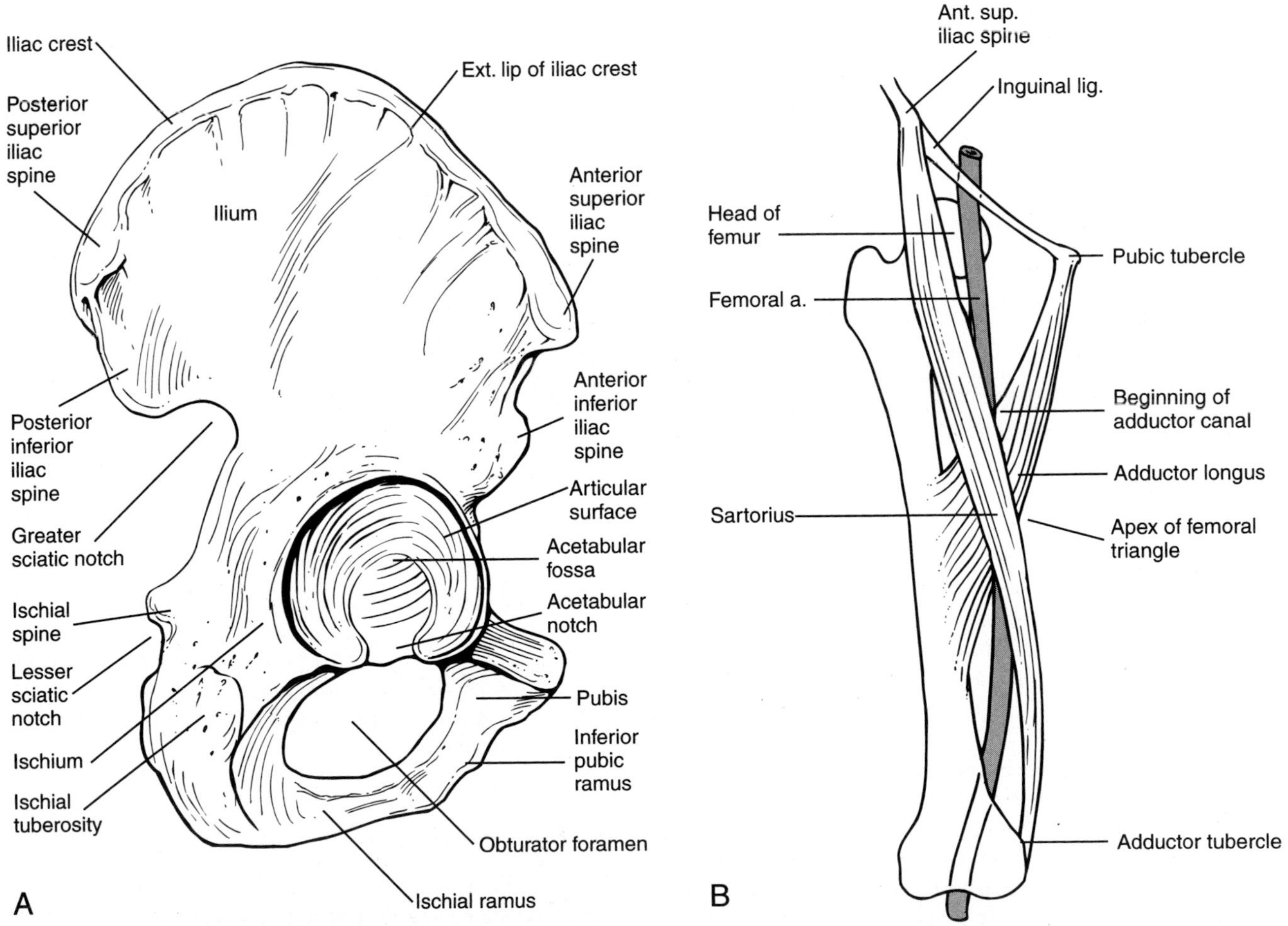

Iliac crest
Ext. lip of iliac crest
Posterior superior iliac spine
Ilium
Anterior superior iliac spine
Anterior inferior iliac spine
Posterior inferior iliac spine
Greater sciatic notch
Articular surface
Acetabular fossa
Ischial spine
Acetabular notch
Lesser sciatic notch
Pubis
Ischium
Inferior pubic ramus
Ischial tuberosity
Obturator foramen
Ischial ramus
A
Ant. sup. iliac spine
Inguinal lig.
Head of femur
Pubic tubercle
Femoral a.
Beginning of adductor canal
Adductor longus
Sartorius
Apex of femoral triangle
Adductor tubercle
B

FIGURE 53.36. Anatomy of the acetabular notch **(A)** and femoral triangle **(B)**.

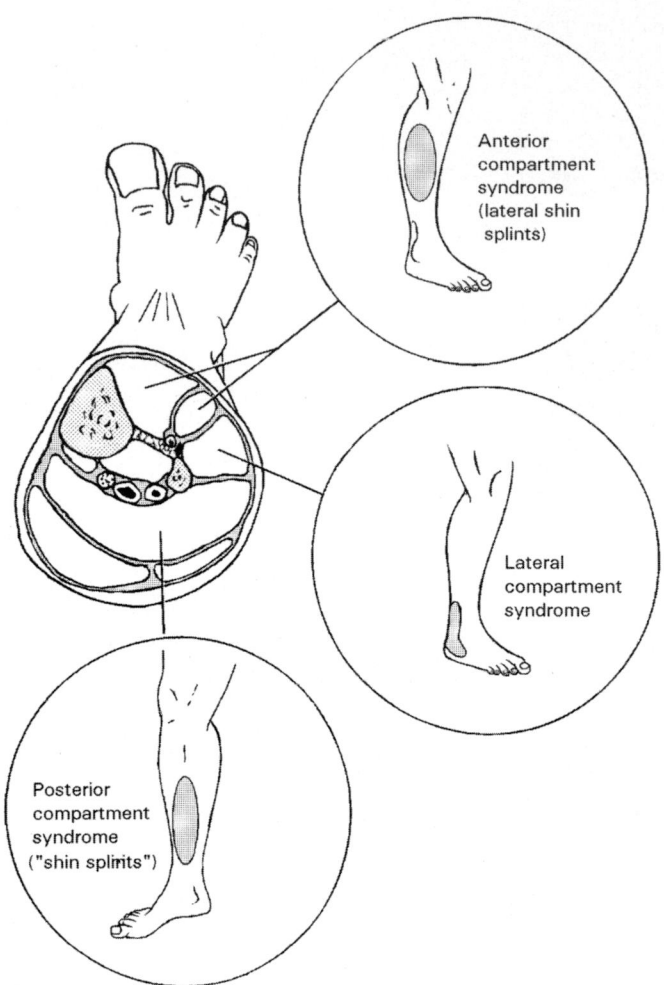

FIGURE 53.37. Fascial compartments of the lower extremity.

The suprapatellar bursa connects to the synovial cavity of the knee joint and can be used in physical diagnosis to determine if knee trauma has caused significant swelling. The physician first milks any fluid in this bursa from medial to lateral. Then, by palpating anteromedially for a fluid wave initiated by a gentle squeeze from the anterolateral side of the suprapatellar tendon, it is possible to detect 10 to 15 mL of effusion in the knee. This bulge test is used for small effusions (Fig. 53.39A). If the effusion is so large that the tissues become turgid, a fluid pulse may not be able to create a bulge and the test may provide a false-negative result. Large effusions are more accurately diagnosed with a ballottement test (Fig. 53.39B) in which the kneecap is tapped gently (ballotted). A palpable transmission of bony contact is palpated if the effusion is large enough to have distanced the patella from the bone behind it.

The superficial and deep infrapatellar bursae are less often involved in clinical problems.

A Baker cyst arises from enlargement of either the semimembranosus bursa or the bursa behind the medial head of the gastrocnemius (Fig. 53.40). The swollen cyst is often painful, especially with flexion of the knee. The swelling is more prominent in the standing position. Both of these bursae commonly communicate

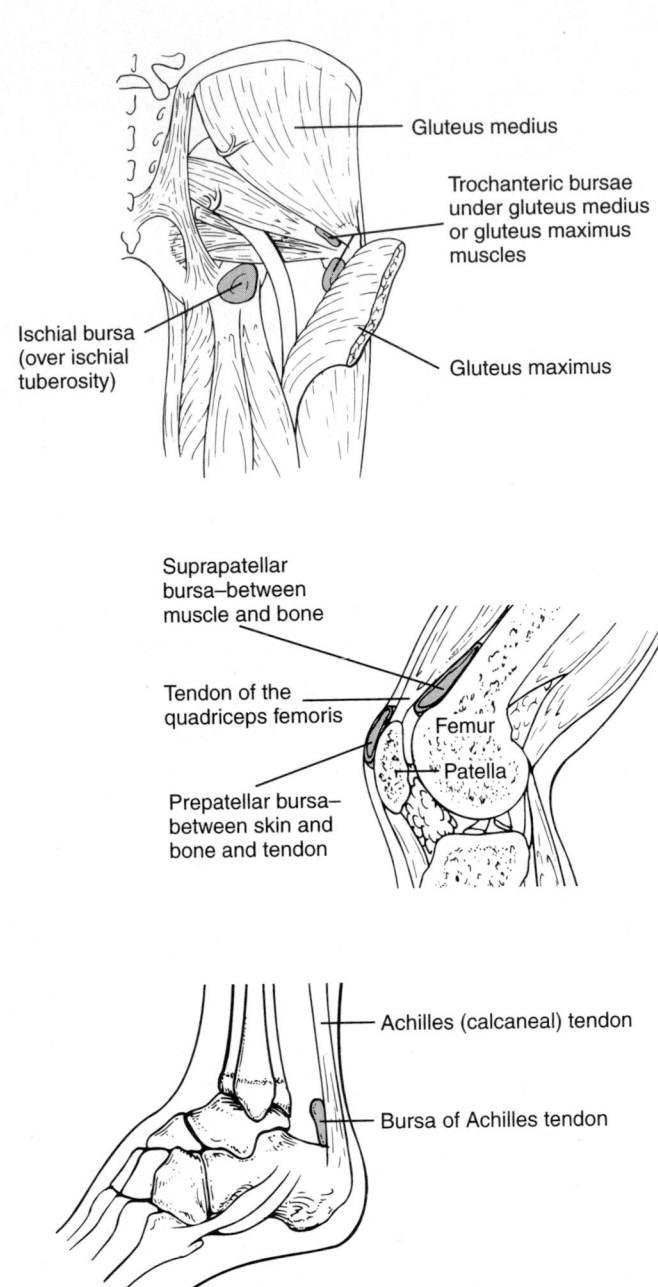

FIGURE 53.38. Bursae of the lower extremity.

with the synovial cavity of the knee. For this reason, knee trauma such as a meniscal tear, or disease such as rheumatoid arthritis, can initiate the cyst. Rupture of a Baker cyst may be misdiagnosed as thrombophlebitis.

Bursa of the Achilles Tendon

In the ankle region, the superficial bursa of the Achilles tendon may be irritated by poorly fitting shoes and may swell. This results in a tender "pump bump."

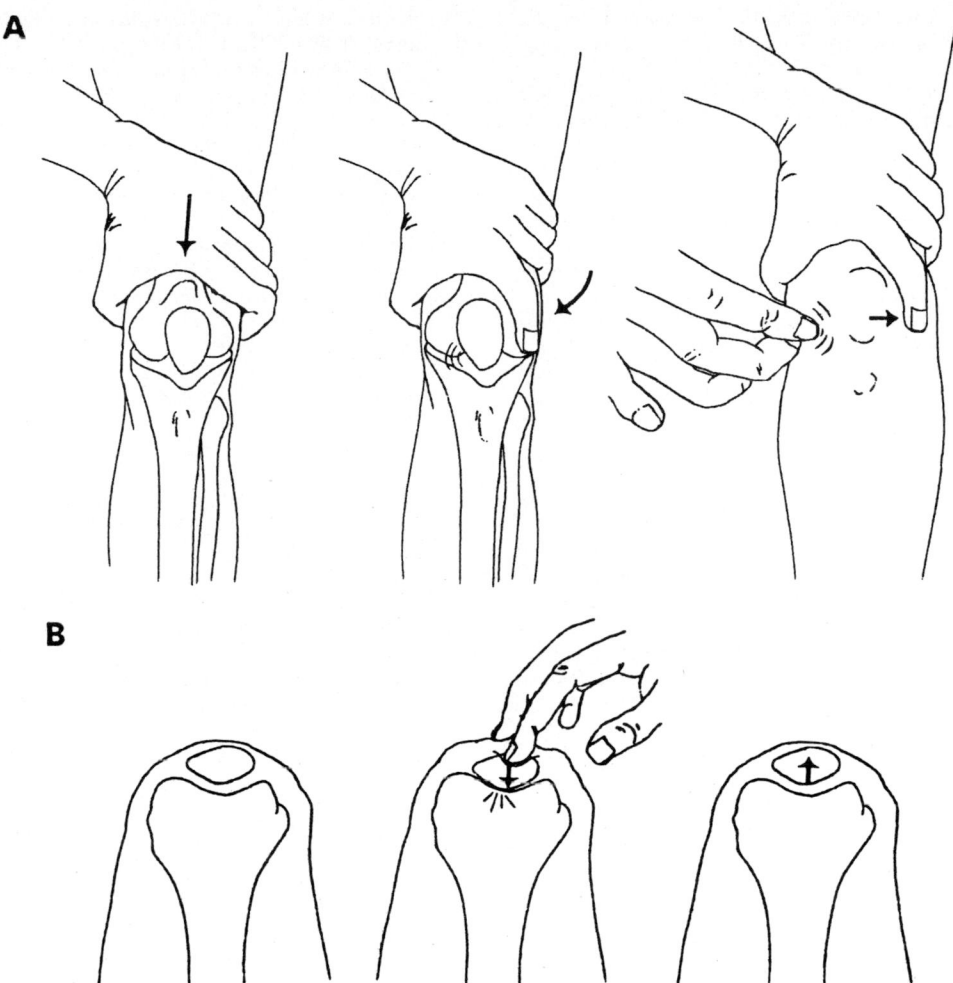

FIGURE 53.39. Tests for effusion in the knee. The bulge test **(A)** is useful for finding a minimal amount of effusion in the knee. The ballottement test **(B)** is positive if there is a large amount of effusion present. (Illustration by W.A. Kuchera.)

CONCLUSION

A thorough understanding of the functional anatomy of the lower extremities establishes a foundation for the osteopathic approach to the lower extremities and their effect on the body unit. Palpation assists in differential diagnosis of a wide range of structural and functional disorders in this region. The osteopathic physician then seeks to balance and improve biomechanical and homeostatic functions to influence a wide range of patient conditions.

From a sports medicine practice to the care of patients with deep vein thrombosis in an internal medicine practice, the osteopathic approach to the lower extremities offers an effective approach to diagnosis, prevention, and/or treatment.

REFERENCES

1. Irvin RE. Suboptimal posture: the origin of the majority of idiopathic pain of the musculoskeletal system. In: Vleeming A, Mooney V,

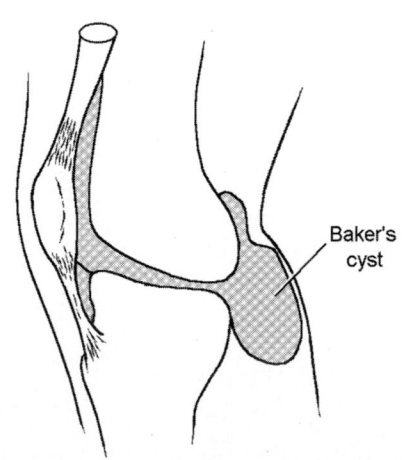

FIGURE 53.40. Bursae of the knee and Baker cyst.

Baker's cyst

Dorman T, Snijders C, eds. *Movement, Stability, and Low Back Pain: The Essential Role of the Pelvis.* New York: Churchill-Livingstone; 1997:133–155.

2. Cyriax JH, Cyriax PJ. *Cyriax's Illustrated Manual of Orthopaedic Medicine,* 2nd ed. Oxford, England: Butterworth-Heinemann Ltd; 1993:6–8.

3. Dorman TA. Refurbishing ligaments with prolotherapy. *Spine*: State of the Art Reviews. 1995;9(2):509–516.

4. Moore KL. *Clinically Oriented Anatomy,* 2nd ed. Baltimore, MD: Williams & Wilkins; 1985:403.

5. Christmann OD. Biomechanical aspects of degenerative joint disease. *Clin Orthop.* 1969;64:77–85.

6. Gofton JP, Trueman GE. Studies in osteoarthritis of the hip, Part II: osteoarthritis of the hip and leg-length disparity. *Can Med Assoc J.* 1971;104:791–799.

7. Brody DM. Running injuries. *CIBA Clin Symp.* 1980;32(4):25.

8. Kuchera WA, Kuchera ML. *Osteopathic Principles in Practice,* 2nd ed. rev. Columbus, OH: Greyden Press; 1994.

9. Cyriax JH, Cyriax PJ. *Cyriax's Illustrated Manual of Orthopaedic Medicine,* 2nd ed. Oxford, England: Butterworth-Heinemann Ltd; 1993:81.

10. Ombregt L, ter Veer HJ. Disorders of the inert structures: capsular and non-capsular patterns. In: Ombregt L, Bisschop P, ter Veer HJ, Van de Velde T, eds. *A System of Orthopaedic Medicine.* London, England: WB Saunders; 1995:783–800.

11. Blood SD. Treatment of the sprained ankle. *JAOA.* 1980;79:680–692.

12. Inman VT. *Joints of the Ankle.* Baltimore, MD: Williams & Wilkins; 1976:42.

13. Inman VT, Mann RA. Biomechanics of the foot and ankle. In: *DuVries' Surgery of the Foot,* 3rd ed. St. Louis, MO: 1973:17.

14. Levens SA, et al. Transverse rotation of the segments of the lower extremity in locomotion. *J Bone Joint Surg.* 1948;30A:859–872.

15. Hicks JH. The mechanics of the foot, I: the joints. *J Anat.* 1953;87:345–357.

16. Kuchera WA, Kuchera ML. *Osteopathic Principles in Practice,* 2nd ed. rev. Columbus, OH: Greyden Press. 1994.

17. Roy S, Irvin R. *Sports Medicine: Prevention, Evaluation, Management, and Rehabilitation.* Englewood Cliffs, NJ: Prentice-Hall; 1983:380.

18. Greenman PE. *Principles of Manual Medicine,* 2nd ed. Baltimore, MD: Williams & Wilkins; 1996:411–446.

19. Travell JG, Simons DG. *Myofascial Pain and Dysfunction: The Trigger Point Manual. The Lower Extremities.* Vol II. Baltimore, MD: Williams & Wilkins; 1992.

20. Hackett GS. *Ligament and Tendon Relaxation Treated by Prolotherapy,* 3rd ed. Springfield, IL: Charles C Thomas; 1958.

21. Travell JG, Simons DG. *Myofascial Pain and Dysfunction: The Trigger Point Manual.* Vol II. The Lower Extremities. Baltimore, MD: Williams & Wilkins; 1992:28–88.

22. Travell JG, Simons DG. *Myofascial Pain and Dysfunction: The Trigger Point Manual.* Vol II. The Lower Extremities. Baltimore, MD: Williams & Wilkins; 1992:23–27.

23. Walsh PC, ed. *Campbell's Urology,* 7th ed. Philadelphia, PA: WB Saunders; 1998:2698.

24. *Travell and Simons' Myofascial Pain and Dysfunction: The Trigger Point Manual.* Vol I. Upper Half of Body. Baltimore, MD: Williams & Wilkins; 1999.

25. Janda V. Muscle weakness and inhibition (pseudoparesis) in back pain syndromes. In: Grieve GP, ed. *Modern Medicine Therapy of the Vertebral Column.* Edinburgh, Scotland: Churchill-Livingstone; 1986:197–200.

26. Kuchera ML. Treatment of gravitational strain pathology. In: Vleeming A, Mooney V, Dorman T, Snijders C, eds. *Movement, Stability, and Low Back Pain: The Essential Role of the Pelvis.* New York, NY: Churchill-Livingstone; 1997:477–499.

27. Basmajian JV. *Grant's Method of Anatomy,* 9th ed. Baltimore, MD: Williams & Wilkins; 1975:327–328.

28. Kuchera ML, Kuchera WA. *Osteopathic Considerations in Systemic Dysfunction,* 2nd ed. rev. Columbus, OH: Greyden Press; 1994:159–167.

54

SOFT TISSUE TECHNIQUES

WALTER C. EHRENFEUCHTER
DAVID HEILIG
ALEXANDER S. NICHOLAS

KEY CONCEPTS

- Soft tissue techniques and classification as direct or indirect techniques
- Goals attainable with soft tissue techniques
- Three basic mechanisms used in soft tissue techniques
- Manner in which soft tissue techniques can be used alone or in combination with other manipulative techniques
- Objective, patient positioning, physician positioning, and implementation of soft tissue techniques for following regions:
  —Cervical
  —Thoracic
  —Lumbar
  —Sacrum
  —Upper extremity
  —Lower extremity

Soft tissue techniques are defined as direct techniques that address the muscular and fascial structures of the body and associated neural and vascular elements. Soft tissue techniques may be applied in a number of different ways to:

1. Relax hypertonic muscles
2. Stretch passive fascial structures
3. Enhance circulation to the local myofascial structures
4. Improve local tissue nutrition, oxygenation, and removal of metabolic wastes
5. Improve abnormal somato-somatic and somatovisceral reflex activity
6. Identify areas of somatic dysfunction
7. Observe tissue response to the application of manipulative technique

8. Improve local and systemic immune responsiveness
9. Provide a general state of relaxation
10. Provide a general state of tonic stimulation

The choice of technique is based on the treatment goals. There are three basic mechanisms used in applying soft tissue technique to muscular structures and their associated fascial elements:

1. Tractional technique, also called stretching, in which the origin and insertion of the myofascial structures being treated are longitudinally separated.
2. Kneading, a rhythmic, lateral stretching of a myofascial structure, in which origin and insertion are held stationary and the central portion of the structure is stretched like a bowstring.
3. Inhibition, sustained deep pressure over a hypertonic myofascial structure.

Other mechanisms used on more superficial fascial structures include variants on techniques developed in the European massage movement:

- Effleurage
- Petrissage
- Tapotement
- Skin rolling

Soft tissue techniques may be used alone or in combination with any other manipulative technique. Many of the positions used for soft tissue techniques readily lend themselves to conversion to other techniques such as the following:

- Articulatory
- Muscle energy
- Counterstrain
- Functional
- Cranial
- High velocity/low amplitude (HVLA) thrusting

CERVICAL TECHNIQUES

Suboccipital Inhibition

Objective

Decrease in suboccipital muscle tone.

Position

Supine (Fig. 54.1).

Procedure

1. Sit at the head of the table.
2. Place the pads of your fingers just inferior to the superior nuchal line in the suboccipital tissues.
3. Lift the head so that the patient's weight is entirely supported on the pads of your fingers. The head is slightly above, but not resting on, your palms.
4. Maintain this position until you achieve the desired relaxation of the suboccipital soft tissues.

Note: This technique is similar in position to the method used by A.T. Still when he created a rope sling to relieve his own headaches.

Rotation

Objective

Increase cervical rotation.

Position

Supine (Fig. 54.2).

Procedure

1. Sit at the head of the table.
2. Use your hands to cradle the head, taking care not to occlude the ear canals.

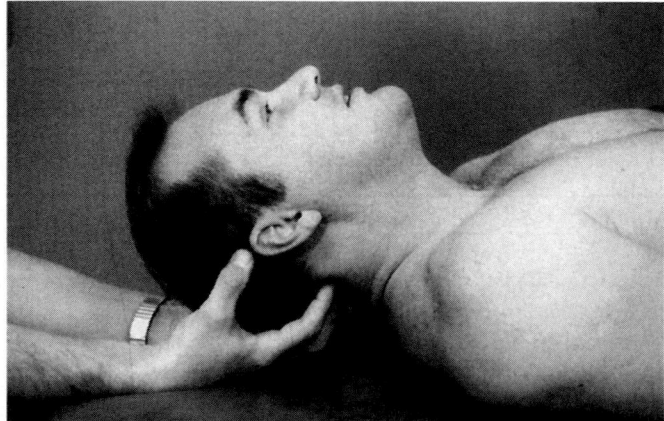

FIGURE 54.1. Suboccipital inhibition.

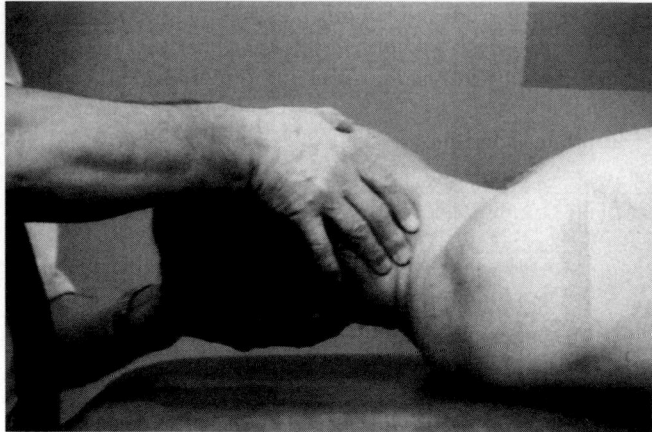

FIGURE 54.2. Cervical rotation.

3. Rotate the patient's head away from you slowly until tissue tension restricts you from further motion.
4. Gently increase the tension by rotating into the restrictive barrier, hold the tension for 12 seconds, and then slowly release it.
5. Repeat as many times as necessary to achieve the desired effect.

Note: This neck position allows for conversion to a muscle energy cervical range of motion technique or for an HVLA thrust for atlantoaxial segmental dysfunction.

Traction

Objective

Stretch paravertebral muscles.

Position

Supine.

Procedure

1. Sit behind the patient at the head of the table.
2. Place one hand cradling the occiput between the thumb and index finger. Place your other hand across the patient's forehead.
3. Exert a gentle axial traction with your occipital hand.
4. Use your hand on the forehead to prevent forward tilt of the patient's head, also applying slight traction.
5. Apply the tractional force slowly; release it slowly.
6. Repeat as many times as necessary to achieve the desired effect.

Forward Bending

Objective

Stretch posterior cervical soft tissues.

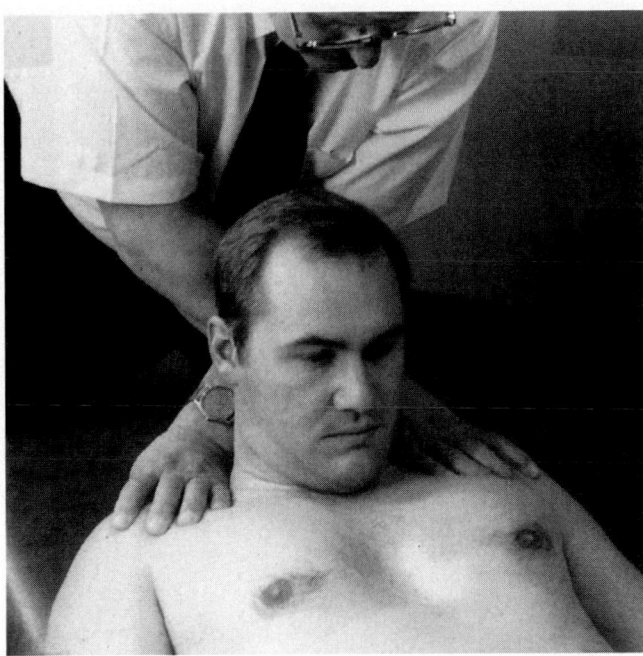

FIGURE 54.3. Cervical forward bending.

Position

Supine (Fig. 54.3).

Procedure

1. Sit or stand at the head of the table.
2. Cross your forearms and place them behind the patient's head with your hands on the patient's shoulders.
3. Exert a slow, forward bending stretch until a restrictive barrier is engaged.
4. Gently, slowly increase the stretch; then release it just as slowly.
5. Repeat as many times as necessary to achieve the desired effect.

Note: This position allows use of a range-of-motion muscle energy technique, and it may also be used to treat anterior counterstrain tender points.

Contralateral Traction

Objective

Relax the cervical paravertebral muscles.

Position

Supine.

Procedure

1. Stand at the side of the head of the table.
2. With your caudad hand, reach across the patient and under the opposite side of the neck to grasp the paravertebral muscles with the pads of your fingers.

3. Grasp the forehead lightly with your cephalad hand.
4. With your caudad hand, draw the paravertebral muscles laterally and anteriorly until you reach the initial restrictive barrier.
5. Increase the anterolateral traction slightly to take the tissues slightly beyond the barrier.
6. Repeat as many times as necessary to achieve the desired effect.

Note: By increasing the rotational force, this technique may be converted to a deep articulatory technique. By adding more of a milking motion, it may be used to enhance lymphatic drainage in the cervical lymph node chains.

Longitudinal Traction

Objective

Relax the cervical paravertebral muscles.

Position

Supine (Fig. 54.4).

Procedure

1. Sit at the head of the table.
2. Bring the palmar surfaces of the fingers of both hands under the neck near the spinous processes.
3. Lift the cervical paravertebral musculature and draw it cephalad.
4. Slowly releasing the musculature, carry the hands caudally.
5. Repeat as many times as necessary to achieve the desired effect, shifting position along the length of the cervical spine.

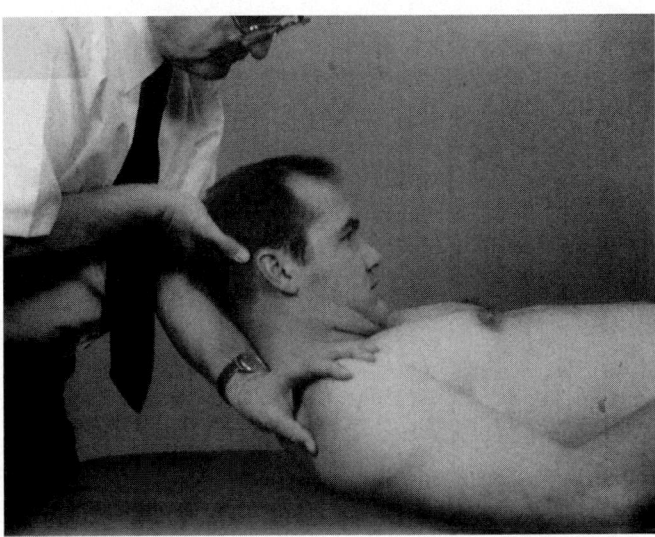

FIGURE 54.4. Cervical contralateral traction.

THORACIC

Prone Pressure

Objective

Relax the thoracic paravertebral muscles.

Position

Prone (Figs. 54.5 and 54.6).

Procedure

1. Stand at the side of the patient, whose head is turned away from the side to be treated.
2. Place your thumb and thenar eminence of one hand on the far side of the thoracic spine between the spinous and transverse processes.
3. Place your other hand reinforcing the first or working in tandem with it along the spine.
4. Exert an anterolateral pressure on the soft tissues, directed away from the spine.
5. You may maintain the pressure as a sustained, inhibitory pressure or use it in an intermittent kneading fashion.
6. Repeat as many times as necessary at various levels to achieve the desired effect.

Note: Additional downward vertical pressure converts this into a deep articulatory technique.

Prone Thumb Pressure

Objective

Decrease paravertebral muscle hypertonicity.

Position

Prone.

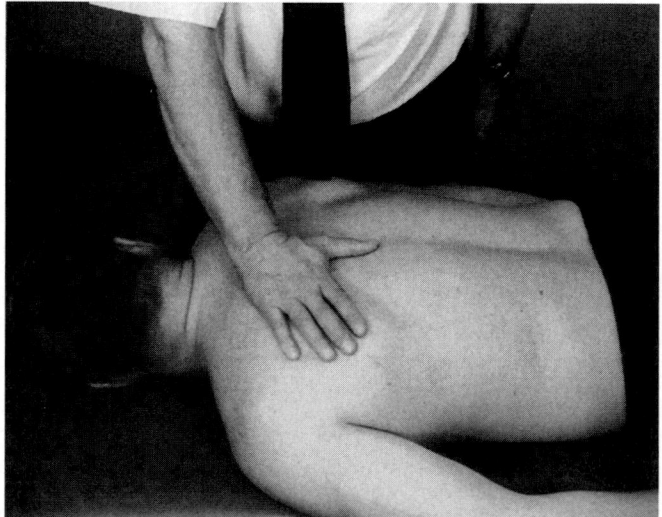

FIGURE 54.5. Placement of thumb for thoracic thumb pressure.

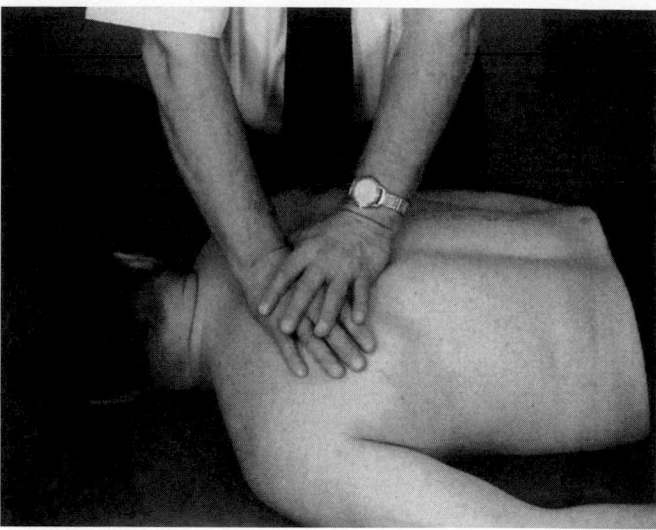

FIGURE 54.6. Caudad hand reinforcing thumb pressure for thoracic thumb pressure.

Procedure

1. Stand at the head of the table.
2. Place the thumbs of both hands just lateral to the spinous processes, on the paravertebral muscles, with your fingers fanned out.
3. Exert a caudad, anterior pressure, allowing muscle to relax and stretch, finishing with a lateral sweeping motion.
4. A kneading motion or inhibitory pressure may be used.
5. The technique is repeated at as many spinal levels as is desired, as many times as necessary to achieve the desired effect.

Prone Pressure with Counterpressure

Objective

Relax deep intrinsic spinal muscles.

Position

Prone.

Procedure

1. Stand at the side of the table.
2. Have the patient turn his or her head toward you.
3. Place one hand on the far side of the spine, over the transverse processes, with your fingers pointing cephalad.
4. Place your other hand on the near side of the spine with your fingers pointing caudad.
5. Exert simultaneous longitudinal and anterior pressure with both hands, imparting a side-bending motion to the thoracic segments under the treating hands. The degree of vertical pressure exerted is varied according to the patient's condition and the degree of vertebral and costal articulation desired.

6. Use a repetitive kneading motion.
7. Repeat as many times as necessary to achieve the desired effect.

Note: This technique can be used as a deep articulatory technique or can readily be converted to a thrust technique directed at thoracic segmental dysfunction.

Upper Thoracic: Lateral Recumbent

Objective

Relax upper thoracic paravertebral muscles.

Position

Lateral recumbent (Fig. 54.7).

Procedure

1. Stand at the side of the table facing the patient.
2. Pass your caudad hand under the patient's arm, grasping the upper side paravertebral muscles just lateral to the spinous processes with the pads of your fingers.
3. Contact the anterior portion of the shoulder with your cephalad hand to provide an effective counterforce.
4. Draw the paravertebral muscles laterally away from the spine until restriction is palpated.
5. Continue to apply lateral traction until the tissues relax, soften, and lengthen. The lateral traction is then slowly released.
6. Work your way up and down the spinal column from the cervicothoracic junction to about the midthoracics.
7. Repeat as many times as necessary to achieve the desired effect.

Lower Thoracic: Lateral Recumbent

Objective

Relax the lower thoracic paravertebral muscles.

Position

Lateral recumbent, treatment side up.

Procedure

1. Stand at the side of the table.
2. Reach both hands under the patient's arm, contacting the paravertebral muscles just lateral to the spinous processes with the pads of your fingers.
3. Pull the pads of your fingers toward the center of the body, drawing the musculature laterally like a bowstring.
4. Slowly release this lateral traction, and reposition your hands along the spine to treat other levels as desired.
5. Repeat as many times as necessary to achieve the desired effect.

Lateral Recumbent Thumb Pressure

Objective

Relax the thoracic paravertebral muscles.

Position

Lateral recumbent, treatment side down (Fig. 54.8).

Procedure

1. Stand at the side of the table, facing the patient.
2. Reach across the back of the patient until your thumbs are contacting the paravertebral tissues just lateral to the far side of the spinous processes.
3. Exert pressure with your thumbs toward the center of the body and down toward the table.
4. You may use an intermittent kneading or sustained inhibitory pressure.
5. Repeat as many times as necessary to achieve the desired effect.

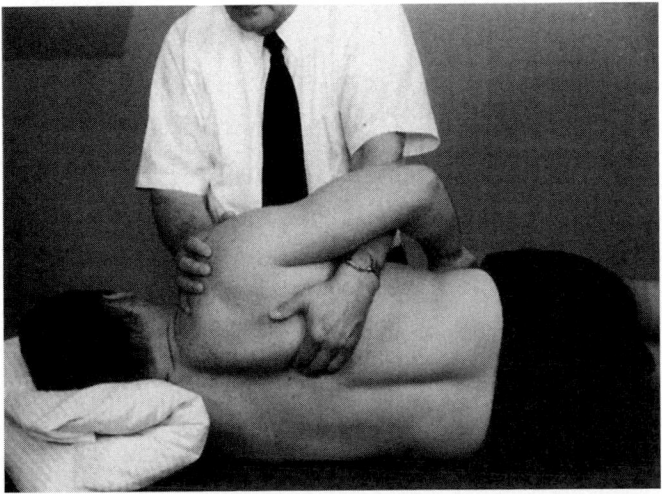

FIGURE 54.7. Lateral recumbent position for upper thoracic technique.

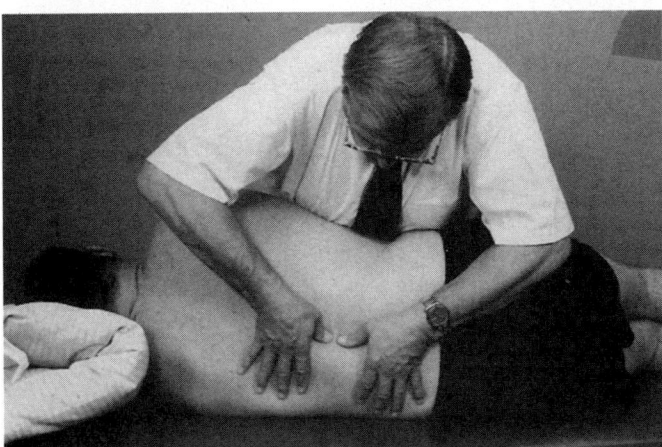

FIGURE 54.8. Lateral recumbent thumb pressure for thoracic technique.

Side Leverage

Objective

Relax thoracic paravertebral muscles.

Position

Lateral recumbent, treatment side down (Fig. 54.9).

Procedure

1. Sit at the side of the table, facing the patient.
2. Position your caudad arm so that the patient's shoulder is in your axilla, with your thumb medial to the paravertebral muscles on the far side of the spine.
3. Lift the patient's head away from the table, introducing a cervical and upper thoracic side-bending force.
4. Simultaneously, your caudad thumb exerts a downward pressure on the upper thoracic paravertebral musculature. This may be applied as a combination of intermittent traction and kneading or with a sustained inhibitory pressure.
5. Repeat as many times as necessary to achieve the desired effect.

Note: This technique can be converted to either a deep articulatory technique or an HVLA thrust with minimal repositioning of the physician's caudad hand.

Seated, Over/Under

Objective

Relax upper thoracic paravertebral muscles.

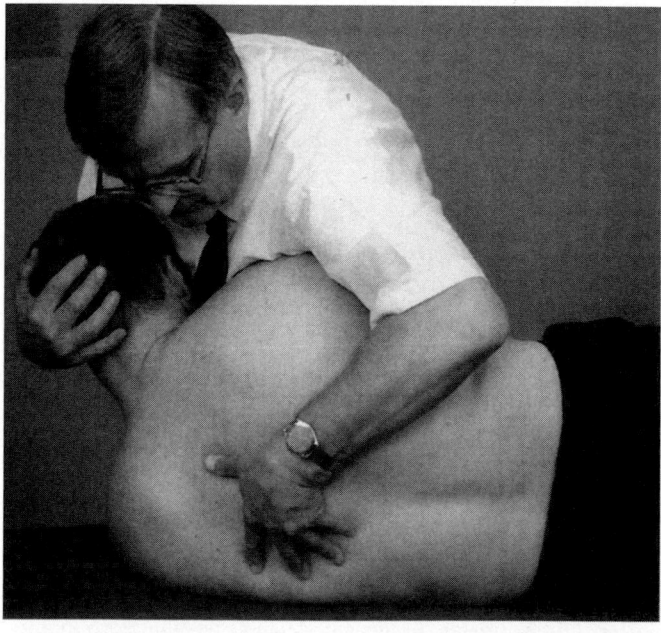

FIGURE 54.9. Side leverage for thoracic technique.

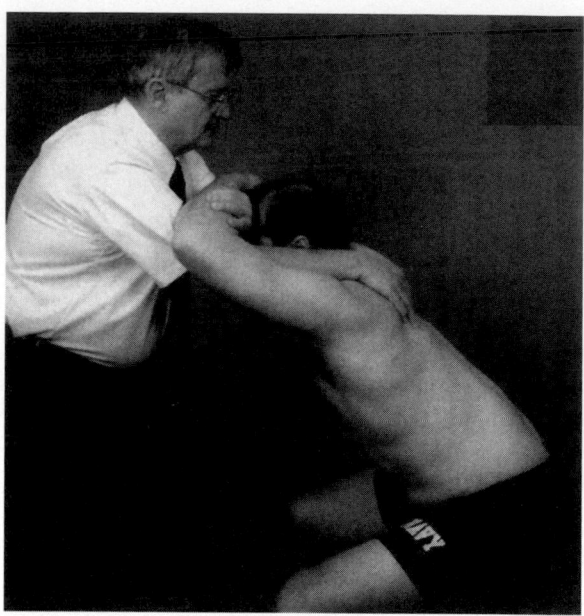

FIGURE 54.10. Seated position using over/under method for thoracic technique.

Position

Seated (Fig. 54.10).

Procedure

1. Stand facing the patient. Have the patient cross his or her arms, hooking the patient's thumbs in the antecubital fossae.
2. Reach under the patient's forearms and over his or her shoulders.
3. Contact the paravertebral tissues over the upper thoracic transverse processes with your fingerpads.
4. Lean back, drawing the patient toward you as you simultaneously exert an upward leverage on the forearms.
5. Exert a downward pressure into the soft tissues with the pads of your fingers; then draw them cephalad with a kneading motion.
6. Repeat as many times as necessary to achieve the desired effect.

Note: This technique may be converted to a deep articulatory technique by increasing the amount of inward pressure on the pads of the fingers, producing thoracic backward bending.

Supine Extension

Objective

Relax the thoracic paravertebral muscles.

Position

Supine (Fig. 54.11).

Procedure

1. Sit at the side of the table.

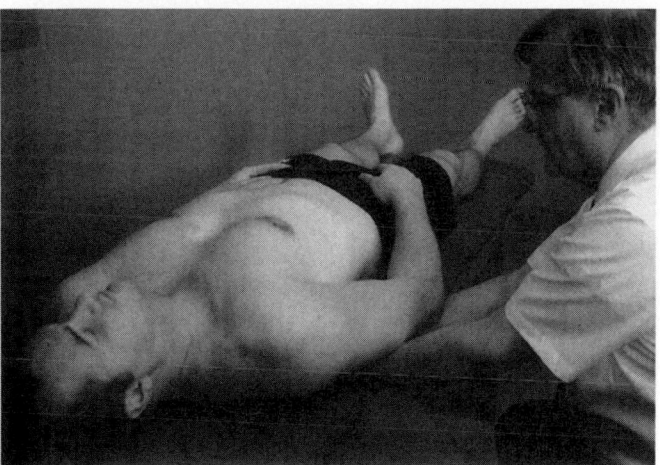

FIGURE 54.11. Thoracic extension in supine position.

2. Slide your hands under the patient until the pads of your fingers contact the paravertebral soft tissues on the near side.
3. By leaning down onto the elbows, you create a fulcrum, transmitting pressure upward into the paravertebral soft tissues.
4. Simultaneously draw your fingerpads toward you.
5. This may be performed in a kneading fashion or with deep inhibitory pressure.
6. Repeat as many times as necessary to achieve the desired effect.

Note: This technique is commonly used in the postoperative setting to prevent and/or treat postoperative paralytic ileus. In this setting, the technique has been referred to as rib raising.

Midthoracic Extension

Objective

Relax the midthoracic paravertebral muscles.

Position

Seated (Fig. 54.12).

Procedure

1. Stand behind the patient, and have the patient clasp their hands behind the neck.
2. Grasp the patient's arms under the elbows.
3. Place your other hand so that it is straddling the spine, with fingers pointed cephalad.
4. Elevate the patient's elbows, applying tractional force as you simultaneously press forward with the hand straddling the spine.
5. Repeat as many times as necessary to achieve the desired effect.

Note: This technique may be converted to a deep articulatory technique by varying the amount of anterior pressure applied through your posterior hand.

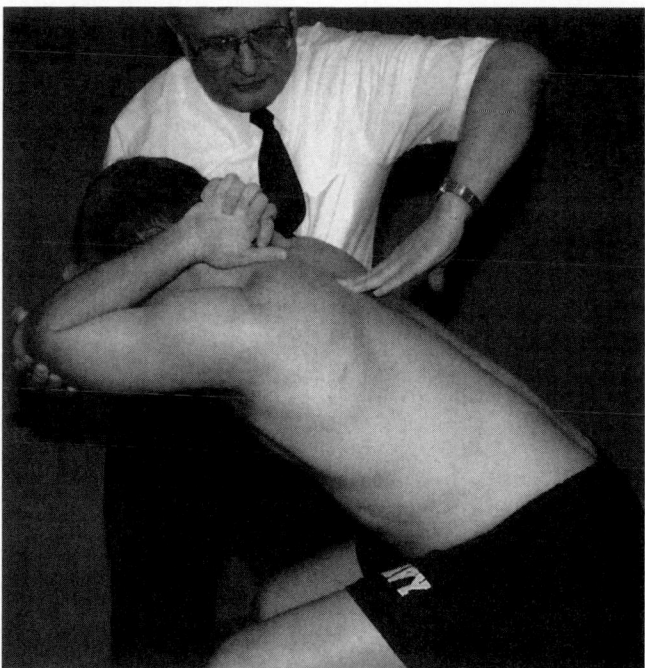

FIGURE 54.12. Seated position for midthoracic extension.

LUMBAR

Supine Flexion

Objective

Relax the lumbar paravertebral muscles.

Position

Supine.

Procedure

1. Stand at the side of the table.
2. Have the patient flex both hips, drawing the knees up toward the chest.
3. Grasp the patient's knees, further flexing the hips until the pelvis begins to follow, exerting a tractional force on the lumbar paravertebral muscles.
4. Continue the tractional stretch in an intermittent or continuous fashion.
5. Additional traction may be brought to bear on either side of the spine by adding side bending away from the side to be treated.
6. Repeat as many times as necessary to achieve the desired effect.

Supine Rotation with Counterleverage

Objective

Relax lumbar paravertebral muscles.

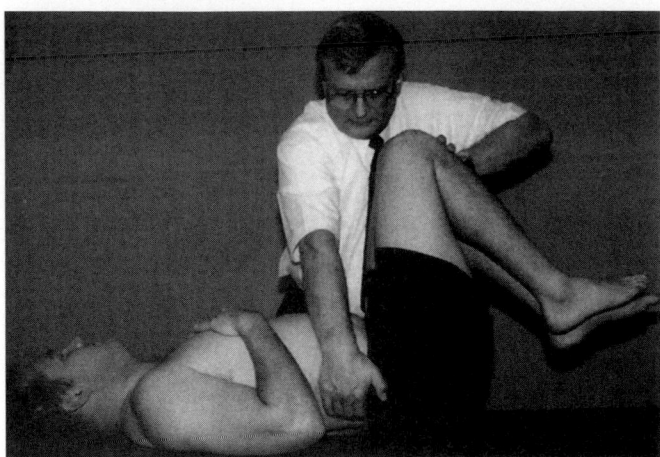

FIGURE 54.13. Supine rotation with counterleverage for lumbar technique.

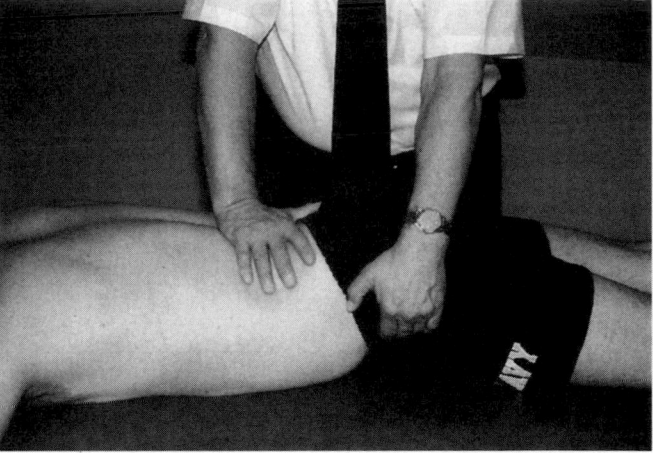

FIGURE 54.14. Prone pressure with counterleverage for lumbar technique.

Position

Supine (Fig. 54.13).

Procedure

1. Stand at the side of the table and have the patient flex the knees and hips.
2. Draw the patient's knees toward you with your caudad hand while the cephalad hand reaches under the lumbar region to grasp the paravertebral tissues with your fingerpads.
3. Pull your cephalad hand upward toward the ceiling.
4. Produce a rotational counterforce by simultaneously pushing the knees away from you.
5. Apply the technique in either a kneading manner or with deep inhibitory pressure.
6. Repeat as many times as necessary to achieve the desired effect.

Prone Pressure with Counterleverage

Objective

Relax lumbar paravertebral muscles.

Position

Prone (Fig. 54.14).

Procedure

1. Stand at the side of the table.
2. Contact the lumbar paravertebral musculature on the opposite side of the spine with the heel of your cephalad hand.
3. Grasp the anterior superior iliac spine with your caudad hand, pulling upward toward the ceiling.
4. Apply a simultaneous anterior and lateral force, stretching the lumbar paravertebral tissues like a bowstring.
5. Use either a kneading motion, or deep inhibitory pressure.
6. Repeat as many times as necessary to achieve the desired effect.

Prone Scissors Technique

Objective

Relax lumbar paravertebral muscles.

Position

Prone (Fig. 54.15).

Procedure

1. Stand at the side of the table.
2. Grasp the patient's opposite leg just above the knee with your caudad hand, lifting the leg far enough to cross it behind the nearer leg. Your hand is now between the patient's knees.
3. Contact the lumbar paravertebral muscles (on the far side) with the heel of your cephalad hand.
4. Apply an anterior and lateral pressure with the cephalad hand, while simultaneously increasing the amount of scissoring with the legs.
5. Use an intermittent kneading motion, or sustained inhibitory pressure.

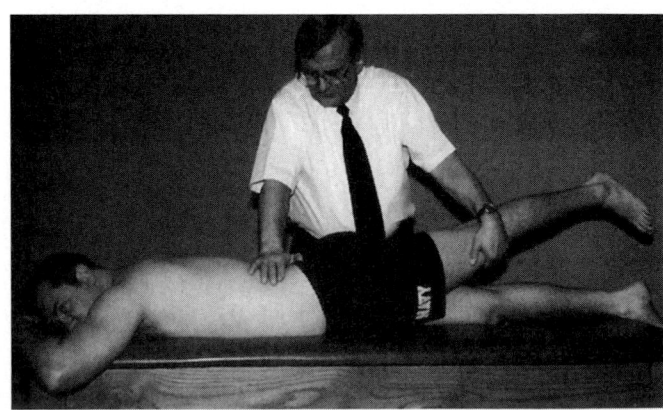

FIGURE 54.15. Prone scissors technique.

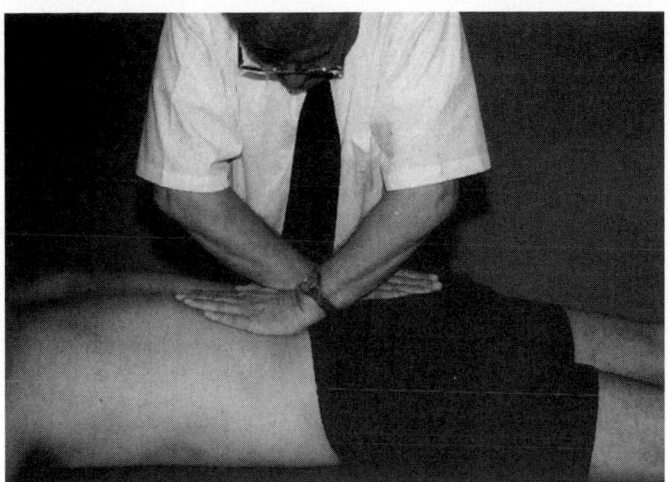

FIGURE 54.16. Prone traction technique.

6. Repeat as many times as necessary to achieve the desired effect.

Prone Traction

Objective

Relax lumbar paravertebral muscles.

Position

Prone (Fig. 54.16).

Procedure

1. Stand at the side of the table.
2. Place your cephalad hand over the base of the sacrum, with the fingers pointing toward the coccyx.
3. Place your other palm straddling the spinous processes of the lumbar vertebrae, with your fingers pointing cephalad.
4. Exert a separating tractional force in the directions in which the fingers point.
5. Use either intermittent traction or sustained inhibition.
6. The position of the caudad hand may be altered by placing it to one side of the spine, thus bringing more force to bear on the paravertebral soft tissues on that side.
7. Repeat as many times as necessary to achieve the desired effect.

Bilateral Thumb Pressure

Objective

Relax lumbar paravertebral muscles.

Position

Prone.

Procedure

1. Stand at the side of the table, near the patient's knees.
2. Place the thumbs of both hands on the paravertebral muscles overlying the transverse processes, with the fingers fanned out over the lateral abdominal muscles.
3. Apply bilateral pressure anteriorly and cephalad until the limits of tissue motion are reached.
4. Sweep your thumbs in a lateral direction.
5. Reposition your thumbs at a different lumbar segment.
6. Repeat steps 4 and 5 in a kneading fashion, as many times as necessary to achieve the desired effect.

Supine

Objective

Relax lumbar paravertebral muscles.

Position

Supine.

Procedure

1. Sit at the side of the table.
2. Reach under the lumbar region with both hands, contacting the ipsilateral paravertebral tissues overlying the transverse processes with the pads of your fingers.
3. Lean down into the elbows, producing an upward leverage at the wrists and hands, simultaneously drawing your hands toward you.
4. Use either a kneading motion or sustained inhibitory pressure.
5. Repeat as many times as necessary to achieve the desired effect.

Lateral Recumbent

Objective

Relax lumbar paravertebral muscles.

Position

Lateral recumbent, treatment side up (Fig. 54.17).

Procedure

1. Stand at the side of the table.
2. Have the patient flex their hips and knees; place your thigh against the infrapatellar region.
3. Reach over the back and grasp the paravertebral muscles of the lumbar region, drawing them toward you and away from the spine simultaneously.
4. Your thighs against the patient's knees may simply be used for bracing or they may also be simultaneously flexed to provide a combined bowstring and longitudinal traction force on the paravertebral musculature.
5. Use either a kneading motion or sustained inhibitory pressure.
6. Repeat as many times as necessary to achieve the desired effect.

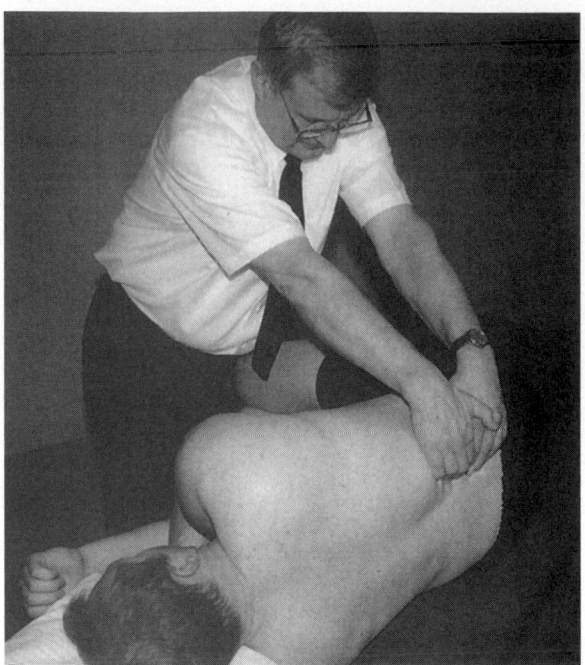

FIGURE 54.17. Lateral recumbent position for lumbar technique.

Seated

Objective

Relax lumbar paravertebral muscles.

Position

Seated (Fig. 54.18).

Procedure

1. Stand behind the patient, opposite the treatment side.

2. Have the patient place their hand on the side to be treated behind the neck. The opposite hand grasps the elbow of the first hand.

3. Reach under the near axilla, grasping the far arm just proximal to the elbow.

4. Place the heel of your posterior hand over the paravertebral tissues on the far side of the spine.

5. Have the patient allow their weight to drop forward onto your arm.

6. Rotate the patient toward you with your anterior hand.

7. Your posterior hand provides a lateral force on the lumbar paravertebral muscles, away from the spine.

8. Repeat as many times as necessary to achieve the desired effect.

Note: This technique may also be used for deep articulation. It is also readily converted to muscle energy and HVLA thrust techniques.

SACRUM

Sacral Rock

Objective

Relax the muscles at the lumbosacral junction.

Position

Prone (Fig. 54.19).

Procedure

1. Stand at the side of the patient's pelvis.

2. Place the heel of your cephalad hand on the sacral base, with your fingers pointing toward the coccyx.

3. Place your caudad hand on top of the first hand, with your fingers pointing in the opposite direction.

4. Exert a gentle pressure straight down toward the table.

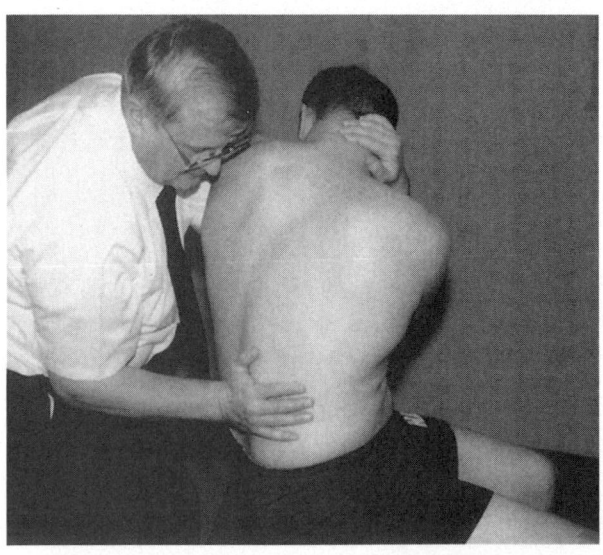

FIGURE 54.18. Seated position for lumbar technique.

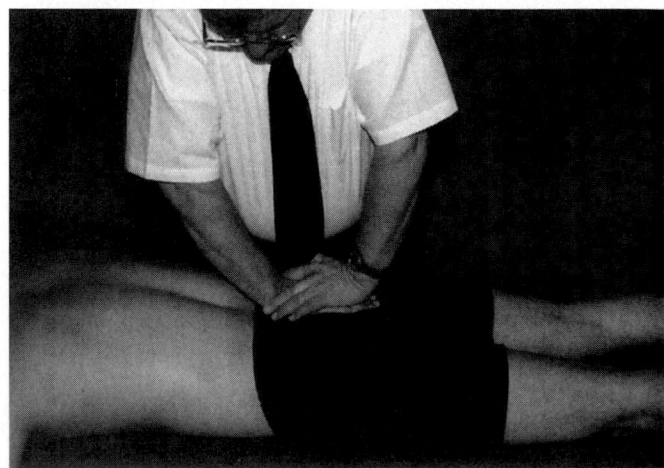

FIGURE 54.19. Prone position for sacral rock.

5. Alternate the direction of your pressure to synchronize it with and augment the natural motion accompanying respiration, rocking the sacrum into flexion and extension.
6. Repeat as many times as necessary to achieve the desired effect.

Note: This technique may be converted to a craniosacral technique by following the cranial rhythmic impulse rather than pulmonary respiration.

Sacral Inhibition

Objective

Inhibit sacral motion, altering parasympathetic nervous system balance.

Position

Prone.

Procedure

1. Stand at the side of the patient's pelvis.
2. Place the heel of your cephalad hand on the sacral base, with your fingers pointing toward the coccyx.
3. Place your caudad hand on top of your other hand, with fingers pointing in the opposite direction.
4. Direct deep pressure straight down toward the table.
5. Maintain this pressure (without rocking motion) for 30 seconds to 2 minutes.

Note: This technique may be converted to a craniosacral technique by following the cranial rhythmic impulse to a still point. This is sometimes referred to as a sacral CV4.

UPPER EXTREMITY

Pectoral Traction

Objective

Relax the anterior muscular attachments of the upper extremity.

Position

Supine (Fig. 54.20).

Procedure

1. Stand at the head of the table.
2. Hook the pads of your fingers into both anterior axillary folds.
3. Apply an anterior cephalad traction.
4. Have the patient inhale.
5. With inhalation, increase your cephalad and anterior traction, and maintain it as the patient exhales.
6. This cycle of inhalation/traction/resisted exhalation may be repeated until no further stretch of the pectoral muscles or

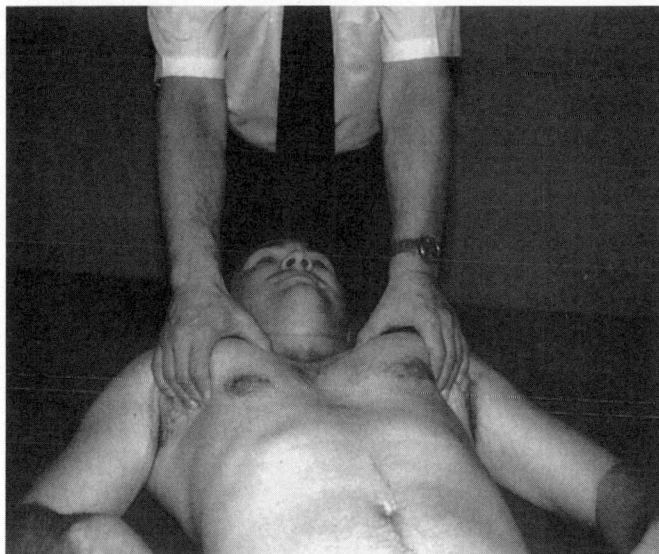

FIGURE 54.20. Upper extremity pectoral traction.

expansion of the rib cage is noted or until you achieve the desired effect.

Note: This technique is often applied following thoracic pump technique to relieve a patient's sense of chest compression. It may also be used as a lymphatic pump by increasing inhalation excursion of the upper seven ribs, thus increasing inhalation negative pressure.

Posterior Axillary Folds

Objective

Relax the posterior muscle attachments to the upper extremity.

Position

Supine, treatment arm palm down on abdomen (Fig. 54.21).

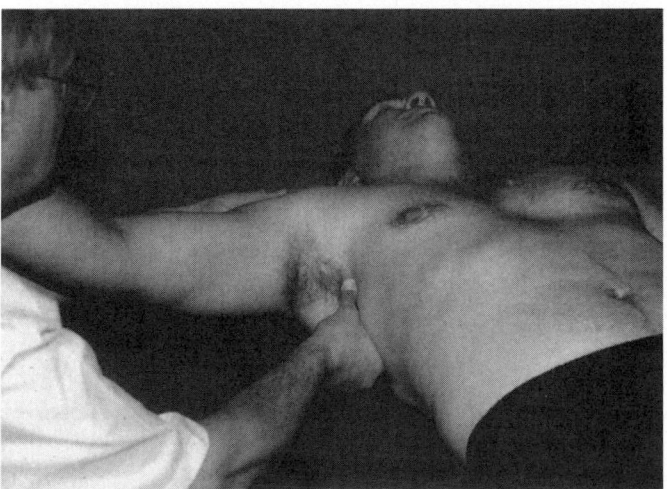

FIGURE 54.21. Upper extremity posterior axillary folds technique.

Procedure

1. Sit at the side of the table, facing the patient's head.
2. Using the hand closest to the patient, grasp the posterior axillary fold between your thumb and fingers.
3. Starting near the trunk, apply a milking motion, rolling along the fold toward the thorax.
4. Gradually, as the muscle softens, work your way away from the trunk, including more of the posterior axillary fold in the sequential rolling motion until the entire fold has been treated.

Note: A similar approach may be applied to the anterior axillary fold.

Interosseous Membrane of Forearm

Objective

Relax the interosseous membrane and soft tissues of the forearm.

Position

Seated.

Procedure

1. Stand facing your patient.
2. Grasp the hand of the arm to be treated, as if to shake hands.
3. Wrap your other hand over the top of the forearm.
4. Slowly induce pronation through the patient's hand.
5. Use your other hand to apply a gentle, opposing wringing motion to the soft tissues of the forearm, stretching and relaxing the muscles.
6. Apply similar treatment in the opposite direction, inducing supination to stretch and relax the muscles.
7. Repeat as many times as necessary to achieve the desired effect.

Rhomboids

Objective

Relax the rhomboid muscles.

Position

Lateral recumbent, treatment side up (Fig. 54.22).

Procedure

1. Stand at the side of the table, facing the patient.
2. Grasp the shoulder with your cephalad hand to control tension in the rhomboid and trapezius musculature.
3. Grasp the rhomboid muscles with your caudad hand, just medial to the vertebral border of the scapula.
4. Gently pull up toward the scapula, drawing the scapula slightly away from the ribs.

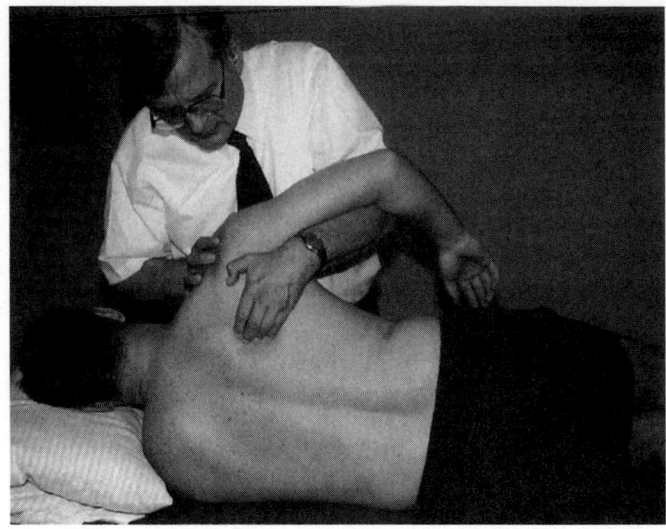

FIGURE 54.22. Upper extremity rhomboids technique.

5. Use either a kneading motion or sustained inhibitory pressure.
6. Repeat as many times as necessary to achieve the desired effect.

LOWER EXTREMITY

Fascia Lata (Method 1)

Objective

Relax the fascia lata.

Position

Prone (Fig. 54.23).

Procedure

1. Stand at the side of the patient, opposite the side to be treated.
2. With your caudad hand, grasp the leg to be treated just above the knee.

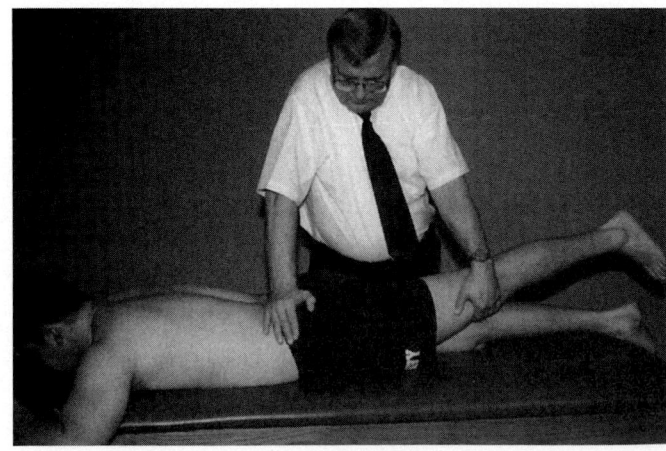

FIGURE 54.23. Lower extremity fascia lata technique.

3. Anchor the pelvis against the table with your cephalad hand.
4. Extend the hip of the leg being treated and adduct the hip across the midline until the desired tension is developed in the lateral soft tissues of the thigh.
5. Apply either intermittent or sustained traction as in a direct myofascial release technique.
6. Repeat as many times as necessary to achieve the desired effect.

Fascia Lata (Method 2)

Objective

Relax the lateral soft tissues of the thigh.

Position

Lateral recumbent, treatment side up (Fig. 54.24).

Procedure

1. Sit on the side of the table behind the patient's knees.
2. Place the thigh to be treated just in front of the other leg with the foot on the table, so that there is a downward slope to the thigh.
3. Apply pressure against the iliotibial band just caudad to the greater trochanter, using the flats of the middle phalanges of your closed fist.
4. Maintaining this inward pressure, drag your fist down the length of the iliotibial band to the level of the knee.
5. Repeat as many times as necessary to achieve the desired effect (i.e., stretch in the lateral fascial structures of the thigh).

Fascia Lata (Method 3)

Objective

Relax and stretch the iliotibial band.

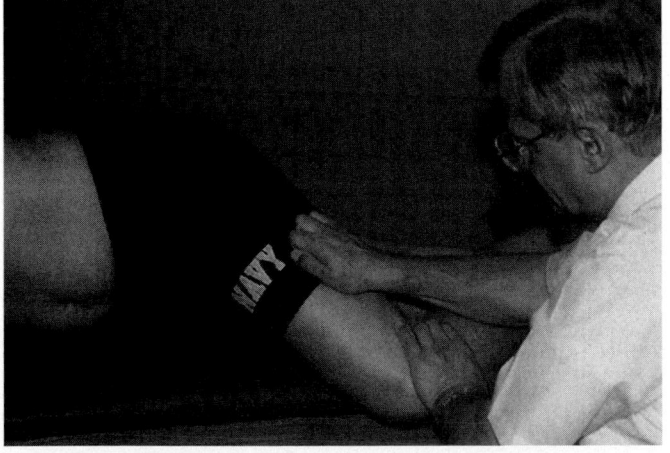

FIGURE 54.24. Lower extremity fascia lata technique.

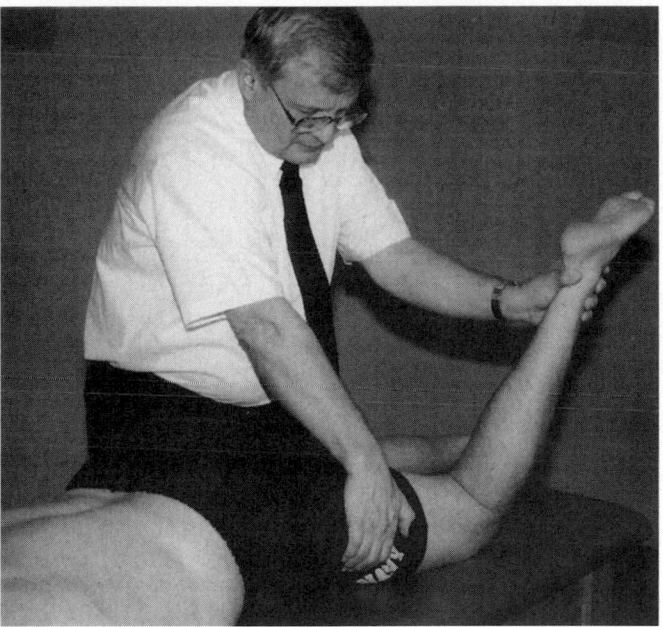

FIGURE 54.25. Lower extremity fascia lata technique.

Position

Prone (Fig. 54.25).

Procedure

1. Stand at the side of the table, opposite the thigh to be treated.
2. Flex the patient's knee to 90 degrees and grasp it with your caudad hand.
3. Use the pads of the fingers on your cephalad hand to hook the iliotibial band and pull upward toward yourself.
4. Simultaneously carry the foot of the same leg away from the midline, increasing the tension on the iliotibial band.
5. Continue with a kneading motion.
6. Repeat as many times as necessary to achieve the desired effect.

Piriformis

Objective

Relax the piriformis muscle.

Position

Prone (Fig. 54.26).

Procedure

1. Stand at the side of the table, opposite the muscle dysfunction.
2. Beginning near the sacrum, apply double thumb pressure into the piriformis muscle, rolling toward the trochanteric insertion. (The piriformis muscle may be accessed on a line beginning midway between the posterior superior iliac spine and the inferior lateral angle of the sacrum, extending to the posterosuperior pole of the greater trochanter.)

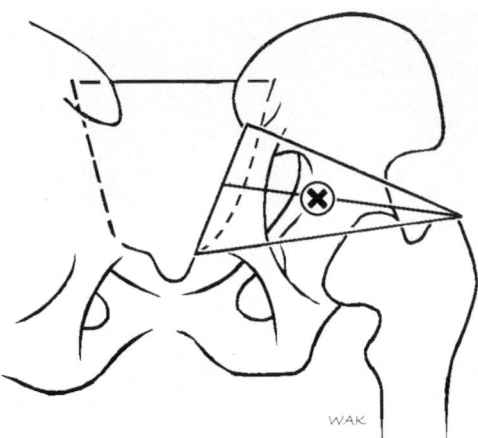

FIGURE 54.26. Location of piriformis tender point.

3. Move sequentially along the muscle toward the trochanter, taking care not to exert too much pressure directly over the sciatic nerve.
4. For heavier patients, you may use your elbow rather than double thumb pressure.
5. Use either a kneading motion or sustained inhibitory pressure.
6. Repeat as many times as necessary to achieve the desired effect.

Plantar Fascia

Objective

Relax and stretch the plantar fascia.

Position

Supine (Fig. 54.27).

Procedure

1. Sit at the foot of the table.

2. Use the proximal phalanges of your closed fist to contact the sole of the patient's foot just posterior to the metatarsal heads.
3. While applying pressure toward the dorsum of the foot, drag your fist over the plantar fascia toward the heel.
4. Repeat as many times as necessary (toes to heel) to achieve the desired effect.

Arch Springing

Objective

Relaxation of the muscles of the arch of the foot.

Position

Supine (Fig. 54.28).

Procedure

1. Sit at the foot of the table.
2. Grasp the foot with both hands, with your thumbs under the arch and fingers on the dorsum of the foot.
3. Move the middle of the foot toward supination, using your proximal hand, while simultaneously moving the forefoot toward pronation with your distal hand. (This wringing motion tends to stretch the fasciae of the foot toward a position of reestablishing the longitudinal arch of the foot.)
4. Repeat as a kneading type of motion, as many times as necessary to achieve the desired effect.

Note: This could also be considered a deep articulatory technique for the arch.

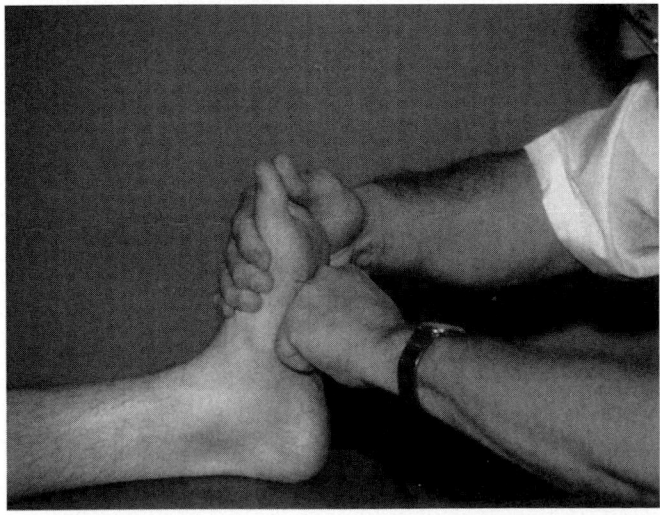

FIGURE 54.27. Lower extremity plantar fascia technique.

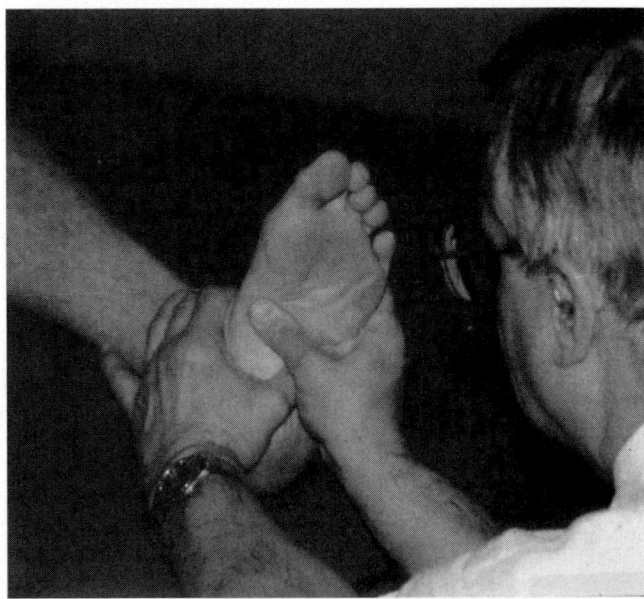

FIGURE 54.28. Lower extremity arch springing technique.

CONCLUSION

Soft tissue direct techniques address the muscular and fascial structures of the body and associated neural and vascular elements. They can relax and stretch structures and muscles, enhance circulation and nutrition, improve reflex activity and immune response, identify areas of change or dysfunction, and provide a state of relaxation and tonic stimulation.

SUGGESTED READINGS

Nicholas NS. *Atlas of Osteopathic Techniques*. Philadelphia, PA: Philadelphia College of Osteopathic Medicine; 1981.

Rubinstein S, Eimerbrink JH, Heilig D, Pratt W. *Osteopathic Techniques*. Philadelphia, PA: Osteopathic Publications; 1949.

Zink JG. Holistic approach to homeostasis. In: Barnes MW, ed. *American Academy of Osteopathy Yearbook*. Indianapolis, IN: American Academy of Osteopathy; 1973.

ARTICULATORY TECHNIQUES

DAVID A. PATRIQUIN
JOHN M. JONES, III

KEY CONCEPTS

- Design of articulatory, or springing, technique
- Uses of and additions to articulatory activation
- Diagnostic findings suggesting use of articulating technique
- Special cases suitable for application of technique
- Contraindications
- General instructions of design of technique
- Rib raising and Spencer techniques
- Specific articulatory techniques by region, including cervical, cervicothoracic, thoracic, costal, lumbar, pelvic, and the extremities

Articulatory technique, also called springing technique, is a direct technique. The physician gently and repetitively forces the part of the body being treated against the restrictive barrier (generally maintained by tight muscles and connective tissues acting as restrainers), with the intent of reducing the resistance or changing the position of that barrier and improving physiologic motion. This form of osteopathic treatment is also called low-velocity/moderate- to high-amplitude, or long-lever, technique. Rib raising with the patient supine, or the Spencer series of techniques for articulating all ranges of motion of the dysfunctional shoulder are examples of this type of technique.

DESIGN AND USE OF ARTICULATING TECHNIQUE

Articulating activation can help resolve a simple problem with a single restrictive barrier or a complex problem with multiple joint and tissue restrictive barriers. This type of technique is particularly useful where the application of slow, gentle, controlled movements is a requirement. Postoperative patients and older patients suffering from arthritis or osteopenia find this type of direct treatment more acceptable than more vigorous ones.

Respiratory cooperation (inhalation to accentuate tissue tension or exhalation to relax tissue tension further) and active muscle contraction or relaxation are frequently added. These addi-

tions enhance the effect of passive articulating motion by resisting it or permitting increased range of motion. The standard technique is modified to increase the range of motion while limiting the amount of discomfort induced by the procedure.

As an example, a direct articulating treatment can be applied to a vertebral unit restricted in right rotation. The physician makes repeated attempts to increase right rotation of the vertebra by slowly, gently encouraging the affected vertebra into right rotation against the restrictive motion barrier. The physician increases the force or induces a wider range of motion on each cycle. Finally, once the barrier to motion is firmly engaged, the patient is instructed to take as deep a breath as comfortable. The positive increased intrinsic force generated by this action markedly augments the stretching, mobilizing forces applied by the physician. The added intrinsic force opposes those forces the physician has already induced. The combination of operator and intrinsic forces results in more tension in soft tissues and produces greater stretching and lengthening in them than would result from physician force alone.

The repetitive application of gentle force may be directed to the reduction of one barrier at a time, in successive steps, or the physician may engage two or more barriers with one movement. The principles of technique design apply in the case of motion restriction in multiple planes, but the actual directions and forces used may be so complex as to defy accurate description in a text. There are many possible combinations of vectors of motion and sequences during one treatment when applying this type of manipulation to multiple-plane restrictions. The simple, passive physician efforts strongly reinforce the addition of intrinsic forces, such as respiratory cooperation or isometric muscle energy activity.

COMMON QUESTIONS
Diagnosis

What diagnostic findings suggest the therapeutic use of articulating technique? The cardinal clinical indicator for applying an articulating technique is limited or lost articular motion. The most common cause for this loss of articular motion is a dysfunction in the local (periarticular) supporting tissues or in the longer muscles or ligaments associated with the articulation. There are also secondary indicators for the application of an articulatory technique. These include a need to increase the frequency or amplitude of motion in a body region. An example of this is the need to increase the frequency and amplitude of motion in the chest of a person with respiratory disease. Accomplish this by applying thoracic lymphatic pump treatment. Expect increased amplitude and efficiency of chest motion to follow this treatment.

Special Cases

Are there special cases most suitable for the application of articulating technique? Very young and very old patients respond well to this type of treatment. They also suffer less reaction in terms of discomfort and post-treatment stiffness than if a high-velocity/low-amplitude technique is employed. Articulating technique permits accurate dosage of force and duration of treatment. It also permits careful and accurate localization of forces. The amount and direction of force can be altered during the course of treatment because movements are slow, deliberate, repeated, and constantly monitored by palpation through the physician's hands. Because the treatment is applied slowly and patient response is sensed, adjustments can be made immediately.

Contraindications

Are there contraindications to the use of articulating technique? There are general cautions that apply to the use of any manual procedure in the treatment of a patient (see Chapter 74, Efficacy and Complications). Because articulating technique consists of repetitive applications of force, it can be quickly modified between applications of force in response to the reaction of the patient. For example, in treating the upper cervical region, it is wise to avoid simultaneous hyperrotation and extension. Repeated application of force to the upper cervical area positioned in extension and hyperrotation may damage the vertebral arteries. It is also not appropriate to use forceful, repetitive motion on an acutely inflamed joint, especially one where the cause of inflammation may be infection or reaction to a fracture.

Instructions For Design

What are the general instructions for the design of an articulating technique?

Patient Position

Use any comfortable position that permits the problem area to be passively moved completely through all ranges of motion.

Physician Position

Use a comfortable position that permits the application of passive motion through the complete range of motion of the affected articulation.

Procedure

Move the affected joint to the limit of all ranges of motion. As the restrictive barrier is reached, slowly and firmly continue to apply gentle force against it to the limit of tissue motion or the patient's tolerance to pain or fatigue. Then return the articulation slowly toward the neutral portion of its motion. Repeat this process several times, each time gaining range and improved quality of motion. Cease repetition of motion when no further response is achieved.

Enhancement

Intrinsic forces, such as respiratory assistance or a muscle energy technique may be added once maximum range of motion has been achieved by positioning alone. Similar modifications can measurably increase motion range and quality.

SAMPLE CLINICAL APPLICATION
Rib Raising
Diagnosis and Findings

A patient has viral pneumonia with a resistant or noncompliant chest wall in which the motion of all ribs is reduced in both inspiration and expiration. There is paraspinal soft tissue tenderness to light pressure, with decreased rib motion and accompanying increased soft tissue tightness (tension/tone) throughout the posterior thorax, especially at the level of the upper five thoracic vertebrae and ribs.

Patient Position

Supine, with the thorax and head slightly elevated as necessary for patient comfort.

Procedure

1. Stand at the head of the treating table facing the patient.
2. Reach under the patient's back, extending the forearms and hands palms upward, so that the finger tips can, on flexion, engage paired upper ribs near their angles on each side of the midline. This is a bilateral treatment technique.
3. Gently pull cephalad. This attempts to mobilize the costotransverse and costovertebral articulations and stretch the intercostal and more superficial thoracic tissues.
4. Hold, then slowly release.
5. Rib raising (articulatory) technique is markedly augmented with patient inspiration after full cephalad tension is applied to the ribs.
6. When repetition of this treatment no longer produces increased range of motion at this level, move your hands to the next inferior group of ribs and repeat the articulating treatment process. Treat groups of two to four ribs progressively, from above downward, until all ribs on both sides are moving freely.
7. Then move to the side of the table, beside the patient's hips, and face the head of the table.
8. Extend your forearms and hands palms up, placing them under the upper thorax of the patient, with your finger tips

engaging the superior surface of the upper ribs at their angles. (This is a unilateral rib articulating procedure.)

9. Pull caudally, attempting to move the ribs inferiorly in relation to other thoracic structures.

10. Repeat the process until there is no increase in motion. Treat successive lower groups of ribs in the same fashion.

11. Rib raising (articulatory) technique is markedly augmented in this phase of treatment by the addition of a deep inhalation by the patient after full caudad tension is applied to the ribs.

Alternate Technique

Patient Position

Supine.

Procedure

1. Stand facing the foot of the treatment table at the level of the patient's shoulder on the side of the rib cage to be treated.

2. Hold the patient's forearm between your arm and chest while grasping the patient's midarm with your hand.

3. Place your other arm obliquely downward under the patient's rib cage. Flex your fingers so that the fingertips engage the caudad edges of the angles of the upper ribs.

4. Pull cephalad on the rib angles with your fingers, reinforced by an augmenting pull on the patient's arm (generated by a cephalad sway of your entire upper body).

5. Hold the tension for approximately 3 to 5 seconds before releasing. After a few seconds of rest, repeat the process, hold 3 to 5 seconds, and release.

6. Repeat this cycle until increased motion results or patient fatigue or discomfort suggests termination of the treatment.

7. When repetition of this treatment no longer produces increased range of motion at this level, move your hands to the next inferior group of ribs and repeat the articulating treatment process. Treat groups of two to four ribs progressively, from above downward, until all ribs on both sides are moving freely.

This technique may be modified by adding the patient's inspiration to produce more tension and therefore induce increased range of motion. Direct the patient to take a deep breath after you have generated maximum tension. Instruct the patient to exhale and relax as the tensions diminish. Then release the passive external traction.

Note that the above techniques may be modified by starting on the lower ribs and progressing cephalad, rather than starting on the upper ribs and progressing downward. In this case, traction is in the caudad direction. Exhalation might enhance this procedure.

SHOULDER TREATMENT: SPENCER TECHNIQUE

This is a classic clinical application of stepwise articulating technique. Seven different but related articulating procedures are car-

ried out in sequence in this treatment. Separate ranges of motion are consecutively engaged, beginning with those least likely to be disturbed (flexion/extension) and progressing to those most commonly restricted (internal/external rotation). It is easy to perform an articulatory technique to increase one or more ranges of shoulder joint motion, using the arm as a long lever against a shoulder girdle fixed to the patient's thorax by the other hand of the physician. Each step of the treatment may be enhanced by the addition of muscle energy activation and/or respiratory force after the barrier has been engaged.

For example, once the lateral traction, stretching, and fluid pumping of the initiating stage of Spencer have been completed, carry the patient's arm, flexed at the elbow, slowly but firmly into extension against the resistance of a fixed scapula and clavicle. After release of the tension, repeat the process until no increase in motion results from application of this phase of the treatment.

ARTICULATORY TECHNIQUES BY REGION

Reminders

1. An articulatory technique may be used to increase motion generally in all joints in that region, or it may be used more specifically at a particular joint by repetitively engaging a specific motion restriction. Most of the force is applied at the end-range of motion.

2. Articulatory techniques use passive, smooth, rhythmic motions designed to stretch contracted muscles, ligaments, and capsules—and, to a lesser extent, move fluids.

3. Articulatory techniques decrease tissue tension, enhance lymphatic flow, and stimulate increased joint circulation. We do not know the effects in the associated autonomic and central nervous system components.

4. Articulatory techniques are especially useful in treating spinal transitional zones (e.g., cervicothoracic, thoracolumbar, and lumbosacral areas).

5. Articulatory techniques may be used to pave the way for high-velocity/low-amplitude (HVLA) treatment.

6. Discomfort during treatment is usually expected. As a rule, pain is not acceptable, except, for example, during the treatment of "frozen shoulder" using the Spencer techniques when discomfort is expected but limited to patient tolerance.

7. Although the treatment is directed to a restriction on one side, some physicians prefer to apply these treatments bilaterally, so as not to induce an imbalance in the tonicity of the musculature or cause nervous system dysfunction/imbalance.

Indications

1. Restriction of joint motion.

2. Myofascial shortening (primary or secondary).

3. Bilateral or unilateral somatic dysfunction in a region or at a segmental level.

4. Preparation for HVLA-specific thrust.

Contraindications (Relative)

1. Advanced bone-wasting diseases.
2. Fractures.
3. Acute local inflammatory condition.
4. Acute localized infection.
5. Neurologic signs elicited during pretest or treatment means that you must stop treatment by this method and reevaluate the patient.

CERVICAL TECHNIQUES

Flexion

Diagnosis

Reduced cervical flexion.

Objective

Increase cervical flexion.

Patient Position

Supine.

Procedure

1. Sit above the head of the patient (Fig. 55.1).
2. Place one hand on the patient's shoulder.
3. Place the other hand cradling the occipital region.
4. Lift the head until full flexion is obtained.
5. Hold in full flexion for 3 to 5 seconds or until no further response is palpated or observed; then return toward neutral.

6. Repeat slowly in a smooth, rhythmic fashion until there is improved motion (or to the tolerance of the patient).

Alternative Procedure

1. Cross both forearms and place your hands on the patient's shoulders to support the head.
2. Raise your arms to flex the head and neck.

Extension

Diagnosis

Decreased cervical extension.

Objective

Increase cervical extension.

Patient Position

Supine. Caution: Do not perform this technique on a patient with neurologic signs on cervical extension or a patient who reports symptoms of vertebrobasilar insufficiency.

Procedure

1. Sit above the head of the patient (Fig. 55.2).
2. Place one hand under the patient's neck.
3. Use your thumb and forefinger as a fulcrum by pressing them against the posterior aspects of a cervical vertebra.
4. Grasp the patient's chin with your other hand and lift it to extend the neck. In patients with temporomandibular joint (TMJ) dysfunction, grasp the patient's forehead instead.
5. Using smooth, rhythmic motion, repeat several times.
6. Shift your fulcrum to another vertebra and repeat until you have treated all of the cervical vertebrae.

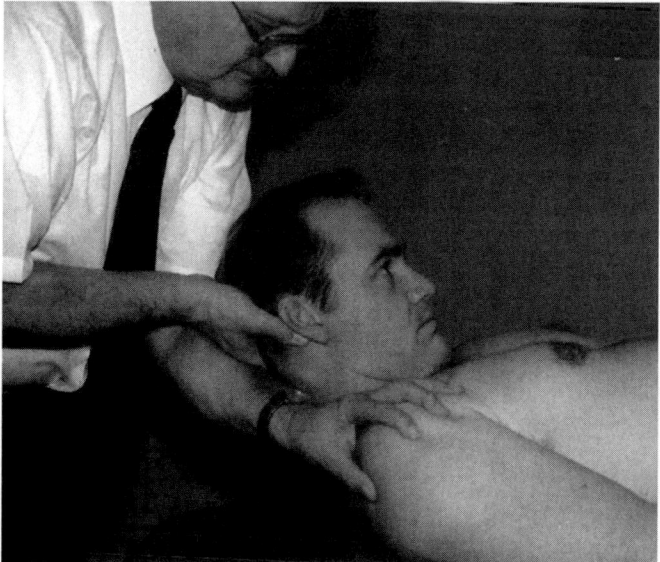

FIGURE 55.1. Cervical flexion technique.

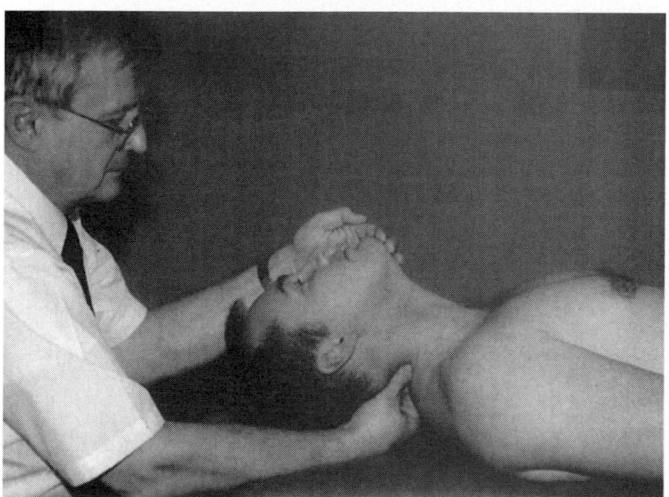

FIGURE 55.2. Cervical extension technique.

Rotation

Diagnosis

Decreased cervical rotation.

Objective

Increase cervical rotation.

Patient Position

Supine. Caution: Do not perform this technique on a patient who demonstrates neurologic signs on cervical rotation or a patient who reports symptoms of vertebrobasilar insufficiency.

Procedure

1. Sit above the head of the patient.
2. Grasp the patient's chin with your hand, with your forearm contacting the patient's zygoma.
3. Cup the patient's occiput with your other hand.
4. Rotate the head toward the side of decreased motion.
5. Hold, then return toward neutral.
6. Repeat slowly in a smooth, rhythmic fashion until there is improved motion (or to the tolerance of the patient).

Alternative Procedure

1. You may rotate one direction, go through neutral, and rotate the other direction if you are treating a patient with bilateral decrease due to myofascial shortening. (This may require change in hand position.)
2. You may also do this rotation procedure with the patient in flexion.
3. *DO NOT DO IT IN EXTENSION!*

Regional Side-Bending

Diagnosis

Decreased cervical side-bending (lateral flexion).

Objective

Increase cervical side-bending.

Patient Position

Supine.

Procedure

1. Sit above the head of the patient (Fig. 55.3).
2. Place one hand on the shoulder opposite the side of restricted side-bending, using the other hand to cradle the occipital region.

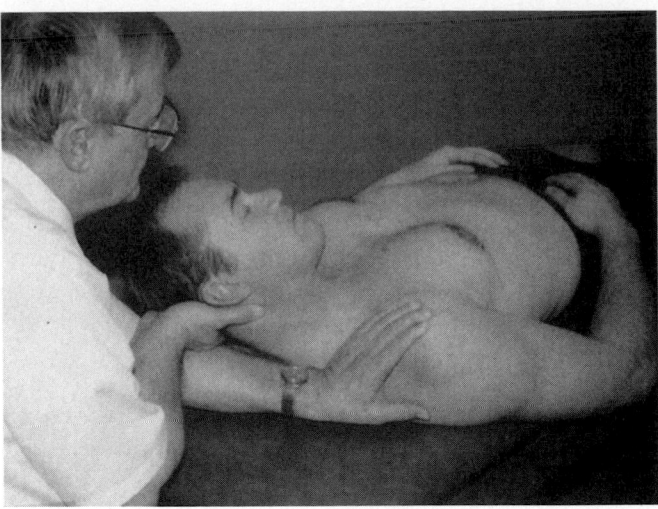

FIGURE 55.3. Cervical regional side-bending technique.

3. Firmly side bend the neck away from the restriction. You may reinforce this lateral movement by gently leaning against the head (with your abdomen). Do not use inferior vertical pressure on the vertex, especially if the patient has any signs of nerve root compression.
4. Hold, then return toward neutral.
5. Repeat slowly in a smooth, rhythmic fashion until there is improved motion (or to the tolerance of the patient).

Segmental Side-Bending Restriction

Procedure

1. Place the medial aspect of your middle phalanx or the pad of your distal phalanx against a specific joint level as a fulcrum. This should be done on the side opposite the restriction.
2. Grasp the posterior aspect of the head with the palm and fingers of your opposite hand.
3. Use lateral translation to induce side-bending toward the restriction with your localized digit. At the same time, use lateral translation of the head in the opposite direction, achieving side-bending around the fulcrum.
4. Hold, then return toward neutral.
5. Repeat slowly in a smooth, rhythmic fashion until there is improved motion (or to the tolerance of the patient).

CERVICOTHORACIC TECHNIQUE

Flexion, Extension, Side-Bending

Diagnosis

Decreased regional flexion, extension, side-bending (lateral flexion), or rotation.

Objective

Introduce motion where it has been inappropriately restricted.

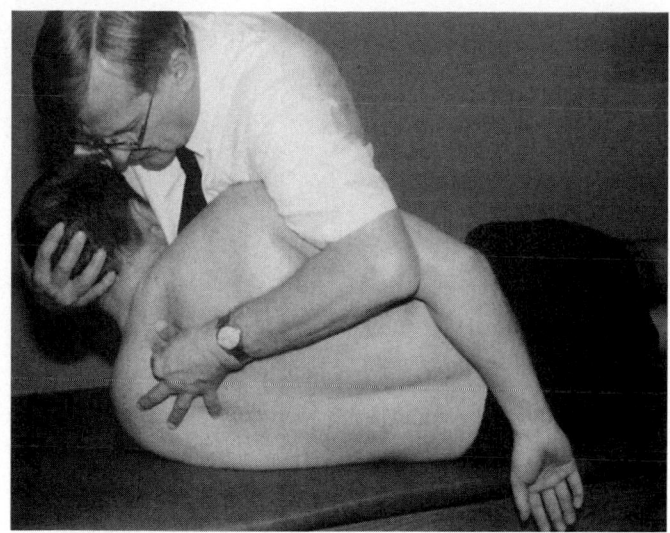

FIGURE 55.4. Cervicothoracic side-bending technique.

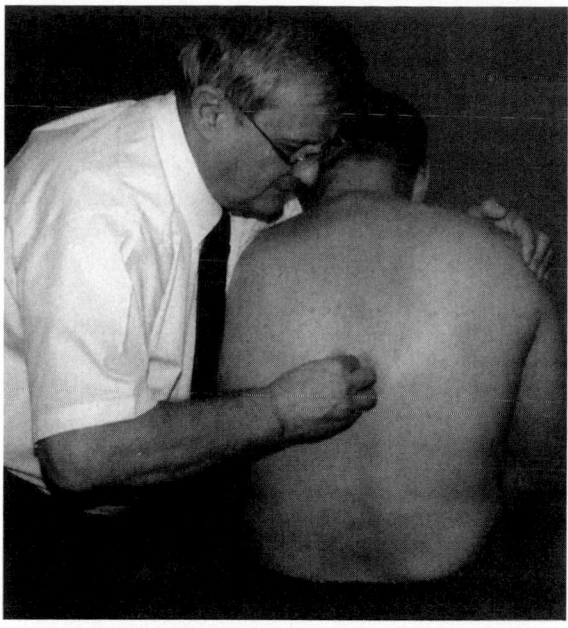

FIGURE 55.5. Thoracic flexion technique.

Patient Position

Lateral recumbent (restricted side up).

Procedure

1. Stand in front of the patient (Fig. 55.4).
2. Support the patient's head and neck with your hand and forearm. The patient's arm nearest the table should be flexed at the shoulder and elbow while the opposite arm is adducted on the lateral thorax and hip area.
3. Grasp the spinous process of T1 with your caudal hand to stabilize it against forces applied from above.
4. Use your other hand to extend, side-bend, or rotate the head and neck to the restriction of motion at the joint level you are treating.
5. Hold, then return toward neutral.
6. Repeat slowly in a smooth, rhythmic fashion until there is improved motion (or to the tolerance of the patient).
7. Move sequentially to the next inferior joint and repeat the process.

THORACIC TECHNIQUES

Flexion

Diagnosis

Decreased flexion.

Objective

Increase thoracic flexion.

Patient Position

Seated.

Procedure

1. Stand behind the patient (Fig. 55.5).
2. Put your arm over the patient's shoulder across his or her chest and place your hand on the patient's opposite shoulder. The patient hooks his or her hands over your arm.
3. Stabilize the lower of the two vertebrae being treated by grasping and fixing the spinous process with your fingers and thumb.
4. Use your other arm to flex the upper thorax of the patient to the level of your stabilizing hand, achieving maximal flexion stretch at the joint space above.
5. Hold, then return toward neutral.
6. Repeat slowly in a smooth, rhythmic fashion until there is improved motion (or to the tolerance of the patient).
7. Move your stabilizing hand to the next inferior vertebra and repeat the process until you have treated all the involved segments.

Extension

Diagnosis

Decreased thoracic extension.

Objective

Increase thoracic extension.

Patient Position

Seated.

Procedure

1. Stand behind the patient.
2. Put your arm over the patient's shoulder across his or her chest and place your hand on the patient's opposite shoulder. The patient hooks his or her hands over your arm.
3. Stabilize the lower of two vertebrae with the thenar eminence of your other hand or by grasping and fixating the spinous process with your fingers and thumb. You also use this hand as a fulcrum.
4. Introduce extension by anterior translation of your stabilizing hand as your other arm bends the upper thorax backward around the fulcrum, achieving maximal extension stretch at the joint space above.
5. Hold, then return toward neutral.
6. Repeat slowly in a smooth, rhythmic fashion until there is improved motion (or to the tolerance of the patient).
7. Move your stabilizing hand to the next inferior vertebra and repeat the process until you have treated all the involved segments.

Note: This technique is contraindicated in a patient with facet arthritis, because increased pressure exerted on the facets by the use of extension can aggravate that problem.

Rotation

Diagnosis

Decreased thoracic rotation.

Objective

Increase thoracic rotation.

Patient Position

Seated.

Procedure

1. Stand to the right, slightly behind the patient. Place your right arm across the front of the patient's thorax, grasping the interior left shoulder (Fig. 55.6).
2. Place your thumb and fingers on both sides of the spinous processes to stabilize the vertebra below the restricted segment.
3. Use your hand on the shoulder to induce rotation to the right, to the point that you feel the rotation at the joint space above your stabilizing hand.
4. Hold, then return toward neutral.
5. Repeat slowly in a smooth, rhythmic fashion until there is improved motion (or to the tolerance of the patient).
6. Move your stabilizing fingers to the next inferior vertebra and repeat the process until you have treated all the segments desired.

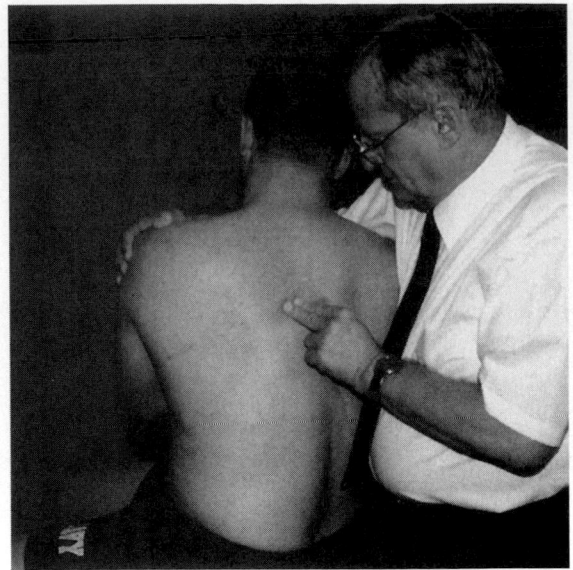

FIGURE 55.6. Thoracic rotation technique.

Side-Bending

Diagnosis

Decreased thoracic side-bending.

Objective

Increase thoracic side-bending.

Patient Position

Seated.

Procedure

1. Stand to the right, behind the patient, who is seated with arms folded across his or her chest.
2. Pass your right arm over the patient's right shoulder and across the chest. Put your hand into the left axilla, palm against the thoracic wall.
3. Apply a stabilizing pressure with your index and long fingers and thumb on the sides of the spinous process at the vertebra below the segment you wish to treat. An alternative is to use the thenar eminence placed against the side of the spinous process as a fulcrum.
4. Introduce right side-bending by applying a downward pressure through your axilla on the patient's right shoulder and an upward lift of the patient's left shoulder with your right hand. This forms a convexity on the left, side-bending the spine to the right. You should feel maximal stretch at the joint space above your stabilizing hand (fulcrum).
5. Hold, then return toward neutral.
6. Repeat slowly in a smooth, rhythmic fashion until there is improved motion (or to the tolerance of the patient).
7. Move your stabilizing hand to the next inferior vertebra and

repeat the process until you have treated all the involved segments.

COSTAL ARTICULATORY TECHNIQUES

Reminder: For a patient who has difficulty breathing, whether because of chronic obstructive pulmonary disease or any other reason, you may need to adjust the timing of these techniques to minimize interference with the already limited breathing cycle. It is generally best to treat the ribs on both sides, even if restriction is most apparent on one side.

Anterior Approach

Diagnosis

Decreased costal motion during the breathing cycle.

Objective

Enhance or optimize costal motion.

Patient Position

Supine.

Procedure

1. Stand on the restricted (right, in this example) side of the supine patient (Fig. 55.7). Grasp his or her right wrist with your cephalad (left) hand. Stretch the patient's arm upward to the point where it is fully extended at the elbow and flexed at the shoulder superior to the head.

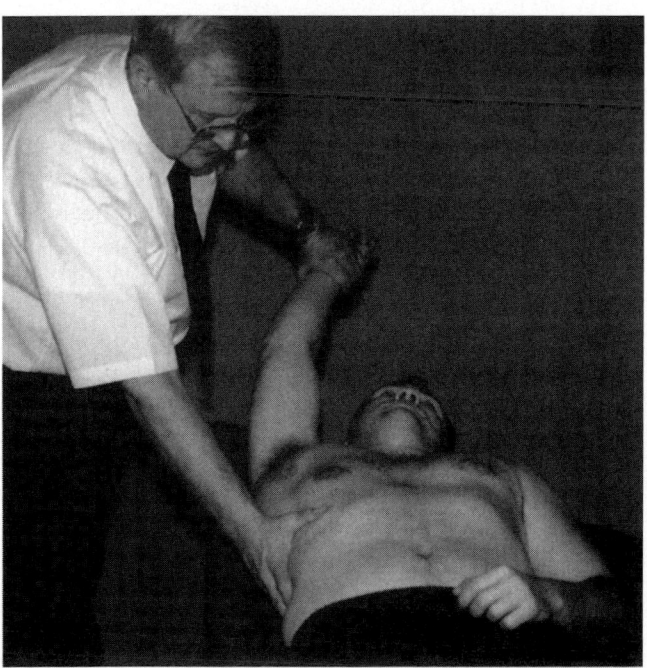

FIGURE 55.7. Costal technique, anterior approach.

2. Stabilize the anterior right ribs with your caudad (right) hand. Use the hypothenar eminence and little finger, the thumb and thenar eminence, or group the fingertips in a row along the superior border to stabilize the lower of the two ribs being treated.
3. Use the patient's right arm to stretch soft tissues in the intercostal space superior to your stabilizing hand. Have the patient breathe in deeply, synchronizing your stretch with full inspiration.
4. Hold, then return toward neutral.
5. Repeat slowly in a smooth, rhythmic fashion until there is improved motion (or to the tolerance of the patient).
6. Move your stabilizing hand to the next superior costal border and repeat the process until you have treated all the ribs desired.

Posterior Approach

Diagnosis

Decreased costal motion during the breathing cycle.

Objective

Enhance or optimize costal respiratory motion.

Patient Position

Prone.

Procedure

1. The patient lies prone with head facing to the left (Fig. 55.8). Stand to the left at the head of the table and use your right hand to grasp the patient's left arm just proximal to the elbow, stretching the arm into full abduction with a slight posterior angle and external rotation.
2. Stabilize the inferior of the two ribs being treated with your left thumb and thenar eminence at the superior border of the lower rib near the angle.
3. Achieve a stretch of the latissimus dorsi and the intercostal muscles by using the arm as a long lever (with abduction/extension) at the same time that you stabilize the inferior rib.
4. Hold, then return toward neutral.
5. Repeat slowly in a smooth, rhythmic fashion until there is improved motion (or to the tolerance of the patient).
6. Move your stabilizing hand to the next superior rib and repeat the process until you have treated all the restricted (or involved) ribs.

Lateral Recumbent

Diagnosis

Decreased bucket-handle excursion during the breathing cycle.

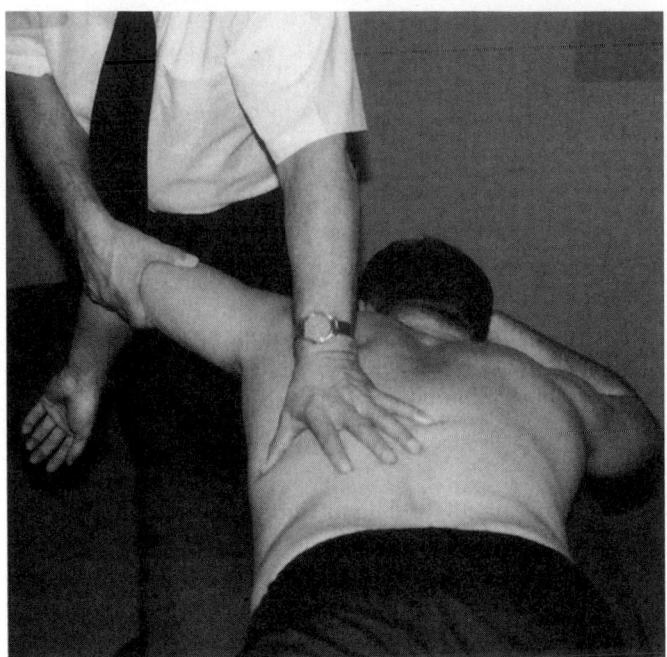

FIGURE 55.8. Costal technique, posterior approach.

Objective

Enhance or optimize costal respiratory motion.

Patient Position

Lateral recumbent (restricted side up; left in this example).

Procedure

1. Stand in front of your right lateral recumbent patient (Fig. 55.9). The patient's left elbow should be flexed.
2. Grasp the patient's left elbow with your left arm and place the shoulder in full abduction.

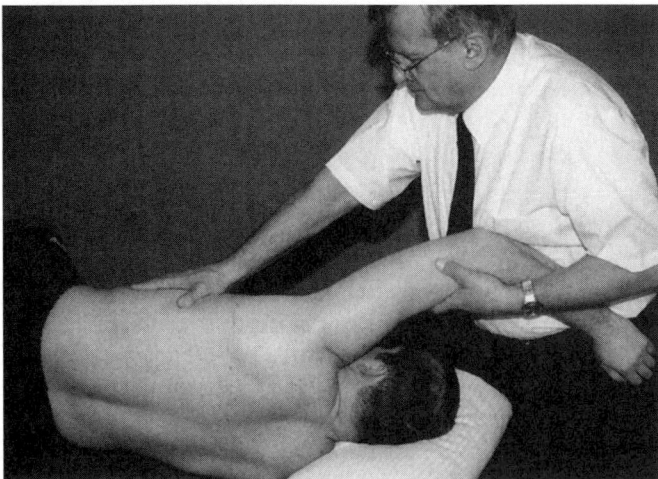

FIGURE 55.9. Costal technique, lateral recumbent.

3. Stabilize the inferior of the two ribs being treated in the mid-axillary line with your right thumb and thenar eminence.
4. Achieve a stretch/separation of the soft tissues between the ribs by abducting the arm as a long lever at the same time that you stabilize the inferior rib. Synchronize this with the patient's full inspiration.
5. Hold, then return toward neutral.
6. Repeat slowly in a smooth, rhythmic fashion until there is improved motion (or to the tolerance of the patient).
7. Move your stabilizing hand to the next superior rib. Repeat the process until you have treated all involved ribs.

Posterior Rib Raising

Diagnosis

Decreased costal motion during the breathing cycle.

Objective

Enhance or optimize costal respiratory motion.

Patient Position

Supine.

Procedure

1. Stand on the restricted side of your supine patient (Fig. 55.10).
2. Place the patient's arm in full abduction, holding the wrist with the operator's right hand.
3. Place your caudal hand under the patient's thorax. Press the tips of your fingers firmly against the inferior surface of the

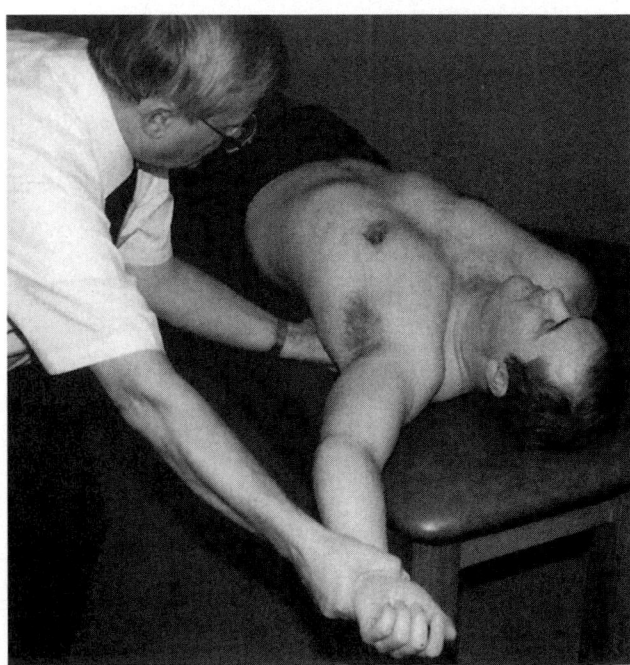

FIGURE 55.10. Costal technique, posterior rib raising.

angles of the patient's ribs and at the same time, extend and abduct the patient's arm (long lever stretch). Synchronize this with the patient's full inspiration. You may need to bend your knees slightly to do this comfortably.

4. Hold, then return toward neutral.
5. Repeat slowly in a smooth, rhythmic fashion until there is improved motion (or to the tolerance of the patient).
6. Move your (fulcrum) hand to the inferior border of the angle of the next inferior rib and repeat the process until you have treated all the involved ribs.

LUMBAR ARTICULATORY TECHNIQUES

Flexion (Seated)

Diagnosis

Decreased lumbar flexion.

Objective

Increase lumbar flexion.

Patient Position

Seated.

Procedure

1. Stand behind and to the side of your patient, who is seated on or straddling the table (Figs. 55.11 and 55.12).
2. Put one arm over his or her near shoulder and across his or her

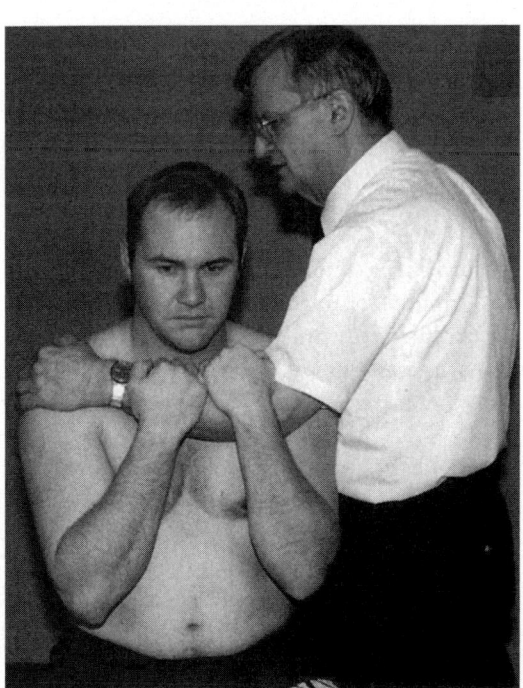

FIGURE 55.11. Lumbar flexion technique, anterior view.

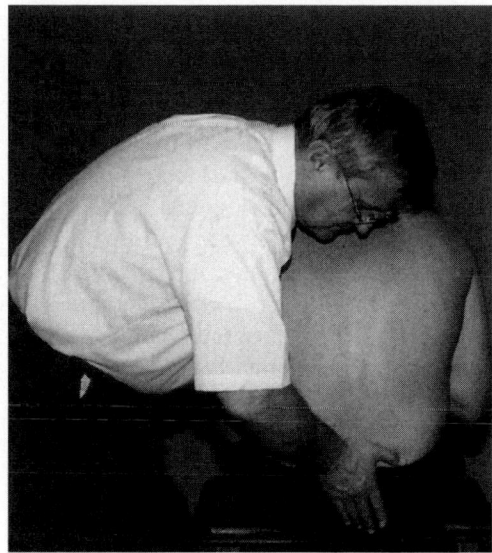

FIGURE 55.12. Lumbar flexion technique, posterior view.

chest with your hand on the opposite shoulder. The patient hooks his or her hands over your arm.

3. With the thenar eminence of your other hand, stabilize one vertebra in the lumbar spine. With your forearm against the patient's sternum, direct the force of flexion straight through the patient toward your stabilizing hand, gapping the joint above it.
4. Hold, then return toward neutral.
5. Repeat slowly in a smooth, rhythmic fashion until there is improved motion (or to the tolerance of the patient).
6. Move your stabilizing hand to the next inferior vertebra and repeat the process until you have treated all the involved segments.

Flexion (Lateral Recumbent)

Diagnosis

Decreased lumbar flexion.

Objective

Increase lumbar flexion.

Patient Position

Lateral recumbent.

Procedure

1. Stand in front of the patient.
2. Face the patient and flex his or her knees and rest them together against your anteromedial thigh or inguinal area.
3. Bend forward at the waist and flex your own knees. Gently flex your patient's lumbar spine by swinging your pelvis with the patient's knees toward the head of the table area.

4. Use your caudal hand to pull the inferior lumbar vertebra in a caudal direction as you induce flexion to the joint space above it. Your cephalad hand should stabilize the superior lumbar vertebra.
5. Hold, then return toward neutral.
6. Repeat slowly in a smooth, rhythmic fashion until there is improved motion (or to the tolerance of the patient).
7. Move your stabilizing hand to the next superior vertebra and repeat the process until you have treated all the involved segments.

Flexion (Supine)

Diagnosis

Decreased lumbar flexion.

Objective

Increase lumbar flexion.

Patient Position

Supine.

Procedure

1. Stand to the side of your supine patient and flex his or her hips and knees. Resting your pectoral area on the knees, place your hands below the patient's lumbar region, one on each side of the spine.
2. Press toward the table through the patient's knees and thighs, in a superior anteroposterior fashion, to spring the lumbar joint space in flexion. Use your hands to pull caudally, stretching the joint space above.
3. Hold, then return toward neutral.
4. Repeat slowly in a smooth, rhythmic fashion until there is improved motion (or to the tolerance of the patient).
5. Move your stabilizing hand to the next superior vertebra and repeat the process until you have treated all the involved segments.

Extension (Seated)

Diagnosis

Decreased lumbar extension.

Objective

Increase lumbar extension.

Patient Position

Seated.

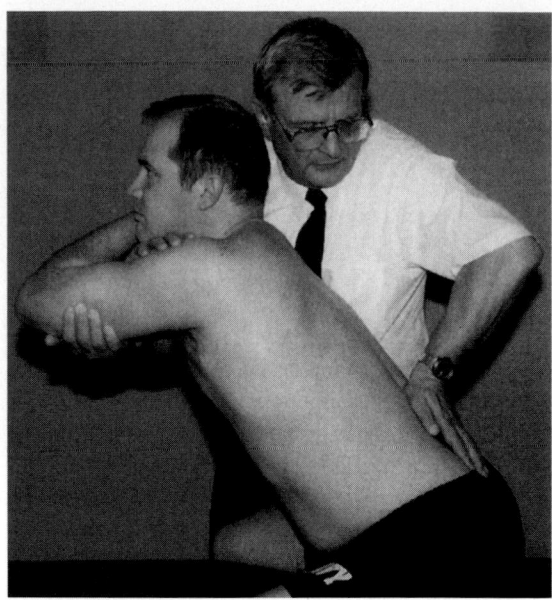

FIGURE 55.13. Lumbar extension technique, seated.

Procedure

1. Stand behind and to the right side of your patient, who is straddling the table (Fig. 55.13). Have the patient cross arms in front, with each hand grasping the opposite shoulder. As the patient leans slightly forward, place your right arm under his or her arms with your hand under the opposite axilla.
2. Place your left thenar eminence against the spinous process of a lumbar segment as a fulcrum around which you extend the lumbar spine.
3. Use your right hand or arm to lift the patient's elbows, introducing thoracolumbar extension to the joint space/segment above your fulcrum. Accentuate this extension with your left thenar eminence, applying an anterior translatory force at the segment level.
4. Hold, then return toward neutral.
5. Repeat slowly in a smooth, rhythmic fashion until there is improved motion (or to the tolerance of the patient).
6. Move your stabilizing hand to the next inferior vertebra and repeat the process until you have treated all the involved segments.

Extension (Lateral Recumbent)

Diagnosis

Decreased lumbar extension.

Objective

Increase lumbar extension.

Patient Position

Lateral recumbent.

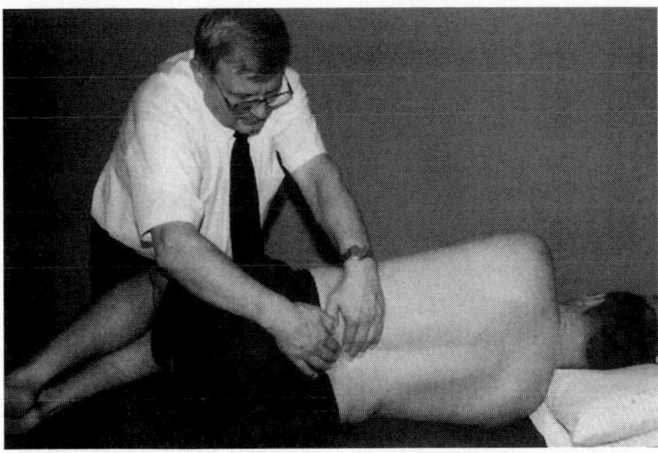

FIGURE 55.14. Lumbar extension technique, lateral recumbent.

Procedure

1. Stand in front of and facing the patient in the right lateral recumbent position (Fig. 55.14). Flex the patient's knees and hips to 90 degrees, resting the knees against your anteromedial thigh or inguinal area.

2. Place your hands posterior to two adjacent lumbar vertebral segments so that your fingertips meet at the joint space.

3. Bend forward at the waist and flex your own knees. By inducing posterior and caudad motion through the patient's knees, extend your patient's lumbar spine. Localize motion to the joint space at which your fingers meet. Pull the inferior lumbar vertebra in an inferoanterior direction as your cephalad hand pulls the superior vertebra in a superoanterior direction.

4. Hold, then return toward neutral.

5. Repeat slowly in a smooth, rhythmic fashion until there is improved motion (or to the tolerance of the patient).

6. Move your stabilizing hand to the next superior vertebra and repeat the process until you have treated all the involved segments.

Side-Bending (Seated)

Diagnosis

Decreased lumbar side-bending (lateral flexion, right in this example)

Objective

Increase lumbar side-bending (lateral flexion).

Patient Position

Seated.

Procedure

1. Stand behind and to the right side of your seated patient (Fig. 55.15). Your right axilla overlies the patient's right

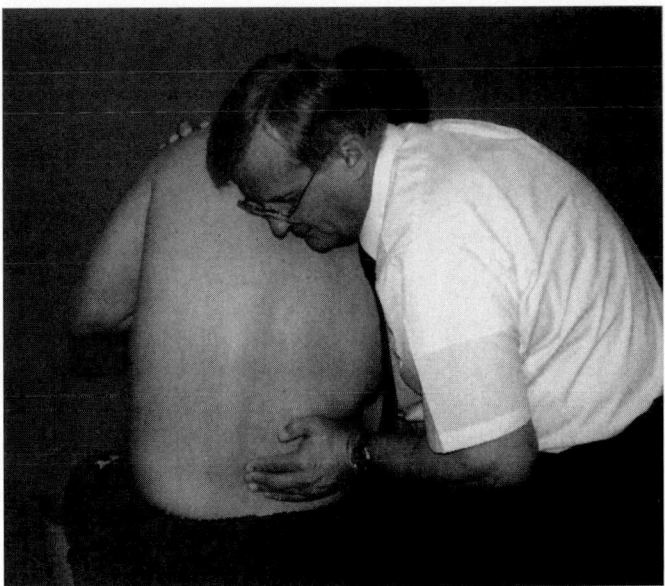

FIGURE 55.15. Lumbar side-bending technique, seated.

shoulder, and your right hand grasps his or her opposite shoulder or axilla.

2. Place your left hand (thenar eminence, or the pads of several fingers) on the right side of a vertebra in the patient's lumbar spine, just lateral to the spinous process.

3. Use your left hand as a fulcrum to induce left lateral translatory force as you create right side-bending by depressing the patient's right shoulder. Repeat in a rhythmic manner to all segments, side-bending more for the lower lumbar segments.

4. Introduce right side-bending by applying a downward pressure through your right axilla on the patient's shoulder and an upward lift of the patient's left shoulder with your right hand. This forms a convexity on the left, side-bending the spine to the right. You should feel maximal stretch at the joint space above your stabilizing (fulcrum) hand.

5. Hold, then return toward neutral.

6. Repeat slowly in a smooth, rhythmic fashion until there is improved motion (or to the tolerance of the patient).

7. Move your stabilizing hand to the next inferior vertebra and repeat the process until you have treated all the involved segments.

Side-Bending (Lateral Recumbent)

Diagnosis

Decreased left lumbar side-bending (lateral flexion).

Objective

Increase left lumbar side-bending (lateral flexion).

Patient Position

Right lateral recumbent (right side down).

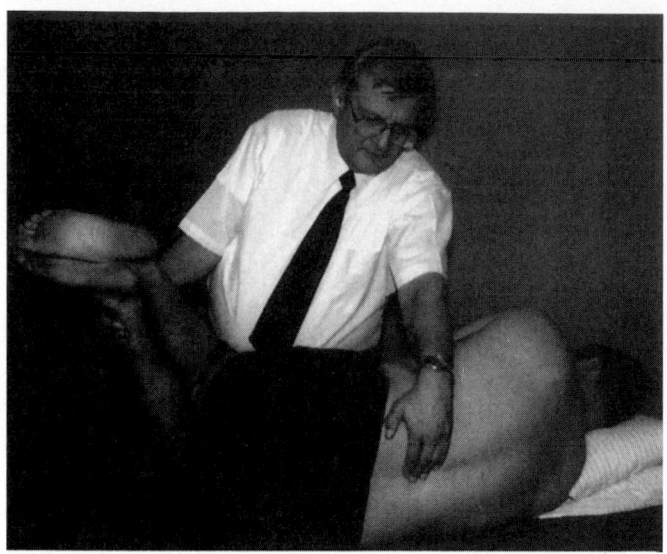

FIGURE 55.16. Lumbar side-bending technique, lateral recumbent.

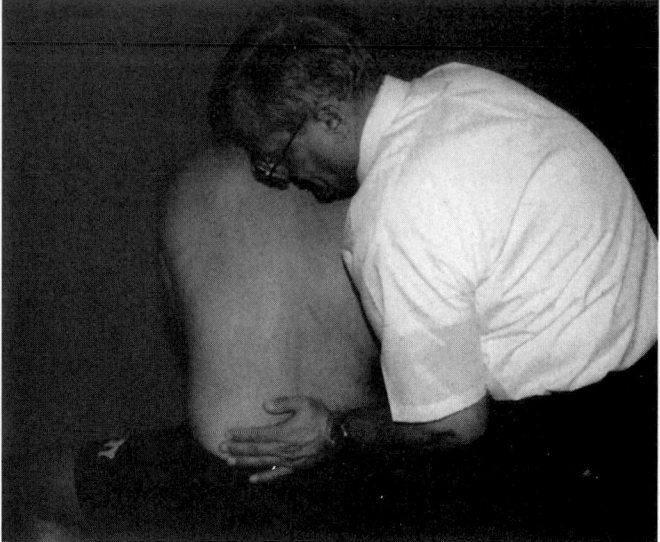

FIGURE 55.17. Lumbar rotation technique, seated.

Procedure

1. Stand at the side of the table, in front of and facing the patient (Fig. 55.16).
2. Flex his or her knees and hips to approximately 90 degrees.
3. Place your left hand so that your fingers are palpating the spinous processes of the lumbar spine.
4. Place your right hand and forearm under the patient's ankles and lift them toward the ceiling until your left hand palpates that you have introduced left side-bending in the lumbar region at the desired level.
5. Hold this stretch, then return toward neutral.
6. Repeat slowly in a smooth, rhythmic fashion until there is improved motion (or to the tolerance of the patient).
7. If you are performing this as a regional motion, complete the treatment by treating the other side in the same manner.
8. If you are attempting to induce more specific articulatory treatment to a particular segmental level, your left hand placement is such that your thumb and fingers hold the spinous process of a particular vertebra, stabilizing it as you induce side-bending to the joint below via the long lever moved by your right hand. When you have achieved the desired effect at a particular level, move to the next superior level to be treated.

Rotation (Seated)

Diagnosis

Decreased right lumbar rotation.

Objective

Increase right lumbar rotation.

Patient Position

Seated.

Procedure

1. Stand behind and to the right of the patient, who is straddling or sitting on the table (Fig. 55.17). Your right axilla overlies the patient's right shoulder and your right hand grasps the opposite shoulder or axilla. The patient hooks his or her hands over your arm.
2. Regional: Place your left hand just to the right of the spinous processes and encourage right rotation by applying a left lateral force to the spinous processes.
3. Segmental: If you want to be more specific in your treatment, stabilize a particular spinous process with your thumb and fingers, and resist the rotation you induce with the other hand or arm, confining the stretching, rotational forces to the joint above the segment you are stabilizing.
4. Induce right rotation to the lumbar spine by rotating the patient's thorax to the right with your right arm and hand.
5. Hold, then return toward neutral.
6. Repeat slowly in a smooth, rhythmic fashion until there is improved motion (or to the tolerance of the patient).
7. Move your stabilizing hand to the next inferior lumbar region or segment and repeat the process until you have treated the lumbar region or the specific involved segments.

Note: For decreased left lumbar rotation, make the appropriate adjustments to treat the other side.

PELVIC ARTICULATORY TECHNIQUES
Rotation to Innominate

Diagnosis

Posteriorly rotated innominate.

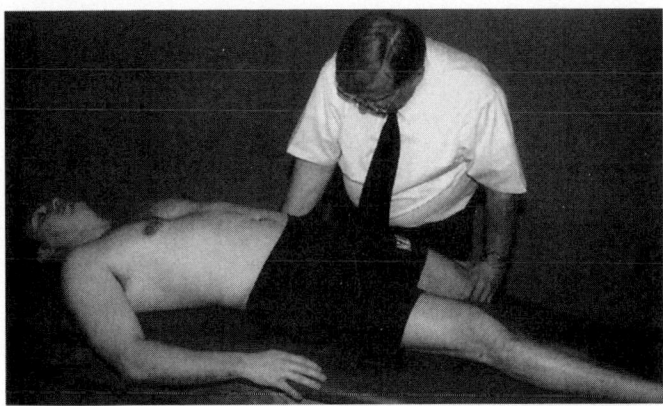

FIGURE 55.18. Pelvis technique, anterior rotation of innominate.

Objective

Normalize innominate position and motion.

Patient Position

Supine, with the leg of the posteriorly rotated innominate hanging over the side of the table, inducing hip extension.

Procedure

1. Stand on the dysfunctional side of the patient (Fig. 55.18).
2. Place your cephalad hand behind the posterior superior iliac spine (PSIS), cupping it.
3. Place your caudad hand on the anterior surface of the distal thigh to induce further hip extension.
4. Induce further hip extension by pressing down on the distal thigh while simultaneously pushing the PSIS anteriorly, inducing anterior rotation to the innominate.
5. Hold, then return toward neutral.
6. Repeat slowly in a smooth, rhythmic fashion until there is improved motion (or to the tolerance of the patient).

Note: This technique can easily be adapted to the lateral recumbent position, with the physician standing behind or in front of the patient and treating the upper hemipelvis.

Rotation to Innominate

Diagnosis

Anteriorly rotated innominate.

Objective

Normalize innominate position and motion.

Patient Position

Supine.

Procedure

1. Stand at the side of your patient's anteriorly rotated innominate (dysfunctional side), facing the patient's head (Fig. 55.19).
2. Flex the patient's knee and hip, grasping the knee between your caudal arm and pectoral area.
3. Place your cephalad hand on the anterosuperior iliac spine (ASIS).
4. Use your caudad hand to grasp the ischial tuberosity.
5. Apply a posterior rotational torque with both hands by exerting downward pressure on the ASIS while pulling upward on the ischial tuberosity. You may slightly adduct the thigh to gap the sacroiliac (SI) joint.
6. Hold, then return toward neutral.
7. Repeat slowly in a smooth, rhythmic fashion until there is improved motion (or to the tolerance of the patient).

Note: This technique can easily be adapted to the lateral recumbent position, with the physician standing behind the patient and treating the upper hemipelvis.

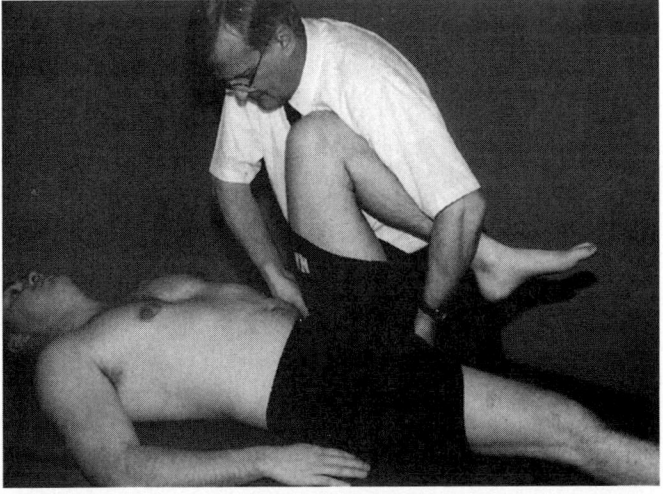

FIGURE 55.19. Pelvis technique, posterior rotation of innominate.

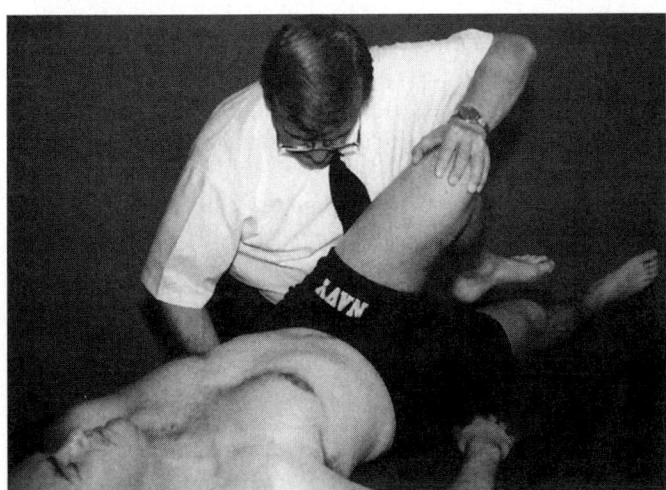

FIGURE 55.20. Pelvis technique, innominate outflare.

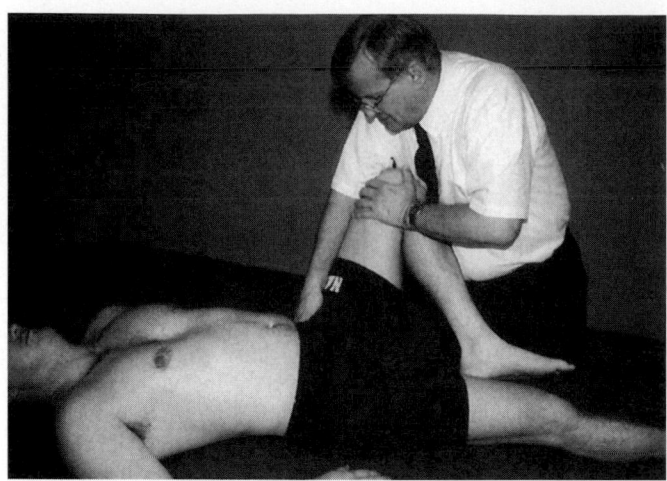

FIGURE 55.21. Pelvis technique, innominate inflare.

Sacroiliac Joint Gapping

Diagnosis

Innominate outflare or inflare.

Objective

Normalize innominate position and motion.

Patient Position

Supine.

Procedure

1. Stand at the patient's dysfunctional side (Figs. 55.20 and 55.21).
2. Grasp the patient's flexed knee with your caudal hand.
3. Grasp the patient's ASIS (inflare) or PSIS (outflare) with your cephalad hand.
4. Inflare: Pull the ASIS laterally and toward the table as you abduct the hip by pulling laterally on the knee.
5. Outflare: Pull laterally on the PSIS as you adduct the hip by pushing medially on the knee.
6. Hold, then return toward neutral.
7. Repeat slowly in a smooth, rhythmic fashion until there is improved motion (or to the tolerance of the patient).

ARTICULATORY TECHNIQUES IN THE EXTREMITIES

The same principles that apply to the spinal segments can be used to treat the extremities. In the extremities, the techniques are particularly useful when a degree of restriction or fibrosis has developed in the surrounding soft tissues during a period of inactivity after injury. This problem often follows a healed capsular tear or immobilization in a cast. These techniques should be used with caution and gentleness on patients who have tissue contractures. Remember to inform your patients that some discomfort during treatment is normal. With that knowledge, they can give you the feedback you need to adjust the force applied in these techniques.

An example of extremity treatment using articulatory technique is the treatment of the shoulder with techniques described and improved by Spencer (1–3). They are useful in diagnosing and treating musculoskeletal dysfunction of the shoulder, and are outlined here as they are presently being taught in most osteopathic colleges.

Spencer's original techniques have undergone some modification with use. An important modification is the addition of muscle energy and the use of compression or traction.

Stage 1: Stretching Tissues and Pumping Fluids with the Arm Extended

Note: This technique is performed as Stage 1 to "pump fluids and stretch tissues" (see Fig. 55.28, pg. 85).

1. Position the patient's arm on your shoulder, elbow extended (an alternate patient positioning and hold is shown in Fig. 55.7).
2. Grasp the patient's proximal humeral area as close to the humeral head as possible with both hands.
3. Pull the patient's humerus toward you (traction), gently and slowly, holding tension on the periarticular tissues. Do not press on the medial neurovascular bundle with your thumbs. Release traction force slowly.
4. Compress the articular area (shoulder) by guiding the humerus toward the glenoid fossa with both hands. Release compression. The traction and compression can be done rhythmically or in a random on-and-off manner.
5. Repeat steps three and four in sequence until motions are freer.
6. Move the patient's shoulder in translatory directions anterior/posterior, medial/lateral, and cephalad/caudal to the limits of motion. Hold, release forces, and repeat until motions are freer.

Stage 2: Glenohumeral Extension/Flexion with the Elbow Flexed

Patient Position

Lateral recumbent (affected shoulder up).

1. Neutral position of the patient's arm with the elbow flexed (operator to side of table facing the patient). Grasp the patient's elbow using the caudal hand. The cephalic hand compresses the scapula and clavicle (shoulder girdle) against the thorax (a critical component) (Fig. 55.22).
2. Move the patient's arm (elbow flexed) into extension in the horizontal plane while holding the shoulder girdle firmly against the superior thorax. Move slowly against the resistive barrier and repeat until no further range of motion (ROM) is achieved.

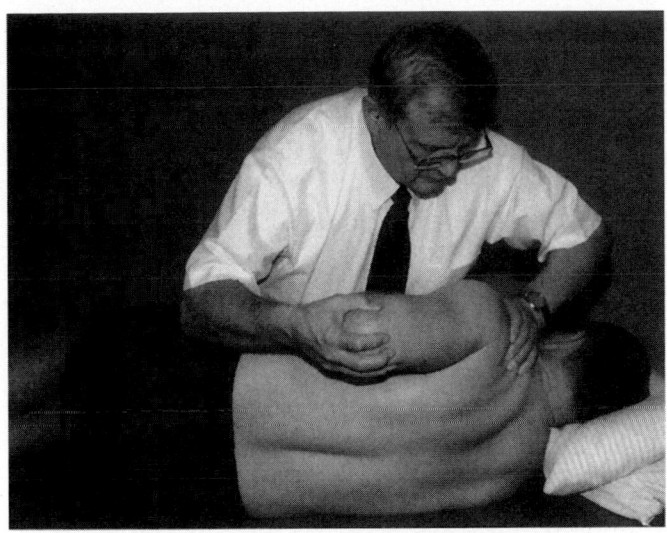

FIGURE 55.22. Extension with elbow flexed.

3. Muscle energy activation: Engage the barrier and instruct the patient to "push your elbow toward the physician" (flexion). Resist isometrically until effective contraction is localized at the shoulder. At that point, ask the patient to relax the muscular contraction and simultaneously "take up the slack motion," then slowly release the isometric resistance.

4. Take the elbow from its new position of resistance to extension and repeat step three until no further ROM is achieved.

Spencer recommended this technique be repeated in flexion—with the elbow flexed.

Stage 3: Glenohumeral Flexion/Extension with the Elbow Extended

1. Neutral position of the patient's arm with elbow flexed. Grasp the patient's forearm using the cephalic hand. The caudal hand compresses the scapula and clavicle against the thorax (Fig. 55.23).

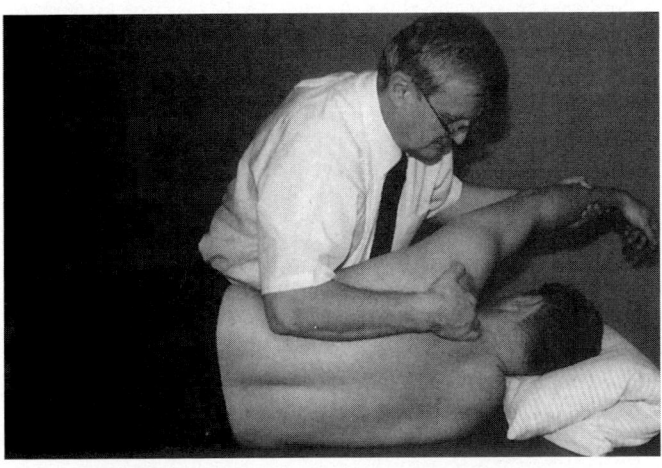

FIGURE 55.23. Flexion with elbow extended.

2. Move the patient's arm into flexion (elbow extended) in the horizontal plane while holding the shoulder girdle firmly against the superior thorax. Move slowly against the resistive barrier and repeat until no further ROM is achieved.

3. Muscle energy activation: Engage the barrier and instruct the patient to "pull your elbow toward your feet." Resist isometrically until effective contraction is localized at the shoulder. At that point, ask the patient to relax the muscular contraction and simultaneously "take up the slack motion," then slowly release the isometric resistance.

4. Take the arm from its new position of resistance to flexion and repeat steps three and four until no further ROM is achieved.

Spencer recommended this procedure be repeated—in extension with the elbow flexed.

Stage 4: Circumduction and Slight Compression with the Elbow Flexed/Extended

1. With the elbow flexed, the patient's arm is abducted to 90 degrees. Grasp the patient's elbow with caudal hand. The cephalic hand compresses the scapula and clavicle (shoulder girdle) against the thorax (Fig. 55.24).

2. Move the patient's arm through full clockwise circumduction with slight compression on the glenohumeral joint. Move slowly and firmly and repeat several times to gain ROM. This step evaluates circumduction ROM with the elbow flexed and also assesses the comfort of moving the articular surface of the humeral head over the articular surface of the glenoid fossa.

3. Move the patient's arm through full counterclockwise circumduction. Move slowly and firmly, repeating several times to gain ROM.

4. A muscle energy activation does not apply in this step.

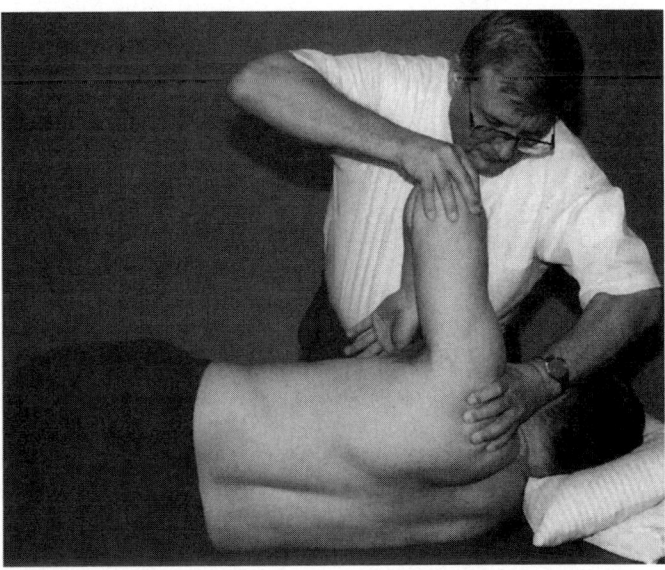

FIGURE 55.24. Circumduction with slight compression and elbow flexed.

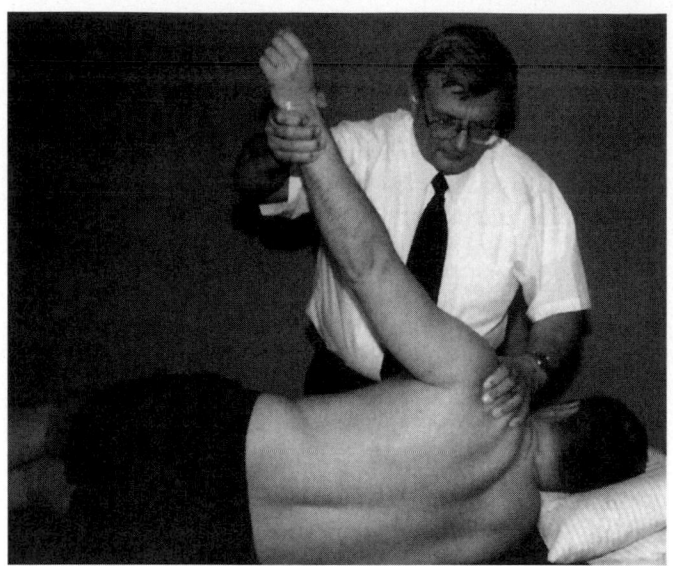

FIGURE 55.25. Circumduction with traction with the elbow extended.

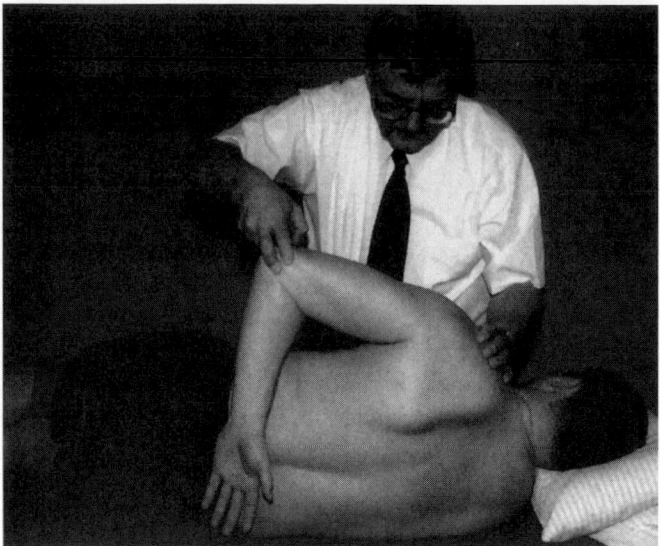

FIGURE 55.26. Abduction and internal rotation with the arm behind the back.

Stage 4 (Continued): Circumduction and Traction with the Elbow Extended

1. With the elbow extended, the patient's arm is abducted to 90 degrees. Grasp the patient's forearm with the caudal hand. The cephalic hand compresses the scapula and clavicle (shoulder girdle) against the thorax (Fig. 55.25).

2. Move the patient's arm through full clockwise circumduction with slight traction. Move slowly and repeat several times to gain ROM. This step evaluates circumduction ROM with the arm extended and also assesses the comfort of applying tension to the capsule of the glenohumeral joint.

3. Move the patient's arm through full counterclockwise circumduction with traction. Move slowly and repeat several times to gain ROM.

4. A muscle energy activation does not usually apply in this step.

Stage 5: Adduction and External Rotation with the Elbow Flexed

1. Neutral position of the patient's arm with the elbow flexed. With the caudal hand, grasp the patient's elbow. The cephalic hand compresses the scapula and clavicle (shoulder girdle) against the patient's thorax. The patient's hand (of the arm being treated) is resting palm down on the wrist of your cephalic hand to stabilize the patient's arm.

2. With your caudal hand, move the patient's elbow in an arc toward his or her face and toward the floor; this produces adduction and external rotation at the shoulder.

3. Muscle energy activation: At the resistive barrier (barrier engagement), instruct the patient to, "pull your elbow toward your waist." Resist isometrically until effective contraction is localized at the shoulder. At that point, ask the patient to relax the muscular contraction, "take up the slack," then release the isometric resistance.

4. Move the elbow to its new resistive barrier (to abduction and

external rotation) and repeat steps three and four until no further ROM is achieved.

Stage 6: Abduction with Internal Rotation with the Arm Behind the Back

1. With the arm abducted and the elbow flexed, position the patient's hand behind the back (to the extent permitted by the patient's comfort with this positioning), observing if the dorsal surface of the hand can be placed against the dorsal surface of the ipsilateral flank area (Fig. 55.26).

2. Grasp the patient's elbow (or place your index and middle fingers around the elbow) and slowly move the elbow ventrally (toward you). Repeat to gain abduction and especially internal rotation.

3. Muscle energy activation: Position the patient at the resistive barrier, then instruct the patient to "pull your elbow away from me." Resist isometrically until effective contraction is localized at the shoulder. At that point, ask the patient to relax the muscular contraction, "take up the slack," slowly release the isometric resistance.

4. Move the elbow to its new position of resistance to abduction and internal rotation and repeat steps three and four until no further ROM is achieved.

Stage 7: Stretching Tissues and Pumping Fluids with the Arm Extended

This stage is a repeat of Stage 1 (Fig. 55.27).

COMMENTS ON SPENCER SHOULDER TECHNIQUES

Spencer used his shoulder treatment program to increase pain-free range of motion by pumping fluids and stretching tissues

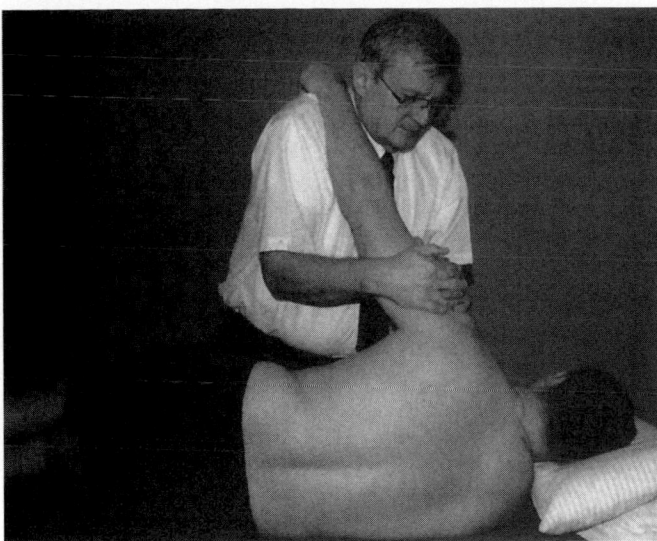

FIGURE 55.27. Stretching tissues and pumping fluids with the arm extended; stretching tissues and pumping fluids with the extremity extended and the elbow flexed.

around the shoulder. Spencer would treat the patient with the elbow flexed and then repeat the stage with the arm extended. He stated that in this way the lever arm was short for initial testing and treatment and was then increased by arm extension, stretching the shoulder and elbow flexors in the extended state. The modified Spencer motion techniques add compression and traction to steps three and four. They also add muscle energy to the applicable steps to enhance treatment possibilities. Experienced physicians report that the Spencer techniques do not seem to have rapid results in patients with metabolic or other debilitating disease, such as poorly controlled diabetes.

Treatment of the shoulder using the seven motions of Spencer (2,3) in their original form or in their modified form provides objective diagnostic tests and articulatory treatment for soft tissue restrictions and gives objective evidence supporting the clinical prognosis of a patient undergoing treatment for shoulder dysfunction.

CONCLUSION

Articulatory technique consists of movements against a diagnosed barrier to (limitation of) motion in an articular structure. These movements are:

Controlled
Slow
Repetitive
Passive

Pressure against the resistant barrier is held long enough in each cycle to allow a stretching of the tissues controlling and limiting the motion of the joint. These techniques are designed to deal with one or several ranges of motion, as indicated by the diagnosis and the nature of the articulation being treated. Passive force against the barrier may be augmented by incorporating patient generated (intrinsic) force, such as that found in the final stage of muscle energy technique or in respiratory cooperation.

Articulatory technique may be the principal component of a treatment program. It is also used to prepare an articular area for other forms of manipulative treatment. It may be preferred to high-velocity treatment in infants, postoperative patients, compromised or debilitated patients, and older patients. Articulating technique is often applied to support general body functions, such as respiratory efficiency.

REFERENCES

1. Spencer H. Shoulder technique. *J Am Osteopath Assoc.* 1916;15:218–220.
2. Spencer H. Treatment of bursitis and tendonitis. *J Am Osteopath Assoc.* 1926;25:528–529.
3. Patriquin DA. The evolution of osteopathic manipulative technique: the Spencer technique. *J Am Osteopath Assoc.* 1992;92:1134–1146.

THRUST (HIGH-VELOCITY/LOW-AMPLITUDE) TECHNIQUES

ROBERT E. KAPPLER
JOHN M. JONES, III

> ### KEY CONCEPTS
>
> - Definition and development of thrust technique
> - Indications and uses for thrust technique
> - Quantity and quality of motion loss with somatic dysfunction
> - End-feel at restrictive barrier and barrier engagement
> - Accumulation of force and corrective force velocity and amplitude
> - Patient relaxation
> - Exaggeration technique
> - Mechanism of thrust technique action
> - Effect of technique on unstable, hypermobile joints
> - Dose, precautions, and contraindications for thrust technique
> - Guidelines for safety and benefits of technique
> - HVLA treatment technique examples by regions and diagnosis

Thrust technique is defined as a type of direct technique that uses high-velocity/low-amplitude forces (1). "Thrust techniques" are a collection of direct method manipulative treatments that use high-velocity/low-amplitude (HVLA) activation to move a joint that is exhibiting somatic dysfunction through its restrictive barrier so that when the joint resets itself, appropriate physiologic motion is restored. The term direct refers specifically to positioning the restricted joint(s) toward the restrictive barrier. Simply stated, you move the restricted joint in the direction it won't move. After precise positioning against the restrictive barrier, the final force is a short (low-amplitude), quick (high-velocity) thrust. Greenman (2) described the force as impulse. Ordinarily, a click or pop is heard at the time the force is applied. There is an immediate increase in the range of motion and the freedom of motion.

HISTORIC PERSPECTIVE

Thrust technique has been the major type of technique taught in colleges of osteopathic medicine and has been practiced by osteopathic physicians for years. In the 1970s, the osteopathic medical school curricula began to include other types of techniques. Until recently, however, osteopathic manipulation and high-velocity technique were essentially synonymous. Graduates are now exposed to a complete spectrum of direct and indirect techniques; therefore, osteopathic manipulation is no longer synonymous with thrust technique.

A. T. Still used very little thrust technique. Instead, he used what we now describe as myofascial release and indirect techniques (see Chapters 58, 60, and 70). It is interesting to speculate why osteopathic manipulative techniques taught in the colleges evolved into the exclusive domain of thrust techniques and remained that way for so many years. Faculty may have been responsible for the change. Students, in the early days, assisted in the teaching of techniques. These students may have played a major role in moving the curriculum to thrust techniques. Thrust techniques can be taught by precisely describing the nature of the restriction and providing techniques for treating the dysfunction. These techniques can be practiced. In contrast, fascial release and indirect techniques require skill in assessing motion patterns in the tissues. The technique is difficult to describe because the physician is responding to tactile and proprioceptive input from his or her hands. Faculty find release techniques difficult to teach, and students may perceive them as abstractions. Thrust techniques are easier to teach and to learn. However, although thrust techniques can be described in a precise manner, the motor coordination necessary to use these techniques effectively requires extensive practice and experience.

MOTION LOSS AND SOMATIC DYSFUNCTION

Somatic dysfunction is impaired or altered function of related components of the somatic system (1):

Skeletal
Arthrodial structures
Myofascial structures
Related vascular lymphatic and neural elements

Diagnostic tests for somatic dysfunction include TART:

T: Tissue texture change (feel)
A: Asymmetry or positional change (look)
R: Restriction of motion (move)
T: Tenderness

Somatic dysfunction exhibits a change in quantity and quality of motion. Quantity of motion involves the following general principles:

1. Motion beyond the anatomic barrier damages anatomic structures. It is also the end point of permitted passive motion.

2. The range of normal active motion occurs between the physiologic barriers.

3. With motion loss in somatic dysfunction, the restrictive or pathologic barrier is the end point of permitted motion.

4. A normal joint has a midline or neutral point within its range of motion.

5. In somatic dysfunction, there is frequently a positional change (or asymmetry) in the joint that shifts its neutral to a new midline.

6. Motion loss occurs in the range of normal physiologic motion.

7. The range between the physiologic barrier and the anatomic barrier is not as finite as the illustration depicts. There is some flexibility of the boundaries.

These principles describe motion loss in somatic dysfunction and a new position that is identified on examination as asymmetry or positional change. Inappropriate lay terminology is sometimes used to describe this positional change, for example, out of place. This kind of term may lead to a misunderstanding of the nature of motion loss in somatic dysfunction and the positional change associated with this motion loss. Inappropriate lay terms to describe treatment as an adjustment (of position) or putting it back further complicate understanding. Thrust technique is designed to remove motion loss in somatic dysfunction. A positional change from the somatic dysfunction position (Fig. 56.1) to the normal neutral or midline is the result of effective treatment. Treatment involves the dynamics of motion, not static positional change.

Quality of Motion

To the experienced examiner, these qualitative changes are the clue to evaluating motion characteristics of somatic dysfunction. Motion is asymmetric with restriction in one direction and freer motion in the other direction. The terms ease and bind are sometimes used to describe the asymmetric motion. Movement toward the restrictive barrier exhibits bind, and moving away from the barrier exhibits ease.

The qualitative aspects of motion can be depicted on the same graph (Fig. 56.1) used to illustrate quantity, with the x axis defining joint position and the y axis defining operator force to move

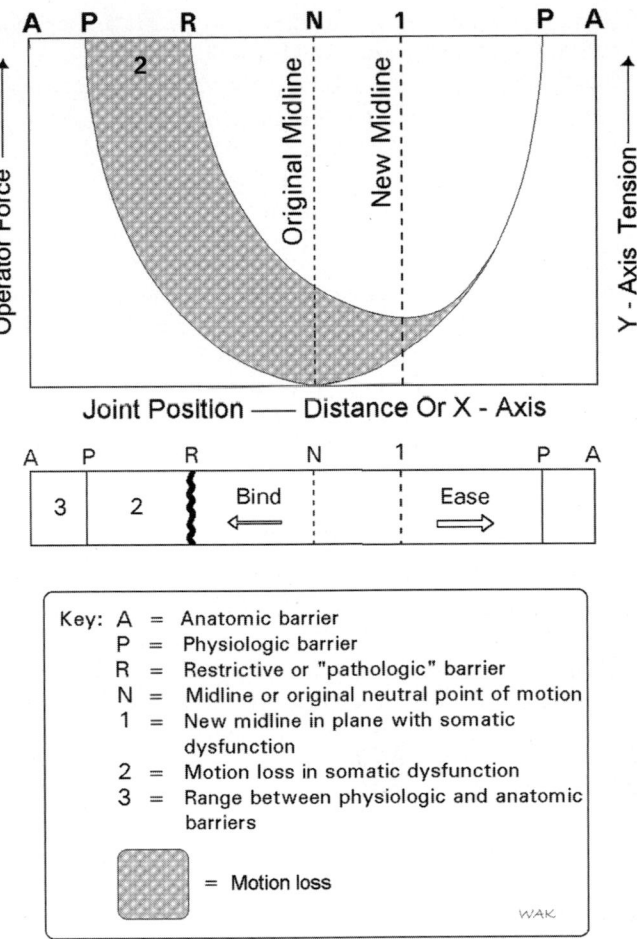

FIGURE 56.1. Somatic dysfunction: quality and quantity of joint motion.

the joint through a range of motion. A joint with somatic dysfunction exhibits an asymmetric quality of motion. If the y axis of the graph is changed to tension rather than force, it emphasizes a different component of motion in somatic dysfunction. There is increased tension in the dysfunctional joint, as if both agonist and antagonist are too tight. Motion in a direction of balanced tension is the basis of functional technique, which is described elsewhere (3).

Motion characteristics using an example of rotational restriction of the atlas can be described as:

1. AA = R_R (the atlas on the axis is rotated right, i.e., position)

2. Freer rotation right

3. Restriction of left rotation

Somatic dysfunction can be described in three ways:

1. Where is it? ("The posterior aspect of the transverse process of the atlas is more prominent on the right." This is static position that describes an asymmetry, and is not sufficient for providing a HVLA technique.)

2. What will it do? (AA = R_R. Active or passive motion testing indicates the direction of the ease of motion for the joint. Example: The atlas is rotated to the right. Set-up for a HVLA

technique would be to rotate the axis to the left, i.e., opposite the diagnosis, to the restrictive barrier.)

3. What won't it do? (AA = restricted R_L. Active or passive motion testing indicates the direction in which the joint is restricted. Set-up for a HVLA technique would be to rotate the axis to the left, i.e., the same direction as the "restriction" diagnosis, to the restrictive barrier.)

These examples illustrate that somatic dysfunction can be named in two ways. The common, classic method states the motion that the joint prefers (i.e., AA = R_R). The second method states the restricted motions that are present. When using this second method, the formula or description must be preceded by the word "restricted" or "restricted in" (i.e., AA = restricted R_L).

Unstable Hypermobile Joint

Some joints are unstable and hypermobile. Within the numerous joints of the spine, a pattern of alternating hypomobility and hypermobility may exist. The loose, hypermobile joints are overworked while the stiff, hypomobile joints escape excess motion.

A normal physiologic reaction to a painful hypermobile joint is for muscles surrounding the joint to splint the joint and protect it from excess motion. Physical examination reveals restriction of motion. Underneath that protective muscle splinting is an unstable joint.

A high-velocity thrust technique may work, as evidenced by a decrease in pain and improvement in motion. Unfortunately, the treatment contributes to the joint instability. The more HVLA technique is used, the looser the joint becomes.

There are some spinal joints that tend to be loose. C5 and C6 become hypermobile (and arthritic). This process is maintained by a stiff, flexed upper thoracic spine requiring a compensatory cervical lordosis. In the lumbar spine, the lumbosacral (LS) region tends to become hypermobile. A flexed upper lumbar spine associated with chronic psoas tension maintains LS dysfunction (4).

Be aware of the possibility of unstable joints. Reevaluation of motion after treatment will reveal excess freedom of motion. Management involves modifying the activity that contributes to instability, mobilizing adjacent hypomobile joints, and prescribing active rehabilitation exercises.

HIGH-VELOCITY/LOW-AMPLITUDE TREATMENT CLASSIFICATION AND MECHANISMS

1. Direct method of treatment
2. Requires specific diagnosis of the joint dysfunction before each treatment
3. Set-up: motion is carried in the direction of its restriction to the restrictive barrier in all planes
4. Activation: high-velocity/low-amplitude thrust

MECHANISM OF THRUST TECHNIQUE ACTION

The mechanism of thrust technique action is shown in Figure 56.2. The answer to the question of what maintains restriction of joint motion has been and is being explored by osteopathic physicians and scientists. In some cases, a joint gets stuck

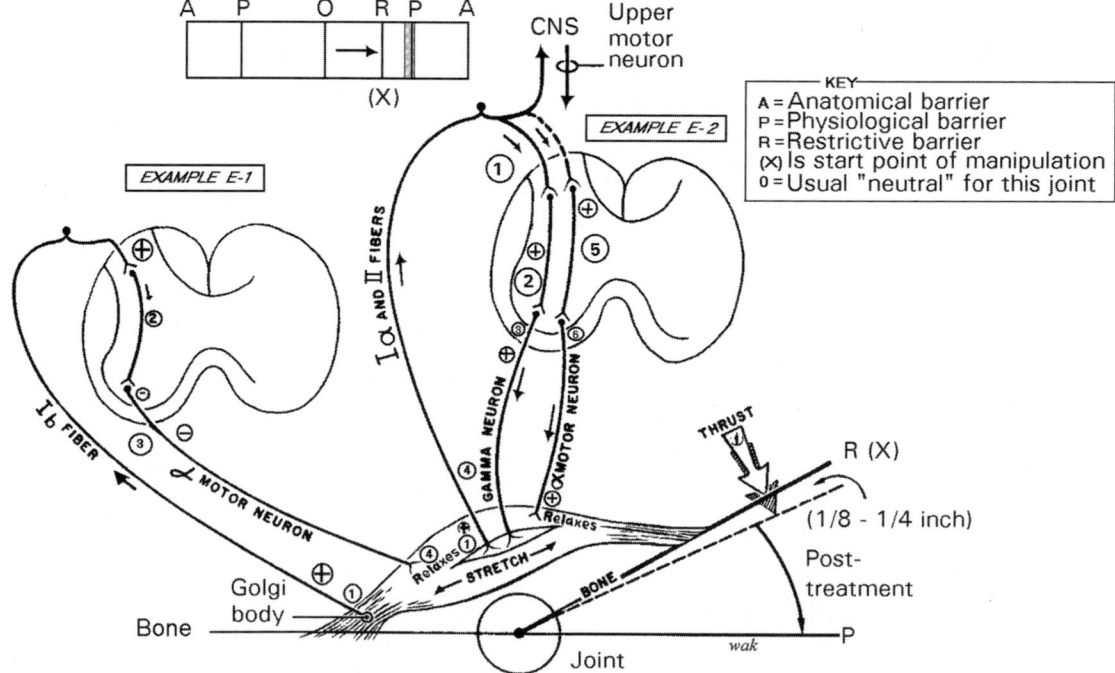

FIGURE 56.2. Proposed mechanism of HVLA thrust technique action.

the same way an old loose window or drawer may get stuck: half open and half closed, in a position no longer parallel to the track. The sacroiliac joint is a good example of this type of restriction. A properly directed mechanical force frees the joint. As with the stuck drawer, the proper force is not directly in or out, which is the major motion of the drawer. The proper force is an oblique or side force. Remember this in extremity techniques, where the minor motions or restoration of joint play is the object, not a direct force against the major motion of a joint. For example, if a wrist is restricted in extension, treatment might involve anterior or posterior translation of the carpal bones.

For mechanisms maintaining joint restriction, abnormal muscle activity is usually involved. Muscles maintain joint restriction. The palpatory findings in somatic dysfunction include tissue texture abnormality. Muscles are hypertonic and sometimes boggy and stringy. When the joint restriction is treated, there is an immediate change in the muscles and an immediate change in the quality and quantity of motion. This change means an immediate change in neural activity. How does the thrust change neural activity? A likely answer lies in the mechanoreceptor in the joint capsule. A sudden stretch or change of position of the joint alters the afferent output of these mechanoreceptors, resulting in release of muscle hypertonicity. This is discussed in the osteopathic and scientific literature on proprioceptors and somatic dysfunction (5–9).

Pop or click: Numerous studies have focused on the pop. One widely held hypothesis states that the sudden distraction of joint surfaces produces a nitrogen bubble, along with noise and increased freedom of motion (10). Osteopathic physicians prefer to focus on joint function and dysfunction and not on the noise. The objective of thrust technique is to overcome joint restriction. Always retest motion after the treatment. Although the pop or click is usually indicative of success, it is possible that an unrelated joint made the noise and the restricted joint remained unaltered. It is also possible to have a successful treatment without any noise. Keep your focus on the patient and the joint restriction.

CLINICAL APPLICATION OF HIGH-VELOCITY/LOW-AMPLITUDE MANIPULATIVE TREATMENT

Indications

Thrust technique is a method of specific joint mobilization. Proper use of thrust technique requires an assessment of restriction of joint motion before each manipulative treatment procedure is performed, along with the conclusion that treatment of this joint restriction will benefit the patient (for example, reduce pain, free motion, improve biomechanical function, reduce somatovisceral reflex).

The performance of thrust technique requires an understanding of somatic dysfunction and the barrier concept. Thrust technique is indicated for treatment of motion loss in somatic dysfunction. Thrust technique is ordinarily not indicated for treatment of joint restriction due to anatomic/pathologic changes, such as traumatic contracture, advanced degenerative joint disease, or ankylosis.

End-Feel at Restrictive Barrier

The use of direct technique requires engaging the barrier. The final activating force is a physician force: high-velocity/low-amplitude.

Figure 56.1, depicting the force necessary to move a joint to the barrier, is a graphic illustration of end-feel. As the barrier is engaged, increasing amounts of force are necessary and the distance decreases. The term barrier may be misleading if it is interpreted as a wall or rigid obstacle to be overcome with a push. As the joint reaches the barrier, restraints in the form of tight muscles and fascia serve to inhibit further motion. We are pulling against restraints rather than pushing against some anatomic structure.

The barrier involves a three-dimensional matrix, not just a single plane of motion. We can define motion in the three cardinal planes as flexion-extension, rotation, and side-bending. To be complete, there are components of translatory motion that should be considered. These are fore-aft translation, side-to-side translation, and compression-distraction. All of these single motions are combined into a single force vector when executing the technique. However, for purposes of diagnosis, each of these components can be tested separately.

For a high-velocity technique to be effective, the barrier must feel solid. If the barrier feels rubbery and indistinct, thrust technique may be ineffective.

Barrier Engagement

Experienced physicians develop skills to engage the barrier quickly. They sense how the tissues are responding to the force being applied and make subtle alterations in the direction of force to effectively engage the barrier in all planes. The novice takes more time by engaging one plane at a time. Engaging the barrier with accuracy and confidence is a skill acquired with practice and experience.

Accumulation of Force at Restriction

With a proper diagnosis, initial positioning engages the barrier. Forces must be applied so that they accumulate at the restricted joints. In the spinal area, the reference is a vertebral unit: two bones and the connections (joints) between them. Forces applied from above to the superior vertebra meet forces applied to the inferior vertebra. Forces from above and from below meet at the restricted joint.

Depending on the technique, force may be applied at one site; the opposing counterforce is resistance of inertia of body mass, resistance of the table, or other resistance. In all cases, direct the force at the restriction. Specificity of a technique is a measure of how accurately the force accumulates at the restriction. Force that does not accumulate at the lesion is dissipated through other parts of the body. This could result in iatrogenic side effect. The greater the specificity, the lesser the force needed, and the potential for untoward side effects is minimized.

Final Corrective Force Velocity and Amplitude

HVLA thrust techniques use a short, quick thrust. High velocity does not mean high force, and it does not mean high amplitude. Once the barrier is engaged, the final force is applied from that position. Do not back off before delivering the corrective thrust. Likewise, do not carry the force through a great distance. Amplitude means distance. The amplitude is low, a small fraction of an inch. High amplitude defeats proper localization of force and decreases the likelihood of achieving the desired effect.

Do not be overly tentative and apply a low-velocity force with an increase of force and amplitude. These efforts are often unsuccessful. The proper application has been described as a tack hammer blow, sudden but not forceful. The term impulse applied to HVLA technique recognizes that the force is a sudden acceleration and deceleration. Experience and practice are very helpful in knowing how to apply the force.

Some thrust techniques are not executed at high velocity. Consider an experience where you set up the patient to treat a joint restriction, the joint goes click, and the restriction is released as you are positioning the patient and localizing forces. Sometimes you tease a joint with carefully and slowly applied forces. Again, experience is very beneficial in applying the proper force. Although we describe HVLA thrust technique, the actual force may be modified to fit the patient's needs.

Methods Used to Improve Effectiveness of High-Velocity/Low-Amplitude Techniques

Patient Relaxation during Thrust Technique

The patient should be as relaxed as possible when applying the corrective force. The more tense the patient, the greater the force necessary, and the greater the risk of side effect or failure to overcome the motion restriction. If the patient feels comfortable and secure with the physician's hands, relaxation is not a problem. If the patient feels insecure, muscles will be tight rather than relaxed. If the technique is hurting the patient, muscles will involuntarily tighten. Nonverbal clues, such as a facial grimace, can alert the physician to a problem. A skilled physician senses when the patient is relaxed and when he or she is not. The exhalation phase of respiration is the relaxation phase, and the final force is often applied during exhalation.

Divert the Patient's Attention

When using a thrust technique to treat cervical somatic dysfunction, some practitioners divert attention by instructing the patient to cross his or her legs. This may help in some cases, but it is not an adequate substitute for the physician's hands transmitting a sense of control, comfort, and confidence. This skill comes with practice and experience. It is possible to distract a patient and apply a corrective force when the patient does not anticipate it. However, if the technique is applied too quickly, forces may not be properly localized. A patient who has experienced a painful thrust in the past cannot be fooled.

Dose of Thrust Technique

The compassionate physician may err on the side of overdose. Give the patient time to respond to the treatment; the sicker the patient, the less the dose. Older patients respond more slowly; young patients respond more quickly (11).

For hospitalized patients, daily osteopathic manipulative therapy (OMT) may be appropriate, but daily thrust technique may be an overdose. When treating hospital patients on a daily basis, Larson (N. J. Larson, personal communication, 1967, 1978) would vary the technique so he did not repeat the same technique on a given area. With the spectrum of techniques available, there should be no reason to overdose a patient on high-velocity technique. The more specific and precise the technique is, the less iatrogenic the side effect.

Precautions and Contraindications

Most of the published precautions about OMT imply forceful HVLA thrust. Instead of presenting a list of absolutes, think in terms of risk/benefit relationships. If the risk of harming the patient exceeds the potential therapeutic benefit, the technique is not indicated. Risk also relates to the skill of the physician. There is more risk with an unskilled physician. If forceful, direct techniques may harm the patient, gentle indirect release techniques might be safe.

Neurologic complications from thrust manipulation can be fatal or result in permanent neurologic impairment. Cervical manipulation has been associated with vertebral basilar thrombosis (12). Dislocation of the dens associated with rupture or laxity of the transverse ligament of the atlas can cause death or quadriplegia. In the low back, massive protrusion of a disc can produce cauda equina syndrome with loss of bowel, bladder, and sexual function.

Pathologic fractures can result from osteoporotic or metastatic bone. Excess force may injure fragile tissues. Joints could be sprained. Arthritic spurs could be broken off.

There may be psychological contraindications to the use of HVLA. Apprehension on the part of the patient is a relative contraindication. Make sure the patient understands what is expected during and after treatment.

Exaggeration Thrust Technique

Some practitioners of manual medicine use a form of thrust technique in which the direction of force is away from the restrictive barrier. An example of this method follows: If T3 is extended, extension is free (freer motion), and flexion is restricted. The exaggeration method (technique) involves thrusting on T3 to extend it suddenly and forcibly. This form of technique is potentially damaging to the ligamentous structure, producing hypermobility. In addition, the patient may experience an increase of symptoms with a prolongation of somatic dysfunction. This is especially true for patients with extended thoracic dysfunction that is misdiagnosed as flexed dysfunction, and an extension force is applied. The exaggeration thrust technique is not taught in U.S. colleges of osteopathic medicine.

Guidelines for Safety

1. Be aware of possible complications.
2. Make a diagnosis.
3. A palpatory examination is a prerequisite for treatment.
4. Listen with your hands and fingers. If it doesn't feel right, back off and collect more data.
5. If the barrier doesn't feel right, don't thrust, but select an alternate technique.
6. Emphasize specificity, not force.
7. Ask permission to treat.
8. If response to treatment does not meet your expectations, reevaluate the patient.
9. Somatic dysfunction with joint restriction is the indication. Pain is not an indication for high-velocity manipulation.
10. Somatic dysfunction often coexists with orthopedic disease (spondylosis, disc degeneration, spondylolysis).
11. Be aware of the total picture.

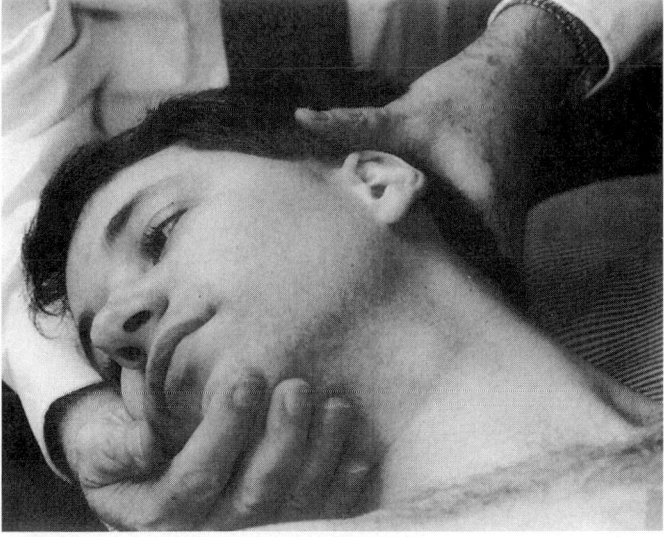

FIGURE 56.3. Occipitoatlantal technique with side-bending focus.

Beneficial Use of High-Velocity/Low-Amplitude Thrust Technique

Thrust technique is a very efficient use of physician's time in treating a patient, as long as the physician has met the prerequisite of an effective skill level. When a patient is able to tolerate thrust technique, the results are long lasting rather than temporary. The patient usually experiences immediate relief, with decreased pain and increased freedom of motion. For years, osteopathic physicians have treated patients using thrust techniques, and these patients continue to seek the services of an osteopathic physician.

HIGH-VELOCITY/LOW-AMPLITUDE TREATMENT TECHNIQUES BY REGION AND DIAGNOSIS

Cervicals

Atypical Cervicals: Occipito-Atlantal Joint, Side-Bending Focus

Diagnosis

The occiput is side bent right, rotated left in relationship to the atlas (posterior occiput on the left).

OA = $S_R R_L$ or CO = $S_R R_L$
OA = restricted $S_L R_R$ or CO = restricted $S_L R_R$

Position

The patient is supine, and the physician stands to the left of the patient at the head of the table (Fig. 56.3).

Procedure

To restore range of motion to the occipital-atlantal (OA) joint so that in resetting itself, appropriate physiologic motion is restored:

1. The physician's right hand cups the patient's chin with the palm at the zygomatic process.
2. The physician's metacarpophalangeal (MP) joint or proximal

interphalangeal (PIP) joint of his or her left index finger is placed on the bony calvaria (left occiput), taking care to avoid the mastoid portion of the temporal bone.

3. Mild extension is added and is limited to the O-A joint, taking care to avoid hyperextension.
4. The physician side bends the patient's head to the left by translation downward (caudally) with the left MP (or PIP) joint and slightly upward with the right hand. The restrictive barrier in left side-bending and right rotation is localized.
5. The patient is asked to take a big breath in and exhale.
6. At the end of exhalation, a high-velocity/low-amplitude thrust to increase the side-bending component is directed through the left MP (or PIP joint) by translation of the occiput toward the patient's right eye.
7. Retest the range of motion.

Atypical Cervicals: Atlanto-Axial Joint, Neutral

Diagnosis

The atlas is rotated right in relationship to the axis and moves more easily in this direction

AA = R_R
AA = restricted R_L

Position

The patient is supine, and the physician stands to the right of the patient at the head of the table (Fig. 56.4).

Procedure

To restore physiologic range of motion to the atlanto-axial (A-A) joint so that in resetting itself, there is a physiologic increase in left rotation:

1. The fingers and palm of the physician's left hand grasps the patient's chin with the palm or the forearm at the patient's left zygomatic process.

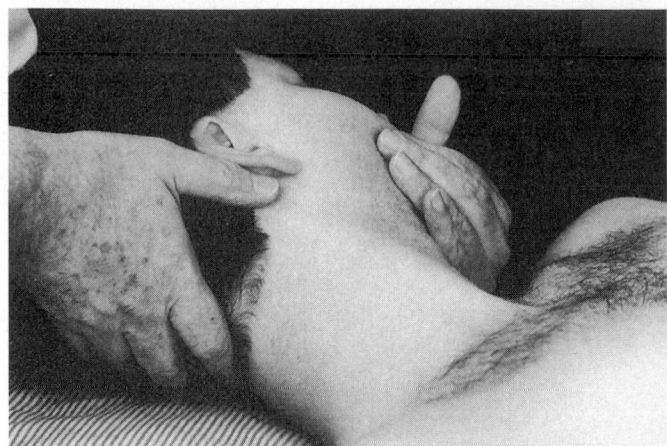

FIGURE 56.4. Atlanto-axial technique.

2. The proximal phalanx of the physician's right index finger is placed by the soft tissue next to the patient's A-A joint, with the thumb contacting the patient's lateral aspect of the face in the region of the right zygomatic process, avoiding the mandible.

3. The patient's head is rotated to the left with enough flexion-extension and/or side-bending to engage the restrictive barrier. (Note the resilience of the end-feel.)

4. The patient is asked to inhale and exhale.

5. At the end of the patient's exhalation, the physician applies a high-velocity/low-amplitude thrust in a left rotational pattern, focusing the force with the right index finger as a fulcrum.

6. Retest the range of motion.

Typical Cervicals (C2-7), Side-Bending Focus

Diagnosis

C3 is flexed, side-bent to the left, rotated left in relationship to C4, and moves more easily in these directions.

C3 = F $S_L R_L$

C3 = restricted E $S_R R_R$

Position

The patient is supine, and the physician stands to the right side of the patient at the head of the table (Fig. 56.5).

Procedure

To restore physiologic range of motion to the C3-4 vertebral unit so that in resetting itself, appropriate physiologic motion is restored:

1. The physician's left palm and fingers cup the patient's chin with the palm or forearm supporting the patient's head in the area of the zygomatic process.

2. The MP or PIP joint of the physician's right index finger is placed at the soft tissue next to the articular pillar of C3.

3. The physician flexes the patient's head and neck down to the C3-4 joint space.

4. To address the sagittal plane restriction, the physician introduces a mild extension by adding a small amount of anterior translation through the C3 fulcrum contact.

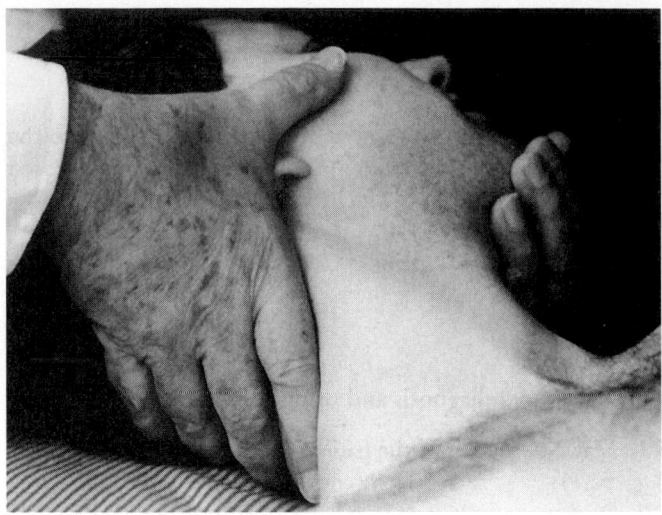

FIGURE 56.5. Technique for cervicals C2-7 with side-bending focus.

5. The physician side bends the patient's head and neck to the right until localized at the C3-4 joint space.

6. The physician rotates the head and neck to the left down to C3 to obtain a facet lock down to the somatic dysfunction, continually adjusting the side-bending and extension to maintain localization at C3.

7. The physician applies a high-velocity/low amplitude right side-bending thrust by translatory motion toward the left through the right index finger MP or PIP joint contact, aiming the thrust in a vector toward the opposite shoulder.

8. Retest the range of motion.

Typical Cervicals (C2-7), Rotational Focus

Diagnosis

C6 is flexed, side-bent right, rotated right in relationship to C7, and moves more easily in these directions

C6 = F $S_R R_R$

C6 = restricted E $S_L R_L$

Position

The patient is supine, and the physician stands to the right of the patient at the head of the table (Fig. 56.6).

Procedure

To restore physiologic range of motion to the C6 vertebral unit so that in resetting itself, appropriate physiologic motion is restored:

1. The physician's palm and fingers of the left hand cup the patient's chin with the palm and forearm supporting the patient's head in the area of the zygomatic process.

2. The MP or PIP joint of the physician's right index finger is placed at the soft tissue next to the articular pillar of C6.

3. The physician flexes the patient's head and neck down to C6 and then induces a small amount of extension by applying an anterior translation of C6 at the index finger (fulcrum contact).

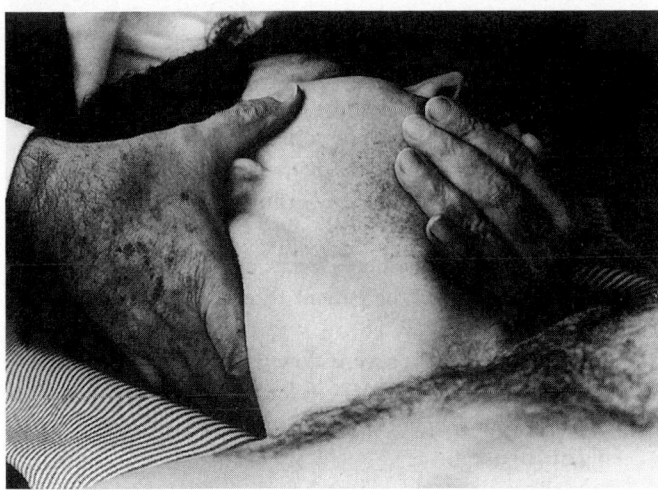

FIGURE 56.6. Technique for cervicals C2-7 with rotation focus.

4. The physician rotates the head and neck to the left (down to and including the C6 segment) to the restrictive barrier. Side bending left is achieved by keeping the patient's left temple close to the table.

5. The physician applies a high-velocity/low amplitude left rotational thrust with the vector aimed at the opposite eye and in the plane of the facets using the right hand contact.

6. Retest for motion.

Thoracic

Thoracic Single Plane: Flexion

Diagnosis

T6 is flexed relative to T7 and flexes more easily

T6 = F

T6 = restricted E

Position

The patient is supine, and the physician stands on either side of the patient, facing the head (Fig. 56.7).

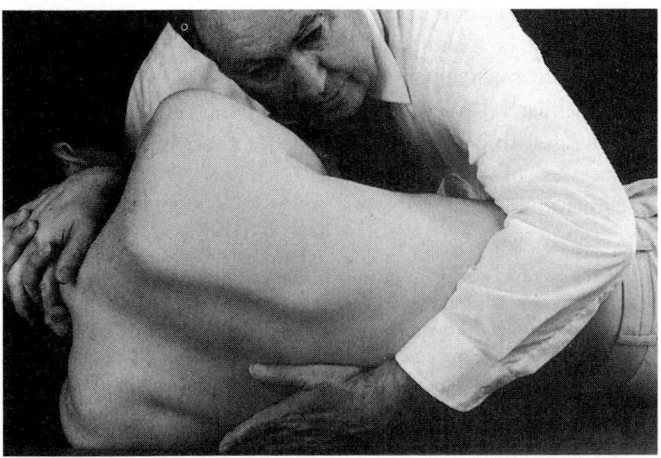

FIGURE 56.7. Hand placement for thoracic supine technique.

Procedure

To restore physiologic range of motion to the T-7 joint so that in resetting itself, appropriate physiologic extension is restored:

1. The physician asks the patient to cross his or her arms over the chest, with the arm on the opposite side opposite the physician superior, and to grasp the lateral portion of each shoulder.

2. The physician supports the patient's head and neck with the cephalad hand and flexes the patient to a point where the caudad hand can palpate motion at the dysfunctional vertebra and the joint space below it.

3. The physician makes a bilateral fulcrum with his or her thenar eminence and flexed fingers of his or her caudad hand. This fulcrum straddles the spinous processes and is placed to contact the soft tissues overlying both transverse processes of the dysfunctional vertebral unit.[1]

4. The physician positions the patient's elbows in his or her epigastric area (or a small pillow is placed between the patient's elbows and the physician's epigastric area). The physician localizes the flexion force to the midline by transferring a portion of his or her body weight until motion is focused over the caudad, fulcrum hand.

5. The patient is asked to inhale and exhale.

6. The physician applies a high-velocity/low-amplitude thrust by momentarily dropping his or her body weight with a bending of the knees, producing force with a vector straight toward the fulcrum (usually straight down toward the floor).

7. Retest the range of motion.

Thoracic Single Plane: Extension

Diagnosis

T6 is extended relative to T7 and extends more easily.

T6 = E

T6 = restricted F

Position

The patient is supine, and the physician stands on either side of the patient facing the head.

Procedure

To restore physiologic range of motion to the T6-7 joint so that in resetting itself, appropriate physiologic flexion is restored:

---

[1]Use of the hand as a fulcrum (at spinal segment level) depends on the thrust itself. In a flexion somatic dysfunction, some physicians will have the bilateral fulcrum at the level of the dysfunctional segment. This places the effective fulcrum at the level of the joint space as they roll the patient over it during the thrust maneuver. Other physicians will stabilize the segment below the dysfunctional vertebra and obtain the same effect with their thrust by less cephalad motion during the roll. Either way, the biomechanics of the thrust necessitate a confrontation of the barrier, with a gapping action at the dysfunctional joint level, reestablishing normal motion.

1. The physician asks the patient to cross his or her arms over the chest, with the arm on the opposite side of the physician superior, and to grasp the lateral portion of each shoulder.

2. The physician supports the patient's head and neck with the cephalad hand and flexes the patient to a point where the caudad hand can palpate motion at the dysfunctional vertebra and the joint space below it.

3. The physician makes a bilateral fulcrum with his or her thenar eminence and flexed fingers of his or her caudad hand. This fulcrum straddles the spinous processes and is placed to contact the soft tissues overlying both transverse processes.[2]

4. The physician positions the patient's elbows in his or her epigastric area (or a small pillow is placed between the patient's elbows and the physician's epigastric area). The physician localizes the flexion force to the midline by transferring a portion of his or her body weight until motion is focused over the caudad, fulcrum hand.

5. The patient is asked to inhale and exhale.

6. The physician applies a high-velocity/low-amplitude thrust by momentarily dropping his or her body weight with a bending of the knees, producing force with a vector approximately 45 degrees cephalad and posterior at the fulcrum.

7. Retest the range of motion.

Thoracic Multiple Plane: Type I

Diagnosis

Dextroscoliosis (left convexity) with left side-bending and right rotation

T7 is at the apex of the curve, side-bent left, rotated right in relationship to T8, and moves more easily in these directions

$T7 = N\ S_L R_R$

$T7 = \text{restricted } N\ S_R R_L$

Position

The patient is supine, and the physician stands on the left side of the patient (the side opposite the posterior transverse process) (Fig. 56.8).

Procedure

To restore physiologic motion to the T7-8 joint:

1. The physician has the patient cross his or her arms over the chest, with the arm on the opposite side of the physician superior, and grasp the lateral portion of each shoulder.

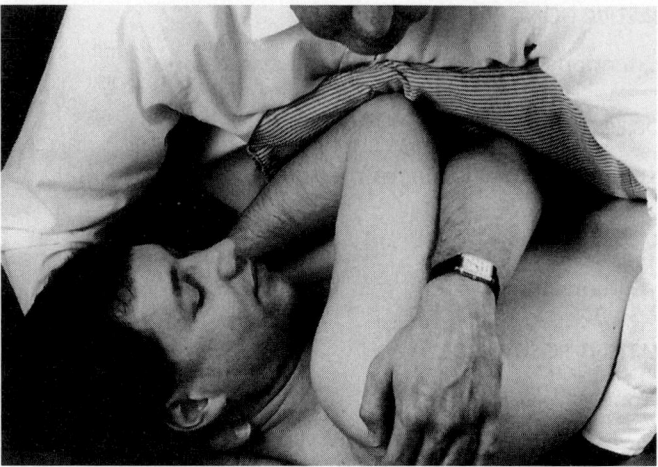

FIGURE 56.8. Thoracic multiple plane technique, type I.

2. The physician's cephalad hand rotates the patient's opposite shoulder and thorax toward him or her.

3. The physician reaches across the patient and places the thenar eminence of the open flat caudad hand on the patient's right T7 transverse process (this is the transverse process that is relatively posterior in position). This is to be used as the fulcrum.

4. The physician supports the patient's head, neck, and shoulders with the cephalad hand and flexes the patient through T7 to the dysfunctional joint space (T7-8).

5. The physician positions the patient's elbows in his or her epigastric area (or a small pillow is placed between the patient's elbows and the physician's epigastric area).

6. The physician side bends the patient's spine right, down to the T7 to T8 junction, and the side-bending, flexion, and rotation forces are localized at the T7 fulcrum by adjusting his or her body weight through his or her epigastric region and the patient's elbows.

7. The patient is asked to inhale, and the physician increases the localization as the patient exhales.

8. At the end of exhalation, the physician applies a high-velocity/low-amplitude thrust through the epigastric contact, aimed straight down toward the fulcrum hand (usually straight down toward the floor). This vector passes through the patient's elbows, around the thorax, and to the T7 fulcrum. This is accomplished more by a momentary drop of the physician's weight then a squeezing or compression of the patient.

9. Retest the range of motion.

Note: These techniques are sometimes referred to by their colloquial name, the Kirksville Krunch.

Thoracic Multiple Plane: Type II, Flexion

Diagnosis

T5 is flexed, side bent right, and rotated right in relationship to T6, and moves more easily in these directions

$T5 = F\ S_R R_R$

$T5 = \text{restricted } E\ S_L R_L$

---

[2]Use of the hand as a fulcrum (at spinal segment level) depends on the thrust itself. In a flexion somatic dysfunction, some physicians will have the bilateral fulcrum at the level of the dysfunctional segment. This places the effective fulcrum at the level of the joint space as they roll the patient over it during the thrust maneuver. Other physicians will stabilize the segment below the dysfunctional vertebra and obtain the same effect with their thrust by less cephalad motion during the roll. Either way, the biomechanics of the thrust necessitate a confrontation of the barrier, with a gapping action at the dysfunctional joint level, reestablishing normal motion.

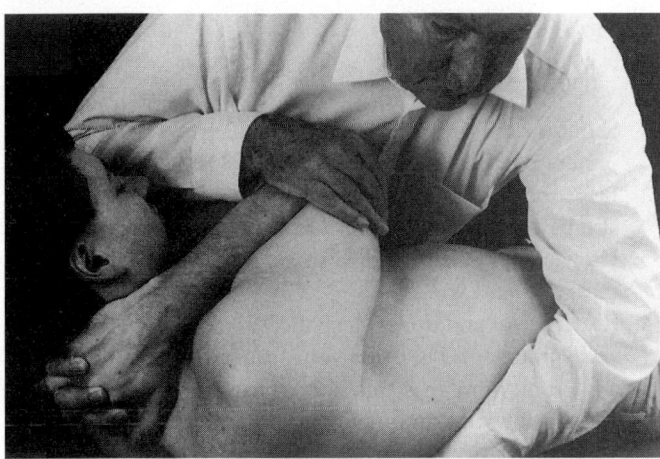

FIGURE 56.9. Thoracic multiple plane technique, type II, flexion.

Position

The patient is supine, and the physician stands at the left side of the patient (the side opposite the posterior transverse process of the somatic dysfunction) (Fig. 56.9).

Procedure

To restore physiologic motion to the T5-6 joint:

1. The physician asks the patient to place his or her hands behind the neck with fingers interlaced. This can also be done by asking the patient to cross his or her arms over the chest, with the arm on the opposite side of the physician superior, and to grasp the lateral portion of each shoulder.
2. The physician uses his or her cephalad hand to rotate the patient's opposite shoulder and thorax toward him or her.
3. The physician reaches across the patient and places the thenar eminence of the open, flat caudad hand on the patient's right T5 transverse process (this is the transverse process that is relatively posterior in position). This is to be used as the fulcrum.
4. The physician supports the patient's head, neck, and shoulders with the cephalad hand and flexes the patient through T5 to the dysfunctional joint (T5-6).
5. The physician positions the patient's elbows in his or her epigastric area (or a small pillow is placed between the patient's elbows and the physician's epigastric area).
6. The physician places the cephalad hand under the patient's neck and cervicothoracic junction to induce a component of left side-bending at the T5-6 joint space. The side-bending, flexion, and rotation forces are localized at the T7 fulcrum (thenar eminence) by adjusting his or her body weight through his or her epigastric region and the patient's elbows.
7. The patient is asked to deeply inhale and exhale. The physician increases localization as the patient exhales.
8. At the end of exhalation, the physician applies a high-velocity/low-amplitude thrust through the epigastric contact, aimed straight down toward the fulcrum hand (usually straight down toward the floor). This vector passes through the patient's elbows, around the thorax, and to the T7 fulcrum. This

is accomplished more by a momentary drop of the physician's weight than a squeezing or compression of the patient.
9. Retest the range of motion.

Multiple Plane: Type II, Extension

Diagnosis

T7 is extended, side-bent right, rotated right in relationship to T8, and moves more easily in these directions

$$T7 = E\ S_R R_R$$
$$T7 = \text{restricted}\ F\ S_L R_L$$

Position

The patient is supine, and the physician stands on the left side of the patient (the side opposite the posterior transverse process (Fig. 56.10).

Procedure

To restore physiologic range of motion to the T7-8 joint:

1. The physician asks the patient to interlace his or her hands behind the neck. (This can also be done with the arms crossed over the chest.)
2. The physician's cephalad hand is used to rotate the patient's opposite shoulder and thorax toward him or her.
3. The physician reaches across and under the patient with his or her caudad hand to contact the right transverse process of T8 with the thenar eminence. This will be used as a fulcrum. Note that this is the transverse process of the segment below the dysfunctional joint space.
4. The patient's head, neck, and shoulders are supported by the physician's cephalad hand, and the patient's spine is flexed down through T7 to the dysfunctional joint space (T7-8).
5. The physician localizes the forces over the fulcrum (thenar eminence) by adjusting his or her weight over the patient's elbows through the epigastric contact.
6. The cephalad hand under the patient's neck and cervicothoracic junction is used to induce a component of left side-bending at the T7-8 joint space.

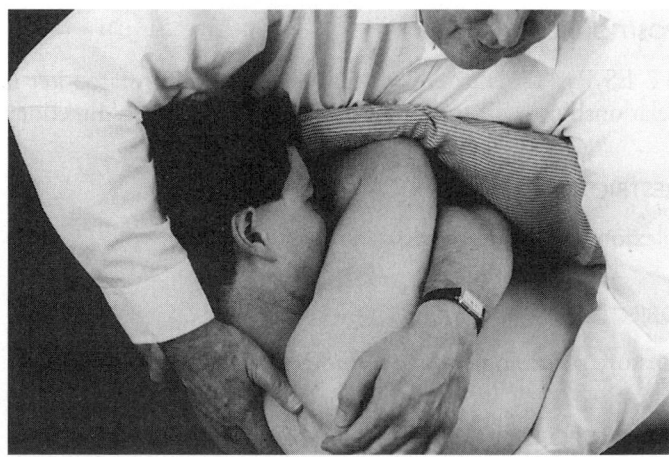

FIGURE 56.10. Thoracic multiple plane technique, type II, extension.

7. The patient is instructed to deeply inhale and exhale. The physician increases localization as the patient exhales.

8. A high-velocity/low-amplitude thrust toward your fulcrum is applied at the end of exhalation. The thrust is in a vector aimed 45 degrees between the floor and the patient's head. The thrust is produced more by a momentary drop of your body weight than by squeezing or compression of the patient.

9. Retest the range of motion.

Multiple Plane: Crossed Hand, Midthoracic

Diagnosis

T8 is flexed, side-bent right, rotated right in relationship to T9, and moves more easily in these directions

T8 = F $S_R R_R$

T8 = restricted E $S_L R_L$

Position

The patient is prone, and the physician stands on the right side of the patient (the side of the posterior transverse process) (Fig. 56.11). Note: A pillow may be placed under the under the thorax to increase thoracic kyphosis.

Procedure

To restore physiologic range of motion to the T8-9 joint:

1. The patient is supine with his or her arms at the sides.

2. The physician places his or her caudad hand over the T8 vertebra, fingers pointing toward the patient's head, and the hypothenar eminence or pisiform region contacting its right transverse process (this transverse process is posterior), and moves the contact into a more cephalad position.

3. The left (opposite) transverse process of the segment (T9) below the dysfunctional joint space is contacted with the thenar eminence of the physician's cephalad hand, fingers point toward the patient's feet, and moves this contact into a more caudad position. This establishes the crossed-arm technique.

4. The patient is asked to inhale, then exhale, through more

than one cycle as you localize your forces. Pressure through the hand over the posterior transverse process is in a cephalad and downward (toward the floor) direction. Pressure through the T9 hand is caudad and downward (toward the floor).

5. Rotation is induced by the posteroanterior forces. A translatory force is also induced to the entire region by moving the hands toward you, therefore decreasing the dysfunctional side-bending.

6. A high-velocity/low-amplitude thrust in the directions already specified is applied by using a momentary drop of the physician's body weight to transmit the force through wrists and elbows that are held rigid.

7. Retest the range of motion.

Note: This commonly used thoracic technique has earned the sobriquet of the Texas Twist.

Multiple Plane: Crossed Hand, Upper Thoracic (T1-4)

Diagnosis

T1 is flexed, side-bent left, rotated left in relationship to T2, and moves more easily in these directions

T1 = F $S_L R_L$

T1 = restricted E $S_R R_R$

Position

The patient is prone, and the physician stands on the left side of the patient at the head of the table (Fig. 56.12).

Procedure

To restore physiologic range of motion to the T1-2 joint:

1. The physician side bends the patient's neck to the right (side of restricted side-bending) through the level of T1 to the dysfunctional joint space, and places the patient's chin on the table.

2. The physician's right hand slightly rotates the patient's head to the left to obtain ligamentous tension locking.

3. The right hand of the physician is on the left side of the

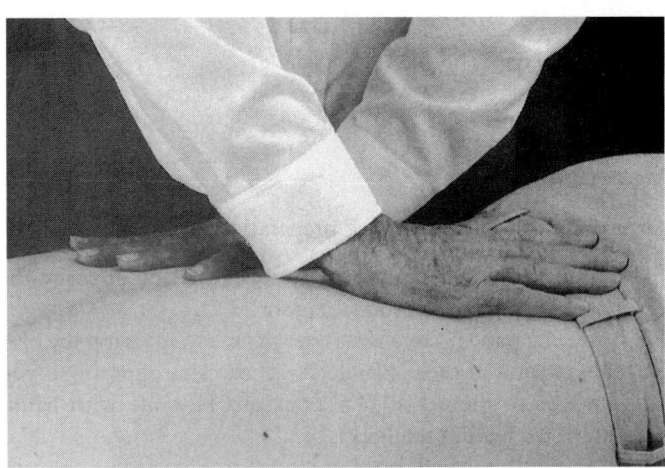

FIGURE 56.11. Thoracic technique with crossed hand.

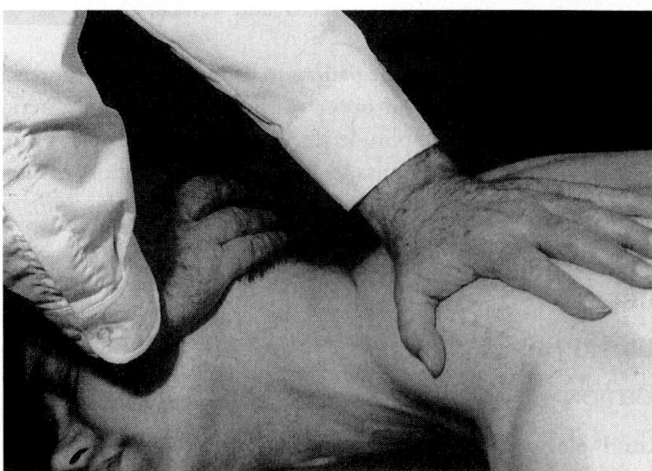

FIGURE 56.12. Upper thoracic technique with crossed hand.

patient's head and the hypothenar eminence (pisiform region) or thenar eminence of his or her left hand is placed over the left transverse process of T1. This is the crossed hand position.

4. The patient is asked to inhale and exhale several times as the physician takes up the tissue slack, localizing forces.

5. A high-velocity/low-amplitude thrust is applied through the pisiform with its vector directed in a lateral, posteroanterior (toward the floor), and caudad direction. This side bends the patient in a direction opposite the dysfunctional side-bending. The hand on the head is used to stabilize it as the thrust is being applied and transmitted through the T1 transverse process. The posteroanterior force on the patient's left transverse process of T1 induces right rotation while the stabilizing hand on the head effects a slight relative rotation in an opposite direction.

6. Retest the range of motion.

Multiple Plane, Pillow Fulcrum: Flexion

Diagnosis
T4 is flexed, side-bent right, rotated right in relationship to T5, and moves more easily in these directions

T4 = F $S_R R_R$
T4 = restricted E $S_R R_R$

Position
The patient is seated (or standing), and the physician stands behind the patient (Fig. 56.13).

Procedure
To restore physiologic range of motion to the T4-5 joint:

1. The patient places his or her hands behind the neck with the fingers interlaced.

2. To control the movements of the patient, the physician places one arm under the axilla on one side of the patient and places the fingers of that extremity on the dorsal aspect of the patient's wrist.

3. The physician places a small pillow between his or her epigastric region (or chest) and the right transverse process of T4.

4. The physician puts his or her other arm under the patient's other axilla and places the fingers of that hand on the dorsal aspect of the patient's wrist. Note: Do not use the hand contacts to pull down and induce spinal flexion (the hand only rests on the patient's wrists).

5. Extension is induced down to and including T4, using your epigastric region and the pillow as your fulcrum.

6. The physician induces left side-bending through right translatory motion at the level of the pillow fulcrum. The pressure of the pillow itself will direct rotation of the patient's vertebra to the left.

7. The patient is asked to inhale and exhale, relax the shoulders and back, and "let the tummy hang." As the patient relaxes, the localization at the fulcrum must be retained.

8. At the end of expiration, ask the patient to bring the elbows

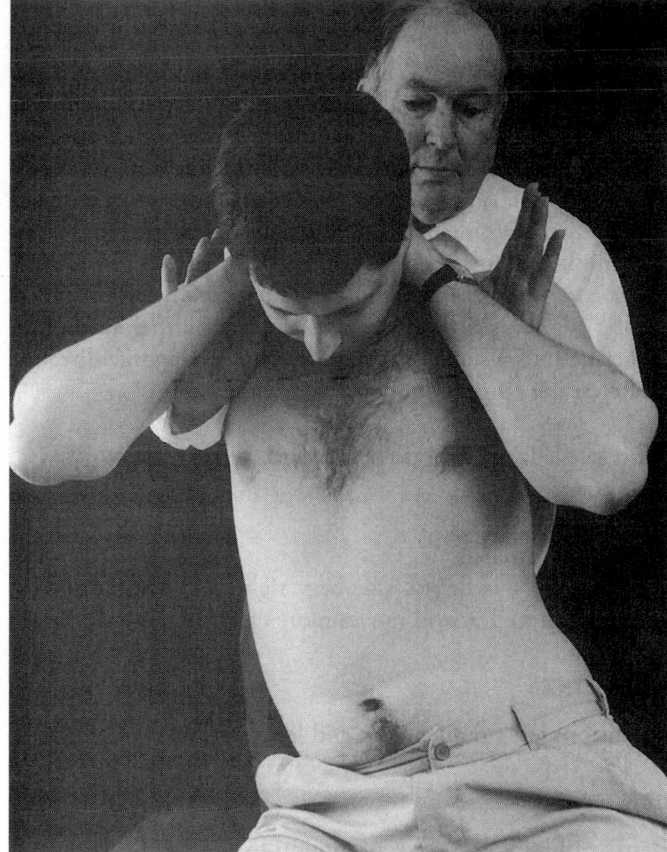

FIGURE 56.13. Thoracic multiple plane technique, flexion.

together. As you feel localization occur in the tissues at the fulcrum, use an anterior and superior high-velocity/low-amplitude thrust through your epigastrium and the pillow. Simultaneously induce superior and posterior traction through your arms (a lifting motion). Some physicians have developed an epigastric muscular contraction that they use to direct the thrust.

9. Retest the range of motion.

Multiple Plane, Pillow Fulcrum: Extension

Diagnosis
T6 is extended, side-bent left, rotated left in relationship to T7, and moves more easily in these directions

T6 = E $S_L R_L$
T6 = restricted F $S_R R_R$

Position
The patient is seated (or standing), and the physician stands behind the patient (Fig. 56.14).

Procedure
To restore physiologic range of motion to the T6-7 joint:

1. The patient places his or her hands behind the neck with the fingers interlaced.

2. To control the movements of the patient, place one arm under

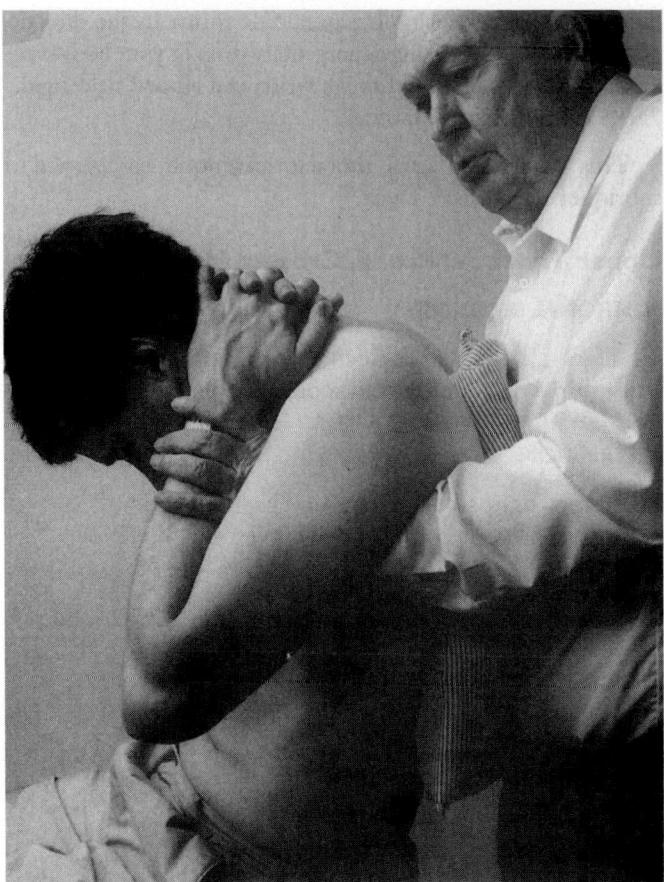

FIGURE 56.14. Thoracic multiple plane technique, extension.

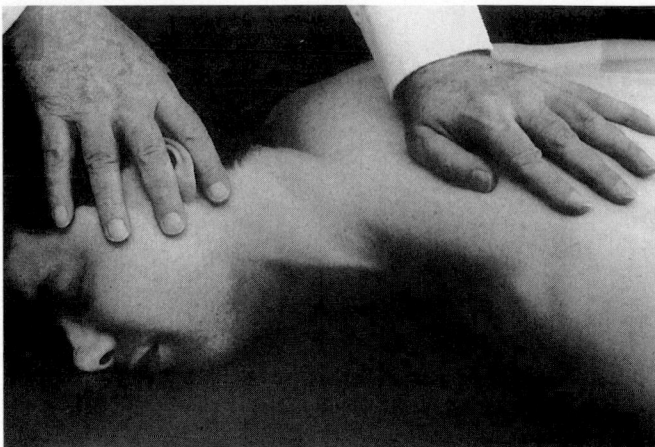

FIGURE 56.15. Rib 1 technique, prone.

the axilla on one side of the patient and place the fingers of that extremity on the dorsal aspect of the patient's wrist.

3. The physician places a small pillow between his or her epigastric region (or chest) and the segment to be treated (T6 vertebral unit).

4. The physician puts his or her other arm under the patient's other axilla and places the fingers of that hand on the dorsal aspect of the patient's wrist. Note: Do not use the hand contacts to pull down and induce spinal flexion (the hand only rests on the patient's wrists).

5. The physician induces flexion of the patient's spine by posterior translation at T6. This is accomplished when the patient slumps forward, letting the "tummy drop toward the floor," and when the physician pulls the patient's upper body backward over the pillow fulcrum.

6. The physician induces right side-bending through left translatory motion at T6. The pressure of the pillow contact itself will induce right rotation.

7. The patient inhales and exhales, relaxes the shoulders and back, and "lets the tummy drop toward the floor."

8. At end-expiration, the physician asks the patient to bring the elbows together. As localization occurs in the tissues anterior to the pillow fulcrum, an anterior and superior high-velocity/low-amplitude thrust through the epigastrium and the pillow is applied. Simultaneously, the physician lifts

upward and backward where the arms contact the patient's axilla (a lifting motion).

9. Retest the range of motion.

Ribs

Rib 1: Prone

Diagnosis

Rib 1 elevated on the left (superior shear, superior translation)
Posterior portion (tubercle) of left rib 1 appears elevated, with surrounding tissue texture changes and tenderness
Cervicothoracic junction is usually side-bent right[3]
Elevated left rib 1
Caudad motion of right rib 1 tubercle is restricted when pressure is applied

Position

The patient is prone, and the physician stands to the right side of the patient at the head of the table (Fig. 56.15).

Procedure

To restore physiologic range of motion to the T1/rib 1 costovertebral joint:

1. The physician places his or her right hand on the left side of the patient's head and the thenar eminence or hypothenar eminence (pisiform region) of his or her left hand over the tubercle of the left rib 1. Note: The physician's arms are crossed, with the right arm superior.

2. Using the chin as a pivot, the patient's head is rotated left to obtain ligamentous tension locking.

3. The physician then side bends the patient's head and neck to the right through the level of T1 to the dysfunctional joint space.

---

[3]These same findings are also present with a fascial dysfunction involving presence of left side-bending and rotation at the cervicothoracic junction (thoracic inlet).

4. The patient is asked to inhale and exhale several times. The physician takes up the tissue slack as the patient exhales, localizing the forces.

5. The physician applies a high-velocity/low-amplitude thrust through his or her left thenar eminence contact with the vector directed in a posteroanterior and caudad direction. The hand on the head stabilizes it as the thrust with the other hand is transmitted through the tubercle of the patient's first rib. A small amount of right rotation to T1 is induced by slight opposite rotatory motions through the pisiform or thenar eminence on the left transverse process of T1 while the hand on the head induces slight rotation in an opposite direction.

6. Retest the range of motion.

Rib 1: Supine

Diagnosis
Rib 1 elevated on the right (superior shear, superior translation)

Posterior portion (tubercle) of right rib 1 appears elevated, with surrounding tissue texture changes and tenderness

Cervicothoracic junction is usually side bent left[4]

Elevated right rib 1

Caudad motion of right rib 1 tubercle is restricted when pressure is applied

Position
The patient is supine, and the physician stands at the head of the table (Fig. 56.16).

Procedure
To restore physiologic range of motion to the T1/rib 1 costovertebral joint:

1. The physician places the MP or PIP joint of his or her right index finger on the upper surface of the tubercle of the right first rib.

2. The physician's left hand cups the left side of the patient's head.

3. The physician rotates the patient's head and neck left to the level of the T1/rib 1 joint space.

4. The patient's head and neck are then side bent right to the level of the tubercle.

5. The patient's head and neck are then flexed to the level of T1.

6. The patient is asked to inhale and exhale. The physician localizes the forces as the patient exhales.

7. A high-velocity/low-amplitude thrust with the physician's right hand contact is directed medially, inferior, and posterior. The index finger of this hand is the fulcrum that side bends the head and neck to the right by using a component of flexion and slight rotation to the left.

8. Retest the range of motion.

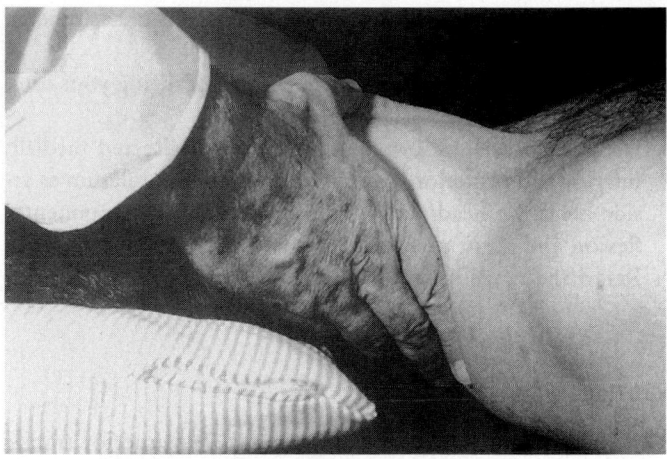

FIGURE 56.16. Rib 1 technique, supine.

Rib 1: Seated

Diagnosis
Right rib 1 is elevated on the right (superior shear, superior translation)

Posterior portion (tubercle) of right rib 1 appears elevated, with surrounding tissue texture changes and tenderness

Cervicothoracic junction is usually side bent left[5]

Elevated right rib 1

Caudad motion of right rib 1 tubercle when pressure is applied

Position
The patient is seated, and the physician stands behind the patient (Fig. 56.17).

Procedure
1. The physician places his or her left foot on the table and drapes the patient's left arm over a pillow that has been placed on the physician's left knee or thigh.

2. The physician's left elbow is placed in front of the patient's shoulder with the forearm contacting the left side of the patient's face and the hand over the top of the head.

3. The physician's right palm is placed on the patient's right shoulder with the first metacarpophalangeal joint contacting the tubercle of rib 1.

4. The patient's head and neck are slowly rotated and side bent right to the level of the rib, with simultaneous downward pressure on the rib. A slight translatory movement of the patient left and posteriorly (using the physician's left knee contact) may aid in localization.

5. The patient is asked to inhale and exhale. The physician localizes the forces as the patient exhales. Sometimes a slight rotation of the head and neck to the left may further free the first rib head.

---

[4]These same findings are also present with a fascial dysfunction involving presence of right side-bending and rotation at the cervicothoracic junction (thoracic inlet).

[5]These same findings are also present with a fascial dysfunction involving presence of left side-bending and rotation at the cervicothoracic junction (thoracic inlet).

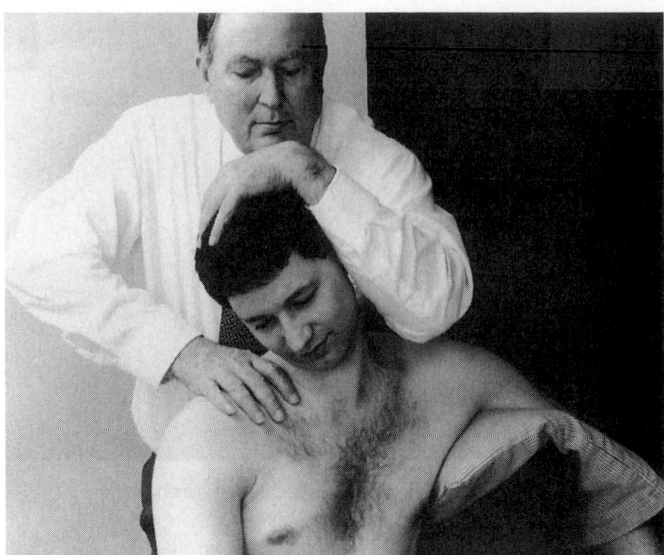

FIGURE 56.17. Rib 1 technique, seated.

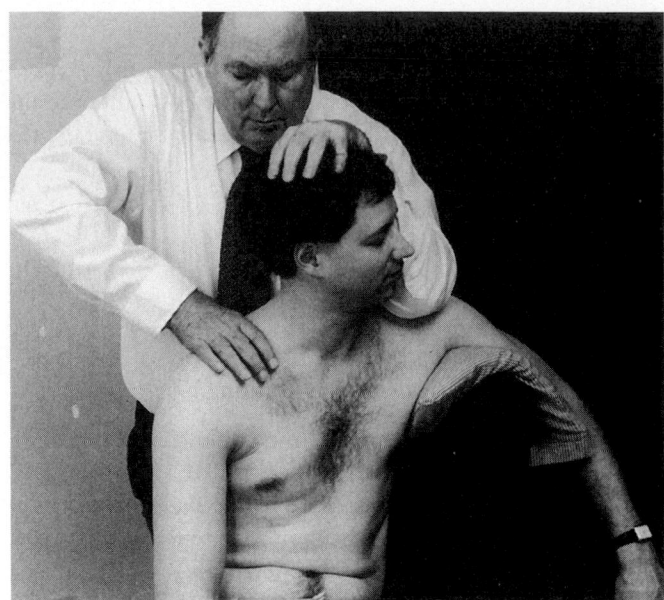

FIGURE 56.18. Rib 2 technique, seated.

6. A high-velocity/low-amplitude thrust is performed through the physician's right MP joint, with a vector directed posteroinferiorly and medially while right side-bending/rotation of the neck is slightly increased.

7. Retest the range of motion.

Rib 2: Seated

Diagnosis

Right rib 2 is elevated on the right

Posterior portion (tubercle) of right rib 2 appears elevated, with surrounding tissue texture changes and tenderness

Right rib 2 is elevated

Caudad motion of right rib 2 tubercle when pressure is applied

Position

The patient is seated, and the physician stands behind the patient (Fig. 56.18).

Procedure

To restore physiologic range of motion to the rib 2 costotransverse joint:

1. The physician places his or her left foot on the table and drapes the patient's left arm over a pillow that has been placed on the left knee or thigh of the physician.

2. The physician places his or her left elbow in front of the patient's left shoulder with the forearm contacting the left side of the patient's face and places the hand over the top of the patient's head.

3. The physician's right hand (dorsum up) is placed on the patient's right shoulder with the thumb contacting the tubercle of the patient's rib 2. The thumb contact is the fulcrum.

4. The patient's head and neck are slowly rotated left, disengaging the rib head as T1 rotates away from it. The region is side bent

to the right to the level of the rib (reducing influence of the scalenes) while exerting simultaneous downward pressure on the patient's right first rib with the fulcrum. The rotation movement ceases when the rib exhibits less resistance to this downward pressure.

5. The patient is asked inhale and exhale. The physician localizes forces as the patient exhales.

6. A high-velocity/low-amplitude thrust applied through the physician's right MP joint contact is directed inferiorly and medially with a small posterior vector.

7. Retest the range of motion.

Ribs 2–10, Inhalation or Exhalation: Supine

Diagnosis

Exhalation lesion: the posterior inferior border of the rib angle is more prominent

Inhalation lesion: the posterior superior border of the rib angle is more prominent

Exhalation rib

Inhalation rib

Rib restricted in exhalation (If an inhalation lesion, exhalation motion is restricted)

Rib restricted in inhalation (If an exhalation lesion, inhalation motion is restricted)

Position

The patient is supine, and the physician stands on the opposite side of the patient's dysfunctional rib.

Procedure

To restore physiologic range of motion to the costovertebral joint:

1. The physician asks the patient to cross his or her arms with the opposite arm superior and the hands on the lateral aspects of

the shoulders. (This can also be accomplished with the hands interlaced behind the neck.)

2. The physician's cephalad hand rotates the patient's opposite shoulder and thorax toward him or her.

3. The physician reaches across and under the patient, placing the thenar eminence of his or her caudad hand posterior to the posterior angle of the dysfunctional rib.[6]

4. With the patient's head, neck, and shoulders supported by the physician's cephalad hand, the patient's spine is flexed toward, and slightly side bent away from the dysfunctional rib.

5. Forces are localized by rolling the patient's body over the fulcrum, past the midline, focusing the weight between the epigastrium and the thenar eminence. A pillow between the physician's epigastric region and the patient's elbows may be used if desired.

6. The patient is asked to deeply inhale, and the physician increases the localization as the patient exhales.

7. A high-velocity/low-amplitude thrust at the end of exhalation is delivered through the physician's epigastric contact and the patient's thorax. The thrust has a vector that is directed straight down and is produced more by a momentary drop of your body weight than by squeezing or compression of the patient.

8. Retest the rib angle for tenderness and for motion during breathing.

Ribs 2–10: Crossed Hand, Prone

Diagnosis

Rib 8 on the right is held in exhalation

Lateral or anterior elevation (during inhalation) in comparison with the corresponding contralateral rib

(Rib 8 major motion = bucket-handle mechanics; minor motion = pump-handle mechanics)

Exhalation right rib 8

Right rib 8 restricted in inhalation

Position

The patient is prone, and the physician stands on the side of the patient's dysfunctional rib (Fig. 56.19).

Procedure

To restore physiologic range of motion to the rib at the costovertebral articulation, allowing free lateral and anterior elevation of the rib during the inhalation phase:

1. Ask the patient turn his or her head away and place arms at the sides.

2. The physician moves the patient's torso and, if necessary, hips

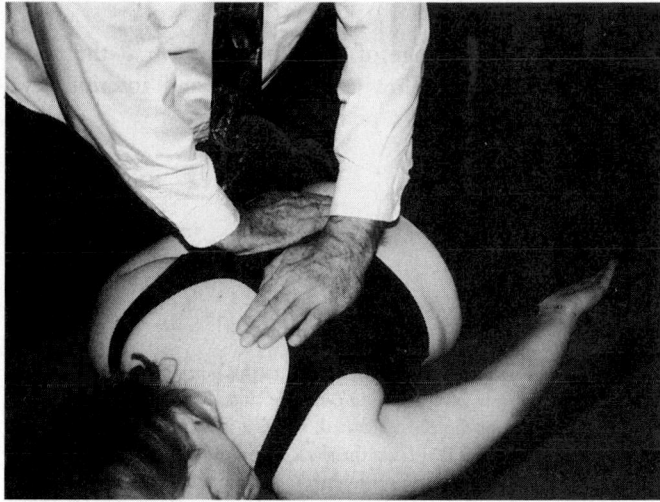

FIGURE 56.19. Ribs 2-10 technique, prone.

away from him or her to induce left side-bending, with the apex at the level of the dysfunctional rib.

3. The physician's hypothenar eminence or pisiform region of the right hand contacts the posterior right eighth rib, with fingers pointing caudad.

4. The palmar surface of the physician's left hand contacts the paravertebral area over the opposite rib (left rib 8), with fingers pointing toward the patient's head. This hand will serve as a stabilizing force. (This is a crossed-arm technique.)

5. The patient is asked to inhale, then exhale through more than one cycle as the physician localizes the forces.

6. Pressure is applied in a caudad and anterior vector with the physician's right hand and toward the floor over the rib and paravertebral area with the left hand.

7. At end of exhalation, a high-velocity/low-amplitude thrust is applied with the physician's right hand contact and has a vector that is directed caudally and anteriorly.

8. Retest the range of motion.

Ribs 11 and 12: Prone

Diagnosis

Rib 11 on the right is held in inhalation; its position is more posterior than that of the opposite rib

The tenth intercostal space is decreased in comparison to the contralateral side

Inhalation right 11th rib

Right 11th rib is restricted exhalation (anterior caliper motion on exhalation but it will rotate backward on inspiration) and decreased lowering during exhalation (bucket-handle motion)

Position

The patient is prone, and the physician stands to the left side (opposite the dysfunctional rib) of the patient, at the level of the patient's hip (Fig. 56.20).

---

[6]The actual contact and vector of force applied to this portion of the rib to engage the barrier benefits from applying pump-handle mechanics (where, in inhalation, the anterior portion of the rib is elevated while it is depressed in back). Apply your contact in a manner that takes the slack out of the soft tissues and posterior costal articulations, drawing inferiorly on the superior rib border for exhalation somatic dysfunction, or pushing superiorly on the inferior border for inhalation somatic dysfunction.

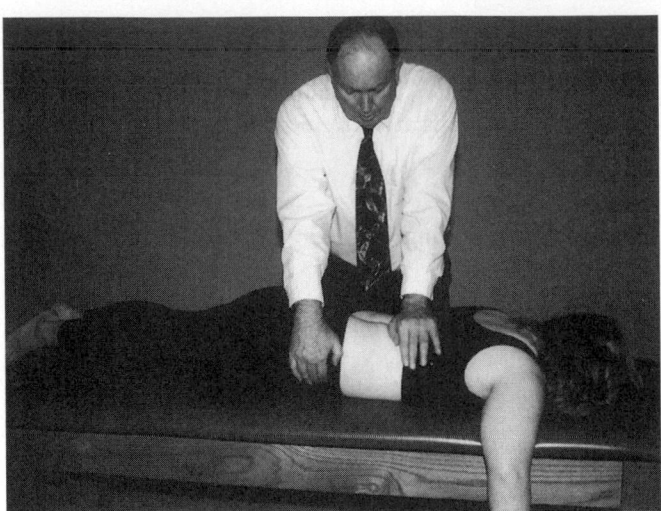

FIGURE 56.20. Ribs 11-12 technique, prone.

Procedure

To restore physiologic range of motion to the rib at its costovertebral articulation so that it will exhibit both anterior and posterior rotatory caliper motion and increased lateral depression (bucket handle) during exhalation:

1. The physician side bends left the patient's thorax by pulling first the feet, then the shoulders, to the left. The convexity has its apex at the dysfunctional rib.
2. For this *inhalation* rib treatment, the patient's right arm is at his or her side. (If this were treatment for a right *exhalation* right 11th rib, the right arm would be hyperabducted to the side of the patient's head.)
3. The physician contacts the most medial aspect of the patient's right rib 11 with the thenar eminence of the cephalad hand.
4. The physician's caudad hand grasps the patient's opposite anterior superior iliac spine.
5. A longitudinal stretch is applied between the hand contacts sufficient to take the slack out of the tissues. This will usually lift the hip off the table by a few inches.
6. The physician's cephalad hand pushes the right 11th rib anterior, lateral, and superior, localizing the disengagement force on the rib.
7. The patient is asked to inhale and then exhale. The physician further localizes the forces as the patient exhales.
8. At end of exhalation, a high-velocity/low-amplitude thrust is applied through the thenar eminence of the physician's cephalad hand with a vector directed anteriorly, laterally, and superiorly. Alternative: Ask the patient to cough instead of applying the thrust.
9. Retest the range of motion.

Note: The hip is used to pull the lateral aspect of the rib posteroinferiorly through stretch of the quadratus lumborum muscle and associated fascia. The cephalad hand's superior thrust will torque the medial aspect of the rib around an effective fulcrum, which is slightly lateral to your hand.

Thoracolumbar Region

Type I: Lateral Recumbent (Posterior Transverse Process Down) (T10-L5)

Diagnosis

L3 is at the apex of a left side-bending group curve (dextrorotoscoliosis), side-bent left, rotated right in relationship to L4, and moves more easily in these directions

$$L3 = N\ S_L R_R$$
$$L3 = \text{restricted } N\ S_R R_L$$

Position

The patient is lateral recumbent, posterior transverse process down, and the physician stands in front of the patient (Fig. 56.21).

Procedure

To restore left side-bending and left rotation with the patient in a (sagittal) neutral position:

1. The physician flexes the patient's legs until motion is palpable at the L3-4 joint space.
2. The inferior leg (the leg next to the table) is straightened. The foot of the superior leg is placed behind the knee of the inferior leg.
3. The physician anteriorly rotates the patient's torso by pulling anteriorly on the right (lower) arm until rotatory motion is palpable at L3.
4. That same arm is then pulled caudad to induce right side-bending down to the L3-4 joint space.
5. The physician's caudad forearm is placed over the area inferior to the patient's iliac crest.
6. The physician's cephalad forearm is placed in the patient's uppermost axilla.
7. The fingers of one or both hands monitor the forces localized at the L3-4 articulation.
8. The patient is asked to inhale and exhale. The physician continues to localize the forces as the patient exhales and observes

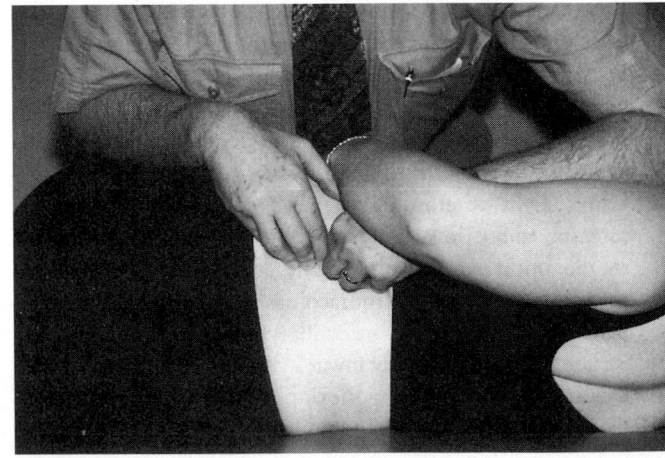

FIGURE 56.21. Lumbar type I technique, posterior transverse process down.

the direction in which the pelvis moves with exhalation. The structure of the patient's facets determines the optimal direction of thrust. If the primary motion observed is rotation, then the thrust will have more of a rotatory component. If the primary motion is side-bending, then the thrust should have more of a side-bending component.

9. A high-velocity/low-amplitude thrust is applied with the physician's caudad forearm contact and has a vector toward the physician's knees. The thrust is by momentarily dropping the patient's body weight, thereby rotating the lumbar region left and side-bending right up through L3. Although the cephalad arm mainly serves as a stabilizing force, it may simultaneously add a small component of left rotation and right side-bending. Note: Too much torsion by opposite motions can injure the patient's shoulder region.

10. Retest the range of motion.

Type I: Lateral Recumbent (Posterior Transverse Process Up) (T10-L5)

Diagnosis

L3 is at the apex of a left side-bending group curve (dextro-rotoscoliosis), is side-bent left, rotated right in relationship to L4, and moves more easily in these directions

L3 = N $S_L R_R$

L3 = restricted N $S_L R_R$

Position

The patient is lateral recumbent with the posterior transverse process of the dysfunctional unit "up." The physician stands in front of the patient (Fig. 56.22).

Procedure

To restore physiologic range of motion to the L3-4 joint:

1. The physician flexes the patient's legs until motion is palpated at the L3-4 joint space.
2. The inferior leg is straightened, and the foot of the superior leg is placed behind the knee of the other leg.
3. The physician pulls the patient's left arm superiorly and slightly forward to reduce left side-bending (and/or induce right side-bending).

4. The physician places the forearm of his or her caudad arm over an area inferior to the iliac crest.
5. The physician places his or her cephalad forearm in the patient's uppermost axilla.
6. The fingers of one or both hands monitor motion at the L3-4 articulation.
7. Using slight anterosuperior pressure through his or her caudad forearm, the physician rotates the patient's hips and lumbar spine to the left to the point where rotation at L4 is palpated. Simultaneously, the thoracolumbar spine is rotated to the right by light pressure through the forearm that is contacting the patient's axilla.
8. The physician slightly rotates the patient toward him or her while maintaining the localization (side-bending, flexion, rotation).
9. The patient is asked to inhale and exhale. The physician takes up tissue slack and maintains localization during exhalation.
10. A high-velocity/low-amplitude thrust through the physician's caudad forearm, by momentarily dropping his or her body weight, is directed toward the table, producing right side-bending. The physician's cephalad arm mainly stabilizes the patient's torso, although a slight simultaneous component of left rotation and right side-bending may occur.
11. Retest the range of motion.

Type II, Extension: Lateral Recumbent (Posterior Transverse Process Up) (T10-L5)

Diagnosis

L3 is extended, side-bent right, rotated right in relationship to L4, and moves more easily in these directions

L3 = E $S_R R_R$

L3 = restricted F $S_L R_L$

Position

The patient is left lateral recumbent, and the physician stands in front of the patient (Fig. 56.23).

Procedure

To restore physiologic range of motion to the L3-4 joint:

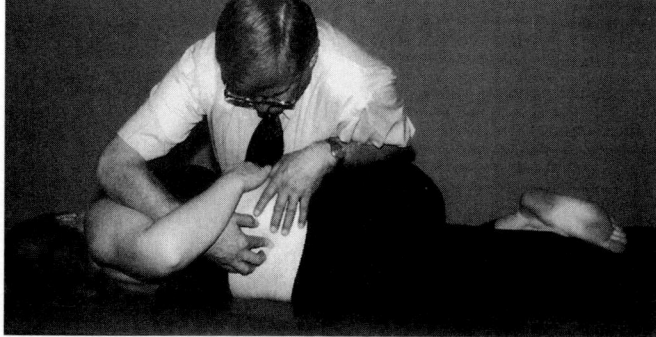

FIGURE 56.22. Lumbar type I technique, posterior transverse process up.

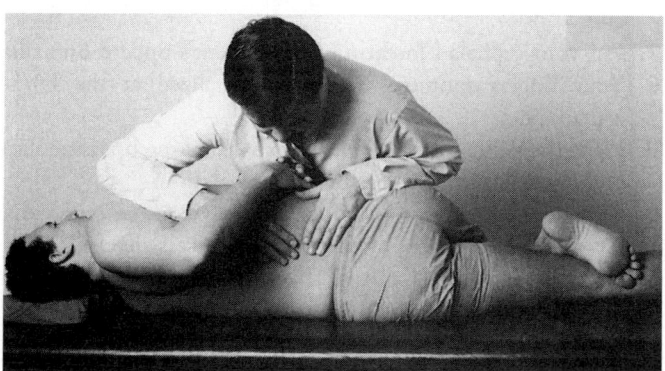

FIGURE 56.23. Lumbar type II technique, posterior transverse process up.

1. The physician flexes the patient's legs until motion is palpated at the dysfunctional transverse process (L3).
2. The inferior leg is straightened and the superior (upper most) foot is hooked into the lower leg's popliteal fossa.
3. The physician rotates the patient's torso (by pulling the left arm) down to, but not including, the dysfunctional vertebral segment as the caudad hand monitors the posteriorly rotated transverse process.
4. The physician places his or her caudad forearm on the patient's iliac crest just superior to the posterior superior iliac spines (PSIS). At least one finger continues to monitor the dysfunctional segment.
5. The physician's cephalad arm is placed in the patient's axilla beneath the patient's upper arm to stabilize the thorax.
6. The patient is slightly rotated toward the physician while localization is continued (side-bending, flexion, rotation).
7. The patient is asked to inhale and exhale. The physician takes up tissue slack and maintains localization during exhalation.
8. The physician performs a high-velocity/low-amplitude thrust through the caudad forearm by momentarily dropping his or her body weight toward the floor, thereby side bending the lumbar region to the left. The physician's cephalad arm mainly stabilizes the torso, although a slight simultaneous component of right rotation and right side-bending may occur.
9. Retest the range of motion.

Type II, Extension: Lateral Recumbent (Posterior Transverse Process Down) (T10-L5)

Diagnosis
L3 is extended, side-bent right, rotated right in relationship to L4, and moves more easily in these directions

$$L3 = E\ S_R R_R$$
$$L3 = \text{restricted } F\ S_L R_L$$

Position
The patient is right lateral recumbent (posterior transverse process down), and the physician stands in front of the patient (Fig. 56.24).

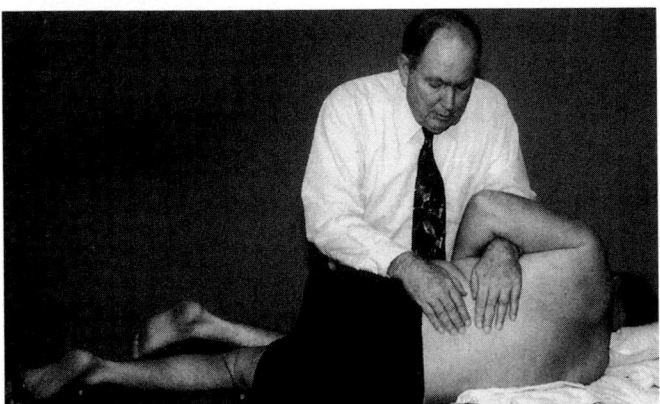

FIGURE 56.24. Thoracolumbar type II technique, posterior transverse process down.

Procedure
1. The patient's legs are flexed until motion is palpable at the L3-4 joint space.
2. The inferior leg is straightened and the foot is placed behind the knee of the other leg.
3. The physician pulls the patient's right arm cephalad and upward to induce left side-bending to the L3-4 joint space. If additional flexion is desired, the thoracic area may be brought anteriorly through a pull on the shoulder.
4. The physician places his or her caudad forearm inferior to the patient's iliac crest.
5. The physician's cephalad forearm is placed in the patient's uppermost axilla.
6. The patient is asked to inhale and exhale. The physician monitors motion at the L3-4 articulation while taking up tissue slack and maintaining localization during exhalation.
7. A high-velocity/low-amplitude thrust through the physician's caudad forearm contact is directed toward the patient's head and downward to encourage L3 side-bending. The patient's cephalad arm functions as a stabilizer of the patient's upper torso during the thrust.
8. Retest the range of motion.

Note: This produces left side-bending and right rotation of the pelvis (rotation toward the physician). The rotation of the pelvis is transmitted through L4, giving a relative left rotation to L3.

Type II, Flexion: Lateral Recumbent (Posterior Transverse Process Down) (T10-L5)

Diagnosis
L1 is side-bent right, rotated right in relationship to L2, and moves more easily in these directions

$$L1 = F\ S_R R_R$$
$$L1 = \text{restricted } E\ SL\ RL$$

Position
The patient is right lateral recumbent (posterior transverse process down), and the physician stands in front of the patient (Fig. 56.25).

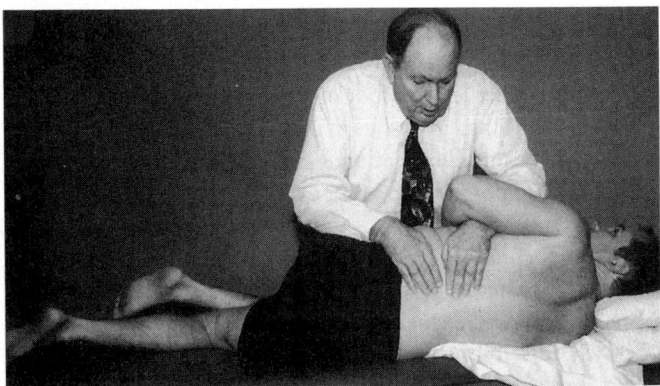

FIGURE 56.25. Lumbar type II technique: flexed, posterior transverse process down.

Procedure

To restore physiologic range of motion to the L1-2 joint:

1. The physician flexes the patient's legs until motion can be palpated at the L1-2 joint space. This locks the lower lumbar facets.
2. The inferior leg is straightened, and the foot of the superior leg is placed behind the other leg.
3. The physician induces extension to the L1-2 joint space by pushing his or her elbow of the caudad arm in a posterior direction while palpating the L1 area for motion using the caudad hand.
4. The physician then pulls the patient's right arm cephalad and upward to induce left side-bending and rotation down to the L1-2 joint space. Be sure not to rotate below L1.
5. The physician places his or her caudad forearm inferior to the patient's iliac crest.
6. The cephalad forearm is placed in the patient's uppermost axilla.
7. The patient is asked to rotate his or her head to the left to rotate the neck and trunk to the left.
8. The patient is asked to inhale and exhale. The physician monitors motion at the L3-4 articulation while taking up tissue slack and maintaining localization during exhalation.
9. The physician performs a high-velocity/low-amplitude thrust with his or her caudad forearm contact. Direction of the vector of force is toward the patient's head and downward. This rotates the patient's pelvis toward the physician, producing left lumbar side-bending and right rotation of the pelvis. The rotation of the pelvis is transmitted through L2, giving a relative left rotation to L1. The physician's cephalad arm functions as a stabilizer of the upper torso.
10. Retest the range of motion.

Pelvis

Anterior Sacrum, Right (Left Rotation on Left Oblique Axis)

Diagnosis

The sacral sulcus is deep on the right, with associated tissue texture changes and tenderness

The left inferolateral angle is posterior (the sacrum is effectively rotated left, side-bent right)

Right anterior sacrum

(or) Sacrum rotated left on a left oblique axis

Posterior motion at the right sacral sulcus is restricted when anterior pressure is applied to the left inferolateral angle

Sacrum restricted in rotating right on a left oblique axis

Position

The patient is left lateral recumbent, and the physician stands in front of the patient (Fig. 56.26).

Procedure

To restore physiologic range of motion to the sacroiliac joint:

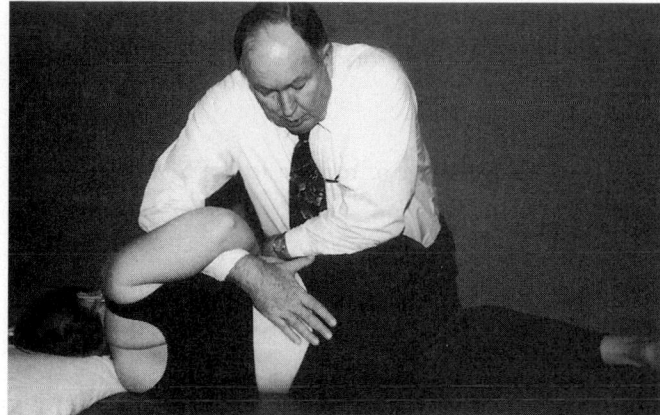

FIGURE 56.26. Anterior sacrum right technique.

1. The physician flexes the patient's hips until motion is palpated at the patient's right sacral sulcus.
2. The physician drops the patient's upper leg and foot off the side of the table to induce left side-bending.
3. The flexor surface of the physician's caudad forearm is placed parallel to the lower spine, posterior to and crossing the iliac crest. This will brace the pelvis.
4. The physician's cephalad forearm is placed through the patient's uppermost axilla, with the hand posterior and inferior to the patient's shoulder and the elbow braced against the anterior portion of the patient's shoulder. The shoulder is rotated posteriorly to stabilize the patient.
5. The patient is asked to inhale and exhale. The physician monitors the localization of forces at the end of exhalation.
6. A high-velocity/low-amplitude thrust with the physician's caudad arm is performed and follows a circular motion with the ilium, rotating it anteriorly from behind.
7. Retest the range of motion.

Posterior Sacrum, Left (Left Rotation on Left Oblique Axis)

Diagnosis

Tissue texture change and tenderness at the left inferior pole of the SI joint

The sacral sulcus is deep on the right

The left inferolateral angle is posterior (the sacrum is effectively rotated left, side-bent right)

Posterior sacrum, left

(or) Left sacral rotation on a left oblique axis

Restricted: Cephalad and downward motion at the left inferior pole of the SI joint when anterior pressure is applied to the left inferolateral angle

(or) Restricted in rotation right on a left oblique axis

Position

The patient is supine, and the physician stands on the right side of the patient (Figs. 56.27 and 56.28).

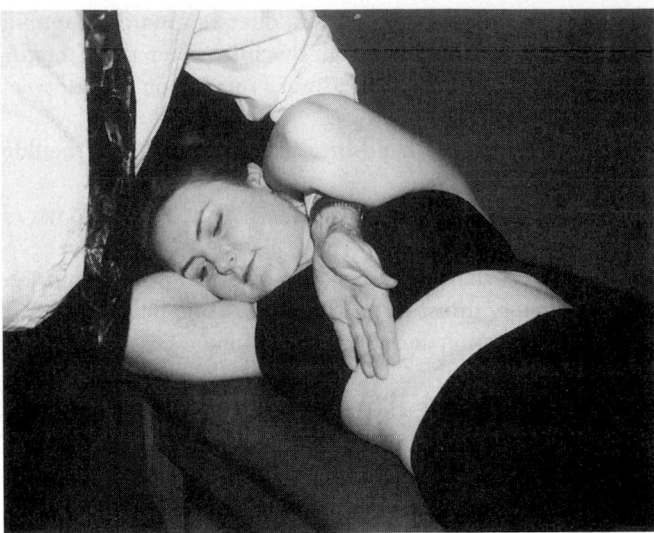

FIGURE 56.27. Posterior sacrum left technique showing hand placement on the patient's chest.

Procedure

To rotate the sacrum right and side-bend it left by applying force from above down through the sacrum with a counterforce on the left ilium, localizing force to the left sacroiliac joint:

1. The physician moves the patient's shoulders so that his or her upper torso is side-bent left and the shoulder closest to the physician is in the center of the table.
2. The patient is asked to interlace his or her fingers behind the neck.
3. The physician inserts his or her cephalad hand through the posterior aspect of the opposite axilla so that the dorsum of the hand is contacting the sternum (Fig. 56.27).
4. Right rotation of the patient is introduced through the physician's cephalad arm, pivoting the patient around the shoulder closest to him or her. Do not flex the patient. The caudad

hand may need to be used to stabilize the shoulder during this rotation to avoid flexion.

5. The physician's caudad hand is placed over the left iliac crest.
6. Right rotation is continued from above until the force is felt to accumulate at the left iliac crest.
7. A high-velocity/low-amplitude rotatory thrust with the physician's cephalad arm rotates the opposite shoulder anteriorly from behind while a small counterforce is exerted on the far ilium through the physician's caudad hand. Note: increased force at the ilium will rarely increase the effectiveness of this technique.
8. Retest the range of motion.

Note: A posterior sacrum (right) has the same motion description as an anterior sacrum (left) (rotated right, side-bent left), but the restriction and tissue change is dominant on the posterior sacrum side. The technique localizes force to the posterior sacrum side.

Anteriorly Rotated Ilium (Innominate)

Diagnosis

Standing flexion test is positive on the side of dysfunction

The anterior superior iliac spine (ASIS) is more caudad on the dysfunctional side

The ipsilateral pubic ramus is more caudad (not always detectable)

The ipsilateral PSIS is more cephalad

Anterior innominate (or) Innominate anterior

Restricted in backward rotation (posterior) of the ilium about a transverse axis

Position

The patient is lateral recumbent, and the physician stands facing the patient (Fig. 56.29).

Procedure

To mobilize the ilium in a posterior rotatory fashion to eliminate the restriction of motion:

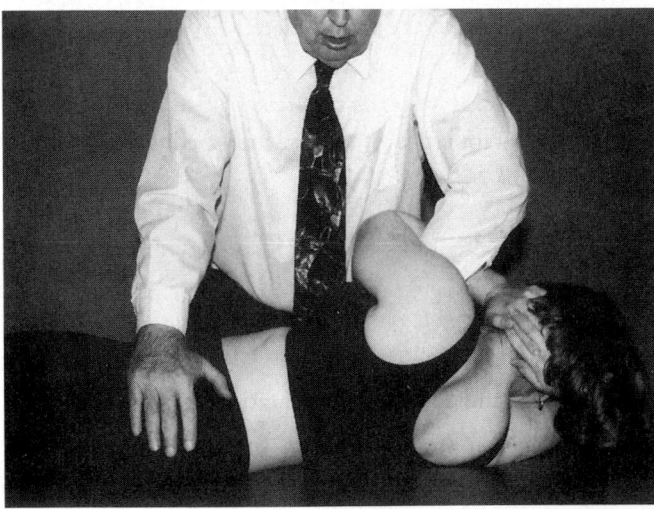

FIGURE 56.28. Posterior sacrum left technique showing hand placement on the ASIS of ilium (hip bone).

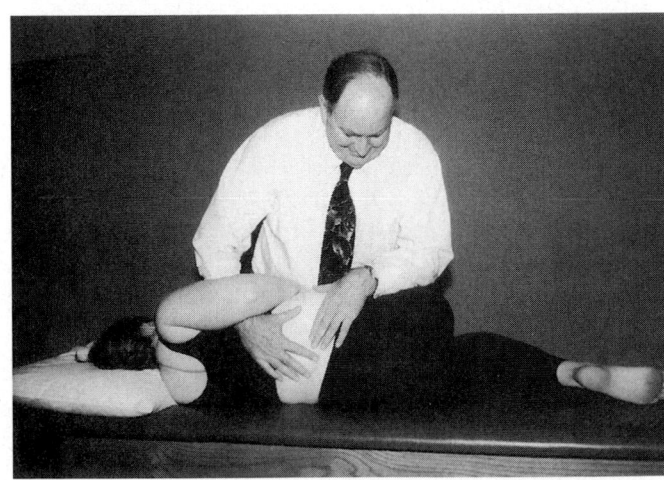

FIGURE 56.29. Anteriorly rotated ilium technique.

1. The physician flexes the patient's legs to 90 degrees and then drops the upper leg off the table in front of the lower leg.

2. The physician contacts the ilium with his or her caudad forearm on a line between the PSIS and the greater trochanter; the thenar eminence of the physician's cephalad hand is placed on the anterior surface of the ASIS.

3. Firm pressure is applied with the physician's caudad hand contact in a direction that follows the line of the upper femur. The physician should feel as though this force is posteriorly rotating the entire innominate (i.e., backward rotation on the transverse axis).

4. The physician's cephalad hand places a force on the upper shoulder, carrying the shoulder backward until force is localized to the SI joint.

5. The patient is asked to inhale and exhale. The physician localizes forces as the patient exhales.

6. At end-exhalation, a high-velocity/low-amplitude anterior rotatory thrust is applied that is directed down the shaft of the femur. Because the thrust is below the axis of rotation, the ilium rotates posteriorly.

7. Retest the position and range of motion.

Posteriorly Rotated Ilium (Innominate)

Diagnosis

Standing flexion test is positive on the side of dysfunction

The ASIS is more cephalad

The ipsilateral pubic ramus is more cephalad (may not be detectable)

The ipsilateral PSIS is more caudad

Posterior innominate (or) Innominate posterior

Restricted anterior rotation of the ilium about a transverse axis

Position

The patient is lateral recumbent, dysfunctional side up, and the physician stands facing the patient (Fig. 56.30).

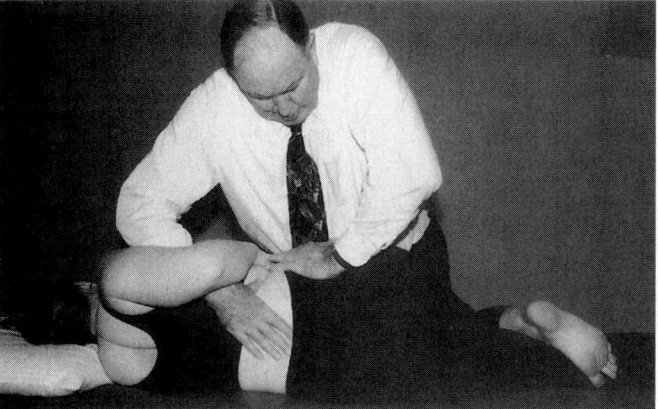

FIGURE 56.30. Posteriorly rotated ilium technique.

Procedure

1. The physician straightens the patient's lower leg and flexes the hip and knee of the upper leg. The foot of that leg is placed in the popliteal fossa of the lower leg.

2. The physician contacts the PSIS of the upper ilium with the palmar surface of his or her caudad forearm (or thenar eminence).

3. The physician's cephalad hand or forearm is placed on the patient's upper shoulder to stabilize the patient.

4. The physician applies firm pressure on the PSIS with his or her caudad hand contact, directed toward the patient's umbilicus. The physician should sense this force is anteriorly rotating the entire innominate (i.e., forward rotation on the transverse axis).

5. The patient is asked to inhale and exhale. The physician localizes forces as the patient exhales.

6. At end-exhalation, apply a high-velocity/low-amplitude anterior rotatory thrust directed toward the umbilicus.

7. Retest the position and range of motion.

Superior Iliac Shear (Upslipped Innominate)

Diagnosis

The standing flexion test is positive on the dysfunctional side

The ASIS, pubic ramus, and PSIS are all superior on the dysfunctional side

Superior innominate shear

(or) Upslipped innominate

Restricted downward motion of the innominate

Position

The patient is supine, and the physician stands at the feet of the patient (Figs. 56.31 and 56.32).

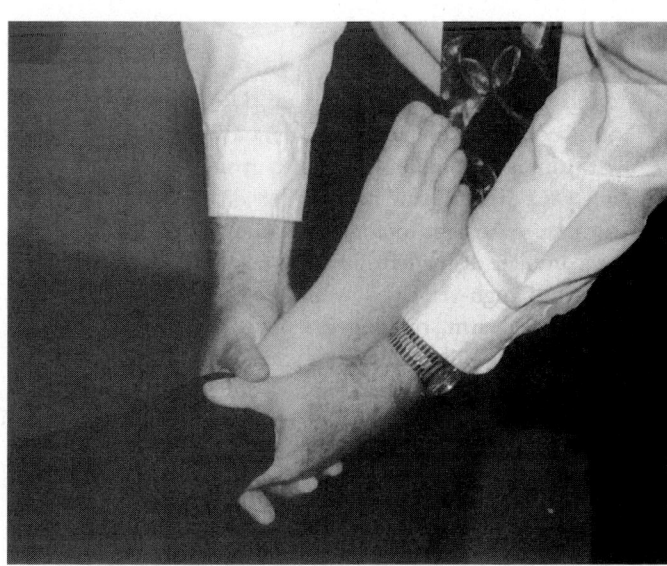

FIGURE 56.31. Superior iliac shear technique.

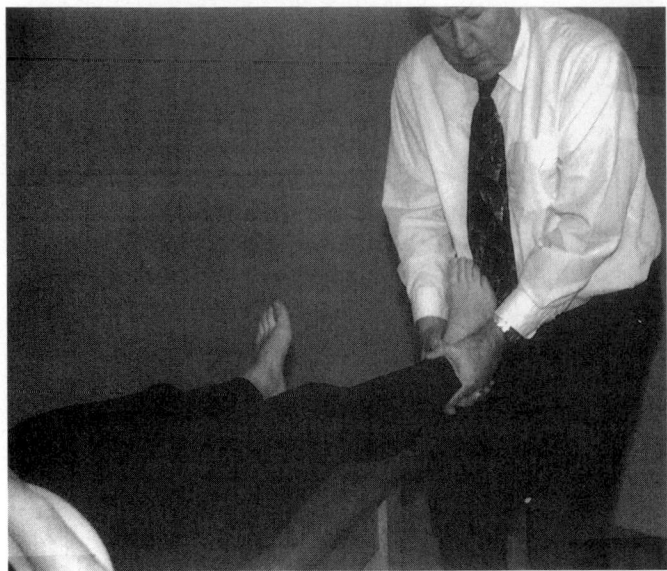

FIGURE 56.32. Superior iliac shear technique.

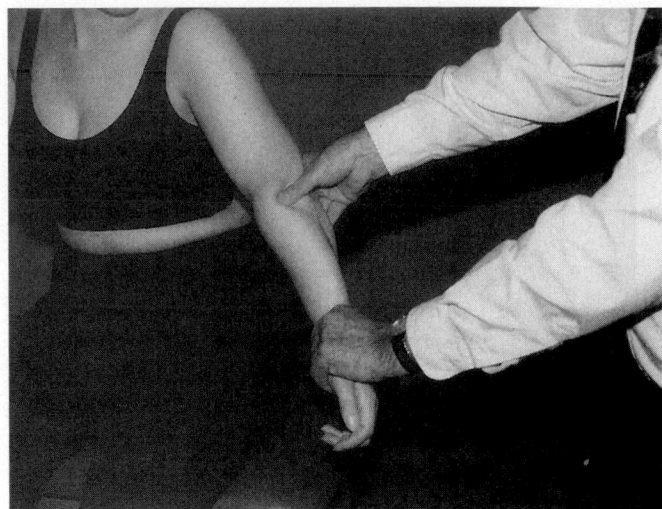

FIGURE 56.33. Posterior radial head technique.

Procedure

To mobilize the SI joint so that increased downward motion is possible:

1. The physician grasps the patient's leg on the dysfunctional side superior to the ankle.

2. The patient's leg is flexed slightly, and traction and internal rotation of the leg are applied.

3. The patient is asked to relax the knee and then the hip. The physician instructs the patient to inhale and exhale as he or she localizes the traction forces to the ilium.

4. On end-exhalation, the physician applies a high-velocity/low-amplitude tractional force (tug) to the leg.

5. Retest the range of motion.

Upper Extremity

Posterior Radial Head

Diagnosis

Tenderness over the radial head
Posterior glide of the radial head is free
Posterior radial head (or) Radial head posterior
Radial head restricted in anterior glide

Position

The patient is seated, and the physician stands on the dysfunctional side of the patient (Fig. 56.33).

Procedure

To increase the range of anterior glide:

1. The physician grasps the patient's flexed elbow with one hand, placing his or her thumb over the posterolateral aspect of the radial head.

2. The physician grasps the wrist with his or her other hand so that the thumb is over the patient's dorsum of the distal ulna.

3. The physician supinates the patient's wrist with his or her distal hand while extending the elbow with his or her proximal hand.

4. Just before reaching complete extension, a high-velocity/low-amplitude thrust is applied on the radial head through the physician's thumb and is directed in a ventral direction. Simultaneously with this thrust, the physician's distal hand provides a slight increase in the supination of the patient's forearm.

5. Retest the range of motion.

Alternate method: If the radial head restriction is greater in pronation, treat with the forearm pronated.

Abducted Elbow (Humeroulnar)

Diagnosis

The angle between the ulna and humerus is increased (increased carrying angle)
Abduction places pressure on the proximal radius, forcing it distally in relation to the ulna and producing radiocarpal adduction
Abducted elbow
(or) Ulnar abduction with medial glide
Restricted ulnar adduction and radiocarpal abduction

Position

The patient is seated, and the physician stands on the dysfunctional side in front of the patient (Fig. 56.34).

Procedure

To increase adduction of the elbow and radiocarpal abduction:
Note: Elbow restriction should be treated before wrist restrictions.

1. The physician places the patient's wrist of the dysfunctional extremity between his or her arm and lateral chest wall.

2. The physician grasps the elbow with both hands, thumbs in the antecubital region over the proximal radius and ulna, avoiding direct pressure over the ulnar nerve.

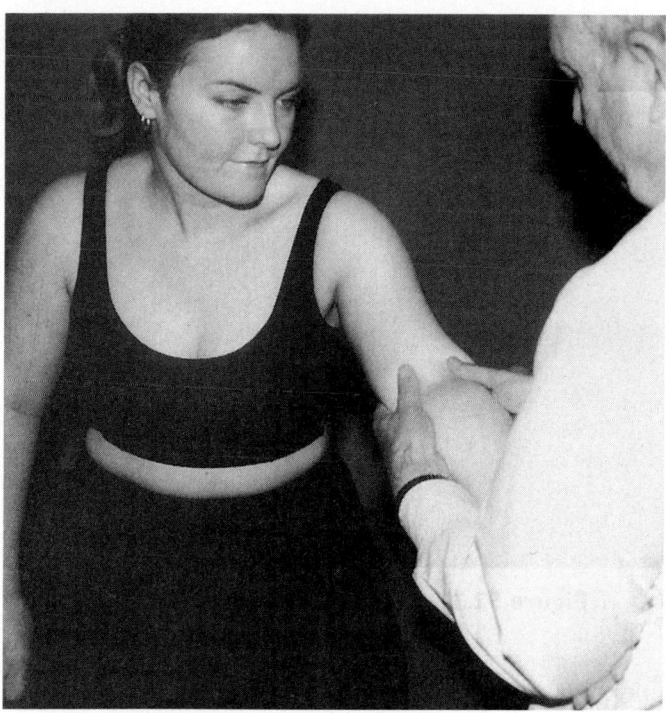

FIGURE 56.34. Abducted elbow technique.

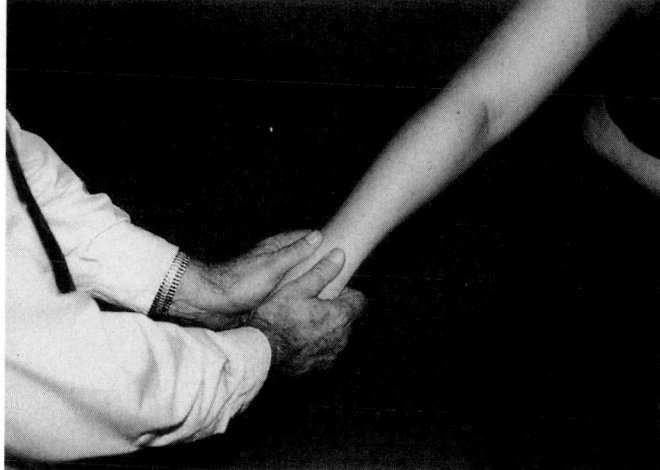

FIGURE 56.35. Wrist technique.

3. With the elbow close to full extension (slight flexion is required to avoid extension locking), the physician applies a lateral translatory force to take the ulna into adduction (a varus force).
4. A high-velocity/low-amplitude thrust is applied in the same vector when the physician reaches the restrictive barrier.
5. Retest the range of motion.

Wrist

Diagnosis

Increased adduction, abduction, flexion, or extension of the wrist

The position of the involved bones may not be demonstrably altered, but motion will be freer in one direction and restricted if attempted in the opposite direction

Wrist abducted, adducted, flexed, or extended

Radiocarpal abduction with medial carpal glide (or) radiocarpal adduction with lateral carpal glide, (or) radiocarpal flexion with dorsal carpal glide, (or) radiocarpal extension with anterior carpal glide

Wrist or radiocarpal joint restricted in motion opposite to the increased or free motion

This example: wrist flexed

(or) Radiocarpal joint flexed with dorsal carpal glide

Position

The patient is seated or supine, and the physician sits or stands facing the patient (Fig. 56.35).

Procedure

To restore physiologic range of motion to the radiocarpal joint:

Note: Elbow restriction should be treated before wrist restrictions.

1. The physician grasps the patient's dysfunctional wrist with both hands, with the fingers under the palm of the hand on the medial and lateral sides.
2. The physician's thumbs are on the dorsal surface of the patient's hand, with the pads over the dorsal surface of the carpal bones. (Usually the lunate has the somatic dysfunction.)
3. The physician applies traction and continues it while producing circumduction of the patient's wrist.
4. The physician continues the traction and completes the motion by dorsiflexing the wrist as the thumbs press firmly downward (anteriorly) on the carpal bones.
5. Retest the range of motion.

Note: This is actually an articulatory technique that usually works smoothly, especially if the traction is steady and continuous throughout. If the physician feels it is necessary, a thrust with minimal force can be added as the restrictive barrier is reached. This technique may be modified to treat the restrictions of motion of other individual carpal bones by superimposing the thumbs over the involved carpal bone and exerting the final manipulation (see step four above) that will mechanically reverse the glide that is present, as determined by the diagnosis.

Lower Extremity

Posterior Fibular Head

Diagnosis

Palpable muscle/connective tissue tension in the interosseous region between the tibia and fibula

Possible posterior displacement of the fibular head; posterior glide is free

Posterior fibular head (with posterior glide of fibular head)

(or) fibular head posterior

Fibular head restricted in anterior glide

This example: posterior right fibular head (with posterior glide of fibular head)

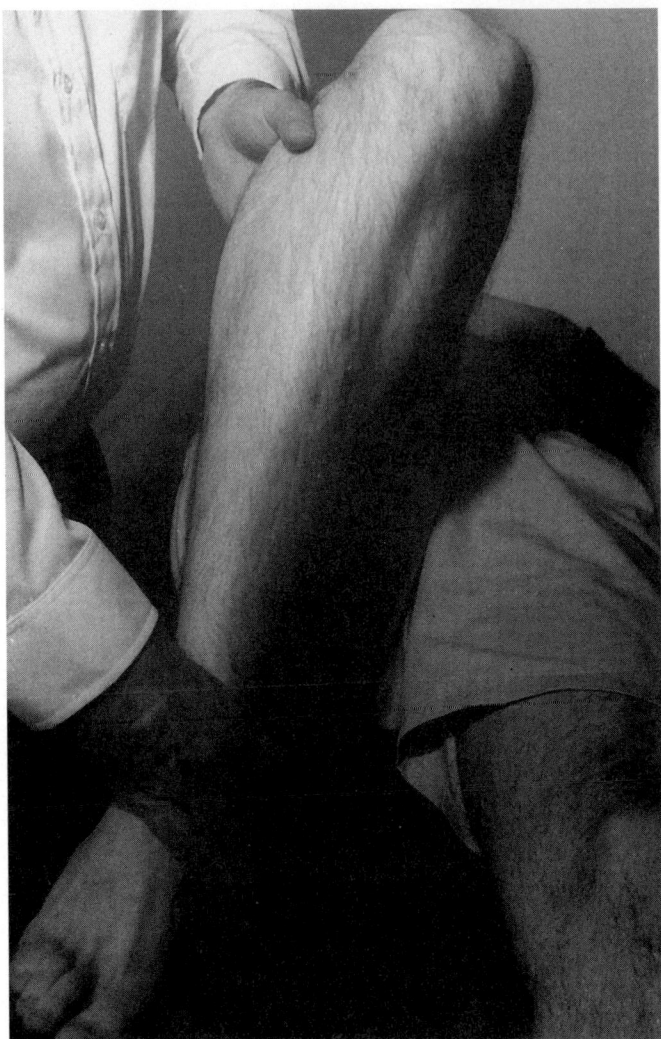

FIGURE 56.36. Posterior fibular head technique.

Position
The patient is supine, and the physician stands by the table on the dysfunctional side of the patient (Fig. 56.36).

Procedure
To increase the anterior glide of the fibular head:

1. The physician flexes the dysfunctional hip and knee.
2. The physician's cephalad hand is placed in the patient's popliteal space, palm upward, with its first MP joint posterior to the fibular head. (Avoid direct pressure over the common peroneal nerve.)
3. The physician grasps the patient's leg proximal to the ankle with his or her caudad hand.
4. The patient's knee is flexed to the point where the physician feels pressure of the fibular head on his or her first MP joint. The physician simultaneously externally rotates the ankle using the caudal hand contact at the ankle to further localize at the fibular head.
5. The physician applies a high-velocity/low-amplitude thrust by flexing the leg with his or her caudad hand while applying

an anterior counterforce to the fibular head with the first MP joint of the cephalad hand.

6. Retest the range of motion.

Note: This technique can be done prone with slight modifications.

Anterior Fibular Head
Diagnosis
Palpable muscle/connective tissue tension in the interosseous region between the tibia and fibula
Possible anterior displacement of the fibular head; anterior glide is free
Anterior fibular head
(or) Fibular head anterior
Fibular head restricted in posterior glide
This example: anterior right fibular head

Position
The patient is supine, and the physician stands at the foot of the table on the side opposite the dysfunction (Fig. 56.37).

Procedure
To increase the posterior glide of the fibular head:

1. The physician places a pillow below the patient's dysfunctional knee to avoid locking it in extension.
2. The physician grasps the leg immediately proximal to the ankle with his or her caudad hand.
3. The thenar eminence of the physician's cephalad hand is placed on the anterior aspect of the patient's fibular head.
4. The physician internally rotates the patient's ankle to draw the distal fibula anteriorly (and move the fibular head to its restrictive barrier through the reciprocal motion principle).
5. The physician's cephalad hand applies a high-velocity/low-amplitude thrust in a posterolateral vector to the fibular head while the caudad hand simultaneously applies a slight internal rotation counterforce to the ankle.
6. Retest the range of motion.

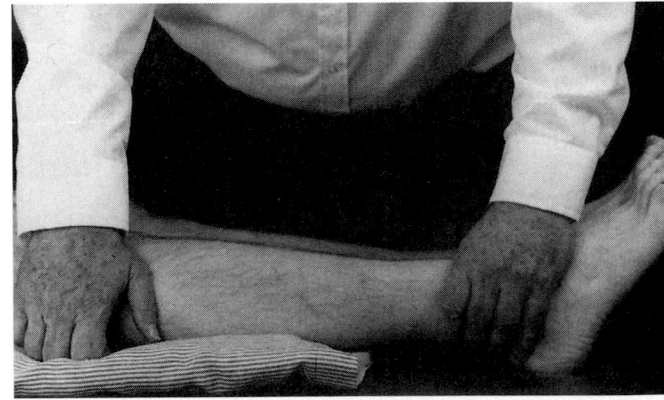

FIGURE 56.37. Anterior fibular head technique.

Anterior Lateral Malleolus

Diagnosis

The lateral malleolus (distal fibula) has free anterior glide relative to the distal tibia
The distal medial border of the talus is more prominent
Anterior lateral malleolus
Lateral malleolus restricted in posterior glide
This example: Anterior right lateral malleolus

Position

The patient is supine, and the physician stands at the foot of the table (Fig. 56.38).

Procedure

To increase posterior motion of the lateral malleolus:

1. The physician grasps the heel with the cupped fingers of the lateral hand. The physician's palm is on the lateral aspect of the heel and the thumb is in contact with the anterior surface of the lateral malleolus.
2. The physician's other hand grasps the medial side of the ankle, reinforcing the first thumb by placing its thumb on top of it.

3. The physician accumulates posterior force on the lateral malleolus by dorsiflexing the foot and applying posterior pressure with the thumbs.
4. Prior to full dorsiflexion, the physician applies a high-velocity/low-amplitude posterior thrust through his or her thumbs to the patient's lateral malleolus.
5. Retest the range of motion.

Posterior Lateral Malleolus

Diagnosis

The lateral malleolus (distal fibula) has free posterior glide relative to the distal tibia
The anterior portion of the talus is displaced in a lateral direction
Posterior lateral malleolus
Lateral malleolus is restricted in anterior glide

Position

The patient is prone, and the physician stands at the foot of the table (Fig. 56.39).

Procedure

To increase anterior glide of the lateral malleolus:

1. The physician grasps the dorsum of the patient's foot with the cupped fingers of his or her lateral hand. The thumb is in contact with the posterior surface of the patient's lateral malleolus.
2. The physician's other hand grasps the medial side of the ankle, reinforcing the first thumb by placing its thumb on top of it.
3. The physician accumulates an anterior force on the patient's lateral malleolus by plantar flexing the foot and applying anterior pressure with the thumbs.
4. Prior to full plantar flexion, the physician applies a high-velocity/low-amplitude anterior thrust through his or her thumbs to the patient's lateral malleolus.
5. Retest the range of motion.

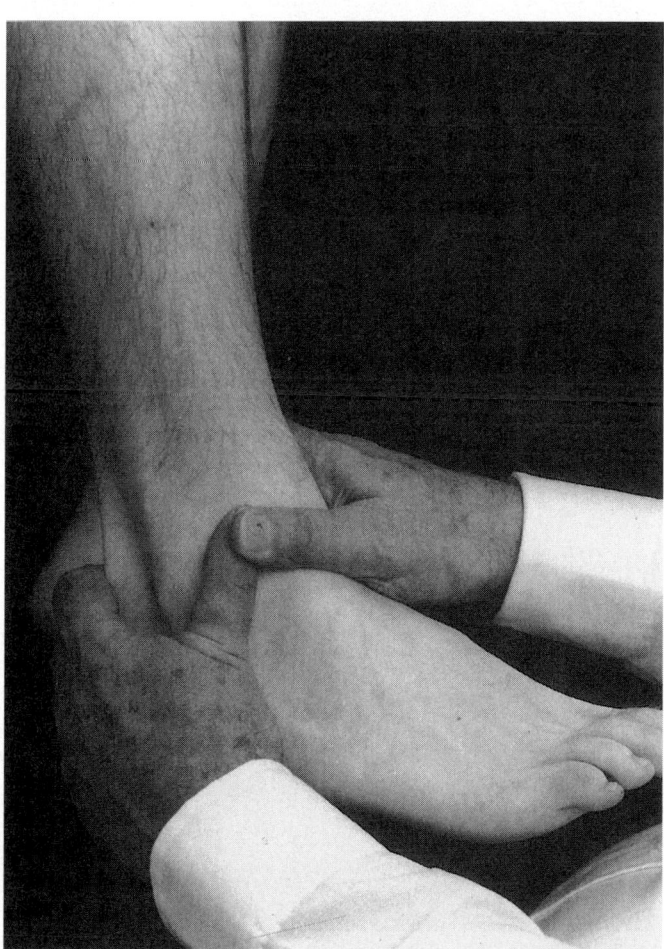

FIGURE 56.38. Anterior lateral malleolus technique.

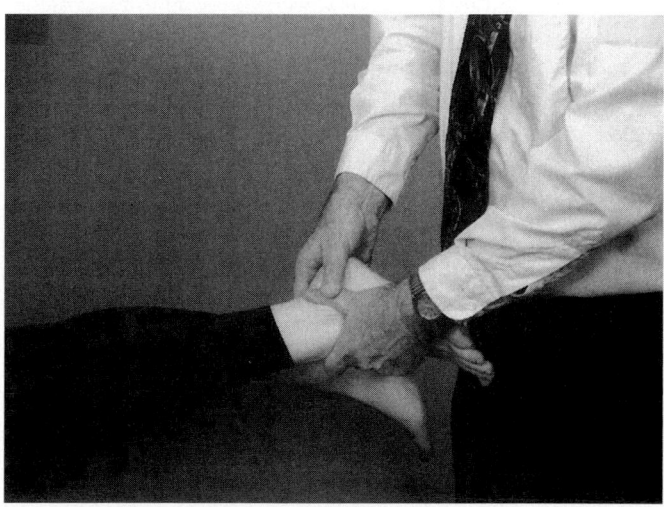

FIGURE 56.39. Posterior lateral malleolus technique.

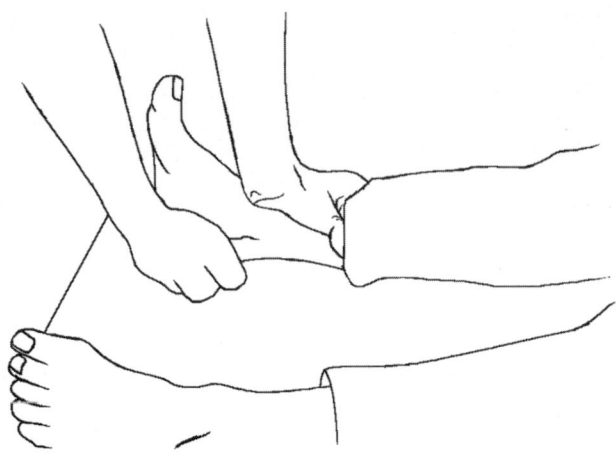

FIGURE 56.40. Anterior tibia on talus.

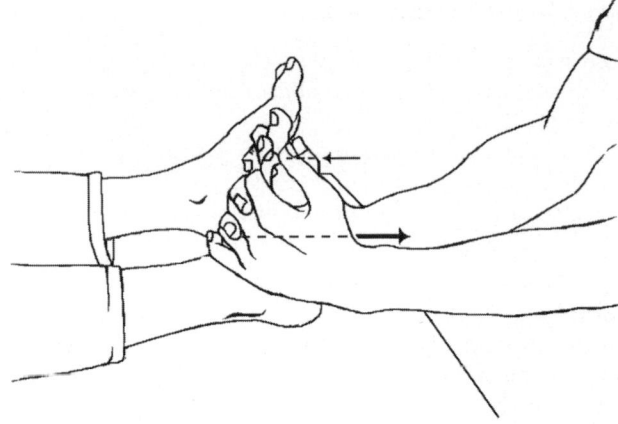

FIGURE 56.41. Inverted talus (plantar flexion of talus).

Talotibial Joint: Anterior Tibia on Talus

Diagnosis

Tibia is anterior on the talus

The ankle prefers dorsiflexion

Anterior tibia on talus

Talus restricted in gliding posteriorly on the talus (the ankle is restricted in plantar flexion)

Position

The patient is supine, and the physician stands at the foot of the table to the side of the somatic dysfunction (Fig. 56.40).

Procedure

To restore physiologic range of motion to the tibiotalar joint (true ankle), specifically to restore full plantar flexion of the ankle (posterior glide of the tibia over the talus):

1. The physician grasps the patient's heel and applies traction to it, dorsiflexing the ankle.
2. The physician's other hand grasps the distal end of the tibia, palm over its anterior surface near the talotibial joint, and applies posterior pressure (down, toward the table).
3. The physician applies a high-velocity/low-amplitude posterior thrust posteriorly through his or her distal tibial contact as the foot is dorsiflexed with the other hand on the heel.
4. Retest the range of talotibial motion.

Talus in Plantar Flexion: Ankle Tug

Diagnosis

Tibia is posterior on the talus

The ankle prefers plantar flexion

Talus in plantar flexion

(or) Talus plantar flexed with anterior glide

Tibia is restricted in gliding anteriorly on the talus

The ankle is restricted in dorsiflexion

Position

The patient is supine, and the physician stands at the end of the table (Fig. 56.41).

Procedure

To restore physiologic range of motion to the tibiotalar joint (true ankle), specifically to restore full dorsiflexion of the ankle (anterior glide of the tibia over the talus):

1. The physician grasps the patient's foot, curling his or her fifth or fourth finger over the dorsal surface of the head of the talus. The physician also grasps the foot with the other hand and clasps his or her fingers so that the fifth or fourth finger supports the same finger of the opposite hand (over the talar head).
2. The physician's thumbs are placed over the ball of the foot and the patient's foot is dorsiflexed at the ankle. This dorsiflexion of the ankle is maintained throughout this technique.
3. Traction is applied with continued dorsiflexion and slight eversion at the ankle, until all joint play is out of the ankle joint.
4. The physician applies a high-velocity/low-amplitude tug to re-seat the talus in the mortise of the ankle.
5. Retest the range of talotibial motion.

Note: This type of somatic dysfunction may be accompanied by tissue congestion and spasm of the peroneus muscles and/or fibular head somatic dysfunction.

Hiss Plantar Whip: Cuboid

Diagnosis

The cuboid is displaced inferiorly with the medial edge gliding laterally, flattening the lateral longitudinal arch

There is palpable tenderness on the plantar surface of the cuboid

Cuboid everted with plantar glide

Cuboid is restricted in dorsal glide (motion toward the dorsal surface of the foot)

Position

The patient is prone, and the physician stands at the foot of the table, or the patient is standing, and the physician stands or sits behind the patient (Fig. 56.42).

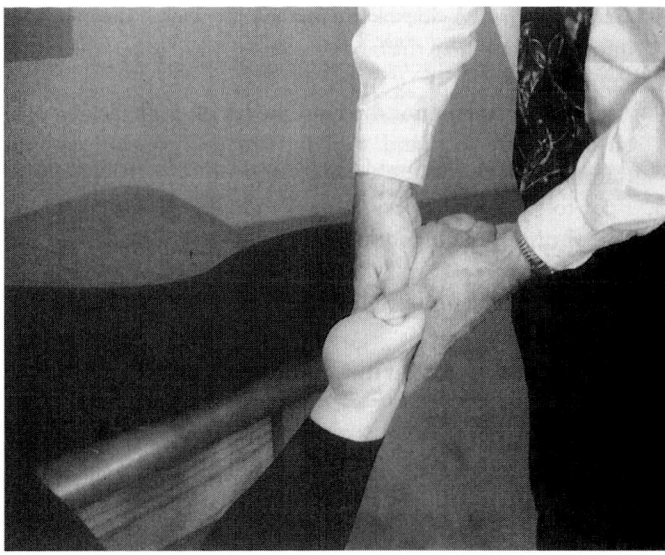

FIGURE 56.42. Hiss plantar whip technique.

Procedure

To restore the cuboid to its appropriate position:

1. In the patient prone position: The physician moves the dysfunctional leg off the table. In the patient standing position: The physician asks the patient to flex the knee on the dysfunctional side.
2. The physician grasps the patient's foot with both hands. The thumb of the hand on the lateral side of the patient's foot is placed on the soft tissues over the medial plantar edge of the patient's cuboid bone, and the thumb of the other hand lies over the first thumb for reinforcement.
3. The physician induces a series of oscillating motions, swinging the foot to produce plantar flexion.
4. A high-velocity/low-amplitude thrust is applied by performing a whip-like motion in the same direction as above (i.e., the foot is pulled toward the physician in the final motion while the thumbs impart a sudden downward and lateral motion, thrusting the cuboid toward the dorsolateral surface of the patient's foot).
5. Retest the range of motion.

Note: This same technique may be used with variations for other somatic dysfunction of the foot (navicular, cuneiforms, metatarsal bases), as follows.

Hiss Plantar Whip: Navicular

Diagnosis

The navicular bone is displaced inferiorly, with the lateral edge gliding medially, flattening the lateral longitudinal arch

There is palpable tenderness on the plantar surface of the navicular bone

Navicular inverted with plantar glide

Navicular is restricted in dorsal glide (motion toward the dorsal surface of the foot)

Position

Same as for the cuboid technique.

Procedure

1. The physician places his or her thumb on the lateral margin of the plantar surface of the navicular bone and reinforces that thumb with the other thumb.
2. The whip-like thrust is directed straight down. The thumb position will direct the force medially. (For preparation, see Hiss Whip: Navicular.)

Hiss Plantar Whip: Cuneiforms

Diagnosis

The cuneiform bone glides inferiorly (toward the plantar surface, usually the second of the three bones

Position

Same as for the cuboid or navicular techniques.

Procedure

1. The physician places his or her thumb on the plantar surface of the appropriate cuneiform.
2. The whip-like thrust is directed straight down toward the floor. (For preparation, see Hiss Whip: Navicular.)

CONCLUSION

The ultimate effective use of these techniques demands considerable knowledge, skill, and experience. The general principles of HVLA thrust technique are to:

1. Identify the motion restriction of somatic dysfunction.
2. Engage the barrier.
3. Apply the activating force, a HVLA thrust.
4. Reevaluate.

Careful execution of high-velocity/low-amplitude thrust techniques in the areas presented can help patients and bring them healing from dysfunction.

REFERENCES

1. The Glossary Review Committee of the Educational Council on Osteopathic Principles. Glossary of Osteopathic Terminology. In: Allen TW, ed. *AOA Yearbook and Directory of Osteopathic Physicians.* Chicago, IL: American Osteopathic Association; 1994.
2. Greenman PE. *Principles of Manual Medicine.* Baltimore, MD: Williams & Wilkins; 1989:94.
3. Bowles CH. Functional technique: a modern perspective. In: Beal MC, ed. *The Principles of Palpatory Diagnosis and Manipulative Technique.* Newark, OH: American Academy of Osteopathy; 1992: 174–178.
4. Hargrove-Wilson. Symposium: manipulative treatment. *Med J Aust.* 1967;24:274–280.
5. Kappler R. Role of psoas mechanism in low back pain. *J Am Osteopath Assoc.* 1973;72.

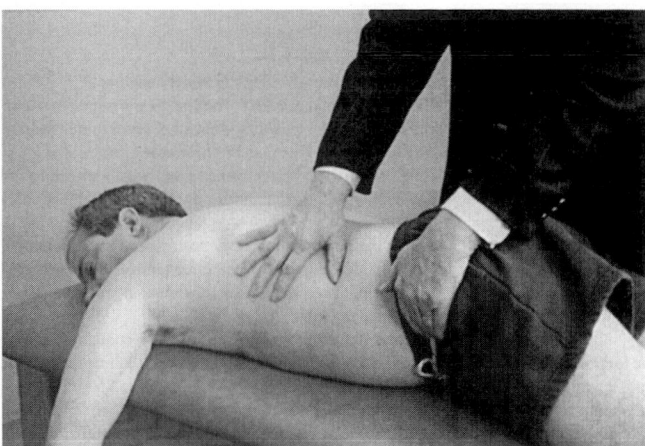

FIGURE 57.17. Treatment for ribs 11 and 12, depressed.

Type of Muscle Energy
Post-isometric relaxation (quadratus lumborum).

Treatment Position
Patient: Prone.
 Physician: Standing on the side of the patient opposite the dysfunctional rib.

Procedure
1. Draw the patient's legs approximately 15 to 20 degrees away from the side of the dysfunctional rib.
2. The physician places the heel of the cephalad hand inferior and medial to the angle of the dysfunctional rib.
3. The physician's caudad hand grasps the ipsilateral anterior superior iliac spine and lifts toward the ceiling.
4. The patient is instructed to "pull your hip down toward the table."
5. This contraction is held for a full 3 to 5 seconds.
6. Direct the patient to relax, simultaneously ceasing your counterforce.
7. Wait 2 seconds for the tissues to relax, and then exert a cephalad and lateral pressure with the hand contacting the angle of the rib.
8. Steps four, five, six, and seven are repeated three to five times.
9. Success of the technique is determined by retesting motion of the dysfunctional rib.

Rib Dysfunction—Ribs 2–9 Held Anterior (Fig. 57.18)

Diagnosis
Position: Anterior rib; rib held anterior.
 Restriction: Rib resists moving posteriorly.

Type of Muscle Energy
Joint mobilization using muscle force.

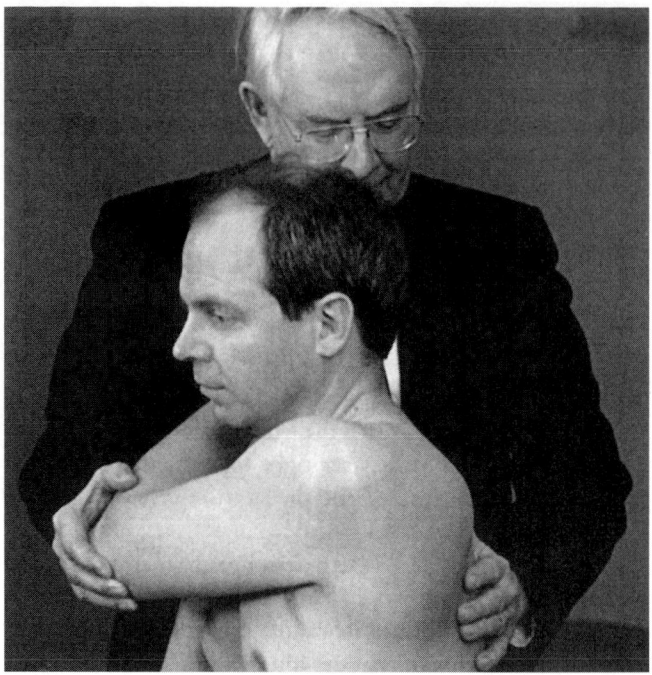

FIGURE 57.18. Treatment for ribs 2–9, held anterior.

Treatment Position
Patient: Seated.
 Physician: Standing on the side opposite the dysfunctional rib.

Procedure
1. Place the patient's hand ipsilateral to the dysfunction on the opposite shoulder.
2. Place your anterior hand on the patient's elbow.
3. Place the heel of your posterior hand medial to the angle of the dysfunctional rib and exert a continuous lateral pressure.
4. Use your anterior hand to pull the patient's arm toward you. Raise or lower the arm until your posterior hand feels the forces localize to the dysfunctional rib.
5. Instruct the patient to "pull your elbow away from me."
6. This contraction is held for a full 3 to 5 seconds.
7. Direct the patient to relax, simultaneously ceasing your counterforce.
8. Wait 2 seconds for the tissues to relax, and then increase the lateral pressure against the angle of the dysfunctional rib.
9. Steps five, six, seven, and eight are repeated three to five times.
10. Success of the technique is determined by retesting motion of the dysfunctional rib.

Innominate Dysfunction

Dysfunction of the innominate bones is due to faulting of the biomechanics of the sacroiliac joint. Due to the irregular surface of the sacroiliac joints, this necessarily results in a separation of the joint surfaces and a drawing taut of the anterior and posterior sacroiliac ligaments. It is this ligamentous tension that maintains the presence of the somatic dysfunction. Muscle energy

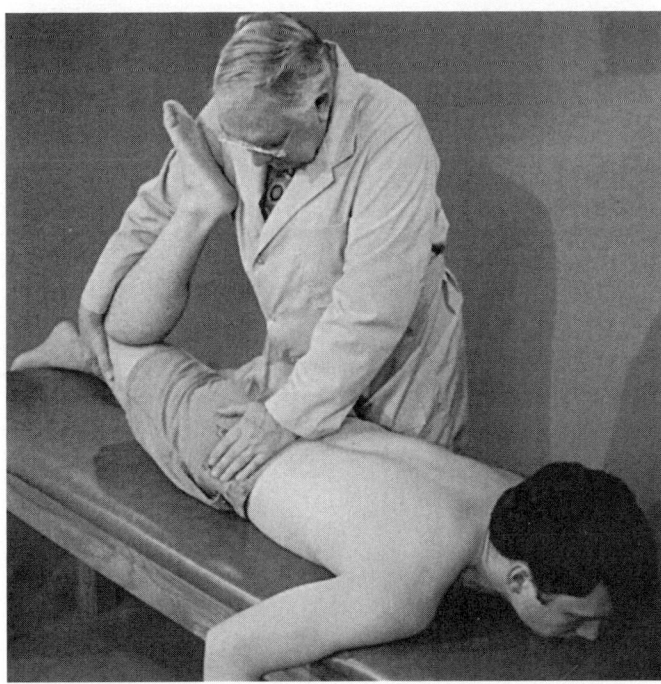

FIGURE 57.19. Treatment for posteriorly rotated innominate.

technique is directed at restoring normal articular relations across the sacroiliac joint.

Pubic symphysis dysfunction is also considered to be innominate dysfunction, but with the greatest positional distortion of the innominate bones (and usually the symptomatology as well), located at and about the pubic symphysis.

Innominate Dysfunction—Posterior Rotation (Fig. 57.19)

Diagnosis
Position: Innominate rotated posteriorly.
  Restriction: Innominate restricted in anterior rotation.

Type of Muscle Energy
Joint mobilization using muscle force.

Treatment Position
Patient: Prone with the knee on the side of the dysfunction flexed 90 degrees.
  Physician: Standing on the side opposite the dysfunction.

Procedure
1. Physician's caudad hand grasps the patient's ipsilateral knee just proximal to the patella. The dorsum of the patient's foot rests against the anterior aspect of the physician's shoulder.
2. The heel of the physician's cephalad hand is placed over the posterior superior iliac spine (PSIS) on the side of dysfunction.
3. The patient's hip is passively extended until forward motion is sensed at the PSIS.

4. The patient is instructed to "pull your knee down toward the table."
5. This contraction is maintained for a full 3 to 5 seconds.
6. Direct the patient to relax, simultaneously ceasing your counterforce.
7. Wait 2 seconds for the tissues to relax, and then further extend the hip until a new restrictive barrier for the innominate is engaged.
8. Steps four, five, six, and seven are repeated three to five times or until a sudden release of the innominate dysfunction is palpated.
9. Effectiveness of the technique is assessed by retesting iliosacral motion.

Innominate Dysfunction—Anterior Rotation (Fig. 57.20)

Diagnosis
Position: Innominate rotated anteriorly.
  Restriction: Innominate restricted in posterior rotation.

Type of Muscle Energy
Joint mobilization using muscle force.

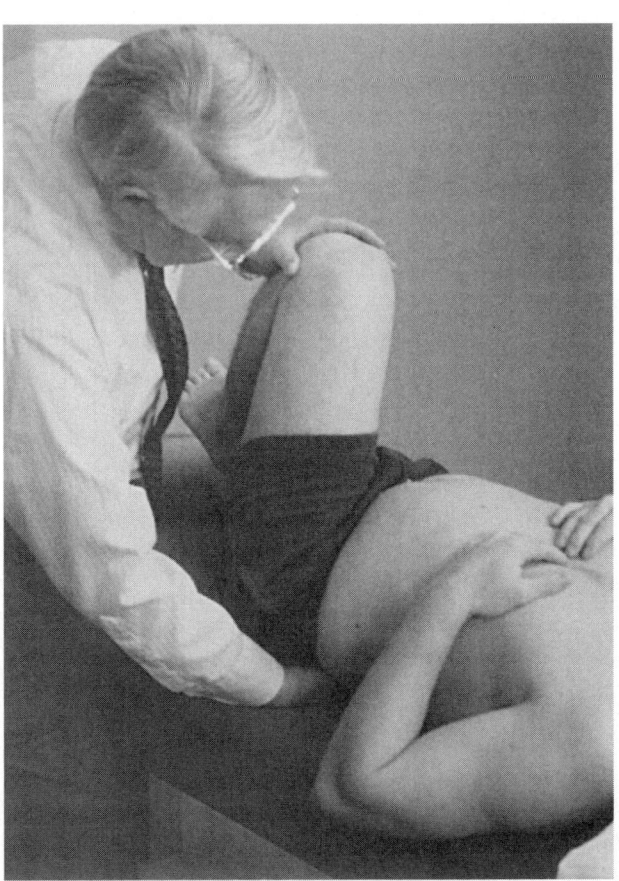

FIGURE 57.20. Treatment for anteriorly rotated innominate.

Treatment Position

Patient: Supine.

Physician: Seated on the table on the side of dysfunction.

Procedure

1. The patient's leg on the side of dysfunction is flexed at the hip and the knee, and the foot is placed on the physician's shoulder.
2. The physician's hands are placed against the hamstring muscles just proximal to the popliteal region.
3. The patient is instructed to "push your thigh against my hands."
4. This contraction is held for a full 3 to 5 seconds.
5. Direct the patient to relax, simultaneously ceasing your counterforce.
6. Wait 2 seconds for the tissues to relax, and then reposition the innominate into further posterior rotation by further flexing the hip until the new restrictive barrier is engaged.
7. Steps three, four, five, and six are repeated three to five times or until a sudden release of the innominate dysfunction is palpated.
8. Effectiveness of the technique is assessed by rechecking iliosacral motion.

Pubic Symphysis—Fixed Compression (Adducted Pubic Bones) (Fig. 57.21)

Diagnosis

Position: Pubic bones are compressed medially; there is typically bulging and tenderness of the symphysial cartilage.

Restriction: Normal pubic symphysis motion is restricted.

Type of Muscle Energy

Joint mobilization using muscle force.

Treatment Position

Patient: Supine with hips flexed to 45 degrees, knees flexed 90 degrees, and the feet flat on the table.

Physician: Standing on either side of the patient.

Procedure

1. The patient's knees are separated to allow insertion of the physician's forearm (elbow to heel of hand) between them.
2. The patient is instructed to "try to pull your knees together."
3. This contraction is sustained for a full 3 to 5 seconds.
4. Direct the patient to relax.
5. Wait 2 seconds for the tissues to relax. There is no need for repositioning in this technique.
6. Steps two, three, four, and five are repeated three to five times or until a sudden release of the pubic symphysis is felt by the patient.
7. Success of the technique is determined by reexamining the symphysial cartilage.

Pubic Symphysis—Fixed Gapping (Abducted Pubic Bones) (Fig. 57.22)

Diagnosis

This is often suspected based on the patient's history of recent childbirth or surgery performed in the lithotomy position. Due to the fascial stresses placed on the urethra, some patients experience urinary frequency and urgency suggestive of infectious cystitis; however, laboratory studies do not support this diagnosis.

Position: Pubic bones are distracted laterally; there is typically a deeper than normal sulcus overlying the symphysial cartilage, which is extremely tender.

Restriction: Normal pubic symphysis motion is restricted.

Type of Muscle Energy

Joint mobilization using muscle force.

Treatment Position

Patient: Supine with hips flexed to 45 degrees, knees flexed to 90 degrees, and feet flat on the table.

Physician: Standing on either side of the patient.

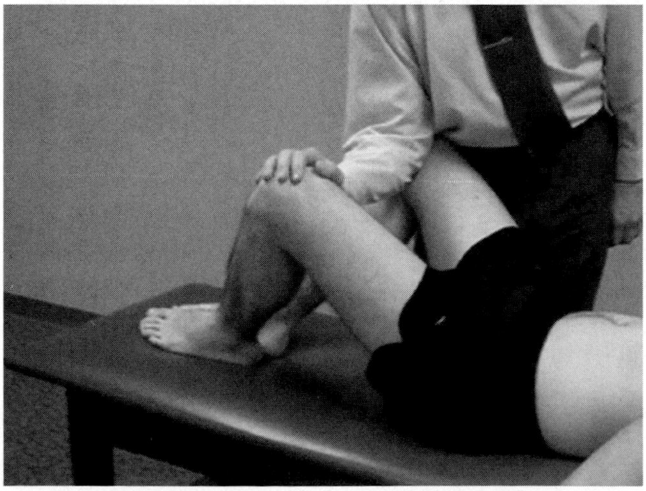

FIGURE 57.21. Treatment for adducted pubic bones.

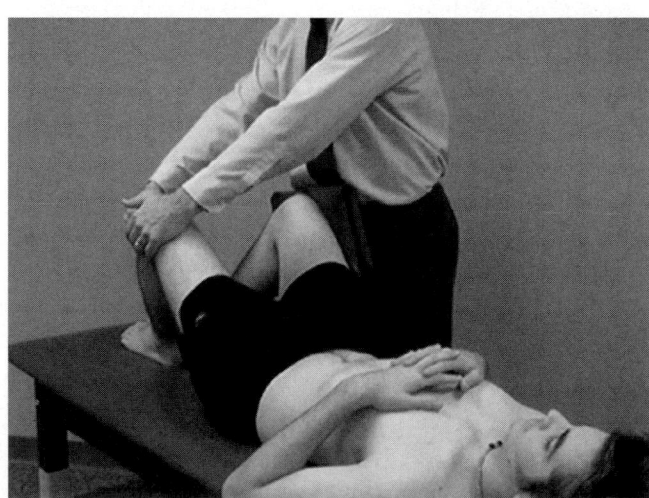

FIGURE 57.22. Treatment for abducted pubic bones.

Procedure

1. The patient's knees are separated about 18 inches.
2. The lateral aspect of the knee closest to the physician is placed against the physician's abdomen (often a pillow is used to protect the physician).
3. The physician reaches across to the other knee and grasps the lateral aspect of that knee with both hands.
4. The patient is instructed to "pull your knees apart as hard as you can."
5. This contraction is maintained for a full 3 to 5 seconds.
6. Direct the patient to relax, simultaneously ceasing your counterforce.
7. Wait 2 seconds for the tissues to relax, and then pull the knees slightly closer together.
8. Steps four, five, six, and seven are repeated three to five times.
9. Success of the technique is determined by reexamining the prominence of the symphysial cartilage.

Sacrum

The diagnosis of sacral dysfunction generally requires just two types of information:

1. *The relative position of the two sacral sulci and the two inferior lateral angles (ILAs)* (Fig. 57.23). The two sacral sulci are designated as feeling either deep or shallow compared with each other. The inferior lateral angles are designated as being posterior/inferior or anterior/superior relative to each other. For unilateral sacral dysfunction, when the deep sulcus and the posterior/inferior ILA are on opposite sides of the sacrum, you have torsion. When the deep sulcus and the posterior/inferior ILA are on the same side of the sacrum, you have a unilateral sacral flexion (shear) or extension.
2. *A motion test.* Several different motion tests have been devised over the years to assess unilateral sacroiliac dysfunction.

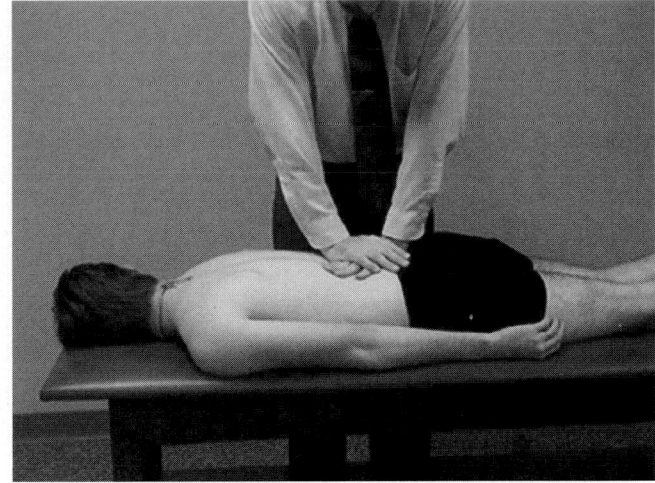

FIGURE 57.24. Lumbar spring test.

- *Lumbar spring test* (Fig. 57.24). In this test, the patient is prone, and a springing force is directed anteriorly into the lumbar spine. Normal spring (negative spring test) indicates the presence of an anterior torsion or a unilateral flexion. Increased resistance to pressure (positive spring test) indicates the presence of either a posterior torsion or a unilateral extension.
- *Sphinx test* (Fig 57.25), also called lumbopelvic hyperextension, employs observation in changes in asymmetry at the sacral sulci. When going from the prone position to the sphinx position, if the sacral sulci become more symmetric, you have an anterior torsion or a unilateral flexion. If the sacral sulci become more asymmetric, you have a posterior torsion or a unilateral extension.
- Seated flexion test (see Chapter 52).
- *Seated assessment of ILA asymmetry* (Fig 57.26 and 57.27). This is performed in a manner similar to a seated flexion test (see Chapter 52, Special Tests of the Pelvis), but the ILAs are monitored. As in the sphinx test, if the asymmetry increases, you

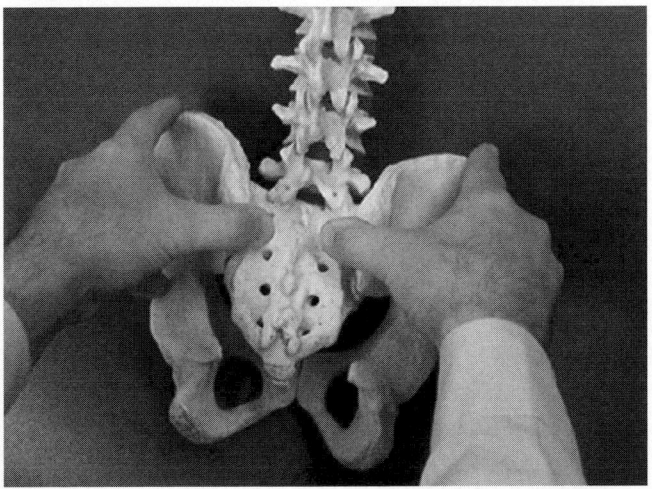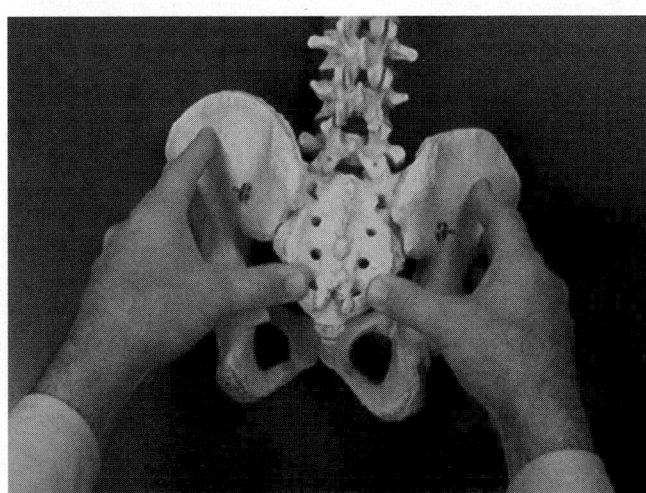

A   B

FIGURE 57.23. Sacral landmarks. **A:** the sacral sulci and **(B)** the inferior lateral angles.

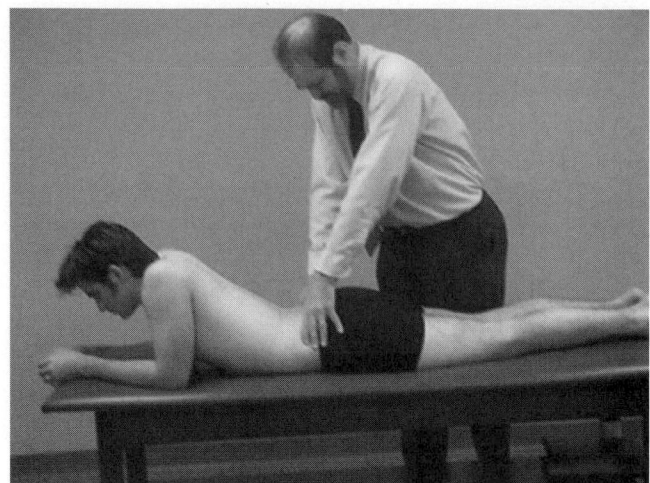

FIGURE 57.25. Sphinx test.

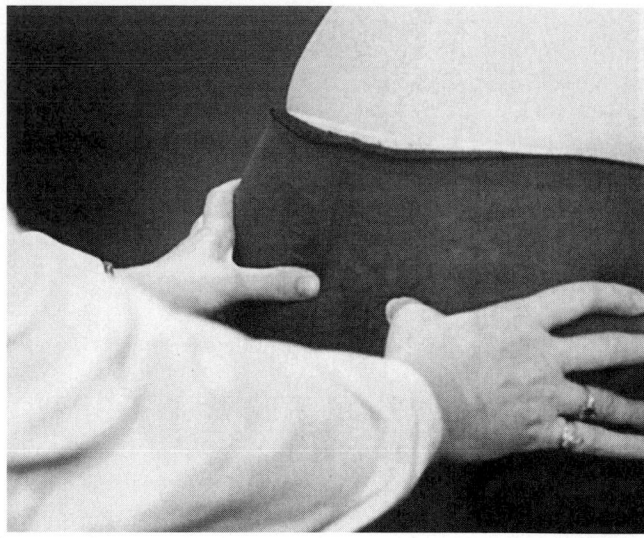

FIGURE 57.27. Test for inferior lateral angle symmetry—at end of flexion.

have a posterior torsion or unilateral extension. If the asymmetry decreases or stays the same, you have an anterior torsion or unilateral flexion.

■ *Four digit contact* (Fig. 57.28). Contact the four corners of the sacrum as depicted. Assess motion of the sacrum by direct pressure on the sacrum, moving it about its various axes, or quietly palpate sacral motion while the patient respires.

Sacral Dysfunction—Anterior Torsion (Fig. 57.29)

Diagnosis

Example: A left on left sacral torsion.

Position: Anterior torsion about a left oblique axis; a L on L sacral torsion (the first L designates the direction of sacral rotation, the second L designates the oblique axis on which this rotation is occurring).

Restriction: Posterior rotation about the left oblique axis is restricted. The oblique axes are not free to alternate during the gait cycle.

Type of Muscle Energy

Complex: the experts are still debating exactly what happens during this technique, but it is likely a combination of multiple muscles simultaneously going through post-isometric relaxation.

Treatment Position

Patient: Left lateral modified Sims' position (lying on the side of the axis).

Physician: Stands at the side of the table facing the patient.

Procedure

1. The patient's right shoulder is pressed as close to the table as it will go. Post-isometric relaxation technique may be used to obtain optimal positioning.
2. The physician's cephalad hand palpates over the right sacral sulcus.
3. The patient's hips and knees are flexed to 90 degrees. Both legs are then dropped off the side of the table. A pillow may be necessary to cushion the distal thigh against the table edge.

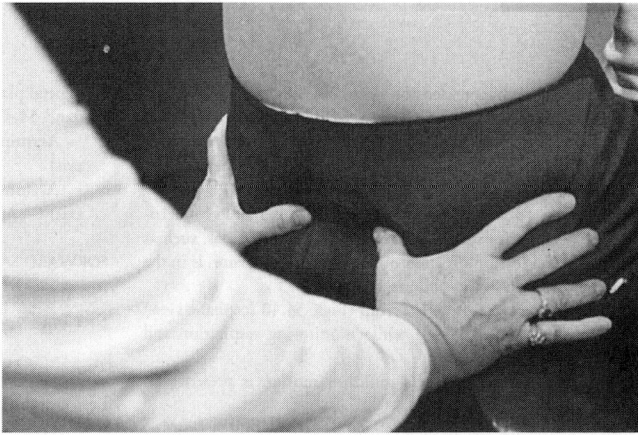

FIGURE 57.26. Test for inferior lateral angle symmetry—starting position.

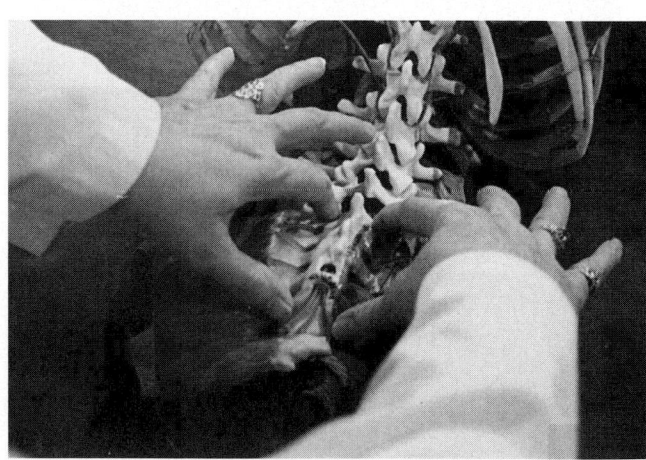

FIGURE 57.28. Four digit contact.

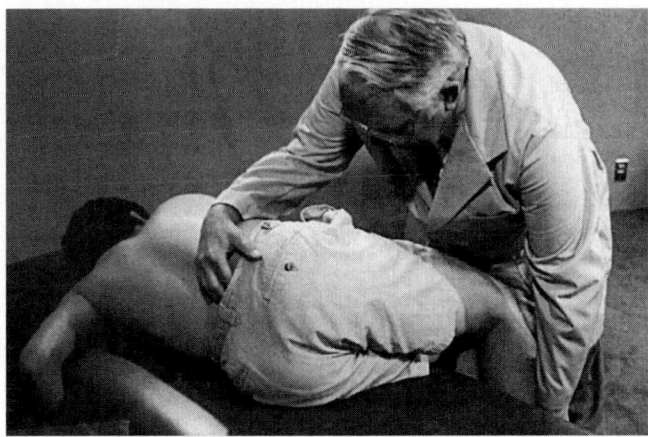

FIGURE 57.29. Treatment of anterior sacral torsion.

4. The physician's caudad hand is placed just proximal to the lateral malleolus of the upper leg.
5. The patient is instructed to "lift your legs straight up toward the ceiling."
6. This contraction is held for a full 3 to 5 seconds.
7. Direct the patient to relax, simultaneously ceasing your counterforce.
8. Wait 2 seconds for the tissues to relax, and then press both legs toward the floor until a new restrictive barrier is reached.
9. Steps five, six, seven, and eight are repeated three to five times.
10. Success of the technique is determined by rechecking the symmetry of the sacral sulci and ILAs, and by retesting sacral motion.

Sacral Dysfunction—Posterior Torsion (Fig. 57.30)

Diagnosis
Example: a left on right sacral torsion.

Position: Posterior torsion about a right oblique axis; a L on R sacral torsion (the L designates the direction of sacral rotation, the R designates the oblique axis on which this rotation is occurring).

Restriction: Anterior rotation about the right oblique axis is restricted. The oblique axes are not free to alternate during the gait cycle.

Type of Muscle Energy
Complex: the experts are still debating exactly what happens during this technique, but it is likely a combination of joint mobilization using muscle force and post-isometric relaxation.

Treatment Position
Patient: Right lateral recumbent position (lying on the side of the axis).

Physician: Stands at the side of the table facing the patient.

Procedure
1. The patient's left shoulder is carried posteriorly until the initial restriction is sensed.

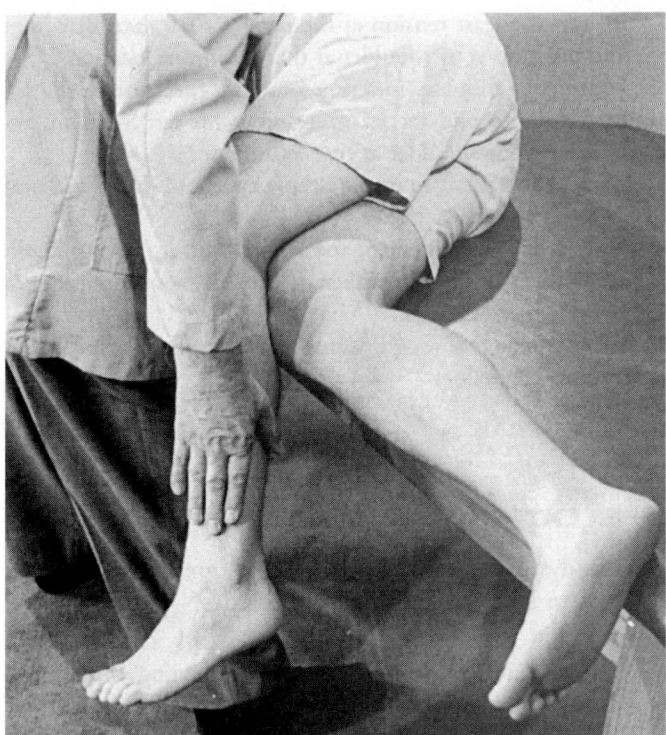

FIGURE 57.30. Treatment of posterior sacral torsion.

2. The physician's cephalad hand palpates over the left sacral sulcus.
3. The patient's hips are flexed to 45 degrees and the knees to 90 degrees.
4. The patient's upper leg is flexed further at the hip and dropped off the table cephalad to the lower leg.
5. The physician grasps this leg just above the lateral malleolus.
6. The patient is instructed to "lift your ankle up toward the ceiling as hard as you can."
7. This contraction is maintained for a full 3 to 5 seconds.
8. Direct the patient to relax, simultaneously ceasing your counterforce.
9. Wait 2 seconds for the tissues to relax, and then press the leg further toward the floor until a new restrictive barrier is reached.
10. Steps six, seven, eight, and nine are repeated three to five times.
11. Success of the technique is determined by rechecking the symmetry of the sacral sulci and ILAs, and by retesting sacroiliac motion.

Sacral Dysfunction—Unilateral Flexed Sacrum (Fig. 57.31)

Diagnosis
Example: Unilateral flexed sacrum, right.

Position: Unilateral flexed sacrum—right; right sacral shear.

Restriction: Right sacroiliac joint is restricted in extension.

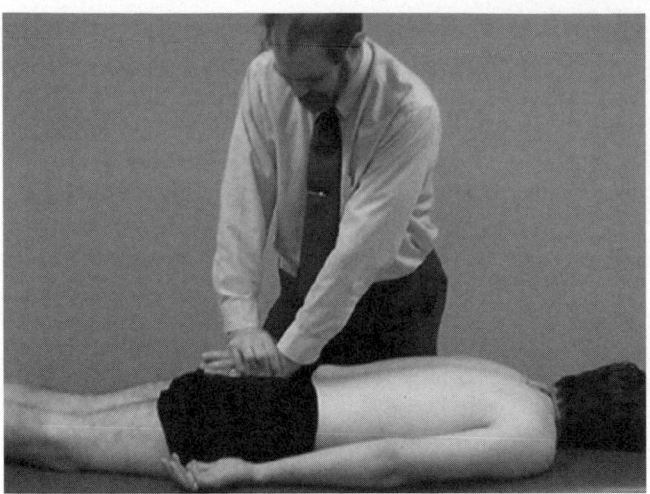

FIGURE 57.31. Treatment of unilateral flexed sacrum.

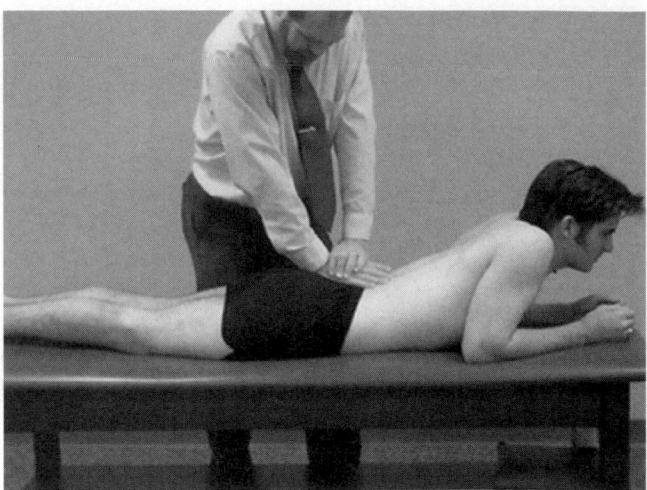

FIGURE 57.32. Treatment of unilateral extended sacrum.

Type of Muscle Energy
Respiratory assistance.

Treatment Position
Patient: Prone.
   Physician: Standing beside the patient on the side opposite the side of dysfunction.

Procedure
1. The hypothenar side of the heel of the physician's left hand is placed on the right ILA of the sacrum and exerts a steady pressure caudad and toward the table. It is reinforced with the physician's right hand.
2. The patient is instructed to, "take a deep breath."
3. During inhalation, the physician follows posterior nutation of the sacrum.
4. The patient is instructed to, "exhale slowly."
5. During exhalation, the physician exerts increased pressure against the ILA to prevent return of the sacrum toward a flexed position.
6. Steps two, three, four, and five are repeated three to seven times.
7. Success of the technique is determined by rechecking symmetry of the sacral sulci and inferior lateral angles, and by retesting sacral motion.

Sacral Dysfunction—Unilateral Extended Sacrum (Fig. 57.32)

Diagnosis
Example: Unilateral extended sacrum—right.
   Position: Unilateral extended sacrum—right.
   Restriction: Right sacroiliac joint restricted in flexion.

Type of Muscle Energy
Respiratory assistance.

Treatment Position
Patient: Sphinx position (prone with the elbows supporting the upper body).
   Physician: Standing at the side of the patient opposite the side of dysfunction.

Procedure
1. The hypothenar side of the heel of the physician's right hand is placed in the region of the right sacral sulcus exerting a steady pressure directed toward the table. It is reinforced by the physician's left hand.
2. The patient is instructed to "inhale and then exhale quickly."
3. During exhalation, the physician follows forward nutation of the sacrum.
4. During inhalation, the physician resists posterior nutation of the sacrum.
5. Steps two, three, and four are repeated three to seven times.
6. Success of the technique is determined by rechecking symmetry of the sacral sulci and the ILAs, and by retesting sacroiliac motion.

The Extremities

When muscular restrictions affect the motion of a peripheral joint, the most common method used is a simple range of motion technique combined with post-isometric relaxation. Examples of this are given for the hip girdle. For similar treatment of the shoulder, the reader is referred to the section on Spencer technique in Chapter 55.

   Muscle energy protocol can readily be added to many of the stages of this common technique. This same type of thinking can be applied to the elbow, wrist, knee, and ankle, as well as the digits. Representative examples of commonly used techniques are given.

   On occasion, muscles will be contracted to move articulations. Examples of this type of technique are the elevated proximal clavicle and the posterior and anterior proximal fibula.

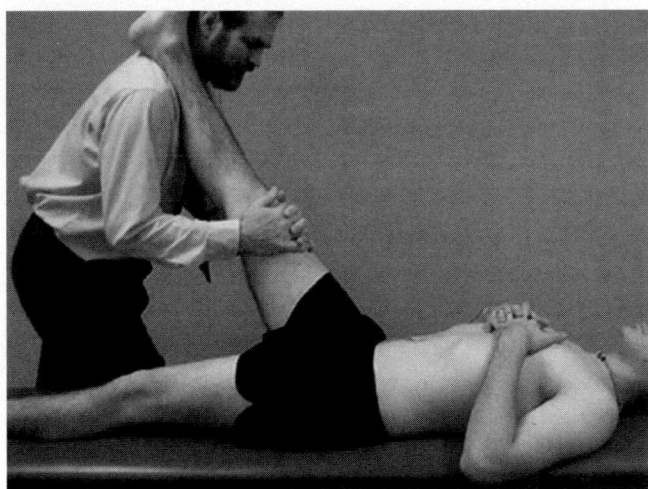

FIGURE 57.33. Treatment of hypertonic hamstring muscle.

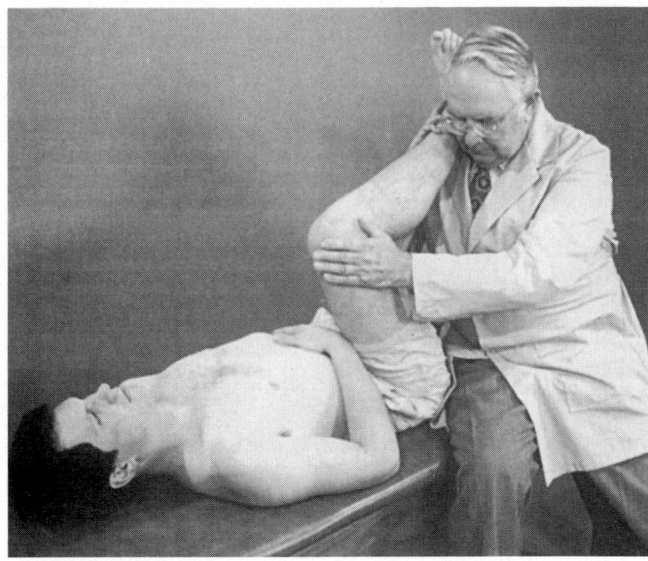

FIGURE 57.34. Treatment of hypertonic gluteus maximus muscle.

Hip Girdle Dysfunction—Hamstring Muscles (Fig. 57.33)

Diagnosis

Position: The hip joint is held extended by hypertonic hamstring muscles.

Restriction: The hip joint is restricted in flexion by hypertonic hamstring muscles.

Type of Muscle Energy

Post-isometric relaxation.

Treatment Position

Patient: Supine.

Physician: Seated on the side of the table on the side of dysfunction at the level of the patient's knee.

Procedure

1. The patient's hip is flexed to the initial resistance while keeping the knee in extension.
2. The patient's leg is then placed on top of the physician's shoulder.
3. The physician's hands are placed on top of the patient's thigh to maintain the knee in extension throughout the technique.
4. The patient is instructed to "push your leg gently down into my shoulder."
5. This contraction is held for a full 3 to 5 seconds.
6. Direct the patient to relax, simultaneously ceasing your counterforce.
7. Wait 2 seconds for the tissues to relax, and then further flex the hip until a new restrictive barrier is met.
8. Steps four, five, six, and seven are repeated three to five times or until no additional motion can be gained.
9. Effectiveness of the technique is assessed by retesting hip range of motion in flexion with the knee extended.

Hip Girdle Dysfunction—Gluteus Maximus Muscle (Fig. 57.34)

Diagnosis

Position: The hip joint is held extended by hypertonic gluteal muscles.

Restriction: The hip joint is restricted in flexion by hypertonic gluteal muscles.

Type of Muscle Energy

Post-isometric relaxation.

Treatment Position

Patient: Supine.

Physician: Seated on the side of the table on the side of dysfunction at the level of the patient's knee.

Procedure

1. The patient's hip is flexed to the initial resistance while keeping the knee in a flexed position.
2. The physician's hands are placed on the posterior thigh just proximal to the popliteal fossa.
3. The patient is instructed to "push your leg gently against my hands."
4. This contraction is held for a full 3 to 5 seconds.
5. Direct the patient to relax, simultaneously ceasing your counterforce.
6. Wait 2 seconds for the tissues to relax, and then further flex the hip until a new restrictive barrier is met.
7. Steps four, five, six, and seven are repeated three to five times or until no additional motion can be gained.
8. Effectiveness of the technique is assessed by retesting hip range of motion in flexion with the knee flexed.

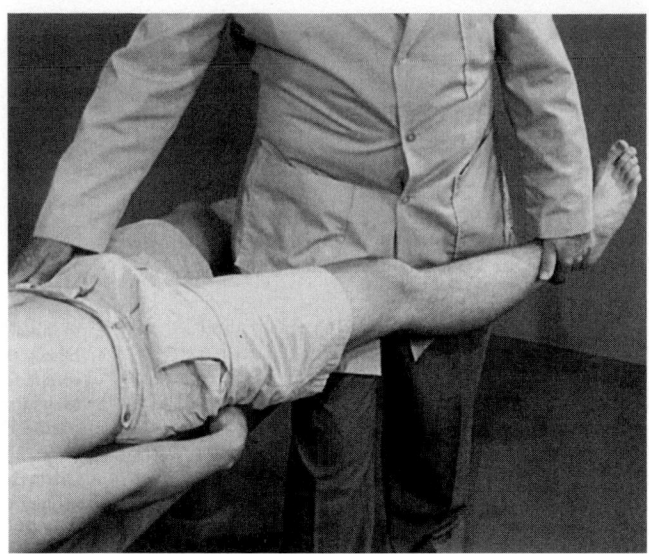

FIGURE 57.35. Treatment of hypertonic hip adductor muscles.

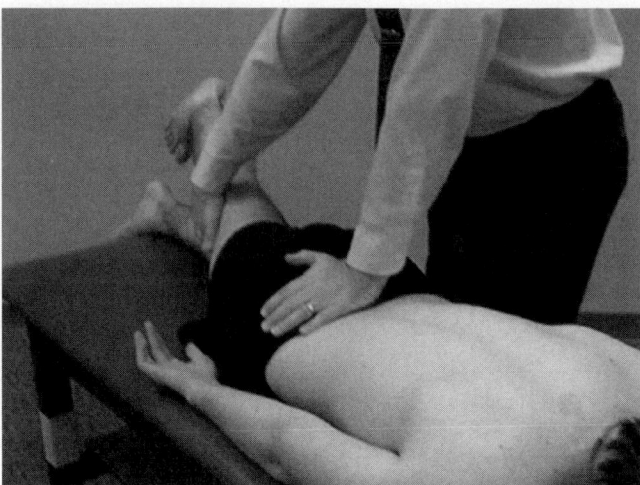

FIGURE 57.36. Treatment of hypertonic hip abductor muscles.

Hip Girdle Dysfunction—Adductor Muscles (Fig. 57.35)

Diagnosis
Position: The hip joint is held adducted by hypertonic adductor muscles.

Restriction: The hip joint is restricted in abduction by hypertonic adductor muscles.

Type of Muscle Energy
Post-isometric relaxation.

Treatment Position
Patient: Supine.

Physician: Standing at the side of the patient between the patient's abducted thigh and the table.

Procedure
1. The patient's hip is abducted until initial resistance is met.
2. The physician's cephalad hand is placed on the contralateral anterior superior iliac spine. The physician's caudad hand is placed on the patient's ipsilateral ankle.
3. The patient is instructed to "pull your leg gently against my thigh."
4. This contraction is held for a full 3 to 5 seconds.
5. Direct the patient to relax, simultaneously ceasing your counterforce.
6. Wait 2 seconds for the tissues to relax, and then further abduct the hip until a new restrictive barrier is met.
7. Steps four, five, six, and seven are repeated three to five times or until no additional motion can be gained.
8. Effectiveness of the technique is assessed by retesting hip range of motion in abduction.

Hip Girdle Dysfunction—Abductor Muscles (Fig. 57.36)

Diagnosis
Position: The hip joint is held abducted by hypertonic abductor muscles.

Restriction: The hip joint is restricted in adduction by hypertonic abductor muscles.

Type of Muscle Energy
Post-isometric relaxation.

Treatment Position
Patient: Supine.

Physician: Standing at the end of the table.

Procedure
1. The patient's hip is flexed until it can clear the other leg and then adducted until initial resistance is met.
2. The physician's hand is placed on the lateral aspect of the patient's ankle.
3. The patient is instructed to "pull your leg gently against my hand."
4. This contraction is held for a full 3 to 5 seconds.
5. Direct the patient to relax, simultaneously ceasing your counterforce.
6. Wait 2 seconds for the tissues to relax, and then further adduct the hip until a new restrictive barrier is met.
7. Steps four, five, six, and seven are repeated three to five times or until no additional motion can be gained.
8. Effectiveness of the technique is assessed by retesting hip range of motion in adduction.

Hip Girdle Dysfunction—Psoas Muscle (Fig. 57.37)

Diagnosis
Position: The hip joint is held flexed by a hypertonic psoas muscle.

Restriction: The hip joint is restricted in extension by a hypertonic psoas muscle.

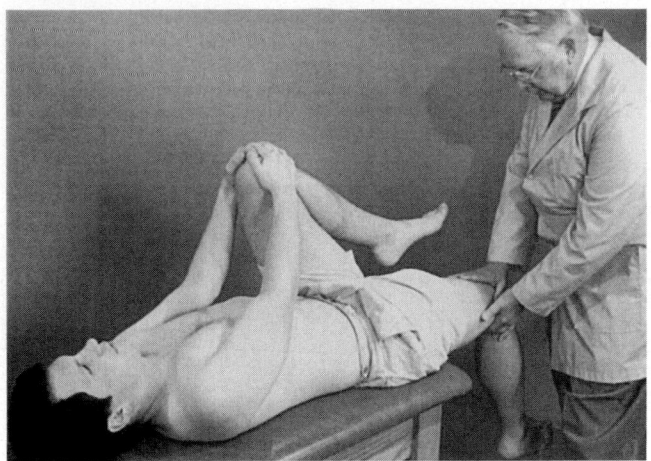

FIGURE 57.37. Treatment of hypertonic psoas muscle.

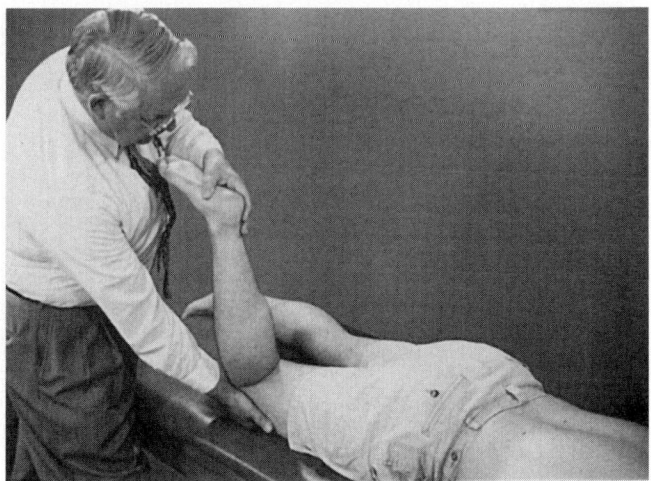

FIGURE 57.38. Treatment of hypertonic hip external rotator muscles (piriformis muscle).

Type of Muscle Energy
Post-isometric relaxation.

Treatment Position
Patient: Supine with legs extended off the end of the table.
> *Physician:* Standing at the end of the table.

Procedure
1. The patient's hips are flexed while keeping the knees in a flexed position.
2. The patient's leg on the side of dysfunction is dropped down off the end of the table while the patient holds the contralateral hip in a flexed position.
3. The physician's hand is placed on the anterior thigh just proximal to the knee.
4. The patient is instructed to "lift your leg gently against my hand."
5. This contraction is held for a full 3 to 5 seconds.
6. Direct the patient to relax, simultaneously ceasing your counterforce.
7. Wait 2 seconds for the tissues to relax, and then further extend the hip until a new restrictive barrier is met.
8. Steps four, five, six, and seven are repeated three to five times or until no additional motion can be gained.
9. Effectiveness of the technique is assessed by retesting hip range of motion in extension.

Hip Girdle Dysfunction—External Rotator Muscles (Piriformis) (Fig. 57.38)

Diagnosis
Position: The hip joint is held in external rotation.
> *Restriction:* The hip joint is restricted in internal rotation.

Type of Muscle Energy
Post-isometric relaxation.

Treatment Position
Patient: Prone.
> *Physician:* Standing at the side of the table.

Procedure
1. The patient's knee is flexed to 90 degrees.
2. The patient's hip is internally rotated until the initial resistance is palpated.
3. The physician's hand is placed on the medial side of the ankle.
4. The patient is instructed to "press your leg gently against my hand."
5. This contraction is held for a full 3 to 5 seconds.
6. Direct the patient to relax, simultaneously ceasing your counterforce.
7. Wait 2 seconds for the tissues to relax, and then further internally rotate the hip until a new restrictive barrier is met.
8. Steps four, five, six, and seven are repeated three to five times or until no additional motion can be gained.
9. Effectiveness of the technique is assessed by retesting hip range of motion in internal rotation.

Hip Girdle Dysfunction—Internal Rotator Muscles (Fig. 57.39)

Diagnosis
Position: The hip joint is held in internal rotation.
> *Restriction:* The hip joint is restricted in external rotation.

Type of Muscle Energy
Post-isometric relaxation.

Treatment Position
Patient: Prone.
> *Physician:* Standing at the side of the table.

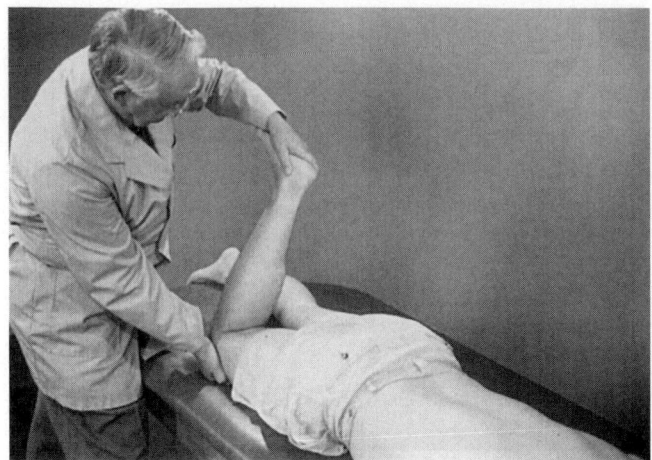

FIGURE 57.39. Treatment of hypertonic hip internal rotator muscles.

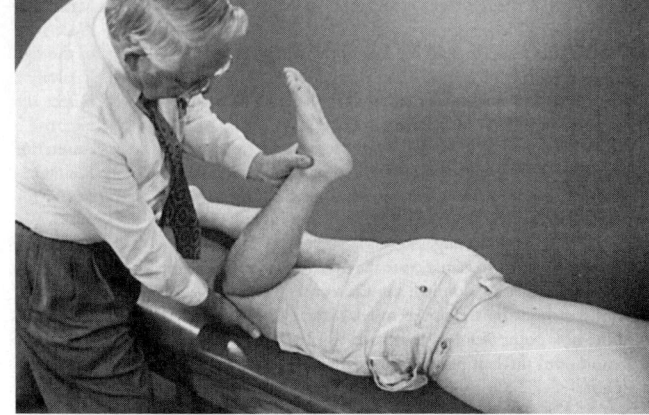

FIGURE 57.40. Treatment of hypertonic rectus femoris muscle.

Procedure

1. The patient's knee is flexed to 90 degrees.
2. The patient's hip is externally rotated until the initial resistance is palpated.
3. The physician's hand is placed on the lateral side of the ankle.
4. The patient is instructed to "press your leg gently against my hand."
5. This contraction is held for a full 3 to 5 seconds.
6. Direct the patient to relax, simultaneously ceasing your counterforce.
7. Wait 2 seconds for the tissues to relax, and then further externally rotate the hip until a new restrictive barrier is met.
8. Steps four, five, six, and seven are repeated three to five times or until no additional motion can be gained.
9. Effectiveness of the technique is assessed by retesting hip range of motion in external rotation.

Knee Dysfunction—Rectus Femoris Muscle (Fig. 57.40)

Diagnosis

Position: The hip joint is held in flexion with the knee extended.
   Restriction: With the hip held in neutral, the knee is restricted in flexion.

Type of Muscle Energy

Post-isometric relaxation.

Treatment Position

Patient: Prone.
   Physician: Standing at the side of the table.

Procedure

1. The patient's knee is flexed until the initial resistance is palpated.
2. The physician's hand is placed on the ankle.
3. The patient is instructed to "press your leg gently against my hand."

4. This contraction is held for a full 3 to 5 seconds.
5. Direct the patient to relax, simultaneously ceasing your counterforce.
6. Wait 2 seconds for the tissues to relax, and then further flex the knee until a new restrictive barrier is met.
7. Steps four, five, six, and seven are repeated three to five times or until no additional motion can be gained.
8. Effectiveness of the technique is assessed by retesting knee range of motion in flexion with the hip in neutral.

Knee—Proximal Fibula Posterior (Fig. 57.41)

Diagnosis

Position: The proximal fibula is posterior.
   Restriction: The proximal fibula is restricted in anterior glide.

Type of Muscle Energy

Joint mobilization using muscle force.

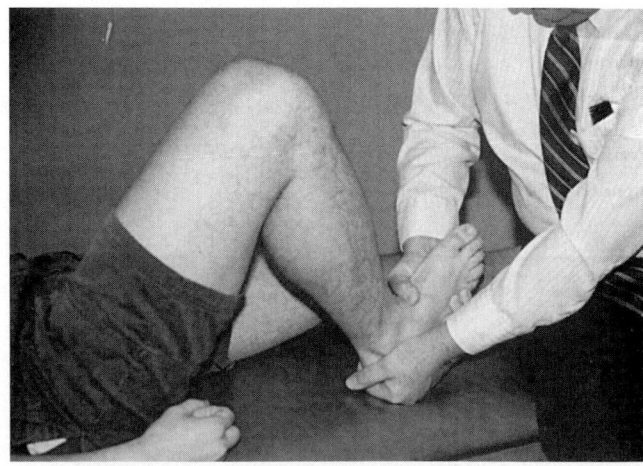

FIGURE 57.41. Treatment of proximal fibula posterior.

Treatment Position

Patient: Supine with hip flexed 45 degrees and knee flexed 90 degrees.

Physician: Standing at the foot of the table facing the patient.

Procedure

1. The physician's medial hand is placed on the dorsum of the foot with his or her thumb on the lateral aspect and the fingers on the medial aspect.
2. The physician's lateral hand anchors the calcaneus.
3. The ankle is inverted to the initial resistance.
4. The patient is instructed to "push your foot sideways into my thumbs and up into my hand." This eversion/dorsiflexion of the ankle is thought to contract the extensor digitorum longus and the tibialis anterior muscles, drawing the fibula forward.
5. This contraction is held for a full 3 to 5 seconds.
6. Direct the patient to relax, simultaneously ceasing your counterforce.
7. Wait 2 seconds for the tissues to relax, and then further invert the foot until a new restrictive barrier is met.
8. Steps four, five, six, and seven are repeated three to five times or until no additional motion can be gained.
9. Effectiveness of the technique is determined by retesting motion at the proximal tibiofibular articulation.

Knee—Proximal Fibula Anterior (Fig. 57.42)

Diagnosis

Position: The proximal fibula is anterior.

Restriction: The proximal fibula is restricted in posterior glide.

Type of Muscle Energy

Joint mobilization using muscle force.

Treatment Position

Patient: Supine with hip flexed 45 degrees and knee flexed 90 degrees.

Physician: Standing at the foot of the table facing the patient.

Procedure

1. The physician's medial hand is placed on the dorsum of the foot with thumb on the lateral aspect and the fingers on the medial aspect.
2. The physician's lateral hand anchors the calcaneus.
3. The ankle is inverted to the initial resistance.
4. The patient is instructed to "push your foot sideways into my thumbs and down into my hand." This eversion/plantar flexion of the ankle is thought to contract the fibularis longus and soleus muscles, drawing the fibula backward.
5. This contraction is held for a full 3 to 5 seconds.
6. Direct the patient to relax, simultaneously ceasing your counterforce.
7. Wait 2 seconds for the tissues to relax, and then further invert the foot until a new restrictive barrier is met.
8. Steps four, five, six, and seven are repeated three to five times or until no additional motion can be gained.
9. Effectiveness of the technique is determined by retesting motion at the proximal tibiofibular articulation.

Ankle—Soleus Muscle (Fig. 57.43)

Diagnosis

Position: The ankle is held plantar flexed by a hypertonic soleus muscle.

Restriction: The ankle is restricted in dorsiflexion by a hypertonic soleus muscle.

Type of Muscle Energy

Post-isometric relaxation.

Treatment Position

Patient: Prone with the knee flexed 90 degrees.

Physician: Standing at the side of the foot of the table.

Procedure

1. The physician's hand grasps the patient's heel with the wrist and distal forearm contacting the sole of the foot right down to the toes.

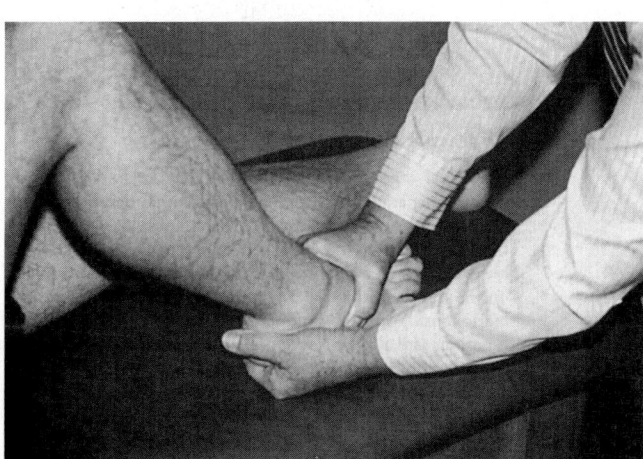

FIGURE 57.42. Treatment of proximal fibula anterior.

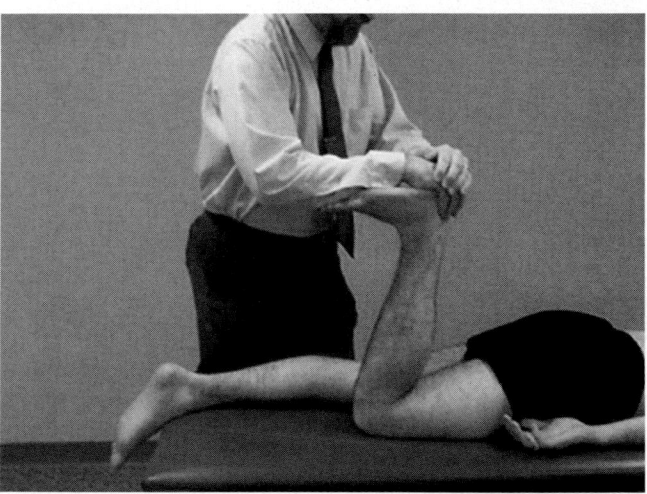

FIGURE 57.43. Treatment of hypertonic soleus muscle.

2. The sole of the foot is maintained parallel to the floor as the ankle is dorsiflexed and the knee is flexed. This motion is continued until the initial resistance is met.

3. The patient is instructed to "push the ball of your foot up into my arm."

4. This contraction is held for a full 3 to 5 seconds.

5. Direct the patient to relax, simultaneously ceasing your counterforce.

6. Wait 2 seconds for the tissues to relax, and then further dorsiflex the ankle until a new restrictive barrier is met.

7. Steps three, four, five, and six are repeated three to five times or until no additional motion can be gained.

8. Effectiveness of the technique is assessed by retesting ankle range of motion in dorsiflexion.

Clavicle—Anterior Rotation (Fig. 57.44)

Diagnosis
Position: The clavicle is rotated anteriorly.
   Restriction: The clavicle is restricted in posterior rotation.

Type of Muscle Energy
Post-isometric relaxation.

Treatment Position
Patient: Seated.
Physician: Standing behind the patient.

Procedure
1. The physician grasps the patient's wrist.

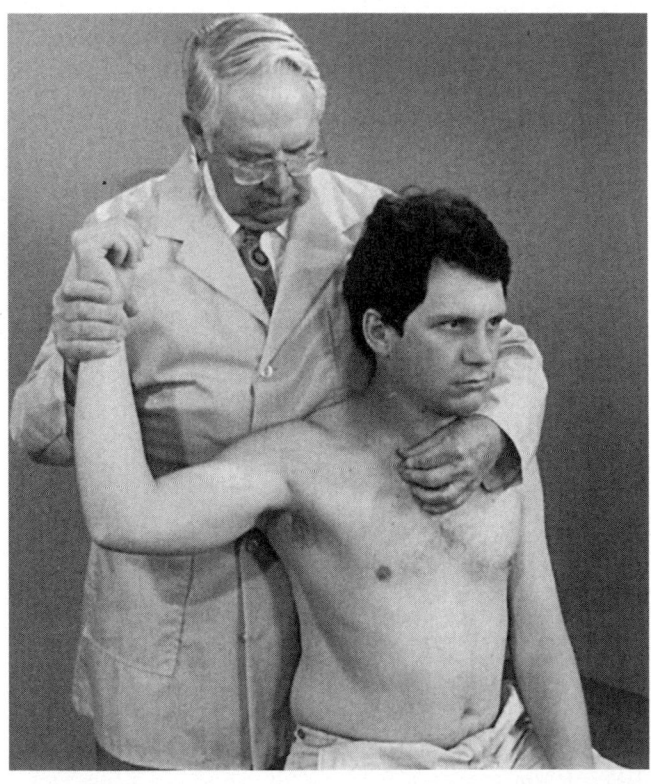

FIGURE 57.44. Treatment of anteriorly rotated clavicle.

2. The shoulder is abducted 90 degrees and then externally rotated until initial resistance is met.

3. The patient is instructed to "gently press your wrist forward and toward the floor." This force would normally internally rotate the humerus in a horizontal position.

4. This contraction is held for a full 3 to 5 seconds.

5. Direct the patient to relax, simultaneously ceasing your counterforce.

6. Wait 2 seconds for the tissues to relax, and then further externally rotate the shoulder until a new restrictive barrier is met.

7. Steps three, four, five, and six are repeated three to five times or until no further clavicular motion can be gained.

8. Effectiveness of the technique is assessed by retesting clavicular motion.

Clavicle—Superior Sternal End (Fig. 57.45)

Diagnosis
Position: The proximal clavicle is displaced medially and cephalad.
   Restriction: The proximal clavicle is restricted in motion laterally and caudad.

Type of Muscle Energy
Joint mobilization using muscle force.

Treatment Position
Patient: Supine with shoulder abducted 45 degrees.
   Physician: Standing at the side of the table.

Procedure
1. The physician grasps the extended wrist, externally rotates the arm, and gently presses it down toward the floor until initial resistance is met.

2. The physician's other hand palpates the sternal end of the clavicle.

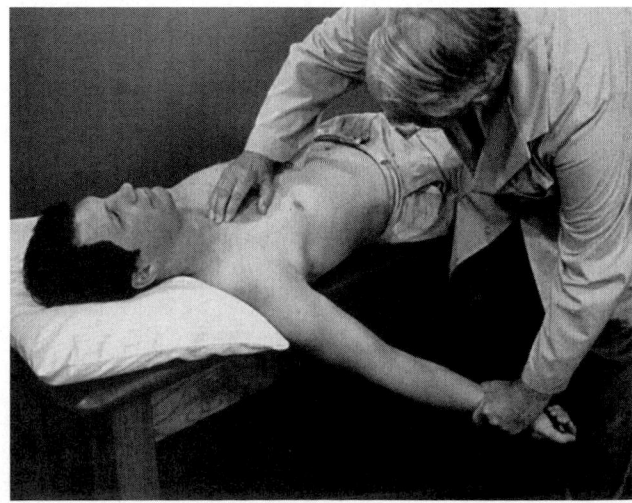

FIGURE 57.45. Treatment of superior displacement of the proximal clavicle.

3. The patient is instructed to "lift your arm up toward the ceiling."

4. The pectoralis muscles pull the clavicle laterally and inferior.

5. This contraction is held for a full 3 to 5 seconds.

6. Direct the patient to relax, simultaneously ceasing your counterforce.

7. Wait 2 seconds for the tissues to relax, and then press the patient's arm further toward the floor.

8. Steps three, four, five, and six are repeated three to five times or until no additional sternoclavicular motion is gained.

9. Effectiveness of the technique is assessed by retesting sternoclavicular motion.

REFERENCES

1. Mitchell Sr FL. Structural pelvic function. In: Barnes MW, ed. *Yearbook of the Academy of Applied Osteopathy.* Indianapolis, IN: American Academy of Osteopathy; 1958:79.

2. Ruddy TJ. Osteopathic rhythmic resistive duction therapy. In: Barnes MW, ed. *Yearbook of the Academy of Applied Osteopathy.* Indianapolis, IN: American Academy of Osteopathy; 1961:58.

3. Guyer AF. Proprioceptive neuromuscular facilitation for vertebral joint conditions. In: Grieve GP, ed. *Modern Manual Therapy of the Vertebral Column.* New York, NY: Churchill Livingstone; 1986:626.

4. Lewit K, Simons DG. Myofascial pain: relief by post-isometric relaxation. *Arch Phys Med Rehabil.* 1984;65:453–456.

5. Travell JG, Simons DG. *Myofascial Pain and Dysfunction: The Trigger Point Manual,* vol. 2. Baltimore, MD: Williams & Wilkins; 1992:10.

6. Mitchell Jr FL, Moran PS, Pruzzo NA. *An Evaluation and Treatment Manual of Osteopathic Muscle Energy Procedures.* Valley Park, MO: Mitchell, Moran, and Pruzzo; 1979.

7. Mitchell Jr FL. *The Muscle Energy Manual.* East Lansing, MI: MET Press; 1999.

8. Goodridge, JP. Muscle energy technique: definition, explanation, methods of procedures. *J Am Osteopath Assoc.* 1981;81:249–254.

9. Mitchell Jr FL, Moran PS, Pruzzo NA. *An Evaluation and Treatment Manual of Osteopathic Manipulative Procedure.* 2nd ed. Kansas City, MO: Institute for Continuing Education in Osteopathic Principles, Inc; 1973:325.

10. Jull GA, Janda V. Muscles and motor control in low back pain; assessment and management. In: Twomaey LT, Taylor JR, eds. *Physical Therapy for the Low Back.* New York, NY: Churchill Livingstone; 1987:272.

FASCIAL-LIGAMENTOUS RELEASE: INDIRECT APPROACH

ANTHONY G. CHILA

KEY CONCEPTS

- Relevance of osteopathic philosophy to the technique of fascial-ligamentous release
- Location and function of fascia (superficial, subserous, and deep), aponeurosis, and tendon
- Indirect techniques of functional release and strain/counterstrain as manipulative models, and how they are incorporated into the technique of fascial-ligamentous release
- Basic procedures involved in fascial-ligamentous release
- Hysteresis and creep, how they allow for relaxation of tissues, and why the relaxation may be temporary
- How fascial-ligamentous release allows for sustained relaxation and resolution of chronic dysfunction via central nervous system desensitization
- Supine treatment model
- Three components of the doctor–patient relationship in making a diagnosis
- Benefits of using a fulcrum in treatment
- Positioning for the following areas: sacrum and pelvis, sacrum, iliosacrum, lower lumbar, abdominal fascia, upper lumbar, psoas muscle, liver, lower extremity (abduction phase, adduction phase, and foot), rib cage, lower and upper thorax, cervical, upper extremity (scapula, axilla, thoracic apertures, clavicle, radius, ulna, hand, and fingers), occipitoatlantal joint and basilar axes of the skull

Classic osteopathic thought has assigned importance to the role of the connective tissue system of the body in health and disease. In his writings, A.T. Still emphasized the connective tissue system in the diagnosis and treatment of dysfunction. Although manipulative approaches based on fascial-ligamentous considerations have enjoyed a reawakening in recent years, they are in fact representative of early osteopathic methods. This chapter offers a synthesis of the thoughts of various representative osteopathic authors on this subject. Other sources provide further detail about fascial-ligamentous release (1–8).

PHILOSOPHY OF MANIPULATION

A philosophy of manipulation is central to, and not synonymous with, the practice of osteopathy. Osteopathic theory holds that when the anatomic-physiologic tendency of a human being is toward a state of health, all functions of the body have an optimal performance capacity. Still made reference to a philosophy of manipulation that was based on absolute knowledge of form and function proceeding from a perfect image of the normal articulations. In Still's view, the adjustment of tissues of the body according to form, function, and image was the basis of treatment. Still indicated equally clearly that diseases could be regarded as effects occurring in regions of the body when optimal performance capacity became compromised.

CONNECTIVE TISSUE CONTINUITY

Fascia of the human body can be described as a sheet of fibrous tissue that envelops the body beneath the skin; it also encloses muscles and groups of muscles, separating their several layers or groups. An aponeurosis is a fibrous sheet or expanded tendon that gives attachment to muscular fibers and serves as the means of origin or insertion of a flat muscle. It sometimes performs the office of a fascia for other muscles. A tendon is a fibrous cord or band that connects a muscle to bone or some other structures. It consists of fascicles of densely arranged collagenous fibers, tendon cells, and a minimum of ground substance.

In addition to extensive attachment for muscles, the fascia of the human body is provided with sensory nerve endings and is thought to be elastic as well as contractile. Fascia supports and stabilizes, helping to maintain balance. It assists in the production and control of motion and the interrelation of motion of related parts. Many of the body's fascial specializations have postural functions in which stress bands can be demonstrated. Finally, the dura mater is a special connective tissue surrounding the central nervous system. Bony anchors for this tissue exist in the skull and at the sacrum.

Fascia in the human body is described as being superficial, deep, or subserous. The superficial and deep layers are found everywhere in the body as complete ensheathments. The subserous layer lies innermost on the deep layer anywhere there is a body cavity. The deep layer of fascia is the most complicated of the three, being two-layered with intervening septa.

Clinically, it is possible to conceptualize such wrapping as being a big bandage of the body. Such an analogy is implied in osteopathic literature. One can find reference to the idea that the body retains form even if everything except the connective tissue framework is removed. If this is so, then it is also reasonable that form permits the consideration of motion. The continuity of this arrangement and considerations of structural-functional interrelationships make it possible to discuss biomechanical attributes of fascia in relation to manipulative treatment.

MANIPULATIVE MODELS

The study of the application of force in osteopathic manipulative treatment (OMT) has led to the development of several manipulative models. In particular, those who seek to reduce the possibility of microtrauma to tissues and joints have built on considerations of fascial distribution and specialization. This is especially so in those models which require refinement of palpatory skills to appreciate subtleties of stress patterns and motion characteristics.

The corrective forces underlying these models are generally approaches in which the dysfunctional component of resistance to motion is carried to a point of simultaneous balance and decreased tension. The focus of procedures in such models is on the quality of movement, particularly on initiation of motion. Emphasis is reduced on the range of motion and the end point of motion. The correct gauging of force and velocity provides infinite variation in the delivery of technique. Control minimizes force. The effective physician should be able to vary the applications of force during a single manipulative treatment or over time for continuing manipulative management. Appropriate use of a fulcrum and leverage can refine the physician's diagnostic touch and treatment effectiveness.

The emphases peculiar to the various manipulative models can be selectively used in preparing the individual patient's manipulative prescription. Sequencing the diagnosis and treatment allows the physician to improve the quality of office records. The level of the patient's response to manipulative treatment can be better documented. Longitudinal assessment of the patient's progress is facilitated. In general, such models are hypothesized to reduce the flow of abnormal afferent impulses into the central nervous system by reprogramming for more normal function. The following three paragraphs illustrate the variable dynamic of fascial-ligamentous release in relation to the functional release and strain and counterstrain approaches.

Functional Release

In functional release, the manipulative procedure is guided by palpation at the dysfunctional segment (spinal or appendicular) for continuous feedback information about the patient's physiologic response to motion. Operator-induced motion compares relative degrees of compliance or resistance of component parts. It does so in opposing directions. The motions introduced are those that lead to an increased sense of compliance (decreased resistance) of component parts.

Strain and Counterstrain

In strain and counterstrain, passive movement away from the area of resistance to motion is induced toward and into planes of increased motion, always searching for the position of greatest comfort. The body is folded around the tender point. A position of mild but asymptomatic strain is induced, which is thought to produce the most efficient reflex release of joint dysfunction within a prescribed period of time.

Fascial-Ligamentous Release

Elements of each of the preceding models are incorporated when using fascial-ligamentous release. The patient provides breath assistance and/or muscular assistance in the corrective procedure. The establishment of a fulcrum is sought within the physician's body to match or balance the fulcrum within the patient's body; this facilitates a continuum of reflex release from within the patient's body. Once local and regional dysfunction have been addressed by the establishment of an appropriate fulcrum, expanding leverage is achieved through torsion and traction applied to the extremities. It is the ongoing analysis of dysfunction within this continuum that makes possible the integration of multiple manipulative approaches through variable applications of force.

TREATMENT CONSIDERATIONS

In performing manipulative procedures, the body responds comprehensively to an externally applied force. From the moment of contact with the skin, avenues for the implementation of variations of force are provided by palpatory clues. In the sense of a body covering, the skin may be regarded as a mass adrenergic medium that is useful in the facilitation and amplification of proprioceptive interchange between unique persons, the patient and the physician.

Osteopathic diagnosis and treatment does not concern itself simply with the performance of a single manual procedure. The particular treatment, as well as the construction of a management program, often requires variation in technical approaches. Visualization and synthesis of messages received through the fingers are the basis for clinical behavior. Conceptualization of anatomic-physiologic dysfunction peculiar to a given patient is the key to maximizing manipulative responses. The sustained effective response following treatment is contingent on selective and controlled variation of force from an appropriate fulcrum. When these conditions are met, inherent neuroregulatory mechanisms acting in accordance with the capacity of the patient will facilitate the resolution of dysfunction.

Generally speaking, the body's connective tissues are under some degree of load and extension. The increase and subsequent reversal of extension produces a degree of tissue response less than the relatively unloaded state. This phenomenon is referred to as hysteresis. It implies the occurrence of some flow and dissipation of energy throughout the loaded tissue. Hysteresis occurs less with successive cycles of extension, indicating stabilization of response.

Connective tissues under sustained load will extend in response to the load. In biomechanical terms, this continued extension is referred to as *creep*. An imposed constant load will result in relaxation, as the extension remains constant. In either situation, the tissue displays less subsequent resistance to extension than in the original state.

Behaviors of connective tissues depend on previous mechanical history. Extension effects revert to their preextension responses. This observation may be useful in appreciating recurrence of dysfunctional complaints. The principle of timed release of tissues associated with the fascial-ligamentous release model of manipulative treatment considers these factors. The sequential and expanding progression of this approach permits the patient to tolerate central nervous system modulation. The lowering of afferent inputs is gradually facilitated. If the patient's capacity to respond is appropriate, the model seeks to ensure the significant reduction or elimination of sensitization. This view is attuned to the idea that central nervous system conditioning over time may be the vehicle for the retention as well as the reduction of dysfunctional states. The physician's role is that of a facilitator. By appropriate facilitation, the physician is able to observe the capacity for change while the patient is enabled to expand the power of the change. The standard for the successful outcome of this interchange is the motivation of the patient.

SUPINE TREATMENT

Observation and Palpation

With the patient lying in the supine position, observational and systemic palpatory findings help to establish a diagnosis related to the mechanical forces associated with body position. With the head unsupported and the legs fully extended, note the increased mechanical stresses impacting the cervical and lumbar lordotic curves. Compromised respiratory-circulatory effectiveness is the result of generalized fascial-ligamentous tension throughout the body. For that reason the character of respiration provides information about such tension. Observe four factors about respiration:

1. *Type of respiration:* diaphragmatic, costal, or mixed
2. *Abdominal wall motion:* visible to the level of the umbilicus; visible to the level of the symphysis pubes
3. *Rate:* slow, rapid; documented before and after treatment
4. *Duration of cycle:* inspiration and expiration equal, inspiration shorter in duration than expiration, inspiration longer in duration than expiration, dilation of the nares during respiration

Diagnostic Touch

Diagnosis is an important component in patient care. There are three central elements in an encounter between a physician and a patient:

1. The patient's ideas and beliefs of what the problem could be
2. The physician's concept of what the problem could be
3. That which the anatomic-physiologic wholeness of the patient's body knows the problem to be

With respect to the last of these aspects, OMT must allow the physiologic function within to manifest its own potency rather than use blind external force and overpower its assistance. This is accomplished through the use of a fulcrum, which is the support or point of support on which a lever turns in raising or moving something.

The establishment of an appropriate fulcrum facilitates diagnostic touch. The placing of the hands and fingers on the tissues under examination is done with the idea that the fingers can mold themselves to the patient's body. The initiation of the pattern within the area of complaint is realized by a slight compression at the fulcrum points. The application of the principle of the fulcrum is as varied as the list of complaints brought to the physician's office. The use of this method is not a time-consuming process. Mechanisms already in action are used. It is necessary only to contact them and to sense them speaking for themselves. There are no techniques. The point or points are listening posts. Let the tissues tell the story; be quiet and listen. Biokinetic (dysfunctional) energies or forces are always at work in all physiologic and pathologic processes. With the appropriate use of diagnostic touch, the biodynamic (healing) intrinsic force within is allowed to manifest itself.

The findings noted on observation and palpation contribute to the evaluation that governs the administration of OMT. The clinical diagnosis and the tolerance of the patient govern the application of forces in OMT. Any sequence for treatment adopted by a physician should have two intentions:

1. The alleviation or elimination of effects of disease processes that have occurred or are occurring in the various regions of the body
2. The restoration of the patient's ability to resume command of the clinical situation

Positions for diagnostic touch of various areas of the body using the principle of fulcrum are outlined below.

Lower Body

The patient's knees are flexed, and the feet placed flat on the table. Lateralization of the feet, with inversion of the toes, helps to stabilize the pelvis.

Sacrum and Pelvis

1. Mold with the patient's sacrum with one hand (Fig. 58.1).
2. Place the fingertips of this hand at the level of the spinous process of the fifth lumbar segment (L5). The opposite arm and hand bridge the anterior superior iliac spine (ASIS) on each side of the pelvis (Fig. 58.2).
3. The fulcrum is established by the elbow, which is leaning on the treatment table.

Sacrum, Iliosacrum, Lower Lumbar

1. Mold with the patient's sacrum with one hand (Fig. 58.3).
2. Place the opposite hand under the iliosacral articulation. The fingertips of this hand contact the spinous process of the lower

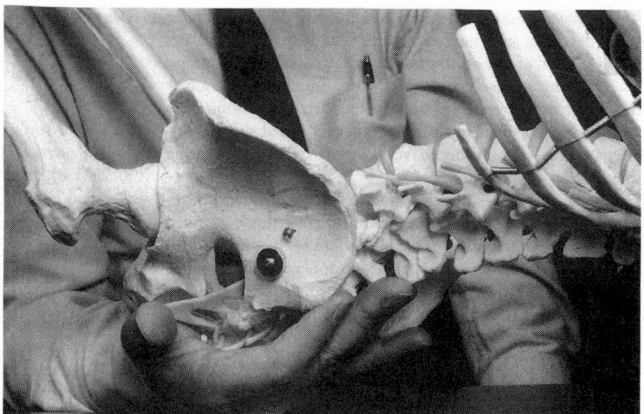

FIGURE 58.1. Sacrum and pelvis. One hand molds with the sacrum.

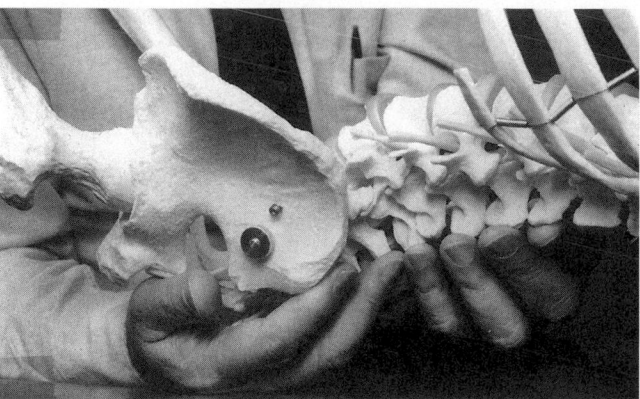

FIGURE 58.3. Sacrum, iliosacrum, lower lumbar.

lumbar segments (L3, L4, L5). Both elbows establish the fulcrum: one leaning on the treatment table (sacrum), the other leaning on the physician's knee (iliosacrum; lower lumbar).

Abdominal Fascial Tension

Mold with the sacrum with one hand. The opposite hand accomplishes multiple assessments: the abdominal quadrants, costal margins, and linea alba; tension of the inguinal ligaments; and shear dysfunctions at the pubic symphysis. Both elbows establish the fulcrum: one leaning on the treatment table (sacrum), and the other being the elbow of the exploring arm (abdomen).

Upper Lumbar, Psoas Muscle

Place one hand under the upper lumbar area (Fig. 58.4). The opposite arm and hand bridge the flexed knees. The fulcrum is established by the elbow on the knee (upper lumbar area).

Liver

Place one hand under the lower ribs beneath the liver. Place the opposite hand over the anterior surface of the liver. The fulcrum is established by the elbow on the knee (lower ribs).

Lower Extremity

Selectively employ torsion (rotation) and traction in two phases to release muscular, fascial, ligamentous, and articular dysfunction. The fulcrum is established by the elbows of the physician's arms in supporting the motions of the patient's foot, lower leg, and knee.

Abduction Phase (Lower Leg)
Invert the plantar surface of the foot (Fig. 58.5). Introduce torsion between the ankle and the knee. Advance the effect of torsion by slowly moving the knee across the lower abdomen, resulting in progressive abduction of the lower leg. The torsion will be felt in the lateral malleolar area, the medial compartmental area of the knee, the tensor fascia lata area, and the trochanter area. Upon completion of this phase, gradually extend the lower extremity and slowly return it to the tabletop.

Adduction Phase (Lower Leg)
Evert the plantar surface of the foot (Fig. 58.6). Introduce torsion between the ankle and the knee. Steadily advance the effect of torsion by slowly moving the knee away from the lower abdomen, resulting in progressive adduction of the lower leg. The torsion will be felt in the medial malleolar area, the lateral compartmental area of the knee, the medial thigh area, and the inguinal

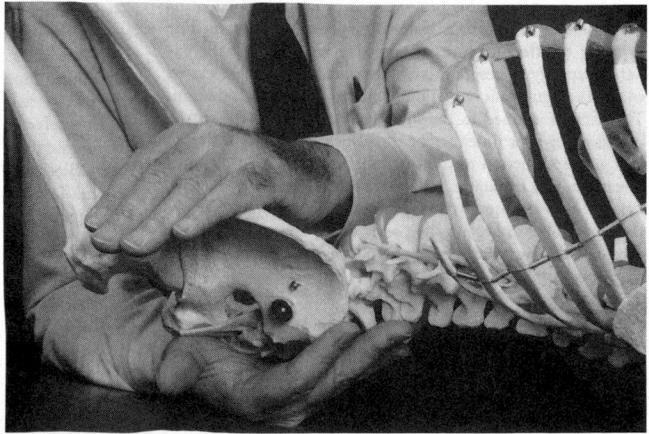

FIGURE 58.2. Sacrum and pelvis. Bridge anterior superior iliac spine.

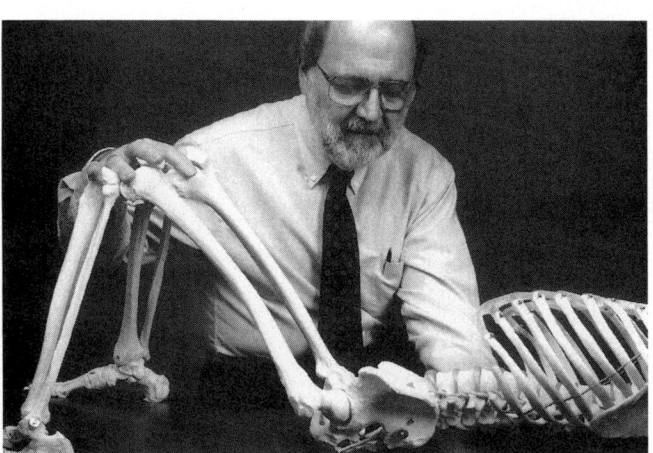

FIGURE 58.4. Upper lumbar, psoas muscle.

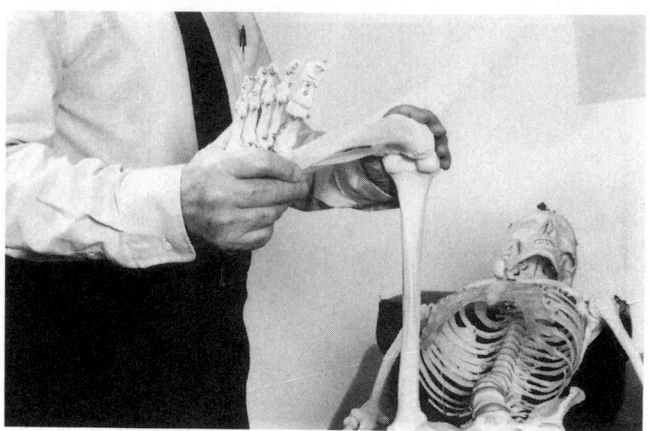

FIGURE 58.5. Lower extremity, abduction phase.

area. Upon completion of this phase, gradually extend the lower extremity and slowly return it to the tabletop.

Foot

Note tenderness to palpation in the plantar myofascial tissues. Give particular attention to such findings along the medial longitudinal arch. The contour of the foot can be analogized to the spinal complex:

The calcaneus represents the sacrum

The tarsal bones represent the lumbar region

The tarsometatarsal area represents the thoracolumbar junction

The metatarsal area represents the thoracic region

The metatarsophalangeal area represents the cervicothoracic junction

The phalangeal area represents the cervical region

Tender points can be analogized to the ipsilateral spinal level, including paraspinal tissues

Treatment is by increased plantar flexion of the foot about the point of greatest tenderness (Fig. 58.7)

Perform articulatory release of the small joints of the toes in sequence, from the great toe to the small toe.

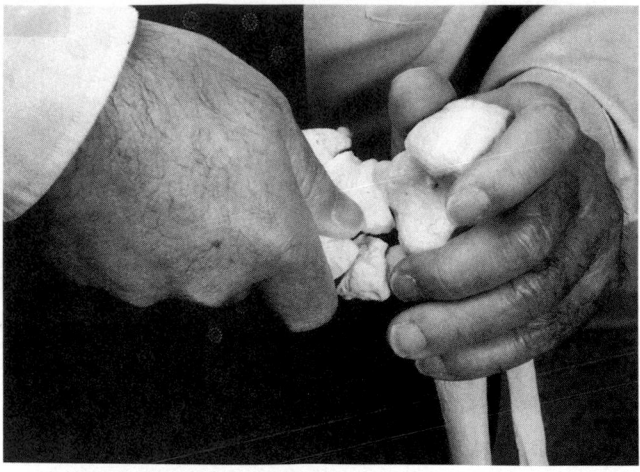

FIGURE 58.7. Foot.

Upper Body

Rib Cage

1. Place one hand beneath the rib cage, with the fingertips just beyond the spinous processes of the associated thoracic vertebrae (Fig. 58.8).
2. Place the other hand on the anterior ends of the ribs. The fulcrum is established by the elbow on the knee.

Lower Thorax

Place both hands beneath the patient at the level of the 12th thoracic segment (T12) (Fig. 58.9). This area corresponds to the level of the insertion of the trapezium muscles bilaterally. The fulcrum is established bilaterally by the elbows resting on the tabletop.

Upper Thorax

The patient's head rests on a pillow. One hand and arm contact the upper thoracic spinous processes, with the fingers spread slightly to contact the ribs on each side (Fig. 58.10). Place the opposite

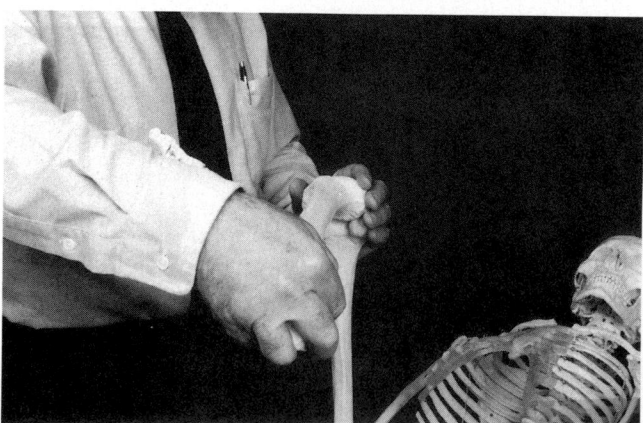

FIGURE 58.6. Lower extremity, adduction phase.

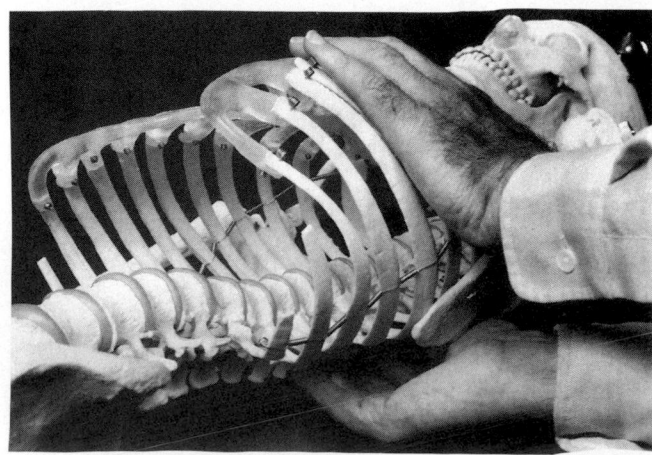

FIGURE 58.8. Rib cage.

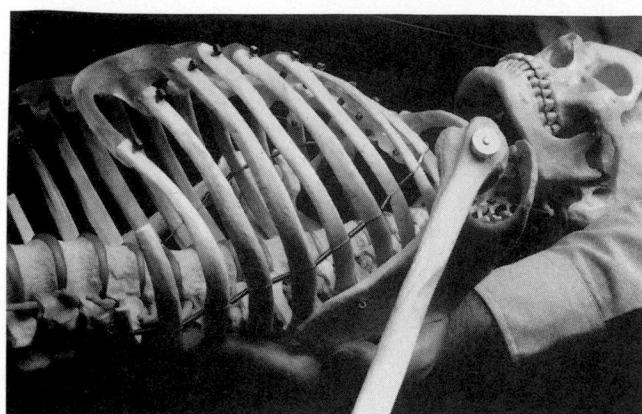

FIGURE 58.9. Lower thorax.

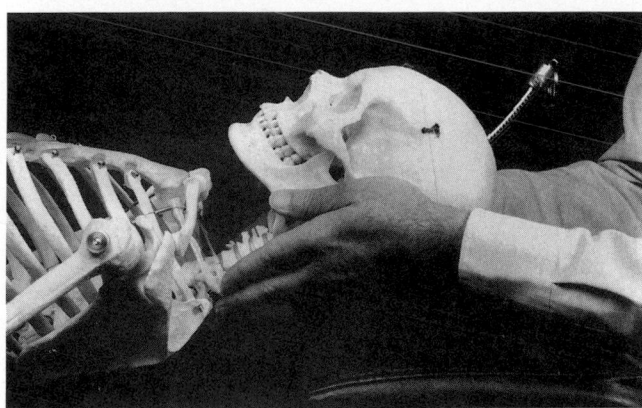

FIGURE 58.11. Cervical area.

hand on the sternum. The fulcrum is established by the elbow on the tabletop, beneath the patient's head.

Cervical Area

Both hands bridge the entire cervical area from the base of the skull to the upper thorax (Fig. 58.11). The fulcrum is established bilaterally by the elbows and forearms resting on the tabletop.

Upper Extremity

Scapulofascial Release

Accomplish this by exploring ease and resistance to motion in several planes: cephalad, caudad, medially, laterally, clockwise, and counterclockwise (Fig. 58.12). Both hands are used to grasp the scapula completely, both medially and laterally.

Axillary Release

Accomplish this by manual decongestion of the posterior axillary tissues and the pectoral tissues.

Expansion of the Inferior Thoracic Aperture

Accomplish this by supporting the elbow region with one hand and the wrist region with the other hand. For this and all subsequent procedures, the fulcrum is established by the elbows of the physician's body in support of the motions of the patient's

upper extremity. Bring the extended upper extremity of the patient closer to the side of the body. Sustained supination as the upper extremity is carried toward the posterior thorax facilitates release of the thoracolumbar junction. Sustained pronation as the upper extremity is carried toward the xiphoid process facilitates musculofascial release along the costal margin. The cumulative effect of these forces contributes to ligamentous articular release of the elbow region.

Clavicular and Glenohumeral Release

Accomplish this by placing the extended upper extremity in a neutral position, with respect to the side of the body, and abducting to the point where a continuum exists between the upper extremity and the position of the clavicle. Sustained pronation as the upper extremity is carried toward the manubrial region facilitates release of the manubrial area and the sternoclavicular articulation. Sustained supination as the upper extremity is carried toward the posterior thorax facilitates release of the acromioclavicular articulation and the glenohumeral area.

Radioulnar, Wrist, Hand, and Fingers Release

Accomplish this by sustained alternating supination and pronation. This facilitates the release of fascial ligamentous tension along the course of the interosseous membrane to the flexor retinaculum (Fig. 58.13).

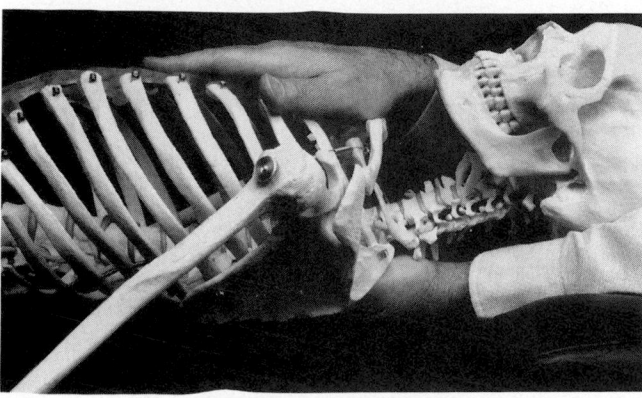

FIGURE 58.10. Upper thorax.

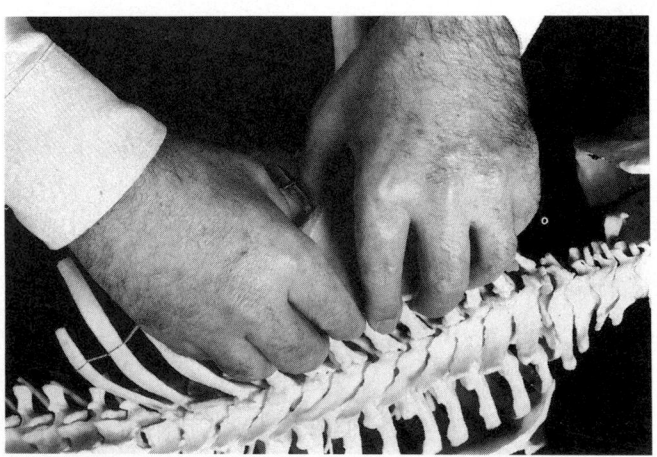

FIGURE 58.12. Upper extremity, scapulofascial release.

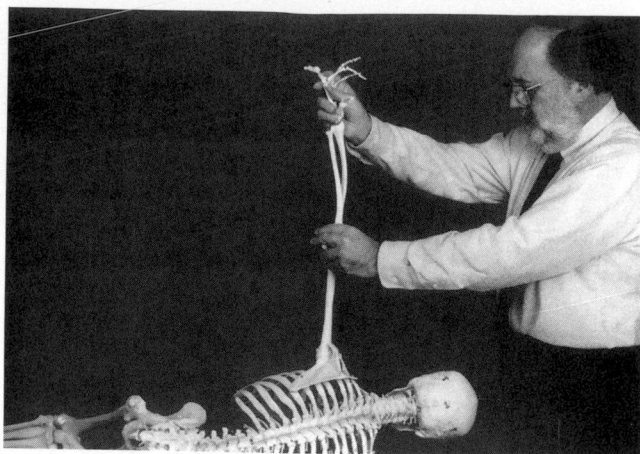

FIGURE 58.13. Upper extremity, radioulnar.

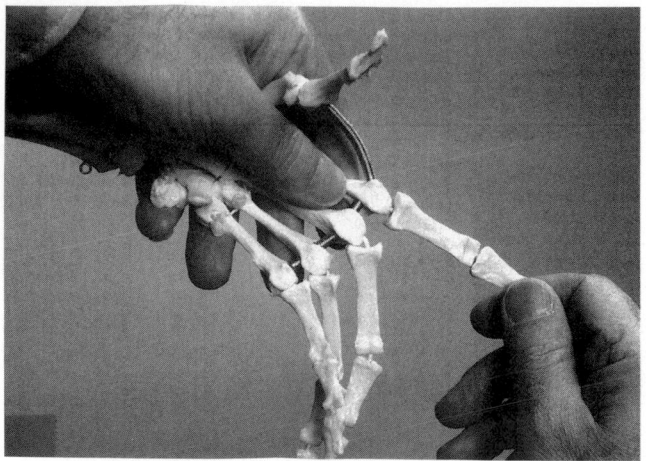

FIGURE 58.15. Upper extremity, hand and fingers.

The addition of alternating flexion and extension of the wrist facilitates the release of articular dysfunctions of the carpal bones (Fig. 58.14). Fascial ligamentous release of the palmar area precedes articulatory release of the small joints of the fingers and thumb. The progress of the sequence is from the small finger to the thumb (Fig. 58.15).

Expansion of the Superior Thoracic Aperture

Accomplish this by grasping the deep webbing between the index finger and thumb of the patient's extended upper extremity. Sustained alternating supination and pronation facilitates the release of congestion in this area and contributes to release of the cervicothoracic junction.

Cranium

Occipitoatlantal Articulation

1. One hand contacts the posterior tubercle of the atlas (Fig. 58.16).
2. The opposite hand contacts the vertex of the patient's head.

The fulcrum is established by the placement of the elbow on the tabletop.

Basilar Axes of the Skull

The patient's head rests on the interlaced or overlapped fingers of the physician. The physician's thumbs extend above the ears toward the forepart of the head. The fulcrum is established by the placement of the elbows on the tabletop.

CONCLUSION

Osteopathic treatment does not concern itself simply with the performance of a single manual procedure. The particular treatment requires variation in technical approaches. Visualization and synthesis of messages received through the fingers are the basis for a keen clinical behavior. Conceptualization of anatomic-physiologic dysfunction peculiar to a given patient is the key to maximizing manipulative responses. The sustained effective response following treatment is contingent upon selective and controlled variation of force from an appropriate fulcrum. When these conditions are met, inherent mechanisms acting in

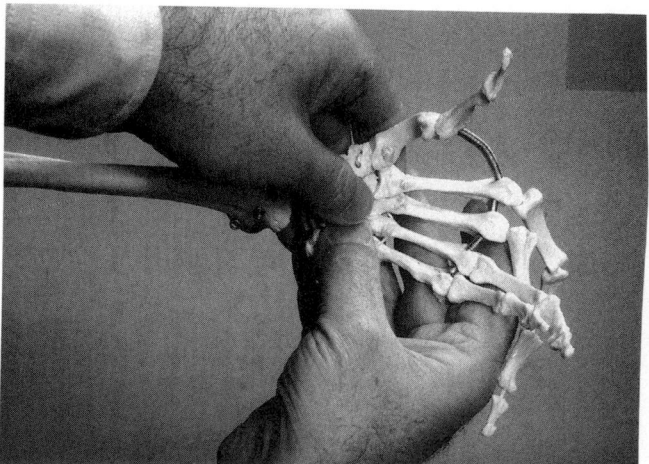

FIGURE 58.14. Upper extremity, wrist.

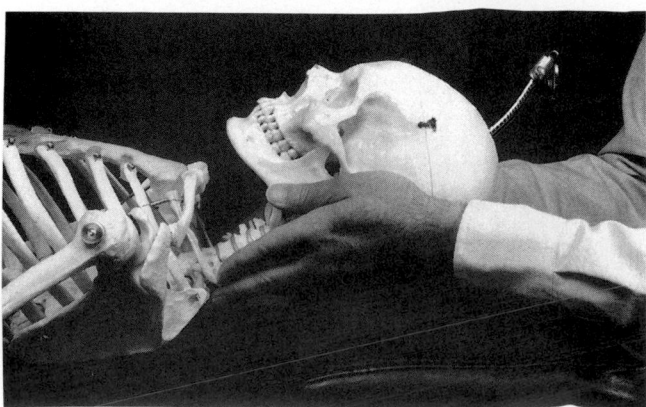

FIGURE 58.16. Occipitoatlantal articulation.

accordance with the capacity of the patient will lead to a state of health.

REFERENCES

1. Becker RE. Diagnostic touch: its principles and application. In: Barnes MW, ed. *Academy of Applied Osteopathy Yearbooks.* Indianapolis, IN: American Academy of Osteopathy; Part I. 1963:32–40. Parts II and III. 1964:153–166. Part IV. 1965:165–177.
2. Becker RF. The meaning of fascia and fascial continuity. *Osteopath Ann.* 1975;3(6):186/35.
3. Cathie AG. Fascia of the body in relation to function and manipulative therapy. In Barnes MW, ed. *Academy of Applied Osteopathy Yearbook.* Indianapolis, IN: American Academy of Osteopathy, 1960:74.
4. Greenman PE. *Principles of Manual Medicine,* 2nd ed. Baltimore, MD: Williams & Wilkins; 1996.
5. Hubbard RP. Mechanical behavior of connective tissue. In: Greenman PE, ed. *Concepts and Mechanisms of Neuromuscular Functions.* New York, NY: Springer-Verlag; 1984:47–54.
6. Jones LH. *Strain and Counterstrain.* Colorado Springs, CO: The American Academy of Osteopathy; 1981.
7. Lippincott HA. The osteopathic technic of Wm. G. Sutherland D.O. In: Northup TC, ed. *Academy of Applied Osteopathy Yearbook.* Indianapolis, IN: American Academy of Osteopathy; 1949:124.
8. Zink JG, Lawson WB. An osteopathic structural examination and functional interpretation of the soma. *Osteopath Ann.* 1979;7(12):433–440.

BALANCED LIGAMENTOUS TENSION TECHNIQUES

JANE E. CARREIRO

KEY CONCEPTS

- Understand the principles of balanced ligamentous and balanced membranous articulatory mechanisms
- Understand the principles of diagnosis and treatment of balanced ligamentous and balanced membranous articulatory mechanisms as described by William Sutherland, DO
- The concept of using the inherent forces within the body as activating forces for manipulative treatment

INTRODUCTION

Balanced ligamentous and balanced membranous tension techniques were first described by William G. Sutherland, DO. Dr. Sutherland graduated from the American School of Osteopathy and was a student of Andrew Taylor Still, MD. Dr. Sutherland described balanced ligamentous tension technique (BLT) as an approach to diagnosis and treatment of the living human body. His model was initially presented to a small group of students between 1942 and 1944, and then subsequently published as the "Osteopathic Technique of Wm. G. Sutherland" in the 1949 *Year Book of the Academy of Applied Osteopathy* (1).

Ligamentous Articular Mechanisms

The principles of BLT are formulated around an understanding of ligamentous articular mechanisms. Ligaments regulate and guide the movement in all the articulatory mechanisms of the body. In most joints they act as checks to the voluntary actions of muscles. The clearest example of this idea occurs in the wrist. There are no muscular forces acting directly upon the carpal bones yet we can flex, extend, circumduct, and move our wrists in all sorts of configurations. Each of these movements occurs as a result of small rotations, twistings, and turnings of the carpal bones. The flexor and extensor carpi ulnaris and radialis, as well as some of the muscles of the digits will initiate motion; the mechanics of carpal bone movement, however, are governed by the nonelastic properties and position of the carpal ligaments. The placement of the carpal

ligaments creates various fulcrums and checks within which the complex movements of the carpal bones occur (2–4). For example, the carpi radialis muscles move the proximal phalanx of the thumb toward the radial side of the forearm. As the phalanx approximates the radius, the trapezium, trapezoid, and scaphoid accommodate this change in spatial relations by moving toward the midline of the wrist. The positions of the other carpal bones will adjust accordingly. None of the carpal bones are directed by muscular efforts, rather they respond to distal muscular forces. This complicated movement is orchestrated and guided by the small ligaments lying between and around the carpal bones. All movements of the wrist are accomplished through a similar mechanism. Consequently, the carpal ligaments can be viewed as levers and pulleys and straps guiding the bones and the articular relationships. Dr. Sutherland described this arrangement as a ligamentous articular mechanism. Furthermore while the positions of the carpal bones may change, the tensions on the carpal ligaments do not. In other words, when the wrist is flexed, the dorsal ligaments are not stretched, nor do the palmar ligaments go slack. As long as the wrist is moved within its physiologic range of motion, the tensions within the carpal ligaments remain balanced. Sutherland called this a balanced ligamentous articular mechanism.

Other obvious examples of ligamentous articular mechanisms are the forearm (radial and ulnar intraosseous membrane), the tibia and fibula (again via the intraosseous membrane), and the foot.* While the range of motion is much less than the wrist, the ligaments of the foot are responsible for creating a system that is capable of weightbearing and mobility. Movements of the forefoot and hind foot are dictated by the ligamentous arrangement. The sacroiliac (SI) joint is yet another example of a ligamentous articular mechanism. Designed for weightbearing and mobility, the SI joints must also be able to accommodate large changes in size (e.g., during labor and delivery), while maintaining stability. The ligaments of the SI and lumbosacral areas function with a reciprocal tension mechanism, responding to the moment-to-moment changes induced by gait (5–7). According to Sutherland's model, all of the joints in the body are

---

*Dr. Sutherland also considered the internal dura as the intraarticular ligaments of the cranium and referred to the principles of balanced membranous tension to describe the mechanics in this area.

balanced ligamentous articular mechanisms. The ligaments provide proprioceptive information that guides the muscle response for positioning the joint, and the ligaments themselves guide the motion of the articular components.

Reciprocal Tension

Sutherland coined the terms "reciprocal tension ligaments" and "reciprocal tension mechanism" to describe the role of ligaments in joints (8). According to Sutherland's model, throughout the physiologic range of motion of any given joint, the associated ligaments maintain a constant level of tension. They do not stretch, nor do they become lax. The motion mechanics between the bones of a joint are a result of a change in the shape of the joint space, not because one set of ligaments becomes taut while another becomes slack. Think of the wrist moving in flexion and extension. As the wrist moves into flexion there is a displacement of the distal row of carpal bones toward the dorsal surface of the arm. During extension these same bones move toward the palmar surface. Accompanying these movements are rotations of individual bones. The sum total of these movements acts to maintain the tension of the carpal ligaments at a consistent level. This is a key concept in Dr. Sutherland's approach.

The type of motion which may occur at any given articulation is determined by the shape of the joint surfaces, the position of the ligaments, and the forces of the muscles acting upon the joint. Ligaments do not stretch and contract as muscles do; consequently, the tension in a ligament has very little variation. The tension distributed throughout the ligaments of any given joint is balanced. In normal movements, as the joint changes position, the relationships between the joint's ligaments also change, but the total tension within the ligamentous articular mechanism does not. The distribution of tension between the ligaments is altered, however, when the joint is affected by injury, inflammation, and/or mechanical forces. This is what happens in somatic dysfunction. The distribution and vector of tension within any given ligament will change according to the position of strain in the joint. However, the shared tension within the ligamentous articular mechanism of any given joint remains constant as long as the ligament is not damaged. This has been called a reciprocal tension mechanism. Of course, the balance within the ligamentous articular mechanism can be strained if the joint is inappropriately moved beyond its physiologic range of motion. In the former case, it is the balance of tension, which is distorted. In the latter case, the fibers of the ligament are subjected to microscopic tears and stretch. While this (the latter case) will most assuredly result in a strain to the balance of the articular ligaments, the ligaments do not need to be disrupted for the balance to be distorted. The distortion in balance is a mechanical strain, which may or may not involve an anatomical one. In any somatic dysfunction, there is always a strain in the balanced ligamentous articular mechanism.

APPLICATION OF THE PRINCIPLES

Within most articulatory mechanisms of the body, there are tissues under voluntary and involuntary control. Dr. Sutherland recommended using the inherent forces within the body such as respiration, fluid mechanics, and postural changes to correct the strain.

In the spine, vertebral balanced ligamentous articular strains can be corrected using a variety of manipulative techniques such as high velocity/low amplitude (HVLA), muscle energy, counterstrain, and so forth, which indirectly address the ligamentous component through muscles or bones. However, when the principles of BLT are used in manipulative treatment, fulcrums and levers are applied directly to direct changes to the ligamentous articular strains. These principles can be used to make corrections in all ligamentous and membranous articulatory mechanisms. In general, the technique combines a fulcrum introduced by the physician with an activating force provided by the patient. The physiologic movements and forces are generated in the body through position and respiration.

The body is always in motion. The physiologic motion of respiration, fluid pressure changes, and postural adjustments occur on a moment-to-moment basis. These motions, however subtle they may appear, affect the entire musculoskeletal system. During deep inspiration the diaphragm contracts, increasing intraabdominal pressure. The abdominal muscles also contract, increasing tension on the thoracolumbar fascia. The thoracolumbar fascia is firmly attached to the supraspinous and interspinous ligaments. When the abdominal muscles are tensed, a posterior force is placed on these ligaments through the thoracolumbar fascia, resulting in a flattening of the lumbar lordosis. As the ribs elevate with inspiration the thoracic kyphosis opens and flattens. The scalene muscles contract as well. Their anterior attachment to the cervical vertebrae acts to flex the cervical spine. Thus the "simple" act of respiration results in a response throughout the body (Fig. 59.1). This is an example of an inherent force, a physiologic force acting within the body. The inherent forces within the body can be used as activating forces to assist the physician in the manipulative procedure. This is a very safe and effective method of treatment.

The same principles that are used to successfully execute a balanced ligamentous manual operation are used for all osteopathic manual procedures. The physician must skillfully position the joint so that all forces within the articular mechanism converge on one specific point. This point becomes the fulcrum around which the shift or change will occur. When performing an HVLA manual operation, the physician needs to place the joint so that all forces converge. The more skilled the operator, the more specific the convergence and the less force needed to correct the dysfunction. Very skilled physicians will merely ask the patient to exhale, or will flex the patient's head to articulate the joint. To be successful with balanced ligamentous and balanced membranous techniques, the physician must balance all forces within the ligamentous structures of the joint so that a fulcrum is established. The inherent forces within the body can then be used to correct the strain.

PRINCIPLES OF DIAGNOSIS

A strain in the balanced ligamentous articular mechanism of a joint creates an alteration in the permitted motion of that joint.

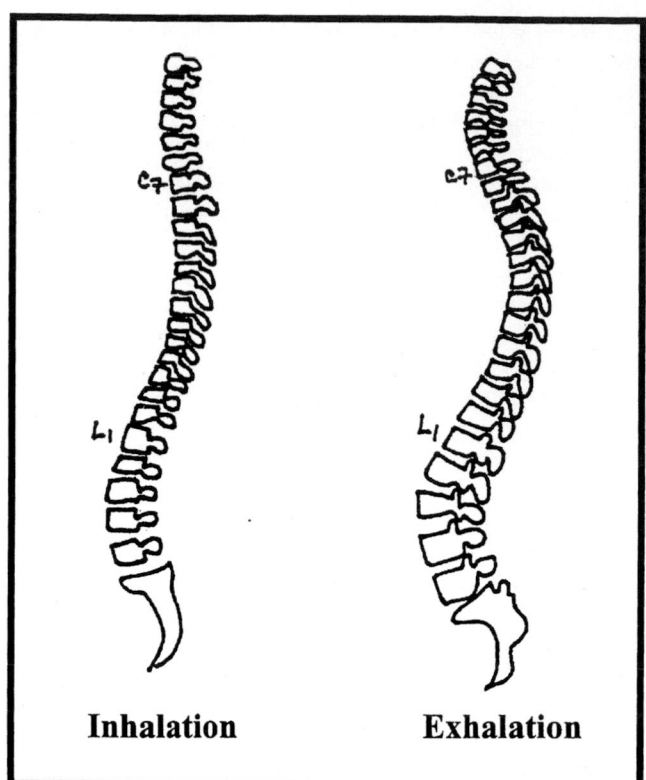

Inhalation   **Exhalation**

FIGURE 59.1. Schematic diagram depicting alterations in spinal curves with respiration.

This includes the normal motion accompanying respiration and postural changes. Consequently, by observing the motion of a given joint during respiration or active motion, the observer can ascertain the position of the articular surfaces. This observation is usually performed through palpation. The physician uses involuntary motion to determine the degree of restriction and the specifics of dysfunction. For example, we know that the thoracic kyphosis flattens slightly during inspiration. We can say that the upper thoracic vertebrae move toward extension (or backward bending) and the lower thoracic vertebrae move toward flexion as the anterior concavity straightens. Thus, if T3 is in a flexed lesion position (i.e., does not want to move into extension), what will happen to T3 during inspiration? If we palpate T2, T3, and T4 during inspiration, will there be equal excursion? What will happen during exhalation? Suppose during exhalation T3 rotated toward the left and side bent toward the left, what would this tell us?

If the ligaments on the left side of the joint are under more tension than the ligaments on the right side of the joint, the vertebrae will resist rotation to the right. If the ligaments that restrict extension are tighter than the ligaments that restrict flexion, the vertebrae will move into flexion more easily. Thus, T3 would resist motion during inspiration and move toward the direction of ease (i.e., exhalation/flexion with rotation and side bending toward the left). We could describe the position of T3 as flexed, rotated, and side bent left. A strain in the balance of a ligamentous or membranous articular mechanism will produce exaggerated motion toward the position of the strain and restricted motion toward the neutral position. While this motion is readily apparent with respiration, gentle motion testing may also be employed.

Assessing the motion mechanics at a joint requires gentle tactile discrimination. Large motions are not necessary, nor are they useful when working with the ligamentous components. Patients may be examined sitting, supine, or prone. The supine position is most effective and is the position that will be used to illustrate the point. With the patient supine and the physician sitting at the patient's side, the physician gently slides their hands under the thorax, placing the fingerpads on the spinous processes of the midthoracic vertebrae. *Do not lift your fingers up into the spine;* rather allow the respiratory motion of the patient's thoracic cage to move your fingers. Observe the flexion/extension movement of these vertebrae during inhalation and exhalation. Is there any lateral movement occurring? The physician can apply a gentle pressure on the spinous processes, using them as handles, to encourage the vertebrae into flexion and extension with the appropriate respiratory cycle. The physician may also apply a gentle pressure to encourage the vertebrae into right and left rotation. (Remember that the spinous process will move to the left when the vertebra moves to the right.) With attentive observation, the physician will be able to diagnose the positional strain within the joint.

Principles of Treatment

The first and most important step in treatment is establishing BLT in the articular mechanism so that the body's inherent forces can resolve the strain. The point of BLT is *the point in the range of motion of an articulation where the ligaments and membranes are poised between the normal tension present throughout the free range of motion and the increased tension preceding the strain . . . which occurs as a joint is carried beyond its normal physiology* (5).

All tensions within the ligaments are reduced to the absolute minimum. As a joint reaches the extremes of its range of motion, the tensions within its ligaments increase; as the joint moves toward neutral, the tensions decrease so that *in the neutral position the ligaments have the minimal amount of tension* (Fig. 59.2A). When a joint is strained and normal motion restricted, the position of minimal tension within the joint is no longer its physiologic neutral (Fig. 59.2B). Consequently, the point of balance for the ligaments will change in relation to the strain that is present. This new point of balanced tension exists somewhere between the tension created by the strain and the physiologic neutral of the joint. We can look at this from a linear model (Fig. 59.2C). When the articular mechanism is held at the precise (new) neutral position, all ligaments will be under the least possible strain. The physiologic forces within the body then become the activating forces to resolve the dysfunction.

Initially the physician can learn to establish a neutral in a strained articular mechanism by assessing the degree of permitted motion in all planes. This is done by gently encouraging the joint first in one direction and then another. For example, to assess the degree of permitted motion in T3 extended and rotated right, the physician would encourage flexion then extension. Next, the physician would assess rotation right then rotation left by applying a slow discriminating pressure to the spinous process. There will be a difference in the *freedom of rotation* in one direction as contrasted with another. The physician will easily discern a point in the motion of the joint where the tension in the articular mechanism is poised between the increased tension felt as the extremes of range of motion are approached. This is the point of BLT. The

FIGURE 59.2. A: Schematic diagram depicting ligamentous tension in a normal joint. **B:** Schematic diagram depicting ligamentous tension in a normal joint. **C:** Linear model representing the point of balanced ligamentous tension.

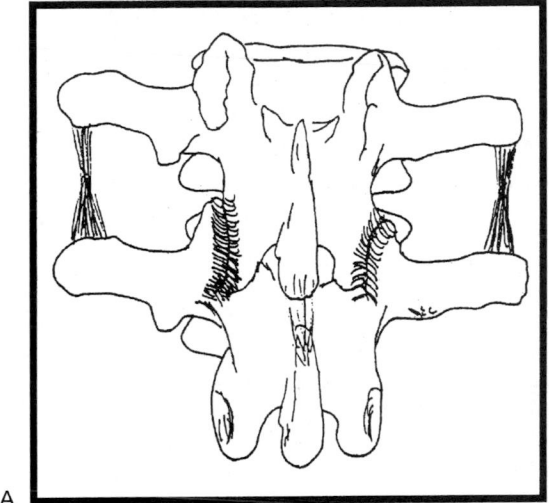

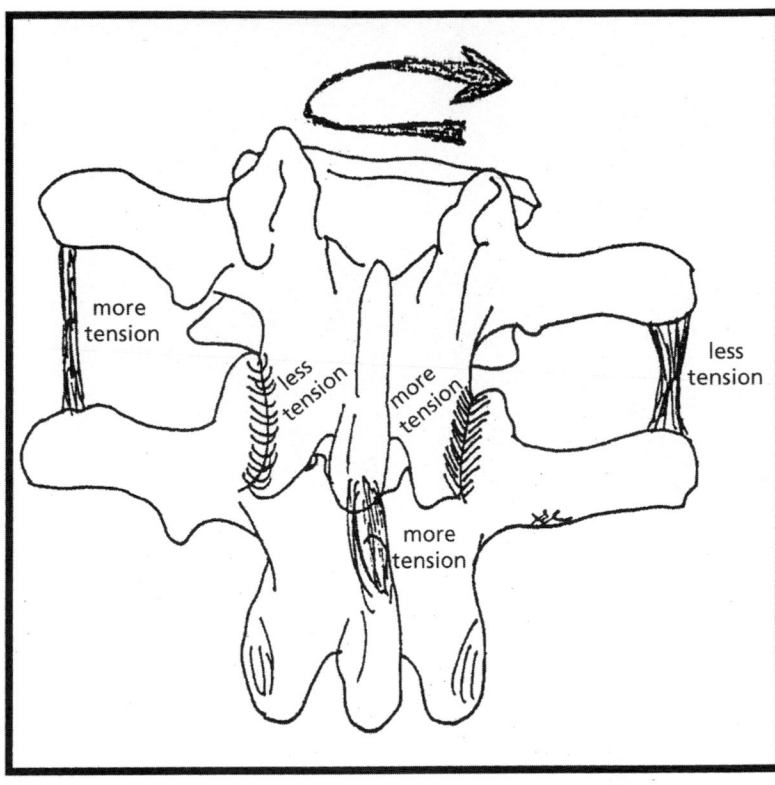

more tension

less tension

more tension

less tension

more tension

A

B

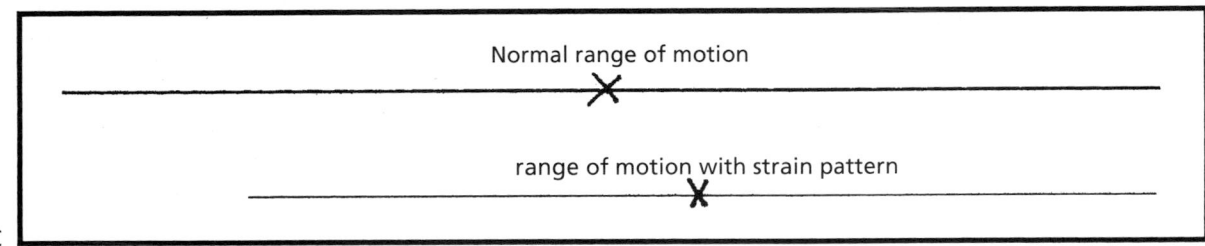

Normal range of motion

X

range of motion with strain pattern

X

C

physician will hold this position while the activating forces within the body, such as breathing, resolve the strain. When the strain corrects, the physician will feel a shift or change in the tension in the joint such that the neutral created is no longer the point of minimal tension. In other words, the physician will often feel an increase in tension as the joint spontaneously moves toward its physiologic neutral.

To establish the point of BLT, the physician will need to assess the tension within the ligaments in all directions of motion. It is the most neutral position possible under the influence of all the factors responsible for the existing strain pattern. Thus, the balance point will change according to the pattern of the strain.

SPECIFIC TECHNIQUE APPROACHES

Remember the degree of motion required is very small. Be precise.

Pelvis: The Differential Technique

The goal of treatment is to normalize movement within the pelvic mechanism, including the SI joints and hips. This approach addresses the iliosacral and SI components. It provides a general approach to the area.

Diagnosis

The physician will evaluate and treat the pelvis by using the patient's legs as long levers. The patient sits squarely on their ischial tuberosities facing the physician. The physician grasps the patient's ankles under the calcaneus and lifts the lower leg until the entire leg is almost straight, taking care not to shift the patient's center of gravity (Fig. 59.3A–C). Using the leg as a long lever, the physician motion tests the SI joint by compressing one leg and distracting the other in an attempt to turn or pivot the innominate on the ischial tuberosity. The tissue resistance is noted. Then the procedure is repeated with the other leg. The side of greater ease is noted (Fig. 59.3D).

Treatment

The legs are used as levers to bring the pelvis to a point of balance (i.e., the position of ease as determined by the previous test). Leg lengths are noted. (Typically, the long leg will be on the same side as the increased resistance.) The physician then asks the patient to turn away from the long leg while maintaining the position of the pelvis through the legs. The patient turns until the tension in the involved ligamentous structures feels balanced. (This usually occurs in the range of 45 degrees

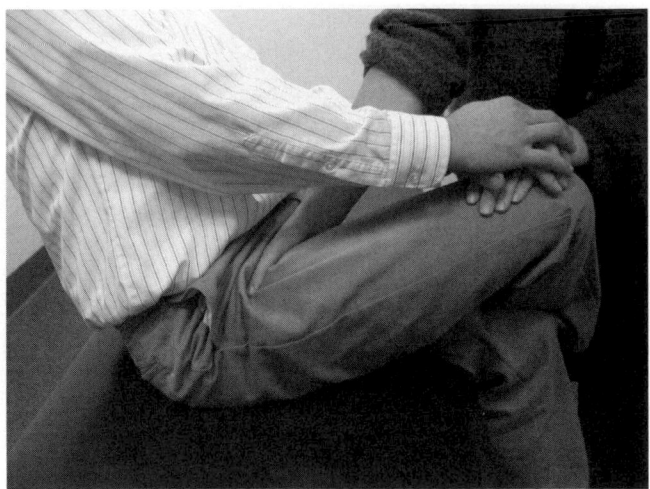
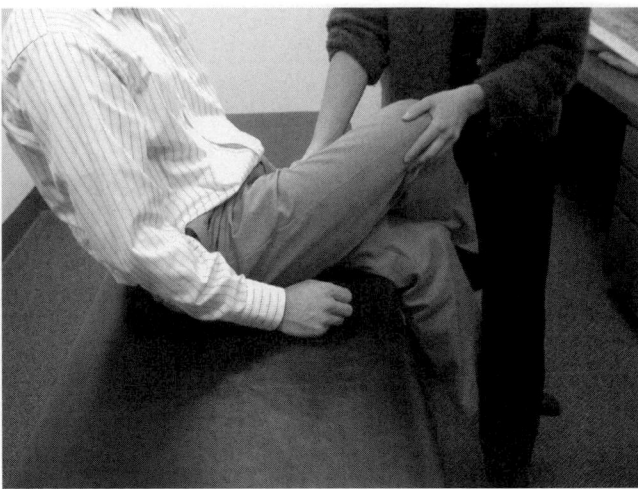

A

B

FIGURE 59.5. A: Position for treatment of externally rotated hip. **B:** Hand position for treatment of internally rotated hip. Note: Patient's hands should be placed on the knee similar to **(A)**.

point of balance between the femoral head and the acetabulum. The patient also places his or her hands upon his or her knee. The patient holds the knee down and laterally while rotating the body away from the leg and backward.

Treatment for Internally Rotated Legs (Fig. 59.5B)

In this instance, the physician's handhold is more proximal so that there is less torque at the acetabulum. The physician establishes a point of balance between the femoral head and the acetabulum. The patient draws the knee medially and upward while rotating forward and toward the affected side.

The Sacral Ala Technique

This technique addresses the prevertebral and presacral fasciae, the obturator fascia, sacral nutation, and restricted SI joints. The patient sits on a table facing the physician who is positioned slightly lower. The physician's knees are placed outside the patient's, thereby internally rotating and adducting the patient's legs. This maneuver acts to spring open the innominates posteriorly, which decompresses the SI joint. The patient his or her places their hands on the physician's shoulders. The physician places their thumbs along the iliac crest at the junction between the rectus abdominus and abdominal oblique muscles. The patient is asked to breathe slowly and deeply, with each exhalation the physician moves his or her thumbs posteriorly along the iliac crest and deeper into the pelvic basin toward the anterior aspect of the sacral ala. The patient may slump forward to further reduce the tension in the anterior tissues (Fig. 59.6). This procedure is continued until the physician's thumbs are deep enough into the tissues that they can act as fulcrums for establishing BLT in the involved tissues. At this point the patient is instructed to sit up slowly starting at the sacrum and curling up through the lumbar and thoracic spines to the cervical area. The patient is instructed to inhale while doing this.

Costovertebral Arches/Twelfth Rib

There are two lumbocostal arches or arcuate ligaments, one medial and one lateral. The lateral ligament is a thickened band in the fascia that covers the quadratus lumborum muscle. It spans from the front of the transverse process of the first lumbar vertebra to the lower margin of the 12th rib near its midpoint. The medial arcuate ligament is a tendinous arch in the fascia over the psoas muscle. It is continuous with the lateral crus of the diaphragm and attaches to the transverse process of the first lumbar vertebra. Displacement of the 12th rib inferiorly will stretch the lateral arcuate ligament and compress the quadratus beneath it. This may also irritate the iliohypogastric and ilioinguinal nerves. When irritated, the patient may complain of pain in the lateral buttocks, pain in the groin or inguinal area, or pain in the medial thigh or scrotum.

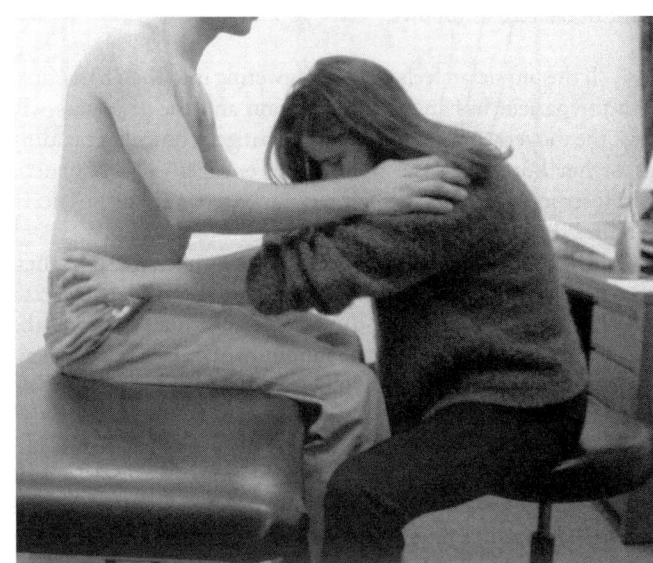

FIGURE 59.6. Patient and physician position for sacral alar technique.

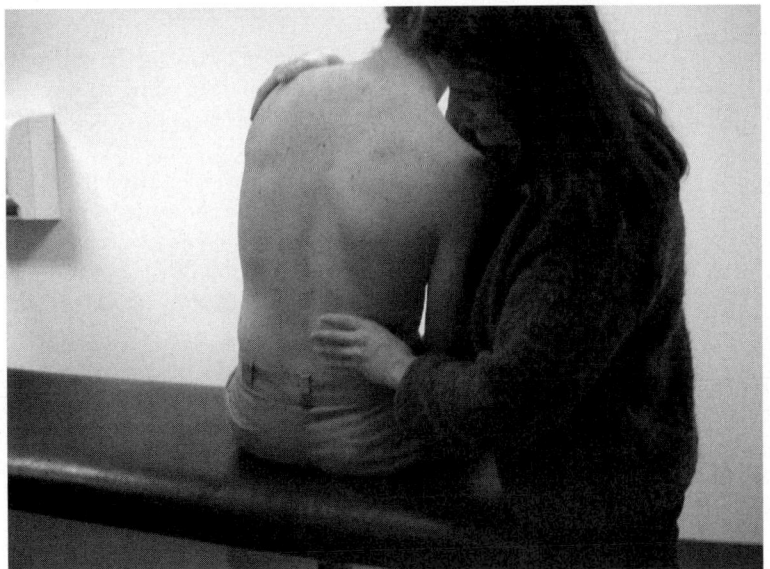
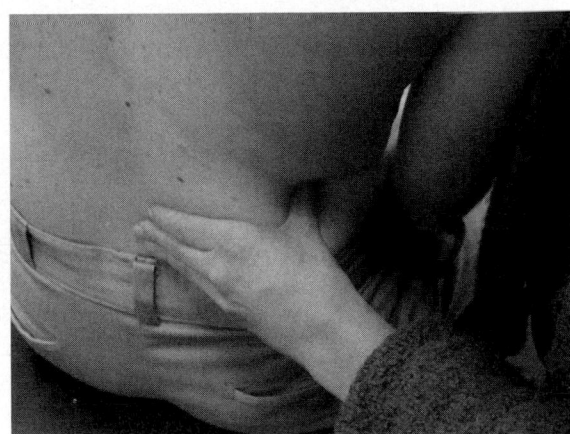

FIGURE 59.7. A: Patient and physician position for costovertebral arches ligaments and 12th rib technique. **B:** Close-up of hand position.

Diagnosis

The tip of the 12th rib is palpated for motion with respiration, as described previously (during exhalation it should rise). Typically, it is found quite posterior and angled more inferiorly than laterally.

Treatment

Treatment is directed at the arcuate ligament. (The right side is used as an example in Fig. 59.7 A and B.) The patient is seated with the affected side facing the physician. The physician places the left thumb just lateral to the erector spinae muscle mass under the 12th rib. The patient bends the trunk over the physician's thumb, which gradually and gently advances upward and posteriorly each time the patient exhales. The position is

held during inhalation and advanced during exhalation until the thumb meets the resistance of the ligament. Once this position has been reached, balanced tension is established between the ligament and the rib. The thumb is then drawn laterally with a rolling motion as the patient inhales. Motion of the 12th rib is then rechecked.

Alternative Treatment

Alternate treatment is directed at the 12th rib. Diagnosis is performed the same way. The patient is supine and the physician sits on the affected side. The physician places one hand under the back and establishes a firm contact on the tip of the 12th rib. The other hand is placed beneath the contact hand and is used to lift the rib anteriorly (Fig. 59.8 A and B). A steady lateral traction

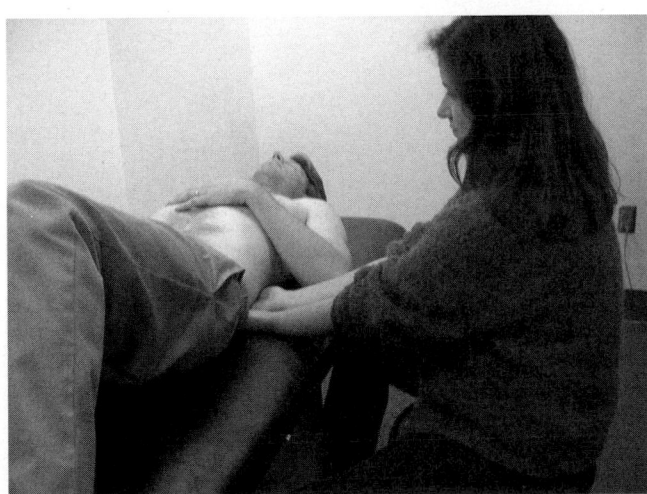
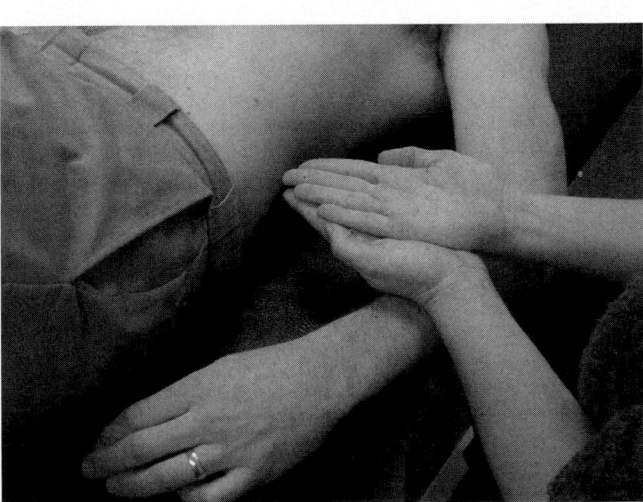

FIGURE 59.8. A: Patient and physician position for alternate approach, to the 12th rib. **B:** Close-up of hand position.

is then placed upon the rib at a vector of 90 degrees from the spine to establish BLT, which integrates the articulation between the rib and the vertebra through the arcuate ligaments and the costovertebral ligaments. The patient breathes slowly and deeply as the physician continues to traction the rib and takes up any slack. This position is held until the rib is felt to slip superiorly with exhalation.

Thorax

Diagnosis

This technique is especially effective in patients with chronic degenerative processes in the vertebral column. Patients may be examined sitting, supine, or prone. The supine position is most effective. With the patient supine and the physician sitting at his or her side, the physician gently slides his or her hands under the thorax, placing the fingerpads on the spinous processes of the midthoracic vertebrae (Fig. 59.9). *Do not lift your fingers up into the spine;* rather allow the respiratory motion of the patient's thoracic cage to move your fingers. Observe the flexion/extension movement of these vertebrae during inhalation and exhalation. Is there any lateral movement occurring? The physician can apply a gentle pressure on the spinous processes, using them as handles, to encourage the vertebrae into flexion and extension with the appropriate respiratory cycle. The physician may also apply a gentle pressure to encourage the vertebrae into right and left rotation. (Remember that the spinous process will move to the left when the vertebra rotates to the right.)

Treatment

The physician uses the spinous process to direct the vertebra into a position of balance in relation to the vertebra below. Side bending, rotation, flexion, and extension can be gently introduced through the spinous process. Postural cooperation may be used to augment positioning as follows:

1. Side bending right in the lower thoracic spine or thoracolumbar junction would be augmented by asking the patient to dorsiflex the ipsilateral foot. Above T6, side bending right would be augmented by asking the patient to elevate the left shoulder toward the ear or side bend the head to the right.

2. Flexion above T8 is augmented by asking the patient to exhale; extension is augmented by asking the patient to inhale. Below T8, inhalation will exaggerate flexion and exhalation will exaggerate extension. This is based on the fact that the spinal curves relax during inhalation. (If in doubt, motion test by asking the patient to inhale and exhale.)

Once a point of balance is established, the position is held through a few respiratory cycles until there is a change in the point of balance and the tension in the ligaments.

Ribs

Diagnosis

Rib restrictions can be diagnosed by palpating rib excursion through a cycle of respiration. It is important to remember that when a vertebral lesion occurs the rib is usually affected.

Treatment (Figs. 59.10A and B)

The patient is supine with the physician sitting beside the affected side. One hand is placed under the back to contact the rib to be treated. The other hand is placed under the back such that a finger contacts the transverse process of each vertebra attached to the rib. The rib is gently tractioned anterolaterally while the physician uses the spinous processes to establish balance between the vertebra-rib unit. The vertebral rib unit includes the rib and both involved vertebrae. Embryologically the rib is an extension of the articular disc, consequently the entire unit needs to be brought to a point of balance. Once found, the position of balance is held through a series of respiratory cycles until a change in tension is felt. Postural and respiratory cooperation may be used.

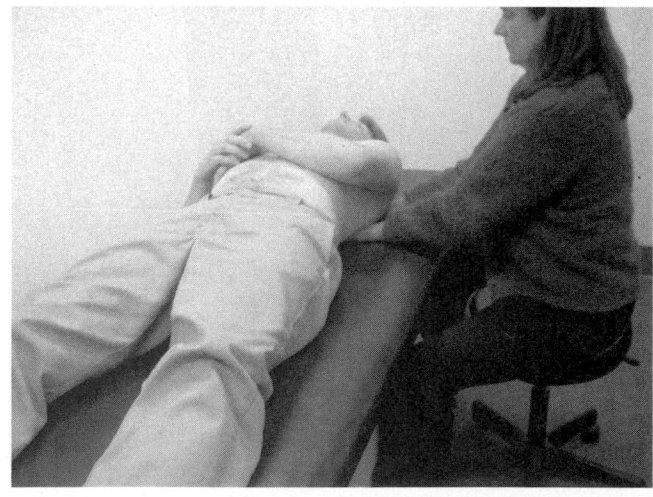
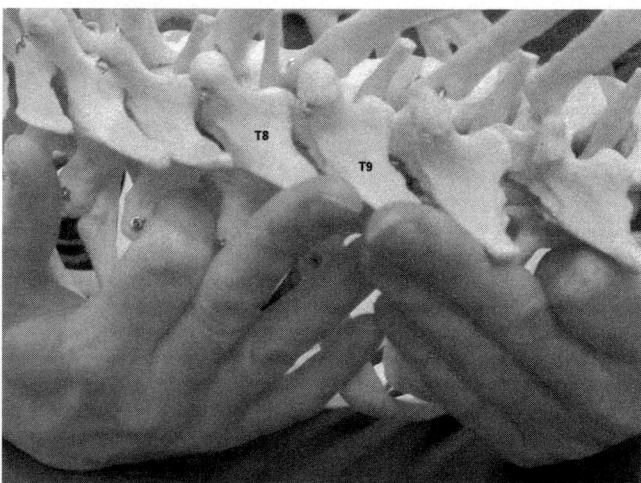

FIGURE 59.9. A: Patient and physician position for treatment of thoracic vertebra. **B:** Hand position demonstrated on thoracic spine model.

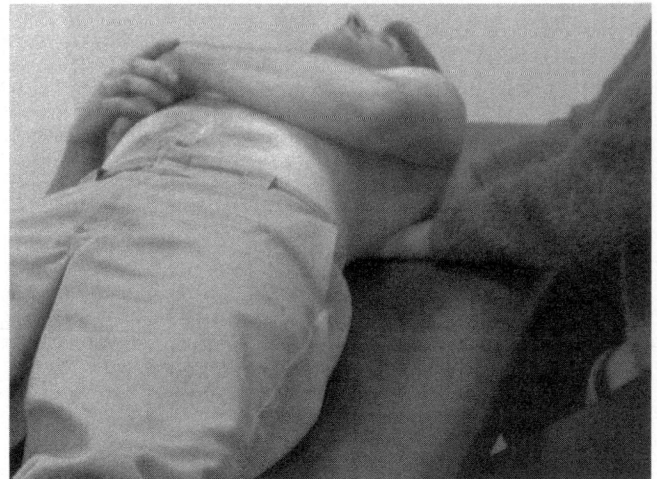

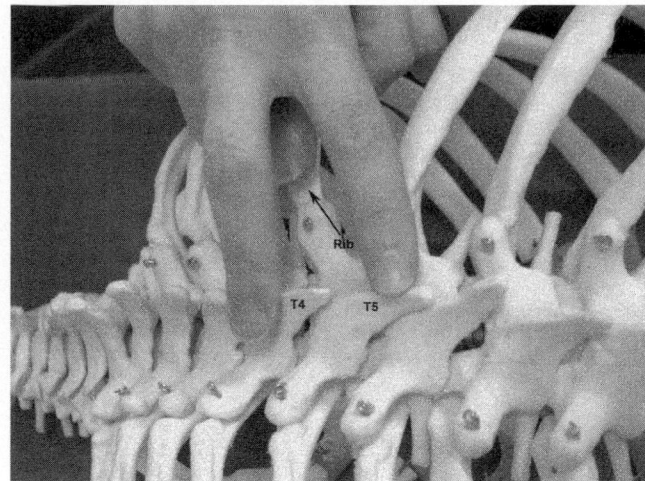

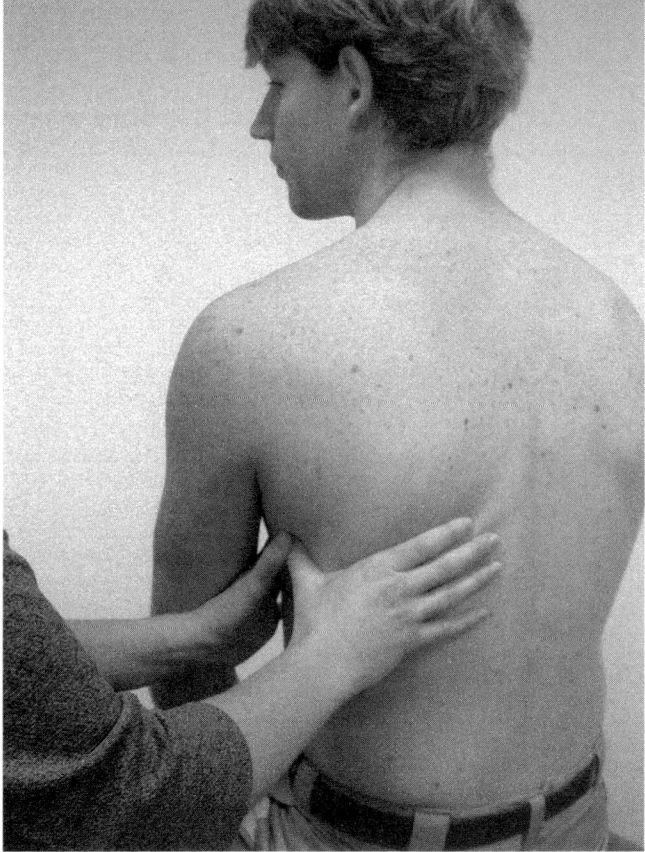

FIGURE 59.10. A: Patient and physician position for supine approach to the ribs. **B:** Hand position demonstrated on thoracic spine model. **C:** Patient and physician position for sitting approach to the ribs.

Alternate Treatment (Fig. 59.10C)

The patient is sitting with the affected side toward the physician. The physician grasps the shaft of the rib using one hand anteriorly and one hand posteriorly. The physician stabilizes the rib as the patient slowly rotates his or her body toward the affected side. The physician monitors the rib for movement. Once a point of balance has been reached, the patient holds that position and inhales and holds the breath. The physician monitors for a change in tension. The second rib is done using one hand under the axilla.

First Rib

Diagnosis

Diagnosis is made by assessing mechanics during deep respiration. The elevated first rib is treated. The physician's thumb is placed lateral to the trapezius muscle and advanced medially along the rib with each inhalation until contact is made with the posterior surface of the rib (Fig. 59.11). The physician should attempt to work the thumb under the trapezius as this is the most effective position. The patient is instructed to slowly turn the neck toward

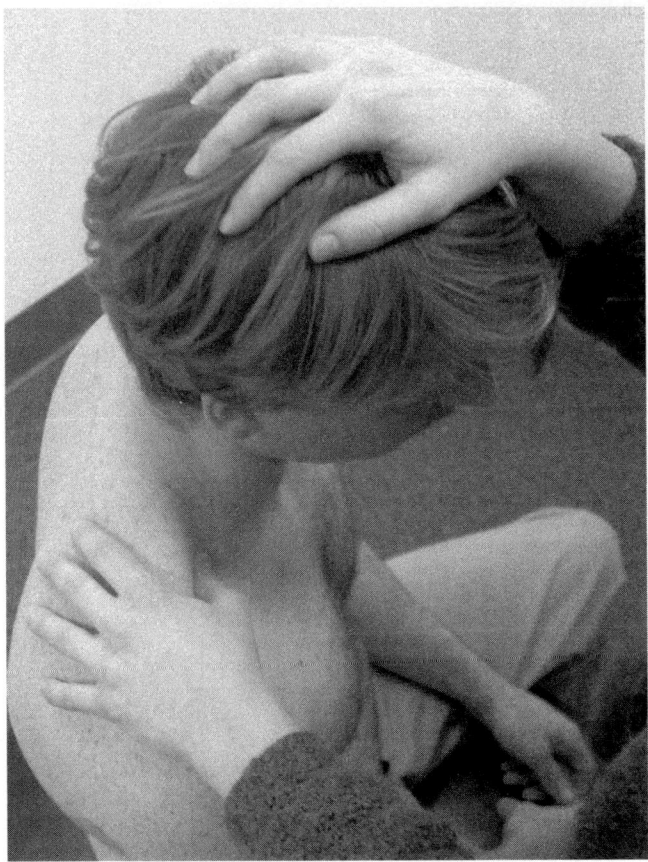

FIGURE 59.11. Patient and physician position for treatment of the first rib.

the affected side as the physician resists movement of the rib to establish a point of balance at the costovertebral articulation. The patient then inhales deeply and holds the breath until a change in tension is noted.

Scapulothoracic Joint

In this technique, the serratus anterior, rhomboid, and teres major muscles are viewed as the functional ligaments of the joint.

Diagnosis

The physician assesses position of scapula on thorax (i.e., scapulothoracic joint). A hypertonic serratus anterior will produce elevation and lateral displacement of scapula.

Treatment

The physician stands on the side of the shoulder to be treated, placing the pad of the thumb on the ribs at the midaxillary line as superior as possible. The physician then slides the thumb posterior along the patient's ribs until it is under the scapula with the pad of the thumb on the thoracic cage and thumbnail against the scapula (Fig. 59.12A).

The physician asks the patient to lean toward him or her so that the thumb slides further under the scapula until the resistance of the serratus anterior is reached. The thumb will act as a fulcrum

for movement of the scapula. The physician places the other hand on top of the scapula, grasping the spine of the scapula with the fingers (Fig. 59.12B). An inferior traction is placed on the scapula to achieve balance between the serratus anterior, rhomboids, and teres muscles. The physician holds this position until a relaxation of the serratus anterior is achieved.

Clavicle

The physician assesses the position of the clavicle by comparing the proximal ends at the sternoclavicular joints. The inferior clavicle is treated first.

Treatment (Fig. 59.13)

The fulcrum for superior-inferior movement of the clavicle is the costoclavicular ligament, located approximately 1-inch lateral to the sternoclavicular joint. To treat the clavicle, the patient sits facing the physician. The physician contacts the distal end of the clavicle with one hand, resting the fingers across the acromioclavicular joint (A–C) and the pad of the thumb under the distal clavicle. The other thumb is placed under the proximal end of the clavicle, just lateral to the sternoclavicular joint.

The patient is asked to lean forward onto the physician's thumbs. The physician applies a gentle pressure to the shoulder at the acromial end until a subtle disengagement or "give" is felt at the A-C joint. The patient is then asked to carry the contralateral shoulder posteriorly, thereby disengaging the sternal end. These two movements are performed to establish a balance in the ligaments at the articulation. This position is held as the patient breathes until a slight "shift" in the clavicle is felt. The patient is then asked to slowly carry the contralateral shoulder forward, and then sit upright. The operator maintains contact with the clavicle until the patient is upright and all weight is removed from the thumbs. The other clavicle is then treated.

Humerus/Glenohumeral Joint

Freedom of rotation of the humerus in the glenoid cavity is tested with the arm at an angle of 45 to 90 degrees laterally from the body, and the elbow flexed. Comparison of the motion on the two sides is made by carrying the hand laterally and upward to test external rotation of the humerus, and medially and downward for internal rotation. Restricted motion in one direction indicates a lesion in the opposite position (Fig. 59.14).

Correction is made with the patient seated. The physician stands on the side of lesion, facing the patient. The physician's hand, which is toward the back of the patient, palpates the shoulder joint. The other hand is placed under the axilla, against the ribs and as close to the head of the humerus as possible. This hand acts as a fulcrum for disengagement of the humeral head (Fig. 59.15). The patient reaches the hand of the involved side across the chest to the distal third of the opposite clavicle and holds that shoulder. If the patient elevates the elbow, the internal rotation lesion is exaggerated. If the patient lowers the elbow, external rotation is exaggerated. The physician directs the elbow to the degree necessary to arrive at the point of balanced tension. The patient is instructed to move the uninvolved

FIGURE 59.12. A: Schematic diagram of hand placement for scapula technique. **B:** Patient and physician position for scapula technique.

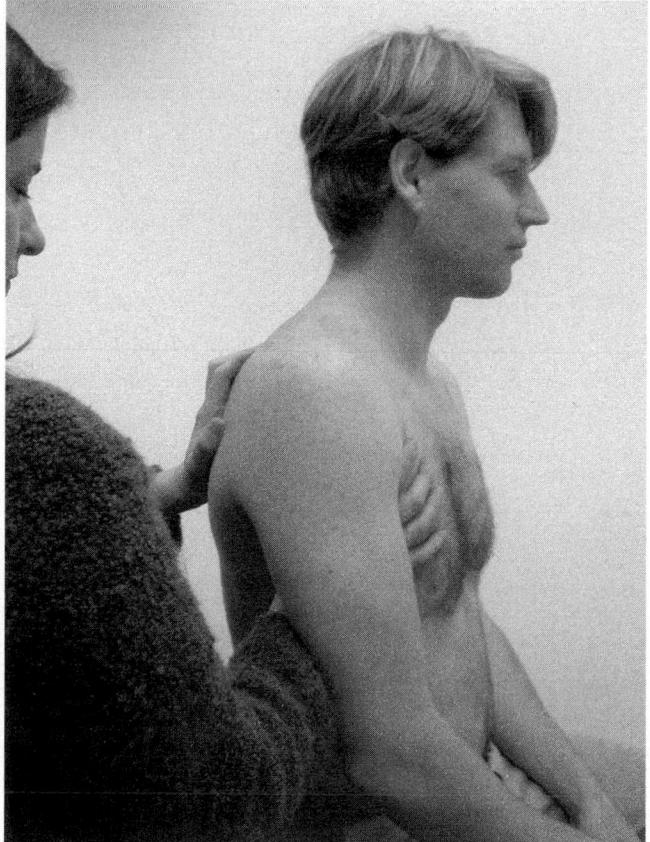

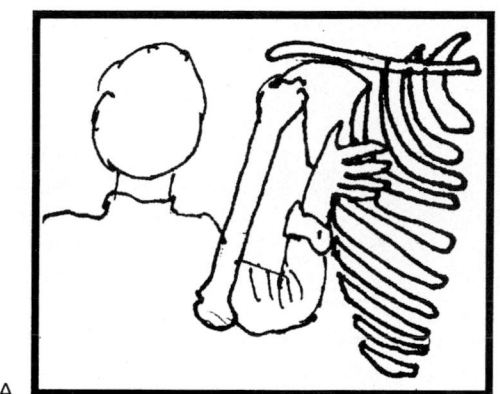

A

B

shoulder posteriorly, carrying with it the hand of the lesioned side. This draws the lower end of the humerus across the chest in order that the leverage over the fulcrum provided by the physician's hand disengages the head of the humerus. BLT is then established by gently internally or externally rotating the humerus. This position is held until there is a change in tissue tension. Respiratory cooperation may be employed to correct the lesion.

The Sacroiliac Joint

The SI joint is a ligamentous mechanism that can be assessed and treated using the same principles that are used in the spine. To assess mechanics at the SI joint, the physician sits at the side of the supine patient. One hand is placed under the pelvis so that the fingerpads lie along the medial aspect of the SI joint. (It is easiest to use the left hand to assess the right SI joint.) The other hand is placed on the innominate over the ASIS (Fig. 59.16 A and B). While monitoring the SI joint posteriorly, the innominate is gently rotated anteriorly and posteriorly by applying pressure to the ASIS. The tension in the articular mechanism of the SI joint is assessed. Then the joint is placed in a position of BLT using the innominate position to establish the neutral. Decompression of the joint is sometimes needed to facilitate the neutral position. This is accomplished by applying an anterior pressure on the sacrum with the posterior hand. Once the point of BLT is found, it is held until the patient's inherent forces correct the strain.

As with treatment of the spine, respiration may also be used to augment the neutral position.

The Lower Cervical Spine

To assess and treat the T1/C7 articular mechanism, the physician sits at the head of the supine patient and cradles the neck between the hands. The physician places the pads of the index or middle fingers along the articular pillars of the lower cervical vertebrae. The left middle finger is placed under the left articular pillar of C7 and the right under the right transverse process of T1 (Fig. 59.17 A and B). The physician slowly applies a gentle anterior pressure to the left articular pillar of C7 to encourage C7 to rotate to the right while stabilizing T1 with the other hand. The hands are then switched so that the left rests on the transverse process of T1 while the right fingerpad contacts the articular pillar of C7. A slow, gentle, anterior pressure is applied to C7 to encourage it to rotate toward the left while T1 is stabilized from below. The physician compares the tension created within the articular mechanism during the two procedures.

If there is greater tension created when C7 is encouraged into right rotation, then the ligaments that limit right rotation are restricted. Left rotation would be "easier" and we could say that C7 was rotated left. The physician would then assess freedom of motion with respiration.

To correct the strain the physician positions the hands to encourage C7 into the direction of ease. If C7 was rotated to the left,

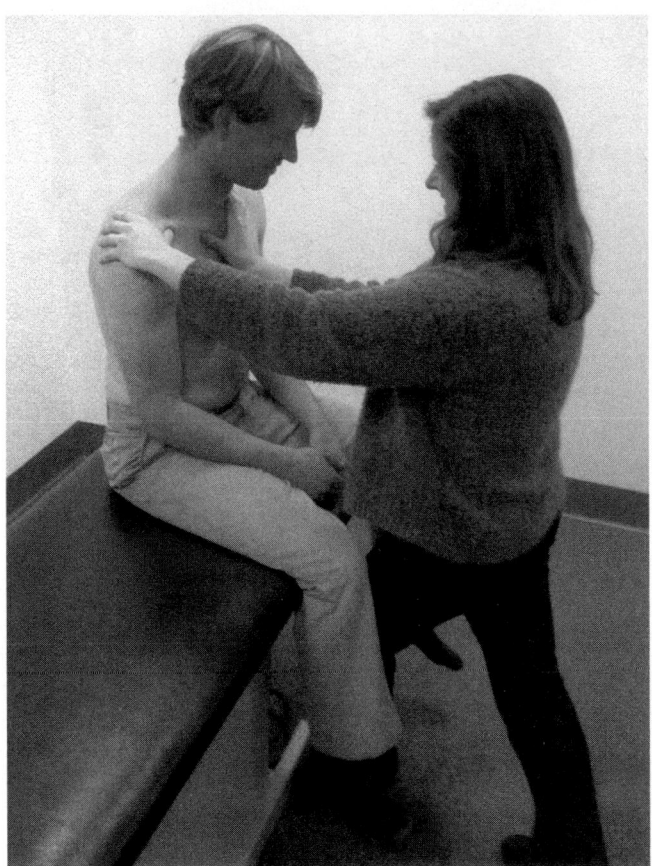

FIGURE 59.13. Patient and physician position for clavicle technique.

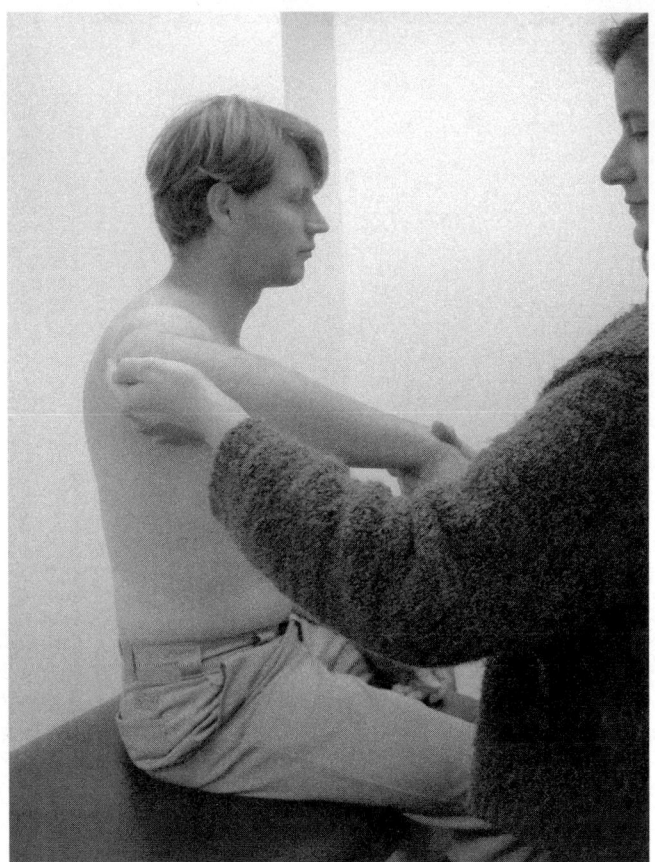

FIGURE 59.14. Position for assessment of rotator cuff.

the pad of the right middle finger would be placed on the right articular pillar of C7 and the pad of the left on the transverse process of T1. The physician then applies a gentle anterior pressure to the right articular pillar encouraging C7 to rotate toward the left, paying close attention to the changing ligamentous tension between the two vertebrae. *The articular mechanism is only rotated to the point where the tension within the ligaments is felt to be in a point of balance—a neutral point.* The physician then holds the joint in this position of BLT while the patient quietly breathes. The patient's breathing is the activating force and it will correct the strain.

The remainder of the cervical spine can be treated in the same manner. The physician can "walk the fingers" up on the articular processes assessing the mechanics of each vertebra and treating the findings. The occipital-atlantal (O-A) joint is treated with a different approach and is discussed subsequently.

Occasionally, the physician needs to employ respiratory cooperation from the patient. In this situation, the physician will ask the patient to inhale and hold his or her breath or exhale and hold his or her breath, in order to fine-tune the point of BLT.

The Upper Cervical Spine

The O-A joint is a ligamentous articular mechanism. The proprioceptive role of the short muscles and ligaments of this area is particularly important to balance and posture. While techniques

such as the O-A release may relieve suboccipital soft tissue congestion, a more specific approach to the O-A mechanism is needed to "address" the ligamentous component.

BLT can be established between the occiput and atlas through subtle, gentle guiding forces. The physician cradles the occiput in one hand so that the pad of the middle finger slides inferiorly toward the opisthion. The index and ring fingers are placed slightly lateral to the midline, approximating the plane of the

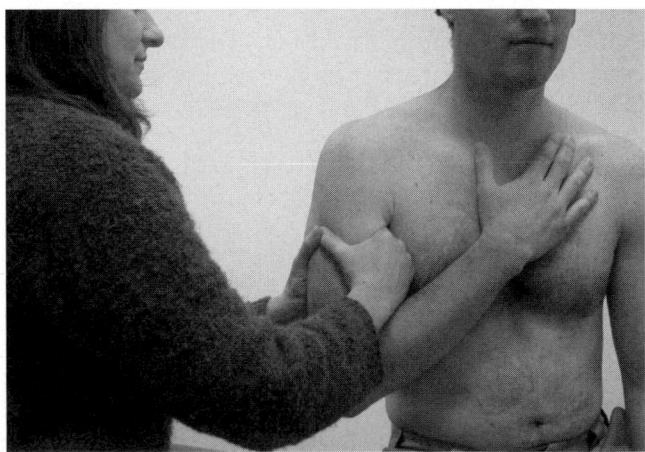

FIGURE 59.15. Patient and physician position for treatment of the glenohumeral joint.

FIGURE 59.16. A: Photograph of patient and physician position for treatment of the sacroiliac joint. **B:** Schematic diagram of hand placement.

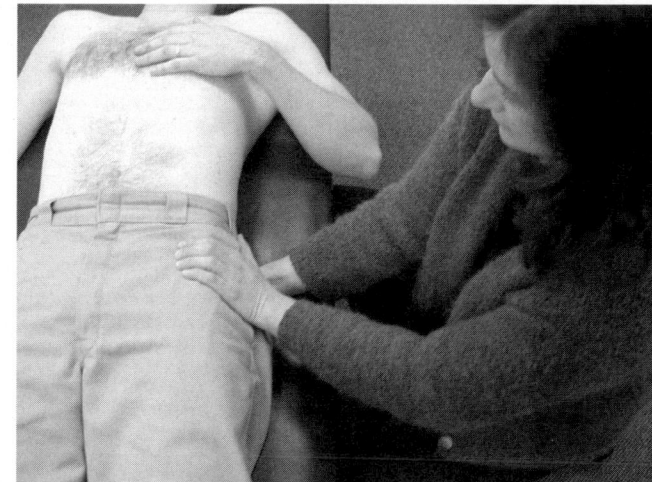

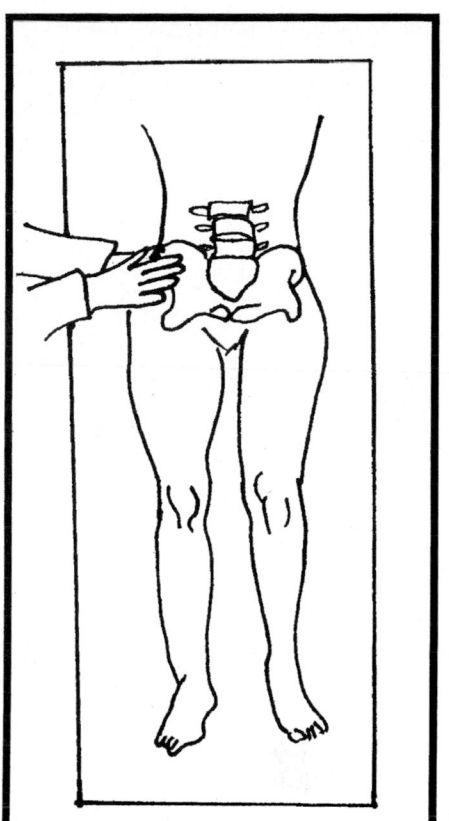

A B

FIGURE 59.17. A: Patient and physician position for treatment of the cervical spine. **B:** Schematic diagram of hand placement.

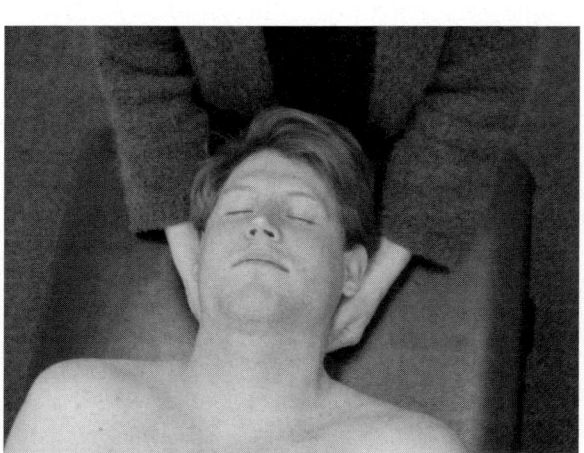

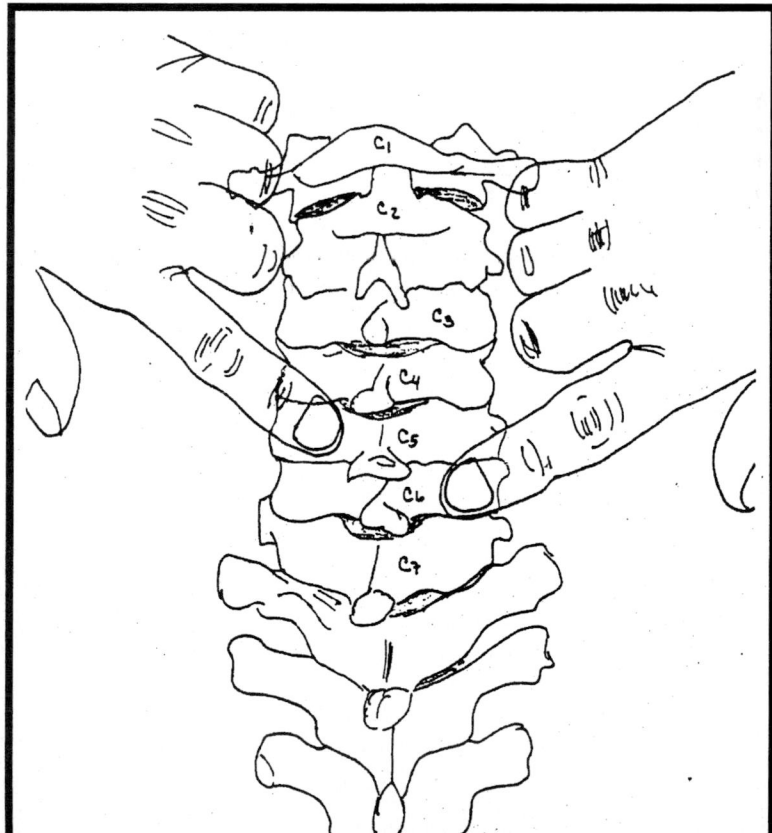

A B

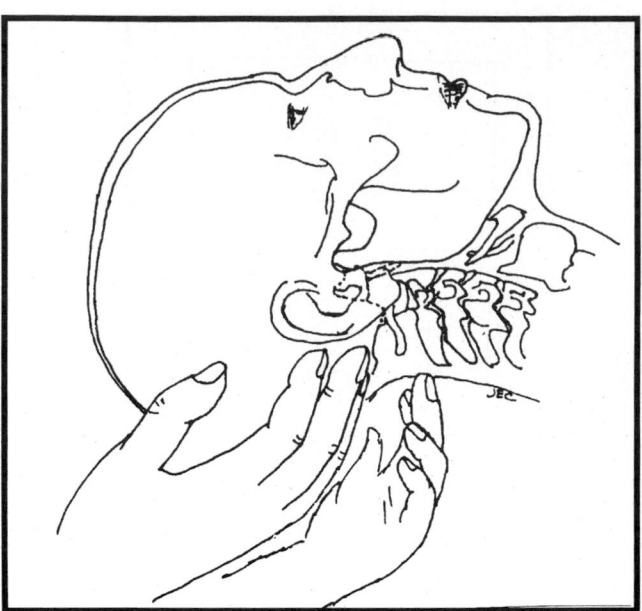

FIGURE 59.18. Schematic diagram for treatment of the occipital-atlantal joint.

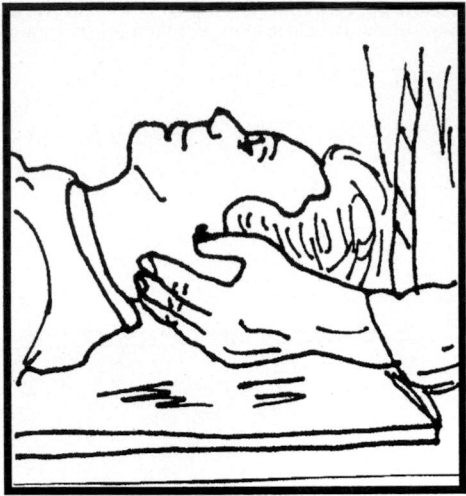

FIGURE 59.19. Schematic of hand placement for treatment of the atlantal-axial joint.

occipital condyles. The other hand is placed under the upper cervical complex with the pad of the middle finger just above the spinous process of C2 (Fig. 59.18). The head must rest, relaxed upon the physician's hands. The physician then asks the patient to dorsiflex the feet. The physician will feel a change in the tension under their hands. The patient is then asked to tuck the chin toward the chest all the while keeping his or her head in the physician's hand until BLT is established between the occiput and atlas. The physician will feel their finger, which is above C2, slide superiorly and come in contact with the tubercle of C1. This finger is creating an anterior vector stabilizing C1 as the patient flexes the occiput. The physician monitors the resistance in the tissues by comparing the tension between the hands. The physician may further augment the procedure by asking the patient to hold his or her breath in either inhalation or exhalation. The release is often felt just as the patient can no longer hold his or her breathing.

Atlantal-Axial

According to Dr. Sutherland's model, the occiput, atlas, and axis act as a unit of function. Assessment and treatment of atlantal-axial (A-A) strains are done using the same principles as the lower cervical spine. However, the hand position is quite different. The physician places the hands in the position assumed for treatment of the O-A, but the pad of the finger of the lower hand maintains contact with C2, while the upper hand stabilizes C1. If the physician's hands are large enough, they may be able to contact each of the articular pillars of C2 (Fig. 59.19). A point of BLT is established between C1 and C2. This position is held as the patient goes through several respiratory cycles. Positional and

respiratory cooperation may be used to augment the point of balance. The A-A joint is often treated after rebalancing of the O-A joint.

ACKNOWLEDGMENTS

In the production of this manuscript the author is indebted to Anne Wales, DO, for supervision and guidance; Michael Burruano, DO, Andrew Goldman, DO, and Hugh Ettlinger, DO, for critical reading; and osteopathic manipulative medicine predoctoral fellows Lynette Bassett, Derek Libby, and Kim Corneal for technical assistance.

REFERENCES

1. Lippincott HA. The osteopathic technique of Wm. G. Sutherland, D.O. In: *Academy of Applied Osteopathy, 1949 Yearbook.* Academy of Applied Osteopathy; 1949.
2. Nordin M, Frankel VH. *Basic Biomechanics of the Musculoskeletal System.* Philadelphia, PA: Lea & Febiger, 1989.
3. Norkin CC, Levangie PC. *Joint Structure and Function.* Philadelphia, PA: FA Davis Co; 1992.
4. Steinberg BG, Plancher KD. Clinical anatomy of the wrist and elbow. *Clin Sports Med.* 1995;14:299.
5. Magoun HIS. *Osteopathy in the Cranial Field,* 3rd ed. Kirksville, MO: The Journal Printing Company; 1976.
6. Vleeming A, Snijders CJ, Stoeckart R, Mens JMA. A new light on low back pain: the selflocking mechanism of the sacroiliac joints and its implication for sitting, standing and walking, In: Vleeming A, Mooney V, Snijders CJ, Dorman T, eds. *The Integrated Function of the Lumbar Spine and Sacroiliac Joints.* Rotterdam: European Conference Organization; 1995.
7. Snijders CJ, Vleeming A, Stoeckart R. Transfer of the lumbarsacral load to iliac bones and legs. *Clin Biomech* 1993;8:285.
8. Sutherland WG. *Teachings in the Science of Osteopathy.* Portland, OR: Rudra Press; 1990.

INTEGRATED NEUROMUSCULOSKELETAL RELEASE AND MYOFASCIAL RELEASE

ROBERT C. WARD

KEY CONCEPTS

- The meaning of the term myofascial release (MFR)
- The meaning of the term integrated neuromusculoskeletal release (INR)
- A theoretic basis for using MFR and INR concepts
- Some of the science that supports INR/MFR ideas
- How the neuromusculoskeletal system responds to mechanical forces
- How integrated peripheral and central neuroreflexive activities influence myofascial functions
- General INR and MFR applications
- To gain an understanding of and apply general MFR and (INR) techniques

Integrated neuromuscular and myofascial release approaches and treatment processes are used to diagnose and modify altered reflex and mechanical patterns anywhere in the body. Applying this form of treatment depends on one's ability to palpate and interactively respond to shifting reflex and mechanical changes as they occur. Recognition of active and passive elements influencing both local and general myofascial and skeletal patterns are important elements in the process. The key to clinical success is the systematic development and application of the MAN acronym— *M*echanics, *A*natomic relationships, and interdependent *N*eural influences.

As Viidik writes:

> The structure of most biological materials (tissues) is to some extent influenced or modified by the in vivo generated mechanical forces which act upon them under physiologic (and pathophysiologic) conditions. The mechanical properties of all materials, living tissues as well as dead are dependent on their structural configurations from the molecular level to the macroscopic (1).

A significant integrated neuromusculoskeletal release (INR)/myofascial release (MFR) concept acknowledges that all human activities are mechanical at many levels—macroscopic to microscopic. In the course of these activities, behavioral patterns both affect and are affected by myriad neuroreflexive and neurovascular activities. Inevitably, both fixed and temporary three-dimensional

patterns arise from a variety of factors such as genetics and age; behavioral characteristics, such as elation and depression; and lifestyle factors, such as good health, effects of accidents, nutrition, drug use, and physical fitness. The clinical challenge is to assess and appropriately treat interdependent "MAN" factors to the extent possible.

INR and MFR ideas have been a part of American osteopathic thinking from early in the profession's history. Until recently, they were commonly referred to as isometric and isotonic methods, fascial release, and functional techniques. Oral traditions over four or five generations suggest that A.T. Still used reflex-based stretch and relaxation procedures without referring to them as such. Pictures of Still performing one or two procedures suggest that he used both functional indirect and articulation methods. Both are described elsewhere in this text (see Chapter 70, "Still Techniques"). Unfortunately, his descriptions lack detail, but Still's writing heavily emphasizes both functional anatomy and related mechanics (2).

This author has been using combinations of isometric, isotonic, functional indirect, and MFR concepts since the early 1950s. At that time, Wilbur Cole and Esther Smoot introduced these procedures to osteopathic medical students attending the Kansas City (Missouri) College of Osteopathy and Surgery. Dr. Cole taught preclinical osteopathic manipulative treatment (OMT) skills, neuroanatomy, and clinical neurology. He was also a neuroanatomy researcher and published two early papers concerning motor end plates on striated muscles (3,4). Dr. Smoot, with a full-time practice in the Osteopathic Hospital of Kansas City, said she learned her methods from several osteopathic pioneers, but she never specifically described her experiences or teachers.

Along with Still and Smoot, William Neidner, who practiced in both Massachusetts and Michigan, was an early proponent of fascial twist maneuvers but wrote little about his work (F.L. Mitchell, Sr., personal communication, 1970; R. Hruby, personal communication, 1989). No doubt there were others.

DEFINITION

INR and MFR techniques are combined procedures (5) designed to stretch and reflexively release patterned soft tissue and joint-related restrictions. Both direct and indirect methods are used interactively. (See "osteopathic manipulative treatment" and its methods in the Glossary at the end of this text.)

GOAL

Three-dimensional neuromusculoskeletal movement patterns are determined by every aspect of biology and behavior. Because of this, a fundamental treatment goal is to interactively assess and modify maladaptive patterns within the ability of the patient to adapt. The process is more effective when the operator uses simultaneously applied, two-handed palpation, much like playing a two-handed musical instrument.

By searching out *tight and loose end-feels* (described in the Glossary), patterned soft tissue and joint-related movements are assessed and treated simultaneously. As both static and dynamic movement barriers are encountered, they are released by sequentially loading areas of tightness using combined compression, traction, and twisting maneuvers. (*Static barrier* is defined as any soft tissue or bony impediment to passively induced motion by an operator. *Dynamic barrier* is defined as any soft tissue or bony impediment to inherent tissue motion.)

Reflexively modulated releases, occurring as varieties of direct and indirect maneuvers, stress and strain the neuromusculoskeletal networks from the skin to the deepest spinal joints and their attachments. A working knowledge of musculoskeletal mechanics is essential (see Chapters 44 to 53). Additional discussion of neutral and nonneutral spinal mechanics including vertebral dysfunctions can be found in Greenman's text (6).

By integrating *patient-assisted release-enhancing maneuvers,* the treatment process is accelerated.

FUNCTIONAL ANATOMY AND CLINICAL PROBLEM SOLVING

The Tight-Loose Concept

Tight-loose patterns involve not only the bony skeleton, but also superficial and deep soft tissue structures of all types. Looking for three-dimensionally related tightness and looseness is essential to the process. For example, patterned three-dimensional changes can be sensed as large or small areas of myofascial and bony positional asymmetry that are tight and loose relative to one another. Assessing tightness and looseness between and among layers of tissue is often helpful.

Some examples:

One shoulder commonly tight and the other loose
Tight left hip and sacroiliac mechanics, loose right
Tight left cervicothoracic junction, loose right
Tight right sternocleidomastoid, loose right scalenes
Tight right sternocleidomastoid, tight left scalenes
Tight lumbodorsal fasciae, loose second layer muscles, tight third and fourth layer muscles

MECHANICS AND FORCES

Patterns can be mechanically assessed by noting effects of multidirectional forces on both local and distant joints and soft tissues.

The definitions of many common patterns, provided by the American Academy of Orthopedic Surgeons' Glossary, follow (7).

Definitions

Motion segment:	A vertebra, its disc, and associated ligaments.
Stress:	Force normalized over the area on which it acts. Normal stress is perpendicular to the cross-section, and sheer stress is parallel to it.
Strain:	Change in shape as a result of stress.
Stiffness:	The ratio of a load to the deformation (strain) it causes (the "tight" concept).
Compliance:	The inverse of stiffness (the "loose" concept).
Creep:	The continued deformation (increasing strain) of a viscoelastic material under constant load over time. Direct MFR methods create creep by using combinations of traction, compression, and twist.
Viscoelastic material:	Any material that deforms in relation to the rate of loading and deformation.

Force Effects

All tissues exhibit nonlinear, stress-strain responses that are functions of their densities and viscosities. For example, tendons deform at different rates than muscle fibers, ligaments, and bone.

Many mechanical components of the body are composed of water-absorbing collagen and supporting ground substances. Chemically, they include glycoproteins, glycosaminoglycans, and other low-molecular-weight material. It is on this background that mechanical forces exert their effects (1).

Inevitably, a number of mechanical principles interdependently affect neurologic and anatomic functions. Palpatory diagnosis and manipulative treatment apply many of these concepts. Examples are: *Wolff's Law, Hooke's Law,* and *Newton's Third Law:*

Wolff's Law:	states that bones tend to deform along the lines of force placed upon them. This is also true for soft tissues (8).
Hooke's Law:	states that any strain (deformation) placed on an elastic body is in proportion to the stress (force) placed upon it (8).
Newton's Third Law:	states that when two bodies interact, the force exerted by the first on the second is equal in magnitude and opposite in direction to the force exerted by the second on the first (8).

Passive and Active Patterns

Mechanical patterns are both passive and active.

Passive external factors such as body conformation are easily recognizable. Passive internal factors, such as asymmetric structural supports, muscle inhibition, and bony asymmetries, are less evident.

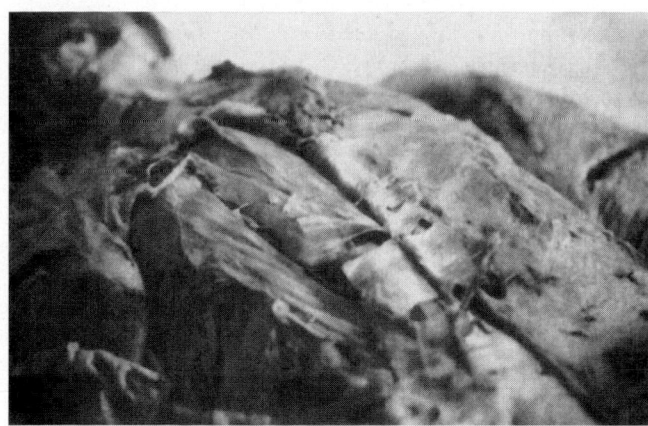

FIGURE 60.1. Fascia in gross dissection. (From Basmajian JV, Nyberg R. *Rational Manual Therapies*. Baltimore, MD: Williams & Wilkins; 1993:230.)

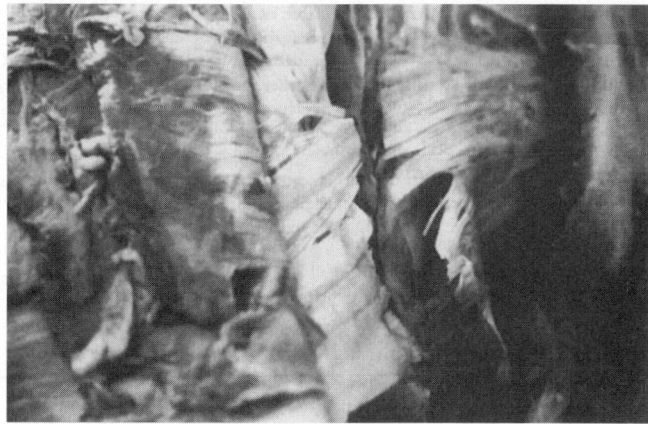

FIGURE 60.3. Sharp dissection difficulties resulting from muscle and fascia being inseparable. (From Basmajian JV, Nyberg R. *Rational Manual Therapies*. Baltimore, MD: Williams & Wilkins; 1993:231.)

Active patterns, that is, those arising from neurally mediated activities, are superimposed on the passive system. Examples include:

- Sitting
- Standing
- Walking
- Sleeping
- Working
- Sporting activities

Figures 60.1 to 60.4 demonstrate a 1987 soft tissue dissection done by Frank George, DO, in the anatomy laboratories of Michigan State University. From this work, we learned that fascia and muscle are anatomically inseparable. Earlier authors like Cathie (9) and Becker (10) suggested that fasciae move independently. George's work suggests that fasciae probably move in response to complex muscle activities acting on not only bones and joints but also ligaments, tendons, and fasciae.

This view is reinforced by other research highlighting the importance of fascia in maintaining general proprioception. Since proprioception is ultimately controlled by interdependent neural and muscular elements, after joint and muscle spindle activity is accounted for, 75% of remaining proprioception occurs in fascial

sheaths (11). Such responses were actually demonstrated in the 1960s by Earl (12) and Wilson (13) in their work with muscles under stretch.

Palpation to Develop Haptic Skills

Palpation is the key to successful use of any manipulative method. Some untrained observers occasionally suggest that the ability to palpate is inborn and difficult to teach. This may be true in a few instances, but all health care professionals are regularly challenged to develop palpation skills when performing physical examinations and myriad medical and surgical procedures.

Haptic neuroscience analyzes both sensory and motor aspects of hand activities. Palpatory diagnosis, technically, is a high-level haptic skill. In an almost literal sense, skilled palpating hands learn to "see" anatomic and mechanical detail, much like a blind person senses the environment. As improvements appear, appreciation for seemingly obscure, but important, subtleties emerge.

Sensing Positional and Movement-Related Asymmetries

One key to success is the ability to identify tethering effects that persistently create and maintain pathologic asymmetries. *Tightness suggests tethering, while looseness suggests joint and/or soft tissue*

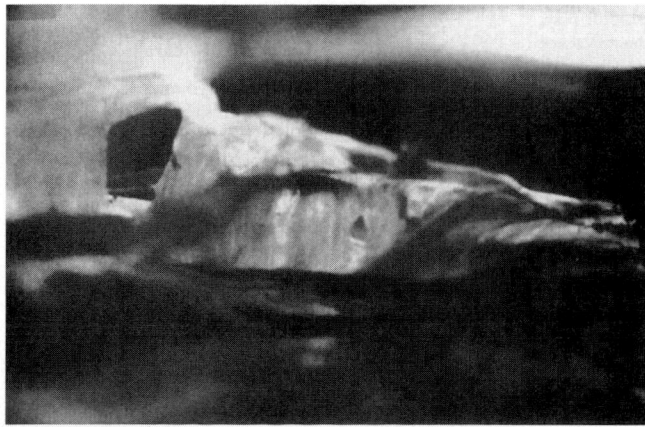

FIGURE 60.2. Closer view of fascia in gross dissection. (From Basmajian JV, Nyberg R. *Rational Manual Therapies*. Baltimore, MD: Williams & Wilkins; 1993:230.)

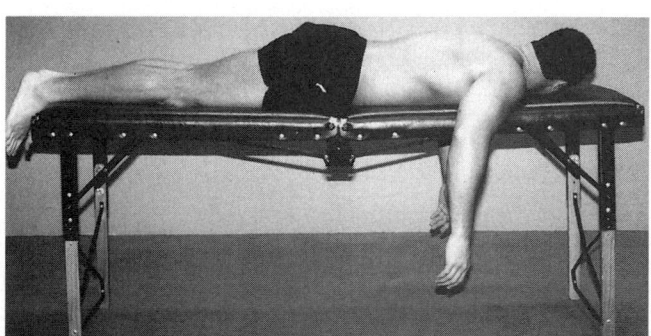

FIGURE 60.4. Position for thoracolumbar release: head to most comfortable side with arms off table.

laxity with or without neural inhibition. Sometimes tethering relates directly to changes in coupled vertebral motions and altered joint play; the motion segment is altered. Knowing the difference between neutral and nonneutral vertebral mechanics is essential (see Chapters 41, 43–50, 52). Both local soft tissue and neuroreflexive and neurocirculatory changes, such as viscerosomatic reflex changes, are common contributors to tethering. Tethering arises from many sources:

The spine, with altered coupled vertebral motions from any source

The synovial joints and their influences on joint play

Altered soft tissue mechanics (remembering that all tissues and their inherent motions are intrinsically asymmetric)

Asymmetric neural inputs arising from:

Multiple levels of the central nervous system, including cranial nerves, brainstem, midbrain, thalamus, and cortex

Limbic system and reticular activating system

Primary spinal cord sources

Peripheral nervous system sources at any level

Viscerosomatic reflexes

Somato-somatic reflexes

Neurohumoral activities of all kinds

Lowered reflex thresholds from sites of disease, injury, and degeneration

Biobehavioral and sociocultural factors are common sources of "tethering" and somatic dysfunction

Awareness of individual beliefs, perceptions, biases, and expectations in relation to expected outcome is an essential requirement for both clinician and patient. Importantly, patients commonly seek professional help when environmental stressors trigger undesirable symptoms. Difficulty coping with overwhelming events is a common presentation in any neuromusculoskeletal practice. Medicalization of nondisease-related problems is frequent. Unwitting encouragement of dependent and co-dependent behaviors, including requests for manipulative treatments, is common under these conditions.

Monitoring Inherent Tissue Motion

Inherent tissue motions are palpably evident, asymmetrically patterned, neuroreflexive activities in the soft tissues. They constantly move, often at variable rates. Palpation that focuses on these motions should readily identify patterns of shifting asymmetric tightness and looseness. Asymmetrically perceived end-feels are commonly referred to as direct and indirect barriers. As a rule, inherent movements are easier in some directions, less so in others. Myofascially, shifting tightness and looseness identifies unevenly distributed direct and indirect barriers. Many are independent of joint mechanics. Others are tightly linked to joint mechanisms.

TREATMENT SKILLS

Treatment skills improve as one learns to apply well-directed forces interactively against direct and indirect barriers. A common example occurs when restrictions involving one side of the pelvis

affect the opposite lower limb, lower costal cage and trunk rotators, the opposite shoulder, the cervical spine, and cranial base.

In some cases, it is likely that successful treatments link as yet unclear intrinsic body movements of both the patient and operator at some level. How this occurs is unknown, but it is likely that both conscious and subconscious brain-mediated factors are at play. Experienced practitioners and patients often comment that a treatment went especially well or not as well on a particular day. Some research indirectly suggests how this occurs.

In 1989, Grinberg-Zylerbaum and Ramos reported on their studies of nontouching, silent communication between two or more individuals. Electroencephalography (EEG) was used as a means for studying silent communication patterns between two individuals. Partners who reported feelings of being blended with one another altered their EEG patterns to the point of being virtually identical (14).

This author and others have repeatedly identified similar blending effects during MFR and craniosacral treatment encounters. Whether these experiences are in any way similar to the Grinberg-Zylerbaum and Ramos work has not been investigated.

Other hypotheses and experiments point out subtle cranial bone movement changes that may be involved. In one instance, Norton hypothesized a model for quantitatively assessing pressure variations in soft tissues of both the subject and examiner. His study is completely theoretical, however, and lacks experimental data (15). Adams and colleagues, on the other hand, made parietal bone movement measurements in cats that suggest the presence of neurally generated waveforms that create 1- or 2-μm movements across the parietal suture (16). Individual abilities to palpate these subtle changes have been carried out in a number of experiments (17,18).

Tight-Loose Concept Exercise (Figs. 60.86 and 60.87)

A simple laboratory exercise readily demonstrates the tight-loose concept. With the patient lying supine, the operator grasps the patient's wrists. By slowly raising the upper limb toward full overhead extension, one gets a sense of shifting three-dimensional tightness or looseness that begins at the wrists and eventually involves the whole of the patient's body. By carefully attending to both the quality and amplitude of these passively induced operator forces, clearly defined mechanically asymmetric sites of tightness and looseness become apparent.

As each limb is moved separately and together, tight-loose relationships vary considerably and their end-feels are different. Some are abrupt, almost like hitting a wall. Others are soft, like either falling into or fluffing a pillow. Importantly, these asymmetric shifts rarely follow classic anatomic patterns. With practice, variable tensions and loads are readily sensed from the hands and wrists distally into the lumbodorsal fascia and pelvis.

Pain at Loose Sites

Painful sensations are common at loose sites, particularly in chronic cases. Typically, there is little muscle spasm or tightening. Under these conditions, associated muscles are commonly weak and inhibited. Some practitioners refer to these sites as hypermobile, implying that ligamentous laxity and joint instability are the fundamental problems. An alternative idea concludes that loose, painful muscles are weak and inhibited over large, often ill-defined areas, including vertebral mechanics.

From a clinical perspective, whole body effects are the rule rather than an exception. Loosened sites are often vulnerable to injury under relatively trivial circumstances. Repeated ankle and lumbosacral sprains, as well as neck and shoulder problems arising from altered lumbopelvic and lower limb mechanics, are common examples.

CLINICAL ASSESSMENT

Tightness and looseness should be evaluated from a patterned three-dimensional context that includes:

Skeletal and soft tissue configurations
Upper and lower motor neuron influences
Effects of mechanical modeling and remodeling of bones, joints, and soft tissues
Effects of general skeletal factors
Injury history
Effects of repetitive daily activities
Psychoemotional states
Limiting psychosocial and socioeconomic factors

Locating direct and indirect barriers is a useful method for understanding tightness, looseness, and tethering effects.

Tightness of any kind suggests tethering and direct barriers. It also implies the presence of direct barriers and "bind" (see Glossary at the end of this text). Some are of bony origin, but many are not. Whether these tethers and areas of bind should be removed requires careful assessment.

One form of tethering is acute muscle spasm, which is almost always self-limited. Another relates to generally tight muscles, which are not always sources of pain and altered function. Stressful lifestyles and personality issues are common in this group. True spasticity, centrally mediated neural tethering, arises from upper motor neuron pathologies. Cerebral palsy, central spinal stenosis, strokes, and effects of head injuries are common examples.

Scar tissue implies the presence of passive mechanical tethering that may actually stabilize an otherwise unstable site.

Acute localized muscle tension and tethering generally imply peripheral neural involvement. A history of direct trauma is common for this group.

Looseness generally occurs in association with indirect barriers, neural inhibition, and painful sites. Since inhibition often accompanies neural injury and Wallerian degeneration, pain reports and muscle weaknesses are a common theme with this group.

THREE-DIMENSIONAL PATTERNS

Three-dimensional vertical, horizontal, and wraparound patterns are the rule and can be identified with some practice. Looking for three-dimensionally related areas of tightness and looseness is the key.

For example, in the prone position, right hip extension should create left lumbar, latissimus dorsi, and shoulder movements, and vice versa. Well-conditioned individuals will extend the hip with minimum use of contralateral back extensors and shoulder groups. The pattern often changes when the head is sequentially changed from left to center to right. A common prone wraparound pattern is as follows:

Tight posterior left hip, sacroiliac joint, lumbar erector spinae, and lower costal cage
Loose posteriorly on the right
Tight anterior and right lateral costal cage
Tight right upper anterior costal cage
Tight left thoracic inlet, posteriorly
Tight right scalenes, and cervical flexors
Tight left craniocervical attachments, including sternocleidomastoid, jaw, and facial mechanics

TREATMENT GOALS

The general goal is to release tightness and restore three-dimensionally patterned functional symmetry to the extent possible without aggravating hypermobility. As forces against direct and indirect barriers are sequentially applied, an experienced operator can efficiently treat the whole body in a reasonably short time.

Direct and Indirect Techniques

Simultaneous direct and indirect two-handed techniques are used. With practice, direct and indirect maneuvers can be applied simultaneously, with one hand performing direct release while the other performs indirect release.

Release-Enhancing Maneuvers and Integrated Neuromuscular Release Processes

Starting from the skin and working inward, varieties of traction, twist, shear, and compression are applied three-dimensionally while inherent tissue and joint motions are simultaneously monitored for shifting tightness and looseness. Inherent tissue movements have been described as "wormlike" activities beneath the palpating hands and fingers. The clinical assumption is that these perceived activities are neuroreflexive responses to the externally applied forces.

Direct Myofascial Release

Direct MFR maneuvers strain (deform) areas of tightness. By holding firmly against the soft tissue resistance (i.e., the direct myofascial barriers) releases are triggered. By making tightness even tighter, releases occur rather quickly, often in multiple directions at the same time. When this happens, the tissues often feel as though they are quivering in multiple directions at the same time.

Indirect Myofascial Release

For every area of perceived tightness, there are one or more areas of three-dimensionally related looseness. Commonly, the looseness is in exactly the opposite direction from the tightness. This mirroring concept is similar to those identified using functional indirect methods described in Chapters 61, 64, and 70.

Experienced operators locate these interdependent relationships quite readily, finding it easier to follow gently behind releases as they occur.

Integrated Neuromuscular Release

Patient assistance with release-enhancing maneuvers helps speed the treatment process. A few enhancers are listed below:

1. Breath holding during phases of inhalation and exhalation changes. The goal is to alter both intrathoracic and intraabdominal pressures using costodiaphragmatic, shoulder girdle, and lumbopelvic interactions.
2. Prone and supine simulated swimming and pendulum arm swing maneuvers use the arms as direct and indirect barriers are released.
3. Right, center, and leftward head turning in any body position is often helpful.
4. Isometric limb and neck movements against the table or chair create post-isometric muscle relaxations at various sites. For example, in the prone position, stubborn lumbopelvic problems often persist until proximal thoracolumbar and iliopsoas attachments are stressed by alternately forcing the knees, thighs, and iliopsoas hip flexors against the table. This can be easily done both prone and supine.
5. For reasons as yet unclear, varieties of patient-invoked cranial nerve activities, such as eye, tongue, jaw, and oropharyngeal isometric and kinetic movements are also helpful. Apparently, progressively engaged cranial nerve activities create central and peripherally mediated neural activities that alter abnormal patterns as external forces are applied. It is also probable that distraction plays a role, similar to the Jendrassik maneuver used to enhance the patellar jerk reflex.

POSTTREATMENT EVALUATION

Posttreatment evaluation is essential for a number of reasons:

1. To know whether appropriate and helpful changes have occurred
2. To help the patient understand what to expect from the treatment
3. To help design an appropriate individualized exercise program
4. To help develop an appropriate pharmacologic program, should it be necessary
5. To identify and accurately record changes for the medical record

POSTTREATMENT DISCOMFORT

Patients commonly experience a temporary worsening of discomfort following the first treatment or two. This possibility should be identified before the patient leaves the office. The phenomenon is similar to postexercise muscle soreness, but does not occur with everyone. Older age groups and general deconditioning are common contributors to the problem. Usually the experience

occurs only once, but those with rheumatologic disorders such as lupus erythematosus and fibromyalgia can experience repeated flare-ups.

ROLE OF EXERCISE IN MAINTAINING CHANGES

It is essential that a simple, time-efficient exercise program be worked out. The program should stretch areas of tightness without aggravating pain or instability. Restoring adequate proprioception by using one-leg standing activities is essential for long-term success. Looseness, or areas of inhibited individual and patterned muscle activities, requires strengthening and toning. For example, identification of weak, inhibited muscle groups, such as altered gluteus maximus and hamstring firing sequences, helps develop a clear rehabilitation focus. In this example, back pain patients often fail to fire one or both gluteus maximus muscles during prone straight leg hip extensions.

CONCLUSION

This section introduces a few basic myofascial and integrated neuromusculoskeletal release concepts. Keys to diagnostic and treatment successes lie in the ability to sort out interdependent mechanical, anatomic, and neurologic problems contributing to altered three-dimensional movement patterns. Hallmarks for identifying these patterns lie in the ability to assess and treat interactive areas of tightness, looseness, and tethering. A well-designed, individualized, easy-to-follow exercise program is essential for long-term success. The following sections of this chapter present a few useful techniques.

INTEGRATED NEUROMUSCULOSKELETAL TECHNIQUES FOR SPECIFIC AREAS

There are many ways to approach neuromusculoskeletal problems manually. For the sake of practicality, descriptions are limited to a few methods used with relative ease that have stood the test of time. Those familiar with muscle energy terminology can record and monitor INR/MFR processes by superimposing functional anatomy descriptors. For example, bony positional changes, such as unilateral left sacral flexion (also called sacral shear), left on right sacral torsion, and L4 nonneutral extension–rotation–side bending left, easily combine with these methods.

Lumbosacral Spine and Pelvis

The general goal is to three-dimensionally balance lumbopelvic mechanics, keeping in mind that the costal cage and lower limbs play major roles in the process.

Thoracolumbar Release

Figures 60.4 to 60.11) illustrate this process.

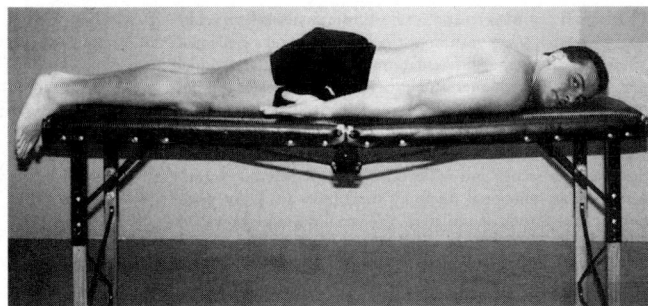

FIGURE 60.5. Position for thoracolumbar release: head to most comfortable side with arms on table.

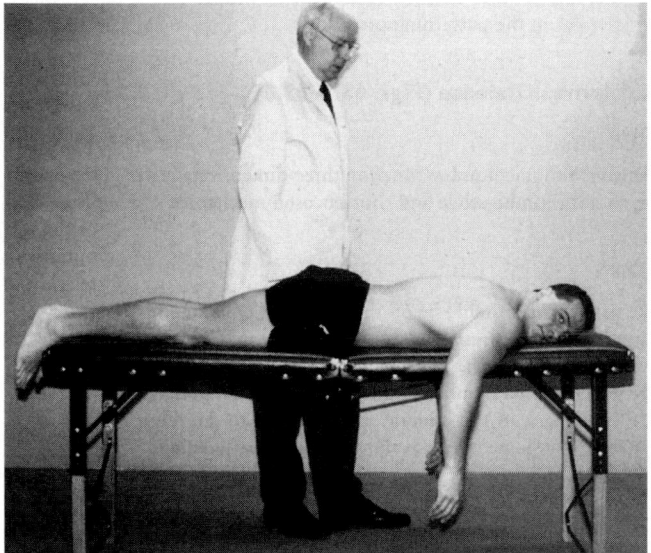

FIGURE 60.6. Position for thoracolumbar release: head comfortable, feet and arms off table.

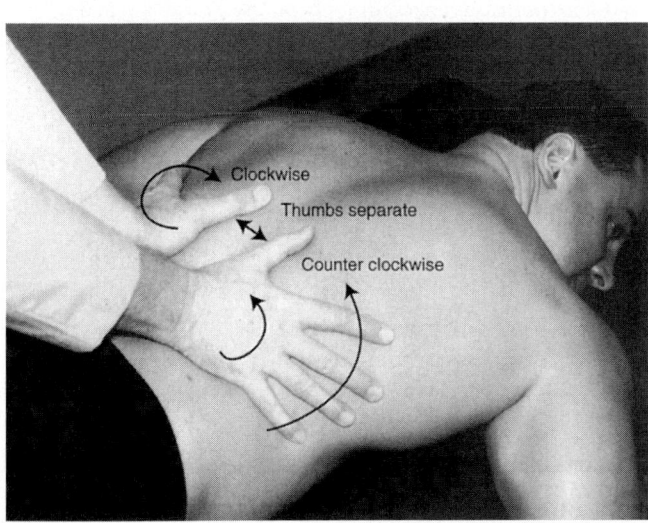

FIGURE 60.7. Operator stands beside patient's hip, with head to side.

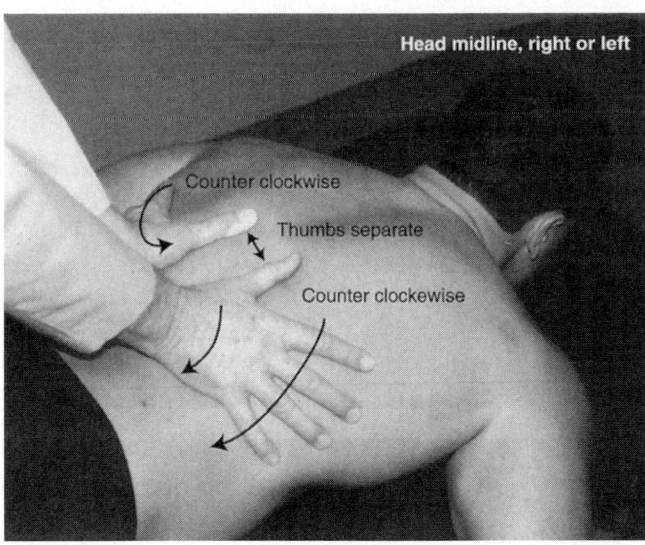

FIGURE 60.8. Hands placed at thoracolumbar junction, with head in midline.

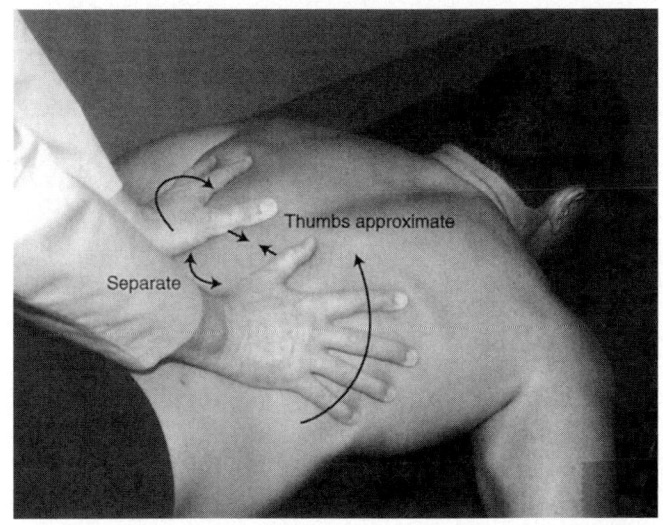

FIGURE 60.9. Head midline.

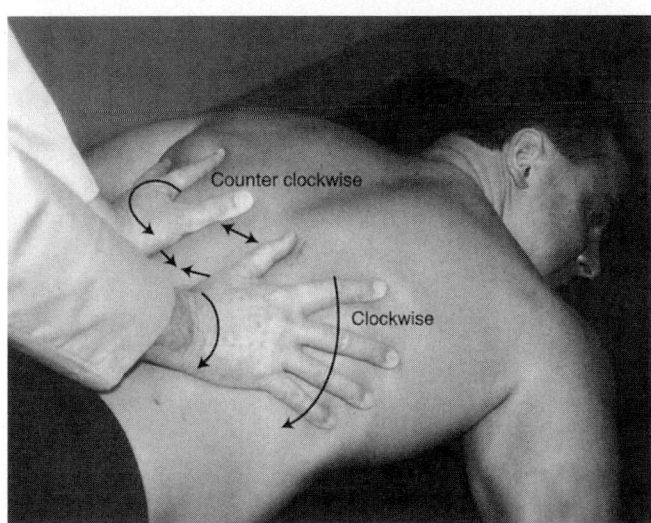

FIGURE 60.10. Head right.

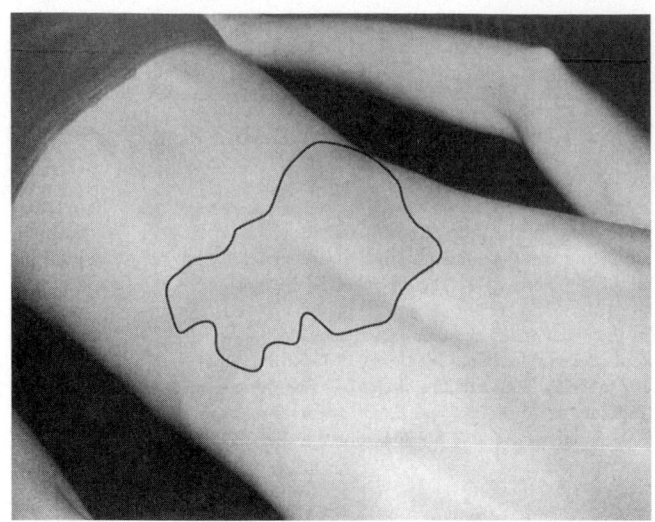

FIGURE 60.11. Blush sign. After blanching, areas receiving major stressing commonly become reddened and warmer.

Objective

To balance the thoracolumbar junction three-dimensionally in relation to lumbopelvic, thoracocostal, and diaphragmatic mechanics.

Review

Review cervical, trapezius, shoulder girdle, and costal cage anatomy for their three-dimensional perspectives and functional relationships to the area.

Procedure

Prone

1. The patient's feet should be off the end of the table to minimize lower limb stresses in relation to the pelvis and low back (Figs. 60.4 to 60.7).

2. Initially, the patient's head should be turned to the most comfortable side. Holding it exclusively in the midline, as many wish to do, often obscures tight-loose effects at the thoracolumbar junction.

3. The hands and arms are comfortably placed either over the sides of the table, or on the table beside the hips and thighs.

4. Stand beside the patient's hip, facing cephalad (Fig. 60.6).

5. Place your hands at the thoracolumbar junction, covering posteroinferior rib, trunk rotator, and diaphragmatic sites (Figs. 60.7 to 60.11).

6. Place hands widely open with the thumbs pointed cephalad along either side of the spinous processes while the remainder of each hand spreads over the posteroinferior costodiaphragmatic and upper lumbar areas.

7. Identify superficial and deep tightness and looseness patterns three-dimensionally.

8. Firmly separate the thumbs across the midline as the left hand creates clockwise and the right hand creates counterclockwise traction. The hands should not slide on the skin.

9. As the skin is stretched between the thumbs, it will initially blanch. As compression, traction, and twist are maintained, tissues begin to relax both reflexively and mechanically in accordance with principles discussed earlier in this chapter. After initial

blanching, the site of major soft tissue tension commonly becomes reddened and warmer, the so-called "blush phenomenon" (Fig. 60.11).

10. Typical releases occur three-dimensionally with sustained traction and twist, and they can occur singly or in multiples. The latter often creates a wormlike sensation under the palpating hands. As multiple releases continue, so-called unwinding phenomena often occur, as shifting patterns of tightness and looseness alter three-dimensional relationships. With practice, one learns to feel deeply into the areas surrounding facet joints. Symmetric segmental movements to passive three-dimensional stressing suggest that the procedure is complete. Treatment is complete when repetitive stressing of selected sites no longer creates release activity.

Combined Sacroiliac, Sacral Base, and Lumbopelvic Releases

This process is shown in Figs. 60.12 to 60.19.

Objective

The goal is to establish symmetric sacral nutation and counternutation movements in relation to the innominates, lumbar spine, and lower limbs. Nutation is anterior nodding (flexion) of the sacral base in relation to the lumbar lordosis; counternutation is posterior nodding (extension) of the sacral base in relation to the lumbar lordosis.

Review

Review three-dimensional anatomy of the sacroiliac joint, sacral base, and lumbopelvic mechanics, including proximal and distal erector spinae and iliopsoas relationships, quadratus lumborum, multifidus, and deep layer, hip rotator, and pelvic diaphragm relationships. Also be aware of congenital anomalies, and iliolumbar-innominate-sacral base influences.

Diagnosis

With practice, sacral torsions, flexions (in some cases called sacral shears), and innominate positions become readily apparent. Innominate positions are commonly referred to as "anterior," "posterior," or "shear." Most typically, they are diagnosed using muscle energy nomenclature.

Procedure

Prone

1. The feet should be off the end of the table to minimize lower limb stresses in relation to the pelvis and low back.

2. The head should be turned to the most comfortable side. Holding it in the midline, as many wish to do, often obscures tight-loose effects in the thoracolumbar regions.

3. The hands and arms are comfortably placed either over the sides of the table, or on the table beside the hips and thighs.

4. Stand at the patient's left shoulder facing caudad.

5. Place your proximal left hand longitudinally over the thoracolumbar junction, with the long finger covering the upper lumbar spinous processes. For best results, place the metatarsophalangeal joint of the long finger precisely at the T12-L1 junction (Fig. 60.12).

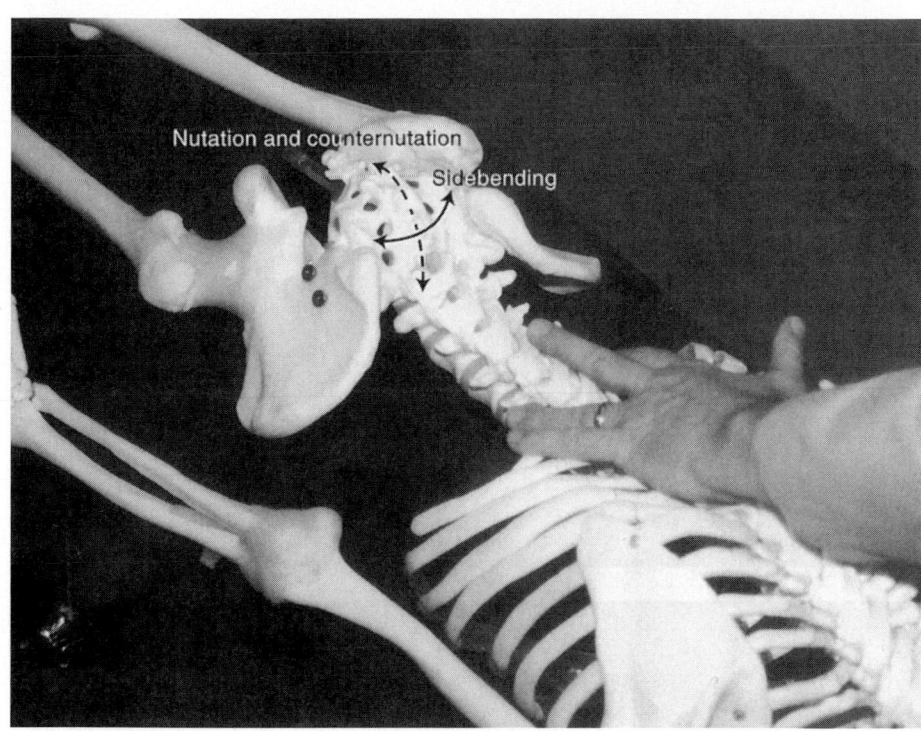

FIGURE 60.12. Position for combined sacroiliac, sacral base, and lumbopelvic releases.

6. The distal right hand covers the sacrum between the two innominates with the index finger overlying the right sacroiliac joint and inferior lateral angle while the ring finger covers the left. The long finger will fall naturally over the sacral spines and sacral hiatus (Fig. 60.13).

7. Evaluate patterns of tightness and looseness:
    a. Proximally and distally, by distracting the sacrum and lumbar spine in the long axis of the spine (Fig. 60.15).
    b. Circumferentially, by transversely translating each hand in opposite directions across the lumbopelvic system (Figs. 60.16 to 60.19).

8. Induce lumbosacral distraction by assertively moving the left

hand proximally up and over the thoracic curve while forcing the right hand distally up and over the natural curve of the sacrum (Fig. 60.15). Importantly, one must respect both the sacral base angle and the natural configuration of the sacral curve. Some are in a more or less straight-line relationship with the back, while others are acutely angled, demonstrating more or less perpendicular relationships with the spine and pelvis.

9. Both heavy-handed and, in some cases, light-handed loads mechanically induce reflexively controlled inherent tissue and sacral movements. Learning both methods takes some practice.

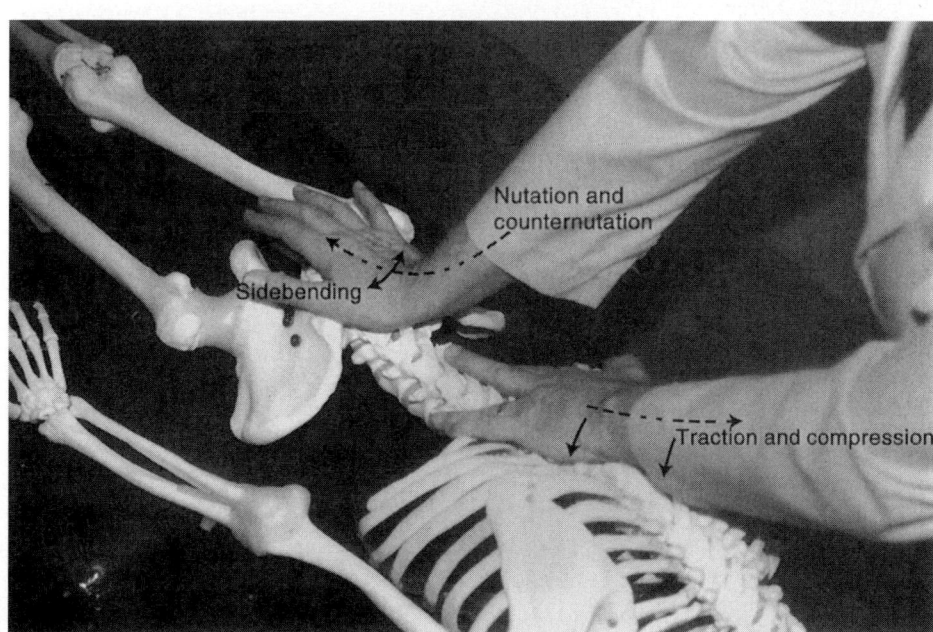

FIGURE 60.13. Position for combined sacroiliac, sacral base, and lumbopelvic releases.

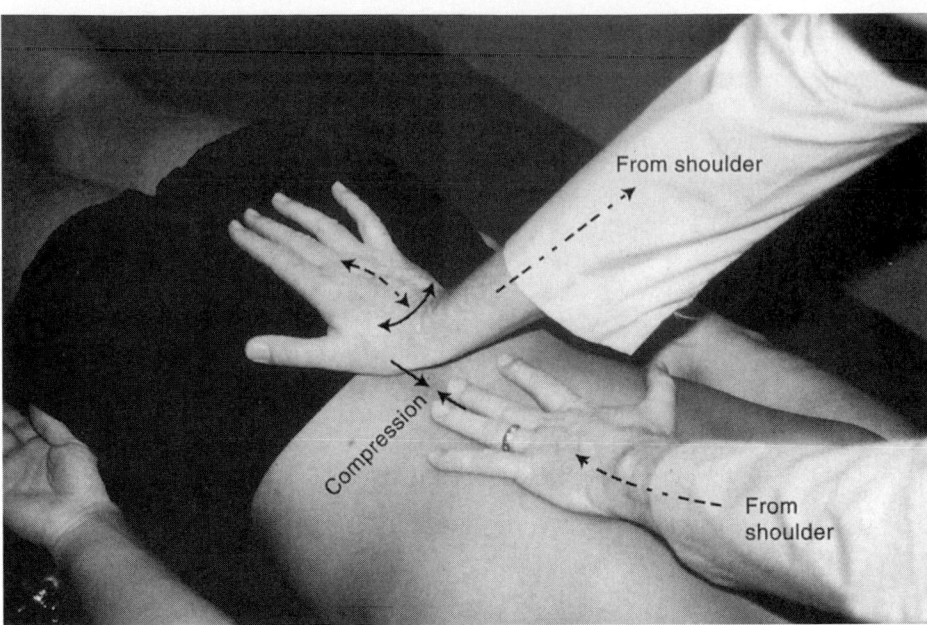

FIGURE 60.14.

10. As loading develops, varieties of three-dimensional tight-ness and looseness become apparent. Sacral torsions, flexions (shears), innominate changes, and sacroiliac joint factors, such as close and loose packing, are noted.

11. By using combinations of distraction and compression (Figs. 60.14 and 60.15) while monitoring inherent tissue movements, sacroiliac positional and movement changes commonly give way and become more symmetric.

12. As the lumbopelvic complex passively drifts right and left, it often helps to change the hands perpendicular to the spine to induce further movement in a crosswise fashion (Figs. 60.18 and 60.19).

13. Treatment is complete when sacroiliac joint and general lumbar movements are as symmetric as can reasonably be expected.

Focused Prone Sacral Base Release: Two-Handed Technique

This process is shown in Figs. 60.20 and 60.21.

Objective

The goal is to three-dimensionally balance the sacral base in relation to L4-5 mechanics, the iliolumbar ligament, and positional innominate asymmetries.

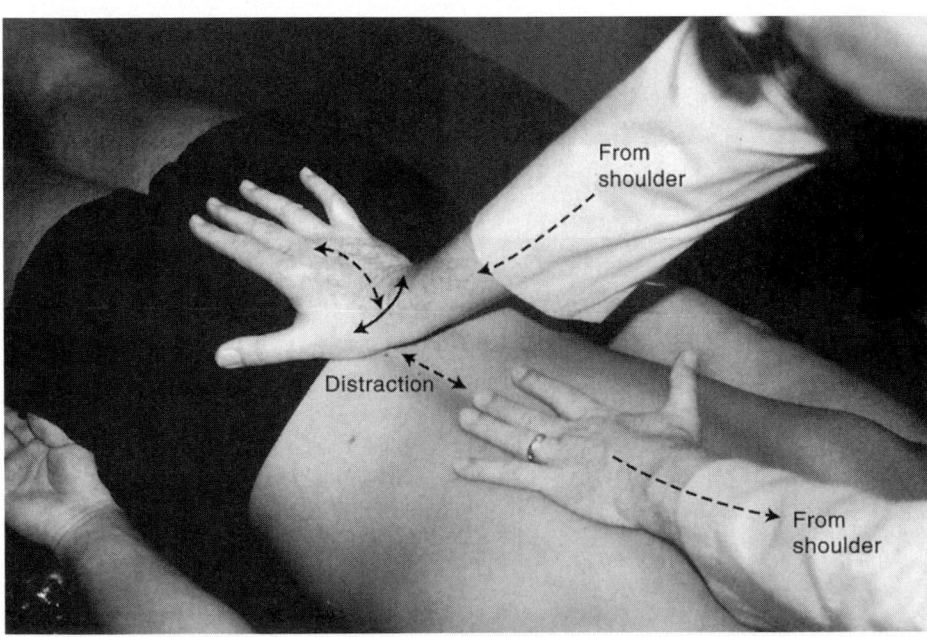

FIGURE 60.15.

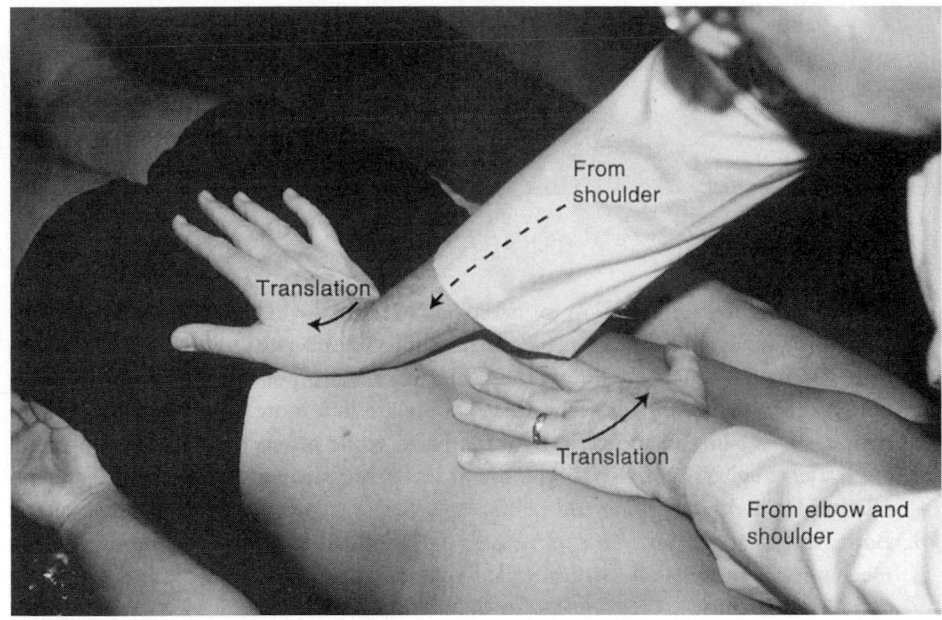

FIGURE 60.16.

Review

Review lumbopelvic anatomy, L4-5 mechanics in relation to the sacrum and pelvis, iliolumbar ligament, and innominate, hip rotator, and pelvic diaphragm relationships, including distal iliopsoas and piriformis muscle influences.

Diagnosis

See "Sacroiliac Release: Supine" later in this chapter.

Procedure

Prone

1. The feet should be off the end of the table to minimize lower limb stresses in relation to the pelvis and low back.

2. The head should be turned to the most comfortable side.

3. The hands and arms are comfortably placed either over the sides of the table or on the table beside the hips and thighs.

4. If right-handed, stand at the patient's left shoulder, facing caudad.

5. Place one hand either horizontally, or transverse to the sacrum, contacting the posterior superior iliac spines and medial gluteus maximus attachments bilaterally.

6. Place the other hand over the bottom hand along the long axis of the sacrum between the two innominates, with the index finger overlying one sacroiliac joint and inferior lateral angle as the ring finger covers the other. By using this hand placement, the long finger falls naturally over the sacral spines and sacral hiatus.

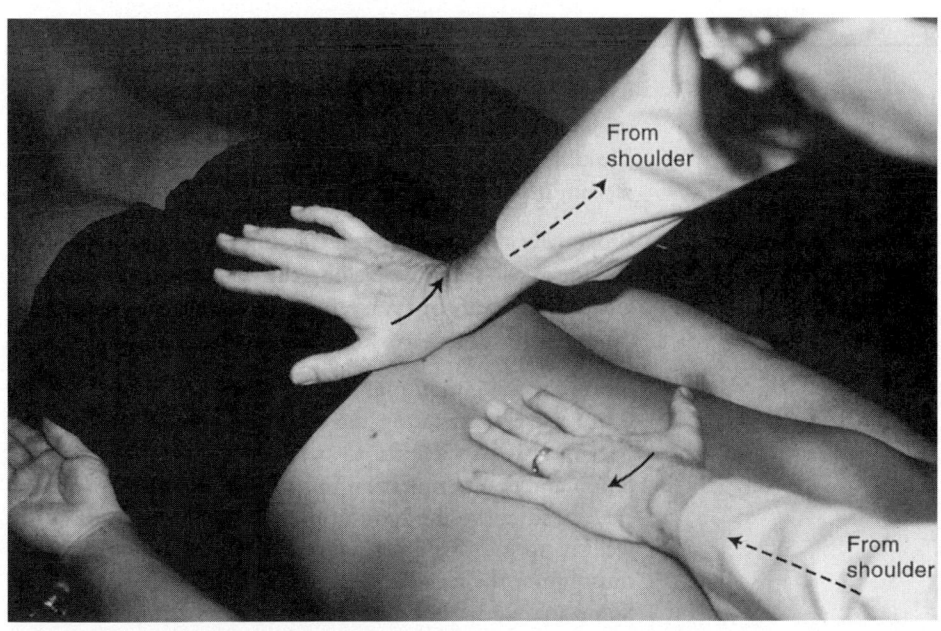

FIGURE 60.17.

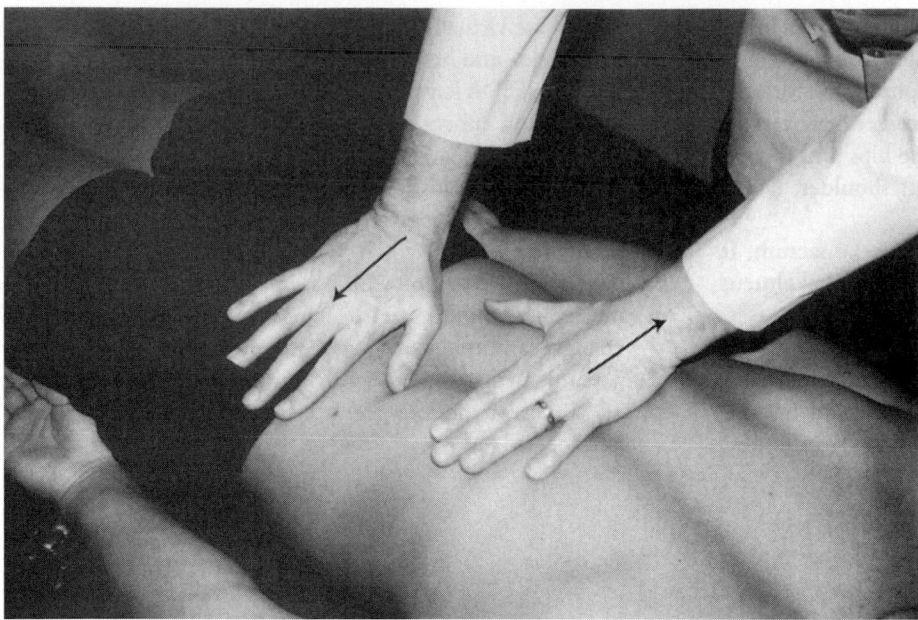

FIGURE 60.18.

7. Evaluate patterns of tightness and looseness by rocking the sacrum in multiple planes:
   a. Proximally and distally, by distracting the sacrum and lumbar spine at the sacral base along the long axis of the spine.
   b. Circumferentially, by transversely translating each hand across the pelvis in opposite directions.
8. Using a rocking nutation-counternutation gapping motion, induce lumbosacral joint distraction (Fig. 60.21). Be sure to create the motion by moving the distal hand caudally as well as up and over the natural curve of the sacrum. (See step no. 8 under "Sacroiliac, Sacral Base, and Lumbopelvic Releases Combined Technique" earlier in the chapter.) Some sacrums

are in a more or less straight-line relationship with the spine. Others are sometimes acutely angled with the plane of the sacral base virtually perpendicular to the flow of the operator-imposed forces.

9. Both light- and heavy-handed force can be used, depending on your skill. A key to success is the ability to monitor, induce, and enhance both inherent tissue and craniosacral activities.

10. As both static and dynamic loading is applied, inherent tissue movement-related tightness and looseness usually becomes apparent. Static forces load the system against direct and indirect barriers without superimposing oscillating movements. Dynamic forces load the system with subtle

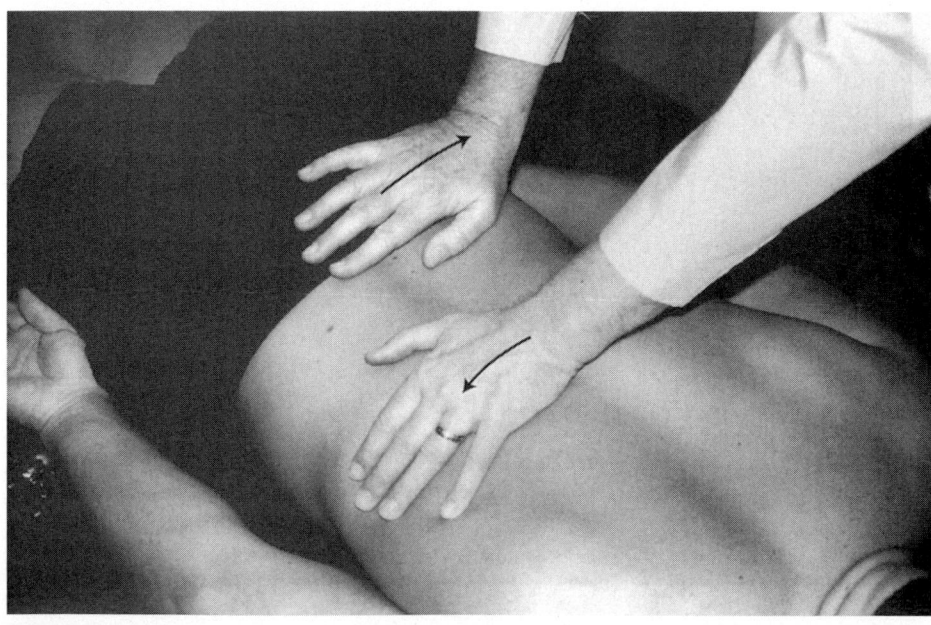

FIGURE 60.19.

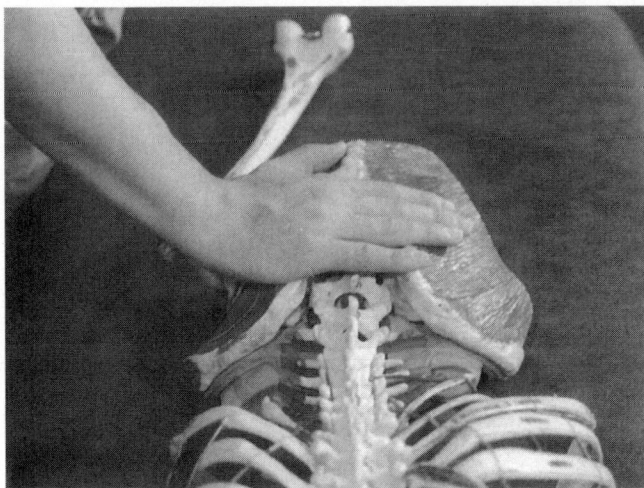

FIGURE 60.20.

operator-induced forces that:
a. Follow along behind inherent tissue and craniosacral movements
b. Systematically seek out three-dimensional shifts of direct and indirect barriers as releases occur

11. Success is more apt to occur when special attention is given to the sacral base in relation to L4-5 mechanics, iliolumbar ligament anomalies, degenerative changes, and nonneutral vertebral mechanics. (See entries for ERs and FSR in the Glossary.)

12. Treatment is complete when L5 and sacral base mechanics and associated inherent motions are as symmetric as can reasonably be expected.

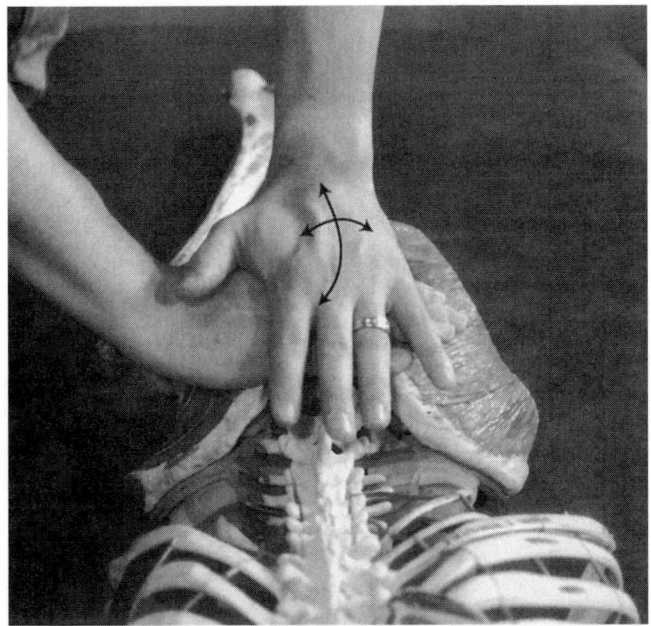

FIGURE 60.21. Using a rocking motion, induce lumbosacral joint distraction.

Sacrotuberous Ligament Release

Objective
The goal is to balance three-dimensional sacrotuberous and sacrospinous ligament factors affecting lumbopelvic, lower limb, and pelvic diaphragm mechanics.

Review
Review functional anatomy of pelvic diaphragm, ligaments of the sacrum, sacrotuberous-sacrospinous ligament relationships, pelvic diaphragm, and proximal adductor-hamstring relationships.

Procedure
Prone
1. The patient's feet should be off the end of the table to minimize lower limb stresses in relation to the pelvis and lower limb.
2. The patient's head should be turned to the most comfortable side.
3. The hands and arms are comfortably placed either over the sides of the table, or on the table beside the hips and thighs.
4. Stand beside the patient's left knee, facing cephalad.
5. Identify inferior and posterior sacral surfaces near the apex (Figs. 60.22 and 60.23).
6. Identify the medial surface of the sacral tuberosity where the sacrotuberous-sacrospinous system attaches (Figs. 60.24 and 60.25).
7. With a firm grasp on each buttock, place the thumbs halfway between the sacral apex and each sacral tuberosity, pressing firmly anteriorly and superiorly toward the symphysis pubis (Figs. 60.26 and 60.27).
8. By shifting the system three-dimensionally, identify tightness and looseness: areas of direct and indirect barriers.

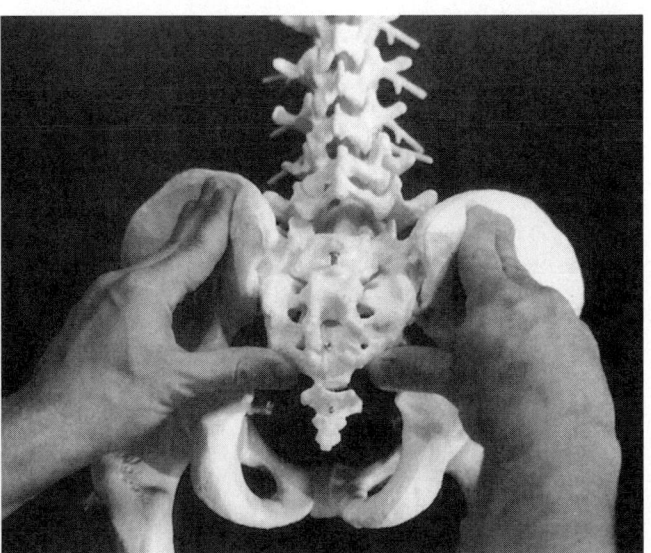

FIGURE 60.22. Inferior sacral surface.

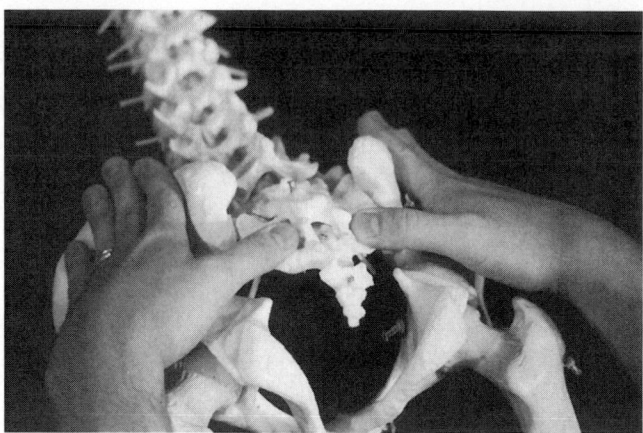

FIGURE 60.23. Posterior sacral surface.

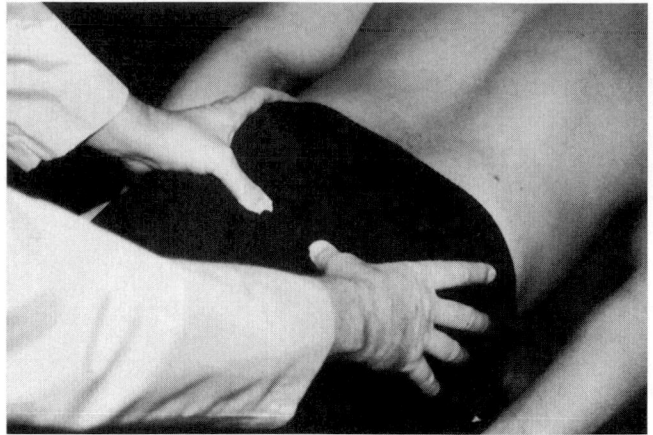

FIGURE 60.26. Place thumbs halfway between the sacral apex and each sacral tuberosity.

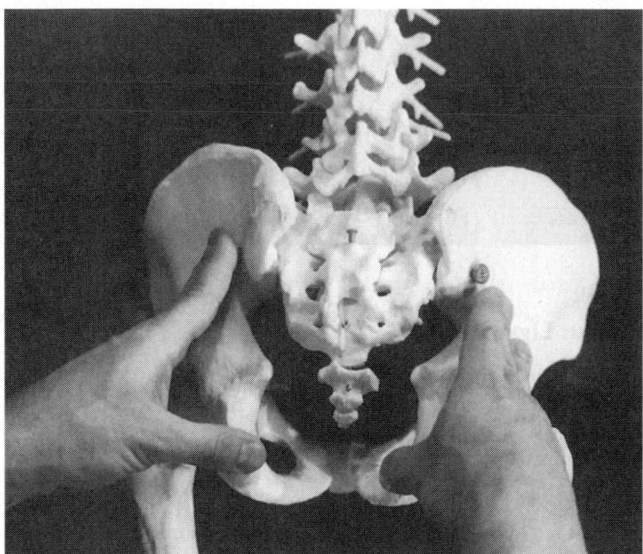

FIGURE 60.24. Medial surface of the sacral tuberosity.

9. This is accomplished by firmly pressing anteriorly and superiorly into the pelvic diaphragm and its attachments while turning the thumbs systematically against either tightness or looseness. Tightness and looseness in both the ligaments and pelvic diaphragm should become quickly apparent (Fig. 60.28). *Hint:* Think of turning a steering wheel with the thumbs.

10. Using each hand interactively, sequentially induce forces against tightness and looseness, stressing both direct and indirect barriers until releases occur.

11. Treatment is complete when sacrotuberous-pelvic diaphragm mechanics and related inherent motions are as symmetric as can reasonably be expected.

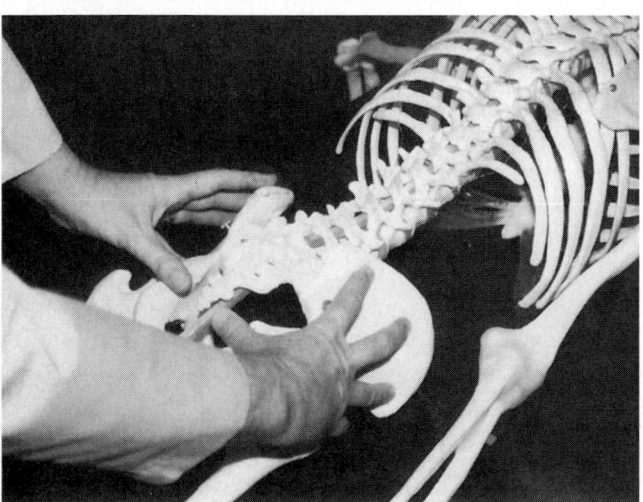

FIGURE 60.25. Medial surface of the sacral tuberosity.

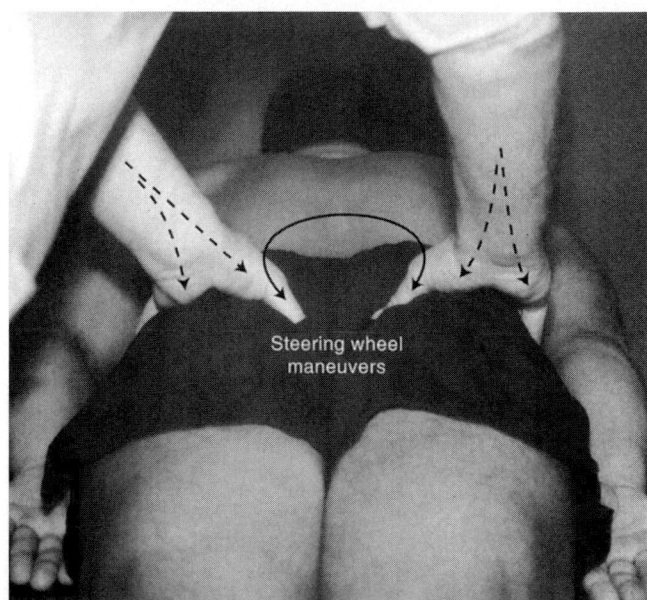

FIGURE 60.27. Place thumbs halfway between the sacral apex and each sacral tuberosity.

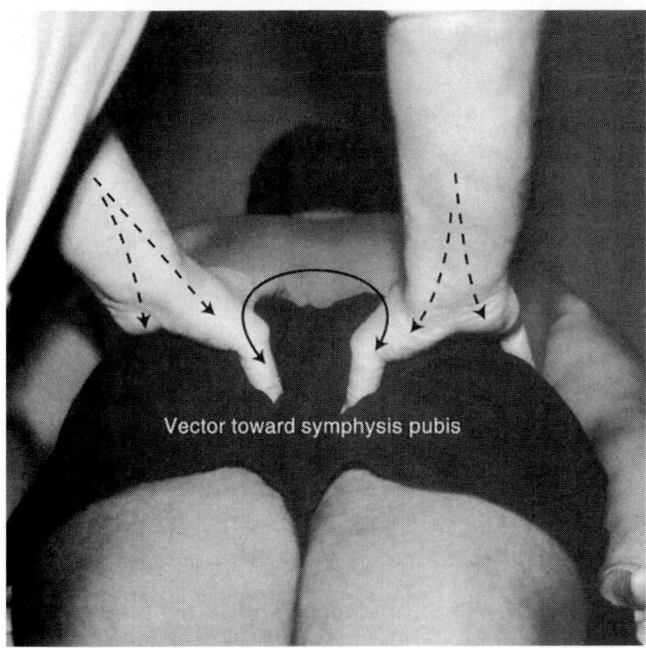
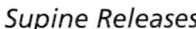

Vector toward symphysis pubis

FIGURE 60.28. Press anteriorly and superiorly while turning thumbs systematically against either tightness or looseness.

Supine Releases

Even after prone maneuvers are successful, lumbopelvic mechanics commonly remain asymmetric during supine assessment. As a result, one should learn to release the lumbopelvic, diaphragm, trunk rotator, pelvis, and hip rotator mechanics from this position. Primary focus is on the sacrum, pelvis, trunk rotators, and thoracolumbar junction.

Pubic Symphysis Release

Objective
The goal is to restore symmetry to the pubic symphysis.

Review
Review the functional three-dimensional relationships among the proximal thigh adductors, anterior and posterior innominates and their asymmetries, as well as changes involving the rectus sheath and transverses abdominis muscles, where they attach to the pubic symphysis.

Procedure
Supine
1. The patient lies supine with heels on the table and the arms comfortably at the sides or on the abdomen. Short-armed individuals should keep the arms on the table to avoid stressing shoulder and thoracolumbar systems. This more or less assures that unusual mechanical stresses transmitted through the Achilles tendons and ankles will be neutralized. For those with significant kyphosis, it is helpful to use a large pillow to minimize cervical and thoracolumbar problems.
2. Facing cephalad, the practitioner sits or stands beside the patient's right thigh, near the knee.
3. First, assess for symphyseal shear and positional asymmetry

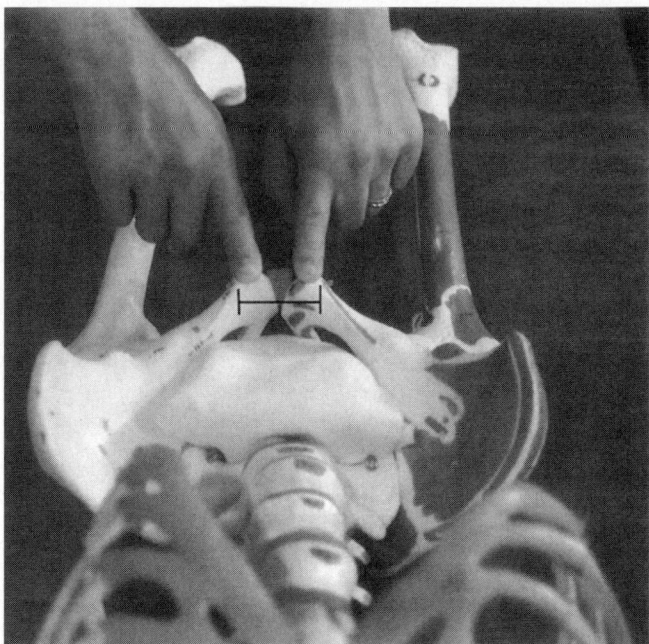

FIGURE 60.29. Assess for symphyseal shear and positional asymmetry.

(Figs. 60.29 and 60.30). Some prefer visual analysis, while others prefer a combination of palpation and vision. Tightness and looseness in the rectus sheath often identify the most problematic site. Sometimes tightness will be on the inferior side, sometimes the superior. Usually there are strong correlations with innominate positioning, but there are enough exceptions that one must be alert.

4. Place the thenar eminences on either side of the symphysis pubis, thumbs pointed superiorly and anteriorly. Proximal adductor and iliacus tendon attachments should be palpably evident under the thenar muscles (Figs. 60.31 and 60.32).

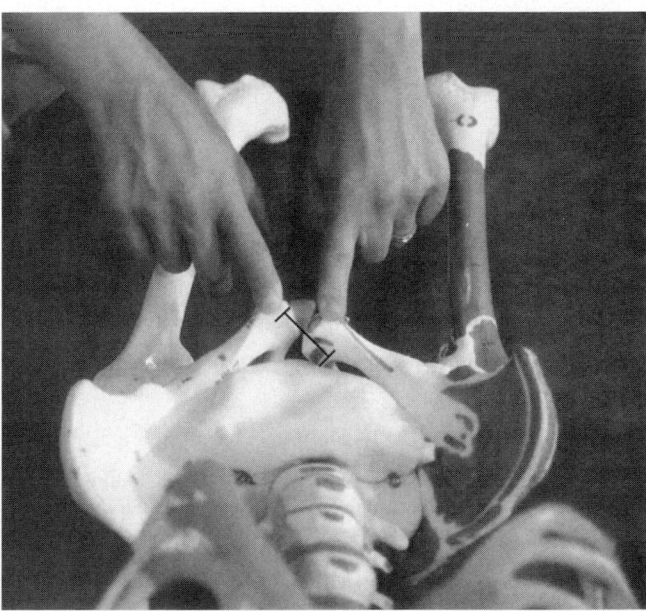

FIGURE 60.30. Assess for symphyseal shear and positional asymmetry.

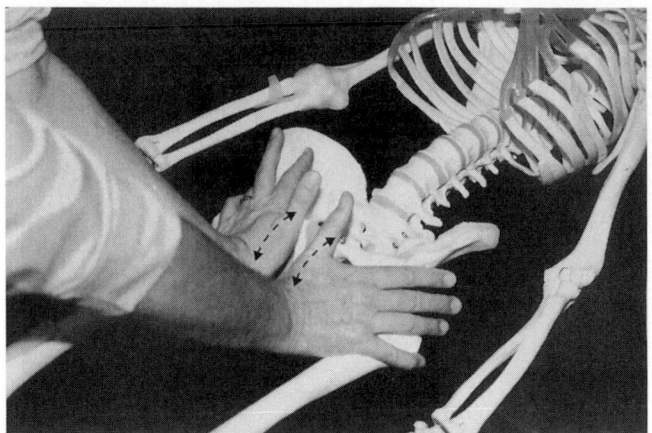

FIGURE 60.31. Symphysis release. Thenar eminences are placed on either side of symphysis pubis, thumbs pointed superiorly and anteriorly.

5. Induce firm, slow forces that either exaggerate (indirect barriers) or decrease (direct barriers) symphysis asymmetry. Direct rocking back and forth, similar to an articular maneuver, is often effective. Hold against the barriers until releases occur. Mild oscillations usually become evident as the rectus fasciae, boay pelvis, pelvic diaphragm, trunk rotators, and thigh adductors become more symmetric.

Anterior Pelvic-Innominate Release

This process is shown in Figs.60.33 to 60.38.

Objective

The goal is to reduce functional obliquity between the two innominates in relation to one another.

Review

1. Review posterior and lateral functional relationships among distal erector spinae groups, gluteus maximus, quadratus lumborum, trunk rotators, lumbodorsal fascia, latissimus dorsi, serratus posterior inferior, diaphragm, and lower rib cage.

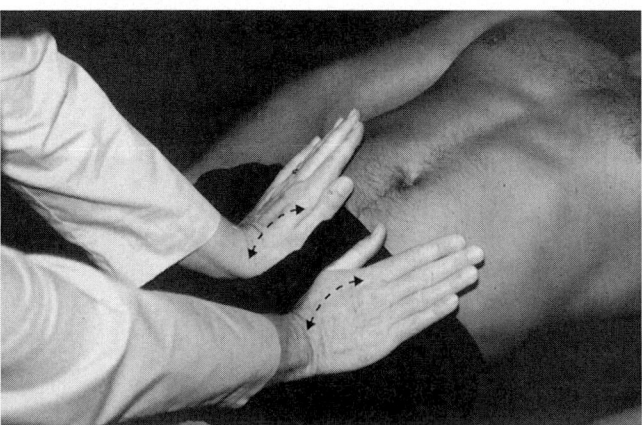

FIGURE 60.32. Thenar eminences are placed on either side of symphysis pubis, thumbs pointed superiorly and anteriorly.

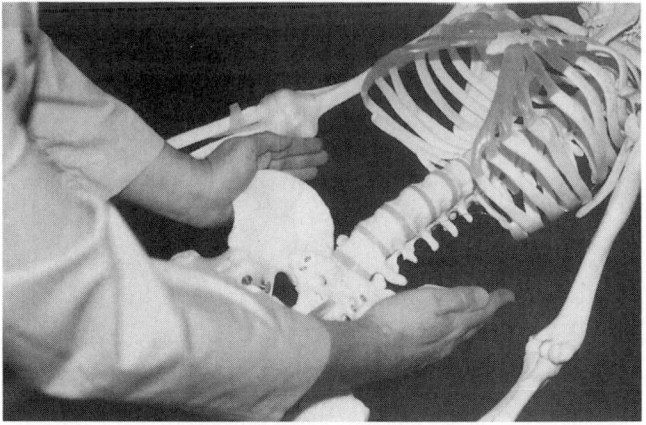

FIGURE 60.33.

2. Review anterior proximal and distal iliopsoas, diaphragm, and pelvic diaphragm elements, including piriformis and quadratus femoris relationships. Remember that distal iliopsoas relationships can be evaluated as they pass beneath the inguinal ligaments on their way to proximal attachments on the lesser trochanters of the femurs.
3. Review lateral hip abductor and knee relationships in relation to gluteus medius and minimus, gluteus maximus, tensor fasciae latae relationships with trunk rotators, and quadratus lumborum.
4. Review lower limb mechanics of all types and their potent effects on innominate asymmetries.

Procedure
Supine

1. The patient lies supine with heels on the table, arms comfortably at the sides. This basically assures that unusual mechanical stresses transmitted through the Achilles tendons and ankles will be neutralized. For those with significant kyphosis, it is helpful to use a large pillow to minimize cervical and thoracolumbar problems.
2. Face cephalad, standing beside the patient's right thigh.
3. Place the palms across the anterior superior iliac spines, being sure to cover the inguinal ligament medially. Include the

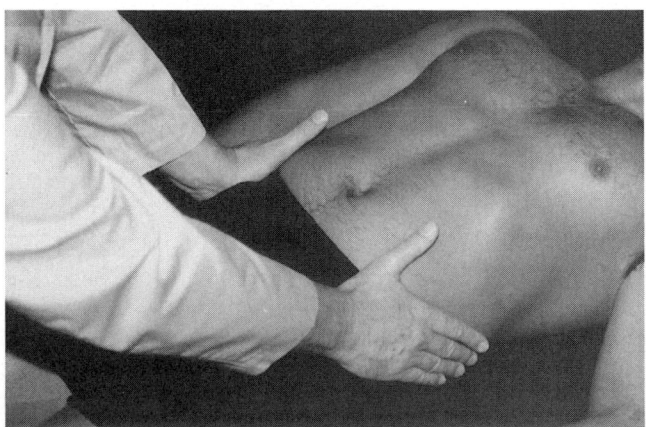

FIGURE 60.34.

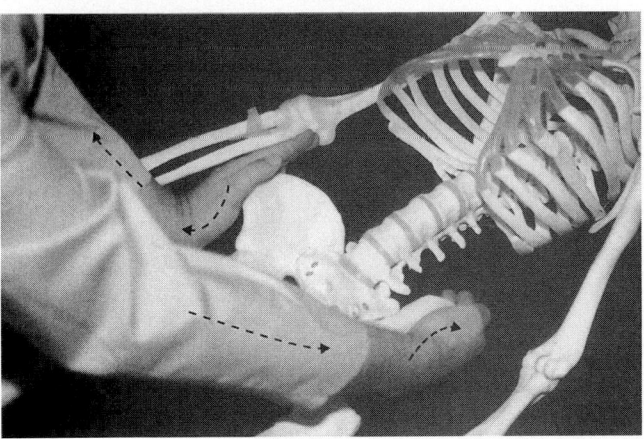

FIGURE 60.35.

iliopsoas muscles as they pass beneath the ligament toward their attachments on the lesser trochanter of the femur (Figs. 60.33 and 60.34).

4. Assess pelvic obliquity both positionally and functionally. Usually the right innominate is more anterior and resists practitioner-imposed posterior displacements. Commonly, the left innominate is positionally more posterior. Typically, this positioning resists operator-induced anterior displacements (i.e., direct barriers are apparent). Conversely, operator-induced posterior displacements assess indirect barriers (Figs. 60.35 and 60.36).

5. Barriers can be stressed both directly and indirectly at the same time by holding one innominate in each hand and three-dimensionally exaggerating pelvic obliquity (Figs. 60.37 and 60.38). As both direct and indirect barriers are approached, a sense of increasing tension occurs. Shifting direct barriers seem to firmly disrupt passively induced shifts, while indirect barriers impose a softer, pillowlike palpatory sensation.

6. Hold against the imposed barriers until release(s) occurs. Usually there are several release sequences, so you must be alert.

7. Remember to assess sequential changes involving both the bony pelvis and ilioinguinal sites.

8. Treatment is complete when positional and tight-loose barrier-related asymmetries are resolved.

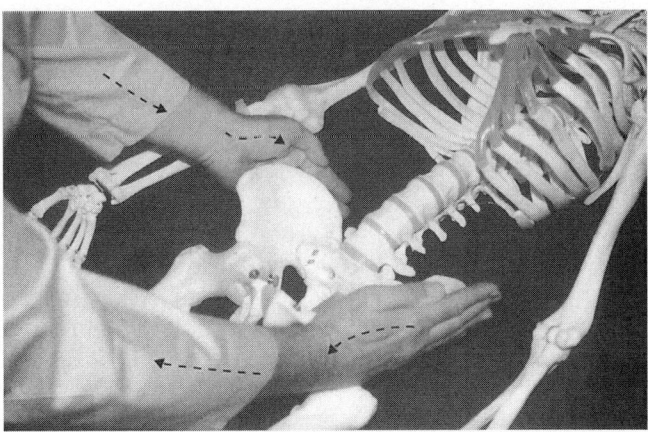

FIGURE 60.37.

Sacroiliac Release: Supine

This process is shown in Figs. 60.39 to 60.46.

Objective

The goal is to create both positional and movement symmetry by creating nutation and counternutation in the sacroiliac system, with particular attention to sacral base asymmetries and associated iliolumbar ligament, L4 and L5 relationships.

Review

Review functional relationships throughout the pelvis, and sacrum, including L4-5 elements and erector spinae influences through the four layers of back muscles. In addition, review posterior sacral relationships in relation to the gluteus maximus system and hip rotators, including distal iliopsoas and piriformis quadratus femoris elements. Be aware of relative sacral positioning between the ilia and in relation to both L5-S1 factors as well as pelvic diaphragm mechanics.

Procedure

Supine

1. The patient lies supine with heels on the table, arms comfortably at the sides. This basically assures that unusual mechanical stresses transmitted through the Achilles tendons and ankles

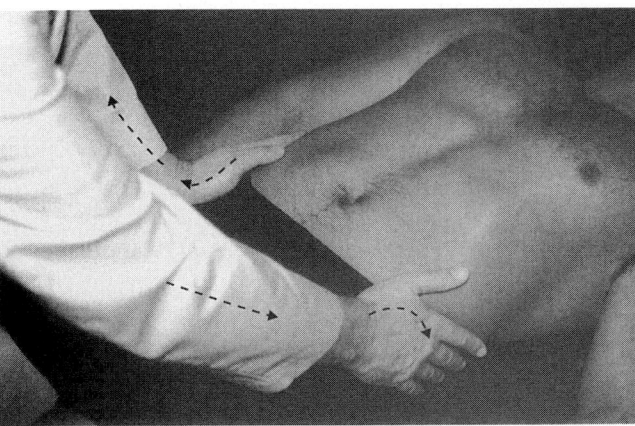

FIGURE 60.36.

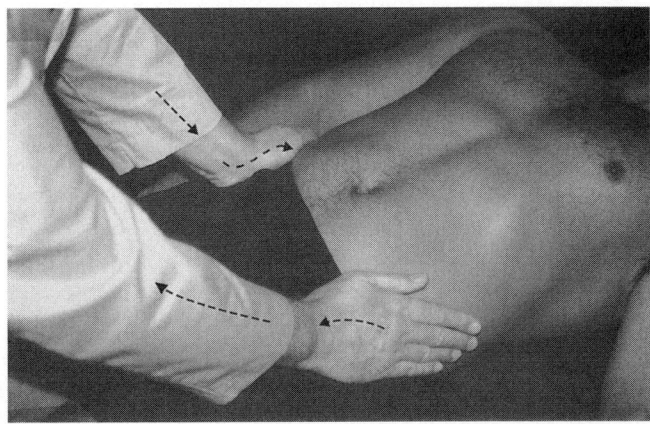

FIGURE 60.38.

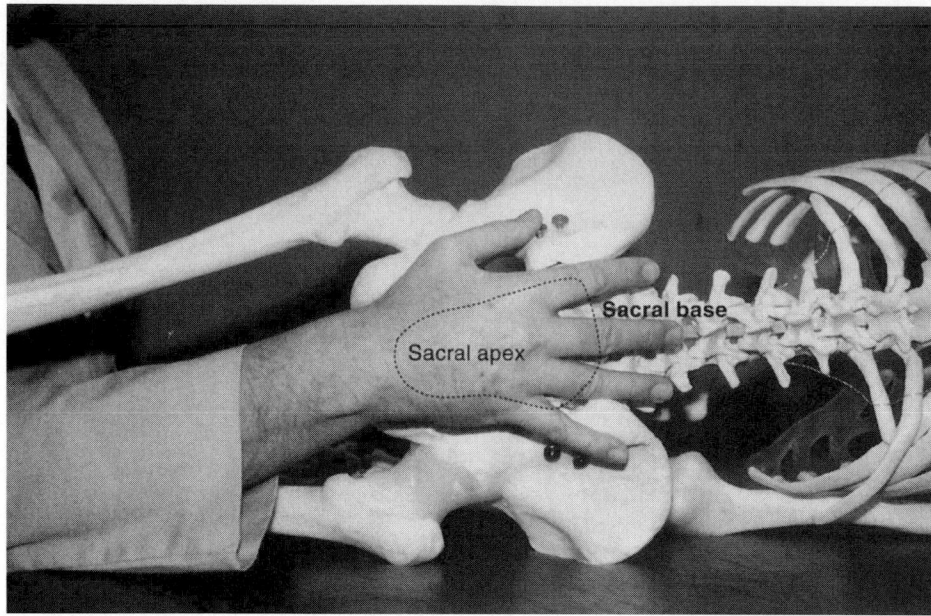

FIGURE 60.39. Hand position for sacroiliac release.

will be neutralized. For those patients with significant kyphosis, it is helpful to use a large pillow to minimize cervical and thoracolumbar problems.

2. Sit beside the patient's right knee.

3. Resting comfortably on the right forearm, place the right hand behind the sacrum so that each sacroiliac joint is covered by an index and ring finger. The apex should easily cover the metatarsophalangeal joints. Notably, some practitioners prefer to place the whole sacrum in the palm. As a practical matter, this positioning is not really necessary because sacral movements are readily palpated with either method (Fig. 60.39).

4. For recording purposes, use muscle energy terminology to identify sacral flexions and torsions. Identify the following:

a. Three-dimensionally related positional and movement asymmetries in relation to the innominates.

b. General tight-loose active and passive movement asymmetries.

c. Sacral nutation and counternutation capabilities as side-bending, and axial twisting movements are induced.

d. Positional and movement asymmetries in relation to the pelvic diaphragm and lower limb.

e. Sacral movements associated craniosacral rhythms.

5. Using distraction, compression, and twisting movements, simultaneously stress direct and indirect barriers (Figs. 60.40 to 60.46). Sustained forces of this type create both mechanical and neurologic releases.

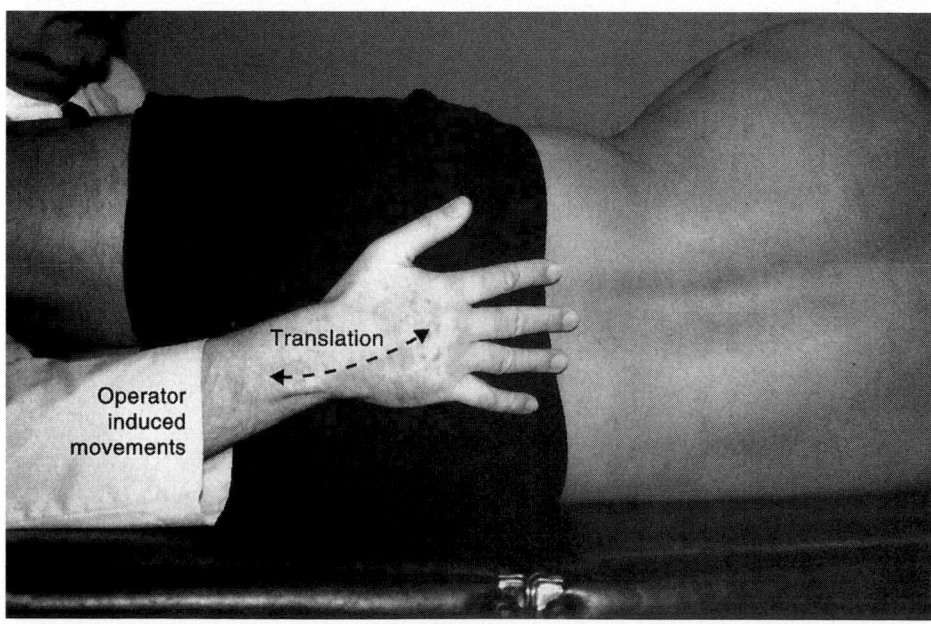

FIGURE 60.40. Hand position for sacroiliac release.

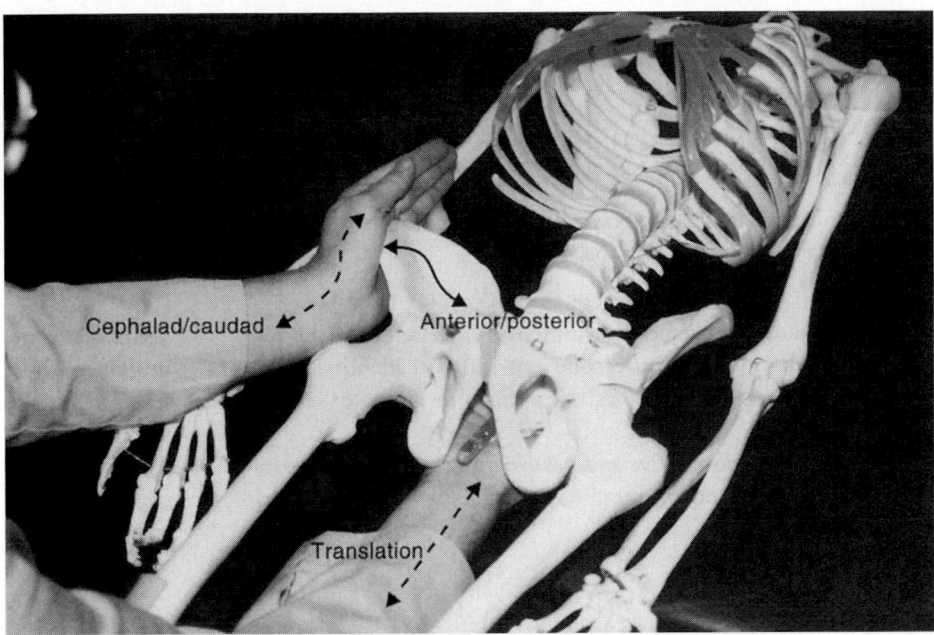

FIGURE 60.41.

6. After general myofascial and sacral balancing have occurred, monitor sacral nutation and counternutation (craniosacral flexion and extension) until the rhythm is smooth and symmetric.

Thoracic Cage and Diaphragm

Objective

The goal is to three-dimensionally balance the thoracic cage and related spinal mechanics in relation to the upper limbs, diaphragm, trunk rotators, and lumbopelvic mechanisms.

Review

Important three dimensionally related functional relationships involve:

1. The shoulder girdle anatomy and innervations
2. Scapulothoracic, omohyoid, costal cage, diaphragm, and trunk rotator interactions
3. Erector spinae elements
4. Cervical-mediated phrenic nerve activities
5. Multiple, autonomically mediated viscerosomatic and somatovisceral reflex factors

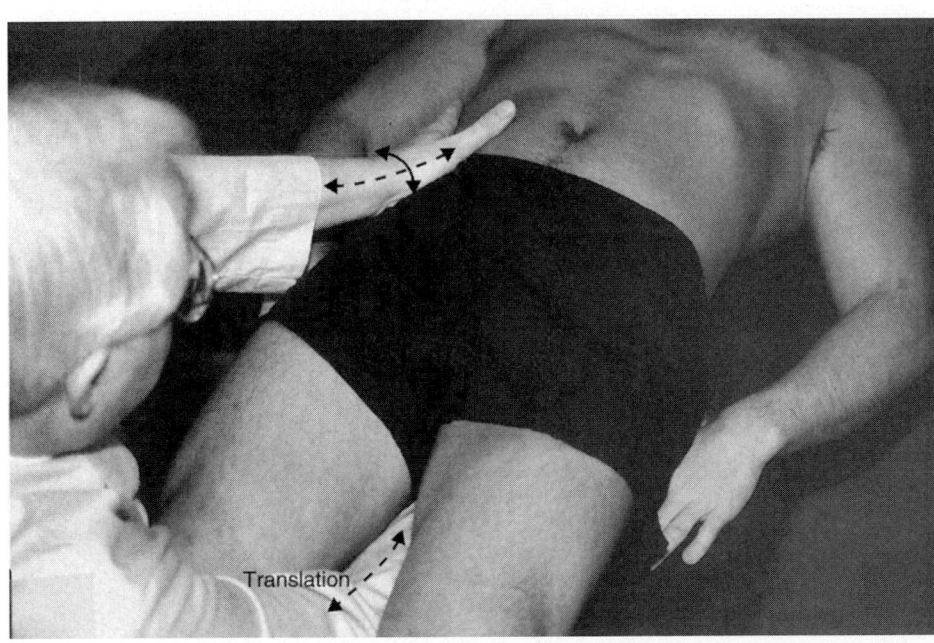

FIGURE 60.42.

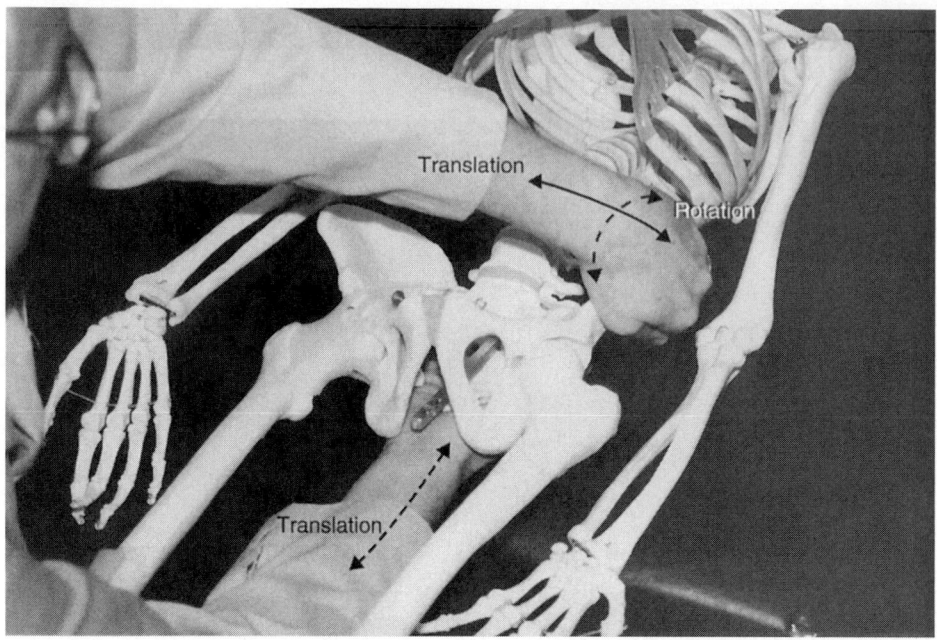

FIGURE 60.43.

6. Cardiopulmonary, upper gastrointestinal, renal, and splenic elements are considered along with lumbopelvic influences, such as proximal iliopsoas, quadratus lumborum, and rectus abdominis organization and function

Procedure
Prone
This technique is virtually identical to the prone, basic, thoracolumbar junction release described previously. The only difference is the movement of the practitioner's hands cephalad between the scapulae. The major differences between the two are tight-loose functional relationships associated with trapezius, rhomboids, subscapularis, iliocostalis, and thoracic attach-

ments of posterior and lateral cervical muscles. It is important to remember that primary cervical mechanisms commonly create significant sites of somatic dysfunction into the middle thoracic spine by way of the splenius cervicis muscles. It is also important to remember that shoulder girdle and costal cage mechanisms are primarily innervated through cervical and brachial plexus mechanisms, as well as local spinal and autonomic components.

Thoracic Cage, Spine, Diaphragm, and Lower Costal Cage: Supine

This process is shown in Figs. 60.47 to 60.53.

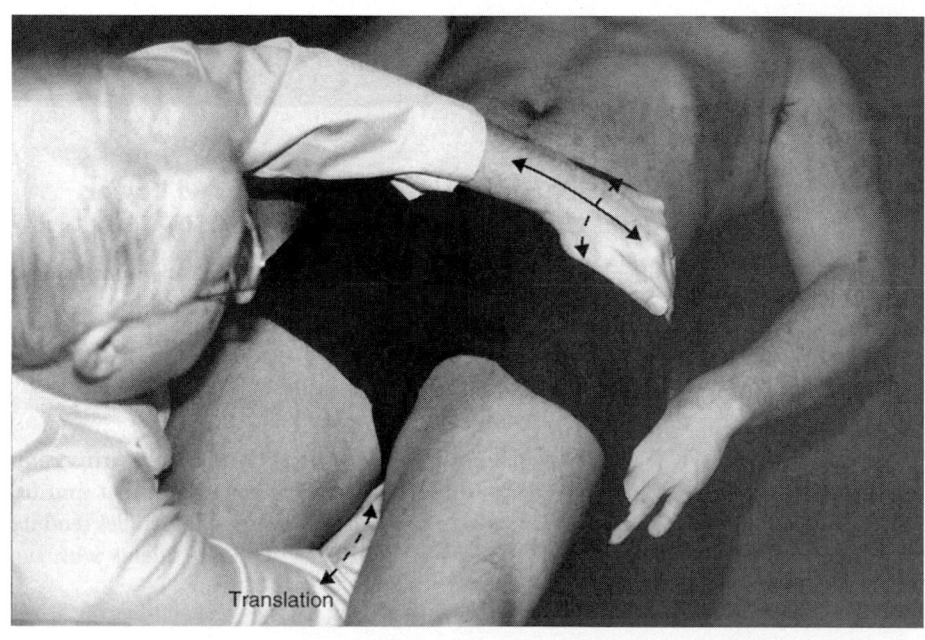

FIGURE 60.44.

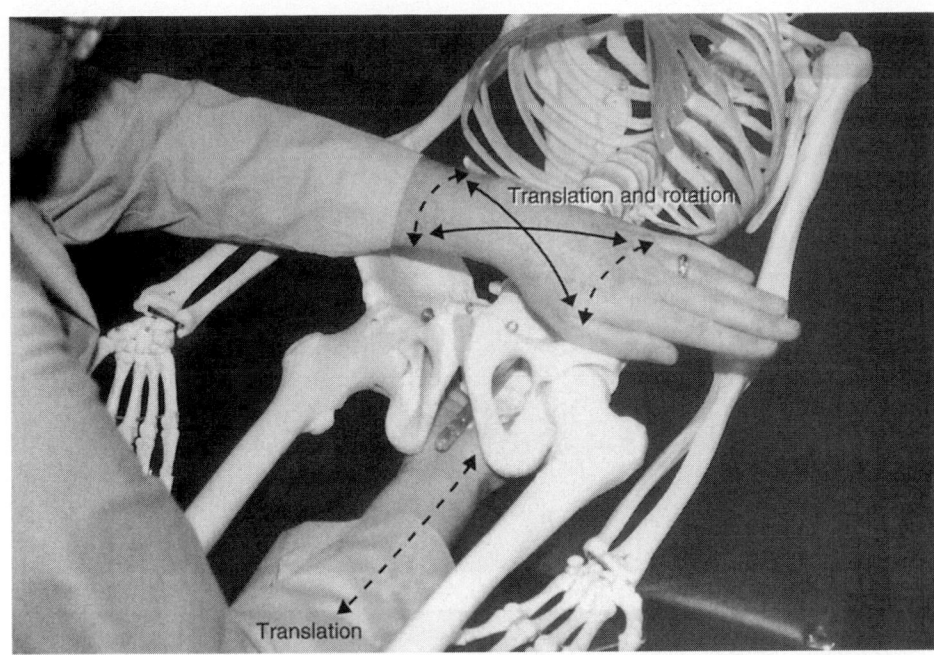

Translation and rotation

Translation

FIGURE 60.45.

Objective

The goal is to three-dimensionally balance scapulothoracic, thoracic spine, and costodiaphragmatic relationships.

Review

See preceding "Prone" procedure.

Procedure

Supine

1. The patient lies supine with heels on the table, arms comfortably at the sides. This basically assures that unusual mechanical stresses transmitted through the Achilles tendons and ankles will be neutralized. For those patients with significant kyphosis, it is helpful to use a large pillow to minimize cervical and thoracolumbar problems.

2. Sit at the head of the table.

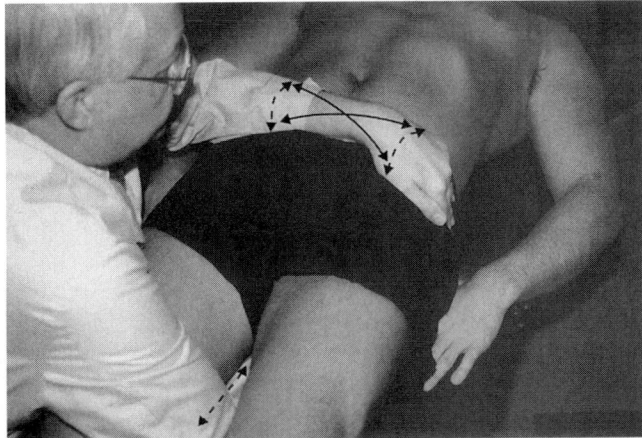

FIGURE 60.46.

3. Resting your elbows on the table, reach under the patient and place the hands firmly against inferior costothoracic attachments on either side of the thoracic spine. Be sure to maintain whole hand contact across and along the erector spinae as well as around the costal cage (Figs. 60.47 and 60.48).

4. Both positional and movement-related tight-loose asymmetries will become apparent.

5. Focus on the following:
   a. Diaphragmatic asymmetries that become apparent as the patient slowly but deeply inhales and exhales (Fig. 60.49)
   b. Upper limb asymmetries which occur as the patient actively moves the upper limbs in a variety of directions (Figs. 60.50 to 60.53)
   c. Repeat the procedure by passively moving each arm and shoulder with one hand remaining behind the patient.
   d. Thoracolumbar junction asymmetries are assessed by having the patient move the lower limbs in a variety of directions; focus on the proximal iliopsoas as well more distal, lumbopelvic relationships as they respond to active patient movements.

6. As inherent tissue movements become apparent, gently, but firmly, lift the thoracolumbar attachments anteriorly and laterally. Shifting sites of tightness and looseness are balanced against each other until inherent movements become quietly symmetric. Sometimes considerable traction and twist are needed to release asymmetrically tight areas.

7. As tightness releases, varieties of release-enhancing activities are helpful. Examples are:
   a. Three-dimensional upper and lower limb movements
   b. Breath holding at neutral, during moderate and deep inhalation, and then during moderate and deep exhalation, that can be combined with three-dimensional upper and lower limb movements.

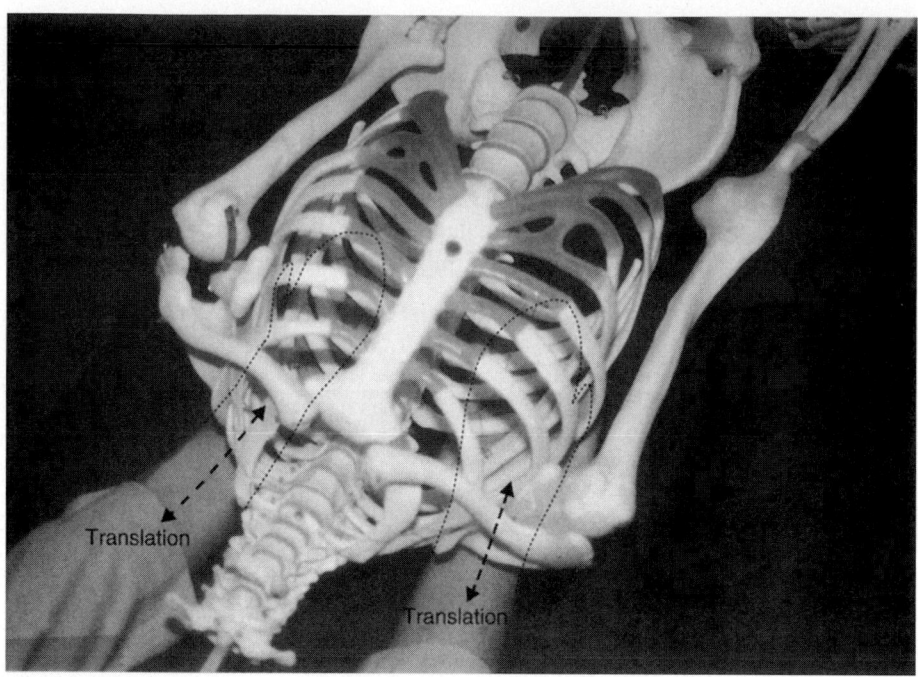

FIGURE 60.47.

8. Treatment is complete when thoracocostal movements are as functionally symmetric as can be expected.

Craniocervical Spine

Seated Position

This procedure is shown in Figs. 60.54 to 60.57.

Goal
The goal is to increase cranial, craniocervical spine, upper ribs, upper thoracic spine, and shoulder girdle ranges of motion.

Review
Review the following:

1. Craniosacral concepts.
2. Craniocervical functional anatomy including scalene, trapezius, anterior and posterior cervical influences.

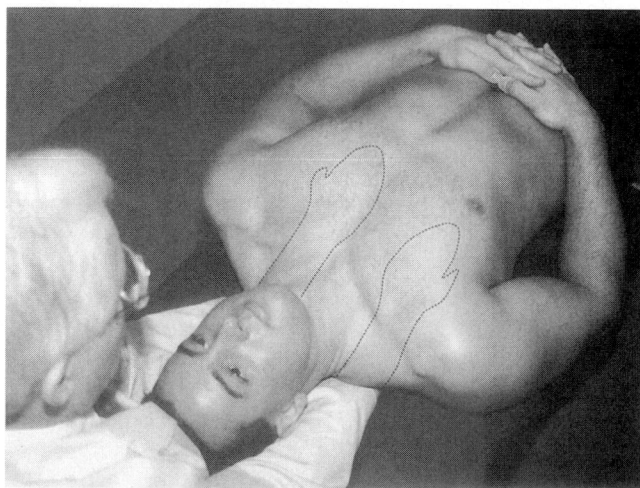

FIGURE 60.48.

3. Three-dimensional costosternal, costovertebral, and cervico-costal relationships including scalene, trapezius, omohyoid, rotator cuff, scapulocostal, and anterior chest wall factors such as pectoralis major and minor influences on cervical mechanics.
4. Functional neurologic relationships, including cranial nerve innervations to the neck and shoulder girdle, as well as autonomic and phrenic nerve/diaphragmatic elements.
5. Remember that intrinsic cardiopulmonary as well as many other medical problems have significant and long-lasting cervical consequences.

Procedure
Note: Palpably apparent tissue and movement-related differences at the same sites during passive and active movements are common with this procedure.

Patient Seated
1. The patient sits with relaxed posture.
2. Stand behind the patient.
3. With each hand, assess lateral, thoracic inlet and posterior cervicothoracic mechanisms for tightness and looseness (Fig. 60.54).
4. Combinations of active and passive operator- and patient-induced neck movements usually improve treatment quality (Figs. 60.55 and 60.56).
5. Commonly tightness occurs in upper and middle thoracic sites where cervical muscles attach to the upper and middle back. For example, trapezius, splenius cervicis, levator scapulae, and semispinalis capitis often exhibit tightness as low as T6-7.
6. Tight-loose asymmetries involving deep cervical rotators and side-benders, as well as sternocleidomastoids and scalenes factors, are common.

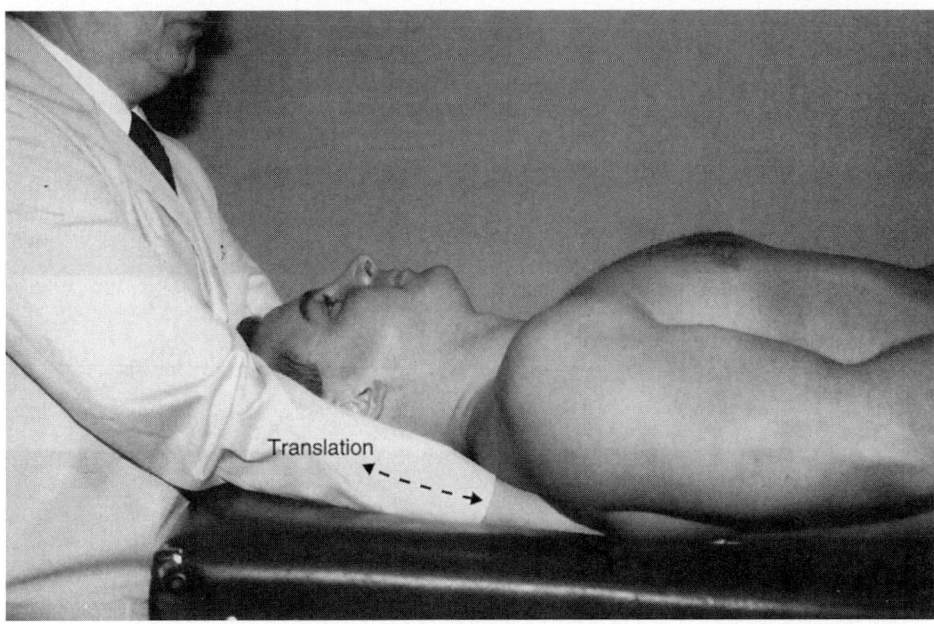

FIGURE 60.49.

7. Place the hands around lateral and posterior cervicothoracic attachments. Be prepared to move anteriorly and laterally as releases get under way. Cranial nerve and upper limb integrated release-enhancing maneuvers are particularly helpful (Fig. 63.57). Mild head nodding and rotations are often powerful release inducers.

8. Simultaneous bilateral, anterior, inferior, and circumferential twist and stress are induced across and around the cervicothoracic junction. Three-dimensionally related direct and indirect barriers quickly appear.

9. Generally, releases begin fairly quickly. Once underway, inherent tissue movements are followed until three-dimensional symmetry occurs.

10. It is particularly important to assess changes that combine varieties of active and passive head, cervical spine, upper limb, and respiratory efforts.

11. Treatment is complete when three-dimensional symmetry has been established in relation to active and passive cervicothoracic, upper limb, respiratory, and costal cage mechanisms.

Patient Supine

This process is shown in Figs. 60.58 to 60.64. The goal is to establish three-dimensional movement symmetry in the cervical spine from basiocciput to upper thoracic influences. Particular

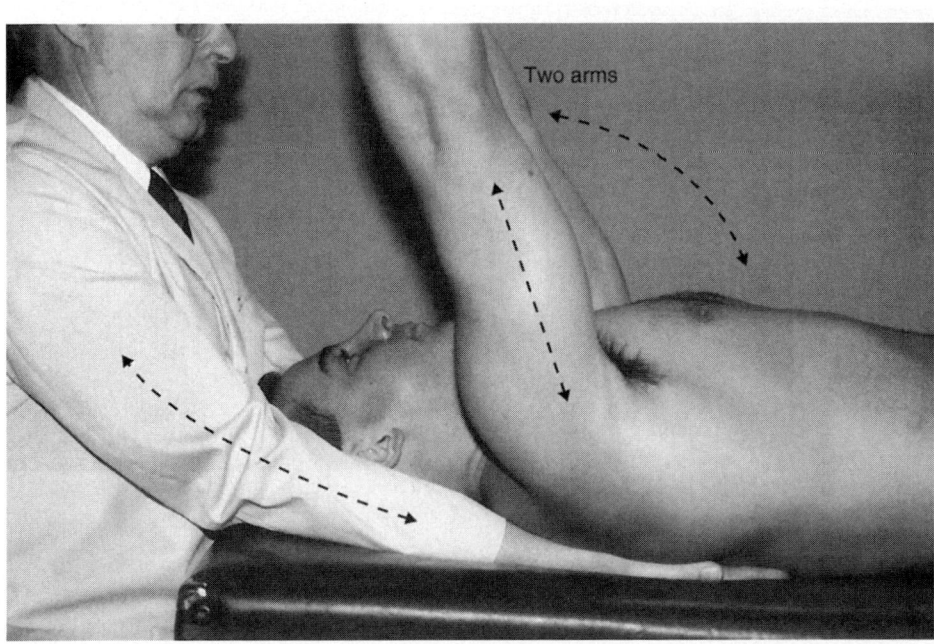

FIGURE 60.50.

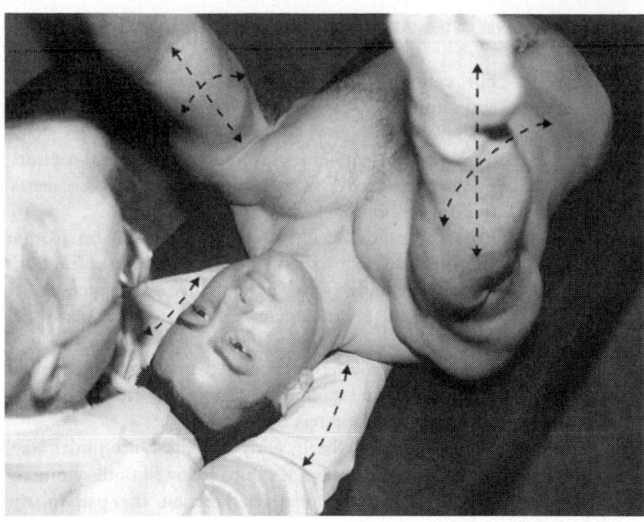

FIGURE 60.51.

emphasis is placed on restoration of adequate side bending and rotation, both generally and in relation to single segment mobility. This technique is usually more effective after lower cervical, cervicothoracic junction, and upper thoracic, upper limb factors have been released beforehand (Figs. 60.58 to 60.60).

Note: To protect the vertebral arteries, take particular caution to avoid simultaneous side-bending and extension maneuvers. *While important for all age groups, most injuries have occurred under age 35.*

Review
See preceding "Seated" description.

Procedure
1. The patient lies supine with heels on the table, arms comfortably at the sides. This basically assures that unusual mechanical

stresses transmitted through the Achilles tendons and ankles will be neutralized. For those patients with significant kyphosis, it is helpful to use a large pillow to minimize cervical and thoracolumbar problems.

2. Sit at the patient's head.
3. Two hand positions, among many possibilities, are particularly useful:
   a. One hand overlapping the other—this permits carefully controlled and focused, twist, traction, and side-bending maneuvers. The maneuvers are used both separately and with patient cooperation (Figs. 60.61 and 60.62).
   b. By grasping the basiocciput with the palms of each hand, the fingers are left free to sort out both superficial and deep mechanisms (Figs. 60.63 and 60.64).
4. From either hand position, traction, turning, and side-bending maneuvers assess myofascial and joint-related tightness and looseness.
   a. Pay particular attention to tightness, remembering that loose joints with surrounding inhibited muscle groups are common sources of pain and disability. In more acute situations, on the other hand, loose joints are usually associated with tight muscles as they work to protect and stabilize the system. The opposite findings are also common, such as tight joints with accompanying inhibition of overlying muscles.
   b. Facet joints are often tight on one side, loose on the other. Side-to-side motion testing with only a little rotation will determine which facets are failing to effectively open or close (see Chapter 59)
   c. The procedure's focus is to carefully, but persistently, apply well-focused stress against tight sites with and without patient assistance.
   d. INR cranial nerve and upper limb activities such as finger tapping and hand rolling are commonly helpful. They also save the practitioner time.

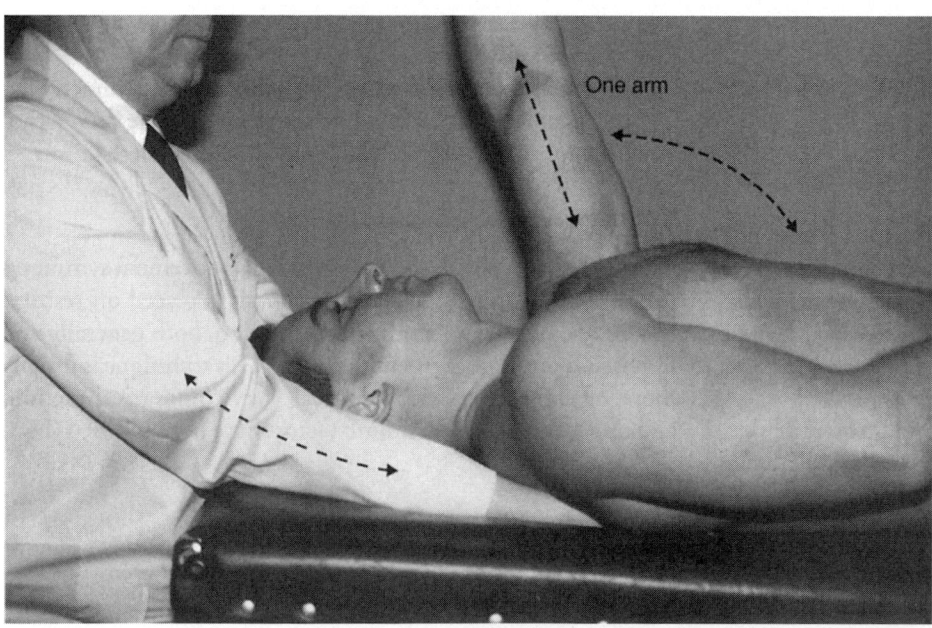

One arm

FIGURE 60.52.

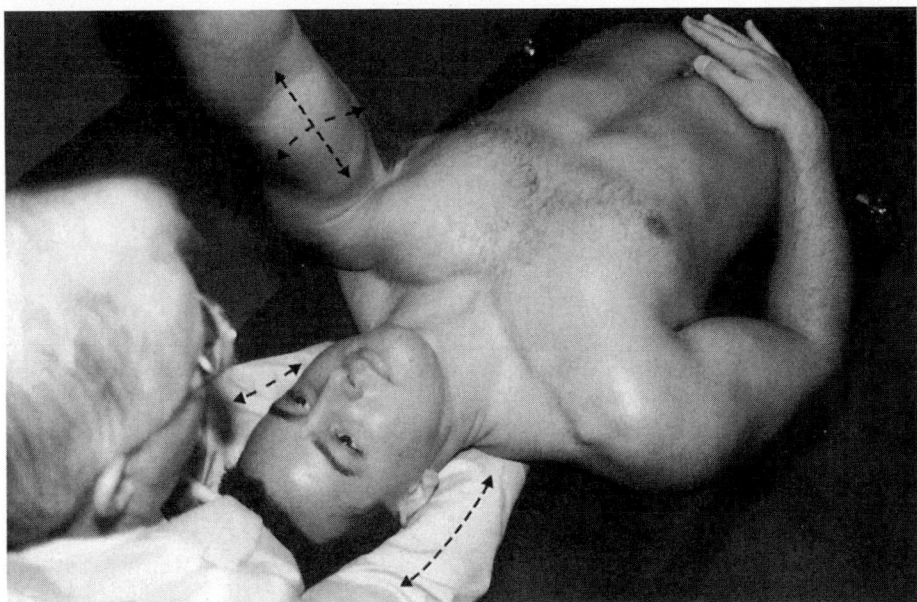

FIGURE 60.53.

5. Linking subtle translatory maneuvers (e.g., combinations of distraction and extension with flexion, extension, side-bending, and rotation) is usually helpful. In particular:

a. Release deep upper cervical muscles by combining cranial nerve (CN) activities with occipitoatlantal nutation and counternutation. Remember that sternocleidomastoid (SCM), trapezius (CN XI), and scalene mechanics are easily accessible primary neck stabilizers that are often asymmetric in relation to each other. For example, the left SCM mechanism is typically tighter than the right from origin to insertion. Commonly, the underlying scalene system is looser (i.e., tightness and looseness occur among ipsilat-

eral layers as well as from side-to-side, front-to-back, and circumferentially).

In the process:

6. Atlantoaxial joints and surrounding attachments are carefully rotated against tightness.

7. Middle and lower cervical attachments and coupled joint movements are stressed using translatory movements with combinations of side bending, flexion, and extension that avoids a lot of rotation. (Remember the vertebral arteries!)

8. Treatment is complete when symmetric movements are restored to facet joints and surrounding soft tissues within the ability of the patient to adapt.

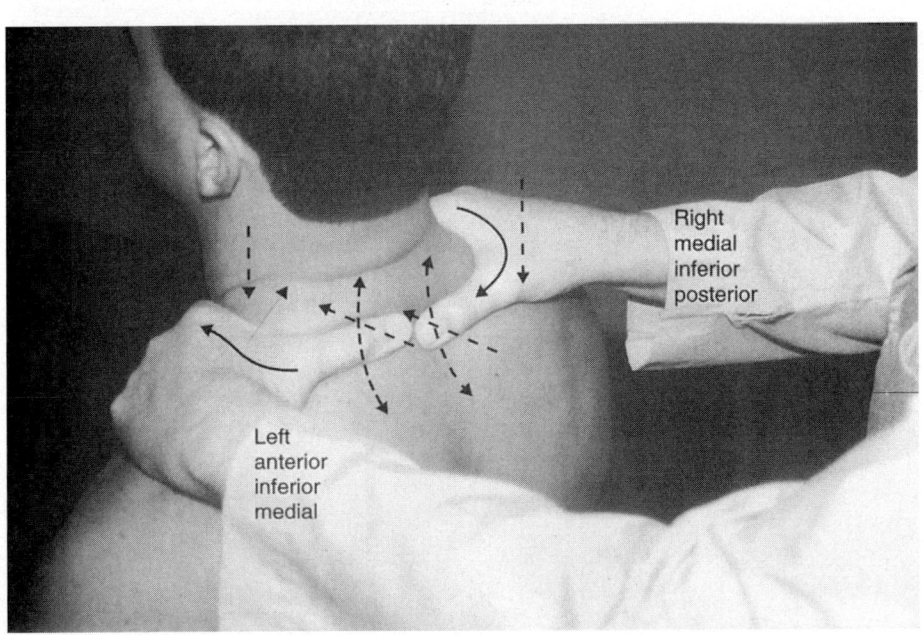

Right medial inferior posterior

Left anterior inferior medial

FIGURE 60.54.

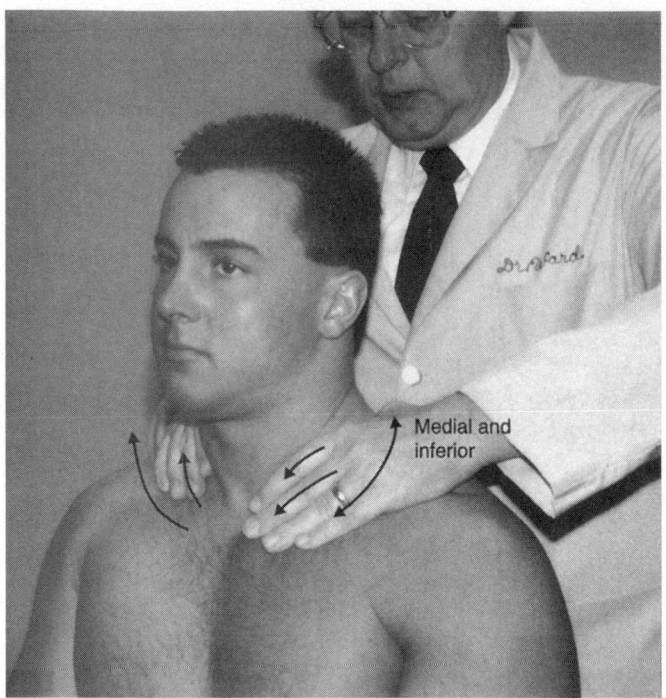

FIGURE 60.55.

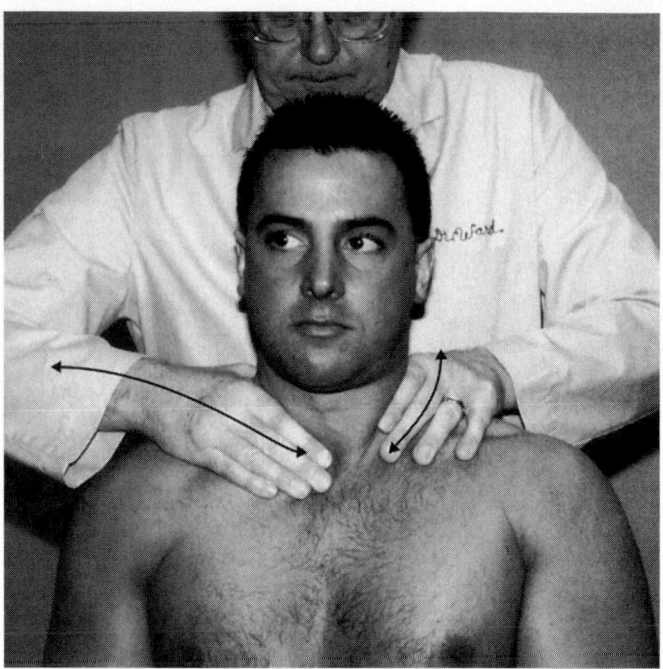

FIGURE 60.57.

Lower Limb

Treatment procedures for the lower limb are shown in Figs. 60.65 to 60.68.

Goal
The goal is to release each lower limb from lumbopelvic and hip rotator attachments to the foot and ankle.

Review
Review the following:

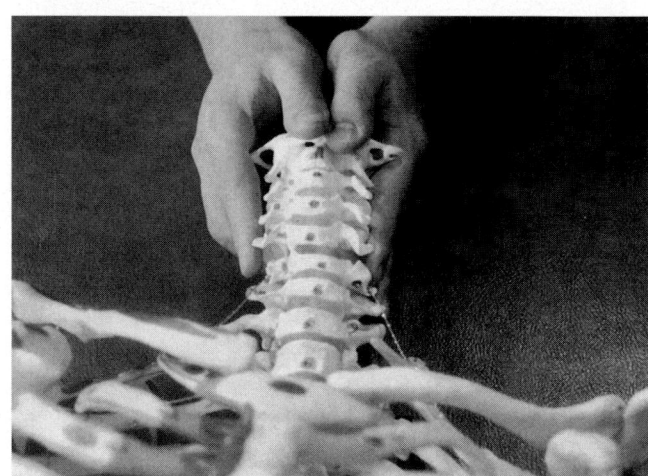

FIGURE 60.58.

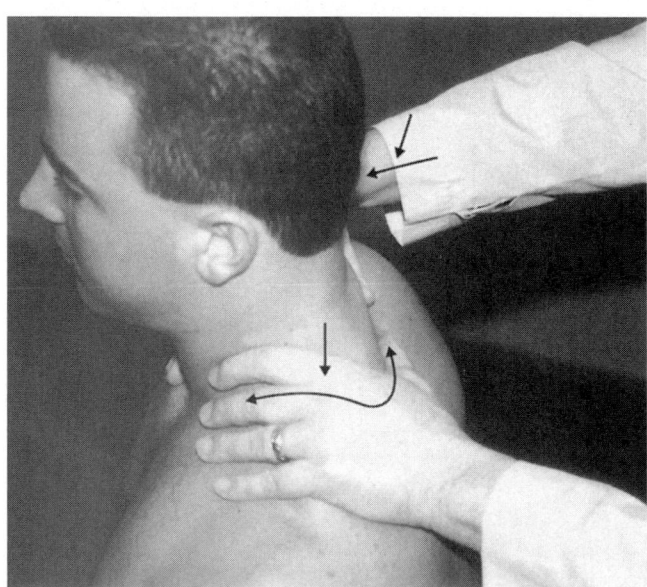

FIGURE 60.56.

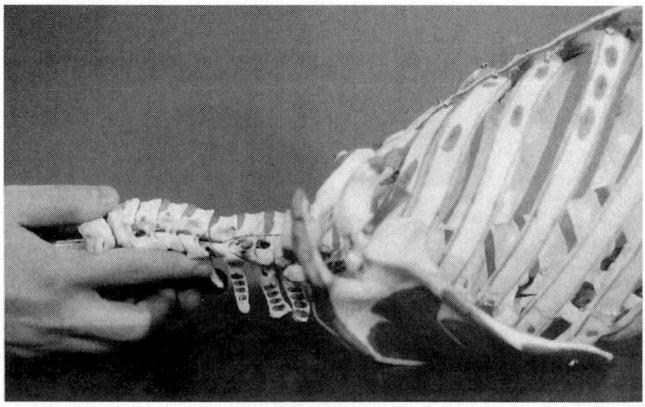

FIGURE 60.59.

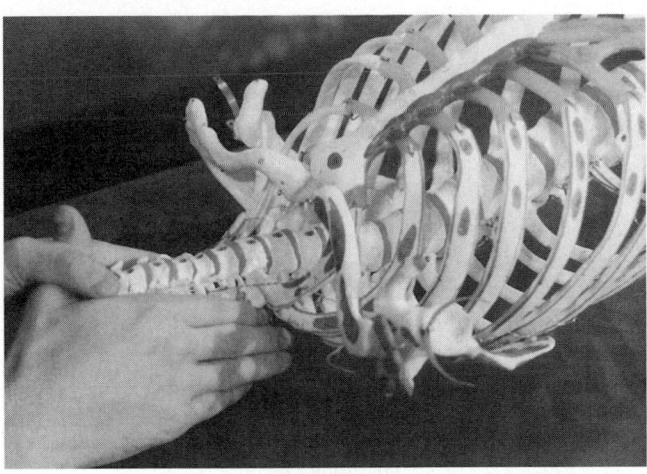

FIGURE 60.60.

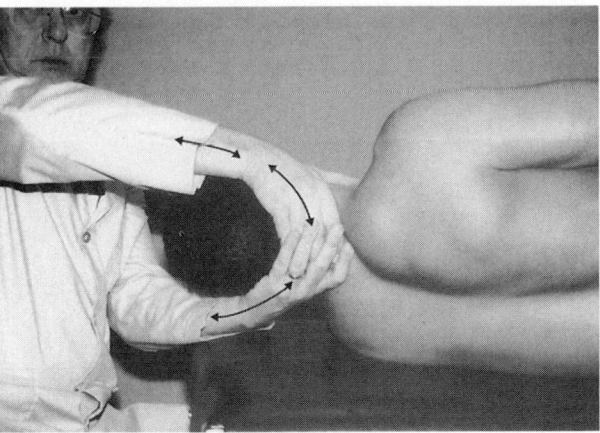

FIGURE 60.62.

1. Functional neurology of the lower limb, including pelvic girdle, low back, trunk rotators, and lumbodorsal fascia, latissimus dorsi, scapulocostal stabilizers in relation to the low back, brachial plexus influences through shoulder girdle structures, as well as diaphragmatic-phrenic influence. Remember that the limbs are precisely represented in cerebellopontine functions as well as in multiple areas of the homunculus and precentral gyrus, among many.

2. Functional neuromuscular anatomy of the foot, ankle, knee, and their myofascial elements.

3. Functional neuromuscular anatomy of the hips and upper leg.

4. Circulatory anatomy of both the lumbopelvic system and lower limbs.

5. The effects of common medical problems, such as arthritis, diabetes, and effects of trauma and surgery.

Note 1: Smoking-related circulatory problems, arthritis, and diabetes are among the most common sources of lower limb dysfunctions.

Note 2: Proprioceptive instability on one leg is a common signal of unilateral muscle weakness and neural inhibition anywhere

from the low back to the plantar surface of the ipsilateral foot. Pain is a common presenting complaint.

Procedure

Supine

1. To begin, the heels should be on the table with knees extended to minimize lower limb stresses. The head and neck should be comfortable with minimal stress on the spine and pelvis.
   Note: Remember to check for leg length inequalities and altered hip mechanics both prone and supine. It is common to find differences supine, prone, and seated. Pelvic obliquities are common when these inconsistencies occur.

2. The hands and arms are comfortably placed either on the abdomen or at the sides.

3. Sit or stand beside the patient.

4. Grasp distal femur and distal patellar/proximal tibial attachments (Fig. 60.65).

5. Using firm, passive, circumferential movements, assess each fully extended knee for three-dimensional tightness and looseness (Figs. 60.65 to 60.68). Particular care is taken in assessing

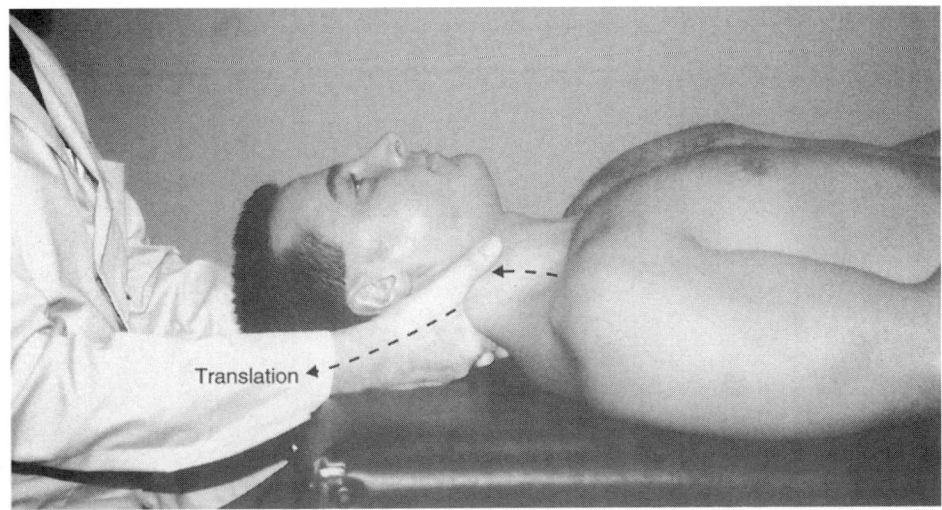

Translation

FIGURE 60.61.

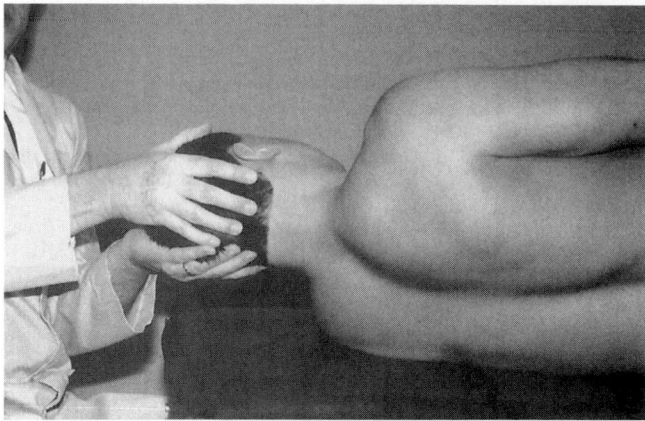

FIGURE 60.63.

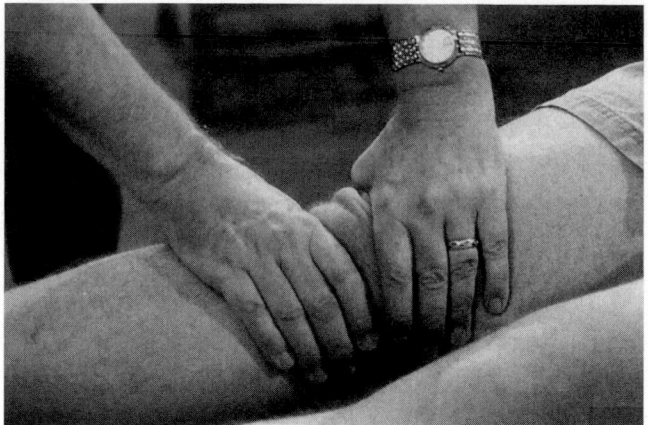

FIGURE 60.65.

medial hamstring as well as lateral hamstring/iliotibial band/proximal fibular head tight-loose relationships.

Note: Myofascially, this is a fairly ambiguous area to assess and treat, so one must subjectively rely on tight-loose end-feels. Remember that both lumbopelvic and foot-ankle mechanics significantly influence the system.

6. Assess hip function in the same way, with the leg in full extension and then with varieties of flexion, internal and external rotation, abduction, and adduction.

7. Passively twist the knee in opposite directions (axial twist), being sure that the hand and fingers are firmly in contact with areas of maximum tightness. Usually maximum tightness is in two places:
   a. Laterally around distal iliotibial band attachments and proximal fibular head
   b. Medially and posteriorly near and around distal hamstring attachments.

8. Asymptomatic lateral knee/fibular head problems (tightness) in response to medial complaints where the knee is generally

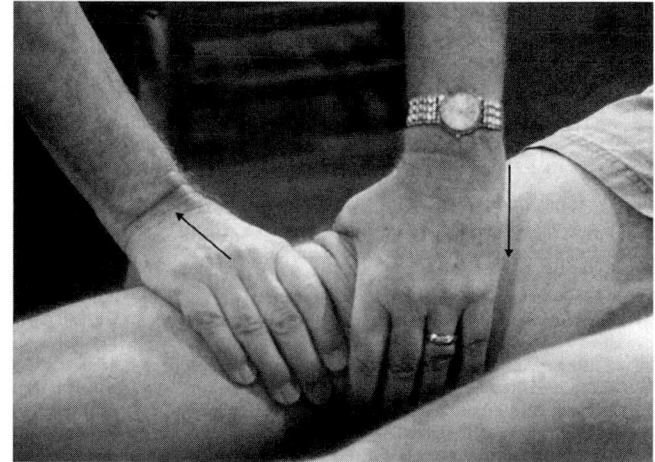

FIGURE 60.66.

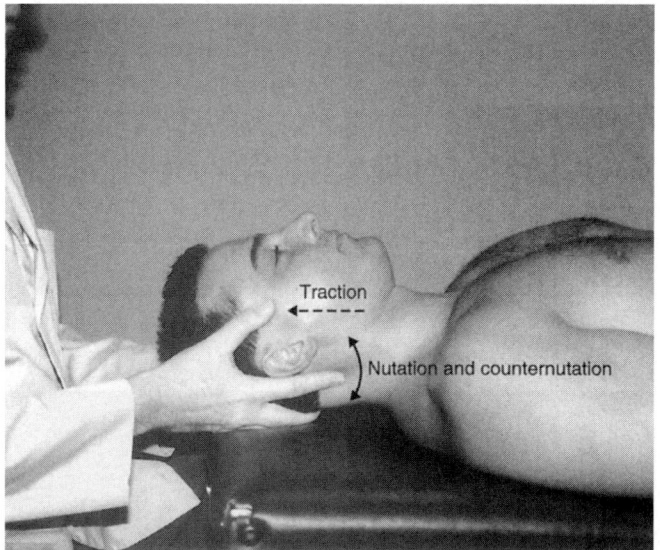

FIGURE 60.64.

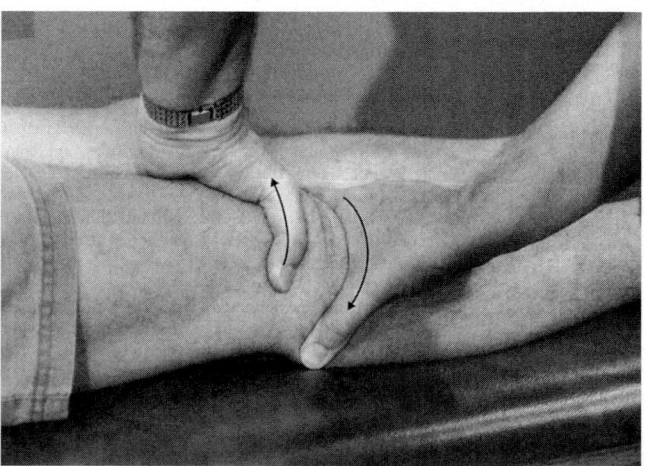

FIGURE 60.67.

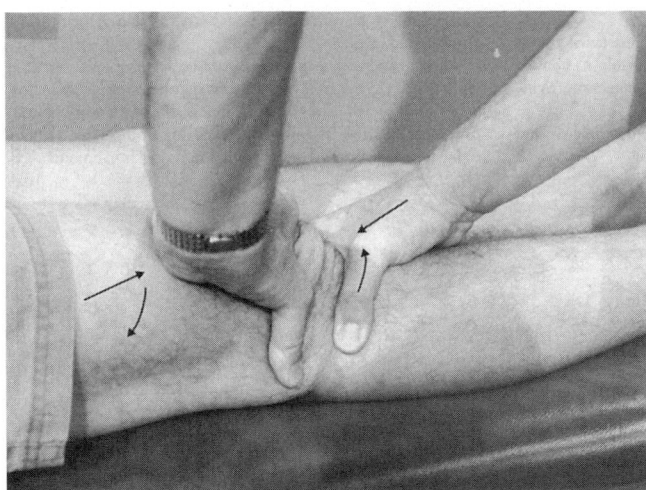

FIGURE 60.68.

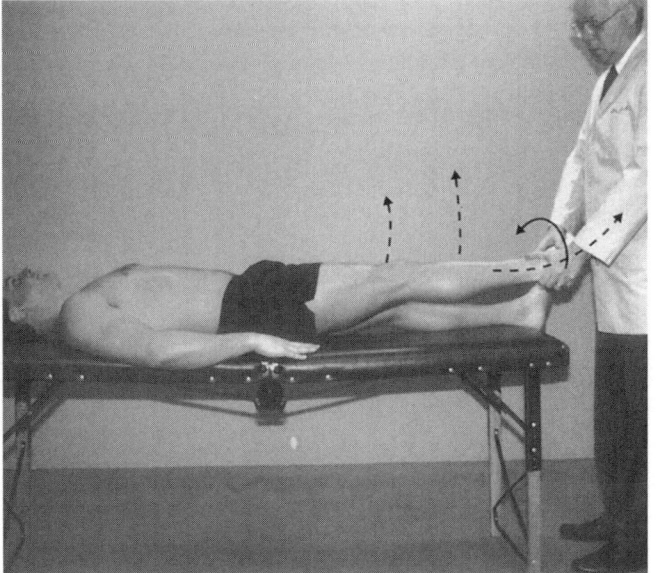

FIGURE 60.70.

more mobile are common. Distal tensor fasciae latae problems are also common in this group in conjunction with ipsilateral gluteus medius weakness. A positive standing Trendelenburg test is the most common signal of gluteus medius weakening.

a. Remember that proximal sacroiliac joint and sacrotuberous-sacrospinous ligamentous factors are also common sources of distal difficulties, and vice versa.

Alternative Treatment

The process for alternative treatment is shown in Figs. 60.69 to 60.76. After assessing and releasing compromised knee mechanics, one commonly encounters proximal hip rotator, abductor, and adductor problems.

1. With knee fully extended, lift each leg off the table, creating slight hip flexion.
   a. Simultaneously focus on both single and bilateral tight-loose hip rotator-lumbopelvic factors. Search out tight-

loose elements by carrying the extended limb into varieties of rotation, abduction, and adduction. This can also be done with both limbs simultaneously.

b. Hold against either the direct or indirect barrier, while focusing attention on associated tight-loose relationships.
   Note: It helps to remember that sites of looseness commonly signal neural inhibition, along with the possibility of absolute or relative hypermobility. Also, they often correlate with pain reports.

c. Releases occur as twist, traction, compression, and shear

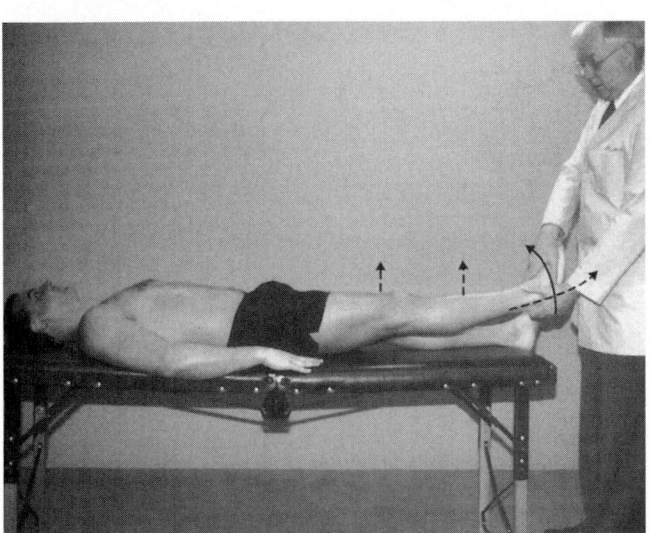

FIGURE 60.69.

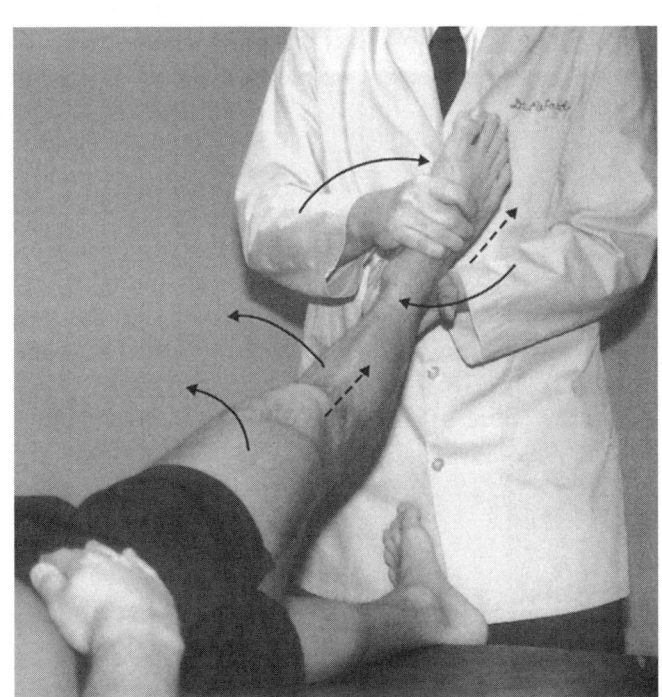

FIGURE 60.71.

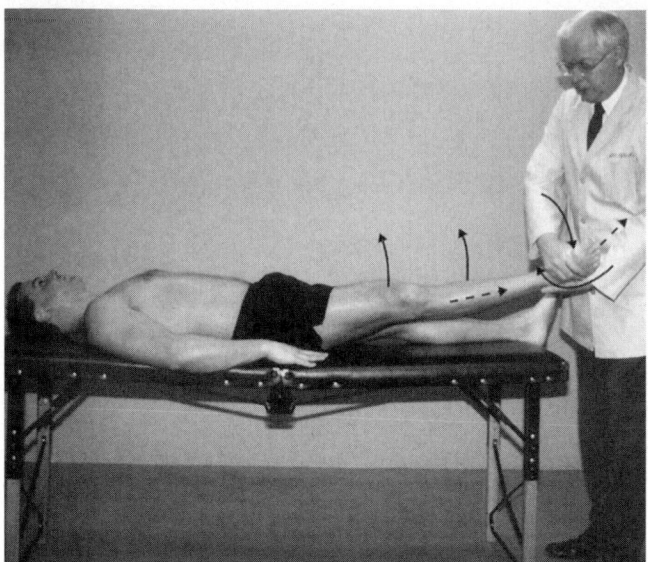

FIGURE 60.72.

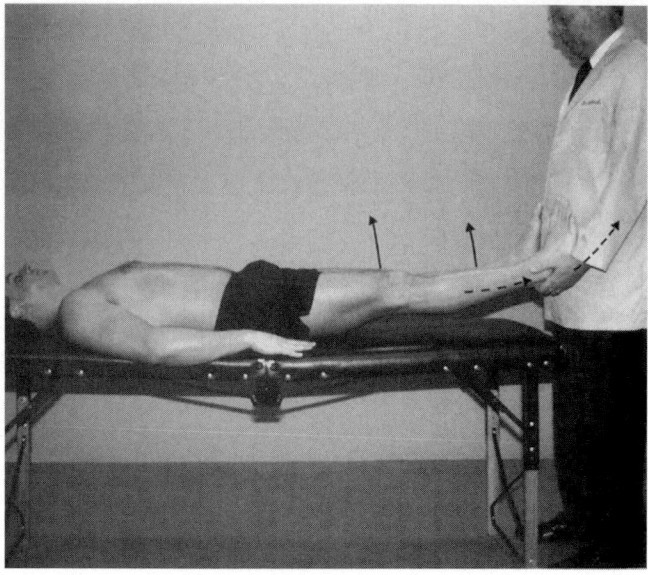

FIGURE 60.74.

against direct and indirect barriers and are used interactively. Compression is often surprisingly useful.

Unwinding Maneuvers

The process for unwinding maneuvers is shown in Figs. 60.69 to 60.76.

Background

Unwinding methods refer to operator-induced spontaneous bending and twisting maneuvers affecting both upper and lower limbs. Their osteopathic origins are unclear. These procedures have been described for decades by many osteopathic practitioners. At times, the patient's whole body takes part. Single and multiple operators sometimes participate together.

Goal

From the foot of the table, long lever unwinding maneuvers release the whole lower limb, including the foot and ankle, in relation to the lumbar spine and pelvis. With practice, one can learn to work through the whole body from the foot of the table. Both rapid and slow-moving releases become apparent as operator skill improves.

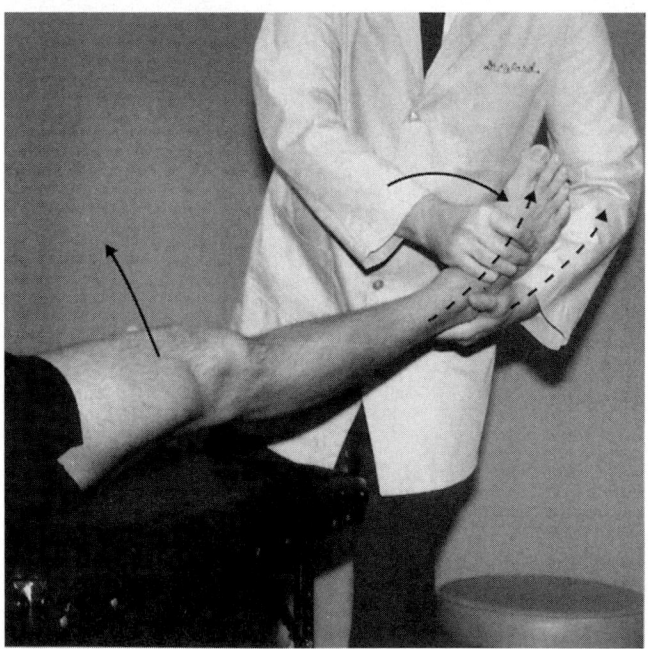

FIGURE 60.73.

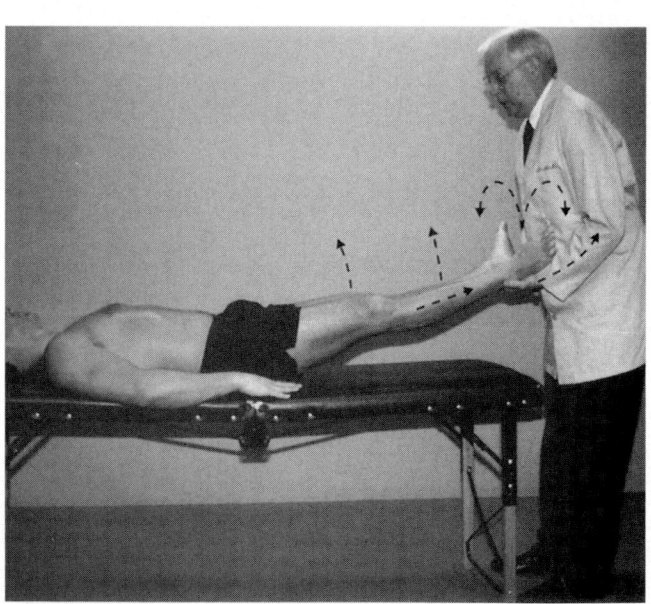

FIGURE 60.75.

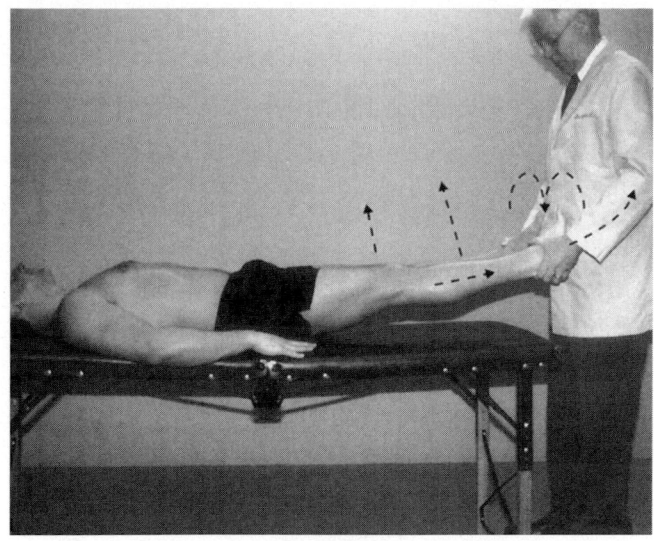

FIGURE 60.76.

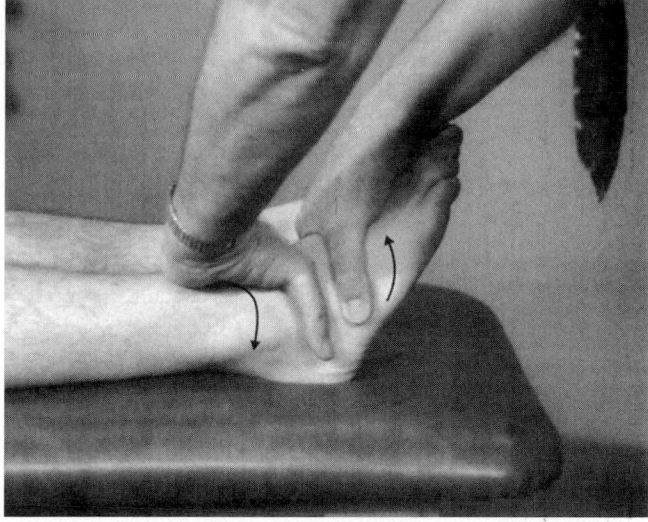

FIGURE 60.78.

Procedure

Combinations of traction, compression, twisting, and bending are used to sequentially follow shifting release activities. Sometimes the limb(s) move rapidly, sometimes slowly. As treatment progresses, seemingly chaotic random movements are apt to occur. Then, suddenly, they stop temporarily as a "still point" occurs, similar to entering the eye of a hurricane. The process then starts again. Presumably, these seemingly random movements reflect a variety of interacting electromechanical events affecting central, peripheral, autonomic, and even psychologic functions. Amid much speculation, satisfactory scientific descriptions for the events are lacking.

Foot and Ankle

Treatment of the foot and ankle (Figs. 60.77 to 60.80) is virtually identical to knee approaches. For example, lateral ankle looseness is commonly associated with medial foot tightness involving the

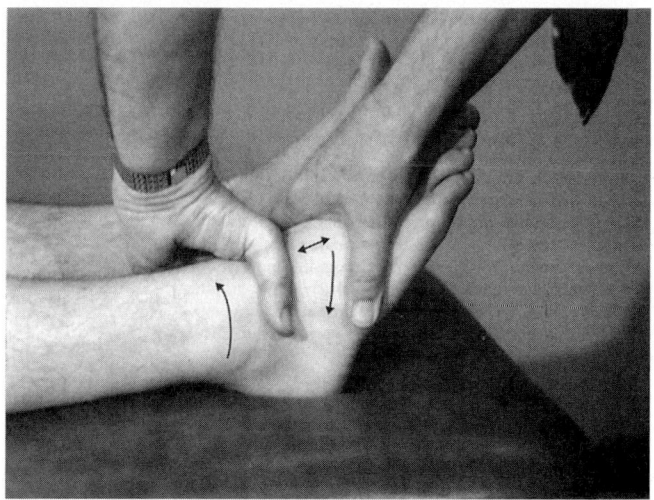

FIGURE 60.79.

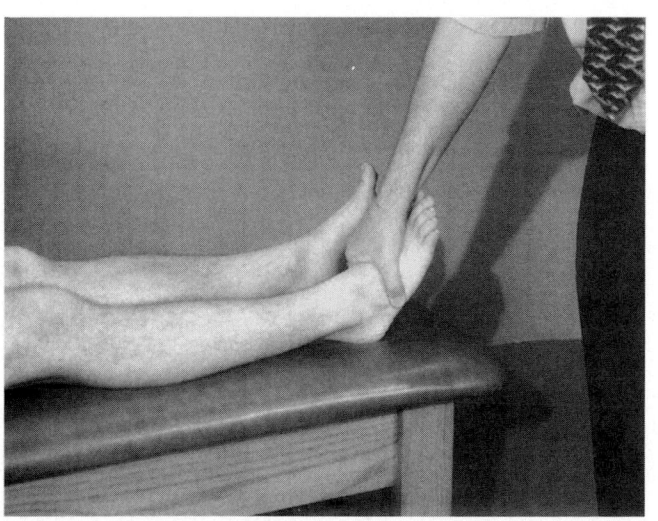

FIGURE 60.77.

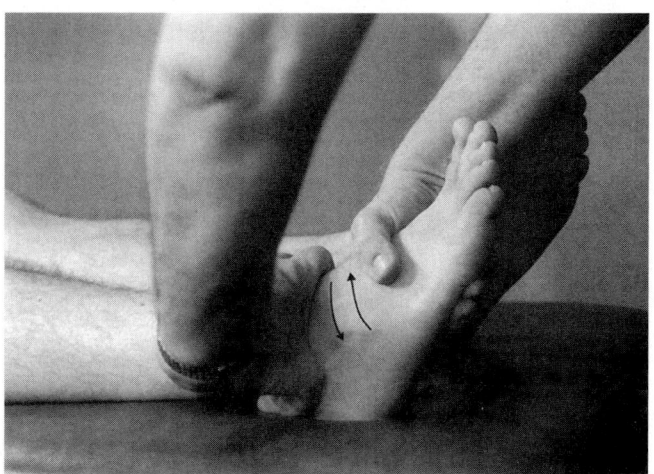

FIGURE 60.80.

deltoid ligament. *Whether release of the tightness is helpful is a matter of clinical judgment, because plantar surface, heel, and tarsal-metatarsal factors play such important roles.*

Upper Limb and Shoulder

Rotator Cuff and Partially Frozen Shoulder Dysfunctions

Goal

The goal of this treatment is to three-dimensionally balance cervical, shoulder, scapulocostal, anterior chest wall, rotator cuff-glenohumeral, upper arm, elbow, wrist, and hand influences.

Review

Review the following:

1. Functional neurology of the neck in relation to the upper limb, including brachial plexus and cervical autonomic elements, as well as cranial nerve sensory and motor functions.
2. Rotator cuff, glenohumeral, elbow, wrist influences.
3. Craniocervical spine relationships with particular reference to large and small muscle influences from basiocciput to upper thoracic and related scapulothoracic, scapulocostal influences.

Procedure

The procedure is carried out with the patient prone, with their arm and shoulder off table (Figs. 60.81 to 60.85). Most of the time this position is used to deal directly with compromised shoulder and scapulocostal mechanics (see also "Spencer Techniques," Chapter 55). Direct myofascial stressing occurs across and around the rotator cuff, acromioclavicular joint, distal glenohumeral attachments, and inferior subscapularis, latissimus dorsi, infraspinatus, teres major and minor attachments.

1. The patient's feet should be off the end of the table to minimize lower limb stresses in relation to the pelvis and lower limb.
2. The patient's head should be turned to the most comfortable side. Note the effect of head turning on tightness and looseness across the shoulder in question. Proximal and superior

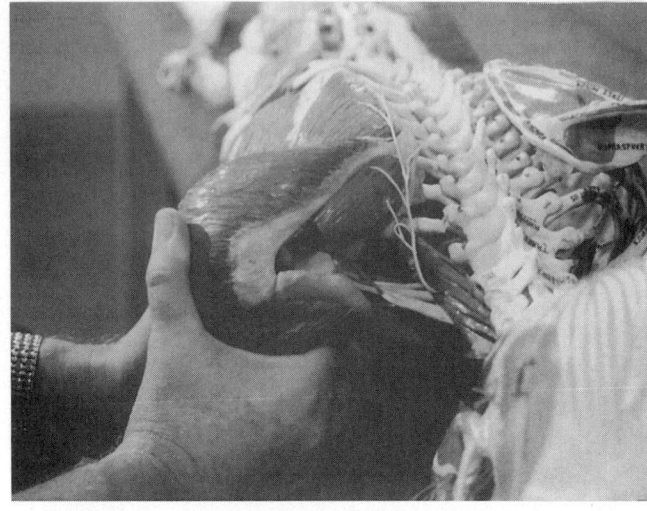

FIGURE 60.82.

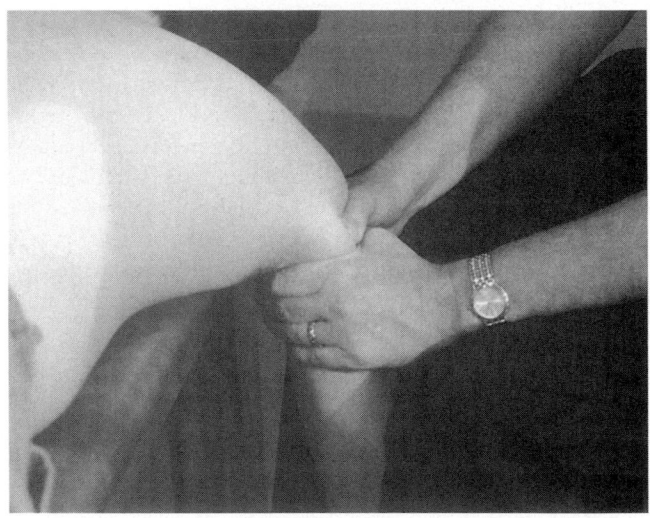

FIGURE 60.83.

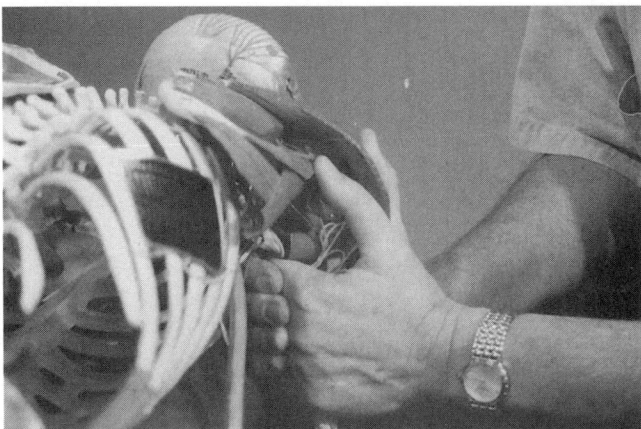

FIGURE 60.81.

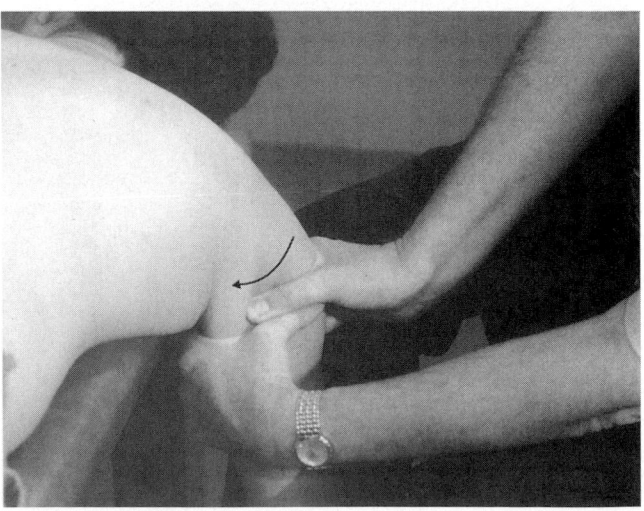

FIGURE 60.84.

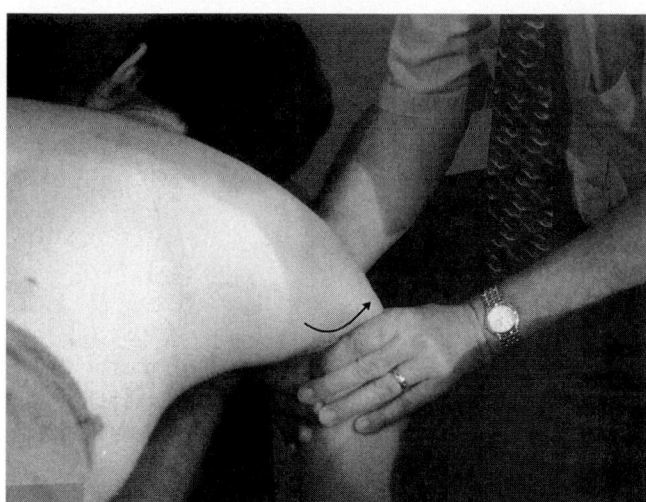

FIGURE 60.85.

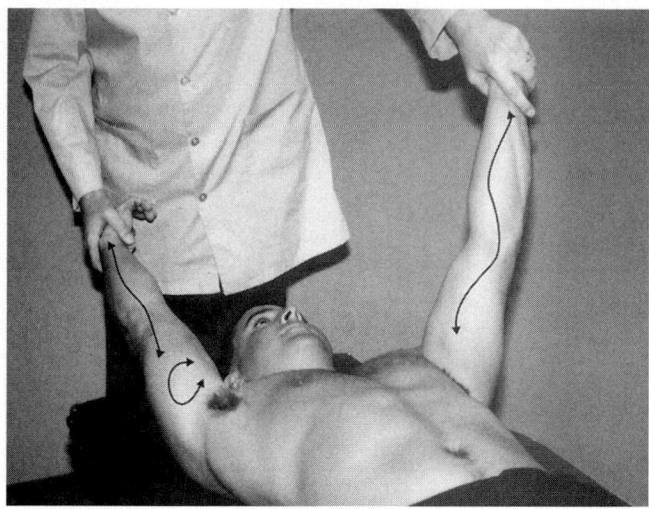

FIGURE 60.86.

cervical attachments are often compromised and need to be released along with the shoulder.

Note: Keeping the head in the midline readily neutralizes craniocervical asymmetries, but also reduces the chance that significant tight-loose asymmetries will be missed.

3. The patient's hands and arms are comfortably placed either over the sides of the table or on the table beside the hips and thighs. If the hands are over the sides of the table, be sure to note any asymmetric scapulocostal effects (see "Note" above).

4. The operator sits on a rolling stool that allows movement in response to shifting sites of tightness and looseness.

5. Holding the affected arm between the knees allows the operator use of the rolling stool to guide movements as specific stressing against tight barriers occurs.

6. Initially, place both hands firmly around the glenohumeral attachments immediately lateral to the acromioclavicular joint. The fingers of one hand firmly contact pectoralis major attachments anteriorly, while the other hand contacts teres/infraspinatus attachments posteriorly (Figs. 60.81 to 60.83).

7. Assess tightness and looseness by three-dimensionally stressing the system using distraction, compression, twist, and shear (Figs. 60.84 and 60.85).

8. Direct and firm stressing against tightness gets the process under way. For example, approximately 5 to 15 pounds of load are common before initial releases begin.

9. Pay particular attention to posterior and inferior glenohumeral restrictions close to the scapula.

10. Long-term problems usually require firmly held movements that assertively stretch the area without interfering with neurocirculatory functions.

11. A well-organized home exercise and/or physical therapy program is usually needed to maintain improvement.

12. Side-lying techniques using a similar approach are also helpful.

Supine

This process is shown in Figs. 60.86 and 60.87.

Goal

The goal is to generally mobilize the shoulder and its relationships with the cervical spine and thorax.

Review

Same as prone.

1. This positioning is less helpful for frozen shoulder situations than prone or side-lying.

2. This position is usually more helpful for lower craniocervical-upper thoracic components affected by the shoulder problem. Mobilizing C6-8 costovertebral mechanics as well as first, second, and third rib mechanics are particular keys to success.

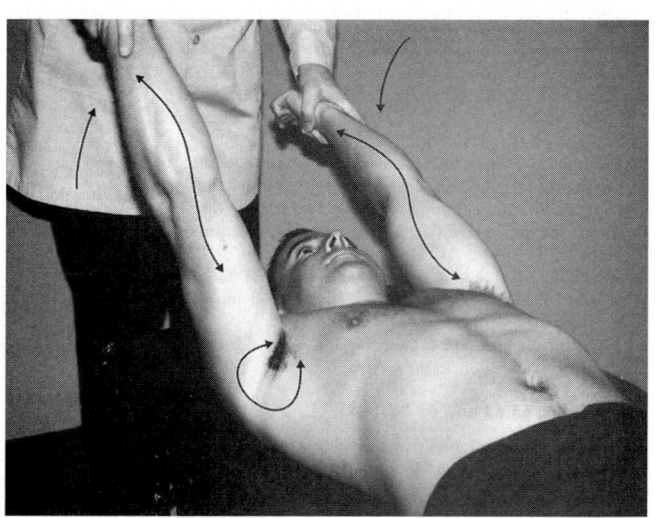

FIGURE 60.87.

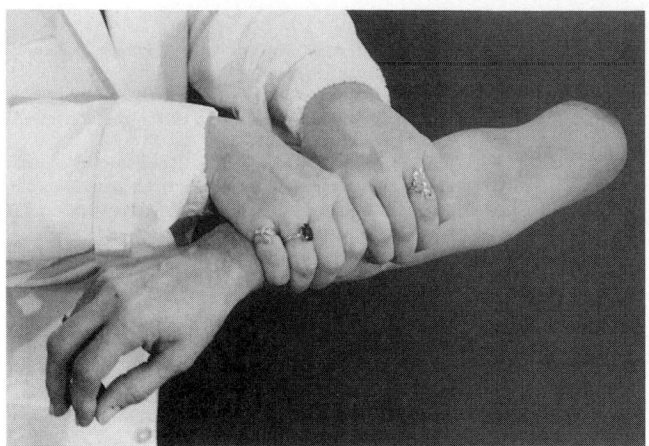

FIGURE 60.88.

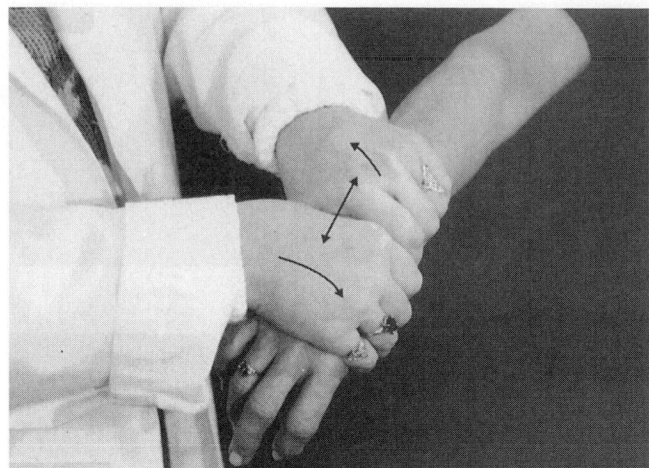

FIGURE 60.89. Forearm-elbow-wrist release, direct technique, transverse approach.

Procedure

1. The patient is supine with heels on the table, arms comfortably at the sides. This basically assures that unusual mechanical stresses transmitted through the Achilles tendons and ankles will be neutralized. For those patients with significant kyphosis, it is helpful to use a large pillow to minimize cervical and thoracolumbar problems.

2. Stand at either the side or head of the table. Choice of position is dictated by scapulocostal-glenohumeral ranges of motion, as well as influential tight-loose factors.

   Note: In addition to primary joint involvement, compromised glenohumeral functions commonly involve pectoralis major mechanics near attachments at the intertubercular groove of the humerus. They also commonly affect posterolateral teres and infraspinatus elements.

3. Grasp the patient's wrists.

4. Progressively apply distraction, compression, and twist to assess end-feels, potential ranges of motion, and barrier-related properties (Figs. 60.87 and 60.88).

5. Use alternating direct and indirect barrier stresses to trigger an unwinding process (see discussion on page 961). As soft tissue and joint barriers release, overall ranges of motion commonly improve. This is particularly true when intrinsic joint mechanics are minimally compromised (i.e., degenerative and calcification changes are minimal).

Forearm, Elbow, and Wrist Release

Direct Technique, Transverse Approach

This technique is shown in Figs. 60.88 to 60.91. The goal is to generally release the forearm, elbow, and wrist by transversely straining direct myofascial barriers along the forearm, elbow, and wrist in a stepwise fashion.

Historical note: This is the first direct MFR technique developed for this system of treatment. In 1976, it came about accidentally while treating a patient with a particularly difficult case of scleroderma. The patient's skin was generally thickened by pannus (inflammatory granulation tissue) that had severely restricted most available myofascial and joint movements about the head, neck, face, chest wall, and upper limbs. Facial restric-

tions were so marked, she could open her mouth about 1.5 cm rather than the expected 4 to 5 cm. Facial expressions were mask-like and almost immobile. There was also anterior abdominal wall involvement. Swallowing was an increasing problem because of the myofascial changes. Fortunately, visceral involvement was minimal. Raynaud phenomenon was severe, with marked flexion contractures of the palmar fasciae and finger flexors. The patient had previously been placed on penicillamine and had physical therapy without substantial success.

After working with her for several visits, it was clear that standard osteopathic manipulative approaches were not helpful. Having had considerable experience with muscle energy techniques as well as fascial twisting maneuvers advocated by Ruddy in the early 20th century (see Chapter 57) and Neidner, the patient was asked if assertive twisting movements of the forearms, elbows, wrists, and hands could be performed. She readily agreed, and, to everyone's surprise, the skin and underlying tissues gave way under the firmly assertive torsional and compressive loads.

From this beginning, a series of assertive, very direct release maneuvers were designed to restore soft tissue resilience anywhere

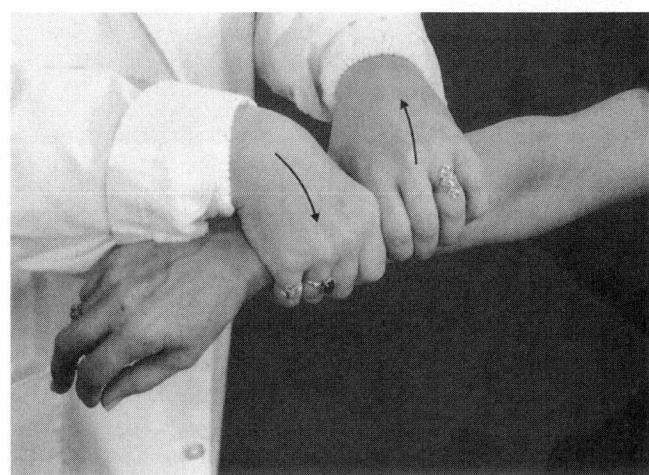

FIGURE 60.90. Forearm-elbow-wrist release, direct technique, transverse approach.

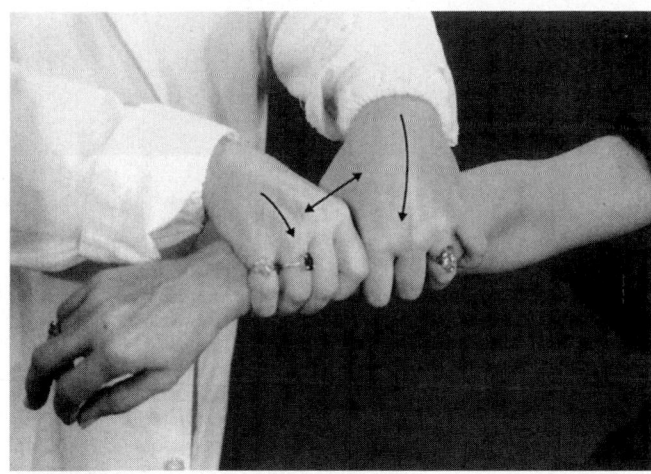

FIGURE 60.91. Forearm-elbow-wrist release, direct technique, transverse approach.

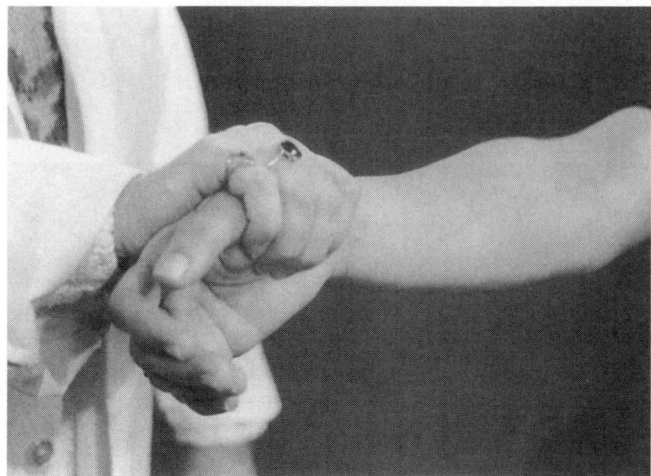

FIGURE 60.92.

on the body. In this particular instance, family members were taught the maneuvers. They turned out to be of great help, and after about 18 months, most of the patient's flexibility was restored. This included the upper limbs, facial muscles, and craniomandibular mechanics. At the time of this writing, she was carrying on a normal lifestyle with minimal need for further attention.

Review
Review the following:

1. Upper limb functional anatomy, including kinesiologic, scapulohumeral, scapulocostal, and craniocervical relationships.
2. Upper limb functional neurology, including cervical innervations, autonomic elements.
3. Upper limb myofascial and ligamentous anatomy, including ulnar nerve-elbow relationships, retinaculum of the wrist, and carpal tunnel and transverse carpal ligament influences.

Procedure
1. The patient is seated, standing, supine, or prone. Stand or sit comfortably for easy access to the forearm.
2. With a light hold on the skin, place the hands transversely across the forearm or wrist, with the knuckles of each index finger touching one another (Figs. 60.88 and 60.89).
3. Induce deformation against the direct barrier by twisting the skin and underlying soft tissues in opposite directions. Then twist in the opposite directions (Figs. 60.90 and 60.91).
4. When barriers are encountered, hold firmly until they give way under the load. Sometimes considerable force is needed to create a release, sometimes not.
5. Treatment is complete when as much free and easy inherent soft tissue motion occurs as can be reasonably expected.

Note: What the release event represents is unknown. Functionally, the phenomenon presumably represents a combination of viscoelastic rebound and a combination of peripheral and centrally controlled neurovascular changes.

Wrist-Forearm-Elbow

Direct Technique: Long-Axis Approach

This technique is shown in Figs. 60.92 to 60.95.

Goal
The general goal is to release forearm flexors and extensors in relation to distal wrist and hand mechanics, as well as proximal lateral and medial elbow to shoulder mechanics. As the release process unwinds the system, special attention is paid to sequential releases affecting both superficial and deep myofascial and joint mechanics.

Review
Review the following:

1. Upper limb functional anatomy
2. Upper limb functional neurology, including central, peripheral, and autonomic influences
3. Cervical spine anatomy and its relationships with shoulder and arm functions

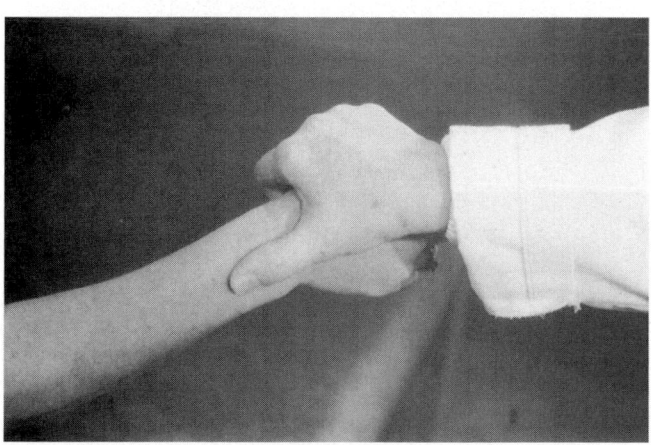

FIGURE 60.93.

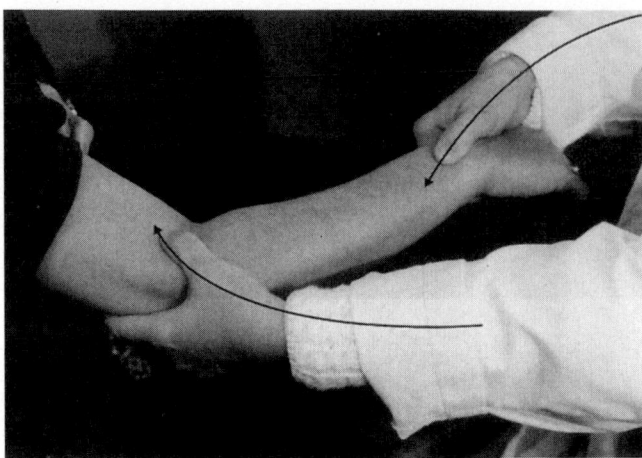

FIGURE 60.94. Wrist-forearm-elbow, direct technique, long-axis approach.

Procedure

1. The patient is standing, seated, or supine.
2. Firmly grasp the thenar eminence with four fingers as shown in Fig. 60.92. The index and long fingers should contact the area of the transverse carpal ligament.
3. Place the grasping thumb on the extensor surface of the hand and wrist pointing proximally along the long axis of forearm as demonstrated in Figs. 60.93. Figure 60.96 shows an alternative hand position.
4. With the other hand, firmly grasp the patient's forearm at elbow.
5. With elbow firmly held, turn the wrist until a tight barrier is noted at either side of the elbow, or within the mechanics of the wrist and hand. (Fig. 60.94 shows twist in one direction, Fig. 60.95 twists in opposite direction.)
6. Hold the tightness firmly for a few seconds until mechanical release is induced. At this point, the limb can be safely released and retested for soft tissue resilience and joint ranges of motion.
7. An alternative option is to continue holding firmly to induce unwinding. Sometimes the movements are slow and arclike,

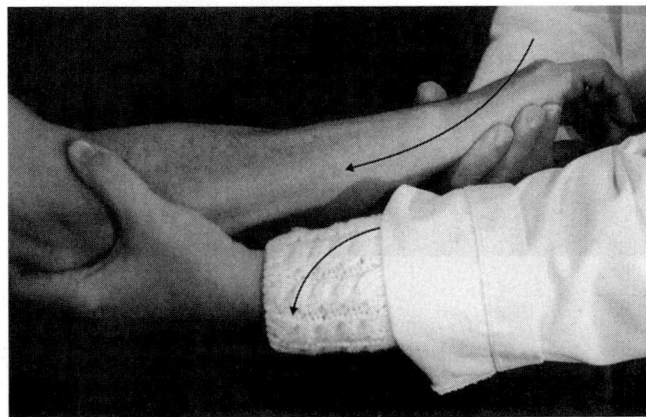

FIGURE 60.95. Wrist-forearm-elbow, direct technique, long-axis approach.

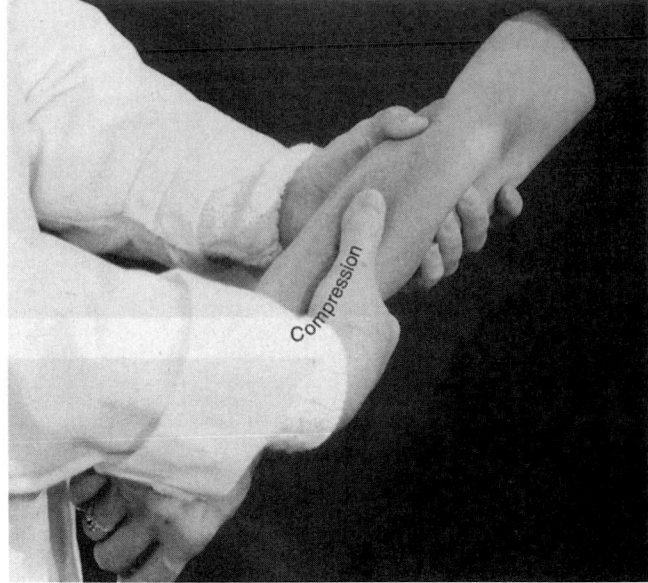

FIGURE 60.96. Wrist-forearm-elbow, direct technique, long-axis approach.

involving the whole limb. At other times they are rapid, even jerky, like a spring suddenly and rapidly uncoiling.

8. Treatment is complete when as much soft tissue motion occurs as can be reasonably expected.

Carpal and Palmar Tunnel Release

Direct Technique, Transverse Approach

This technique is shown in Figs 60.97 to 60.101.

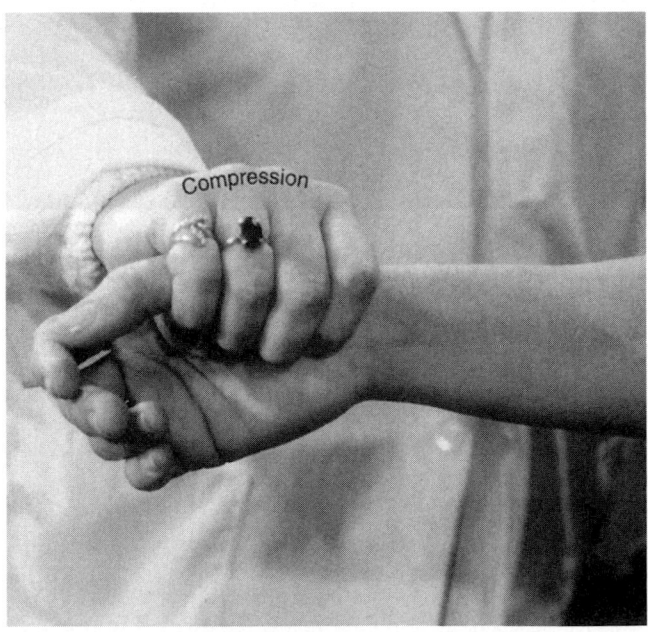

FIGURE 60.97. Wrist-carpal tunnel release.

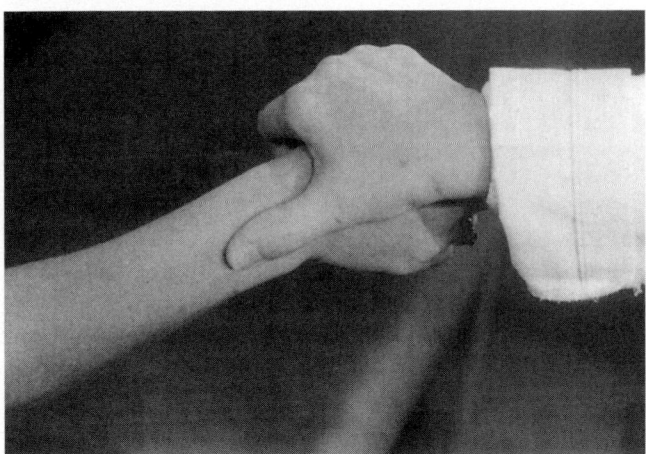

FIGURE 60.98.

Goal

The goal is to restore freedom of movement within the carpal and palmar tunnels by simultaneously releasing the soft tissues of the wrist, the carpal bones, and the palmar-carpal tunnel, and the transverse carpal ligament.

Review

Review the following:

1. Functional anatomy of the hand, wrist, and elbow
2. Functional neurology of the hand, wrist, and elbow

Procedure

1. The patient is seated, standing, or supine.
2. Stand comfortably in front or beside the patient.
3. With the distal hand, grasp the thenar, palmar tunnel transverse carpal ligamentous attachments (Fig. 60.97).

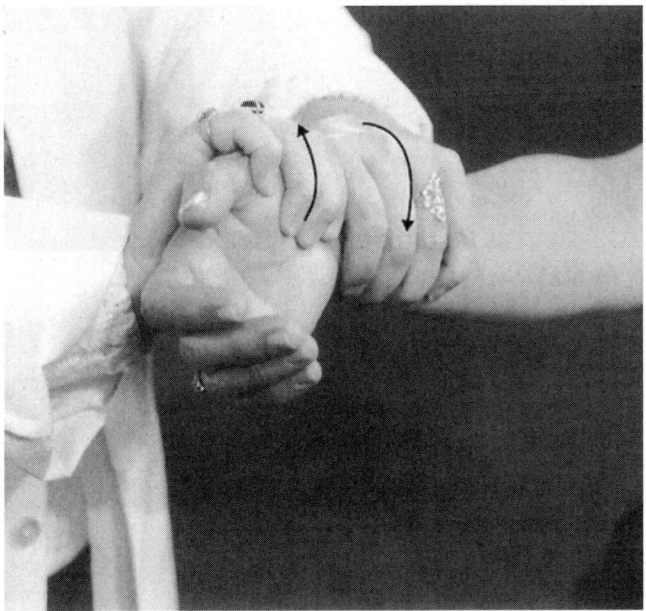

FIGURE 60.99. Wrist-carpal tunnel release

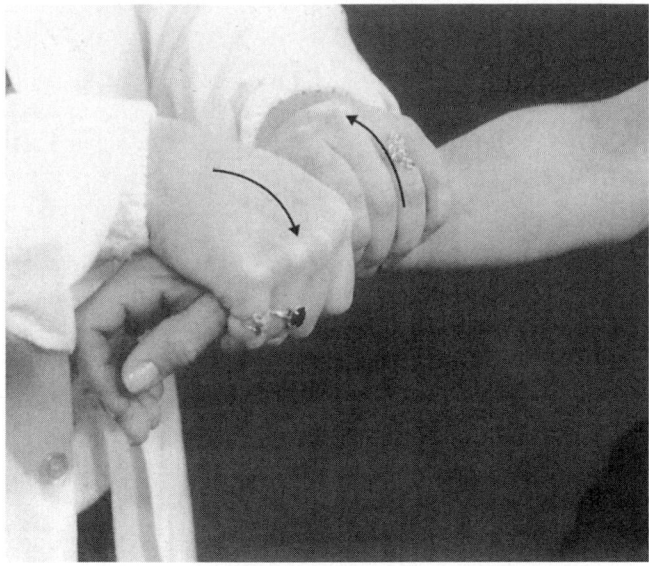

FIGURE 60.100. Wrist-carpal tunnel release.

4. The distal hand thumb points along the long axis of forearm as described above (Fig. 60.98).
5. With the proximal hand, grasp the wrist with specific attention to carpal-metacarpal and palmar tunnel-carpal tunnel tight-loose relationships.
6. Twist in supination until the myofascial barrier separates and opens the carpal tunnel (Fig. 60.99).
7. Then twist in pronation to further release the radiocarpal attachments (Fig. 60.97).
8. Hold firmly against the tightness for a few seconds until release occurs.
9. A second option is to continue holding firmly to see what happens as unwinding occurs.
10. Treatment is complete when as much soft tissue motion occurs as can be reasonably expected.

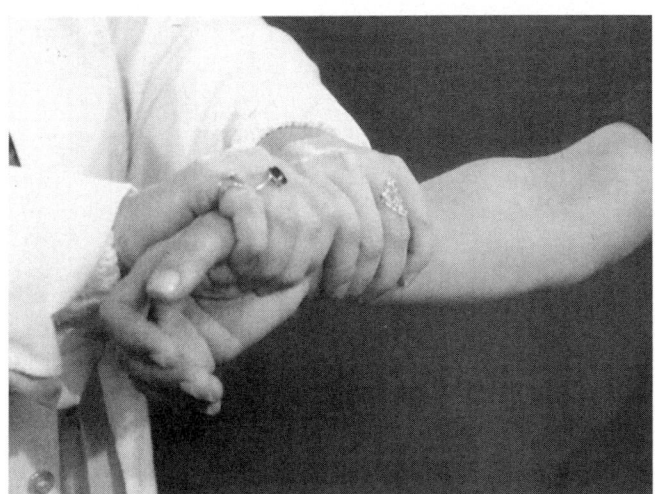

FIGURE 60.101.

CONCLUSION

These rudimentary MFR and INR techniques can help ease any number of neuromusculoskeletal problems. Having stood the test of time, they are easily learned and can be applied with relative ease.

REFERENCES

1. Viidik A. Interdependence between structure and function in collagenous tissues. In: Viidik A, Vuust J, eds. *Biology of Collagen.* New York, NY: Academic Press; 1987:257.
2. Still AT. *Philosophy of Osteopathy.* Kirksville, MO: Journal Printing Co; 1899.
3. Cole WV. Some histological aspects of the motor end plate. *J Osteopath.* 51:7:1820:44.
4. Cole WV. A gold chloride method for motor end plates. *Stain Technol.* 1946;21:2325.
5. The Glossary Review Committee of the Educational Council on Osteopathic Principles. Glossary of osteopathic terminology. In: Allen TW, ed. *AOA Yearbook and Directory of Osteopathic Physicians.* Chicago, IL: American Osteopathic Association, 1996.
6. Greenman PE. *Principles of Manual Medicine,* 2nd ed, Baltimore, MD: Williams & Wilkins; 1996:65–73
7. Woo S-L, An K-N, Arnoczky SP, et al. Anatomy, biology, and biomechanics of tendon, ligament, and rotation. In: Simon SR, ed. *Orthopedic Basic Science.* American Academy of Orthopedic Surgeons; 1994: 45–88.
8. *The New Lexicon Webster's Dictionary of the English Language.* New York, NY: Lexicon Publications; 1988.
9. Cathie AG. The fascia of the body in relation to function and manipulative therapy. In: *The American Academy of Osteopathy Yearbook.* Indianapolis, IN: American Academy of Osteopathy; 1974: 81–87.
10. Becker RF. The meaning of fascial and fascial continuity. *Osteopath Ann.* 1975;3:8–32.
11. Bonica JJ. *The Management of Pain,* 2nd ed. Philadelphia, PA: Lea & Febiger; 1990:66.
12. Earl E. The dual sensory role of muscle spindles. *Phys Ther J.* 1965;45:4.
13. Wilson VJ. Inhibition in the central nervous system. *Sci Am.* 1966;5:102–108.
14. Grinberg-Zylerbaum J, Ramos J. Interpersonal communication: an experimental approach. *Int J Neurosci.* 1989;36:41–52.
15. Norton JN. A tissue pressure model for the palpatory perception of the cranial rhythmic impulse. *JAOA.* 1991;10:975–994.
16. Adams TA, Heisey RC, Briner BA. Parietal bone mobility in the anesthetized cat. *JAOA.* 1992;5:599–622.
17. Upledger JE. Reproducibility of craniosacral examination findings: a statistical analysis. *JAOA.* 1977;6:746.
18. Upledger JE, Karni Z. Mechanoelectric patterns during craniosacral osteopathic diagnosis and treatment. *JAOA.* 1978;11:782–791.

FUNCTIONAL TECHNIQUE: AN INDIRECT METHOD

WILLIAM L. JOHNSTON

KEY CONCEPTS

- History of indirect methods
- Historic principles behind functional technique
- Motion-function test pattern
- Palpable motor dysfunction: descriptive research
- Functional technique as a distinctive indirect method
- Diagnosis in a functional approach, including tissue compression and motion testing stages
- Criteria for judgment during functional procedures
- Functional guidelines for application of an indirect manipulative method
- "Response information" guides functional technique
- Conceptual basis of functional technique
- Practical application of functional technique for the body, including thoracic, lumbar, and sacral regions, cervical region, costal region, thoracic cage, innominate, and appendicular regions
- Spinal motion dysfunction: regarding the differential in palpatory diagnosis for reflex manifestations of somatic and visceral inputs

HISTORICAL PERSPECTIVES

To engage the term *functional technique,* one needs to sense the stimulus driving its initial development in the early 1950s. Within the osteopathic discipline, there was a growing recognition that *motor function* had a broader conceptual framework than just bony relationships, with their structural configuration relatively confined to joints, and to concepts for motion of one bone on the bone below. To open up this conceptual model, it was necessary to give increasing attention to the physiologic aspects and clinical manifestations of motor control. For a mobile system, specific directions of regional motion tests were becoming effective in delineating positive diagnostic signs of dysfunctional behaviors, both regional and segmental. Within these broader functional parameters, motion tests would supply promising tools for application in clinical practice and osteopathic research.

To engage the term *indirect* as a method of manipulation, one needs to refer back to the early 1900s. In the history of osteopathy, information derived from palpatory examination had led to the development of a classification for methods of manipulation. Development of the terms *direct* and *indirect* gave recognition to the specific directions of motion forces used in osteopathic manipulative procedures. A brief look at 100 years of professional history indicates a significant struggle regarding the issue of terminology. The controversy involves two areas:

1. Verbalizing palpatory findings in the musculoskeletal system, and
2. Conceptualizing models for palpable findings, for example: the use of bony malposition at a joint, to depict a local area of segmental dysfunction (referred to in the past as a lesion, the Still lesion, or osteopathic lesion).

Difficulties with terminology create problems for communication about the clinical signs of musculoskeletal dysfunctions. To describe a direct manipulative technique for segmental dysfunction, initial concepts of somatic dysfunction focused on joint restriction and direct forces to encounter and overcome restriction; this fit the layperson's concept of "putting the bone back in place." Other techniques did not directly encounter the restriction yet still overcame restricted movement. Such manipulative procedures did not fit the concept of the direct method. They did use motion and maneuvers in the opposite direction of the restriction effectively, however, and were given the term indirect. Owing to the fact that they seem to defy positional relationships and joint concepts, indirect methods are often set aside. Since they do not fit with those earlier models of thought, they continue to present a special challenge for instruction.

Several early osteopathic practitioners expressed these issues. Edythe F. Ashmore, a faculty member at the American College of Osteopathy in Kirksville, Missouri, wrote the first textbook on the mechanics of osteopathy in 1915. She stated:

There are two methods commonly employed by osteopathists in the correction of lesions the older of which is the traction method, the later the direct method or thrust.* Those who employ the traction method secure the relaxation of the tissues about the articulation by what has been termed exaggeration of the lesion, a motion in the direction of the forcible movement which produced the lesion, as if its purpose were to increase the deformity. The exaggeration is held, traction made upon the joint, replacement initiated and then completed by reversal of the forces.†

The direct method consists in the application of a precisely directed force toward a bony prominence during the process of putting the articulation or lesion through the spinal movement which is the reversal of that which produced the lesion.

*The term "direct" is preferred for the reason that the imitators of osteopathy have given the word "thrust" an objectionable meaning of harshness.

† This method is the more difficult of the two and for the instruction of students does not find favor with the author (1).

Ashmore's footnotes about terminology and instructional problems are particularly illuminating. The limited concepts implied by the expressions *"exaggerating the lesion"* and *"reversal of that* [movement] *which produced the lesion"* remained in use for many years. The direction of restricted movement was even then becoming a determinant for methods of manipulative technique and their classification as direct and indirect.

Carl P. McConnell, DO, was another osteopathic pioneer who actively contributed to osteopathic literature from 1905 to 1938. He commented:

So, striving to get the bones in normal position, per se, or perhaps to keep them in position, is simply hopeless. In this regard, the bony item is simply an idol, and a similar idol could be made of the muscles, and so forth (2).

McConnell also wrote:

Precision of method follows definiteness of diagnosis. It is evident that there are many ways of applying the same mechanical principles. But ease and effectiveness should be the goal of operative activity. In adjusting lesions it is obvious that a method which retraces the path of the lesion with a minimum of irritation is highly desirable (3).

McConnell's orientation was still on *"the path of the lesion,"* but this was tempered by a growing discomfort with using bony position or any single anatomic structure as the key to conceptualizing about areas of musculoskeletal dysfunction.

By 1923, in *Principles and Practice of Osteopathy,* C. Harrison Downing (4) went a step further in describing restriction at a lesioned segment. He referred to the fact that, when testing a physiologic motion, the lesioned segment becomes more restricted going in one direction. He added that the restriction decreases in the opposite direction, and *"apparently disappears."* Keeping his motion testing procedure as a frame of reference, Downing provided palpatory information about the restriction *decreasing* in a direction opposite to the direction of restricted motion. These new facts sometimes supported the concepts centered on the joint and bony description of malposition, and sometimes did not.

By 1949, Howard A. Lippincott reported on the osteopathic technique of William G. Sutherland as follows:

The articulation is carried in the direction of the lesion, exaggerating the lesion position as far as is necessary to cause the tension of the weakened elements of the ligamentous structure to be equal to or slightly in excess of the tension of those that were not strained. This is

the point of balanced tension. When the tension is properly balanced, the respiratory or muscular cooperation of the patient is employed to overcome the resistance of the defense mechanism of the body to the release of the lesion (5).

This described an indirect method of treatment, but the anatomic construct was more *"ligamentous."* The *"point of balanced tension"* (also referred to as *"the point of balanced ligamentous tension"*) became the significant phrase used to describe techniques where the physician palpated throughout the procedure and continually adjusted treatment to the changing tissue tensions. Descriptive terminology still relied mainly on a positional orientation to express this important feedback of palpable information during motion. "Balance and hold" became another phrase to describe indirect techniques, but this phrase fails to point out the continued balancing carried out by the physician in response to the tissues changing.

In the early 1940s at the Chicago College of Osteopathy, indirect diagnostic skills were a part of students' formal training. This involved instructing students regarding the diagnosis of directions of motion that would initially relax the tissues, and their application in combined techniques. In Boston, by 1944, some very prominent physician teachers in the New England area had already been applying indirect methods extensively in their practices; however, the difficulty in communicating these skills was still a problem.

In the 1940s, the Academy of Applied Osteopathy (now known as the American Academy of Osteopathy) initiated a national program of education to improve the clinical skills of physicians, for those proficiencies in practice that can be achieved with continual application of Still's principles. This was done through the implementation of postgraduate instruction. Harold Hoover was a part of this effort. His classification of direct and indirect manipulative methods included the following:

1. Direct technique: the method of moving one bone or segment of the articular lesion directly to a normal relationship with its neighbor. This is accomplished against the resistance of tissues and fluids maintaining the abnormal relationship.
2. Indirect technique: the method of moving one bone or segment slightly in the direction away from the direction of correction until the resistance of holding tissues and fluids is partially overcome and the tensions are bilaterally balanced, then allowing the released ligaments and muscles themselves to aid in pulling the part toward normal. Other body forces, including that of respiration, may be employed (6).

Hoover's experiences with both of these methods of manipulation were beginning to channel his major interest toward the indirect (7). Recognizing a functional model, he was reporting on his use of palpatory tests, palpable findings, and manipulative procedures, especially those of the clinically effective indirect method. He often introduced his functional approaches in seminars. His presentation in New England in 1951 initiated an era of development in the New England Academy of Osteopathy. Biannual study sessions, led by Charles Bowles, resulted in a series of three publications entitled "A Functional Orientation for Technic."

In his initial report, Bowles wrote:

This was not the birth of a new entity in osteopathy, but simply a new type of measuring stick for evaluating the Still lesion as a process of aberrated function . . . our functional investigation had become formalized by using the pattern of a demand-response transaction, instituting motion demands (which could be named) with a motive hand, down to, and through a given segment, while assessing the motion response of this given segment through a palpatory listening hand. To best understand, follow, and control this demand-response transaction therapeutically at a segmental level, certain specific insights seem necessary, namely:

1. An understanding of typical motion-demands and a system of annotation that makes them easily communicable between operators,
2. An understanding of responses which allows an accurate reporting and a useful evaluation of the specific demand-response transaction taking place currently under the fingertips of the palpating or "listening hand" during manipulation, and
3. An understanding of criteria for lesioned and non-lesioned performance, i.e., in terms of functional adequacy.

Thus the significant functional information about vertebral motion or restriction is not so much that there is motion or restriction, but rather how these motions and restrictions change, and under what circumstances, and in response to what demands.

It is the response information that eventually guides functional technic (8).

It should be noted that these comments by Bowles are in contrast to guides based on anatomic *concepts*, and bony, muscular, or ligamentous relations.

By 1961, Lippincott was expressing educational concerns similar to those of Ashmore. He reported student confusion, as well as practice trends, that were leading him to analyze and clarify the various methods of correcting lesions. In "Basic Principles of Osteopathic Technique," he reported:

It is evident that Dr. Still treated his patients carefully, with due consideration for the delicacy and the welfare of the tissues beneath his fingers. It is also evident that he imparted to the students who came under his supervision this wholesome respect for the tissues, the structures, and their functioning. Then, after the turn of the century, it became popular with many of the vigorous and enthusiastic young doctors to treat with vigor and enthusiasm. They developed techniques that would produce a "pop" regardless of the force required to produce it. This gave them a sense of accomplishment but it also gave osteopathy a reputation for being rough, painful, and even dangerous, a stigma that still persists among the uninformed. Within a decade or two the trend turned back toward more careful and intelligent, but perhaps less spectacular methods. The result is a wealth of technical procedures representing varied approaches to the correction of osteopathic lesions. It is a decided advantage for the physician to have at his command a variety of methods whereby he can meet the needs of each individual patient (9).

During the 1960s and 1970s, the steadfastness of positional concepts continued to be reflected in the development of new techniques. In 1964 Lawrence H. Jones published his original article, "Spontaneous Release by Positioning," introducing the technique for manipulative treatment called strain/counterstrain. Dr. Jones questioned:

Is the muscular tension arranged so as to splint this joint, to prevent it from moving back into its eccentric position? No! The muscular tension resists any position away from the extreme position in which the lesioning occurred. Even the severest lesions will readily tolerate

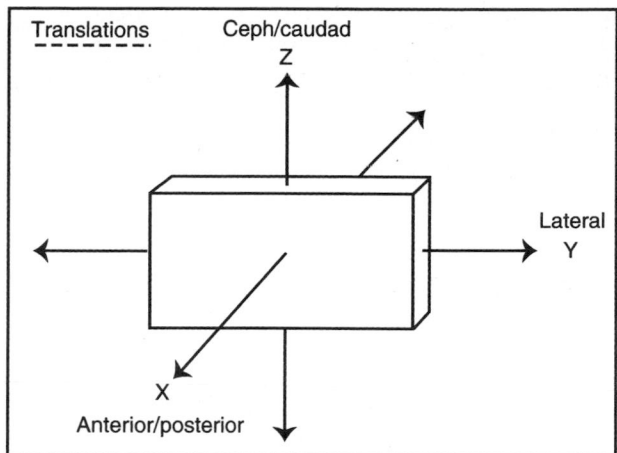

FIGURE 61.1. Coordinate system to illustrate straight-line directions of movement used to describe translatory motion tests. (From Johnston WL. Segmental definition, part I: a focal point for diagnosis of somatic dysfunction. *JAOA.* 1988;88:99–105, with permission.)

being returned to the position in which lesion formation originally occurred, and only to this position. When the joint is returned to this position (indirect), the muscles promptly and gratefully relax (10).

Since 1969, and possibly starting during the Bowles initiative in New England in 1955, interest has grown in relation to motor function, with a focus on the application of motion tests and palpable findings for descriptive clinical research. A test pattern of passive gross motions evolved with standards relevant to the six elementary directions of the body's movement (Figs. 61.1 and 61.2). These motions are:

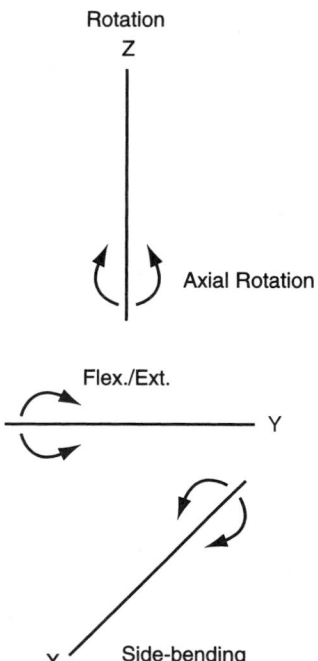

FIGURE 61.2. Coordinate system to illustrate directions of movement about axes used to describe rotary motion tests. (From Johnston WL. Segmental definition, part I: a focal point for diagnosis of somatic dysfunction. *JAOA.* 1988;88:99–105, with permission.)

- Flexion/extension
- Side bending
- Rotation
- Translation from side to side
- Translation anteriorly/posteriorly
- Translation cephalad/caudad (traction/compression)

This test pattern allows implementation of an organized diagnostic process for describing the motor characteristics of neuromusculoskeletal dysfunctions. Investigations (11) using this test pattern have been advancing our knowledge about functional aspects of both regional and segmental somatic dysfunction, as follows:

1. Passive gross motion tests provide a means to attain baseline palpatory information in medical problem solving for a mobile system:

> Examining *regional* motor performance (12)
> Locating *segmental* motor defects (13,14)
> Characterizing *the specifics of a segment's motor dysfunction* as a basis for designing manipulative interventions to address somatic dysfunction (15–17)

2. Segmental somatic dysfunction is a complete asymmetry of its elementary motion functions: three rotary, three straight-line translatory, and respiratory (18). (Respiratory was the seventh function, and takes under consideration the demands of inhalation and exhalation on motor function.) Palpable recordable cues evident in response to these motion tests provide seven possible descriptors for the motion characteristics of each motor defect.

3. A fundamental unit of segmental somatic dysfunction (16,19) consists of a three-segment complex, as illustrated in Fig. 61.3. A central asymmetric segment is the primary defect. Mirror-image (opposing) motion asymmetries are present at the adjacent segments, above and below. (These are secondary and adaptive, implying a basis in somato-somatic reflex activity.)

4. A different organizational principle operates when primary defects are identified at a midline vertebra and an adjacent rib at the same spinal level with *identical* motion asymmetries; this contrasts with the *opposing* asymmetries presented by mirror images (20). An example is illustrated in Fig. 61.4 at T2 and left rib 2. Accompanying this primary defect at the T2 level, note that there still are secondary mirror-image asymmetries at the adjacent segments above and below in both the midline vertebral and left costal columns. Clinical research (21) has supported the premise that visceral afferents contribute to this characteristic configuration of two segmental units, vertebra and rib, *linked* in similar primary motion asymmetries at the same spinal level.

This preceding historical perspective puts one in mind of the classic tale of the blind men and the elephant, with each man describing the elephant according to the part being touched. From clinical palpatory experience, asymmetry *(A)* of joint position, restriction *(R)* of motion, and tissue texture changes *(T)* are expressed in the mnemonic acronym ART. Tenderness (T) has recently been added to the acronym, making it TART, with the first "T" representing tenderness. Each of the last three has emerged as a palpable sign of segmental somatic dysfunction, where motor function is asymmetric and its manifestations are

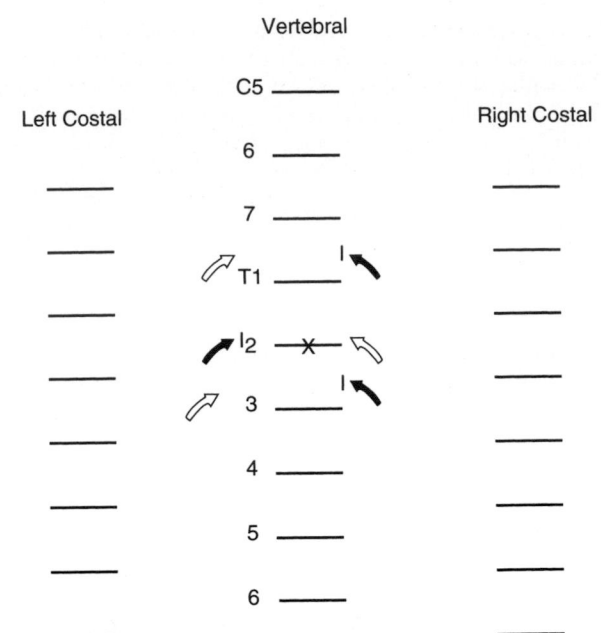

FIGURE 61.3. Schematic representation of three mobile columns in thoracic region, with a three-segment unit of dysfunction in vertebral column. *X*, location of primary functional defect at T2, with resistance to shoulder/trunk rotation to right (*short, solid arrow, with bar representing sense of resistance*). In adjacent T1 and T3 segments, mirror-image resistance to left rotation is secondary (*short, solid arrows with bars*). *Longer, open arrows without bars* at each level represent sense of compliance with motion and a greater range of motion in directions opposite to directions of limited mobility. (From Johnston WL. Somatic manifestations in renal disease: a clinical research study. *JAOA.* 1987;87:22–35, with permission.)

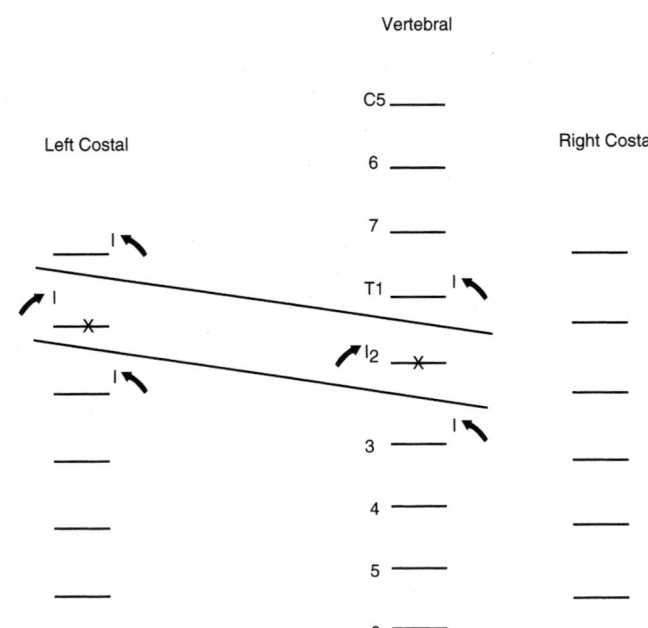

FIGURE 61.4. Schematic representation of two primary motor asymmetries at T2 spinal level, indicated by *X* in vertebral and adjacent left costal columns. *Arrows with bars* at T2 spinal level indicate resistance in both columns to right rotation of shoulders/trunk. Secondary mirror-image asymmetries of restricted motor function are indicated at T1 and T3 spinal levels by *bars on arrows* for left rotation that is (again) present in both columns.

present in structure, motion, and tissue. The functional characteristics of motor asymmetry emerge primarily from motion tests. These characteristics provide detailed descriptors to implement differential diagnosis and also establish basis for the classification of methods of manipulation as direct and indirect.

FUNCTIONAL TECHNIQUE

The term *"functional technique"* refers to osteopathic manipulative procedures that apply palpatory information gained from tests for motor function, although the term is often applied inappropriately as a general synonym for "indirect." To be specific, in functional manipulative procedures the palpable information regarding all six degrees of freedom and respiration are used to address the dysfunctional aspects of segmental behavior. Passive gross motion testing identifies motion symmetry/asymmetry at an individual mobile segment. If you can, temporarily set aside the interpretation of palpatory information about mobility in a format for static concepts of joint position–for example, a posterior transverse process. Instead, criteria for determining a mobile segment's behavior and its resistance to or compliance with opposing directions of specifically induced passive *regional* motion tests are applied. The demonstration in Fig. 61.5 illustrates a

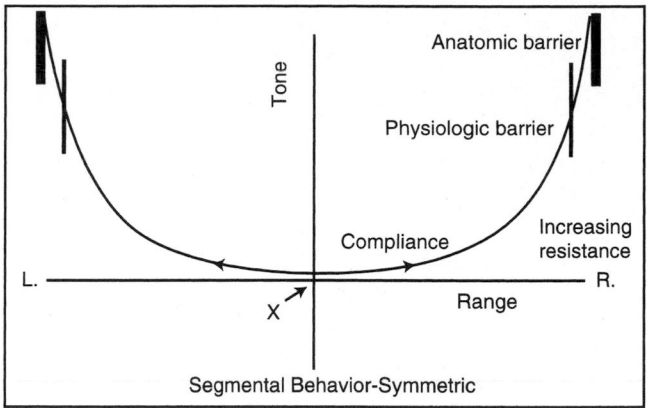

FIGURE 61.6. Symmetric response to motion at a nonlesioned thoracic segment where only axial rotation is represented. Shown are equal initial compliance to right *(R)* and left *(L)*, and then increasing resistance toward an equidistant final anatomic end point. (From Johnston WL. Segmental definition, part I: a focal point for diagnosis of somatic dysfunction. *JAOA.* 1988;88:99–105, with permission.)

single axial motion test introduced through the shoulders and trunk in rotation to the right. With the patient seated and arms folded, right rotation of shoulders and trunk is introduced by the physician's right hand at the patient's right elbow. The fingers of the left hand monitor bilaterally the *immediate* response of paravertebral tissues overlying T6 transverse processes. To compare for response to rotation left, the operator stands to the left and the hand positions are reversed. Finding asymmetric behavior at T6, one can report resistance encountered at T6, for example, during shoulder trunk rotation right. (The test and the criterion are explicit, and the finding becomes clear in relation to the test used to elicit it, thereby attending to scientific method for first-order reporting.) This is in contrast to applying *local* pressure prone at T6, encountering increased resistance to pressure on the left versus the right, and then reporting a posterior left transverse process, with limited rotation to the right of T6 on T7 within the concept of a joint.

As illustrated in Fig. 61.6 for symmetric behavior, the initial resting level of minimal muscle tone or tension at point X reflects the natural palpable resistance that the operator's fingertips sense as they lightly contact tissues overlying the bony segment at rest. Point X also illustrates there is palpable symmetry in a segment's initial compliance to move right and left with no rise on the tone scale at the initiation of movement. Indicated also is the normally increasing resistance to range as motion approaches a physiologic and an anatomic barrier.

Start with a compression test. The compression test is the application of pressure through the fingers to sense any *increased* tissue tension at one segment compared with adjacent segments. Even at rest, a compression test of a *dysfunctional* segment will register the local increased resistance of that segment's deep musculature; this can be illustrated as an elevation to X1 on a tone scale (Fig. 61.7). The fingertips mark the site of the increased resistance to pressure.

The segment's tissue tension in the marked area changes *immediately* on initiation of each passive motion test. Palpatory cues reflect the immediately increasing resistance to pressure in one direction (in this example, to the right), while in the

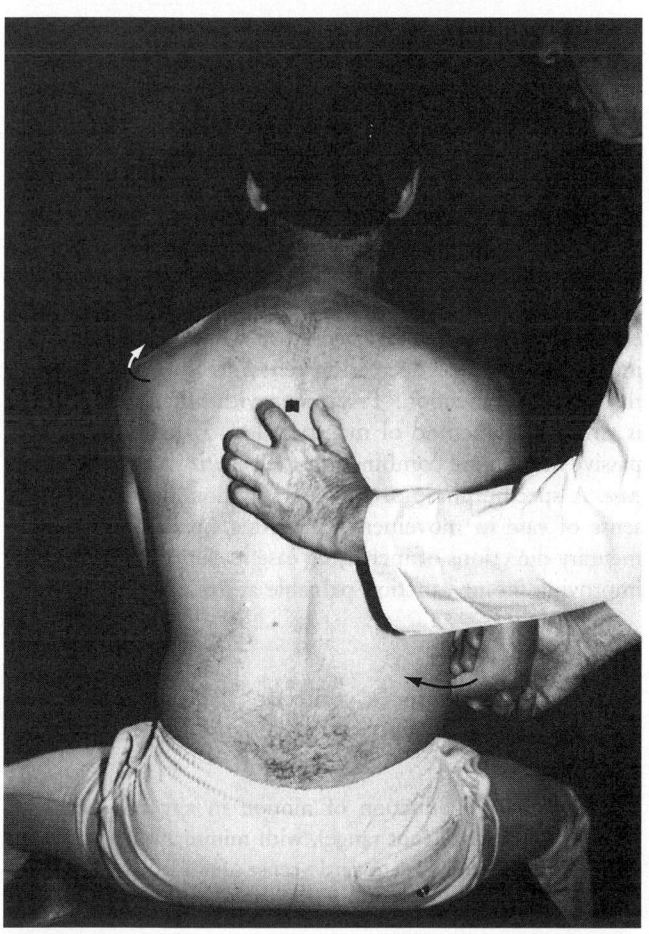

FIGURE 61.5. Single axial motion test of shoulders and trunk in rotation to right. (From Johnston WL. Segmental definition, part I: a focal point for diagnosis of somatic dysfunction. *JAOA.* 1988;88:99–105, with permission.)

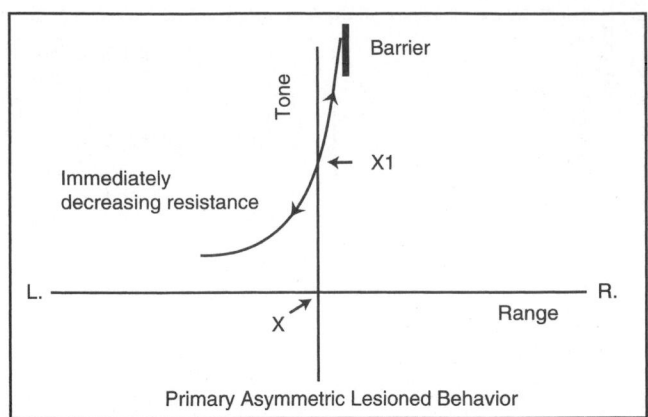

FIGURE 61.7. Asymmetric behavior at a dysfunctional (lesioned) segment. (From Johnston WL. Segmental definition, part I: a focal point for diagnosis of somatic dysfunction. *JAOA.* 1988;88:99–105, with permission.)

opposing direction they reflect an immediate sense of decreasing resistance to pressure (i.e., a decreasing tension with increasing ease of motion). These palpable changes provide an indicator of asymmetric motor function, to monitor not only during diagnosis to guide accuracy, but also during treatment to guide efficacy in the return to symmetric motor function. Treatment with functional technique is a distinctive application of an indirect method of manipulation. Well-defined directions of passive motion are combined *in their initial stages of increasing ease.* A particular phase of active respiration also increases this sense of ease in movement. As the responses to each precise elementary direction of increasing ease are summed up, the reduced tissue tension signals a rapidly improving motor function palpable at the fingertips.

Guidelines

Certain procedural aspects of functional technique help to ensure success in the application of an indirect method of manipulation for segmental dysfunction (22).

1. The initial introduction of motion in any one elementary direction is small (not range), with minimal forces applied.
2. Motion directions are toward a sense of *immediately increasing ease.* This response manifests a decreasing sense of resistance to pressure at fingers monitoring the tense dysfunctional segment (at the same time, motions are away from the opposing direction in which increasing resistance is encountered).
3. Single elements of rotary and translatory directions are combined, effecting the control of an eventual smooth torsion arc for body movement. The order of introduction of these elements is not important.
4. The final step of the functional procedure involves request for a specific direction of active respiration, whichever direction (inhalation or exhalation) contributes further to the increasing ease. For example, if inhalation, the request is for the subject to take a deep breath *slowly* and hold it briefly.
5. This respiratory interval, adding to a continuous feedback of decreasing resistance, allows the operator to fine-tune the

combination of translatory and rotary directions. The objective is to reach a sense of release of tissue tension at the fingertips, which are continually monitoring response at the dysfunctional segment.
6. The release of restraint in the motor mechanism allows a return to midline resting, unobstructed by any sense of the resistance previously encountered in the return direction.

A successful outcome is signaled by a sensed release of the segmental tissues' holding forces, which then allows a free return to a resting position, and a new tissue tone at rest. The segment's new functional symmetry is evident in the responses to further motion retesting. Increased resistance in response to directions previously limited is no longer encountered.

Examples of applying this functional method of palpatory diagnosis and manipulative treatment are presented under "Examples of Functional Technique" later in this chapter. To memorize any technique for use as a manipulative procedure, without recreating each of the steps outlined above, this would be inappropriate and probably clinically ineffective. Bowles (23) stated, "It is ... the response information that eventually guides functional technic." Therefore, at a mobile segment, focus attention on the following:

1. The criteria for symmetric and asymmetric motor function
2. The orientation of motion testing to the palpable findings of bony and tissue tension expressed at a dysfunctional mobile segment
3. The way that response at your fingertips, to each direction of motion test, guides not only diagnosis but also the development of each individual manipulative procedure

Conceptual Basis

The following phrases reveal the static positional concepts that emerged during osteopathy's early professional history:

Describing the lesion as a bone out of place,
Exaggerating the lesion position,
Retracing the path of the lesion,
Noting the position in which the lesion occurred, and
Stacking positions to balance the tension.

Bowles' comments about demand/response transactions and the motor coordination necessary for each bone to be in the right place at the right time during demands for body movement strongly indicate that he was moving beyond static positional concepts. His conceptual bias for motor function called for the recognition of a mobile system and mobile segments, patterned to act in concert with one another. Each mobile segment is a bone with articular surfaces for movement, and adnexal tissues under motor control; together, they respond to precise functional demands to:

1. Maintain postural position,
2. Carry out active movements, and
3. Allow passive movement.

For Bowles, functional diagnosis and technique were "unique in accuracy and universal in nontraumatic application" (24).

Currently there is widespread recognition, but still limited understanding, of the neural control of these motor dynamics. In 1978, Stein (25) reviewed principles emerging from studies of the properties of interneurons and their application to the organization of the body's motor patterns. Fundamental concepts of command neurons and pattern generators furnished a baseline for continuing research in this field. This growing knowledge about neural networks and motor control systems has been reviewed by Getting (26). Atsuta and colleagues' research presents an ongoing example (27). In areas where motion tests detect signs of segmental motor asymmetry, somatic proprioceptive and nociceptive afferents (sensory impulses) acting through feedback loops effect adaptive changes in motor patterns. These changes are palpable as a three-segment unit of segmental dysfunction, which describes a basic unit of defective and adapted function.

During functional technique, the release of holding forces (using minimal force) and the return to motor symmetry have been expressed as follows (28):

> At the moment when the release of resistance forces is sensed, the response (conceptually) appears to be the result of a matching in movement function, in which the local segmental control becomes appropriate to the current, overall movement—a matching of adequacy in physiologic response to specific motion demand. The return to local controlled compliance of the mobile segment within the whole complex movement restores the opportunity for adequate part-to-whole functional relations of this segment within the mobile system.
>
> Basic knowledge about proprioceptor and nociceptor stimuli as a source of reflex communication from somatic tissues to other somatic tissues is well established (29). Even at rest, in response to only gravity and positional demands, the palpable findings of bony irregularity and increased resistance of muscular tissue to pressure at dysfunctional segments reflect ongoing stimulation of proprioceptor sensors. During movement, these palpable cues to the traffic on afferent pathways are highly erratic, since in some directions of ease they decrease whereas in opposing directions of resistance they increase.
>
> The sheer immediacy of the changes palpated during motion testing and treatment suggests the moment-to-moment afferent monitoring by numerous muscle spindle stretch receptors and the resulting efferent control of muscle contraction/relaxation as a physiologic basis for interpreting the response to osteopathic manipulation being reported here (28).

At vertebral levels where segmental motion asymmetry is present, the physical stress of daily demands for movement and positioning accounts for a major increase in somatic sensory afferent impulses reaching the spinal cord (30). A concept of *afferent reduction* has application where the palpable sense of decreasing resistance, monitored throughout a functional manipulative procedure, successfully restores symmetric motor function.

EXAMPLES OF FUNCTIONAL TECHNIQUE

Thoracic, Lumbar, and Sacral Regions: Seated

The method described in the following example of functional technique (17) is applicable in the thoracic, lumbar, or sacral spinal regions.

Findings

This patient has a dysfunctional T6 segment, locally resisting regional rotation of shoulders and trunk to the right. Additional findings on shoulder/trunk rotation tests indicate that the increasing *ease* in rotation left at T6 is accompanied by *resistance* to rotation left at T5 and T7. Other rotary motion tests reveal initial increasing ease at T6 to side bending left and to extension, and to initial *inhalation* on respiratory testing. These directions are resisted at T5 and T7. In the next test (Fig. 61.8A), the physician initiates right side bending of the trunk with moderate caudally directed force through the right hand, which is on the patient's right shoulder. The fingers of the physician's left hand monitor the response at T6. In the second test (Fig. 61.8B), trunk flexion and extension are initiated, being careful not to introduce translatory aspects of movement (e.g., the patient is maintained in midline of the intersection of midcoronal and sagittal planes). Slightly relaxed slumping supported by the physician's left arm initiates flexion. Reversal of this rotary direction (about the y axis of Fig. 61.2) initiates extension. The physician's right fingers compare responses to these opposing directions of motion.

Position

The patient is in the seated position. As indicated in Fig. 61.9, the physician's left arm is over the left shoulder and under the right shoulder of the patient to allow easy introduction of side bending left and rotation left in the following functional application of an indirect method of manipulation.

Treatment Procedure

1. Hold the patient to provide control in side bending left, rotation left, and extension in a smooth torsional arc. Each of these directions will begin to diminish the local tissue resistance being monitored at T6 during the manipulative procedure.

2. Using slight shifting of postural forces to control movement of the patient's body, three translatory tests can be completed. In Fig. 61.10A, with patient's hips relatively fixed by sitting position, a slight shift in the physician's body weight to the right and then to the left allows comparison of response of T6 to lateral translations of the patient's trunk. In Fig. 61.10B, a slight shift in the physician's weight controls patient's shoulders and trunk, relative to the pelvis, to initiate anterior and then posterior translation motions for testing response at T6. In Fig. 61.10C, for testing cephalad/caudad directions, the physician initiates slight lifting cephalad through the patient's shoulders and trunk, and then caudad by applying mild body compression; the segment's responses to opposing directions are monitored by the physician's right hand.

In this example, movements are added with increasing ease in translations to the left, anterior, and cephalad. Testing had indicated increasing resistance in each opposing translatory direction. Initial introduction of each appropriate direction is more important than extent of range in any one direction alone.

3. The final component is to direct a slow inhalation by the patient. The additional element of increasing ease promotes an eventual release of the holding tensions at the dysfunctional

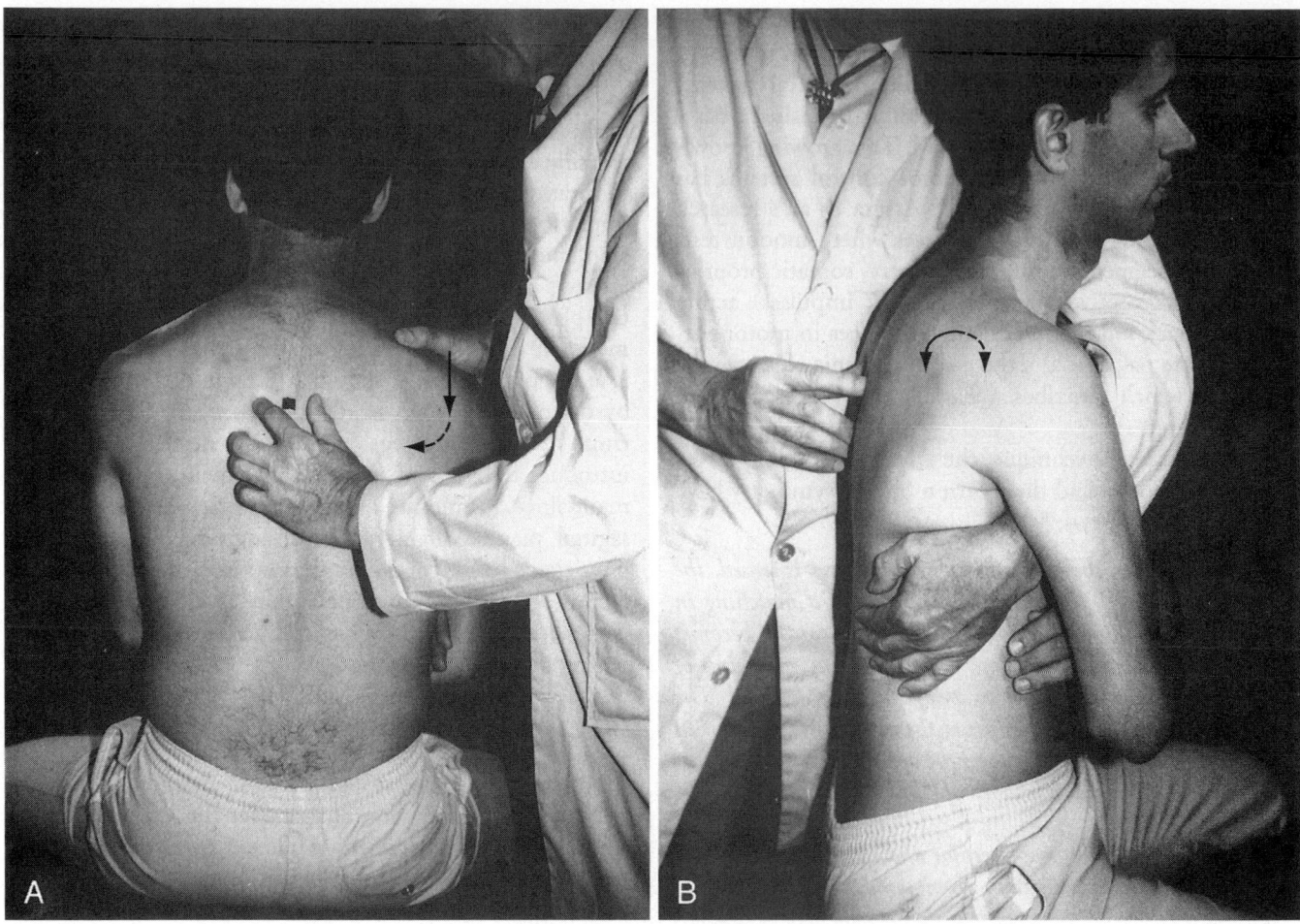

FIGURE 61.8. Additional rotary motion tests. **A:** Physician initiates right side bending of trunk. **B:** Trunk flexion and extension. (From Johnston WL. Segmental definition, part II: application of an indirect method in osteopathic manipulative treatment. *JAOA.* 1988;88:211–217, with permission.)

segment. The release allows return to a central resting position without encountering the previous resistance in these opposing directions.

4. Following successful release, retesting confirms a return to compliance and symmetry in response throughout the T5-7 area.

Cervical Region

In this example, the cervical region is examined initially in the seated position, followed by treatment in the supine position.

Findings

The first cervical vertebra (atlas) is limited in head and neck rotation left.

Diagnostic Procedure

Position No. 1
The patient is seated; the practitioner stands behind the patient.

1. With the left hand, contact the frontal-parietal region, palm frontal, with fingerpads at the right, thumb at the left.

2. For the rotation test, introduce motion with the left hand. The right hand monitors for restricted motion response to the rotation left, with the third fingerpad of the right hand at the right, thumb at the left, and overlying the facet processes. (Hand placements are reversed to monitor the associated limitations in rotation right at occiput and at C2.)

Position No. 2
The patient is supine; the physician sits at the head of the table as shown in Fig. 61.11.

Positioning of the physician's arms with elbows supported on the knees provides comfortable support of the patient's occiput in the palms of the physician, who then monitors response to introduced motion. The third fingertips overlie cervical articular facets at C1 bilaterally to monitor response. As rotary motion tests continue, C1 responds with initial increasing ease in side bending right and flexion. During respiration, exhalation is easier.

Treatment Procedure

1. (the patient is supine) To small amounts of each of the three directions of rotary ease, add translatory components (of the

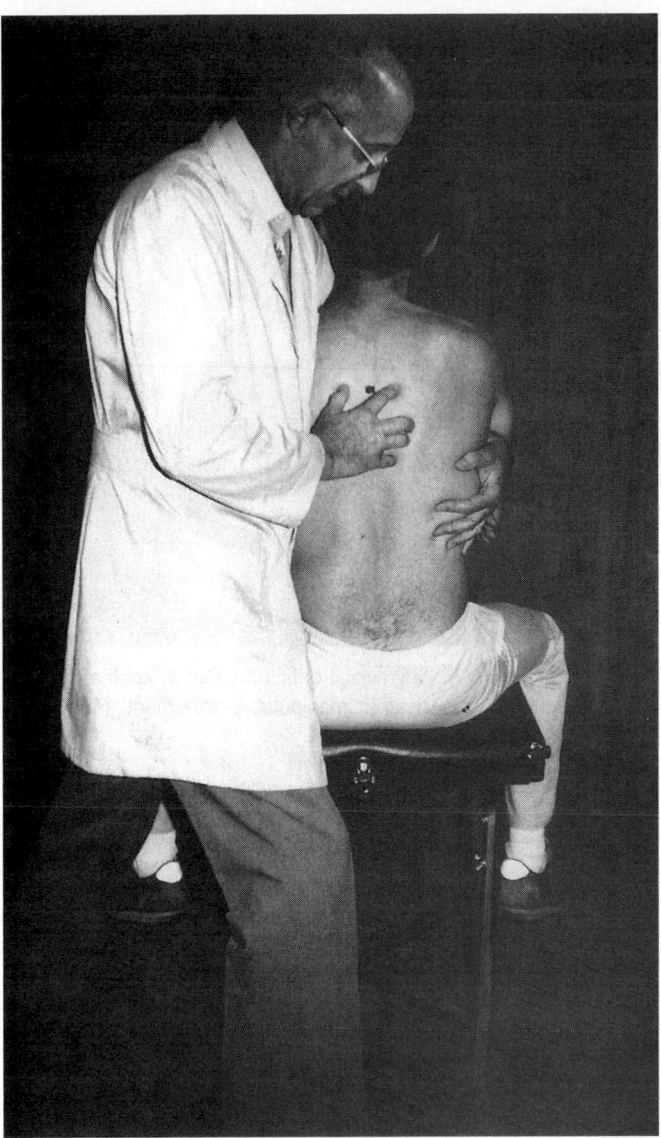

FIGURE 61.9. Positioning of patient and physician to facilitate initial introduction of combined three rotary components toward a sense of increasing compliance (ease) in extension, left side bending, and left rotation. (From Johnston WL. Segmental definition, part II: application of an indirect method in osteopathic manipulative treatment. *JAOA.* 1988;88:211–217, with permission.)

Costal Region

When diagnosing the motor functions of ribs, it is significant to recognize that their elementary function is respiratory. Ribs also function, however, within the context of routine gross body movements that involve the thoracic spine and cage. Therefore, rib function is examined with the patient in the seated position with fingertip contact over the rib angle to monitor a rib's response to the spinal test pattern of elementary passive gross movements (rotations and translations), as well as active respiration. In principle, costal mobile units also function in association with movement of the upper extremities. Recognizing their intermediary role in so much of the body's movement suggests that costal dysfunctions may show more complex characteristics of motor asymmetry because they have one major motor function (inspiratory/expiratory) and two subsidiary motor roles active in trunk and appendicular movement.

This complexity becomes evident when the palpatory characteristics of costal motor asymmetries are identified. There appears to be an element of simplicity, however, in the manner in which that asymmetry is organized. The primary movement of the ribs occurs in inhalation and exhalation. It is this respiratory primacy that appears to dictate the remaining characteristics of the total motor asymmetry when a rib becomes dysfunctional.

For example, if a primary costal defect is freer during exhalation and resists inhalation, this respiratory feature distinctively patterns the motor dysfunction of that rib. This becomes apparent when tested through the shoulders and trunk, with the patient seated, and through the ipsilateral arm with the patient in the lateral recumbent position. However, if the dysfunctional rib is freer during inhalation and resists exhalation, then the asymmetric pattern of this rib's motor function is largely reversed from that of the preceding (exhalation) example.

Ribs are also involved in asymmetric motor function associated with afferent input from visceral disease. This distinctive category of a viscerosomatic component needs consideration separate from the two dysfunctions to be detailed here. They arise more strictly from the physical stresses incurred in this somatic region.

The following two examples illustrate the most common kinds of dysfunction in the rib cage (essentially somatic in origin, rather than visceral). One shows elementary limitation on exhalation; one is limited in inhalation. The predominance of bucket-handle or pump-handle motion during the inspiratory and expiratory function varies throughout the rib cage and is not considered in these examples. Instead, each example is concerned with monitoring a rib's response to specific demands for rotary and translatory aspects of passive motion tests. These are introduced through the shoulders and trunk of the seated patient and through the ipsilateral upper extremity when the patient is in the lateral recumbent position. Each example of treatment has two procedural components, one seated and one side lying.

Findings in Example 1

The right rib 3 resists *exhalation*. It predictably resists shoulder/trunk rotation left and side bending left in the seated position,

head in relation to the trunk) in straight-line directions of increasing ease to the left, posterior, and caudal approximation. (Translatory testing in this example has indicated increasing resistance in each opposing direction.)

2. The increasing ease accumulating at C1 during the initial introduction of these six specific elements of motion is enhanced during a directed exhalation.

3. The smooth torsion pathway for final release of tissue tension allows an easy return to a central resting position.

4. Reexamination in the seated position should reveal a return to symmetry in response to head/neck rotation tests including the occiput, C1, and C2.

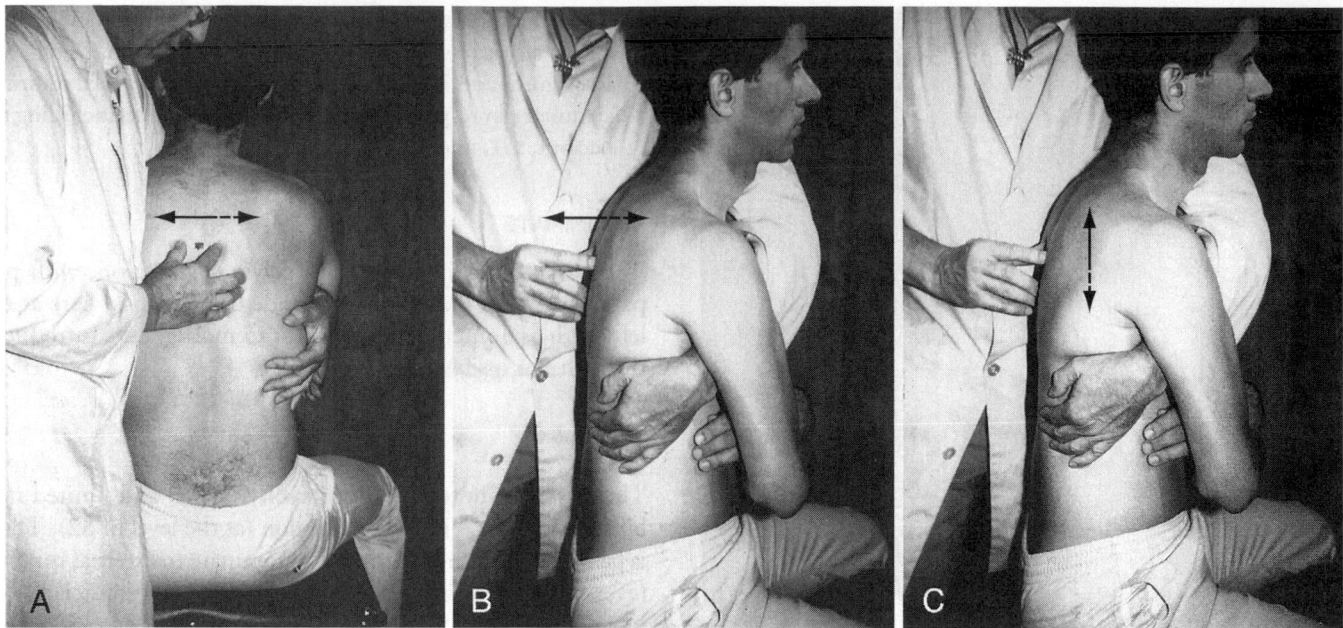

FIGURE 61.10. Translatory motion tests. **A:** Patient in sitting position for comparison of response of T6 to lateral translations of trunk. **B:** Shift in physician's weight initiates anterior and then posterior motion testing at T6. **C:** Testing cephalad/caudad directions. (From Johnston WL. Segmental definition, part II: application of an indirect method in osteopathic manipulative treatment. *JAOA*. 1988;88:211–217, with permission.)

monitored with the right fingertips overlying the rib angle. Testing adjacent ribs above and below demonstrates mirror-image asymmetries if right rib 3 is the primary functional defect.

Procedure No.1: Concurrent Diagnosis and Treatment: Through the Trunk

1. Standing at the right of the seated patient, monitor directions of increasing ease of motion with the left fingers.

2. The right arm is over the patient's right shoulder and under the left to control initiation of motions through shoulders and trunk during side bending and rotation to the right (Fig. 61.12A).

3. Tissue tension and limited mobility continue to improve during initial introduction of backward bending and translations

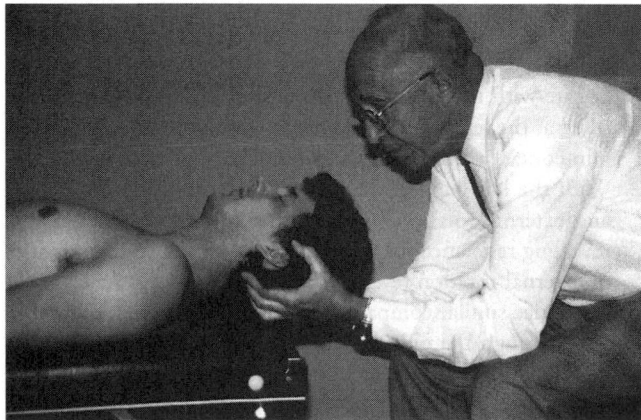

FIGURE 61.11. Supine position for cervical technique.

to the right and anterior. (They worsen during flexion and translations to the left and posterior.)

4. Direct the patient to inhale slowly and hold the inhalation phase momentarily as directions of motion are carefully combined in a smooth torsion arc of movement. This promotes a release and return to a central resting position.

5. Retest shoulder/trunk movements, seated, to assess return to symmetry of these motion components.

Procedure No. 2: Concurrent Diagnosis and Treatment: Through the Upper Extremity

1. The patient is in a left lateral recumbent position. Stand in front of the patient with the patient's right upper arm supported just cephalad to the elbow, as shown in Fig. 61.12B, on the physician's left forearm. The patient's right hand hangs toward the floor.

2. The right fingers overlie the tissue tension/restriction identified at the rib angle and monitor respiratory motion to confirm continuing resistance to exhalation.

3. Palpate for response to motion tests introduced through the patient's right arm. Typical findings include resistance to external rotation (about the long axis of the humerus), abduction, and cephalad movements.

4. In the treatment procedure, monitor increasing ease to internal rotation, adduction, and caudad movements during a directed slow inhalation phase of the patient.

5. Following a successful release, retest the arm motion components in the side-lying position.

6. Following successful release in each of these two treatment components at right rib 3 resisting exhalation, retesting

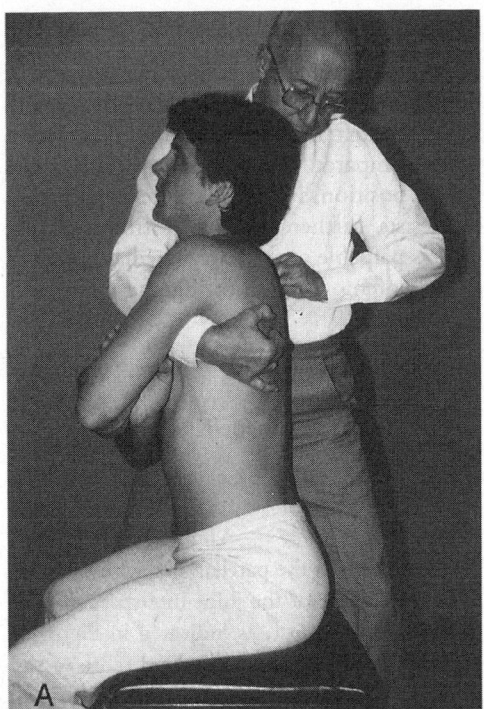

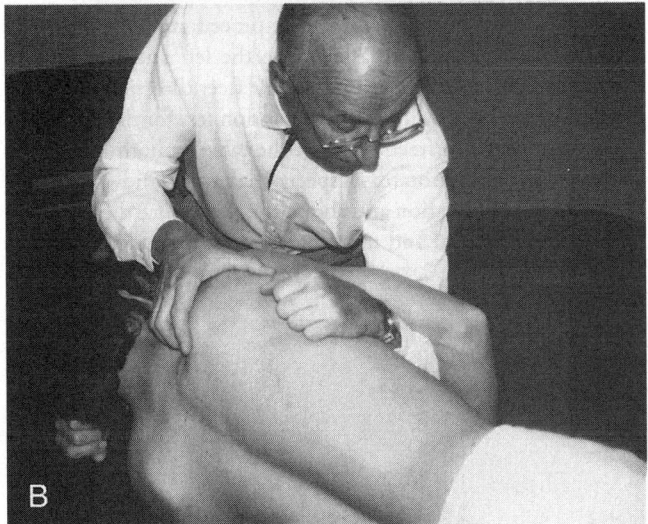

FIGURE 61.12. Example I: Right rib 3 resists exhalation. **A:** In seated position, motions introduced through the shoulder/trunk. **B:** In left side-lying position, motions introduced through the right arm.

throughout right ribs 2, 3, and 4 confirms return to functional symmetry in this area of the rib cage.

Findings in Example 2

Right rib 3 resists *inhalation*. During diagnostic testing, stand on the right to test rotation to the right, and on the left to test rotation to the left. The right rib 3 resisting inhalation predictably resists shoulder/trunk rotation right and side bending right. This is monitored with the left fingertips overlying the rib angle. Testing adjacent ribs above and below demonstrates mirror-image motion asymmetries, if the right rib 3 is the site of the primary dysfunction.

Procedure No.1: Concurrent Diagnosis and Treatment: Through the Trunk

1. Standing at the left of the seated patient, monitor directions of increasing ease of motion with the right fingers.
2. The left arm is over the patient's left shoulder and under the right shoulder to control initiation of motions through the shoulders and trunk during side bending left and rotation to the left, as shown in Fig. 61.13A.
3. Tissue tension and limited mobility continue to improve as you allow initial slouched flexion over the left arm support and translate to the right and posterior. (They worsen during backward bending and translations to the left and anterior.)
4. Direct the patient to exhale slowly and hold the exhalation phase momentarily as directions of motion are carefully combined in a smooth torsion arc of movement to promote a release and return to a central resting position.
5. Retest shoulder/trunk motions in the seated position.

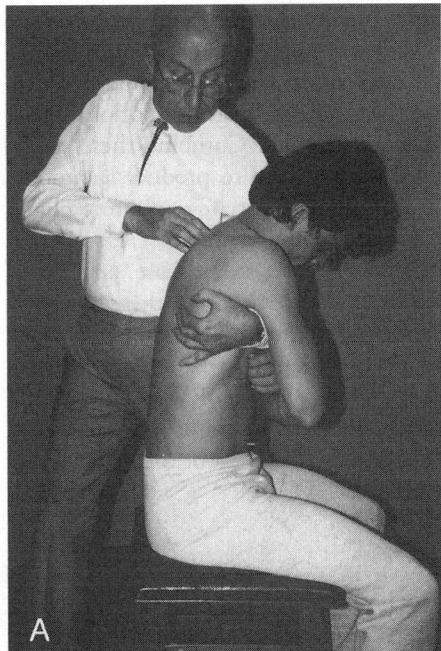

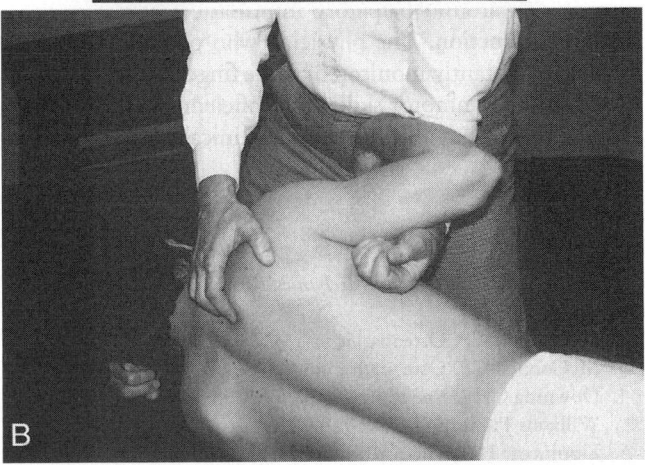

FIGURE 61.13. Example 2: Right rib 3 resists inhalation. **A:** In seated position. **B:** In left side-lying position.

Procedure No.2: Concurrent Diagnosis and Treatment: Through the Upper Extremity

1. The patient is in a left lateral recumbent position. Stand in front of the patient. With the left forearm, support and introduce motion through the patient's right arm, having it relaxed and folded at the elbow as seen in Fig. 61.13B.

2. The right fingers overlie the tissue tension/restriction identified at the rib angle and monitor response to respiratory tests to confirm continuing resistance to inhalation.

3. Palpate for response to motion tests introduced through the patient's right arm. Typical findings include resistance to internal rotation (about the long axis of the humerus), adduction, and caudad movements.

4. In the treatment procedure, monitor increasing ease to external rotation, abduction, and cephalad movements, during a directed slow exhalation phase of the patient.

5. Following release, retest arm motion components in the side-lying position and retest inhalation and exhalation throughout right ribs 2, 3, and 4.

Although the description of these two examples of rib technique (exhalation restriction and inhalation restriction) begin with the seated phase followed by the side lying, the order is not necessarily important and can be optional.

The physician's approach in functional technique is important. Evaluate immediately as each direction of motion is introduced. Combine these minor ranges in each direction, as described, to produce a smooth torsion arc of motion during the appropriate final respiratory phase. This complements the continually monitored response of increasing ease. The palpable tension decreases to a sense of release, and the patient is returned to a resting state. Although these aspects of rib technique are presented as specific directions patterned to inhalation or exhalation restrictions, they should not be applied as if to copy a technique procedure. Rather, test each direction to promote appropriate summation of increasing ease, and monitor decreasing tension throughout each manipulation.

Thoracic Cage: Differentiating Somatic and Visceral Inputs

The spinal cord provides communication pathways that conduct impulses from sensory receptors in both musculoskeletal and visceral tissues. When noxious stimuli are persistent, the afferent bombardment contributes to palpable somatic manifestations of spinal dysfunction. Segmental motion asymmetries develop individuality in their dysfunctional behavior depending on the afferent source, somatic or visceral.

From functional methods in descriptive research, Fig. 61.3 illustrates a three-segment configuration of vertebral motion asymmetries that characterizes somato-somatic reflex activity. The primary dysfunction at the central segment demonstrates a complete asymmetric behavior in response to motion tests introduced through the shoulders and trunk in the seated position; the secondary dysfunctions at adjacent segments display mirror-image (opposing) motion asymmetries. The reflex basis for these secondary mirror images becomes apparent when all three seg-

ments return to motion symmetry following successful response to a functional manipulative procedure that addresses only the central (primary) dysfunctional segment.

In Fig. 61.4, the mirror-image phenomenon is still evident. However, this time it accompanies central segments that present a different primary orientation. The primacy relates to a vertebra and one adjacent rib at the same spinal level presenting *identical* motor asymmetries, rather than opposing. The term *linkage* applies to this phenomenon, because both vertebra and rib respond to motion tests in identical fashion, as if they were now linked together as a single mobile unit. This dysfunctional unit's motion asymmetry is typically complete in rotary, translatory, and respiratory tests; secondary mirror images exist at the adjacent coupled segments, as indicated.

Clinical data from interexaminer (31) and longitudinal (32,33) studies with hypertensive subjects, as well as a controlled clinical trial with renal, hypertensive, and normotensive subjects (21) have supported the presence of linkage as a somatic manifestation of visceral disease. The characteristic motion asymmetries at several linkage sites are reproducible, and have been reported (20).

Manipulative treatment at a linkage site requires attention to two aspects of the motion behavior disturbed at such a dysfunctional costovertebral level. The segmental locus demonstrates not only asymmetry to spinal motion tests in the seated position induced through the shoulders/trunk, but also in recumbent positions to motion tests introduced through the lower extremities. A manipulative approach to address the former behavior has been detailed for both diagnostic and treatment procedures, seated, in the preceding thoracic section of "Examples of Functional Technique." However, maximum response at a linkage site also demands attention to motion behaviors related to the lower extremities (34). An example of diagnostic and treatment procedures follows.

Findings

Examined in the seated position, the patient has segmental dysfunction at spinal level T5, with linkage to left rib 5, and resistance to inhalation locally (and to exhalation at adjacent segments above and below). There is also resistance to anterior translation, monitored at tissues overlying the transverse processes at T5 and the angle of left rib 5. Under these circumstances, positioning the patient prone (rather than supine) enhances posterior translation and begins to decrease the palpable tension locally, as a first step in a functional procedure (35). The physician now stands at the left of the prone patient, as illustrated in Fig. 61.14. With both legs initially resting on the table, begin with the right leg resting semiflexed. With plantar contacts of your right hand at the patient's right heel, control for the introduction of inversion and eversion motion tests of the whole right limb. Monitoring responses with the left hand in contact at the T5 left linkage site will reveal immediately increasing resistance to *both* directions initiated. Similar testing with the left leg will reveal *asymmetric* behavior; for example, with eversion there is once again resistance, while with inversion there is increasing compliance.

Note: For linked segments in the thoracic region, this characteristic behavior during lower extremity tests is typical, in that

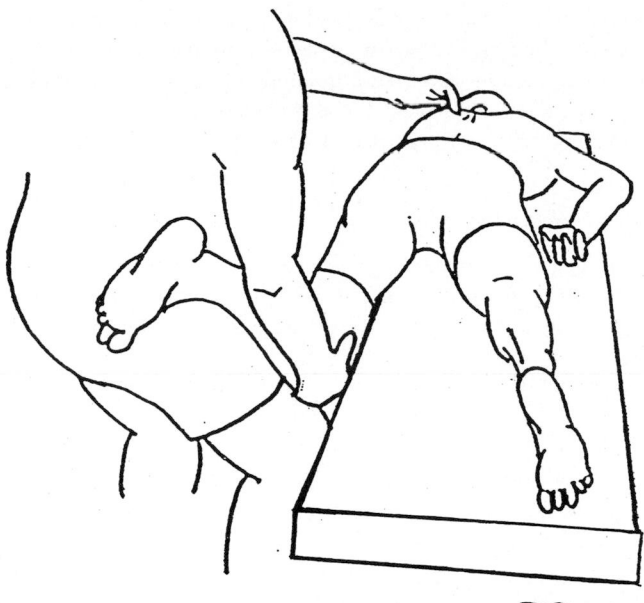

FIGURE 61.14. Examination of linkage left site at T5 spinal level leads to treatment, prone, involving specific motion directions introduced through the ipsilateral lower extremity. With appropriate control by right hand support at the left knee, the operator monitors response at the left hand contacting the linked costovertebral segments. (From Johnston WL. Segmental definition, part IV. Updating the differential for somatic and visceral inputs. *JAOA.* 2001;5:278–283, with permission.)

responses are asymmetric to tests with the leg ipsilateral to the linked costal component, while resistance is present in both responses to tests with the contralateral leg.

Procedure: Concurrent Diagnosis and Treatment of Costovertebral Linkage

Engage support at the knee for control of the patient's left leg semiflexed as illustrated in Fig. 61.14. Maintaining slight inversion freedom, monitor responses at the T5 linkage site to compare inversion with eversion, flexion with extension and cephalad with caudad directions of the limb. Select and combine initial aspects of these other elementary directions of increasing ease. In Fig. 61.14, abduction of the limb laterally from the table, flexion, and caudad directions are combined. With the finding of resistance to inhalation, the final decrease in palpable tension is maximized during a slow exhalation phase to release, followed by return of the leg to natural positioning on the table. When successful, repeating the diagnostic tests involved with each leg will reveal a return to symmetry in these aspects of the dysfunctional behavior at T5.

Note: Apart from the linkage phenomenon, as recognized in the costovertebral region, an additional distinctive characteristic of visceral input is now applicable for those spinal levels lacking costal components, that is, in cervical, lumbar, and sacral regions. Our continuing interest in examination of viscerosomatic linkage sites has led to a descriptive study. The following excerpt details that characteristic:

For example, consider any non-linked dysfunctional vertebral or costal segment that shows increased resistance to the seated test for

sidebending right as compared with left, introduced through the shoulders/trunk. In such an instance, an expectation also exists for increased resistance to sidebending right compared with left when introduced through the head/neck. However, segments involved in linkage do not show accord in response to these two apparently similar sidebending tests. Instead, segmental resistance to sidebending *right* through the shoulders/trunk will accompany resistance to sidebending *left* introduced through the head/neck. *This lack of accord serves as a convenient tool for use in differential diagnosis of active visceral influence in any spinal region dysfunction* (34) [author's italics added for emphasis].

Comment: Regarding Somatic Manifestations of Visceral Input

When spinal analysis identifies a site with palpable signs positive for visceral input, the search for the source of the visceral input narrows somewhat, based on the known distribution of visceral afferent pathways via dorsal routes (36,37). Further, the palpable characteristics of the spinal tissue changes presented at a site of visceral input bear directly on the time element involved. When historically connecting possibly relevant incidents of illness, recent/current paravertebral soft tissue changes trend toward aspects of local prominence and congestion. On the contrary, when related illness is long-standing/recurrent, there is a depressed area of the spinal musculature overlying the transverse processes at the vertebral site central to the visceral input. This sparse, deep, horizontal band of markedly increased tissue tension reflects the hypoxia associated with tissues that are subjected to prolonged, concentrated reflex action. In time, this action will be both primary visceral and secondary somatic, since the spinal dysfunction once initiated continues as a focus for motion stress, and becomes self-maintaining within continuing demands of the motor system.

Innominate

The patient has an elementary kind of pelvic dysfunction, one with palpatory findings localized to one side of the pelvis, with asymmetric response to motion tests introduced through only the ipsilateral lower extremity (and no resistance encountered with tests introduced through the contralateral limb).

Findings

There is a tissue texture abnormality (TTA) and limited mobility at the left ilium/gluteal region (at the level of S2). There is palpable resistance at the left innominate to external rotation (eversion) of the left lower limb.

Diagnostic Procedure

1. The patient is supine, with the left knee semiflexed and the foot resting on the table; the physician stands at the patient's left.
2. Locate with the right hand the area of TTA and limited mobility at the left ilium/gluteal region, at the S2 level, and maintain contact throughout the procedure.

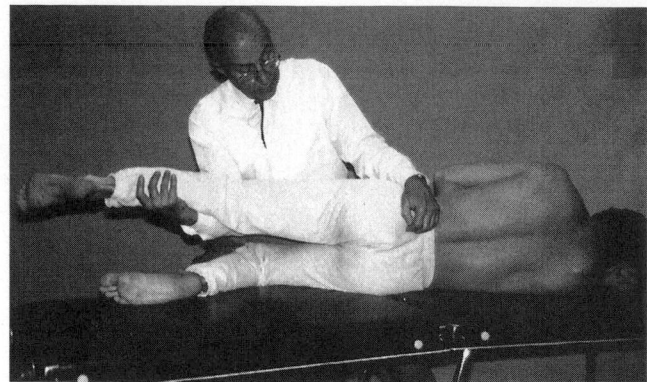

FIGURE 61.15. Right lateral recumbent position for left innominate technique.

3. With the left hand at the patient's left knee, initiate internal and external rotation (moving knee toward right, then left), revealing resistance palpated at the right hand to the initiation of external rotation (eversion).

4. Introduce similar comparison of internal and external rotation tests through the right semiflexed limb, but monitor it at the right hand, revealing left innominate compliance to both directions of the test.

Treatment Procedure

1. Position the patient right lateral recumbent. Stand in front, with left hand contact at the innominate, TTA at level S2 (Fig. 61.15). Direct the patient to shift the pelvis slightly in anterior translation relative to the shoulders. Maintain this positional shift if this direction decreases tension at the S2 level, compared with posterior translation.

2. With your right hand supporting the patient's knees, introduce flexion through both legs together to localize action at the S2 sacral level monitored by the left hand.

3. Now alter your support to the left leg only (Fig. 61.15), with the right hand/forearm to monitor (in this example) the increasing ease at your left hand in response to abduction of the limb (versus adduction), backward bending (versus flexion), and caudal traction (versus cephalad). Each of these components is combined during introduction of internal rotation (external rotation is resisted).

4. Direct the patient in inhalation (the direction of ease of the TTA).

5. During the final component of directed inhalation ease, combine these directional elements appropriately to achieve a palpable sense of decreasing tension and then a release by the holding forces. Return the limb to its resting position with the patient in lateral recumbency.

6. Reexamining the motion tests supine indicates a return to symmetry of response at the left innominate, with reduced tissue tension of the left gluteal musculature.

Variations in the findings from those described for this example simply require application of elementary motion testing procedures at a diagnosed focus of TTA, and restricted mobility, wherever these are evident on pelvic structural examination (35). Specific directions of positioning and motion are then applied in a controlled manner to the pelvic location diagnosed, to ease increasingly the holding forces of restricted motor function.

Appendicular Regions

Note: There is a continuing application of principle here as the physician maintains use of the six elementary motions and respiration as functional tools for testing and reducing specific dysfunction in an appendage.

Findings

In this example, the left knee fails to hyperextend. On examination in the supine position with the physician standing at the left side, the left knee lies slightly raised from the table surface when compared with the right. In this uncomfortable, slightly flexed position, it is tenser to palpation than the right and resists further passively introduced extension. A prominence is palpable at the anteromedial border of the joint interspace (tibiofemoral), indicating the edge of the medial semilunar cartilage.

Position

The patient is supine and the left knee is flexed; stand by the left side of the table.

Procedures: Concurrent Diagnosis and Treatment

1. The right palm spans the patellar area with the thumb following the lateral aspect of the joint interspace. The third finger follows the medial aspect, as indicated in Fig. 61.16. This hand is keyed sharply to the distorted sense of rigid binding resistance

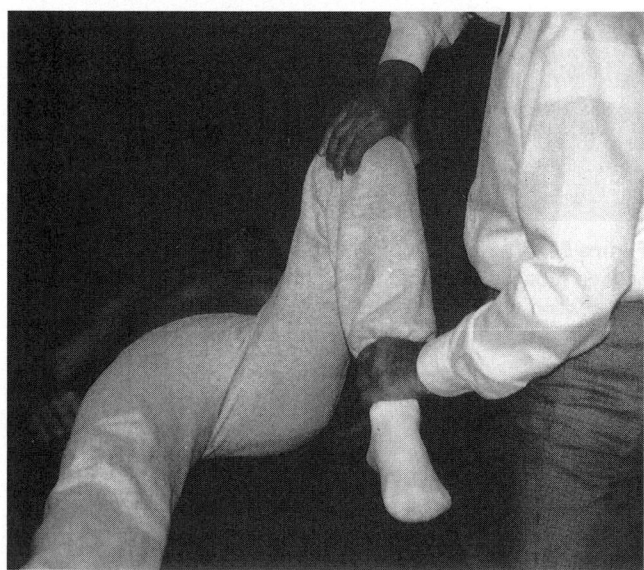

FIGURE 61.16. Appendicular example at the left knee. Right hand monitors and supports. Left hand introduces major motions in testing and treatment.

where it is most apparent. Keep the contact light enough to appreciate this palpable marker, yet firm enough in grasp to assist in the manipulative procedure.

2. The left hand firmly grasps above the left ankle to assist in slowly bringing the knee up into the freer direction of flexion.

3. Explore additional directions of motion test for the limb while it is supported in freedom from the table by both hands: these motions address the other rotary aspects, which are found to be freer in medial rotation and abduction. Begin the introduction of these motions with the left hand and monitor response with the right.

4. Maintain the initial introduction of rotary components.

5. While still monitoring response at the knee, the tests using translatory directions for the limb indicate increasing ease anterior, above the table (binding posterior), increasing ease to the left (compared with right), and cephalad (with binding in caudal traction). The respiratory test indicates easier response to inhalation.

6. In the final maneuver, the right hand contact at the knee guides the lifting support anteriorly to the left, while the left hand controls the amount of each rotary motion in a cephalad direction via the distal tibiofibular contact. There is a proportionately larger amount of flexion introduced, guided by the sense of continuing increasing ease. (This aspect of the knee's template of motion has the greatest range.)

7. Direct the patient to slowly exhale to promote the final release of holding forces. Mobility then allows an easier return into improved extension range as the leg is guided back down onto the table.

CONCLUSION

The term functional technique applies to an indirect method of osteopathic manipulation in which the treatment procedure is organized around palpatory information gained from tests for motor function. By paying attention to the feedback constantly monitored by the fingertips, the physician will experience improved psychomotor skill and proficiency in the use of this treatment method, and in many other clinical procedures as well.

REFERENCES

1. Ashmore EF. *Osteopathic Mechanics.* Kirksville, MO: Journal Printing Co; 1915:72.
2. McConnell CP. Osteopathic art, V. *JAOA.* 1935;34:369–374.
3. McConnell CP. Osteopathic studies, IV. *JAOA.* 1931;31:206–212.
4. Downing CH. *Principles and Practice of Osteopathy.* Kansas City, MO: Williams Publishing Co; 1923:162.
5. Lippincott HA. The osteopathic technique of Wm. G. Sutherland, D.O. In: Northup TL, ed. *Yearbook of the Academy of Applied Osteopathy.* Ann Arbor, MI: Edwards Brothers Inc; 1949:124.
6. Hoover HV. Fundamentals of technique. In: *Yearbook of the Academy of Applied Osteopathy.* Ann Arbor, MI: Edwards Brothers Inc; 1949:25–41.
7. Hoover HV, Nelson CR. Basic physiologic movements of the spine. In: *Academy of Applied Osteopathy Year Book.* Ann Arbor, MI: Cushing-Malloy Inc; 1950:65.
8. Bowles CH. A functional orientation for technic. In: Page LE, ed. *Yearbook of the Academy of Applied Osteopathy.* Carmel, CA: Academy of Applied Osteopathy; Indianapolis, IN: American Academy of Osteopathy; 1955:177–191.
9. Lippincott HA. Basic principles of osteopathic technique. In: Barnes MW, ed. *Yearbook of the Academy of Applied Osteopathy.* Carmel, CA: Academy of Applied Osteopathy; Indianapolis, IN: American Academy of Osteopathy; 1961:45–48.
10. Jones LH. Spontaneous release by positioning. *The DO.* 1964;4:109–116.
11. Johnston WL. Interexaminer reliability studies. Spanning a gap in medical research. *JAOA.* 1982;81:819–829.
12. Johnston WL. Passive gross motion testing, part 1: its role in physical examination. *JAOA.* 1982;81:298–303.
13. Johnston WL, Hill JL. Spinal segmental dysfunction: incidence in cervicothoracic region. *JAOA.* 1981;81:67–76.
14. Johnston WL, Kelso AF, Hollandsworth DL, Karrat J. Somatic manifestations in renal disease: a clinical research study. *JAOA.* 1987;87:22–35.
15. Kelso AF, Grant RG, Johnston WL. Use of thermograms to support assessment of somatic dysfunction or effects of osteopathic manipulative treatment. *JAOA.* 1982;82:182–188.
16. Johnston WL. Segmental definition, part I: a focal point for diagnosis of somatic dysfunction. *JAOA.* 1988;88:99–105.
17. Johnston WL. Segmental definition, part II: application of an indirect method in osteopathic manipulative treatment. *JAOA.* 1988;88:211–217.
18. Johnston WL. Segmental behavior during motions, 1: a palpatory study of somatic relations. *JAOA.* 1972;72:352–361.
19. Johnston WL, Hill JL. Spinal segmental dysfunction: incidence in cervicothoracic region. *JAOA.* 1981;81:22–28.
20. Johnston WL. Segmental definition, part III: definitive basis for distinguishing somatic findings of visceral reflex origin. *JAOA.* 1988;88:347–353.
21. Johnston WL, Kelso AF, Hollandsworth DL, Karrat J. Somatic manifestations in renal disease: a clinical research study. *JAOA.* 1987;87:22–35.
22. Johnston WL, Friedman HD. *Functional Methods: A Manual for Palpatory Skill Development in Osteopathic Examination and Manipulation of Motor Function.* Indianapolis, IN: American Academy of Osteopathy; 1995:44–45.
23. Bowles CH. A functional orientation for technic. In: Page LE, ed. *Yearbook of the Academy of Applied Osteopathy.* Carmel, CA: Academy of Applied Osteopathy; 1955:177–191.
24. Bowles CH. Functional technique: a modern perspective. *JAOA.* 1981;80:326–331.
25. Stein PSG. Motor systems, with specific reference to the control of locomotion. *Ann Rev Neurosci.* 1978;1:61–81.
26. Getting PA. Emerging principles governing the operation of neural networks. *Ann Rev Neurosci.* 1989;12:185–204.
27. Atsuta Y, Garcia-Rill E, Skinner RD. Characteristics of electrically induced locomotion in rat in vitro brain stem-spinal cord preparation. *J Neurophysiol.* 1990;64:727–735.
28. Johnston WL. Segmental definition, part II: application of an indirect method in osteopathic manipulative treatment. *JAOA.* 1988;88:211–217.
29. Henneman E. Organization of the spinal cord and its reflexes. In: Mountcastle VB, ed. *Medical Physiology,* 14th ed. Vol 1. St. Louis, MO: CV Mosby; 1980:762–786.
30. Johnston WL. Osteopathic clinical aspects of somatovisceral interaction. In: Patterson MM, Howell JH, eds. *The Central Connection: Somatovisceral/Viscerosomatic Interaction.* Indianapolis, IN: American Academy of Osteopathy; 1992.
31. Johnston WL, Hill JL, Elkiss ML, Marino RV. Identification of stable somatic findings in hypertensive subjects by trained examiners using palpatory examination. *JAOA.* 1982;81:830–836.
32. Johnston WL, Kelso AF, Babcock HB. Changes in presence of a segmental dysfunction pattern associated with hypertension, part I: a short-term longitudinal study. *JAOA.* 1995;4:243–255.
33. Johnston WL, Kelso AF. Changes in presence of a segmental dysfunction pattern associated with hypertension, part II: a long-term longitudinal study. *JAOA.* 1995;5:315–318.

34. Johnston WL, Golden WJ. Segmental definition, part IV: updating the differential for somatic and visceral inputs. *JAOA.* 2001;5:278–283.

35. Johnston WL, Friedman HD. *Functional Methods: A Manual for Palpatory Skill Development in Osteopathic Examination and Manipulation of Motor Function.* Indianapolis, IN: The American Academy of Osteopathy; 1995:83–91.

36. Beal MC. Viscerosomatic reflexes: a review. *JAOA.* 1985;12:786–801.

37. Johnston WL, Friedman HD. *Functional Methods: A Manual for Palpatory Skill Development in Osteopathic Examination and Manipulation of Motor Function.* Indianapolis, IN: The American Academy of Osteopathy; 1995:135–137.

OSTEOPATHY IN THE CRANIAL FIELD

HOLLIS H. KING
EDNA M. LAY

KEY CONCEPTS

- History of osteopathy in the cranial field, including the contribution of William G. Sutherland
- The primary respiratory mechanism
- Research indicative of primary respiratory mechanisms
- The mechanics of physiologic motion
- Strains
- Diagnosis via history, observation, and palpation
- Clinical problems requiring treatment
- Principles of treatment

During my years in practice as an osteopathic physician, there never has been one regret for having chosen this field for my life's work. Professional experience daily demonstrates the truth that the Science of Osteopathy includes the key to the great physiological chemical laboratory, the human body, unlocking the living potent forces that heal. To the student looking forward to a professional field of scientific research, and with the desire in his or her heart to render beneficial service to humanity, let me truly say: Osteopathy Provides The Golden Opportunity.

—W.G. SUTHERLAND, DO

Osteopathy is a philosophy, a science, and an art. The study of osteopathy in the cranial field (OCF) offers a unique perspective on all three areas. Through persistent study of the intricate osseous armor that protects the brain and spinal cord, keen observation, and a compassionate dedication to relieve human suffering, William Garner Sutherland, DO, made a significant discovery about the central nervous system that is important in osteopathy today.

HISTORY

William G. Sutherland, DO, DSc (Hon) (1873–1954) was an early student of Dr. A.T. Still. Sutherland graduated from the American School of Osteopathy in Kirksville, Missouri in 1899. While a student, he observed a mounted disarticulated skull. The sphenoid and the squamous portions of the temporal bones caught his attention, and he remembers:

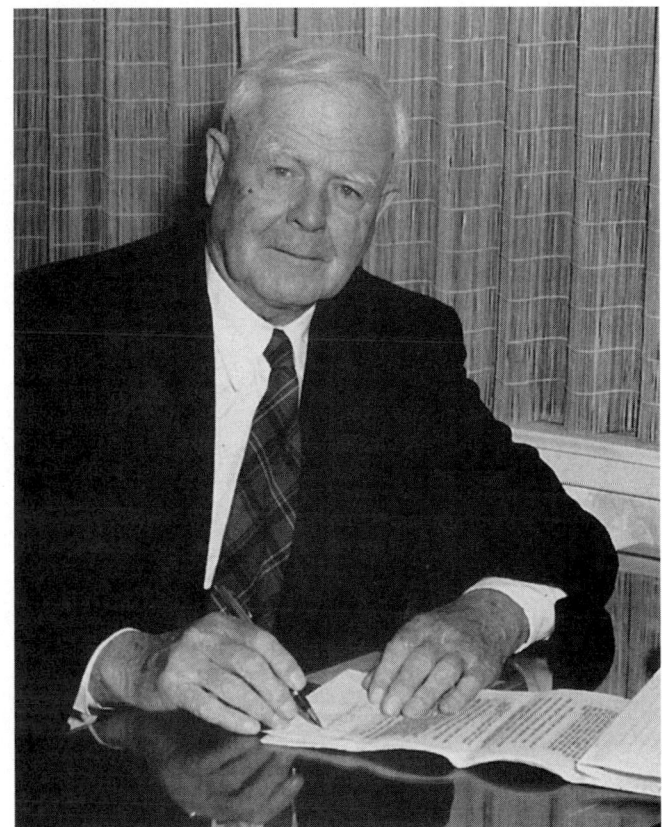

William G. Sutherland, DO, DSc (Hon)

As I stood looking and thinking in the channel of Dr. Still's philosophy, my attention was called to the beveled articular surfaces of the sphenoid bone. Suddenly there came a thought; I call it a guiding thought—beveled like the gills of a fish, indicating articular mobility for a respiratory mechanism (1).

He dismissed the thought but it kept returning, as if goading him to study the details of the various articulations of the skull.

Sutherland was an original thinker, and his application of Still's philosophy is recognized as "one of the most innovative ideas to be advanced by a member of the osteopathic profession" (2). Anatomy books at that time stated that the sutures of the cranium were immovable. This, however, did not deter Sutherland. He was determined to understand why the articular surfaces have such a unique design, and he persevered until he understood that the design was accommodative to the function of the central nervous system (CNS), cerebrospinal fluid (CSF), and dural membranes, all of which function as a unit. He named this functional unit the primary respiratory mechanism (PRM).

Sutherland established his practice in Minnesota and devoted 30 years to study, original research on himself, and observation of his patients before he began to share his discovery with his colleagues. The remarkable results he obtained with patients aroused the interest of other physicians. They prevailed on him at his home to teach them his method of treatment. The classes and the interest grew, slowly but steadily, because those who were able to learn the concept and apply this method of osteopathic diagnosis and treatment had similar results of relieving patients of pain and distressful conditions when other forms of treatment failed to help.

As more physicians studied and practiced this method of osteopathic treatment, they formed an organization, the Osteopathic Cranial Association, for the purpose of joining together to promote further study, support research, and publish literature to help educate physicians and laypersons. This membership organization later changed its name to the Cranial Academy and became a component society of the American Academy of Osteopathy.

In 1953 Dr. Sutherland, with Drs. C. Handy and H. Magoun, Sr, established the Sutherland Cranial Teaching Foundation, Inc., for the purpose of continuing the teaching of the cranial concept. Dr. Sutherland had established that an accurate diagnosis and successful treatment required sensitive and proficient palpation that could not be learned from a book; expert instructors using hands-on teaching and repeated verification were needed.

Dr. Still's teachings also provided these basic principles:

- The body functions as a unit
- The body possesses self-regulatory and self-healing mechanisms
- Structure and function are reciprocally interrelated
- Rational treatment is based on application of these three principles

Dr. Sutherland's discovery and teachings have supplied knowledge and methods that clarify and expand on the science of osteopathy. Prior to Dr. Sutherland's work, the body was treated as if the head was incapable of having somatic dysfunction.

OCF is osteopathy of the entire person because the inherent force that manifests from within the head region functions throughout the body; therefore, this form of diagnosis and treatment affects the whole person rather than being limited to the cranium. Furthermore, the position of the head atop the vertebral column affects the postural balance of the entire neuromusculoskeletal system. For example, if the cranial bone structures have been brought into a state of imbalance through trauma, the cranium will cause compensatory changes throughout the neuromusculoskeletal system in order to keep the equilibrium apparatus efficient in its function.

The insights and techniques derived by Dr. Sutherland's expansion of basic osteopathic principles are increasingly integrated into osteopathic teaching and care (3–5). *The International*

Classification of Disease, Ninth Revision (ICD-9) delineates coding for somatic dysfunction of the cranium. Competency testing of osteopathic manipulative treatment (OMT) to treat this dysfunction is available to nonspecialists and specialists alike. In recent years, the American Osteopathic Association (AOA) has received numerous research grant proposals from both clinicians and basic scientists to study the mechanisms and/or efficacy of this approach; the AOA has funded several of these projects (6–10).

Instruction in OCF, also commonly referred to as cranial osteopathy (CO), has been a part of standard training in departments of osteopathic principles, practice, and manipulative medicine in all osteopathic medical schools. Concepts and terminology pertaining to OCF/CO have been developed and defined by the Educational Council on Osteopathic Principles (ECOP) of the American Association of Colleges of Osteopathic Medicine (AACOM). They have been published in the Glossary of Osteopathic Medical Terminology which appears annually in AOA's *Yearbook and Directory of Osteopathic Physicians* (11).

As the federally recognized accrediting body for residency training programs within the osteopathic medical profession, the AOA has approved the *Basic Standards for Residency Training in Neuromusculoskeletal Medicine and Osteopathic Manipulative Treatment*. OCF/CO is one of the OMT models within these basic standards. The AOA also is the federally recognized body charged with approval of certifying boards within the osteopathic medical profession. The AOA has chartered the American Osteopathic Board of Neuromusculoskeletal Medicine. This certifying board administers written, oral, and practical examinations that include items relating to OCF/CO.

PRIMARY RESPIRATORY MECHANISM

Primary refers to first in importance; Dr. Sutherland considered thoracic respiration secondary to the PRM. By this he meant that the physiologic centers that control and regulate pulmonary respiration, circulation, digestion, and elimination are located in the floor of the fourth ventricle and depend on the function of the CNS (12). Respiratory refers to the exchange of gases and other metabolites at the cellular level. Mechanism implies an integrated machine, each part in working relationship to every other part. The PRM is described as having five anatomic-physiologic components, described in the following sections.

Inherent Motility of Brain and Spinal Cord

The inherent motion of the CNS is a subtle, slow, pulse-wavelike movement. It is described as having a biphasic cycle, which may have a rhythmic nature. The entire CNS shortens and thickens during one phase and lengthens and thins during the other (12). As the cerebral hemispheres develop in fetal life, they grow, lengthen, and curl or coil within the developing cranium in the shape of a pair of ram's horns. This embryologic development may account for the anatomic and physiologic processes producing the specific motion characteristics described as the PRM is palpated. In words still relevant today Lassek described the brain as being "vibrantly alive ... incessantly active ... dynamic

...highly mobile, able to move forward, backward, sideward, circumduct and to rotate." He further stated:

> The normal, human brain is a wondrous, enormously complex, master organ which can be only made by nature. There are probably approximately twenty billion neurons in the central nervous system of man and it runs on a mere 25 watts of electrical power (12).

Fluctuation of Cerebrospinal Fluid

The CSF is formed by the choroid plexuses and circulates through the ventricles, over and around the surface of the brain and spinal cord through the subarachnoid spaces and cisternae. Thus, the CSF is inside and outside of the CNS, bathing, protecting, and nourishing it. Fluctuation is defined as a wavelike motion of fluid in a natural or artificial cavity of the body observed by palpation or percussion (13). From the perspective of Sutherland's concept of the PRM, as the CNS shortens and lengthens in a biphasic rhythmic motion, the ventricles of the brain change shape slightly and the fluid moves concurrently. Furthermore, the combined motility of the CNS and the fluctuation of CSF manifests as a hydrodynamic activity as well as a bioelectric interchange throughout the body. Stated simply, this combined activity of the CNS and CSF functions both as a pump and as an electric generator.

Mobility of Intracranial and Intraspinal Membranes

The meninges surround, support, and protect the CNS. The dura mater, the outermost of the three coverings, is composed of two layers of tough fibrous tissue. The outer layer of dura mater lines the cranial cavity, forming a periosteal covering for the inner aspect of the bones, and extends through the sutures of the skull to become the periosteum on the outer surface of the skull.

The inner layer of dura mater covers the brain and spinal cord and has reduplications named the falx cerebri and the tentorium cerebelli. These sickle-shaped structures arise from a common origin along the straight sinus and invest the various bones of the cranium. The two layers of dura mater are blended or fused in certain areas and are separated in other areas, forming the intradural venous sinuses.

The dura mater extends down the spinal canal with firm attachment around the foramen magnum, to C2 and C3, and to the lower lumbar and sacrum at the level of the second segment. The falx cerebri arises from the straight sinus, attaching to the occiput, parietals, frontals, and the crista galli of the ethmoid. The two halves of the tentorium cerebelli arise or originate at the straight sinus and attach to the occiput, temporals, and sphenoid bone.

The spinal and cranial dura and its reduplications respond to the inherent motion of the CNS and fluctuation of CSF and move through the biphasic cycle, influencing the bones of the cranium and the sacrum. Sutherland named this functional anatomic unit, consisting of the dura mater within the cranium and spinal canal, the reciprocal tension membrane (RTM) (12). It has also been referred to as the core link (12) because it transmits forces by linking the cranium to the sacrum. Influences such as trauma and postural strains that affect one part of the mechanism have been clinically observed to affect the entire unit of function.

Articular Mobility of Cranial Bones

The most dramatic and debated phenomenon of the PRM has been the articular mobility of the cranial bones. Careful study of the design of the various articulations of the cranium and face and the RTM and its influence on the motion of the bones led Sutherland to an understanding of the mechanical design and relationship of the inherent motility of the CNS and CSF. At birth, the cranial bones are smooth-edged osseous plates with membrane and/or cartilage between them. With growth and motion the edges of the plates develop sutures between them that develop in a way that allows for a minimal amount of motion and yet provides protection for the brain. The debate and research are reported subsequently.

Involuntary Mobility of Sacrum Between Ilia

The cranial dura is continuous with the spinal dura; the spinal dura extends through the vertebral canal into the sacral canal, attaching at the level of some lumbar segments and the second sacral segment. Careful study of the design of the articular surfaces reveals that the sacrum may move on one or several postural axes in relation to the ilia (pelvic bones). In addition to these voluntary or postural movements, the sacrum also responds to the inherent motility of the CNS, to the fluctuation of the CSF, and to the pull of the intracranial and intraspinal membranes with an involuntary movement that can be observed by palpation in the living body. This slight rocking motion occurs around a transverse axis (called the respiratory axis). Normally, the involuntary motion of the sacrum is synchronous with the involuntary motion of the occiput, each bone being influenced by the rhythmic pull of the spinal and cranial dura mater.

Appreciation of the five phenomena of the PRM in theoretical and practical terms requires an integration of the anatomic and physiologic factors substantiated by empirical research, and experience-derived applications discussed subsequently. Try to visualize this physiologic unit of function with all five components moving slightly but steadily in the living body from before birth until death. Becker (14) summarizes its influence on the total body economy as follows:

> Health requires that the PRM have the capacity to be an involuntary, rhythmic, automatic, shifting suspension mechanism for the intricate, integrated, dynamic interrelationships of its five elements. It is intimately related to the rest of the body through its fascial connections from the base of the skull through the cervical, thoracic, abdominal, pelvic, and appendicular areas of the body physiology. Since all of the involuntary and voluntary systems of the body, including the musculoskeletal system, are found in fascial envelopes, they, too, are subjected to the 10 to 14 cycle-per-minute rhythm of the craniosacral mechanism in addition to their own rhythms of involuntary and voluntary activity. The involuntary mobility of the craniosacral mechanism moves all the tissues of the body minutely into rhythmic flexion of the midline structures with external rotation of the bilateral structures and, in the opposite cycle, extension of the midline structures with internal rotation of the bilateral structures 10 to 14 times per minute throughout life.

RESEARCH INDICATIVE OF THE PRIMARY RESPIRATORY MECHANISM

Inherent Motility of Brain and Spinal Cord: Research

Since Lassek's time, much research has confirmed the inherent motility of the brain and spinal cord. Greitz and colleagues (15) offer diagrams of the brain movement and describe motion in certain areas in the range of 1.0 mm to 1.5 mm. While their concern, in part, was how this motion affects the clarity of magnetic resonance imaging, the evidence of substantial motion is well documented. Feinberg and Mark (16) report the velocity in the anterior cortex and corpus callosum as 0.4 ± 0.25 mm/sec and in the basal ganglia and foramen of Monro as 0.63 ± 0.5 mm/sec. Poncelet and co-workers state, "In summary, brain motion appears to consist of a single displacement in systole followed by a slow return to the initial configuration in diastole. This displacement includes a descent of the midbrain and brain stem toward the foramen magnum, with velocities increasing with proximity to the foramen magnum (≤ 2 mm/sec) and medial compression of the thalami on the third ventricle (≤ 1.5 mm/sec)" (17). Enzmann and Pelc report, "Peak brain displacement was in the range of 0.1 mm to 0.5 mm for all structures except the cerebellar tonsils, which had greater displacement 0.4 mm ± 0.16" (18).

Basic science research by Wolley and Shaw (19), Clark (20), and Hyden (21) was cited by Magoun (12). Wolley and Shaw report rhythmic contractions of the of oligodendroglial cells of the CNS. Clark reports research on cats which showed "waves or cycles of 8–12 per minute occur ... not related to the respiratory rate or heart rate." Hyden shows that glial cells, grown in tissue culture, pulsate continuously. Magoun cites this research as supportive of the concept of the motility of the brain and spinal cord. This line of research, central to the PRM concept, has continued to be of great interest to physiologists, radiologists, and neurologists. The majority of the mass of the brain is composed of nonneural cells called glia. Glia cells contain actin and myosin, which are capable of contractile motility. Examination of fetal human astroglia by immunofluorescence staining was carried out by Abd-El-Basset and Federoff who found, "contractile units, suggesting that the stress fibers in astroglia may be contractile. Contractile stress fibers would enable astroglia to exert tension on the matrix surrounding them, thus facilitating rapid changes in cell shape" (22). Related research by Dani and associates (23) shows active waves of astrocytic Ca^{2+} in the rat hippocampus in response to neural activity. Propagation of the calcium wave was usually within 5 to 6 seconds from the beginning of neural stimulation, and under constant stimulation produced waves at the rate of 2 per minute. These findings are indicative of a regular periodicity propagated by biochemical activity of astroglia.

Fluctuation of Cerebral Spinal Fluid: Research

That the CSF fluctuates is no longer controversial. It is the nature of production of the fluctuations that has not been completely determined by scientific research. A comprehensive review of the extrinsic factors affecting CSF was made by DuBolay and colleagues (24). They cited research correlating heart rate with pulsatile CSF in dogs going back to 1896 (25) and discussion on the relationship between CSF and blood flow going back to 1877 (24). In 1971 DuBolay summarized the vascular-CSF relationship issue thusly, "The majority of workers throughout these seven decades have become convinced that the 'cardiac' CSF pressure rise measured in the ventricles, at the cisterna magna and in the lumbar theca, is caused by the rhythmic arterial input of blood to the cranial cavity. Their conclusions are based upon: [1] Timing in relation to the carotid pulses and ECG and various venous pulses and heart sounds ... [2] Upon the character of the pulse wave ... [3] Upon its alteration by obstruction elsewhere in the vascular system. ... A very few have suggested as a result of their experiments that the 'cardiac' CSF pulse has a venous rather than arterial characteristics" (24). DuBolay further states, "Most authors, e.g. Becher, (27) had envisaged the arterial inflow to the head as causing an expansion of the brain and of the vessels within the basal cisterns. O'Connell (28) suggested that the brains' [*sic*] expansion, *by compressing the third ventricle, might constitute a CSF pump* [authors' italics added for emphasis]. The observations of Falkenheim and Naunyn (29), of Knoll (30), and of Becher (27)—in dogs for the most part—drew attention to the effects of respiration upon CSF pressure" (24).

DuBolay's summary has not been modified or challenged and appears to be current today, though much more research with more refined instrumentation has been done. DuBolay's discussion of relationships between respiration and CSF pressure, and that the third ventricle might in some way be a CSF pump appeared to support Sutherland's formulation of the PRM.

Mobility of Intracranial and Intraspinal Membranes

That this anatomy indeed exists as described has never been disputed, but few, other than practitioners of OCF/CO, have examined the physiologic implications or even carried out research pertaining to this phenomenon of the PRM.

In a study of spinal cord motion, Levy and associates (31) compared normal subjects with patients who had tethering of spinal cord structures due to spinal dysraphism (e.g., spina bifida), cord compression, or tumor. Their data were in velocity dimensions but based on empirical displacement of spinal dura tissue. Their data showed healthy subjects to have a spinal CSF flow rate of 12.4 ± 2.92 mm/second, subjects with spinal dysraphism 2.12 ± 1.69 mm/second, and subjects with cord compression 1.87 ± 1.4 mm/second. They further elaborate their findings with the nature of CSF flow, "The origin of cord pulsations is compatible with a direct transfer of motion from brain pulsations. In our cases, the timing of cord impulse coincided with the onset of the caudal phase of flow in the spinal canal. This is in agreement with the observation that the caudal motion of the brain leads to reversal of CSF flow by expulsion of cranial CSF, thereby generating a wave of CSF that propagates and descends into the spinal canal" (31). That these phases of flow, based on analysis of brain and spinal dural tissue displacement, were empirically demonstrated, is suggestive of continuity of motion in these structures and the reciprocal nature of the connection between intracranial and intraspinal membranes.

An unusual approach was taken by Kostopoulos and Keramidas (32) on a male cadaver that had been embalmed for 6 months. The brain tissue was removed through two cut windows, leaving intact the three divisions of the dural membranes. The measurement used was a piezoelectric element attached to the falx cerebri with the motion recorded by oscilloscope. Application of the frontal lift cranial treatment maneuver then produced a 1.44-mm elongation of the falx cerebri and a parietal lift produced a 1.08-mm elongation. Even on embalmed tissue, application of the sphenobasilar compression maneuver produced a −0.33-mm movement, and the sphenobasilar decompression maneuver a +0.28-mm movement of falx cerebri. The observable motion of dural membrane tissue by cranial bone pressure is a unique demonstration of the continuity of cranial bone and dural-fascial structures, and supports Sutherland's formulation of the PRM with regard to the core link.

Articular Mobility of Cranial Bones: Research

Despite modern statements that the cranial bones do not move (33), there is ample evidence demonstrating that cranial sutures are constructed in such a way to allow for motion, and other studies that have measured some degree of cranial bone motion (Fig. 62.1).

Those who hold that there is no cranial bone motion cite evidence that cranial sutures ossify by a certain age, and are not capable of motion (33,34). However, Pritchard and colleagues (35) studied the histology of cranial sutures in humans and five other species, and were among the earliest researchers to seriously question the complete ossification of cranial sutures. "Obliteration of sutures and synostosis of the adjoining bones, *if it happens at all* (author's italics added for emphasis), occurs usually after all growth has ceased. In the great apes synostosis of all sutures occurs immediately after growth has ceased, but in man and most laboratory animals sutures may never completely close. These differences have been attributed to the differences in the degree of development of the masticatory apparatus" (35).

Retzlaff, with collaborators in a number of studies confirmed, and refined the Pritchard study. Retzlaff and associates state, "Gross and microscopic examination of the parieto-parietal and parieto-temporal cranial sutures obtained by autopsy from 17 human cadavers with age range of 7 to 78 years shows that these sutures remain as clearly identifiable structures even in the oldest samples" (36). Other studies by Retzlaff and colleagues (37) delineated sutural elements contraindicating ossification and demonstrated the presence of vascular and neural structures in the sutures. These studies also showed the presence of nerve and vascular tissue substantial enough to supply the needs of connective tissue activated beyond mere bony sutural adhesions and ossification. Additionally, Retzlaff and colleagues (38) traced nerve endings from the sagittal sinus through the falx cerebri and third ventricle to the superior cervical ganglion in primates and mammals.

Empirically demonstrated cranial bone motion in animals is well documented. Michael and Retzlaff (39) demonstrated cranial bone (parietal) mobility in the squirrel monkey. In significant work, Heisey and Adams (40,41) and Adams, Heisey, and others (42) demonstrated parietal bone mobility in cats as a function of laboratory-induced fluctuation in CSF volume.

Demonstration of human cranial bone motion is suggestive of support for the PRM phenomena, but has involved studies with few subjects. In 1971, Frymann (43) reported cranial bone excursions ranging 0.0005 to 0.001 inches. She used an electronic, spring-loaded, strain-gauge apparatus and was able to show dyssynchrony between cranial bone motion and thoracic respiratory motion. Heifitz and Weiss, using technology similar to Frymann's found, "A definite increase in the bitemporal dimension of the intact skull was associated with the rise in ICP [intracranial pressure] over 15 mm Hg in our two comatose patients. This increase was detectable with ordinary strain-gauge technology" (44). Using force transducers, Tettambel and associates (45) showed differences between heart rate, respiratory rate, and a third rhythm which appeared to be associated with the PRM of 30 subjects between the ages of 16 to 71.

In a substantial body of work, yet to be replicated, Zanakis and co-workers (46) demonstrated human parietal bone motion. The objective measure used was infrared reflectors on acupuncture needles "anchored" in the parietal bones, and movement was measured by a camera in a "kinematic system." Regular repetitive motion frequencies ranged from 7 to 12 cycles per minute, and the total excursion ranged 20 to 200 microns, with the absolute diameter of the skull changing by 2.2 millimeters over a 10-second period (46). The rate and amplitude characteristics were replicated and a further conclusion that "motion of cranial bones is not a simple 'hinge' operation, but a complex motion involving more than one axis of movement" was reached (47). Lewandowski and associates (48) concluded, "Movement of the parietal bones therefore appears to be movement about the cranial sutures alone."

Among the more promising ongoing research on cranial bone motion is that of Moskalenko and colleagues (49–51). A recent publication speaks not only to cranial bone motion but also to intracranial fluid volume characteristics suggestive of changes inconsistent with a rigid calvarium. Moskalenko and co-workers state:

It has been shown that the cranial dimensions in healthy people undergo continuous changes in the frontal and sagittal sections with a mean amplitude 0.38 0.21 mm (N = 18) and a maximum deviation of up to 1 mm. Two-channel bioimpedence [*sic*] imaging (60 kHz)

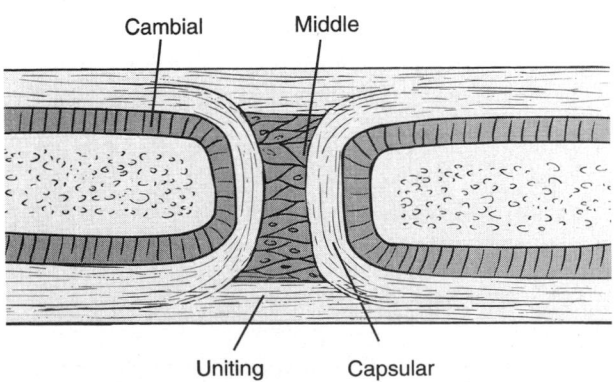

FIGURE 62.1. Histology of cranial sutures. (From Magoun HI. *Osteopathy in the Cranial Field*, 2nd ed. Kirksville, MO: Journal Printing Company; 1966, with permission.)

Cambial Middle

Uniting Capsular

of the human head, with electrodes placed in fronto-occipital and bitemporal positions and with further analysis of the resulting curves in the two-dimensional X (one channel)-Y (another channel) coordinate system, revealed the ellipsoid shape of the recorded data with a 0.23 0.16 axis ratio (N = 26) characteristic of the presence of an antiphase, or reciprocal, component. Owing to this the cranial cavity volume increases by 12–15 mL under natural elevation of the intracranial pressure. The prevalence of periodic movements with a frequency of 6–14 cycles per minute was observed by means of spectral analysis of 3-minute sections of continuous recording in one of the channels (50).

Moskalenko and colleagues (51) further describe an interaction between intracranial hemodynamics and CSF circulation which combined to give a frequency of 6 to 12 cycles per minute. "It was found that slow oscillations of the bio-impedance [*sic*] (BIM) in the frequency range 0.08–0.2 Hz were of intracranial origin and were related to the mechanisms of regulation of the blood supply to and oxygen consumption by cerebral tissue, as well as with the dynamics of the CSF circulation" (51).

Utilizing laser-Doppler flowmetry, Nelson and co-workers (52) demonstrated that the Traube-Hering-Meyer (THM) oscillations were highly correlated with PRM rhythmicity. They report PRM and THM rates of 5 to 10 cycles per minute, and state, "The results of this study indicate that the PRM oscillation occur simultaneously, though they may not represent the exact same phenomenon" (52).

Involuntary Mobility of Sacrum Between Ilia: Research

Empirical research by Weisl has substantiated this phenomenon of the PRM (53). Further research by Mitchell (54), Pruzzo (55), and Mitchell and Pruzzo (56) demonstrates a horizontal axis of sacral motion located anterior to the second sacral segment. Their research also reports sacral movement characteristics consistent with Weisl's findings. The S2 axis has become known as the respiratory axis of the sacrum. This "southern pole" of the PRM awaits the type or research effort applied in the demonstration of cranial bone motion.

MECHANICS OF PHYSIOLOGIC MOTION

The overall shape of the skull is that of a relative sphere with its inferior surface indented. The terminology used to describe the directions of motion of the various bones is similar to that for the motions of the spine and extremities. Midline bones move through a flexion phase and an extension phase during their biphasic cycle. Paired bones move through external rotation and internal rotation during the cycle. The flexion phase of midline bones is simultaneous with external rotation of paired structures. The extension/internal rotation phase occurs reciprocally.

The sphenoid and occiput (midline bones) form the key articulation at the sphenobasilar symphysis (or synchondrosis) in the base of the skull. This is a cartilaginous union up to the age of 25 years and thereafter has the resiliency of cancellous bone (57). This articulation is slightly convex on its superior surface. With flexion of this joint there is slight increase in this convex-

ity. The motion of each midline bone occurs around a transverse axis. The other midline bones of the mechanism are the ethmoid, vomer, and sacrum. They are moved through the biphasic cycle in response to the pull or influence of the dural membranes that are influenced by the coiling and uncoiling of the CNS and the fluctuation of the CSF. The motion is initiated from within the living body and is referred to as inherent motion or involuntary motion.

The overall motion of the cranium is similar to the motion of the chest during respiration, but the two do not occur simultaneously. Thoracic respiration occurs 12 to 16 cycles per minute in adults and up to 44 cycles per minute in newborns (58); the most frequently encountered motion of the PRM normally occurs 10 to 14 cycles per minute (12). During flexion of the midline bones, palpation senses that the head widens slightly in its transverse diameter and shortens slightly in its anteroposterior diameter. The area where the coronal and sagittal sutures join, called bregma, descends. This widening occurs as the paired bones move toward external rotation.

With extension of the midline bones, the head narrows and lengthens slightly as the bregma ascends, and all paired bones move toward internal rotation. During the biphasic cycle, the osseous cranium changes shape slightly but its volume remains essentially constant; the research of Heisey and Adams (40) and Moskalenko (50) suggests there is enough cranial bone compliance and "sutural stretch" to allow as much as a 15-mL intracranial fluid volume change.

During flexion, the sacrum is influenced by the spinal dura and core link and moves posterosuperiorly at its base while the apex moves anteriorly toward the pubes. During extension, the base moves anteriorly and the apex moves posteriorly. This motion occurs around a transverse axis in the area of the second sacral segment posterior to the sacral canal and is called the respiratory axis of the sacrum. The other axes of sacral motion are postural axes (Fig. 62.2).

The inherent motion of the cranium is not visible but it is palpable. This motion is perceived as a subtle, soft, slight movement of fluid (CSF) and semifluid (CNS) inside an osseous case. The first attempts at this palpatory exercise may not reveal anything, or you may feel the subject's thoracic respiration transmitted through the neck to the head. If the breathing is a distraction, ask the patient to hold their breath for a moment. If you can still sense the rhythmic motion in the head, the inherent motion is coming from within the cranium. With palpatory experience, one learns to distinguish between these different motions.

Follow these steps to palpate this rhythmic motion:

1. Position the patient supine, with the head 8 to 10 inches from the head of the table.
2. Sit comfortably at the head of the table with your forearms resting on the table and your hands placed on the sides of the patient's head. Have the patient move up or down on the table to comfortably accommodate to your relaxed posture (see Fig. 62.8).
3. Contact the patient's head lightly, allowing the fingers and part of the palms to gently conform to the curvature of the head. (It is essential that the palmar surface of all the fingers, not the thumbs, contact the head because the nerve endings

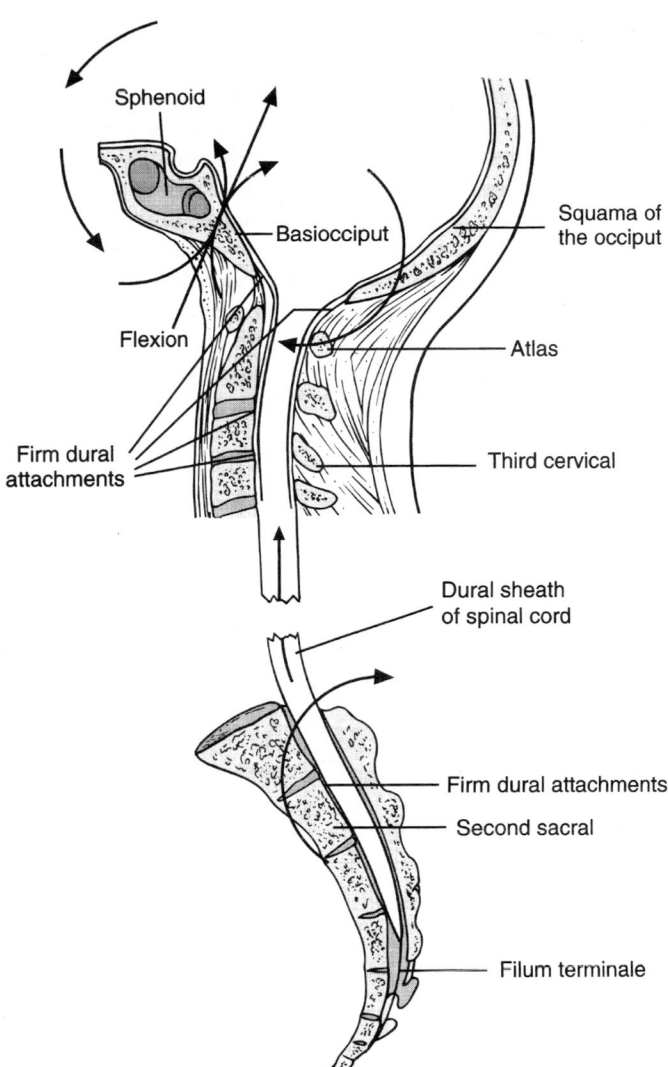

FIGURE 62.2. Craniosacral mechanism with *arrows* indicating direction of motion during flexion phase of physiologic motion. (From Magoun HI. *Osteopathy in the Cranial Field*, 2nd ed. Kirksville, MO: Journal Printing Company; 1966, with permission.)

that sense the subtle cranial motion are proprioceptors located in tendons and around joints. The numerous tactile sensors in the fingerpads are not as receptive to this motion. Even though a gentle and light contact is essential, it is not a fingertip contact.)

4. Allow your mind to become quiet and direct your attention to the space between your hands, allowing what is sensed by your proprioceptors to be perceived by your brain. (Continue to stay relaxed; do not try to feel something. If the patient's head has fairly normal motion, you may feel a slow, rhythmic swelling or widening followed by a receding or narrowing. This constitutes one cycle of inherent motion. This cycle is usually steadily repeated. The motion is so mild and subtle that it may actually feel as if the head is breathing.)

Subtle motion is easier for some physicians to palpate than for others. Some find this difficult to sense because they try too hard. Their intensity is so set, their effort so strong, that they block their

own sensorium. It is essential to be relaxed, physically, mentally, and emotionally. Your attitude should be similar to one who is trying to hear a minor sound—complete attention is given to listening.

Keep the hand contact light. Pressure by the hands will suppress the inherent motion and/or distract the sensors (proprioceptors) in the hands. If excessive hand pressure is continued, the patient may get a headache.

If you have difficulty perceiving the motion in one patient, try other patients. The cyclic characteristics of the motion and its amplitude (strength or power) usually vary from one individual to another.

The biphasic cycle of motion of the PRM most often encountered occurs 10 to 14 times per minute. When observing the rate, allow one full minute and count the number of cycles (one flexion phase plus one extension phase equals one complete cycle). Evaluating the amplitude of the PRM in patients who have clinical problems requires experience, but has been found to be statistically possible (59) and may reveal the most useful clinical data about the patient. After palpating five or ten individuals, one can determine that the strength or vitality of the rhythm is stronger in one or two individuals, fair or medium in some, and weak or poor in others. With experience in palpation and clinical knowledge of the patient's history and symptoms, the rate and amplitude become an additional diagnostic indication of their state of health and is helpful in determining a prognosis.

The rate and quality of the PRM may be increased slightly:

- Following vigorous physical exercise
- With systemic fevers
- Following effective OMT of the craniosacral mechanism

The rate and quality of the PRM may be decreased with:

- Stress (mental, emotional, physical)
- Chronic fatigue
- Chronic infections
- Mental depression and other psychiatric conditions (60)
- Chronic poisoning
- Other debilitating conditions

The cyclic, biphasic motion originating within the PRM, is most evident to palpation in the head region but is palpable in every part of the body. The impulse moves longitudinally through the body and extremities, with midline structures moving through flexion/extension and paired structures moving through external/internal rotation. Its presence or absence and its deviation from normal direction are useful diagnostic signs.

The body is subject to stresses and strains from before birth until death. Pressures and forces affect the developing fetus, the neonate during birth, and the individual through childhood, adolescence, and adulthood. These forces cause minor to major distortions of the cranium that result in strains of the sphenobasilar synchondrosis (SBS). With induced strain, the efficiency of the PRM is compromised. The compromise may be minor to major in its effect on the health of the individual.

- Cyanosis
- Convulsions
- Fever
- Tremors

Abnormal habits such as lying with the head turned to one side only, head banging, or constant rubbing of the back of the head against the sheet are indicative of strains of the cranium.

Diagnosis by Observation

Look for symmetry or distortion of the osseous structure beneath the soft tissues. Observe the face and head: the shape and contours of the head and face show hereditary influences as well as the combined effect of the forces of labor on the bones. At birth the sphenoid, temporals, and occiput are made up of several osseous parts with cartilage between parts and between bones to allow for compression and molding of the head during birth. Strains within a bone may occur and are called intraosseous strains.

The flexion type of skull is round in shape with a wide transverse and a shortened AP diameter, with the temporals in relative external rotation (flared laterally). In this type of skull, the frontals are wide and sloping upward, the cheek bones are wide, and an open mouth view of the maxillary region of the hard palate reveals it to be wide and with a low arch to the vault. All paired structures are in a position of relative external rotation.

The extension type of skull is long and narrow with temporals in relative internal rotation, frontals narrow with the brow appearing more vertical, orbits and face narrow, and maxillae (hard palate) narrow with a high arched vault. All paired structures are in a position of relative internal rotation.

Note the positioning of the bones. The position of the sphenoid bone influences the position of the peripheral bones of the anterior cranium, which includes the frontals and all bones of the face except the mandible. The position of the occiput influences the position of the bones of the posterior cranium (the parietals and temporals) and in turn influences the position of the mandible.

With torsion and side bending/rotation of the SBS, the facial structures tend to appear asymmetric as they assume a position of relative external rotation on the side of the high wing and a position of relative internal rotation on the side of the low wing. If the sphenoid is rotated on an AP axis, the eyes and orbits will appear unlevel. Compare the relative positions of the cheekbones and the maxillae.

Note the relative positioning of landmarks. It is sometimes difficult to determine if the occiput has rotated on the AP axis because it is hidden by hair. As the occiput tilts on this axis, it carries the temporals with it. The temporal on the low side of the occiput is positioned toward relative external rotation, and the temporal on the high side of the occiput is positioned toward relative internal rotation. Therefore, the relative position of the ears gives an indication of the tilt of the occiput. Compare right and left ear lobes to see if they are level; note flaring of the ears. A temporal positioned toward external rotation tends to be more flared; a temporal positioned toward internal rotation tends to be more flat. By combining the findings of the anterior and posterior

cranium, the observer is able to arrive at a tentative or working diagnosis of torsion or side bending/rotation of the SBS.

Viewing the midline of the face, noting the nose, mouth, and center of the chin, provides additional information. Nasal deviation may indicate the relative position of the maxillae and sphenoid or may indicate past trauma or fracture. The chin (mandible) tends to deviate to the side of the externally rotated temporal bone. Heredity also influences facial characteristics and is a significant consideration for establishing a prognosis.

Strains of the cranial base occur during birth or from trauma. If trauma is induced into a prior strain pattern, the findings of observation are not reliable for diagnosis.

Diagnosis by Palpation

To become expert at the art of palpation for diagnosis and treatment requires repeated experience, patience, and perseverance. These guidelines help improve palpatory skill:

1. Use a light hand contact. If your contact is stronger than the force of the inherent motion, you interfere with the mechanism you are attempting to diagnose or treat. Do not interject yourself into the patient's PRM.

2. Have a clear visualization of the structure(s) beneath your hands. This requires a detailed study of the anatomy and physiologic motion of each of the bones of the body, including the cranium and face. The design of the articulations between bones and their mechanical and physiologic relationship is a complex study, but it is essential to providing accurate diagnosis and successful treatment. (Space constraints do not permit such detailed study in this chapter.)

3. Understand that the job of the physician is to assist the patient to obtain or maintain optimal health. The physician does not do the healing; healing comes from within the patient. With knowledge and experience, one learns to tune in to and be guided by the PRM of the patient to facilitate this healing process, assisting the patient's own inherent healing capacity to release biomechanical impediments. The automatic processes that promote healing are much more intelligent and efficient in the management of the health of the individual than any external force or person can be.

CLINICAL PROBLEMS REQUIRING OSTEOPATHIC MANIPULATIVE TREATMENT
Neonatal

OMT of infants and children can be a rewarding experience for the patient and the doctor. Children respond to treatment faster than adults.

Compromised function of the PRM is a cumulative process beginning *in utero* or during birth, combined with the various traumatic incidents of growing up, as well as one or more traumatic events sustained as an adult. The physician must keep this in mind when taking the history.

Consideration of the trauma of the birth process deserves further explanation. The base of the skull is formed in cartilage and the vault is formed in membrane. At birth, the sphenoid is in three parts, the temporal is in three parts, and the occiput is in four

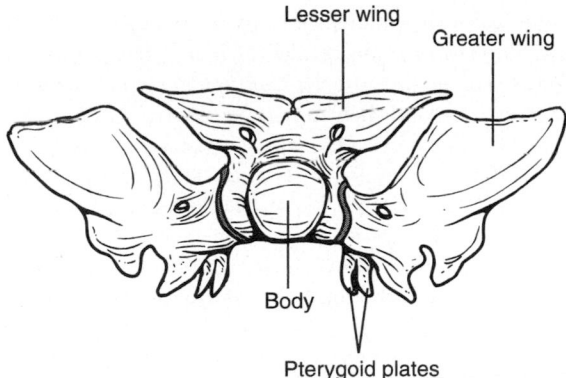

FIGURE 62.5. Sphenoid at birth in three parts. Cartilage intervenes between body-lesser wing unit and greater wing-pterygoid units. (From Sutherland WG, Wales AL. *Teachings in the Science of Osteopathy*. Portland, OR: Rudra Press; 1990, with permission.)

parts, with cartilage intervening between the osseous elements (61). The frontal and mandible are in two parts and each maxilla is in two parts. This is nature's way of protecting the CNS and providing for compressibility of the head as it passes through the birth canal. The bones of the vault are osseous plates that overlap at the edges. The cartilaginous base tends to compress, bend, twist, or buckle depending on the amount and direction of compression and rotational forces of labor and birth. These various parts are vulnerable to misalignment; the brain, cranial nerves, and intracranial membranes are subject to possible injury or malfunction. One or more of the strain patterns of the SBS generally has its beginning during the birth process (Figs. 62.5 and 62.6).

The infant's first breath and subsequent crying with deep breathing, kicking, squirming, and suckling assist with decompression of the cranium, face, and pelvis (61). Decades of clinical experience have shown that if the activities of the neonate are not strong enough to open up the entire PRM to its optimal function, these neonates benefit from the assistance of an osteopathic physician trained in the cranial concept and in treatment procedures. Examination and treatment are best given during the first few days of life, at which time a great deal is accomplished by releasing the compressive forces of birth. If no treatment is provided, as time passes and growth progresses, the strains become more established. In time, the formative parts of the various bones of the base change from cartilage to osseous tissue. If overlapping of the osseous plates of the vault is allowed to remain, the plates grow together, forming a synostosis. Osteopathic physicians utilizing OCF have found that when synostosis pervades the vault, the osseous case cannot grow and expand at the same rate as the brain inside, and the brain function of that individual appears to be compromised. Expert treatment given early in the life of an individual can be one of the most important therapeutic measures in preventive medicine. Treatment given later is beneficial, but more can be accomplished in less time and with less effort and expense if treatment is given soon after the stresses and strains occur.

An example of disturbance of function directly related to the compressive forces of birth concerns the posterior part of the cranial base. The four parts of the developing occiput are the:

- Basilar process
- Two condylar parts along the lateral sides of foramen magnum
- Squama extending from the posterior border of the foramen magnum to the lambdoid suture

The medulla oblongata rests on the basilar part, and the spinal cord extends through the space within the four parts. Cranial nerves IX, X, and XI and the jugular veins pass through the jugular foramina at the anterolateral border of each condylar part. Cranial nerve XII passes through the anterior condylar canals located within the condylar parts near the junction between the condylar parts and basilar part. Compression with rotation of the posterior cranium during birth with distortion, displacement, and jamming of these four osseous plates and intervening cartilage is easily visualized (Fig. 62.6). The symptoms manifested in the newborn or young infant that indicate the presence of abnormal mechanical stress in this area include:

- Respiratory distress
- Excessive crying
- Inability to suckle or weak suckling
- Vomiting
- Bradycardia
- Tachycardia
- Tremors
- Spasticity or flaccidity of the limbs
- Cyanosis
- Torticollis

This abnormal mechanical stress on the brainstem, cranial nerves, and venous drainage is treated by gentle application of mild, sustained spreading of the formative parts of the base of the skull by a physician trained to apply OMT in this manner.

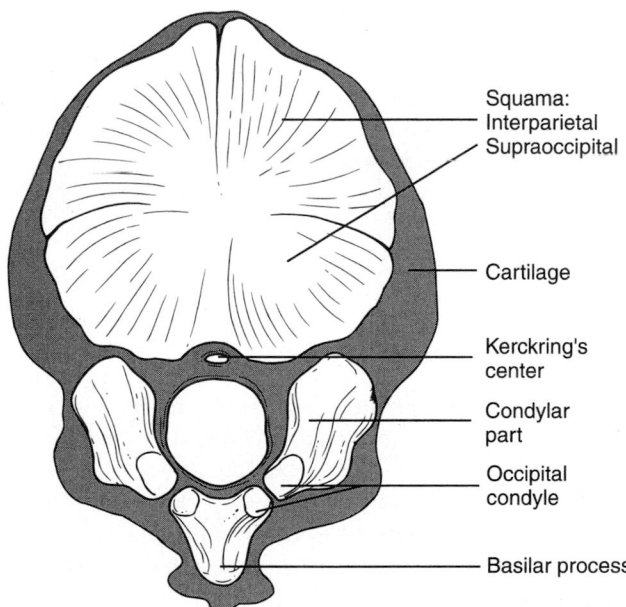

FIGURE 62.6. Occiput at birth in four parts within a cartilaginous matrix. Articular condyles receive contributions from both condylar and basilar parts of the occiput. (From Sutherland WG, Wales AL. *Teachings in the Science of Osteopathy*. Portland, OR: Rudra Press; 1990, with permission.)

The relative position and motion of the temporal bones affect drainage from the middle ear through the pharyngotympanic tube; their somatic dysfunction is clinically capable of resulting in tinnitus, dizziness, and decreased auditory acuity. Treatment is aimed at releasing membranous strains of the cranial base, temporal bones, and upper cervical spine to help reestablish equal and synchronous motion to the temporals as well as the entire PRM. Consider these factors:

1. Without normal motion present, stasis of fluids and lack of oxygen provide an ideal medium for microorganisms.
2. When the inherent motion throughout the cranium and face is optimal, the movement of fluids and mucus is enhanced (a provision of nature for emptying the ethmoid, sphenoid, and maxillary sinuses).
3. The autonomic nerve supply to the nasal mucosa by way of the sphenopalatine ganglion is vulnerable to impinging adnexa.
4. Middle ear infections, sinusitis, pharyngitis, and other acute inflammatory processes are often associated with altered cranial functions (62).

Vascular Supply

Consider the vascular supply to the brain. The internal carotid arteries enter the petrous portions of the temporal bones, extend forward and medially within those bones, exit from the tips of the petrous, and turn superiorly along the sides of the basisphenoid to enter the cranial cavity. Disturbance in physiologic motion, in which the petrous portion of the temporal articulates with the basiocciput and the basisphenoid, compromises the optimal function of these arteries through related dural tension. The vascular interchange between the choroid plexus and the CSF (occurring within the ventricles of the brain) is affected by the widening and narrowing of the ventricles, which occurs with each biphasic motion of the PRM.

The venous drainage from the brain is by way of the various intracranial veins emptying into the venous sinuses, which are channels between layers of dura mater. The great cerebral vein enters the straight sinus, which joins the transverse sinus to become the sigmoid sinus. That sinus becomes the jugular vein, which passes through the jugular foramen to exit the skull. The jugular foramen is an aperture between the occiput and temporal bones. Ninety-five percent of the venous blood from the brain exits the skull through these two apertures (12). This area is extremely vulnerable to trauma to the back or side of the head. Impaired venous drainage leads to venous stasis. The movement of venous blood along the various venous sinuses directly depends on the biphasic motion of the RTM and the bones to which it attaches (62). Consider venous stasis as a causative factor for headache, decreased cerebral function, and depression.

The pituitary body is located in the sella turcica on the superior surface of the sphenoid bone just anterior to the SBS. This neuroendocrine gland, an extension of the brain, secretes a number of hormones that affect all the glands of the endocrine system. A reduplication of dura, the diaphragma sella, encircles the stalk of the pituitary like a collar. The hormones secreted by the pituitary pass into the vascular plexus surrounding it. Pituitary function is compromised if the inherent motility of the CNS or the movement of blood through the cranial vascular system is impaired (5).

The dura mater lines the skull and spinal canal, and extensions of it continue beyond the various apertures as the sheaths of the cranial and spinal nerves. Entrapment neuropathy describes the localized injury or irritation to nervous tissue from the mechanical effect of impinging adnexa. There are multiple examples (62–64) of entrapment of cranial and spinal nerves and their branches throughout the body, all of which are amenable to osteopathic treatment by releasing membranous and/or ligamentous articular strains.

The interstitial fluids of the entire body are constantly influenced by the biphasic cycle of the PRM. This movement of fluids is slow, steady, and efficient even at the cellular level with the exchange of metabolites across the cell membrane. In that sense, the CNS functions as a pump. Sutherland compared this fluid motion in the body to the tide of the ocean (12). It is a major factor in the repair of damaged tissue from contusions, sprains, strains, and inflammatory processes (12). Knowledge of the PRM and its effects on the health of the total being broadens our understanding of the self-healing and self-regulatory mechanisms taught by Dr. Still.

Trauma

Trauma is by far the major cause of disruption and malfunction of the PRM. The force of trauma is extreme in vehicular accidents. The force from a fall is transmitted from the feet or ischial tuberosities upward through the body into the base of the skull. The vector of force established through the body or head is palpable (65,66) and is an important diagnostic sign. The direction of motion of the CSF and CNS is disrupted, and the function of the PRM is mildly to severely impaired, depending on the severity of the trauma and the response of the patient.

Trauma to the PRM can occur from mild, sustained force such as wearing a spring type of headset or from orthodontic appliances on the teeth (67); wearing a tight hat or swim cap will augment or create or alter existing patterns. Trauma occurs in various degrees and in innumerable forms.

The PRM functions as a unit; trauma to one area affects the entire RTM. The PRM does its best to continue to function, but the quality of that function decreases with the passage of time and additional trauma. The rate and amplitude of the PRM is a most valuable diagnostic and prognostic indicator of the severity of the compromise and response to treatment (68). A slow rate and a low amplitude are dependable indicators of a long-standing and/or overwhelming problem during which the patient's vitality has been depleted, indicating more treatment over a longer period of time will be required (68). The reciprocal is also true. In the course of treatment, improvement is associated with a rate and amplitude increase toward a more normal pattern.

Dentistry

OCF is especially pertinent to the practice of complete dentistry (69). Improperly directed forces of extraction, fillings, setting of crowns, and improperly fitted dentures alter the occlusion of maxillary and mandibular teeth and disturb the PRM (70).

Resultant symptoms include:

- Headaches
- Vertigo with its attendant gastrointestinal symptoms
- Cervical syndromes
- Temporomandibular joint dysfunction syndrome

Clinical enigmas of the head and neck (such as atypical facial pain) require evaluation of dental problems and the effects of dental procedures and orthotics on the PRM (71). Satisfactory therapeutic response depends on evaluation and treatment by both the dentist and the osteopathic physician.

PRINCIPLES OF TREATMENT

The aim of treatment, as with any osteopathic procedure, is to normalize structure and function. The optimal function of the PRM affects not only the CNS but also every cell and tissue in the body. Regardless of which method or procedure a physician elects to use, this constant cyclic motion is at work behind the scenes every minute of every hour of every day of every year of an individual's life.

Goals of Treatment

The goals of treatment include:

- Normalizing nerve function, including all cranial and spinal nerves as well as the autonomic nervous system
- Counteracting stress-producing factors by normalizing function of the cerebrum, thalamus, hypothalamus, and pituitary body
- Eliminating circulatory stasis by normalizing arterial, venous, and lymphatic channels
- Normalizing CSF fluctuation
- Releasing membranous tension
- Correcting or resolving cranial articular strains
- Modifying gross structural patterns

Some hindrances to treatment are myofascial strains from below the cranium or the sacrum, local or general infections, nutritional deficiencies, and organic poisons (12). Removal of nonstructural hindrances must be addressed as well as OMT in the management of the patient's health problems. To use the power or potency of the inherent activity of the PRM within the patient to assist with the release of strains (somatic dysfunctions), it is necessary to understand balanced ligamentous tension and balanced membranous tension. Balanced ligamentous tension is used in treating any articulation supported and protected by ligaments. Balanced membranous tension refers to the dura mater (RTM) and is used to treat the articulations of the cranium, face, and sacrum.

The point of balanced membranous tension is defined as that point in the range of motion of an articulation where the membranes are poised between the normal tension present throughout the free range of motion and the increased tension preceding the strain or fixation that occurs as a joint is carried beyond its normal physiologic range (12). Thus, it is the most neutral position possible under the influence of all the factors responsible for the

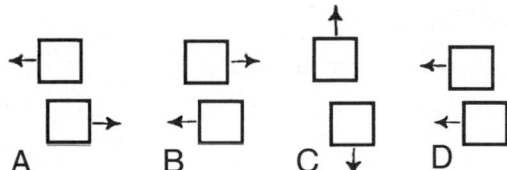

FIGURE 62.7. Methods for arriving at the point of balanced membranous tension. **A:** Indirect action (exaggeration). **B:** Direct action. **C:** Disengagement. **D:** Opposite physiologic motion. (From Magoun HI. *Osteopathy in the Cranial Field*, 2nd ed. Kirksville, MO: Journal Printing Company; 1966, with permission.)

existing pattern, all attendant tensions having been reduced to the absolute minimum.

This point is unique for each strain that occurs. It is the point at which the inherent force can move through the involved tissues at its maximum efficiency. The operator seeks to position the bones making up the articulation at the point of balanced membranous tension by keen, sensitive, knowledgeable palpation. Dr. Sutherland expressed this as palpating with seeing, feeling, thinking, knowing fingers.

Figure 62.7 illustrates arriving at the point of balanced membranous tension by positioning the components. The squares indicate two bones making up an articulation, and the arrows represent the directions the operator employs for positioning (12).

Figure 62.7A illustrates indirect action or exaggeration. This procedure is commonly employed from the age of 5 through adulthood. It is not used in acute trauma to the head when exaggeration of misalignment may produce or increase intracranial hemorrhage. To employ this method, increase the abnormal relationship at the joint by moving the articulation slightly in the direction toward which it was lesioned.

Figure 62.7B illustrates direct action. This treatment method is employed when exaggeration is not desirable, as in acute trauma and in young children in whom the sutural pattern has not yet developed. This treatment is also used when there are overriding sutures. The components are gently guided back toward their normal position.

Figure 62.7C illustrates disengagement. This treatment method is used when force or excessive membranous tension impacts the osseous components. Disengagement technique merely separates the opposing surfaces within the anatomic and physiologic limits of permitted motion.

Figure 62.7D illustrates opposite physiologic motion. This method is seldom used, but when needed it is employed to release a strain when a traumatic force has severely violated the physiologic pattern. One component is influenced by direct action; the other is influenced by indirect action.

The physician selects the method of choice according to the patient's age and history, as well as by palpatory diagnosis.

Respiratory cooperation may be used to enhance the effort of inherent motion. The patient is asked to hold their breath in full inhalation or exhalation after the physician has positioned the articulation at balanced ligamentous or membranous tension. Holding the breath at full inhalation is more commonly used, but if the articulation is held toward extension or internal rotation, holding the breath at full exhalation is more effective.

Example One

An example of treatment follows.

Diagnosis

Somatic dysfunction of the midcervical spine (C4 E R$_R$ S$_R$).

Treatment

Treatment is indirect method, using balanced ligamentous tension, exaggeration, and inherent force.

Procedure

1. Position the patient supine.
2. Sit at the head of the table.
3. Place the fingerpads of the two index fingers at the lateral border of the articular pillars of C5. The long (third) fingerpads are at the articular pillars of C4. This gives you optimum contact for precise positioning of the two bones and for maximum sensing of the soft tissues over the articulation.
4. Slowly and gently position the two segments so that C4 is side bent right, rotated right, and slightly extended to the point of balanced ligamentous tension. Note that the tension on the involved muscles and ligaments eases, softens, and cannot be perceived as tension. The joint is not in physiologic neutral, but is in neutral for this ligamentous strain in all three planes.
5. Maintain this position and allow the inherent force to work. Keep your sensing apparatus alert so that it perceives the slow cyclic movement of the PRM. This movement feels like a longitudinal ebb and flow or a subtle pumping effect up and down the spine.
6. Continue to maintain the positioning and to observe this cyclic motion; the inherent force is working through the tissues that are maintaining the somatic dysfunction. As they accomplish their task for this articulation at this time, the amplitude of the inherent rhythm lessens and the pumping decreases, and the tissues beneath your palpating fingers seem to soften or melt.
7. At this time, cease to hold the articulation in the treatment position. Gently recheck the motion of the articulation to ascertain the therapeutic response. Physiologic motion is restored to varying degrees.

A strain of the cranial base can be treated using the inherent forces and positioning for balanced membranous tension of the reciprocal tension membranes. This technique is applicable for an uncomplicated strain of the SBS. If a strain of the cranial base is complicated by additional traumatic strains such as a frontosphenoidal or occipitomastoid strain, the technique as described will probably not be successful. The complicating strains from induced trauma are treated before treating the sphenobasilar strain.

Example Two

Diagnosis

Somatic dysfunction of the sphenobasilar symphysis is side bending/rotation right (SBS is SBR$_R$).

The sphenoid and occiput have rotated on an AP axis so that the right side of the cranium is relatively inferior (caudad) and the left side is relatively superior (cephalad). Concomitant with that position, the greater sphenoid wing and the lateral angle of

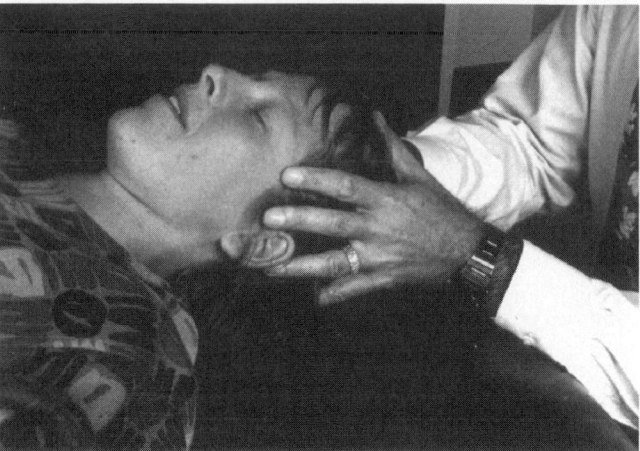

FIGURE 62.8. "Vault hold" for contact of the cranium (From Hruby R. *Craniosacral Osteopathic Technique: A Manual,* 2nd ed. Okemos, MI: The Institute for Osteopathic Studies; 1996:33, with permission.)

the occiput on the right side are slightly spread and the greater sphenoid wing and the lateral angle of the left occiput are slightly approximated.

Treatment

Treatment is indirect method, balanced membranous tension, with exaggeration and inherent forces to balance the RTM.

Procedure

1. Position the patient supine.
2. Sit at the head of the table.
3. Place your hands on the lateral sides of the patient's head with the index fingers contacting the greater wings of the sphenoid and the little fingers contacting the lateral angles of the occiput (vault contact) (Fig. 62.8).
4. Gently palpate the rhythmic activity of the patient's PRM and RTM.
5. The right hand slowly moves slightly caudad with index and fifth fingers spreading slightly while the left hand moves slightly cephalad and fingers approximate slightly. This positioning is slight and must be accurate, being guided by the ease of tension in the membranes within the cranium. With the ease of membranous tension, the inherent forces begin to manifest with increased vigor. The amplitude of the primary respiratory mechanism (PRM) automatically increases.
6. Maintain the positioning and carefully and continuously observe the increased activity of the inherent forces at work within the patient's mechanism. As the inherent forces work through the membranous strain, they gradually cease the increased activity and become quiet. This cessation of the inherent rhythm is called a still point (61).
7. After the still point occurs, cease to maintain the positioning of the bones and membranes and continue to observe the fluctuant activity by light palpation. The quiet period passes, the rhythmic fluctuation resumes, increasing slowly and steadily in amplitude until it has returned to a more normal flexion-extension of the SBS.
8. Gently remove your hands.
9. There is no substitute for thorough training and practice

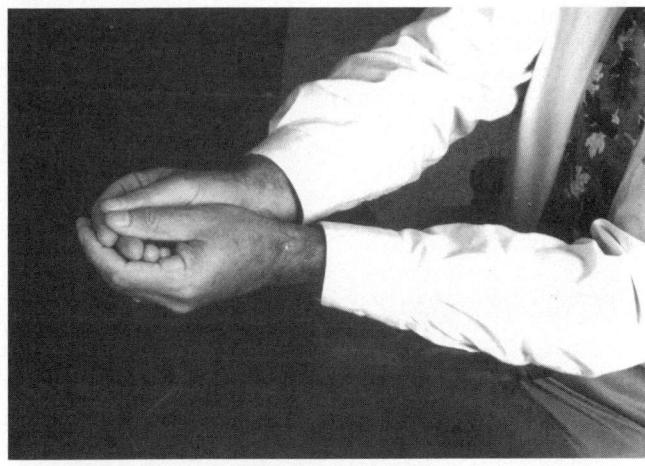

A

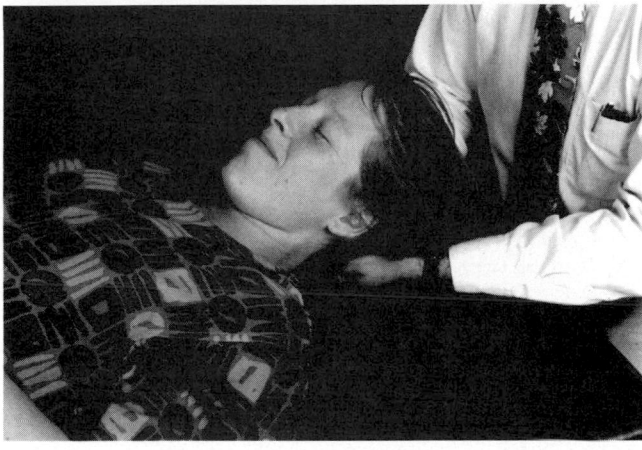

B

FIGURE 62.9. Compression of forth ventricle (CV₄). **A:** Hand position for CV₄ technique. **B:** CV₄ technique. (From Hruby R. *Craniosacral Osteopathic Technique: A Manual,* 2nd ed. Okemos, MI: The Institute for Osteopathic Studies; 1996, with permission.)

in the development of skill in OMT based on the principles of OCF/CO. Well-known and typically utilized treatment procedures based on the principles of OCF/CO are the compression of the forth ventricle (CV₄) and the V-spread procedures.

The CV₄ (Fig. 62.9 A and B) is typically used to stimulate the body's inherent therapeutic capacity to deal with whatever dysfunction is present. By inducing extension (or internal rotation) of the PRM the inherent capacity for self-regulation and healing is facilitated by a stimulation of CSF flow. The technique is as follows:

1. Operator at head of table.
2. Patient supine.
3. Place one hand in the palm of the other so that the thenar eminences lie uppermost and parallel to each other. Then slip them under the head, permitting the lateral angles of the occiput medial to the occipitomastoid suture to rest on them. The thenar eminences provide a cushion for the occiput that should be comfortable for the patient and operator. The fingers are free and not pressing on the neck. The weight of the head rests on the thenar eminences and thereby gently compresses the lateral angles.

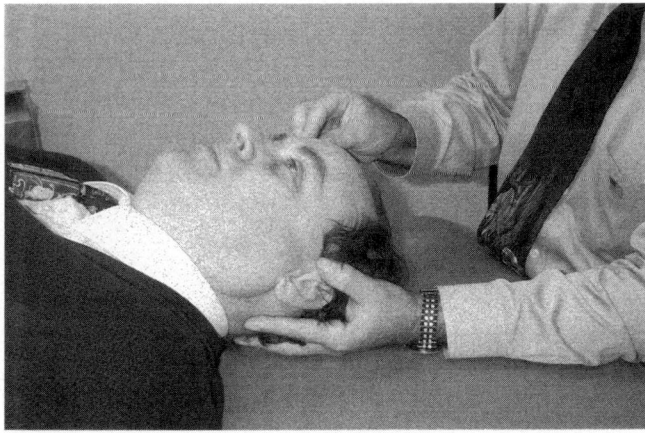

FIGURE 62.10. V-spread of occipitomastoid suture. (From Hruby R. *Craniosacral Technique: A Manual,* 2nd ed. Okemos, MI: The Institute for Osteopathic Studies; 1996, with permission.)

4. Become aware of the cyclic motion of the occiput. Follow it toward extension (i.e., as the hands rock gently toward the operator). Discourage flexion (hands moving away). The amplitude of the motion will get progressively smaller until the still point is reached. This may pass so swiftly it may not be detected, but it is followed by a sense of softening and warmth in the occiput and a gentle rocking motion of flexion/extension. At the same time thoracic respiration should become primarily diaphragmatic and approximate the same cycle as the PRM.

5. Observe the cranial activity to be sure that it remains quiet and then very gently remove your hands and put the patient's head on the table. Figure 62.9 demonstrates the CV₄ via the occiput, it is possible to accomplish a CV₄ via the temporals, parietals, and sacrum.

The V-spread (Fig. 62.10) is a very simple, safe technique for releasing any peripheral suture such as frontonasal, nasomaxillary, or occipitomastoid. The technique is as follows:

1. Place the index and middle fingers of the ipsilateral hand on either side of the suture. For a linear suture like the occipitomastoid, use the palmar surface of the length of two fingers. For a small suture like the frontonasal, use the fingertips.

2. Place the palm of the other hand on the patient's head at the other end of the longest diameter of the head from the suture (e.g., for the left occipitomastoid [Fig. 62.10]), place the hand on the right frontal only. You will soon perceive a gentle impulse coming into the palm of this hand. Now cluster the fingers at the site of that impulse. You have thereby localized the optimum place from which to direct a palpatory sensation of a "fluid wave" to the restricted suture. As long as the suture is restricted, the fluid sensation will "bounce" back, but as soon as it releases, you will feel a gentle, easy motion between your hands.

Treatment procedures of the cranium should be used only by physicians experienced with palpation of the subtle activity of the PRM. Guidance by a physician experienced with the function of the PRM and the inherent forces is essential to learning this technique.

CONCLUSION

Much research remains to demonstrate the exact mechanisms involved in craniosacral dysfunction and recovery. However, more than 50 years of clinical experience has indicated that the use of OCF/CO has given relief to many patients in whom no other treatment was effective.

REFERENCES

1. Sutherland AS. *With Thinking Fingers.* Indianapolis, IN: Cranial Academy. Originally printed by Journal Printing Company, Kirksville, MO; 1962:1213.
2. Northrup GW, ed. *Osteopathic Research: Growth and Development.* Chicago, IL: American Osteopathic Association; 1987:40.
3. DiGiovanna EL, Schiowitz S. *Osteopathic Approach to Diagnosis and Treatment.* New York, NY: JB Lippincott Co; 1991.
4. Greenman PE. *Principles of Manual Medicine.* Baltimore, MD: Williams & Wilkins; 1991.
5. Kuchera ML, Kuchera WA. *Osteopathic Considerations in Systemic Dysfunction,* 2nd ed rev. Columbus, OH: Greyden Press; 1994.
6. Heisey SR, Adams T. Effects of cranial bone mobility on cranial compliance. In: *Thirty-sixth Annual AOA Research Conference Abstracts, 1992,* part 2; 1992. Also in: *JAOA.* 1992;92(9):1284.
7. Heisey SR, Adams T, Smith MC, Briner B. The role of cranial suture compliance in defining intracranial pressure. In: *Thirty-seventh Annual AOA Research Conference Abstracts, 1993,* part 2; 1993. Also in: *JAOA.* 1993;93(9):951.
8. Norton JM, Sibley G, Broder-Oldach RE. Quantification of the cranial rhythmic impulse in human subjects. In: *Thirty-sixth Annual AOA Research Conference Abstracts, 1992,* part 2; 1992. Also in: *JAOA.* 1992;92(9):1285.
9. Sibley G, Broder-Oldach E, Norton JM. Inter-examiner agreement in the characterization of the cranial rhythmic impulse. In: *Thirty-sixth Annual AOA Research Conference Abstracts, 1992,* part 2; 1992. Also in: *JAOA.* 1992;92(9):1285.
10. Norton JM. Failure of a tissue pressure model to predict cranial rhythmic impulse frequency. In: *Thirty-sixth Annual AOA Research Conference Abstracts, 1992,* part 2; 1992. Also in *JAOA.* 1992;92(9):1285.
11. *2000/2001 Yearbook and Directory of Osteopathic Physicians.* Chicago, IL: American Osteopathic Association; 2000:865.
12. Magoun HI. *Osteopathy in the Cranial Field,* 2nd ed. Kirksville, MO: Journal Printing Company; 1966.
13. *Dorland's Illustrated Medical Dictionary,* 26th ed. Philadelphia, PA: WB Saunders; 1981.
14. Becker RE. Craniosacral trauma in the adult. *Osteopath Ann.* 1976;4:43–59.
15. Greitz, D, Wirestam R, Franck A, et al. Pulsatile brain movement and associated hydrodynamics studied by magnetic resonance phase imaging: the Monro-Kellie doctrine revisited. *Neuroradiology.* 1992;34:370–380.
16. Feinberg DA, Mark AS. Human brain motion and cerebrospinal fluid circulation demonstrated with MR velocity imaging. *Radiology.* 1987;163:793–799.
17. Poncelet BP, Wedeen VJ, Weisskoff RM, Cohen MS. Brain parenchyma motion: measurement with cine echo-planar MR imaging. *Radiology.* 1992;185:645–651.
18. Enzmann DR, Pelc NJ. Brain motion: measurement with phase-contrast MR imaging. *Radiology.* 1992;185:653–660.
19. Wolley DW, Shaw EN. Evidence for the participation of serotonin in mental processes. *Ann N Y Acad Sci.* 1957;66:649–665.
20. Clark LC. Discussion of evidence for the participation of serotonin in mental processes. *Ann N Y Acad Sci.* 1957;66:668.
21. Hyden H. Satellite cells in the central nervous system. *Sci Am.* 1961;205:62.
22. Abd-El-Basset EM, Federoff S. Contractile units in stress fibers of fetal human astroglia in tissue culture. *J Chem Neuroanat.* 1994;7:113–122.
23. Dani JW, Chernjavsky A, Smith SJ. Neuronal activity triggers calcium waves in hippocampal astrocyte networks. *Neuron.* 1992;8:429–440.
24. DuBolay GH, O'Connell J, Currie J, et al. Further investigations on pulsatile movements in the cerebrospinal fluid pathways. *Acta Radiol Diagnost.* 1971;13:496–523.
25. Ziegler P. Über die Mechanik des normalen und pathologischen Hirndruckes. *Langenbecks Arc. Klin Chir.* 1896;53:75.
26. Salathè. Recherches sur les mouvements du cerveau. Travaux du Laboratoire de Maray 2, 1876. Paris, 1877.
27. Becher E. Untersuchungen über die Dynamic der "Cerebrospinalis". *Mitt Grenzgeb Med Chir.* 1922;35:329.
28. O'Connell JEA. Vascular factor in intracranial pressure and maintenance of cerebro-spinal fluid circulation. *Brain.* 1943;66:204–228.
29. Falkenheimer H, Naunyn B. Über Hirndruck. *Naunyn-Schmeideberg's Arch Exp Path Pharmak.* 1887;22:261.
30. Knoll PW. Über die Druckschwankungen in der Cerebrospinalflussigkeit und den Wechsel in der Blutfülle des centralen Nervensystems. *S.-B. Akad Wiss Wein, math-nat Kl.* 1886;93/94 B:217.
31. Levy LM, DiChiro GD, McCollough DC, et al. Fixed spinal cord: diagnosis with MR imaging. *Radiology.* 1988;169:773–778.
32. Kostopoulos DC, Keramidas G. Changes in elongation of falx cerebri during craniosacral therapy techniques applied on the skull of an embalmed cadaver. *J Craniomand Pract.* 1992;10:9–12.
33. Ferre JC, Barbin JY. The osteopathic cranial concept: fact or fiction? *Surg Radiol Anat.* 1991;13:165–170.
34. Rohan AJ, Golombek SG, Rosenthal AD. Infants with misshapen skulls: when to worry. *Contemporary Pediatr.* 1999;16(2):47–70.
35. Pritchard JJ, Scott JH, Girgis FG. The structure and development of cranial and facial sutures. *J Anat.* 1956;90:73–86.
36. Retzlaff EW, Upledger J, Mitchell FL Jr, Walsh J. Aging of cranial sutures in humans. *Anat Rec.* 1979;193:663(abst).
37. Retzlaff EW, Mitchell FL Jr, Upledger J, et al. Neurovascular mechanisms in cranial sutures. *JAOA.* 1980;80:218–219(abst).
38. Retzlaff EW, Jones L, Mitchell FL Jr, Upledger J. Possible autonomic innervation of cranial sutures of primates and other animals. *Brain Res.* 1973;58:470–477(abst).
39. Michael DK, Retzlaff, EW. A preliminary study of cranial bone movement in the squirrel monkey. *JAOA.* 1975;74:866–869.
40. Heisey SR, Adams T. Role of cranial bone mobility in cranial compliance. *Neurosurgery.* 1993;33(5):869–876.
41. Heisey SR, Adams T. A two compartment model for cranial compliance. *JAOA.* 1995;95(5):547.
42. Adams T, Heisey RS, Smith MC, Briner BJ. Parietal bone mobility in the anesthetized cat. *JAOA.* 1992;92(5):599–622.
43. Frymann VM. A study if the rhythmic motions of the living cranium. *JAOA.* 1971;70:1–18.
44. Heifitz MD, Weiss M. Detection of skull expansion with increased intracranial pressure. *J Neurosurg.* 1981;55:811–812.
45. Tettambel M, Cicora RA, Lay EM. Recording of the cranial rhythmic impulse. *JAOA.* 1978;78:149(abst).
46. Zanakis MF, Cebelenski RM, Dowling D, et al. The cranial kinetogram: objective quantification of cranial mobility in man. *JAOA.* 1994;94(9):761(abst).
47. Zanakis MF, Morgan M, Storch I, et al. Detailed study of cranial bone motion in man. *JAOA.* 1996;96(9):552(abst).
48. Lewandowski MA, Drasby E, Morgan M, Zanakis MF. Kinematic system demonstrates cranial bone movement about the cranial sutures. *JAOA.* 1996;96(9):551(abst).
49. Moskalenko YE, Kravchenko T, Chervotok A, Sharapov K. Bioengineering support of the cranial osteopathic treatment. *Med Biol Eng Comput.* 1996:34[Suppl 1, Part 2]:185–186.
50. Moskalenko YE, Kravchenko TI, Gaidar BV, et al. Periodic mobility of cranial bones in humans. *Hum Physiol.* 1999;25(1):51–58.
51. Moskalenko YE, Frymann V, Weinstein GB, et al. Slow rhythmic oscillations within the human cranium: phenomenology, origin, and informational significance. *Hum Physiol.* 2001;27(2):171–178. Translated from *Fiziologica Cheloveka.* 2001;27(2):47–55.
52. Nelson KE, Sergueff N, Lipinski CM, et al. Cranial rhythmic impulse

related to the Traube-Hering-Mayer oscillation: comparing laser-Doppler flowmetry and palpation. *JAOA.* 2001;101(3):163–173.

53. Weisl H. The movements of the sacro-iliac joint. *Acta Anat.* 1955;23:80–91.

54. Mitchell FL Jr. Voluntary and involuntary respiration and the craniosacral mechanism. *Osteopath Ann.* 1977;5:52–59.

55. Pruzzo NA. Lateral lumbar spine double-exposure technique and associated principles. *JAOA.* 1970;69:84–86.

56. Mitchell FL Jr, Pruzzo NA. Investigation of voluntary and primary respiratory mechanisms. *JAOA.* 1971;70:149–153.

57. Williams PL, Warwick R, Dyson M, Bannister LH. *Gray's Anatomy,* 37th ed. Edinburgh, Scotland: Churchill-Livingstone; 1988.

58. Bates B. *A Guide to Physical Examination,* 3rd ed. Philadelphia, PA: JB Lippincott Co; 1983:149.

59. Drengler KE, King HH. Inter-examiner reliability of palpatory diagnosis of the cranium. *JAOA.* 1998;98(7):387(abst).

60. Woods JM, Woods RH. A physical finding related to psychiatric disorders. *JAOA.* 1961;60:988–993.

61. Sutherland WG, Wales AL. *Teachings in the Science of Osteopathy.* Portland, OR: Rudra Press; 1990.

62. Magoun HI. Entrapment neuropathy in the cranium. *JAOA.* 1968;67:643–652.

63. Magoun HI. Entrapment neuropathy of the central nervous system, part II. *JAOA.* 1968;67:779–787.

64. Magoun HI. Entrapment neuropathy of the central nervous system, part III. *JAOA.* 1968;67:889–899.

65. Magoun HI. Whiplash injury: a greater lesion complex. *JAOA.* 1964;63:524–535.

66. Harakal JH. An osteopathically integrated approach to the whiplash complex. *JAOA.* 1975;74:941–955.

67. Lay EM. In: Gelb H, ed. *Clinical Management of Head, Neck and TMJ Pain and Dysfunction.* Philadelphia, PA: WB Saunders; 1977;17.

68. Becker RE. *Lecture: Sutherland Cranial Teaching Foundation Basic Course.* Colorado Springs, CO; 1985.

69. Magoun HI. Dental equilibration and osteopathy. *JAOA.* 1975;74:981–991.

70. Magoun HI. Osteopathic approach to dental enigmas. *JAOA.* 1962;62:110–118.

71. Magoun HI. The dental search for a common denominator in craniocervical pain and dysfunction. *JAOA.* 197;78:1–6.

63

STRAIN AND COUNTERSTRAIN TECHNIQUES

JOHN C. GLOVER
PAUL R. RENNIE

KEY CONCEPTS

- History
- Theoretical physiologic basis
- Treatment
- Instructions to patients
- Clinical pearls
- Specific treatments by body region

HISTORY

Counterstrain began as an unexpected discovery in 1955. A young, athletic-looking man visited Lawrence H. Jones, DO, FAAO (1) because he had developed a condition 2 months prior that left him unable to stand erect. The injury was not caused by trauma, but it gradually worsened over the 2 months. Since the onset, the man had received treatment by two chiropractors with no substantial improvement. Jones treated the man several times over the course of 6 weeks with no better results.

At one visit, the man reported difficulty sleeping due to pain. Jones worked with the patient to find a comfortable position for the man to sleep in. After finding the position, Jones left the young man in the position and went to treat another patient. When Jones returned 20 minutes later, he assisted the young man to a standing position and to their mutual surprise, the patient stood erect and pain free for the first time in 4 months. Jones was impressed by the results and decided to investigate these findings.

Jones experimented by treating patients with positions of comfort. He had frequent success, but wanted to shorten the waiting time of the treatment position. He observed that paravertebral areas that were tender to palpation prior to positioning were pain free after placing the patient in a position of comfort for a period of time. Dr. Jones then began positioning only the affected region of the body, and this reduced the time in the treatment position. Ninety seconds in the position of comfort proved to be the optimal time required to benefit the patient. Shorter periods of time

did not always produce lasting relief, and longer periods did not necessarily yield greater benefit. He also began mapping the discrete areas of tenderness and correlating them to specific somatic dysfunction identified by the methods he learned in osteopathic medical school.

However, Jones found that he could only find the discrete paravertebral areas of tenderness in half of the patients. More answers came when Jones saw a patient with a groin injury. Although the examination revealed no inguinal hernia, there was a discrete area of tenderness. Jones placed the man in a position of comfort and palpated the tender area. To their surprise, it was no longer tender. Jones slowly returned the patient to a neutral position and palpated the area of complaint again. He found no evidence of tenderness.

Jones discovered that there were anterior, as well as posterior, tender points. Jones began to search for tender points in the anterior tissues (2). This observation is consistent with the osteopathic principle of the body as a unit. The emphasis on spinal function and posterior diagnostic evaluation had eclipsed this connection.

Other treatment approaches to the musculoskeletal system have identified discrete areas of tense, tender tissue. Travell (3) developed an approach and used the term *trigger point* to describe tense areas. Jones (1,4) initially used the same term, but later referred to these areas as *tender points*. Jones described over 200 specific tender points, and new tender points continue to be found. Through correspondence, Travell and Jones identified similarities and differences between their diagnostic and treatment approaches.

Initially, Jones referred to his new treatment approach as *spontaneous release by positioning* (5), but found this term to be cumbersome. Jones decided to use a shorter term, *counterstrain*, describing what Jones believed happened when his technique was used to treat somatic dysfunction. The initial injury produces a sudden "panic" lengthening of the antagonistic muscle to the originally strained and painful agonist muscle. Jones treats the tender point associated with the antagonistic muscle by shortening this muscle, which also places the originally strained and painful muscle back into a stretched position—the position of the original strain.

Dr. Jones made two important discoveries that contributed to manual medicine:

1. Placing the body into a position of maximum comfort can treat somatic dysfunction.
2. The anterior aspect of the patient must be evaluated, as well as the posterior, to effectively diagnose and treat somatic dysfunction.

THEORETICAL PHYSIOLOGIC BASIS OF COUNTERSTRAIN

Physicians have demonstrated the clinical benefits of counterstrain for almost 50 years (6–14,19,22). However, research to confirm the physiologic basis of manual techniques has been limited. Therefore, we must draw on physiologic studies to shed light on how counterstrain works.

Because tender points are found in myofascial tissue, understanding muscle physiology provides some answers. This includes the palpatory changes in the myofascial tissue, as well as hypertonic muscles associated with somatic dysfunction. The neural system is another key component in the development and maintenance of somatic dysfunction. A third element important to understanding counterstrain is the role of the circulatory system.

At the time Jones was formulating his ideas about counterstrain, Korr (15) published an article on proprioceptors and somatic dysfunction. The article helped explain the role of the proprioceptors in muscle tone and the response to injury. Another important part of the model is the gamma system and its role in muscle tone. Van Buskirk (16) described the important role of nociception in somatic dysfunction. The role of the circulatory system has not been adequately explained.

One of the most important characteristics of the counterstrain model is the relationship between tender points and somatic dysfunction. The location of a specific tender point is constant from one patient to another. This suggests a strong anatomic basis for their location. Different myofascial structures, including tendons, ligaments, and muscle bellies have all been found to contain tender points. Myotomal, dermatomal, and sclerotomal relationships have been proposed to explain the relationship between a specific anatomic segment and the related tender points (17,18,20). Another interesting anatomic correlation is the close location of tender points in areas where motor points are found. A motor point is the site where the motor nerve pierces the investing fascia and enters the muscle it innervates.

Mapping the pathways of afferent nerves and the central system is important to understanding the role of the afferent nervous system. The bulk of afferent input comes from the soma (as opposed to the viscera). This difference is so great that nociceptive messages from the viscera are typically interpreted as being of somal origin. This unequal distribution can also be seen with the illustration of the homunculus in the cerebral cortex. The homunculus illustrates the proportional area in the cortex devoted to sensing and interpreting afferent input from different locations in the periphery. The neuronal "crosstalk" in the central nervous system between sensory and motor nerves is the source of the various reflexes between the viscera and the soma. It also provides an explanation for why counterstrain treatment can have an effect on visceral function and circulatory flow.

Normal function of the gamma efferent system is responsible for the change in muscle tone with changing demand. Jones proposed that the gamma system is responsible for the development of an inappropriate proprioceptive reflex associated with somatic dysfunction. A rapid shortening, then lengthening of the myofascial tissue sets up the inappropriate reflex. An event occurs that produces rapid lengthening of a muscle. Afferent feedback indicates possible myofascial damage from a strain. The body tries to prevent the myofascial damage by rapidly contracting the myofascial tissue that may be strained. This produces a rapid lengthening in the antagonist muscle. It is proposed that the rapid shortening, then lengthening of the antagonist produces the inappropriate reflex, and this is manifest as a tender point. The theory is that the nociceptive feedback from the antagonist is interpreted as a muscle strain (although a strain has not occurred). The end result is hypertonic myofascial tissue and restricted motion. A guarding reflex by the patient, without actual mechanical trauma, can also produce the inappropriate reflex. Although this model does explain the development of some tender points, it does not explain all of them.

Trauma produces change in myofascial tissues at microscopic and biochemical levels (21). The force of the trauma causes damage to myofibrils and their microcirculation. Myofibril damage interferes with the actin-myosin bridges and changes the chemistry around them. Nociceptive information is carried to the central nervous system to alert the body to the tissue damage. The tissue disruption and subsequent chemical changes cause the tissue to become more sensitive to touch and may be part of the reason for the formation of a tender point. The damage to the microcirculation changes intramuscular pressure and muscle function. A small increase in intramuscular pressure can produce muscle fatigue due to decreased cellular metabolism (21). This change in metabolism changes the chemical matrix around the myofibrils and can produce nociceptive activity, resulting in tenderness (21).

A tender point is sensitive to palpation and therefore must be related to nociceptive activity. The position of comfort used to treat a somatic dysfunction with counterstrain is a very specific, three-dimensional position in space. When the optimal position of comfort is established, the tenderness of the tender point disappears or becomes insignificant. This seems to indicate a neural relationship between the tender point and the somatic dysfunction. Neural messages are rapidly transmitted and used by the body when quick responses are needed. If counterstrain treats the neural component of somatic dysfunction, why did Jones determine 90 seconds as the optimal time to maintain the position of comfort? Palpation of changes at the tender point and in the surrounding tissue suggests that in addition to the neural component, the position of comfort also produces changes in the myofascial tissue and small circulatory vessels.

A clue for the treatment time comes from the palpation of a pulsation, the therapeutic pulse, at a tender point location. The frequency of the pulsation is the same as the cardiac cycle and would therefore indicate a circulatory relationship. Another important fact is that the pulsation is not present before positioning, develops only when the patient is moved close to the position of comfort, and disappears after myofascial tissue relaxation. This process takes approximately 90 seconds to occur. The pulsation phenomenon does not occur with every tender point but when it is palpated, it does correlate with markedly improved treatment response.

TREATMENT

Counterstrain is a very gentle technique that is well tolerated by most patients. The patient is not subjected to any external force other than gentle positioning. In addition, patients do not generate force from their own muscle contraction to produce effective treatment. It is an indirect technique, with positioning away from restrictive barriers; therefore, it is tolerated in both acute and chronic problems.

Counterstrain is based on identifying tender points associated with a somatic dysfunction and positioning the patient to eliminate the tenderness of the point. Counterstrain is easy to understand and apply, but mastery requires time to learn the location of tender points; skill in fine-tuning the treatment position for maximum results; and clinical experience to understand the correlations between symptoms, structural findings, and associated tender points. The basic steps for treating with counterstrain are:

1. Find a significant tender point.
2. Position the patient for maximum comfort.
3. Maintain the position for 90 seconds.
4. Slowly return the patient to a neutral position.
5. Recheck the tender point.

Find a Significant Tender Point

Tender points are typically located in tendinous attachments or on the belly of a muscle. Additional tender points are found in other myofascial tissues (often ligaments) associated with the joint dysfunction. Tender points are typically discrete, small, tense, and edematous. The areas are about the size of a fingertip, and they are exquisitely tender. A significant tender point is at least four times more tender than the adjacent tissue. Tissue changes of the tender points may range from several inches to virtually nonexistent. The tissue of the tender point is found to be tenser than the surrounding tissue.

It is essential to identify the most significant tender point associated with the somatic dysfunction rather than just finding a point that is tender. Due to the exquisite tenderness of significant tender points, a patient will typically wince, guard, or push your hand away when you press the tender point. Patients are often surprised with the amount of tenderness, especially when they were unaware of the existence of the tender point. In rare cases, a patient does not perceive tenderness when a tender point is pressed. These patients are referred to as stoics and can be treated with counterstrain by monitoring tissue changes that occur during treatment.

Palpate for a tender point with the pad of your finger or thumb. The pads of the fingers are profoundly more sensitive to tactile input and are better at identifying the location of tender points. Avoid using the fingertips, especially if you have long fingernails. Fingertips are less sensitive and can elicit iatrogenic tenderness.

Palpation should be firm but gentle. The pressure used to elicit a tender point is typically a few ounces and not strong enough to elicit tenderness in normal tissue. Jones recommended using the amount of force needed to blanch the nail bed of the palpating finger. The vector of pressure is also important. Typically, the tissue of the tender point is pressed onto more rigid tissue like bone or cartilage. Do not forget to check for other pathology that might produce tenderness that is not related to neuromusculoskeletal tender points, such as infection, inflammation, or viscerosomatic referred pain.

Verify the presence of a tender point by asking the patient if the area is tender while the potential tender point is pressed. The tenderness of a tender point is an objective sign elicited by physically palpating the dysfunctional area. In contrast, pain is a subjective symptom that the patient may experience without undergoing palpation. Again, Jones found that often pain and weakness are found in areas away from where tender points may be found.

One method to determine where tender points may be found is to perform an osteopathic structural examination, noting any alteration of movement, asymmetry of paired landmarks, or tissue texture changes. Palpating these areas for tender points is how Jones originally found many of the tender points he described. Evaluate the patient for variations from ideal posture and palpate those areas for tender points. For example, a patient presenting with flattening of the normal thoracic kyphotic curve is likely to have one or more posterior thoracic tender points associated with the extension in this region. Tender point locations can also be suggested based on clinical history and presenting complaints. The most likely places for significant tender points can be deduced from knowing the position in which the original injury occurred. Many myofascial pain patterns have been described by Travell (3) and may provide additional correlation.

A significant tender point results in the patient attempting to obtain a comfortable posture to alleviate the functional distress. This is an unconscious attempt by the patient to shorten and relieve tense myofascial tissues. Patients tend to bend around tender points. That is, tender points tend to be at the apex or focal point of the concavity of the postural adaptation. If the patient is forward bent, tender points tend to be anterior. If a patient is backward bent, tender points tend to be posterior. Jones found that a patient who presents side-bent to the right usually has tender points on the left side of the spine. Conversely, a patient who is side-bent to the left usually has tender points on the right (Jones LH. Personal communication, 1993).

Tender points are frequently found in areas other than the area of pain or discomfort. The primary or key strain may induce a secondary or compensatory strain elsewhere, which may be more symptomatic. Treatment of the primary dysfunction often alleviates symptoms reported elsewhere. For example, when the psoas muscle chronically stays in spasm, patients seldom complain of abdominal or anterolateral hip pain. Instead, they complain of pain in the lumbosacral or sacroiliac regions, due to the strain and compensation of those regions by the psoas spasm. Tender points are frequently found 180 degrees around the body from the site of the presenting pain. For example, in a patient with pain between the shoulder blades, the tender point is often on the sternum. It is also possible to have both anterior and posterior or right and left tender points associated with the same anatomic segmental level. This is because tender points are mediated through the nervous system and can result in multiple points for a single somatic dysfunction. If there are multiple tender points in a given area, ask the patient which is the tenderest. Treat the most severe tender point first. Associated but less significant tender points often disappear after successful treatment of the tenderest point.

If the tender point results from a viscerosomatic reflex, tenderness returns within minutes or hours. When this happens, a thorough review of the patient's medical history and more careful physical examination is needed. Be sure all of the possible causes of the original tenderness have been considered. For more information about viscerosomatic reflexes, refer to the discussion of viscerosomatic reflexes in the basic science section of this book, or read Beal's article (18). This information is also important when treating patients in the hospital. Refer to the article by Schwartz (19) on the treatment of hospital patients with counterstrain.

Position the Patient for Maximum Comfort

One of the advantages of counterstrain is that treatment is always in a position of comfort. The position of comfort correlates with the same position in which the patient suffered the original injury. If an adequate history is elicited, the position in which to treat the patient can frequently be deduced and used for treatment. For example, if the patient was injured attempting to lift an object while bending forward at the waist and side bending to the right, then the treatment position would be with the patient forward-bent and side-bent to the right.

By placing the patient in a position of comfort, discomfort is avoided and further injury is unlikely to occur. Counterstrain can be used for patients with a wide variety of medical conditions, unless gently moving the patient into the specific treatment position is contraindicated. A word of caution: Medical judgment must always be used to determine the appropriateness of any treatment. Counterstrain may be contraindicated for some patients with metastatic carcinoma, uncontrolled infection, and some other conditions. Every patient needs to be evaluated on an individual basis. The only absolute requirement is that the patient must be relaxed while the physician places the dysfunctional area of the body into the treatment position.

The optimal position of comfort is a very specific position in space. The position is similar for the same tender point in different patients, but the exact position is unique for each patient. To find the optimal position, the physician uses a combination of palpation and feedback from the patient. To test the tender point, press this area and immediately release the pressure, but maintain light contact with the myofascial tissue. Then ask the patient for the level of tenderness. Maintaining continuous light contact with the tender point during treatment is important for maximum effectiveness.

To facilitate the communication between physician and patient, it is important to establish a means of monitoring the level of tenderness of the tender point. Physicians typically use a tenderness scale to enhance verbal feedback with the patient. Several scales have been used effectively. The one most commonly used is a 0-to-10 scale, with 10 being equal to the level of tenderness prior to positioning for treatment and 0 representing the absence of tenderness. The scale allows the patient to communicate changes in tenderness and is correlated with palpatory changes. The same amount of pressure should be used each time the physician attempts to elicit tenderness of the point. It should be emphasized to the patient that this is not acupressure or a form of massage. Firm pressure is applied only when trying to determine the level tenderness. At other times, only light contact is maintained. This feedback provides a means for monitoring the effectiveness of positioning and treatment for both patient and physician.

The first step in positioning is to approximate the position expected. The expectation may be from previous clinical experience, patient history, or from looking at an illustration of the positioning in a counterstrain book. The purpose of the positioning is to reduce the tension on the dysfunctional myofascial structures.

Slowly move the patient toward the described or expected position of comfort while monitoring the tender point for relaxation of the tissue. When relaxation of the tender point is palpated, stop moving the patient. Press the tender point and ask for the level of tenderness. If the level of tenderness is greater than 3 on the 10-point scale, continue to move the patient in the same direction. Then, as further relaxation is palpated, stop movement and test again. Repeat this process until the tenderness level is three or less. If the number increases, return in the direction just traveled and retest. It may be necessary to change direction or add other directions to find the correct position.

As you get close to the optimal position, fine tuning the position with small motions is required. A small change in position at this point in the treatment markedly reduces tenderness. For example, several inches of movement close to the neutral position may reduce the tenderness by one on the scale. Whereas, it may take only one-quarter inch of movement close to the optimal position to reduce the tenderness the same amount. Slow, small movements, constant light contact of the tender point for monitoring, and retesting the tender point for reduction of tenderness with each new position all allow the practitioner to find the precise position of optimal comfort. If the optimal position is overshot, the level of tenderness will increase. Fine-tune the position until the tenderness has been reduced by at least 70% (3 on the scale), preferably 100%. The position of comfort must be at least 70% improved over the initial tenderness, or the technique is ineffective. Jones recommended a reduction of two-thirds, and other practitioners have suggested three-fourths. An effort should be made to maximally reduce the tenderness. The extra time spent trying to eliminate the tenderness will significantly increase the effectiveness of the treatment.

A common mistake is to use constant firm pressure on the tender point throughout the treatment sequence. Instead, constant light contact should be maintained. Once the optimal treatment position has been determined, be sure to maintain only light contact with the myofascial tissue of the tender point. There are three important reasons for maintaining contact:

1. Tissue changes that occur in the tender point can be monitored more easily and can aid in determining the end point of treatment.

2. The tender point can continue to be fine-tuned while maintaining the optimal position of comfort, because the position may change slightly during treatment.

3. Both the patient and the practitioner can be confident of the location of the tender point.

The third reason may seem unimportant, but when contact with the tender point is lost, the patient may question whether the same point is being pressed. Also, the practitioner may have difficulty reestablishing contact with the point with enough confidence to allow an accurate recheck.

At times, a pulsation in the tender point may be palpated. This is referred to as the therapeutic pulse. Although its intensity may vary, it is often close to the intensity of the radial pulse. In fact, palpating the patient's radial artery with the other hand typically shows it to be synchronous with the therapeutic pulse. For this reason, it is postulated that the position of release results in a sympathetic vasodilation of the small arterioles in the myofascial tissue. At times, the therapeutic pulse can be palpated while attempting to find the optimal position of comfort, enabling the practitioner to establish the position more accurately. At other times, the therapeutic pulse will not be palpated until the treatment position has been maintained for 90 seconds. In either case, the appearance of the therapeutic pulse can be used to enhance the treatment.

As a rule, the closer tender points are to the midline, the more flexed or extended is the patient's presenting posture, and more flexion or extension is required for the treatment position. With tender points more lateral to the midline, more side bending and rotation are usually required for treatment. Side-bending and/or rotation of the body away from the tender point are the most common positions needed for effective treatment.

Maintain the Position for 90 Seconds

Once the position of comfort has been established, hold it for 90 seconds. It is important to remember that the patient must remain relaxed without contracting the affected myofascial tissue. The 90 seconds does not begin until the patient is completely relaxed.

It may be necessary to remind the patient to stay relaxed several times during the 90 seconds, because often the patient contracts muscles unconsciously. Patients who are not comfortable will not be able to relax for the entire 90 seconds. Also, if the practitioner is not comfortable, it is difficult to hold the patient in the treatment position for 90 seconds. You may need to experiment to find the best way to remain comfortable during treatment. Each patient and clinical setting offers different challenges. It may be necessary to invent a new treatment position to enable both the patient and yourself to remain comfortable. This is especially true with pregnant patients, patients with some degree of paralysis, and hospitalized patients.

Feel for tissue changes in the tender point and surrounding tissue. As time in the treatment position increases, the tissue relaxes and can feel like melting butter. The myofascial tissue around the tender point may begin to move in a seemingly random pattern. This sensation is due to the relaxation of myofascial tissue in different planes. Once the tissue changes that signal the end of treatment can be palpated with confidence, watching a clock is no longer needed.

The ability to palpate myofascial release patterns enhances counterstrain treatment and can also be used to improve palpatory skills needed for myofascial release techniques. As discussed earlier, you may also feel the therapeutic pulse. Once the random motion has stopped or the therapeutic pulse disappears, it is time to move the patient back to the starting position.

Slowly Return the Patient to Neutral

After maintaining the position of comfort for 90 seconds, it is time to slowly return the patient to neutral. The first few degrees of motion during return are the most critical. Before starting to move, ask the patient to remain passive and not assist you by actively moving. Patients may unconsciously try to help.

A common error when learning counterstrain is to move the patient too quickly. Watch the patient for signs of flinching or other guarding gestures. Palpating for muscle contraction could also provide a sign. An apparent decrease in the patient's weight as you support them in the treatment position is another indication that the patient is contracting muscles. If the patient starts to help or move, stop the return and remind the patient not to help. When the patient has relaxed, start moving again, more slowly.

Recheck the Tender Point

Once the patient has been returned to a relaxed position, recheck the tender point for tenderness. To consider the treatment successful, no more than 30% of the original tenderness should remain. Ideally, all of the tenderness will have resolved. If more than 30% of the tenderness remains, several possible reasons may exist. The patient may not have been optimally positioned or may have moved during the 90-second holding time. Repeat the positioning, with particular attention to obtaining and maintaining the optimal position with the patient completely relaxed.

Another cause for failure may be that another tender point is the primary problem and, therefore, the most significant point was not treated. Evaluate the area around the tender point to see if another, more significant tender point is present. Consider the possibility that the primary tender point is distant from the area evaluated or on the opposite side of the body from the reported problem. More than one treatment may be necessary to completely resolve a tender point. Also, failure to completely resolve the tenderness does not necessarily indicate an ineffective treatment. Although treatment time may not always be exactly 90 seconds, it is important to maintain the treatment position for 90 seconds when learning counterstrain.

Recheck the original structural findings to evaluate the effectiveness of the treatment. You are treating a somatic dysfunction, not a tender point, so rechecking cannot be overstated. Motion restrictions should disappear and tissue texture changes should start to return to normal after effective treatment. With chronic somatic dysfunction, the tissue changes may be slower to return to normal.

INSTRUCTIONS TO PATIENTS

It is most prudent to start instructions before the patient gets off the treatment table. Patients are curious to see if the treatment eliminated the presenting complaint. Warn the patient not to test previously restricted motions and to avoid extremes of motion for several days. This is especially true if the movement approximates the original position of injury, because it may reproduce the inappropriate reflex just treated. Active movement that reproduces the position of injury is different from the careful positioning performed by the physician while the patient is passive.

The patient should stay well-hydrated for several days after treatment. This helps with the elimination of increased metabolic waste products that may be released into circulation after relaxation of the tense myofascial tissue. Water is recommended over other fluids, which may contain sugar and other dissolved chemicals.

Although counterstrain techniques are well tolerated, a treatment reaction may occur. Approximately 30% of patients experience a generalized soreness or a flu-like reaction 1 to 48 hours after treatment. This usually is experienced by the patient on the morning after treatment and may last 1 to 5 days, although 1 day is most typical. The reaction usually happens only after the first treatment but may occur for several treatments. The cause of the reaction is unclear, but may be related to the washout of metabolic waste products from the dysfunctional myofascial tissue. There also is a correlation with treating dysfunctions where the therapeutic pulse is palpated during treatment. In any case, the patient should be alerted to the possibility of a treatment reaction. Prescribing an analgesic for one or two days may help reduce the reaction. This possibility of a treatment reaction also provides a reason for caution in using counterstrain to treat some severely ill patients.

Patients want to know how often they need to be treated and how long it will take to resolve the complaint. As with all forms of manipulative treatment, there is no single, definitive answer. One treatment may eliminate some somatic dysfunction, although other dysfunction requires treatment over a more extended period of time. On average, the patient is asked to return 3 to 7 days after the initial treatment. As the somatic dysfunction resolves, the time between treatments is increased. The end point of treatment depends on the cause of the problem, the underlying tissue damage, preexisting medical problems, the response of the patient, cooperation by the patient to avoid painful positions, and the skill of the physician.

CLINICAL PEARLS

- Examine the patient thoroughly.
- A single somatic dysfunction may have more than one associated tender point.
- Test for tenderness with the same amount of pressure each time.
- Use less pressure to monitor a tender point than to test it.
- Your palpatory abilities are more reliable than a patient's tenderness report.
- Anterior points typically require flexion, although posterior points typically require extension.
- Midline points typically require pure flexion (if anterior) or pure extension (if posterior), whereas the more lateral a point is from midline, the more rotation and/or side-bending is required.
- Treat the most significant tender point first.
- If several tender points of equal tenderness occur in a row, treat the middle one first.
- Spend a little extra time to fine tune and completely eliminate the tenderness of a tender point.
- The optimal position of comfort is obtained when the tender point is no longer tender.

- Monitor myofascial changes and adjust the treatment position for maximum results.
- Maintain light contact with the tender point throughout the treatment.
- For maximum results, the patient must be completely relaxed (passive) during treatment.
- Recheck the tenderness of a point several times while in the treatment position.

SPECIFIC TREATMENTS BY BODY REGION

General Comments

The after illustrations are intended as an introduction to counterstrain technique. Because this presentation is aimed at the introductory level, primary focus has been placed on the review of vertebral and pelvic dysfunction with limited coverage to the extremities. More in-depth counterstrain reference texts are available for complete coverage of the techniques (1,4,17,20).

The treatment positions presented may be modified as appropriate for the comfort of the physician and the patient. Therefore, knowledge of the three-dimensional position that is typically used to treat a tender point site could be used to treat the patient, for example, while seated, supine, or side-lying. As long as the treatment can be successfully performed, modifications may be helpful adaptations to these techniques.

The following figures are presented by permission of Rennie PR, Glover JC, Carvalho C, Key LS. *Counterstrain and Exercise: An Integrated Approach.* Williamston, MI: RennieMatrix; 2001.

Cervical Spine

The cervical spine has several maverick tender points (points where the position of comfort is different from what might be expected). Anterior tender points are typically located on the most lateral aspect of the lateral masses or slightly anterior on the lateral masses. Posterior tender points are found on the occiput or associated with the tip of the spinous processes or lateral to the spinous processes.

Anterior First Cervical (AC1) (Fig. 63.1)

Tender Point Locations
Found on the posterior surface of the ascending ramus of the mandible approximately a finger width above the angle of the jaw.

Treatment Position
Rotate the head approximately 90 degrees away. Slight side bending away may further reduce the sensitivity by applying a slight caudal force on the contralateral parietal aspect of the cranium. Do not apply extension and do not maintain this position if discomfort increases.

Anterior Second to Sixth Cervical (AC2-6) (Fig. 63.2)

Tender Point Locations
Found at the anterior surface of the transverse processes of the named vertebrae. The sternocleidomastoid muscle crisscrosses over this line of tender points.

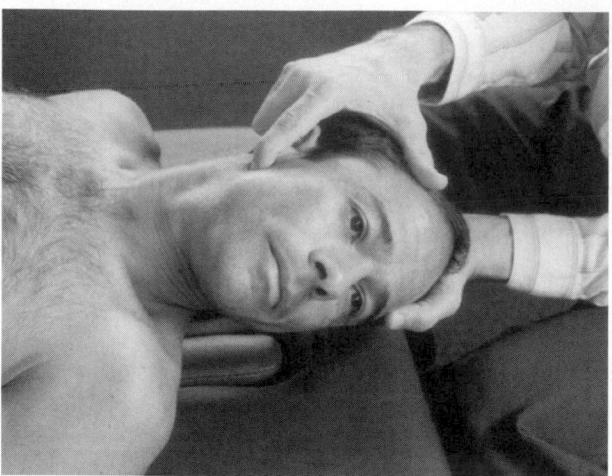

FIGURE 63.1. From Rennie PR, Glover JC, Carvalho C, et al. *Counterstrain and Exercise: An Integrated Approach.* Williamston, MI: RennieMatrix; 2001, with permission.

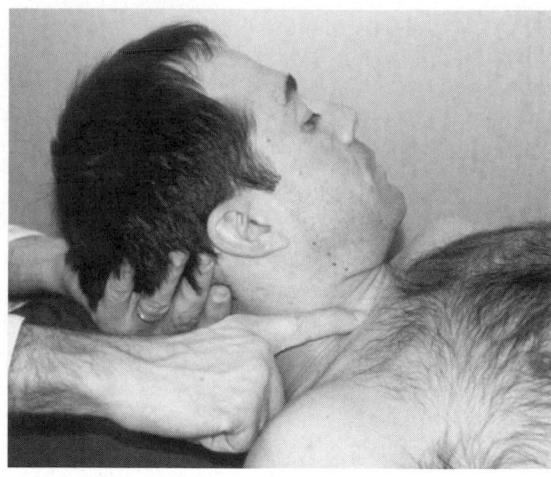

FIGURE 63.3. From Rennie PR, Glover JC, Carvalho C, et al. *Counterstrain and Exercise: An Integrated Approach.* Williamston, MI: RennieMatrix; 2001, with permission.

Treatment Position

Flexion of the head and upper neck (by approximately 45 degrees) to the segment involved. Side bend and rotate the head and upper neck away from the tender point side.

Anterior Seventh to Eighth Cervical (AC7-8) (Fig. 63.3)

Tender Point Locations

AC7: 2 to 3 cm lateral from the medial portion of the clavicle at the origin of the clavicular division of the sternocleidomastoid muscle.

AC8: at the medial end of the clavicle at the sternal notch and involves the sternal division of the sternocleidomastoid muscle.

Treatment Position

Marked flexion of the head and neck by lifting from the middle of the neck. Rotate the head away and side bend the neck toward (away for AC8) from the tender point side.

Posterior Second Cervical (PC2) (Fig. 63.4)

Tender Point Locations

Within the semispinalis capitis in association with the greater occipital nerve (which pierces this muscle near the tender point site). Another tender point can be found at the superior lateral surface of the C2 spinous process.

Treatment Position

Mild extension of the head at the occiput with simultaneous mild caudal push on the vertex of the head to create slack in the occipital muscles.

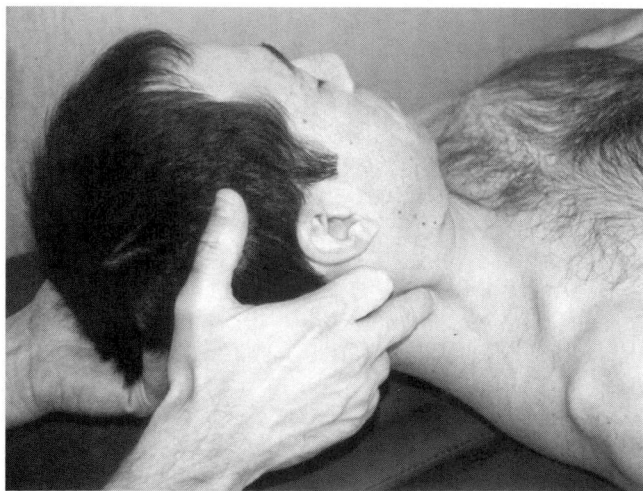

FIGURE 63.2. From Rennie PR, Glover JC, Carvalho C, et al. *Counterstrain and Exercise: An Integrated Approach.* Williamston, MI: RennieMatrix; 2001, with permission.

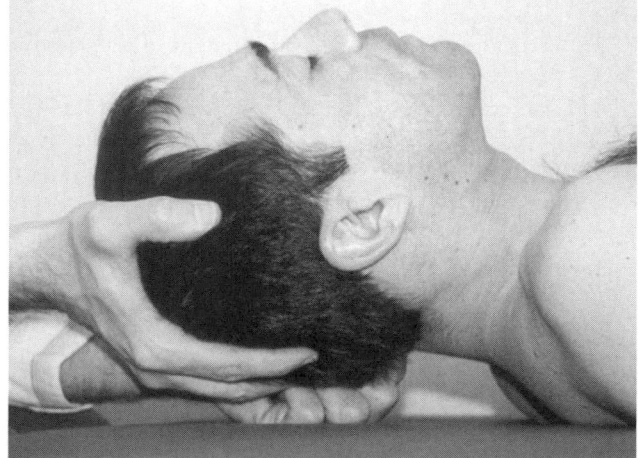

FIGURE 63.4. From Rennie PR, Glover JC, Carvalho C, et al. *Counterstrain and Exercise: An Integrated Approach.* Williamston, MI: RennieMatrix; 2001, with permission.

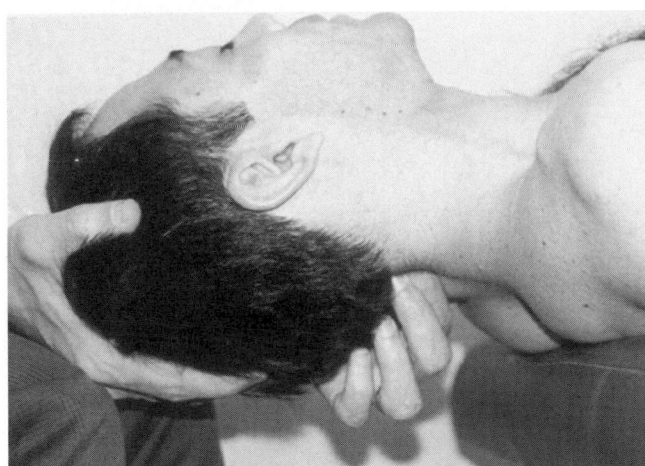

FIGURE 63.5. From Rennie PR, Glover JC, Carvalho C, et al. *Counterstrain and Exercise: An Integrated Approach.* Williamston, MI: RennieMatrix; 2001, with permission.

Posterior Fourth to Eighth Cervical (PC4-8) (Fig. 63.5)

Tender Point Locations
The C4 tender point is at the inferior portion of the C3 spinous process (named for the spinal nerve associated with this level). The remaining inferior tender points at each cervical segment follow this nomenclature.

Treatment Position
Extension of the segment involved with side bending and rotation to the opposite side.

Thoracic Spine

Anterior thoracic spine tender points are located in two major areas. The first group of tender points, AT1-6, are located midline on the sternum. They can be located by palpating for tense, tender tissue overlying the sternum. The second group is located in the abdominal wall. Most are located in the rectus abdominis muscle and can be found an inch or two lateral to midline on the right or left. Posterior thoracic tender points are found on two parts of each vertebra. One location is associated with the spinous process, typically on either side. The second location is on either transverse process.

The treatments described here are given for different spinal levels, but are not hard and fast requirements. Extension, side-bending, and rotation to any level can be introduced either from above or below the segment. The physician's choice is based on the flexibility of the patient, patient comfort, and the relative size of the patient and physician.

Anterior First to Sixth Thoracic (AT1-6) (Fig. 63.6)

Tender Point Locations
AT1: apex of the sternal notch.
    AT2: middle of the manubrium.
    AT3 to AT6: on the sternum at the same numbered costal level.

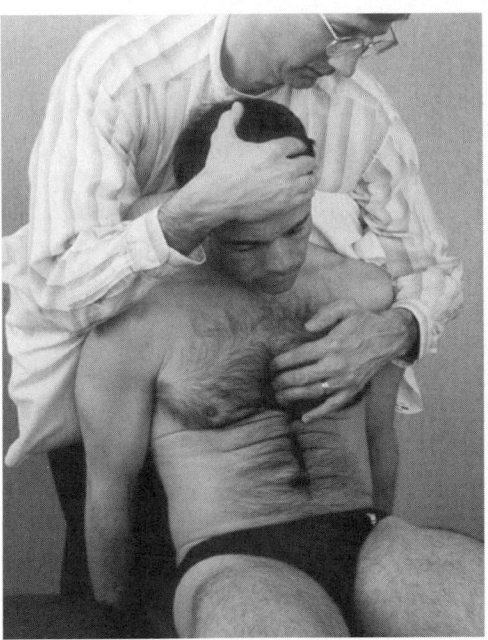

FIGURE 63.6. From Rennie PR, Glover JC, Carvalho C, et al. *Counterstrain and Exercise: An Integrated Approach.* Williamston, MI: RennieMatrix; 2001, with permission.

Treatment Position
Flexion of the involved vertebrae by placing a vector force from the top of the shoulders to enhance the flexion. The arms are internally rotated.

Anterior Seventh to Ninth Thoracic (AT7-9) (Fig. 63.7)

Tender Point Locations
AT7: under the costochondral margin, lateral, and inferior to the xiphoid process.
    AT8: approximately 3 cm below the xiphoid process.
    AT9: 1 to 2 cm above the umbilicus, 2 to 3 cm lateral to the midline.

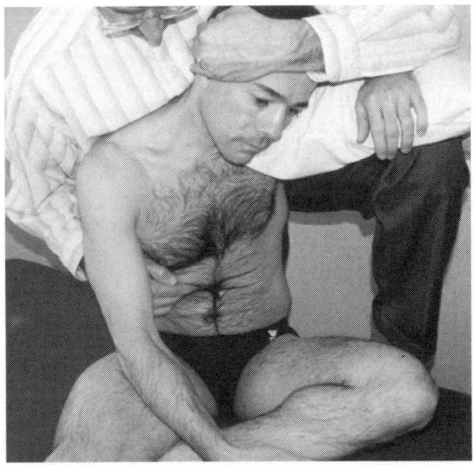

FIGURE 63.7. From Rennie PR, Glover JC, Carvalho C, et al. *Counterstrain and Exercise: An Integrated Approach.* Williamston, MI: RennieMatrix; 2001, with permission.

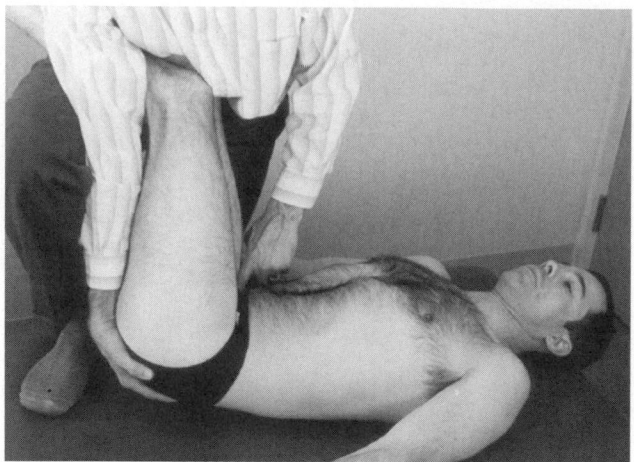

FIGURE 63.8. From Rennie PR, Glover JC, Carvalho C, et al. *Counterstrain and Exercise: An Integrated Approach.* Williamston, MI: RennieMatrix; 2001, with permission.

Treatment Position

Flexion of the involved vertebrae by placing a vector force from the top of the shoulders to enhance the flexion. Flexion is also enhanced at the hips, more as the lower thoracic levels are involved. Add side bending toward and rotation away from the tender side.

Anterior Tenth to Twelfth Thoracic (AT10-12) (Fig. 63.8)

Tender Point Locations

AT10: 1 to 2 cm below the umbilicus, 2 to 3 cm lateral to the midline.

AT11: 5 to 6 cm below the umbilicus, 2 to 3 cm lateral to the midline.

AT12: inner surface of the iliac crest at the midaxillary line.

Treatment Position

Hips are placed in marked flexion while the legs are pulled to the same side to create slight side-bending toward the tender side. Rotation is typically minimal, rolling the pelvis toward the tender side.

Posterior First to Ninth Thoracic (PT1-9) (Figs. 63.9 and 63.10)

Tender Point Location

On the inferolateral side of the deviated spinous process of the named vertebra. This signifies vertebral rotation of this segment to the opposite direction.

Treatment Position

PT1-4: extend the involved vertebral level, avoiding extension of the occipitoatlantal region. Side bend and rotate the involved segment away from the tender side.

PT5-9: ask the patient to turn their head opposite to the tender side. Side bend the trunk away from the deviated side of the spinous process by pulling the opposite shoulder in a caudal and posterior direction. This creates extension with rotation and side-bending away from the deviated side.

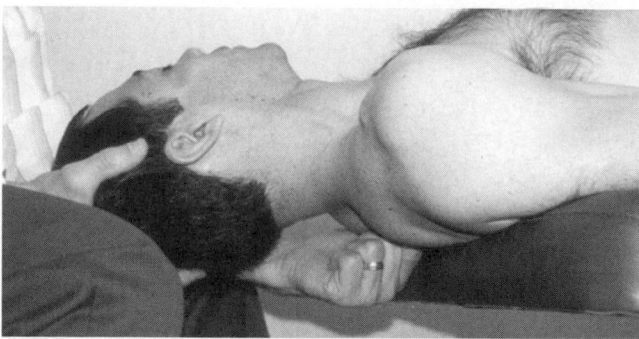

FIGURE 63.9. From Rennie PR, Glover JC, Carvalho C, et al. *Counterstrain and Exercise: An Integrated Approach.* Williamston, MI: RennieMatrix; 2001, with permission.

Posterior Tenth to Twelfth Thoracic (PT10-12) (Fig. 63.11)

Tender Point Location

On the inferolateral side of the deviated spinous process. This signifies vertebral rotation of this segment to the opposite direction.

Treatment Position

Extend the trunk on the ipsilateral side of the deviated spinous process by lifting the pelvis in a posterior direction. This creates extension with the needed rotation of the lower vertebrae toward the tender point side.

Lateral Posterior First to Twelfth Thoracic (LPT1-12) (Fig. 63.12)

Tender Point Location

These points are found more along the transverse process.

Treatment Position

Side-bending is the main action away from the tender site. Rotate the head toward the tender side. Side bend the trunk away from the tender side by pulling the ipsilateral shoulder in an abducted direction without placing pressure or inducing pain in the axilla.

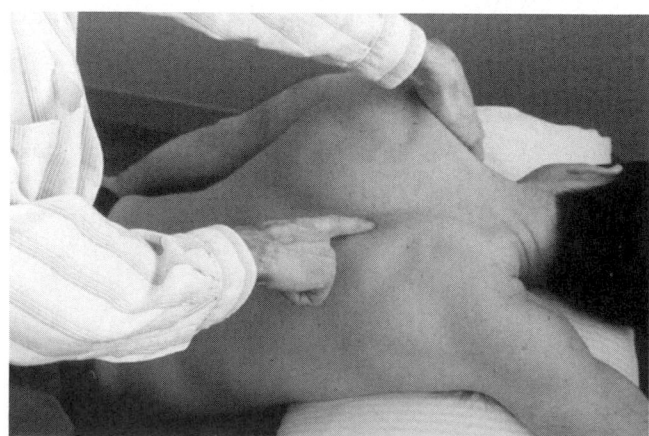

FIGURE 63.10. From Rennie PR, Glover JC, Carvalho C, et al. *Counterstrain and Exercise: An Integrated Approach.* Williamston, MI: RennieMatrix; 2001, with permission.

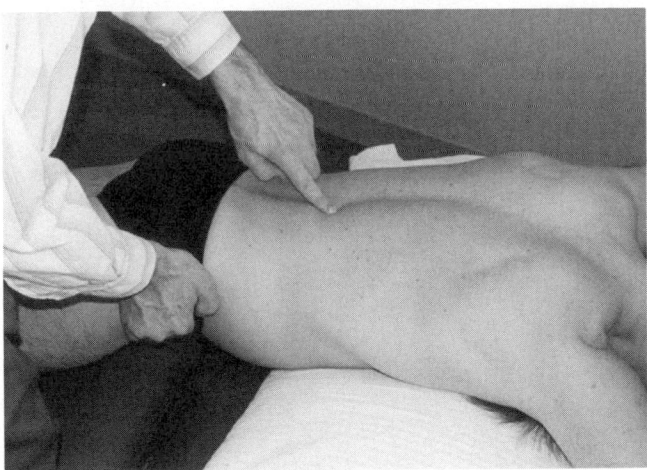

FIGURE 63.11. From Rennie PR, Glover JC, Carvalho C, et al. *Counterstrain and Exercise: An Integrated Approach.* Williamston, MI: RennieMatrix; 2001, with permission.

This creates extension with rotation toward and side-bending away from the tender side.

Ribs

Jones used the terms depressed and elevated to refer to the tender points associated with rib somatic dysfunction. This was done to emphasize what needed to be done with the patient to find a position of maximum comfort. The convention in current use is to name the tender points for their location on the body. In the examples used here, both conventions have been combined.

Anterior tender points correspond to depressed ribs, although posterior tender points correspond to elevated ribs. The anterior rib tender points start just below the medial end of the clavicle where the first rib attaches to the sternum, and move laterally in an arc to the anterior axillary line. Most of the anterior rib tender points are on the ribs along the anterior axillary line. It is not common to find tender points below the sixth rib, but

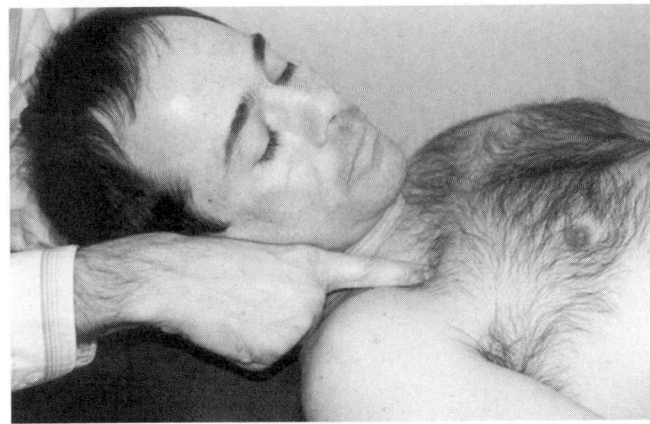

FIGURE 63.13. From Rennie PR, Glover JC, Carvalho C, et al. *Counterstrain and Exercise: An Integrated Approach.* Williamston, MI: RennieMatrix; 2001, with permission.

they do occur. The posterior tender points are located on the angle of the ribs.

Anterior (Depressed) Second Rib (AR1-6) (Figs. 63.13 and 63.14)

Tender Point Location
AR1: on the first rib where it articulates with the manubrium.
 AR2: on the second rib in the midclavicular line.
 AR3-6: on the numbered rib in the anterior axillary line.

Treatment Position
AR1-2: neck flexion, rotation toward, side bending toward.
 AR3-6: flexion of the thoracic cage, head, and neck with elevation of the shoulder and translation away from (side bend toward) the tender point. Rotate toward tender point. Side-bending can be increased with patients legs placed the table opposite the elevated shoulder. The elevated shoulder is usually supported on the physician's thigh.

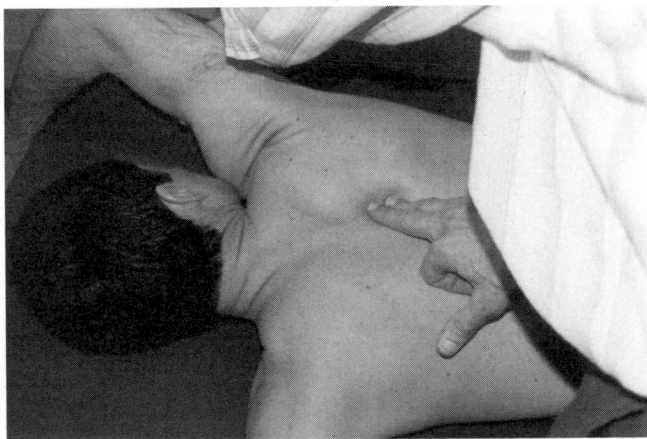

FIGURE 63.12. From Rennie PR, Glover JC, Carvalho C, et al. *Counterstrain and Exercise: An Integrated Approach.* Williamston, MI: RennieMatrix; 2001, with permission.

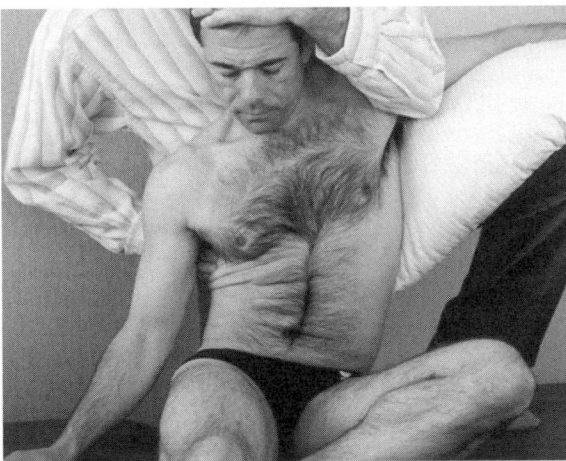

FIGURE 63.14. From Rennie PR, Glover JC, Carvalho C, et al. *Counterstrain and Exercise: An Integrated Approach.* Williamston, MI: RennieMatrix; 2001, with permission.

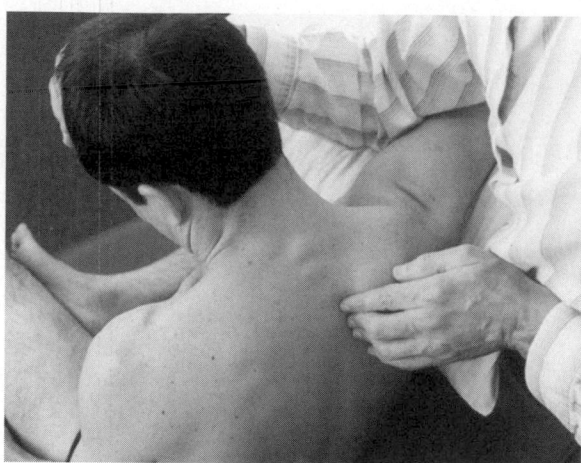

FIGURE 63.15. From Rennie PR, Glover JC, Carvalho C, et al. *Counterstrain and Exercise: An Integrated Approach.* Williamston, MI: RennieMatrix; 2001, with permission.

Posterior (Elevated) Second to Sixth Ribs (PR2-6) (Fig. 63.15)

Tender Points

On the posterior aspect of ribs 2 through 6 at the rib angles.

Treatment Position

Flexion of the thoracic cage, head, and neck with elevation of the shoulder and translation toward (side-bent away from) the tender point. Rotate away from tender point. Side-bending can be increased by placing the patient's legs on the side of the table opposite the elevated shoulder. The elevated shoulder is usually supported on the physician's thigh.

Lumbar Spine

Anterior lumbar spine tender points are mostly located around the rim of the pelvis anteriorly. They can be found in association with the anterior superior iliac spine (ASIS), anterior inferior iliac spine (AIIS), and anterior surface of the pubic rami. Posterior lumbar tender points are found mostly in the same places as in the thoracic spine, although the tender points found on the tips of the transverse processes need to be approached by pressing anteromedially at about a 45 degree angle.

The naming convention used for describing spinal dysfunction in the osteopathic profession is to describe the dysfunctional segment relative to the segment below it. If motion is introduced from below the dysfunctional segment, the vertebral segment below it moves first, producing a position relative to the dysfunctional segment that can seem confusing. As an example, if the vertebra below the dysfunctional segment is rotated to the right, then the relative position of the dysfunctional segment to the vertebra below is described as rotated left. This is important to understand when reading the treatment descriptions for this section.

Anterior First to Fifth Lumbar (AL1-5) (Fig. 63.16)

Tender Point Location

AL1: medial side of the ASIS, press laterally (Fig. 63.16).

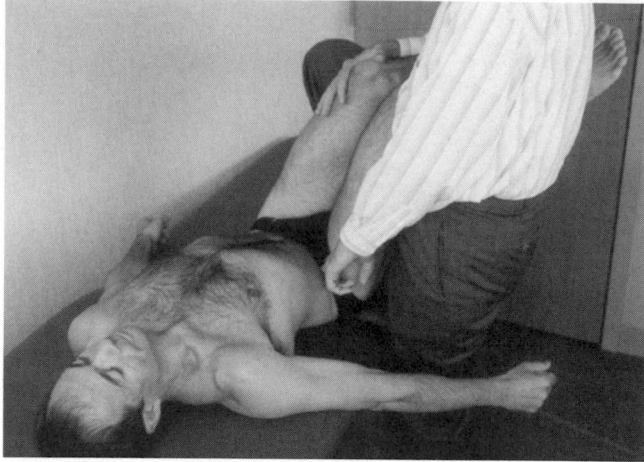

FIGURE 63.16. From Rennie PR, Glover JC, Carvalho C, et al. *Counterstrain and Exercise: An Integrated Approach.* Williamston, MI: RennieMatrix; 2001, with permission.

AL2: medial side of the AIIS, press laterally (Fig. 63.17).

AL3: lateral side of the AIIS, press medially (Fig. 63.17).

AL4: inferior side of the AIIS, press cephalad (Fig. 63.17).

AL5: anterior surface of the pubic rami about 1 cm lateral to the symphysis, inferior to the pubic tubercle, press posteriorly (Fig. 63.18).

Treatment Position

AL1: marked *flexion* of the hips to the level of the L1 vertebrae. The feet are pulled *toward* the tender point side to side bend the lumbar spine. The knees are pulled slightly *toward* the tender side to induce lumbar rotation of the L1 segment *away* from the tender point side.

AL2-4: Stand on the opposite side as the tender point. Moderate *flexion* of the hips and lumbar spine to the level of the named vertebrae. Rotate knees away from tender side, with the amount varying at different levels. Side bend by moving feet away from the tender point side.

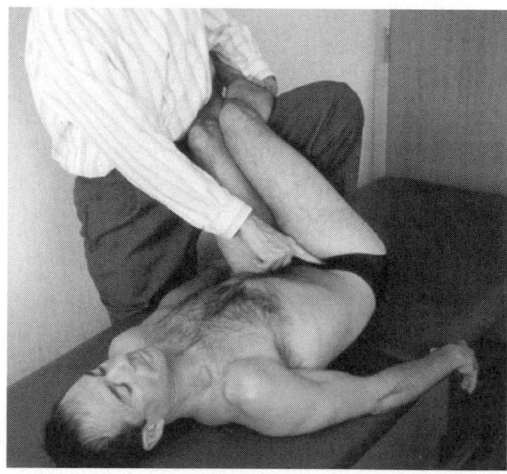

FIGURE 63.17. From Rennie PR, Glover JC, Carvalho C, et al. *Counterstrain and Exercise: An Integrated Approach.* Williamston, MI: RennieMatrix; 2001, with permission.

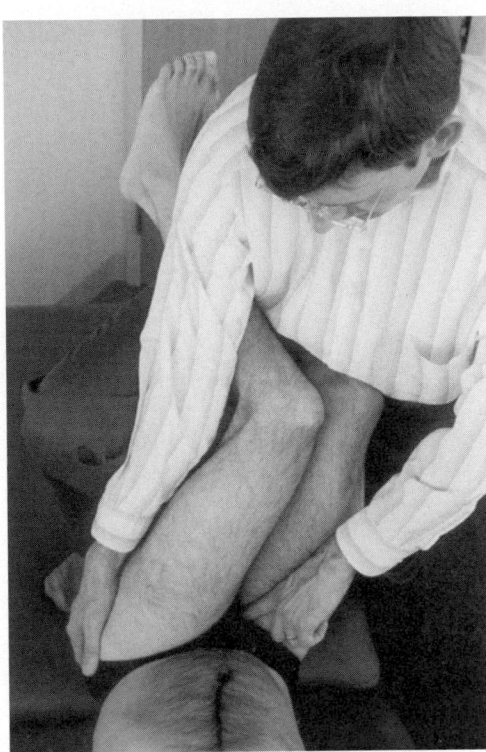

FIGURE 63.18. From Rennie PR, Glover JC, Carvalho C, et al. *Counterstrain and Exercise: An Integrated Approach.* Williamston, MI: RennieMatrix; 2001, with permission.

AL5: Marked *flexion* of the hips up to the level of L5. Pulling the knees *toward* the tender side and the feet toward the *opposite* side produces the side-bending *away* and torso rotation *away* from the tender side.

Posterior First to Fifth Lumbar (PL1-5) (Fig. 63.19)

Tender Point Location
On the inferolateral side of the deviated spinous process. This signifies vertebral rotation of this segment to the opposite direction.

Treatment Position
Extend the trunk on the ipsilateral side of the deviated spinous process by lifting the pelvis in a posterior direction. This creates extension with the needed rotation of the lower vertebrae toward the tender point side.

Pelvis

There are several anterior tender points and several posterior tender points that are important for diagnosis and treatment of pelvic somatic dysfunction. The anterior points typically require flexion. Rotation of varying amounts is also needed and, to a lesser degree, side-bending. Posteriorly, tender points are associated with sacral problems and muscles of the pelvis. Extension is the predominant motion associated with the posterior tender points, although several points require some degree of flexion.

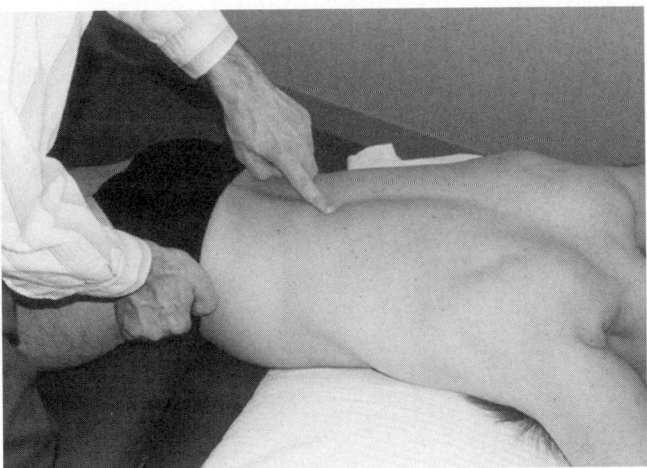

FIGURE 63.19. From Rennie PR, Glover JC, Carvalho C, et al. *Counterstrain and Exercise: An Integrated Approach.* Williamston, MI: RennieMatrix; 2001, with permission.

Iliacus (Fig. 63.20)

Tender Point Location
Half way between the midline and the ASIS about 7cm deep in the abdomen toward the iliacus.

Treatment Position
Marked *flexion* of the hips bilaterally to shorten the iliacus muscles. Both hips are *laterally rotated* with the knees *abducted* from the center of the body.

Lower Pole Fifth Lumbar (LPL-5) (Fig. 63.21)

Tender Point Location
Found 2 cm below the PSIS of the ilium, pressing cephalad.

Treatment Position
Flexion of the ipsilateral hip to approximately 90 degrees to enhance posterior rotation of the innominate. Slight *medial rotation* and *adduction* of the hip is also added. Treatment can be performed in the prone or supine positions.

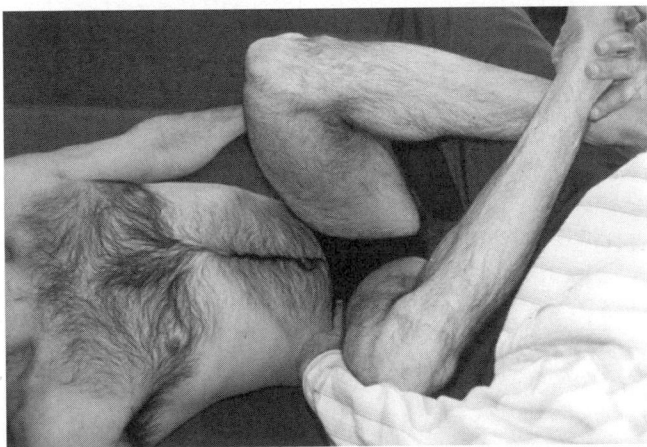

FIGURE 63.20. From Rennie PR, Glover JC, Carvalho C, et al. *Counterstrain and Exercise: An Integrated Approach.* Williamston, MI: RennieMatrix; 2001, with permission.

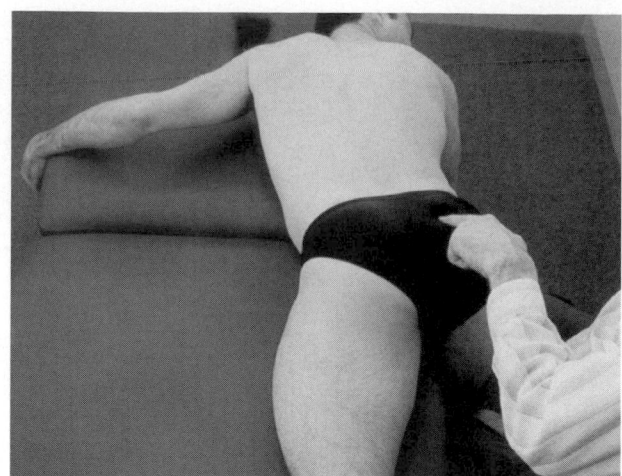

FIGURE 63.21. From Rennie PR, Glover JC, Carvalho C, et al. *Counterstrain and Exercise: An Integrated Approach.* Williamston, MI: RennieMatrix; 2001, with permission.

Piriformis (Fig. 63.22)

Tender Point Location
In the middle of the piriformis muscle, half way between the greater trochanter and where it attaches to the lateral side of the sacrum.

Treatment Position
Marked flexion of the ipsilateral hip to about 135 degrees and marked *abduction. Lateral rotation* of the hip may also be required, particularly if tenderness is found more lateral on the piriformis muscle.

Upper Extremity

The after three tender point locations and treatments demonstrate the counterstrain approach to the upper extremity. Because there are many tender points in the upper extremity, it is rec-

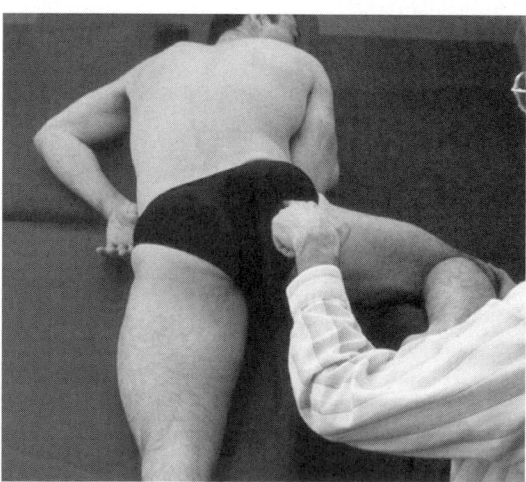

FIGURE 63.22. From Rennie PR, Glover JC, Carvalho C, et al. *Counterstrain and Exercise: An Integrated Approach.* Williamston, MI: RennieMatrix; 2001, with permission.

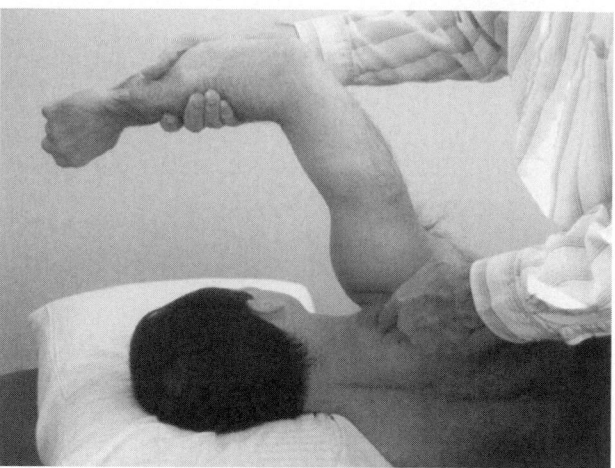

FIGURE 63.23. From Rennie PR, Glover JC, Carvalho C, et al. *Counterstrain and Exercise: An Integrated Approach.* Williamston, MI: RennieMatrix; 2001, with permission.

ommended that a text devoted to counterstrain (1,4,17,20) is consulted for more extensive discussion of the tender points associated with this body region.

Supraspinatus (Fig. 63.23)

Tender Point Location
In the middle of the supraspinatus muscle, superior to the spine of the scapula.

Treatment Position
Flexion and abduction to 45 degrees and external rotation of the humerus.

Subscapularis (Fig. 63.24)

Tender Point Location
On the anterior and lateral surface of the scapula.

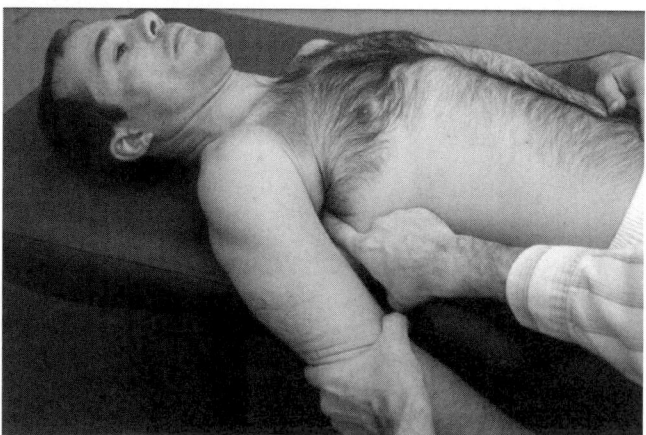

FIGURE 63.24. From Rennie PR, Glover JC, Carvalho C, et al. *Counterstrain and Exercise: An Integrated Approach.* Williamston, MI: RennieMatrix; 2001, with permission.

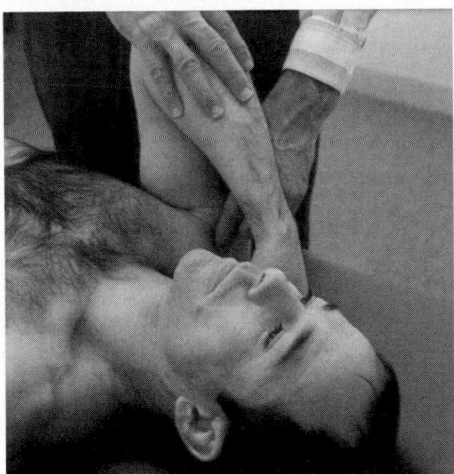

FIGURE 63.25. From Rennie PR, Glover JC, Carvalho C, et al. *Counterstrain and Exercise: An Integrated Approach.* Williamston, MI: RennieMatrix; 2001, with permission.

Treatment Position
Extension, internal rotation, and slight abduction of the humerus.

Biceps (Fig. 63.25)

Tender Point Location
On the tendon of the long head of the biceps in the bicipital groove.

Treatment Position
Flexion of the elbow to shorten the biceps followed by adduction and internal rotation of the upper arm.

Lower Extremity

The after two tender point locations and treatments demonstrate the counterstrain approach to the lower extremity. Because there are many tender points in the lower extremity, it is recommended

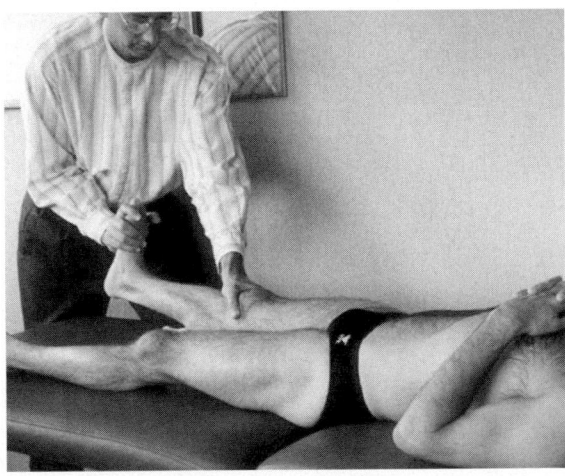

FIGURE 63.26. From Rennie PR, Glover JC, Carvalho C, et al. *Counterstrain and Exercise: An Integrated Approach.* Williamston, MI: RennieMatrix; 2001, with permission.

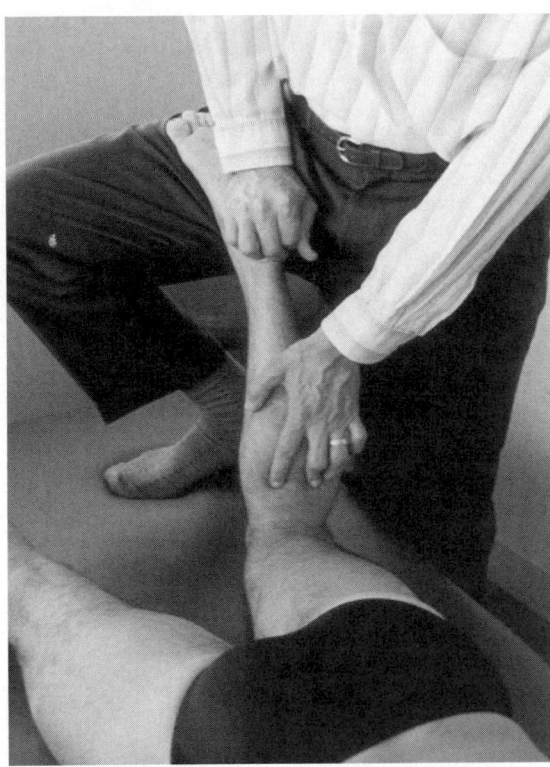

FIGURE 63.27. From Rennie PR, Glover JC, Carvalho C, et al. *Counterstrain and Exercise: An Integrated Approach.* Williamston, MI: RennieMatrix; 2001, with permission.

that a text devoted to counterstrain (1,4,17,20) is consulted for more extensive discussion of the tender points associated with this body region.

Rectus Femoris (Fig. 63.26)

Tender Point Location
Tenderness can be found at the musculotendinous region at the distal end, above the patella, and at the patellar ligament.

Treatment Position
Mild hyperextension of the knee and slight internal rotation of the hip.

Gastrocnemius (Fig. 63.27)

Tender Point Location
Within the two bellies of the gastrocnemius at the lower popliteal margin.

Treatment Position
Marked plantar flexion of the ankle.

ACKNOWLEDGMENTS

Appreciation to Charlene James, DO, PhD and Gabriele Rennie for their editorial review of this chapter and to Claudio Carvalho, DO, for his help in modeling the treatment positions.

REFERENCES

1. Jones LH. *Strain and Counterstrain*. Newark, OH: American Academy of Osteopathy; 1981.
2. Jones LH. Missed anterior spinal lesions. A preliminary report. *The DO*. 1966;6:75–79.
3. Travell JG, Simons DG. *Myofascial Pain and Dysfunction: The Trigger Point Manual*, vol. 1. Baltimore, MD: Williams & Wilkins; 1999.
4. Jones LH, Kusunose R, Goering E. *Jones Strain-Counterstrain*. Boise, ID: Jones Strain-Counterstrain; 1995.
5. Jones LH. Spontaneous release by positioning. *The DO*. 1964;4:109–116.
6. Brandt Jr B, Jones LH. Some methods of applying counterstrain. *J Am Osteopath Assoc*. 1976;75(9):786–789.
7. Jones LH. Foot trauma without hand trauma. *J Am Osteopath Assoc*. 1973;72(1):87–95.
8. Ramirez MA, Haman J, Worth L. Low back pain: diagnosis by six newly discovered sacral tender points and treatment with counterstrain. *J Am Ostepath Assoc*. 1989;89(7):905–906, 911–913.
9. Anonymous. Reader's thoughts on treating low back pain with counterstrain technique. *J Am Osteopath Assoc*. 1989;89(11):1379, 1384, 1387 passim.
10. Jacobson EC, Lockwood MD, Hoefner Jr VC, et al. Shoulder pain and repetition strain injury to the supraspinatus muscle: etiology and manipulative treatment. *J Am Osteopath Assoc*. 1989;89(8):1037–1040, 1043–1045.
11. Cislo S, Ramirez MA, Schwartz HR. Low back pain: treatment of forward and backward sacral torsions using counterstrain technique. *J Am Osteopath Assoc*. 1991;91(3):255–256, 259.
12. Bailey M, Dick L. Nociceptive considerations in treating with counterstrain. *J Am Osteopath Assoc*. 1992;92(3):334, 337–341.
13. Radjieski JM, Lumley MA, Cantieri MS. Effect of osteopathic manipulative treatment of length of stay for pancreatitis: a randomized pilot study. *J Am Osteopath Assoc*. 1998;98(5):264–272.
14. Luckenbill-Edds L, Bechill GB. Nerve compression syndromes as models for research on osteopathic manipulative treatment. *J Am Osteopath Assoc*. 1995;95(5):319–326.
15. Korr IM. Proprioceptors and somatic dysfunction. *J Am Osteopath Assoc*. 1974;74:638–650.
16. Van Buskirk RL. Nociceptive reflexes and the somatic dysfunction: a model. *J Am Osteopath Assoc*. 1990;90(9):792–794, 797–809.
17. Yates HA, Glover JC. *Counterstrain: A Handbook of Osteopathic Technique*. Tulsa, OK: Y Knot Publishers; 1994.
18. Beal MC. Viscerosomatic reflexes: a review. *J Am Osteopath Assoc*. 1985;85(12):786–801.
19. Schwartz HR. The use of counterstrain in an acutely ill in-hospital population. *J Am Osteopath Assoc*. 1986;86(7):433–442.
20. Rennie PR, Glover JC, Carvalho C, et al. *Counterstrain and Exercise: An Integrated Approach*. Williamston, MI: RennieMatrix, 2001.
21. Mense S. Pathophysiologic basis of muscle pain syndromes: an update. *Phys Med Rehabil Clin N Am*. 1997 8(1):23–53.
22. Woolbright JL. An alternative method of teaching strain/counterstrain. *J Am Osteopath Assoc*. 1991;91(4):370, 373–376.

FACILITATED POSITIONAL RELEASE

STANLEY SCHIOWITZ
EILEEN L. DIGIOVANNA
DENNIS J. DOWLING

KEY CONCEPTS

- Technique of facilitated positional release
- Possible mechanisms for effectiveness of facilitated positional release
- Benefits of using facilitated positional release
- History of facilitated positional release
- Diagnosis of any form used with this technique
- Two levels of facilitated positional release and treatment programs appropriate to each level
- Specific treatments for these tissue texture changes and intervertebral motion restrictions
- Cervical soft tissue
- Cervical segmental somatic dysfunction
- Thoracic, seated
- Thoracic, prone
- First rib
- Lumbar soft tissue
- Lumbar extension somatic dysfunction
- Lumbar flexion somatic dysfunction
- Sacroiliac discogenic pain syndrome
- Gluteal and hip soft tissue

Facilitated positional release (FPR) is an indirect positional method of treatment of either abnormal muscle tension or somatic dysfunction. The physician initially places the region or somatic dysfunction into a position between flexion and extension to approach the neutral position defined by Fryette (1). An activating force is then applied to facilitate immediate release of tissue tension, joint motion restriction, or both. The goal of treatment is to decrease the tissue hypertonicity that maintains somatic dysfunction, and the technique can be modified to influence deep muscles involved in joint mobility.

The modality is easily applied, nontraumatic, effective, and efficient. When properly performed, patients report immediate relief of point tenderness and restoration of function. If complete normalization is not achieved, the treatment can be repeated or other methods of treatment can be applied immediately.

THEORY OF EFFECTIVENESS

A neurophysiologic explanation that may explain the effectiveness of this method of treatment was first suggested by Korr (2), who wrote that the immobility of a lesioned segment was initiated or maintained by an increased gain in gamma motor neuron activity of that segment. Subsequently, Bailey (3) proposed that an inappropriately high gain-set of the muscle spindle results in changes characteristic of somatic dysfunction.

When using FPR, the region of somatic dysfunction is first placed into its neutral position to unload the joints' articulating surfaces, which allows the area of dysfunction to respond easily and rapidly to the applied motion and force. In the case of the spine, the articular facets are placed into an idling position between the flexed and extended extremes. This most often involves flattening of the spinal region. A facilitating force (compression and/or torsion) is applied and maintained, followed by decreasing the length of the involved muscle and/or further positioning of the somatic dysfunction into all three planes of relative freedom. The whole application of the positioning into neutral, engaging all directions of relative freedom, and then return to the original position takes only a few seconds. The dysfunction is then reassessed. This method may result in an immediate effect on the muscle spindle-gamma loop, which then allows the extrafusal muscle fibers to lengthen to their normal relaxed state.

In discussing the feedback mechanism of the muscle spindle stretch reflex, Carew (4) stated that shortening the muscle more than intended caused a decrease in spindle output and lowered the afferent excitatory input to the spinal cord through the Ia nerve fibers. This results in a decrease in gamma motor gain to the spindle and, by reflex action, decreases tension of the extrafusal muscle fibers. As a result, hypertonicity of the muscle mass is reduced.

Joint motion asymmetry decreases after treatment with FPR if its mobility was impaired by muscle hypertonicity. If the asymmetry of joint motion is caused by other factors, such as meniscus or synovial impingement or degenerative arthritis, mobility is not restored; the joint remains restricted. This may account for the need to repeat the application or use other modalities of osteopathic manipulation to complete treatment of the dysfunction.

HISTORY

FPR was developed by Stanley Schiowitz, DO. Because of his busy practice and limitation on providing time-intensive treatments, he sought treatment methods for providing fast and effective relief for patients that were soundly based on anatomic and physiologic principles. Other practitioners had already used some of the components employed in FPR, which probably date back to the time of Andrew Taylor Still. In 1977, he was able to further develop and systematize the principles of this form of treatment. Over time, faculty members in many colleges of osteopathic medicine have added FPR to the curriculum.

DIAGNOSIS

Many publications have described diagnostic methods. Methods may consist of:

Skin rolling described by Mennell (5)
Testing for thoracic/lumbar rotoscoliosis in the method of Mitchell and colleagues (6)
Palpatory motion testing as described by Johnston (7)
Other direct or indirect tissue or motion testing procedures described in the literature

Diagnosis of somatic dysfunction is described in other chapters in this text. The use of FPR treatment procedures does not require special diagnostic tests unique to FPR. However, diagnosis is a prerequisite to treatment.

TREATMENT

FPR treatments are classified into two categories: a) one directed at normalization of palpable abnormal tissue texture, and b) the other modified to influence deep muscle involved in joint mobility. Sometimes it is difficult to make a clear diagnostic distinction as to which one of these is primarily involved in the somatic dysfunction.

If in doubt, the palpable tissue changes should be treated first. If motion restriction persists after this treatment, the technique can be adapted to treat the deep muscle component involved in the specific joint motion restriction.

Tissue Texture Change Treatment

1. The anteroposterior spinal curve of the area to be treated is flattened. This position places that region of the spine into its position of ease of motion, which shortens and softens the associated muscle.
2. A facilitating force is applied. This may be compression, torsion, or a combination of the two.
3. The physician places the patient's involved myofascial structures into a shortened, relaxed position. This softens the tissues and reduces stretch receptor activity.
4. The position is held for 3 to 5 seconds and then released.
5. The patient's condition is reevaluated.

Intervertebral Motion Restriction Treatment

The same procedures used for tissue changes are used to address intervertebral motion restrictions, with the additional requirement that the physician place the vertebra into a position that allows freedom of motion in all planes. In the following example, with a restriction at C3 ESRRR, the fourth cervical vertebra moves more easily into extension, right rotation, and right sidebending.

1. The cervical lordosis is flattened.
2. Place the third cervical vertebra into a position of extension, right lateral flexion, and right rotation with respect to the fourth cervical vertebra.
3. Apply a facilitating force: compression, torsion, or a combination.
4. Hold the position for 3 to 5 seconds; release should be palpable.
5. Reevaluate the patient.

SUMMARY

FPR is easily applied, nontraumatic, effective, and efficient. When it is properly performed, the patient reports immediate relief of point tenderness and restoration of function. If complete normalization is not achieved, it can be repeated or other methods of treatment can be applied immediately.

FACILITATED POSITIONAL RELEASE TECHNIQUES

Cervical

Soft Tissue Treatment

Findings
Posterior cervical muscle hypertonicity (soft tissue texture abnormalities).

Patient Position
Supine on the table; the patient's head is beyond the end of the table, resting on a pillow on the physician's lap (Fig. 64.1).

Procedure
1. Sit at the head of the table.
2. Cup the patient's neck in the palm of your hand with the pad of the index or other finger acting as both monitoring finger and fulcrum on the contralateral tense tissue to be treated. Your thumb rests on the other side of the neck.
3. Use your non-monitoring hand on the top of the patient's head to straighten the cervical lordosis by slightly forward bending the neck.
4. Use the same hand to apply a compressive facilitating force to the neck through the patient's head until felt at the monitoring finger.
5. Maintain the compressive force and introduce extension of the neck to the level of the monitoring finger. (If the tissues being

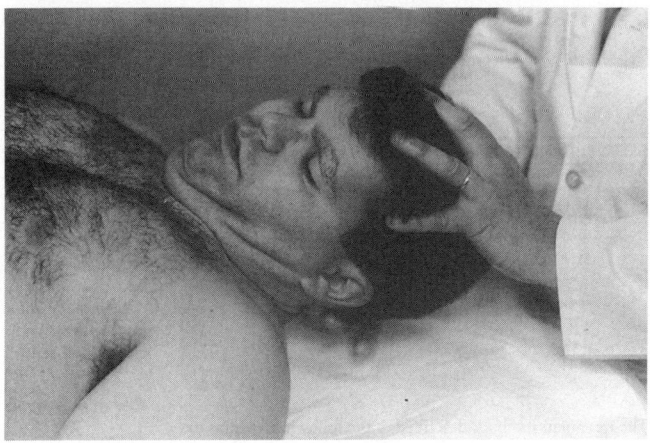

FIGURE 64.1. Cervical soft tissue technique.

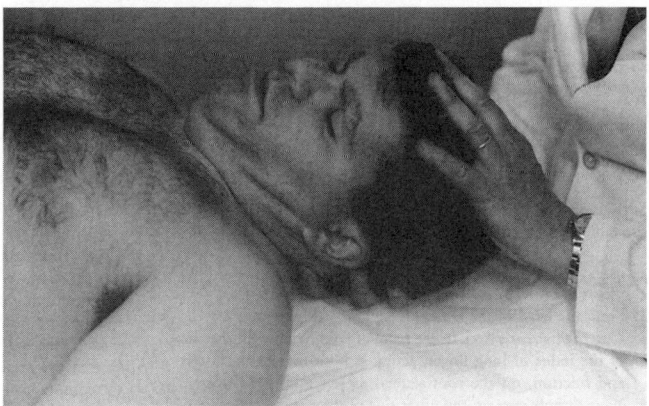

FIGURE 64.2. Typical cervical C3 ESLRL technique.

treated are anterior rather than posterior, introduce flexion rather than extension.) This should cause a palpable softening of the tissue being treated.

6. Add side-bending and rotation (usually toward the side of the tense tissues) to the point that the tissues continue to soften.
7. Hold in this position for 3 to 5 seconds and then return the neck slowly to a neutral position.
8. Reevaluate the tissue being treated.

Note: If tissue changes are found anteriorly, forward bending is usually required. Some muscles have a contralateral side-bending, a rotary component, or both. Those muscles must be placed in their individual shortened positions determined by palpation and tissue response. Careful localization of the component motions of forward/backward bending, side-bending/rotation, and compression to the area of tissue texture change will result in faster and more efficient results.

Cervical Segmental Somatic Dysfunction

Findings
C3 ES$_L$R$_L$.

Patient Position
Supine, with the patient's head beyond the end of the table resting on a pillow on the physician's lap (Fig. 64.2).

Procedure
1. Sit at the head of the table.
2. Cup the patient's neck in the palm of your right hand with the pad of the index or other finger on the left articular pillar of C3.
3. Use your left hand on the top of the patient's head to straighten the cervical lordosis by forward bending the neck to the monitoring finger on C3.
4. Add a compressive force through your left hand, directed through the head to the neck. The force should be sufficient enough to be felt with the monitoring finger. It should not exceed this.
5. Extend the neck through the level of C3 while maintaining the compression.

6. Side bend C3 to the left by adding a translatory force through your monitoring finger, pulling C3 to the right.
7. Add a slight left rotation of the head and neck through the level of C3. This places C3 in all three planes of freedom of motion.
8. Hold this position for 3 to 5 seconds then slowly return the neck to neutral.
9. Reevaluate C3 motion.

Note: If the diagnosis is flexion rather than extension (C3 FS$_L$R$_L$), step four is replaced by adding flexion through the level of C3 rather than adding extension. Similarly, if the diagnosis is one of right side-bending and right rotation, the appropriate adjustments should be made.

When applying this procedure to dysfunction of the suboccipital area or to the occipito-atlantal articulation, localize the flexion-extension using a slight nodding motion to the skull (not total flexion-extension of the cervical spine). Also, the occipito-atlantal (O-A) joint side bends in one direction and rotates in the opposite direction. The appropriate motions should be added to the positioning to place the O-A joint into its relative freedoms.

Thoracic

Thoracic Spine, Seated

Findings
T6 FS$_L$R$_L$.

Patient Position
Seated on the edge of the table (Fig. 64.3).

Procedure
1. Stand behind and to the left of the patient.
2. Ask the patient to sit up as straight as possible and push his or her chest forward. This will straighten the thoracic kyphosis.
3. Monitor the transverse process of T6 with your right index or other finger.
4. Place your left axilla over the patient's left shoulder as close to the cervicothoracic junction as possible, with your forearm in front of the patient and your left hand in the patient's right axilla or grasping the patient's right shoulder.

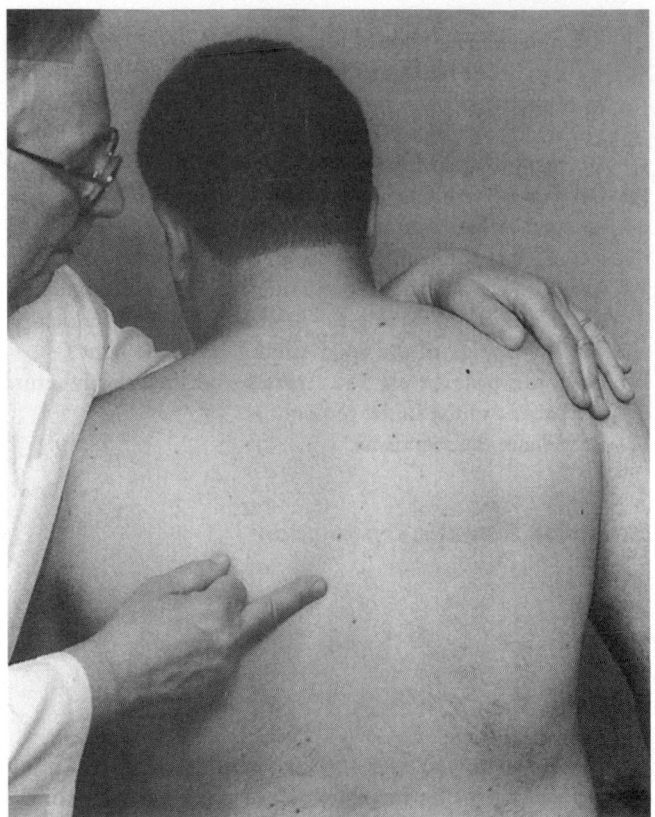

FIGURE 64.3. Thoracic spine T6 FSLRL technique, seated.

5. Add a compressive force through your left axilla downward (toward the table), causing left side-bending down through the level of the monitoring finger at T6.
6. Add flexion to the level of T6 by pulling forward on the patient's shoulders while maintaining the side-bending.
7. Rotate the thoracic spine to the left down through the level of T6 by pulling the patient's right shoulder forward.
8. Hold this position for 3 to 5 seconds and then slowly return the patient to a neutral position.
9. Reevaluate.

Note: If the diagnosis is extension rather than flexion (T6 ES_LR_L), replace step 6 by creating extension through the level of T6, pulling back on the shoulders. Similarly, if the diagnosis is side-bending and rotation is to the right, make appropriate adjustments. If the somatic dysfunction is neutral, do not induce flexion or extension and adjust so that side-bending and rotation are achieved in the appropriate directions.

Thoracic Spine, Prone

Findings
T7 ES_LR_L.

Patient Position
Prone, with pillows beneath the abdomen and head. The patient's arms are at his or her side (Fig. 64.4).

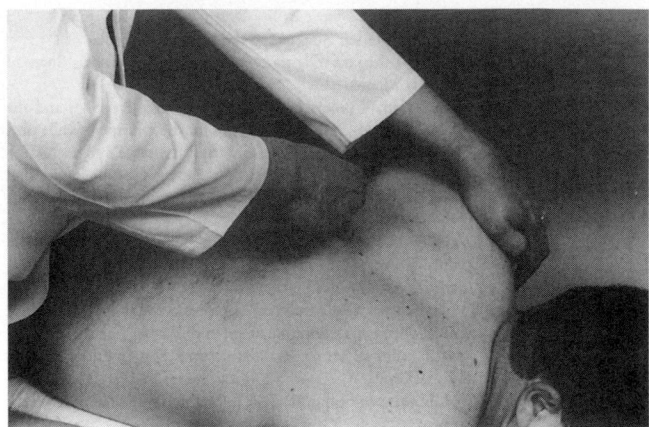

FIGURE 64.4. Thoracic spine T7 ESLRL technique, prone.

Procedure
1. Stand at the right side of the patient.
2. Palpate the T7 posterior transverse process (right) with the fingers of your right hand.
3. With your other hand, grasp the patient's left shoulder. The patient's entire shoulder should be held with your fingers on the upper and outer surfaces.
4. Pull the patient's left shoulder medially toward the spine (this flattens the spine in the anteroposterior plane) then toward the patient's feet (this compressive force creates left side-bending).
5. Extend the spine through the level of T7 by maintaining traction on the shoulder as you step further down the table until motion can be palpated at the level of your monitoring fingers.
6. Stand up straighter, pulling the patient's shoulder posteriorly and creating left rotation down through the level of T7.
7. Hold this position for 3 to 5 seconds then slowly return to the neutral position.
8. Reevaluate T7 motion.

Note: If the diagnosis is flexion rather than extension (T8 ES_RR_R), FPR is more easily accomplished with the patient in the seated position.

First Rib

Soft Tissue Treatment

Findings
First rib elevated on left.

Patient Position
Supine (Fig. 64.5).

Procedure
1. Stand to the left of the patient facing the head of the table.
2. Place the monitoring finger of your left hand over the posterior portion of the left first rib. The finger should contact the tensest tissue overlying the superior posterior part of the rib.
3. With your right hand, grasp the patient's left elbow, flex the upper arm to approximately 90 degrees, and abduct the upper arm to the position in which the tissues soften maximally.

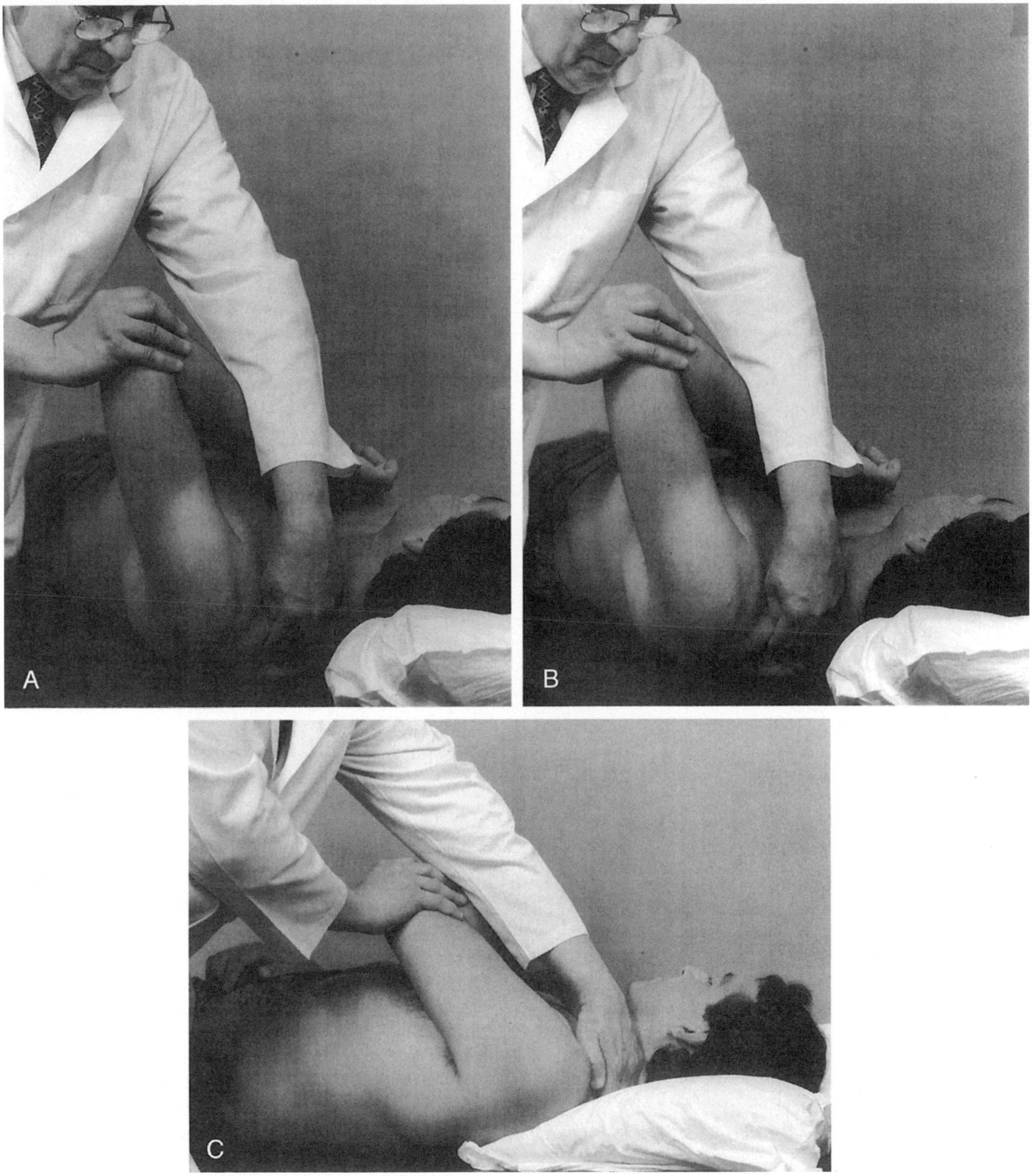

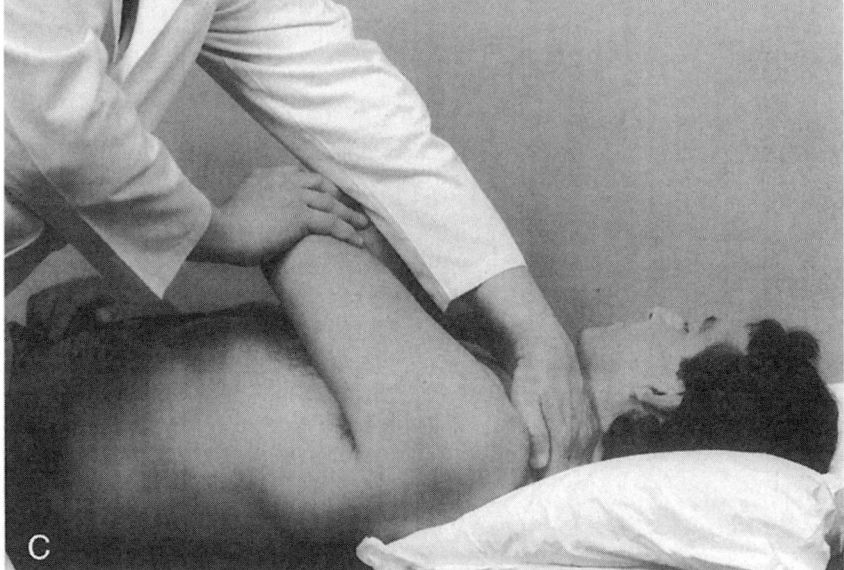

FIGURE 64.5. Treatment for first rib. **A:** First rib elevated on left. **B:** Internal rotation and flexion introduced. **C:** Adduction and circumduction added.

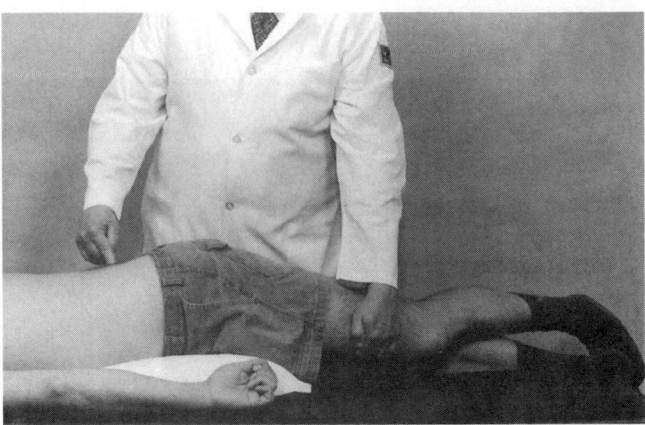

FIGURE 64.6. Lumbar soft tissue technique.

4. Create a compressive force through the left elbow downward, directed toward the monitoring finger.
5. Press the volar surface of your left forearm against the dorsal surface of your patient's left forearm. This will act as a fulcrum for the additional movements. Increase the amount of shoulder flexion. This also causes an internal rotation of the humerus.
6. Hold this position for 3 to 5 seconds.
7. Maintain the compressive force and internal rotation, adduct the upper arm across the patient's chest, swing it down through a curving motion, and finally into a neutral position.
8. Reevaluate the motion of the first rib.

Lumbar

Soft Tissue Treatment

Findings

Hypertonic right paravertebral lumbar muscles.

Patient Position

Prone, close to the right edge of the table, with a sufficient number of pillows beneath the abdomen to cause flattening of the lumbar lordosis (Fig. 64.6).

Procedure
1. Stand at the right side of the table facing the patient.
2. Monitor the tissue tension with a finger of the right hand.
3. Place your left knee on the table next to the patient's pelvis. This acts as a fulcrum to position the patient's legs.
4. With your left hand, grasp the patient's left knee.
5. Pull the patient's legs toward you to induce right lumbar side-bending until you feel motion and/or softening at your monitoring finger.
6. Remove your knee from the table.
7. Cross the patient's legs by placing the left ankle over the right.
8. With your left hand, reach around the left thigh from the lateral surface and place your fingers between the patient's thighs so that your palm is on the anterior and medial left thigh.

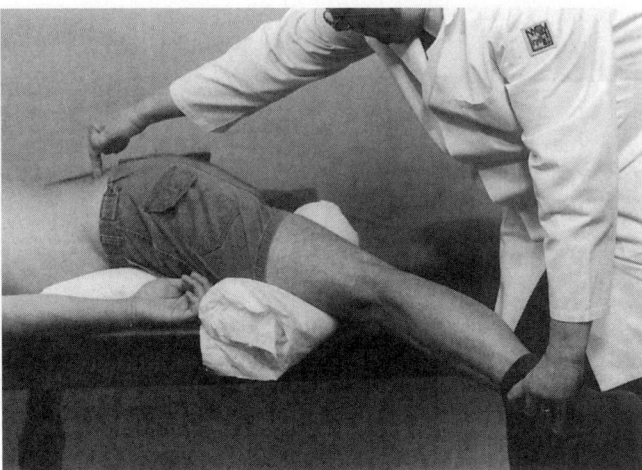

FIGURE 64.7. Lumbar extended L3 ESLRL technique.

9. Lift it slightly toward you so that the dorsal surface of your left hand is against the back of the right thigh. This creates a slight increase in adduction of the left leg.
10. Stand upright with your arm straight, using postural rather than arm muscles to pull the left leg further toward the dysfunctional side. Adduct it and induce external rotation. At the same time, extend the lumbar region and induce a relative rotation of the upper trunk toward the right.
11. Hold this position for 3 to 5 seconds then slowly return the patient to the initial position.
12. Reevaluate the soft tissue.

Extension Somatic Dysfunction

Findings

L3 ES_LR_L.

Patient Position

Prone, close to the left edge of the table with a sufficient number of pillows beneath the abdomen to cause flattening of the lumbar lordosis (Fig. 64.7).

Procedure
1. Stand at the left side facing the head of the table.
2. Monitor the posterior transverse process (left) with a finger of the right hand.
3. Place a small pillow between the patient's left thigh and the table. This will provide a fulcrum for the treatment while protecting the thigh from the pressure of the table's edge.
4. Use your left hand to abduct the right leg, creating left lumbar side-bending, and stand between the table and the patient's abducted leg.
5. Grasp the patient's left lower leg or ankle and internally rotate the leg until you feel motion at the monitoring finger (this creates relative rotation of the trunk to the left).
6. Move the patient's abducted leg toward the floor (hip flexion) until you palpate motion at the monitoring finger. With the thigh pillow acting as a fulcrum, lift the pelvis from the table and introduce lumbar extension.

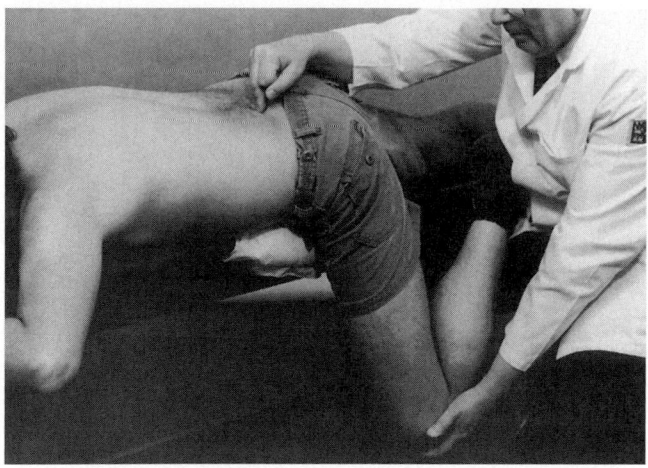

FIGURE 64.8. Lumbar flexed L4 FSLRL technique.

7. Hold this position until there is a sudden release of the somatic dysfunction (usually in about 3 to 5 seconds), then slowly return the patient to a neutral position.
8. Reevaluate L3 motion.

Flexion Somatic Dysfunction

Findings
L4 FS_LR_L.

Patient Position
Prone, close to the left edge of the table with a sufficient number of pillows beneath the abdomen to cause flattening of the lumbar lordosis (Fig. 64.8).

Procedure
1. Sit on a rolling stool (thighs parallel to the table) on the left side of table at the level of the patient's pelvis, facing the patient's head.
2. Monitor the posterior transverse process (left) with a finger of your right hand.
3. Flex the patient's left leg at the knee and hip, with the lower leg coming to rest between your knees to create a relative amount of flexion of the spine to the point where you feel motion at your monitoring finger.
4. Use your left hand to grasp the patient's left knee, and adduct it toward and under the edge of the table until you feel motion at the monitoring finger. Hold and support the knee during the rest of the technique. Rotate your body clockwise (This induces left rotation, because internal rotation of the leg causes pelvic rotation to the contralateral side, and relative lumbar rotation toward the posterior transverse process.) Some compression may be added through the patient's knee.
5. Hold this position until there is a sudden release of the somatic

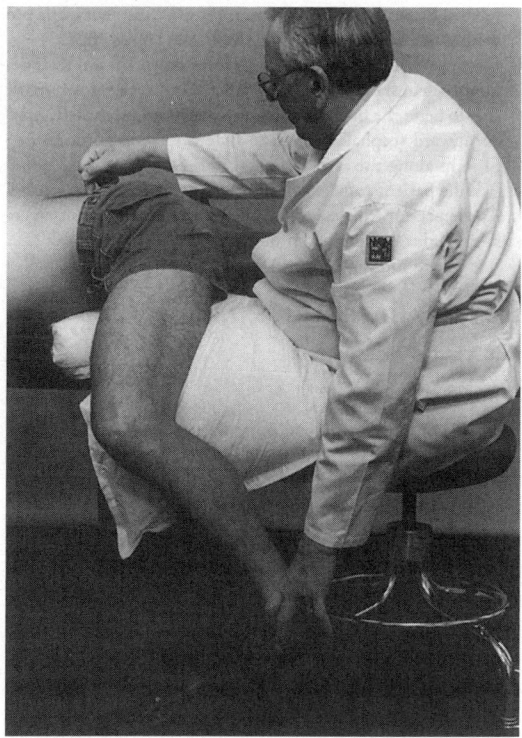

FIGURE 64.9. Discogenic pain syndrome treatment.

dysfunction (usually in about 3 to 5 seconds) then slowly return the patient to a neutral position.
6. Reevaluate L4 motion.

Discogenic Pain Syndrome Treatment

Findings
Left lumbar disc pathology with left radiculopathy.

Patient Position
Prone, close to the left edge of the table with a sufficient number of pillows beneath the abdomen to cause flattening of the lumbar lordosis (Fig. 64.9).

Procedure
1. Sit on a rolling stool at the left side of table (thighs parallel to the table) at the level of the patient's pelvis, facing the patient's head.
2. Use a finger of your right hand to monitor the area of documented or suspected disc pathology.
3. With your left hand, flex the patient's left hip and knee.
4. Place the upper leg across your anterior thighs, moving to create abduction and external rotation.
5. Localize motion to the involved segment by moving the patient's leg in a cephalad direction. It is easiest to do this by rolling the stool closer to the head of the table.
6. Raise your left knee by lifting your heel off the floor. Push the lateral part of your knee into the popliteal fossa of the patient's knee. Create a traction force that can be modified (as you further raise and move your knee laterally) until you

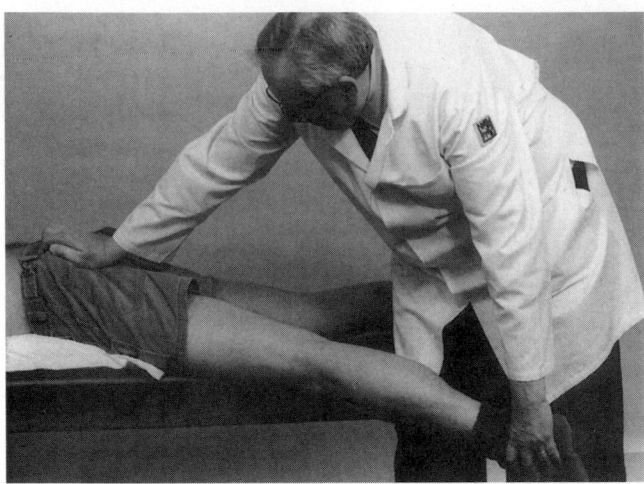

FIGURE 64.10. Motion restriction treatment for the sacroiliac joint.

palpate motion at your monitoring finger. Your knee is now at the medial surface of the popliteal fossa. The lateral surface of your knee acts as a fulcrum for the rest of the technique.

7. Use your left hand to push the patient's left lower leg toward the floor until you palpate motion at your monitoring finger. Note a slight amount of initial tension at the monitored location.

8. Maintain this position until a release is noted, generally in 3 to 5 seconds, and then slowly return the patient to a neutral position. The patient generally experiences some relief of his or her radicular symptoms with this treatment.

9. Reevaluate the lumbar region.

Sacroiliac Joint

Motion Restriction Treatment

Findings
Left sacroiliac motion restriction.

Patient Position
Prone, with a sufficient number of pillows under the abdomen to flatten the lumbosacral junction (Fig. 64.10).

Procedure
1. Stand on the left side of the table facing the head of the table.
2. Place a small pillow between the patient's left thigh and the table. This will provide a fulcrum for the treatment while protecting the thigh from the table's edge.
3. Monitor the left sacroiliac (SI) joint with a finger of your right hand and place your right hypothenar eminence on the left inferior lateral angle (ILA) of the sacrum.
4. Use your left hand to abduct the left leg until the thigh is over the edge of the table.
5. Use your left hand to press the left leg down toward the floor. Simultaneously press your hypothenar eminence down on the ILA to bend the base of the sacrum backward on the left. Apply an upward (cephalad) force to slide the sacral portion of the SI joint along the ileal portion.

6. Ask the patient to take a deep breath and hold it for 3 to 5 seconds.
7. As the patient exhales, return the leg to a neutral position and release your pressure from the ILA.
8. Reevaluate motion of the SI joint.

Gluteal and Hip

Soft Tissue Treatment

Findings
Right hip muscles or gluteal musculature hypertonicity.

Patient Position
Prone, close to the edge of the table with a sufficient number of pillows under the abdomen to flatten the lumbar lordosis.

Procedure
1. Sit on a rolling stool at the right side of table (thighs parallel to the table) at the level of the patient's pelvis, facing the patient's head.
2. With a finger of your left hand, monitor the soft tissue to be treated.
3. Use your right hand to slightly abduct the patient's right leg and flex the hip and knee until you feel motion at your monitoring finger. The patient's lower leg will come between your knees, and the ankle will rest on your lap. Insert a small pillow between the patient's inner thigh and the table edge for comfort and to provide a fulcrum.
4. Push the patient's flexed knee into adduction beneath the table until you palpate motion at the monitored location.
5. Induce internal rotation of the thigh with your hand on the knee. This can be further accentuated by swiveling your own body and right shoulder forward, causing adduction and internal rotation of the lower leg.
6. Place your right palm and fingers so that they encompass the patient's knee.
7. Direct a compressive force upward along the long axis of the femur toward the hip and gluteal region.
8. Maintain this position until a release is noted, generally in 3 to 5 seconds, then slowly return the patient to a neutral position.
9. Reevaluate the soft tissue.

CONCLUSION

Although axial procedures have primarily been described here, it is possible to use FPR for other regions of articular and soft tissue dysfunction. Rather than describe these in detail, it is left to the reader to apply these principles to the individual region.

REFERENCES

1. Fryette HH. *Principles of Osteopathic Technic.* Carmel, CA: Academy of Applied Osteopathy; 1980:19.

2. Korr IM. Proprioceptors and somatic dysfunction. *J Am Osteopath Assoc.* 1975;75:638–650.

3. Bailey HW. Some problems in making osteopathic spinal manipulative therapy appropriate and specific. *J Am Osteopath Assoc.* 1976;75:486–499.

4. Carew TJ. The control of reflex action. In: Kandel ER, Schwartz JH, eds. *Principles of Neural Science,* 2nd ed. New York, NY: Elsevier Science; 1985:464.

5. Mennell JM. *Back Pain: Diagnosis and Treatment Using Manipulative Techniques.* Boston, MA: Little, Brown and Company; 1960:75.

6. Mitchell Jr FL, Moran PS, Pruzzo NA. *An Evaluation and Treatment Manual of Osteopathic Muscle Energy Procedures.* Valley Park, MO: Mitchell, Moran & Pruzzo Assoc; 1979:229–253.

7. Johnston WL. Segmental definition, Part 1: A focal point for diagnosis of somatic dysfunction. *J Am Osteopath Assoc.* 1988;88:99–105.

PROGRESSIVE INHIBITION OF NEUROMUSCULAR STRUCTURES TECHNIQUE

DENNIS J. DOWLING

KEY CONCEPTS

- Technique of progressive inhibition of neuromuscular structures
- History of development of progressive inhibition of neuromuscular structures
- Review of other modalities of point diagnosis and/or treatment
- Diagnostic considerations
- Method of applying the progressive inhibition of neuromuscular structures technique
- Proposed mechanisms of action
- Possible side effects and contraindications
- Considerations for inclusion in treatment

More than 20 years ago, I had several years in which I suffered from headaches. Most of the treatments offered had a limited impact or undesirable side effects. Other, apparently related symptoms accompanied the cephalgia, including a boring pain of the right eye, increased lacrimation, right-sided facial pain, nasal congestion, and scalp sensitivity. Suboccipital pain occurred, which appeared to be related to the periorbital pain, although no direct connection was apparent. Precipitating events leading to the symptoms included excessive reading, eyestrain due to exposure to bright sunlight, and dehydration. There were no sensory deficits. Some symptoms occurred independently and were usually worsened by stress. With little knowledge of anatomy at the time, early attempts at self-treatment involved the application of manual pressure to various locations of the head. Pressing painful sites appeared to bring about temporary relief when any were pressed singly. However, the pain recurred almost immediately after release of the pressure. Sometimes other adjacent regions of the scalp developed pain during or after release of pressure. Eventually, some patterns seemed to develop as secondary and even subsequent points appeared. The most successful approach, more so than addressing any individual or pair of points, was the treatment of a sequence of points.

As an osteopathic student and physician, I began to integrate knowledge of osteopathic manipulative medicine theory along with my personal clinical observations. The method of self-treatment was used with patients and taught to other students of osteopathy. Gradually, the rationale, as well as further expansion of use of this inhibitory technique beyond treatment of headaches, became clearer (1). Some similarities and differences were noted in relationship to other manipulative methods of point or applied pressure techniques.

INHIBITION

Progressive inhibition of neuromuscular structures (PINS) is most closely related to the osteopathic modality of inhibition. The Glossary of Osteopathic Terminology defines inhibition as " . . . a term that describes steady pressure to soft tissues to effect relaxation and normalize reflex activity" (2). The "steady pressure to soft tissues" is perhaps one of the oldest methods of manual treatment, regardless of the name applied. Classically, inhibition is a constant mild-to-moderate amount of force exerted by the fingers, elbow, knee, or foot on regions of hypertonic muscle. Although the patient's presenting complaint may be of pain or decreased function, the objective of the treatment is to decrease the tonicity of the muscles. Any symptom the patient has is assumed to be directly related to this increased dysfunctional muscular tone (3). The larger, more superficial muscles are the most easily identified, whether they are in the normal-relaxed or hypertonic states. Regional muscles can be selected and treated individually or in pairs. Positioning the patient either supine or prone may facilitate the process, because these positions do not usually require the use of some muscles for positional support of the trunk and neck. A muscle, such as the trapezius, can be easily located in the cervical, shoulder, and upper thoracic regions. Some portion of the muscle can be grasped, pressed, or pinched. A hypertonic muscle is commonly found to be firmer than the same muscle on the opposite side and perhaps more firm than its antagonist. An increase in the firmness and perhaps greater sensitivity are noted as the pressure is introduced. As long as the pressure remains constant, the structures should relax. Attempts should be made to avoid altering the position or amount of pressure, because these will more likely be stimulatory.

The relationship between musculoskeletal structures and the underlying visceral organs is also of consideration. These organs receive innervations from the same spinal cord segments that serve the skin, bones, joints, ligaments, and muscles. The sympathetic chain lies just anterior to the rib heads, and dysfunction of the vertebral or rib joints may result in increased stimulation to related structures, visceral and musculoskeletal (4). Acute response to increased sympathetic activity is the same as to any new injury: redness (rubor), pain (dolor), swelling (tumor), heat (calor), and decreased function (funcio laesa) (5). More superficial structures, such as the skin and subcutaneous tissue, may have a "doughy" consistency, and the pain noted by the patient would be typically sharp and throbbing. With continued hyperactivity in the absence of adequate treatment and/or recovery, the signs and symptoms demonstrated are altered. The muscles may feel fibrotic ("ropy"). The skin is thinner, paler, and cooler. Pain responses can range from relative insensitivity ("anesthetic") to altered sensitivity ("paresthesia") to hypersensitivity. The pressure provided by the application of modalities (such as inhibition) may result in a transitory increase in the palpatory findings or symptoms. Almost inevitably, subsequent reduction of some or all of these components can be readily appreciated. When the visceral organs are the primary dysfunction, the persistence or recurrence of a musculoskeletal somatic dysfunction may indicate the underlying problem. When a musculoskeletal injury is the etiology, any other reflexive activity or manipulative treatment may result in a more persistent reduction or elimination of all pathologic components.

Inhibitory techniques have a different visceral focus in the suboccipital and sacral regions. Rather than reacting to external danger as the sympathetic system does, the parasympathetic system modifies the body's own reconstructive processes. Increased parasympathetic activity influences such elements as increased gastrointestinal motility, decreased sphincter closure, reduction of heart rate, constriction of pupils, and sleepiness. Somatic dysfunction of the upper cervical, occipital, and sacral regions may reflect or result in inappropriate parasympathetic activity. Inhibitory treatment results in reduction of increased regional musculoskeletal tone and congestion, and theoretically downregulates the more internal mechanisms.

A thorough understanding of the structure and function of the factors related to somatic dysfunction should guide accurate treatment. Inhibitory and PINS treatments may be moved about several locations with the intent of reducing all relevant related dysfunction.

When Andrew Taylor Still (6) was a young man suffering from chronic headaches, he treated himself with a rope-swing by lowering the rope to a few inches above the ground. A blanket was slung across it. He positioned himself on the ground with the contraption supporting his neck at the base of the skull, and subsequently fell asleep. He awakened refreshed and pain free. Whether intentionally or inadvertently, the method he employed appears to represent inhibition as much as positional intervention. Despite his usual tendency to avoid specific types of treatment in his writings, Dr. Still included some descriptions of both inhibition and stimulation methods (7).

Some of Still's early students likewise described inhibitory techniques, as well as the rationale for their use. In *A Manual of Osteopathy*, Goetz (8) described and illustrated inhibition for various conditions, both somatic and visceral. The accompanying photographs in this small handbook clearly demonstrate and detail inhibitory treatment of several regions. Of special note are the orbital and suboccipital regions of the head. A few minutes of pressure applied individually to each of these points is recommended.

A more extensive description appears in Tasker's *The Principles of Osteopathy* (9). Tasker describes reasoning as to the effectiveness of inhibitory techniques, especially because inhibition is a natural phenomenon. Bodily functions, such as defecation and urination could not come under conscious and unconscious control without the adapted or learned ability to perform inhibition. In discussing the effectiveness of externally applied inhibitory pressure directed toward decreasing hyperactivity (as is applied by an osteopathic physician), he states that it is not the surface pressure that is effective but the initiation or alteration of the reflex arc that subsequently occurs. Observation reveals that the initial response to the placing of a pressure is, in effect, a form of stimulation, because it impacts the soft tissue. However, the inhibitory process of applied steady pressure sets in motion a removal of the lesion and brings about some alterations both deep to and distant from the location of the applied pressure. In citing the Hilton law "that the skin, muscles, and synovial membrane of a joint, or the skin, muscles of the abdomen, and contents covered by peritoneum are innervated from the same segment of the cord," Tasker states that the "overstimulation" caused by inhibition results in diminution or elimination of the overreactivity.

OSTEOPATHIC POINT AND/OR PRESSURE TECHNIQUES

Many types of passive direct and indirect systems of osteopathic treatment of somatic dysfunction exist. Some standard points and diagnoses are used as fulcrums and/or monitoring locations in practically all of these modalities. Monitoring by constant palpation at the points is one of the best means for an osteopathic physician to experience feedback and monitor the success of the treatment when performing Jones strain-counterstrain treatment (10–12). The patient can likewise appreciate the alteration. The muscle spindle sensory organ is embedded into the larger extrafusal muscle. The sensory ends of nerve fibers to these small muscles are stimulated by stretch of any kind, whether it is static or dynamic. The result is a single spinal segment increase in alpha motoneuron activity, which results in contraction of the whole muscle. It is quite successful as a means of preventing overstretching, and should decrease as soon as the danger retreats. Sometimes the reflex persists longer than is appropriate. The signals from the spindle continue to fire as if the tissue were being too rapidly overstretched, although the overall length may be fairly short. The sensitivity of a tender point reflects increased activity. The external pressure at the tender point elicits the complaint while the positioning during strain-counterstrain technique shortens the whole muscle. This allows the spindle reflex mechanism to be reset, and the sensitivity disappears.

Facilitated positional release (FPR) (13) is similar in many respects to strain-counterstrain. It differs in its use of an activating force (usually compression or torsion) after initially positioning the region in neutral. Strain-counterstrain is a form of positional release, whereas FPR uses an additional facilitating force. Both strain-counterstrain and FPR theoretically use the same neurophysiologic mechanism, the muscle spindle. Van Buskirk (14) has recently contributed what he describes as the Still technique. It shares many similar applications to strain-counterstrain and FPR. Van Buskirk based his recovery of components of the technique on the writings of Hazzard (15), as well as Still himself. The techniques use palpatory diagnosis of dysfunction followed by therapeutic motion into the freedoms. Finally, the osteopathic physician introduces movement past the neutral point into the barrier directions. This low-velocity, relatively low-amplitude articulatory movement toward the barriers follows the positional treatment into the freedoms.

Functional technique (16) uses diagnostic points to define the somatic dysfunction that exists at that level relative to its two adjoining vertebrae: the one above and the one below. Detection of somatic dysfunction is typically made by percussion and more specific testing to scan and screen the regions. Wallace developed torque unwinding (17), and has taught it on a limited basis. She uses a theoretical construct whereby the body is imagined as a collection of adjacent or overlapping cubes. Injuries direct forces into a whole "cube." When the patient is twisted, the initial vector force may be straight. Because of bodily composition, motion, or twists, the resultant pathway becomes arced or more twisted as the person straightens. Memory of the force in the form of adaptation adversely affects the tissues, especially the fascia. Torque unwinding treatment involves the introduction of direct and rhythmic balancing pressures directed centrally from two opposing imaginary cube faces. The intent is for the therapeutic forces to negate the residual traumatic ones. Other variations of myofascial or fascial release techniques (18,19) that use point contacts as references, contact points, and/or diagnostic reflections occur in the osteopathic literature. Trigger band technique, described by Typaldos (20), is a method of changing the pathologic cross-linkages of fascial bands. Either instruments or fingers are used to exert significant deep pressure along certain connective tissue pathways. Chaitow (21,22) describes neuromuscular technique consisting mostly of point localization. Reflected dysfunction is treated by pressure followed by deep stroking and/or rolling of the tissue.

Chapman point treatment (23) reflects a neurologic/endocrine/lymphatic alteration reflected to specific points on the surface. Although they may not be tender or sensitive to pressure, the location of a Chapman point should raise suspicion of a possibly latent visceral correlate. Some of the specific mapped points are similar in location and correlation to those of acupuncture. The treatment consists of the application of circular pressures applied rhythmically by the pad of the physician's finger(s) to the nodular findings.

NON-OSTEOPATHIC POINT AND/OR PRESSURE SYSTEMS

Cyriax method (24), trigger point therapy (25,26), acupressure (27,28), reflexology, Rolfing, and shiatsu (29,30) bear some similarities to typical inhibition techniques, as well as to some other manual medicine systems of treatment. In each, the practitioner provides the treatment by pressing the patient's soft tissue. The overall intent is to bring about a persistent alteration. Each builds on a foundation of a system of diagnosis and/or treatment points.

Cyriax, a medical orthopedist, practiced joint mobilization and massage. He used a pinching technique on several locations. Trigger point therapy, developed by Travell, maps out the relationship between a remote referral region and a damaged myofascial nexus. The methods of treating these findings can include manual pressure, dry needling, or a combination of anesthetic and/or steroid agents injected into the trigger point. A vapocoolant spray is directed from the trigger point toward the referral zone in another form of the treatment. If used, the pressure applied to the selected points must be deeply administered. An apparent variant of the trigger point concept, Prudden myotherapy, consists of primary points, as well as satellite points. Both of these points are treated for short intervals several times per day over several sessions (31,32). Stretching may also be incorporated in either Prudden myotherapy or trigger point therapy.

Acupressure uses similar surface points that represent reflections of energy or chi forces within the body. Traditional oriental concept meridians align the specific point locations. Although several points may be treated within a session, the practitioner generally treats one or two points at any given time. The technique generally involves the application of pressure, as well as circular motions.

Rolf (33) developed the eponymous system called Rolfing. Sometimes called "Dr. Elbow" because of her use of it to apply pressure, she proposed using deeply applied forces on regions of the body as a tool to reestablish symmetry and normal function. The actual amount of force applied in this modality exceeds that commonly employed in osteopathic inhibition. There is a great deal of emphasis placed on approximating ideal symmetry and alignment. Followers of Rolf made some alterations to the technique and integrated them into other modalities involving movement patterns (Hellerwork, Aston-Patterning).

Shiatsu, one of the oldest forms of manual therapy, also usually involves relatively heavier pressures applied for short intervals. Improvements are reflected by the resultant reduction of the tissue tension. Although brief, the amount of force can be quite intense (especially in the hands of a traditional practitioner). Specific treatment patterns are used for certain conditions Reflexology relates energetic or visceral components to resonant areas located on the hands, feet, and ear. In theory, as with acupuncture, the name of the organ has more to do with the functional contribution to the integrity or energy component of the organ than the actual physical structure of the viscera.

PROGRESSIVE INHIBITION OF NEUROMUSCULAR STRUCTURES METHOD

The PINS method requires the localization of points and the application of pressure in a logical fashion to treat persistent or resistant dysfunction. The PINS system of treatment allows for versatility that is based on the osteopathic physician's capability to use anatomic and clinical knowledge to determine involved structures and sequence of treatment. The osteopathic physician must have a thorough knowledge of the typical and variant courses of nerves, fascial bands, and muscles, and this knowledge must be augmented by clinical decision-making skills for efficacy and accuracy. This may involve the treatment of contiguous muscles, dealing with the overlapping zones where more than one nerve, muscle, or fascial tissue may be contributing to the persistence of somatic dysfunction, as well as the development of a sequence of PINS treatment. It is not as simple as locating a sensitive point. Any patient can do that. An example would be the assumption that shoulder pain originates in the glenohumeral joint. If the treatment is successful in increasing mobility and decreasing discomfort, further investigation is halted. However, when that is unsuccessful, more of the same treatment is not the answer. This may prove frustrating to both the patient and the doctor. If the restrictions of motion of the shoulder involve the combination of flexion, abduction, and external rotation, as well as reduction of scapulothoracic motion, then this indicates something outside of one of the shoulder joints. The latissimus dorsi, which attaches in the bicipital groove of the humerus, pulls the arm into extension, internal rotation, and adduction, the motions directly opposite the restrictions. Treatment may have to go beyond this focus by including the upper ribs, pectoralis muscles, lower cervical spine, clavicle, thoracic spine, lumbar spine, pelvis, and lower extremity in the process. Fascial planes, and therefore fascial stresses, must also be considered.

With PINS, patients can offer feedback. They participate in the treatment by describing the amount of pain or other sensitivity at the palpated areas. As the treatment proceeds, the osteopathic physician takes note of the changes that occur, as well as the comparison of patient's subjective experience. The PINS method does not have to be the only treatment modality employed. It can be used before or after other methods of treatment (manipulative or otherwise).

Procedure

The development of an appropriate and specific diagnostic and treatment protocol using PINS requires:

1. In most cases, the patient should be supine or prone to allow postural muscles to be in a fairly relaxed state.

2. Stand or sit near the region to be treated. The fingers of both hands should be able to contact the patient comfortably and accurately.

3. Examine the patient. Determine any relationship between the patient's symptoms, somatic dysfunction, and the soft tissue findings.

4. Determine the components of the somatic dysfunction. The mnemonic "S.T.A.R." (34) can be used to track the different aspects:

■ Inquire about *(S) sensitivity changes.* These are the patient's subjective responses to palpation, and can include tenderness, numbness, radiation, warmth, irritation, throbbing, and so on.

■ Locate *(T) tissue texture changes.* They can be chronic (prolonged blanching of the skin, ropy or fibrous texture of the muscles and fasciae, coolness, dryness, vascular changes) or acute (increased redness, swelling and edema, moist, and/or increased temperature). Palpation may initially worsen this component.

■ *(A) asymmetry* can be noted by visual inspection or by palpatory examination. The so-called nondysfunctional side is used as the standard of expected form. Theoretically, an imaginary line down the middle of the body should reveal symmetry of one side to the other in a nondysfunctional condition.

■ Perhaps the most important determinant of somatic dysfunction is *(R) restriction of motion.* Restriction can be measure by quantity (degrees of motion) or quality (i.e., stiffness, tremors, cogwheel rigidity, extraneous movement, etc.).

5. The site of subjective complaints of pain can be deceptive and may not help in the actual localization of the true problem, but it is fairly reliable as an indicator that a problem exists. Tight muscles on one side may be relatively pain free while the contralateral stretched muscles may be more "attention-seeking." Symptoms may distract treatment from the more needy locations. Pain or any other symptom indicates a problem, but may or may not correlate with the dysfunction.

6. Locate a "primary sensitive" point by examination of the tissue in the region of the patient's complaint. If a significant point is not found, then use your knowledge of anatomic relationships to widen the search to adjacent areas.

7. Use knowledge of anatomic structures to locate another point. This may be designated as the "end point" for treatment purposes. It is located either distally or proximally to the primary point in a structure that links the two points. A thorough working knowledge and understanding of muscle origins/insertions, nerve pathways, and ligamentous attachments is a good beginning in determining this pair of points. If the primary point is at a muscular origin, the end point may be at the insertion, or vice versa. Sometimes one or the other point is located in the belly of the muscle. In that case, exploration of both ends of the attachments to bone may reveal the location of an end point. Ligaments, which are generally shorter and more fibrous, have points that are probably also fairly close to one another. Keep in mind that fascia encompasses all structures, and the path between one point and another may seem to cross other structures. The more specialized the fascia, the more palpable and tendinous it is. Tracing superficial and deep pathways of nerves is useful when determining paths that apparently do not correlate with the other structures. Primary and end points may be found where a nerve passes out of a foramen, between or through muscles, or around bony protrusions. If more than one nerve innervates a region, the primary point can sometimes be found at the beginning of one nerve and the end point or the beginning of the other. In the case of nerve distribution of an extremity, one point will typically be found closer to the body while the other will be closer to the end of the extremity. There are no exhaustive maps of points and sensitive point locations, and there is no substitution for an excellent working knowledge of anatomy. The designated primary point will most likely be nearer to the symptoms. The end point may also elicit the presenting symptoms, but usually to a lesser extent. As part of the reason for the maintenance of the dysfunction, all intervening points between the primary and the end points must be addressed. In any case, the first steps are to make a determination of the two ends of the pattern. A patient's complaints of apparently unrelated regions of the body being related may give a clue as to the location of some components.

TABLE 65.1. EXAMPLES OF PRIMARY POINTS AND END POINTS

Primary Point	End Point	Connection	Figure No.[a]
Surpaorbital notch	Sub-occipital region	Frontalis and occipitalis muscles	1A
		Trigeminal and greater occipital nerves	1B
Superior medial scapular border	Base of occiput	Levator scapula	2
Greater trochanter of femur	Fibular head	Iliotibial band	3
Sternum at 2nd rib	Coracoid process	Pectoralis minor	4
Gluteal region	Greater trochanter	Piriformis muscle	5
	Popliteal region	Sciatic nerve	6
Xiphoid process	Pubic ramus	Rectus abdominus	7
Antecubital region	Wrist	Median nerve	8

[a]See Appendix II (pp. 1258–1261) for figs.

Assuming that their knowledge of anatomy is small, it is left to you to draw conclusions necessary to begin treatment. These are indications that there is a problem.

8. For the purpose of proceeding in a logical fashion, the point that is more sensitive is designated as "primary." Put this in more easily understood language by referring to it as the "first point" with the patient. Both you and the patient can consider the other point, which is found on the other extreme, as the "end point." See Table 65.1 for a few examples of some primary and end points.

9. Determine a muscular, fascial, and/or neurologic pathway between the primary point and the end point. The line may be curved rather than straight. The direction of treatment may be from distal to proximal, or vice versa.

10. Understand the connection between the two points using knowledge of anatomy, especially:

Nerve innervation:

- Direct connections (e.g., the connection of a point near the antecubital region of the elbow at the elbow to a point along the middle of the forearm near the wrist—median nerve).
- Consider overlap or "watershed regions" of innervation (e.g., the ophthalmic division of the trigeminal nerve travels from the supraorbital notch over the frontal region to the top of the head. The greater occipital nerve exits the suboccipital region in the occipital sulcus and travels over the occiput to the top of the head. They overlap in the scalp near the vertex).

Muscle origins and insertions:

- Typical (e.g., a sensitive point may be found at the medial aspect of the clavicle and another found at the mastoid process representing involvement of the sternocleidomastoid muscle).
- Overlap (e.g., the location of a sensitive point on the superior anterior chest may involve the intercostal muscles, pectoralis major, and/or pectoralis minor).
- Contiguity (e.g., the tensor fascia latae and iliotibial band actually form a continuity for two possible tender points located at the greater trochanter and the fibular head, respectively. If a terminal point was actually found near the lateral malleolus instead of the fibular head, then there might be a tensor fascia latae, iliotibial band, peroneal muscle connection).

Fascia:

- Specialized (e.g., interosseous ligaments are actually specialized fasciae connecting the radius and ulna in the arm and the fibula

and tibia in the leg. Consider their involvement if a pattern appears to overlie their locations).

- Septums (e.g., although it is mostly muscular, the diaphragm has fascial components, including the central tendon and crus of the diaphragm. It supports and separates. Points found around the lower costal cartilage, the twelfth rib, and T10-12 and may represent diaphragmatic involvement).
- Overlaps (e.g., the common thoracolumbar fascia acts an attachment for muscles, such as the latissimus dorsi, and overlaps muscles, such as the quadratus lumborum, iliocostalis, and other erector spinae muscles. Points may be found anywhere within the region and may extend to the lateral edge of the 12th rib [quadratus lumborum], or even to the bicipital groove of the humerus [latissimus dorsi]).

Ligamentous attachments:

- Typical (e.g., the attachments of either end of the collateral ligaments in the elbow and knee can be considered).
- Relationships to muscles (e.g., specific points can be found on the superior or lateral C7 spinous process, and the base of the occiput may represent spinalis muscles or the nuchal ligament).
- Relationships to nerves (e.g., the flexor retinaculum and palmar aponeurosis of the hand are related to the median nerve in the forearm. These structures, in turn, are related to attachments with at least four [pisiform, hamate, scaphoid, and trapezium] carpal bones by means of the flexor retinaculum).

Bones (the bones and their components should also be considered connective tissue):

- Construction of joints (e.g., joint capsules represent connections between two or more bones. At the elbow and the knee, the capsules are stronger and reinforced on their medial and lateral surfaces by collateral ligaments. The anterior and posterior surfaces are relatively weaker and may tighten or loosen in one extreme of motion or the other. Points may occur in the middle of the capsule and at the bony attachments).
- Lever action (e.g., muscle, tendons, and ligaments attach to bony prominences. Because of the forces placed on them, they enlarge into tubercles, trochanters, and other processes. Points located at tendinous insertions may also theoretically represent a contribution from the bony attachments).

11. Press both the primary point and the end point simultaneously using the pad region of a finger on each hand (Fig. 9,

Appendix II). (Again, for the sake of simplicity, identify the primary point as the "first point" for the patient.) The pressure exerted is a few ounces. It should be enough to elicit the patient's symptoms, and should be and of equal amount on both points. The patient may initially experience a mild to moderate increase in sensitivity. Also note the soft tissue response to the pressure:

- Acute dysfunction may be more sensitive than chronic. A muscle that has been hypertonic will usually be more sensitive to pressure than the same muscle on the contralateral side.
- Chronic hypertonic muscles will usually be larger than those on the contralateral side:
  —Larger muscles do not necessarily indicate dysfunction. Asymmetric use (where there is preference with one side being used more) will result in the dominant side becoming typically larger. An enlarged muscle does not indicate dysfunction.
  —Whether dysfunctional or not, frequently used muscles or ones in chronic dysfunction may not be quite so sensitive to pressure. This may due to the chronicity of usage.
- Both sides can be dysfunctional. One side may be more symptomatic than the other. Treat the more dysfunctional tissue first; re-examine, and then the lesser-involved side can also be treated.
- A firmer muscle is probably in greater dysfunction.

12. Exert the same amount of pressure on both the primary and end points.

- Patients may assume that a more sensitive location is being pressed harder. They should be reassured that the reason for the asymmetry is the greater dysfunction or hyperactivity of the involved tissue.
- Patients may indicate to the practitioner that they can tolerate greater pressure. This does not accelerate the treatment. It is not necessary to increase, and may even be counterproductive.
- Pain or tenderness may not be the only sensations experienced from the applied pressure. The patient may report other sensations that occur alone or in combination with pain.

13. Maintain constant pressure on the end point throughout the treatment. Initiate pressure on the point with greater sensitivity (primary point). Ask the patient to report what they are feeling. When inhibition is used properly, any increase in sensitivity at a point will most probably be transient. Also, a typical, rapid decrease in sensitivity occurs as the tissue accommodates the irritation of the inhibition. Ultimately, it may totally disappear. The duration can vary from several seconds to minutes.

14. Maintain contact with the primary point for 20 to 30 seconds before seeking any subsequent points.

- One finger remains on the primary point. Use another finger of the same hand to locate a "secondary point." If the middle finger is on the primary point, then use the index finger to palpate the secondary point (Fig. 10, Appendix II).
- Search for a secondary point approximately 2 to 3 cm away from the primary point. An imaginary line connecting the primary and end points gives the approximate direction. This will

typically follow the predicted course of an anatomic structure (innervating nerve, along the direction of the muscle fibers, or following fascial planes).
- Identify the secondary point as "the second point" for the patient.

15. Exert equal pressure onto both the primary and secondary points while maintaining the constant pressure on the end point.

16. Ask the patient to determine which of the two points (primary vs. secondary or "first versus second") is more sensitive.

- To make it simpler for the patient, use a phrase such as, "I am pressing on two points that are close together. Please tell me which of the two, the 'first' or the 'second,' is more sensitive?"
- If the second point is more sensitive or equally as sensitive as the first:
- Relieve the pressure from the first (primary) point and then remove it entirely.
- Maintain constant pressure on the new, second (secondary) sensitive point for an additional 20 to 30 seconds.
- It is not necessary to wait for the sensitivity at any point to be completely gone before moving on to the next point. It is more important that each subsequent point is more sensitive than the prior one.
- Both increased tension and sensitivity can be found in the new secondary point. With practice, the "secondary" points can be located by palpatory sense of tension alone. A return to a lower level of sensitivity and response baseline usually occurs after a few seconds. The amount of time depends on the soft tissue response.

Certain points may require further inhibition before progress can be made. After doing so, a new secondary point may be located where previously there was less sensitivity. If the original or a subsequent "first point" persists as the more sensitive of the two points:

- Maintain pressure at the location of the primary point for an additional 20 to 30 seconds; and/or
- Move the finger that was locating the secondary point more laterally or medially from the connecting line. A located new secondary point should have at least the same sensitivity, if not more, as the primary point. (The anatomic structure, whether muscle, nerve, or fascia, that is being inhibited may have slight variations in the specific course in this individual.)
- Once a secondary point that is equally or more sensitive is located, relieve pressure from the primary point and maintain on the new secondary point as described above.
- The secondary point then becomes the new "first" point in the continuing sequence of treatment toward the end point.

17. Inhibit the end point with constant pressure with a finger of the other hand throughout. The patient will often forget that this point is being treated. As the anchor for the dysfunctional tissue, continuous treatment is necessary. It may lose sensitivity during the course of treatment.

18. Repeat the process until an ultimate "second" point is located 2 cm from the end point.

19. Once the two final points have been treated with inhibition, determine the amount of dysfunction that persists, especially

at the end point location. It may have become significantly reduced or may completely disappear.

20. Another modality of treatment can be used if the dysfunction (including the end point) remains persistent. The end point and overall dysfunction may now be easier to treat than they were previously. Facilitated positional release, strain-counterstrain, muscle energy, balanced ligamentous tension techniques, or some other modality may be used. The use of high-velocity/low-amplitude (HVLA) techniques that were difficult to perform before may now be easier. Guidelines for determining the choice include:

- The persistence of the dysfunction or related components after treatment.
- The ability of the practitioner to perform other modalities of treatment.
- The need or capability of the patient to tolerate additional treatment.

21. The conclusion of manipulative treatment for the session should be based on the findings for the individual. It should not be based solely on the patient's subjective complaints. Overtreatment can cause as many problems as undertreatment.

22. Patients may limit types of treatment based on prior experience or misconceptions. They may have had a reaction to previous treatments or they may have had no previous difficulties but have developed a dislike for a particular modality (i.e., "popping" secondary to HVLA). Attempting to coerce a patient to allow certain forms of treatment would be counterproductive to the therapeutic relationship. In many locales, it could also be considered illegal (i.e., battery).

23. The somatic dysfunction is always reassessed.

24. Despite a relatively comfortable treatment, a post-treatment reaction may occur. Inform the patient that some treatment reactions can include transient soreness, aches, and fatigue. In patients prone to bruising, when certain other predisposing factors exist (e.g., medication), or if excessive pressure has been used, ecchymoses can occur. Generally, all such side effects resolve in 24 to 48 hours.

Possible Mechanism of Action

One important component that distinguishes an inhibitory contact from a stimulatory one is the use of a low level, but constant amount of pressure applied to dysfunctional tissue. Although the initial effect may be irritating, a contact of this type may initiate accommodation or habituation over time. At first, the patient may be acutely sensitive with complaints of increased pain, sensitivity, pressure, or some other sensation. These reactions decrease and may disappear altogether as the system adapts (35). Part of this reduction in awareness may be from the screening mechanisms provided by the reticular formation. The body accommodates to other stimuli, such as body contact with eyeglasses, tight belts, stiff clothing, uncomfortable shoes, as well as constant background auditory and visual stimuli. This sensory filtering process may also involve the spinal cord acting as a mediator or "brake" when sensory overload (36) occurs. Some stimuli remain relatively subliminal if not of sufficient quality, duration, or quantity.

Effects may include pressure or contact as a counterirritant. Instead of actually inhibiting, they act as stimulation to the neighboring tissue, thus reducing the sensitivity of the original tender point. Scratching in the region of an itch would be one such example. Rapid conducting, large-nerve afferent fibers may gate transmission in the dorsal horn of the spinal cord with collateral fibers in the substantia gelatinosa or adjacent interneurons inhibiting the transmission of pain to the central nervous system via the spinothalamic tract (37).

Relative ischemia has also been proposed as a theory. Muscle maintained in prolonged contraction produces metabolites and waste products from the local tissue damage (38). Impaired circulation also occurs concomitantly with hyperemia and congestion. Some of the substances have vasoactive effects, which theoretically may have the purpose of reacting to tissue injury. Trophic and fibrotic changes may occur if the injury persists. Normally, the overlying skin shows a brief blanching followed by redness, which also fades when normal, but may persist when the tissue is damaged for a prolonged time. It appears that the use of therapeutic pressure may add to the ischemia. Initially, this does not make intuitive sense when considering the amount of nutrient deprivation. However, the increased ischemia may reduce the capacity of the nociceptive receptors to process information. Hyperemia may also occur once this pressure is removed, resulting in the flushing of the waste products from the location.

A muscle in dysfunction may appear to be in its neutral position, but may still be hypertonic. Further stretch from the relatively shortened length increases activity of the muscle spindle mechanisms, and will result in a reflexive and prolonged contraction. This is a means of protection (39–42). If stretching is used, slow stretching is the type. Pressure applied during inhibition introduces a gentle stretch while allowing the re-setting of the stretch receptors (43). Only a small amount of the tissue may be challenged without upsetting the whole structure. Once the small, localized component is overwhelmed, any affected adjacent area can subsequently be inhibited with similar results. Inhibition in general and PINS in particular may be very effective methods to deal with a series of irritated pieces. The osteopathic physician may treat the entire dysfunction by progressively treating all of the involved elements.

The Golgi tendon organ is a sensory mechanism that becomes relatively stretched during muscular contraction (where the overall length of the muscle does not change). When a critical amount of tension occurs, increased Golgi tendon organ activity brings about reflex relaxation of the muscle as a whole. An inhibitory interneuron between the afferent nerve ending in the spinal cord and the alpha motoneuron bring about sudden, almost complete muscular relaxation. The pressure from the osteopathic physician's fingers may create an initial stretch that results in further contraction. This is then followed by resultant relaxation (44).

Contraindications and Side Effects

There appear to be few contraindications and side effects with the use of PINS. Pressure should not be exerted onto localized inflammation, abscess, or infection, as the integrity of the skin or walled infection may be compromised.

CONCLUSION

PINS represents a unique variant of the more traditional approach to using inhibition, as well as a means of discovering the ways in which dysfunction occurs and is maintained. It can be used solely or in combination with other methods of osteopathic manipulation. The effect of other treatment modalities can be enhanced by the use of PINS.

Using PINS does require an investment of time. When it appears that other typical interventions are of limited success with recalcitrant dysfunction, alternative means must be used. However, when this occurs, the time necessary to perform PINS would be worth the effort.

REFERENCES

1. Dowling DJ. Progressive inhibition of neuromuscular structures (PINS) technique. *J Am Osteopath Assoc.* 2000;100(5),285–286,289–298.
2. *Glossary of Osteopathic Terminology.* AOA Yearbook and Directory of Osteopathic Physicians, 1998.
3. Dowling DJ, Scariati PD. Neurophysiology relevant to osteopathic principles and practice. In: DiGiovanna EL, Schiowitz S, eds. *An Osteopathic Approach to Diagnosis and Treatment,* 2nd ed. Philadelphia, PA: Lippincott-Raven Publishers; 1997:33.
4. Ehrenfeuchter WC. Soft tissue techniques. In: Ward RC, ed. *Foundations for Osteopathic Medicine.* Baltimore, MD: Williams & Wilkins; 1997:781–794.
5. Robbins SL, Cotran RS, Kumar V. *Pathologic Basis of Disease,* 3rd ed. Philadelphia, PA: WB Saunders; 1984:40.
6. Still AT. *Autobiography of A. T. Still,* rev. ed. Kirksville, MO: Published by the author; 1908:32.
7. Still AT. *The Philosophy and Mechanical Principles of Osteopathy.* Kansas City, MO: Hudson-Kimberly Publishing Co; 1902:101.
8. Goetz EW. *A Manual of Osteopathy,* 2nd ed. Cincinnati, OH: 1905.
9. Tasker DD. *Principles of Osteopathy,* 4th ed. Los Angeles, CA: Bireley & Elson Printing Co; 1916:354–370.
10. Jones LH. *Strain and Counterstrain.* Newark, OH: American Academy of Osteopathy; 1981.
11. Jones LH, Kusenose R, Goering E. *Jones Strain-Counterstrain.* Boise, ID: Jones Strain-Counterstrain; 1995.
12. Glover JC, Yates HA. Strain and counterstrain techniques. In: Ward RC, ed. *Foundations for Osteopathic Medicine.* Baltimore, MD: Williams & Wilkins; 1997:809–818.
13. Schiowitz S. Facilitated positional release. In: DiGiovanna EL, Schiowitz S, eds. *An Osteopathic Approach to Diagnosis and Treatment,* 2nd ed. Philadelphia, PA: Lippincott-Raven Publishers; 1997:91.
14. Van Buskirk VL. A manipulative technique of Andrew Taylor Still as reported by Charles Hazzard, DO, in 1905. *J Am Osteopath Assoc.* 1996;96(10):597–602.
15. Hazzard C. *The Practice and Applied Therapeutics of Osteopathy.* 1905.
16. Johnston WL. Functional technique: An indirect method. In: Ward RC, ed. *Foundations for Osteopathic Medicine.* Baltimore, MD: Williams & Wilkins; 1997:795–808.
17. Dowling DJ. Myofascial release techniques. In: DiGiovanna EL, Schiowitz S, eds. *An Osteopathic Approach to Diagnosis and Treatment,* 2nd ed. Philadelphia, PA: Lippincott-Raven Publishers; 1997:381–383.
18. Chila AG. Fascial-ligamentous release: An indirect approach. In: Ward RC, ed. *Foundations for Osteopathic Medicine.* Baltimore, MD: Williams & Wilkins; 1997:819–830.
19. Ward RC. Integrated neuromusculoskeletal release and myofascial release: An introduction to diagnosis and treatment. In: Ward RC, ed. *Foundations for Osteopathic Medicine.* Baltimore, MD: Williams & Wilkins; 1997:846–849.
20. Typaldos S. Introducing the fascial distortion model. *Am Acad Osteopath J.* 1994;4(2).
21. Chaitow L. *Neuro-muscular Technique.* Wellingborough, Northamtonshire, England: Thorsons Publishers Ltd; 1980.
22. Chaitow L. *Modern Neuromuscular Techniques.* New York, NY: Churchill Livingstone; 1996.
23. Owens C. *An Endocrine Interpretation of Chapman's Reflexes,* 2nd ed. Chattanooga, TN: Chattanooga Printing and Engraving Co; 1937.
24. Cyriax J. *Text-book of Orthopaedic Medicine Volume II: Treatment by Manipulation and Massage,* 6th ed. New York, NY: Harper & Row; 1959.
25. Travell JG, Simons DG. *Myofascial Pain and Dysfunction: The Trigger Point Manual: The Upper Extremities,* vol I. Baltimore, MD: Williams & Wilkins; 1983.
26. Chaitlow L. *Osteopathic Self-Treatment.* Wellingborough, England: Thorsons Publishing Group; 1990:105–119.
27. Kenyon J. *Acupressure Techniques: A Self Help Guide.* Rochester, VT: Healing Arts Press; 1988.
28. Cerney JV. *Acupuncture Without Needles.* West Nyack, NY: Parker Publishing Company, Inc; 1974.
29. Shultz W. *Shiatsu: Japanese Finger Pressure Therapy.* New York, NY: Bell Publishing Company; 1976.
30. Weil A. *Spontaneous Healing.* New York, NY: Ballantine Books; 1995.
31. The Burton Goldberg Group. *Alternative Medicine: The Definitive Guide.* Puyallup, WA: Future Medicine Publishing, Inc; 1994:106–108.
32. Prudden B. *Pain Erasure: The Bonnie Prudden Way.* New York, NY: Ballantine Books; 1980.
33. The Burton Goldberg Group. *Alternative Medicine: The Definitive Guide.* Puyallup, WA: Future Medicine Publishing, Inc;1994:102–103.
34. Dowling DJ. S.T.A.R.: a more viable alternative descriptor system of somatic dysfunction *Am Acad Osteopath J.* 1998;8(2):34–37.
35. Bailey HW. Some problems in making osteopathic spinal manipulative therapy appropriate and specific. *J Am Osteopath Assoc.* 1976;75:486–499.
36. Patterson MM. A model mechanism for spinal segmental facilitation. *J Am Osteopath Assoc.* 1976;76:62–72.
37. Ganong WF. *Review of Medical Physiology.* Upper Saddle River, NJ: Prentice Hall; 1995:130–131.
38. Stoddard A. *Manual of Osteopathic Practice.* London, UK: Hutchinson Medical Publications; 1969:238.
39. Buzzell KA. The potential disruptive influence of somatic input. *The Physiological Basis of Osteopathic Medicine.* The Postgraduate Institute of Osteopathic Medicine and Surgery. New York, NY: Insight Publishing Company; 1967:39–51.
40. Ganong WF. *Review of Medical Physiology.* Upper Saddle River, NJ: Prentice Hall; 1995:113–117.
41. Becker RF. The gamma system and its relation to the development and maintenance of muscle tone. *1976 Year Book of the American Academy of Osteopathy.* Colorado Springs, CO: American Academy of Osteopathy; 1976:26–40.
42. Korr IM. Proprioceptors and somatic dysfunction. *1976 Year Book of the American Academy of Osteopathy.* Colorado Springs, CO: American Academy of Osteopathy; 1976:41–50.
43. Korr IM. Proprioceptors and somatic dysfunction. *J Am Osteopath Assoc.* 1974;74:638–650. Reprinted in *The Collected Papers of Irvin M. Korr.* Colorado Springs, CO: American Academy of Osteopathy; 1979:200–207.
44. Ganong WF. *Review of Medical Physiology.* Upper Saddle River, NJ: Prentice Hall; 1995:117–118.

MYOFASCIAL TRIGGER POINTS AS SOMATIC DYSFUNCTION

MICHAEL L. KUCHERA
JOHN M. McPARTLAND

KEY CONCEPTS

- Similarities and differences between various myofascial points
- Definitions of active and latent Travell trigger points
- Postulated physiologic mechanisms of referred pain
- Trigger points as somatic dysfunction
- Effect on somatic function, venous-lymphatic drainage, and autonomic function
- Relationship to somatovisceral and viscerosomatic reflexes
- Commonalities in palpatory diagnosis, signs and symptoms
- Osteopathic clinical approach to trigger points
- Incidence in healthy populations and those seeking medical care
- Addressing contributing and perpetuating factors
- Techniques for treatment, including osteopathic manipulative treatment, soft tissue techniques, spray and stretch, deep massage, injection, and others

Throughout the history of medicine, tender points in myofascial tissues have been observed and mapped. They figure prominently, for example, in several ancient eastern patient care systems, including acupuncture. Increasingly, various western physicians have correlated palpable myofascial points with patient histories and their accompanying symptoms. Today, many myofascial point systems are found in the modern physician's differential diagnosis and treatment armamentarium.

MYOFASCIAL POINT SYSTEMS

Myofascial points have certain common clinical characteristics (1); by meeting *t*enderness/*a*symmetry/*r*ange of motion/*t*issue texture changes (TART) diagnostic criteria, all are definable forms of somatic dysfunction. All are subjectively tender with moderate to deep palpation, and all are characterized and recognized as palpably small, circumscribed, hypersensitive myofascial thicken-

ings. Often they are associated with local or referred autonomic disturbances (2,3). They may exhibit localized tenderness alone, or they may also have a referred pain pattern to a reference zone that may or may not have an obvious neurologic distribution.

Although many of these myofascial points have overlapping characteristics, they also have unique factors (2) related to the perspective and philosophy of the physician mapping them. Over time, many clinicians have correlated tender points, reflex points, and trigger points with visceral pathology. In 1893, both Head (4) and Mackenzie (5) associated dermal and myofascial tender points with internal pathology. In the 1920s, Chapman found useful clinical correlations between palpable tender points and visceral complaints (6); his system of viscerosomatic reflexes is discussed further in Chapter 67. Beginning in the 1940s, an internal medicine physician, Janet Travell, spent over 50 years researching and documenting the myofascial genesis of pain patterns and their role in clinical diagnosis and treatment (2,7,8).

Myofascial Trigger Points in Osteopathic Practice

Travell and Simons (2,8) developed the most widely recognized myofascial point system used in diagnosis and treatment. These physicians devoted their careers to the understanding of myofascial pain and dysfunction, and the clinical application of the trigger point system for their treatment. Travell's prominence in using this system in the care of President John F. Kennedy, and the excellent two-volume text, *Travell & Simons' Myofascial Pain and Dysfunction: The Trigger Point Manual* (2,8) brought worldwide recognition to this form of somatic dysfunction, which might otherwise have been overlooked. Diagrammatic summaries of trigger point maps affecting different regions are shown in Figure 66.1. When a patient complains of pain in a particular region, consider examining these points.

A myofascial trigger point (TP) is a specific form of impaired or altered myofascial function with distinctive clinical and pathophysiologic characteristics; these characteristics are extremely well documented in the literature (1). A TP is defined as "a hyperirritable spot in skeletal muscle that is associated with a hypersensitive palpable nodule in a taut band. The spot is painful on compression and can give rise to characteristic referred pain, referred

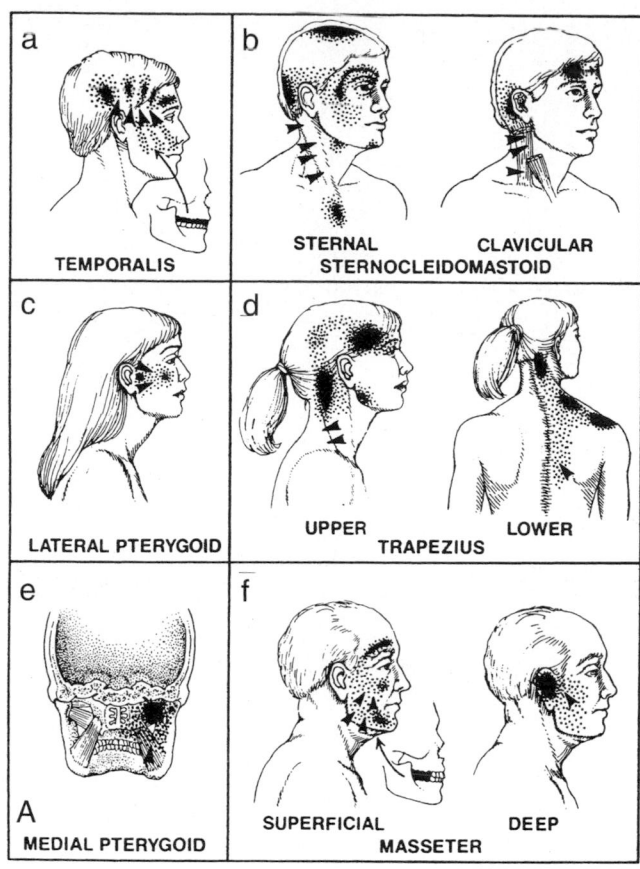

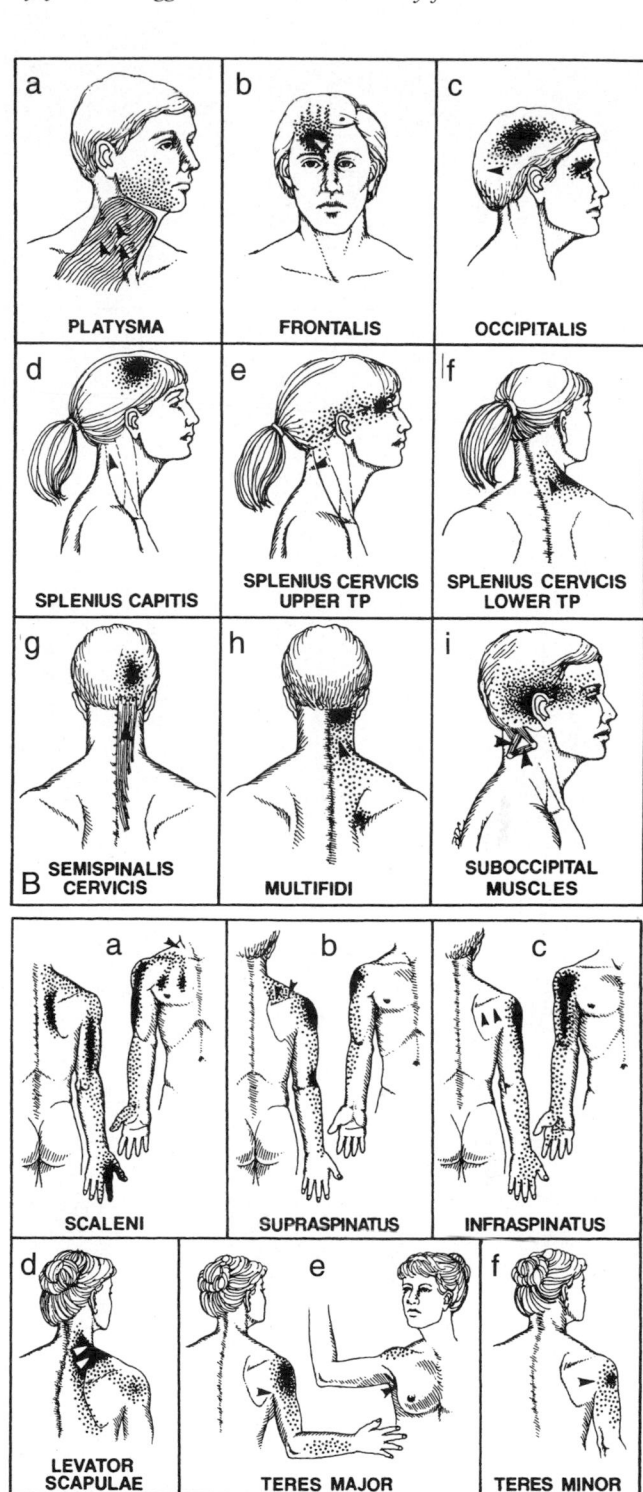

FIGURE 66.1. Regional depiction of Travell myofascial trigger points; referred pain patterns *(black stippled area)* and location of trigger points *(arrows)*. **A:** Masticatory and two neck muscles, **(B)** several head and neck muscles, **(C)** neck muscles (scaleni) that refer pain in the upper extremity and for many shoulder girdle muscles, **(D)** arm and several forearm muscles, **(E)** forearm and intrinsic hand muscles, **(F)** shoulder girdle, chest, and iliocostalis paraspinal muscle, **(G)** superficial paraspinal, several deep paraspinal, quadratus lumborum back muscles, and two abdominal wall muscles, **(H)** pelvic girdle muscles and three parts (vastus medialis, rectus femoris, and vastus intermedius) of the quadriceps femoris muscle, **(I)** vastus lateralis of quadriceps femoris, several muscles of leg, and selected intrinsic foot muscles. (From Wall PD, Melzack R, eds. *Textbook of Pain,* 2nd ed. Edinburgh, Scotland: Churchill Livingstone; 1989:368–385, with permission.)

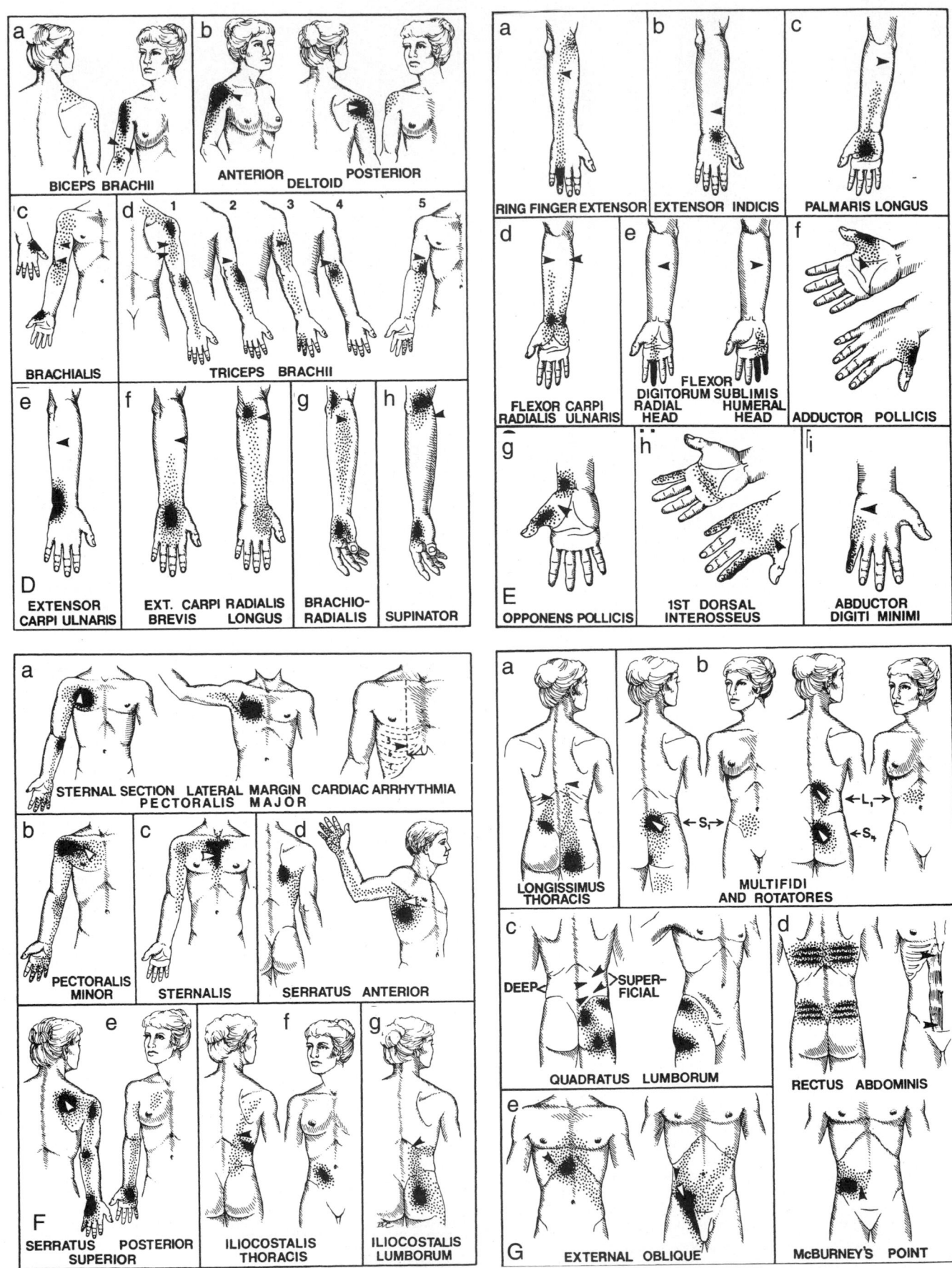

FIGURE 66.1. (*continued*)

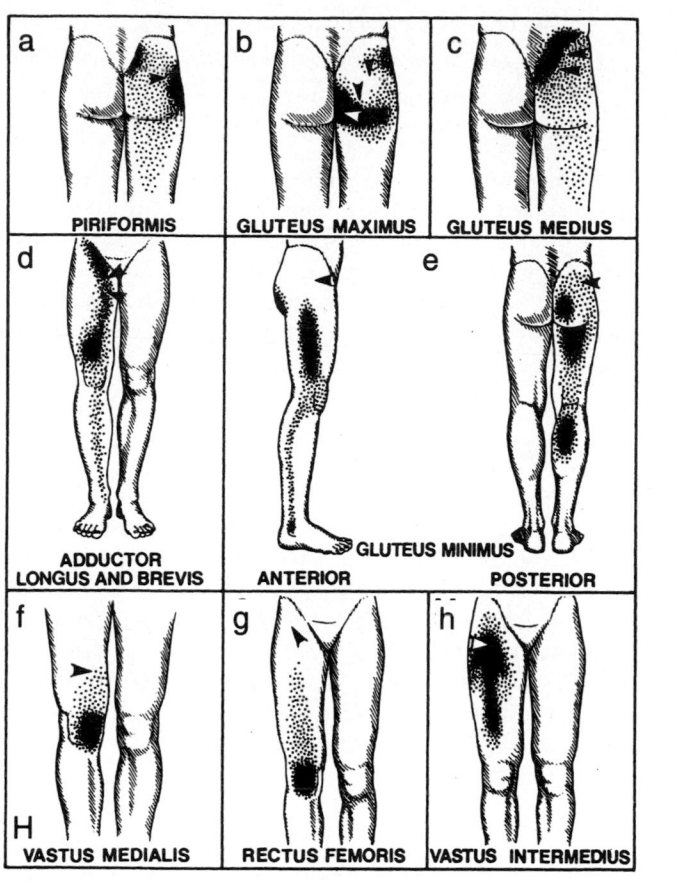

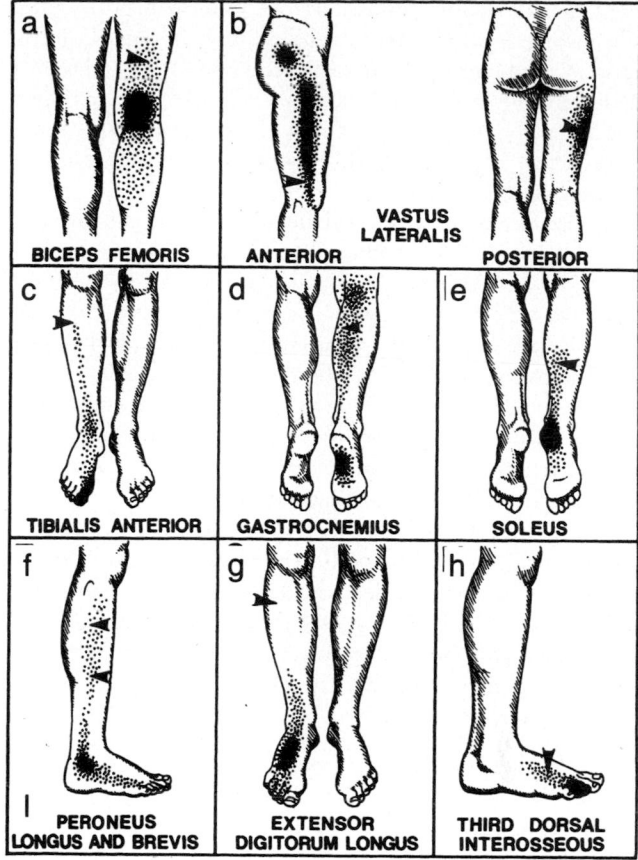

FIGURE 66.1. *(continued)*

tenderness, motor dysfunction, and autonomic phenomena" (2). In short, a TP is a specific form of somatic dysfunction.

The term TP is reserved for a point that has the potential to refer ("trigger") pain in a certain predictable distribution. TPs are classified as "active" or "latent" depending on their ability to refer pain into the characteristic distribution empirically mapped for each point. Active points refer pain at rest, with muscular activity, or with palpation. Latent points produce pain only when probed with more steady pressure. Unless a skilled palpatory examination is conducted, latent points are often overlooked, and the true cause of dysfunction may be misdiagnosed.

In several ways, this system is distinct from that described by Jones (see Chapter 63), in which locally tender myofascial points do not typically refer pain beyond the location being compressed. In general, however, Simons (9) describes a significant overlap in location between TPs and several systems of tender points. Chaitow (10) believes their distinction is arbitrary. He notes that tender points can develop referral capabilities by the simple introduction of a chill or strain to the affected muscle. Similarly, Bennett (11) suggests that tender points become trigger points as a result of enhanced patient pain perception. Comparing yet another system, Melzack (12) reported a 71% correspondence between published locations of TPs and classic acupuncture points used in the relief of pain.

Myofascial TPs are only one manifestation of somatic dysfunction, but they provide significant osteopathic insights. This type of somatic dysfunction has far-reaching implications in the differential diagnosis and treatment of:

Pain syndromes and disability
Repetitive strain injuries and overuse syndrome
Reduced muscle functions
Fibrositis, fibromyalgia, myofasciitis, and chronic fatigue syndrome
Disrupted visceral homeostasis

Diagnosing, interpreting, and treating myofascial points as a form of somatic dysfunction provides a better understanding of the osteopathic perspective. It expands our interpretation of structure-function relationships and offers possible mechanisms for treatment of other somatic tissues. It also enhances our clinical diagnostic and treatment skills. In return, osteopathic medicine continues to contribute greatly to the documentation, interpretation, and treatment of myofascial tender points and trigger points.

Incidence

There are more than 200 pairs of muscles in the human body, with myofascial structures constituting approximately half of the body's mass. Not surprisingly then, these soft tissues are a common source of patient complaints. Different centers have reported the incidence of various primary myofascial syndromes: for example, the documented prevalence in a general internal medicine outpatient practice was 30% (13) compared with 55% of 296 patients admitted for chronic head and neck pain (14) and

85% of 283 consecutive admissions for chronic pain (15). Often misdiagnosed, a specific myofascial syndrome, fibromyalgia, has a reported incidence of 2% in the general population and 6% to 10% in general internal medicine clinics (16,17). Interestingly, in one study, about 72% of patients with fibromyalgia syndrome also had active TPs, and 20% of those with active TPs also had fibromyalgia (18).

The specific documented incidence of latent TPs also varies. It has been reported (19) as 54% and 45%, respectively, in asymptomatic 19-year-old female and male Air Force recruits. Of 61 consecutive patients presenting to an internal medicine practice, 10% with general medical symptoms and 31% with the chief complaint of pain had TPs as the primary cause (20). Trigger points are most likely to develop in the upper trapezius muscle (19). Overall, however, trigger points in the quadratus lumborum muscle are reported to be the most common, and most commonly overlooked, cause of myogenic low back pain (21).

TPs are both more likely to occur and, once present, are more likely to remain in patients with perpetuating factors. Postural and other mechanical disorders, including articular somatic dysfunction (1,2,8,22,23), are reported to be some of the most pervasive perpetuating factors. An osteopathic structural analysis is therefore warranted in any patient with myofascial TPs. Other contributing factors include:

Hypothyroidism, hypoglycemia, and various metabolic/endocrine dysfunction (11)
Nutritional deficiencies (2)
Chronic infections (2)
Allergic rhinitis (2)
Psychological stressors (2,24)

Systemic perpetuating factors may include any structural or functional disorder that compromises homeostasis of the local energy supply to the involved muscle(s).

Referred Pain Mechanisms and Causation

Regardless of the exact mechanism or mechanisms proposed, afferent information to the central nervous system from peripheral somatic and visceral structures figures prominently in the proposed origin of all myofascial points. In the Travell system, overuse of somatic structures, especially chilled muscle, is often implicated (2). Although primary visceral dysfunction related to facilitated segments is more frequently associated with Chapman reflex points (25), Travell and Simons also note the association of segmentally related visceral dysfunction in TP initiation and/or perpetuation (1,2). Proponents of Chapman points (26), Jones points (27), and Travell TPs (2) all recognize the importance of segmentally related somatic dysfunction in the interpretation and treatment of each myofascial point system.

Unless physicians recognize and understand the basis for referral phenomena, appropriate diagnosis and treatment may result from mislocalization or misinterpretations of the true origins of the pain. Several mechanisms are postulated to play a role in TP referral phenomena:

1. Convergence-projection
2. Convergence-facilitation
3. Activity of the sympathetic nervous system
4. Convergence or image projection at the supraspinal level
5. Peripheral axon branching from certain dorsal root ganglion cells to two different muscles

Most of the central mechanisms applied to understanding TPs suggest that pain referral may result from nociceptive information being misdirected in the spinal cord to reach somatotopically inappropriate dorsal horn neurons. The first and fifth mechanisms relate to the structure of the nervous system, although the others relate to functional factors. (Further discussion of referred pain may be found in Chapter 15.)

Central Nervous System

The central integration of afferent data with generalized, predictable modification of efferent responses is a neurologic model used to explain causation and maintenance of somatic dysfunction (including TPs), referred pain, and several reflexes between the soma, the viscera, and the sympathetic systems (1,28,29). This view is consistent with Korr's observations (30) that the spine can be viewed as an "organizer" of disease and dysfunctional processes, and may harbor a segmentally related "neurologic lens" for a wide variety of stressors (Fig. 66.2).

Peripheral Local Conditions

Local conditions resulting from or accompanying the development of myofascial points have also been studied (1,31). These conditions suggest that palpatory tenderness and TPs are increased by endogenous tissue sensitizing and pain-producing substances (bradykinins, serotonin, histamine, substance P, prostaglandin E2, etc.) (1,31). Branching axon subpopulations, as well as local microtrauma and/or macrotrauma are also implicated in the wider release of these substances. Somatic dysfunction alters the local biochemical milieu and impairs or alters neural, vascular, and lymphatic mechanisms, preventing removal of these sensitizing and/or pain-producing substances (3,32).

Physiologically, there appears to be local metabolic crisis in the presence of impaired circulation, a factor that leads to tissue texture abnormalities that aid in finding the myofascial point by palpation. Palpatory findings in the area of a TP include an alteration of cutaneous temperature and humidity. There is a small nodular or spindle-shaped thickening of the tissues, representing the myofascial point itself. The point is extremely tender to the patient and usually invokes a generalized "jump sign" or some other patent response of discomfort. In the case of myofascial trigger points, there is a "local twitch" of the taut muscle band containing the point when the muscle is palpated perpendicular to its long axis. There may be localized goose flesh or trophic changes at the site. A summary of these palpatory findings is proposed in Figure 66.3.

Biomechanical Conditions

The activation of a TP is usually associated with some degree of mechanical abuse of the muscle. This may be associated with:

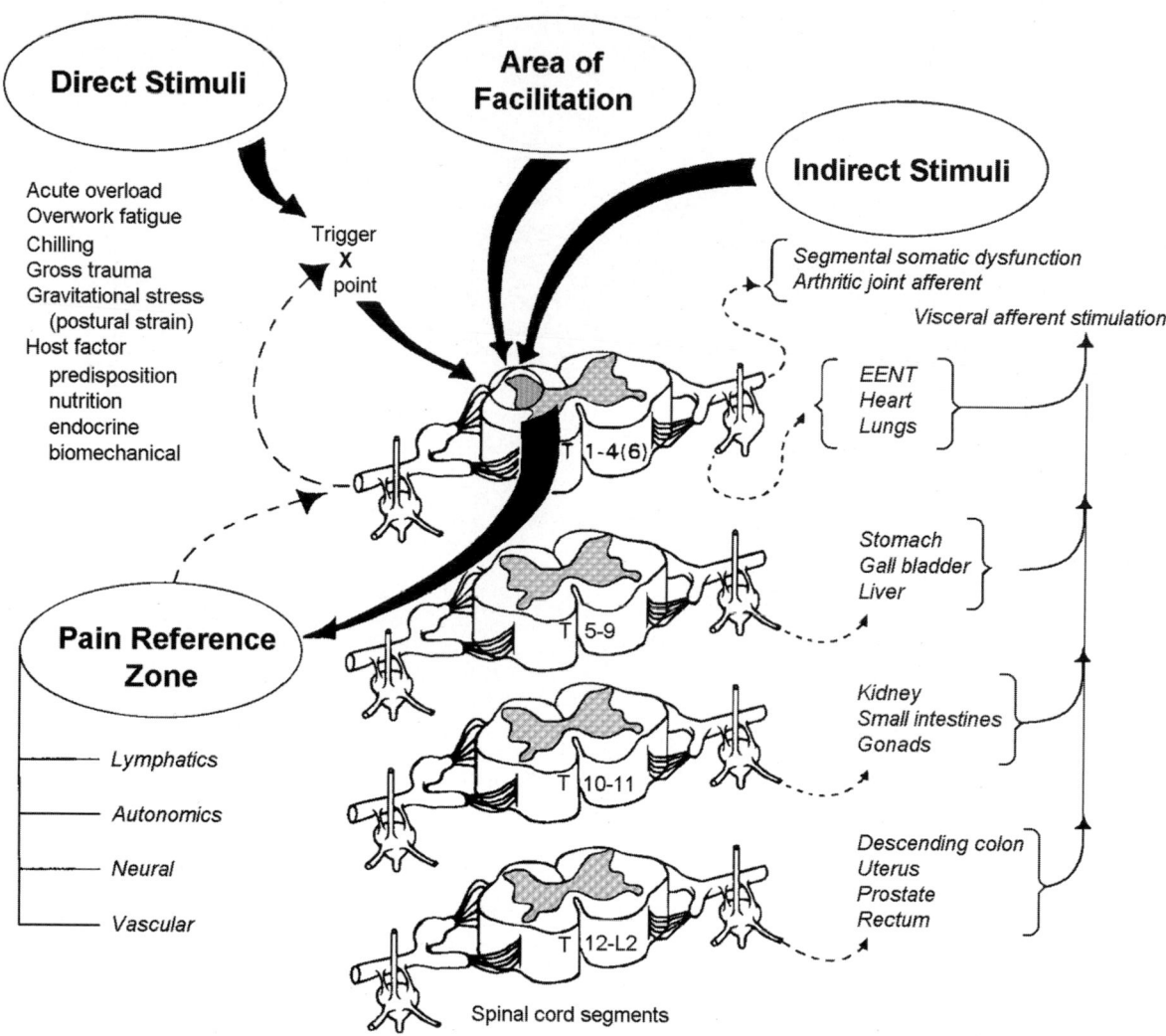

FIGURE 66.2. The spinal cord as a neurologic lens for a variety of stressors to initiate somatic and/or visceral symptoms.

Muscle overload (acute, sustained, and/or repetitive)
Myofascial postural stress
Leaving a muscle in a prolonged shortened position (especially if the muscle is then contracted while in the shortened position)
Muscle chilling

Furthermore, dysfunction in a given muscle places additional biomechanical demand on other muscles in the functional myotatic unit. (A "myotatic unit" is made up of muscles sharing the same functional responsibilities.) Functional overuse may result in associated TPs in a given myotatic unit. "Satellite trigger points," on the other hand, may develop in muscles covered by the referred pain pattern of another myofascial TP.

An understanding of the structure-function relationships and physiologic mechanisms involved in instigation and perpetuation of TPs leads to a more accurate diagnosis of the patient. Successful treatment of that patient depends on removing the primary myofascial TP, its associated and satellite TPs, related articular dysfunction, and any underlying or perpetuating factors. Failure to address all of these elements usually results in the full return of the dysfunctional myofascial situation.

DIAGNOSIS

Diagnosis of myofascial TPs depends on distinctive palpatory findings (local spot, palpable band, and twitch response); muscle testing (strength and range-of-motion); distribution of the pain pattern; and the patient's history. TPs are locally very tender. They are palpated as small nodular or spindle-shaped thickenings within a taut band of tissue.

Each suspicious muscle is examined. A muscle contains a myofascial TP when fingertip pressure across the long axis of the muscle produces a generalized "jump sign" by the patient and a "local twitch" of the taut band. The two findings are not synonymous. (The jump sign is a general patient pain response characterized by wincing or a voluntary withdrawal response; the local twitch is a transient contraction of the taut band of fibers housing the TP.) The local twitch response is clinically significant because it is usually absent in the fibromyalgia syndrome but present in myofascial pain syndromes due to TPs (19).

Precise localization of the TP is required for accurate diagnosis, as well as in accomplishing many of the specific treatments. Depending on the muscle examined, use either flat palpation or

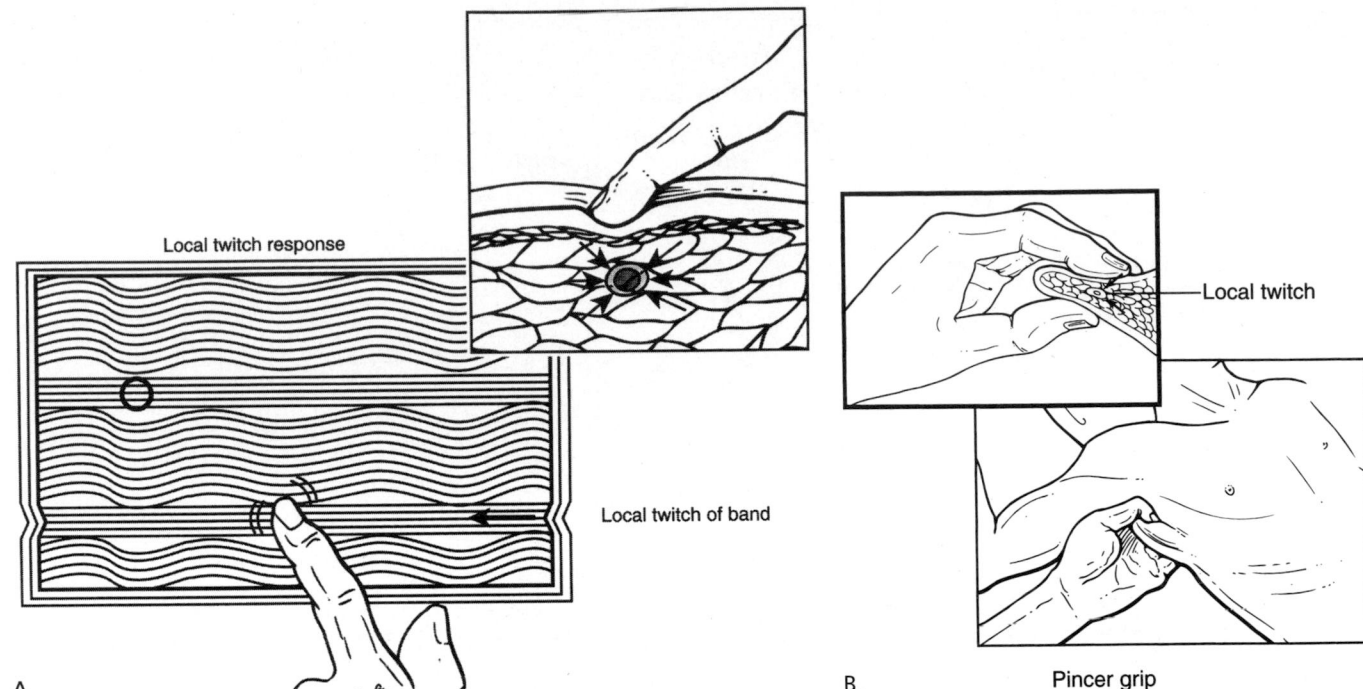

FIGURE 66.3. Palpation for myofascial trigger points. **A:** Draw fingertips across large, flat muscles, **(B)** use pincer grip for muscles like trapezius or those in axillary folds. (From Travell JG, Simons DG. *Myofascial Pain and Dysfunction: The Trigger Point Manual. Volume I. The Upper Extremities.* Baltimore, MD: Williams & Wilkins; 1983:60, 61, 398, with permission.)

palpation with a pincer type grip (Fig. 66.3). In large, flat muscles like the quadratus lumborum, fingertips can be drawn across the muscle perpendicular to its fibers. Some muscles, like the trapezius or those in the axillary folds, are better palpated with a pincer grip. The most appropriate palpation for a TP is that which permits pressure to be applied perpendicular to the long axis of the muscle suspected of harboring the point.

Joints controlled by muscles with myofascial TPs may show restricted ranges of motion in the direction of stretch, and the muscles are painful with either active or passive stretching. Patchy weakness during muscle testing may result from a conscious or unconscious desire to avoid pain. If present, attention to the precise pain patterns is extremely important in the diagnosis, because the empirically mapped patterns for each given muscle are fairly consistent among patients (Fig. 66.1). Histories of activities leading to the onset of pain and dysfunction or detailed descriptions of the muscular activities no longer comfortable for the patient are often sufficient to identify specific muscles that need to be examined for TPs.

Interrater reliability tests demonstrate the need for all examiners to be trained and experienced to perform reproducible examinations (2). Experienced examiners who were pretrained to conduct and interpret findings similarly were able to generate good to excellent kappa values (33). Although no one diagnostic examination is considered a satisfactory criterion for diagnosing a TP, the combination of local spot tenderness and the finding of a palpable, taut band are essential elements in defining an active or latent TP. Current recommended diagnostic criteria are summarized in Table 66.1.

Laboratory, imaging, and neuroelectrodiagnostic tests are not diagnostic for primary myofascial TPs or for most other forms of somatic dysfunction. They may prove useful, however, in identifying factors that perpetuate trigger points or in ruling out a variety of clinical conditions from which secondary myofascial TPs may arise. For example, in the presence of nerve compression sufficient to create peripheral electromyographic changes, an increased number of active TPs will be found in the affected muscles (34).

TREATMENT

Myofascial TPs have been treated in several ways, ranging from needles to manual techniques to medication. Treatment is directed toward inactivation of the trigger points in the involved muscles and toward identification and resolution of contributing and perpetuating factors. Lasting success depends on:

Correction of associated somatic dysfunction
Patient education to prevent recurrences
Appropriate self-stretch exercise programs
Correction of underlying perpetuating and facilitating factors

Specific treatment of myofascial TPs can be accomplished with (2):

Inhibition soft tissue technique
Vapocoolant spray or other intermittent cooling with stretch
Deep massage

TABLE 66.1. CRITERIA AND COMPARATIVE RELIABILITY FOR TRIGGER POINT DIAGNOSIS

A. Recommended criteria for identifying a latent trigger point or an active trigger point

Essential criteria
1. Taut band palpable (if muscle accessible).
2. Exquisite spot tenderness of a nodule in a taut band.
3. Patient's recognition of current pain complaint by pressure on the tender nodule (identifies an active trigger point).
4. Painful limit to full stretch range of motion.

Confirmatory observations
1. Visual or tactile identification of local twitch response.
2. Imaging of a local twitch response induced by needle penetration of tender nodule.
3. Pain or altered sensation (in the distribution expected from a trigger point in that muscle) on compression of tender nodule.
4. Electromyographic demonstration of spontaneous electrical activity characteristic of active loci in the tender nodule of a taut band.

B. Comparative reliability of diagnostic examinations for trigger points, estimate of the relative difficulty performing the examinations, and estimated relative diagnostic value of each examination by itself, regardless of other findings

Presence of	No. of studies	Mean kappa	Difficulty	Diagnostic value alone
Spot tenderness	3	0.70	+	+[a]
Pain recognition	3	0.59	++	+++
Palpable band	3	0.54	+++	++[a]
Referred pain	4	0.47	+++	+
Twitch response	3	0.23	++++	++++

[a] The combined presence of these two will likely have a high diagnostic value for sufficiently skilled examiners.
From Simons DG, Travell JG, Simons LS. *Travell and Simons Myofascial Pain and Dysfunction: The Trigger Point Manual*, vol. I. Upper Half of Body, 2nd ed. Baltimore, MD: Williams and Wilkins, 1999, with permission.

Injection
Jones counterstrain
Isometric muscle energy techniques
Myofascial release
Other osteopathic manipulative treatment (8,35)

Other adjunct neuromusculoskeletal therapies may be added as needed.

Successful TP treatment addresses the central nervous system's response to nociceptive information or modifies peripheral input. These techniques may be ineffective if the patient is unable to relax and involuntary tensing takes place. If the operator releases the pressure too soon or too quickly, or if perpetuating factors are not addressed, reoccurrence or incomplete resolution of the TPs may result.

Neuroplastic structural and functional changes in the central nervous system arise from prolonged nociceptive input, and may not be reversible with time alone (36,37). Thus, much suffering from chronic pain is preventable if nociception is controlled promptly and effectively (1). The earlier the treatment of somatic dysfunction (myofascial and articular), the less likely the patient is to develop central processing dysfunctional patterns, and the more likely it is to have a favorable outcome. Outcomes and number of treatments required were directly related, for example, to

the time between injury and onset of treatment in patients with pectoralis minor TPs from whiplash injuries (38). In this study, the longer it took to start treatment, the more treatments that were required and the less likely that complete symptom relief could be achieved.

Cooling with Stretching

Intermittent cooling with a vapocoolant spray followed by myofascial stretch (spray with stretch) is reported to be the "single most effective noninvasive method" to inactivate acute TPs (2). Stroking with plastic-covered ice followed by passive stretching is also effective, however. These techniques are believed to act through Wall and Melzack's (1) gate theory (Fig. 66.4). The cooling activates Kraus receptors, which report centrally through fast fibers. The afferent volley of neural impulses conveyed through these fast fibers reflexively block the TP nociceptive impulses conveyed by slow fibers at the substantia gelatinosa. Blocking this neurologic reflex allows the operator to restore the muscle containing the TP to its normal resting length with full range of motion without producing pain or reflex muscle contraction. The common adage is "spray is the distraction, stretch is the action" (2).

Vapocoolant spray is best applied to the skin at an angle of 30 degrees at a rate of approximately 4 inches per second. Adjusting the distance for different coolant products permits the physician to stimulate cold receptors in the skin without chilling the underlying muscle. For example, apply Fluori-Methane from a distance of 18 inches, but the "colder" ethyl chloride spray (or Gebaur Pharmaceutical's vapocoolant spray) at a distance of 12 inches. Apply cooling in unidirectional parallel sweeps over the entire length of the muscle in the direction of its fibers, passing over the TP. Gently stretch the muscle by "taking up the slack" rather than forcibly stretching it.

Subsequent passes of the spray should include similar application continuing over the TP's reference zone. Again, follow this by a gentle stretch of the muscle. Care should be taken to activate the cold receptors of the skin while carefully avoiding chilling the muscle. Chilling of the underlying muscle will often activate a TP and prevent the effective muscle stretch needed to eliminate that TP. After intermittent cooling with stretch, warm the area with moist heat and take the muscle through its full active range of motion.

Injection

Injection is sometimes necessary to inactivate a TP (2). Although dry needling of the TP has been reported to be successful by some operators, most inject procaine. Some mix the procaine with a steroid preparation. Aspirate before injecting. The needle should be placed directly into the TP (Fig. 66.5) for the greatest effect. This will often be intensely uncomfortable and reduplicate the patient's pain pattern, so warn the patient of this. Successful penetration of the TP will create a local twitch response that correlates highly with a successful injection. Injection of a TP may fail if:

Primary or secondary trigger points are missed by the needle
The injected solution causes irritation of the tissues

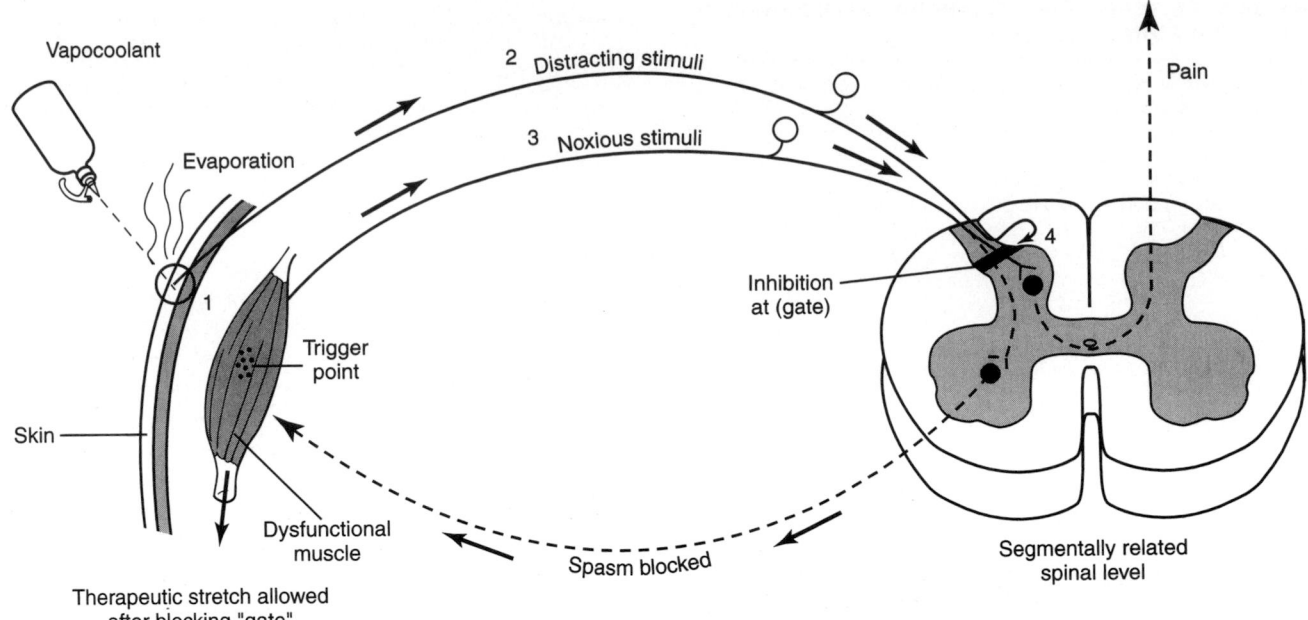

FIGURE 66.4. Spray-with-stretch technique. Cooling **(1)** must occur at rate that significantly activates Kraus (cold) receptors in skin but avoids chilling underlying muscle. Cold is conveyed centrally by fast afferents **(2)** that block noxious afferent information **(3)** from dysfunctional muscle at the substantia gelatinosa **(4)** or gate. (From Travell JG, Simons DG. *Myofascial Pain and Dysfunction: The Trigger Point Manual. Volume I. The Upper Extremities.* Baltimore, MD: Williams & Wilkins; 1983:72, with permission.)

Local bleeding acts as an irritant to reinitiate a trigger point
Perpetuating factors are not addressed

If injection of a TP with a radicular or peripheral nerve distribution is attempted, omit steroids to avoid accidental injection into the nerve itself.

OSTEOPATHIC APPROACH

Somatic dysfunction is present when there is "impaired or altered function of the somatic system and its related neural, lymphatic, and circulatory elements" (39). Travell and Simons' description of myofascial (TP) dysfunction also includes:

Neural entrapment
Arterial entrapment
Venous entrapment
Lymphatic entrapment
Autonomic sequelae
Viscerosomatic-somatovisceral reflex phenomena resulting from myofascial dysfunction

With such inherent overlap, TPs can easily be integrated into the diagnostic and treatment considerations of an osteopathic physician as a subset of somatic dysfunction. Professional collaboration has ensured that this insight is growing exponentially. As recently as 1991, Simons reported that the interface between (myofascial pain syndromes) and somatic dysfunction was one of the "greatest voids" in our knowledge (28). However, the following year, Basmajian ( ) remarked that second major text on myofascial pain and dysfunction opened up "new ground in sen-

sitizing clinicians to the important interfaces between myofascial pain syndromes and articular (somatic) dysfunction."

Since that time, extensive interactions have taken place with practitioners of manual medicine worldwide, embracing the contributions of Simons and Travell. The new, second edition of *Travell & Simons' Myofascial Pain and Dysfunction: The Trigger Point Manual* (2), includes chapters with extensive correlation between articular somatic dysfunction and TPs, especially in chapters detailing the posterior cervical and suboccipital muscles. It also extensively discusses the use of several manual medicine techniques to effectively treat TPs. Lewitt (40), a neurologist in the Czech Republic, has also described the close relationship between articular somatic dysfunction and myofascial trigger points. The increased tension of the TP and facilitation of motor activity can maintain articular stress while abnormal sensory input from articular dysfunction can reflexively activate TP dysfunction. For this reason, he emphasizes the importance of treating both the muscular and articular components of somatic dysfunction when both are present (40).

Trigger Points Affecting Regional Somatic Functions

TPs typically result in weakness and/or dysfunction of the muscle harboring them (2). Overuse in the myotatic unit because of this primary myofascial point may cause secondary associated myofascial points, resulting in further weakness and reduced function. If the point is latent (2), it may be clinically silent unless it is palpated directly or the muscle harboring it is functionally stressed. If the point is active (2), it weakens and prevents full lengthening of the muscle. It may produce referred

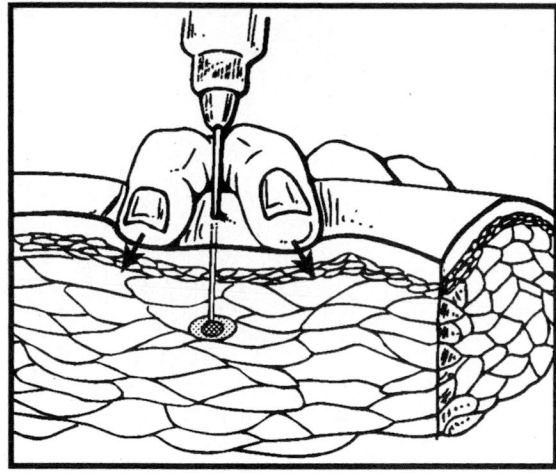

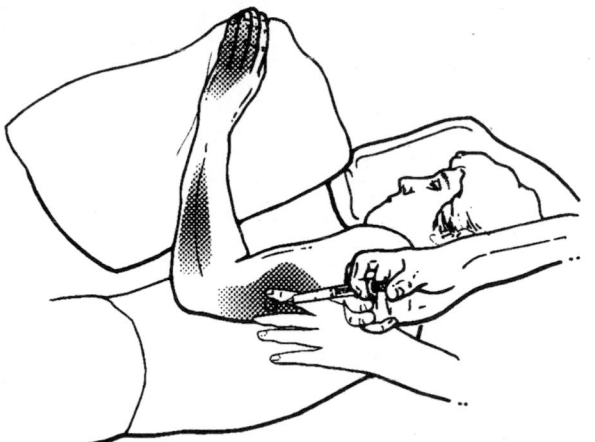

FIGURE 66.5. Triceps TP3 and injection-precipitated pain pattern. (From Travell JG, Simons DG. *Myofascial Pain and Dysfunction: The Trigger Point Manual. Volume I. The Upper Extremities.* Baltimore, MD: Williams & Wilkins; 1983:83, 473, with permission.)

TABLE 66.2. LIMITATIONS OF SHOULDER RANGE OF MOTION (ROM)

Motion restricted[a]	Myofascial point found
Flexion	Triceps
Abduction	Subscapularis
	Infraspinatus
	Supraspinatus
	Teres major (levator scapulae)
Internal rotation	Teres minor
	Infraspinatus
External rotation	Subscapularis
	Pectoralis minor

[a]Stage of Spencer that is restricted. Note: The majority of muscles are rotator cuff muscles.

pain and/or autonomic phenomena in a predictable trigger or reference zone. These zones are characteristic for each muscle and have been empirically mapped and documented (Fig. 66.1) (2,8,19,31).

Altered somatic function that has been noted includes (2,19):

Disturbed proprioceptor and motor coordination (2)
Temporomandibular joint dysfunction (2)
Depressed deep tendon reflexes (19)
Muscular stiffness and weakness (2)
Diminished ranges of motion (2)

The patient often complains of these symptoms, as well as dysesthesia, paresthesia, and pain. The pain is described as steady, deep, and achy in nature. Symptoms are often aggravated by:

Use of the muscle
Chilling
Psychogenic stress
Viral infection
Prolonged shortening of the muscle
Pressure over the trigger point

Chronic pain may lead to secondary depression, sleep disturbance, and chronic pain behavior (2).

Diminished range of motion caused by myofascial TPs should be differentiated from structural limitations of the joints, such as occur in osteoarthritis, and functional arthrodial limitations, such as occur in other forms of somatic dysfunction. In particular, Travell myofascial points should be distinguished from fibromyalgia syndrome (2,11) and other rheumatologic disorders (41). Appropriate recognition and treatment of TPs have provided dramatic restoration of function in numerous patients previously misdiagnosed with these other conditions.

Similarly, as a component element of somatic dysfunction, myofascial TPs must sometimes be specifically addressed to allow complete resolution of the joint dysfunction (2,40). Clinically, this is often the case in recurrent exhalation somatic dysfunction of rib 12 related to quadratus lumborum TPs. The presence of trigger points must be considered when the usual treatment for shoulder dysfunction fails to respond fully to manipulative techniques, such as the seven stages of Spencer (see Chapter 47). Table 66.2 delineates the trigger points associated with Spencer technique.

Many clinical diagnoses have associated myofascial trigger points in which the dysfunctional trigger zone overlaps with the structural symptoms profile. Although a cause-and-effect relationship has not been demonstrated, treatment of those myofascial elements contributes significantly to patient management and symptom reduction. This point is very well illustrated by two common clinical diagnoses: lateral epicondylitis and carpal tunnel syndrome.

In lateral epicondylitis, or tennis elbow syndrome, TPs in the supinator, wrist, and finger extensor muscles, anconeus, and triceps are all capable of referring symptoms to the lateral epicondyle (2). Conversely, all become significantly stressed with the altered biomechanics adopted in a true inflammatory process of the lateral epicondyle.

In carpal tunnel syndrome (CTS), TPs are found in the pronator teres, and wrist, finger, and thumb flexors (42). Here also, triggered referral zones from the myofascial points overlap with the wrist pain, finger and thumb paresthesias, grip weakness, and referred forearm pain perception common to patients with CTS. Forearm muscles also become significantly stressed with the altered extremity mechanics adopted by patients with CTS.

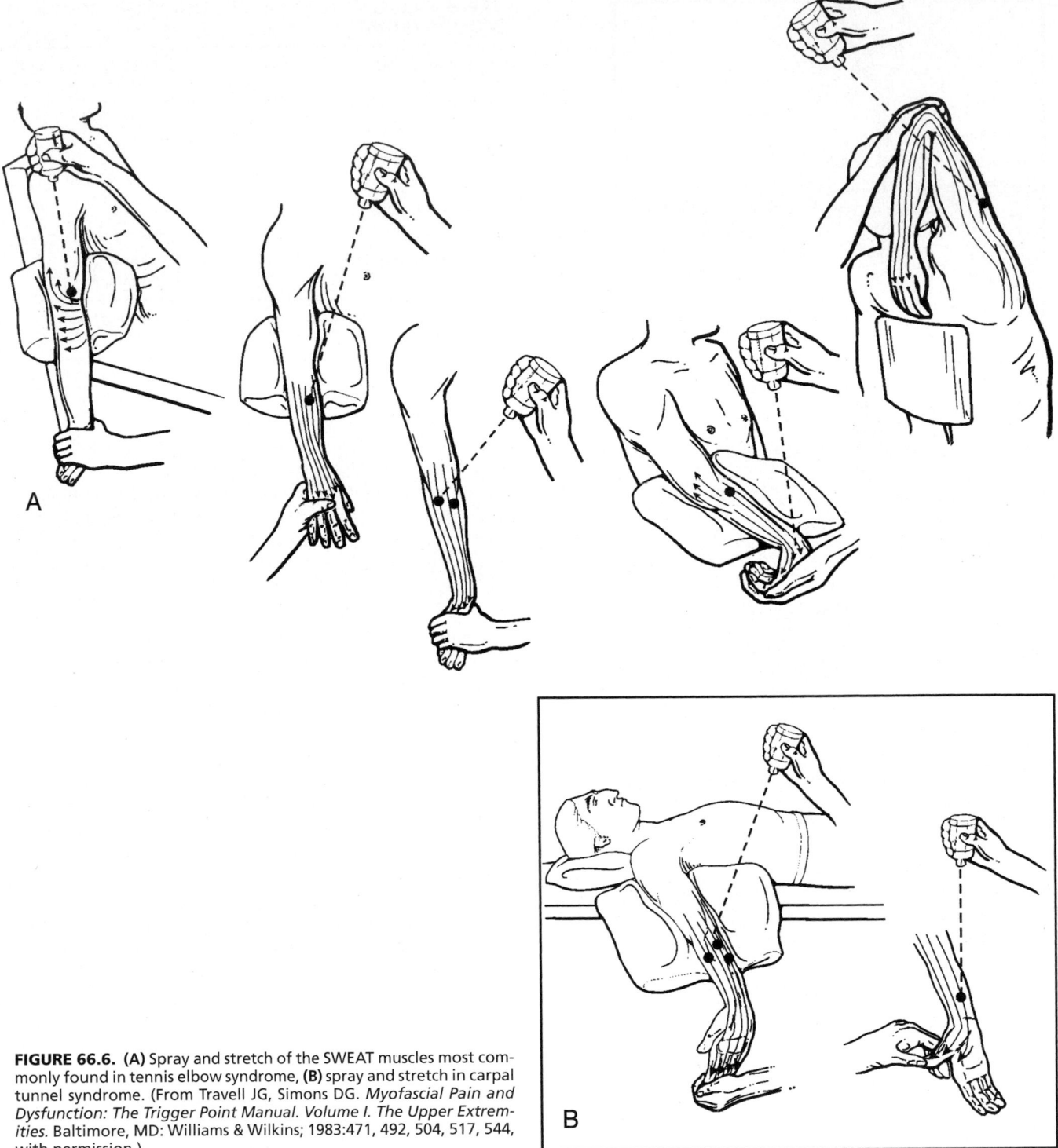

FIGURE 66.6. (A) Spray and stretch of the SWEAT muscles most commonly found in tennis elbow syndrome, **(B)** spray and stretch in carpal tunnel syndrome. (From Travell JG, Simons DG. *Myofascial Pain and Dysfunction: The Trigger Point Manual. Volume I. The Upper Extremities.* Baltimore, MD: Williams & Wilkins; 1983:471, 492, 504, 517, 544, with permission.)

Failure to address TPs results in failure to help a significant number of these patients. For example, in CTS, osteopathic treatment protocols that specifically address treatment of these myofascial structures in addition to traditional conservative care have been more effective than wrist splints and medication alone (43). The stretch component addressing each of these conditions is pictured in Figure 66.6. Note in Figure 66.6A that the same general position is modified to localize the supinator, wrist, and finger extensors, in turn, with a separate position for the anconeus and triceps. In Figure 66.6B, general positioning with slight localization modifications during the stretch component effectively, and in a time-efficient manner, addresses the ventral forearm muscles most commonly involved in patients with CTS or its symptoms.

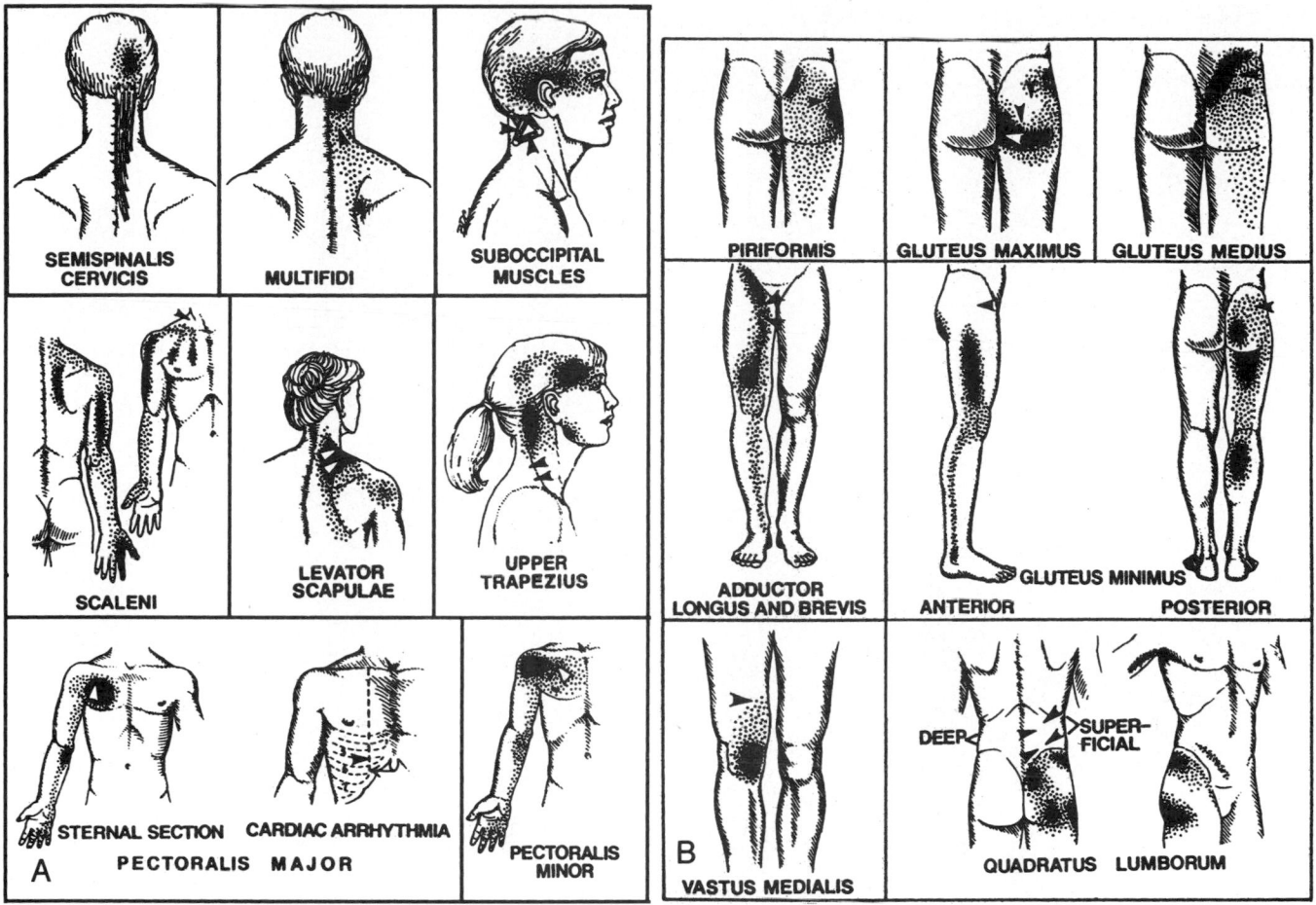

FIGURE 66.7. Trigger points commonly precipitated by poor posture. Referred pain patterns *(black stippled area)*, location of trigger points *(arrows)*. (From Wall PD, Melzack R, eds. *Textbook of Pain*, 2nd ed. Edinburgh, Scotland: Churchill Livingstone; 1989:371, 372, 376, 377, with permission.)

Trigger Points and Posture

TPs may result from and/or contribute to postural disorders (1,22,23,44). Patterns of recurrent TPs in various combinations should alert the clinician to an underlying postural disorder. Likewise, all patients with postural disorders should be evaluated for patterns of TPs to address in the postural treatment regimen.

Patients with postural decompensation have a higher propensity to develop patterns of recurrent somatic dysfunction, TPs, facilitated segments, and related visceral dysfunction (45). (See Chapter 43 and Figure 66.7, depicting muscles most commonly contributing to postural patterns.) For this reason, numerous clinicians (1,2,44,46,51,52) cite postural disorders as one of the primary precipitating and/or perpetuating factors of myofascial TPs, even stating that "postural training should be one of the first parts, if not the first part, of the treatment program" (8).

The so-called "short leg syndrome" (see Chapter 43) has been implicated in causing multiple TPs, including those in the paraspinal (19), sternocleidomastoid (19), and quadratus lumborum (8) muscles. Quadratus lumborum TPs have already been implicated as an extremely common primary cause of myogenic low back pain (21). Conversely, TPs in this muscle are capable of producing a false short leg syndrome caused by muscular at-

tachments to the iliac crest (8). This situation is likely to result in compensatory postural charges, recurrent somatic dysfunction, and TPs in local and distant areas. It also may lead to lift therapy being incorrectly or inappropriately instituted.

Impairment of Venous and Lymphatic Drainage

Optimal venous and lymphatic drainage depends on unobstructed myofascial pathways through which these circulatory vessels pass, and on respiratory-circulatory mechanisms efficiently creating pressure differentials. Zink (47,48) stated the relevance of this perspective to the osteopathic clinician. Travell and Simons have also documented the effect of certain myofascial points in creating lymphatic dysfunction and have reported improvement of congestive sequelae by removing this type of somatic dysfunction. The osteopathic profession and Travell (2) emphasize the importance of proper and effective respiration and attention to the somatic factors involved.

The scalene muscles are often referred to as the entrappers (19) because of their clinical tendency to entrap structures passing through the superior thoracic aperture (thoracic inlet). The

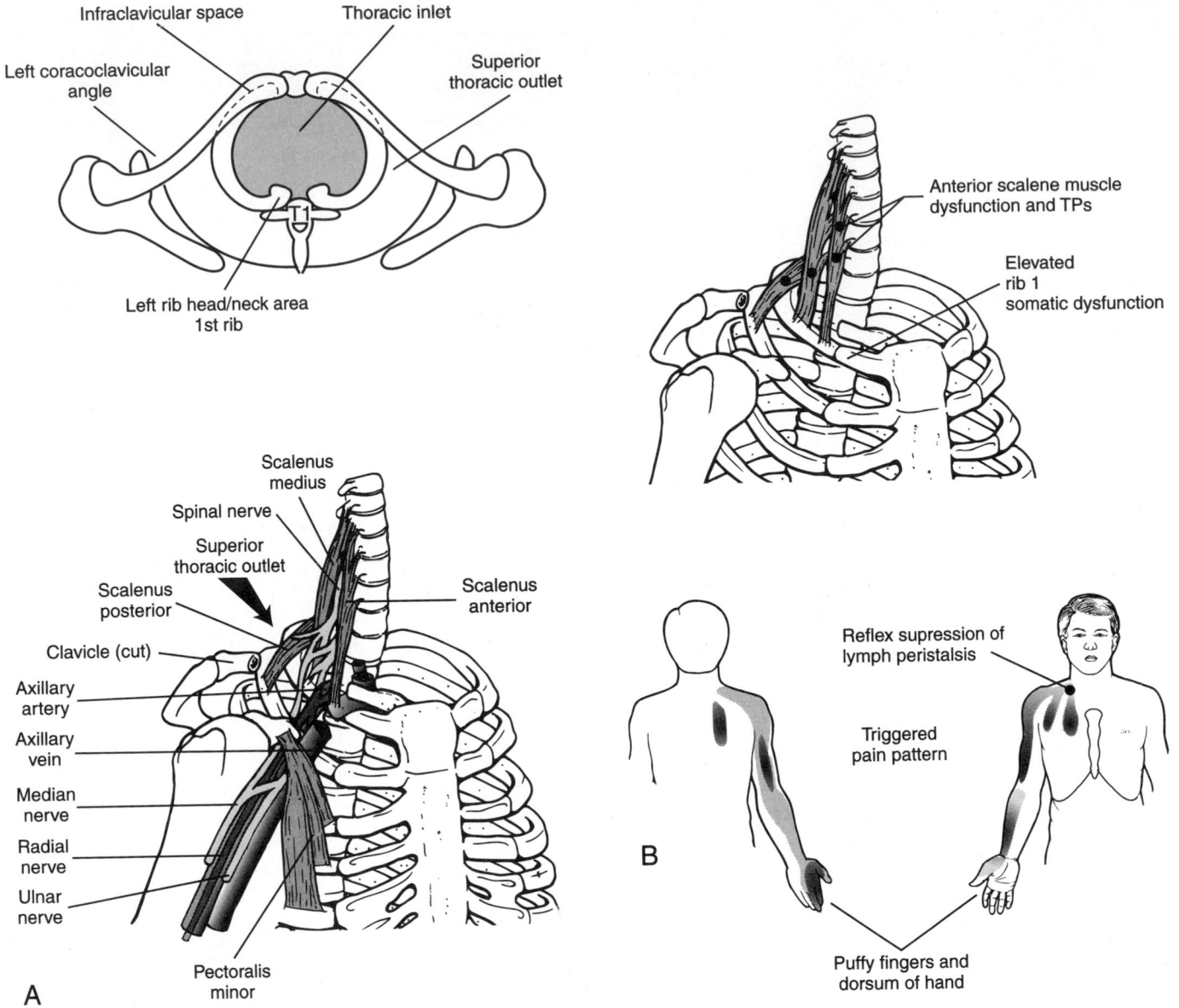

FIGURE 66.8. A: Entrapment of vascular and lymphatic structures in the thoracic inlet, **(B)** anterior scalene muscle referred pain and lymphatic/venous congestion in affected extremity. (From Travell JG, Simons DG. *Myofascial Pain and Dysfunction: The Trigger Point Manual. Volume I. The Upper Extremities.* Baltimore, MD: Williams & Wilkins; 1983:345, 356, with permission; **A:** top illustration by W. A. Kuchera.)

subclavian lymphatic trunk and the subclavian vein are particularly susceptible to muscular compression caused by TPs in the anterior scalene muscles (Fig. 66.8). This compression is further aggravated by elevation of the first rib, which may result from a variety of dysfunctional phenomena, including TPs in the anterior or middle scalene muscles. Somatic dysfunction of the first rib and other parts of the functional superior thoracic inlet should also be treated because of their effect on this region (2). Scalene TP activity has been implicated in reflex suppression of lymphatic duct peristaltic contractions in the affected extremity (19).

Palpation of the posterior and anterior axillary folds for evidence of myofascial dysfunction is clinically important in assessing the degree of lymphatic dysfunction affecting the upper extremities and/or breasts. The posterior axillary fold is the location of palpable myofascial points in the subscapularis, teres major, and latissimus dorsi muscles. It is also the site of terminal lymphatic drainage dysfunction for the upper extremities (Fig. 66.9). Zink (49) discusses diagnosis and treatment of this region to relieve lymphatic congestion in the upper extremity. Those findings closely parallel the palpatory and clinical findings described independently by Travell and Simons, using myofascial points located in the posterior axillary fold (2). Figure 66.9B shows that points higher in the posterior axillary fold correlate predominantly with shoulder referral, although lower points refer distally. Zink and Travell () both report that treatment of myofascial dysfunction in this area results in reduction of swelling, joint dysfunction, and dysesthesia (Fig. 66.10). Likewise, appropriate treatment of anterior axillary fold dysfunction results in

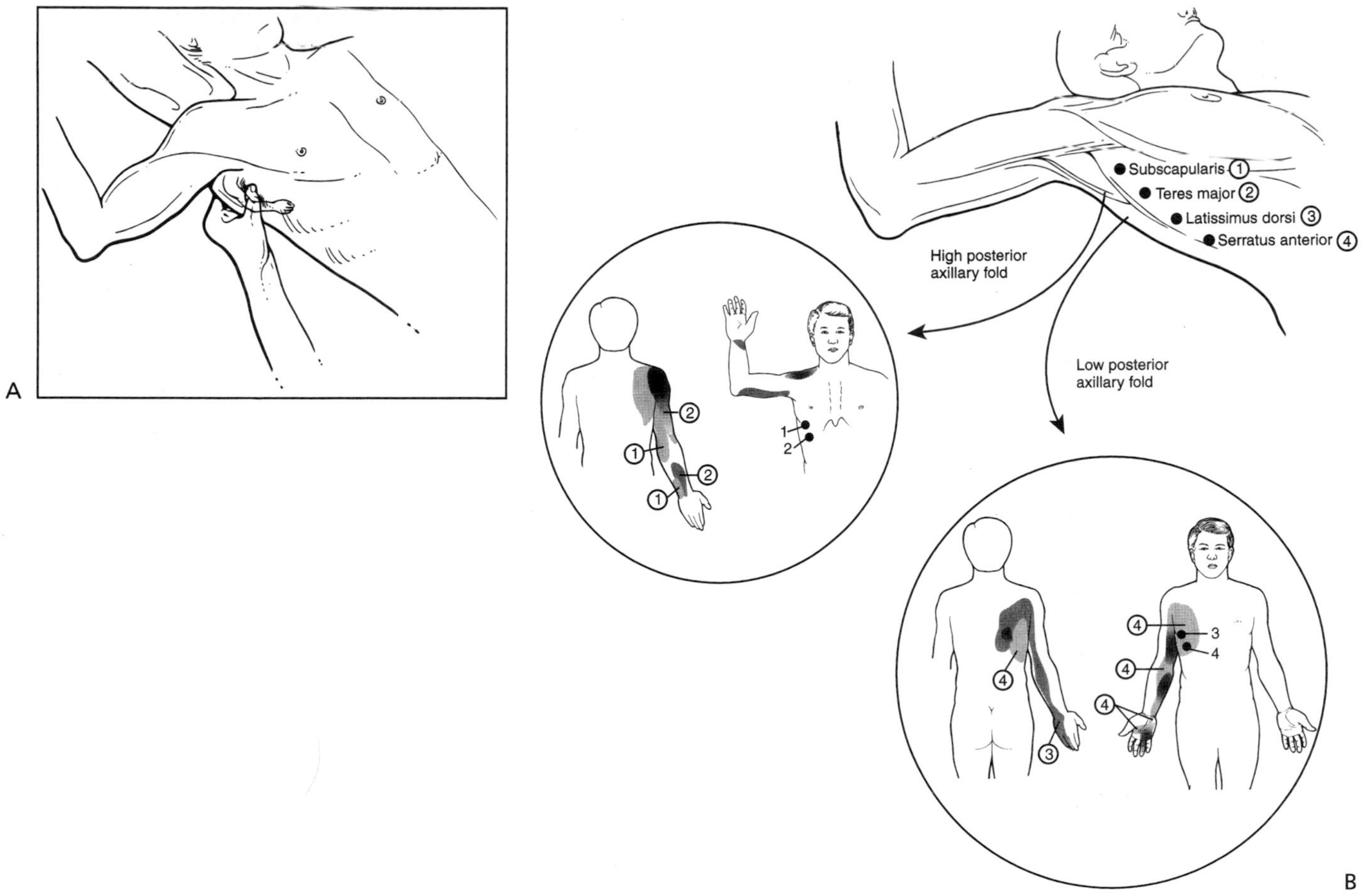

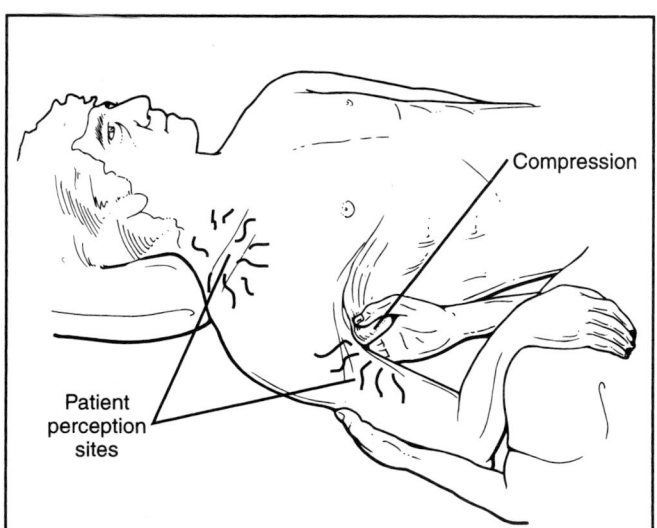

FIGURE 66.9. **A:** Zink's posterior axillary fold technique, **(B)** location and overlapping patterns of Travell and Simons' trigger points located in the posterior axillary fold. *(1),* subscapularis; *(2),* teres major; *(3),* latissimus dorsi; *(4),* serratus anterior. Overlapping patterns between *(1)* and *(2)* and between *(3)* and *(4)* are shown in black. (Grom Travell JG, Simons DG. *Myofascial Pain and Dysfunction: The Trigger Point Manual. Volume I. The Upper Extremities.* Baltimore, MD: Williams & Wilkins; 1983:398, with permission.)

FIGURE 66.10. Compression of the posterior axillary fold at the palpatory site of each thickened tender point. (From Travell JG, Simons DG. *Myofascial Pain and Dysfunction: The Trigger Point Manual. Volume I. The Upper Extremities.* Baltimore, MD: Williams & Wilkins; 1983:418, with permission.)

reduction of breast tenderness and congestive changes attributed to entrapment of breast lymphatics traveling around and through the pectoralis muscle toward the subclavicular lymph nodes (19).

Autonomic Effects of Travell Myofascial Points

Clinically, autonomic effects of myofascial dysfunction are common (2,11). Travell's term "referred autonomic phenomena" (2) refers to the vasoconstriction (blanching), coldness, sweating, pilomotor response, ptosis, and/or hypersecretion that is caused by activity of a trigger point in a region separate from the trigger point. The phenomena usually appear in the same area as the pain referral for that TP (19).

Travell and Simons (19) and Korr (30) have postulated an organizing role for the spinal cord by relating somatic and visceral input to palpatory and symptomatic findings in both systems (Fig. 66.11). Afferent input to the spinal cord may facilitate the segment at the spinal level it enters. Efferent consequences include sympathetic changes to somatic and visceral tissues at the same spinal level, and palpable somatic dysfunction, including tissue texture changes. A series of reflexes and referred symptoms result.

of students of osteopathic medicine. In the end, all of our patients benefit.

REFERENCES

1. Mense S, Simons DG. *Muscle Pain: Understanding its Nature, Diagnosis, and Treatment.* Philadelphia, PA: Lippincott Williams & Wilkins; 2001.
2. Simons DG, Travell JG, Simons LS. *Travell and Simons' Myofascial Pain and Dysfunction: The Trigger Point Manual. Volume I: Upper Half of Body,* 2nd ed. Baltimore MD: Williams & Wilkins; 1999.
3. Hubbard DR, Berkoff GM. Myofascial trigger points show spontaneous needle EMG activity. *Spine.* 1993;18(13):1803–1807.
4. Head H. On disturbance of sensation with especial reference to the pain of visceral disease. *Brain.* 1893;16:1–133.
5. Mackenzie J. Some points bearing on the association of sensory disorders and visceral disease. *Brain.* 1893;16:321–354.
6. Owens C. *An Endocrine Interpretation of Chapman's Reflexes,* 2nd ed. Chattanooga, TN: Chattanooga Printing & Engraving Co; 1937.
7. Travell J, Rinzler SH. The myofascial genesis of pain. *Postgrad Med.* 1952;11:425–434.
8. Travell JG, Simons DG. *Myofascial Pain and Dysfunction: The Trigger Point Manual. Volume II. The Lower Extremities.* Baltimore, MD: Williams & Wilkins; 1992:547.
9. Simons DG. Muscle pain syndromes. *J Man Med.* 1991;6:3–23.
10. Chairow L. *Soft Tissue Manipulation.* Ellington, Great Britain: Thorston Publishing; 1987.
11. Bennett RM. Myofascial pain syndrome and the fibromyalgia syndrome: a comparative analysis. *J Man Med.* 1991;6:34–45.
12. Melzack R, Stillwell DM, Fox EJ. Trigger points and acupuncture points for pain: Correlations and implications. *Pain.* 1977;3:3–23.
13. Skootsky SA, Jaeger B, Oye RK. Prevalence of myofascial pain in general internal medicine practice. *West J Med.* 1989;151:157–160.
14. Fricton JR, Kroening R, Haley D, et al. Myofascial pain syndrome of the head and neck: A review of clinical characteristics of 164 patients. *Oral Surg Oral Med Oral Pathol Oral Radiol Endod.* 1985;6:615–623.
15. Fishbain DA, Goldberg M, Meahger BR, et al. Male and female chronic pain patients categorized by DSM-III psychiatric diagnostic criteria. *Pain.* 1986;26:181–197.
16. Wolfe F, Ross K, Anderson J, et al. The prevalence and characteristics of fibromyalgia in the general population. *Arthritis Rheum.* 1995;38:19–28.
17. Campbell SM, Clark S, Tindall EA, et al. Clinical characteristics of fibrositis. I. A "blinded" controlled study of symptoms and tender points. *Arthritis Rheum.* 1983;26:817–824.
18. Gerwin RD. A study of 96 subjects examined both for fibromyalgia and myofascial pain. *J Musculoske Pain.* 1995;3(Suppl 1):121(abst).
19. Travell JG, Simons DG. *Myofascial Pain and Dysfunction: The Trigger Point Manual. Volume I. The Upper Extremities.* Baltimore, MD: Williams & Wilkins; 1983.
20. Skootsky SA, Jaeger B, Oye RK. Prevalence of myofascial pain in general internal medicine practice. *West J Med.* 1989;151:157–160.
21. Simons DG, Travell JG. Low back pain, Part 2: torso muscles. *Post Grad Med.* 1983;73(2):81–92.
22. Kuchera ML. Gravitational stress, musculoligamentous strain and postural alignment. *Spine State Art Rev.* 1995;9(2):463–490.
23. Kuchera ML. Gravitational strain pathophysiology, Parts I and II. In: Vleeming A, ed. *Low Back Pain: The Integrated Function of the Lumbar Spine and Sacroiliac Joints.* Proceedings of the 2nd Interdisciplinary World Congress, November 1995.
24. McNulty WH, Gevirtz RN, Hubbard DR, et al. Needle electromyographic evaluation of trigger point response to a psychological stressor. *Psychophysiology.* 1994;31:313–316.
25. Kuchera ML, Kuchera WA. *Osteopathic Considerations in Systemic Dysfunction,* 2nd ed. rev. Columbus, OH: Greyden Press; 1994:200–201.
26. Kuchera ML, Kuchera WA. *Osteopathic Considerations in Systemic Dysfunction,* 2nd ed. rev. Columbus, OH: Greyden Press; 1994:79–84.
27. Jones LH. Missed anterior spinal lesions. A preliminary report. *The DO.* 1964;4:109–116.
28. Simons DG. Muscle pain syndromes. *J Man Med.* 1991;6:3–23.
29. vanBuskirk RL. Nociceptive reflexes and the somatic dysfunction: a model. *J Am Osteopath Assoc.* 1990;90(9):792–809.
30. Korr IM. The spinal cord as organizer of disease processes. In: Peterson B, ed. *The Collected Papers of Irvin M. Korr.* Newark, OH: American Academy of Osteopathy; 1979:207–221.
31. Simons DG. *Myofascial Pain Syndrome Due to Trigger Points.* (International Rehabilitation Medicine Association Monograph Series Number 1). Cleveland, OH: Rademaker Printing; 1987.
32. Gilliar WG, Kuchera ML, Giulianetti DA. Neurologic basis of manual medicine. *Phys Med Rehabil Clin N Am.* 1996;7(4):693–714.
33. Gerwin RD, Shannon S, Hong C-Z, et al. Interrater reliability in myofascial trigger point examination. *Pain.* 1997;69:65–73.
34. Wu C-M, Chen H-H, Hong C-Z. Inactivation of myofascial trigger points associated with lumbar radiculopathy: surgery versus physical therapy. *Arch Phys Med Rehabil.* 1997;78:1040–1041.
35. Greenman PE. *Principles of Manual Medicine.* Baltimore, MD: Williams & Wilkins; 1989:106–122.
36. Yaksh TL, Abram SE. Focus article: preemptive analgesia: a popular misnomer, but a clinically relevant truth? *Am Pain Soc J.* 1993;2:116–121.
37. Patterson MM, Steinmetz JE. Long-lasting alterations of spinal reflexes: a basis for somatic dysfunction. *Man Med.* 1986;2:38–42.
38. Hong C-Z, Simons DG. Response to treatment for pectoralis minor myofascial pain syndrome after whiplash. *J Musculoske Pain.* 1993;1(1):89–131.
39. The Glossary Review Committee of the Educational Council on Osteopathic Principles. In: Allen TW, ed. *Glossary of Osteopathic Terminology.* AOA Yearbook and Directory of Osteopathic Physicians. Chicago, IL: American Osteopathic Association; 1991:678–690.
40. Lewit K. *Manipulative Therapy in Rehabilitation of the Locomotor System,* 2nd ed. Oxford, UK: Butterworth-Heinemann; 1991.
41. Wolfe F, Smythe HA, Yunus MB, et al. American College of Rheumatology 1990 criteria for the classification of fibromyalgia: Report of the Multicenter Criteria Committee. *Arthritis Rheum.* 1990;33:160–172.
42. Melchior DE, et al. A study of the components of somatic dysfunction in relationship to the carpal tunnel syndrome. Residency paper accepted by the Osteopathic Manipulative Medicine Department, Kirksville College of Medicine, Kirksville MO, 1990.
43. Strait B, Kuchera ML. Osteopathic manipulation for patients with confirmed mild, modest, and moderate carpal tunnel syndrome. *J Am Osteopath Assoc.* 1994;94(8):673.
44. Janda V. Muscles, central nervous motor regulation, and back problems. In: Korr IM, ed. *The Neurobiologic Mechanisms in Manipulative Therapy.* New York, NY: Plenum Publishing; 1978:27–41.
45. Korr IM, Wright HM, Chace JA. Cutaneous patterns of sympathetic activity in clinical abnormalities of the musculoskeletal system (1964). In: Peterson B, ed. *The Collected Papers of I. M. Korr.* Newark, OH: American Academy of Osteopathy; 1979:66–72.
46. Jungmann M. *Backaches, Postural Decline, Aging and Gravity Strain.* Lewiston, ME: Penmor Lithographers; 1988.
47. Zink JG. Respiratory and circulatory care: the conceptual model. *Osteopath Ann.* 1977;5(3):108–112.
48. Zink JG, Lawson WB. An osteopathic structural examination and functional interpretation of the soma. *Osteopath Ann.* 1979;7(12):433–440.
49. Zink JG, Fetchik WD, Lawson WB. The posterior axillary folds: a gateway for osteopathic treatment of the upper extremities. *Osteopath Ann.* 1981;9(3):81–88.
50. Kuchera ML, Kuchera WA. *Osteopathic Considerations in Systemic Dysfunction,* 2nd ed. rev. Columbus, OH: Greyden Press; 1994:87.
51. Irwin R. Reduction of lumbar scoliosis by use of heel lift to level the sacral base. *J Am Osteopath Assoc.* 1991;91(1):34, 37–44.
52. Hench PK. Myofascial pain syndromes in clinical insights into musculoskeletal problems. *Myology.* 1980;5(1):5.

CHAPMAN REFLEXES

DAVID A. PATRIQUIN

KEY CONCEPTS

- General uses of anterior and posterior Chapman reflex points, and the relationship between them
- Distinguishing characteristic of Chapman reflexes
- Importance of treating the whole person when using this reflex technique
- Importance of resolving pelvic dysfunction before treating Chapman reflexes
- Locations and uses of Chapman reflexes
- How to treat Chapman reflexes

Most physicians and basic scientists have never heard of Chapman reflexes, yet these particular viscerosomatic reflexes are an osteopathic entity dating from the 1920s. They are described as a viscerosomatic reflex mechanism that has diagnostic and therapeutic importance.

Chapman described the reflex as a gangliform contraction that blocks lymphatic drainage, causing inflammation in tissues distal to the blockage. Current thinking links this involvement of the lymphatic system with concurrent sympathetic nervous system dysfunction. Regardless of the mechanism, both somatic and visceral tissues suffer from the presence of this reflex.

Chapman did not write about his reflex system, but his brother-in-law, Charles Owens, and Chapman's wife, Ada Hinckley Chapman, published the only reference text on this subject. Their book (1) discusses using the anterior and posterior points for diagnosis and treatment and for evaluation of the outcome of treatment. Today, physicians tend to use these reflexes as a diagnostic indicator of which organ is most likely to be dysfunctional.

In current clinical practice, Chapman reflex points are used more for diagnosis than for treatment. Treatment of the somatic representations of visceral dysfunction is a part of a complete osteopathic health management plan. Many posterior Chapman reflexes are located in the paraspinal areas near the transverse processes. Those reflexes may be treated incidentally as "standard" soft tissue treatment is applied to the area. Chapman reflexes may thus be treated by design or inadvertently. Treatment of these somatic points still remains an additional procedure for enlisting the patient's body in its own recovery from dysfunction.

PALPATORY CHARACTERISTICS

On palpation, Chapman reflexes are located deep to the skin and subcutaneous areolar tissue, most often lying on the deep fascia or periosteum. For the most part, they are found paired on both the dorsal and ventral surfaces of the body. For example, an anterior point found next to the sternum at the fifth intercostal space has a corresponding posterior point between the transverse processes of T5 and T6, adjacent to the costotransverse junction. Both reflex points represent the same viscus (Fig. 67.1).

A Chapman reflex point is fixed in its anatomic location. It may have a characteristic palpatory quality that makes its identification positive. When an anterior Chapman point is gently compressed, the patient's response is one of greater pain than expected. Attempts to microscopically describe the reflex change have failed; biopsy attempts have provided no information concerning the tissue or pathology of the reflex change. Still, Chapman reflexes have good interexaminer reliability and correlate well with final hospital diagnoses (2).

Distinguishing Characteristics

What are the distinguishing characteristics of a Chapman reflex? They are nodules that are:

Small
Smooth
Firm
Discretely palpable or grouped in irregular patches
Approximately 2 to 3 mm in diameter when found alone

Sometimes they are described as feeling like small pearls of tapioca lying, partially fixed, on the deep aponeurosis or fascia. The masses are dense but not hard. One gets the impression of a circumscribed area of firm edema. They move slightly but are otherwise firmly moored in place and cannot be displaced. Occasionally, they are confluent and then thought to represent longstanding visceral reflexes of greater magnitude, or chronicity, than those palpable as a single, discrete mass.

Once a Chapman reflex point is identified and isolated by the examiner's fingertip, gentle but firm pressure usually causes a deep, disagreeable pain response in the patient. The pain is

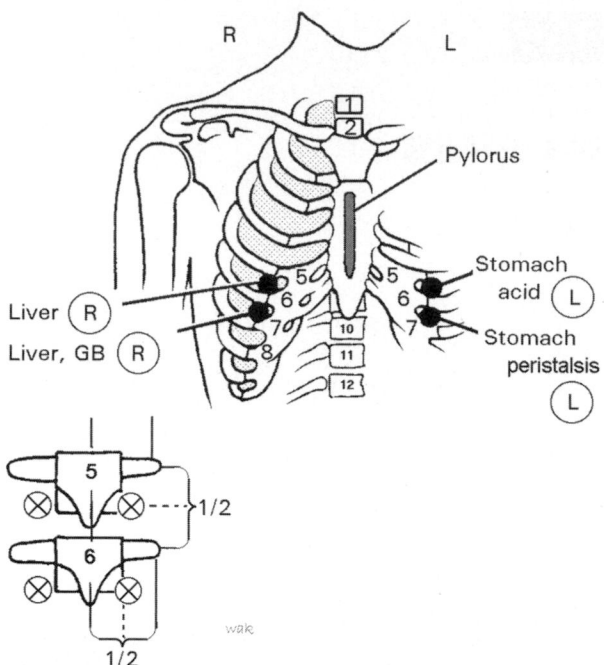

FIGURE 67.1. Often, anterior Chapman reflex points have corresponding posterior points. (From Kuchera ML, Kuchera WA. *Osteopathic Considerations in Systemic Dysfunction*, 2nd ed. rev. Columbus, OH: Greyden Press; 1994, with permission.)

characteristically:

Pinpoint
Located under the finger
Nonradiating
Sharp
Exquisitely distressing

Patients invariably wince or complain while stating that they did not know they had such a sore spot. Equivalent deep pressure on any adjacent normal tissue will produce only vague, mild, local distress.

Locating Reflexes

How are these reflexes found? Owens' personal commentary on Chapman's work suggests that the novice practitioner should refer to the book early and often. When a differential diagnostic dilemma exists, look in the book for the location of reflexes related to the items on the differential diagnostic list. Then find the reflex locations identified on the chart as relating to the organs to be considered. The subsequent identification of a reflex can help to call into question or reduce the number of diagnostic items on the list.

HISTORY AND PHILOSOPHY

This systematized method of diagnosis and treatment is an empirical system developed from the observations recorded by Chapman, an osteopathic physician who practiced in Chattanooga, Tennessee. Ada Hinckley Chapman, Charles Owens, and W. F. Link collected his notes, arranged them, and, in 1932, published the only reference text material on the subject (1). Owens notes in a later edition of the book that he only became convinced of

the efficacy of the reflex system after Chapman's death, by using it in his practice.

Osteopathic physicians who use Chapman reflexes select from the many reflex points they have frequently found to be helpful to them in their practice. They refer to Chapman charts if they wish to search for a less common point. For example, one pathologist palpated the tip of the right 12th rib to identify the typical appendix reflex. Some physicians learn the location of the Chapman reflex for the appendix during their internship. The presence of this particular reflex point for the appendix helps to direct the differential diagnosis of lower right quadrant abdominal pain in children or in women of childbearing age toward acute appendicitis more than toward acute mesenteric lymphadenitis, acute right salpingitis, ruptured right ectopic pregnancy, or chronic appendicitis. This sort of focal push-button diagnosis has great appeal to any physician faced with the dilemma of undiagnosed abdominal pain. This noninvasive examination is performed quickly and without altering the position of the patient.

The whole-person approach is critical in the application of Chapman's system just as it is the basic principle of all osteopathic treatment. Chapman's description of the pelvic-thyroid-adrenal syndrome (PTAS) confirmed his dedication to the concept of the interconnectedness and interrelatedness of all parts of the body. It also suggests a connectedness via the autonomic nervous system. He insisted that treatment of reflex points should not begin until the pelvis is made to function properly. This requires an accurate diagnosis of pelvic function or dysfunction with proper and successful pelvic treatment before these local reflexes are dealt with. Chapman emphasized the important relatedness of the endocrine components, the thyroid and adrenals, by including them in his acronym for treatment of neuroendocrine dysfunction. A physician using Chapman reflex treatments finds that a much enhanced response follows a complete Chapman reflex treatment, especially when all pelvic dysfunction is successfully resolved as the initiating step of the treatment protocol (see Chapter 52, Pelvis and Sacrum).

CURRENT CLINICAL USE

Today, Chapman reflexes are more likely to be used as an integral part of an osteopathic physical examination than as a specific therapeutic intervention. They are more likely to contribute to the differential diagnosis and implicate dysfunction of an organ system rather than be the basis of a specific pathophysiologic diagnosis. They are more likely to be used selectively than as a complete systematized diagnostic process.

Specific Reflexes to Seek and Treat

What specific reflexes might be sought and treated frequently or advantageously in practice? The reflex for appendicitis can be valuable in the differential diagnosis of lower abdominal pain. We need all the help we can find when we are faced with the lower right quadrant dilemma. The presence of Chapman reflex for appendicular involvement can help in differential diagnosis of this vexing complaint.

The presence of colon reflexes aids in the clinical identification of chronic constipation or irritable bowel syndrome (IBS). Such reflexes are easily identified by palpatory examination along the

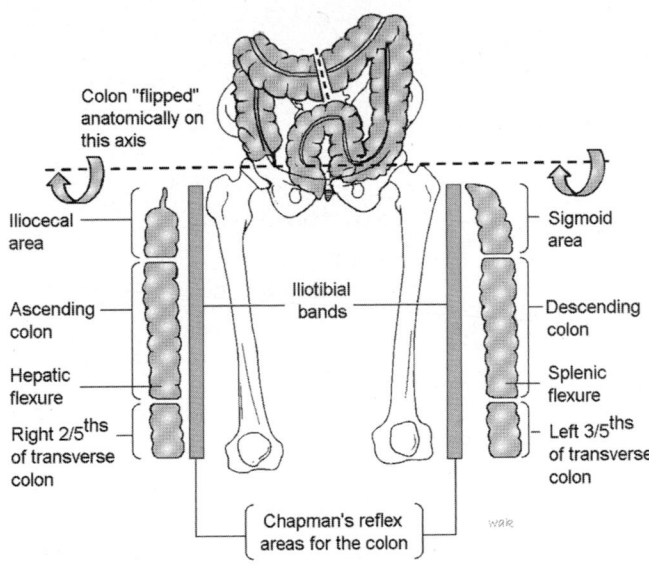

FIGURE 67.2. Anterior Chapman reflexes for the colon.

The palpatory finding of tissue texture changes consistent with Chapman reflexes alerts the practitioner to screen the lower gastrointestinal system even more carefully. It also leads to seeking and correlating more thorough history, abdominal and rectal examination findings, and other musculoskeletal reflex clues with the Chapman findings. Because of the proximity of this reflex to those associated with the prostate or broad ligament, clinicians should carefully screen these viscera as well.

Other reflex points that are clinically useful in a general practice include those in the upper respiratory system (sinus, pharynx, middle ear), the upper gastrointestinal system (stomach, gallbladder), and the genitourinary system (kidney, gonads, prostate/broad ligament). Figures 67.3 and 67.4 show anterior and posterior Chapman points, as summarized from Chapman's book by the College of Osteopathic Medicine (3).

anterior aspect of the iliotibial fascial tract from the trochanter to within 1 inch of the patella on one or both legs. Those reflexes lie just superficial to the deep fascia and are slightly adherent to it. The reflex gangliform masses may be single, multiple, or in chronic or severe cases, coalescent mats or even "strings of pearls." Owens suggests that the anatomic location of the Chapman reflexes on the iliotibial tracts correlates with specific portions of the colon (Fig. 67.2):

Starting with the trochanter on the right side, a gangliform contraction in the tissues of the upper fifth shows inflammation within the mucous membrane of the cecum or a spastic state of the circular fibers of the cecum.

The next succeeding three-fifths show a similar state of the ascending colon. The last fifth has the same indication as the first two-fifths of the transverse colon.

Starting on the left thigh just above the knee, the first fifth corresponds to the last three-fifths of the transverse colon, indicating the same condition explained regarding the right side.

The middle three-fifths show a similar state of the descending colon. The last fifth corresponds with the sigmoid. More especially, the extreme upper end of the trochanter on the left side effects the junction of the sigmoid with the rectum, which will often cause a stricture to form, almost closing the lumen of the bowel (1).

The reflexes for the colon are distributed along the lateral thigh, lateral to the shaft of the femurs. It is as if the upper portions of the large bowel were removed from the abdomen and rotated ventrally around a transverse axis through the cecum and low sigmoid regions so that the transverse colon lies on the ventral surfaces of the two legs extended side by side. The ascending colon then lies over the proximal and midportion of the right femur. The hepatic flexure and right half of the transverse colon lie over the distal right femur. The left half of the transverse colon and the splenic flexure both lie in relation to the distal left femur. The descending colon lies along the midshaft of the left femur, and the sigmoid and rectum are represented on the proximal left femur in order (Fig. 67.2).

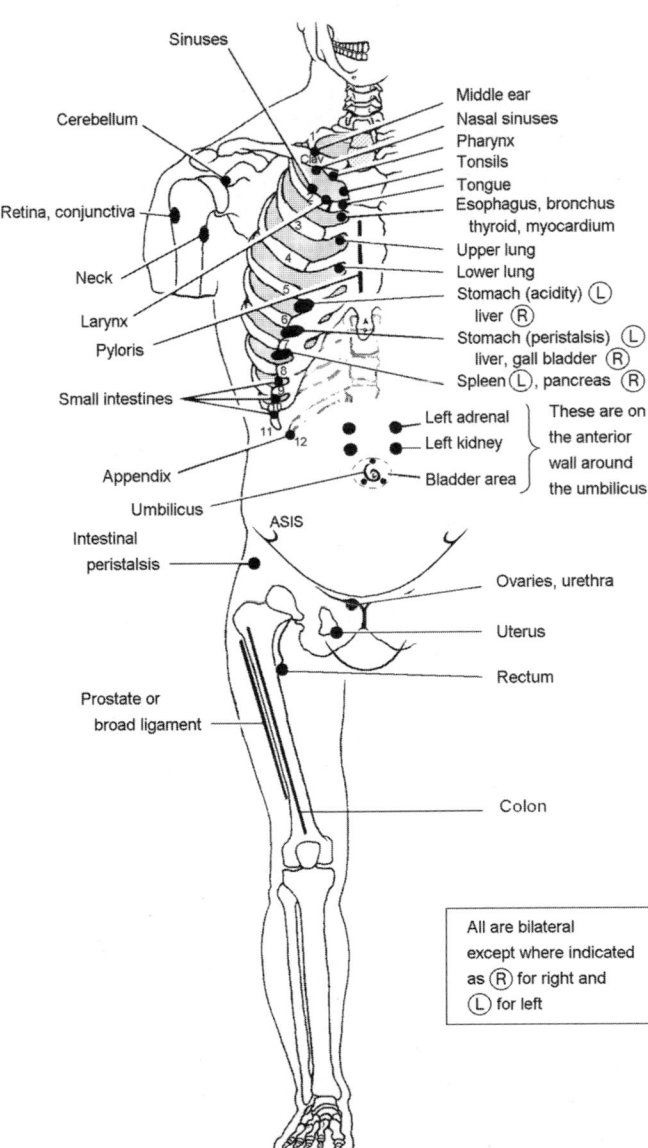

FIGURE 67.3. Chapman reflexes: anterior points. (From Kuchera ML, Kuchera WA. *Osteopathic Considerations in Systemic Dysfunction*, 2nd ed. rev. Columbus, OH: Greyden Press; 1994, with permission.)

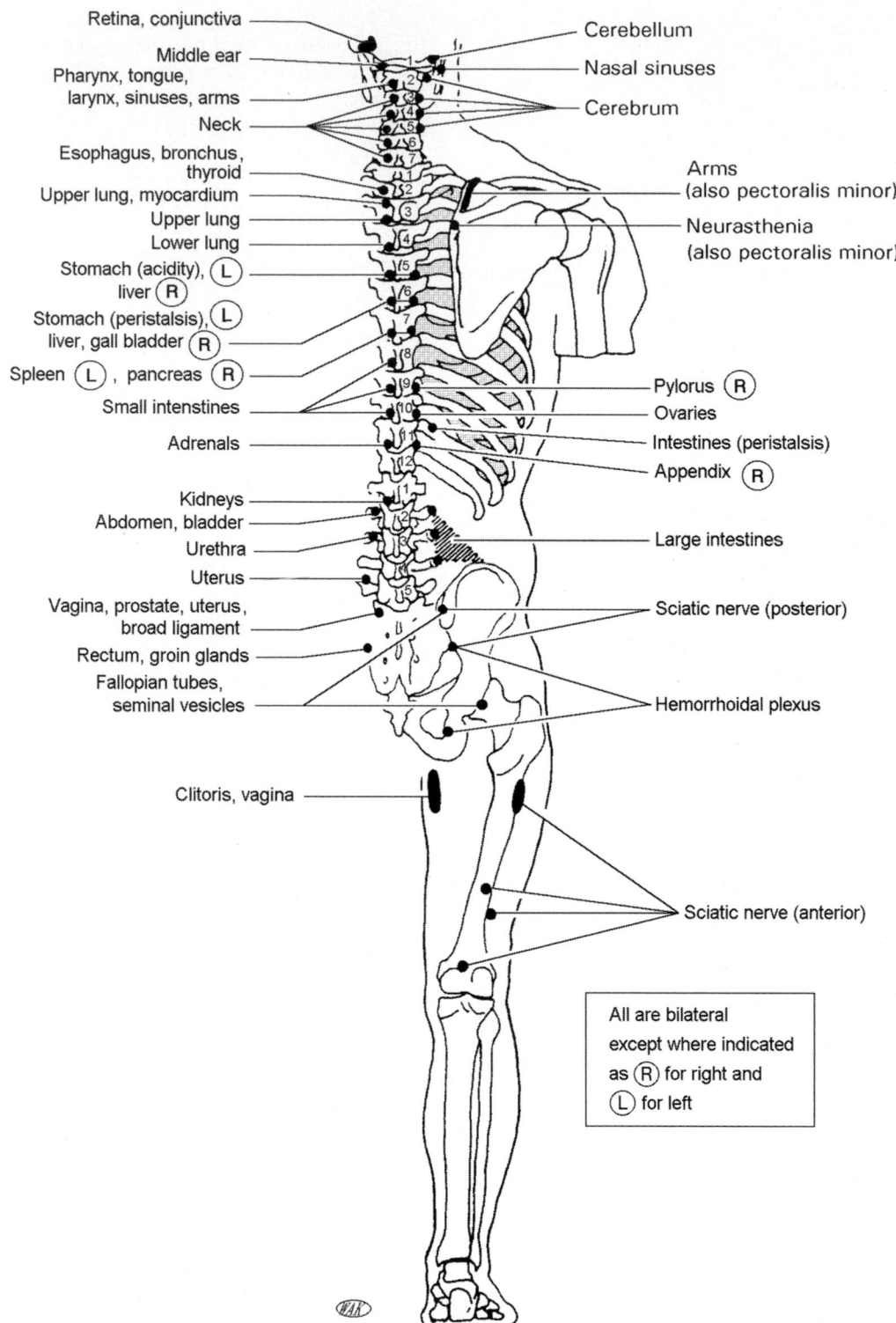

FIGURE 67.4. Chapman reflexes: posterior points. (From Kuchera ML, Kuchera WA. *Osteopathic Considerations in Systemic Dysfunction,* 2nd ed. rev. Columbus, OH: Greyden Press; 1994, with permission.)

Use of Chapman Reflexes

How do we use Chapman reflexes? In some clinical situations, the differential diagnosis hinges on whether the cause is visceral dysfunction or primary musculoskeletal dysfunction. Palpating for Chapman reflexes provides clinical evidence of the presence or absence of visceral disease. It suggests the possible cause of abdominal pain to the physician. The clinical ability to better differentiate a pathologic condition in the urinary bladder from that in the uterus or prostate can be critical.

Chapman reflex diagnosis is highly efficient in these days of expensive diagnostic, medical, and surgical care. Imagine how useful it is to have evidence that a patient's abdominal pain more likely arises from the colon than from the ovary.

Chapman reflexes can also be clinically manipulated to specifically reduce adverse sympathetic influence on a particular organ or visceral system. Improved function of the disturbed organ often follows treatment of its corresponding Chapman point. For example, patients with frequent bowel movements from the effects of irritable bowel syndrome report that they have more normal bowel movements for days to months after soft tissue treatment over the iliotibial bands and/or the lumbosacral paraspinal tissues and associated Chapman reflexes.

Research into the efficacy of Chapman reflex treatment has been limited. One study of hypertensive patients, in whom posterior points to the adrenals were treated, reported a blood pressure drop of 15 mm Hg systolic and 8 mm Hg diastolic pressure, and decreased serum aldosterone levels 36 hours after Chapman treatment (4).

Treatment

How does one treat Chapman reflexes? Treat these reflex points with firm pressure on the volar-distal finger pad of one finger. Assuming that the pelvis has been normalized first, apply somewhat heavy and even uncomfortable pressure to the gangliform mass. Slowly move the tip of the finger in a circular fashion and attempt to work (flatten) the mass as if to mobilize a localized fluid accumulation. Continue the moving pressure for 10 to 30 seconds. Cease treatment when the mass disappears or the patient or physician can no longer tolerate the procedure.

CONCLUSION

Chapman reflexes have particular value in the differential diagnosis of visceral disease and should be integrated with historic and other physical examination findings. Most of these reflexes are found loosely attached to the deep fascia near the costotransverse structures posteriorly and in the intercostal spaces near the sternum anteriorly. These anatomic sites are typically viscerosomatic representations in or on somatic structures. The reflex itself is described as a neurolymphatic gangliform structure. The few histopathologic studies of biopsies of Chapman reflexes have identified nothing. Although its cellular structure has yet to be described, the anatomic location of a Chapman reflex is predictable and consistent. This suggests that the sympathetic nervous system may play an important role in the generation and maintenance of the reflexes. It further suggests that treatment of the reflexes may alter sympathetic influences on any related viscus. Other important reflex sites include the iliotibial tracts overlying the femora and in several locations related to the pubic symphysis.

A Chapman reflex treatment includes general and specific components. The general component deals with management of postural factors, as well as the care of short-term and long-term pelvic dysfunction. Specific treatment consists of deep rotary finger pressure applied to one or a series of Chapman reflexes. The combination of general and specific treatment supports and assists the self-regulating and self-healing capabilities of the patient.

REFERENCES

1. Owens C. *An Endocrine Interpretation of Chapman's Reflexes.* Carmel, CA. Reprinted by the American Academy of Osteopathy; 1932.
2. Byrnes TR, Kuchera ML, Guffey JM, et al. Correlation of palpatory findings with visceral diagnoses. *J Am Osteopath Assoc.* 1992;92(9):1177.
3. Kuchera ML, Kuchera WA. *Osteopathic Considerations in Systemic Dysfunction,* 2nd ed. rev. Columbus, OH: Greyden Press; 1994:65, 90–92, 119, 124, 200–201, 231, 233.
4. Mannino JR. The application of neurologic reflexes to the treatment of hypertension. *J Am Osteopath Assoc.* 1979;79(10):607–608.

ADDITIONAL READING

Brown EA. Clinical aspects of the Chapman's reflexes. In: Northup TL, ed. *Academy of Applied Osteopathy Yearbooks, 1949.* Ann Arbor, MI: Edwards Brothers, Inc; 1949:212–214. (Brown discusses the possible physiologic basis of the reflexes with more attention paid to patterns of reflexes and their possible mechanism of action.)

Patriquin DA. Viscerosomatic reflexes. In: Patterson MM, Howel JN, eds. *The Central Connection: Somatovisceral Interactions. 1989 International Symposium.* Athens OH: University Classics, Ltd; 1992:418. (Patriquin introduces Chapman reflexes as a model of osteopathic diagnosis and treatment of visceral dysfunction. He suggests that the somatic changes termed Chapman reflexes, which clinicians find by palpation, represent specific visceral dysfunction and that the sympathetic nervous system is most likely the connecting link.)

Soden CH. Lecture notes on Chapman reflexes. In: Northup TL, ed. *Academy of Applied Osteopathy Yearbooks, 1949.* Ann Arbor, MI: Edwards Brothers, Inc; 1949:201–211. (Soden reviews Chapman's work from a theoretical and practical perspective. Several pages contain labeled diagrams much like those found in Owens' book.)

Young MD. Osteopathy unlimited. In: Northup TL, ed. *Academy of Applied Osteopathy Yearbooks, 1947.* Ann Arbor, MI: Edwards Brothers, Inc; 1947:34–35. (Young presents Chapman reflexes integrated into osteopathic practice.)

LYMPHATIC SYSTEM: LYMPHATIC MANIPULATIVE TECHNIQUES

ELAINE WALLACE
JOHN M. MCPARTLAND
JOHN M. JONES, III
WILLIAM A. KUCHERA
BOYD R. BUSER

KEY CONCEPTS

- Anatomy of the lymphatic system
- Physiology and pathophysiology of the lymphatic system
- Theories of treatment
- Diagnostic techniques and treatment approaches to lymph-related problems
- Techniques to remove impediments to lymphatic drainage

We strike at the source of life and death when we go to the lymphatics.
—A. T. STILL (1)

The lymphatic system is known as the second circulatory system of the body and as the great integrator for all body fluids. If this system were to stop functioning, the patient would be dead within 24 hours as a result of massive edema and the effects from retention of toxic metabolic wastes. The lymphatic system is a passive system whose functioning can be greatly influenced and altered by extrinsic forces. Of all the systems of the body, osteopathic manipulative treatment (OMT) can exert perhaps its greatest influence on lymphatic function.

This chapter reviews the anatomy, physiology, pathophysiology, and theories of treatment of the lymphatic system. Diagnostic techniques, as well as treatment approaches and techniques are presented.

When Harvey solved the circulation of the blood, he only reached the banks of the rivers of life. —A. T. STILL (1)

In the field of lymphatics, osteopathic physicians have made brilliant advances that parallel the osteopathic advances in the cranial field. William Harvey's student, Olaf Rudbeck, a Professor of Medicine and Botany at Uppsala University, first described the lymphatic system in 1653. More than 200 years later, Andrew Taylor Still became the first medical researcher to emphasize treatment of the lymphatic system for maintaining health and treating disease. The next major contribution to

thought was made by Frederic P. Millard, who was a student of Dr. Still alongside William Sutherland. Beginning in 1904, Millard researched the structure and function of the lymphatic system. In 1922, he published *Applied Anatomy of the Lymphatics* (2), with contributions from 15 authors constituting a veritable "Who's Who" of early 20th century osteopathy, including Evelyn R. Bush, Edwin Martin Downing, George M. Laughlin, and T.J. Ruddy. They addressed controversial issues, such as the effects of vaccines and surgery (tonsillectomy!) on the lymphatic system. Millard's brilliant anatomic illustrations grace many pages of the text; the beauty and precision of these illustrations has never been surpassed.

The editor of Millard's text, A. G. Walmsley, practiced in Bethlehem, Pennsylvania. Another osteopath from Bethlehem, C. Earl Miller, first described the lymphatic pump technique in 1926 (3). Three years later, in nearby Philadelphia, William Galbreath developed the well-known Galbreath technique, a method for mobilizing lymphatic fluid in the mandibular region, and for draining accumulated fluid from the middle ear (4).

Frank Chapman, another student of Still, elucidated a series of neurolymphatic reflexes, which became popularized as "Chapman reflexes" in the 1930s. His work is highlighted in the *Foundations* chapter authored by David Patriquin. J. Gordon Zink, a self-professed "lymphomaniac," contributed a myofascial approach to treatment of the lymphatic system. His work is described later in this chapter.

EMBRYOLOGIC DEVELOPMENT

The lymphatic system and the immune system both begin developing at approximately 20 weeks of fetal age. The lymphatic system is immature at the time of birth and continues to undergo changes until approximately puberty. In infancy, lymphoid tissue is plentiful and actually increases in amount until approximately 6–9 years of age. At that time, a regression in the system begins, and by the age of 15 or 16, stable adult levels of lymphoid tissue remain.

COMPONENTS

The lymphatic system comprises approximately 3% of the total body weight (5). It can be divided into three distinct components:

Organized lymph tissues
Collecting ducts
Lymph fluid

Organized Lymph Tissues

Organized lymph tissues consist of the spleen, the thymus, the tonsils, the vermiform appendix, the visceral lymphoid tissues located in the gastrointestinal (GI) and pulmonary systems, and the liver. These are structures of lymphoid material that are not located along the course of the lymph ducts and that do not directly function in the filtration of lymph. Each organ serves a specialized and ancillary function in the immune system.

The spleen is the largest single mass of lymphoid tissue in the body. Located deep to ribs 9, 10, and 11 on the left side of the thorax, the superior surface of the spleen abuts the abdominal surface of the diaphragm, and its inferior surface extends to the area just cephalad to the left costal margin. In the normal physiologic state, the spleen is approximately 12 cm long and 7 cm wide and is generally nonpalpable. The spleen serves important ancillary services for the lymphatic system by destroying deformed or damaged red blood cells and synthesizing immunoglobulins. The spleen is also a clearance site for particulate antigens and microorganisms, especially poorly organized bacteria. The liver also clears bacteria; this is one reason why the liver is sometimes considered an organ of the lymphatic system.

The thymus is located in the superior mediastinum, anterior to the great vessels of the heart and extending upward into the neck. In infancy, the thymus is a relatively large structure that continues to develop, reaching its greatest size at the age of 2 years. The thymus provides immunologically potent cells that appear to be essential to the development of mature immune functions. It is the preprocessing site for the T lymphocyte immune cells. After puberty, the thymus undergoes involution, and by adulthood, most of the gland has been replaced by fatty tissue. It is presently believed that the minimal tissue that does remain serves little or no function in the adult.

The tonsils are a ring of lymphoid tissue lying at the posterior oropharynx. The palatine tonsils line the lateral aspects of the pharynx at the base of the tongue and are continuous with the lingual tonsils, which cover the posterior one-third of the tongue. The pharyngeal tonsils, known as the adenoids, lie in the mucosa at the nasopharyngeal border of the tonsillar ring. The tonsils, like the thymus, provide cells that appear to influence and build immunity early in life but appear to be nonessential contributors to adult immunologic function.

The vermiform appendix is a long, tapered structure, 2 to 20 cm in length at the medial surface of the cecum. Although the exact function of the appendix is unknown, it is richly imbued with lymphoid tissue and presumably offers support to the immune system. However, like the thymus and the tonsils, we know that this support is nonessential to the adult patient.

Visceral lymphoid tissue is also located in the respiratory and GI systems. The lymphoid tissue of the respiratory system aids filtration of toxins from the lungs. The lymphoid tissues located in the mucosa of the small intestine are the most highly organized of all visceral tissues. In the small intestines, both Peyer patches and lacteals can be identified. Peyer patches are nonencapsulated areas of lymphoid tissue that are most highly concentrated in the distal ileum. Lacteals are small lymphatic capillaries located centrally in each small intestinal villus. These capillaries converge to form a lymphatic capillary plexus in the submucosal layer. Both Peyer patches and the lacteals are the structures by which fats in the digestive system enter the circulatory system. These tissues drain into the superior and inferior mesenteric lymphatic trunks and ultimately into the thoracic duct.

Autonomic regulation of Peyer patches and the lacteals are controlled by the enteric nervous system (ENS). The ENS contains an enormous number of neurons (2×10^8), nearly equaling the number of neurons in the central nervous system (6). Many neurotransmitters associated with the brain also function in the ENS, including acetylcholine, dopamine, glycine, norepinephrine, serotonin, endogenous opioids, and endogenous cannabinoids. The discovery of these neurotransmitters and their receptors in the gut offers new insights concerning psychosomatic diseases of the GI system, such as irritable bowel disorder. The proximity and interaction between Peyer patches and ENS tissues (such as Auerbach and Meissner plexi) suggest the potential benefit of lymphatic treatment for functional bowel disorders.

Lymph nodes are perhaps the most highly organized of all lymphoid tissues. Lymph nodes differ from other organized lymphoid tissues in that they are dispersed along the course of the lymph vessels and are involved primarily in the filtration of lymph. The nodes can be divided into two categories: the superficial nodes, located in the subcutaneous connective tissues accompanying the superficial veins; and the deep nodes, which lie beneath the fascia and muscle layers and are adjacent to the deep veins. A normal, young adult body contains some 400 to 450 lymph nodes (7). Aggregates of lymphocytes intermeshed with lymphatic sinuses are supported in a framework of reticular tissue and encased in a connective tissue capsule. These structures vary in size from a few millimeters to a few inches in diameter. They serve a dual function of filtration and synthesis (production). Afferent lymph vessels deliver lymph to the node wherein reticuloendothelial cells phagocytize bacteria, particulate matter, and fragments of cells. In the germinal centers of the nodes, lymphocytes are manufactured and enter into the lymph as it passes through the node.

The superficial lymph nodes receive lymph from the skin, as well as from the deeper tissues of the upper extremities, lower extremities, head, and neck. Superficial nodes drain into three main groups of nodes located in the cervical, axillary, and inguinal regions. The cervical nodes receive lymph from the head and areas superior to the clavicle and send it on to the jugular nodes. Lymph from the superficial areas between the clavicle and the umbilicus drain into the axillary nodes that drain into the deeper subclavian nodes; superficial areas caudal to the umbilicus drain into the inguinal nodes and eventually into the right and left lumbar nodes in the deep tissues. Deep nodes drain into a system of collecting channels.

Lymph Channels

The second component of the lymphatic system is the lymph channels. These channels perfuse all tissues of the body with the exception of the central nervous system (brain and spinal cord), the epidermis (including the hair and the nails), the endomysium of muscles and cartilage, the bone marrow, and selected portions of the peripheral nerves. Although these tissues are devoid of lymph channels, they are perfused by minute interstitial conduits or by direct diffusion.

The anatomic arrangement of the lymph channels mirrors that of the lymph nodes in that there are both superficial and deep vessels. The superficial lymph vessels follow the course of the superficial veins and the superficial nodes. The deep lymphatic vessels, as in the case of the deep nodes, follow the course of the deep veins and drain the deep structures of the thorax, the abdomen, the pelvis, and the perineum. Deep lymph channels lie around all major organs of the body.

The structure of the lymphatic system differs significantly from all other fluid flow systems in the body. It begins in the tissues as lymphatic capillaries or blind endothelial tubes composed of a single layer of leaky squamous epithelium (Fig. 68.1).

These thinly walled capillaries are supported by anchoring filaments that are attached to the endothelial cells and extend into the surrounding interstitium. These filaments bind the endothelial tubes to the proteinaceous fibers in the interstitial matrix. They also function to open spaces between the endothelial cells as fluid accumulates, and prevent collapse of the thinly walled lymph capillaries.

At the level of the arterial capillaries, filtration of intravascular fluid occurs, allowing for the passage of fluid, proteins, and particles from the vascular system directly into the interstitium. This fluid then diffuses along the connective tissue fibers and the anchoring filaments in the interstitium, where it actively mixes with extracellular fluids. More fluid gets into the interstitial spaces than is removed by the capillaries, even when all is normal. Because the simple squamous epithelium of the lymphatic capillaries contains no basement membrane, it possesses a greater permeability than do the blood capillaries. This promotes ready passage of

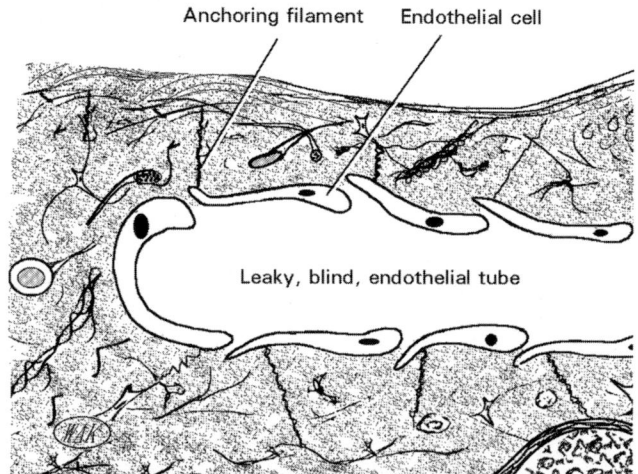

FIGURE 68.1. The beginnings of the lymphatic system. (Illustration by W. A. Kuchera.)

the excess transudate from the interstitium back into the closed circuit of the lymphatic system.

Peripheral lymphatic capillaries join to form capillary plexus that, in turn, form larger trunks. In the superior portion of the body, the chest wall and the pleural spaces are drained by the intercostal trunks. The mediastinal trunks drain the thoracic viscera. The internal jugular trunk drains the left side of the head and neck, and the subclavian trunk drains the left arm and shoulder. The pelvis is drained by the internal iliac trunk, and the lower extremities are drained by the external iliac trunk. The lumbar trunk drains the lumbar area; the small intestine trunk drains the small intestine, the lacteals, and Peyer patches. The colon and the mesentery are drained by the superior and inferior mesenteric trunks. The gastric trunk receives drainage from the liver, spleen, stomach, and pancreas. All of these trunks eventually drain into two main trunks that empty into the venous system in the cervicothoracic area, either the right lymphatic duct (RLD) or the thoracic duct, also called the left lymphatic duct (LLD).

The trunks of the abdomen, pelvis, and lower limbs drain into the cisterna chyli, a saccular dilation of the thoracic duct that lies on the anterior right side of the Ll and L2 vertebral bodies at the level of the renal vessels. The cisterna chyli lies behind the right crus of the diaphragm next to the abdominal aorta and represents the distal portion of the thoracic duct. In some cases, the lumbar trunks unite above the level of the L2 vertebra, forming a plexus of vessels that drain directly into the thoracic duct, in which case the cisterna chyli is absent.

All of the aforementioned trunks (from the left side of the head and neck, the left arm and thorax, left and right portions of the lower body, and the thoracic viscera) drain into the LLD. Only the right side of the head, the right side of the neck, the right arm, and the right chest (inclusive of the heart and portions of the lungs) drain into a separate main duct, the RLD. Sodeman and Sodeman (8) state that sometimes the posterior portion of the left upper lobe of the lung drains into the thoracic duct.

The thoracic duct is the largest lymph vessel in the body, typically measuring 36 to 45 cm in total length. The thoracic duct lies directly against the vertebral column as it courses cephalically. It passes through the aortic hiatus of the diaphragm and traverses the posterior mediastinum between the aorta and the azygos vein, passing in front of the phrenic nerve and behind the vagus nerve. At the level of the sternal angle (T4), it inclines to the left of midline and enters the superior aperture of the thorax behind the aortic arch and to the left of the esophagus. At this juncture, it passes laterally across the carotid sheath and then arches caudally and anteriorly to the subclavian artery. The thoracic duct terminates at its junction with the venous system. It empties into the venous circulation in the region of the junction between the left subclavian and left brachiocephalic vein.

The RLD is formed by a merger in the right jugular trunk, the right subclavian trunk, and the right transverse cervical trunks. This short duct courses the medial border of the anterior scalene muscle and terminates in the jugulosubclavian junction in the anterior neck. A distinct RLD, approximately 1 cm in length, is present in only 20% of patients (8). Usually, the three main contributing trunks of the duct empty separately via two or three separate openings.

The terminal points of both main trunks are protected by valves that prevent the back flow of blood into the lymphatic system. These are one-way valves under sympathetic autonomic control. In addition, the lymph vessels possess a series of one-way valves situated in the vessels every few millimeters that prevent regression of lymph as it returns to the central lymphatic collection sites. All lymph moves unidirectionally. Each segment between valves acts independently, filling and emptying on fluid demand. The larger lymph vessels contain smooth muscle, which is also innervated by the sympathetic nervous system. The extent of sympathetic innervation suggests that response to stress may hinder optimal decongestion of tissues via the lymphatic system.

Lymph

Lymph is the final component of the lymphatic system. Lymph is the substance that leaks out of the arterial capillaries, into the interstitium, and into the single-cell lymphatic vessels. Lymph is usually clear in color and contains proteins (2 to 6 gm%) (9) and salts. After a meal, the lymph in the thoracic duct becomes richly laden with emulsified water-soluble fats, and its color may actually change to yellow. The primary cells of lymph are lymphocytes. Lymphocytes have been found in quantities of 2,000 to 20,000/mm in the thoracic duct (10). Lymph also contains clotting factors; it clots on standing. Finally, large particles, such as bacteria and smaller viruses, are found in the peripheral lymph before filtration through a lymph node or one of the organized lymphoid tissues. These larger particles are brought into close contact with lymphatic cells that have immune functions.

PHYSIOLOGY

Let the lymphatics always receive and discharge naturally, if so we have no substance detained long enough to produce fermentation, fever, sickness, and death. —A. T. STILL (1)

Function

The lymphatic system has four basic functions:

> Maintaining fluid balance in the body
> Purification and cleansing of tissues
> Defense
> Nutrition

Fluid Balance

One of the most important functions performed by the lymphatic system is that of fluid balance. At least 50% of all plasma proteins that diffuse out of the vascular system within a 24-hour period return to the body by way of the lymphatic system (5). On a daily basis, approximately 30 liters of fluid filters out of the capillaries and into the interstitial spaces (10). Of this 30 liters, approximately 90% (27 liters) drains back into the blood capillaries, but the remaining 10% (3 liters) drains into the lymphatic channels. In addition to absorption of this 3-liter volume, the system has a capacity to absorb a limited amount of excess fluid from the cavities of the pleura, the peritoneum, the pericardium, and the

joints. Although 10% is a proportionately small amount of fluid that is returned to the circulation by way of the lymphatics, this lymph flow is vital because proteins and other substances of high molecular weights that are unable to pass easily into the pores of the vascular capillaries because of their large size are able to enter the lymphatic capillaries with relative ease. In the case of significant fluid overload, it is the lymphatic system that provides the homeostatic reserve to resist or forestall damage (10).

Purification and Cleansing

The lymphatic system serves important functions in cleansing the body, both within the structure of the lymphatic conduits and without. Because lymph forms as a filtrate from the arterial capillaries into the extracellular spaces, lymph actually bathes all of the organs of the body. Before passing into the capillaries of the lymphatic system, it cleanses the extracellular spaces of particulate matter, exudates, and bacteria. Once inside the lymphatic system, it readily delivers all of these substances to the lymph nodes, which act as purifying filters for removal of this waste matter from the circulation.

Defense

Intimately associated with the cleansing and purification functions of lymph are the defensive properties of the lymphatic system. Because of the pervasive quantities and locations of lymphoid tissues in the body, lymph comes in fairly immediate contact with any toxins, bacteria, and viruses entering the system. The lymphatic system provides the first line of defense against this invasion. Acquired immunity does not develop until the body has first exposure to these invading antigens. All of these substances contain proteins, polysaccharides, or lipoprotein complexes, and these are the essential substrates by which the body is able to develop acquired (adaptive) immunity. The lymphatic system's importance is underlined by the fact that any individual who genetically lacks lymphoid tissue or who has had chemical or radiation obliteration of the body's lymphoid tissue cannot defend against antigenic invasion and will die. The lymphatic defense system is broken down into two separate divisions, both embryologically derived from lymphocytic stem cells in the bone marrow. The T-lymphatic division contains those sensitized lymphocytes that have been processed through the thymus gland and function to provide cellular immunity. The majority of this preprocessing occurs before birth of the infant, and the remainder shortly thereafter. Cellular immunity, also known as lymphocytic immunity, is the capability of the sensitized lymphocyte to attach to a foreign substance and to destroy it.

The B-lymphocytic division is named for the bursa of Fabricius, a structure not found in mammals but found in birds, where B lymphocytes were first identified. These B lymphocytes are believed to be processed in the liver or the spleen in humans (although the exact location is unknown) and give rise to humoral immunity. Humoral immunity is the capability of the body to produce globulin molecules known as antibodies, which possess the specific capability of attacking the invading antigens.

The lymphatic system is not only responsible for the production and maintenance of these two essential defensive armies;

the free flow of lymph is also vital for direct contact of the invading agents with the defense factors. Whenever injury occurs, the subsequent inflammation brings increased vascular perfusion, increased capillary filtration, and increased lymph production to the area. This is the body's obvious mechanism for increasing contact between antigens and antibodies, as well as phagocytes. The greater the lymphatic flow through the body, the greater the contact of body defenses with all toxins, particulate matter, and other foreign substances.

Nutrition

As stated earlier, 50% or more of all plasma proteins are carried by the lymphatic system back to the vascular system after their efflux from the arterial capillaries into the extracellular spaces. Many of these proteins are capable of binding nutrients that the cells need. Long-chain fats, chylomicrons, and cholesterol are absorbed in large quantities from the lacteals in the villi of the small intestine. After a large and fatty meal, the thoracic duct may contain up to 2% fat. With fat absorption, the lymph of the gastrointestinal tract changes from its normal clear appearance to a yellow or milky color. This particular kind of lymph is called chyle.

Mechanisms of Flow

Several factors determine the rate of lymph flow in the body. Interstitial fluid pressure is one important factor. Normally, interstitial fluid pressure is maintained at −6.3 mm Hg. Any increase in this pressure increases the absorption of lymph into lymph capillaries. An increase from −6.3 mm Hg to 0 mm Hg increases lymphatic flow approximately 20 times its normal rate of 120 ml/hr (10).

At 0 mm Hg, a ceiling of efficiency is reached. Above that level, interstitial fluid pressure becomes greater than the pressure inside of the lymph channels, causing them to collapse and obstructing the pathways; drainage ceases.

Several elements increase interstitial pressure:

Increased arterial capillary pressure (such as in systemic hypertension)

Decreased plasma colloid osmotic pressure (as in cirrhosis of the liver, in which there is a decrease of plasma protein synthesis)

Increased interstitial fluid protein (as in plasma hypoalbuminemia associated with starvation)

Increased capillary permeability (associated with toxins such as rattlesnake poisoning)

A second factor affecting lymph flow is the lymphatic pump. As stated earlier, each section between the valves of the lymph channels functions as an independent unit. This provides the lymphatic vessels with an intrinsic, active pumping mechanism. When lymph enters a segment of the lymph vessel, distension of that individual section occurs. In the larger vessels, this distension causes contraction of the smooth muscle within the walls of the lymph channel and effectively pumps the lymph to the next independent segment, where the dilation and pumping process is repeated. A similar process occurs in the lymph capillaries. Although there is no smooth muscle in the lymph capillary, the endothelial cells contain contractile fibers (myoendothelial fibers) that respond to fluid distension in the same way. This lymphatic

pumping at the capillary level also creates a slight degree of suction as the capillary passes from relaxed to distended to relaxed states, and it is this suction that helps pull fluids from the interstitium.

In the extremities, the rhythmic motility of lymphatic vessels has an intrinsic rate of 6 to 8 seconds per cycle (11). This duration equals a frequency of 7.5 to 10 cycles per minute, similar to that of the cranial rhythmic impulse (CRI). Indeed, the CRI may be a palpable harmonic wave ("summation signal" in the language of chaos theory) that integrates the lymphatic rhythm with other biologic oscillations, such as heart rate, respiration rate, Traube-Hering modulation, and oscillating fluctuations in cerebral blood volume (12). The pacemaker responsible for the rhythmic contractility of lymphatic vessels has not been identified. Pacemaker activity in the gut, which drives peristalsis and secondarily propels lymphatic fluid, appears to be stimulated by the interstitial cells of Cajal (13). A hypoplasia of these pacemaker cells leads to intestinal dysmotility (14). Pacemaker cells are influenced by autonomic nerve function, which suggests that OMT directed at dysfunctional autonomic tone will provide therapeutic effects (12).

Finally, in the same way that lymph flow is pumped by intrinsic mechanisms, extrinsic pressures on the lymph channel also promote passive filling of lymphatic segments with subsequent pumping effect.

Direct external pressure on a lymph channel increases the flow of lymph. Internally, wherever pressure is exerted over the lymph vessel, flow increases. Wherever arteries with their rhythmic contractions cross lymph channels, flow increases.

The diaphragm is considered by many to be an extremely important extrinsic pump for the lymphatic system. Movements of the diaphragmatic crura exert a pumping influence on the cisterna chyli. All movements of internal organs, such as respiration and abdominal peristalsis, as well as movements of the extremities, exert an effective external pump. Not only does the diaphragm directly massage the lymphatics, but respiration produces pressure gradients between the chest and the abdomen. These pressure gradients, along with the one-way valves, help to pull lymph toward the venous circulation. If a person breathes 12 breaths per minute, this produces 17,280 pressure changes per day. Therefore, rate and depth of breathing can increase or decrease lymphatic flow.

The overall effect of the extrinsic pump is best underlined by the fact that vigorous exercise, with its movement of extremities, organs, and the diaphragm, may increase lymph flow 15 to 20 times the normal resting flow amount.

Other functional diaphragms, such as the pelvic diaphragm, normally work in synchrony with the abdominal diaphragm. When this happens, there is optimal movement of interstitial fluids from the pelvis and optimal pressure gradients from abdominal diaphragmatic contractions. The pelvic organs predominantly rest on the soft tissues of the perineal floor, in contrast to the abdominal contents that rest against the large iliac fossae. The soft tissues that form the urogenital diaphragm, pelvic diaphragm, and other perineal ligaments and tissues close the pelvic outlet. They form a solid, yet elastic floor that also allows for periodic opening to occur for excretion and, in females, for childbirth.

The abdominal viscera constitute a dynamic column that rests on the iliac fossa and the edge of the ischiopubic rami. In spite of these supports, some pressure is still exerted on the pelvic inlet from above. The pelvic organs themselves add their weight and, along with the effects of gravity, add to the load that must be supported by the perineal floor.

To completely fulfill its function, the pelvic floor needs to provide elasticity in addition to its supportive function. If the floor were rigid, thoracic inhalation would compress the pelvic organs from above. Compensation by the pelvic floor must dissipate or alleviate the permanent, cyclic respiratory pressure and also the transient or temporary increased pressures produced by coughing, sneezing, hiccups, pregnancy, and so on. This synchronized contraction of the abdominal diaphragm and descent of the relaxed pelvic diaphragm, as well as the reciprocal motions with exhalation, produce a mechanical pump for the lymphatic vessels and venous sinuses in the pelvis and around the rectum and perineum.

Within the perineal floor are openings for the urogenital tract and rectum. These orifices are anatomic weak points, and because of the number and size in women, the female perineum is much more fragile than the male perineum. Structurally, these orifices provide a weakness that may allow herniation or ptosis in the adult. Because of these weak areas where the urinary and vaginal tracts exit, the body has developed a second layer of reinforcement distal to the shelf of the levator ani muscles. This is called the urogenital diaphragm.

The pelvic diaphragm needs to act as a support and yet remain elastic. Distension of the pelvic diaphragm must be in phase with the continual movements of the thoracic diaphragm and also with the transient changes in intrapelvic pressure. This helps assure that the pelvic organs escape undue pressure and that there is a free flow of fluids within the vascular and lymphatic channels of the pelvic region.

PATHOPHYSIOLOGY

The consequence of a poorly functioning lymphatic system is congestion or frank edema from the build-up of interstitial fluids. Edema is the result of too much fluid getting into the interstitium or too little fluid getting out. Its presence signifies that the body's compensatory mechanisms have already failed. Conditions that overload the interstitium produce congestion and edema by overriding the absorptive capabilities of the lymphatic system. Excessive interstitial fluid produces excessive interstitial pressure, which, in turn, is associated with collapse of the lymph capillaries, resulting in further interstitial congestion and edema. Edema has a second deleterious effect of dilating the lymphatic capillaries. With dilation, the endothelial cells separate and the flap valves of the capillaries become nonfunctional. This is associated with a shutdown of the intrinsic lymphatic pumping of the capillaries.

Conditions of high venous pressure are associated with increased capillary filtration rates and have an increased tendency to produce edema. These conditions include congestive heart failure, incompetent heart valves, venous obstruction, and the effects of gravity. Arteriolar dilation and venous constriction are also associated with increased capillary permeability, as are the effects of substances such as cytokines and histamines.

Conditions of starvation and cirrhosis of the liver, as well as other states of abnormal protein metabolism, affect interstitial fluid gradients by altering the osmotic effect of plasma protein levels. Decreased osmotic pressure gradients across the capillary, which occur with decreased plasma protein level or the accumulation of osmotically active substances in the interstitium, promote increased accumulation of fluid in the extracellular spaces with all the ramifications that go along with the edematous state.

Inadequate drainage also results in the development of edema because of the relative imbalance created in pressure gradients, even in the face of normal capillary filtration. Posttraumatic or postsurgical scarring may cause mechanical obstructions to absorptive flow and mechanical blockages, such as those produced by filariasis or intraluminal carcinoma, creating absorptive insufficiency that will eventually lead to edema.

The results of edema are pervasive and profound to all surrounding tissues. Edema causes compression not only on the lymphatic channels but also on the nearby vascular and neurologic structures, thus potentially diminishing their function. Edema is associated with increased tissue congestion. Stasis of interstitial fluids promotes changes in the pH of tissues and organs, which further compromises function. This promotes inflammation that, in turn, produces greater edema and continuation of the cycle. It also is associated with infiltration of fibroblasts, which can lead to fibrosis and contracture of tissues. Edema also affects the delivery of nutrients to the affected sites and is associated with even greater changes in tissue function and healing abilities. Finally, edema affects bioavailability of drugs and hormones, hampering not only medical management of the primary fluid build-up but also, because of tissue congestion, decreasing the efficacy of any pharmacologic treatment.

PRINCIPLES OF TREATMENT

Goals

The goal for treatment of the lymphatic system is to have a balanced, well-functioning system in which no edema occurs. The fact that the lymphatic system is a passive system underlines the importance of motion and adequate drainage of lymph. OMT has long provided an extra measure of movement that promotes proper fluid dynamics. Manipulation is associated with:

Increased resorption of fluids
Increased circulation and respiration
Decreased proteins in the interstitium
Facilitation from a more beneficial pH balance

Fascial Pattern Diagnosis (Zink)

Although there was previous talk about the fasciae of the body having rotatory preferences, Zink (15) was the first to provide a written, understandable, and clinically useful explanation for treatment, with a method of diagnosing and manipulative methods of treating the fascial patterns of the body. Fasciae form the pathways for lymphatic vessels, as well as for arteries, veins, and nerves. Torsion of these pathways can hinder the flow of lymph through the lymphatic vessels. Zink identified four areas of the body as cross-over sites where fascial tension could occur (15):

Occipito-atlantal (O-A)
Cervicothoracic (CT)
Thoracolumbar (TL)
Lumbosacral (LS)

He tested the fascial preference for rotation and side-bending of those regions of the body. Zink had observed that almost all people who thought they were well and healthy had alternating patterns of rotatory preference at the key sites. When testing rotation from the O-A to the LS regions, he found that approximately 80% of these people had the body pattern of L/R/L/R, and the other 20% had R/L/R/L, so he named the former pattern the common compensatory pattern (CCP). Zink reasoned that, ideally, there should be equal motion to the right or to the left in all of these reference zones, but apparently the stress of gravity and living produced the alternative patterns.

People in the hospital tend to have patterns that do not alternate; this is also true for people who are easily stressed, who get sick easily, and who have low levels of wellness. When reference zones do not indicate equal or alternating patterns of rotational preference among the four regions of the body, Zink called these uncompensated fascial patterns, and they need OMT. The goal of treatment for these people is to return their fascial patterns to ideal so that their bodies can establish more efficient fascial patterns, usually of the compensated form. Because fascia attaches to bone, direct (thrust or muscle energy) or indirect methods of OMT can be performed to normalize the fascial preferences. Zink's diagnostics and treatment for the fascial regions of the body improved the pathway for lymph flow.

Types of Treatment

Lymphatic treatments are essentially divided into two broad categories: those techniques that remove restrictive impediments to lymphatic flow, and those that promote and augment the flow of lymph. A thorough treatment regime usually includes techniques from both categories, in that sequence. A sequence for a basic lymphatic treatment program includes:

1. Rib raise and/or use paraspinal inhibition (T1-L2). This is designed to reduce hypersympathetic activity to the lymphatic vessels in the area of concern and around the major lymphatic duct that anatomically drains that area or region. Mobilizing the ribs also enhances respiration.
2. Diagnose and treat any thoracic inlet somatic dysfunction. The thoracic inlet is the common obstruction to lymphatic flow from anywhere in the body.
3. Dome (relax) the abdominal diaphragm. This improves the ability of this major fibromuscular diaphragm to produce effective pressure gradients between the thoracic and abdominal cavities.
4. Apply some additional form of lymphatic pump and/or techniques to further promote lymphatic flow. This may be optional in a basic plan but would further enhance lymphatic flow.

More than one type of treatment affects the lymphatic system. For instance, use of high-velocity/low-amplitude treatment

alters muscle tone and neural reflexes that affect structures such as the diaphragm, adding to the efficiency of the system. Muscle energy, deep articulatory, or other direct techniques do the same thing. An example of a deep articulatory technique is rib raising in a repetitive fashion, freeing the ribs and diaphragm to have a more relaxed, efficient performance and normalizing sympathetic autonomic activity from the thoracolumbar sympathetic chain ganglia. Conversely, myofascial release techniques are particularly effective in eliminating inappropriate tension in tissues surrounding lymphatic channels that tend to be constrictive in nature. Cranial techniques are thought to have a balancing effect on the sympathetic/parasympathetic nervous system, leading to deeper diaphragmatic breathing, as well as promoting appropriate cranial venous fluid return.

Treatment Plan (One Example)

Treatment of the lymphatic system should begin with the removal of all restrictions resulting from tissue hypertonicity that may be affecting lymph flow. Release of the central lymphatic system should be accomplished first, followed by release of the periphery. This decreases the likelihood of exceeding the system's innate 7 mm Hg maximum increase in capability of handling increased flow.

Treatment begins by releasing the central lymphatic system: the area of the thoracic inlet, then the abdominothoracic diaphragm, and the pelvic diaphragm. Release of the peripheral lymphatic systems should include drainage techniques of the head and neck, as well as the extremities (in each case beginning centrally and progressing peripherally). Lymphatic treatment should be accompanied by a release of all respiratory restrictions (rib or clavicular somatic dysfunctions), as well as restrictions of the muscles, joints, and abdomen. Rib raising and treatment of any spinal somatic dysfunction are also prudent to optimize autonomic activity. Attention should also be given to dysfunction of the cranium (including the temporals, the occiput, and the sphenoid) to promote optimal functioning of the cranial nerves, particularly the vagus nerve (cranial nerve X).

Contraindications of Lymphatic Treatments

Contraindications of individual treatments are included along with the following individual techniques. Relative contraindications for lymphatic treatment techniques include osseous fracture, bacterial infections with a temperature over 102° F (38.8° C, in which case antibiotic control should first be implemented to reduce the chance of seeding and encouraging a generalized body infection) and certain stages of carcinoma.

LYMPHATIC MANIPULATIVE TECHNIQUES

Even under normal conditions, more blood gets to the tissues than can be removed by the venous system. This amount is even greater when there is dysfunction or inflammation. An important principle in the efficient care of patients with dysfunction or disease is to be sure that the lymphatic drainage is as efficient as possible. This can be performed by diagnosing impediments to flow and then designing osteopathic manipulative techniques to remove those impediments, improve the pumps, and directly promote decongestion of an organ or region of the body. The lymphatic system has no intrinsic pump and must rely heavily on the production of efficient pressure gradients between the thoracic and abdominal regions, produced by the efficient action of a well-domed abdominal diaphragm. Recent studies reveal that there are sympathetic fibers innervating muscle fibers in the larger lymphatic vessels, implying that sympathicotonia may reduce the amount of lymph that the lymphatic vessels can carry.

TECHNIQUES TO REMOVE IMPEDIMENTS

Open Thoracic Inlet Fascia

Anatomically, the thoracic inlet (Fig. 68.2) is the first ribs, the first thoracic vertebra, and the manubrium. Clinically, the thoracic inlet is the first two ribs, the first four thoracic vertebrae, and the manubrium of the sternum. Fascia from the scalenus and the longus coli muscles joins together to produce a functional fascial diaphragm for the superior thoracic inlet. Lymphatic fluid returning from any site outside the thorax must pass through this diaphragm.

The thoracic fascial inlet is a common diaphragm for both the right and the left lymphatic ducts. The LLD (thoracic duct) passes through this diaphragm twice. The tissues of the thoracic inlet are frequently subjected to the stresses associated with carriage of the head on the shoulders, as well as the muscular pull of the shoulders themselves. Some physicians evaluate the thoracic inlet fasciae by examining first rib motion during respiration and then determining the direction of fascial ease or restriction to the application of traction in all directions at the cervicothoracic junction. This is an organized method of determining preference of the tissues at the cervicothoracic junction:

1. The patient may be supine or seated, and the physician may approach the patient from either the anterior or the posterior position.
2. Place the fingertips at the superior aspect of the shoulders in the region of the first rib (Table 68.1).

The fasciae at the inlet tend to pull the cervicothoracic region into side-bending and rotation to the same side. Opening the thoracic inlet relieves obstruction to lymphatic flow at this level.

TABLE 68.1. THORACIC INLET DIAGNOSIS: STATIC AND MOTION TEST FINDINGS

	Inlet fascia rotated and side-bent left	Inlet fascia rotated and side-bent right
First rib	Left rib ↓ /right rib ↑	Left rib ↑ /right rib ↓
Infraclavicular space	Left deep	Right deep
Coracoclavicular angle	Left posterior	Right posterior
Spring upper ribs	Left spring/right resist	Right spring/left resist

Thoracic Inlet: Two-Step with Muscle Energy Activation

Patient Position
Supine.

Physician Position
Sitting or standing at the head of the table (to treat side-bending restriction).

Procedure
1. Side bend the neck to the side of restricted side-bending, using IP joints of the index finger of one hand as a fulcrum at the cervicothoracic junction on that side (Fig. 68.3).
2. Rotate the patient's head to the opposite side to lock out the cervical spine above the cervicothoracic junction.
3. Ask the patient to attempt side-bending the head to the side opposite the fulcrum hand as you isometrically resist the effort.
4. Ask the patient to completely relax and repeat step 3 three or four times.
5. Place the head and neck back to neutral position; now, rotate the head to the restrictive barrier of rotation (without side-bending) using your hand on the side of the head and the fingers of the IP joints of the index finger of that hand at the cervicothoracic junction (the fulcrum) (Fig. 68.4).
6. Ask the patient to attempt to rotate the head and neck toward your fulcrum hand as you isometrically resist the effort.
7. Ask the patient to completely relax, and repeat Step 6 three or four times.
8. Recheck the fascial preference at the thoracic inlet.

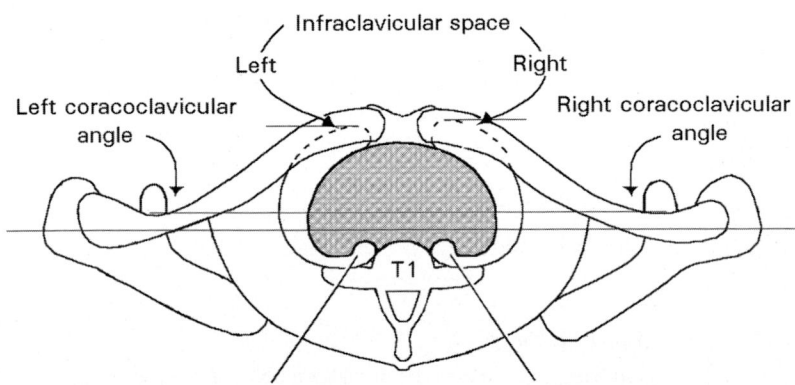

Left rib head/neck area: First rib   Right rib head/neck area: First rib

FIGURE 68.2. Thoracic inlet: static landmarks. (Illustration by W. A. Kuchera.)

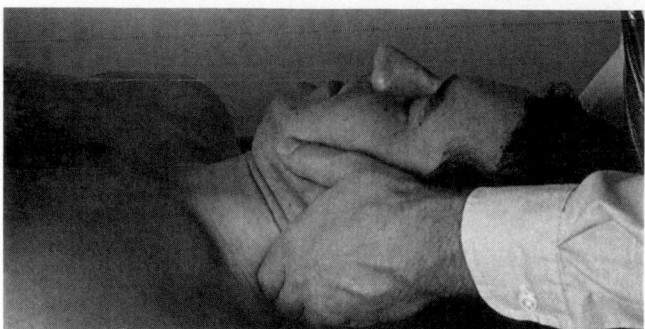

FIGURE 68.3. Thoracic inlet: side-bending.

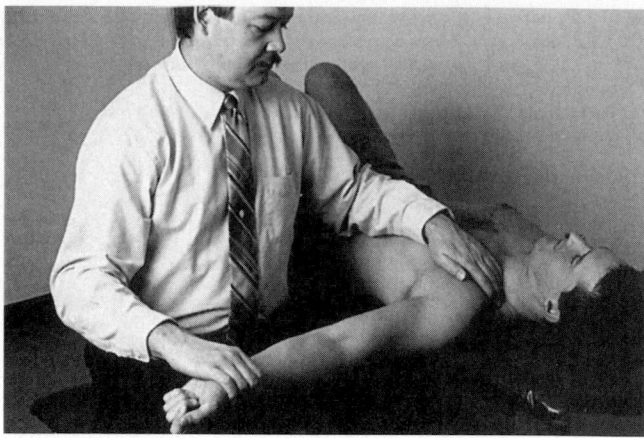

FIGURE 68.5. Thoracic inlet: direct myofascial release.

Thoracic Inlet: Direct Myofascial Release

Patient Position
Supine with arm abducted 90 degrees from the body.

Physician Position
Seated at the side of the patient.

Procedure
1. Use your knee to support the patient's elbow and cephalad hand to support the patient's wrist.
2. With caudal fingers placed on the superior aspect of the supraclavicular fossa, apply downward pressure to the patient's wrist (Fig. 68.5). The caudal fingers apply gentle anterior pressure against the clavicle.
3. Move the patient's wrist superior. The caudal hand follows the rotation of the clavicle posteriorly until tension develops. Hold this until some relaxation is noted.
4. Repeat this two or three times.

Note: This technique can be uncomfortable to those who need it the most. Please be aware of your whole patient and not just the clavicle.

Normalize Sympathetic Activity

Treatment by rib raising reduces constriction of larger lymphatic vessels. Rib raising that raises the rib heads also stimulates the thoracic sympathetic chain ganglia. This initially stimulates regional sympathetic efferent activity to organs related to that spinal level of sympathetic innervation. But in the long run, rib raising results in a prolonged reduction in sympathetic outflow from the area treated. By freeing rib motion, the excursion of the rib cage during respiration is also freed. By freeing the rib heads, the excursion of the chest during breathing is increased, and lymphatic flow is improved.

Rib Raising Seated

Patient Position
Seated on table.

Physician Position
Standing at the side of the table, facing the patient.

Procedure
1. Ask the patient to cross his or her arms and grasp the deltoid muscles.
2. Ask the patient to lean toward you resting his or her crossed arms on your chest. (A variation: patient's arms raised overhead and draped on your shoulders instead of crossed.)
3. Grasp the posterior, inferior rib angles bilaterally in the area you are treating (Fig. 68.6). (Begin cephalad, move caudad, return to cephalad.)
4. Apply a lateral traction bilaterally at the rib angle while pulling the patient toward you.
5. Have the patient breathe deeply to aid the mobilization of the entire rib cage.

Rib Raising Supine

Patient Position
Supine.

Physician Position
Standing or seated at the patient's side.

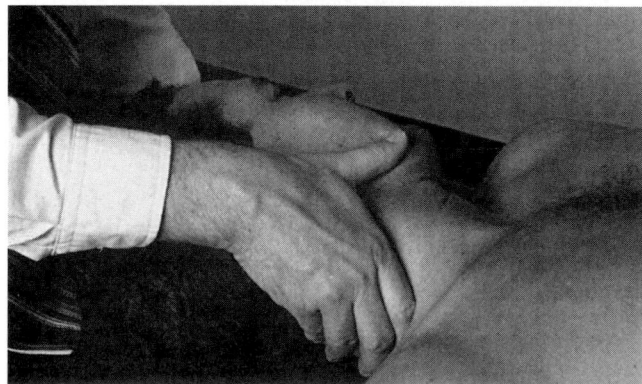

FIGURE 68.4. Thoracic inlet: rotation.

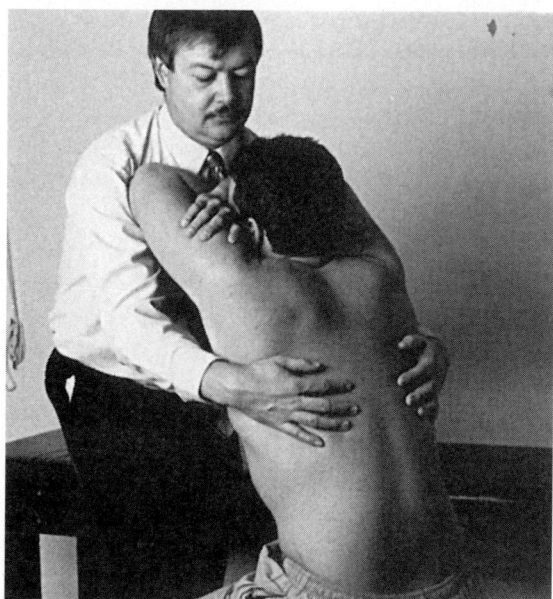

FIGURE 68.6. Rib raising: seated.

Procedure

1. Place your hands (palms) under the patient's thorax, contacting the rib angles with the pads of your fingers (Fig. 68.7).
2. Flex your fingers to achieve contact with the rib angle and the patient's posterior thorax.
3. Apply traction on the rib angle.
4. While maintaining traction, bend your knees and lower your trunk to raise the ribs by moving your hands upward. This is a fulcrum/lever action. Do not bend your wrists. (Particularly if the patient is in a hospital bed, it is easier to move your hands upward if you reciprocally push your forearms down.)
5. Move your hands to subsequent rib angles until all ribs are treated.
6. Treat the opposite side of the rib cage in the same manner.

Note: If you have an assistant, a two-person technique can be used treating both sides of the rib cage at once. Care must be

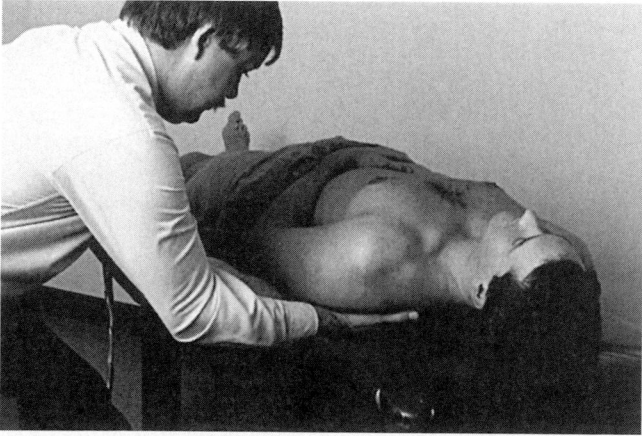

FIGURE 68.7. Rib raising: supine.

taken to treat both sides of the rib cage with equal traction, and motions of the operators must be synchronous.

Improve Extrinsic Lymphatic Pump

Osteopathic manipulative techniques affect diaphragms so that they can more efficiently create alternating pressure gradients. This can usually be done most time-efficiently if the abdominal diaphragm's muscular attachments are first treated for maximal structure-function; cervical somatic dysfunction should also be treated because this is the region associated with the diaphragm's innervation. The thoracoabdominal diaphragm is a strong muscular structure innervated by the phrenic nerve (C3-5). Tension in this structure produces substantial alterations in lymphatic flow.

The body is constructed in such a fashion that lymph flow predominately runs in a longitudinal plane. At several significant regions, however, horizontal tissues transect this pattern. Should these horizontal tissues be placed on tension for any reason, lymph flow could be significantly impeded. Osteopathic physicians have long considered that there are four of these regions:

Abdominal diaphragm: located between the abdomen and the chest cavity, it is muscular and tendinous in nature, forming a continuous sheet interrupted only by the aorta, esophagus, inferior vena cava, and accompanying blood vessels, lymphatics, and nerves.

Thoracic inlet or outlet: these are located in the cervicothoracic region.

Tentorium cerebelli: this diaphragm affects venous return from the brain because the brain has no lymphatic system and relies on the veins to perform both functions.

Pelvic diaphragm: this is a group of muscles and fascia that span the perineum and form a lower border to the abdominal cavity. Some writers describe a fifth diaphragm, the paired arches of the feet; a collapse of the pedal arches can profoundly affect the pelvic diaphragm.

Dome Abdominal Diaphragm

Doming the diaphragm is a term used to refer to relaxing the resting state of the abdominal diaphragm (or the pelvic diaphragm). If the diaphragm can be completely relaxed and well-domed, its contraction and relaxation produce greater pressure gradients between the thoracic and abdominal cavities, along with the one-way valves, and promotes better lymphatic drainage back into venous circulation. The pressure gradients act as an extrinsic pump for the lymphatic system. The doming techniques may also directly engage the inferior surface of the diaphragm and augment its excursion during expiration.

Thoracoabdominal Diaphragm

Diagnosis of Fascial Restriction at the Thoracoabdominal Diaphragm

Procedure

1. Place the palmar surfaces of your hands on the right and left side of the lower rib cage of the patient, with the fingers pointing toward the table (Fig. 68.8).

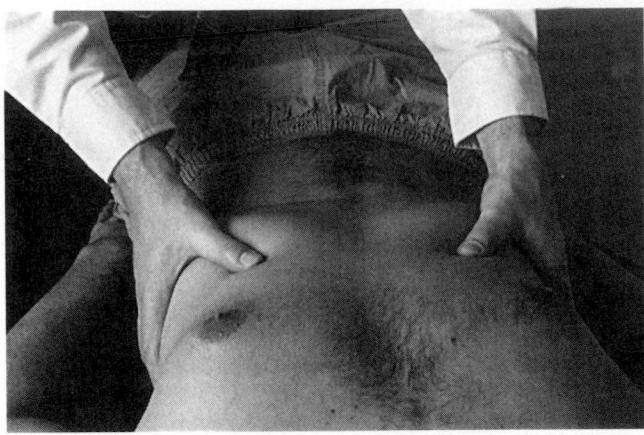

FIGURE 68.8. Diagnosis of thoracoabdominal restriction.

2. Rotate the tissues of the thoracoabdominal cylinder to the right and then to the left about a vertical axis, to test the ease of or restriction to rotatory motion.
3. This region can then also be tested for side-bending preference by inducing translation of the region in each direction.

Treatment examples for thoracic diaphragm dysfunction point out a problem: fasciae at the thoracoabdominal diaphragm prefer to rotate to the left side.

Thoracic Diaphragmatic Fascial Release: Direct Method

Patient Position
Supine on the table.

Physician Position
Standing beside the table.

Procedure
1. Rotate the tissues of the thoracoabdominal region (tube) in the direction of their restriction; rotate to the restrictive barrier (Fig. 68.9).
2. Hold there and ask the patient to take a deep breath in and out through the mouth. Notice the side of greatest movement and the side of least movement.

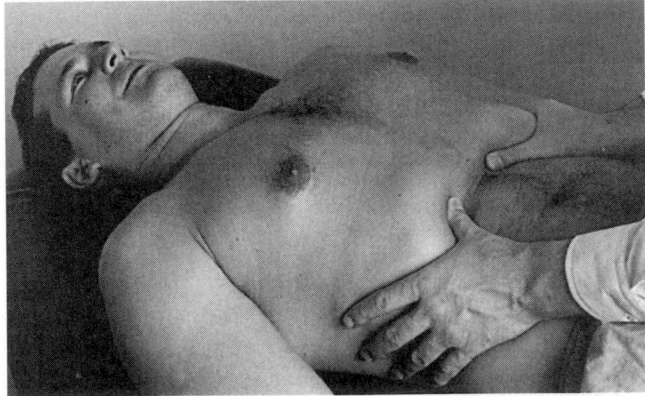

FIGURE 68.9. Direct fascial release of thoracic diaphragm.

3. Maintain the rotation but adjust tension through your hands to produce a vertical shearing force on the thoracoabdominal tube, and ask the patient to repeat the big breath in and out through the mouth.
4. Adjust the tensions through your hands until there is equal excursion produced by the right and the left side of the thoracoabdominal diaphragm.
5. Hold those vectors while the patient breathes deeply two or three times.
6. Return the patient to neutral and retest rotational preference of the tissues of the thoracoabdominal region.

Thoracic Diaphragmatic Fascial Release: Myofascial

Patient Position
Seated, erect and not slumped; the patient may relax but not collapse.

Physician Position
Standing behind the patient.

Procedure
1. Pass your hands around the thoracic cage (under the patient's arms) and gently but firmly introduce your fingers underneath the costal margin.
2. Test for motion by passively rotating the thorax to the left and to the right. Determine (in one cycle of motion testing) in which direction there is greater freedom/ease of motion.
3. Treatment phase: with the fingers on the diaphragm (i.e., underneath the costal margin), carry the thorax in the direction toward which it moves more freely. Hold it in that position. Follow it as it goes through its fascial release (unwinds) and continue until it finally settles down into a free, gentle, rhythmic, vertical motion.
4. Retest the range of motion and evaluate treatment effectiveness.

Dome Abdominal Diaphragm: Direct Mechanical

Patient Position
Supine.

Physician Position
Standing at the patient's side.

Procedure
1. Place fingers on the outer aspect of the inferior border of the ribs with thumbs pointed toward each other medially and positioned directly caudad to the xiphoid process of the sternum.
2. On the first respiration, gently press downward with thumbs toward the table as the patient exhales; follow the diaphragm motion.
3. Hold this end position (barrier); the patient inhales again. (Note: The thumbs will sense resistance to respiration.)
4. On the second exhalation, press in further downward toward the table, following the diaphragm.
5. Repeat step three.

6. On the third exhalation, press the thumbs cephalad following the superior course of the diaphragm.

Dome Pelvic Diaphragm

The pelvic diaphragm is a muscular sling located on the bony floor of the true pelvis that provides support for the pelvic organs. It is composed of two main muscles, the coccygeus muscle and the levator ani muscle. The coccygeus muscle attaches to the ischial spine and then to the sacrum and coccyx. The levator ani muscle is subdivided into two main parts according to its attachments to the innominate bone. The various muscles are as follows:

Iliococcygeus muscle: attaches to the iliac bone and the tendinous arch of the obturator internus to the coccyx and the anococcygeal ligament

Pubococcygeus muscle: attaches to the pubic bone and then to the coccyx and the midline structures of the perineum; it can be divided into three attachments according to attachments to the midline structures

Pubococcygeus proper muscle: pubic bone to the coccyx and anococcygeal ligament

Puborectalis muscle: pubic bone to rectum forming a muscular sling behind the rectum near the anorectal junction

Pubovaginalis or puboprostatic muscle: pubic bone to one of these structures in the midline

Diagnosis of Pelvic Diaphragm Somatic Dysfunction

Procedure

1. To approach the pelvic diaphragm, position the patient supine and sit on the side of the pelvis to be treated. Face toward the patient's head.
2. Flex the patient's knee and hip on this side. Identify the ischial tuberosity with your outside hand. Introduce the fingers of the other hand medial to the ischial tuberosity, letting the pads of the fingers keep contact with the medial surface of the ischium. Your fingers are now pressing into the ischiorectal fossa, the inclined roof of which is the pelvic diaphragm (Fig. 68.10). (See also Chapter 57).

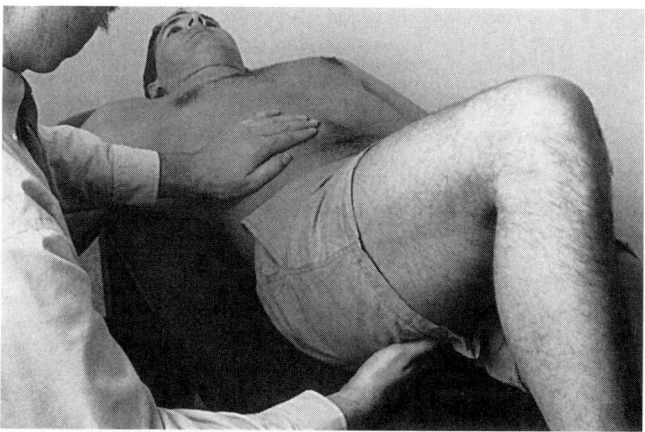

FIGURE 68.10. Dome pelvic diaphragm.

3. As the patient inhales, the pelvic diaphragm should press down on your fingertips. With exhalation, the pelvic diaphragm should move cephalically.
4. If the pelvic diaphragm is unable to descend, it is in an exhalation somatic dysfunction and is restricted in its inhalation phase. If it does not ascend well, it is in an inhalation somatic dysfunction and is restricted in its exhalation phase.

Dome Exhalation Pelvic Diaphragm: Indirect Method

Diagnosis
The pelvic diaphragm is in a cephalad position and does not descend during inhalation.

Patient Position
Supine, with knee and hip flexed on the side to be treated.

Physician Position
Sitting by the table on the side of the pelvis to be treated.

Procedure

1. With the hand closest to the patient, introduce the fingers as described above into the ischiorectal fossa. Place the other hand just below the costal margin on the same side to monitor movement of the thoracic diaphragm.
2. Ask the patient to take a deep inhalation, then exhale to the limit and hold the exhalation until forced to breathe. Repeat this procedure two or three times.
3. Recheck pelvic diaphragmatic tension.
4. Repeat treatment until both the thoracic and pelvic diaphragm come into phase with good amplitude (i.e., descend and ascend together).

Dome Inhalation Pelvic Diaphragm: Indirect Method

Diagnosis
The pelvic diaphragm is in an inferior position and does not ascend in exhalation.

Patient Position
Supine, with knee and hip flexed on the side to be treated.

Physician Position
Sitting by the table on the side of the pelvis to be treated.

Procedure

1. Instruct the patient to hold his or her breath to the limit in inhalation. The pelvic diaphragm begins to ascend a moment before forced exhalation occurs.
2. The procedure may need to be repeated two or three times.

Dome Inhalation Pelvic Diaphragm: Direct Method

Diagnosis
The pelvic diaphragm has descended and is restricted in moving superiorly into an inhalation position.

Patient Position

Supine, with knee and hip flexed on the side to be treated.

Physician Position

Sitting by the table on the side of the pelvis to be treated.

Procedure

1. Use the same hand placements as above.
2. Ask the patient to inhale, then exhale. With exhalation, encourage the diaphragm to move superiorly into its exhalation phase by providing fingertip pressure in a cephalic direction.
3. Maintain this position. Ask the patient to inhale. Be sure to hold ground, not allowing the pelvic diaphragm to descend.
4. As the patient exhales a second time, follow the diaphragm cephalically even more.
5. Repeat the treatment until both the thoracic and pelvic diaphragm come into phase with good amplitude (i.e., descend and ascend together).

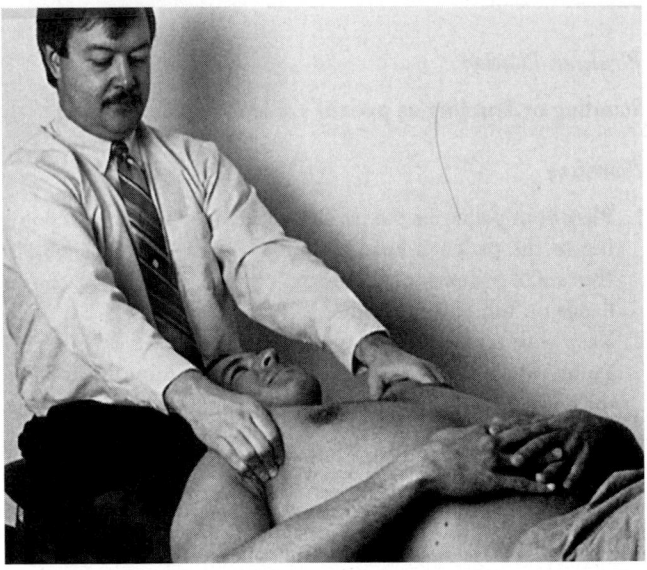

FIGURE 68.11. Pectoral traction.

TECHNIQUES TO PROMOTE LYMPHATIC FLOW

Pump Techniques

Lymphatic pump techniques are techniques designed to augment the pressure gradients that develop between the thoracic and abdominal regions during normal respiration. Some techniques are rhythmic; some are continuous. Some of the techniques influence the negative intrathoracic pressure of the thorax and some affect the abdominal pressure gradient.

Pectoral Traction

Pectoral traction influences lymph flow by means of influencing the pectoralis minor muscle. By exerting a cephalic traction on the pectoralis minor, the range of motion of the first six ribs is augmented during inhalation, thereby increasing the negative pressure in the thorax, as well as the volume of the chest. It is estimated that a 1-cm increase in the diameter of the chest increases the intake of air by 200 to 400 cc (16). This is an efficacious technique that can be used with relative ease for patients with brittle bones, patients in the intensive care unit where multiple tubes and monitoring devices may be in place, and postsurgical patients.

Patient Position

Supine.

Physician Position

Standing at the head of the patient.

Procedure

1. Gently grasp the inferior border of the pectoralis muscles of each anterior axilla in a meat hook fashion, taking care not to gouge with the fingertips (Fig. 68.11).
2. With your arms fully extended, apply a bilateral cephalad traction. (Lean back, using your body to produce the traction.)

3. While maintaining traction, have the patient breathe deeply. The combination of traction and respiratory motion releases the upper thoracic muscle tension.

Thoracic Pump

Thoracic pump techniques, like pectoral traction, affect the intrathoracic pressure gradients by augmenting the thoracic range of motion and also by increasing expiratory efficacy. These techniques are indicated as initial treatments for clearing the thoracic duct region and are also especially effective for patients with chronic obstructive pulmonary disease (COPD), upper and lower respiratory infections, mastitis, or swollen upper extremities, and for postsurgical reduction of respiratory volume. Preliminary studies and a long history of clinical efficacy suggest that lymphatic pump techniques enhance immune function (17).

Contraindications to these (and rib raising) techniques include:

1. Thoracic cage bony derangements: fractures, dislocations, and osteoporosis (relative contraindication).
2. Malignancy of the lymphatic system.
3. Use caution in patients with a decreased cough reflex.

Repetitive (Classic) Thoracic Pump

Patient Position

Supine. Caution: be sure that the patient does not have any food, gum, or foreign body (loose dentures, etc.) in the mouth.

Physician Position

Standing at the head of the table.

Procedure

1. Place your hands on the patient's thoracic wall with the thenar eminence of each hand over the pectoralis muscles, just distal

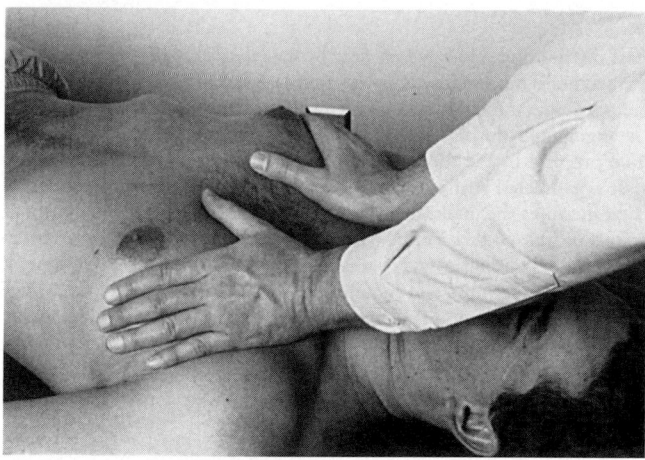

FIGURE 68.12. Thoracic pump.

to the respective clavicle; fingers are spread and angled toward the sides of the patient's body. The heels of the hands are on ribs 2 through 4 (Fig. 68.12). (With females it is important not to apply heavy pressure to the breast, but gentle pressure can assist in lymphatic drainage of congested breasts.)

2. A rhythmic pumping action is induced by alternating pressure and release through the physician's hands at a rate of approximately 110 to 120 times/minute. The motion is generated through a slight extension/flexion of the elbows, with forearm, wrist, and hand acting as a fixed lever.

3. The rate of pumping action should be in sync with the natural response of the patient's body tissues; during this rhythmic treatment, the patient continues to breathe as usual.

Thoracic Pump Variation of Activation

Patient Position
Supine. Be sure that the patient does not have any food, gum, or foreign body (loose dentures, etc.) in the mouth.

Physician Position
Standing at the head of the table.

Procedure
1. Position hands the same as in the first step of the classic pump technique.
2. Have the patient breathe in deeply with the mouth open. As the patient exhales, and with your elbows straight, follow the exhalation motion downward and maintain the end point. This applies a compressive force. With each subsequent breath, follow the exhalation motion downward, increasing the intrathoracic pressure with each exhalation.
3. One-third of the way through the fourth or fifth inhalation, as the patient's inhalation is creating a negative intrathoracic pressure within the thoracic cavity, briskly remove your hands. This will suddenly release the pressure from the chest, and you will hear suction or vacuum release as air rushes into the lungs.
4. The rate of pumping action should be in sync with the natural response of the patient's body tissues.

Abdominal and Pedal Pumps

The abdominal and pedal pumps work by intermittently pushing the abdominal contents up against the diaphragm, therefore indirectly affecting intrathoracic/abdominal pressure gradients. These techniques also indirectly massage the thoracic duct at its origin in the cisterna chyli.

Indications

1. Congestive heart failure (CHF)
2. Infective processes (in these patients, it may increase immune competence)
3. Upper respiratory tract infection, asthma, and COPD
4. Restricted mobility of the lumbar spine and thoracic cage
5. Hiatal hernia
6. Upper and lower GI dysfunction

Contraindications

1. Thoracic cage mechanical derangements: fracture, dislocation
2. Traumatic disruption of liver, spleen, or adjacent organs
3. Recent surgery to gallbladder or other adjacent organs
4. A full stomach (postprandial)

Abdominal Pump

Patient Position
Supine.

Physician Position
Standing or kneeling at patient's side (on table).

Procedure
1. Place your palms on the patient's abdomen with your fingers pointing to the patient's head, thumbs side by side (Fig. 68.13). (For small patients, or for greater control, you may place your hands on top of one another.)
2. Keep your arms extended and elbows locked.
3. Pump in a rhythmic manner. (The pumping motion is similar to the pedal or thoracic pump.) The rate should be 20 to 30 times/minute.

Pedal Pump (Dalrymple Pump)

Patient Position
Supine (or prone).

Physician Position
Standing at the patient's feet.

Procedure
1. Grasp the patient's feet and dorsiflex (Fig. 68.14).
2. Introduce a force that hyperdorsiflexes the feet. Continue the force along the longitudinal axis of the body. The force should send a wave of motion cephalad, which is followed by a

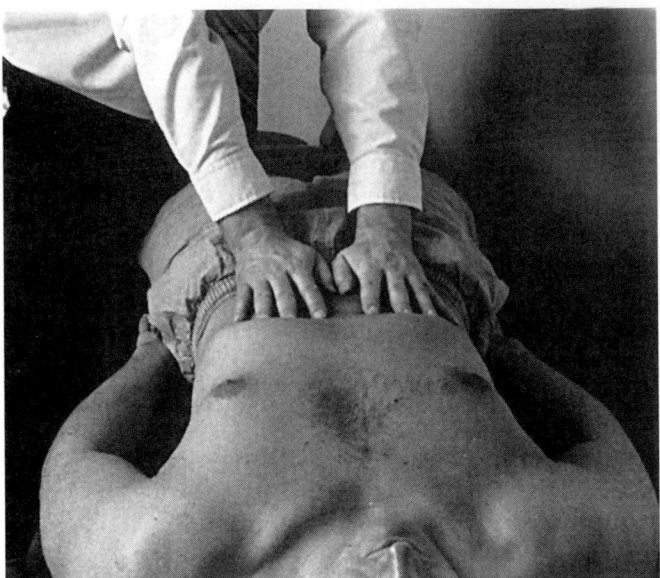

FIGURE 68.13. Abdominal pump.

rebound wave moving caudally. (Note: Use the umbilicus, an osseous landmark, or a dermal lesion to appreciate the wave motion.)

3. As the rebound wave returns to the feet, reapply the dorsiflexion force, thereby creating an oscillatory pump.

4. The above technique may also be combined with the application of force through the plantar flexed feet (Fig. 68.15), thereby stretching the anterior body wall fascial structures.

Liver and Spleen Pump Techniques

Both the liver and spleen are pressure-sensitive organs in the sense that they respond quickly to intermittently changing pressure gradients. The liver has a rich bed of lymphatic vessels, and its decongestion is postulated to aid in detoxification and in relief of visceral congestion (17). The spleen stores red and white blood cells and screens the blood of damaged cells; the spleen pump is most commonly used for patients with systemic infections and for selected anemic patients with low resistance to

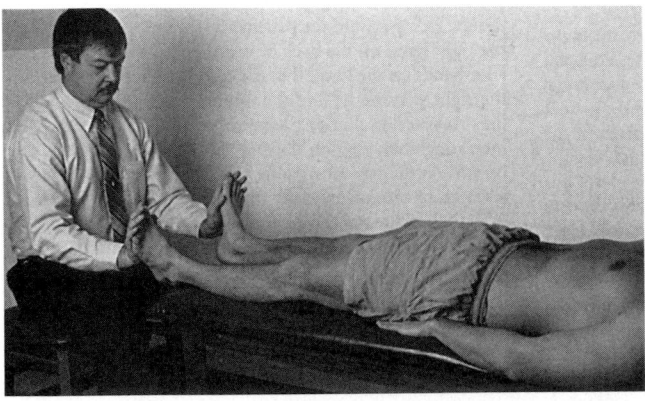

FIGURE 68.14. Pedal pump: dorsiflexion.

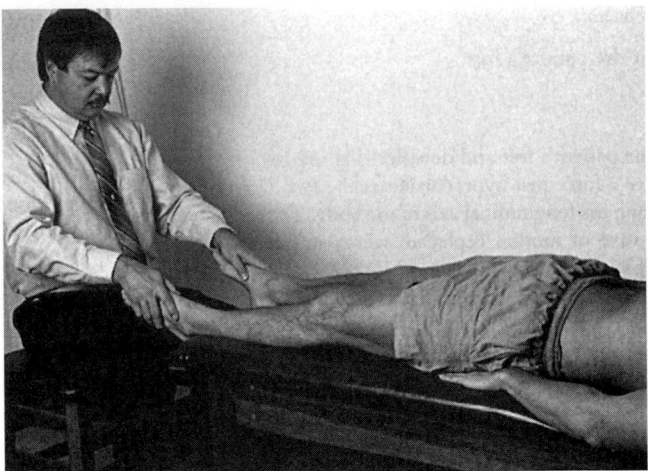

FIGURE 68.15. Pedal pump: plantar flexion.

infection. The proximity of these organs to the diaphragm and their pressure-sensitive nature suggest that this attribute may be important in the homeostatic functional mechanisms associated with these structures. Although other lymphatic pump techniques and diaphragm techniques indirectly or secondarily enhance pressure gradients affecting the liver and spleen, these pumps have long been available in the osteopathic armamentarium and are specifically designed for the liver and spleen.

Indications

1. Passive congestion of liver or spleen
2. Congestive heart failure (especially right-sided failure)
3. Consider in patients with infective processes (may increase immune competence)
4. Consider in patients with parenchymal disease of liver or spleen (may affect disease process by modulating blood and lymph fluid dynamics)

Contraindications

1. Thoracic cage mechanical derangements: fracture, dislocation
2. Lymphatic system malignancy
3. Traumatic disruption of liver, spleen, or adjacent organs
4. Acute hepatitis
5. Friable hepatomegaly, as in infectious mononucleosis

Lymphatic Drainage of the Liver ("Liver Quiver")

Stand on the right side of the supine patient, beside the lower thorax facing the head (Fig. 68.16). Pass the left hand underneath the lower ribs and the right hand on the abdominal wall immediately below the costal margin. Request the patient to take a deep breath and identify the inferior border of the liver with the tips of the fingers of the right hand. As the exhalation occurs, the fingers penetrate over the liver and underneath the thoracic cage. Again, a deep breath; this time, as the breath goes out, use a vibratory motion of the right hand on the liver. This may be

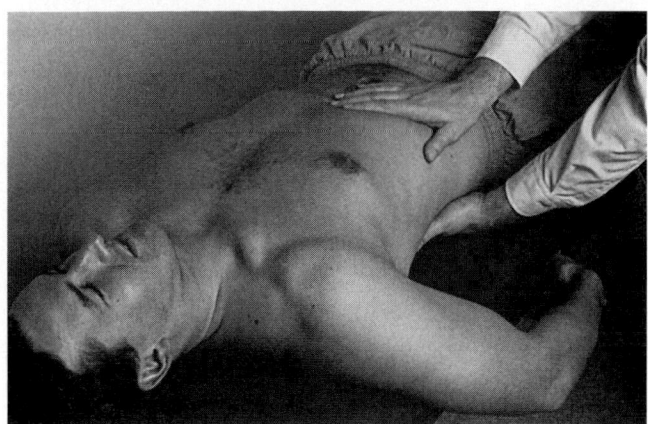

FIGURE 68.16. Liver drainage.

done three or four times; each time penetrate a little deeper into the area underneath the costal margin in relation to the liver.

Liver/Spleen Pump

An alternative technique for the liver pump is performed with the patient lying on the left side with the hips and knees flexed to stabilize the body (Fig. 68.17). Sit on the table behind the thorax, facing the patient's feet. Ask the patient to place his or her right hand on the back of your right shoulder. Place both your hands on the lower thoracic cage, the left hand anteriorly, the right posteriorly, and the thumbs meeting in the axillary line. As you lean slightly backward, open up the rib cage while increasing abduction on the arm, and ask the patient to take a deep breath. As the patient exhales, lean on the thoracic cage with a vibratory motion to apply the pumping action to the liver. A similar technique can be used for the splenic area with the patient lying on the right side while you sit behind the patient on the left side of the table.

Direct Pressure Techniques to Move Lymph

Direct pressure techniques exert their influence by extrinsically increasing pressure on the lymphatic vessels. This extrinsic pressure facilitates movements of lymph into segmental regions of the lymphatic channel that, in turn, dilate the lymph vessel and invoke the intrinsic pressure of the lymphatic conduit via contraction of the smooth muscle within the lymph channel and the myoendothelial fibers within the lymph capillaries. This is especially effective for locally decongesting tissues.

Effleurage is defined in the *Glossary of Osteopathic Terminology* as "light or deep stroking of the skin toward the heart from any place in the body to force fluids through lymphatic vessels." Petrissage is defined as "deep kneading or squeezing action to express swelling."

Head Effleurage Mandibular Technique (Galbraith Technique) (4)

Patient Position
Supine (Fig. 68.18).

Physician Position
Standing beside the patient.

Procedure
1. Rotate the patient's head to face you.
2. With your right hand, place your fingers at the temporomandibular joint and your thenar eminence along the ramus of the mandible as shown in Figure 68.18.
3. Apply a repetitive, downward traction on the mandible. Anterior and medial motion should be done slowly.

Submandibular Technique

Patient Position
Seated.

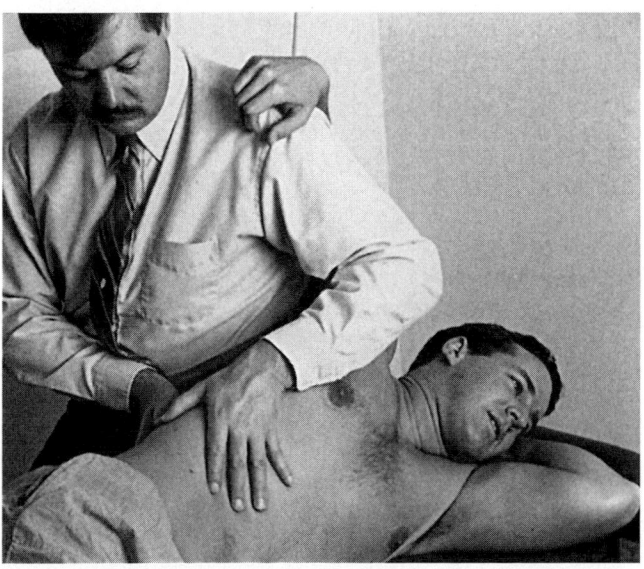

FIGURE 68.17. Liver drainage: alternative method.

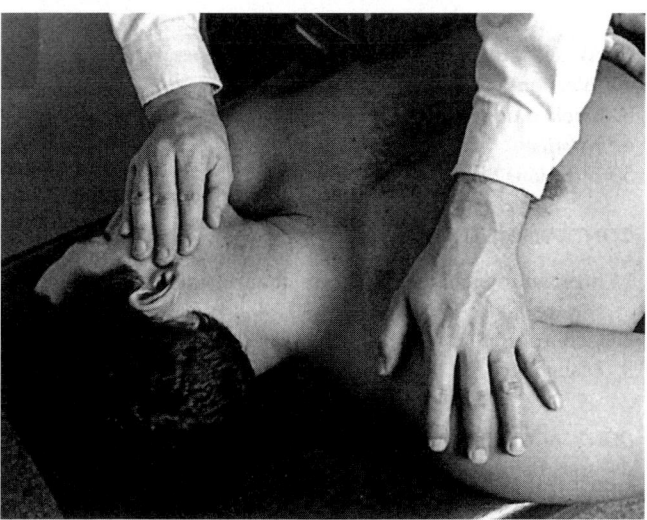

FIGURE 68.18. Mandibular technique: supine.

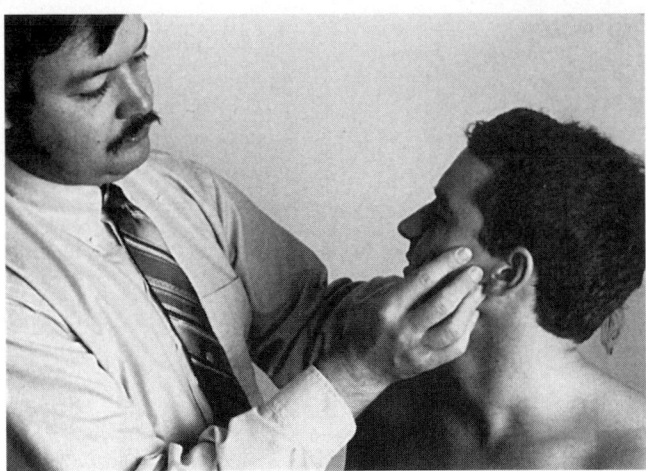

FIGURE 68.19. Mandibular drainage: seated.

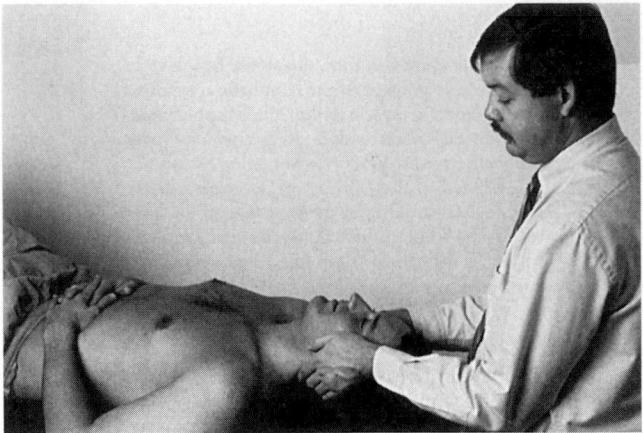

FIGURE 68.20. Cervical stroking.

Physician Position
Standing.

Procedure
1. Start at the angle of the jaw (Fig. 68.19).
2. Use the palmar aspect of the fingertips and walk your fingers medially on the inferior mandibular line until you reach the chin.
3. The fingertips make contact with the submandibular nodes using a gentle vertical karate-chop motion.

Preauricular and Postauricular Node

Patient Position
Seated.

Physician Position
Standing behind patient (may be performed in front of patient).

Procedure
1. The preauricular and postauricular nodes are situated in front of and behind the ear.
2. Spreads your fingers and contact the lateral side of the head so that the index fingers contact the postauricular node and the third fingers contact the preauricular node.
3. Apply a rotary motion both in clockwise and counterclockwise directions over the ear.

Cervical Soft Tissue

Indications

1. As an initial central lymphatic treatment to be followed by peripheral lymphatic treatments
2. As an integrated treatment for an upper respiratory tract infection
3. Swollen upper extremities
4. Mastitis
5. Infections of the HEENT system

Contraindications

1. Structural derangement, bony abnormalities, or fractures in the area to be treated
2. Cervical ribs
3. Malignancy

Cervical Stroking

Cervical stroking is a method of stretching the muscle groups surrounding the cervical vertebrae.

Patient Position
Supine.

Physician Position
Standing or seated at the head of the table.

Procedure
1. Place your hands along the paravertebral muscles (Fig. 68.20).
2. Slowly stroke these muscles in a cephalic direction, not letting the muscles slip, but giving the muscles a good stretch.

Anterior Cervical Traction

Patient Position
Supine.

Physician Position
Standing or seated at the head of the patient.

Procedure
1. Locate the anterior and posterior border of the inferior portion of the sternocleidomastoid (SCM) muscle. Place your thumb along the anterior margin, and second through fifth digits along the posterior margin (Fig. 68.21).
2. Beginning in the lower portion of the SCM and anterior cervical fascia, gently lift anteriorly and laterally until you note relaxation.

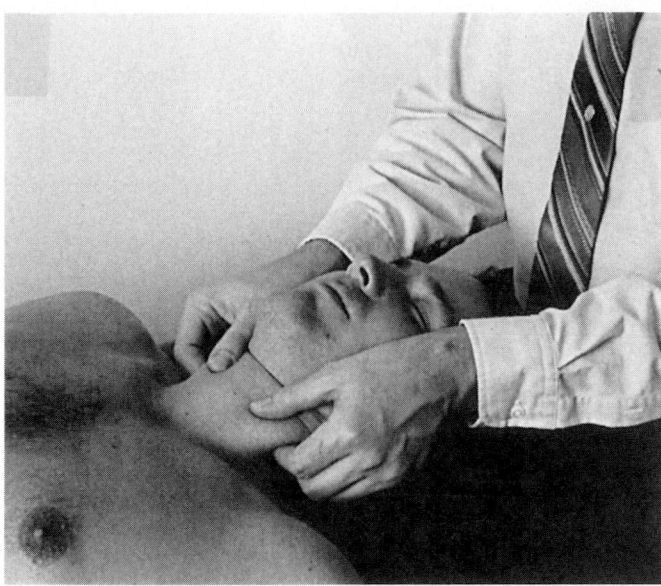

FIGURE 68.21. Anterior cervical traction.

3. Move superiorly to the middle portion, and repeat again on the superior portion. This procedure may be repeated up to three times.

Suprahyoid and Infrahyoid Node Technique

Patient Position
Prone (must allow the hyoid to fall forward off the nodes, which are located superior and inferior to the hyoid bone).

Physician Position
Standing.

Procedure
1. Place your fingers on the lateral aspect of the hyoid bone (Fig. 68.22).
2. Gently move the hyoid bone from side to side four or five times.
3. If notable restriction continues, gently position the hyoid by translating it to the soft tissue barrier and ask the patient to swallow as you maintain the resistance.

Anterior Tracheal Technique

Patient Position
Seated or supine.

Physician Position
Standing in front of the patient.

Procedure
1. Place your fingers along the lateral borders of the trachea. Move the trachea from side to side (Fig. 68.23).
2. Move lymph in the cervical region in a downward fashion toward the thorax.

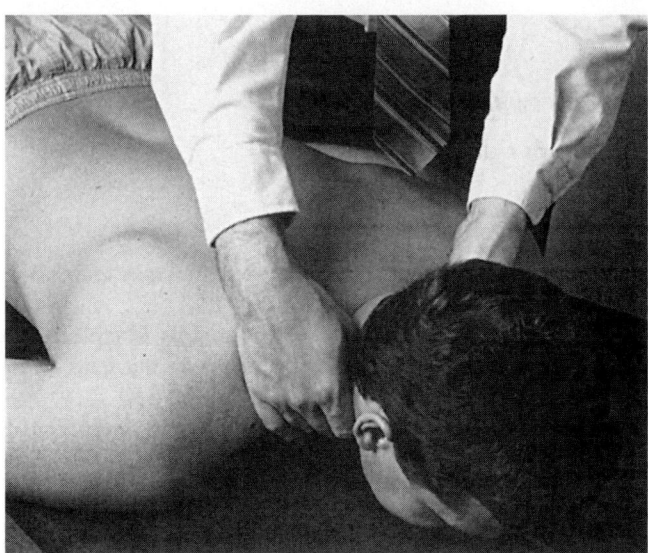

FIGURE 68.22. Suprahyoid and infrahyoid node technique.

Thoracic Soft Tissue

See Chapter 55, Articulatory Techniques, on rib raising.

Abdominal

Manipulative techniques can be used in the abdominopelvic region to reduce congestion and improve circulation to the abdominal and/or pelvic viscera. Mesenteric lift techniques involve careful hand positioning to apply direct pressures in directions that take stress off of the mesenteries and/or ligaments supporting that organ. Barral (18) describes release techniques for each abdominopelvic organ; his work is highlighted in the *Foundations* chapter authored by Ken Lossing. Visceroptosis, most commonly resulting from upright postural problems, is a major cause of congestion in the abdominopelvic organs. Treatment improves organ function and can decrease many functional visceral symptoms, including bloating, constipation, and pelvic or abdominal pain.

Application of this principle can be seen with the following mesenteric lift techniques (17). The small intestines have an

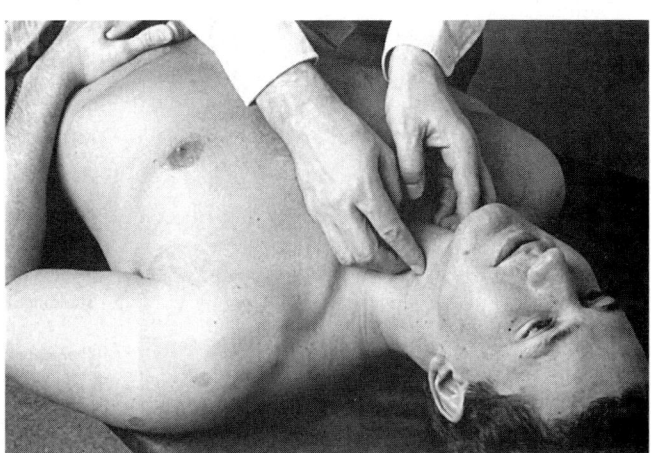

FIGURE 68.23. Anterior tracheal technique.

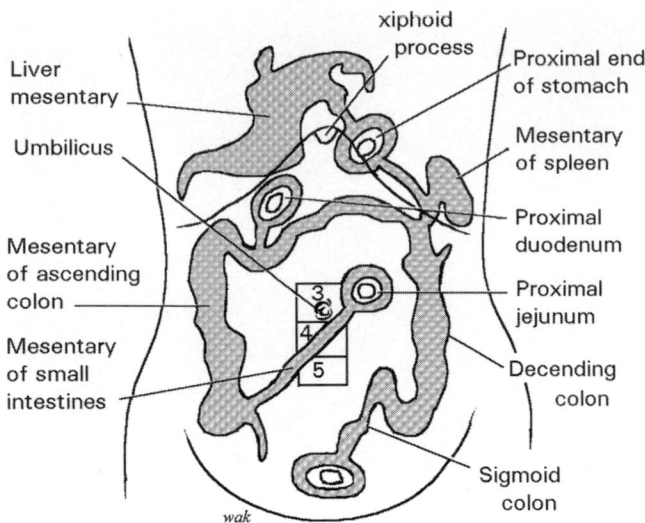

FIGURE 68.24. Mesenteric attachments. (Illustration by W. A. Kuchera.)

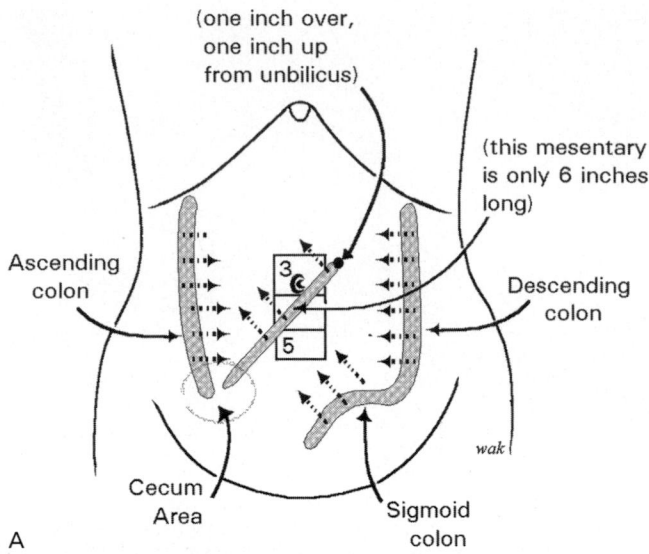

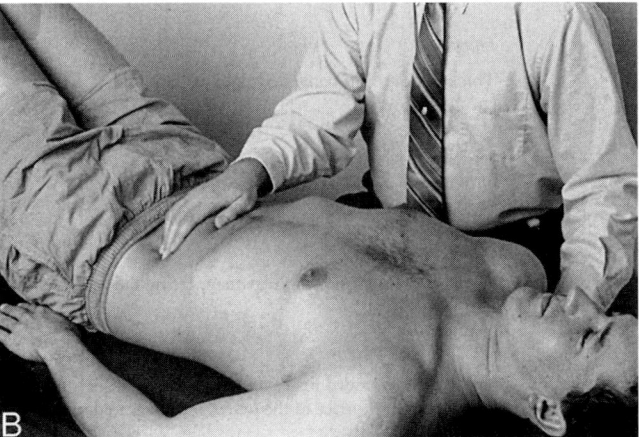

FIGURE 68.25. A: Direction for tissue treatment of intestinal mesenteries. (Illustration by W. A. Kuchera.) **B:** Mesenteric lift: small intestine.

interesting anatomic relationship to its mesentery (Fig. 68.24). The small intestines hang from a 6-inch mesenteric attachment located under a line from a point approximately 1 inch to the left and 1 inch above the umbilicus to the lower right quadrant of the abdomen just anterior to the right sacroiliac joint and the cecum.

Mesenteric Lift: Small Intestines

Patient Position
Supine.

Physician Position
At the patient's right side.

Procedure
1. To relax the abdomen, bend the patient's knees with his or her feet placed on the table or bed.
2. Gently apply your fingers from the middle interphalangeal joints to the finger pads into the left lower quadrant of the abdomen.
3. Gently scoop the abdominal wall and underlying loops of small intestine toward their mesenteric attachment (Fig. 68.25). Do not force tissues or cause pain.
4. It is often helpful to gently turn the tissues in slight clockwise or counterclockwise directions for maximal tissue freedom.
5. Hold the tissues until a sense of relaxation is palpated, or hold for approximately 90 seconds to allow time for visceral tissues to decongest.

Mesenteric Lift: Cecum

Patient Position
Supine.

Physician Position
At the patient's right side.

Procedure
1. To relax the abdomen, bend the patient's right knee with that foot placed on the table or bed.
2. Gently apply the heel of your right hand to the inferior portion of the right lower quadrant of the abdomen.
3. Gently lift the cecum superiorly away from any pelvic entrapment by pushing toward the hepatic flexure of the colon (Fig. 68.26).
4. Hold the tissues until a sense of relaxation is palpated, or hold for approximately 90 seconds to allow time for visceral tissues to decongest.

Petrissage with Cough Activation: Abdominal Scars

Throughout the body, petrissage and deep friction soft tissue techniques can also be used to break down connective tissue impediments to lymphatic drainage and free movement between adjacent fasciae (Fig. 68.27). In the case of an abdominal scar where superficial tissue restricts complete motion between the region of the scar and deeper fascial layers, the fasciae associated

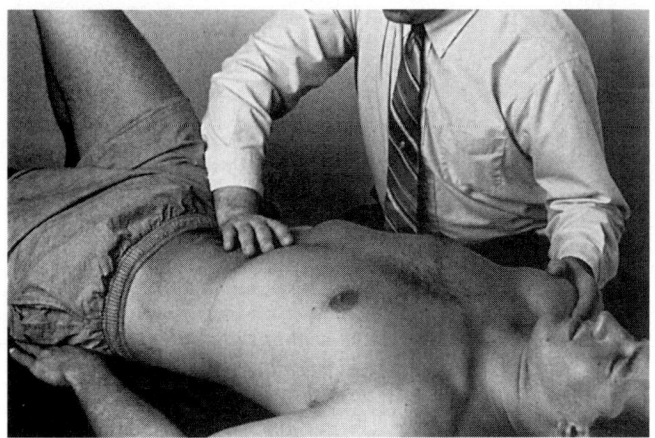

FIGURE 68.26. Mesenteric lift: cecum.

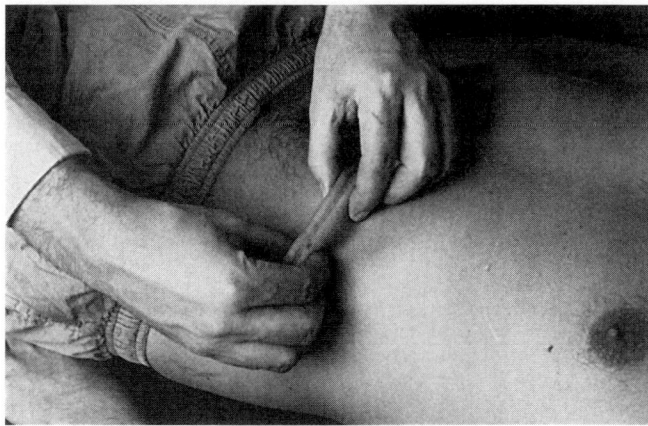

FIGURE 68.28. Abdominal scar: treatment.

with the scar can be treated with gentle petrissage and a cough activation to improve mobility in the region and to subsequently improve lymphatic flow. This technique should be used only in well-healed scars where restriction of motion between fascial layers is noted. This can be evaluated by gently attempting to move the scar in various directions on the abdomen and either sensing restriction or observing fascial dimpling/retraction adjacent to the scar at the end of motion testing.

Patient Position
Supine.

Physician Position
At the patient's side.

Procedure
1. Gently grasp the abdominal scar between the thumb(s) and fingers. Include some of the nearby adjacent superficial tissue.
2. Lift the scar and superficial tissues perpendicularly away from the abdomen to tissue tension (Fig. 68.28).
3. Now take the scar and superficial tissues in the direction of restricted motion to tissue tension.

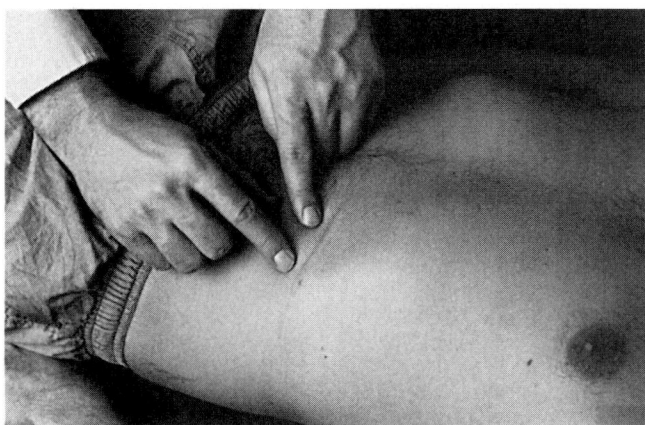

FIGURE 68.27. Abdominal scar: identification.

4. Ask the patient to cough deeply enough to feel the deeper fascia of the abdominal wall pull into the scar that you are holding, but not so deep that you cause discomfort.
5. Recheck and repeat in any other direction where restriction is palpated.
6. This technique can be taught to the patient to perform at home.

Extremities

Indications

1. Edema
2. Infection
3. Lymphatic stripping (especially postmastectomy)

Contraindications

1. Fracture
2. Friable skin or stasis ulcers (for example, from diabetes)
3. Malignancy

Posterior Axillary Fold Technique

This technique is related to ipsilateral upper extremity congestion.

Diagnosis
Thick, tender, and congested right axillary fold.

Patient Position
Supine.

Physician Position
Seated at the right side of the patient facing the patient's head.

Procedure
1. Place the extended fingers of your right hand high up under the posterior surface of the posterior axillary fold with the index finger next to the patient's chest cage. Place your right

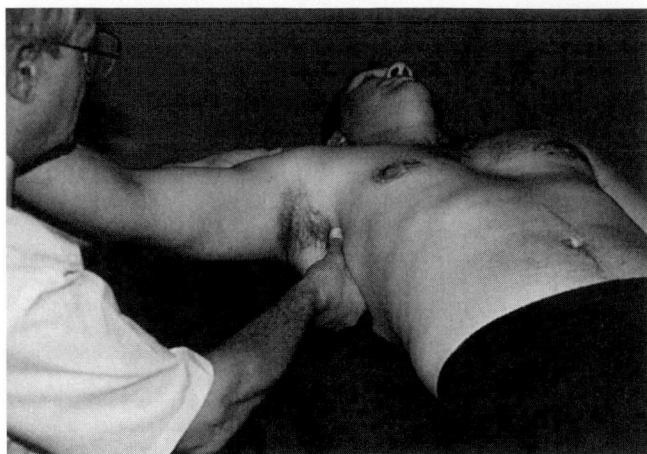

FIGURE 68.29. Posterior axillary fold technique.

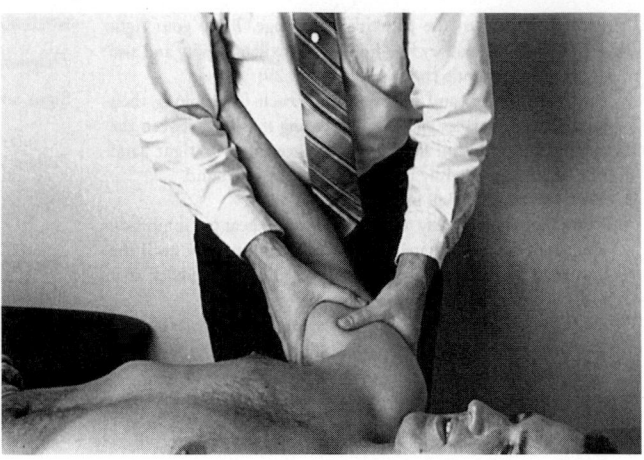

FIGURE 68.30. Effleurage and petrissage: upper extremity.

thumb over the axillary fold high in the axillary cavity and also next to the patient's chest wall (Fig. 68.29).

2. Bring the thumb and fingers toward each other along their longitudinal surfaces chest wall, creating tension between the extended thumb and fingers. The fingers of your right hand can be strengthened by the fingers of your left hand.

3. Hold the compression until the tissues relax.

4. Move the grip inferiorly to a new area and repeat the inhibition if signs of congestion are found. Continue caudally until the border of the latissimus muscle disappears over the back as it progresses medially toward the spine.

Effleurage and Petrissage: Upper Extremity

Diagnosis
Signs and symptoms of a congested right upper extremity.

Patient Position
Supine.

Physician Position
Seated at the right side of the patient facing the patient's head.

Procedure
1. Tuck the patient's right hand into your right axilla and hold it there.

2. Grasp the upper arm close to the shoulder, and with a hand on either side of the limb, apply a wringing motion, moving from proximal to distal (Fig. 68.30).

3. When the second step is completed, start closer to the elbow with the wringing motion, and again move distally.

4. Continue this process of lymphatic movement an additional three or four times or until adequate drainage has been achieved in the arm.

5. When step four is completed, go to the forearm, placing your thumbs on the ventral surface between the flexor and extensor muscle masses and the rest of your digits around the other side. Squeeze the muscle masses simultaneously, and then relax.

6. Repeat this process again, moving from proximal to digital.

Effleurage and Petrissage: Lower Extremity

Diagnosis
Signs and symptoms of a congested right lower extremity.

Patient Position
Supine; the right knee is flexed to a right angle; the lower leg is horizontal, parallel with the table; the thigh is flexed at a right angle with the body.

Physician Position
Seated on the table facing the patient's head.

Procedure
1. Balance the patient's right leg on your shoulder.

2. Place the palmar surface of both hands on opposing sides of the proximal end of the thigh, and perform a rotatory wringing-out type of movement in a clockwise direction.

3. As tissue change takes place, move distally down the thigh toward the knee, one hand's width at a time.

4. Repeat the sequence of motions, going back again to the inguinal area and progressively moving toward the knee.

5. When the tissues have softened and there is less congestion in the thigh, move below the knee.

6. Place the hand on either side of the lower leg; with the thumbs, press deeply between and into the calf muscles, squeezing out the muscles, progressing down from the knee toward the ankle.

7. During each squeezing motion, rock your body forward and backward using your body weight to flex and extend the knee and hip in a rhythmic fashion.

Effleurage: Arms and Legs

Effleurage is the stroking of appendages from distal to proximal. This facilitates the flow of lymph to the axilla and the thorax from the upper limb and facilitates the flow of lymph to the abdomen from the lower limb.

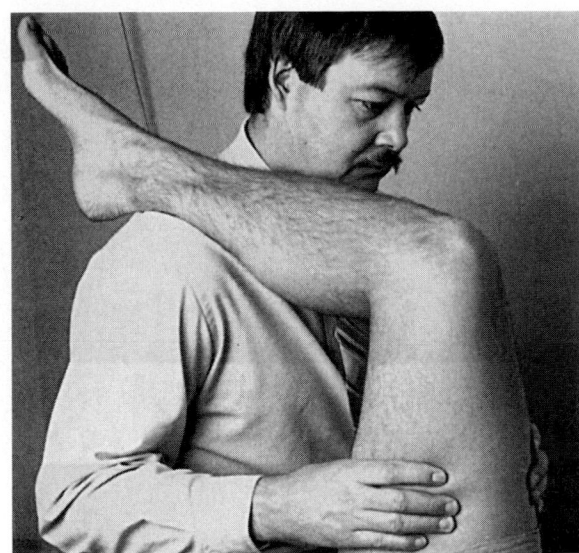

FIGURE 68.31. Effleurage: lower extremity.

Patient Position

Supine.

Physician Position

At the patient's side.

Procedure

With effleurage, you stroke the appendages from distal to proximal (Fig. 68.31) using a milking motion.

Petrissage: Arms and Legs

Petrissage is a method of draining lymph from the extremities into the thoracic duct.

Patient Position

Supine.

Physician Position

At the patient's side.

Procedure

Knead the extremity, starting distally (Fig. 68.32) and proceeding toward the trunk.

CONCLUSION

Because lymphatic function can be critically influenced and altered by extrinsic forces, osteopathic diagnosis, and manipulative treatment, use of the techniques outlined in this chapter can greatly influence lymphatic function.

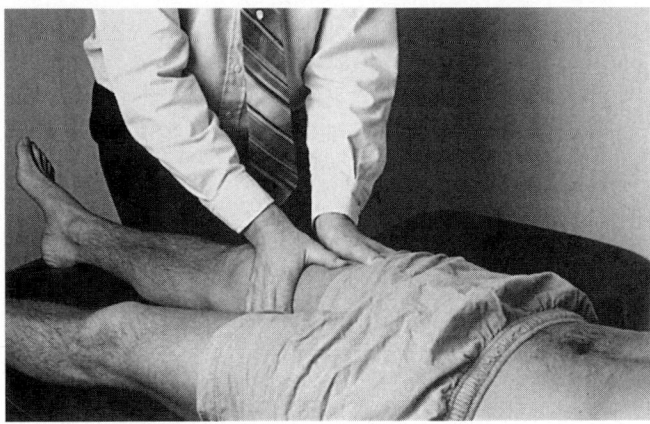

FIGURE 68.32. Petrissage: lower extremity.

REFERENCES

1. Still AT. *Philosophy of Osteopathy.* Kirksville, MO: A. T. Still; 1809:108.
2. Millard FP. *Applied Anatomy of the Lymphatics.* Kirksville, MO: The Journal Printing Company; 1922.
3. Miller CE. The lymphatic pump, its application to acute infections. *J Am Osteopath Assoc.* 1926;25:443–445.
4. Pratt-Harrington D. Galbreath technique: a manipulative treatment for otitis media revisited. *J Am Osteopath Assoc.* 2000;100:635–639.
5. Gangong WF. *Review of Medical Physiology,* 14th ed. Los Altos, CA: Lange Medical Physiology; 1989.
6. Mein EA, Richards DG, McMillin DL, et al. Physiologic regulation through manual therapy. *Phys Med Rehabil: State of the Art Rev.* 2000;14(1):27–42.
7. Williams PL, Warwick R, Dyson M, et al. *Gray's Anatomy,* 37th ed. Edinburgh, Scotland: Churchill Livingstone; 1989:841.
8. Sodeman Jr WA, Sodeman TM. Protective mechanism of the lungs; pulmonary disease; pleural disease. *Pathologic Physiology: Mechanism of Disease,* 6th ed. Philadelphia, PA: WB Saunders; 1979.
9. Guyton A. *Textbook of Medical Physiology.* Philadelphia, PA: WB Saunders; 1976.
10. Woodburne R. *Essentials of Human Anatomy,* 8th ed. New York, NY: Oxford University Press; 1988.
11. Olszewski WL, Engeset A. Intrinsic contractility of leg lymphatics in man: preliminary communication. *Lymphology.* 1979;12:81–84.
12. McPartland JM, Mein EA. Entrainment and the cranial rhythmic impulse. *Altern Ther Health Med.* 1997;3:40–44.
13. Huizinga JD, Thuneberg L, Kluppel M, et al. W/kit gene required for interstitial cells of Cajal and for intestinal pacemaker activity. *Nature.* 1995;373:347–349.
14. Masumoto K, Suita S, Nada O, et al. Abnormalities of enteric neurons, intestinal pacemaker cells, and smooth muscle in human intestinal atresia. *J Pediatr Surg.* 1999;34:1463–1468.
15. Zink G, Lawson WB. An osteopathic structural examination and functional interpretation of the soma. *Osteopath Ann.* 1979;7:12–19, 433–440.
16. Kuchera ML, Kuchera WA. *Considerations in Systemic Dysfunction.* Columbus, OH: Greyden Press; 1994:43.
17. Measel Jr JW. The effect of the lymphatic pump on the immune response: preliminary studies on the antibody response to pneumonococcal polysaccharide assayed by bacterial agglutination and passive hemagglutination. *J Am Osteopath Assoc.* 1982;82(1):22, 28–31, 59–62, 89, 219.
18. Barral JP, Mercier P. *Visceral Manipulation.* Seattle, WA: Eastland Press; 1988.

VISCERAL MANIPULATION

KENNETH LOSSING

KEY CONCEPTS

- History of visceral technique
- Theory of visceral technique
- Mobility, motility
- Visceral diagnosis
- Treatment of thorax, abdomen, and pelvis

A visceral dysfunction is impaired or altered function of related components of the visceral system, including the ligaments, fascia, lymphatic and vascular channels, neural connections, and the skeletal system. Visceral dysfunctions may be associated with local symptoms (e.g., gastroesophageal reflux disease or stress incontinence), distant symptoms (shoulder pain from gallbladder disease), or with presymptomatic strain patterns.

HISTORY

Osteopathic manipulation of the viscera began with Dr. A.T. Still. He described treating many different digestive, respiratory, and urogenital complaints (1). For Dr. Still, almost all medical conditions had an osteopathic treatment, in some cases curative, in some cases supportive. Dr. Still left few descriptions of techniques of any kind, but some of his early students, Carl McConnell (2) and E. Barber (3) did. Gaddis (4), Teal (5), Smith (6), Woodhall (7), Hover (8–10), Young (11,12), Hazzard (13), Riggs (14), Murray (15), Goetz (16), and Sutherland (17) later added to this literature. Hoover called it ventral technique, and addressed only the abdomen. Sutherland had techniques for both the pelvis and the abdomen. Woodhall's applications were gynecologic.

As the case with all clinical sciences, with time and clinical experience the knowledge base increases. The current knowledge base has expanded to include all the organs of thorax, abdomen, and pelvis. Most medical conditions and musculoskeletal pains are found to have a component that is addressable with osteopathic techniques. Other current authors and educators in visceral technique are Bensky (18), Barral (19–24), Lossing (25), Finet and Willame (26), Davidson (27), and Blackman (28).

THEORY

Visceral manipulation applies osteopathic theory and principles to the viscera, in addition to the musculoskeletal and the cranial systems. In all cases, the theory and principles remain the same; only the area of anatomy changes. The implication, of course, is that by also addressing the viscera, the osteopathic physician is able to address a larger range of medical problems.

While structural problems (like tumors) are relatively easy to document on standard medical tests, functional problems (like sustained abnormal mechanical tension) are less easy to document, but are palpable. Sustained abnormal mechanical tension in the tissues adversely affects the exchange of fluids and nutrition, overstimulates the nervous system leading to facilitation, decreases the exchange of pressures, and taxes the homeostatic mechanisms of the body. Conversely, treating the sustained abnormal mechanical tension improves neurologic exchange, improves homeostatic mechanisms, and improves exchange of fluids, nutrition, and pressures. In the case of viscera, the main tissue addressed is the attachments (ligaments, peritoneum, pleura, and mediastinum).

For many years osteopathic literature has expressed the principle that one part of the body may affect another part, and indeed the whole body. Our neurologic model describes somatosomatic reflexes, somatovisceral reflexes, viscerosomatic reflexes, and viscerovisceral reflexes (29).

Traditional osteopathic thought has always contained the idea that the intelligent physician should try to find the most primary problem, address that, and allow the body to do the rest of the job. This being the case, when the viscera are the primary problem, they should be addressed first.

Visceral diagnosis follows Dr. Still's adage that "life is motion." With each inhalation the rib cage raises, while the respiratory diaphragm, thoracic inlet, pelvic floor, and all of the viscera descend. As measured by magnetic resonance imaging (MRI) scan, the respiratory diaphragm and inferior pericardium descend by 1.5 cm with a normal volume inhalation (in approximate-vital-capacity breathing, diaphragmatic excursion increases to over 4 cm), with the inferior pericardium swinging toward the middle line (30). The superior pericardium moves much less, giving an axis of rotation near the attachment of the aorta to the heart. Obviously, this area needs to be stable.

Along with the mechanical displacement of these structures there is a corresponding change in the exchange of fluids. With inhalation, the flow of blood in the superior vena cava increases and the flow of blood in the portal vein decreases.

Respiration-induced motions of the abdominal visceral are well documented (32–34). During respiration the diaphragm and abdominal organs move cephalocaudal (more so laterally than near the midline), and anterior/posterior, as measured by MRI (31). An osteopathic perspective is that abnormal mechanical tension in these structures decreases their respiratory motion and adversely affects their function. Preliminary work has been done measuring the respiratory movements of the abdominal organs in symptom-free and symptom-present states, showing normal and abnormal axis of motion (26). The viscera are found to move, and have potential restrictions, in the same three planes of motion described for all joints and sutures.

VISCERAL DIAGNOSIS

Palpatory diagnosis should be performed both globally (to find the total body pattern), and locally. Appropriate medical tests should be ordered when indicated.

Each organ can be evaluated for motion, like all cranial and musculoskeletal structures, with:

1. Inhalation and exhalation (described as mobility by Sutherland).
2. Motion testing the attachments (see Chapter 39)
3. Sympathetic and parasympathetic connections (viscerosomatic and somatovisceral reflexes; see Chapter 6)
4. Exchange of fluids (lymphatic; see Chapter 68)
5. Inherent motion (described as motility by Sutherland)
6. Temperature changes
7. Associated musculoskeletal structures (rib cage, attachments through the posterior peritoneum to the anterior longitudinal ligament and spine, etc.)
8. Associated cranial structures (e.g., the esophagus attaches to the temporals, occiput, and sphenoid by the pharyngeal constrictor muscles; see Chapter 62)
9. Chapman reflexes (see Chapter 67)

As with all osteopathic diagnosis, the general area of the body in trouble needs to be found. One diagnostic technique (general listening) uses a fascial continuity model (see Chapter 60). Bones, muscles, blood vessels, and viscera are seen as tissues stuffed in a three-dimensional covering, the fascia. The fascia is tighter in an area of abnormal mechanical tension, and pulls into that location. With the patient's body in the standing anatomical position, the physician's hand is placed on the top of the head to feel which direction the fascia pulls. In general, an anterior pull can be from a visceral restriction, anterior rib, or sternal problem. A posterior pull indicates a spinal or dural problem. A lateral pull indicates a problem in the extremities, or the paired bilateral viscera.

Once the general area has been determined, specific localization of the restriction can be found using palpation of tissue pull in the local area (local listening). At that point, a thorough knowledge of anatomy becomes paramount. In the case of suspected visceral restrictions, the specific organ is palpated and evaluated

for motion during respiration, it is named for the direction in which it moves the easiest. Next, motion testing is performed to evaluate the distensibility of all the attachments. Inherent motion (similar, but distinctly different from the cranial rhythmic impulse) is evaluated by palpating the viscera with a hand on its longitudinal axis. The active phase (inspir) is away from the middle line, the passive phase (expir) is toward the middle line. Palpation of the specific spinal segments of sympathetic innervation will reveal any tissue texture changes (29). Areas of parasympathetic innervation, and other mechanically associated structures are also examined for tissue texture changes.

A simple test is then performed to find which of the structures is most primary by palpating two related structures and gently pressing on one to inhibit it, and see if the other responds immediately with decreased fascial tension. If this occurs, the structure is selected as the one to treat. This test is used to determine whether the problem is viscerosomatic, somatovisceral, or viscerovisceral.

TREATMENT

For a visceral problem resulting from a somatovisceral reflex, the somatic structure responsible is treated. If a visceral or somatic problem is caused from a viscerosomatic reflex, the viscera are treated. In the case of viscerovisceral reflex causing a visceral problem, both involved viscera are treated.

Once the area of the most primary problem is found, it may be addressed by a wide variety of principles and techniques, including short lever arm (direct contact), long lever arm (using a body part as a lever), indirect (in the direction of ease), and direct techniques (in the direction of tension), and various activating forces like respiratory assistance. The goal of treatment is achieving a state of balanced ligamentous tension, normal movement with respiration, balanced inherent motion, and normalization of the nervous system, along with fluid, nutrition, and pressure exchange.

ABDOMEN

The Lower Esophagus, Stomach, and Duodenum

The lower esophagus, stomach, and duodenum should be checked in cases of gastroesophageal reflux disease, gastritis, duodenitis, ulcers, hiatal hernia, and gastric ptosis.

Stomach Diagnosis (Fig. 69.1)

Step 1. The patient is supine. The physician stands to the right side.

Step 2. Place your right hand over the stomach, and point your thumb to the pylorus.

Step 3. Palpate through the skin and abdominal wall to the abdominal contents.

Step 4. Check the fascial pull, is it toward the gastroesophageal junction, gastrophrenic ligament, gastrosplenic ligament, the left kidney, splenic flexure, greater omentum, or lesser omentum?

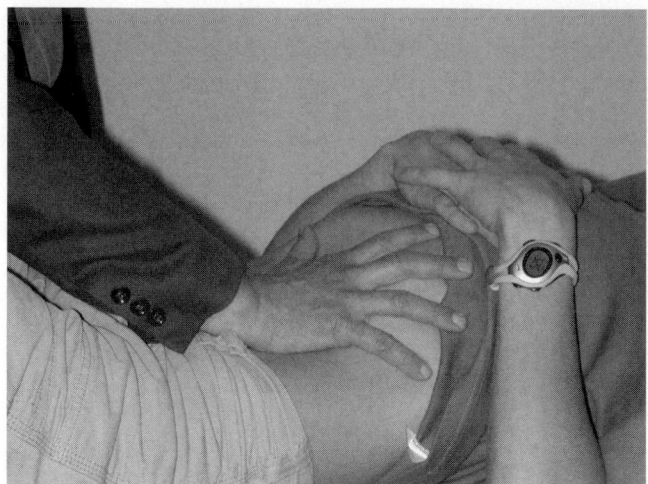

FIGURE 69.1.

Step 5. Have the patient take a deep breath. Does the stomach descend with inhalation and ascend with exhalation?

Step 6. Palpate motility. Inspir is counterclockwise, superior, and posterior. Expir is clockwise, inferior, and anterior.

Sutherland Technique for Stomach (Fig. 69.2)

The 12th rib attaches through the lateral arcuate ligament to the diaphragm, and provides access to the area of the diaphragm around the esophagus.

Test

Right hand on 12th rib, left under the right. Right hand monitors only, left hand provides the traction. Engage rib and traction laterally, feeling for tension.

Treatment

Maintain traction until the rib releases and you can feel the area of the diaphragm.

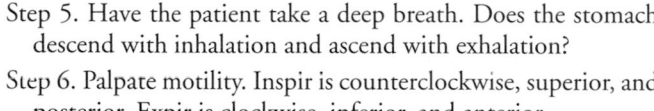

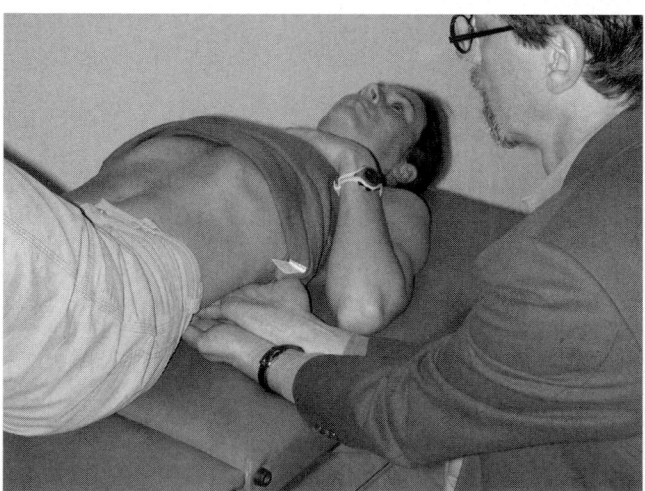

FIGURE 69.2.

Still Stomach Technique (Fig. 69.3)

This technique addresses the upper stomach and lower esophagus.

Test

Step 1. The patient is in a right lateral recumbent position. The physician stands behind.

Step 2. Use both hands on the stomach, your fingers are flat. Pull the stomach inferior and lateral to the left. Appreciate any tension.

Treatment

Maintain the tension on the stomach and slightly lean backward, until the tension releases and you are able to feel up through the esophagus.

Duodenal Diagnosis (Fig. 69.4)

Step 1. The patient is supine. The physician stands on the right with the right hand over the transverse section of the duodenum.

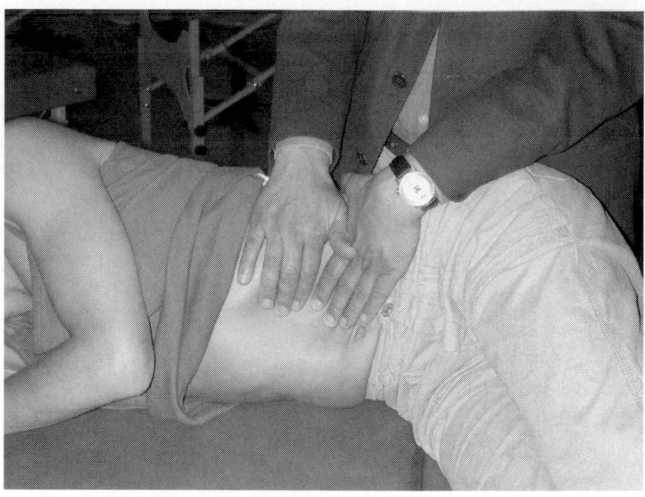

FIGURE 69.3.

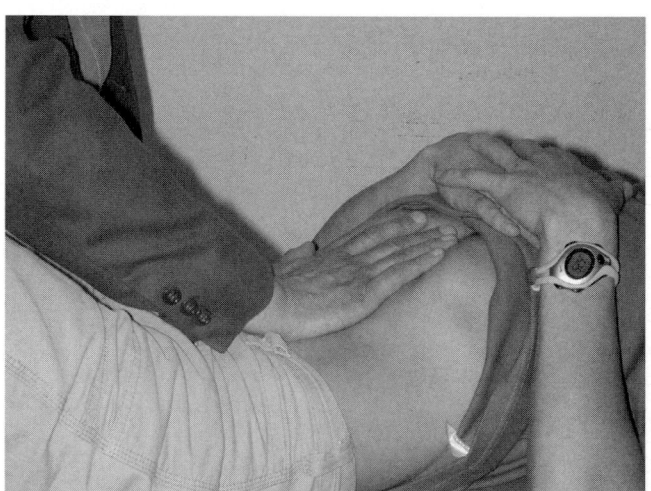

FIGURE 69.4.

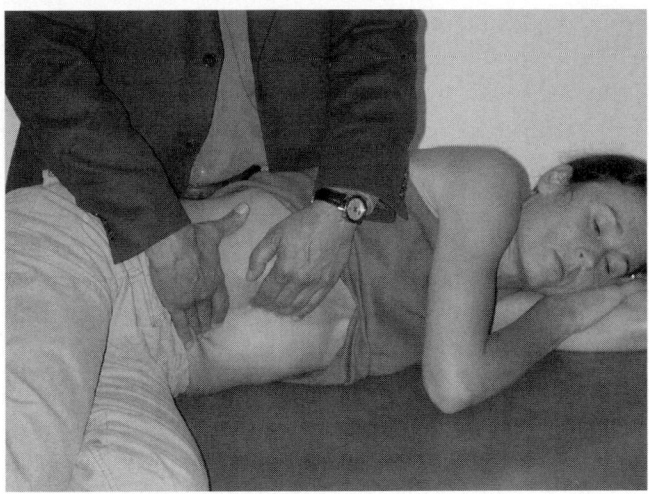

FIGURE 69.5.

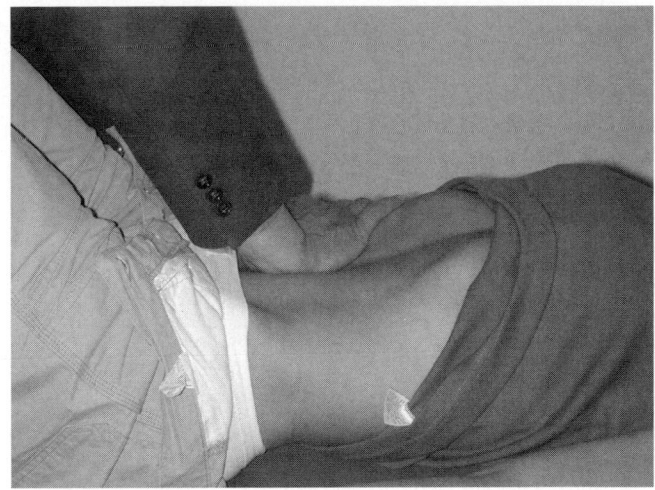

FIGURE 69.6.

Step 2. Palpate through the skin and abdominal wall until you reach the tissues in the abdomen.

Step 3. Check the direction of fascial pull, and think of what attachments might be in that direction.

Step 4. Check movements with respiration (should descend with inhalation, ascend with exhalation).

Step 5. Palpate motility. In inspir, the duodenum opens, and in expir it closes.

Duodenal Manipulation (Fig. 69.5)

Step 1. The patient is in the left lateral recumbent position. The physician stands behind the patient.

Step 2. Palpate with the fingers to the left of the ascending portion of the duodenum and the attachment of the muscle of Treitz.

Step 3. Draw both hands toward the patient's right side, and spread your hands inferiorly and superiorly. To treat the descending and transverse portions, the patient lies on the right, your hands are lateral and draw medially and superior/inferior.

THE SMALL INTESTINE

The jejunoileum should be evaluated in cases of intestinal ptosis, stress urinary incontinence, abnormal stool production, diverticulosis, ulcerative colitis, Crohn disease, asthma, and allergies.

Root of Mesentery Diagnosis (Fig. 69.6)

Step 1. The patient is supine. The physician stands to the right, the base of the right hand is placed over the area of the root of the mesentery.

Step 2. Palpate through the abdominal wall to the abdominal contents.

Step 3. Palpate the direction of fascial pull. If there is no abnormal tension, you will not feel any fascial pull. If there is a fascial pull, is it in the direction of the ileocecal valve, duodenal-jejunal junction, inferior, or superior?

Root of Mesentery Manipulation (Fig. 69.7)

Step 1. The patient is supine, knees bent. The physician stands to the right, near the lower thorax, with the fingers below the root, the thumbs above.

Step 2. Gently palpate deeper, until you feel the tension of the root.

Step 3. Motion test the superior part inferiorly, and the inferior part superiorly.

Step 4. Treat by taking the tissue to tension, then relax and see what speed the tissues come back. Use that speed to rhythmically engage and disengage the tension. When it releases, there will be no more tension.

Small Intestine Motility (Fig. 69.8)

Step 1. The patient is supine. The physician stands to the right. The right is hand over the patient's right side of the small intestine, the left hand is over the left small intestine. In inspir,

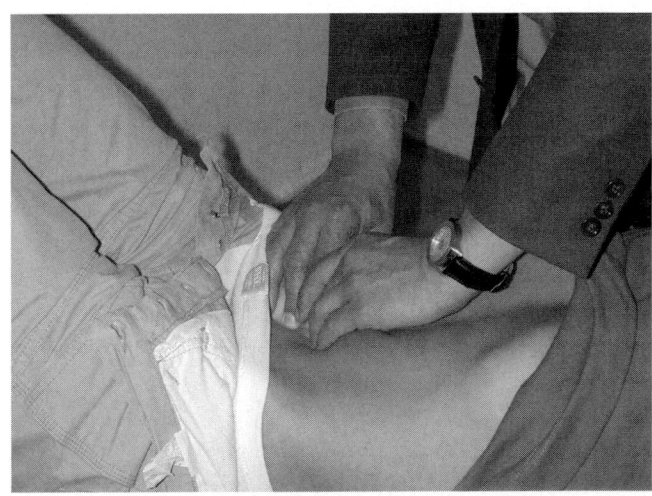

FIGURE 69.7.

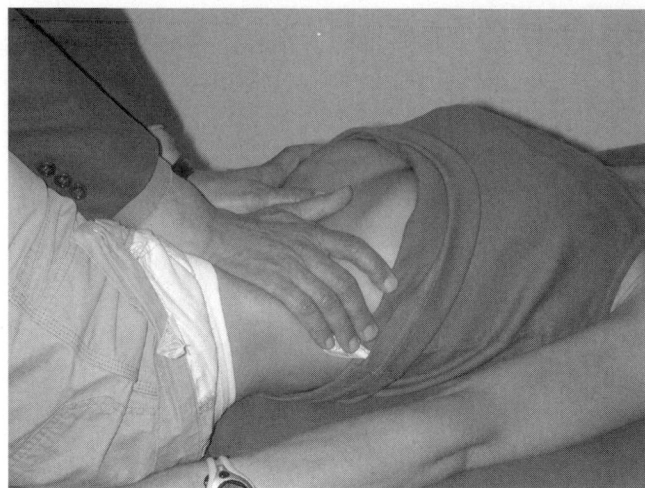

FIGURE 69.8.

the small intestine rotates counterclockwise, in expir the small intestine rotates clockwise.

Step 2. Diagnose the movement.

Step 3. Slightly encourage the better motion until it is even.

THE COLON

The colon should be evaluated in cases of constipation, diarrhea, intestinal prolapse and ptosis, diverticulosis, history of appendectomy, irritable bowel, ulcerative colitis, Crohn disease, hemorrhoids, or anorectal pain.

Cecum and Ascending Colon (Fig. 69.9)

Test

Step 1. The patient is supine with their knees bent. The physician stands to the right, with the right hand over the area of the cecum.

Step 2. Palpate to the abdominal contents.

Step 3. Test by palpating fascial pull.

Step 4. Test motion superior, inferior, medial, and lateral.

Step 5. Palpate motility. Inspir is a counterclockwise inferior movement. Expir is clockwise and superior.

Treatment

Step 1. Take to the direct barrier, relax, and let the tissues come back, noting their speed.

Step 2. Assume that rhythm, taking the tissues to the barrier and coming back until there is no tension left.

Step 3. Treat the motility by gently encouraging the motion that is better.

Transverse Colon and Flexures (Fig. 69.10)

Test

Step 1. The patient is sitting. The physician stands behind, with the fingers placed on the area of the hepatic flexure.

Step 2. Draw the ascending colon superior, and spread your fingers medially and laterally.

Step 3. Repeat on the left side for the splenic flexure.

Step 4. Then, with one hand on each, lift the flexures and the transverse colon superiorly.

Root of Sigmoid (Fig. 69.11)

The root of the sigmoid is a thickening of the peritoneum, extending from the sigmoid to the area of the bifurcation of the iliac vessels. The mechanical tension extends further to the area of the duodenal-jejunal junction.

Test

Step 1. The patient is supine. Place your fingers above, and thumbs below this line.

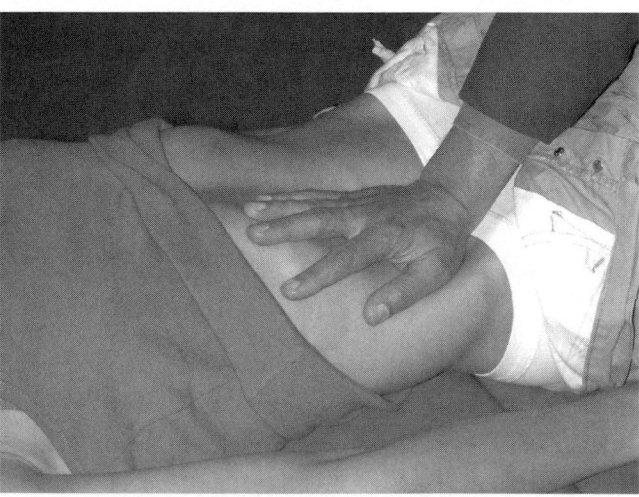

FIGURE 69.9.

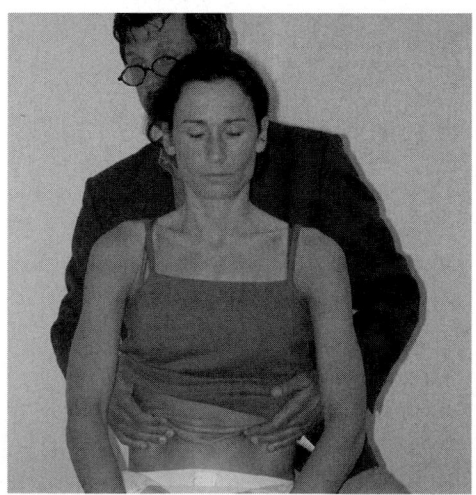

FIGURE 69.10.

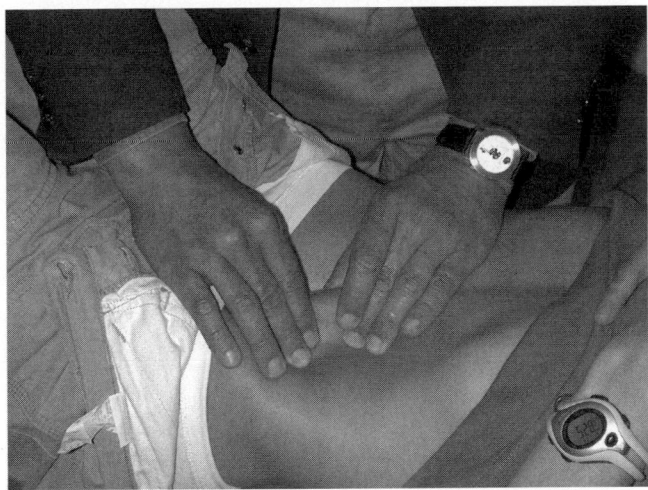

FIGURE 69.11.

Step 2. Move the mesocolon superior-lateral and inferior-medial, checking for tension.

Treatment

Engage the tension, and let the tissue come back, noting the speed the tissue responds. Continue this rhythm until the tissue releases, and there is no more tension.

Sigmoid Colon (Fig. 69.12)

Test

Step 1. The patient is supine. The physician stands on the right, your right hand over the area of the sigmoid.

Step 2. Palpate the direction of fascial pull.

Step 3. Test motion superior-medially and inferior-laterally.

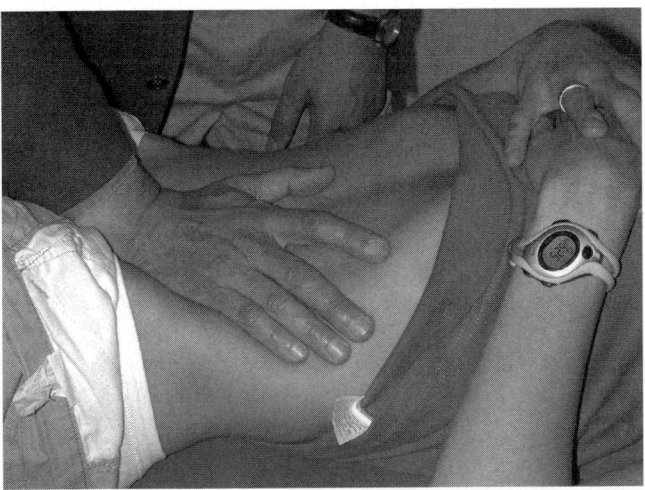

FIGURE 69.12.

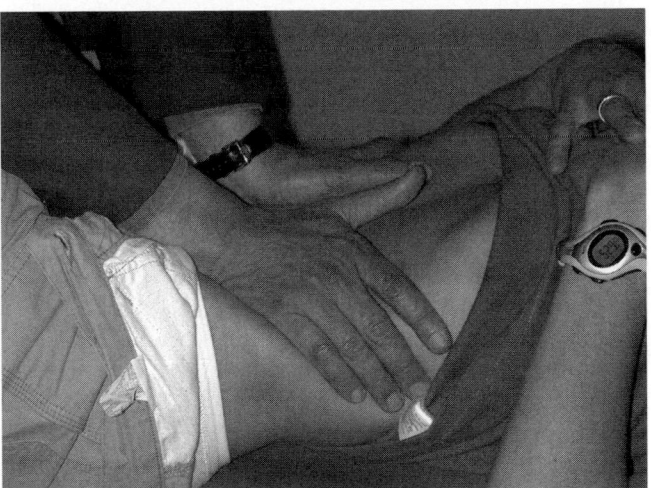

FIGURE 69.13.

Treatment

Step 1. Take the tissues first in the direction they will go (the direction of listening), slightly exaggerating the direction until you perceive a release.

Step 2. Then take the tissues in the direction they will not go. Maintain the barrier and use respiratory assistance.

Colon Motility (Fig. 69.13)

Step 1. The patient is supine. The physician stands on the right, with the right hand on the descending colon and the left hand on the ascending colon. In inspir, the colon will rotate counterclockwise, in expir it will rotate clockwise.

Step 2. Encourage the better motion until it is symmetric.

LIVER

The liver should be evaluated in cases of chronic hepatitis, right shoulder pain, depression, chronic excessive alcohol intake, cholelithiasis, hormonal imbalances, and cirrhosis.

"Frozen" Liver (Fig. 69.14)

Test

Step 1. The patient is supine. The physician stands on the right. Use both hands and engage the liver through the ribs.

Step 2. Translate the liver to the left, noting if there is any resistance to movement.

Treatment

Step 1. Take the liver to tension, taking up the slack through a few exhalations.

Step 2. At the beginning of an inhalation, quickly release your hands. Repeat up to three times as needed. This will free up the bare area of the liver from the diaphragm, which may

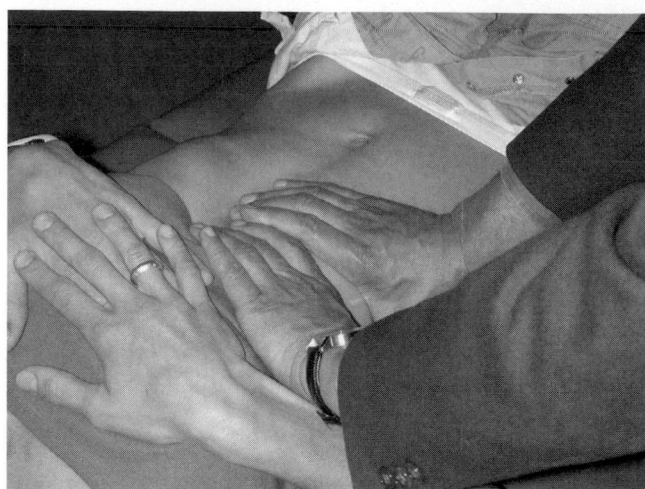

FIGURE 69.14.

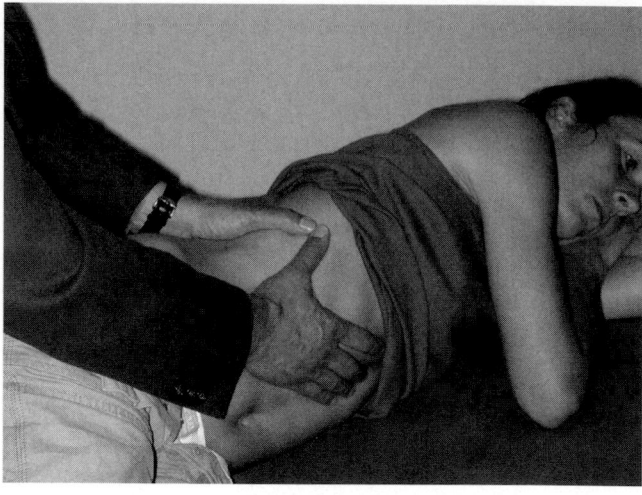

FIGURE 69.16.

be stuck due to metabolic problems, inflammation, or old infections.

Liver and Gallbladder Diagnosis (Fig. 69.15)

Step 1. The patient is supine. The physician stands on the right and places the right hand slightly to the right of midline.

Step 2. Compress through the abdominal wall until you feel the abdominal contents.

Step 3. Check the direction of fascial pull. Does the tissue pull in the direction of the liver, gallbladder, duodenum, pancreas, right kidney, or the colon?

Step 4. Test the structure you believe to be dysfunctional with fascial pull and motion testing.

Liver, Sagittal Plane (Fig. 69.16)

Test

Step 1. The patient is in the left lateral recumbent position. The physician stands behind and near the pelvis.

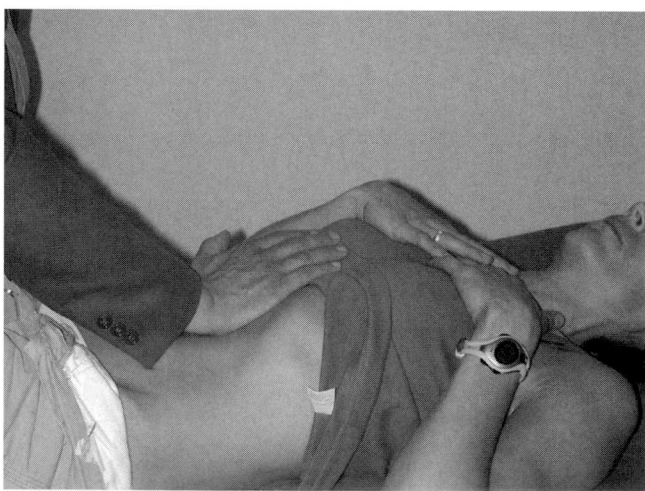

FIGURE 69.15.

Step 2. The right hand engages the liver anteriorly, the left hand is over the lower ribs. Compress the hands slightly to feel the liver.

Step 3. Move the anterior liver inferior and the posterior liver superior, then reverse, noting restrictions in either direction.

Treatment

Take the liver to tension and take up the slack during the phase of respiration where there is some. Maintain the tension through a few phases of respiration, until it releases.

Liver, Transverse Plane (Fig. 69.17)

Test

Step 1. The patient is in a left lateral recumbent position. The physician stands behind the area of the liver. Both hands are used.

Step 2. Bring the area of the liver anterior and toward the midline, then posterior and laterally, noting any restriction to movement.

Treatment

Take the liver to tension, see which phase of respiration gives a little slack, and take out the slack. Repeat this procedure until there is no more resistance.

Liver, Frontal Plane (Fig. 69.18)

Test

Step 1. The patient is in the left lateral recumbent position. The physician stands behind the thoracic area. Both hands are used on the lateral area of the liver.

Step 2. Bring the lateral portion of the liver inferior and medially, then laterally and superior, noting any direction of resistance.

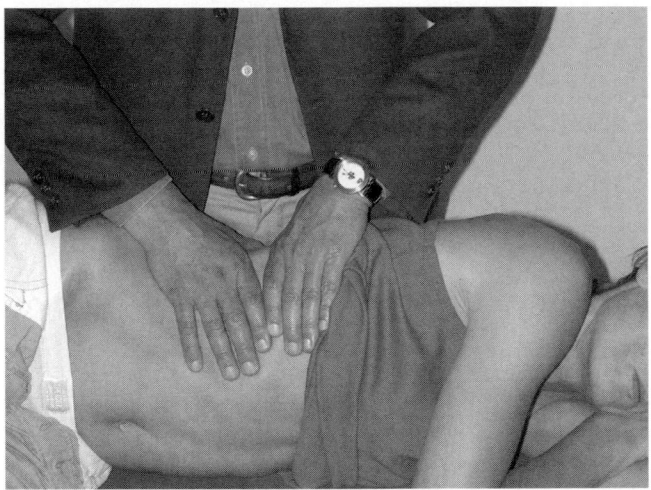

FIGURE 69.17.

Treatment

Take the liver to tension, noting the phase of respiration where there is some slack. Take up the slack. Repeat this until there is no more resistance.

Liver Lift (Fig. 69.19)

Test

Step 1. The patient is seated. The physician stands behind. The inferior border of the liver is palpated with both hands.

Step 2. Lift the liver, noting any resistance to distension, then let the liver drop, noting the speed and how well it drops. Lifting the liver tests the inferior attachments, dropping the liver tests the superior attachments.

Step 3. Test the right side (for colon, kidney, and right triangular ligament).

Step 4. Test the middle (for duodenum, lesser omentum, coronary ligament).

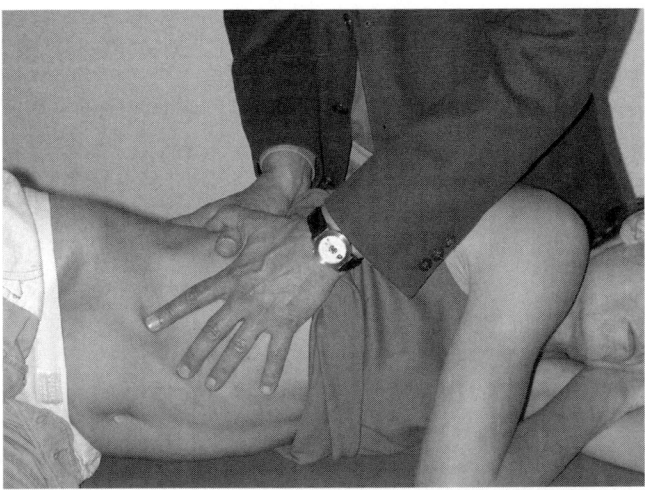

FIGURE 69.18.

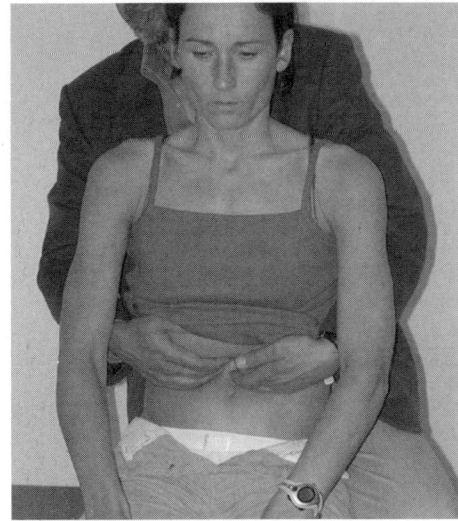

FIGURE 69.19.

Step 5. Test the left side (stomach, descending colon, left triangular ligament).

Treatment

Take the area and direction of the greatest resistance to tension. Take up the slack with the phase of respiration where it is available and maintain it through a few phases of respiration until there is no more resistance. If the tension is in the superior attachments, lift the liver and let it drop a few times until it drops easier.

GALLBLADDER

The gallbladder should be evaluated in cases of cholestasis, cholecystitis, left-sided neck pain, chronic sinusitis, and postcholecystectomy chronic abdominal pain.

Gallbladder (Fig. 69.20)

First treat the sphincter of Oddi, described later.

Test

Step 1. The patient is sitting. The physician stands behind. Bring the fingers under the liver to the area of the fundus of the gallbladder. The right fingers are placed to the right of the gallbladder, the left fingers to the left.

Step 2. Test the distensibility of the tissues medially and laterally, noting resistance.

Treatment

Step 1. Take the tissue to the direction of ease until it softens.

Step 2. Then take the tissues in the direction of tension, until it softens.

Step 3. Press on the fundus, making a sweeping motion in the direction of the cystic duct and common bile duct until you meet resistance. Repeat up to ten sweeping motions until the gallbladder feels empty.

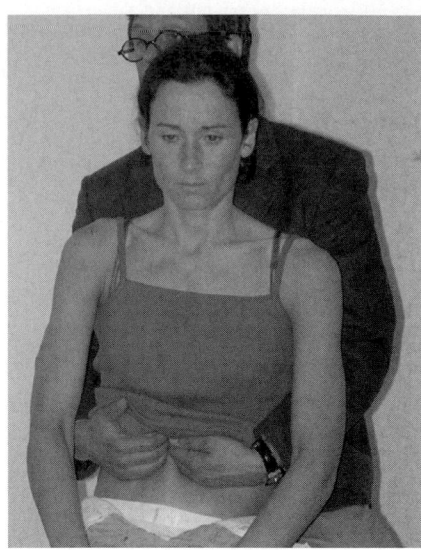

FIGURE 69.20.

Common Bile Duct (Fig. 69.21)

Test

Step 1. The patient is sitting. The physician stands behind.

Step 2. Use your left thumb to fix the sphincter of Oddi posteriorly and inferiorly.

Step 3. Have the patient place their hands behind their neck, elbows together.

Step 4. Use your right hand under the elbows to extend the body, and rotate to the right to tension. Repeat the movements until the resistance is no longer palpable.

Sphincter of Oddi (Fig. 69.22)

Test

Step 1. The patient is supine. The physician stands on the righ

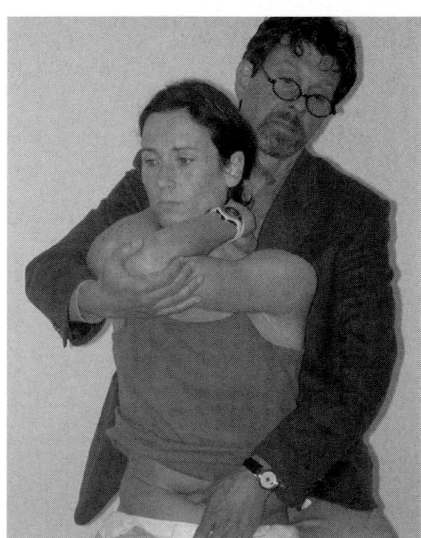

FIGURE 69.21.

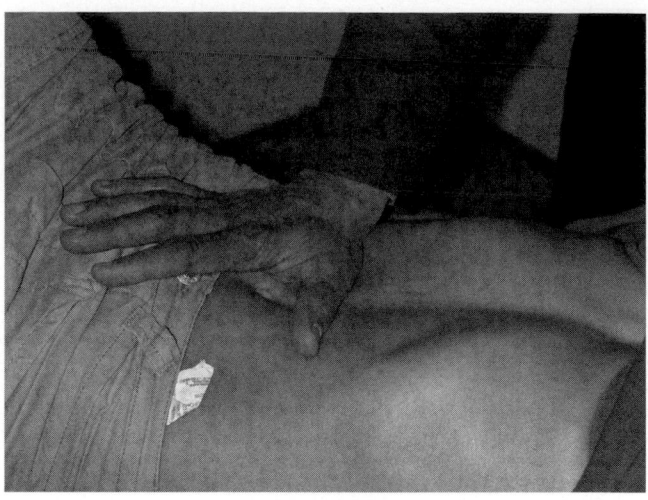

FIGURE 69.22.

side, with the right thenar eminence over the area of the sphincter.

Step 2. Press posteriorly until you feel a small rotational movement.

Step 3. Motion test this area medially, laterally, superior, and inferiorly. Note distance of distensibility and end-feel.

Treatment

Step 1. Take the tissue to the indirect barrier first, until you feel it release.

Step 2. Take the tissues to the direct barrier, and hold until it releases.

Step 3. When all barriers are gone, encourage the direction of the better rotation, until it normalizes. All other sphincter-like areas are treated in a similar fashion, including the gastro-esophageal junction, pylorus, duodenal-jejunal junction, and the ileocecal valve.

KIDNEYS

The kidneys are evaluated in cases of renal ptosis, low back pain, recurrent pyelonephritis, renal lithiasis, sciatica, and inguinal pain.

Kidney (Fig. 69.23)

Test

Step 1. The patient is supine. The physician stands on the side of the kidney that is going to be tested. Description here is for the right kidney.

Step 2. With the left hand, find the space between the 12th rib and the crest of the ilium. The right hand is over the area of the kidney. Press posteriorly until you think you feel the kidney.

Step 3. Lift the posterior hand anteriorly, until you can feel the anterior portion of the kidney with your anterior hand.

Step 4. Palpate fascial pull.

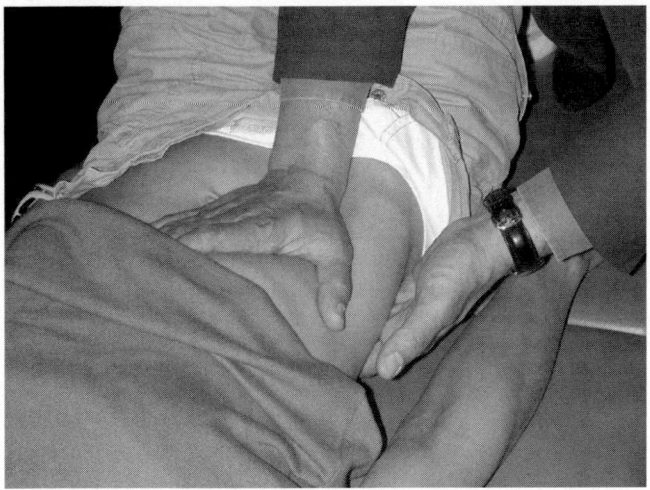

FIGURE 69.23.

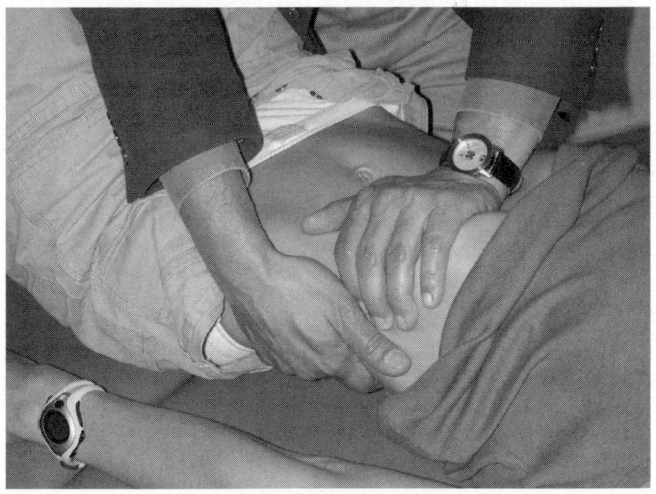

FIGURE 69.25.

Step 5. Motion test the kidney superior, inferior, medially, and laterally, noting any resistance to movement.

Treatment

Step 1. Take the kidney in the direction it moves easiest, until you feel it release.

Step 2. Then, take the kidney in the direction it does not move as easy. Take up the slack in the phase of respiration where it is available, until it releases.

Ureter (Fig. 69.24)

The ureter should be evaluated in any case where there is a history of renal lithiasis.

Test

Step 1. The patient is supine. The physician stands on the side of the dysfunction.

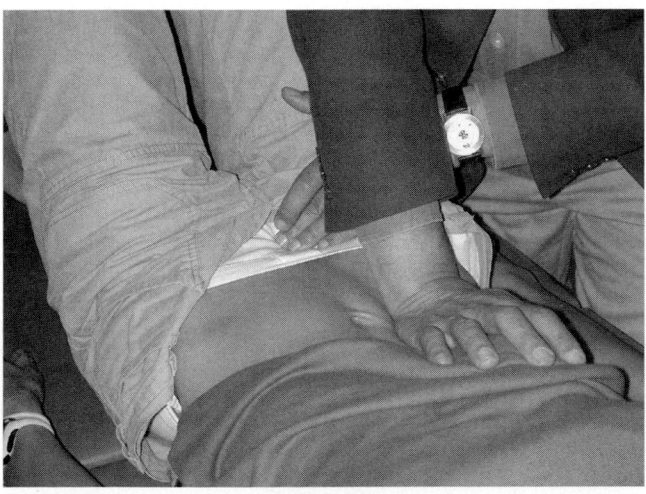

FIGURE 69.24.

Step 2. Lift the kidney superior while palpating above the bladder, if the ureter is tight you will feel a small pull on the bladder.

Treatment

Place your finger on this area (bladder-ureter connection) and lift the kidney while maintaining tension on the area of the bladder.

SPLEEN

The spleen should be evaluated in any case of impaired immunity, chronic fatigue, human immunodeficiency virus (HIV), or chronic infections. Since the spleen is not normally palpable, the attachments are evaluated by assessing the area of the spleen in relation to the diaphragm, pancreas, left kidney, splenic flexure of the colon, and the stomach. If the spleen is palpable, it needs to be worked up medically before any treatment is attempted (Fig. 69.25).

Test

Step 1. The patient is supine. The physician stands on the opposite side. The right hand is behind the lower rib cage, the left hand is in the left upper quadrant of the abdomen. Compress the hands together.

Step 2. Bring the area inferior, then superior, noting any resistance to distension.

Step 3. Palpate fascial pull.

Treatment

Take the tissue to tension and hold. During the phase of respiration that you can get some slack, take it, until you feel the tissues release.

PANCREAS

The pancreas is evaluated, very gently, in cases of chronic pancreatitis (Fig. 69.26).

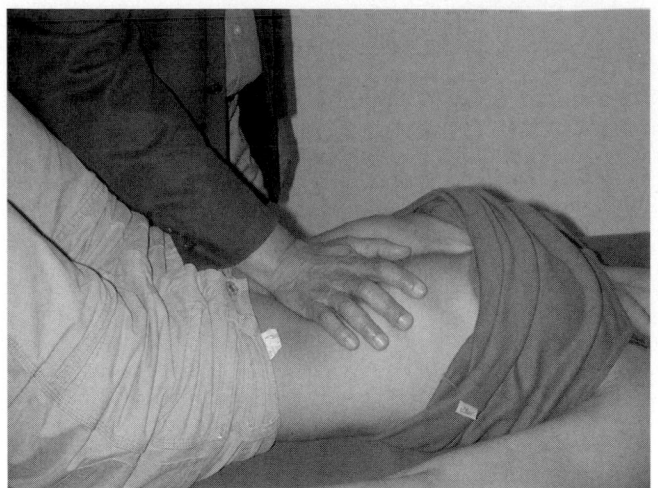

FIGURE 69.26.

Test

Step 1. The patient is supine. The physician stands on the right. The palm of the right hand is over the descending duodenum, fingers pointed toward the spleen. The left hand is posterior to the spine in the same area.

Step 2. Compress through the abdominal wall to the abdominal contents.

Step 3. Palpate fascial pull.

Step 4. Then, compress a little more and take the area inferiorly and superiorly, noting distance and end-feel of distensibility.

Treatment

In the same position, take tissue to indirect barrier until it releases using respiratory assistance.

THORAX

The thorax should be evaluated in any respiratory problems (asthma, pneumonia, pleurisy, chronic bronchitis), heart problems, chronic postural problems, thoracic pain, and when the upper abdominal viscera will not descend with inhalation. Once the side of the dysfunction has been determined, more specific testing can be done to localize the structure in dysfunction.

Thoracic Diagnosis (Fig. 69.27)

Test

Step 1. The patient is supine. The physician stands on the right side near the abdomen.

Step 2. Place your right hand in the middle of the thorax.

Step 3. Palpate the direction of the fascial pull. Is the pull toward the right or the left, toward the mediastinum, lungs, or pericardium?

Step 4. Do further tests on the structures in question.

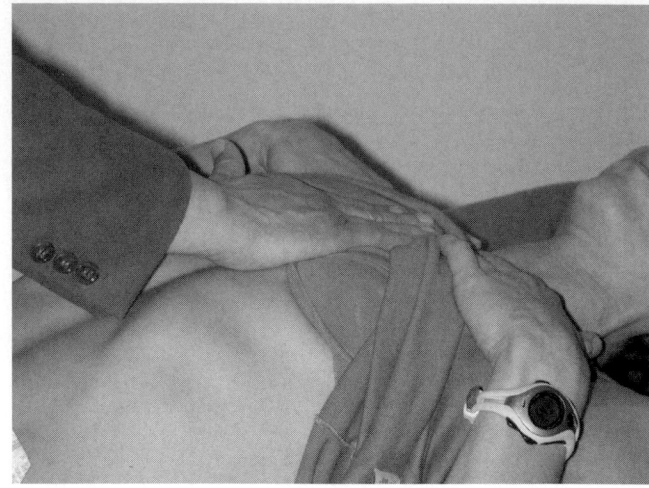

FIGURE 69.27.

Cervical-Pleural Ligaments (Fig. 69.28)

Test

Step 1. The patient is supine. The physician sits near the patient's head.

Step 2. Place a thumb on each dome, have the patient take a deep inhalation. Both domes should descend, if they do not, there is a restriction.

Treatment

Step 1. On the side of the restriction (described here for the left), place your left thumb on the dome, and side bend the patient's neck to the left.

Step 2. Have the patient inhale, and follow the dome inferiorly. Do not allow it to return on exhalation. Repeat until the area softens.

Step 3. Then, maintaining the dome inferiorly, side bend the patient's neck to the right, stretching the fibers of the cervical-pleural ligament.

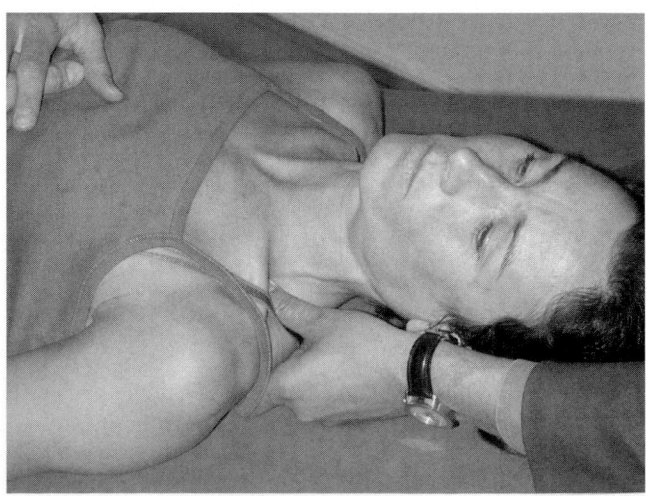

FIGURE 69.28.

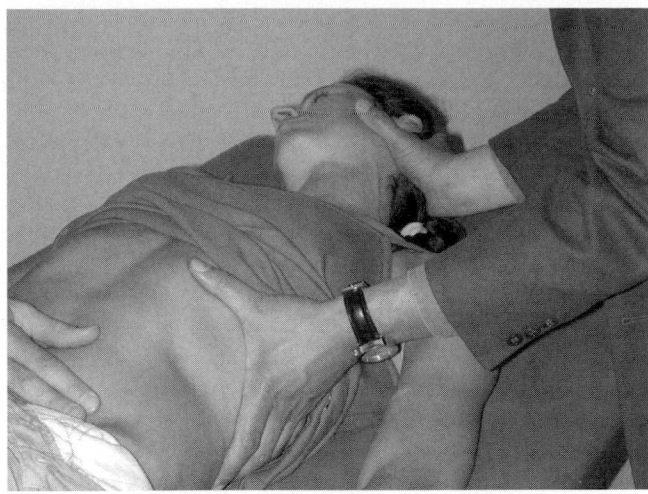

FIGURE 69.29.

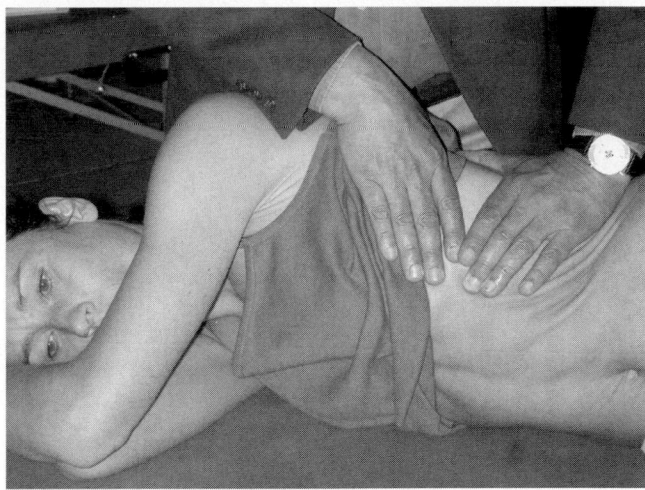

FIGURE 69.30.

Parietal Pleura (Fig. 69.29)

Treatment

Step 1. The patient is supine. The physician stands near the shoulder of side of the restriction. With your right hand contact the upper cervical spine and lower cranium.

Step 2. Place your left hand on the anterior-lateral lower rib cage.

Step 3. Take the cervical spine in rotation and side bending to the opposite side to tension. This hand then remains stationary.

Step 4. The left hand follows the ribs inferiorly with an exhalation, and maintains them inferiorly as the patient continues to breathe.

> Can you afford in treating diseases of the lungs to give your verdict and prescribe drugs or manipulations as a doctor of medicine, an osteopath, or masseur, without first carefully examining the pleura in all divisions and knowing that their blood and nerve supply are perfectly normal? —*A.T. Still (1)*

Lung Fissures (Fig. 69.30)

Test

Step 1. The patient is in the right lateral recumbent position. The physician stands behind the thorax. The left hand is over the fifth rib posteriorly and the seventh rib anteriorly. The right hand is over the fourth rib posteriorly and the sixth rib anteriorly.

Step 2. Palpate through the ribs to the thoracic contents.

Step 3. With an inhalation, follow the lung movement inferiorly. Maintain the tissue inferiorly during an exhalation phase. Translate the upper lobe relative to the lower lobe horizontally, noting direction of ease. Maintain inferiorly until it releases.

Treatment

Remain in this position, and when at maximal tension, have the patient continue to breathe, taking out the slack with each exhalation, until you feel a release. The right fissures are treated in the same way, but with the patient in the left lateral recumbent position. Hand placement is on the same ribs for the oblique fissure, and the fingers move up to over and under the fourth ribs anteriorly for the horizontal fissure.

Bronchi (Fig. 69.31)

Test

Step 1. The patient is supine. The physician stands near the head. Palpate the upper trachea.

Step 2. Traction the trachea superiorly, then to the left and the right. If there is more resistance tractioning to the right, it means the left bronchus is under more tension, and vice versa.

Treatment

Step 1. While tractioning on the trachea, palpate the fascial pull over the area of the mainstem bronchus until you feel where it pulls in. Check both sides.

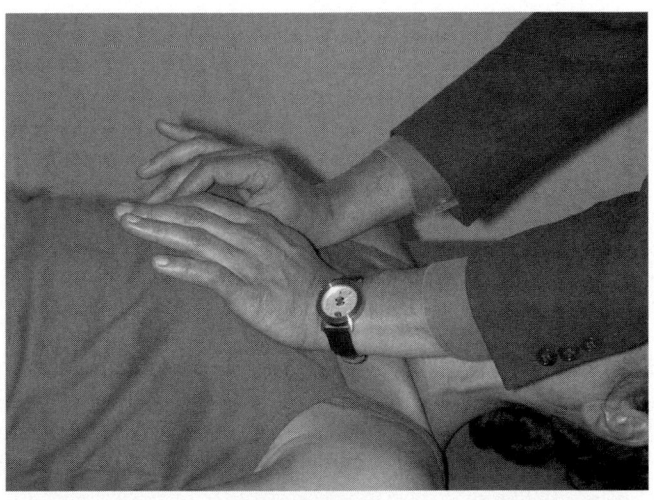

FIGURE 69.31.

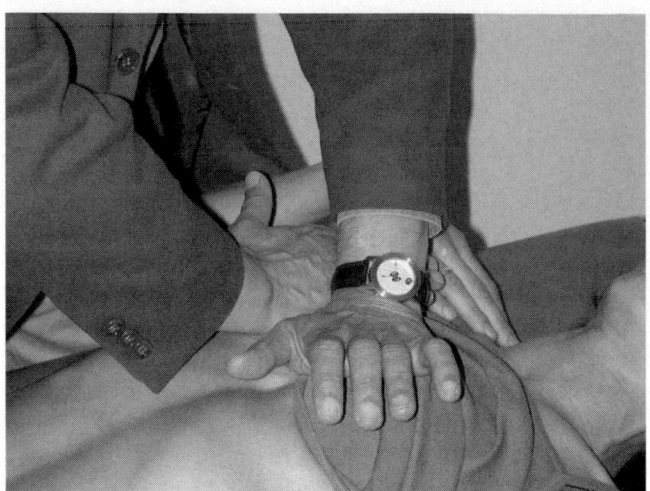

FIGURE 69.32.

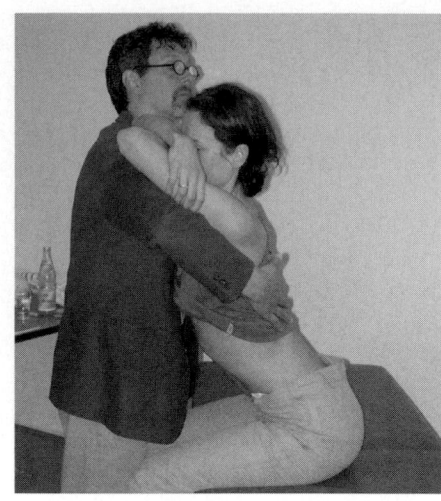

FIGURE 69.33.

Step 2. Then, place one hand over each bronchus, and compress posteriorly to "catch" the bronchus.

Step 3. Traction the bronchus inferior and lateral, taking up the slack with respiration until you feel a release. Retest the distensibility of both bronchi.

Mediastinum, Supine (Fig. 69.32)

Treatment

Step 1. The patient is supine. The physician stands on the side of the tension in the mediastinum (description here is for the right side).

Step 2. The left hand engages the sternum medially. The right hand engages the fourth rib near the articulation with the sternum, and brings it laterally.

Step 3. Take up the slack during the phase of respiration that the tension decreases. At maximum tension, quickly release your hands.

Mediastinum, Seated (Fig. 69.33)

Treatment

Step 1. The patient is seated. The physician stands in front of the patient. The patient folds their arms over each other and rests them on the physician's chest.

Step 2. Reach behind the patient and engage the 12th rib bilaterally. With an exhalation, bring the 12th rib laterally and toward you.

Step 3. Repeat until the 12th rib is free, then move your hand to the 11th rib and repeat.

Step 4. Move up the spine until it feels free. This will increase the distance between the superior mediastinum and its inferior attachments.

PELVIS

Bladder

The bladder should be evaluated in cases of stress incontinence, recurrent cystitis, bladder prolapse, and cystalgia. Structures tested are the pubovesicular ligaments, median umbilical ligament, medial umbilical ligaments, distensibility of the obturator membrane, obturator internus muscle, and the hips. Of course the pubis, pelvic floor muscles, sacrum, and coccyx should also be evaluated. The urethra, pubovesicular ligaments, trigone muscle, and the walls of the bladder itself may be evaluated with an internal examination and treated. Internal treatment can be more effective than external treatment, due to better palpation and treatment access.

Bladder Diagnosis (Fig. 69.34)

Step 1. The patient is supine. The physician stands on the right, with the right hand just superior to the pubis.

Step 2. Palpate the fascia for a direction of pull. If there is a

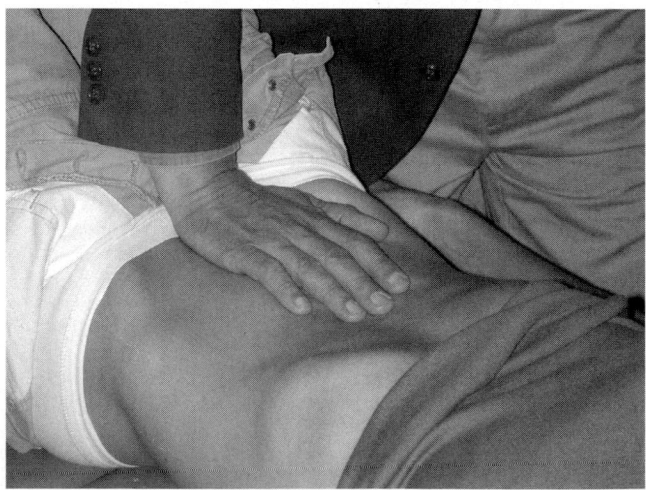

FIGURE 69.34.

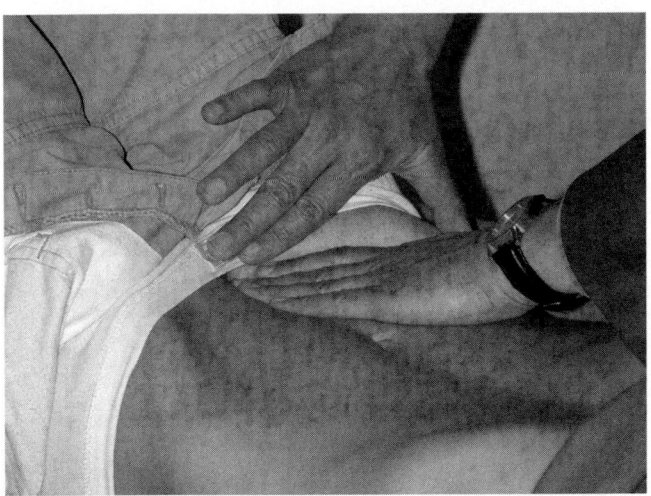

FIGURE 69.35.

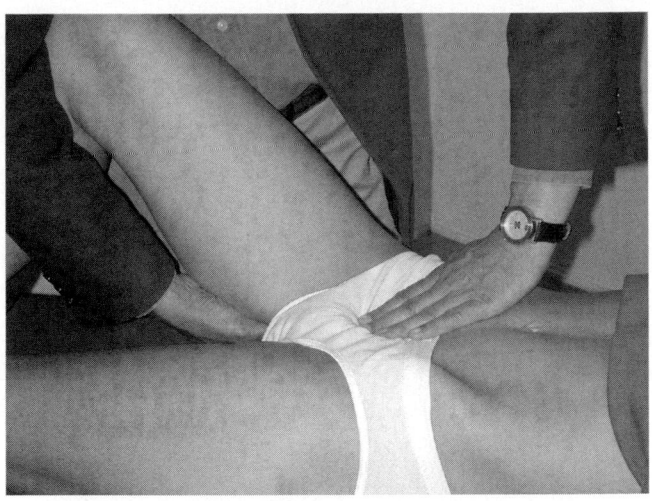

FIGURE 69.36.

problem, the bladder will pull just behind the pubis, in the area of the pubovesicular ligaments, or sometimes laterally toward the hip.

Step 3. Do more specific tests in suspected dysfunctional areas.

Pubovesicular Ligaments (Fig. 69.35)

Test

Step 1. The patient is supine with knees bent. The physician stands on the side to be tested.

Step 2. Palpate the top of the bladder, and gently press it inferiorly.

Step 3. Check the opposite side and compare the distensibility.

Treatment

Take the side that moves inferior better and slightly exaggerate it until it releases and comes back, then treat the other side.

Obturator Foramen (Fig. 69.36)

With bladder dysfunction the obturator foramen is found to be tense, and does not distend properly.

Test

Step 1. The patient is supine with knees bent. Stand on the side to be tested.

Step 2. Place your thumb posterior to the origin of the adductor longus muscle, and palpate into the obturator foramen.

Step 3. Have the patient inhale. The membrane should descend, and with exhalation it should ascend, unless there is a problem.

Step 4. Check the distensibility of the membrane, it should move easily. When you press on it the bladder it should move to the opposite side, if not, it is restricted.

Treatment

Carry the membrane superior with exhalation, and maintain it there with inhalation. Hold until it releases. Recheck by comparing it with the other side.

CERVIX, UTERUS, FALLOPIAN TUBES, AND OVARIES

This area should be evaluated in cases of prolapse, dysmenorrhea, pelvic pain, low back pain, sciatica, menopause, dyspareunia, infertility, and cervical stenosis. External examination can point to the location of the largest tension, but internal examination is required to get more specific information. This area is quite amenable to osteopathic treatment, and the results are often dramatic. The easiest cases may be treated externally. Internal treatment has been found to be more precise, faster, and result in a larger percentage of improvement. Still (1), Woodhall (7), and Barral (21) have described the internal techniques. The external examination is performed by placing your hand in the position used for diagnosing the bladder, but slightly higher. Fascial pull is also palpated over the area of the ovaries.

Cervix (Fig. 69.37)

Test

Step 1. The patient is supine, knees bent. The physician stands on one side, with the foot on the table. The thigh is under the patient's calves.

Step 2. Use your thumb to press posteriorly just above the pubis, until you feel the uterus, press it toward the opposite side, noting distance traveled and resistance at the end of the movement.

Step 3. Then move to the opposite side and test and compare it.

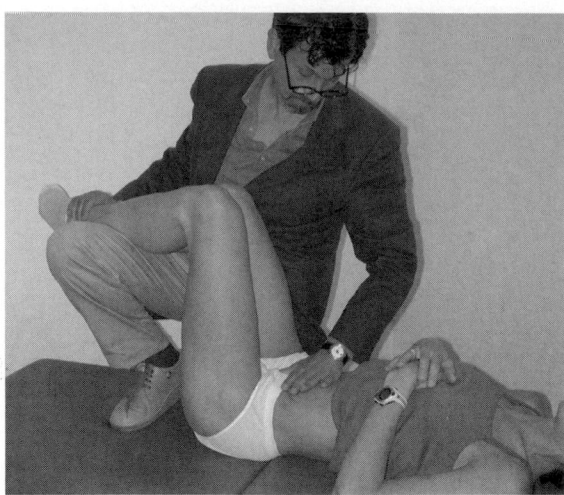

FIGURE 69.37.

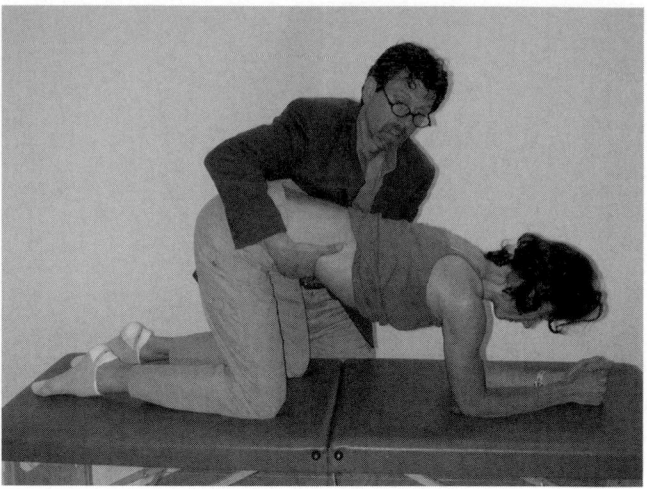

FIGURE 69.39.

Treatment

Maintaining the same position, take the uterus to the indirect side first. When that releases, go to the opposite side and treat the direct barrier. The legs are used as lever arms both to maximize your palpation, and during treatment.

GENERAL TREATMENT POSITIONS

General Lower Abdominal/Pelvic Lift (Fig. 69.38)

This is one of the positions preferred by Still (1), McConnell (2), and Sutherland (17). The patient is supine, with the hips and knee bent. The fingers are flat, with area to be treated engaged. Gently lift the area superiorly until you hit a barrier, then let the tissue respond. Sutherland used one hand to engage the tissue, with the other hand over the first to do the lifting (17). This technique can be used for pelvic organs, colon, ureters, and kidneys.

Knee/Elbow Position (Fig. 69.39)

This is a position preferred by Still and McConnell (1,2). It also can be done with a small stool under the patient's chest. Still and McConnell used this position to "lift" the cecum, sigmoid, pelvic organs, stomach, liver, duodenum, small intestine, kidneys, and ureters. The position uses the effect of gravity to pull the viscera anteriorly, thus taking them to tension. Both hands can also be used to pull the peritoneum anteriorly, and stretching it.

REFERENCES

1. Still AT. *Research and Practice of Osteopathy*, 1911.
2. McDonnell CP. *Selected Writings of Carl Philip McConnell, D.O.* Squirrel's Tail Press, 1994.
3. Barber E. *Osteopathy Complete*, 1898.
4. Gaddis CJ. Bedside technique. *JAOA.* 1922(Jul);21:691.
5. Teal CC. Palpation of the colon with special reference to the cecum. *JAOA.* 1922(Apr);21:492.
6. Smith RK. Mechanical principles of the human body. *JAOA.* 1912(Dec);12:210.
7. Woodhall P. *Intrapelvic Technique,* 1907.
8. Hoover HV. A consideration of an osteopathic lesion of the whole liver and its effects on hepatic dysfunction. In: *AAO Yearbook.* American Academy of Osteopathy, 1948.
9. Hoover HV. Liver and gall bladder technique. In: *AAO Yearbook.* American Academy of Osteopathy: 1947.
10. Hoover HV. Technique for removing still lesion usually found in gall bladder disease. In: *AAO Yearbook.* American Academy of Osteopathy: 1950.
11. Young MD. Head's law and its relation to the treatment of the viscera. *Osteopathic Profession.* 1946(Aug).
12. Young MD. Illustration of visceral technique. In: *AAO Yearbook.* American Academy of Osteopathy: 1948.
13. Hazzard C. *The Practice and Applied Therapeutics of Osteopathy,* 1905.
14. Riggs W. *A Manual of Osteopathic Manipulations and Treatment,* 1901.
15. Murray C. *Practice of Osteopathy: Its Practical Application to the Various Diseases of the Human Body,* 6th ed. 1925.
16. Goetz E. *A Manual of Osteopathy,* 2nd ed. 1909.
17. Sutherland WG. *Teachings in the Science of Osteopathy* . Portland, OR: Rudra Press; 1990.
18. Bensky D. Asthma treated by visceral manipulation. *AAOJ.* 1995 (Spring).

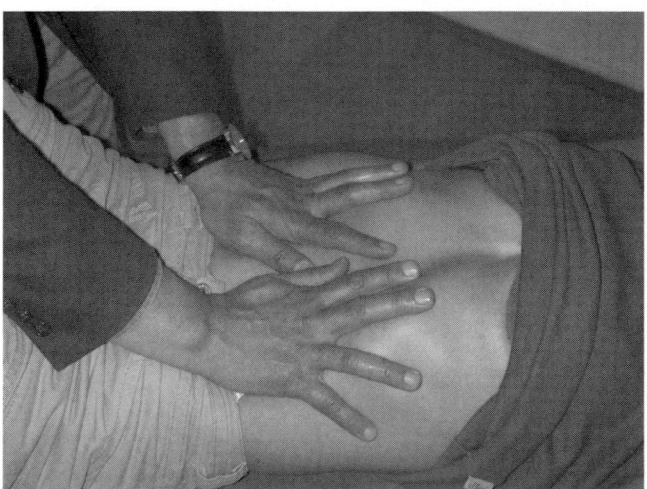

FIGURE 69.38.

19. Barral J, Mercier P. *Viscera Manipulation*. Vista, CA: Eastland Press; 1988.
20. Barral J. *Visceral Manipulation II*. Vista, CA: Eastland Press; 1989.
21. Barral J. *Urogenital Manipulation*. Vista, CA: Eastland Press; 1993.
22. Barral J. *The Thorax*. Vista, CA: Eastland Press; 1991.
23. Barral J. *Manual Thermal Diagnosis*. Vista, CA: Eastland Press; 1996.
24. Barral JP, Croibier A. *Trauma an Osteopathic Approach*. Vista, CA: Eastland Press; 1999.
25. Lossing KJ. *An Osteopathic Approach to Gastroesophageal Reflux Disease* [residency thesis]. Ohio University, Athens, OH, 1997.
26. Finet G, C Willame C. *Treating Visceral Dysfunction*. Portland, OR: Stillness Press; 2000.
27. Davidson SM Vitalize the viscera. Seminar, Phoenix, AZ, January 12, 1992.
28. Blackman E. Posterior midline. Port Richmond, CA, Feb. 23–25, 2001.
29. The Central Connection: Somatovisceral/Viscerosomatic Interaction. Paper presented at the American Association of Osteopathy1989 International Symposium.
30. Fredrickson J. Simultaneous temporal resolution of cardiac and respiratory motion in MRI imaging. *Radiology*. 1995;195:169–175.
31. Gierada D. Diaphragmatic motion: fast gradient-recalled-echo MRI imaging in healthy subjects. *Radiology*. 1995;194:879–884.
32. Moerland M. The influence of respiration induced motion of the kidneys on the accuracy of radiotherapy treatment planning, a magnetic resonance imaging study. *Radiother Oncol*. 1994;30(2):150–154.
33. Davies S. Ultrasound quantitation of respiratory organ motion in the upper abdomen. *Br J Radiol*. 1994;67(803):1096–1102.
34. Korin H. Respiratory kinematics of the upper abdominal organs: a quantitative study. *Magn Reson Med* 1992;23(1):172–178.

TREATMENT OF SOMATIC DYSFUNCTION WITH AN OSTEOPATHIC MANIPULATIVE METHOD OF DR. ANDREW TAYLOR STILL

RICHARD L. VAN BUSKIRK

Knowledge of any of the manipulative methods used by Dr. A.T. Still was severely limited for almost a century. The osteopathic profession was started to develop a cadre of practitioners who would apply Dr. Still's concepts about health and healing and utilize musculoskeletal manipulation to the benefit of patients. In spite of Dr. Still's reported mastery of musculoskeletal manipulation with attendant improvement of health, by the latter half of the 20th century no one could point to any manipulative method and say with any certainty that this was the method used by Andrew Taylor Still. In fact Dr. Still seems to have intentionally prevented the preservation of his methods in favor of the preservation and advancement of the more general concepts underlying osteopathy (1).

The Still technique was redeveloped following the discovery of several quotes describing how Dr. Still performed manipulative treatment. These quotes were found in a text by Charles Hazzard DO (2), a student and colleague of Dr. Still at the American College of Osteopathy in Kirksville, Missouri. The initial discussion of this rediscovered method was an article titled "A Manipulative Technique of Andrew Taylor Still" published in the *Journal of the American Osteopathic Association* (3). The current description has evolved significantly from the original (4):

1. Determine where the dysfunctional joint or tissue moves most easily. This is opposite the direction in which it is restricted.
2. Move the joint and/or tissues in the direction of its ease of motion until the tissue relaxes palpably. It is often useful to slightly exaggerate the position of ease, which further relaxes the dysfunctional tissue.
3. Introduce a vector of force of about 5 pounds (2 kg) into the affected tissue using the operating hand.
4. Using the force vector as a lever and maintaining compression, carry the tissue in the opposite direction toward and through the initial restriction. There will be a palpable and perhaps audible release as one passes through the former restriction.
5. The force vector and its compression is now removed and the tissue passively returned to neutral.
6. The procedure is retested and repeated if necessary.

One of the critical aspects and absolute requirement for the ability to use the Still technique is diagnostic specificity of musculoskeletal evaluation. If the diagnosis is not accurate this musculoskeletal manipulative technique is less likely to be successful, although it is rare that it will worsen a patient's condition.

This chapter presents examples of the Still technique applied to portions of the spine and limbs. No attempt is made to be comprehensive. Many of the diagnostic techniques discussed are shortcuts based on the author's clinical experience. Classic diagnostic procedures can also be used (5–7) (see Chapters 42, 47, 49–56).

CERVICAL SPINE (C2-C7)

Normal and abnormal segmental motion of the cervical spine below the atlanto-axis interface generally involves coupling of side bending and rotation toward the same side. This is thought to result from the existence of four facet-type joints between cervical vertebrae rather than two as seen in the spine below the neck. Two synovial intervertebral facet joints are situated on the posterior-lateral articular columns of the vertebra and the two additional joints (joints of Luschka) are located on the anterior-lateral aspect of the vertebral bodies.

Diagnosis

A typical cervical somatic dysfunction is found by palpating a usually tender prominence of the posterolateral margin of the articular column on one or both sides. The patient may not note pain at that site prior to being examined. The somatic dysfunction is specifically diagnosed by examining for ease/restriction in flexion, extension, side bending, and rotation.

If a segment exhibits a multiple plane, extended somatic dysfunction, the articular pillar on the side toward which it is rotated will be prominent in neutral and flexion and much less prominent in extension. Palpably the vertebra will not move into flexion as easily as it does into extension. The articular pillar on the opposite side of the same vertebra will not change with flexion or extension.

A classic test for cervical segment side bending is lateral translation. This involves pressing the articular pillars of the affected vertebra toward one side and then the other. The side toward which it translates most easily is opposite the side toward which it is side bent. For instance, translation easily to the left means side bending to the right is permitted. The superior segment of the functional unit tilts to the right, the side on which the pressure is exerted. A cervical segment that translates easily toward the left and not as well toward the right is side bent right. Because of the obligatory coupling of side bending and rotation toward the same side in the typical cervical vertebral spine, the vertebral unit will also be rotated toward the right.

To test for cervical rotation the head and neck are held in neutral. The fingertips are maintained on the posterior margins of the segment's articular pillars. The head and cervical spine down to the vertebral unit are rotated to the right and left. The direction in which the segment moves most easily is opposite to the position of rotational restriction. This somatic dysfunction will be named for the position in which the segment moves most easily. This is generally the position in which it is found. In this case it will be extended, rotated, and side bent right ($ER_R S_R$). This naming convention designates the position of ease as well as delineating the side on which the ease is found as a subscript.

An alternate diagnostic method is based on the author's experience. It also begins with assessment of prominence, tenderness, and bogginess on the posterior surface of the articular pillars. A unilateral finding corresponds to the side toward which the dysfunctional segment side bends and rotates most easily. A unilateral finding of prominence, tenderness, and bogginess over the posterior surface of an articular pillar allows one to reduce motion testing to determination of the effect of flexion and extension. One must be careful to distinguish these findings from any tenderness found lateral to the articular pillars or from the deeper exquisite tenderness over the transverse processes that are found on the lateral side of the vertebra about a centimeter anterior to the articular pillar. It is not recommended that the physician who is first mastering cervical segmental diagnosis use this shortcut until comfortable with the traditional diagnostic methods of testing for motion in all three planes and is satisfied that the author's observations are correct.

Cervical Treatment, Supine

Diagnosis: $ER_R S_R$

Position

The patient is supine. The physician sits or stands at the head of the table.

Procedure

1. Physician's left hand (sensing hand) is placed behind the neck with the pad of the index finger on the articular pillar of the affected cervical vertebra. The remainder of the sensing hand supports the head and neck.
2. Physician's right hand (operating hand) is placed on the top of the patient's head.
3. Physician extends and side bends the head and neck to the dysfunctional cervical unit and then markedly rotates the head and neck to the right to the point where the tissues palpably relax (Fig. 70.1).

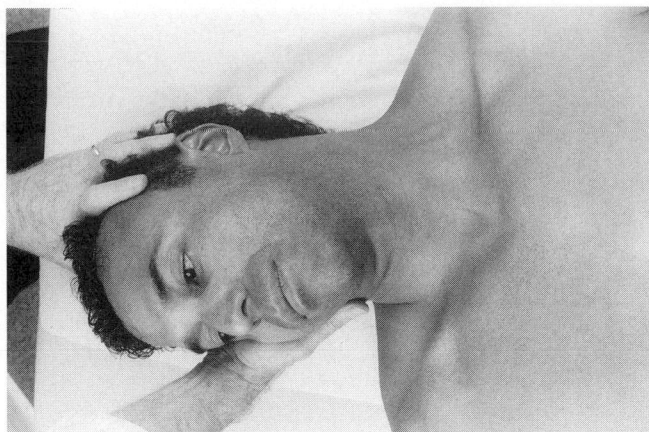

FIGURE 70.1. Initial position for treating typical extended right rotated and side bent cervical dysfunction.

4. Physician's right hand applies compression through the patient's head and neck down to the dysfunctional unit.
5. While maintaining the compression, the physician rotates the patient's head and neck toward the left and carries the head and neck from extension into flexion in a single smooth arc to and through the area of the restrictive barrier (Fig. 70.2). Release will be felt sometime between neutral and full left rotation.
6. Compression is released and the neck is returned to neutral.
7. The procedure is retested and repeated if necessary.

Note: Palpable and/or audible release may or may not be experienced. In some cases a traction force, rather than compression, might work better as a lever. This can be introduced by placing the operating hand under the basiocciput on the side of the dysfunction and applying traction along with rotation and anterior/posterior movement.

OCCIPITAL-ATLAS

An occipital-atlas (O-A) somatic dysfunction is demonstrated by boggy, tense, and tender tissue at the basiocciput at the origin of

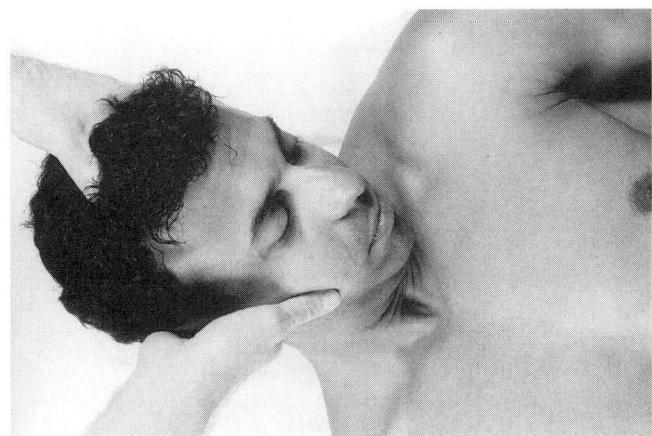

FIGURE 70.2. Final position, typical extended right rotated and side bent cervical dysfunction.

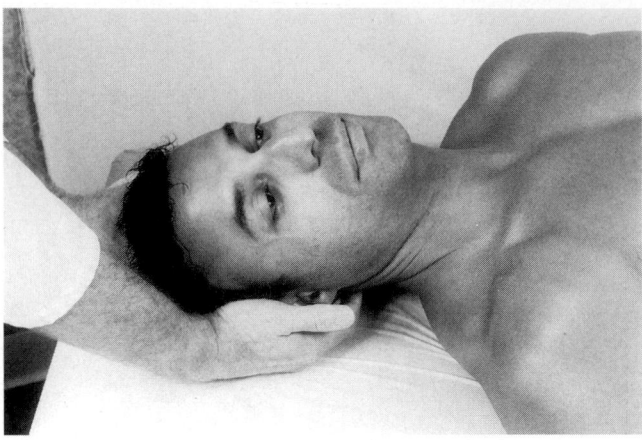

FIGURE 70.3. Initial position, right extended occiputal-atlas dysfunction.

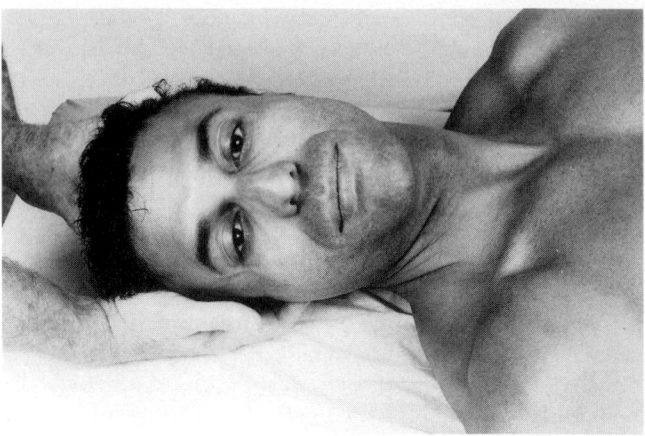

FIGURE 70.4. Initial position, right rotated atlas-axis dysfunction.

rectus capitus, the lateral margin of semispinalis capitus, and the medial margin of splenius capitus. This is roughly at the site of the recurrent occipital nerve foramen. Restriction will be noted in either flexion or extension of the O-A and the overlying tissues will be most relaxed in the opposite direction. For example, if the right O-A is extended and restricted in flexion (OAE$_R$), the tissue will relax with extension of the basiocciput and become more prominent, tight, boggy, and tender with flexion.

Diagnosis: O-A E$_R$

Position

The patient is supine. The physician sits or stands at the head of the table.

Procedure

1. Physician's left hand (sensing hand) is placed under the patient's occiput with the index finger on the affected tender joint and the thumb on the opposite splenius capitus muscle.
2. The physician's right (operating) hand is placed on the dorsum of the head.
3. Physician slightly side bends the patient's head to the right (side of the restricted joint) and extends the patient's head on the atlas.
4. The physician's right hand (operating hand) introduces compression through the dorsum of the head to the right O-A joint (Fig. 70.3).
5. While maintaining compression the physician moves the patient's head into flexion with some right rotation. Movement should be done at a moderate pace.
6. When release is palpated, release compression and return the patient's head to neutral.
7. The procedure is retested and repeated if necessary.

ATLAS-AXIS

The primary movement of the atlas on the axis is rotation. The transverse process of the axis is identified between the angle of the jaw and the mastoid process. If the atlas exhibits somatic dysfunction, its transverse process will be more prominent on the

side toward which it is rotated (the sulcus will be more shallow). Tenderness and tissue bogginess will be noted on the same side. Rotational motion testing will demonstrate easy motion toward the prominent side and restriction toward the opposite side. The somatic dysfunction will be named for the side toward which it rotates most freely. Thus, if the transverse process is tender and boggy on the right, the axis is rotated right (A-AR$_R$).

Diagnosis: A-A R$_R$

Position

The patient is supine. The physician sits or stands at the head of the table.

Procedure

1. Physician's right (sensing) hand is placed under the patient's occiput with the pad of the index finger on the right atlas transverse process. The other fingers of the sensing hand are behind the neck and the palm supports the occiput.
2. Physician's left (operating) hand is placed on the dorsum of the head.
3. Physician rotates the patient's head toward the right to the ease of the tissues.
4. Physician introduces compression through the head to the right A-A joint (Fig. 70.4).
5. The patient's head is rotated to the left toward and through the former restriction.
6. Compression is removed once release is felt and the head is returned to neutral.
7. Retest.

SUPERIOR (ELEVATED) FIRST RIB

No universal convention for naming first rib (R1) dysfunctions has been accepted. The terminology used here names a dysfunction by the ease of movement of the posterior portion most proximal to the spine (e.g., the R1 head). For a superior or elevated R1 the head is tender and presents superior and posterior relative to that of the opposite side. The anterior end of the R1 will be inferior relative to the opposite side and is also generally tender

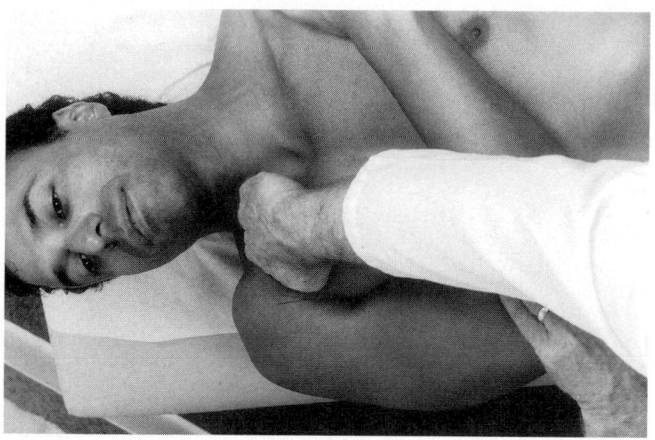

FIGURE 70.5. Initial position, right superior first rib dysfunction.

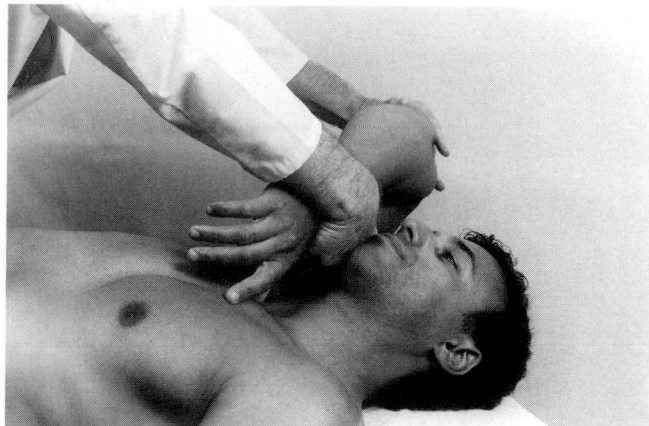

FIGURE 70.6. Intermediate position, right superior first rib dysfunction.

to palpation. Testing the rib for respiratory motions the rib will move easily during inhalation and be restricted during exhalation.

Diagnosis: R1 Superior_R

Position

The patient is supine. The physician stands near the patient's right hip facing the patient's head.

Procedure

1. The physician has the patient flex their right arm at the elbow. The patient's right palm is face down on the left shoulder.
2. The pad of the of the physician's right index finger is placed on the patient's R1 head.
3. The palm of the physician's operating hand is placed on the olecranon of the patient's right elbow.
4. The patient's right elbow is moved medially until it lines up with the head of the R1. The patient's wrist will now be in contact with the physician's sensing arm.
5. The physician introduces compression with the operating hand in a vector toward the head of the affected R1 (Fig. 70.5).
6. The physician brings the patient's elbow superior along a line between the anterior and posterior attachments of the R1 while maintaining compression (Fig. 70.6).
7. The physician now carries the patient's elbow in a backward arc until the patient's arm is passing their ear. Thereafter the motion arcs lateral toward the shoulder.
8. Typically release is felt shortly after the arc starts away from the neck (Fig. 70.7).
9. Compression is reduced.
10. The procedure is retested and repeated if necessary.

INFERIOR (DEPRESSED) FIRST RIB

In an inferior or depressed R1 dysfunction the rib head is inferior and tender relative to the opposite side. The anterior end of the rib will be relatively superior and also tender. The rib will move appropriately during exhalation and not during inhalation.

Diagnosis: R1 Inferior_R

Position

The patient is supine. The physician stands near the patient's waist on the same side as the affected rib.

Procedure

1. The patient's right elbow is flexed with the palm down on the patient's chest.
2. The pad of the physician's right index finger is placed on the rib head.
3. The patient's right elbow is brought into a lateral abducted position. The physician's left hand positions the patient's flexed elbow to maximally relax the right R1 head.
4. With the patient's wrist contacting the underside of the physician's sensing arm the physician's left hand (operating hand) introduces compression through the elbow toward the head of the R1 (Fig. 70.8).
5. The patient's right arm is now swung through an arc superiorly and laterally while maintaining compression toward the rib head (Fig. 70.9).

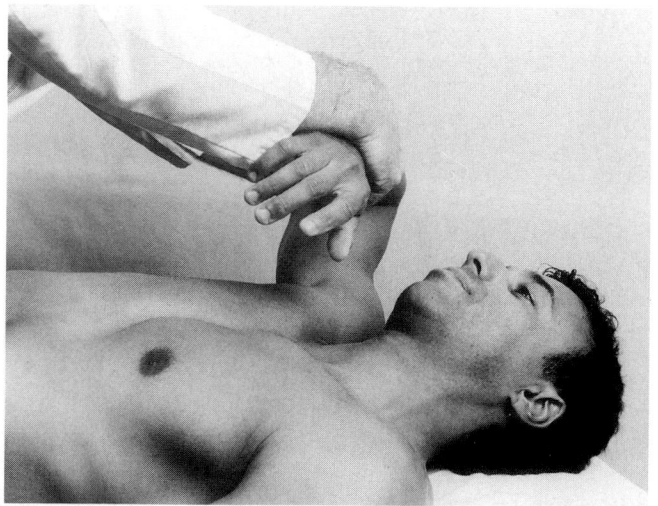

FIGURE 70.7. Final position, right superior first rib dysfunction.

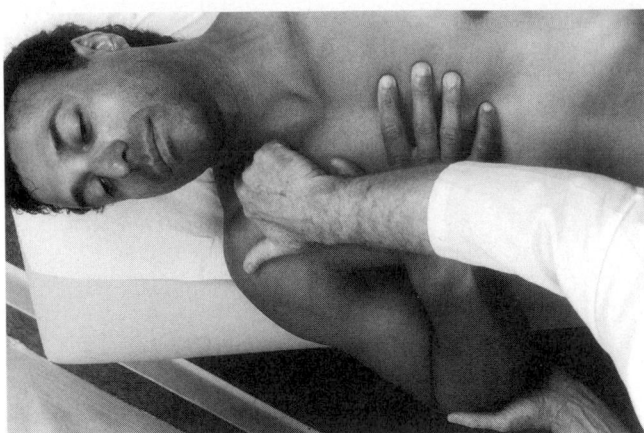

FIGURE 70.8. Initial position, right inferior first rib dysfunction.

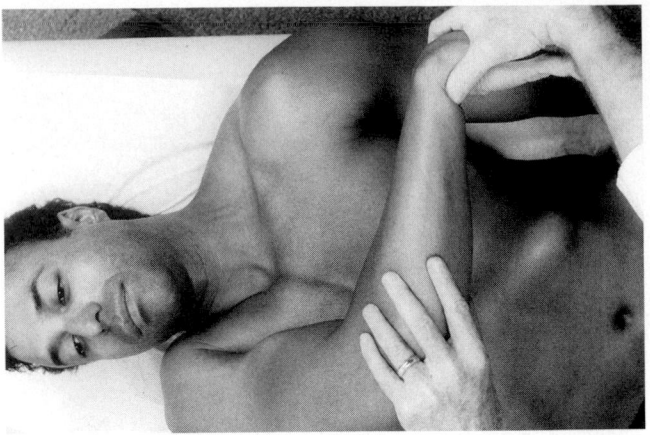

FIGURE 70.10. Final position, right inferior first rib dysfunction.

6. The patient's right elbow is carried anterior-medial. Its final position is below the anterior end of the R1 (Fig. 70.10).

7. As the patient's elbow reaches its apex above the patient's ear, release will be felt. Compression is then released.

8. The physician's sensing finger is removed from the rib head and the sensing hand catches the patient's wrist.

9. The patient's arm is returned to its resting position next to the thorax.

10. The procedure is retested and repeated if necessary.

THORACIC SPINE

The standard thoracic diagnostic method has the physician standing behind the patient. The physician has the patient flex. The physician checks each segment for motion asymmetry in side bending and rotation. The patient is then evaluated in the same manner using extension (5–7) (see Chapters 47 and 51).

An experienced osteopathic physician may use an alternative simple and rapid method for assessing segmental thoracic somatic

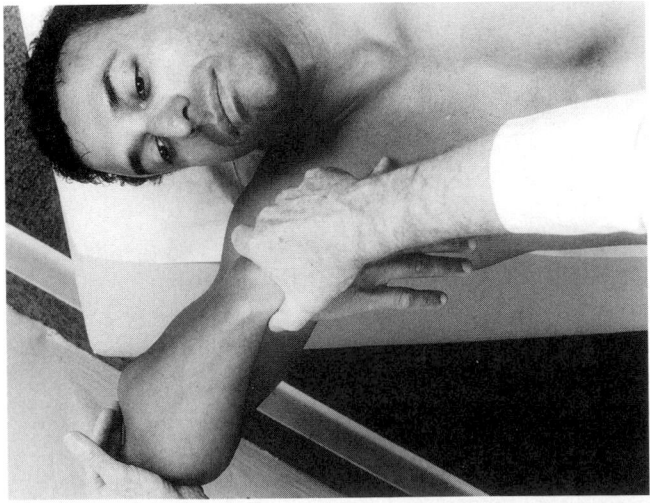

FIGURE 70.9. Intermediate position, right inferior first rib dysfunction.

dysfunctions. The physician stands behind the seated patient and runs their fingertips lightly along two lines parallel to and about 2.5 cm lateral to the spinous processes. This positions the sensing fingers over the transverse processes and facet joints.

Typically one finds a fullness, bogginess, and/or tissue ropiness over the transverse process of a vertebra with somatic dysfunction. If the segment shows type II mechanics the tissue texture changes will be found over the transverse process on the side toward which the segment is side bent and rotated. One can simply proceed to test whether the transverse process on that side becomes more or less prominent when the patient flexes or extends the spine. However, it is my experience that testing is easier and more accurate when the physician induces flexion and extension. If the transverse process and its overlying tissue become more prominent in extension and indistinguishable from its neighbors in flexion, then it is flexed. If it does not improve in either flexion or extension, then it is probably a neutral or type I segmental somatic dysfunction and side bending and rotation will need to be assessed independently.

Upper Thoracic Vertebra Type II Dysfunction

Note: This version is similar to that described by Dr. Still (4). It can be useful down to about T8 on most patients.

Diagnosis: T3FR$_R$S$_R$

Position
The patient sits. The physician stands in front of the patient.

Procedure
1. Physician's arms are placed over the patient's shoulders.

2. Physician's left index finger (sensing hand) is on the right transverse process of the patient's third thoracic vertebra.

3. Physician's arms on the patient's shoulders flex and right side bend the patient's thorax until the tissues under the sensing finger are palpably reduced or softened and the transverse process is no longer prominent (Fig. 70.11). Physician's arms introduce about 5 pounds (2 kg) pressure in a vector through the affected segment.

4. Physician rotates the patient's shoulders and spine to the left,

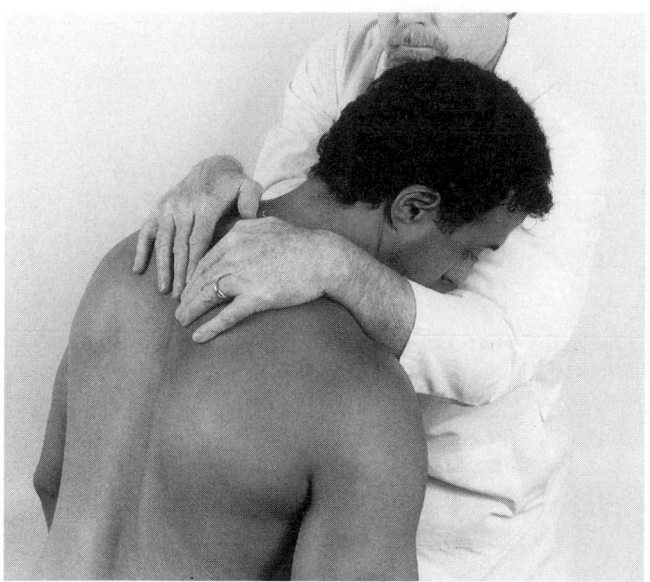

FIGURE 70.11. Initial position, upper thoracic vertebra, flexed, side bent, and rotated right.

reducing flexion until it becomes extension. As the segment is carried into left rotation with mild extension, release of the segmental restriction may be felt (Fig. 70.12).

5. Compression is released and the patient is passively returned to neutral.
6. The procedure is retested and repeated as necessary.

Comment: It is quite easy to couple this treatment technique with diagnosis as was generally done by Dr. Still (1). The only reason I do not typically simultaneously diagnose and treat is that I prefer to write all my diagnoses down before treating so as not to confuse my memory. If one can dictate at the time of treatment or has a very good short-term memory, one could probably diagnose and treat at the same time, as did Dr. Still.

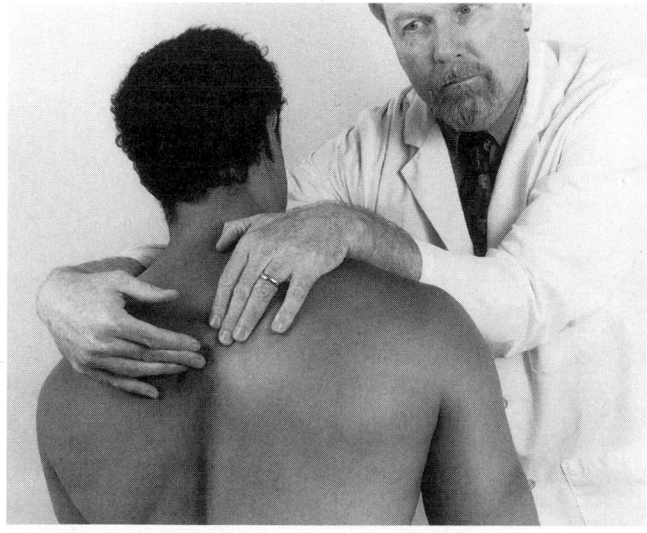

FIGURE 70.12. Final position, upper thoracic vertebra, flexed, side bent, and rotated right.

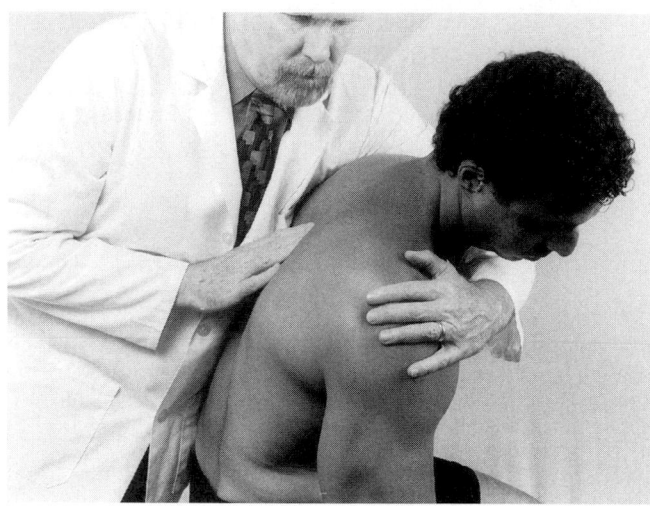

FIGURE 70.13. Initial position, thoracic vertebra, flexed, side bent, and rotated right.

Thoracic Vertebrae Type II Dysfunction

This technique is usable for all thoracic vertebrae below T_1 or T_2.

Diagnosis: $T3FR_RS_R$

Position
The patient is seated with the physician standing behind.

Procedure
1. The pad of the physician's right index finger (sensing hand) is placed over the prominent transverse process of the affected segment.
2. The patient's right hand is placed on their left shoulder.
3. The physician's operating arm (left) is passed over the patient's left shoulder around the patient's superior chest wall and the hand is placed on the patient's right shoulder. This gives the physician adequate leverage to introduce flexion or extension, compression, and rotation.
4. The patient's thorax and spine are flexed and rotated right producing palpable relaxation over the affected segment.
5. The physician introduces compression through the patient's shoulders (Fig. 70.13) vectored toward the affected segment.
6. The physician's operating arm simultaneously reduces the patient's spinal flexion, moves into extension, and rotates the spine through neutral into the previously restricted range of left rotation.
7. Once release is noted compression is removed and the patient passively returned to neutral.
8. The procedure is retested and repeated as necessary.

RIBS (BELOW RIB 1)

Rib motion is typically described based on the dominant axis of motion (pump handle versus bucket handle) and/or whether a rib or ribs move more easily in inhalation or exhalation (5–7)

TABLE 70.1. SINGLE RIB DIAGNOSIS

Diagnosis	"Posterior Rib"	"Anterior Rib"
Rib angle	Posterior and tender	Anterior and tender
Costochondral junction	Posterior and tender	Anterior and tender
Compression	Anterior direction restricted	Posterior direction restricted
	Posterior direction permitted	Anterior direction permitted
Movement permitted	Exhalation	Inhalation
Movement restricted	Inhalation	Exhalation

(see Chapter 52). Although both concepts make sense when examining group restrictions, it has been the author's experience that single rib restrictions are more common and more likely to be symptomatic. To simplify diagnosis I have developed a new terminology for single rib dysfunctions (Table 70.1).

Most single rib dysfunctions can be described in terms of a single plane of motion: anterior-posterior. If the rib crosses under the scapula the patient often reports "something painful" between the chest wall and scapula. Tissue bogginess is present over the rib angle in both types of rib somatic dysfunction and may make palpation of an "anterior" rib angle more difficult. Note that a posterior rib appears to correspond to what is traditionally termed an exhalation rib and an anterior rib appears to correspond to what is traditionally termed an inhalation rib. However, diagnosis as a "posterior" or "anterior" rib is easier, quicker, and responds well with the treatment methods of the Still technique described in the next paragraph.

Solitary Posterior Upper Thoracic Rib

Diagnosis: Rib3P$_L$

Position

The patient is seated on a table or stool. The physician stands behind the patient toward the side of the affected rib.

Procedure

1. Physician places the pad of the right thumb as a sensor on the angle of the patient's left third rib. The palm and fingers of that hand stabilize the patient's upper back.
2. Physician holds the patient's left elbow with the left hand (operating hand). Depending on the relative size of the physician and the patient, the physician may encircle the patient's arm somewhat more proximally to the elbow.
3. Patient's left arm is brought posterior (extended at the shoulder). The patient's elbow will be at about the level of the angle of the affected rib.
4. Physician introduces compression through the elbow vectored toward the dysfunctional rib's head (Fig. 70.14).
5. Patient's left shoulder is articulated in a smooth arc through abduction with partial flexion (to about 110 degrees) (Fig. 70.15) and then into adduction. The final position of the patient's arm is in the area of the patient's right abdomen (Fig. 70.16).
6. Axial compression is released. The patient's arm is returned to a neutral position along the left chest wall.
7. Rib motion and position are reassessed.

Note: To treat ribs 4 through 6, the initial positioning is similar, but with the elbow at the level of the affected rib's angle, the arc of articulation is progressively more lateral with each lower rib. At times the best arc to treat below rib 5 may require the arm being used to end above the level of the opposite shoulder to obtain a full release.

Solitary Posterior Rib

Diagnosis: Rib3P$_L$

Position

The physician stands in front of the seated patient.

Treatment

1. Physician places forearms over the patient's shoulders. A finger of the physician's right hand (sensing hand) is on the angle of the rib.
2. Physician side bends the patient's spine left and rotates the patient's left thorax posterior until the tissues around the rib angle relax (Fig. 70.17).
3. Physician develops compression of 5 pounds or less vectored through the physician's forearms to the rib head.
4. Maintaining compression, the physician side bends the patient toward the right side and simultaneously rotates the patient's thorax to the right.
5. Compression is released and the patient returned to neutral.
6. The rib is retested.

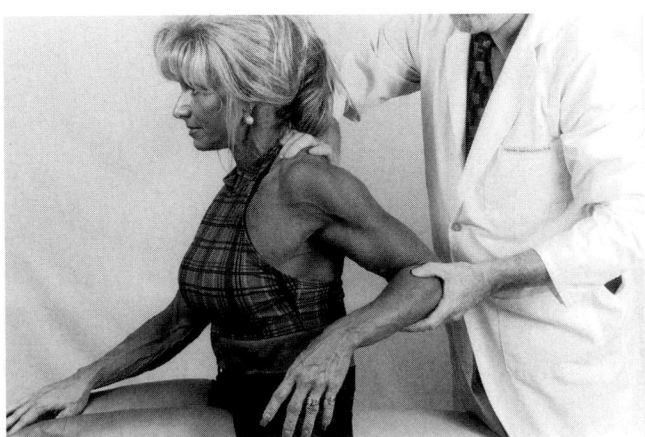

FIGURE 70.14. Initial position, upper rib posterior left.

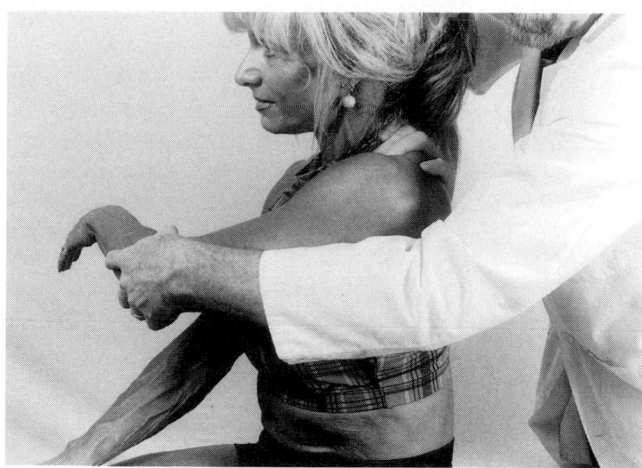

FIGURE 70.15. Intermediate position, upper rib posterior left.

Anterior Rib

The treatment of an anterior rib from in front of the patient starts with the patient's shoulder and thorax anterior on the side of the somatic dysfunction. The treatment of single rib dysfunctions from in front of the patient coordinates well with the thoracic spinal segment techniques approached from in front. The alternative is to treat from behind.

Diagnosis: Rib3A$_L$

Position

The patient is seated on a table or stool. The physician stands behind the patient toward the patient's left side.

Procedure

1. Physician places thumb of the right hand on the affected rib angle with palm and fingers of the hand stabilizing the patient's upper back.
2. Physician's left hand encircles patient's left elbow. The patient's

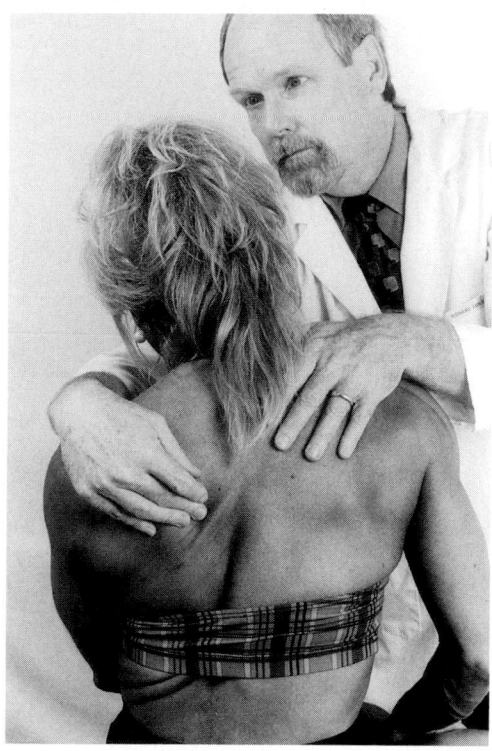

FIGURE 70.17. Initial position, upper rib posterior left, treated from in front.

arm is adducted in the same plane as the affected costochondral junction to produce palpable easing in the tissues over the rib angle (Fig. 70.18).
3. Physician articulates the patient's arm through partial flexion (to 140 degrees) and abduction (Fig. 70.19). Now it is carried into extension in a smooth arc while maintaining compression through the arm toward the rib head (Fig. 70.20).
4. Physician releases compression and returns the arm to a neutral position.
5. The rib is reassessed.

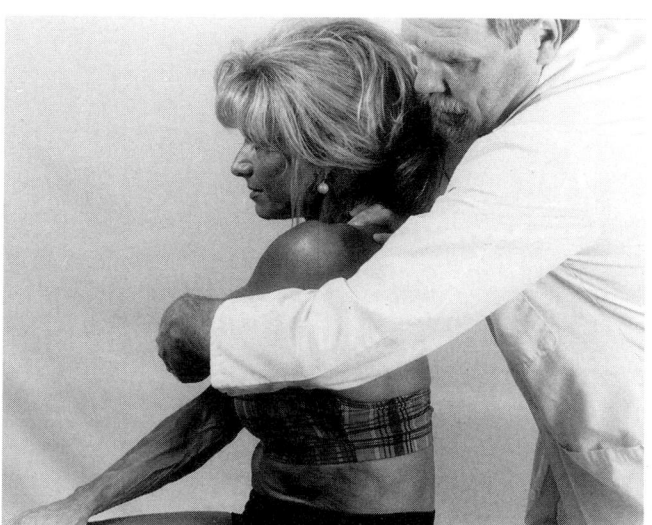

FIGURE 70.16. Final position, upper rib posterior left.

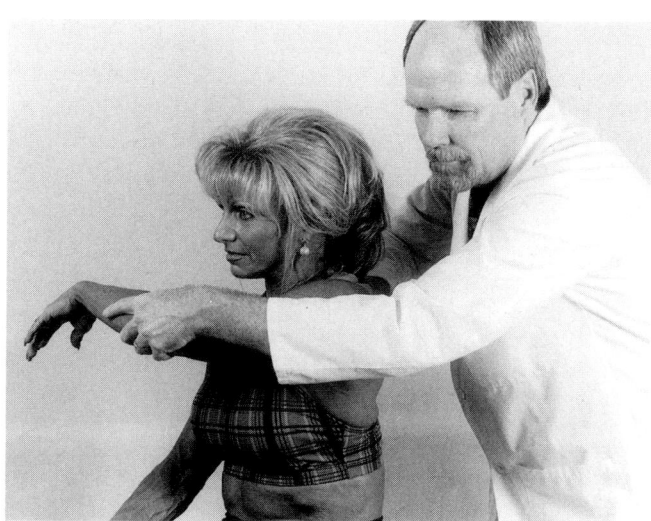

FIGURE 70.18. Initial position, upper rib anterior left.

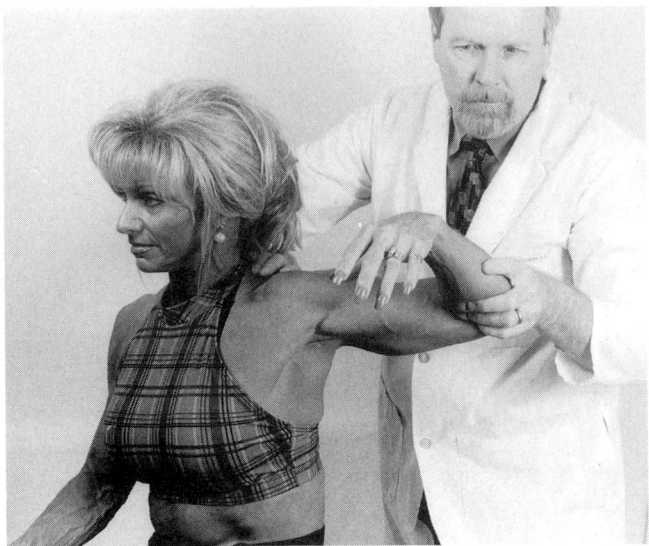

FIGURE 70.19. Intermediate position, upper rib anterior left.

Note: For ribs 4 through 6 the arc is lowered so that correction of a fifth rib will involve an arc that is at the level of the patient's shoulder.

LUMBAR SPINE

Treating the lumbar spine, pelvis (innominates), and sacrum using the Still technique requires a specific order to treatment. Diagnosis can be performed for all three areas prior to treatment. However treatment must begin with the lumbar spine and pelvis with the sacrum being treated last. Doing so vastly simplifies diagnosis and treatment of the sacrum.

Usually, there are five lumbar vertebrae. No ribs are attached to these vertebrae. Generally the lumbar spine exhibits a mild lordotic curve. Normally there is no scoliotic curve. Like the thoracic spine most clinically significant somatic dysfunctions involve type II mechanics (e.g., flexed or extended, and side bent and rotated toward the same side). Palpably the tissues over one of the transverse processes of a type II segmental somatic dysfunction will be prominent and boggy, representing the side toward which it is rotated and side bent. Often there will be tenderness in the same area. The spinous process will be slightly displaced toward the opposite side due to vertebral rotation. To determine whether the segment is flexed or extended the physician passively induces flexion and extension, monitoring the prominent transverse process for palpable relaxation. Thus if the left transverse process of L3 is prominent and if it becomes indistinguishable from its neighbors during induced flexion, the segment is flexed, side bent and rotated to the left.

Flexed Lumbar Segment

Diagnosis: L3FS$_L$R$_L$

Position

The patient is supine. The physician stands at the patient's left side.

Procedure

1. Physician inserts left hand under the patient's lumbar area and a sensing finger is placed on the left transverse process of L3.
2. Physician flexes the patient's left leg at the hip and knee until the sensing finger palpates relaxation. Now the physician's left hand is moved to the patient's left (flexed) knee and the physician's right hand is placed on the patient's left ankle. The patient's left knee is then adducted and the ankle is swung laterally, internally rotating the patient's thigh. This effectively side bends the patient's hip toward the affected side and induces flexion of L3 on L4 (Fig. 70.21).
3. Physician introduces compression vectored toward L3.
4. Physician moves the patient's knee laterally into abduction, slightly rotating the patient's pelvis posterior toward the table on the side of the dysfunction (Fig. 70.22).
5. Physician extends the patient's leg (Fig. 70.23).
6. Physician releases compression and returns the patient's leg to a neutral position.
7. Retest.

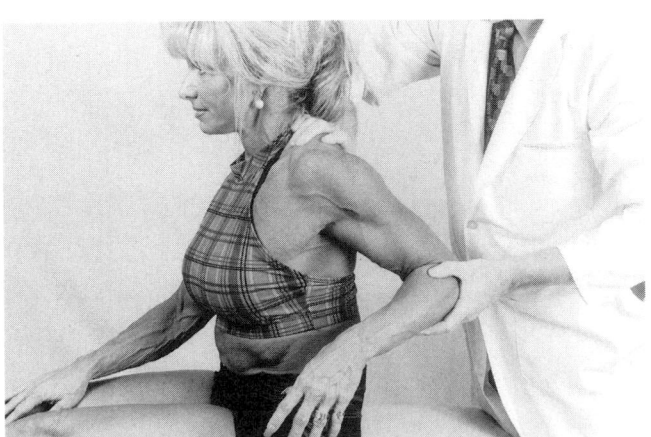

FIGURE 70.20. Final position, upper rib anterior left.

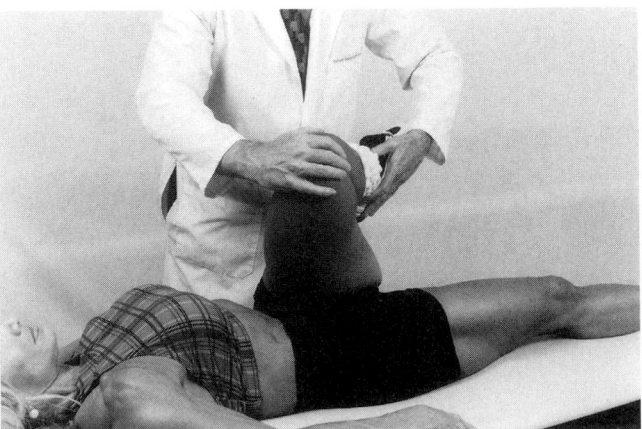

FIGURE 70.21. Initial position, lumbar vertebra flexed, side bent, and rotated left.

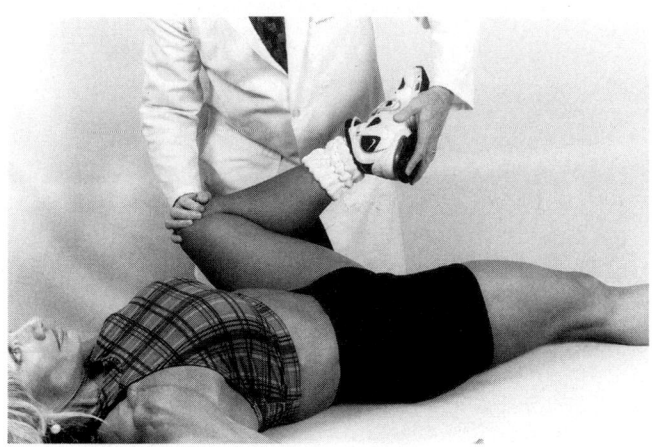

FIGURE 70.22. Intermediate position, lumbar vertebra flexed, side bent, and rotated left.

Extended Lumbar Segment

Diagnosis: L3ES$_L$R$_L$

Position

The patient is supine. The physician stands at the patient's side.

Procedure

1. Physician inserts sensing hand under the patient's lumbar spine with a sensing finger placed on the dysfunctional segment's left transverse process.
2. The patient's knee and hip on the side of the dysfunction are flexed. The physician's operating hand is on the flexed knee. The flexed knee is abducted until the affected segment palpably relaxes.
3. Physician introduces compression vectored from the patient's left knee to the affected segment (Fig. 70.24).
4. Physician adducts patient's left knee across the midline.
5. Physician extends the patient's knee and compression is released.
6. Retest.

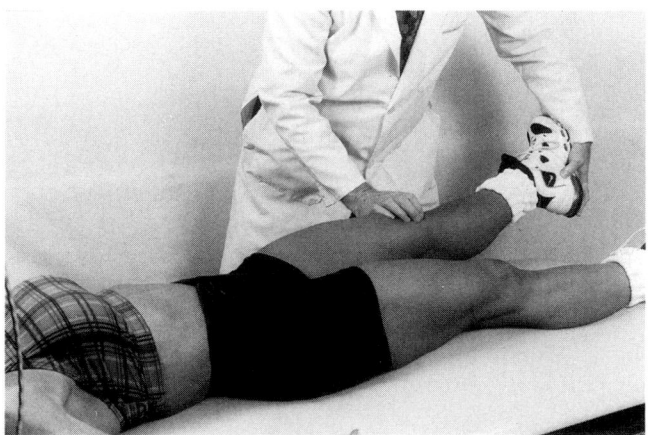

FIGURE 70.23. Final position, lumbar vertebra flexed, side bent, and rotated left.

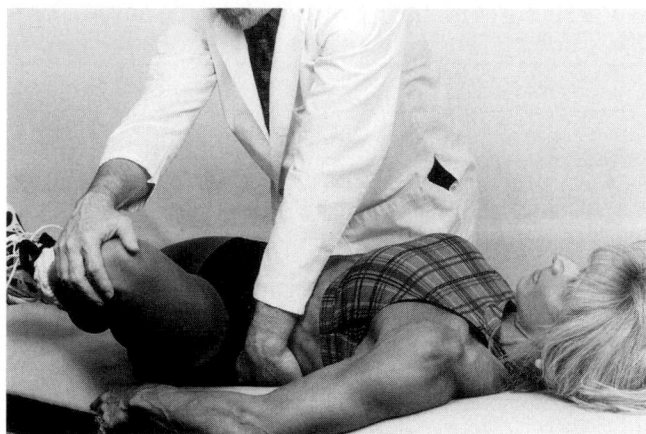

FIGURE 70.24. Initial position, lumbar vertebra extended, side bent, and rotated left.

ILIUM OR INNOMINATE

The relationship between the ilium or innominate and the sacrum is traditionally termed iliosacral. The emphasis is on the orientation of the ilia. Diagnosis of *iliosacral* (IS) somatic dysfunctions is based on combinations of three basic tests and reflects the relative positions and movements of the two hemipelvic bones (innominates).

Two main types of innominate somatic dysfunction are known. Functionally, the ilium or innominate exhibits a cam-like rotation with its primary fulcrum of rotation at the hip joint. Because the hip joint is inferior and anterior to the largest portion of the ilium, as the hip flexes the iliac crest swings posterior, and as the hip extends, the iliac crest rotates anterior. Rotation of the innominate occurs primarily at its joint with the sacrum and normally is restrained anteriorly by the limited elasticity of the pubic symphysis synostosis and posteriorly by the ligaments of the sacroiliac joint. Most iliosacral rotational dysfunction seems to develop in the complex joint between the ilium and sacrum. A vertical shear is the other potential source of somatic dysfunction in iliosacral mechanics. The iliosacral joint has a normal, although minimal, amount of vertical glide. Within its normal short vertical motion range the iliosacral complex appears behave as a shock absorber. Pushed to its limits by excessive or prolonged unilateral force from below and in line with the body's axis, the ilium can shear in a cephalad direction, producing the somatic dysfunction termed an upslipped innominate. Pelvic landmarks and their related tests used in the diagnosis of iliosacral dysfunction are:

1. *Posterior superior iliac spine* (PSIS): Levelness of the PSISs is easily assessed with the patient seated and the physician behind the patient. Although classically it is stated that PSIS position is assessed with the patient prone, standing, or seated, there is little to be gained from testing in multiple positions. The seated test starts with the physician placing the fingers of both hands on the patient's iliac crests. The physician's thumbs slide down the patient's lumbar paravertebral spine about 3 cm lateral to the midline where the superior surfaces of the bony prominences of the PSISs are encountered. One should then follow the PSISs caudad until their inferior margins are discovered. The physician then determines whether one of the thumbs is superior to the other.

TABLE 70.2. TESTS TO DIAGNOSE ILIOSACRAL DYS-FUNCTION

Diagnosis	PSIS	ASIS	Pelvic Translation
Anterior right rotation	^Right	^Left	+Right
Anterior left rotation	^Left	^Right	+Left
Posterior right rotation	^Left	^Right	+Right
Posterior left rotation	^Right	^Left	+Left
Upslipped right innominate	^Right	^Right	+Right
Upslipped left innominate	^Left	^Left	+Left

PSIS, posterior superior iliac spine; ASIS, anterior superior iliac spine.

2. *Anterior superior iliac spine* (ASIS): Levelness of the ASISs can be performed seated (in most cases), standing, or supine. Since most of the IS treatments using the Still technique are performed with the patient supine, the author has routinely performed this test with the patient supine. The physician stands at the patient's side, below the level of the patient's hips. The physician uses their thumbs to locate the inferior edge of the ASIS bilaterally, then judges which, if either, is superior.

3. *Pelvic rocking* or *ASIS compression test:* There are two versions of this very common test. Both work equally well. Both are performed with the patient supine. In the first version the physician places the palms of the hands on the ASIS bilaterally and alternates pressure on each. The side toward which there is less easy movement is positive. The other test involves placing the fingertips of both hands on the lateral surface of both ASIS. Alternating gentle pressure toward the midline will result in small lateral translation of the hips. The side toward which motion is restricted is positive. Table 70.2 shows three tests used in the diagnosis of iliosacral dysfunction.

There is no single test or even a pair of tests that predict the nature of the iliosacral somatic dysfunction. If there is a question about which innominate is dysfunctional, the author has found that there will be tender points just medial to the ASIS on the side of a dysfunctional innominate. The use of tender points for diagnosing somatic dysfunction is not generally a formal part of the diagnostic criteria for either muscle energy or high velocity/low amplitude (HVLA) techniques. However, when there is a high correlation between particular tender points and functional problems the tender point can be used to help settle a diagnosis that is in doubt.

Anterior Right Iliosacral Dysfunction (Right Anterior Innominate)

Position
The patient is supine. The physician stands on the patient's right side.

Procedure
1. Physician's left hand is placed under the patient's pelvis so that a sensing finger can be placed on the lower pole of the sacroiliac joint.
2. Physician's right hand grasps the patient's right knee and partially flexes the patient's leg at the hip to 45 to 60 degrees.
3. Physician slightly abducts or adducts the patient's right knee until the tissues of the sacroiliac joint relax (Fig. 70.25).

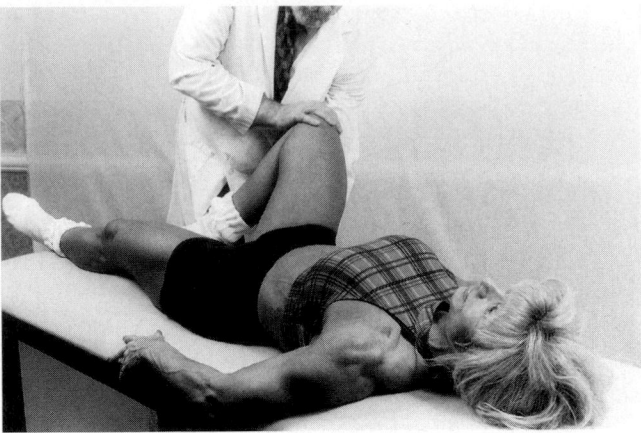

FIGURE 70.25. Initial position, anterior right iliosacral dysfunction.

4. Physician introduces compression through the knee to the lower pole of the sacroiliac joint.
5. Physician moves the patient's knee in an arc through full hip flexion and into flexion with adduction (Fig. 70.26).
6. Physician carries the patient's hip into extension.
7. Physician releases compression at about 30 degrees of hip extension and then completes extension of the patient's leg.
8. Retest.

Posterior Left Iliosacral Dysfunction (Left Posterior Innominate)

Position
The patient is supine. The physician stands at the patient's left side.

Procedure
1. The physician's right hand is placed under the patient's pelvis so that a sensing finger can be placed on the cephalad portion of the sacroiliac joint.
2. The patient's left knee and hip are flexed to more than

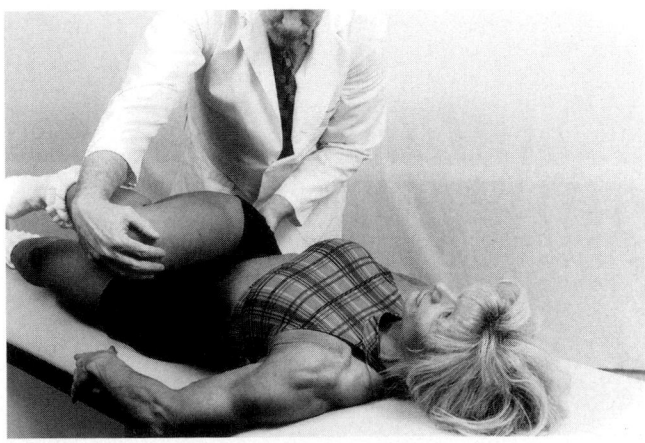

FIGURE 70.26. Intermediate position, anterior right iliosacral dysfunction.

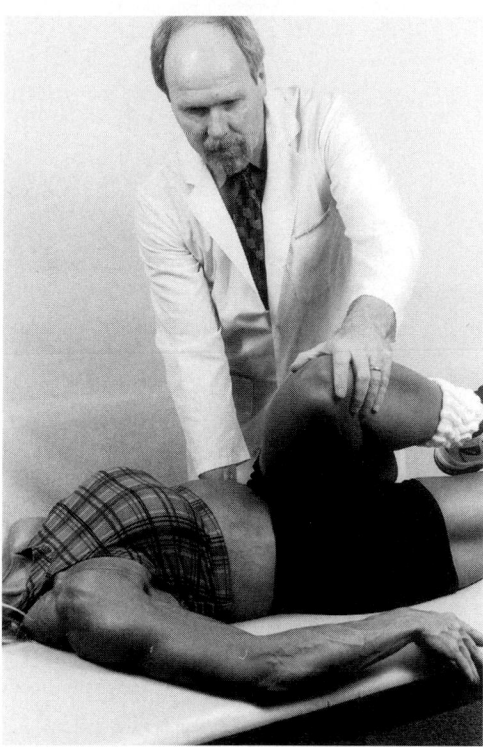

FIGURE 70.27. Initial position posterior left iliosacral dysfunction.

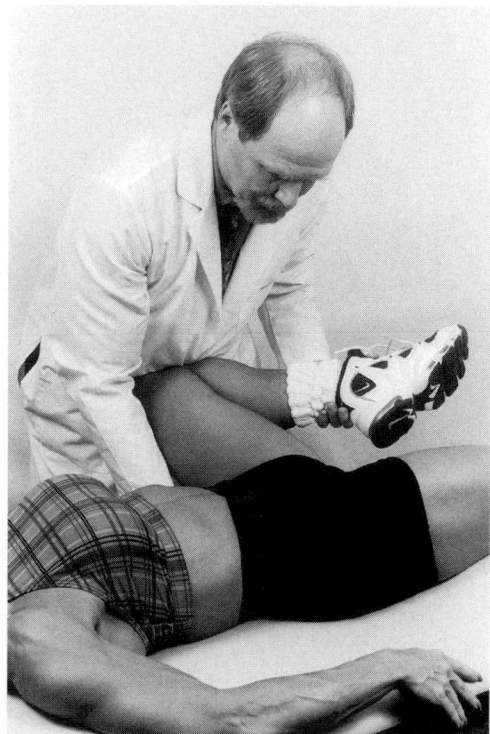

FIGURE 70.28. Intermediate position, posterior left iliosacral dysfunction.

90 degrees and adducted across the midline. Physician's left hand (operating hand) is on the patient's knee.

3. Physician introduces compression in a vector through the upper pole of the sacroiliac joint (Fig. 70.27).

4. Physician abducts the patient's left hip while maintaining compression.

5. As the patient's knee reaches its most lateral point in the arc (as determined by tissue compliance), compression on the patient's knee is transferred from the physician's hand to the physician's abdomen and the operating hand slips down to capture the patient's left ankle (Fig. 70.28).

6. Maintaining compression through the patient's knee, the physician extends the leg.

7. Compression is discontinued after release is palpated or after the hip is extended approximately 30 degrees. The leg is then passively extended.

8. Retest.

Upslipped Innominate

To date no single treatment using the Still technique has been found that resolves all of this dysfunction. Perhaps this is because the innominate shear is not physiologic, making it more of a joint strain than a simple somatic dysfunction. For the most part the Still technique is deployed within physiologic ranges, although the author has used the Still methods to help reduce and properly mobilize ankle sprains to good effect. Whatever the case, an upslipped innominate functionally acts as if limitations at several joints or tissues are defining this dysfunction. The author has provisionally identified three separate restrictions involving

three embryonic remnants of the sacral transverse processes seen within the sacroiliac joint. Although this identification may be useful, it should not be thought of as any more than a focusing tool and should not be taken as an established fact.

Diagnosis: Innominate U_R (Step 1)

Position

The patient is supine on the table. The physician stands at the patient's feet.

Procedure

1. Physician grasps the patient's right ankle with both hands. The ankle and leg are gently externally rotated.

2. Axial compression is introduced toward the right sacroiliac joint (Fig. 70.29).

3. Physician internally rotates the patient's leg.

4. Compression is changed to gentle traction.

5. The leg is released and returned to rest.

6. If the ASIS is assessed at this point it will be found to be level with the opposite side, but motion testing still demonstrates persistence of somatic dysfunction.

Step 2

Use the Still treatment technique for a posterior rotated innominate.

Step 3

Use the Still treatment for an anterior rotated innominate.

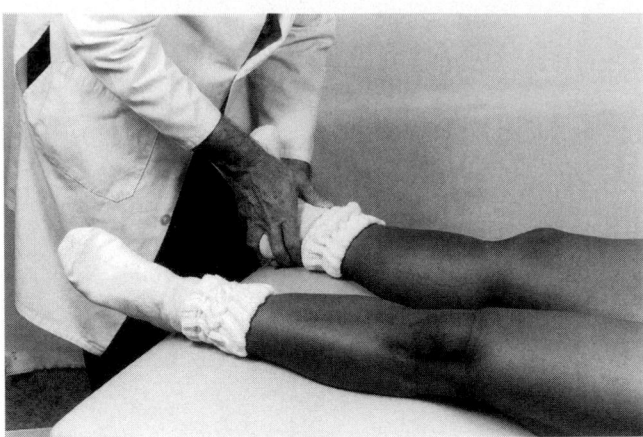

FIGURE 70.29. Initial position, right upslipped innominate dysfunction.

PUBIC RAMUS

The principal somatic dysfunction of the pubic ramus is that one side will be either superior or inferior relative to the other. It is common for the pubic ramus dysfunction to follow the innominate dysfunction. Thus a superior pubic ramus may be seen on the same side as a posterior innominate, or more commonly an upslipped innominate. It is also common to see an inferior pubic ramus on the same side as an anterior innominate. However, this relationship is not obligatory. Presumably any uncoupling of pubic ramus dysfunction from innominate dysfunction reflects the relative flexibility of living bone.

The relative displacement and immobilization of one side of the pubic ramus places considerable strain on the pubic synostosis. It is typically accompanied by tender points at the superior margin of the pubic ramus and/or at the lateral margins of the pubic bones at the insertion of the inguinal ligaments. To evaluate for a possible pubic ramus dysfunction the patient is supine. The physician starts with the fingertips about 2 inches (5 cm) below the umbilicus and about $\frac{1}{2}$ inch (1 cm) out from the midline bilaterally. Using the pads of the fingertips, the physician sweeps downward until the bony prominence of the pubic ramus is palpated. Recognize which side is superior. Note as well the side of tenderness. The tender side generally indicates the side of dysfunction. Sometimes the pubic ramus is just compressed or stretched, in which case both sides would be tender. In every case the manipulative technique would be approximately the same. It should be noted that treatment of innominate dysfunctions often reduces pubic ramus dysfunctions, so the innominates should be treated first.

Pubic Ramus Dysfunction

Position
The patient is supine. The physician stands at the patient's feet.

Procedure
1. Physician bilaterally flexes the patient's hips and knees so that the patient's feet are on the table about 12 inches (30 cm) from the ischial tuberosities. The patient's knees are together and vertical relative to the table.

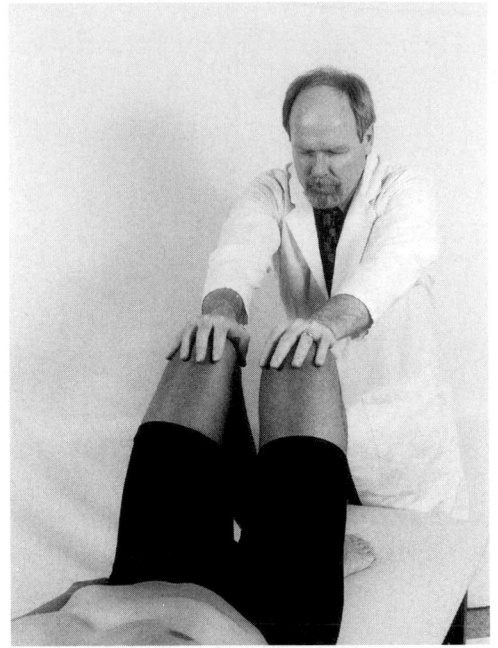

FIGURE 70.30. Initial position, pubic ramus dysfunction.

2. Physician places one hand on each of the patient's knees (Fig. 70.30).
3. Physician introduces compression from the patient's knees toward the pubic ramus.
4. Physician simultaneously brings the patient's knees laterally maintaining compression (Fig. 70.31).
5. Release may be felt through the legs as the knees pass 60 degrees.

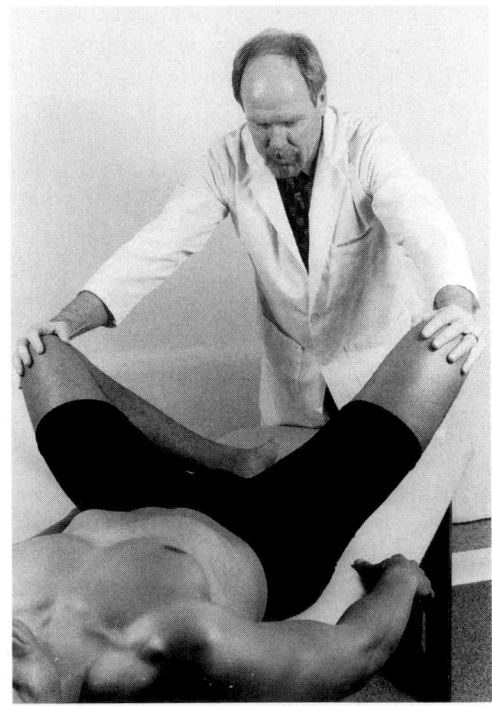

FIGURE 70.31. Intermediate position, pubic ramus dysfunction.

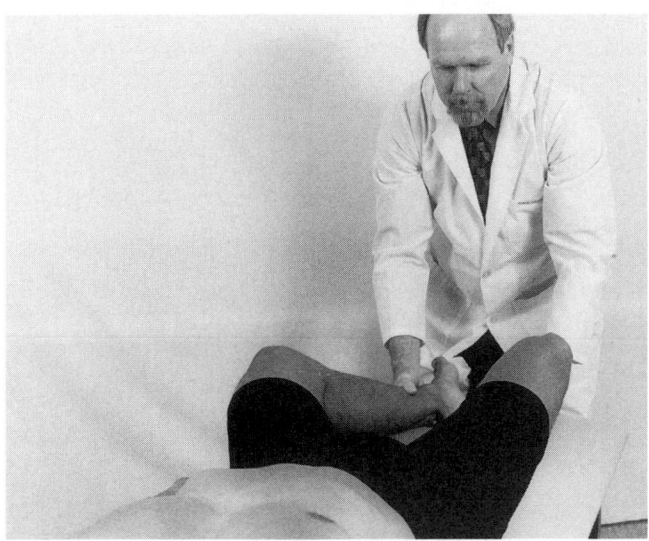

FIGURE 70.32. Final position, pubic ramus dysfunction.

6. Physician removes the hands from the patient's knees and captures both ankles.
7. Keeping the patient's legs at 60 degrees, the physician draws the patient's feet toward the foot of the table until the knees and hips are again extended (Fig. 70.32).
8. Retest.

SACRUM

Sacroiliac motions are classically described as rotatory along two angled planes, and flexion and extension about a transverse axis. The two most common systems for describing, diagnosis, and treating sacral somatic dysfunctions are those from the Chicago school that focused on HVLA methods (7) (see also Chapters 47, 55, and 59), and those developed by Mitchell for the muscle energy methods (5,6) (see also Chapter 60).

During the author's process of redeveloping applications of the Still technique, a great deal of similarity was found between the diagnostic and treatment positions in both HVLA and muscle energy treatment systems. Examples include sacral torsions, unilateral sacral flexions (shears), and the anterior and posterior sacral dysfunctions. For instance, the HVLA treatment for a unilateral flexed left sacrum is virtually identical to that for a left on left dysfunction. Nonetheless, early attempts were made to develop Still applications for each of the sacral dysfunctions described in the Mitchell model. Initially, no particular treatment order was imposed. However, over time, and without consciously deciding on an order of treatment, the author found himself treating the lumbar spine first because the patient was still seated after treating the thoracic spine. Further, when treating innominate and sacral dysfunctions with the patient supine, more often than not the author tended to treat the innominate dysfunctions first.

Surprisingly, it was found that prior treatment of the innominate and lumbar dysfunctions seemed to limit the number and type of sacroiliac dysfunctions that remained untreated. In the years since work began with the Still technique, no bilateral sacral flexions or extensions have been found after treatment of lumbar and iliosacral dysfunctions. Likewise, the backward sacral torsions seemed to resolve after treatment of any concomitant anterior or posterior innominate dysfunction. One obvious reason for the paucity of sacral findings after treatment of lumbar and iliac dysfunctions must be the interdependence of lumbar, sacral, and iliac mechanics. Logically one would expect the sharing of joints, tendons, and muscles to create an interdependence of function. By treating those structures that are engaged with the sacrum, a number of dysfunctions that were due to the relation between the sacrum and its neighbors should be, and in fact are, released. In view of the complexity of sacral diagnosis and mechanics in other systems of analysis, the limitation of sacral findings following treatment of lumbar and innominate dysfunctions has been an unexpected and pleasant side effect.

After treatment of lumbar and innominate somatic dysfunctions only two types of sacral dysfunctions seem to remain. For a number of years, while developing the Still technique, the author tended to identify these two classes of sacral dysfunctions with the names used in the Mitchell model for sacral torsions. This terminology was used even though the method of analysis was severely truncated and the dysfunctions identified did not necessarily meet the criteria of Mitchell's diagnostics. Finally, it became apparent that the terminology was not reflecting either the diagnostic criteria used or the limited number of techniques necessary for successful resolution of sacral dysfunctions following the proposed order of treatment and use of the Still techniques.

Both of the residual sacral dysfunctions observed after successful treatment of lumbar and innominate dysfunctions behave as if the sacrum was fixated at two poles, one superior and one inferior. The two superior poles are inferior to L5 lateral on the sacral base and just medial to the PSISs. Functionally, a restriction of a superior pole seems to correspond to tension in the tendinous insertions of the erector spinae on the superior portion of the sacrum. The two inferior poles are near the origins of the sacrotuberous ligaments on the lower part of the sacrum. Restriction in one of them appears to correspond to tension in the sacrotuberous ligament. Although these residual restrictions are the hallmarks of the only sacral dysfunctions seen after treatment and resolution of lumbar and innominate dysfunctions, the restrictions are identifiable even before treatment. This emphasis on fixation at two sacral poles is different from the models used by both the Chicago and Michigan schools that emphasize single pole dysfunctions. It does not negate the findings of either. It does suggest that any abnormalities of sacral mechanics in isolation from lumbar and thoracic mechanics may be somewhat different than has been previously described.

When the sacrotuberous ligament on one side is fixed or tight and the superior pole on the opposite side is fixed, the sacrum acts as though it can only rotate on the diagonal axis. Its ease of rotation at the sacral base would be in an anterior or posterior direction toward or away from the restricted sacral pole. This type of sacral dysfunction is now being termed a *diagonal sacral dysfunction*. In other cases the sacrum is found to have restrictions at the upper and lower poles on the same side. These are now being termed *unilateral sacral dysfunctions*. It is important to understand that the generation of these new terms is not a gratuitous exercise.

After successful treatment of any lumbar and innominate somatic dysfunctions, all residual sacral dysfunctions seem to fit in one of these two restriction patterns and are treatable with one of two Still techniques. The implication of these findings is that there are two distinct residual restriction patterns in the sacrum following successful treatment of any lumbar and innominate dysfunctions. These residual sacral dysfunctions are quite different from those described by either the Chicago or Mitchell models of sacral dysfunction. Therefore, it would not be appropriate to extend either terminology to these "new" versions of sacral dysfunction.

Sacroiliac somatic dysfunctions can be diagnosed fairly quickly using seated tests. Although it is common to perform many of the tests for sacral dysfunction in a prone position, the author has found that patients with lumbosacral pain have a problem tolerating transfers from one position to another. In particular they have a problem transferring from seated to supine or prone positions and back again. The less position changes required of these patients, the more they appreciate it. The following sacral tests are abbreviated significantly from those used by the Chicago school and the Mitchell model:

1. *The seated flexion test:* This test differs in significant details from the classic seated flexion test (5–7) (see Chapter 47). This modified seated flexion test starts with the patient seated. Weightbearing on the ischial tuberosities should be equal. The tips of the physician's sensing fingers are placed firmly on the sacrum just medial to the PSIS at the level of the sacral base (sacral sulcus). The patient is instructed to bend forward. As the patient flexes the physician notes which side of the sacrum glides superior. The side that moves is noted and is the positive side.

2. *Position of the inferior lateral angle (ILA):* This is checked at the sacrotuberous ligament. This is said to be positive if one ILA is posterior and does not move anterior, if the sacrotuberous ligament is tight on that side, or if the ILA is more inferior on one side. The positive side is that of restriction.

The sacroiliac diagnoses are named for the pattern of free poles (which is the same as the pattern of restricted poles) and the free direction of rotation of the sacral base (Table 70.3).

Diagonal Right Sacroiliac Dysfunction

Position
The patient is supine on a table. The physician stands to the side of the patient.

Procedure
1. Both of the patient's legs are flexed at the hips and knees.

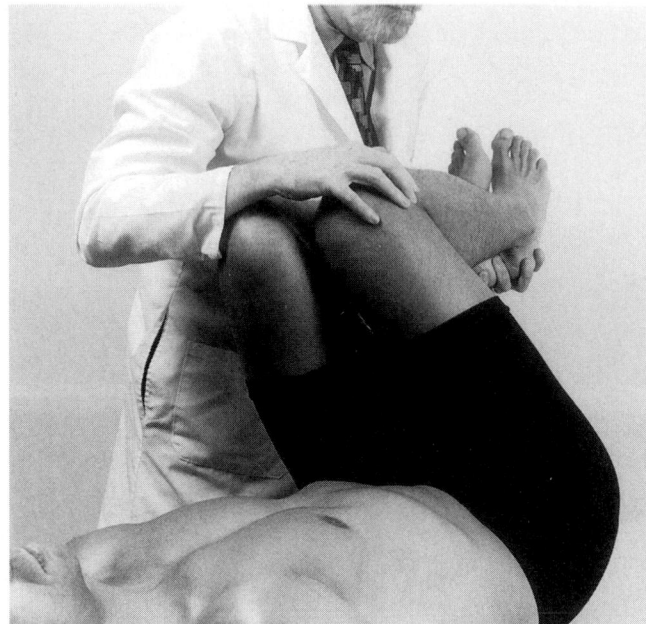

FIGURE 70.33. Initial position, diagonal right sacroiliac dysfunction.

2. The physician's hand closest to the patient's feet picks both feet up and increases the hip flexion to about 90 degrees.
3. The physician's hand closest to the patient's head is placed on the patient's knees and is used to side bend the legs and knees to the left. This provides some anterior rotation to the right innominate that may be slightly lifted off the table. The physician now rotates the patient's feet and lower legs outward away from the midline (Fig. 70.33).
4. The physician introduces compression through the patient's knees vectored toward the sacrum.
5. The physician swings the patient's feet toward the right (away from the midline) at a moderate pace and simultaneously carries the knees across the midline toward the right (Fig. 70.34). When the patient's lower legs are about 30 to 45 degrees off the midline, the legs are carried into extension (Fig. 70.35).

TABLE 70.3. SACROILIAC DIAGNOSES NAMED FOR THE PATTERN OF FREE POLES AND THE FREE DIRECTION OF ROTATION OF THE SACRAL BASE

Diagnosis	Seated Flexion	Inferior Lateral Angle
Diagonal right	+Right	+Left (posterior, tight, long)
Diagonal left	+Left	+Right
Unilateral right	+Right	+Right
Unilateral left	+Left	+Left

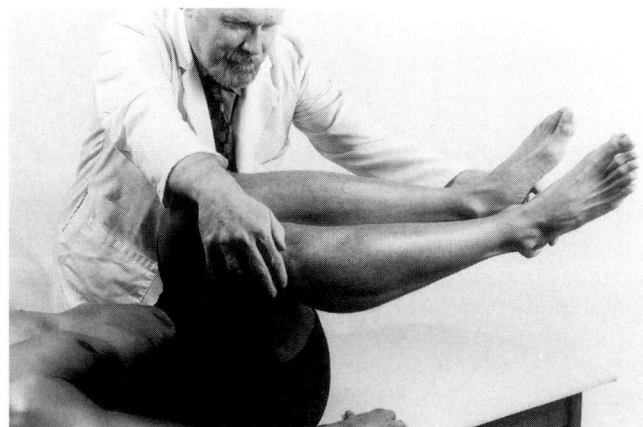

FIGURE 70.34. Intermediate position, diagonal right sacroiliac dysfunction.

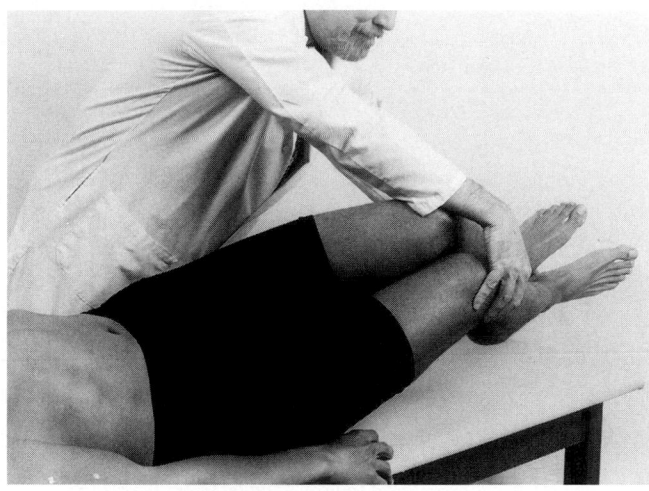

FIGURE 70.35. Final position, diagonal right sacroiliac dysfunction.

6. The physician brings the patient's legs back to neutral (full extension). Since this is an unmonitored technique it is very possible that no release will be felt.

7. Retest.

Unilateral Left Sacroiliac Dysfunction

Position

The patient is supine. The physician stands at the patient's left side.

Procedure

1. Physician's left hand monitors the patient's left sacroiliac joint for relaxation while the physician's right hand flexes the patient's right leg at the knee and hip. The patient's right hip is also abducted until the sacroiliac joint relaxation is palpated (Fig. 70.36).

2. Physician moves the right hand to the patient's right knee and the left hand to the patient's right ankle.

3. Physician carries the patient's right ankle laterally (away from the patient's body), internally rotating the hip. This relaxes the lower pole of the sacrum.

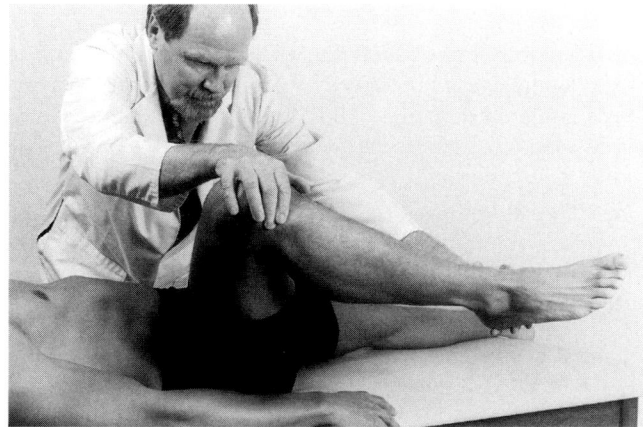

FIGURE 70.36. Initial position, unilateral left sacroiliac dysfunction.

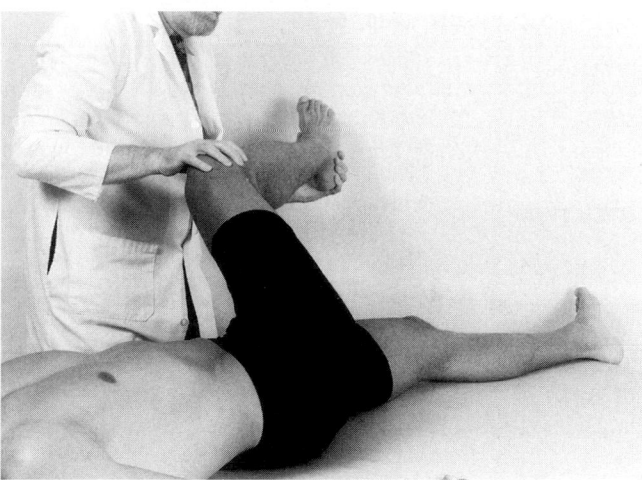

FIGURE 70.37. Intermediate position, unilateral left sacroiliac dysfunction.

4. Physician introduces compression through the patient's right knee vectored toward the patient's sacrum.

5. Maintaining compression, the patient's right knee is carried toward the midline (adducted), bringing the right pelvis slightly off the table. At the same time the right ankle is brought toward the patient's left side, crossing the midline (Fig. 70.37).

6. The right ankle is drawn down toward the foot of the table until the right leg is fully extended (Fig. 70.38). Release will occur during extension of the patient's leg.

7. Retest.

HIP MUSCLES

Five hip muscles are mentioned in Table 70.4.

The sciatic nerve generally passes out of the pelvis just under the piriformis muscle. Occasionally the sciatic nerve exits the greater sciatic foramen over the superior margin of the piriformis. The sciatic nerve may also split so that part of it passes through the belly of the piriformis.

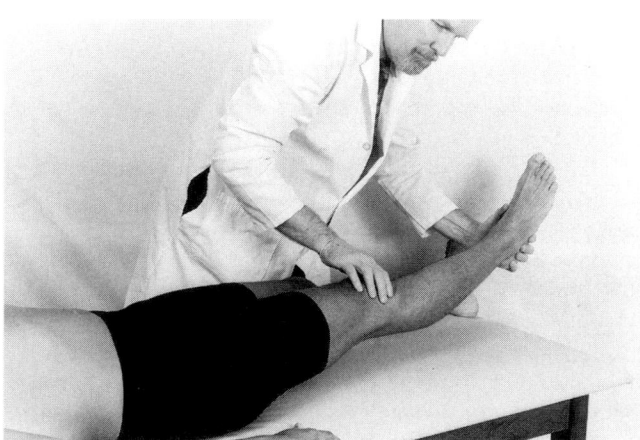

FIGURE 70.38. Final position, unilateral left sacroiliac dysfunction.

TABLE 70.4. PELVIC MUSCLES

Muscle	Origin	Course	Insertion	Action
Psoas	Transverse processes of L1-4 (L5)	Over superior pubic ramus and anterior to the hip joint	Lesser tuberosity of the femur	Hip flexion
Gluteus maximus	Just above and lateral to posterior superior iliac spine (PSIS) down to sciatic foramen		Greater trochanter of the femur and the iliotibial band	Extends hip when flexed; externally rotates hip. Aids in extending knee.
Gluteus medius	Beneath iliac crest to the PSIS		Greater trochanter of the femur	Stabilizes hip during swing phase of opposite hip during walking. Contributes to hip adduction.
Gluteus minimus	Ala of the ilium beneath gluteus medius and lateral to gluteus maximus		Greater trochanter of the femur	Stabilizes hip during swing phase of opposite hip. Contributes to hip adduction.
Piriformis	Anterior lateral sacrum	Passes through the greater sciatic foramen	Posterior medial aspect of femur's greater trochanter	External rotator of the hip. Beyond 20° of hip adduction acts as a hip flexor.

The diagnosis of a somatic dysfunction among these hip muscles is little different from that of any other somatic dysfunction. Typically there will be a decrease in appropriate range of motion. Gait will often be somewhat abnormal. The muscle belly and tendons may be quite tender to palpation. When somatic dysfunction is found in these muscles each will demonstrate significant tender points at its origin and insertion, although these are hard to demonstrate in the case of the piriformis. However, a somatic dysfunction of the piriformis will demonstrate tender points in the muscle as it exits the sciatic notch. This may reflect either tenderness in the muscle itself due to spasms or in the origin of the neighboring and synergistic gemelli muscles.

In the case of restriction and inflammation of the psoas, termed psoasitis or psoas syndrome, the patient stands slightly flexed at the waist and slightly side bent toward the side of the dysfunction. Leg extension is markedly restricted and the foot will tend to be everted.

Similarly, hip flexion and internal rotation will be restricted if the gluteus maximus is dysfunctional. Leg adduction may be somewhat decreased if either the gluteus medius or gluteus minimus are restricted. Leg internal rotation will be restricted if the piriformis group is dysfunctional. If the patient complains of pain in the area of the upper gluteals, asking the patient to stand on the affected leg will worsen spasms if the gluteus medius and minimus are involved.

It is quite common that somatic dysfunctions of the piriformis or one or more of the gluteal muscles will produce numbness, tingling, paresthesia, and perhaps even a burning pain than runs down the back of a patient's leg. As long as there is no evidence that a spinal compression of the sciatic nerve is responsible, this functional sciatica can be relieved, sometimes instantly, by treating those gluteal muscles that are exhibiting signs of somatic dysfunction. (A complete treatment for this condition will also include any sacral and innominate dysfunctions.) Recalling its course through the sciatic notch along with the sciatic nerve, it is easy to see how piriformis spasms and restrictions could produce the symptoms of sciatica. Additionally, because it overlies the sciatic nerve as it travels distal to piriformis, spasm in the gluteus maximus can provoke sciatic-type symptoms. The gluteus minimus, when it is in spasm or chronic activation, can also contribute to functional sciatica because it lies just superior to the piriformis.

Right Psoas Dysfunction

Position
The patient is in a lateral recumbent position with the right side up with the right hip and knee fully flexed. The physician stands behind the patient.

Procedure
1. A finger of the physician's left hand (sensing hand) is on the patient's right L2 transverse process. The remainder of the hand stabilizes the lower lumbar spine and upper pelvis. The physician's right hand is placed on the patient's flexed right knee.
2. The physician introduces compression through the patient's knee vectored toward the right lumbar paravertebral gutter (Fig. 70.39).
3. Maintaining compression, the physician abducts the patient's knee and draws it inferiorly, carrying the hip through neutral and into extension (Fig. 70.40). During treatment no attempt is made by the physician or the patient to extend the knee, although commonly, some extension of the knee seems to develop naturally.
4. As the patient's hip is extended compression is released and the leg is returned to neutral.
5. Retest.

Right Gluteus Maximus Dysfunction

Position
The patient is supine on the table. The physician stands on the right side of the patient.

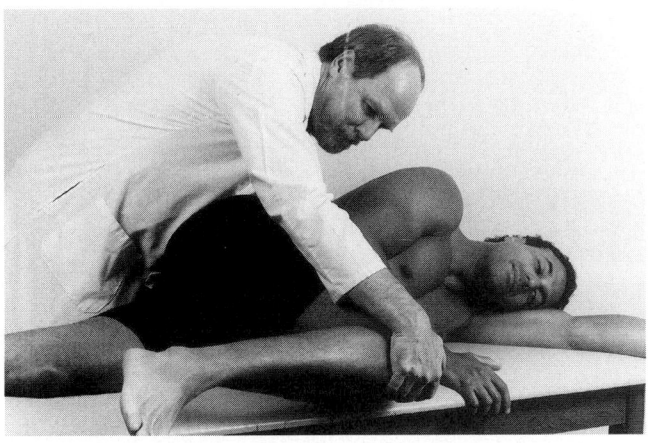

FIGURE 70.39. Initial position, right psoas dysfunction.

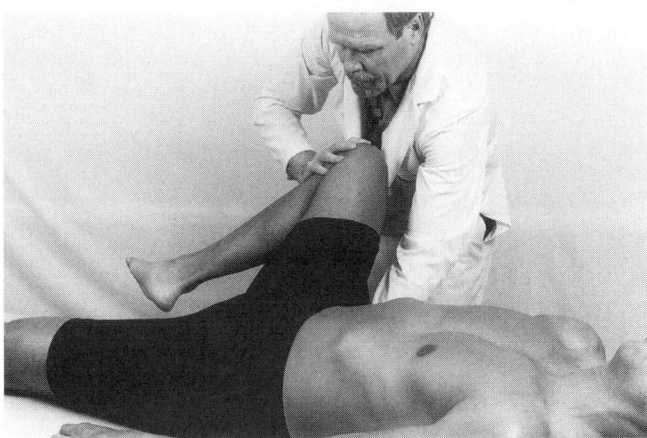

FIGURE 70.41. Initial position right, gluteus maximus dysfunction.

Procedure

1. Physician's left hand is placed under the patient's pelvis with a sensing finger on the tender points in the origin of the gluteus maximus. The physician's right hand is placed on the patient's right knee.

2. Physician flexes the patient's right knee and hip and abducts the patient's thigh until relaxation is palpated at the origin of gluteus maximus (Fig. 70.41).

3. Physician introduces compression through the knee vectored toward the origin of gluteus maximus.

4. Maintaining compression, the physician adducts the patient's thigh in a smooth arc, bringing it across the midline to the point where the right hip is off the table (Fig. 70.42).

5. Physician carries the patient's knee into extension. Release occurs at about 30 degrees of hip flexion (Fig. 70.43).

6. The patient's leg is returned to neutral (full extension) and the patient is retested.

Right Gluteus Medius and Minimus Dysfunctions

Position

The patient is supine on a table. The physician stands by the right side for a right dysfunction.

Procedure

1. Physician's left hand is placed under the patient's pelvis with a sensing finger on a tender spot in the origin of the muscle.

2. Physician draws the patient's right leg and knee into about 100 to 120 degrees flexion for gluteus medius. Gluteus minimus requires somewhat less hip flexion, often only about 70 degrees. Both may require slight adduction.

3. Physician's right hand wraps around the patient's right ankle and externally rotates the patient's hip. The physician's left axilla gently captures on the patient's right knee and supplies compression toward the sensing finger and the muscle origin (Fig. 70.44).

4. Physician draws the patient's ankle toward the patient's right side, internally rotating the hip. Once the patient's hip is internally rotated, the physician maintains compression through the knee while abducting the knee (Fig. 70.45).

5. The physician draws the patient's ankle toward the foot of the table. Release of the somatic dysfunction and compression occurs when the patient's knee clears the physician's axilla (Fig. 70.46).

6. Retest.

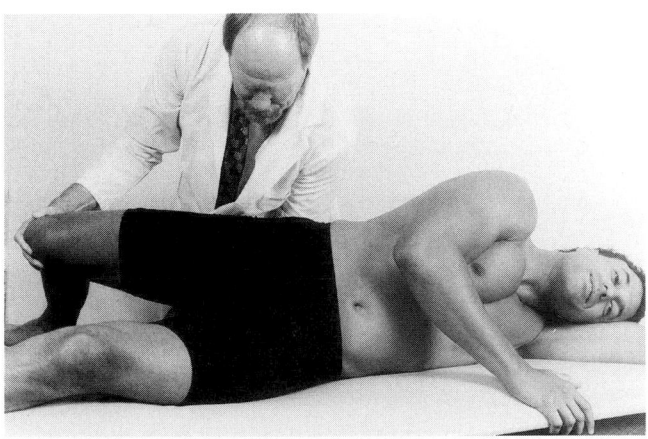

FIGURE 70.40. Intermediate position, right psoas dysfunction.

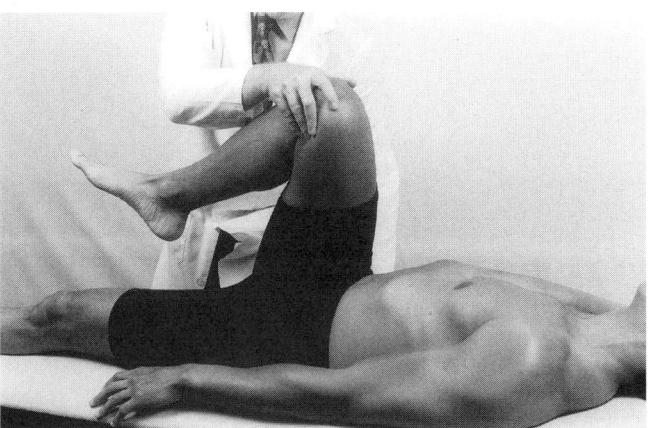

FIGURE 70.42. Intermediate position, right gluteus maximus dysfunction.

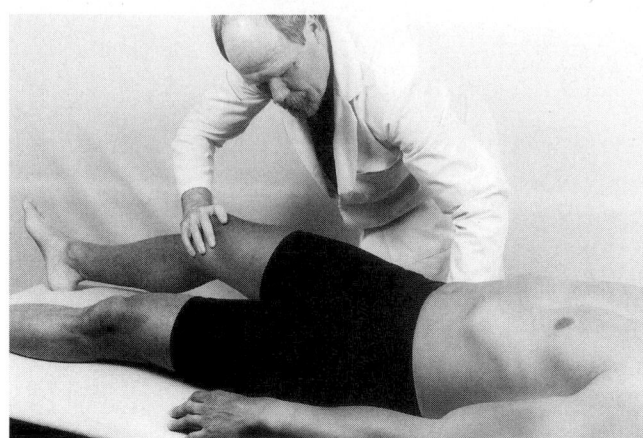

FIGURE 70.43. Final position, right gluteus maximus dysfunction.

Note: If the physician is not so tall as to easily capture the patient's knee with the axilla, this technique can be performed as an unmonitored technique using one hand on the patient's knee and the other on the patient's ankle.

Right Piriformis Dysfunctions

Position
The patient is supine. The physician stands at right side of the patient.

Procedure
1. Physician's left hand is placed under the patient's pelvis and the sensing finger is placed on the piriformis tender point in the area of the sciatic foramen.
2. Physician flexes and fully abducts the patient's right knee. Once the muscles are relaxed the sensing hand is withdrawn and transferred to the patient's right knee. The physician's right hand is placed on the patient's right ankle.
3. Physician develops and maintains a vector of compression through the patient's right knee toward the sciatic foramen (Fig. 70.47).
4. Leading with the patient's right foot the physician carries the

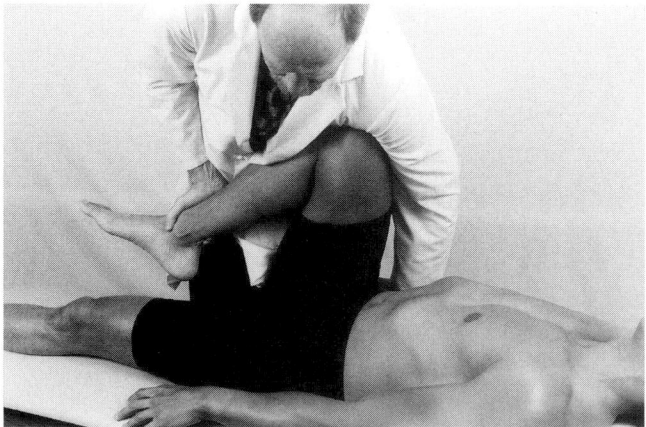

FIGURE 70.44. Initial position, right gluteus medius dysfunction.

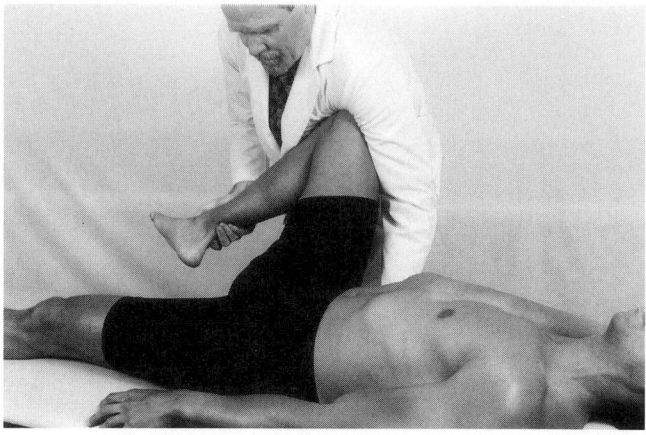

FIGURE 70.45. Intermediate position, right gluteus medius dysfunction.

patient's knee across the midline into adduction. The patient's right foot should pass over the patient's left thigh before the right knee does (Fig. 70.48).
5. Now the physician draws the patient's right foot back across the patient's left thigh, internally rotating the thigh (Fig. 70.49).
6. Thereafter the physician draws the patient's knee and hip into extension and releases compression through the knee (Fig. 70.50).
7. Retest.

THE HAND

Right In-Rotated Scaphoid

Position
The patient is usually seated with the right hand palm up in the physician's right hand.

Procedure
1. Physician's fingers from the right hand are curled around the thenar eminence and one is placed over the scaphoid bone.

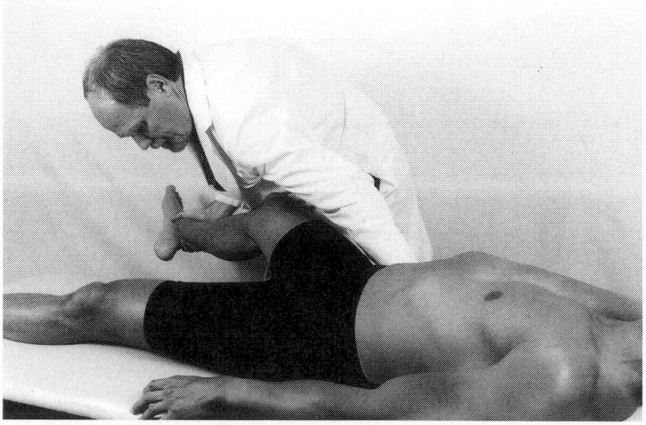

FIGURE 70.46. Final position, right gluteus medius dysfunction.

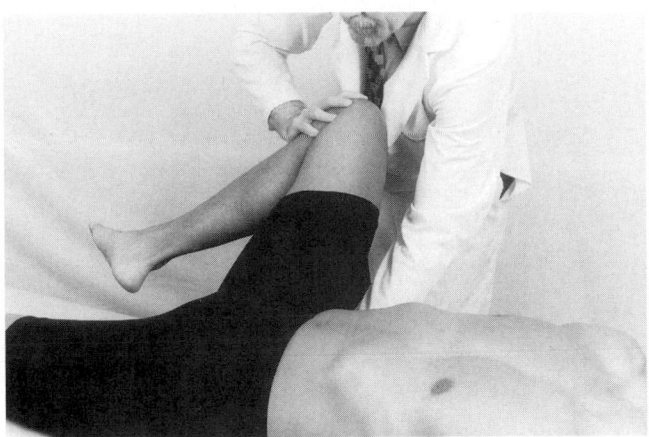

FIGURE 70.47. Initial position, right piriformis dysfunction.

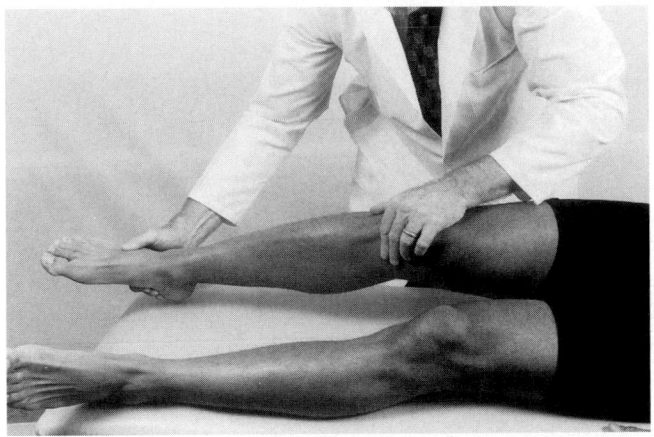

FIGURE 70.50. Final position, right piriformis dysfunction.

2. Physician grasps the patient's thumb with the left hand. The patient's thumb is adducted until the scaphoid is palpably relaxed.
3. Physician introduces compression vectored through the patient's thumb toward the scaphoid (Fig. 70.51).
4. Physician rotates the patient's thumb outward into abduction with extension (Fig. 70.52).
5. Retest.

THE KNEE

Many different possible dysfunctions around the knee are potentially treatable with the Still technique. For purposes of demonstration we will limit ourselves to that involving the fibular head. Typically the fibular head has a limited range involving, at most, a couple of millimeters of anterior and posterior gliding motion. However, if the fibular head is limited from its normal range it can result in a marked pain in the lateral side of the knee, a pain that is poorly localized by the patient. Palpation of the knee demonstrates marked tenderness of the fibular head. The foot is used as a lever to assess restriction and freedom of the fibular

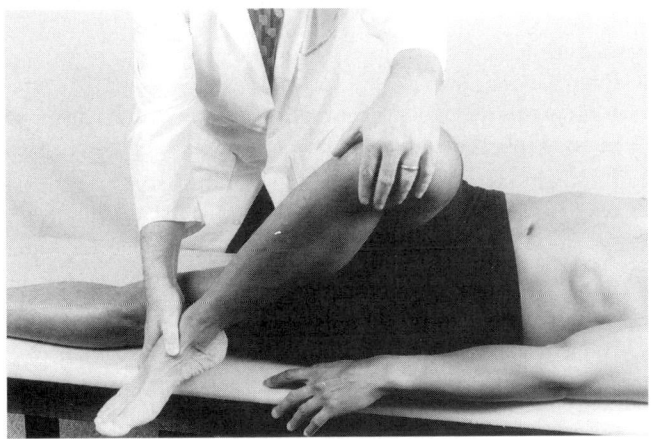

FIGURE 70.48. Intermediate position, right piriformis dysfunction.

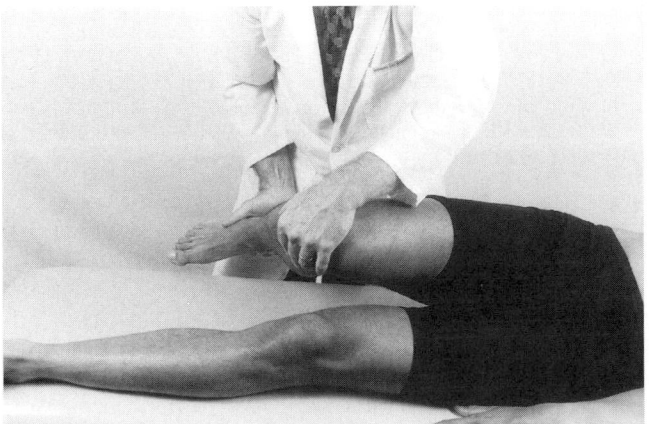

FIGURE 70.49. Late intermediate position, right piriformis dysfunction.

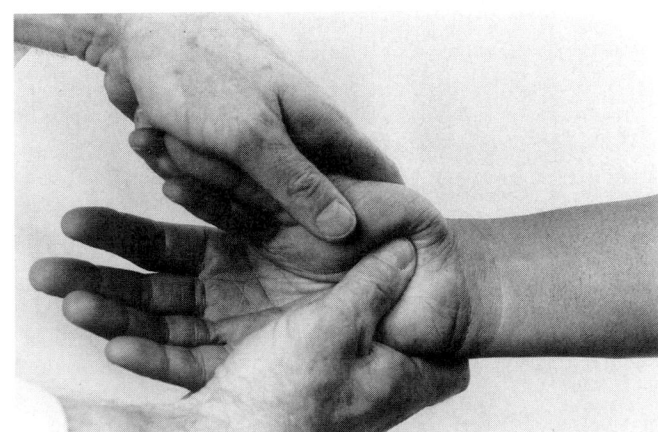

FIGURE 70.51. Initial position, right in-rotated scaphoid.

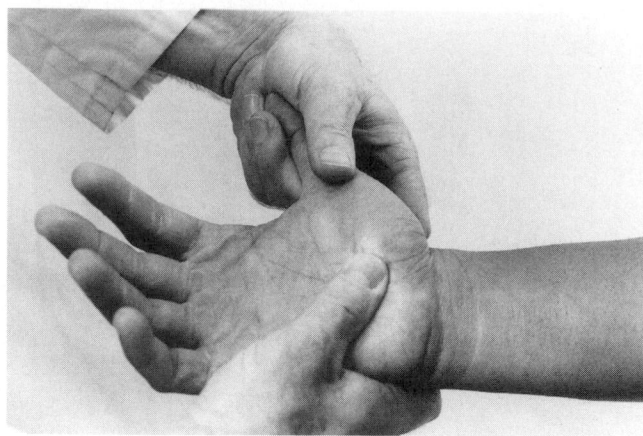

FIGURE 70.52. Final position, right in-rotated scaphoid.

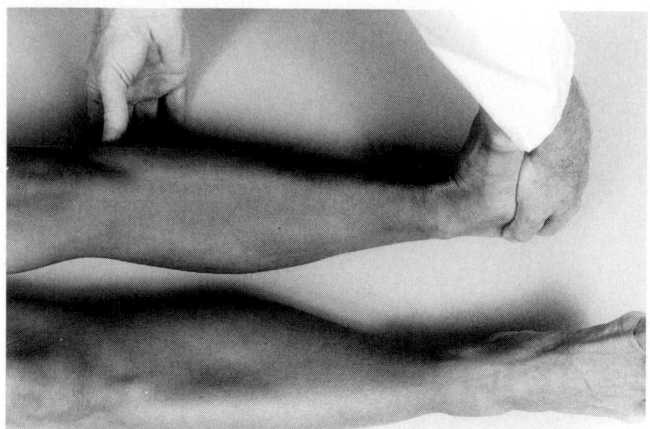

FIGURE 70.54. Final position, anterior fibular head dysfunction.

head. If the fibular head is assessed with the knee flexed, we find that foot dorsiflexion with a little external rotation produces anterior excursion of the fibular head. Likewise foot plantar-flexion coupled with internal rotation produces posterior excursion of the fibular head. Failure to move adequately in either direction is demonstration of dysfunction.

When the author began to assess fibular head dysfunction with the patient supine and the knee extended he found, much to his surprise, that fibular mechanics reversed. That is, with the knee extended, the fibular head moved posterior with foot dorsiflexion and anterior with foot plantar-flexion. Further analysis suggests that the most likely explanation for this discrepancy has to do with the effect of tension in the iliotibial band. Whatever the cause, the author has typically treated fibular head dysfunctions with the patient in the supine position and, thus, the unusual mechanics influence how it is treated.

Anterior Fibular Head Dysfunction

Position
The patient is supine with the physician at the foot of the table.

Procedure
1. Physician monitors the fibular head with one hand. The other hand grasps the patient's foot, plantar flexes it, and adds some internal rotation and supination on the tibial axis.
2. Physician introduces compression from the hand on the patient's foot with a vector through the fibular head (Fig. 70.53).
3. Physician maintains the compression while the patient's foot is passively moved through its range of motion into dorsiflexion, external rotation, and some pronation (Fig. 70.54). The fibular head may be felt to release.
4. Physician discontinues compression and returns the foot to neutral.
5. Retest.

Note: If the fibular head dysfunction is to be treated with the patient's knee flexed, the opposite foot motions would be used.

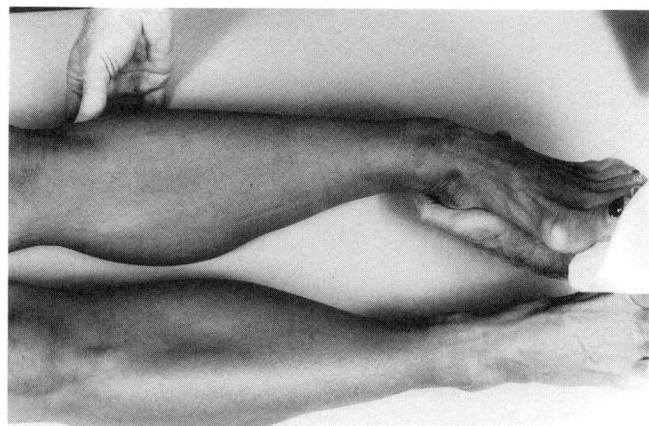

FIGURE 70.53. Initial position, anterior fibular head dysfunction.

REFERENCES

1. Still AT. *Osteopathy, Research and Practice.* Published by the author, Kirksville, MO; 1910. Reprinted by Eastland Press, Seattle, WA; 1992.
2. Hazzard C. *The Practice and Applied Therapeutics of Osteopathy,* 3rd rev. ed. Kirksville, MO: Journal Printing Co; 1905.
3. Van Buskirk RL. A manipulative technique of Andrew Taylor Still. *JAOA.* 1996;96:597–602.
4. Van Buskirk RL. *The Still Technique Manual.* Indianapolis, IN: American Academy of Osteopathy; 2000.
5. Greenman PE. *Principles of Manual Medicine,* 2nd ed. Baltimore, MD: Williams & Wilkins; 1996.
6. Mitchell FL Jr, Moran PS, Pruzzo NA. *An Evaluation and Treatment Manual of Osteopathic Muscle Energy Procedures.* Valley Park, MO: Mitchell, Moran and Pruzzo, Associates; 1979.
7. Walton WJ. *Textbook of Osteopathic Diagnosis and Technique Procedures.* Newark, OH: The American Academy of Osteopathy; 1972.

TREATMENT OF THE ACUTELY ILL HOSPITALIZED PATIENT

HUGH ETTLINGER

KEY CONCEPTS

An osteopathic structural examination:

- Providing clues to the medical/surgical diagnosis of a hospitalized patient
- Directed toward the underlying pathophysiology of the disease process

An individualized osteopathic manipulative treatment plan:

- At each visit
- For each acutely ill hospitalized patient
- Specifically directed toward dysfunction, discovered during a musculoskeletal structural examination
- Appropriate for the patient's condition and directed toward improving physiologic function
- For support and assistance to the patient recovering from an illness or other acute stress

The science of osteopathy is applicable to the full spectrum of medical and surgical problems. Osteopathic evaluation and treatment, integrated into the care of the acutely ill hospital patient, is based on an understanding of the mechanical and functional aspects of the body's viscera and systems, including the respiratory, circulatory, the immune, and autonomic nervous systems. This chapter specifically presents a template for an osteopathic structural evaluation that investigates body physiology related to a patient's disease processes, not just the mechanics of the neuromusculoskeletal system, and as such, becomes an invaluable part of the physical examination. It presents the general principles upon which the treatment plan is based and suggests manipulative treatment techniques that apply these principles. The resulting treatment plan is a natural extension of the structural examination. The osteopathic treatment that is administered supports the patient and assists in their recovery from illness or other acute stress. A unique and individualized treatment plan must be designed for each acutely ill hospitalized patient at each visit.

THE STRUCTURAL EXAMINATION

Accurate diagnosis is the key to appropriate treatment of any patient with any disease process. For this reason, a basic structural examination should be performed on all hospital patients. The structural examination offers the osteopathic physician additional clues that assist in the overall assessment of a patient's condition and the development of an appropriate treatment plan. The hospital structural examination is a variation of the general structural examination described in Chapter 44. The American Osteopathic Association (AOA) has designed a standardized hospital structural examination form for use in all osteopathic services (Fig. 71.1).

This examination consists of required and optional parts. The required section, which includes static symmetry, both anteroposterior (AP) and lateral, and regional screen for tissue tension, fulfills the requirements of a basic musculoskeletal examination. This part of the examination is described in Chapter 44. Adaptations must be made for the condition of the patient; some patients are unable to sit, stand, or walk.

Although listed as optional, this author strongly recommends that the focused examination described herein be carried out in the acutely ill patient, as it will provide clues to the diagnosis and overall condition of the patient. It assesses the function of the patient's major organ systems. Also, if an osteopathic manipulative treatment is to be performed on a hospitalized patient, a focused musculoskeletal examination is required. Notes regarding the focused examination can be recorded in the "optional" region of the standardized form, for later dictation with the physical examination or the progress notes. The aspects of this focused structural examination will be described in detail in this chapter.

Assessing for Segmental Facilitation

Reflex somatic dysfunction provides important clues to the presence of acute and/or chronic disease. The information gathered is combined with the rest of the physical examination to reach a working differential diagnosis. In order to most accurately interpret structural findings as they relate to the systemic diseases they reflect, reflex somatic dysfunction must be differentiated from postural, traumatic, and other purely somatic causes of somatic

Osteopathic Musculoskeletal Examination of the Hospitalized Patient

Examiner: _(print)_ _____

Chief Complaint: **Required** _____

Ant./Post. Spinal Curves	I	N	D	For Coding Purposes Only
Cervical Lordosis	☐	☐	☐	
Thoracic Kyphosis	☐	☐	☐	
Lumbar Lordosis	☐	☐	☐	

I = increased   N = normal   D = decreased

Scoliosis (Lateral Spinal Curves)

☐ None   Sitting ☐

☐ Functional   Standing ☐

☐ Mild   Prone/supine ☐

☐ Moderate   lat. recumbant ☐

☐ Severe   Unable to examine ☐

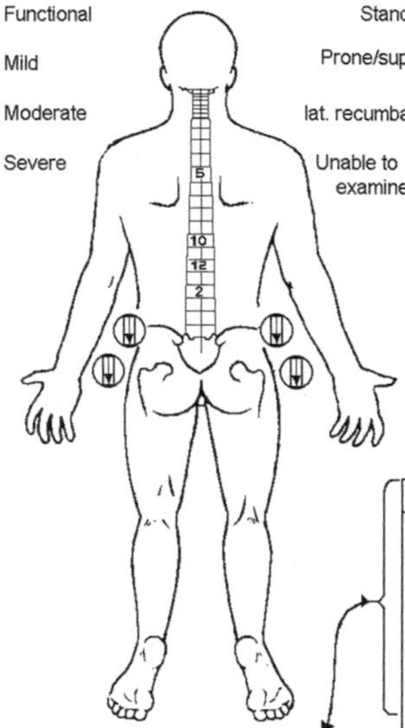

Assessment Tools:

☐ T = Tenderness

☐ A = Asymmetry

☐ R = Restricted Motion
  ☐ Active
  ☐ Passive

☐ T = Tissue Texture Change

Severity Key:

Ø = No SD or background (BG) levels

1 = Minor TART more than BG levels

2 = TART obvious (R & T esp) –/– symptoms

3 = Symptomatic, R and T very easily found, "key lesion"

Optional Worksheet

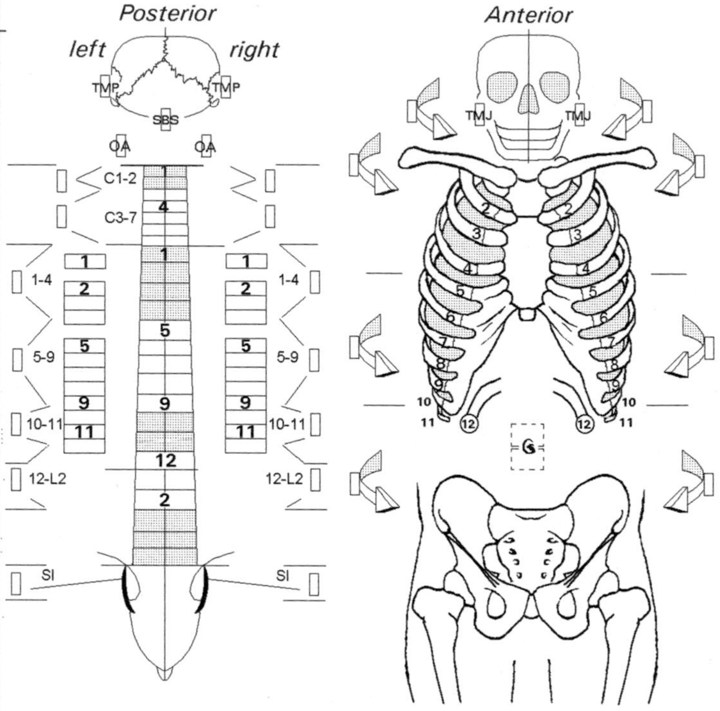

Posterior   Anterior

left   right

Abbreviation Key:

OA = Occipitoatlantal joint   TMJ = Temporomandibular joint
Sympathetic ganglia: TMP = Temporal bone
  C = celiac ganglion   SBS = Sphenobasilar symphysis
  S = superior mesenteric Ganglion
  I = Inferior mesenteric ganglion

Region Evaluated	Severity 0	1	2	3	Specifics of Major Somatic Dysfunctions
Head	☐	☐	☐	☐	
Neck	☐	☐	☐	☐	
Thoracic T1-4	☐	☐	☐	☐	
T5-9	☐	☐	☐	☐	
T10-L2	☐	☐	☐	☐	
Lumbar	☐	☐	☐	☐	
Pelvis / Sacrum	☐	☐	☐	☐	
Pelvis / Innominate	☐	☐	☐	☐	
Extremity (lower) R	☐	☐	☐	☐	
Extremity (lower) L	☐	☐	☐	☐	
Extremity (lower) R	☐	☐	☐	☐	
Extremity (lower) L	☐	☐	☐	☐	
Ribs	☐	☐	☐	☐	
Other /Abdomen	☐	☐	☐	☐	

Major Correlations With:

☐ Traumatic   ☐ Rheumatological

☐ Orthopedic   ☐ EENT

☐ Neurologic   ☐ Cardiovascular

☐ Viscerosomatic   ☐ Pulmonary

☐ Primary Ms-skeletal ☐ Gastrointestinal

☐ Activities of daily living ☐ Genitourinary

☐ Other _____   ☐ Congenital

Other: _____
_____
_____

Signature of the examiner: _____   Date of Examination: _____

Signature of the examiner(s): _____   Date of Examination: _____

O5A2X.PCX   MLK / WAK   VERSION 8:041499   Official form of the American Osteopathic Association and the Educational Council on Osteopathic Principles –1998

FIGURE 71.1. The American Osteopathic Association standardized hospital structural examination form.

dysfunction. There are unique qualities of viscerosomatic reflexes, which are related to the known pathophysiology of the reflex and the unique tissue changes they create. A viscerosomatic reflex is produced by the stimulation of nociceptors (pain carrying sensory fibers) within the diseased viscera or its fascia. Nociceptors are particularly sensitive to inflammation, and their exaggerated response to inflammatory processes may explain the distinct and identifiable tissue changes they produce. For this reason, reflexes are most apparent in diseases associated with acute inflammation, particularly those with a presenting complaint of pain, and may not be evident in a patient with a malignant tumor if the tumor is not causing irritation or inflammation. The nociceptive input travels to interneurons in the dorsal horn of the spinal cord, where it converges with nociceptive inputs from all somatic tissues. These interneurons stimulate both sympathetic efferent fibers and α-motor neurons.

Stimulation of sympathetic outflow nerves produces changes in blood supply and sweat gland activity at the body surface, in addition to visceral motor changes. I.M. Korr measured the cutaneous changes produced by segmental facilitation via alterations in skin resistance (sweat) and temperature (blood flow) (1). These changes are palpable as increased temperature and sweat (moisture and/or skin drag) in the paraspinal tissues, and are excellent and reliable indicators of segmental facilitation at that level of the spinal cord. In a study of the palpatory findings in acute myocardial infarction, Nicholas and colleagues found increased temperature as the second most common tissue finding (2).

Viscerosomatic reflexes initially produce vague, midline, gnawing deep pain (Fig. 71.2). As they progress they involve neuromuscular changes in the segmentally related tissues; this reflex effect on muscle tone is important, as it identifies their spinal segmental level and distinguishes them at a paraspinal level (Fig. 71.3).In his work with Korr, Denslow describes "doughy, boggy" paraspinal myofascial tissues at the levels of facilitation (3). Patriquin describes a "fusiform soft tissue change in the paraspinal muscles" occurring over several segments which "tails out on the

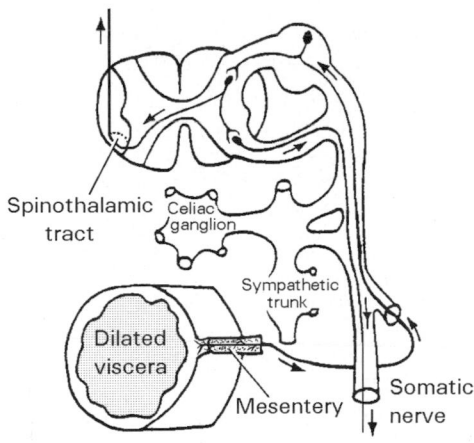

FIGURE 71.3. Viscerosensory pain pathway. This reflex produces the typical segmental viscerosomatic reflex. Palpable tissue texture changes are found over the somatic paravertebral tissues innervated by somatic nerves from the same cord level that supplies sympathetic innervation to the affected organ.

ends" (4). He continues to say, "the multifidus and rotatores are the best place in the spinal region to palpate for changes of viscerosomatic origin" (4). Beal, in his studies of cardiac and pulmonary patients, found a supine compression test to be the most accurate indicator of reflex dysfunction (5,6). Beal's description of the response to the compression test is at the level of joint motion, but is considered secondary to deep muscle splinting. Nicholas and associates, in a study of acute myocardial infarction, most often found "firmness" and warmth (2). Osseous/articular motion changes also occur, but these findings are most likely secondary to the altered muscle tone produced by the acute viscerosomatic reflex processes. William Johnston, DO, describes a "linkage" of thoracic vertebral and rib motion that he considers indicative of a viscerosomatic reflex (7). Once again, this articular motion finding is considered to be secondary to an altered neuromuscular response to a motion challenge. The movement restriction, found at a joint involved in this reflex process, is soft, with a springy feel, which, when palpated, suggests the viscerosomatic reflex. These regions also show unusual resistance to manipulative treatment, especially high velocity/low amplitude, when directed toward primary joint somatic dysfunction. Somatic dysfunction that rapidly recurs after "successful" manipulative treatment also suggests viscerosomatic origin or accentuation. When visceral inflammation involves the parietal peritoneum, the patient's discomfort becomes localized over the viscera involved (Fig. 71.4).

Acute segmental facilitation creates a variety of palpable tissue changes that may be used to identify the presence of an underlying disease process. The most superficial clues, temperature and skin drag or moisture, are among the most useful, and are easy to identify in the seated position. Palpation of the typical boggy, fusiform muscular changes can be performed with the patient either seated or supine. As with articular motion restrictions, viscerosomatic dysfunction is identified by motion restriction *without* a firm, stiff end-point but with a characteristic end-feel. It is likely that the differences between findings expressed by different examiners result from different diagnostic approaches.

The skills required to consistently identify reflexes develop with time and experience. For the practitioner learning to recognize the unique tissue changes of viscerosomatic reflexes, it is

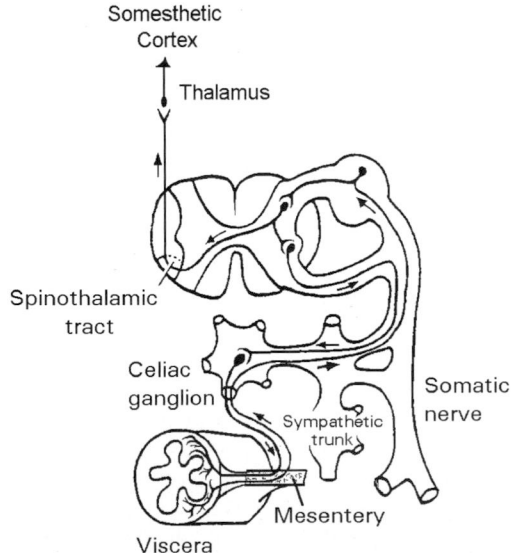

FIGURE 71.2. Visceral pain pathway—vague and periumbilical. Palpable tissue texture change is found in the abdomen over the prevertebral (collateral) sympathetic ganglion associated with that organ.

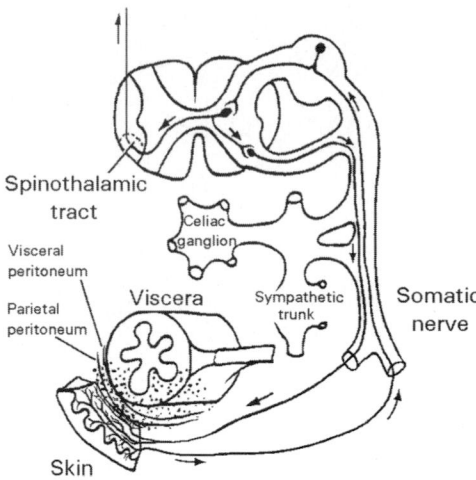

FIGURE 71.4. Peritoneal cutaneous reflex of Morley. The pain is localized over the viscera due to involvement of the parietal peritoneum directly over the organ. Palpable tissue texture change and acute pain is found directly over the organ and segmentally at the innervation level of the peritoneum or pleura.

TABLE 71.1. SEGMENTAL FACILITATION

Type	Characteristics
Acute	Increased temperature (a local chemical physiologic reaction), increased moisture and/or skin drag. Prolonged red reflex. Boggy, fusiform muscular changes. Articular motion restrictions *without* a firm, stiff end point.
Chronic	Thickened skin and subcutaneous tissues. Rapid fading red reflex. Localized muscle contraction (increased muscular tone). Muscles are hard, tense, and hypersensitive to palpation. Stiff joints with articular motion restrictions that are firm with more definite end-feel.
Acute on chronic	Warm, moist, and boggy superimposed on deeper hard, stiff tissues.

Nociceptive input from somatic tissue converges in the dorsal horn → Interneurons stimulate sympathetic efferents and α-motor neurons → Palpable somatic changes are produced.

helpful to evaluate reflex patterns in patients with clearly identified, acute disease processes. In this way the physician develops the skills required to recognize reflexes and to sense their unique qualities.

If a reflex persists, as occurs in a patient with a chronic disease, the tissues, including the joints, become stiff and the qualities palpated become different. Beal states, "The chronic phase of reflex activity is . . . characterized by trophic changes in the skin, increased thickening of the skin and subcutaneous tissues and localized muscle contraction. The muscles are hard and tense and may be hypersensitive to palpation" (8). The chronic muscle spasm ultimately stiffens the joints, giving the articular motion restriction a more firm, definite end-feel that is much closer to a typical postural or somatic problem. When someone with a chronic problem has an acute attack, a warm, moist, boggy tissue reaction will be superimposed on the deeper hard, stiff tissues, leading to a separate tissue diagnosis that may be called an acute on chronic problem. The tissues tell the story. This finding may be helpful in understanding the history of a current problem where the patient may be unaware of previous episodes of the problem (Table 71.1).

Interpretation of Findings

There is a tremendous amount and variety of information available to the osteopathic physician provided through the evaluation for the presence of segmental reflexes. Although practice will obviously improve the accuracy of the examination, 10 years of experience doing structural examinations in the acute care setting has demonstrated to this author that the great majority of cases present with significant, obvious reflex patterns which are easily recognized.

1. *The presence or absence of an acute process* (perhaps the most fundamental difference). Although this information alone should not determine workup and treatment, it can be a factor in how aggressively a patient should be worked up, especially with a

somewhat vague complaint. The presence of an acute reflex indicates an underlying acute process. For example, a right lower quadrant abdominal pain, appendicitis, a ruptured ovarian cyst, or Crohn disease will all produce an acute reflex pattern. Simple cramping or mild gastroenteritis will not.

2. *Identification of visceral disease in the presence of an acute reflex finding.* There are some diseases that may be differentiated by localization of reflexes and some that may not. For example, the heart is innervated by levels T1-5, whereas the stomach is innervated by levels T5-9. Although there is anatomic variation within these levels, it is usually clear if substernal pain has its origin in the heart or the stomach. On the other hand, the gallbladder and the duodenum are both innervated via the right side of the celiac ganglion, and cholecystitis and duodenal ulcer would produce a similar, if not identical reflex pattern. Although many sources identify unique sympathetic innervation levels for each viscus, clinically there are four important groupings which are easy to remember and practical for use (Fig. 71.5).

All structures above the diaphragm are innervated (approximately) by the T1-5 levels. This includes the heart, lungs (often extended to T6 or T7 in the literature), esophagus, and viscera of the head and neck. A vast majority of cardiac problems occur on the left side (left ventricle), and these problems would produce a left-sided somatic reflex. Spinal roots T5-9 (approximately) transmit and receive via the pathway of the greater splanchnic nerve primary sympathetic fiber synapse in the celiac ganglion. The liver, gallbladder, duodenum, and pancreas (head) are innervated from the right side at these levels. The stomach, spleen, and pancreas (tail) are innervated from the left. The inferior border of the scapula can help a physician identify this general spinal region in the seated patient. Spinal roots T10-12 (approximate) transmit and receive via the lesser splanchnic nerve pathway and primary sympathetic fibers synapse in the superior mesenteric ganglion. It should be remembered that these spinal levels include the innervation of kidneys and upper part of the ureters, testes, ovaries, and upper part of the fallopian tubes, as well as the entire small

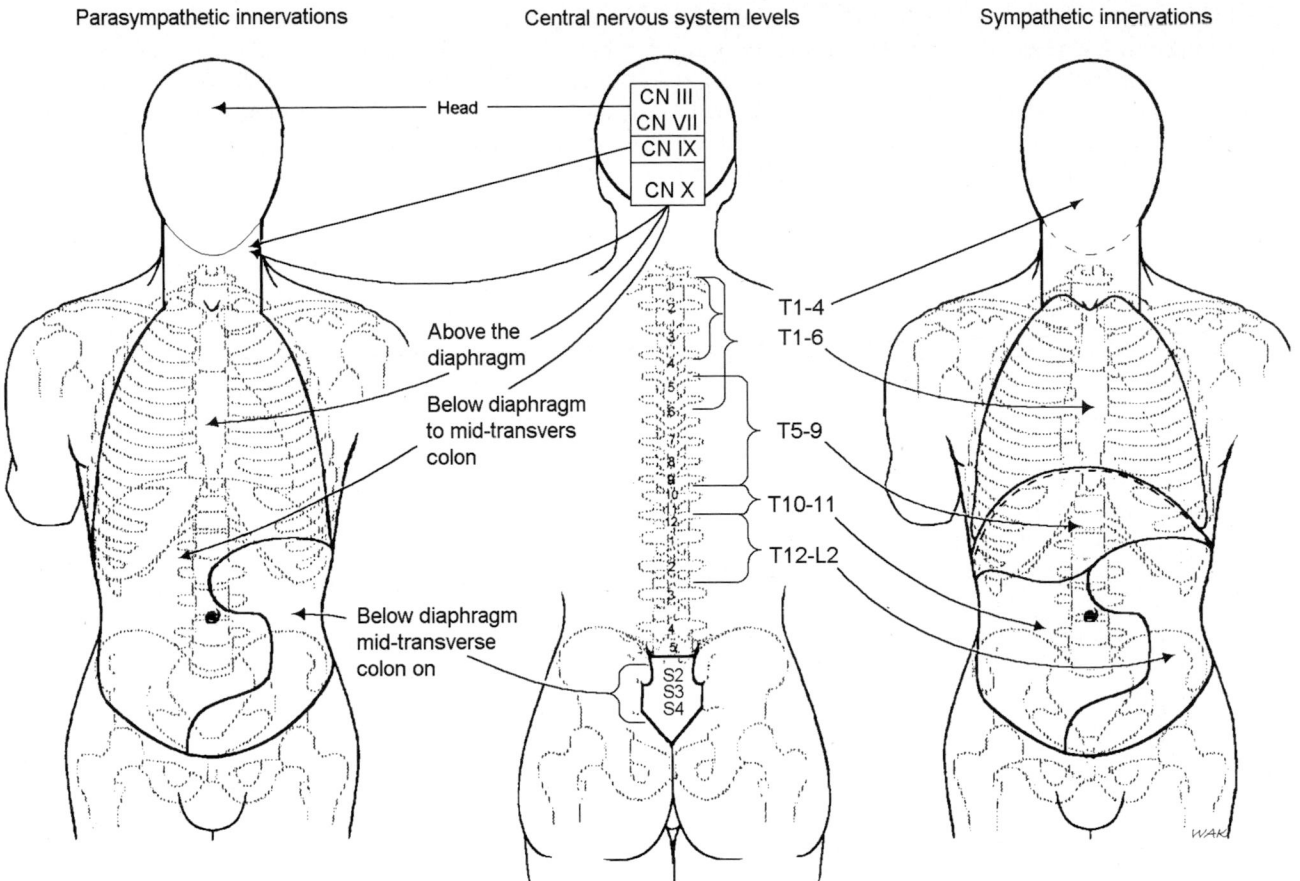

FIGURE 71.5. Sympathetic and parasympathetic innervations.

bowel, ascending colon, and transverse colon to about the splenic flexure (including the appendix). Right-sided organs, including the appendix, cecum, and ascending colon have a right-sided innervation. The T10-11 spinal region is contacted by placing one hand on the spinal region just posterior to the xiphoid process and extending caudad. Spinal roots T12-L2 innervate the lower abdominal and pelvic viscera. Fibers travel in the pathway of least splanchnic nerve and primary sympathetic fibers synapse in the inferior mesenteric ganglion. This level also innervates the lower part of the fallopian tubes and the lower part of each ureter, as well as the uterus (prostate in males) and bladder. The colon here has a left-sided innervation so irritations would produce left-sided paraspinal somatic reflexes. The 12th rib is useful in differentiating the middle from lower abdominal levels. The T12-L2 region can also be approximated by putting one hand over the spinal region at the level posterior to the umbilicus and extending it cephalad.

It is suspected by this author that variations recorded between organs within the same general level may have more to do with individual variation of the populations investigated than with consistent differences in actual innervation. Regardless, this author does not believe it is clinically possible to differentiate between different viscera within a given level if their innervation comes from the same side. Furthermore, grouping the viscera by general level is easy to remember and is clinically useful. In this scheme, it is impossible to distinguish appendicitis from a

right-sided ovarian cyst, but appendicitis can be differentiated from cholecystitis or a left-sided ovarian cyst with a midline pain presentation. Early visceral pain is referred to the midline of the abdomen, often around the umbilicus. It is a good idea to have some way of recalling the basic autonomic innervation to the viscera of the body (Fig. 71.5).

3. *Assessing degree of disease by degree of reflex facilitation.* This is an intriguing thought, but an ill-advised one. Different individuals have different reactivity within their nociceptive nervous systems, and will therefore present with varying degrees of reflex facilitation with the same degree of inflammatory process and/or disease. One particular example from clinical practice would be the patient with diabetic neuropathy, which affects small caliber peripheral nerves. These patients often have blunted reflexes that are more difficult to identify and interpret. Once a baseline level of dysfunction is established, and compared to other clinical indicators of disease severity, it may be possible to follow the progress of the disease by changes in the intensity of the reflex, although this has not been studied. However, it is not uncommon to find a reflex has changed or disappeared, indicating a change in the patient's clinical status before other indicators have changed.

4. *Differentiating acute versus chronic processes.* This can be important in several ways. First, it may allow the identification of a long-standing process in the face of an acute presentation (i.e., the "acute on chronic" tissue changes). Surprisingly, patients do not always recall past episodes of a problem. The examiner can

also identify if a known chronic problem is, in fact, the cause of a present complaint. A chronic reflex pattern, without an acute overlay in that region makes it is unlikely that the chronic organ or system is the source of the acute disease process. This might be useful in the evaluation of chest pain in a patient with a history of ischemia or myocardial infarction, who will undoubtedly demonstrate chronic findings with or without an acute process superimposed.

The Thorax

Breathing is one of the most fundamental processes in human physiology. Respiration is responsible not only for the movement of air, but is also directly involved with venous and lymphatic circulation. A focused evaluation and treatment of the thorax is indicated in all respiratory diseases, such as asthma and pneumonia. Thoracic function also has an impact in less obvious situations, such as the postoperative abdominal surgery patient, whose most likely complication will be pulmonary, or the lower extremity cellulitis patient, whose body depends on diaphragmatic respiration for proper drainage of the infection. There are few, if any, acutely ill patients who do not warrant a focused examination of their respiratory mechanism.

The structural examination of the thorax can reveal a great deal about the underlying condition of the respiratory system. Breathing may be divided into an inhalation and exhalation phase. Restricted motion in one phase may suggest one pathology over another. Pneumonia will reduce the excursion of the thorax toward inhalation locally, over the area of consolidation, whereas asthma and other obstructive diseases will reduce the excursion of the thorax toward exhalation. This finding may help differentiate the patient with a primary asthmatic attack from one whose asthmatic attack was triggered by pneumonia. The difference between restricted inhalation and exhalation may also help differentiate chronic obstructive pulmonary disease (COPD) from congestive heart failure (CHF), which often coexist in the same patient, and may present similarly with shortness of breath and crackles in the lung bases. If the present exacerbation is due primarily to CHF, there will be restriction of the lower thorax to inhalation, and the exhalation phase will be relatively effortless. If the present exacerbation is COPD, the patient will have dramatic limitation to exhalation and the exhalation phase will be active (the patient will work to get the air out). This effort by the patient is easily observed by placing the fingerpads or palm in contact with the patient's skin, just below the costal margin.

Structural examination of the thorax should be performed along with auscultation and percussion in the physical examination of the cardiac and respiratory systems. The structural examination includes evaluation of the entire spine, the pelvis, and sacrum, which move, in addition to the ribs, during respiration and contribute to the overall shape change of the thoracic cavity (9,10). The excursion of the thorax produces the volume and subsequent pressure changes that produce the movement of air and fluids.

Compliance of the thorax is a separate, important functional parameter of respiration related to the structural evaluation of respiration, as it more accurately reflects the work of breathing, especially in obstructive and restrictive pulmonary disease. The clinical difference between excursion and compliance may be understood by comparing the difference between an otherwise healthy patient with COPD, who will have a limited but adequate excursion of a very stiff, noncompliant thorax, to a patient with no preexisting pulmonary disease going into acute respiratory failure due to exhaustion of the respiratory musculature. The latter patient will have a very limited excursion of their thorax, but may have a compliant spine and rib cage. Comparing excursion (by monitoring movement during respiration) to compliance (by motion testing the spine and rib cage) will yield a much more complete picture of the respiratory system than reviewing either of these factors alone.

The length and tone of the respiratory musculature, including the diaphragm, will complete the structural examination of the respiratory system. Evaluate the muscles, both during contraction (inhalation) and at rest (end exhalation). Evidence of respiratory muscle fatigue and failure should be obtained during this part of the examination. Intercostal retractions may be observed during the evaluation of rib excursion. Paradoxic motion of the lower ribs (inward movement during inhalation), an indicator of a flattened, tense diaphragm, may be observed during evaluation of the excursion of the lower rib cage. Paradoxic movement of the abdomen (inward movement of the abdomen during inhalation), a sign of impending respiratory failure, may be observed with a hand below the costal margin. A less obvious sign of diaphragm fatigue may be noted with the same contact, as the effort or force of contraction during inhalation will be reduced as the diaphragm fatigues.

Focused Structural Examination of the Thorax

This is also discussed in Chapter 49, Ribs and Sternum.

Upper Thorax

1. *Sternum.* Evaluate movement of the sternum, both inhalation and exhalation.
2. *Clavicle.* Evaluate a sense of posterior/superior movement of the clavicle with inhalation, and an anterior/inferior movement during exhalation. Also evaluate inferior movement at the sternoclavicular (SC) joint during upward shrug of the shoulders and its relative superior movement during return to resting state. Evaluate rotation on its long axis during forward flexion of the shoulder. Palpate for a normal slight movement of the acromioclavicular (AC) joint during adduction of the arm across the chest. Test for hinge motion of the sternomanubrial joint during inhalation and exhalation.
3. *First rib.* Evaluate when examining the clavicle.
4. *Ribs 2 through 6.* Evaluate pump handle motion of the upper ribs with hands lateral to the sternum; evaluate middle ribs with thumbs approaching the xiphoid and fingerpads over the midaxillary line; evaluate bucket handle motion with hands below the breasts (see Chapter 49, Fig. 49.8).
5. *Musculature.* Evaluate the tension of the scalene, sternocleidomastoid, and trapezius muscles when evaluating the clavicle and first rib. Evaluated the intercostals when evaluating rib motion. Evaluate the paravertebral musculature, particularly those with rib attachments.

Lower Thorax and Diaphragm

1. *Ribs 6 through 10.* Evaluate bucket handle motion at the mid-axillary line, thumbs along the costal margin to evaluate any degree of AP motion.

2. *Costal margin.* Rest thumbs along costochondral margins. Evaluate angle and motion.

3. *12th rib.* Most easily found just lateral to the lateral edge of the erector spinae musculature. Compare the right and left 12th rib angles and motion and note that it should move down with inhalation as opposed to other ribs that move up with inhalation.

4. *Diaphragm.* Direct palpation of the diaphragm can be difficult due to its position under the rib cage. Its motion can be evaluated in several ways.

   a. With a hand just below the costal margin, the superior/inferior motion of the anterior and lateral parts of the diaphragm may be evaluated. This will allow evaluation of the anterior and lateral aspects of the diaphragm, but will not yield information about the posterior aspect. These regions do not necessarily operate together, as in the vomiting reflex, where the anterior and lateral contractions produce the forces for regurgitation; simultaneously the crura must relax to maintain patency of the gastroesophageal junction. The motion of the diaphragm should be differentiated from the motion of the abdominal wall.

   b. The motion of the 12th rib closely parallels the excursion of the posterior part of the diaphragm.

   c. The lumbar spine will reflect the tension in the posterior aspect of the diaphragm through the attachment of the crus to the first three lumbar vertebrae. When tense, the crura will flatten the upper lumbar vertebra. This will be noted as flattening or reversed lordosis statically, and resistance to upward spring or compression, at levels L1-3. This is easily accomplished with the patient in the supine position.

   d. With a hand above and below the lower thorax, the superior/inferior motion of the diaphragm may be distinguished from the lateral excursion of the ribs.

The Abdomen

Evaluation of the container should accompany the classic palpatory evaluation of the abdomen. The shape of a container will affect the function of its contents. The abdomen has a roof, a floor, and anterior and posterior walls.

- The *diaphragm* is the roof of the abdomen; the liver, spleen, and supporting mesenteries are suspended from it.
- The *pelvic diaphragm* is the floor. It, along with the shelf created as the posterior abdominal wall crosses the pelvic brim at the level of the pectinate line, and supports the abdominal and pelvic viscera from below.
- The *iliopsoas and quadratus lumborum* make up the posterior abdominal wall. The insertion of iliopsoas on the lesser trochanter of the femur involves the hip in abdominal and pelvic function.
- The *abdominal wall* is its anterior boundary.

Skeletal Considerations

The sacrum, pelvis, hip joint, lumbar spine, and lower six ribs and thoracic vertebrae form the structural and functional framework to which the soft tissue container of the abdomen is attached and supported. All should be evaluated for motion restriction and/or altered position.

The diaphragm should be evaluated with emphasis on its lower attachments to the 12th rib and lumbar spine. When the diaphragm becomes tense it flattens and carries the 12th ribs inferiorly at their tips. The lumbar spine will become flattened and resist anterior pressure in the supine patient. The same relative positions will be adopted when the diaphragm has a fascial "drag" placed on it, although the resistance encountered will be of a lesser degree and different quality. Rarely will the diaphragm be displaced superiorly from a dysfunction.

The movement of the pelvic diaphragm may be inferred by the magnitude and intensity of the consequent nutation/counternutation movement of the sacrum occurring during respiration (see Fig 71.13). Although this movement may be more obvious with the patient prone, supine evaluation is often necessary in the acutely ill, hospitalized patient. A two-handed contact from the side of the patient, one hand contacting the sacral base and the other on the sacral apex may be used for this evaluation. More direct evaluation of the tension and movement of the pelvic diaphragm may be performed with a contact in the ischiorectal fossae. These are found just medial and slightly posterior to the tip of the ischial tuberosities (Fig. 71.6). The pelvic diaphragm will move inferiorly with inhalation and superiorly with exhalation.

The quadratus lumborum may be palpated anterior and lateral to the erector spinae mass in the lumbar spine. Its edge is usually discernible beginning just below the tip of the 12th rib. The psoas major is a deeper, more medial flank muscle that is more difficult to palpate directly. The increased amount of muscle tone observed and the combination of upper lumbar somatic dysfunction and external hip rotation on the same side may infer tension. The tendon of the iliopsoas is directly palpable just below the inguinal ligament in the floor of the femoral triangle. The iliopsoas tendon is usually tense, full, and tender when the muscle is in spasm. One can often sense the tension in the entire iliopsoas with one hand contacting the tendon in the femoral triangle and the other under the upper lumbar attachments. Only the iliopsoas travels antero-inferolaterally here. Jones has also described anterior abdominal tender points related to spasm of the iliopsoas muscle (see Chapter 73, Counterstrain).

Palpation

Palpation is an essential part of any abdominal examination. However, extra care must be taken to avoid exacerbation of the patient's pain, as the resultant guarding by the patient will interfere with the examiner's ability to gather reliable information.

Light Palpation

It is useful to begin the abdominal examination with light palpation and in a region of the abdomen distant to the patient's chief complaint of pain or discomfort. This will help secure the

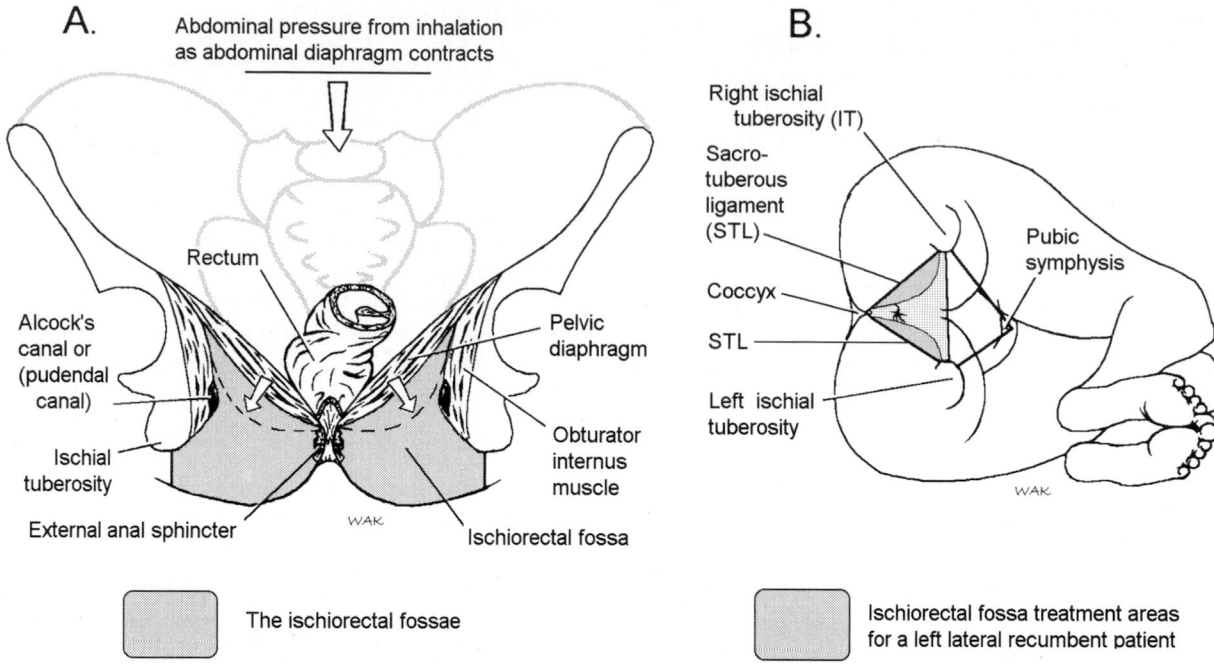

FIGURE 71.6. The ischiorectal fossa and pelvic diaphragm. **A.** The broken line depicts the pelvic diaphragm during inhalation. **B.** The ischiorectal fossa as it would appear in a lateral recumbent patient.

patient's comfort and cooperation, and can yield information not obtainable with deep palpation.

1. *Involuntary guarding by the patient.* Involuntary guarding, present without any actual or perceived stimulation of the discomfort, should be distinguished from voluntary guarding due to actual or perceived exacerbation of pain induced by the examination. This determination is an essential part of the abdominal examination, and is most accurately evaluated with light palpation, as many healthy individuals will guard with deep palpation.

2. *Ptosis.* Dr. Still often taught that there is a sag of the abdominal contents into the pelvis resulting in physiologic consequences. He wrote, "The caecum and the transverse and sigmoid flexure are often forced from their normal positions and piled into the pelvis, dragging the uterus and small intestine down with the caecum and obstructing all possible chance for the fluids of the small intestine to pass through the ileocecal valve and reach the colon" (11). Sag of the abdominal contents and the mesenteries that support them may be evaluated by comparing the resistance to normal limits and with the right and left sides, produced by a gentle lift just superior to each inguinal ligament. This quick test should be part of the light palpatory examination.

3. *Congestion.* A sense of fullness and or congestion will often be evident over areas of acute inflammation, such as cholecystitis or diverticulitis. It may be accompanied by a palpable sense of warmth. This somewhat subtle finding will be much more difficult to identify during deep palpation. There may also be a subcutaneous puffiness palpable over the epigastric region of the abdomen, a terminal drainage site related to the abdomen.

4. *Tenderness.* Tenderness is a subjective symptom but can usually be identified accurately during light palpation. Identifying the tender area early in the examination and leaving that area for evaluation near the end of the examination will help maximize

patient cooperation for the bulk of the early abdominal examination. The area of the patient's tenderness can be evaluated in depth at the end of the abdominal examination.

Deep Palpation

Deep palpation must be carefully performed. Slow, deliberate movements will minimize discomfort and voluntary guarding. Never palpate with your fingertips. Use the fingerpads.

Palpation with one hand over the other may be more comfortable to the patient and enhance palpatory sensing. The fingerpads of a relaxed hand rest on the patient and receive information while the other hand, resting on top, exerts gentle, steady pressure to reach the desired depth. The abdomen is classically divided into four quadrants for palpation (see Chapter 51, Fig. 51.11). The epigastrium and suprapubic areas may be considered separately. The examiner should always keep a clear mental picture of all significant anatomic structures in the area being palpated (see Fig. 51.12). Although many viscera are not palpable in normal conditions, in pathologic situations they may become discernible and offer clues to an accurate working diagnosis. Several examples, that this author has been found to be useful in practice, are presented, but the possibilities of abdominal palpation are far greater than just these examples.

1. The tip of the gallbladder capsule is often palpable in cases of acute cholecystitis, with associated fullness, congestion, and often warmth overlying it. When present, these signs are more accurate than the Murphy sign of right upper quadrant tenderness.

2. The stomach is palpable slightly left and inferior to the xiphoid. Sometimes the physician will note that the stomach resists gentle downward distraction produced with one hand, while the other hand contacts the xiphoid to stabilize the

diaphragm. This resistance is consistently present in patients with hiatal hernia and reflux disease. Fullness, congestion, and warmth are often present in the left upper quadrant in acute gastritis.

3. The motion of the liver with breathing and the tension within the ligaments anchoring the liver to the diaphragm should be evaluated, along with the size and contour of the liver. The movement of the diaphragm is essential for efficient portal circulation (12).

The Fluid (Lymph) Mechanism

The evaluation of the body's circulatory system is an integral part of any physical examination. The evaluation of the status of the lymphatic circulation is indicated in any inflammatory process, as the lymphatic system is responsible for the drainage of inflammatory exudates, and is integral in the progression and resolution of an inflammatory process. Millard was the first osteopathic physician to discuss the evaluation of the lymphatic system in the physical examination. He said, "For every congested tissue there is a corresponding lymph disturbance. Wherever pus is present there is enlargement in the nearest nodes. The lymph stream ebbs and flows according to the amount of blockage and nodular involvement at certain points" (13). Dr. Millard considered it possible to differentiate disease processes by the location, degree, and quality of lymph node enlargement. He also described a principle that is important in the treatment of lymph congestion: "The lymph stream is readily checked in many ways. The lymph vessels are pliable and readily compressed" (13). In the evaluation of lymphatic function, one must investigate tissue tension along the course of lymphatic drainage, with an emphasis on the regions where lymph vessels are most vulnerable to altered tissue tension.

J. Gordon Zink, a student of Dr. Millard, continued to develop methods for the evaluation of lymph function and dysfunction. He called attention to the congestion produced in the regions of lymph nodes when there was dysfunction of the lymph system, with or without frank edema, and the supraclavicular congestion found with dysfunction of the thoracic duct and "terminal lymph drainage from the head and neck." He also described a specific test he used in the evaluation of the lymphatic system, "There is a simple but very practical test to confirm better circulation, because of restored diaphragmatic respiration, when the patient is supine. The hands of the physician are placed high on the patient's abdomen, just below the costal arch. Firm pressure is used downward toward the table and cephalad, as if to 'raise' or 're-dome' the diaphragm. The patient should experience a sensation of 'warmth' or 'heat' in the lumbar and sacral area" (10).

W.G. Sutherland introduced the concept of fluid fluctuation in his description of the primary respiratory mechanism (14). The movement of interstitial fluids is important in the process of cellular respiration (the cellular exchange of gases), as well as the exchange of nutrients and waste products. Motion of the interstitial fluids occurs in response to intrinsic, rhythmic motions of the body, including pulse, respiration, and the primary respiratory mechanism. Interstitial fluid fluctuation may be evaluated passively, by the presence or absence of these inherent forces in the region of the body being evaluated. They can also be actively eval-

uated by assessing the response of the tissue and its fluid matrix to local or general lymph pump techniques aimed at fluctuating the interstitial fluid. The evaluation of the static and dynamic findings of the lymphatic circulation is important in the overall physical evaluation of the circulatory system (Table 71.2).

APPROACHING THE ACUTELY ILL HOSPITALIZED PATIENT

Osteopathic treatment in the hospital setting is most effective when it addresses underlying physiologic mechanisms of the disease and supports the physiologic response of the host who has the disease. Although the manipulative treatment is ultimately based on the findings of the structural examination, these findings should be interpreted with regard to the body's response to the disease process and directed toward supporting the body's physiologic processes. This section will present a variety of conceptual models from which treatment plans should evolve. Techniques will be described to provide examples of how some of the underlying principles may be achieved, but should not be construed as the best or only way to treat an area or problem. One cannot overemphasize the importance of designing treatments to the individual. There is, therefore, no such thing as a technique for asthma, congestive heart failure, or any disease, nor is there a manipulative technique for reducing segmental facilitation, improving respiratory/circulatory function, or any other physiologic process. A variety of techniques can be employed for any of these treatment goals. Any technique is appropriate if it addresses the underlying physiology and mechanics, is appropriate for the present condition of the patient, and brings about the changes a physician expects to see from application of an efficient treatment to accomplish a specific physiologic goal.

Inflammation

Inflammation is the generalized response to injury and disease. It is the hallmark of most acute illnesses. Inflammation involves the vascular system, the immune system, the nervous system, and the connective tissues. It is essential to the initial response of the body to the disease process, as well as the healing process. The lymphatic system is an integral part of the progression and ultimate resolution of inflammation. Besides draining areas of infection and injury, lymphatic drainage carries antigen to the nodes, where immune stimulation takes place and T and B cells are produced. Nodal efferents provide migration routes for these cells to enter the primary circulatory system.

The lymphatics are the only vascular system permeable to large particles, fats, and protein. In normal function, the lymphatics remove the proteins, which leak into the interstitium from the capillaries, maintaining a delicate osmotic balance, and keeping the interstitial environment pristine. During any inflammatory process, increased capillary permeability allows a tremendous efflux of protein into the interstitial spaces, producing an exudative swelling. This exudate can only be drained through the lymphatics. In addition, there is evidence that lymphatic drainage is necessary for the removal and deactivation of the chemical and immune mediators, which control inflammatory processes, making the lymphatics central in the progression and resolution of the

TABLE 71.2. CLINICAL PEARLS

Patient		Findings
Compare:	1. Paradoxic movement of lower ribs	1. Inward movement of these ribs during inhalation; indicates *flattened tense diaphragm*
	2. Paradoxic movement of abdomen	2. Inward movement of abdomen during inhalation; indicates *impending respiratory failure*
Compare:	1. Sign of impending respiratory failure	1. Paradoxic movement of abdomen during breathing
	2. Sign of a *flattened, tense abdominal diaphragm*	2. Paradoxic movement lower ribs
Compliance of the rib cage		The ease with which the rib cage will move
Compare:	1. *Poor excursion*	1. Evaluated by movement of the rib cage during breathing (i.e., poor observed motion)
	2. *Poor compliance*	2. Evaluated by motion testing of rib cage and sternum (i.e., poor motion tests)
Sign: abdominal *diaphragmatic fatigue*		Force of diaphragmatic contraction is reduced during inhalation
Compare:	1. Paradoxic movement lower ribs	1. Dramatic limitation of exhalation; patients uses active effort to exhale
	2. Paradoxic movement of abdomen	2. Restricted lower rib cage during inhalation; relatively free exhalation
Compare:	1. *Congestive heart failure* patient	1. Poor excursion; poor compliance
	2. *Chronic obstructive pulmonary disease* patient in relatively good health	2. Limited excursion but often spine and rib cage compliant
A manipulative technique is appropriate when:		1. It addresses the underlying physiology and mechanics
		2. It is appropriate for the present condition of the patient
		3. It brings about changes expected when applying efficient treatment to accomplish a specific physiologic goal
The work of breathing		A quantitative measure of the energy required by the body to overcome the resistance of the lung parenchyma and chest wall and accomplish inhalation and exhalation
35% to 60% of thoracic duct lymphatic flow is due to:		The response and effects of respiratory movements

process itself (15–18). Diseases including pancreatitis, asthma, rheumatoid arthritis, and even myocardial infarction will depend on lymphatic drainage for resolution.

The large efflux of protein and water from the capillary bed leaves a very high concentration of erythrocytes, which pack into the small venules producing local venous stasis (17). This makes the lymphatic system the only source of fluid drainage from an inflamed tissue. The tissue becomes saturated when the small hydrostatic gradient that produces capillary filtration is met by the increased interstitial pressure that the swelling tissue produces. At this point, the rate of blood supply will equal the rate of lymphatic drainage.

Inflammation and healing are aspects of one continuous process, guided by the same group of cells. Cellular activity will shift from proinflammatory to healing as the proportion of relative controlling mediators shift their activity. Although this progression is related to the production of mediators, one must consider the role of the efficient breakdown and removal of these mediators in the progression and resolution of any inflammatory process. Prolonged inflammation leads to poor healing, smoldering infections, chronic inflammatory processes, and eventually tissue destruction. There is evidence that lymphatic drainage is involved in the removal and breakdown of histamine, bradykinin, prostaglandins, and leukotrienes (including cytokines). Other mediators or the fate of other mediators simply have not been studied.

As proinflammatory mediators are removed, those that stimulate fibroblasts and macrophages will predominate, and the heal-

ing process will ensue. Residual (interstitial plasma) protein from the inflammatory exudate will also stimulate fibroblasts to produce collagen. As with the inflammatory phase, rapid and efficient removal of these elements is essential to a physiologic healing process. A prolonged healing phase will lead to excess collagen production, fibrous adhesions, and eventually to tissue fibrosis. The lymphatic system is responsible for the removal of most, if not all, of the inflammatory exudate. It has been shown that lymphatic drainage is involved with controlling the rate of collagen production, both during the healing process and in the pathogenesis of diseases that result in tissue fibrosis. Diseases such as cirrhosis of the liver, interstitial lung diseases, and atherosclerosis have been linked to impaired lymphatic function (19).

The lymphatic system is vulnerable to somatic dysfunction and its dysfunction is responsive to osteopathic manipulative treatment. The function of the lymphatic system should be evaluated and treated as part of the osteopathic treatment of any patient with an inflammatory process.

Segmental Facilitation

The treatment of acute segmental facilitation is fundamental and a broadly applicable model for the treatment of virtually any acutely ill patient. Reflex facilitation occurs in response to a vast majority of disease processes, and can alter and/or exaggerate the body's response to the disease, interfering with the recovery process. Facilitation is produced by nociceptor input, so that diseases presenting with pain are the most likely to produce significant reflex patterns. Van Buskirk notes that the spinal cord may be activated at a lower level of firing than is necessary to activate the cortex and produce pain perception, so the perception of pain is not necessarily required for a reflex to be present (20). Inflammation has been shown to greatly increase the firing of nociceptors. Therefore, those diseases that involve inflammation and/or a very tense patient are also likely to produce reflex facilitation, with or without the perception of pain (21). The effects of segmental facilitation will vary depending of the spinal cord levels involved and/or the organ systems involved in the disease process.

The heart is extremely responsive to its innervation. Reflexes in the region of the sympathetic innervation of the heart have been shown to occur in ischemic heart disease and acute myocardial infarction (2,6). Increases in sympathetic outflow will increase heart rate and contractility, while simultaneously constricting the coronary vessels, reducing blood flow to the heart. This can produce an increased discrepancy between oxygen demand and supply available to a patient with coronary artery disease or to the ischemic portion of the heart after acute myocardial infarction. Segmental facilitation may also increase the arrhythmogenicity of the heart, a potentially devastating occurrence following a myocardial infarction. Talman writes, "Parasympathetic influence tends to stabilize and adrenergic stimulation tends to increase the ventricle's propensity to develop arrhythmias. Asymmetrical sympathetic activity, particularly that which favors the left-sided sympathetic pathways to the heart, is especially arrhythmogenic" (22). The left-sided, upper thoracic segmental facilitation noted in response to acute myocardial infarction will produce an increase adrenergic influence to the heart that favors left-sided innervation. Finally, Korr noted other, less obvious effects of increased sympathetic activity to the heart, including a prolonged healing time and reduced production of collateral circulation (23). Both are important in the recovery period following a myocardial infarction.

The heart also has a parasympathetic innervation via the vagus nerve. The vagus nerve will reduce heart rate and contractility, and carries information via the baroreceptors concerning blood pressure. Beal reports a less common cervical finding associated with cardiac disease that may reflect a reflex carried by the afferent fibers of the vagus nerve (6). It has been found that firing vagal afferent fibers stimulates the C1 and C2 segments of the spinal cord (24). Kuchera and Kuchera suggest that vagal sensory innervation of the heart is concentrated in the posterior and inferior walls, which explains the greater number of bradyarrhythmias from those infarctions (25). Although this idea has had little study, Rosero and colleagues did find a reduced correlation of upper thoracic somatic dysfunction with posterior/inferior wall myocardial infarction (26). His study did not look at the presence of cervical findings in these patients. The presence of upper cervical and cranial (especially occipitomastoid) somatic dysfunction should be treated in patients with cardiac disease, especially in the presence of a bradyarrhythmia (right vagus) or atrial ventricular block (left vagus). Reducing segmental facilitation in patients with acute cardiac disease is central to the osteopathic treatment of their cardiac processes. However, extreme care must be taken in the treatment of acute cardiac patients, as the heart is extremely sensitive to changes in autonomic firing, which may occur during the treatment if appropriate caution is not exercised. Techniques

that have been found safe and effective are described in the treatment portion of this chapter.

The response of the lungs to the autonomic nervous system is important in a variety of disease processes. Vagal activity is related to the bronchospasm and mucous production in the pathophysiology of asthma. As stated previously, the vagus reflexes with the spinal cord at the C2 level. C2 somatic dysfunction has been consistently noted in diagnostic studies of pulmonary disease (8). Ipsilateral cranial base dysfunction, in particular that of the occipitomastoid articulation, usually is associated with vagal type reflexes. The sensory ganglion of the vagus nerve lies within the jugular foramen, adjacent to the occipitomastoid suture. Though the cervical findings are reported less often than the upper thoracic findings, this may be because the vagus and other parasympathetic nerves will not vasodilate or stimulate sweat glands, producing the associated temperature and skin moisture changes that are among the most common recognizable signs of acute segmental facilitation. It is therefore possible that segments facilitated in areas of parasympathetic innervation are underrecognized. Upper cervical findings in pulmonary disease, especially asthma, may be the most significant structural findings, due to the pathologic effects of segmental facilitation of the vagus nerve in this disease. Wilson also noted that, in asthmatic patients, he consistently found right paraspinal changes at T4-5 and somatic dysfunction of the right fourth or fifth rib (27). He reports significant improvement in acute asthmatic attacks following manipulative treatment of these dysfunctions. Asthma, an inflammatory disease, usually produces a more significant reflex at these levels than COPD.

Recognizing the role of the vagus nerve in producing bronchospasm and secretions, reflex facilitation of the vagus from somatic dysfunction at C2, the occipitomastoid suture, and/or the cranial base will exaggerate the degree of bronchospasm and secretions. Reducing the segmental facilitation may raise the threshold necessary for production of an asthma attack, reduce the need for medication, especially bronchodilators that are prone to overuse, and help reduce the severity of an acute attack. Vagal reflex somatic dysfunction should be identified and treated in patients with pulmonary diseases.

A different type of reflex is present in pneumonia. Pneumonia is accompanied by a local reduction in rib excursion. This dysfunction pattern is described in standard physical diagnosis texts, as well as osteopathic literature (25,28). This phenomenon cannot be a typical viscerosomatic reflex, since the dysfunction levels in lower lobe pneumonia are outside the levels of the sympathetic innervation of the lung. It is more likely they are produced through the parietal pleura, which carries a local, intercostal innervation. These reflex changes are likely involved in the pleuritic chest pain (Fig. 71.4) which often accompanies pneumonia, and are very useful in locating and making the diagnosis of pulmonary consolidation. Treatment of these reflex changes is important in the overall treatment plan of patients with pneumonia.

Upper thoracic findings associated with pulmonary disease (T1-5, and occasionally T6) are commonly found in patients with acute and chronic bronchitis. This is consistent with the notion that the sensory innervation of the large airways travels mostly via the sympathetic nerves, while the sensory innervation of the small airways (asthma, lobar pneumonia) travels predominantly via the vagus. While sympathetic outflow may not be as detrimental to pulmonary function as vagal, the associated thoracic segmental spinal facilitation and somatic efferent outflow results in restriction of the upper ribs, reducing the ability of the patient with bronchitis to expectorate secretions. Somatic dysfunctions in these patients should be treated with osteopathic manipulation.

The gastrointestinal (GI) system has an extensive autonomic innervation, which is involved in a variety of disease processes. The vast majority of nociceptors from the GI tract travel with the sympathetic nervous system, producing reflex somatic dysfunction at approximate spinal levels from T5-L2. Cervical findings are absent in diagnostic studies involving GI diseases (8). Increased sympathetic outflow can have a multitude of detrimental effects on patients with GI diseases. The sympathetic nervous system reduces blood flow to the entire GI tract, making recovery from virtually any problem more difficult. The other major effect of the sympathetic nervous system is to reduce GI motility. This effect may be most noticeable in postoperative ileus, a common complication of abdominal surgery. The skin carries the highest concentration of nociceptors of any tissue in the body. Therefore, the patient, whose dermatomes are affected by a midline incision from the xiphoid to pubes, will have the possibility of having nociceptive reflexes to the entire T5-L2 spinal region. This is also the segmental site for sympathetic innervation of the entire GI tract. The bilateral segmental facilitation produced by a surgical abdominal incision, particularly a large midline incision, can significantly delay the body's ability to return to normal GI motility following abdominal surgery. Osteopathic treatment to reduce segmental facilitation is indicated following abdominal surgery, and in any case of paralytic ileus. Normalization of the sympathetic nervous system by ileus prevention manipulative treatment given before abdominal surgery has been shown to reduce the incidence of paralytic ileus. Alteration in GI motility is also a major part of the pathophysiology of irritable bowel syndrome. Osteopathic treatment to reduce reflex facilitation is indicated in these patients as well.

The sympathetic nervous system also affects the sphincters of the abdominal viscera. This can have an adverse effect in a number of situations. Cholecystitis accompanied by a stone lodged in the common bile duct will produce a reflex in the T6-9 region on the right. This is the origin of the innervation of the ampulla of Vater, whose tone will be increased by the segmental facilitation resulting from this pathophysiology. This, in turn, makes the passage of the stone more difficult. A similar situation may exist with an irritation of the ureter from a ureteral calculus, affecting motility of the ureters, or from the viscerovisceral reflex facilitation from gastritis or a peptic ulcer, affecting the pyloric sphincter, delaying the emptying of the stomach.

Sympathetic outflow will reduce the secretions throughout the GI tract. Of clinical significance is the reflex viscerovisceral facilitation that occurs in patients with either gastritis or a gastric ulcer. This results in reduction of secretions of stomach glands that would normally contribute to a protective bicarbonate barrier to stomach acid and therefore promotes an environment for increased mucosal damage. Finally, in experimental trials, pancreatitis has been found to become much more severe in the face of increased sympathetic outflow (25). Pancreatitis commonly

produces a significant, bilateral reflex that results in increased sympathetic output to the pancreas.

The discussion of reflex facilitation would not be complete without a mention of the pelvic innervation. It is of note that there is no mention of sacral or pelvic findings in the literature in response to diseases of the lower GI or pelvic viscera (8). Similar to the discussion of vagal reflexes at C2, if reflex facilitation occurred via the pelvic nerves, it would not present with sweat gland or cutaneous vascular changes. In the pelvis, there is also the absence of deep, intersegmental musculature and, therefore, somatic muscular findings, the other most common finding associated with acute segmental facilitation, is not evident. If reflex facilitation did occur in the pelvis, it might present with a completely different set of palpatory findings than those occurring elsewhere in the body. Animal studies have demonstrated increases in GI motility with stimulation of the skin of the lower abdomen and pelvis. The sacrum should be included in the evaluation and treatment plan of any viscera that have a pelvic innervation. The sacrum will be presented in this chapter when considering treatment of segmental facilitation.

Often, the consequences of facilitation create physiologic imbalance that interferes with the body's response to a challenge. Segmental facilitation is a consequence of many acute diseases, especially those producing pain and/or inflammation. One osteopathic treatment goal is to remove somatic dysfunctions of related segments to reduce their somatic contribution to the facilitated spinal cord segments. Another goal might be to improve the general function of the nervous system.

Neuroendocrine Immune Considerations

The hypothalamus, and the neuroendocrine immune system that it controls, is at the center of the body's response to the almost unlimited variety of challenges from the body's external and internal environments. It is central to the maintenance of homeostasis in the face of these challenges, and deeply involved in the body's response to virtually all acute illnesses. The hypothalamus exerts immense influence on the central functioning of the autonomic nervous system, the pituitary gland, and through it, by way of the autonomic nervous system and adrenal glands, the entire endocrine system and the immune system. The physiology of the hypothalamic-pituitary axis is also vulnerable to the neurophysiologic effects brought about by the mechanical dysfunctions resulting from somatic dysfunction.

Information about the local functioning within the body is monitored by the hypothalamus in several ways. The ability of the hypothalamus to respond to internal and external changes will depend on the accuracy of its inputs. The hypothalamus receives a large input from the nociceptive system, via the spinohypothalamic tract (29). Spinal cord facilitation will exaggerate this source of input, affecting the degree and quality of the response. The hypothalamus also receives input about levels of inflammation and immune activity in the body from circulating leukotrienes, delivered to the systemic circulation by the lymphatics (18). Levels of circulating leukotrienes are monitored by circumventricular organs in the third and fourth ventricles (30). This system will operate at maximum effectiveness when circulation and fluctuation of cerebrospinal fluid is undisturbed. Reduced rate and

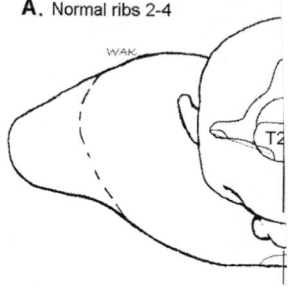

A. Normal ribs 2-4

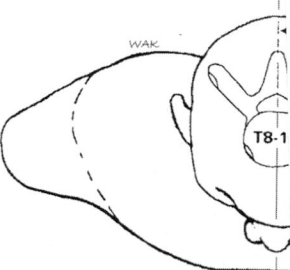

B. Normal ribs 8-10

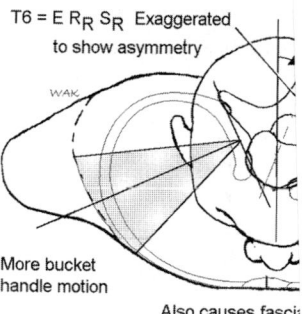

C. T6 with somatic dysfunction

T6 = E R$_R$ S$_R$ Exaggerated
to show asymmetry

More bucket
handle motion

Also causes fascia

FIGURE 71.8. Vertebral rotation
and the movement of that rib pro

associated flattening in acute an
flattening of the diaphragm ma
the movement of the lower rib
doxic rib motion. This will red
chest, and greatly reduce the e
mechanism. In osteopathic lite
and vertical orientation of the d
diaphragm. Doming of a flatten
crease the pressure gradients tha
thoracic and abdominal region:
rib motion and improve the fu
as the respiratory mechanism a
ing the mechanics of breathing,
the compliance of the thorax a
generally, and the function and ∈
culature will have far-reaching :
acute and chronic respiratory di:

The physiologic impact of r
exchange of air. The negative
excursion are important to the fu
as well.

amplitude of the primary respiratory mechanism will reduce the fluctuation of the cerebrospinal fluid.

The pituitary gland sits within the sella turcica of the sphenoid. The hypothalamus is just above, in close relation to the body of the sphenoid and sphenobasilar junction. The pituitary gland has a portal circulation, similar to the portal circulation of the liver. The liver is situated against the undersurface of the diaphragm and is anchored to it, and the respiratory movement of the diaphragm provides the motive power for its circulation. The pituitary gland has a similar anatomic relation to the diaphragma sella. The diaphragma sella continues into the sella turcica. It completely surrounds the pituitary gland and blends with its capsule (31). The diaphragma sella is a continuation of the anterior reaches of the tentorium cerebelli. The movement of the sphenoid and the tentorium cerebelli would, therefore, alternately change the shape of the gland with the phases of the primary respiratory mechanism, pumping the fluid within it. It has been suggested that the portal circulation of the pituitary is bi-directional; the backward movement from the pituitary gland to the hypothalamus is theorized to be important to the feedback regulation of the hypothalamic pituitary axis (31). This is also a possible mechanism for the central distribution of corticotropin-releasing factor (CRF), which has far reaching effects in the central nervous system. The alternating movement of the primary respiratory mechanism would explain the ability of this circulation to move in alternating directions. W.G. Sutherland described the importance of the motion of the sphenoid to the functioning of the pituitary gland (32) It is important to consider treatment of somatic dysfunctions of the cranium, including the sphenobasilar area, in the management of the acutely ill hospitalized patient.

Approach to Thorax

Sutherland writes, "The diaphragm is the 'piston' to the big 'combustion cylinder' of the body. Its crura are the 'legs' that lead down from the piston to the 'crankshaft' in the lumbar vertebrae. Its ligamenta arcuarta are the 'piston rings.' The lungs might represent the 'combustion chamber' to the cylinder while the nasal region the 'carburetor,' while the 'ignition' and 'self starter' might be found somewhere in the 'cranial bowl'." (32)

The thorax contains the heart, lungs, and mediastinum and its contents. These structures are related anatomically by their fascial attachments. The fibrous pericardium blends inferiorly into the central tendon of the diaphragm, this relation is important to diaphragmatic function. The fibrous pericardium attaches to the sternum via the sternopericardial ligaments, and is continuous superiorly with the mediastinal fascia, which blends with the anterior cervical fascia at the inner aspect of the clavicles and manubrium. The anterior cervical fascia, including the pretracheal fascia, has attachment to the hyoid bone and mandible before finally hanging from the cranial base. This continuity must be considered in any approach to manipulative treatment of the thorax, neck, or cranium.

Breathing is largely a mechanical process by which intrathoracic pressure changes are created via the action of skeletal musculature on the spine and bony thorax. It also produces pressure gradients between the thoracic and abdominal cavities. This process is critical to the movement of both air and fluids throughout

the body. A detailed look at the mechanics involved will offer insight as to how osteopathic treatment may improve the efficiency and effectiveness of breathing in the acutely ill patient, an important consideration whether or not the patient is suffering directly from a respiratory problem.

The physical action of producing a negative intrathoracic pressure requires a definable amount of energy, referred to as the work of breathing. Although difficult to quantify, increased work of breathing is clinically relevant, since many pulmonary problems dramatically alter the work of breathing. Restrictive lung diseases, by their very nature, increase the work of breathing. West considers increases in work of breathing an important factor in the pathophysiology of COPD (33). In the pathophysiology of asthma, patients progress to respiratory stage three and ultimately to respiratory failure due to an inability to maintain a state of hyperventilation caused by fatigue and the eventual exhaustion of the respiratory musculature. This failure is directly related to increased work of breathing in the patient with acute asthma. The work of breathing is a quantitative measure of the energy required by the body to overcome the resistance of the lung parenchyma and chest wall and accomplish inhalation and exhalation. Compliance is the ease with which those tissues are stretched (moved). Lung compliance is clearly reduced in all of the above diseases, contributing to the overall increased work of breathing. Restrictive diseases directly alter lung elasticity. Obstructive diseases reduce compliance through increased airway resistance and a variety of other factors.

Somatic dysfunction, by its definition, will reduce the compliance of the bony thorax in patients with pulmonary diseases and increase the work of breathing. Somatic dysfunction of the thoracic spine and ribs has been noted by a number of sources (5). The general shape changes of the thorax in COPD (barrel chest) can produce dramatic changes in chest wall compliance which are obvious on osteopathic structural examination and, in addition to the specific dysfunctions noted in association with pulmonary disease, actually stand out. General techniques will be described to address general compliance issues, as well as more specific techniques for individual somatic dysfunctions. Osteopathic treatment to improve the compliance of the thorax will not necessarily directly alter the parenchymal pathology, especially those with chronic lung disease. However it will improve issues such as exercise tolerance, giving the patient the ability to function with their disease. West notes the effect of the work of breathing on exercise tolerance of the chronic lung patient (34).

In addition to general changes in compliance of the bony thorax, specific somatic dysfunctions may have an effect on the function of the respiratory mechanism that goes beyond the small changes in compliance they invariably produce. The movement of a typical rib during breathing operates in conjunction with the orientation of its costotransverse and costovertebral joints (Fig. 71.7). Rotation of the thoracic vertebrae with somatic dysfunction will not only create resistance to movement, but will change the orientation of the costotransverse and costovertebral articulations, produce thoracic fascial torsions, and further impair the ability of the muscles to move the rib during inhalation. With rotation of thoracic vertebral units involved in somatic dysfunction, a rib with a predominantly bucket handle movement might become oriented to move more in a pump handle movement.

Spinous pro

Transverse
process

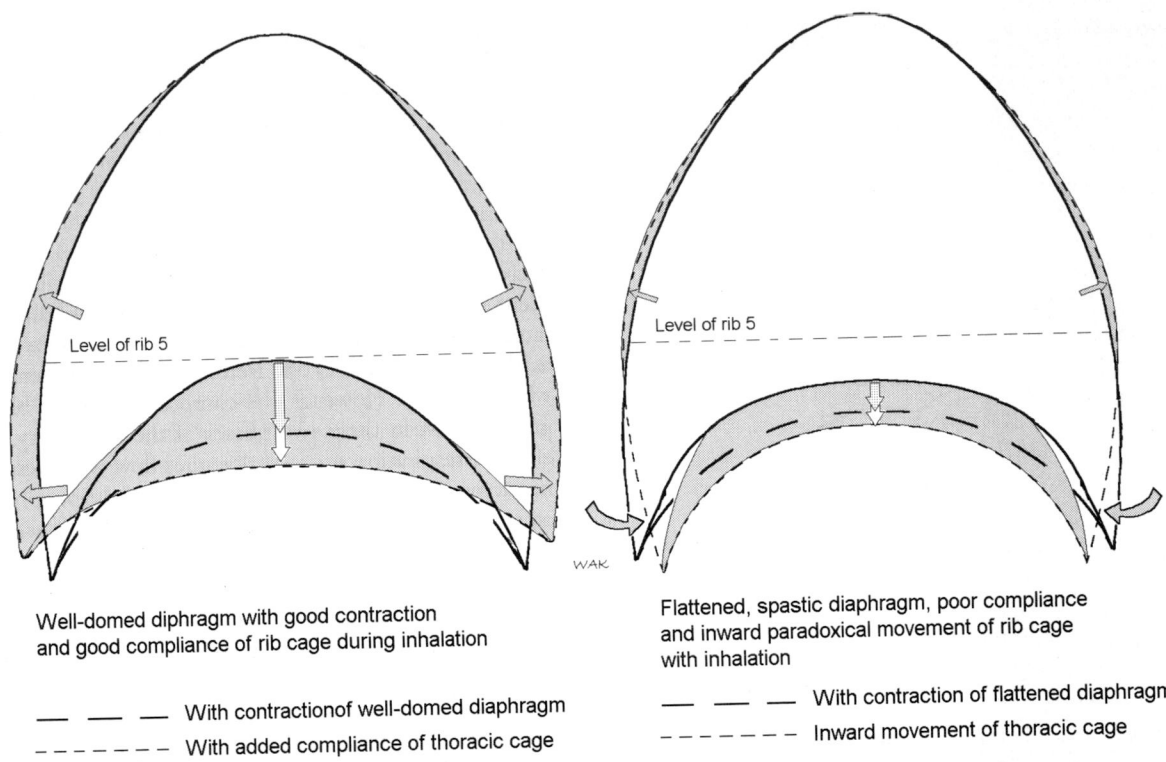

Pump handle
motion

Well-domed diphragm with good contraction
and good compliance of rib cage during inhalation

— — — With contractionof well-domed diaphragm

– – – – – With added compliance of thoracic cage

Flattened, spastic diaphragm, poor compliance
and inward paradoxical movement of rib cage
with inhalation

— — — With contraction of flattened diaphragm

– – – – – Inward movement of thoracic cage

FIGURE 71.9. The mechanical effects of contraction of the diaphragm. **A:** Normal excursion of a compliant thoracic rib cage with contraction of a well-domed diaphragm. **B:** Reduced excursion of thoracic cage and even the possibility of paradoxic motion of the lower rib cage with contraction of a flattened abdominal diaphragm.

(Fig. 71.8). Lumbar somat
per lumbar spine, will alter
and may, thereby, impair t
contraction of the diaphra

Cathie describes moven
tion (9). During inhalation
rotation of the sacrum wi
reverse movement occurs v
anywhere in the body may

Increases in work of brea
fatigue. Respiratory muscle
in the pathophysiology of
structive diseases produce i
the effects of hyperinflation
understood as the immedia
patient with acute asthma.
and the patient can no lon
quate air exchange. Respira
in COPD, and has led to the
muscle fatigue in the pathop
ratory muscle fatigue has als
such as pulmonary edema,
patients off ventilators (36,3
thorax will reduce the load
reduce the likelihood of fati
ditions. Osteopathic treatme
function and efficiency of th

Respiratory muscles, like
the principle of their length-
ship, muscles will develop a
resting tone. Consider the
with exacerbations of obstruc

in the area. The initial lymphatics in the abdomen and pelvis, in particular, respond significantly to respiratory excursions.

The clinical significance of this mechanism is considerable. Lobar pneumonia is an example of an intrapulmonary inflammatory process that will greatly increase the demand on the local lymphatic circulation. The local excursion of the thorax, however, is consistently and significantly reduced in the local region of the consolidation. This discrepancy will reduce the drainage of the exudate produced by the local inflammation, reduce the delivery of antigen to lymph nodes, and ultimately reduce the delivery of immunity and antibiotics to the area as interstitial pressure rises and shunts blood away from the area. Restoring local excursion of the thorax will improve the body's ability to move lymph in this situation; specific lymph pump techniques are also indicated. Asthma is an example of a more generalized inflammatory process of the pulmonary tissues. This disease produces

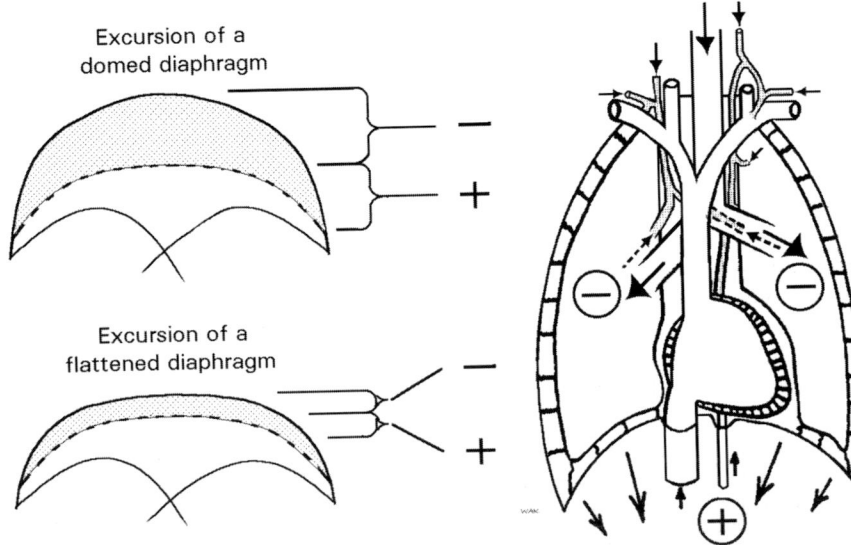

Excursion of a
domed diaphragm

Excursion of a
flattened diaphragm

FIGURE 71.10. The excursion of the diaphragm has a powerful influence on venous and lymphatic return. This effect is reduced when the resting diaphragm is flattened.

a significant, overall restriction of the thorax to the exhalation phase of respiration, reducing both local drainage of lymph from the small airways and central lymph drainage through the thoracic duct. This physiologic model should also be considered in patients who have had a thoracotomy and/or sternotomy. These procedures produce intrathoracic inflammation that simultaneously and dramatically reduces the patient's ability to produce excursion of the thorax in the postoperative period.

The work of breathing, with its mechanical considerations associated with respiration, and its respiratory/circulatory function, with its role in the body's response and recovery from disease (especially inflammatory processes), must be considered in the osteopathic evaluation and treatment of any disease of the thorax. The work of breathing directs one to consider the compliance of the thorax, most easily evaluated by motion testing of the spine and ribs. Respiratory/circulatory function depends on the excursion of the thorax, evaluated by passively observing the patient's respiratory excursion. Although there is an undeniable relationship between compliance and excursion, separate evaluation and consideration of these will lead to a more accurate understanding of the patient and a more appropriate and effective treatment plan. For example, a relatively strong and healthy COPD patient may have a relatively good excursion, but a much reduced thoracic compliance, best seen by motion testing of the ribs and thorax. Alternately, a patient just out of surgery will have a greatly reduced excursion, but the compliance may be relatively good. These two situations will lead to very different treatment programs. The ability to address compliance and excursion of the thorax is an important reason for including osteopathic manip-

ulative treatment in the management program of patients with a wide variety of diseases.

Approach to Abdomen/Pelvis

The abdomen and pelvis form a single space, even though anatomists separate this space into two divisions. The abdomen, viewed as a single space, functionally contains, supports, and influences the function of the GI and the genitourinary viscera (see Chapter 51, Abdominal Region, Fig. 51.1). The lower ribs and their thoracic vertebral attachments, lumbar spine, sacrum, and pelvic bones form the osseous components of this container. The diaphragm, anterior and posterior abdominal walls, and pelvic diaphragm are the myofascial components. The abdominal diaphragm is as integrated to the function of the abdomen as it is the thorax. The diaphragm forms the roof of the abdomen, and suspends the liver, stomach and spleen, and colon via direct ligamentous attachments (Fig. 71.11). Flattening of the diaphragm, which may result from increases in its resting tone, airway obstruction, or sag from fascial strain and drag, will allow sag of these viscera as well as those suspended beneath them. The posterior attachments of the diaphragm, which lie within the abdomen, are mechanically important. They provide the stable fulcrum necessary for effective contraction. The crura blend with the anterior longitudinal ligament of the upper lumbar spine, usually L1-3. Posterolaterally, the lumbocostal arches extend across the posterior abdominal wall to the tips of the 12th ribs on either side. The medial lumbocostal arch is a thickening of the psoas major fascia (Fig. 71.12). Its medial aspect blends with the crus of the

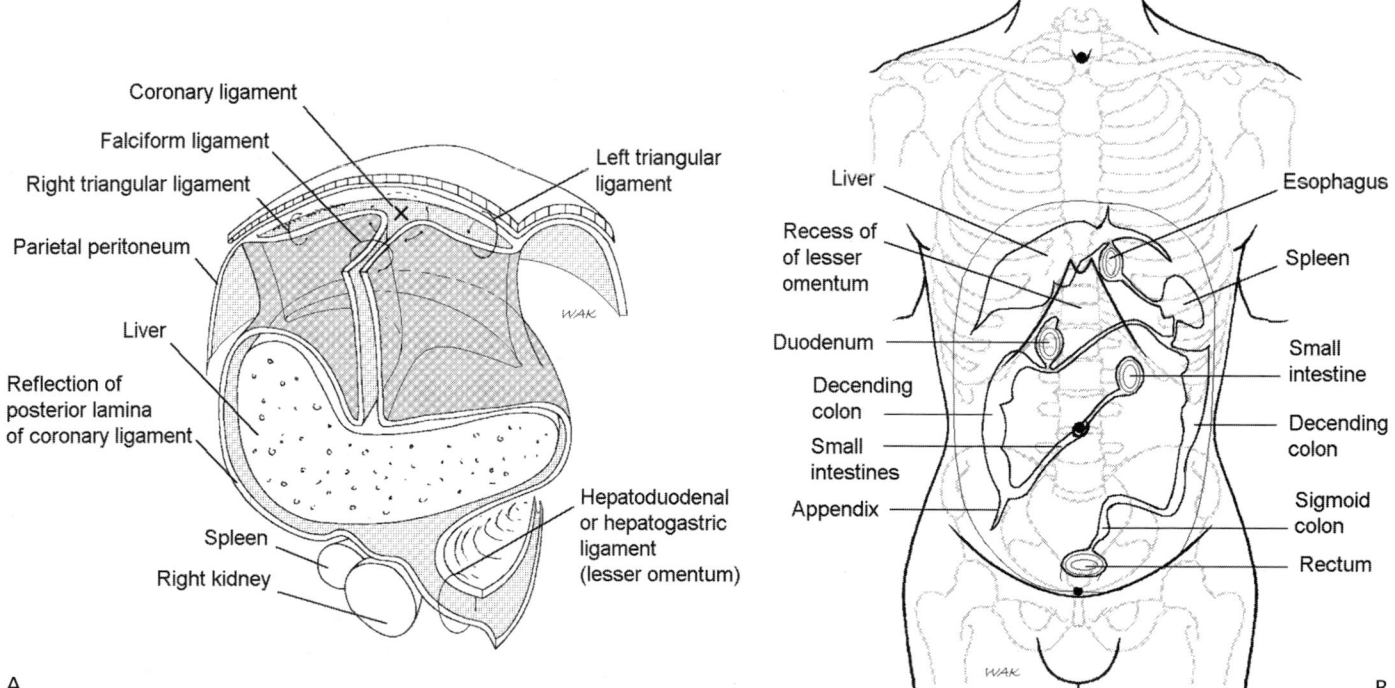

FIGURE 71.11. A: The attachments of the liver to the diaphragm. These are firm and allow the diaphragm to strongly influence portal circulation. **B:** The attachments of the abdominal mesenteries. These provide support for the abdominal viscera as well as providing the pathways for their neurovascular supply.

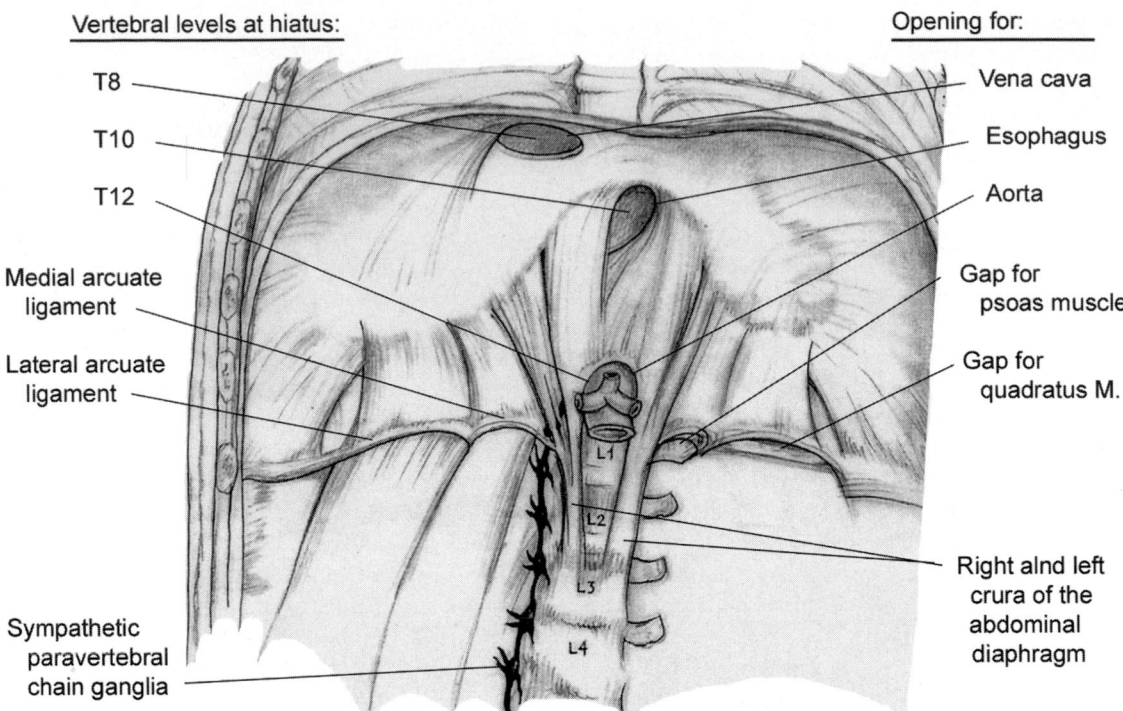

Vertebral levels at hiatus:

T8
T10
T12

Medial arcuate ligament

Lateral arcuate ligament

Sympathetic paravertebral chain ganglia

Opening for:

Vena cava
Esophagus
Aorta

Gap for psoas muscle

Gap for quadratus M.

Right alnd left crura of the abdominal diaphragm

L1
L2
L3
L4

FIGURE 71.12. The abdominal surface of the diaphragm. The crura and lumbocostal arches blend, forming a continuous series of arches which anchors the diaphragm posteriorly to the 12th ribs and lumbar spine.

diaphragm. It then crosses over the psoas muscle and is laterally attached to the front of the transverse process of the first lumbar vertebra near its tip. Here it blends with the lateral lumbocostal arch. The lateral lumbocostal arch is a thickening of the quadratus lumborum fascia. Medially it is attached to anterior surface of the tip the transverse process of the first lumbar vertebra. It then crosses over the quadratus lumborum muscle and is attached laterally to the lower border of the 12th rib. Together, the lumbocostal arches and the right and left crus of the diaphragm, attaching to the lumbar spine, form a continuous series of five arches which integrates the function of the diaphragm and posterior abdominal wall. Mechanical support for the contraction of the diaphragm comes from the crural anchors to the lumbar spine and from the depression and stabilization of the 12th rib through the contraction of the quadratus and tension in the lumbocostal arches. The continuity of the posterior abdominal wall to the pelvic brim and to the lesser trochanter of the hip allows these more remote, but important, mechanical anchors to also be included as supports for diaphragmatic contraction. Evaluation and treatment of somatic dysfunctions of the crura and lumbocostal arches via the 12th ribs and lumbar spine will have a major impact on the excursion and physiologic function of the diaphragm.

The diaphragm has openings for the passage of numerous structures between the thorax and abdomen (Fig. 71.12; and also Chapters 50 and 51). The esophagus passes through a loop in the right crus that acts as the most substantial functional portion of the gastroesophageal sphincter. Dysfunction of the crus is often present in patients with gastroesophageal reflux and hiatal hernia. Osteopathic manipulative treatment directed toward altering tension of the crus may be helpful in the management of

patients with these problems. The aorta and the cisterna chyle, or beginning of the thoracic duct, pass between the right and left crus. The potential effect of the phasic contraction of the crura on the normal central lymph flow, through the thoracic duct as part of an overall effect of respiration, must be considered. Conversely, the potential for obstruction of central lymph flow with increased tension in the crura must be considered as well. The sympathetic chain with its paraspinal ganglia pass through the medial lumbocostal arch. Several authors have implicated that altered tension of the fascia surrounding the chain ganglia has an effect on the function of the sympathetic chain ganglia (4,25,32).

The passage beneath the lumbocostal arch is a small, tight space vulnerable to altered tension of the psoas and/or diaphragm. The inferior vena cava passes through the tendinous portion of the diaphragm near its apex. Unequal tension in the diaphragm, either side to side or front to back can draw the central tendon off center and alter the size, shape, and position of this opening, interfering with passage of blood through the diaphragm. As stated by Dr. Still, "He cannot expect blood to quietly pass through the diaphragm if impeded by muscular constriction around the aorta, vena cava, or thoracic duct. The diaphragm can and is often pulled down on both the vena cava and thoracic duct, obstructing blood and chyle (lymph) from returning to [the] heart" (42). In this regard, one must consider the potential deleterious effects of altered tension in the diaphragm on venous and lymphatic circulation as an additional consideration, using treatment according to the respiratory circulatory model. The diaphragm, on a variety of levels, is intimately involved in the function of the GI system, the circulatory system, and the nervous system.

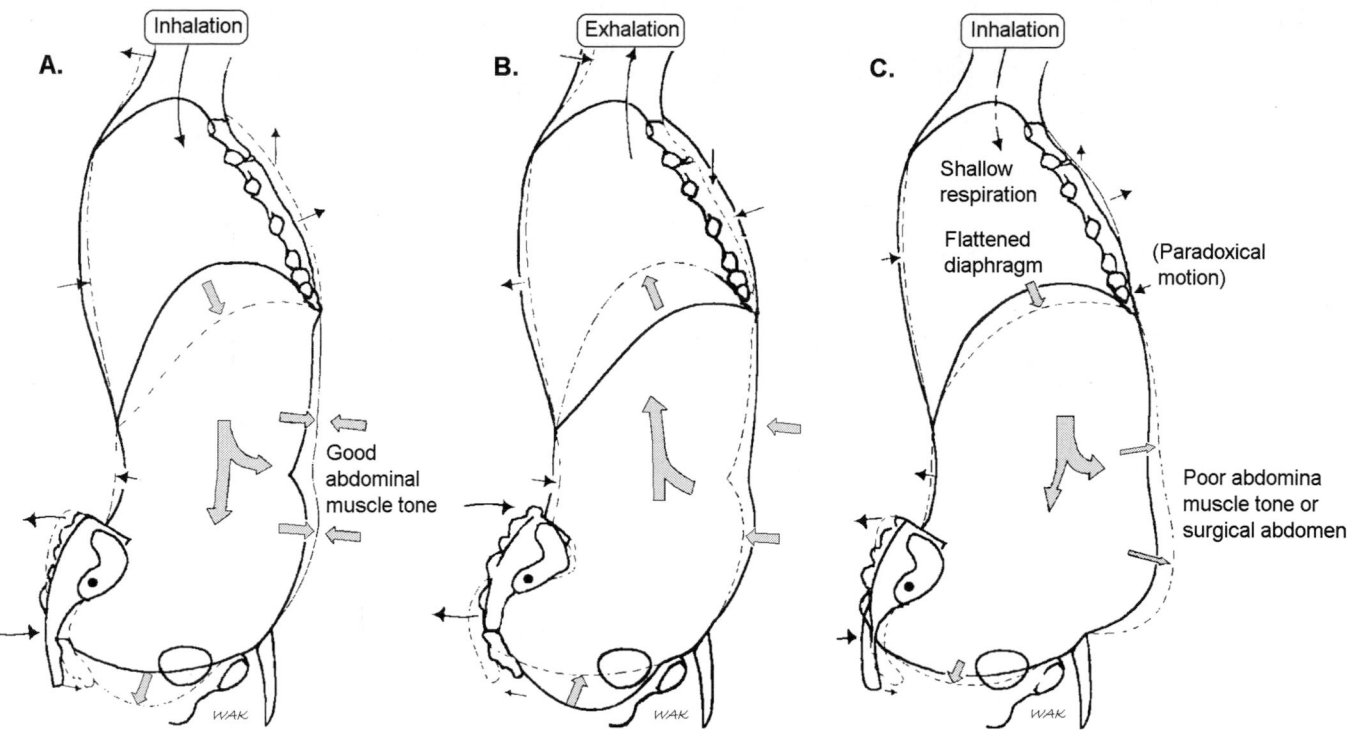

FIGURE 71.13. **A & B:** Relative movements and function of the abdominal diaphragm, pelvic diaphragm, abdominal wall, spine and sacrum occurring during respiration. **C:** The effect of a significant abdominal surgical incision or presence of poor abdominal tone on the physiologic movements occurring during breathing.

The iliacus, psoas, and quadratus lumborum constitute the posterior abdominal wall. The role of the posterior abdominal wall in the mechanical function of the diaphragm has been discussed, particularly the lumbocostal arches. The posterior abdominal wall is also involved in support of the abdominal viscera. The psoas fascia blends with the fascia of the kidney and is the primary support for this organ. The iliopsoas forms a shelf as it crosses the pelvic brim and this helps to support the cecum and sigmoid colon. Increased tension in this region will reduce the overall support of the colon, and may predispose to sag of the viscera and the mesenteries. The posterior abdominal wall is also the site for most of the posterior mesenteric root attachments (see abdominal mesenteries shown in Fig. 71.11), and this further increases its importance as support of the abdominal viscera. The ureter travels along the medial aspect of the psoas in the abdomen. It is not surprising that psoas spasm is a common finding in nephrolithiasis and pyelonephritis. The deep abdominal lymph nodes also travel in relation to the iliopsoas as they ascend from the inguinal area to the diaphragm. The tendon of iliopsoas also forms the floor of the femoral triangle where the inguinal lymph vessels and the femoral veins cross into the pelvis and abdomen.

The pelvic diaphragm forms the floor of the abdominopelvic cavity. Its muscular attachments include the pubic symphysis, the ischial tuberosities, and the coccyx and sacral apex. In addition to supporting the pelvic viscera, including the prostate in the male, the pelvic diaphragm forms the external anal sphincter and has an opening for the passage of the urethra and, in the female, the vagina. Sensory nerves in the pelvic diaphragm are part of the reflex control mechanism for urination. In addition to its roles in the function of the bladder and rectum, the pelvic diaphragm has a role in respiration. The pelvic diaphragm descends with the abdominal diaphragm during inhalation, creating space for the descending abdominal viscera (Fig 73.13). Clinically, there is tension palpable with its descent. The pelvic diaphragm may act in conjunction with the anterior abdominal wall, lengthening under tension to control the descent of the diaphragm and stabilize abdominal pressure. The abdominal diaphragm will lose the important fulcrum created by the resistance of the viscera if abdominal pressure is reduced by poor tone of the abdominal wall or dysfunction of the pelvic diaphragm. If abdominal pressure is allowed to rise, the increased resistance reduces the effectiveness of the diaphragm and reduces inferior vena caval flow. One of the problems occurring after abdominal surgery is the reduced ability of the abdominal wall to participate in this process. The role of the pelvic diaphragm becomes heightened in the postsurgical patient, and freedom of the sacrum and pelvic diaphragm are essential in this situation.

The integrated function of the diaphragm, pelvic diaphragm, and abdomen, occurring as the patient breathes, plays a significant role in the prognosis of the postsurgical patient. The most common complication from abdominal surgery is atelectasis and pneumonia. The patient is predisposed to these complications by the shallow, costal breathing that is so common in postoperative cases. Although usually considered to be one of the effects from pain, it has been shown that intraoperative epidural injection, completely blocking postoperative pain does nothing to alter the limited and dysfunctional diaphragmatic breathing pattern

(43). Other explanations for the pattern of altered postsurgery diaphragmatic breathing include the effects of the somatovisceral reflex produced by the incision and the altered abdominal wall function. A midline abdominal incision extending from the xiphoid to the pubes will produce bilateral reflex facilitation from the T5-7 region (including ribs) all the way to the L2-3 area. This includes the entire attachment of the diaphragm, including the crura, and disproportionately increases the lower thorax workload and limits its excursion. The coordinated action of the abdominal wall and diaphragm is impaired. The abdominal incision alters the tone and reactivity of the abdominal wall, impairing its ability to help control inhalation. Osteopathic treatment of the lower thorax and lumbar spine will improve compliance of these tissues, thereby reducing the resistance against which the diaphragm must push. It will simultaneously reduce sympathetic outflow to the entire GI tract and thereby reduce the chance of postoperative ileus, another common postoperative complication. Treatment of the sacrum and pelvis with a focus on maximizing the excursion of the pelvic diaphragm will help compensate for the reduced ability of the abdominal wall to participate in the coordinated control of inhalation.

Respiration also plays a role in the abdominal lymph circulation. The role of breathing in the central movement of lymph has already been discussed. Respiration also exerts a powerful influence on the formation of lymph in the abdomen (44); only peristalsis is more influential (45). The postsurgical abdomen, particularly when peritonitis is present, responds with a tremendous inflammatory process. At the same time, the two most powerful factors in the abdomen related to the accumulation of lymph and the reduction of lymphatic flow are impaired breathing and the absence of peristalsis. Osteopathic treatment to promote lymph formation and flow is important to the immediate healing process. The inability to clear inflammatory exudate increases the potential to produce the most common long-term complication of abdominal surgery, adhesions. Most diseases of the abdomen are inflammatory, and will respond to osteopathic treatment to promote the formation and propulsion of lymph. Lymph flow may be obstructed at the crura of the diaphragm, and this region must be evaluated and treated if indicated. Lymph vessels exit the peritoneal cavity via the mesenteric roots, and drag on these mesenteries will increase the tension at the root, which may also obstruct the flow of lymph. Mesenteric drag is a common finding in postsurgical and medical problems of the abdomen and pelvis, and may be treated carefully with mesenteric lifts, to promote the flow of lymph.

TREATMENT APPROACHES

General Considerations

First the patient is evaluated and the structural findings are interpreted in relation to the above principles and an understanding of the patient's disease process. Then a treatment plan is developed to address the dysfunctions in such a way as to improve the function of the patient's underlying physiology. Often, a single area will need treatment based on several different models. In most, if not all cases, there will be multiple physiologic issues that can be addressed simultaneously through a treatment process. For example, an area of the thoracic spine and ribs may be

facilitated in a patient who has a dysfunctional breathing pattern and central lymph congestion. In such a case, the ribs need only be treated once to accomplish all three treatment goals, as the choice of technique is one that is consistent with accomplishing all three goals. Furthermore, the techniques described in each of the treatment areas that follow, may or may not be the proper choice for any particular patient, even if they have the same diagnosis. The choice of technique is based on the effect desired and the condition of the patient. Sometimes it is the combination of techniques in a particular sequence that best achieves the desired physiologic effects.

It is important to keep the treatment within the capabilities of the patient. It is often difficult, if not impossible to know what those capabilities are before initiating the treatment. It is also difficult to know in advance which techniques will be effective and well tolerated. Therefore, in the acutely ill patient, it is often best to apply a focused manipulative treatment, in a minimal effective time frame and then recheck later to see how the patient responds. At that time the type and dosage of treatment for that patient can be better formulated. A most effective way to consistently provide a safe and effective treatment is to monitor the effect of a chosen technique on the patient while it is being performed, sensing how the tissues are reacting to the technique, and modifying the technique, as indicated, as it is being applied. A common mistake of the inexperienced practitioner is to place all of their attention on the procedural aspects they are performing, and not sense the dynamic nature of the patient's tissue changes, occurring during the treatment process. By placing attention on the patient and their tissues as the treatment is performed, several things become possible. The technique and the forces involved may be continuously adjusted to the response of the tissue, making the treatment more effective. This is particularly useful in deciding between a direct and indirect method of treatment in a particular area. The initial impression may be to perform a direct method treatment, but, as the tissue barriers are engaged, the response of the tissue may suggest that an indirect approach should be performed instead.

If the initial impression suggests an indirect approach, but as the tissue is positioned into its point of freedom there is no palpatory sense that the tissues are responding to the treatment method, the operator may need to use a direct approach, or at least recheck the diagnosis and/or the original positioning of the patient. The choice between direct and indirect approaches is an important one; indirect approaches are, by their nature, gentler than direct approaches. Since the activating force for the treatment comes from within the patient, it is virtually impossible to give a treatment in excess of the tolerance of the tissue, or the patient as a whole. However, since they require internal forces to generate the therapeutic response, sometimes the sickest patients are unable to generate enough force to accomplish the desired effect from an indirect method and a direct method technique will be the more appropriate and effective one to use.

If the findings on structural examination do not initially suggest a physiologic treatment plan, treatment to arbitrarily reduce somatic dysfunction *should not be initiated*. It is far wiser to repeat the examination over the course of the illness, obtaining added clues as to the relation between the osteopathic findings and the pathophysiology of the disease process. It stands to reason that those somatic dysfunctions involved in the disease will change as the disease progresses, either improving or getting worse with the patient's condition. Once a better understanding of the relationship between the somatic dysfunction and disease process is achieved, a physiologic treatment plan to assist that patient's recovery from their disease will be apparent, and may be initiated.

Segmental Facilitation

A viscerosomatic reflex is produced when nociceptor input from inflamed viscera reaches a level great enough to produce facilitation of the interneurons of the spinal cord on which they converge. Spread of the impulses within the facilitated cord segment to involve the somatic neurons and the resulting muscle spasm produces a palpable, segmental somatic dysfunction, which, in turn, stimulates somatic nociceptors. This somatic nociceptive input converges on the same spinal cord segment and involves the interneurons of the original visceral input, creating a positive feedback loop which further increases the reflex output to segmentally related viscera and soma. The goal of osteopathic treatment is to remove the added somatic input, reduce the overall firing of the segmental interneurons, and remove the potentially devastating, self-perpetuating effects of a positive feedback loop. There is no definitive technique for reducing segmental facilitation; any procedure that normalizes the somatic tissues and reduces the nociceptive input will work. Treatment is based on the condition and responsiveness of the patient. However, several guidelines should be followed when designing a treatment program to reduce segmental facilitation. The remainder of this chapter presents these guidelines and presents manipulative treatment techniques that have been found useful in treating patients with acute segmental facilitation.

Nociception

Viscerosomatic and somatovisceral reflexes are initiated through pain-carrying fibers. Rapid movements at the vertebral unit, and of course painful maneuvers, have been shown to create a sympathetic motor outburst from the related and also distant facilitated spinal cord segments. Pain experienced at the segment will create further facilitation. Vigorous or painful procedures should be avoided when treating to reduce segmental facilitation, especially in acute situations.

Order of Treatment

Neurons in facilitated segments have a low threshold and often fire off, even to signals passing through the spinal cord from other regions. Treatment of the facilitated areas first will help prevent these segments from excessively firing impulses to their related viscera in response to treatment given in another region. Extremely reactive segments may actually require several treatments before other body areas can be effectively treated, although this is unusual. Gentle, deliberate procedures used throughout the entire treatment will minimize this effect.

Frequency of Treatment

Facilitated segments are often the result of acute visceral processes. The underlying disease will reproduce facilitation at the segments, often quite rapidly. Frequent treatment, even more than once

daily, is indicated. As the process improves, treatment frequency may be decreased.

Articular Tissues

Although the most obvious signs of acute segmental facilitation are found in the soft tissues, remember that treatment is directed to those tissues sending somatic nociceptive information back into the spinal cord. Muscle has a low concentration of nociceptors, whereas a joint capsule has the second highest, next to the skin. Treatment directed toward articular tissues may have a greater effect on the segmental facilitation than soft tissue techniques, such as myofascial releases or counterstrain. The techniques presented will all be directed toward the tension in articular segments.

Skeletal/Fascial Relations

Traditional focus has been on the areas immediately surrounding the sympathetic chain ganglia as these have an increased clinical importance in the treatment of segmental facilitation. Patriquin suggests an effect of respiratory motion on the functioning of the chain ganglia (4). Kuchera and Kuchera discuss the fascial relation of the ganglia with the rib head (25). Johnston also focuses on the costovertebral junction in his discussion of the diagnosis of viscerosomatic reflexes (7). Sutherland discusses the relationship between anterior vertebral ligamentous and fascial tension and autonomic function (32). Although the known physiology of reflex phenomena focus on the nociceptor input as the cause of segmental facilitation, and both somatic and visceral motor (via the chain ganglia) as the effects, one cannot deny the improved clinical response when the application of manipulative treatment is directed more specifically to the somatic dysfunctions and paraspinal fascial and ligamentous tissues in the anatomic location of the chain ganglia related to the patient's visceral dysfunction. The sacral plexus lies anterior to the sacrum. The lumbar chain ganglia lie anterior to the bodies of the lumbar vertebrae, medial to the edge of psoas. The thoracic chain ganglia lie anterior to the heads of the ribs. The cervical ganglia lie anterior to the cervical transverse processes.

SPECIFIC MANIPULATIVE TREATMENT TECHNIQUES

All of the techniques described here are direct method; they engage a restrictive barrier and involve the application of an activating force. They are especially applicable in the hospital patient, and may be used to produce a wide variety of physiologic effects. Force should always be introduced gradually, with attention to the patient and to the patient's response, and maintained at the level that matches or balances the resistance or tension felt in the tissues.

Indirect method techniques may also be used in the treatment of acute segmental facilitation, and should be considered especially in patients whose tissues are sensitive or reactive to the application of outside forces. Indirect technique, on the other hand, will not always work, because the acutely ill patient may not be able to generate the inherent forces necessary to affect a good response to the treatment process.

Paravertebral Ganglia Techniques

Direct Rib Release

Position

1. The patient is supine. The operator is seated at the side of the patient.
2. One hand of the physician identifies a single rib to be treated. The other hand extends under the patient to the spinous process and identifies the two segments with which a typical rib articulates. This is most easily done by gently springing the rib medially while monitoring at the spinous process.
3. Contact the two vertebrae at the spinous processes and simultaneously carry the rib and two vertebrae laterally. This will disengage the costovertebral articulation.

First Rib/Stellate Ganglion Technique

The stellate ganglia sit just anterior to the heads of the first ribs.

Position

1. The patient is supine. The operator is seated or standing at the head of the bed.
2. The physician contacts the posterior aspects of the first ribs at the angle with the thumbs of each hand.
3. The physician simultaneously applies gentle lateral traction to both ribs, gradually increasing until the traction force is equal to the resistance found in the tissues.
4. Traction is held at this level until release is felt.

Suboccipital Decompression

The superior cervical ganglion and vagus nerve are related to the occipital-atlantal and suboccipital tissues.

Position

1. The patient is supine. The operator seated at the head of the bed.
2. The physician places the fingerpads in the patient's suboccipital sulcus (groove) on both sides.
3. The physician carries their elbows medially, placing lateral traction on the suboccipital tissues.
4. The physician simultaneously places gentle traction on the occiput. The force of the physician's traction matches the resistance of the tissues.
5. This position is held until release of both sides is felt.

Lumbar Ganglia Technique

Position

1. The patient is supine with their arms crossed over the chest. The operator is seated at the side of the patient.
2. The physician makes a fist with the fingers of the cephalad hand, leaving the thumb extended.

3. The physician slides that hand under the patient's upper lumbar spine, fitting the lumbar spinous processes in the depression between the distal phalanges and the base of the hand.
4. The physician applies a gentle superior lift with the cephalad hand, the knuckles and base of the hand maintaining even pressure on the respective transverse processes.
5. With the caudad hand on the patient's elbows, the physician uses downward pressure into the bed (or treatment table) to closely control the lift of the fingers, balancing the lift to the resistance felt in the tissues.
6. This positioning is held until release is felt.

Sacral Plexus Techniques

Sacroiliac Decompression
Position

1. The patient is supine. The operator is seated at the side of the patient.
2. The physician contacts the medial aspect of the posterior superior iliac spine and associated medial ilium with the fingerpads of one or both hands.
3. The physician leans back, with the arms as straight as possible to create the traction with their shoulders and trunk, rather than with the forearms.
4. The physician's traction equally matches the resistance that is palpated.
5. The physician holds until yielding or release is felt.
6. This process is repeated on the other side.

Sacral Technique
Position

1. The patient is supine with the arms crossed over the chest. The operator is seated at the side of the patient.
2. The physician contacts the sacrum in the midline, with the caudad hand on the inferior lateral angle near the sacral apex and the cephalad hand on the sacral base above the level of S2. Alternately, the physician may use only one hand and spread the fingers so that some rest above and the others rest below the S2 sacral vertebra.
3. The physician's fingers, contacting the patient's sacrum, are gently lifted anteriorly. The physician's arms are resting on the bed or table top and the degree of lift is controlled by applying downward pressure on the elbows and upward pressure with the fingers.
4. This position of lift is held until a yielding or release is felt.

Collateral (Prevertebral) Ganglia Inhibition Techniques

Abdominal Ganglia Inhibition

The celiac and the superior mesenteric and inferior mesenteric ganglia may be treated by the same method, altering the hand position on the abdomen for the different ganglia. The celiac area is below the xiphoid, the inferior mesenteric just above the umbilicus, and the superior mesenteric halfway between.*

Position

1. The patient is supine. The operator stands at the side of the patient.
2. The physician's fingerpads of one or both hands are lined up along the patient's midabdominal line, contacting the skin over the collateral ganglion that is to be inhibited.*
3. The physician applies a gentle, downward pressure until the resistance of the underlying tissues is felt and its resistance is matched.
4. This pressure is held until a softening or release is felt.

Cervical Ganglia Inhibition

Although the cervical ganglia are situated more like the collateral (paravertebral) ganglia, the cervical ganglia function more like prevertebral ganglia, having their spinal origin in the thoracic spinal cord.

Position

1. The patient is supine. The operator is seated at the head of the bed or table.
2. The physician's fingerpads contact the articular pillars of the patient's cervical spine on both sides.
3. The physician gently lifts the finger contacts in an anterior and superior direction until articular (not soft tissue) resistance is perceived and matches the degree of lift.
4. This amount of lift is held until release is sensed.

Thoracic Region Techniques

The treatments described here are designed to increase thoracic compliance and excursion. Choice of method in clinical situations will depend primarily on the condition and tolerance of the patient. One will be confronted with patients limited to the supine position, such as the postoperative thoracotomy patient, and those limited to sitting, such as the patient with COPD. Adaptability in applying treatment techniques is a key to giving an effective treatment. Appropriate caution must always be exercised when working with acutely ill patients. Autonomic and lymphatic considerations should also be applied to the thorax. They are described elsewhere in the chapter.

Seated Techniques

In acute respiratory illness, the patient is sometimes unable to lie down for treatment. Seated techniques are particularly useful in these situations. All procedures described may be done very gently or more forcefully depending on the particulars of the case. Care must always be exercised when using force in an acutely ill hospitalized patient.

---

*This technique should not be attempted in the postoperative patient with a midline abdominal incision.

Translation of the Spine

Since the heads of ribs two through ten articulate with a vertebral unit, rather than a single vertebral segment, the motion of the thoracic spine is intimately involved with rib motion and thoracic compliance.

Position

1. The patient is seated. The operator stands at the left side of the patient.
2. The patient's left hand is placed on the right shoulder.
3. The physician places their left hand over the patient's hand and right shoulder while allowing the left axilla to rest lightly on the patient's left shoulder for patient control.
4. The physician's right palm is placed over the patient's left paravertebral tissues near the T10-12 region.
5. The physician simultaneously leans on the patient's left shoulder and places a right lateral translatory force on the spine via the left axillary and right hand contacts.
6. The physician moves the hand contact and the apex of the translation superiorly and the right lateral translatory force to the spine is repeated until the entire hemithorax is mobilized. A focused effort may be placed on the region with the greatest restriction.
7. The physician then moves to the patient's right side, positions of the patient's arms and the physician's arms and hands are reversed and the other side of the thorax is treated with translation to the left.

Note: This mobilization by spinal translation can also be carried into the lumbar region of the body.

Rotation and Rib Raising
Position

1. The patient is seated. The operator stands at the left side of the patient.
2. The patient's left hand is placed on the right shoulder.
3. The physician places their left hand over the patient's hand and right shoulder while allowing their left axilla to rest lightly on the patient's left shoulder for control of the patient.
4. The physician's right palm is placed over the patient's lower right rib cage with the thenar eminence in the area of the tenth rib angle.
5. The physician simultaneously produces a right anterolateral translatory force as the patient's body is rotated to the left.
6. The right hand contact with the patient's right rib angles is moved superiorly and the right anterolateral translatory force and left rotation of the spine is repeated until the entire hemithorax is mobilized. A focused effort may be placed on the region with the greatest restriction.
7. The physician then moves to the patient's right side, positions of the patient's arms and the physician's arms and hands are reversed and the left side of the thorax is treated in a similar manner.

Rib Raising

Position

1. The patient is seated with arms crossed in front of the chest. The operator stands facing the patient.
2. The patient's arms are supported on the physician's chest and the physician's hands reach around the patient to contact the patient's rib angles on both sides.
3. The physician leans so that gentle extension of the patient's thoracic spine occurs and simultaneously carries the contact with the patient's ribs, anteriorly and superiorly.
4. The physician's hand contacts with the patient's rib angles superiorly and/or inferiorly and the procedure is repeated until all of the patient's ribs have been raised. A focused effort may be placed on any region that that exhibits the greatest restriction.

Supine Techniques

Mobilizing the Ribs

This is rib raising coordinated with patient respiration. If the patient cannot lie completely flat, these procedures may be performed by elevating the head of the bed or emergency room stretcher to a more comfortable angle. These techniques are useful in the acute asthmatic patient, who reacts with further increased difficulty in breathing, even when very light pressure is applied to the rib cage. These techniques may be adapted to both pump and bucket handle motion. It is best to begin in the area of greatest rib restriction and continue up and/or down the entire thorax until all ribs are treated. By coordinating the procedure to the patient's respiratory rhythm, you can avoid any challenge to the patient's breathing. Used in this way, any of these treatment techniques will immediately lessen the patient's work of breathing, and can be used even in patients with the most acute respiratory problems.

Direct Method

Bucket Handle Ribs

This technique is most useful for lower rib restrictions.

Position

1. The patient is supine. The operator is at the side of the table, facing the patient.
2. The physician's fingerpads of the cephalad hand contacts rib angles posteriorly and the fingerpads of the caudad hand contact costochondral junction on the same side. The thumbs make a broad contact with rib shafts across midaxillary line.
3. The physician monitors the patient's breathing with light finger contact until the patient's breathing rhythm is familiar.
4. Then, as the patient begins to inhale, the physician's hands turn in the same direction, moving both thumbs cephalad, exaggerating the inhalation motion of the bucket handle-type ribs.
5. As the patient begins to exhale, the physician's hands also turn in the opposite direction to exaggerate the exhalation motion of these ribs.

Note: The entire hand and palm should be in contact with the rib cage to broaden surface area of contact.

Pump Handle Ribs

Position

1. The patient is supine. The operator is seated at side of the table, facing the patient.
2. The physician's fingerpads of the cephalad hand contacts a pump handle rib posteriorly at its rib angle.
3. The physician's caudad hand contacts the same rib anteriorly with its fingerpads across the rib's costochondral junction. The palm of this hand is lifted to avoid the breast of a female patient.
4. The physician monitors the patient's breathing with light finger contact until the rhythm of the patient's breathing is familiar.
5. As the patient begins inhalation, the physician's caudal fingerpad contacts move superiorly while the fingerpad contacts of the cephalad hand simultaneously move inferiorly to exaggerate the inhalation motion of the pump handle rib.
6. As the patient begins exhalation, there is reversal of the physician's hand movements to exaggerate the exhalation motion of the pump handle rib.

Indirect Method Treatment

Rib Raising

This method is described here for a single rib dysfunction, although it may be applied to a group of ribs.

Position

1. The patient is supine. The operator is at the side of the bed or table, facing the patient.
2. The fingerpads of the index and/or middle fingers of the physician's cephalad hand contact the restricted rib posteriorly across its angle.
3. The physician's index and/or middle fingers of the caudad hand contact the same rib anteriorly across the patient's costochondral junction.
4. The physician's thumb pads should contact the shaft of that rib at its midaxillary line for added control.
5. The patient's inhalation and exhalation is monitored as the physician gently encourages the rib to move in the direction of its freedom. This is carried to the point of ligamentous balance (point of greatest ease) and held there.
6. Adjustments in cephalad/caudad, anterior/posterior, and traction/compression may need to be carried out by passive motion testing and added to bring about the best balanced positioning of the rib.
7. Respiratory cooperation may be added by asking the patient to hold their breath in the direction associated with the greatest freedom.
8. The positioning is held in ligamentous balance until release is felt.

9. The rib motion is reevaluated during active inhalation and exhalation.

Sternal Mobilization

The mediastinal fascia is continuous with the fibrous pericardium of the heart and central tendon of the diaphragm. The fibrous pericardium of the heart is attached to the sternum via the superior and inferior sternopericardial ligaments. A sternal release may be used to mobilize this important fascial mechanism.

Position

1. The patient is supine. The operator is seated at the head of the table.

2. The physician's caudad hand contacts the sternum and manubrium and the palm of their cephalad hand is placed posteriorly across the patient's spinous processes, approximately in the Tl-6 region.

3. The physician's sternal contact moves the patient's sternum through its six motions—superior, inferior, lateral to the right, lateral to the left, clockwise rotation, and counterclockwise rotation—determining its directions of restriction in motion.

4. The hand of the physician's spinal contact will always be moved in the direction that is opposite to the sternal restrictions.

5. As the patient continues to breathe normally, each sternal preference is held at its motion barrier until release occurs. Rather than doing each motion separately, the sternal restrictions can be taken to their restrictive barrier and each "stacked upon the other" and the composite held until release occurs.

Note: This can also be performed as an indirect method technique. To do this, the sternal motions are stacked, or each is separately carried to the point of ligamentous balance and held at that balance while intrinsic forces release the dysfunction. Respiratory force can be added to hasten release by having the patient hold their breath in the phase that produces the most ligamentous relaxation.

Abdominal Treatment Techniques

The abdomen follows the principle that the shape of a container will affect the function of its contents. The abdomen has a roof, a floor, and anterior and posterior walls. The diaphragm is the roof of the abdomen; the liver, spleen, and supporting mesenteries are suspended from it. The pelvic diaphragm is the floor. It supports the abdominal and pelvic viscera, along with the shelf created as the posterior abdominal wall crosses the pelvic brim. The iliopsoas and quadratus lumborum make up the posterior abdominal wall. The insertion of iliopsoas on the lesser trochanter of the femur involves the hip in abdominal and pelvic function. The aforementioned structures are usually treated before directly treating viscera. The autonomic relationships and lymphatic drainage of the abdomen and pelvis should also be considered.

Direct Hip Release

Position

1. The patient is supine. The operator is at the side of the table on the side of the leg to be treated.

2. The physician's cephalad hand contacts the patient's hip behind the greater trochanter for monitoring.

3. The physician's caudad hand holds the leg so it can be maneuvered.

4. The physician's caudad hand induces abduction/adduction and internal/external rotation to find the point of balanced tension of the hip joint.

5. While monitoring with the cephalad hand, the physician's caudad hand places the patient's ankle into the axilla to control the patient's leg position. The caudad hand then moves up to or above the knee to create a fulcrum.

6. The distal part of the patient's extremity is taken medially to create lateral traction at the femoral head and held in that position.

7. When lateral release is felt, the physician applies inferior traction on the patient's leg and holds that until another release is felt.

Pelvic Diaphragm Release

Position (Fig. 71.6)

1. The patient is in the lateral recumbent position with the legs and knees flexed. The operator stands behind patient. This may also be done with the patient in the supine position with the operator standing by the patient on the side that is to be treated. *The operator should explain the procedure to the patient and that a contact will be made near an intimate area before proceeding.*

2. The extended fingers of the physician's caudad hand contact the ischial tuberosity of the patient on the side up off the table. The fingers are then moved at a point that is just medial and slightly caudad to the tuberosity; the fingerpads may stay in contact with the medial aspect of the tuberosity.

3. The physician's fingertips and rigid fingers are then gently but firmly advanced, medial to the sacrotuberous ligaments, into the ischiorectal fossa until the resistance of the pelvic diaphragm (on that side) is initially palpated.

4. At that point the excursion of the pelvic diaphragm is monitored during the patient's respiratory efforts.

5. Then the fingers are held at the point of tissue tension (*not lifted to produce more tension*). They simply resist the downward movement of the pelvic diaphragm that occurs as the patient inhales slowly and deeply.

6. The physician's fingers follow the pelvic diaphragmatic tension cephalad as the patient exhales slowly and completely.

7. Steps 5 and 6 are repeated until the maximal amount of diaphragmatic lift (muscular tension release) has occurred.

8. The patient is turned to the opposite lateral recumbent position. With the physician behind the patient, the other half of the pelvic diaphragm is released in a similar manner.

Posterior Abdominal Diaphragmatic Releases

Releasing the Lumbar Spine/Crura
Position
1. The patient is supine and the operator is at the side of the table facing the patient.
2. The physician evaluates T12 to L3 for somatic dysfunction or increased paraspinal tissue tension.
3. The physician then contacts the spinous processes on either side of the vertebral unit that has somatic dysfunction.
4. The vertebral unit is moved in directions that exaggerate its freedom of motion–flexion/extension, rotation, and right or left side bending.
5. These directions of freedom may be individually held at their point of ligamentous balance or each direction of motion preference might be stacked, one-upon-the other, and released.
6. Release occurs as the tissues are held at their point of ligamentous balance.
7. Respiratory effort of the patient may be added to hasten the release. This is performed by asking the patient to hold their breath in the respiratory cycle that is sensed to be accompanied by the greatest relaxation of the tissues.

Releasing the 12th Ribs/Arcuate Ligaments
Position
1. The patient is supine. The operator is at the side of the patient to be treated.
2. The physician contacts the patient's 12th rib near mid-shaft. *Note:* Doubling the finger contact may provide better control. Remember, the 12th rib does not have a rib angle.
3. The physician applies traction to the 12th rib in a direction between horizontal and the direction of the long axis of the 12th rib; settle on the composite direction that maximizes the perception of "tension in the lumbocostal arches," matching the traction force with resistance found in the tissues.
4. The rib is held in this position of traction until release is felt. This may occur as a change in the long axis of the rib rather than just a simple decompression.
5. The physician walks to the other side of the patient and the technique is repeated for the other 12th rib.

Anterolateral Abdominal Diaphragm Releases
Position
1. The patient is seated. The operator stands behind patient.
2. The physician reaches around the patient and contacts the soft tissues just below the costal margin (chondral masses) with the fingerpads of both hands.
3. The patient is asked to slouch as the physician supports the patient's back with their chest. This allows the physician's fingers to advance medially and superiorly around the costal margin.
4. The excursion of the abdominal diaphragm during respiration is monitored.
5. The physician's finger placements gently resist the downward motion of the diaphragm as the patient inhales and follows the diaphragm superiorly as the patient exhales. Note: *Do not push upward against the diaphragm.*
6. Step 5 is repeated, as the patient continues to take slow, deep breaths, until a release is felt.
7. The fingers of the physician's hands are then moved medially or laterally until the entire anterolateral surface of the diaphragm has been treated.

Abdominal Lifts

Abdominal lifts provide a safe, simple means of addressing ptosis and congestion of the abdominal viscera and its mesenteries. More specific treatment techniques for the viscera should not be attempted until palpatory skill and anatomic familiarity of the abdomen has been studied and achieved.

Position
1. The patient is supine with the knees bent to 90 degrees and the feet are flat on the table. The physician stands at the side of the patient that is to be treated.
2. The physician contacts the lower left quadrant of the abdomen just superior to the inguinal ligament and gently inserts the fingerpads into the patient's abdomen.
3. The physician then gently lifts the patient's abdominal contents obliquely toward the right upper quadrant until slight tension is palpable.
4. The tissues are then held in this position until a release is felt and the contents can be moved slightly further toward the patient's right upper quadrant. *Note:* The physician should be attentive so that the lift occurs to the internal organs and that they are not just lifting the anterior abdominal wall.
5. Steps 3 and 4 are repeated until the patient's maximal release has been accomplished.
6. For the right lower quadrant, repeat steps 1–5, lifting vertically towards the *right* upper quadrant.

Note: A minor vibration may be transmitted to the abdomen by the physician's finger contacts and be substituted for the lift. Also, respiratory force may accentuate and hasten the release of a lift. Respiratory force is instituted by asking the patient to take a partial breath in and hold it until they have to breathe. Just as the patient has to take the breath, the physician will notice a release of the tissues.

Lymph Mobilization

Stimulating the Movement of Lymph

Osteopathic treatment to enhance lymph flow is described elsewhere in this text. In this chapter, the concept of interstitial fluid fluctuation was introduced in relation to lymph formation and flow. Techniques to stimulate the formation of lymph using this principle were taught by Anne Wales, DO, and will be presented here as an addition to those presented in Chapter 70. The respiratory mechanism, as well as any areas of restriction along the course of drainage should be treated before stimulating the formation and movement of lymph.

Osteopathic treatment designed to stimulate formation and movement of lymph is based on an understanding of the physiology and mechanics of lymph formation and propulsion. A limiting factor in lymphatic drainage is the movement of fluid from the interstitium into the initial lymphatic vessels. This is the formation of lymph. There are no inherent hydrostatic or osmotic gradients to drive this process. Fluid fluctuation and rhythmic movement in the immediate environment of the initial lymphatic vessels forms lymph. These actions form the physiologic basis for most of the following lymphatic techniques. Successful treatment depends upon creating a rhythmic fluctuation of extracellular fluid. This movement of fluid can be palpated and monitored from the hand contact on the patient, and must be differentiated from the tissue movements monitored during treatment on the musculoskeletal tissues. The movement of the body's fluids in response to the treatment is the key.

Propulsion of lymph is dependent on several factors. Stretch receptors located in the distal end of lymphatic vessels, responsive to the formation of lymph, begins the peristaltic contraction of smooth muscle in the wall of the lymph vessels. The thin and pliable lymphatic vessels are also responsive to external pressures, such as skeletal muscle contraction in muscle adjacent to the vessel. The relative importance of these factors differs in different areas.

Lateral Fluctuation at the Knee

Position

1. The patient is supine. The physician stands at the side of the patient to be treated.
2. The physician flexes the patient's knee to 90 degrees and the hip to 45 degrees; the patient's foot is resting flat on the table.
3. The physician's caudad hand gently holds the dorsum of the patient's foot and ankle.
4. The physician's cephalad hand rests on top of the patient's knee.
5. The physician gently moves the patient's leg medially and laterally at the knee to find the position of greatest ease.
6. At that point of ligamentous balance, a small medial, lateral excursion is initiated and maintained.

Lateral Fluctuation at the Forearm

Position

1. The patient is seated. The physician sits facing the patient.
2. The physician grasps the hand of the patient on the affected side as if to make a handshake.
3. The physician's other hand supports the patient's elbow, keeping it at 90 degrees.
4. The patient's forearm is supinated and pronated to find the point of greatest ease.
5. From this point of ligamentous balance, a gentle, rhythmic pronation/supination excursion is initiated to fluctuate fluid

Abdominal Lymph Stimulation

The abdominal lymphatics reside in the mesenteries of the abdomen. Dr. W.G. Sutherland described the use of a transmitted

vibration to stimulate the movement of abdominal and thoracic lymph. The effect of the vibration is to produce a wave like that produced by a pebble landing in the center of a pond. The transmitted vibration to the abdomen will also act to lift the mesenteries in a very gentle manner. This can be useful in acute situations, such as the immediate postoperative period. These specific techniques were demonstrated by Dr. Wales and are based on this concept.

Position

1. The patient is supine with knees bent to relax the abdominal wall. The physician stands at the right side of the patient.
2. Physician contacts the patient's left lower abdomen just superior to the inguinal ligament, placing one hand over the other.
3. The tissues are gently lifted superomedially until the first sense of resistance is palpable.
4. A transmitted vibration is directed toward the cisterna chyle–a point that would be approximately posterior to halfway between the xiphoid process and the umbilicus, slightly to the right of center. This point will be approximately perpendicular to the suspension of the mesentery of the descending colon.
5. A palpatory sense of decongestion or lift of the mesenteries indicates successful treatment.
6. The physician walks to the left side of the patient and contacts the right lower abdomen in the same manner and steps 3 through 5 are repeated for the right side of the patient.

Thoracic Duct Technique

Dr. Sutherland likened the thoracic duct to a siphon, indicating a functional significance to the turn located at its superior end, that allows it to drain downward into the superior aspect of the subclavian vein. The thoracic duct may be stimulated with a transmitted vibration at its proximal and distal ends.

Position

1. The patient is supine and the physician stands at the right side of the patient.
2. The physician contacts the patient's abdomen just below the costal margin and to the right of center, in the area overlying the cisterna chyle. Use the contact of one-hand-over-the-other-hand.
3. The physician induces a transmitted vibration directed toward the cisterna chyle.
4. Then the physician contacts the left axilla at the second or third intercostal space, near the midclavicular line, using the one-hand-over-the-other-hand contact.
5. The physician transmits a vibration of tissues directed posteriorly and slightly laterally.
6. A perceived change in the quality of the deep tissues or a sense of decongestion may become apparent as the treatment proceeds.

CONCLUSION

The osteopathic treatment of the acutely ill hospitalized patient is designed to support and enhance the underlying physiology of a patient as they recover from an illness or other severe stress. Care must be taken to insure that the treatment is appropriate and within the physical capabilities of the patient to respond appropriately. Specialist level intervention may be indicated in unusual and challenging cases, but many cases can be treated effectively by osteopathic physicians, residents, and students if the principles described in this chapter are followed. The structural examination findings, along with knowledge of the pathophysiology of the disease process and individual patient's condition, are combined to form a unique treatment plan for each patient, at each visit.

ACKNOWLEDGMENT

Special thanks to the guidance, hard work, valuable suggestions, and drawings from William Kuchera, DO, FAAO. This chapter is better because of his efforts.

REFERENCES

1. Korr IM, et al. Effects of experimental myofascial insults on cutaneous patterns of sympathetic activity in man. *J Transmission.* 1962;23(22):330–355.
2. Nicholas A, et al. A somatic component of acute spontaneous myocardial infarction. *JAOA.* 1983;83(68).
3. Denslow JS, Korr I, et al. Quantitative studies of chronic facilitation in human motoneuron pools. *Am J Physiol.* 1947;150:229–238.
4. Patriquin DA. Viscerosomatic reflexes. In: Patterson MM, Howell JN, eds. *The Central Connection: Somatovisceral and Viscerosomatic Interaction.* Athens, OH: University Classics, Ltd; 1992.
5. Beal MC, Morlock JS. Somatic dysfunction associated with pulmonary disease. *JAOA.* 1984;82:179–183.
6. Beal MC. Palpatory testing for somatic dysfunction in patients with cardiovascular disease. *JAOA.* 1983;82:822–831.
7. Johnston WL. Segmental definition: III. Definitive basis for distinguishing somatic findings of visceral reflex origin. *JAOA.* 1988;88:347–353.
8. Beal MC. Viscerosomatic reflexes: a review. *JAOA.* 85(12):53–68.
9. Cathie A. Physiological motions of the spine as related to respiratory activity. In: *AAO Yearbook.* American Academy of Osteopathy; 1974:59–60.
10. Zink JG. Applications of the osteopathic holistic approach to homeostasis. In: *AOA Yearbook.* American Academy of Osteopathy; 1973:37–47.
11. Still AT. *The Philosophy and Mechanical Principles of Osteopathy.* Kansas City, MO: Hudson-Kimberly Publishing Co; 1902:155.
12. Rabinovici N, et al. The Relationship between respiration, pressure and flow distribution in the vena cava and portal and hepatic veins. *Surg Gynecol Obstet.* 1980;151:753–763.
13. Millard FP. *Applied Anatomy of the Lymphatics.* Kirksville, MO: The Journal Printing Co; 1922:26.
14. Sutherland WG. *Teaching in the Science of Osteopathy.* Portland, OR: Rudra Press; 1990.
15. Hurley JV. Inflammation. In: Staub NC, Taylor AE, eds. *Edema.* New York, NY: Raven Press; 1984:463–488.
16. Atkinson TP. Histamine and serotonin. In: Gallin JI, et al, eds. *Inflammation: Basic Principles and Clinical Correlates.* New York, NY: Raven Press; 1992:196.
17. Movat HZ. *The Inflammatory Reaction.* New York, NY: Elsevier; 1985.
18. Olszewski WL, et al. Lymph drainage from foot joints in rheumatoid arthritis provides insight into local cytokine and chemokine production and transport to lymph nodes. *Arthritis Rheum.* 2001;44(3):541–549.
19. Witte CL, Witte MH. Lymphatics in the pathophysiology of edema. In Johnston MG, ed. *Experimental Biology of the Lymphatic Circulation.* New York, NY: Elsevier; 1985:167–188.
20. Van Buskirk R. Nociceptive reflexes and somatic dysfunction: a model *JAOA.* 1990;90(9):792–809.
21. Schmidt RF. Neurophysiologic mechanisms of arthritic pain. In: Patterson MM, Howell JN, eds. *The Central Connection: Somatovisceral and Viscerosomatic Interaction.* Athens, OH: University Classics, Ltd; 1992.
22. Talman WT. The central nervous system and cardiovascular control in health and disease. In: Low PA, ed. *Clinical Autonomic Disorders.* Boston, MA: Little, Brown and Company; 1993.
23. Korr IM. Sustained sympathicotonia as a factor in disease. In: *The Neurobiologic Mechanisms in Manipulative Therapy.* New York, NY: Plenum Publishing Co; 1978:229–268.
24. Fu QG, et al. Vagal afferent fibers excite upper cervical neurons and inhibit activity of lumbar spinal cord neurons in the rat. *Pain.* 1992;51(1):91–100.
25. Kuchera M, Kuchera W. *Osteopathic Considerations in Systemic Dysfunction,* rev. 2nd ed. Columbus, OH: Greyden Press; 1994.
26. Rosero HO, et al. Correlation of palpatory observations with the anatomical locus of acute myocardial infarction. *JAOA.* 1987;87:118–129.
27. Wilson P. The osteopathic treatment of asthma. *JAOA.* 1946;45(11):491–492.
28. Degowin, Degowin. *Bedside Diagnostic Exam,* 5th ed. New York, NY: Macmillan; 1987.
29. Geisler GJ. Studies of spinal cord neurons that project directly to the hypothalamus. In: Willard FH, Patterson MM, eds. *Nociception and the Neuroendocrine Immune Connection.* Athens, OH: University Classics, Ltd; 1994.
30. Dinarello CA. Role of interleukin-1 and tumor necrosis factor in systemic responses to infection and inflammation. In: Gallin JI, et al: *Inflammation: Basic Principles and Clinical Correlates,* 2nd ed. New York, NY: Raven Press; 1992.
31. Williams PL, ed. *Gray's Anatomy,* 38th ed. London, England: Churchill-Livingstone; 1995:1883.
32. Sutherland WG. *Contributions of Thought,* 2nd ed. Portland, OR: Rudra Press; 1998:339.
33. West JB. *Pulmonary Pathophysiology: The Essentials,* 4th ed. Baltimore, MD: Williams & Wilkins; 1992:74.
34. West JB. *Respiratory Physiology: The Essentials,* 5th ed. Baltimore, MD: Williams & Wilkins; 1995.
35. Roussos C, Macklem PT. Inspiratory muscle fatigue. In: *Handbook of Physiology, Section III,* The Respiratory System, Vol III. The Mechanics of Breathing, Part II. Bethesda, MD: American Physiological Society; 1986:521.
36. Grassino A, et al. Respiratory muscle fatigue and ventilatory failure. *Ann Rev Med.* 1984;35:625–647.
37. Cohen C, et al. Clinical manifestations of inspiratory muscle fatigue. *Am J Med.* 1982;73:308–316.
38. West JB, ed. *Best and Taylor's Physiologic Basis of Medical Practice,* 12th ed. Baltimore. MD: Williams & Wilkins; 1991:95–96.
39. Aukland K, Reed RK. Interstitial mechanisms in the control of extracellular fluid volume. *Physiol Rev.* 1993;73:1.
40. Browse NL, et al. Pressure waves and gradients in the canine thoracic duct. *J Physiol.* 1971;237:401–413.
41. Dumont AE. The flow capacity of the thoracic duct-venous junction. *Am J Med Sci.* 1975;269(3):292–301.
42. Still AT. *Philosophy of Osteopathy.* Published by the author; Kirksville, MO: 1899:36.
43. Simonneau G, et al. Diaphragm dysfunction induced by upper abdominal surgery. *Am Rev Respir Dis.* 1983;128:899–903.
44. Drake RE, Gabel JC. Diaphragmatic lymph vessel drainage of the peritoneal cavity. *Blood Purif.* 1992;10:132–135.
45. Schmid-Schonbein GW. Microlymphatics and lymph flow. *Physiol Rev.* 1990;70(4):987–1026.
46. Sutherland WG. *Contributions of Thought,* 2nd edition. Portland, OR: Rudra Press, 1998:34–35.

EFFICACY AND COMPLICATIONS

MICHAEL L. KUCHERA
EILEEN L. DIGIOVANNA
PHILIP E. GREENMAN

KEY CONCEPTS

- Current state of research on efficacy of osteopathic manipulation, and problems in current studies
- Difficulties of research trials studying effectiveness of osteopathic manipulation on low back pain, and success rates
- Effectiveness of manipulation for patients with systemic disease
- Osteopathic practice guidelines and difficulties for osteopathic physicians trying to follow existing written guidelines
- Difference between symptom exacerbation and true complication
- Incidence of complications, difference between physician-related and patient-related complications, and best ways to avoid complications
- Cervical spine manipulation as source of most serious manipulation complications
- Difficulty in listing absolute contraindications to osteopathic manipulation
- Complications most likely to result from high velocity/low amplitude manipulation
- Discomfort or complications associated with muscle energy, counterstrain, and craniosacral treatments

Manipulation has enjoyed wide usage for many centuries of medical practice in most cultures. In most cases, it has been applied empirically, based on clinical observations. As with many forms of medical treatment, ongoing clinical successes have contributed to its continuous and expanding use.

Osteopathic manipulation uses palpatory diagnosis and manual treatment methods as integrated components of a patient encounter. This modality is an important element of an osteopathic approach to total patient care. Osteopathic manipulation is prescribed not only as care for a variety of musculoskeletal and systemic pathophysiologic problems but also as part of general health maintenance and enhancement strategies. It is directed toward optimizing structure-function relationships and assist-ing the patient's homeostatic mechanisms. Its processes help to strengthen physician–patient relationships, allowing better diagnostic insights and treatment for all aspects of human problems.

Osteopathic manipulative techniques are among the safest medical treatments a physician can provide. Whenever manipulative treatment is carried out, however, certain risks are present, along with potential side effects ranging from mild to severe, including death, when particularly aggressive maneuvers are used. Such risks also occur with pharmaceutical, surgical, and a variety of other mechanical treatments.

Even though osteopathic manipulation has a very low risk-to-benefit ratio, it is necessary that the operator be aware of inherent risks and avoid untoward occurrences while weighing anticipated benefits against the risk of treating or not treating.

EFFICACY OF MANIPULATION

Despite years of successful use of osteopathic and other forms of manipulation, components of the orthodox medical community continued to be critical of its use, often referring to its practitioners as cultists. The reasons are both cultural and scientific. The latter problem arises because of a lack of adequate scientific methods to explore not only clinical efficacy but also basic mechanisms. Researchers with a directed osteopathic focus, such as Louisa Burns, DO; Irvin M. Korr, PhD; J. Stedman Denslow, DO; and Wilbur V. Cole, DO, have been few. Clinically, when osteopathic models were originally proposed, double-blind research methods were yet to emerge. When they were developed, they were more readily applied to pharmacologic and surgical practices. More ambiguously defined clinical processes, such as osteopathic manipulation, remain difficult to evaluate. Progress is occurring, however.

In 1975, the first of several international seminars brought together a group of international basic scientists and clinicians to examine the scientific basis for the use of manipulation (1). The National Institute of Communicative Diseases and Stroke held this conference in Bethesda, Maryland. Attendees were drawn from the osteopathic, allopathic, and chiropractic professions. The goal was to define the current state of research and identify areas for future study; several areas of agreement were reached.

With the exception of the AOA/Rush-Anchor HMO protocol, other large-scale prospective research protocols have not accurately integrated the total patient approach characteristic of osteopathically oriented manipulative interventions. Conversely, the Tillinghast statewide studies of Workmen's Compensation outcomes (26) report the costs associated with total patient approach as delivered by practitioners including osteopathic physicians, allopathic physicians, allopathic surgeons, physical therapists, and chiropractors. However, these do not delineate the extent to which each group may have incorporated a manipulative or mobilization technique. In these latter studies, the osteopathic management of cases in each region studied was reported to be more cost-effective than that delivered by any other group.

Systemic Disease

Controlled trials for manipulation in conditions other than low back and cervical pain are few. Most studies represent pilot observations by experienced osteopathic clinicians. Fitzgerald and Stiles (19) reports reduction in hospital length of stay when osteopathic manipulative care was used for patients with the following:

Asthma:	14%
Pneumonia:	10%
Cholecystectomy:	7%
Hysterectomy:	12%

Fitzgerald and Stiles also reports a reduction in shock, dysrhythmias, and mortality when osteopathically oriented manipulative care was integrated into the care of a group of patients with myocardial infarction (Fig. 72.1). More recently, Cantieri (27) reports on a survey of the use of OMT in 18 osteopathic hospitals. In those diagnosis related groups with documentation of more than 10 patients receiving OMT, a decreased length of stay of one day or more was noted in a number of systemic conditions including:

Noncancerous pancreatic disorders
Psychosis
Upper gastrointestinal procedures
Intestinal obstructions
Transient ischemic attacks
Cardiovascular disorders in acute myocardial infarction patients discharged alive

Complex cardiovascular disorders undergoing cardiac catheterization

There are a greater number of studies in the osteopathic literature documenting the incidence of somatic dysfunction findings in certain systemic diseases. Kelso (28) reports on a double-blind clinical study of osteopathic findings in hospital patients. Student examiners were compared with experienced osteopathic clinicians. In 5,174 separate examinations, somatic findings were significantly more frequent in acute visceral disease than in controls.

Nicholas (29) reports a pilot study that examined 286 hospitalized patients with 73 different diseases. Again, a variety of identifiable somatic patterns were found with different disease entities. The study focused on somatically identified cervical and thoracic spine pattern differences associated with respiratory, gastrointestinal, and genitourinary diseases.

Other osteopathically based observational studies assessed somatic correlations with gastrointestinal diseases. Their findings closely mirror pain pattern discoveries recorded by surgeons at the Mayo Clinic (30).

Several well-controlled studies have identified common somatic dysfunction patterns in patients with coronary artery disease and myocardial infarction (31,32). Somatic findings are primarily located in the left upper thoracic area (Fig. 72.2). Evidence of upper cervical (C2) dysfunction was also found in patients with

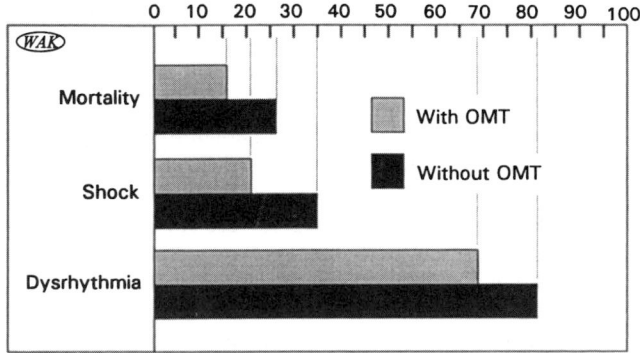

FIGURE 72.1. Response of 50 patients with myocardial infarction. (Adapted from work by Ed Stiles, DO.)

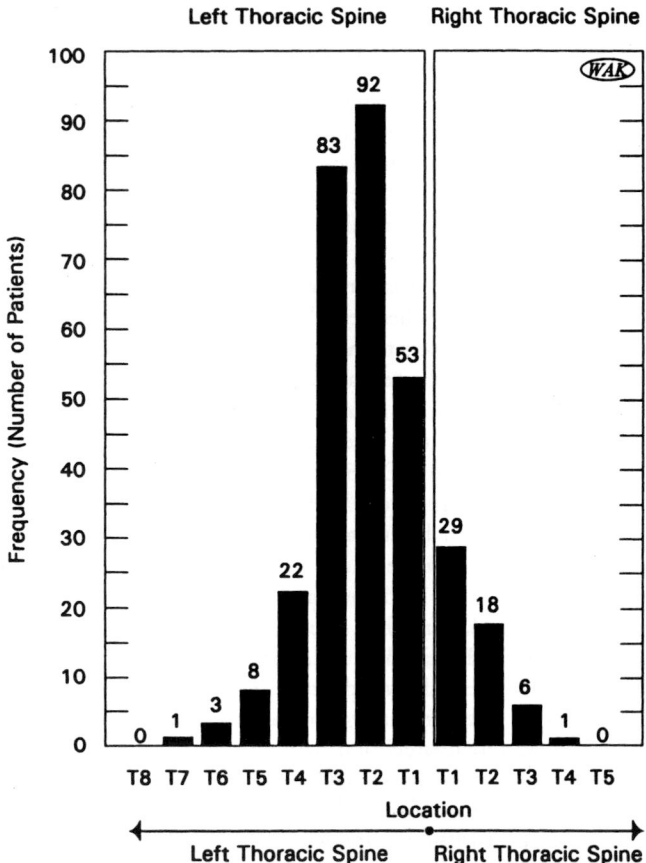

FIGURE 72.2. Location and incidence of thoracic somatic dysfunction in 94 cardiac patients. (From Kuchera ML, Kuchera WA. *Osteopathic Considerations in Systemic Function*, rev. 2nd ed. Columbus, OH: Greyden Press; 1994, with permission.)

certain acute visceral diseases. It is hypothesized that these findings correlate with the anatomy of the proximal vagus nerve in relation to the second cervical vertebra.

Beal and Kleiber evaluated 70 patients prior to angiography. Specificity for both positive and negative cervicothoracic palpatory findings in patients with and without coronary artery diseases was 79% (33).

Many other authors have reported on the efficacy of manipulation in managing coronary heart disease, but no controlled studies have been performed (34,38). Nevertheless, these authors have identified similar clinical findings and results associated with the addition of manipulative treatment to an overall management plan.

Similar studies have been done for spinal levels of somatic findings associated with pulmonary diseases (39,40). Authors report a strong dominance of problems located in the upper thoracic and C2 region of the spine. Many of these authors report beneficial outcomes associated with osteopathic manipulative treatment (OMT).

Howell and associates (41) reported on the efficacy of OMT in 17 patients who showed improvement in the severity score over a 1-year time frame. Miller (42) reported on a study of 23 patients with chronic obstructive lung disease randomly assigned to a treatment or control group. With the exception of OMT, the treatment received by all patients was the same. Although there was a small change in the mean vital capacity of the treated versus the untreated group, this parameter was not considered statistically significant. What did prove to be clinically significant was a clear improvement in functional capacity of the treated group with reduction of cough, increased walking capacity, less dyspnea, and fewer respiratory tract infections.

Numerous other observational studies and pilot projects suggest the value of continuing use of manipulative treatment to enhance self-healing mechanisms in patients with systemic illnesses. For example, two pilot studies suggest that preoperative and postoperative OMT reduce the incidence of atelectasis (43) and ileus, respectively (44). In subsequent randomized, researcher-blinded trials, Sleszynski and Kelso (45) demonstrated similar outcomes using thoracic lymphatic pump OMT compared to using incentive spirometry in prevention of postcholecystectomy atelectasis. Study patients developing atelectasis had earlier recoveries and were quicker return to preoperative forced vital capacity and forced expiratory volume in 1 second values than the incentive spirometry groups. Radjieski and Lumley (46) demonstrated significant length of stay reduction when OMT was added to in a randomized, controlled study to the care of hospitalized patients with pancreatitis (mean reduction, 3.5 days). In another randomized, controlled study, Noll (47) demonstrated that the addition of OMT resulted in shorter length of stay and shorter duration of intravenous antibiotic use in geriatric hospitalized patients with pneumonia.

Some reports suggest that OMT can be effective in decreasing blood pressure and aldosterone levels in hypertensive patients (48–50). Other OMT research reports suggest that fibromyalgia-related tender points can be decreased, with improved quality of life measures (51–53).

The value of OMT as part of health promotion in preventive practices is noted by osteopathic pediatricians and may extend to opportunities to enhance the efficacy of certain immunizations. In respect to the latter, Jackson and co-workers (54) documented data to support enhanced immunologic response in subjects who received lymphatic and splenic pump OMT. Measel had also documented this in earlier studies (55).

The value of promoting health through prevention of degenerative change and maximizing function through reduction of biomechanical risk factors is more fully discussed in Chapter XX.

Simons and Travell document (56) improved visceral functions when related somatic components are corrected with manipulative treatment and other manual neuromuscular release techniques. Problems that improved include:

Supraventricular tachyarrhythmia
Gastrointestinal functioning
Reduced recurrences of peptic ulcer disease

Korr, drawing from his and others' published research, has hypothesized about neurophysiologic factors, such as segmental facilitation and sympathetic nervous system factors that contribute to these phenomena (57).

COMPLICATIONS AND CONTRAINDICATIONS

Although manual treatment methods have been used for centuries, little has been recorded regarding morbidity and mortality arising from their use. The earliest documentations were recorded as case histories in various journals.

Complications associated with various procedures have been reported only recently. Most center on impulsed thrust manipulations and focus on isolated case reports of manipulation of the upper cervical spine. Greater interest in the gathering of data regarding these problems began in the 1980s. Attempts were made to identify the actual incidence, nature, and causes of the injuries.

Any discussion of complications must make a clear distinction between symptom exacerbation and true complication. Even though uncomfortable, symptom exacerbations following manipulative treatments are often normal, temporary outcomes of the treatment process. This is particularly true following changes associated with long-term, chronic tissue texture abnormalities and a resulting short-term acute inflammatory response.

True complications are those that worsen the patient's pathologic condition or result in development of new injury or disorder as a direct result of the manipulative treatment.

When describing manipulative treatment contraindications, one must also differentiate between absolute and relative factors. There are few absolute contraindications, but many are relative. If the condition being treated risks worsening when activating forces of a particular technique are apt to create harm, it constitutes a relative contraindication. Other manipulative techniques that use different activating forces may however be appropriate and useful.

Incidence

A true incidence of complications is difficult to identify. Most studies arrive at similar conclusions: major, serious, or significant complications range from 1 in 400,000 to 1 in 1 million (Table 72.1) (58–69).

TABLE 72.1. POSSIBLE SERIOUS CONSEQUENCES OF MANIPULATION REPORTED IN THE WORLD LITERATURE[a]

Sequelae	Preexisting Condition	Incidence
Vertebrobasilar artery sequelae Locked-in syndrome Wallenberg syndrome Vertigo/dizziness/posterior headache Aneurysm/dissection subintimal tears Intraluminal clot Transischemic attack/stroke Death	Unilateral atresia of vertebral artery Prior neck trauma including prior traumatic cervical manipulation	1:400,000 to 1:1,000,000

Cervical cord compression	Agenesis of odontoid process
	Odontoideum
	Down syndrome with:
	    agenesis of transverse axial ligament
	    odontoid developmental variation
	Ligamentous laxity in:
	    severe rheumatoid arthritis
	    other rheumatologic disorders
	Posterior osteophytes
		1:1,000,000

Exacerbation of disc disease[41,42] sequestration and acute radiculopathy	Disc disease	Rare
Thrombosis anterior spinal artery		Very rare
Dissecting hematoma of internal carotid[43]		Very rare
Paralysis of diaphragm[44]		Very rare
Hearing loss		Very rare
Horner syndrome[45]		Very rare
Herniation of thoracic disc[46]		Very rare
Rib fracture	Osteoporosis/metastasis	1:1,000,000
Spinal meningeal hematoma[47]	Concurrent anticoagulation	Very rare
Thoracic spine fracture/discitis	Alcoholic patient	Very rare
Cauda equina syndrome[48–52]	Disc herniation	1:1,000,000

[a]In a survey of the literature, only approximately 5% of these rare sequelae have occurred as a result of osteopathic physicians using osteopathic manipulative techniques.

Dvorak and Orelli (70) surveyed members of the Swiss Manual Medicine Society in 1981. The survey reports a serious incidence of 1 in 400,000 procedures, most of which were mobilization with impulse (HVLA) with considerable accompanying rotation. Of 1,408 reported complications, 1,255 were associated with cervical procedures. Most were minor complications, such as vertigo. More serious complications included 10 patients with altered consciousness, 12 with loss of consciousness for as long as 5 minutes, and 11 with an undefined neurologic disturbance. Four underwent surgery. The Swiss survey reports less frequent complications relating to the lumbar spine, with most complaints related to an increase in subjective pain.

Although the Swiss survey did not involve U.S. osteopathic techniques, it was among one of the first careful reports on manipulative treatment-related morbidity. It also highlights the low risk involved with these procedures. In addition, in a 1991 lecture to students at the MSU College of Osteopathic Medicine, Dvorak reported a zero incidence of manipulative treatment complications throughout the 1980s when cervical manipulations were modified to principally use muscle energy/postisometric relaxation (MET) procedures.

Patijn (71) identified 93 papers yielding 129 cases of significant manipulation-related complications. He notes that of the reports:

67% (85 cases) involved chiropractors
5% involved physical therapists
5% involved European osteopathic practitioners
2% were unknown
2% were self-induced
2% were performed by unqualified persons
18% (23 cases) were unspecified

The most frequent significant complication (65%) involved vertebral artery injury. Other complications included:

Cauda equina syndrome (12%)
Ruptured lumbar disc (6%)
Cervical fracture and/or dislocation (5%)
Thoracic disc rupture (2%)
Other occurrences (less than 1% each)

All appeared to involve HVLA activations. Vertebral artery complications occurred in a younger group than might be anticipated, with a mean age of 35 to 40 years. Male and female distributions were equal. Despite these occurrences, spontaneous vertebral artery dissection is more likely to occur during normal daily activities, such as looking backward over one's shoulder.

Koss (72) reports on the higher incidence of side effects from medications when compared with manipulative procedures. He notes that 5% of hospital admissions result from adverse drug reactions and that 36% of patients on an internal medicine service had an adverse reaction to a drug or diagnostic or therapeutic procedure.

Choice of Osteopathic Technique

Because a wide variety of mild to assertive impulsed (thrust) manipulative techniques are available to U.S.-educated osteopathic physicians, it is difficult to list or generalize absolute contraindications for the procedures. Rather than rely on one method, one should tailor treatment to the individual patient's circumstances. An essential key is the practitioner's familiarity with the approaches discussed in this text.

Kleynhans (73) divides causes of manipulative complications into two categories: physician-related and patient-related. Physician-related problems include:

Diagnostic errors
Lack of manual skills
Lack of interdisciplinary communication and consultation with those who are specially skilled in manipulative techniques

Kleynhans reports that patient-related problems arise from physical intolerance to the procedures as well as pathologic and structural factors. Other factors are often pertinent:

Personal expectations of both physician and patient
Previous experiences with other practitioners
Subjective pain responses
Other psychological and behavioral factors
Congenital abnormalities
Osteophytes
Atheromatous plaques
Active arthritis
Joint instabilities

Physician examination and diagnostic errors can lead to improper or inappropriate use of manipulation, with complications potentially occurring. For example, using manipulation in the absence of an appropriate physician encounter runs the risk of delayed diagnosis of potentially life-threatening diseases, such as cancer and heart disease. Anecdotal reports of such problems are common. Properly performed history, physical, and testing procedures avoid this pitfall.

Lack of diagnostic and manipulative treatment skills can result in:

Poor choice of manipulative procedures
Use of manipulation in a contraindicated situation
Improper soft tissue preparation
Incorrect patient positioning
Poorly applied techniques that use excessive force

Finally, history of trauma severe enough to raise the suspicion of fracture, dislocation, or neurovascular insult requires that imaging procedures be performed before manipulation is undertaken.

High Velocity, Low Amplitude Thrusting

HVLA thrusting (mobilization with impulse) techniques reportedly cause the most serious complications, occurring in 1 of 400,000 procedures to 1 in 1 million procedures. They are designed to apply low-amplitude planar and rotational forces along planes of both single and multiple joint systems. The most frequent of the severe complications are neurovascular accidents following manipulations of the upper cervical spine. These include:

Occipitobasilar strokes (Wallenberg syndrome)
Vertebral artery compression with thrombosis
Arterial dissections
Cerebellar infarctions

Vascular complications occur primarily with the use of cervical rotational forces with the head extended on the neck. The risk increases when the neck is moved away from the midline. Injuries at C1 and C2 are more prone to create vascular complications than are other cervical regions. Several living and cadaveric studies have shown that during rotation, the extracranial portion of the vertebral arteries can be occluded on the side opposite to the rotation (i.e., rotation right can occlude the left vertebral artery) (74). Fortunately, decreased blood flow to the brain as a result of cervical rotation is a rare complication, arising only in the presence of a significant preexisting compromise of the other vertebral artery, often congenital. Basmajian states, furthermore, "The cervical spine is, without doubt, quite resistant, and the atheromatous vertebral arteries are quite tolerant." (75).

Patients with rheumatoid arthritis and Down syndrome are also at particular risk to cervical direct method manipulation because the odontoid ligament is likely to be weakened and susceptible to rupture.

Severe complications are less frequent in the lumbar and thoracic spine. Increased pain reports are most common in this group. Complications also may include fractures in patients with the following underlying conditions:

Osteoporosis
Metastatic bone disease
Bone infections
Vertebral tuberculosis

Cauda equina syndromes have occasionally been reported in conjunction with the use of HVLA procedures.

Muscle Energy

When indicated, MET procedures are effective direct method alternatives for HVLA. MET is most effective when a specific joint or muscle is involved and when patient cooperation and operator forces can be well controlled. Posttreatment discomfort and complications are uncommon. The most frequent complications are temporary increases of pain. MET is not effective for someone if muscle contracting increases pain or if proper patient positioning cannot be achieved.

Absolute MET contraindications are fractures and severe neuromuscular injuries involving potential treatment sites.

Counterstrain

Counterstrain technique is a gentle, nontraumatic, indirect manipulative treatment. Posttreatment pain can occur several hours after the procedure, particularly in antagonist muscles, but this is usually well accepted by patients who have been informed of this possibility. Take care to avoid combined upper cervical hyperrotation and hyperextension. Stop treatment immediately if the patient reports any unusual neurologic sensations. Anecdotally, one documented case of counterstrain-related stroke has been reported in Europe during formal course teaching. A 38-year-old physical therapist, with unknown vascular disease but with many risk factors including smoking, sustained an internal carotid artery stroke after multiple classroom procedures. The complication was documented by angiography. It had not been previously reported (R. Ward, personal communication, 1993).

Avoid positioning that fails to relieve pain and discomfort, as well as positions that produce dizziness or radicular pain. Osteoporotic patients should avoid positions that require extreme forward bending of the thoracolumbar spine.

Craniosacral

Osteopathically based cranial manipulations, with their potential for providing valuable help in a wide variety of cases, also can create problems when used by the unskilled. For example, unanticipated lassitude and temporary emotional reactions ranging from tears to laughter occur at times. Uncomfortable side effects include:

Nausea
Vertigo
Lightheadedness
Headache
Loss of appetite
Sleep problems

Most are temporary and respond to rest. If problems occur in the clinic, the gentle use of CV4 techniques usually calms the reaction.

In the hands of nonprofessionals, serious complications have occurred. One author (E.L.D.) reports the case of a young man who developed hypopituitarism following an unskilled and forceful cranial treatment. After several months of hormone treatment and osteopathic treatment for the cranial dysfunctions, he had a favorable recovery.

Prevention of Complications

Proper diagnosis and treatment of any kind, including manipulative procedures, occur when one links the patient's background and presenting history with present circumstances. This includes:

Mechanism of injury
Medication use and abuse
Exercise levels
Lifestyle factors
Mental and emotional well being

A well-performed history and physical examination, including a careful, osteopathically oriented history and physical examination, complete this essential process. The application of osteopathic principles associated with functional anatomy, biomechanics, and manipulative skills reduces the potential for complications.

Histories of trauma, joint and soft tissue diseases, infectious diseases, and cancer are major considerations. When appropriate, include blood work and imaging studies.

Another line of defense is the appropriate choice of manipulative procedure. Indirect and neuromuscular-activating methods are typically safe and effective. If HVLA procedures are considered, explore the risk-to-benefit ratio. Most complications have occurred with HVLA maneuvers in the upper cervical spine during combined extension and rotation. Statistically, there is less chance of injury if cervical flexion and side-bending maneuvers are used. Take care to keep the neck in the midline, remembering the basic rule of spinal motion: modification of motion in one plane limits motion in all other planes.

Following manipulative treatment, pain or soreness may be prevented if the patient remains well hydrated and refrains from overexertion.

Finally, the broader the manipulative armamentarium possessed by the clinician, the better the chances for safe and effective outcomes.

OSTEOPATHIC PRACTICE GUIDELINES

Disease and dysfunction-based allopathically designed medical practice guidelines have been created and are under continued development for a wide variety of diagnoses. For example, the American Association of Family Physicians established a guideline for depression after more than a year in development and at a cost of more than $1 million. Such MD-oriented guidelines are often difficult to implement for osteopathically oriented physicians because they do not allow for the wide range of patient responses (i.e., the host). As a parallel but distinctive health care system (76), osteopathic medicine is ill served by directly adopting another group's standard of practice as anything more than partial guidelines in the strictest sense of that word.

In general, osteopathically oriented guidelines consider both the host and the etiologic factors. They should include an appropriate osteopathic diagnosis that incorporates palpatory diagnosis and potential manipulative treatment relatively early in the evaluation and treatment process, respectively. Goals of manipulation within an osteopathic practice guideline may include:

Resolution of primary somatic dysfunction
Resolution of secondary somatic dysfunction
Improvement of homeostatic mechanisms (e.g., respiratory, circulatory, immune, etc.)
Reduction of inappropriate afferent neural stimuli (especially from segmentally related somatic and visceral structures)

Significant somatic dysfunction is that which reduces the body's ability to recover, compensate, and repair itself. Psychologically, it is typically the somatic component that causes the patient discomfort and concern. It is also the somatic component of a problem that prevents the patient from functioning with a high level of efficiency. This is of particular importance for patients such as high-level athletes and ballet dancers.

Functional disorders of other systems affected by a primary disorder need to be a part of osteopathically oriented practice guidelines. The strategy is to reduce or remove identifiable lingering elements of somatic dysfunction to improve the body's ability to:

Compensate
Repair
Recover
Improve health

Finally, osteopathically oriented practice guidelines include all related elements relating to the diagnosis, treatment, and long-term health-enhancing strategies embodied in the application of osteopathic principles.

CONCLUSION

OMT has the potential for complications and side effects, but the risk is low. Properly selected and applied osteopathic procedures are beneficial for a wide variety of human ailments and health-enhancing activities. Palpatory diagnosis and manipulative treatment enlists the patient's cooperation in the process of maintaining health and overcoming the detrimental effects of somatic dysfunction. In general, the benefits far outweigh the rare and usually minor risks. Serious complications have occurred with the work of some practitioners but are only anecdotally documented in the practice of American-trained osteopathic physicians. Osteopathically based manipulative treatment is tailored to the individual patient's needs in a context of total health care that is in the patient's best interests. When osteopathic treatment is appropriate, it should be performed with gentleness, care, and skill.

REFERENCES

1. Goldstein M, ed. *The Research Status of Spinal Manipulative Therapy.* Bethesda, MD: Department of Health, Education and Welfare; 1975. NIH publication 76-998.
2. Korr IM. *The Neurobiologic Mechanisms in Manipulative Therapy.* New York, NY/London, England: Plenum Press; 1978.
3. Greenman PE, ed. *Concepts and Mechanisms of Neuromuscular Functions.* Berlin, Germany: Springer-Verlag; 1984.
4. Beurger AA, Greenman PE, eds. *Empirical Approaches to the Validation of Spinal Manipulation.* Springfield, IL: Charles C Thomas; 1985.
5. Patterson MM, Howell JN. *The Central Connection: Somatovisceral/Viscerosomatic Interaction. Proceedings of the 1989 American Academy of Osteopathy International Symposium.* Athens, OH: University Classics, Ltd; 1989.
6. Willard FH, Patterson MM. *Nociception and the Neuroendocrine-Immune Connection. Proceedings of the 1992 American Academy of Osteopathy International Symposium.* Athens, OH: University Classics, Ltd; 1994.
7. Kwoh K. Development of research protocols to study the efficacy of osteopathic manipulative treatment. In Sirica, ed . *Current Challenges to M.D.s and D.O.s. Proceedings of a Conference.* New York, NY: Josiah Macy, Jr. Foundation; 1996:263–270.
8. Kuchera ML. Global alliances: advancing research and the evidence base. *JAOA.* 2002;102(1):4–7.
9. Parker GB, Tupling H, Pryor DS. A controlled trial of cervical manipulation for migraine. *Aust N Z J Med.* 1978;8:589–593.
10. Sloop PR, Smith DS, Goldenberg E, et al. Manipulation for chronic neck pain: a double-blinded controlled study. *Spine.* 1982;7:532–535.
11. Gross AR, Aker PD, Quartly C. Evidence-based review of the literature: manual therapy in the treatment of neck pain. *Rheum Dis Clin North Am.* 1996;22(3):579–599.
12. Hurwitz EL, Aker PD, Adams AH, et al. Manipulation and mobilization of the cervical spine. A systematic review of the literature. *Spine.* 1996;21(15):1746–1760.
13. Shekelle PA, Adams AH, Chassin MR, et al. Spinal manipulation for low back pain. *Ann Intern Med.* 1992:117:590–598.
14. Koes BW, Assendelft WJJ, von der Heijden GJMG, et al. Spinal manipulation and mobilisation for back and neck pain: a blinded review. *Br Med J.* 1991;303:1298–1303.
15. Blomberg S. A pragmatic approach to low-back pain including manual therapy and steroid injections: a multicentre study in primary health care. 1993. Acta Universitatis Upsaliensis: *Comprehensive Summaries of Uppsala Dissertations from the Faculty of Medicine 394.*
16. Waagen GN, Haldeman S, Cook G, et al. Short-term trial of chiropractic adjustments for the relief of chronic low back pain. *Man Med.* 1986;2:63–67.
17. Gibson T, Grahame R, Harkness J, et al. Controlled-wave diathermy treatment comparison of short wave with osteopathic treatment in nonspecific low back pain. *Lancet.* 1985:1258–1261.
18. Dyer C. Osteopathic vs medical manipulation in clinical trials. *Br Osteopath J.* 1983;15:65–67.
19. Fitzgerald M, Stiles E. Osteopathic hospitals' solution to DRG's may be OMT. *The DO.* November 1984:97–101.
20. Andersson GBJ, Lucente T, Davis AM, et al. A comparison of osteopathic spinal manipulation with standard care for patients with low back pain. *N Engl J Med* 1999;341(19):1426–1431.
21. Blomberg S, Hallin G, Grann K, et al. Manual therapy with steroid injections—a new approach to treatment of low back pain. A controlled multicenter trial with an evaluation by orthopedic surgeons. *Spine.* 1994;19(5):569–577.
22. Koes BW, Bouter LM, van Mameren H, et al. Randomised clinical trial of manipulative therapy and physiotherapy for persistent back and neck complaints: results of one year follow up. *Br Med J* 1992;304(6827):601–605.
23. Pope MH, MacDonald L, Haugh L, et al. A prospective randomized three week trial of spinal manipulation, transcutaneous muscle stimulation, massage and corset in the treatment of subacute low back pain. *J Manip & Physiol Therap.* 1994;17(4):287–288.
24. Cherkin DC, Deyo RA, Battle M, et al. A comparison of physical therapy, chiropractic manipulation, and provision of an educational booklet for the treatment of patients with low back pain. *N Engl J Med.* 1998;339(15):1021–1029.
25. Brodin H. Inhibition-facilitation technique of lumbar pain treatment. *Man Med.* 1987;3:24.
26. Data compiled by Labor and Industry computers in Florida (FCER, 1988, Arlington, VA: FCER; 1988) and Colorado (Denver, CO: Tillinghast; 1993).
27. Cantieri MS. Inpatient osteopathic manipulative treatment: impact on length of stay. Available at: http://www.ohhpf.org/research96.html. Accessed May 31, 2002.
28. Kelso AF. A double-blind clinical study of osteopathic findings in hospitalized patients: progress report. *JAOA.* 1970;70:570–592.
29. Nicholas N. Correlation of somatic dysfunction with visceral disease. *JAOA.* 1975;75:426–428.
30. Smith LA, et al. *An Atlas of Pain Patterns: Sites and Behavior of Pain in Certain Common Disease of the Upper Abdomen.* Springfield, IL: Charles C Thomas; 1961.
31. Nicholas AS, DeBias DA, Ehrenfeuchter W, et al. A somatic component to myocardial infarction. *Br Med J.* 1985;291:13–17.
32. Beal MC. Palpatory testing for somatic dysfunction in patients with cardiovascular disease. *JAOA.* 1983;82:73–82.
33. Cox JM, Gorbis S, Dick LM, et al. Palpable musculoskeletal findings in coronary artery disease: results of a double-blind study. *JAOA.* 1983;82:832–836.

34. Rogers JT, Rogers RC. The role of osteopathic manipulative therapy in the treatment of coronary heart disease. *JAOA.* 1976;76:23–31.

35. Robuck SV. Osteopathic manipulative therapy in organic heart disease. In: *AOA Yearbook.* Indianapolis, IN: American Academy of Osteopathy; 1956:11–25.

36. Patriquin DH. Osteopathic management of coronary disease. In: *AOA Yearbook.* Indianapolis, IN: American Academy of Osteopathy; 1956:75–79.

37. Koch RS. A somatic component in heart disease. *JAOA.* 1961;60:92–97.

38. Stookey JR. OMT for angina. *Osteopathic Symposium.* May 1975:16–18.

39. Beal MC, Morlock JW. Somatic dysfunction associated with pulmonary disease. *JAOA.* 1984;84:179–183.

40. Koch RS. Structural patterns and principles of treatment in the asthmatic patient. In: *AOA Yearbook.* Indianapolis, IN: American Academy of Osteopathy; 1957:71–72.

41. Howell RK, Allen TW, Kappler RE. The influence of osteopathic manipulative therapy in the management of patients with chronic lung disease. *JAOA.* 1975;74:757–760.

42. Miller WD. Treatment of visceral disorders by manipulative treatment. In: *The Research Status of Spinal Manipulative Therapy.* Bethesda, MD: U.S. Department of Health, Education, and Welfare; 1975:295–301.

43. Henshaw RE. Manipulative and postoperative pulmonary complications. *The DO.* 1963;4(1):132–133.

44. Hermann E. Postoperative adynamic ileus: its prevention and treatment by osteopathic manipulation. *The DO.* 1965;6(2):163–164.

45. Sleszynski SL, Kelso AF. Comparison of thoracic manipulation with incentive spirometry in preventing postoperative atelectasis. *JAOA.* 1993;93(8):834–838, 843–845.

46. Radjieski JM, Lumley MA, Cantieri MS. Effect of osteopathic manipulative treatment on length of stay for pancreatitis: a randomized pilot study. *JAOA.* 1998;98(5):264–272.

47. Noll DR, Shores JH, Gamber RG, et al. Benefits of osteopathic manipulative treatment for hospitalized elderly patients with pneumonia. *JAOA.* 2000;100(12):776–782.

48. Northup TL. Manipulative management of hypertension. *JAOA.* 1961;60:973–978.

49. Mannino JR. The application of neurologic reflexes to the treatment of hypertension. *JAOA.* 1979;10:607–608.

50. Mannino JR. The application of neurological reflexes to the treatment of hypertension. *JAOA.* 1979;12:225–231.

51. Lo KS, Kuchera ML, Preston SC, Jackson RW. Osteopathic manipulative treatment in fibromyalgia syndrome. *JAOA.* 1992;9:1177.

52. Rubin BR, Gamber RG, Cortez CA, et al. Treatment options in fibromyalgia syndrome. *JAOA.* 1990;90:844.

53. Rubin BR, Gamber RG, Shores J, et al. The effect of treatment options on perceived pain in fibromyalgia syndrome. *JAOA.* 1991;91:1032.

54. Jackson KM, Steele TF, Dugan EP, et al. Effect of lymphatic and splenic pump techniques on the antibody response to hepatitis B vaccine: a pilot study. *JAOA.* 1998;98(3):155–160.

55. Measel JW. The effect of lymphatic pump in the immune response: I. Preliminary studies in antibody response to pneumococcal polysaccharide assayed by bacterial agglutination and passive hemagglutination. *JAOA.* 1982;82(1):28–31. Also: Measel JW, Kafity A. The effect of lymphatic pump on the B and T cells in peripheral blood. *JAOA.* 1986;86:608.

56. Simons DG, Travell JG, Simons LS. *Travell & Simons' Myofascial Pain and Dysfunction: The Trigger Point Manual.* Vol 1. Upper Half of Body. Baltimore, MD: Williams & Wilkins; 1999.

57. Korr IM. The spinal cord as organizer of disease processes: III. Hyperactivity of sympathetic innervation as a common factor in disease. *JAOA.* 1979;79(4):232–237.

58. Wolff HD. Akute Wurzelkeompression durch zervikalen Bandscheibensequester nach gezielter Handgrifftherapie. *Man Med.* 1989;27:14–15.

59. Hooper J. Low back pain and manipulation. *Med J Aust.* 1973;1:549–557.

60. Beatty RA. Dissecting hematoma of the internal carotid artery following chiropractic cervical manipulation. *J Trauma.* 1977;17:248–249.

61. Heffner JE. Diaphragmatic paralysis following chiropractic manipulation of the cervical spine. *Intern Med.* 1985;145:562–564.

62. Grayson MF. Horner's syndrome after manipulation of the neck. *Br Med J.* 1987;295:1381–1382.

63. Lanska DJ, Lanska MJ, Fenstermaker R, et al. Thoracic disk herniation associated with chiropractic spinal manipulation. *Arch Neurol.* 1987;44:996–997.

64. Darbert O, Freeinna DG, Weis AJ. Spinal meningeal hematoma, warfarin therapy and chiropractic adjustment. *JAMA.* 1970;214:2058.

65. Dan NG, Saccasan PA. Serious complications of lumbar spinal manipulation. *Med J Aust.* 1983;2:672–673.

66. Richard J. Disk rupture with cauda equina syndrome after chiropractic adjustment. *NY J Med.* September 1967:2496–2498.

67. Malmivaara A, Pohjola R. Cauda equina syndrome caused by chiropraxis on a patient previously free of lumbar spine symptoms. *Lancet.* 1982;2:986–987.

68. Schvartzman P, Abelson A. Complications of chiropractic treatment for back pain. *Post Grad Med.* 1988;83:57–61.

69. Quon JA, Cassidy JD, O'Conner SM, et al. Lumbar intervertebral disc herniation: treatment by rotational manipulation. *J Manipulative Physical Ther.* 1989;12:220–227.

70. Dvorak J, Orelli FV. How dangerous is manipulation to the cervical spine? Case report and results of a survey. *Man Med.* 1985;2:1–4.

71. Patijn J. Complications of manual medicine: a review of the literature. *Man Med.* 1991;6:89–92.

72. Koss RW. Quality assurance monitoring of osteopathic manipulative treatment. *JAOA.* 1990;90(5):427–434.

73. Kleynhans AM. Complications of and contraindications to spinal manipulative therapy. In: Haldeman S, ed. *Modern Developments in the Principles and Practice of Chiropractic.* New York, NY: Appleton-Century-Crofts; 1980;359–384.

74. Heinking K, Kappler R, et al. Vertebral artery blood flow during cervical extension and rotation as assessed by color flow duplex ultrasound. *JAOA.* 1995;95(9):548.

75. Basmajian JV. *Grant's Method of Anatomy,* 8th ed. Baltimore, MD: Williams & Wilkins; 1983.

76. Gevitz N. Parallel and distinctive. The philosophic pathway for reform in osteopathic medical education. *JAOA.* 1994;94:328–332.

SOMATIC DYSFUNCTION

H. JAMES JONES

KEY CONCEPTS

- Definition of somatic dysfunction
- Anatomy and physiology of somatic dysfunction
- Facilitation and sensitization
- Mechanoreceptors
- Spinal cord response to nociception
- Somatovisceral and viscerosomatic relationships
- Dorsal horn response to peripheral nociception
- Central descending inhibition of nociception
- Myofascial responses to states of immobilization
- Some proposed effects of osteopathic manipulative treatment (OMT) in relation to somatic dysfunction

INTRODUCTION

The Glossary of Osteopathic Terminology defines somatic dysfunction as "impaired or altered function of related components of the somatic (body framework) system: skeletal, arthrodial, and myofascial structures, and related vascular, lymphatic, and neural elements" (1). The diagnosis of somatic dysfunction is supported by visual and palpable findings of *T*issue texture changes, *A*symmetry of structure, *R*estriction of motion, and *T*enderness to palpation (TART) (1). Palpable temperature changes have also been stated to correlate to areas of somatic dysfunction (2). This chapter will explore the underlying neurophysiologic concepts and theories that support this diagnosis and its treatment by a variety of manipulative procedures. The diagnostic term "somatic dysfunction" was accepted by the *International Classification of Diseases-Abridged, Ninth Revision (ICDA-9)* in 1973. It supplanted the older terms such as "osteopathic lesion" and "osteopathic lesion complex" (2).

In the 19th century, musculoskeletal motion restrictions and visceral disorders were thought to occur due to "anatomical abnormalities followed by physiologic discord." It was reasoned that trauma was a large part of the cause of various disorders. The musculoskeletal dysfunctions that A.T. Still and others found to be amenable to manipulation were thought to be due to an alteration in the position of joints and their mechanics. Manipulating the joints into proper alignment enabled restoration of normal function. Progress in neurologic and biochemical sciences in the 20th century elucidated the nature of musculoskeletal (somatic) dysfunction. Current concepts include the understanding of the role of modulation of central nervous system (CNS) processes as well as changes in the nature of the connective tissues. The effectiveness of osteopathic manipulative medicine can be appreciated in light of this understanding.

ANATOMY AND PHYSIOLOGY OF SOMATIC DYSFUNCTION

Somatic dysfunction consists of neural, vascular, and connective tissue adaptations. The activity and condition of body tissues (the *soma*) are partly influenced via excitation and inhibition of nerves that emerge from the CNS. Joint stiffness, myofascial fibrotic changes, and eventual joint contracture can occur from excessive activity of CNS mediated alpha-motor neurons that may provoke a state of increased contraction (hypertonicity) of muscles innervated by those nerves. Associated with these articular and periarticular changes will be distortions of the body's fascial connective tissue architectural matrix. This can result in alterations of blood and lymphatic flow to the contractured tissues, conceivably eliciting states of relative ischemia and hypoxia and alterations of the local tissue chemical milieu. Osteopathic manipulative treatment (OMT) is designed to alleviate deleterious neurologic processes and connective tissue abnormalities that comprise somatic dysfunction.

Facilitation

In areas of somatic dysfunction, the physiologist Irvin Korr theorized that a large portion of these neurons are kept near their points of depolarization, making them more sensitive to the production of an action potential. The action potential would be conveyed via nerve axons to the final end organ (e.g., in the case of alpha-motor neurons, the end organ would be the myoneural junction of the muscle). This concept has been termed *facilitation* in the osteopathic medical literature (3) and *sensitization* by others (4–6). The facilitated state may then lead to alterations in muscle tone, resulting in myofascial connective tissue stiffness, contracture, and pain. Repeated or strong stimuli tend to elicit a decremental response in most types of nervous receptors (7).

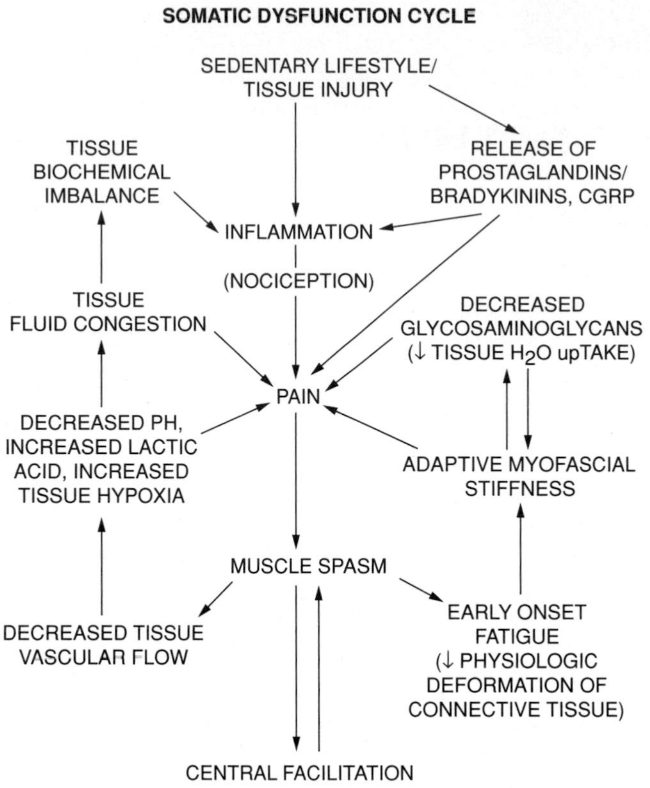

SOMATIC DYSFUNCTION CYCLE

FIGURE 73.1. Somatic dysfunction cycle.

However, in the case of *nociceptors* (nervous receptors that convey a noxious sensation), repeated noxious stimuli appear to lower the activation energy necessary to provoke an action potential that is conveyed along the nerve axon (8). Therefore it is believed that nociceptors play an integral role in the facilitation process.

The volleys of afferent input can be derived from a whole host of somatic and/or visceral insults, including physical or chemical trauma or even the effects of a sedentary lifestyle. With tissue damage there is the elaboration of proinflammatory and neuroir-

ritative chemicals, such as bradykinins, prostaglandins, calcitonin gene-related peptide (CGRP), and so forth, into the surrounding tissue environment, which play an integral role in facilitation and promulgation of somatic dysfunction (9). Associated with these adaptive changes may be local tissue biochemical alterations denoted by the loss of connective tissue lubricants (glycosaminoglycans [GAGS]) that would manifest themselves as further impaired myofascial and joint flexibility (10) (Fig. 73.1).

Mechanoreceptors

In order to understand how manipulation resolves somatic dysfunction, it is necessary to be aware of the anatomy and physiology of the mechanoreceptors and connective tissue involved. Various kinds of mechanoreceptors that respond to noxious stimuli are known as nociceptors. *Cutaneous nociceptors* are described on the basis of their relative size, degree of myelination, and their responsiveness to different kinds of noxious stimuli (11). In primates the most prominent types of nociceptors include A-delta (Aδ) mechanical nociceptors (12), Aδ mechanical heat nociceptors (13), and C polymodal nociceptors (which respond to heat, chemical, and mechanical stimuli) (6).

In 1967, the British neurologist, Barry Wyke, building on the work of Polacek, described an *articular* nervous receptor system (Table 73.1) that is responsive to *mechanical* stimuli (14–16). Subsequently, others have corroborated the existence of mechanoreceptors that exist in the cervical (17), thoracic (18), and lumbar spinal joints (19), as well as the intervertebral discs themselves (20). Mechanoreceptors are also found in ligaments, knee joint menisci, the articular discs of the temporomandibular joint (21), and in the gut (22,23), pulmonary bronchi (24), and cardiac tissue (25).

The nomenclature for mechanoreceptors relates to the *A-afferent and B-afferent systems* originally proposed by Prechtl and Powley (1990) (26). The A-afferent system is characterized by encapsulated nerve endings, large myelinated fibers, low thresholds of depolarization, discriminative touch and proprioception, and a line-labeled system. The B-afferent system is

TABLE 73.1. MECHANORECEPTORS AS DESCRIBED BY BARRY WYKE, MD

Type	Location	Receptor Appearance	Physiologic Function
I	Stratum fibrosum of ligaments and joint capsule	Laminated Ruffini-like corpuscles	Active during movement and at rest Low threshold for activation Slowly adapting
II	Intraarticular and extraarticular fat pads Junction of the synovial and fibrosum of the joint capsule	Laminated, pacinian-like shaped corpuscles	Active at the onset and ending of movement Low threshold for activation
III	Collateral ligaments Absent in interspinous ligaments of the cervical spine region	Golgi-Tendon Organ (GTO)-like corpuscles	Active at end of joint range of motion High threshold for activation Slowly adapting
IV	Joint capsule, ligaments and articular fat pads Absent in synovial tissue	Free nerve endings Lattice-like endings	Active only in response to extreme mechanical or chemical irritation High threshold for activation Slowly adapting

TABLE 73.2. COMPARISON OF THE PRECHTL AND POWLEY SYSTEM OF NOMENCLATURE WITH THE WYKIAN NOMENCLATURE

Prechtl and Powley System	Wykian System
A-Afferent Division	Type I, Aα fibers
Encapsulated nerve endings, larger diameter myelinated fibers, low thresholds of depolarization, discriminative touch, proprioception, line-labeled system	Type II, Aβ fibers
B-Afferent Division	Type III, Aδ fibers
Naked nerve endings, typically smaller diameter unmyelinated nerve endings (except Aδ fibers which *are* myelinated), high thresholds of depolarization, nociception, pain and a frequency-labeled system	Type IV, C-fibers

characterized by naked nerve endings, small unmyelinated nerve fibers, high thresholds of depolarization, nociception, pain, and a frequency-labeled system. The types I and II mechanoreceptors of the wykian system of nomenclature correspond to the A-afferent system, A-alpha (Aα) and A-beta (Aβ) fibers, respectively. The types III and IV mechanoreceptors correspond to the B-afferent system, Aδ and C fibers, respectively (Table 73.2). Afferent nerve fibers from *muscle* that correspond to the types III and IV mechanoreceptors appear to function as nociceptors (26,27). During states of ischemia, some type IV muscle afferents appear to be activated more strongly (28).

The Spinal Cord Response to Nociception

Manipulation has been known to alleviate pain in various musculoskeletal conditions. In order to understand how manipulation intervenes in the nociceptive process, it is necessary to first understand the spinal cord response to acute nociceptive input (which can be symptomatic or asymptomatic). Primary afferent nociceptive fibers (types III, Aδ) reach the spinal cord via the dorsal roots and synapse in the dorsal horn of the spinal cord in Rexed laminae I, II, V, and X (29). C-fiber (type IV) nociceptors synapse primarily in the substantia gelatinosa (lamina II) of the dorsal horn (30). Primary nociceptive afferent fiber terminals contain neuropeptide-laden vesicles. Some of the putative peptides are substance P (SP) and CGRP (31,32). The neuropeptides interact with receptors in the dorsal horn, resulting in the activation of second messenger systems leading to long, slow depolarization (33). These depolarizations then invoke the opening of *N*-methyl-d-aspartate (NMDA) voltage-gated ion channels (34) and transcription factors producing proteins of the endogenous opioid class such as dynorphins (35). These cascade of events lowers the thresholds for activation of certain dorsal horn cells known as *wide dynamic range* (WDR) neurons (36). Additionally, the same nerve endings contain excitatory amino acids (EAA) (glutamate and aspartate) that are believed to cause a rapid excitatory synaptic ion-gated transmission (37).

Wide Dynamic Range Neurons

Three different classes of neurons involved in nociception that reside within the dorsal horn of the spinal cord are *low threshold mechanoreceptors, nociceptive specific neurons,* and *WDR neurons*

(36). Convergence of Aβ, Aδ, and C fibers on the WDR neurons may contribute to the perception of *allodynia* (an ordinarily nonnoxious stimulus is perceived, because of a change in central processing of the stimulus, such as a painful sensation).

Responses to Painful Stimuli

Information conveyed to the CNS by nociceptors includes the activation of both excitatory and inhibitory circuits. The excitatory signals result in transmission of nociceptive input to higher centers via ascending nervous tracts such as the lateral spinothalamic tract (LSTT) neurons (38). Inhibitory circuitry is found in both the dorsal horn of the spinal cord and in more rostral supraspinal control systems activated by discharges in ascending tracts. Local inhibitory circuits are believed to involve interneurons containing inhibitory amino acid neurotransmitters, and γ-aminobutyric acid (GABA) (39). Peptides of the opioid class, such as enkephalin and, as mentioned earlier, dynorphin, are also thought to contribute to the inhibitory circuitry of the dorsal horn (40,41). Serotonin and norepinephrine function as inhibitory neurotransmitters in the terminals of descending pain control systems (42).

Ascending Tracts

Nociceptive information conveyed from the dorsal horn (after synapsing with first order Aδ [III] and C fibers [IV]) to more rostral CNS centers for processing and interpretation include the LSTT (pain and temperature). From the substantia gelatinosa (lamina II), second order axons cross via the ventral (anterior) white commissure and then ascend rostrally via the LSTT. At least a portion of the LSTT tract below the face projects to the ventroposterolateral (VPL) nucleus of the thalamus in primates and humans (11). Pain sensation from the face, cornea of the eye, the sinuses, cranial dura, temporomandibular joint labial mucosa, and cheeks is conveyed via the trigeminal nerve (V) through its sensory ganglion (43). The ganglion is known as the semilunar or gasserian ganglion (44). The central processes of the gasserian ganglion form a descending tract known as the spinal tract of V after entering the pontine brainstem region. Terminals from this tract form synapses with the spinal nucleus of V. Axons from the spinal nucleus of V cross to the contralateral side of the spinal cord and ascend as the ventral (anterior) trigeminothalamic tract to the ventroposteromedial (VPM) nucleus of the thalamus. From the VPM and the VPL, third order axons project to the somatosensory cortex of the parietal lobe of the brain where the full nuance of the nociceptive sensation is experienced as pain (44). Emotional-affective features of pain perception involve other parts of the CNS as well.

Response of Ventral Horn Neurons to Peripheral Nociception

Peripheral nociception induces increased firing rates and sensitivity of α-motor neurons within the ventral horn of the spinal cord (45). Conceivably, this would result in increased hypertonicity of muscle and associated myofascial structures subserved by those neurons leading to states of increased muscle contraction and spasm that will manifest themselves as the palpable changes that osteopathic physicians denote by the TART acronym. Concomitantly, the convergence of somatic primary afferent and visceral afferent fibers onto dorsal horn neurons will result in alterations in sympathetic nervous activity. Aihara and colleagues and Kimura and colleagues demonstrated that nociceptive input conveyed to midthoracic (T6-9) somatic tissues increases sympathetic outflow to the stomach, inhibiting peristalsis (46,47).

Somatovisceral and Viscerosomatic Relationships

Louisa Burns, DO, was one of the first osteopathic researchers to suggest that a connection existed between affectations of the somatic and visceral tissues. In a series of experiments performed primarily on rabbits bred specifically for the purpose, experimentally produced spinal "strains" were induced in her animal population. The strains were described as manually tractioning the anesthetized prone animal by grasping the animal's legs, and while the traction was maintained, hyperextending and rotating the spine until a "slight slipping" or maladjustment of the spinal articular surfaces was readily palpable. Burns reported that the paraspinal muscles in the experimentally lesioned areas of her rabbits were different than those of her controls. She noted an increase in the lactic acid content, edema of the striated muscle fibers, and congestion of small blood vessels and capillaries associated with muscle fibrosis in her lesioned animals (48). In anesthetized animals devoid of emotional factors, Sato demonstrated that somatic afferent nerve stimulation (skin pinching or brush stroking) is capable of regulating visceral functions in a variety of domains. Gastrointestinal motility is inhibited by stimulation of the abdominal skin; cerebral blood flow is increased by stimulation of the hind or forelimb in animal models (49).

Jorgensen and Fossgreen (50) studied 39 patients with complaints of upper abdominal pain without demonstrable organic abnormalities contrasted with 28 healthy control subjects, and compared them blindly with regard to back pain (*P* value less than 0.001). Back pain was reported in 72% of the patients who complained of upper abdominal pain versus 17% of the control subjects. Seventy five percent of the patients with complaints of back pain manifested abnormalities on physical examination localized to the lower thoracic and thoracolumbar regions of their backs; the very same neurologic levels that innervate the gastrointestinal tract. These findings suggest a connection between the abdominal and back pains, based upon the concept of viscerosomatic or somatovisceral reflex loops with reference patterns directed either from or to the viscus or to or from the skin, muscles, tendons, ligaments, and associated myofascial structures. Interestingly, Jorgensen and Fossgreen were able to demonstrate in their study that 51% of the patients experienced symptoms of irritable bowel syndrome and 41% reported heartburn, both of which were strongly correlated to their complaint of back pain. In a blinded controlled clinical trial, palpatory evidence of somatic dysfunction in left upper thoracic vertebral segments were found in 70 of 99 patients with coronary artery disease (CAD) (51).

Frobert and co-workers (52) demonstrated significantly more degenerative bony changes on cervical spine radiographs in symptomatic patients (30 women and 18 men) with chest pain but with normal electrocardiograms, normal echocardiograms, and normal coronary angiograms compared with asymptomatic control subjects (10 women and 8 men). Further, physical examina-

tion demonstrated abnormal palpatory musculoskeletal findings in the anterior and posterior chest wall at thoracic vertebral levels T1-6 and in the muscles of the neck and shoulder girdle of the symptomatic patients.

Response of Dorsal Horn Neurons to Peripheral Nociception

Primary afferent nociceptive input to the dorsal horn results in generator potentials of adjacent terminals of other afferent fibers. Under conditions of peripheral inflammation, action potentials are conducted backwardly (antidromically) along the afferent axons to its parent tissue. This phenomenon is known as a dorsal root reflex (DRR) (53). Antidromic conduction of DRRs may result in the elaboration of neuropeptides (i.e., SP of adjacent nerve terminals contributing to the inflammatory [and hence TART changes] process) (54).

Central Descending Inhibition of Nociception (55)

The descending inhibition of nociception begins at the level of the hypothalamus and prefrontal cortex, which permits hormonal and emotional influences to interact and affect the nociceptive experience. In the rostral pons, in an area known as the periaqueductal gray (PAG), cells in response to nociceptive afferent input elaborate opioid neuropeptides (enkephalin) and the inhibitory amino acid, GABA. Additional inhibitory contributions from the locus coeruleus (LC) consist of norepinephrine (noradrenaline). Descending fibers from the PAG synapse on the nucleus raphe magnus (NRM) and nucleus reticularis paragigantocellularis (NRP) with the resultant elaboration of serotonin (5-hydroxytryptophan). Subsequently these cells activate inhibitory neurons that proceed via the dorsolateral funiculus and terminate in the dorsal horn of the spinal cord. Within the dorsal horn, multiple synapses occur with local inhibitory circuitry with the elaboration of multiple enkephalinergic neuropeptides, GABA, α-adrenoceptor release of norepinephrine (noradrenaline), and glycine. The presence of the inhibitory agents effectively hyperpolarize (makes it more difficult to mount an action potential) any second order neuron transmission of nociceptive information along spinothalamic pathways, blocking the conduction of noxious stimuli to the somatosensory cortex of the brain.

Myofascial Responses to States of Immobilization

The nonfibrous portion of collagen connective tissue is known as the "ground substance." It is composed of linear polymers of repeating disaccharide units collectively known as *glycosaminoglycans (GAGs)* and water.

Within connective tissues there exist several types of GAGs: hyaluronic acid, chondroitin-4-and-6-sulfate, keratan sulfate, dermatan sulfate, and heparin sulfate. Typically GAGs are bound to a protein and are referred to collectively as *proteoglycans* (56). The function of GAGs is to maintain a certain critical collagen interfiber distance owing to their large hydrophilic capacity, thus permitting the expression of normal myofascial flexibility by allowing these collagen fibers to move freely against one another (57). Woo and colleagues (58) and Akeson, Amiel, and others (9,59) provide evidence that physiologic joint motion appears to function as a cell signal (ligand) that stimulates fibrocytes embedded within a connective tissue matrix to elaborate GAG into the surrounding tissue milieu. Saari and associates (60) monitored responses to joint mobilization in patients with rheumatoid arthritis. Utilizing a radiolabeled, hyaluronate-binding assay, they were able to determine that joint mobilization increased the serum concentration of the GAG. As alluded to previously, owing to their large capacity to uptake and bind water, the GAGs function as connective tissue "lubricants" inhibiting the formation of *excessive* adhesive *cross-links* by maintaining a certain critical distance between collagen fibers. However, some cross-linking is necessary to impart physical strength and integrity to the tissue. Cross-links consist chemically of aldol condensations between aldehydes (61). In human collagen, major types of cross-links are: dihydroxylisinonorleucine, hydroxylysinonorleucine, and histidino-hydroxymerodesmosine (56,61).

Histologic evidence suggests that joint fibrosis may occur within as little as 4 days after the onset of joint immobilization (62). This has been seen in states of immobilization, such as would occur with casting an extremity after a fracture, or in bedbound patients who have incurred either orthopedic or neurologic insult and essentially mold to the shape of the bed or wheelchair within which they reside. In the case of individuals who work in sedentary occupations, a dearth of physiologic deformation (and hence loss of cell signal) to the joint and adjacent periarticular connective tissue fibrocytes may have similar effects. With decreased physiologic connective tissue deformation, this will presumably result in a decreased production of GAG, with a decrease in tissue uptake of water, and therefore permits collagen fibers to physically approximate one another. When a certain critical collagen interfiber distance is achieved, excessive cross-linkage adhesions will develop that impair myofascial mobility. If the excessive cross-linking is not subjected to physiologic deformational stresses, it will result in eventual joint and periarticular contracture.

Conceivably, vascular structures, such as blood and lymph vessels traversing an area of TART-associated somatic dysfunction, because of the distortions to the connective tissue architecture, may lead to localized regions of ischemia and hypoxia altering the chemical environment of the tissue, followed by stimulation of nociceptors. Type IV (C) and possibly type III (Aδ) nociceptors embedded within the joint and adjacent soft tissues will be further provoked as the individual attempts to impart normal movement upon a now dysfunctional and adaptively shortened connective tissue matrix. This will result in the cascade of events leading to nociception, pain, and palpable TART changes as described previously.

SOME PROPOSED EFFECTS OF OSTEOPATHIC MANIPULATIVE TREATMENT IN RELATION TO SOMATIC DYSFUNCTION

"Manipulation" is thought to be derived from the Latin term *manus* (hand) or *manipulare* (to use the hands). Manipulation in a generic sense cannot be viewed as the exclusive domain of any particular manual medicine-oriented practitioner in so much as it is practiced on a worldwide basis by osteopathic physicians, chiropractors, physical (physio) therapists and others (63). Some practitioners make a distinction between "mobilization" versus "manipulation" to indicate that mobilization procedures generally refer to an oscillatory, rhythmic type of physical maneuver and manipulation refers to a "thrusting" type of physical maneuver directed against an area of dysfunction of the body (64). OMT is described as the therapeutic application of manually guided forces by an osteopathic physician to improve physiologic function and/or support homeostasis, which is accomplished via a variety of techniques (1). (Fig. 73.2).

A compelling rationale can be mounted that the many myriad forms of manipulative expression practiced by a variety of practitioners simply represent *different points* on a treatment armamentarium *spectrum* and that the putative connective tissue, vascular, biomechanical, and neurophysiologic effects are mediated through final common pathways. Thus practitioners of the manipulative arts tend to describe the various approaches as separate and discrete techniques, possibly because that permits an easier understanding of the complex relationships governing this body of technique. It is probably more likely that manipulative techniques employ multiple interlinking mechanisms, often deployed simultaneously.

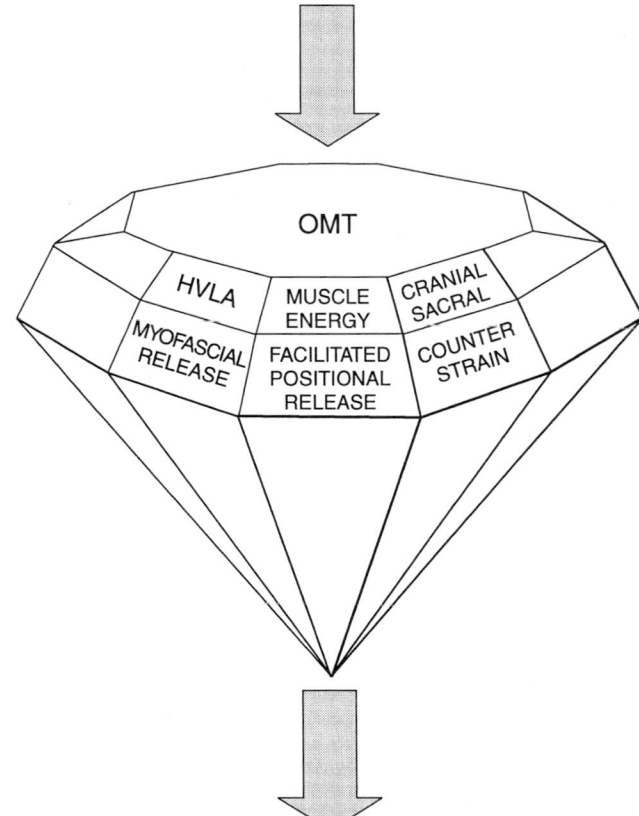

SOMATIC DYSFUNCTION

OMT

HVLA | MUSCLE ENERGY | CRANIAL SACRAL

MYOFASCIAL RELEASE | FACILITATED POSITIONAL RELEASE | COUNTER STRAIN

OPTIMUM HOMEOSTASIS AND FUNCTION

FIGURE 73.2. Somatic dysfunction mediated via osteopathic manipulative technique.

Soft Tissue and Myofascial Release

Thus *soft tissue* and *myofascial release techniques* may function primarily via the interdiction of excessive cross-linkage adhesions by imparting physiologic motion to a given area of TART. This will provoke the fibrocyte imbedded within the dysfunctional tissue to produce more GAG with the resultant uptake of water and restoration of appropriate collagen connective tissue interfiber distance and the full free expression of myofascial flexibility and pliability (9,10,57–62).

During the loading and unloading of a connective tissue, the restoration of the final length of the tissue occurs at a rate and to an extent *less than* during deformation (loading). These differences represent energy loss in the connective tissue system. This difference in viscoelastic behavior (*and energy loss*) is known as *hysteresis* (or "stress-strain") (64). It can be illustrated by a stress-strain or hysteresis curve (Fig. 73.3).

Loading the connective tissue to the point "A" on the hysteresis curve will result in an "elastic" deformation, with the connective tissue upon release of the load returning to near baseline length. Stressing the connective tissue to point "B" and beyond (the "plastic" range) will result in disruption of so many of the connective tissue cross-links that a sustained lengthening of the connective tissue will result. In the case of a contractured myofascial tissue, such as a tendon or ligament, the soft tissue or myofascial manipulative technique may interdict the TART changes associated with somatic dysfunction, at least in part, via this model. Myofascial techniques are divided into *direct* (the operator engaging a TART-associated area of somatic dysfunction with a palpatory sense of *greatest* tissue resistance) and *indirect* techniques (wherein the operator engages the tissues in the direction of *less* palpatory resistance). Even in areas of less palpatory myofascial resistance, this would not imply that there is an *absence* of cross-link formation. Rather it simply indicates that the *end feel* imparted to the operator's palpating hands is perceived as qualitatively less resistant than when engaging a soft tissue or myofascial barrier directly. When the deformational load proceeds to the point "C" on the hysteresis curve, then the design characteristics of a given tissue are exceeded and so many of the cross-links supporting the tissue are disrupted that the tissue loses coherence and structural integrity, resulting in failure of that tissue. If we are talking about a muscle tendon or a ligament, then those tissues are torn. If we are discussing bone, then the bone sustains a fracture (60,61).

Articulatory Techniques

Articulatory techniques are described as low velocity/low, moderate, or high amplitude manipulative techniques that carry a joint and its adjacent soft connective tissue though a range of motion designed to restore mobility (1). These techniques are often referred to as *joint mobilization* by physical therapists. In addition to proposed connective tissue effects, articulatory techniques may function predominantly by the activation of joint mechanoreceptors (types I and II [Aα and Aβ]) within an area of somatic dysfunction. Joint mechanoreceptors of types I and II (Aα and Aβ) are faster conducting fibers compared to type III (Aδ) and IV (C) nociceptors. Conceivably, a preponderance of nonnoxious activity within the faster conducting axons, as they are conducted to the level of the dorsal horn, synapse with local inhibitory circuitry of the enkephalinergic and GABA types. This inhibits the transmission of nociception via second order neurons to the thalamus and subsequently to the somatosensory cortex. This may explain the phenomenon that occurs when an individual inadvertently strikes their thumb with a hammer. The concussive injury activates type III (Aδ) and IV (C) mechanoreceptors within the tissues and joints of the thumb which are conveyed rostrally to the spinal cord and supraspinal centers (thalamus) via the LSTT. Activation of α-motor neurons in the ventral horn produce an action potential conducted to the muscle of the involved digit. In response to the painful stimulus, the individual immediately reflexively withdraws his or her digit and typically shakes it back and forth in a *rhythmic and oscillatory manner*. Presumably this activates the larger and faster conducting mechanoreceptor endings located in the metacarpophalangeal joint of the digit. This generates an action potential that is conducted along large diameter afferent axons to the dorsal horn of the spinal cord with the inhibition of nociception via interactions with the inhibitory dorsal horn circuitry and with contributions from descending central inhibitory systems as discussed previously. The central pain inhibitory pathway also plays a role in this process, but with a larger latency.

Strain-Counterstrain

Lawrence Jones, DO, developed strain-counterstrain techniques (65). Strain-counterstrain is an OMT that is described as a system of diagnosis that considers the somatic dysfunction to be a continuing, inappropriate strain reflex. The dysfunction is inhibited by applying a position of mild strain (typically the joint position of relative comfort), followed after a brief period of sustained positioning, by slowly repositioning the joint in the opposite direction of the initial mild strain (2). Peripheral somatic insults elicit nociceptive input to the spinal cord as previously discussed via type III (Aδ) and IV (C) afferents. Pain provokes the individual to attempt to reflexively withdraw from the noxious stimulus. Synapses with γ-motor efferent fibers cause the muscle spindle apparatus (intrafusal fibers) to shorten, which causes a relative length mismatch between the intra- and extrafusal muscle fibers

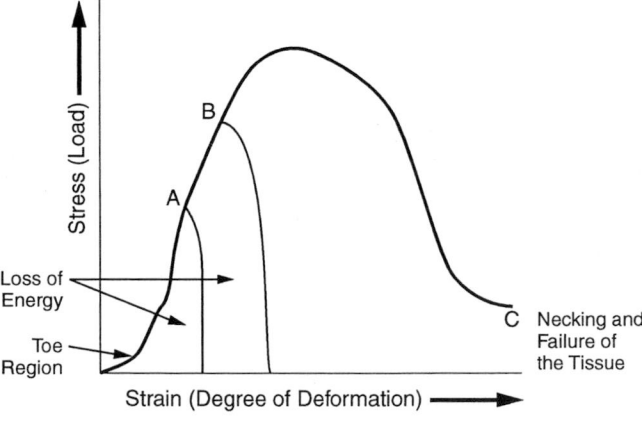

FIGURE 73.3. Hysteresis curve.

in areas of somatic dysfunction. Type Ia and II afferents, sensing the length mismatch between the intra- and extrafusal muscle fibers, generate action potentials mediated via the α motor neurons and axons, which result in hypertonicity of the motor units and hence muscle shortening innervated by particular α-motor neurons. All of these events then perpetuate the cycle of somatic dysfunction. When presented with this scenario, if the individual attempts to lengthen the maximally shortened muscle *rapidly,* it is suggested that the shortened muscle begins to report itself in a position of strain well in advance of achieving a neutral length. Strain-counterstrain techniques then may interdict the pain of somatic dysfunction by initially placing the dysfunctional joint in a position of relative shortening of the muscles that surround and attach to the osseous structures. By placing the muscle in a relative shortened position, it is believed that this inhibits inappropriate proprioceptive input regarding the length mismatch between agonist and antagonist muscles (66). The muscle joint-complex is held in this relative position of comfort for several seconds, then *slowly* repositioned to neutral in order not to provoke a nociceptive proprioceptor response. Van Buskirk (67) and Bailey and Dick (68) have proposed that a purely proprioceptive reflex model to explain the effects of counterstrain techniques appears inadequate. They suggest that *nociceptive* reflexes contribute to the paradigm of somatic dysfunction, probably mediated via type III and IV nociceptors.

Muscle Energy

Muscle energy techniques are osteopathic manipulative interventions first developed by Fred Mitchell, Sr., DO (69). They are described as OMTs in which the patient's joint(s) are positioned against a restrictive motion barrier and held immobile. The patient uses muscular effort against an unyielding operator counterforce to elicit *direct* reflex inhibition of *agonist* muscles or *indirect* reflex inhibition of *antagonist* muscles (70). Muscle energy techniques are often used to mobilize joints, to strengthen weak muscles, to stretch tight muscles and fascia, and to improve circulation.

Guissard and colleagues (71) studied the effects of different types of stretching maneuvers on motor neuron excitability of the human triceps surae muscles (gastrocnemius and soleus) as a function of the Hoffman (H) reflex. The H reflex is an electromyographic representation of the degree of activity of the anterior horn (α-motor neuron) excitability. The H reflex is normally present at birth. After 6 months of age it is present in the gastroc-soleus, flexor carpi radialis, and has been recorded in the hamstring and quadriceps muscles (72). In their study, Guissard and colleagues examined three different types of stretching maneuvers to the triceps surae musculature of their subjects. They were able to determine that a "contract-relax" maneuver (similar in execution to muscle energy technique), in which the subjects contracted their agonist triceps surae against an unyielding counterforce, followed by relaxation of the muscle with the ankle joint repositioned (stretched) to a new range of motion during the relaxation period, and an antagonist-contraction of the tibialis musculature with similar repositioning of the ankle joint during the post-isometric relaxation period, was a *superior* stretching maneuver than simply static passive stretching of the agonist

triceps surae muscles. During the period of stretching, the H reflex was depressed. This indicated that α-motor neuron excitability, which could conceivably contribute to increased states of muscle hypertonicity and hence the TART changes associated with somatic dysfunction that would inhibit any stretching maneuver, were also depressed. In the physical therapy literature, Schenck and co-workers were able to demonstrate significantly improved lumbar extension spine range of motion in a group of 26 volunteers subjected to muscle energy techniques with limited initial lumbar range of motion (73).

High Velocity/Low Amplitude Thrusting

High velocity/low amplitude (HVLA) thrusting techniques (sometimes referred to as *mobilization with impulse* or *thrust*) are described in the osteopathic literature as direct techniques that engage a restrictive joint/connective tissue barrier. A short (low amplitude), quick (high velocity) operator force is then applied to the joint to elicit release of the restriction (1). The exact mechanisms of HVLA techniques remain enigmatic (74). Postulated mechanisms may include alterations in cross-link adhesions that impair joint and myofascial mobility (59,75). In other words, from a connective tissue/biomechanical perspective, perhaps a part of what HVLA techniques do is disrupt the connective tissue adhesions that impair joint arthrokinematics by functioning closer to the "C" region of the hysteresis curve. Other postulated mechanisms include the production of afferent discharges from skin receptors, muscle spindles, mechanoreceptors, and free nerve endings in the zygapophysial joints and adjacent connective tissue of the spine, as well as in peripheral joints (76). The afferent discharges then would synapse on dorsal horn inhibitory circuitry as discussed previously, leading to inhibition of α-motor neuron pools in the ventral horns of the spinal cord. Dishman and Bulbulian conducted a study of 17 subjects (10 men and 7 women) in which spinal mobilization *without* thrust and spinal manipulation *with* thrust were employed. The amplitude of the tibial nerve/gastrocnemius H reflex was suppressed transiently during the mobilization and/or manipulation procedures. This was consistent with attenuation of α-motor neuronal excitability (74). Conceivably, this results in a state of decreased firing of the motor units innervated by those α-motor neuronal pools, ultimately leading to improved myofascial flexibility. As the flexibility of the soft connective tissue architecture is restored, blood and lymph flow may improve within these regions (77).

SUMMARY AND CONCLUSIONS

Somatic dysfunction is a complex paradigm that likely involves interlinking mechanisms from the biomechanical, connective tissue, neurophysiologic, vascular, and affective (emotional/behavioral) domains. Currently the lifestyle foundations that promote somatic dysfunction are beginning to be better elucidated. The role of OMT in ameliorating somatic dysfunction, while not completely understood, appears to function at simultaneous multimodal levels employing a variety of mechanisms.

REFERENCES

1. Educational Council on Osteopathic Principles. *Glossary of Osteopathic Terminology.* Washington, DC: American Association of Osteopathic Colleges; 2001.

2. Denslow JS. Pathologic evidence for the osteopathic lesion: the known, unknown and controversial. In: Beal MC, ed. *Selected Papers of John Stedman Denslow, DO.* Indianapolis, IN: American Academy of Osteopathy; 1993:154–160.

3. Korr I. The neural basis of the osteopathic lesion. In: Peterson B, ed. *The Collected Papers of Irvin M. Korr.* Colorado Springs, CO: American Academy of Osteopathy; 1979:120–127.

4. Beck PW, Handwerker HO. Bradykinin and serotonin effects on various types of cutaneous nerve fibres. *Pflugers Arch.* 1974;347:209–222.

5. Cohen RH, Perl ER. Contributions of arachidonic acid derivatives and substance P to the sensitization of cutaneous nociceptors. *J Neurophysiol.* 1990;64:457–464.

6. Lang E, Novak A, Reeh PW, Handwerker HO. Chemosensitivity of fine afferents from rat skin in vitro. *J Neurophysiol.* 1990;63:887–901.

7. Burgess PR, Perl ER. Cutaneous mechanoreceptors and nociceptors. In: Iggo A, ed. *Handbook of Sensory Physiology.* Berlin, Germany: Springer-Verlag; 1973:29–78.

8. Bessou P, Perl ER. Response of cutaneous sensory units with unmyelinated fibers to noxious stimuli. *J Neurophysiol.* 1969;32:1025–1043.

9. Akeson WH, Amiel D. Immobility effects of synovial joints: the pathomechanics of joint contracture. *Biorheology.* 1980;17:95–110.

10. Akeson WH, Amiel D. The connective tissue response to immobility: a study of the chondroitin 4 and 6 sulfate and dermatan sulfate changes in periarticular connective tissue of control and immobilized knees of dogs. *Clin Orthop.* 1967;51:190–197.

11. Willis WD. *The Pain System. The Neural Basis of Nociceptive Transmission in the Mammalian Nervous System.* Basel, Switzerland: Karger; 1985.

12. Perl ER. Myelinated afferent fibres innervating the primate skin and their response to noxious stimuli. *J Physiol.* 1968;197:593–615.

13. LaMotte RH, Thalhammer JG, Torebjauork HE, Robinson CJ. Peripheral neural mechanisms of cutaneous hyperalgesia following mild injury to heat. *J Neurosci.* 1982;2:765–781.

14. Wyke B. The neurology of joints. *Ann Royal Coll Surg England.* 1967;41(1):25–50.

15. Polacek P. Receptors of the joints. Their structure, variability and classification. *Acta Fac Med Univ Brunesis.* 1966;23:1–107.

16. Dvorak J, Dvorak V. Neuropathophysiology of the apophyseal joints. In: *Manual Medicine Diagnostics.,* New York, NY: Georg Thieme Verlag; 1984:chapter 2.

17. McLain RF. Mechanoreceptor endings in human cervical facet joints. *Spine.* 1994;19(5):495–501.

18. McLain RF, Pickar JG. Mechanoreceptor endings in human thoracic and lumbar facet joints. *Spine.* 1998;23 (2):168–173.

19. Yamashita T, Cavanaugh JM, El-Bohy AA, et al. Mechanosensitive afferent units in the lumbar facet joint. *J Bone Joint Surg.* 1990;72-A(6):865–870.

20. Roberts S, Eisenstein SM, Menage J, et al. Mechanoreceptors in intervertebral discs, morphology, distribution, and neuropeptides. *Spine.* 1995;20(24):2645–2651.

21. Zimny ML. Mechanoreceptors in articular tissues. *Am J Anat.* 1988;182 (1):16–32.

22. Yokoyama S, Ozaki T. Effects of gut distension on Auerbach's plexus and intestinal muscle. *Jpn J Physiol.* 1980;30(2):143–160.

23. Accarino AM, Azpiroz F, Malagelada JR. Selective dysfunction of mechanosensitive intestinal afferents in irritable bowel syndrome. *Gastroenterology.* 1995;108 (3):927–931.

24. Sant'Ambrogio G, Widdecombe J. Reflexes from airway rapidly adapting receptors. *Respir Physiol.* 2001;125(1-2):33–45.

25. Kamkin A, Kiselva I, Wagner KD, et al. Mechanically induced potentials in fibroblasts from human right atrium. *Exp Physiol.* 1999;84(2):347–356.

26. Prechtl JC, Powley TL. B-afferents: a fundamental division of the nervous system mediating homeostasis? *Behav Brain Sci.* 1990;13:289–331.

27. Kumazawa T, Mizumura K. Thin-fibre receptors responding to mechanical, chemical and thermal stimulation in the skeletal muscle of the dog. *J Physiol.* 1977;273:179–194.

28. Mense S, Stahnke M. Responses in muscle afferent fibres of slow conduction velocity to contractions and ischemia in the cat. *J Physiol.* 1983;342:383–397.

29. Light AR, Perl ER. Spinal termination of functionally identified primary afferent neurons with slowly conducting myelinated fibers. *J Comp Neurol.* 1979;186:133–150.

30. Sugiura Y, Lee CL, Perl ER. Central projections of identified, unmyelinated C afferent fibers innervating mammalian skin. *Science.*1986; 234:358–361.

31. Carlton SM, McNeill DL, Chung K, Coggehall RF. Organization of calcitonin gene-related peptide immunoreactive terminals in the primate dorsal horn. *J Comp Neurol.* 1988;276:527–536.

32. De Lanerolle NC, LaMotte CC. Ultrastructure of chemically defined neuron systems in the dorsal horn of the monkey. Substance P immunoreactivity. *Brain Res.* 1983;274:31–49.

33. Liu H, Brown JL, Jasmin JE, et al. Synaptic relationship between substance P and the substance P receptor: light and electron microscope characterization of the mismatch between neuropeptides and their receptors. *Proc Natl Acad Sci USA.* 1994;91:1009–1013.

34. Traub RJ. The spinal contribution of substance P to the generation and maintenance of inflammatory hyperalgesia in the rat. *Pain.* 1996;67:151–161.

35. Coderre TJ, Katz J, Vaccarina AL, et al. Contribution of central neuroplasticity to pathological pain: review of clinical and experimental evidence. *Pain.* 1993;52:259–285.

36. Maixner WR, Dubner DR, Kenshalo MC, et al. Responses of monkey medullary dorsal horn neurons during the detection of noxious heat stimuli. *J Neurophysiol.* 1989;62:437–449.

37. DeBiasi SN, Rustioni A. Glutamate and substance P coexist in primary afferent terminals in the superficial laminae of the spinal cord. *Proc Natl Acad Sci USA.* 1988;85:7820–7824.

38. Carlton SM, Westlund KN, Zhang D, et al. Calcitonin gene-related peptide containing primary afferent fibers synapse on primate spinothalmic tract cells. *Neurosci Lett.* 1990;109:76–81.

39. Carlton SM, Hayes ES. Light microscopic and ultrastructural analysis of GABA-immunoreactive profiles in the monkey spinal cord. *J Comp Neurol.* 1990;300:162–182.

40. LaMotte CC, de Lanerolle NC. Ultrastructure of chemically defined neuron systems in the dorsal horn of the monkey. II. Methionine-enkephalin immunoreactivity. *Brain Res.* 1983;274:51–63.

41. Takahashi O, Shiosaka S, Traub RJ, et al. Ultrastructural demonstration of synaptic connections between calcitonin gene-related peptide immunoreactive axons and dynorphin immunoreactive dorsal horn neurons in a rat model of peripheral inflammation and hyperalgesia. *Peptides.* 1990;11:1233–1237.

42. LaMotte CC, de Lanerolle NC. Ultrastructure of chemically defined neuron systems in the dorsal horn of the monkey. Serotonin immunoreactivity. III. *Brain Res.* 1983;274:65–77.

43. Fix J. *Neuroanatomy,* 2nd ed. Baltimore, MD: Williams & Wilkins, 1995.

44. Gilman S, Newman SW. *Manter and Gatz's Essentials of Clinical Neuroanatomy and Neurophysiology,* 8th ed. Philadelphia, PA: FA Davis Co; 1992.

45. Schaible HG, Grubb BD. Afferent and spinal mechanisms of joint pain. *Pain.* 1993;55:5–54.

46. Aihara Y, Nakamura H, Sato A, et al. Neural control of gastric motility with specific reference to cutaneo-gastric reflexes. In: Brooks C, ed. *Integrative Functions of the Autonomic Nervous System.* New York, NY: Elsevier, 1979.

47. Kimura A, Sato A, Sato Y, et al. Single electrical shock of a somatic afferent nerve elicits A and C reflex discharges in gastric vagal efferent nerves in anesthetized rats. *Neurosci Lett..* 1996;210:53–56.

48. Burns L. Viscero-sensory and somato-visceral spinal reflexes. *JAOA.* 1907;7:51–60.

49. Sato A. Reflex modulation of visceral functions by somatic afferent activity. In: Patterson MM, Howell JN, eds. *The Central Connection: Somatovisceral/Viscerosomatic Interaction, Proceedings of the 1989 American*

Academy of Osteopathy International Symposium. Athens, OH, University Class, Ltd; 1992:53–72.

50. Jorgensen LS, Fossgreen J. Back pain and spinal pathology in patients with functional upper abdominal pain. *Scand J Gastroenterol.* 1990;25(12):1235–1241.

51. Beal MC, Kleiber GE. Somatic dysfunction as a predictor of coronary artery disease. *JAOA.* 1985;85(5):302–307.

52. Frobert O, Fossgreen J, Sondergaard-Pertersen J, et al. Musculoskeletal pathology in patients with angina pectoris and normal coronary angiograms. *J Intern Med.* 1999;245(3):237–246.

53. Sluka KA, Willis WD, Westlund KN. The role of dorsal root reflexes in neurogenic inflammation. *Pain Forum.* 1995;4:141–149.

54. Raja SN, Meyer RA, Ringkamp M, et al. Peripheral neural mechanisms of nociception. In: Wall P, Melzack R, eds. *Textbook of Pain.* Edinburgh, Scotland: Churchill-Livingstone; 1999:36.

55. Cousins M, Power I. Acute and postoperative pain. In: Wall P, Melzack R, eds. *Textbook of Pain.* Edinburgh, Scotland: Churchill-Livingstone; 1999:458–460.

56. Stryer L. *Biochemistry,* 3rd ed. New York, NY: WH Freeman and Co, 1988:chapter 11.

57. Cantu RI, Grodin AJ. *Myofascial Manipulation Theory and Clinical Application.* Gaithersburg, MD: Aspen Publications; 1992.

58. Woo S, Matthews JV, et al. Connective tissue response to immobility. *Arthritis Rheum.* 1975;18:257–264.

59. Akeson WH, Amiel D, et al. Collagen cross-linking alterations in the joint contractures: changes in the reducible cross links in periarticular connective tissue after nine weeks of immobilization. *Connective Tissue Res.* 1977;5:15–19.

60. Saari H, Konttinen YT, Nordstrom D. Effect of joint mobilization on serum hyaluronate. *Ann Med.* 1991;23 (1):29–32.

61. Skinner HCW. Bone: cellular and molecular organization. In: Albright JA, Brand RA, eds. *The Scientific Basis of Orthopaedics.* New York, NY: Appleton-Century-Crofts, 1979:chapter 4.

62. Salter BB. Royal College Lecture: Prevention of arthritis through preservation of cartilage. *J Can Assoc Radiol.* 1981;32: 5–7.

63. Haldeman S, Hooper PD. Mobilization, manipulation, massage and exercise for the relief of musculoskeletal pain. In: Wall PD, Melzack R, eds. *Textbook of Pain,* 4th ed. Edinburgh, Scotland: Churchill-Livingstone; 1999:1399–1418.

64. Nordin M, Frankel VH. *Basic Biomechanics of the Musculoskeletal System,* 2nd ed. Philadelphia, PA: Lea & Febiger; 1989.

65. Jones LH, Kusunose RS, Goering EK. *Strain-Counterstrain.* Boise, ID: Jones Strain-Counterstrain, Inc; 1995.

66. Matthews PBC. Proprioceptors and the regulation of movement. In: Towe AL, Luscher ES, eds. *Handbook of Physiology, Section 1, The Nervous System,* Vol II, Part 1. Bethesda, MD: American Physiological Society; 1981.

67. Van Buskirk RL. Nociceptive reflexes and the somatic dysfunction: a model. *JAOA.* 1990;90 (9), 792–809.

68. Bailey M, Dick L. Nociceptive considerations in treating with counterstrain. *JAOA.*1992;92(3):334–341.

69. Mitchell F. *The Muscle Energy Manual,* Vol I. Lansing, MI; 1995.

70. Goodridge JP. Muscle energy technique: definition, explanation, methods of procedure. *JAOA.* 1981;81(4):249–253.

71. Guissard N, Duchateau J, Hainaut K. Muscle stretching and motoneuron excitability. *Eur J Appl Physiol.* 1988;58:47–52.

72. DeLisa JA, Mackenzie K, Baran EM. *Manual of Nerve Conduction Velocity and Somatosensory Evoked Potentials,* 2nd ed. New York, NY: Raven Press, 1987.

73. Schenck RJ, MacDiarmid A, Rousselle J. The effects of muscle energy technique on lumbar range of motion. *J Man Manipulative Ther* 1997;5(4):179–183.

74. Dishman JD, Bulbulian R. Spinal reflex attenuation associated with spinal manipulation. *Spine.* 2000;25(19):2519–2525.

75. Enneking W, Horowitz M. The intraarticular effect of mobilization on the human knee. *J Bone Joint Surg.* 1972;54(A): 973–985.

76. Vandeenenabeele F, Creemers J, Lambrichts I, et al. Encapsulated ruffini-like endings in human lumbar facet joints. *J Anat.* 1997;191:571–573.

77. Sucher BM. Thoracic outlet syndrome—a myofascial variant: Part 1. Pathology and diagnosis. *JAOA.* 1990;90(8):686–696.

BASIC AND CLINICAL RESEARCH FOR OSTEOPATHIC THEORY AND PRACTICE

INTRODUCTION

ALBERT F. KELSO
BERNARD R. RUBIN

Osteopathic philosophy suggests a broader basis in the 21st century for continued advancement of its theory and practice. A. T. Still's experience with deaths in his family initiated his search for a new treatment to replace medicine. His search identified manipulative techniques used to restore the body's capacity to heal itself. The philosophy that the body behaves as an integrated unit is derived from the application of his findings. His practice, based on treating the osteopathic lesion as the intervention to restore the body's inherent capacity to heal itself, assumed that the treatment affected the entire person. The principle of the body behaving as an integrated unit is evident in the research throughout osteopathic history. The same question faces osteopathic philosophy, theory, and practice that faces the chicken and the egg, "which came first?"

The introduction of the osteopathic lesion (somatic dysfunction) and treatment of the whole person initiated Smith's use of the skiagraph (a forerunner to the radiograph) to study circulation (1). Still's research focused on reflex mechanisms contributing to the integration of the somatic system functions with other body structures and functions.

Osteopathic philosophy and principles assume that somatic dysfunction or its components (segmental, cranial, appendicular, and visceral) have a response to treatment that involves the whole person. This assumption is difficult to support with some scientific methods, although they can provide detailed explanations. Structural and functional mechanisms are altered at multiple sites during progression from an acute to a chronic condition, and only longitudinal studies provide data on changes occurring during the course. The acceptance in both clinical and basic sciences that the body behaves as an integrated unit to the presence of somatic dysfunction or the body's response to its treatment needs longitudinal, evidence-based support.

BACKGROUND FOR A RESEARCH MODEL

Models of a system to be studied increase the efficiency of research. Advancement of osteopathic health care is supported by documenting patients' health outcomes obtained in epidemiologic studies; mechanisms of integration are supported by basic or clinical research contributions to knowledge.

The earliest clinical explanations for manipulative treatment of somatic dysfunction (initially identified as an osteopathic lesion) attributed favorable responses to the whole-body response. Satisfied osteopathic patients in the 19th and 20th century supported the founding and early development of the osteopathic profession. Their experience with osteopathic treatment influ-

enced state legislatures to approve establishment of osteopathic schools, colleges, and universities, and acceptance of osteopathic physicians into government positions. It is a continuing challenge to explain the patients' change in health status as an outcome of osteopathic health care. Patients, students admitted to osteopathic schools of medicine, and state or federal government positions manned by osteopathic medical graduates expect advances in osteopathic theory and practice to keep the profession abreast of scientific knowledge.

In 1892, The American School of Osteopathy (now the Kirksville College of Osteopathic Medicine or KCOM) included William Smith, a physiologist, in its faculty. Smith added his discipline to the basic science curriculum. His reputation in using xerography to investigate circulation is widely recognized. The A. T. Still Research Institute and early osteopathic faculty researchers supported the osteopathic somato-somatic and viscerosomatic reflex concepts by application of neurophysiologic information. Beginning in 1919, Sutherland published his search for information and an anatomic and physiologic explanation for the effects of cranial manipulative treatment. In the middle of the 20th century, Denslow and the KCOM faculty made major basic science contributions to osteopathic theory and concepts in reflexive and behavior research.

Subsequent osteopathic research has strengthened the knowledge base created by these early contributors. However, evidence on the course of somatic dysfunction remains a continuing challenge. Development of a model for research efforts is proposed to focus and facilitate research that advances osteopathic theory and practice.

DEVELOPMENT OF A MODEL

Some clinical and most basic science research on somatic dysfunction provides cross-sectional data on single and multiple interactions of a stimulus (environmental change), the body's reactions to the dysfunction, and its response to interventions (experimental variables). Outcome variables are observed or measured in molecular, cellular, or organ systems, or as behavior. *In vivo* research in man or animals that uses longitudinal rather than cross-sectional studies identifies a sequence of responses to a stimulus. The stimulus site remains constant but may develop, as indicated by local changes accompanying a stimulus.

Effects of the stimulus on other body sites involve observed or measured responses to multiple molecular, cellular, organ, and systemic reactions. Reactions to stress are observed or measured as changed function, behavior, or structure. Cannon's triple response in the skin is an example of a stressor (change in environment) that elicits local changes in skin. The stressor and associated local responses create neural and humoral signals that initiate reactions at remote sites. Selye's syndrome (2), produced by diverse noxious reactions, is the beginning of extensive research, including many theories and applications to health care. This reference provides information to develop an osteopathic model for research on the osteopathic principle that humans behave as an integrated unit.

A PROPOSED MODEL FOR RESEARCH TO ADVANCE OSTEOPATHIC THEORY AND PRACTICE

An osteopathic model similar to the Selye model can be used to investigate osteopathic philosophy, theory, and practice. Immediate success is likely to require years of effort, but less than the seventy-five years thus far devoted to early physiologic stress models.

The suggested model to advance osteopathic theory assumes that observations of a total body response include:

- Internal or external environmental stress that initiates reactions at remote sites and that can be reliably observed or measured.
- A reliable course description for the stimulus and integrated responses, which also requires standard, clinically observed descriptions and guidelines to enable data from collaborating scientists or other research reports to be pooled.
- The philosophy that the body behaves as an integrated unit requires knowledge of the role of somatic dysfunction as a stimulus and research on the sequence of responses beginning with the acute changes and continuing in subsequent reactions.

CONSIDERATIONS RELATING TO THE PROPOSED MODEL

The nature of a stimulus is an important factor. Is the site and reaction stable and unchanging? Some stressors, Cannon triple response in the skin to a nociceptive stimulus, for example, release neural and humoral signals that target multiple structures and functions distributed throughout the body. However, local changes in skin characterize a "triple response" that follows the response to the noxious insult. A cutaneous red reaction, axon reflex, and local vascular changes appear almost instantaneously and occur as local responses. Neural and humoral signals generated during these local changes initiate the neural reflexive and endocrine or humoral controlled behavioral and metabolic responses. Whether the whole-body response will undergo the same or similar course to Selye's stress response depends on the validity of assuming similarity between the two models.

Published information on disturbances in any system, organ, cell, or molecular reaction to a known stressor provides information for formulating a model and research design.

Progress from Cannon's and Selye's stressor and stress reactions to our current knowledge of stress provides a large body of evidence to support integrated adaptation to stress. It will be a challenge to initiate and develop a similar body of evidence-based knowledge. Acceptance of evidence-based support for the clinical aspects may require answers to questions about somatic dysfunction. When is somatic dysfunction a sign that the stressor is directly related to the somatic dysfunction? When is somatic dysfunction a response stressor initiated by some other internal or external environmental change? Are the whole-body responses to interventions used for treating the somatic dysfunction different for the dysfunction's direct and indirect relationship to the stressor?

AUTHORS AND THEMES

In the following chapters, the authors discuss the history of osteopathic medical research and introduce reviews of methods of basic and clinical research, discussing how they specifically relate to current and future osteopathic physicians. Historic and methodological information is important to create a sound research plan, protocol, and subsequent publication. Each of the authors in this section reviews research methods that are practical and applicable to understanding the types of osteopathic research that has been done in the past and what challenges lie ahead. The details of what hypotheses, methods, and types of analyses are needed for a given project may change frequently, so knowledgeable consultants assist researchers in keeping current and timely.

Five chapters in this section are devoted to clinical investigation. These five chapters review and discuss fundamental principals of research and offer ways that each type of research has relevance to osteopathic medicine. Heath and Gevitz review somatic dysfunction and relevant osteopathic research efforts over the last 20 years. Patterson explains the basic science approach to designing and implementing research projects that have been used to try to explain the theoretical basis for osteopathic medicine. Snow, Licciardone, and Gamber have written a timely chapter dealing with outcomes research, which is designed to study clinical end results of a given therapy. The authors review the existing data to assess the efficacy of osteopathic manipulative therapy in one specific entity—low back pain. Rubin introduces the concepts of clinical research in the context of pharmaceutical research. Good clinical practice guidelines are explained as a method to show osteopathic physicians the methods used to produce rigorous research studies. Foresman, D'Alonzo, and Jerome have written a chapter dealing with biobehavioral research in osteopathic medicine—research involving mechanisms of disease modification thorough mind-body interaction. Lastly, Patterson has predictions for future developments and challenges facing osteopathic medical research. His long career in osteopathic medical research uniquely positions him to note that the future of the profession is linked to research advances.

CONCLUSION

The osteopathic profession has embraced research from the beginning of its existence. Basic, clinical, biobehavioral, and outcomes research provide evidence regarding the nature and importance of osteopathic medicine to health. Research must involve all parts of the osteopathic health care system. Therefore, practicing osteopathic physicians, clinical faculty members at osteopathic medical schools, and basic and clinical researchers all share the responsibility to investigate the unique aspects of osteopathic medicine.

Clinical research must adhere to accepted practice, including the ethical standards regarding the protection of research subjects as governed by an institutional review board. Therefore, osteopathic physicians must be knowledgeable of these requirements and adhere to them.

The future of osteopathic medical research has never been brighter. Researchers who read this section will note great detail paid to the role of research design, methods, and ideas, as well as the use of statistics to analyze data. These areas are important whether one is discussing basic research, outcome research, clinical pharmaceutical research, or biobehavioral research. In investigating osteopathic theory and practice, it is critical to develop sound research protocols. Research collaboration among all interested parties serves to promote advances in osteopathic medicine based on a solid research framework.

REFERENCES

1. Cole WV. Historical basis for osteopathic theory and practice. In: Northrup GW, ed. *Osteopathic Research: Growth and Development.* Chicago, IL: American Osteopathic Association; 1987.
2. Selye H. The general adaptive syndrome and the diseases of adaptation. *J Clin Endocrinol Metab.* 1946;6:117–173.

FOUNDATIONS FOR OSTEOPATHIC MEDICAL RESEARCH

MICHAEL M. PATTERSON

mature research efforts into the
the profession. It should help attr
collaboration within the osteopat

Thus, the next phase of resea
pathic profession has begun. Thi
tion on the basics for conceptuali
to osteopathic medicine and som
vestigators designing research in

WHAT IS OSTEOPATHIC R
WHO DOES IT?

A definition for osteopathic rese
osteopathic researchers since its i
tion be asked? It is often asked
project should be funded by an o
as the AOA Bureau of Research
whether research should be inclu
It can be a condition for wheth
in a research project. Whether
has both political and practical i
eral definitions of osteopathic re
various times.

Research Under Osteop

Perhaps the broadest definition
any research done under osteo|
implies that any research, basic
subject matter, is osteopathic wh
institution or under the contro
Under this rubric, research on
osteopathic. This is obviously to

Research on Topics of S
to the Profession

Some topics in biomedicine hav
terest to the osteopathic professic
actions of the nervous system in
functions and the effects of mar
function have been topics of ir
times, efforts have been made to
oncs that define osteopathic res
new avenues of inquiry are cons
the clinical and theoretical topi
list can be devised that will cove

Research on Osteopath
Manipulative Treatmen

Definitions of osteopathic resea
to those studies attempting to c
teopathic treatment. This appro
mechanism inquiry that seeks t
efficacy. Obviously, this is too n

KEY CONCEPTS

- The forces that have shaped the research programs of the osteopathic profession
- What constitutes osteopathic research?
- Who does research in the osteopathic profession?
- Ethical considerations in doing osteopathic research in animals and humans
- Mechanisms underlying osteopathic concepts and their research basis
- Types of research design and their uses
- Considerations in osteopathic clinical research
- The question being asked is the most important part of osteopathic research
- Characteristics of good osteopathic clinical research
- Potential pitfalls in osteopathic research

DEVELOPMENT OF RESEARCH IN THE OSTEOPATHIC MEDICAL PROFESSION

Early Research (1874 to 1939)

Research began in the osteopathic profession before the formal inception of the profession itself. A. T. Still was a true researcher, practicing observation, questioning his observations, trying new ways of thinking, and refining his hypotheses about his practice. He did not do what would now be regarded as organized research, but in fact, he did research at the basic level in a way that is still at the basis of almost all medical research. He observed, studied, questioned, and constructed testable hypotheses. The ideas and philosophy that have become the osteopathic profession and that undergird much of the research in the profession today came out of his questioning.

Soon after Still founded the first school in Kirksville in 1892, his students began to do formal research into the concepts he espoused. At first, these research endeavors were mainly devoted to inquiries into the anomalies that became known as the "osteopathic lesion," which is now called somatic dysfunction. Skiagraphy, a crude form of x-ray, was used before 1900 to try to find

evidence of the structural abnormalities attributed to the osteopathic lesion. Soon after, animal models were used to determine the actual physiologic effects of the palpatory findings that made up the "lesion" (1). In 1906, the American Osteopathic Association (AOA) formed a research center, the A. T. Still Postgraduate College of Osteopathy, and called for donations to fund it. The name was changed to the A. T. Still Research Institute in 1909, and about $16,000 was raised to support its efforts. It was not until about 1913, when the Institute opened in a dedicated building in Chicago, that research under Wilborn J. Deason began. Funding continued to be a problem, even after Louisa Burns was appointed Director, and the Institute struggled to meet its modest needs, despite calls from the AOA for more research and support. Over the ensuing years, Burns produced a body of work investigating the effects of spinal "lesions" in a rabbit model. The results of her studies indicated that artificially produced strains of specific vertebral segments produced a somewhat reproducible constellation of changes in function of organs and tissues innervated from the area of strain. These changes were later substantiated by Wilbur Cole using various neural stains (2). Burns published four books (3–6), a collected work (7), and several reports from the Institute that, unfortunately, are not widely available today but that contain much of value to the modern researcher. She continued her work until the early 1950s.

During the first third of the 1900s, research in the profession was encouraged at several osteopathic schools (8). This research included studies on basic neural and physiologic mechanisms underlying somatic dysfunction and the effects of osteopathic treatment on symptoms and immune function. Much of this research would only be considered suggestive by today's standards, but formed the basis for lines of study produced later within the profession.

The Second Period of Research (1940 to 1969)

In 1938, J. S. Denslow began a path of inquiry that would lead to a program of research that literally defined the modern research era in the profession. He became convinced that to bring increased credibility to the profession, research based on the latest research standards and published in highly recognized journals would have to be done. This research would have to show the basic mechanisms underlying the osteopathic lesion (9). He

received training from internat
tists, including Ralph Gerard,
aimed at understanding the ch
relation to palpatory diagnosis.
by several others at Kirksville, tl
facilitated segment (10–12). T
dominate much of the osteopa
palpation and treatment to the

During the 1950s and 196(
sion did not expand greatly. Th
the AOA in 1939 to fund resear
forts at several schools, but exc
no research efforts of a full pi
studies, such as those on joint
published (13), but in genera
gressed slowly during this tim
sion was busy training a flood
to the new post-war world.

However, in the late 1950
fession emerged. Culminating
Osteopathic and Medical Assc
the profession would be eradic
years from 1960 to 1969 were
fession's future. In 1969, a ne
in Pontiac, Michigan, as the
between 1969 and 1980. The
and the profession began a peri
prosperity unparalleled in its l

Unfortunately, it was duri
threat that the profession mis
sion of biomedical research fac
World War II. The expansion
(NIH), with its emphasis on b
of new laboratories and progr
the biomedical research com
osteopathic profession was ur
expansion. By the time new
established in the 1970s, thi
expansion was over.

The Third Period of R

With the founding of new scr
inal schools remaining after
Chicago, Kansas City, Philac
fession finally achieved a base
research. The schools began t
and the political arms of the
encourage research endeavor:
ing research through the Bur
search Conference. Awards
productivity, such as the Lou
sohn/Denslow Award (1984)
Student research efforts were
encouraged more actively, fo
the Burnett Osteopathic Stu
tantly, the basis of research p
the new schools and rejuven

Experience in learning and receiving manipulative treatment is also an enlightening experience. However, researchers are trained to investigate new areas of knowledge and to ask questions of those areas. Basic scientists and others within the profession can easily access books and journals relevant to their osteopathic understanding. This book is a good start in that journey. A second source is the *Journal of the American Osteopathic Association,* where reviews, original research articles, and case studies are available. Other sources, such as A. T. Still's *Autobiography* (14) or his *Osteopathy Research and Practice* (15), are useful. Other books, such as Northup's books on the profession (16) and research (2), are useful in helping the basic scientist understand the profession.

As much as the researcher must be expected to find and read materials pertinent to his or her understanding, so must those knowledgeable in the profession be willing to help promote the necessary understanding. Osteopathic physicians and students must be willing to discuss their beliefs and clinical observations with often skeptical scientists. The experience of the 1989 AAO symposium (17) is illustrative of this point. Several internationally known basic scientists were assembled for 2 days of discussion prior to the symposium itself. They questioned the attending osteopathic physicians about the experiences of the profession, and consented to having osteopathic manipulative treatment. Rather than being antagonistic to the largely anecdotal clinical observations, they were uniformly supportive and excited by them. Several altered their prepared talks to reflect their new understanding and have maintained active contact with the profession since. In fact, one is actively training DO students in his laboratories. Active and open communication about ideas most often leads to exciting opportunities. Thus, the development of basic scientists who understand the osteopathic profession is a two-way street.

Although much has been accomplished in this area, the cadre of trained clinical and basic science investigators must be expanded to those who understand the principles and clinical experiences of osteopathy so that they can frame their research questions in the light of osteopathic clinical experience and theory. Without this understanding, data will not be examined from the perspective of osteopathic treatment and insight.

ETHICAL CONSIDERATIONS IN OSTEOPATHIC RESEARCH

Human Subjects Protection

Since the end of World War II, there has been a growing understanding of the problems associated with the ethical considerations of research on both human and animal subjects. The horrible experiments performed by physicians on prisoners in the Nazi concentration camps sparked reforms and regulations to control human medical experimentation. Coming out of the Nuremberg Trials and codified in the 1964 Declaration of Helsinki, these regulations have been the subject of continuing review, refinement, and discussion since then (18–20). The researcher who contemplates doing research in osteopathic topics must be aware of and abide by the current human subject regulations. Not only is this the law, but it is the moral and just thing to do. In fact, no reputable journal will publish results of a human study without evidence that applicable human subject guidelines have been scrupulously followed.

The novice investigator must be familiar with not only the principles of ethical treatment of subjects, but also with the procedures in effect in the institution where the research will be done. In the event that a private physician wishes to conduct human subject research in a private office, the research must first be approved by an appropriate human subjects review board, usually known as the institutional review board (IRB). The IRB is a governmentally sanctioned body whose members are appointed by the institutional executive in charge of research and the President or CEO of the institution, and must include individuals with specific interests, including a person who has no other affiliation with the institution.

INSTITUTIONAL REVIEW BOARD AUTHORITY

The IRB has the authority to deny or approve any research proposal involving human subjects. The main purpose of the IRB is to protect the safety of the subjects. It can stop ongoing research if it deems protection not sufficient or uncovers problems in the research. When applications for research are submitted to the IRB, the application can receive expedited review if certain conditions are met, such as that the research uses only data collected in the normal course of office practice and that are not identified with a patient. However, it is not up to the investigator to determine whether the research is exempt, can have expedited review, or must undergo full review. Case reports and retrospective reviews of cases (see discussion below) seen in the routine office practice do not generally need IRB approval unless the patient is identified or if written permission is given prior to release of any information.

MAJOR INSTITUTIONAL REVIEW BOARD CONSIDERATIONS

The major factors in human subject research include:

Informed consent
Confidentiality
Risk
Absence of coercion

One of the cornerstones of human subject protection is the principle of informed consent. This idea holds that the subject be informed of the study fully and completely and be able to give free consent to participation. If the subject be a minor, incapable of giving consent due to mental or other disability, or a prisoner, special and specific protections are specified.

The principle of subject confidentiality is another vital concern. The subject's confidentiality is to be protected and not divulged without the subject's written consent. Thus, medical and research data are considered private matters when linked to an identifiable subject. Data are usually coded in such a way that they cannot be linked to a particular patient and great care must be taken that no such link can be inferred.

Risk to the patient is another factor in human research. Risk to a patient runs from essentially nonexistent to grave. If the risk is anything but incidental, the subject must be fully informed of that risk and have every option to decline participation. The risk must also be justified by potential gain, perhaps not to the individual subject, but to the field. This assessment is difficult to make, and the investigator must therefore justify the study well.

Absence of coercion is a complex topic that is often debated in study design. Is providing a monetary incentive to a subject for time taken by the study coercion? Is the investigator using force of personality or doctor–patient relationship to coerce the subject to enter the study? These questions are difficult to quantify, and the committee and investigator must consider them carefully.

IRBs are usually in existence in osteopathic medical schools and in many hospitals. Each IRB is allowed operating discretion within established NIH guidelines as to how it reviews protocols. Some IRBs meet on a regular basis and others are on call. The potential investigator is responsible for finding the protocols used by the appropriate IRB and fully following these regulations.

It cannot be overemphasized how important it is to be cognizant of current guidelines for human subject protection and to fully adhere to them. For current and full information, including downloadable human subjects research guidelines, go the NIH web site at: *http://ohsr.od.nih.gov.*

Animal Protection

No less important in research on human subjects is the protection of subjects in animal research. As is evident from the media, animal rights have become a volatile issue in much of the world. Some of the emotion surrounding animal rights obviously stems from the fact that animals cannot give informed consent or judge risk in a study. In addition, by its nature, animal research often ends in the subject's death. For these and other reasons, some groups use violence to attempt to stop animal research.

Not unlike human subject protection, a well-defined, protective structure has been implemented by the NIH and other groups, such as the American Association for Assessment and Accreditation of Laboratory Animal Care (AAALAC), have promulgated guidelines and rules for the proper use of animals in research studies. The Animal Care and Use Committee (ACUC), a governmentally mandated body enforces these rules at research institutions. Like the IRB, the ACUC has the authority to shut down research not in compliance with applicable regulations and must approve all animal research prior to its start. The osteopathic researcher who wishes to use animals in research must first successfully seek ACUC approval. As with the IRB, each ACUC has latitude in its procedures about which the investigator must be informed. Again, as with human research, the investigator must be meticulous in following animal care and use guidelines: first and foremost, for moral and ethical reasons but also because humanely treated and well cared for animal subjects provide more reliable information. For more information on animal care and use guidelines, visit the NIH Office of Animal Care and Use site at *http://oacu.od.nih.gov/.* Another useful site is the American Association for Laboratory Animal Science site at *www.aalas.org* or the AAALAC site at *www.aaalac.org.*

Applying for Institutional Review Board or Animal Care and Use Committee Approval

The process for applying for research approval for either human or animal research is determined by each committee. Some commit-

tees meet monthly or more often; others meet on call. However, at the least, each protocol submitted for IRB or ACUC approval will have to contain the following elements:

> Background literature review
> Justification for the project
> Hypothesis to be tested
> Complete description of the methods to be used
> For human research:
> - Informed consent form
> - Confidentiality statements
> - How subjects will be obtained and paid for service
> For animal research:
> - Evidence that animals will be legally obtained and humanely housed
> - Evidence that precautions will be taken to minimize any necessary pain or suffering
> - Evidence that other alternatives to animal use are not available
> Data to be collected
> Statistical methods for analysis
> Any pilot data available

These items represent a fair amount of work that must be done prior to submitting a protocol for review. It also means that the investigator will find it necessary to think through the studies prior to getting approval. The appropriate approvals are also necessary before funds are awarded for the proposed research from government agencies.

TYPES OF RESEARCH IN OSTEOPATHIC MEDICINE

Basic Science

Within the purview of osteopathic research, there are several valid types of studies. Perhaps the most basic is research that flows from basic science studies. This research includes studies designed to define the basic functions of the body and mind, and explain how they interact with the environment. These studies are mainstream biomedical research. An increased understanding of the human organism and its function is invaluable in validating osteopathic practice. The osteopathic profession must therefore nurture the basic sciences.

Basic Research in Other Institutions and Professions

Basic science has been performed for many years in most biomedical facilities and research institutes. Most basic research relevant to the osteopathic profession is done not in the educational institutions of the profession but in other biomedical settings. The amount of research that can be supported directly by the profession is small compared with the amount of such research performed around the world. The total amount of funding available from within the osteopathic profession for support of its research programs is less per year than the annual budgets of many individual laboratories outside the profession. This suggests two things. First, maximal use must be made of data from laboratories outside the profession. Osteopathic researchers and clinicians must cultivate interactions with biochemical researchers at other institutions who can supply data and interpretations. Second, the limited resources of the profession must be put into research endeavors that provide the greatest return in explaining osteopathic experience and theory. This requires, as stated above, that investigators within the osteopathic profession understand the unique and defining concepts of osteopathy within which to interpret their findings. Without this understanding, the investigator is unable to interpret the findings in ways that are useful to the profession, and a large part of the research investment is lost.

The use of data from laboratories outside the profession is certainly a very useful and fruitful endeavor. We have made use of this mechanism in proposing mechanisms for the facilitated segment (21). However, care must be taken in using data generated in studies not specifically designed to answer the question to which the data are now being applied. Unless the limitations and specifics of the data are well known, implications can easily be made that are beyond the scope of the data and hence potentially misleading. It is important to realize these limitations, but to use data and sources from outside the profession whenever possible. Such was the case when the AAO commissioned two international symposia held in 1989 and 1992, which resulted in proceedings publications (17,22) that have been very useful in informing the profession of possible mechanisms for clinical phenomena and the results of manipulative treatment.

Integrative Model Building

Integrating Basic Science and Clinical Observation

A second type of research activity necessary within the profession is the integration of basic science knowledge and clinical observation. This endeavor is extremely valuable and potentially dangerous. A recent article by Van Buskirk (23) illustrates such research. In this article, Van Buskirk builds a theoretical model of somatic dysfunction based on nociceptive input. He marshals an impressive array of basic science data and synthesizes it in a unique way from his clinical understandings and observations. The result is a well-grounded look at one of the central concepts of the osteopathic philosophy of health and disease. This is the valuable aspect of the article.

The dangerous part is that the model will be taken as fact. Van Buskirk goes to great lengths to point out that the model seems to be explanatory but still needs to be subjected to rigorous research verification and clinical observation before it can be accepted as proven. Unfortunately, the pioneering models that came out of the research of Korr and Denslow (11,24) suffered from being taken as factual explanation rather than as models in need of experimental verification. Once a model has been accepted as truth, the perceived need for further research or theory is impeded or stopped, and the model becomes accepted as truth. This can be disastrous if the model is then shown to be erroneous or incomplete because there are then no alternatives to take its place. Integrative model building provides much needed direction for both basic and clinical research but must not be taken at face value without verification and experimental testing.

Thus, the osteopathic profession must continually examine its theories and subject its explanations to close scrutiny. The vast body of clinical evidence demonstrates that the precepts of the osteopathic profession are sound. However, often the profession embraces explanations that are not solidly research based. The result is theory taken for fact with further exploration of alternative theory or factual basis effectively stymied.

Synthesis and Meta-Analysis Research

Two types of scholarly activities that can be of immense benefit to any area are the synthesis review and the meta-analysis. Synthesis papers are efforts to review and critically analyze an area or field of study. In this type of work, the author would select a topic area for analysis and review all available work in that area. Although the review is in itself important, a synthesis then analyzes the work that has been done and attempts to find common themes, areas of agreement or disagreement, and then builds a hypothesis as to what the accumulated knowledge of the area is saying. This type of paper can often point to why seeming contradictions between studies exist, what studies should be done to finalize questions in the field, and so forth. Early in my career, we did such a synthesis for the field of spinal cord learning (25). The insights from that activity directed spinal cord plasticity research for many years—not only in our laboratories, but in other laboratories (26). Often, a good synthesis of an area will open the area for more intensive study and can be an impetus for real advances in an area that was seemingly uninteresting or filled with conflicting data.

The meta-analysis is another useful tool for research. This analysis attempts to accumulate all studies in a field that are deemed sufficiently rigorous and determine the combined power of the results. In this way, by statistically combining smaller studies that are not particularly convincing by themselves, it is often possible to achieve sufficient statistical or analytical power to have confidence in the phenomenon being investigated. Such an analysis was done on the area of spinal manipulation for low back pain and resulted in acceptance of that modality as effective treatment for acute low back pain (27). An analysis of spinal palpatory procedure validity and reliability is currently under way at the Center for Complimentary and Alternative Medicine at the University of California Irvine College of Medicine, and is sponsored by the trust fund acquired by that school when the California College of Osteopathic Medicine became the University of California Irvine College of Medicine in 1962. More information on procedures of meta-analysis can be found in many statistical texts (28).

Qualitative Studies in Osteopathy

Valuable information can often be gathered by means of surveys and interviews. Such studies, although not experimental, are often the only way to find trends in populations, practice distributions, or to gather the collected thought of experts in a field. Often, surveys seem simple and easy to perform. The investigator must only write down a few questions on a topic and send them out to some selected individuals and wait for the returns. Such simplicity is illusory. Good surveys must be well planned and executed. The topic must be carefully framed and the questions prepared with precision. Pitfalls in the use of surveys include poorly framed questions, problems in determining to whom the survey should be sent, poor return rates, and others (28). Prior to instituting a survey, an investigator must consult texts and/or experts in survey design and procedure. Within the osteopathic profession, Johnson and Kurtz have performed several surveys addressing such issues as student interests and the use of manipulative treatment (29–31). These studies have provided a baseline for the use of osteopathic manipulation in the profession and are invaluable in charting future direction within the profession. These surveys are excellent examples of well-done and analyzed survey studies.

Another instrument that can provide valuable information is the collection and analysis of expert interviews or writings of often long-departed authors. These methods also often seem deceptively simple. In fact, as with surveys, interviews with experts require extensive preparation and careful planning. Both directed and open-ended questions may be asked and answers recorded for later transcription, or the expert may be asked to write on predetermined topics. In any event, the answers must be carefully analyzed for content and other information. The analysis of writings by departed authors can be valuable in translating what may now seem to be arcane jargon into terms understandable in today's terminology. For example, why did Andrew Taylor Still put so much emphasis on the fasciae of the body? What did he mean by such terms as "fluids of life?" To understand these ideas in the way in which Still did, it would be necessary to find the meaning of those terms in the late 1800s, as well as to look at the context in which he used them. Various means of content analysis are available to help in such a task (32). Both interview analysis and writing analysis can be of great value to osteopathic understanding.

Epidemiology and Outcomes Studies

Epidemiologic studies have not been widely used in the osteopathic profession. It should be noted, however, that there are some very important epidemiologic topics awaiting study. Because epidemiology refers to the study of patterns of health and disease and what influences these patterns, those influences on health and loss of health that are of particular interest to osteopathic medicine should be subjected to such studies. One of the most important such study would be the incidence and natural history of somatic dysfunction in normal populations and various subpopulations with defined illness. As with most studies, epidemiologic studies of this entity would require careful planning and execution. However, it could reveal very important information on the potential uses for manipulative treatment modalities. The interested investigator can find more information in such references as *Medical Epidemiology* (33).

Outcome studies are a very important type of research that bridges both epidemiology and at times, experimental studies. In the usual such study, outcome measures are taken or reviewed for patient populations, and the outcomes of one type of treatment outcome, cost, patient satisfaction, and so on are reported. Outcome studies usually require large patient populations to gain sufficient data to be meaningful.

Research on Manipulation

As one of the key elements of osteopathic care, manipulative treatment should be the subject of increasing amounts of research in the profession. In research aimed at investigating the usefulness of manipulative treatment, there is much confusion about proper research methodology. However, the researcher approaching osteopathic manipulation as an independent variable must decide which of the following is to be evaluated:

A treatment or manipulative technique
Osteopathic manipulative treatment (OMT)
Osteopathic health care

Depending on the aspect of manipulation to be studied, different experimental designs will be employed. Too often, investigators fail to distinguish between these three entities and hence have difficulty determining the correct experimental design for their study.

MANIPULATIVE TECHNIQUES

One of the most illustrative studies of manipulative technique is the Irvine study, performed by Buerger and colleagues at the School of Medicine at the University of California, Irvine, in the late 1970s and early 1980s (34,35). They wished to determine the effects of a single lateral recumbent roll (high-velocity/low-amplitude thrust) on low back pain. The study was elegantly designed and executed, with a result that showed an immediate effect of the lateral recumbent roll on certain measured variables; simply positioning the patient for a lateral recumbent roll and omitting the thrust did not provide the same changes. After a few weeks, however, no differences between the experimental and control groups remained, probably the result of the nature of the presenting complaint, which has a natural history of relief in a few weeks. Nonetheless, an immediate effect of the thrust was seen. The point missed by many readers was that the investigation was not of OMT but of a treatment technique.

THE IRVINE STUDY COMPARED WITH CLINICAL TRIALS OF MEDICAL INTERVENTIONS

In many ways, the Irvine study was similar to drug studies. One specific manipulative technique was used on each patient in the experimental group (and not in the control group), the patients were blinded to whether they received manipulation, and measurable variables were used. In the typical drug trial, the specific effects of a certain chemical compound on the course of a specific set of symptoms are studied. The design of the study controls for other factors that might cause a change in the outcome. This is a legitimate model for the study of a specific technique within manipulative treatment. If the intent of the study is to determine the effect of a specific and repeatable manipulation, the research design should emulate the design of a drug trial, including attempts to blind the patient to whether the technique was delivered. Such studies are useful in instances where there may be reason to suspect that a specific manipulative technique would change a particular condition. Great care must be taken to control for:

The actual presenting complaint
Whether the patient has knowledge of manipulation

The actual delivery of the technique to make certain that it is given in the same way to each patient

Such studies can be useful as long as it is recognized that the study's purpose is to evaluate the effect of a specific, single, or small group of physical manipulations on a specific condition. Another recent example of this design was published by Wells and colleagues (36), who looked at the effects of a set of standard manipulative techniques on gait parameters of patients with Parkinson disease. They found that the standardized techniques produced increased performance in various aspects of gait in these individuals. Such designs, performed correctly, give information on the effects of a technique on some aspect of patient function.

STUDIES OF MANIPULATIVE TREATMENT

This type of research is used to study the effects of OMT on one or more measurable patient parameters. The research design and the goals are somewhat different from those used in technique studies. Korr (37) has elegantly reviewed these differences. Osteopathic theory and practice holds that the full treatment of an individual by an osteopathic physician entails an interaction between the physician and the patient that is not static but dynamic, changing from treatment to treatment and instant to instant as the treatment progresses. The physician responds to the dynamic changes in the patient's function; the patient responds to the attitudes and touch of the physician. The treatment is not a prearranged set of movements and thrusts given to each patient, but an ongoing stimulus/response synergism between the physician and patient, with the patient's response guiding the actions of the physician.

In this case, the manipulation cannot be predetermined or prescribed by the research protocol but must "go with the flow" in response to the reactions of both physician and patient. The manipulative treatment is properly a "black box." The physician/patient interaction determines what manipulative treatment is performed. The physician is free to do what is deemed best for the interaction. Because one of the basic axioms of osteopathy is that each person responds differently to stress and treatment, this freedom of interaction cannot be removed from the physician without changing the research to a technique investigation. To investigate manipulative treatment rather than a manipulative technique, manipulative treatment must be used.

The recent study on the effects of osteopathic treatment on low back pain by Andersson and colleagues (38), comparing manipulation with standard of care is a case in point. In this study, treating osteopathic physicians were allowed to use any manipulative techniques necessary for the patient. The study found that there were no differences in outcomes, but that the group treated with manipulation required less medication and physical therapy. In this study, unlike in a technique study, the physician chose the treatment that was indicated for the patient.

Technique Versus Manipulative Treatment

Once the difference between these two basic types of research on manipulation is realized, many of the other problems associated with investigating manipulation can be much more easily resolved. Both types of research are valuable and valid. Research on techniques gives information on specific techniques; research on treatment gives information on what the osteopathic physician does in practice. Both are necessary and essential for the future of the profession. Their differences must be recognized and appreciated for appropriate studies to be designed.

Subtypes of Manipulative Treatment

Within the general types of research on manipulative treatment, there can be several subtypes. One aims at the effect of manipulative treatment in general on some aspect of a disease or body function. This could be called the nonspecific design. It is done to improve body function without identifying specific somatic dysfunction in patients with some clinical presenting complaint. The treating physician provides a general manipulative treatment without specifying areas of somatic dysfunction or specific areas to be addressed. By contrast, in specific treatment designs, the physician applies manipulative treatment to specific somatic dysfunction as defined by palpatory diagnosis and documented with such signs as asymmetric motion, tissue texture changes, and so forth. This type of treatment is designed to restore function or ameliorate functional difficulties and may or may not be related to actual presenting complaints (the patient may not be aware of some somatic dysfunction). In each of these study types, appropriate data on what is done must be collected, and specific measures of outcome must be made.

Effectiveness Studies

A third type of study incorporates either of the first two: the effectiveness study, in which manipulative treatment is given to alleviate a specific presenting complaint. The patient is selected for a particular complaint, such as low back pain; the treating physician gives appropriate manipulative treatment. The effect of the treatment on the complaint (e.g., low back pain) is measured. This study type may or may not require the delineation of somatic dysfunction during treatment. Efficacy studies are the most usual in the literature because the measure of results is the most straightforward.

Functional Outcomes of Manipulative Treatment

In the fourth design subtype, the functional outcome design, the effect of manipulative treatment on general physiologic function is assessed. In the philosophy of the osteopathic profession, the origin of disease is believed to be some loss of normal function in the body that then allows for the development of clinical symptoms. This type of study is accomplished on clinically disease-free subjects with somatic dysfunction who are addressed with specific treatment. Measures of outcome are such things as:

Immune system function
Tolerance to stress
General activities of daily living assessments (in older subjects)
Other measures of normal function that assess general health and function

Presumably, such studies would find increases in the functional ability or capacity of treated subjects.

TOTAL OSTEOPATHIC CARE STUDIES

Another general study design takes into account the total care given by the osteopathic physician; it is not limited to manipulative treatment. This study type assesses the health status of patients given care by osteopathic physicians and presumably, but not necessarily, includes manipulative treatment over the course of care. Such studies are longitudinal or cross-sectional in nature and include as data such things as disease episodes and measures of total body function and activities of daily living. If the osteopathic philosophy of health is taken seriously, there is a heavy component of preventive care that would include periodic manipulative treatment to correct somatic dysfunction as it occurs. Such care should prevent a least some of the acute disease episodes seen in nonmanipulated subjects. A study of this kind would be expensive and long-term, and could be approached in various ways. Research of this type could show whether the application of osteopathic principles to health care is differentiated from disease care. Practitioners applying total osteopathic care to their patients would be used to determine if their outcomes in terms of patient health were different from physicians not using osteopathic care. Obviously, there would be many potentially confounding factors that would have to be analyzed. Interesting results, such as cost/benefit ratios, quality of life issues, and others, could be addressed.

DESIGNING AND CONDUCTING OSTEOPATHIC RESEARCH

Understanding the basics of what type of study is to be done is an important step in beginning osteopathic research. Realizing the importance of ethical considerations and data confidentiality is vital. The next steps in a research project are also vital. These steps can be characterized as follows:

Observation
Literature search
Hypothesis building
Study Design
Data Collection
Data Analysis
Discussion of results
Publication

These steps are all necessary and important in the conduct of research in any field. We will briefly discuss each.

Observation

Virtually all biomedical research stems from clinical observation. The clinician observes patients and their response to illness and treatment. He or she often conducts impromptu "experiments" to see if there is any effect on a patient's outcome. Such observations are valuable, but rarely conclusive. Observations are usually subject to too many uncertainties, called biases, to lead to definitive conclusions about what actually occurred or whether there was really an effect of a certain treatment on a condition. The realization over many years that observation by itself was rarely useful in establishing reliable cause and effect relationships in fact led to the art of research design. However, observation is the beginning point for investigation. The investigator should begin with observation of his or her practice. What is of special interest to the investigator? One of the most important aspects of doing research is to pick a topic that piques the interest. Once that is accomplished, the basis of a research project is laid. A prime example of observation being the basis for a lifetime of research is that of Larry Jones (39). He made the observation of a patient with severe muscle spasm that was relieved by placing the patient into an extremely awkward position to alleviate the pain. Instead of dismissing the result as spurious or inconsequential, Jones pursued the observation and developed the area of strain/counterstrain.

Literature Search

The next step in developing a research project is the literature search. This is a very important step and one that is often either slighted or done without sufficient diligence. The first steps in a literature search are to examine texts and other reference works easily available. Do they show that the problem interesting the investigator has already been thoroughly researched? Is there an abundance of literature already available? Or does a preliminary search reveal little or no information? Texts and reference books are called secondary literature because they report second hand on research articles (primary literature). Hopefully, something will easily be found in the secondary literature that will lead to primary research articles or even reviews of the topic.

The search for information will almost invariably lead to the primary literature; to journals in which research findings are presented. The search for primary literature can be greatly simplified by using one of the many computer resources now available. The National Library of Medicine (NLM) has the largest compilation of medical literature in the world. This resource is available to anyone with World Wide Web access. The "search engines" for the NLM database may be accessed free through services like PUBMED or by fee-for-service engines, such as PaperChase. These search engines make searching the many millions of articles in MEDLINE and its associated databases easy and fast. However, the search must be done with some skill in selecting appropriate search terms or author names, or the result may be a return of thousands of often irrelevant articles. Hopefully, the search will be productive in producing several articles and papers on the topic at hand. The investigator may then proceed to acquire the articles through libraries or by ordering them on-line, and begin to read about what is known about his or her topic.

The search can be both a time-consuming and strenuous task. In osteopathic medicine, there is only one journal included in the NLM databanks: the *Journal of the American Osteopathic Association* (JAOA). Because the NLM Medline database only goes back to 1966, it is also important to review articles in earlier issues of the JAOA (as it often is for other journals). Thus, the investigator may have to actually go to a library with holdings of the journal and search back issues, or ask the librarian to review an index of the journal for relevant topics. In addition, other osteopathic source materials should be searched. The AAO has an important collection of osteopathic articles in its Yearbook collection and has now released a CD-ROM with its bibliography in searchable form. This listing should be included in any search. Other osteopathic collections, such as the *Osteopathic Annals* (no longer published), are also valuable sources of information.

Many of the on-line databases available to the investigator are listed in Table 74.1. We are grateful to Willard and Swartzlander (40) for granting permission to use this table. When using any database, it is advisable to keep careful records of articles read and what was in each. A computer database program, such as Reference Manager or Endnote *(www.isiresearchsoft.com),* is excellent

for this purpose, and such programs also allow easy construction of bibliographies when writing papers.

What should be looked for during a literature search? Obviously, the primary goal is to find articles and information on the topic of interest. What has been found about the topic? What research or observations have already been made? It is also important to find how others have looked at the area. If research has been done, how was it done, and what measures did the investigators use in the studies? What techniques and research designs were used? If other research has been done, it is best to find how it was done, what pitfalls were encountered, and how they were overcome.

TABLE 74.1. MAJOR REFERENCE SOURCES FOR THE MEDICAL AND LIFE SCIENCES[a]

Print	CD-ROM	Online
Index Medicus (1879+)	Medline (1966+) OVID Cambridge Scientific Abstract DIALOG SilverPlatter	Medline (1966+) OVID NLM DIALOG DataStar
Excerpta Medica (1946+)	EMBASE (1974+) OVID SilverPlatter	EMBASE (1974+) OVID DIALOG
Biological Abstracts (1926+)	Biological Abstracts (1985+) OVID SilverPlatter	BIOSIS Previews (1969+) OVID DIALOG DataStar
Cumulative Index to Nursing α Allied Health (1960+)	CINAHL (1983+) OVID SilverPlatter Cambridge Scientific Abstracts	CINAHL (1983+) OVID DataStar
Chemical Abstracts (1907+)		CA Search (1967+) OVID DIALOG DataStar ORBIT
Science Citation Index (1961+)	SCISEARCH Institute for Scientific Information (ISI)	SCISEARCH (1974+) DIALOG DataStar
Hospital Literature Index (1945+)	Health Planning and Administration OVID	Healthline (1975+) NLM Health Planning and Administration (1975+) OVID DIALOG
Current Contents-Clinical Medicine (1973+) Current Contents-Life Sciences (1958+)	Current Contents on Diskette Institute for Scientific Information (ISI)	Current Contents OVID DIALOG
Psychological Abstracts (1894+)	PsycLIT (1974+) OVID SilverPlatter	PsycINFO (1967+) OVID DIALOG
Nutrition Abstracts (1931+)	CAB Abstracts SilverPlatter	CAB Abstracts (1972+) OVID DIALOG CHIROLARS (1900+) OVID
Physician's Desk Reference (PDR) Merck Manual	Physician's Desk Reference Medical Economics with or without Merck Manual	

(continued)

TABLE 74.1. (*continued*)

Print	CD-ROM	Online

Martindale: The Extrapharmacopoeia	Martindale CD-ROM Microindex	Martindale Online
		  DIALOG
		  DataStar

		Comprehensive Core Medical Library (CCML) (1982+) OVID (full text)

		National Library of Medicine (NLM)
		  MEDLINE
		  AIDSLINE
		  AIDSDRUGS
		  AIDSTRIALS
		  BIOETHICSLINE
		  CATLINE
		  AVLINE
		  CHEMLINE
		  HEALTH
		  CANCERLIT
		  TOXLINE
		  TOXLIT
		  DIRLINE
		  SERLINE
		  HSTAR
		  SPACELINE
		  PDQ

[a]The underlined terms represent specific databases; nonunderlined terms represent the vendors carrying the databases.
MEDLINE, produced by the U.S. National Library of Medicine (NLM), is one of the premier sources of biomedical literature. MEDLINE corresponds to three print indexes: Index Medicus, Index to Dental Literature, and International Nursing Index. More than 3,700 journals are indexed and more than 70% of the records contain author abstracts.
EMBASE, the Excerpta Medica database, is a leading source for biomedical and pharmaceutical literature. It contains citations and abstracts to more than 3,500 international journals.
BIOSIS Previews is one of the world's most comprehensive databases in the life sciences. More than 6,500 serials, 2,000 international meetings as well as books and monographs are monitored for inclusion.
CINAHL provides bibliographic access to important nursing and allied health journals in the fields of cardiopulmonary technology, emergency services, laboratory technology, medical assistants, occupational therapy, physical therapy, physician's assistants, radiologic technology, respiratory therapy, and surgical technology.
CA SEARCH database includes more than 10 million citations to the literature of chemistry and its applications.
SCISEARCH is a multidisciplinary index to the literature of science and technology prepared by the Institute for Scientific Information (ISI). Cited reference searches are possible in this database.
Health Planning and Administration contains references to nonclinical literature on all aspects of health care planning and facilities, health insurance, the aspects of financial management, personnel administration, manpower planning, and licensure and accreditation that apply to the delivery of health care.
Current contents is a weekly service that reproduces the tables of contents from current issues of leading journals in clinical medicine and life sciences and five other subsets.
PsycINFO database provides access to the international literature in psychology and related behavioral and social sciences, including psychiatry, sociology, anthropology, education, pharmacology, and linguistics.
CAB Abstracts is a comprehensive file of agricultural and biologic information and contains all records in the 26 main abstract journals published by CAB International.
CHIROLARS is a health care database that emphasizes health promotion, prevention, and conservation care. More than 700 periodicals are included from medical, osteopathic, physical therapy, chiropractic, and other disciplines.
National Library of Medicine computer files contain approximately 15 million records covering its holdings of books, journal articles, and more. With GRATEFUL MED software, health professionals in even the most rural areas can access the files listed in this table.

Thus, the literature review is a vital and often very poorly done part of any study. Careful literature review will often save the investigator much work and even embarrassment. It is not good to find, after doing a study, that someone else has already done it or one similar.

The literature search allows the investigator to go to the next step of research design: the formation of the research hypothesis.

The Hypothesis

One of the most important aspects of designing any research project, be it quantitative or qualitative, experimental or observational, is forming the hypothesis. The hypothesis is the statement of the question being asked by the study. The hypothesis must be clear and concise. It must state exactly what the research is to investigate. Most beginning researchers try to make the hypothesis too complex or design a hypothesis that is simply not testable. For example, the hypothesis "osteopathic treatment is good for headaches" is not a good hypothesis. Although we would like to think that the statement is true, can we test it? The answer is no. What is "osteopathic treatment?" What does "good" mean? What type of headache is to be studied? A good experimental hypothesis is simple, precise, and well defined.

The Hypothesis Dictates the Study Design

The hypothesis also will dictate the design of the study to be done. Too often, an investigator produces an imprecise hypothesis and then has difficulty designing the appropriate study because the actual question and its implications are not clear. If the hypothesis is clear and simple, the design of the study will not only be much more evident, but it will be defensible to others. For example, in the Irvine study referenced above (41), the hypothesis was simple and straightforward: "What is the effect of a lateral recumbent roll thrust on measures of well-defined, acute low back pain?" This hypothesis defined the study as a technique study on a well-defined problem, acute low back pain (which was very precisely specified).

Thus, the hypothesis, not a preconceived notion of design, must dictate the study design. Too often, it is assumed that one type of study design is the only one appropriate for some type of research, such as manipulative medicine, when in actuality, the design flows from the question being asked. If the investigator has the question clearly in mind, the research design can be chosen and refined to reflect that question, not some other question that is not being asked.

Once the hypothesis is determined, it is usually converted to the "null hypothesis." The null hypothesis simply states the negative of the experimental hypothesis. Thus, if the experimental hypothesis was that "a lateral recumbent thrust will have an effect on acute low back pain," the null hypothesis would be that "a lateral recumbent thrust will have no effect on acute low back pain." The null hypothesis can be disproved by a study showing an effect, but a study showing no effect does not necessarily prove that no effect exists. Rather, it shows only that an effect was not observed in the present study. Thus, the null hypothesis is the preferred statement with the intent of the study to disprove it. In fact, many study designs provide both null and experimental hypotheses.

Study Design

The design of a research project is vital to the success and value of that project. In osteopathic research, there are many types of studies that can be done, as outlined above in this chapter. Once the investigator has chosen the topic of the study and has at least stated the hypothesis, if not completely refined it, the choice of research designs must be made. Is the research to be:

Observational
Epidemiologic
Descriptive
Experimental

Each of these types of research has particular requirement for design components (28,32,42). The investigator must consult with experienced clinical research designers for appropriate help.

In the area of research on manipulative techniques or treatment, the most usual type of study is either a descriptive or experimental study. In descriptive studies, patients are simply treated, and the results of the treatment are reported.

CASE STUDIES
Case Report

A case study is the report of a single, supposedly unique case, or of a unique treatment of a case. In case studies, a patient's history

is given, the treatment is described, and the results are reported. The case study was the staple for medical research many years ago, but is now only infrequently used. Many medical journals will no longer publish case studies except under the most stringent circumstances. Case studies are useful as observations leading to more complete studies, but rarely stand on their own. The limitations of case studies include poor recording of findings, incomplete history and physical reporting, and in many cases, unconfirmed diagnosis. If the investigator believes that a case is sufficiently unique to warrant publication, a very complete literature review must be done prior to attempted publication to assure that no such findings have been previously reported. Kaprow and Sandhouse recently reported on the treatment of a case by osteopathic manipulation, an example of a relatively unique treatment of an uncommon complaint (43).

Case Series: Retrospective

Case series are of two types. The first is the retrospective case series. In this design, the investigator searches the office files for all cases of a similar type and attempts, through reviewing the cases, to find commonalities in symptoms, treatment, or outcomes that warrant publication. The retrospective case series brings together similar cases to add credibility to a unique or new clinical entity or treatment regime. The retrospective case series may add weight to an argument that a new or unrecognized clinical syndrome is emerging, or that a new treatment technique is effective, but suffers the same problems as the single case study; the data are usually not uniform and diagnoses may be lacking. In addition, there is little assurance in a retrospective case series that all patients of the targeted type have been included; it is possible that only selected cases have been reported, making the results seem more beneficial than is actually the case.

Case Series: Prospective

Prospective case series studies are usually done after the realization that some treatment has a greater impact than thought or can be used on some unique condition. In this study type, nothing new is introduced, but only usual and standard practices may be used in a different manner. However, the means of identifying prospective patients, the data to be collected, and the methods of treatment are clearly specified in advance. All patients that meet the predefined criteria are treated and the data recorded uniformly. Thus, there is some assurance that the patients actually had the specified condition and the data gathered are uniform.

In most cases, case series do not have to be approved by an IRB unless a new treatment is being tried or data not usually collected in the course of practice are being collected. Although somewhat more indicative of effect, the prospective case series fall short of providing convincing arguments for effectiveness, because there is no comparison with other treatments or subjects.

OTHER OBSERVATIONAL STUDY DESIGNS

As mentioned above, various other types of designs, such as interview, epidemiologic, survey, and outcomes designs, are useful for many aspects of osteopathic research and can bring powerful and useful data to bear on such questions as:

How do the attitudes of osteopathic students toward the profession change over their training?

How satisfied are the patients of osteopathic physicians?

What did statements of pioneers in the profession mean?

How do patients of osteopathic physicians choose their doctors?

What is the incidence of somatic dysfunction in the normal population?

These and many other questions are awaiting well-planned studies and would produce information valuable for planning the future of the profession.

Experimental Design

The proof of cause and effect relationships is very difficult. Humans are very good at recognizing what seem to be correlations between two events, a trait that has undoubtedly been honed over thousands of years. The rustle of grass on a dark night correlates well with the approach of a tiger intent on finding a meal, and quickly becomes a signal for retreat to a safe cave. However, the rustle does not cause the cat to eat the unwary human. The human (and other animal) nervous systems are well adapted to recognizing correlation, but poorly designed to establish cause and effect. The art (and some would say, science) of experimental design has been developed to find ways to be able to assign cause and effect relationships in all areas of science.

Medical science is one of the most difficult areas in which to assign cause and effect relationships. The human organism is very complex, and what may seem like cause and effect relationships may be nothing more than random variation in function or disease state, or even the patient's own perception of how they are feeling. For example, the drug Laetrile was for years thought to produce good results for advanced cancer patients, but was finally shown to be useless and perhaps harmful (44). Patients and doctors alike thought that there was a cause-effect relationship between cancer outcomes and Laetrile therapy (that Laetrile cured cancer); in fact, there was neither a cause-effect relationship, nor even a decent correlation.

In experimental studies, a treatment group of some sort is compared with a control group. Ideally, the experimental and control groups differ in only one way; the treatment is given to the experimental group and not to the control group. Although this seems a simple task at first, in reality it is very difficult, especially in medical areas. As the complexity of this task unfolds, remember that when designing a research project, there is no such thing as the perfect design. Research designs always mean making compromises and choices that open the results to other interpretations. The problem is not that the design is not perfect; the problem is in not recognizing the imperfections and dealing with them.

Types of Experimental Designs

Experimental designs for osteopathic research can take several forms, depending on the question being asked. These include:

Between-subject designs
Within-subject designs
Crossover designs
Variations

The hallmark of an experimental design is the comparison of the treated or experimental group of patients with a group receiving no, or some other, treatment. The experimental study is always prospective, that is, it is planned in advance and must always be approved by an IRB.

BETWEEN-SUBJECT DESIGNS

The simplest experimental design is that comparing a treated group with a historical control. Historical controls would be patients from the practice or from other practices that had received some other form of treatment than the one being investigated. This design is considered to be weak in its ability to define cause-effect relationships. It is only one step above the prospective case series design, because the control subjects may or may not be comparable to the experimental subjects. However, in some cases, such as very severe disease states or when it is considered unethical to withhold a putative treatment, it may be the only way to attempt to determine the effect of a new or altered treatment regimen.

The most usual of the experimental designs is the two or more group direct comparison design. In this study design, patients fitting the criteria for inclusion in the study are randomly assigned to one group or the other. If the design is an experimental and control group design, the subjects in the experimental group receive the treatment and the subjects in the control group receive either no treatment or some alternative (perhaps community standard) treatment. The results of the two groups are then compared on one or more measures.

Independent and Dependent Variables

The treatment given to the experimental group is the "independent variable," and the measures taken to judge results in both groups are the "dependent variables." Thus, in a study comparing the lateral recumbent thrust, such as the Irvine study, the independent variable was the thrust given to the experimental group, but not the control group. The dependent variables included straight leg raising and judgment of pain before and after the treatment. One of the hardest aspects of research on osteopathic manipulative treatment is finding good dependent variables or measures of results.

Random Assignment to Groups

In experimental studies, it is very important that the two groups of patients be as much alike as possible. For example, if some systematic difference between the groups existed at the beginning of the study, such as the mean age of the experimental group being 24 and the control group being 56, a better result in the experimental group may well be due not to the treatment provided, but to the superior health of the younger patients. The comparability of the groups is usually achieved by "random assignment" of the patients to the groups. The patients are assigned to the groups completely at random, so that neither the investigator's bias nor other factors will result in patients in one group being different in any systematic way from the other group. There are many ways to do random assignment (44), but it is vital that it be done; how it is to be done must be specified prior to the study. Randomization can be as simple as flipping a coin to determine the group a patient is assigned to, but more reliable means are available, such as random number tables in books or on computers.

Blinding

One of the most important aspects of experimental research is the principle of blinding. It is well known that even the most honest investigator can unwittingly affect the results of a study by judging the results of a treated patient as better than an untreated patient. This often slight and unconscious bias or systematic error has often resulted in faulty and unreliable results from an otherwise well-designed study. To preclude this type of error, it is almost always necessary to make sure that the person measuring the outcome of a treatment does not know whether the patient received the experimental treatment (independent variable) or not. If the observer is blind to the patient's group, the study is called a single blind study. If the patient is also blinded to the treatment given, the study is a double-blind study. At times, it is also desirable to have others in the study blind to patient group. However, at the absolute least, the observer must be blind to the patient's treatment status. If blinding of this sort cannot be shown or is not feasible, the study has a very serious problem that almost always will make the results suspect. This subject will be further discussed in the section on Special Considerations on Osteopathic Clinical Research, below.

WITHIN-SUBJECT AND CROSSOVER DESIGNS

The research types reviewed above include mainly those that use planned comparisons between experimental and control groups, or long-term determinations of health status that are then compared with the general population. Many variations on these study types exist. Another group of study types should receive careful attention when the effects of manipulative techniques or treatment are studied. These designs are within-subject designs; they essentially use the same subject as both the control and experimental group. Keating et al. (45) have summarized this type of design in some detail.

The within-subject study usually involves following a patient for a period of time to determine the baseline symptoms and whether they are fairly stable or changing in some fairly predictable fashion. After the baseline measurement, treatment is introduced and the measurements continued. The measured variables can be compared before and after treatment to see if the treatment had an effect. The baseline measurement period will vary among several subjects, allowing the treatment to be introduced at different times, assuring that there was no peculiar effect of time on treatment intervention. This is known as the variable baseline, within-subject study design. Frymann (46) used this design type in her study of the effects of osteopathic care of children with neurologic and developmental deficits.

Crossover designs usually use experimental and control groups, but after the control group has finished, these patients are "crossed over" to receive the experimental treatment. Crossing over sometimes meets objections that the control group will not get the benefit of a supposedly effective treatment. This design is useful if the illness or disease being studied is not particularly severe and can wait to receive the experimental treatment.

Crossover and within-subject studies are not especially effective if the measurements and symptoms are not fairly stable for a period of time that can be used as the control condition. In addition, there is some problem with establishing whether the manipulative intervention actually did cause any change in the symptoms being measured. However, these designs allow treatment for every subject in the study, whereas the control group does not receive treatment in traditional experimental and control group studies.

The study designs considered here have many variations that must be considered before final design elements are determined. Some of the major issues in design of osteopathic research are considered below in the Special Considerations section of this chapter. The investigator is also urged to consult design experts and/or reference texts (28,32).

Data Collection

The actual work of doing the study comes only after careful planning, written statement of the study, and IRB approval. It is absolutely necessary to do the preliminary steps carefully and completely, or the study will almost certainly be useless due to problems of design, execution, or data collection. The entire procedure of the study design must be written out so that all those involved in the study will fully understand every step. When writing or reviewing a clinical study protocol, I do not consider the design to be complete until the informed reader of the protocol will know from reading the document what happens to the patient all the way through the study.

Data collection is the actual performance of the study. The patients are recruited, assigned to groups, treated (or not), and measurements performed. The data are collected by the appropriate study participant, including measures of somatic dysfunction, functional tests, laboratory results, and so forth. All data must be kept confidential until the study is over (unless it is agreed to look at preliminary data earlier). The study group should meet frequently during the study itself to discuss any problems or concerns. Data analysis is the next step.

Data Analysis

Once data collection has been completed, the task of data analysis begins. Data from most studies must be subjected to some form of statistical analysis as a help in decision making. At most, statistical analysis is a way to help the investigator make informed decisions about the meaning of the data. Statistical tests are of three basic types:

Descriptive statistics
Nonparametric statistics
Parametric statistics

Descriptive statistics give information about the basic attributes of the collected data, such as the mean, median, and standard deviation. These numbers tell the investigator how each group performed on the dependent variables used. However, to obtain information about whether there might be a difference between the performance means of the experimental and control groups, some form of nonparametric or parametric statistical tests are used. The decisions about whether the independent variable caused a change in the experimental group's responses (dependent variables) rely on the results of tests of significance.

Statistical tests to determine differences between group data rely on the assumption that the experimental or independent variable caused a change in the experimental group that resulted in an actual difference being created between the groups, as measured by the dependent variable(s). According to this view, if the measure was the distance moved by the leg in a straight leg raising test, both groups would have the same average movement prior to treatment, but the treated group would have more movement after treatment. Thus, the treated group would now be a different group or population, as measured by straight leg raising tests. The treatment changed them from what they were before to a group able to perform straight leg raising to a greater level.

Several things determine how well the statistical test is able to indicate this difference. Two of the most powerful of these are the amount of variability in the initial measurements of the groups, and the number of subjects in each group (subject numbers are discussed below, under Power). If all subjects initially had exactly the same movement distances, then a very small increase in all the treated subjects would be detected by the statistical test as a significant effect. However, if there was a great deal of variability among the subjects, then a much larger average increase due to the treatment would be necessary before the statistical test could predict that the treatment had produced an effect. Thus, variability is best kept as small as possible between subjects in any study.

Parametric statistical tests, such as the t test or analysis of variance (ANOVA), make some assumptions about the distributions of the data and the population of subjects, in effect relying on the data to have a "normal" or bell-shaped distribution. If the data do not have roughly such a distribution, it is best to use nonparametric statistics, such at the Mann-Whitney test, to determine whether the results of the study show a difference due to the independent variable (47).

Many fairly simple computer programs are now available to help with statistical analysis. Such programs as Kaleida-Graph *(www.synergy.com)*, Instat *(www.graphpad.com)*, GB Stat *(www.gbstat.com)*, the SPSS packages (such as SYSTAT at *www.spssscience.com/SYSTAT*), and others are available for both Apple and IBM-compatible computers (see also, for example, *http://ebook.stat.ucla.edu/*). However, statistical assistance should be sought to avoid mistakes in analysis.

STATISTICAL SIGNIFICANCE

Tests for differences between groups provide an estimate of whether differences in the dependent measures seen between the groups after the study can be relied on to have actually been produced by the independent variable, or whether the differences are

more likely to have been the result of random or chance fluctuations. The reliability of the difference is called the significance of the test, or the level of statistical significance. By tradition, and some logic, the usual standard value that must be reached for a difference between the experimental and control groups to be considered significant is $p = 0.05$. This is the so-called p value, and is a measure that takes into account the variability of the data and the numbers of subjects in the study, among other things. The p value is essentially an estimate of the probability that the study would show a difference as great as or greater than the observed difference purely by chance.

Thus, a p value equal to 0.05 means that only one time in 20 or five in 100 would a difference as great or greater than that observed happen by chance alone, if the experimental variable actually had no effect. Thus, p values greater than 0.05 are considered probably due to chance fluctuations in measurement or to weak effects of the experimental variable. If the p value is 0.05 or less, it is assumed that the chances of finding the observed differences by chance are so small that the differences can be accepted as due to the experimental variable.

It is a mistake, however, to assume that if the data show a p value "approaching" 0.05 ($p = 0.056$, for example), that the data are "almost" significant. In many cases, the addition of additional subjects or other refinements of the study produce no more significant results. If the data are close to significance, consider ways to redo the study with less variable data or stronger treatment.

The investigator must generally consult with a biostatistician before finalizing a study design. The statistician will give advice on what data can be successfully analyzed and how the data can best be collected. In addition, due to the number of different statistical tests available, the methods of analysis should be specified before the study is undertaken.

Discussion

Once the data are analyzed, the investigator can undertake a discussion of the results and the study. The results must be considered in light of the background of the study, the results themselves, and the interpretation of those results by the investigator.

Data are only data; they are nothing until interpreted. The results of any study can be looked at in various ways. Consider what happened in the Irvine study. Osteopathic physicians looked at the data and basically said that the study was not important because the independent variable, the thrust, was not osteopathic treatment or spinal manipulation, but only a thrust. Allopathic physicians viewed the results as insignificant because the thrust and nonthrust groups showed no differences 3 weeks later. However, immediately after the technique, there was a significant difference. Presumably, the thrust patients would have been able to return to work sooner, an important difference to an insurance company paying for time off work. Thus, if the study had been correctly interpreted as a technique study and the immediate effects recognized as important, the study would have made more of an impact.

The discussion or interpretation of the data is where the investigator can state his or her opinion of the outcomes, link them to other data, and interpret them for the osteopathic profession. The discussion should not be too grandiose, claiming that the study had proven everything in the universe (unless it really has), but the investigator should legitimately link the study to the areas of interest and suggest to the reader how the data are important. This is another reason that a good literature review is necessary; without that background, the investigator will not be able to properly interpret the results.

Writing and Publication

If it is not documented, it did not happen. This statement is true for data gathering, observations during a study, orders given for participants of a study, and for publication of the results of a study. If a study is done but not published, it did not happen. It is vital to write a report of a study and publish it in some format. There are numerous books available for the novice scientific writer (48). However, the investigator can follow basically the same format as that given above in the design of a study for writing a scientific paper.

The parts of a research paper, although varying to some extent, are basically:

Abstract
Introduction
Methods
Results
Discussion
Conclusions (sometimes not included)
References

The abstract of any paper should present a concise and informative overview of the paper. Where the idea came from should be stated; this can be an overview of the literature review or observations that led to the idea for the study. The major methods should be given along with the major findings. The import of these findings finishes the abstract. Such statements as "The results are found below" or "The results will be discussed" are inappropriate. The abstract is the only thing that many people will read, so it must immediately tell the reader why they should look at the rest of the paper. Seeing it as unimportant, many writers dash off an abstract although it is a very important part of the paper.

The introduction is basically the background of the study. It gives an overview of the literature and other information about why the study was conceived. It provides the reader with the rational for the hypothesis of the study. In fact, the introduction can be conceived of as a funnel with the hypothesis being at the bottom, small end. The introduction starts from the big picture overview and comes down to the hypothesis. The reader can see immediately why the hypothesis makes sense, given the background. Of course, some reports, such as case histories, have no hypothesis, but nonetheless, should have the background presented in the introduction.

The methods section is a fully detailed report of the procedures, tests, manipulative procedures, subject selection criteria, and so forth of the study. The methods section should allow a reader knowledgeable in the field to reproduce the study. The methods section should present sufficient detail that the reader can make judgments about the validity and usefulness of the study results.

The results section presents the actual data from the study and the analyses of the data. It gives tables and graphics to clearly show the reader the outcomes of the study. Graphs should be presented in formats that clearly show differences, data trends, and group data descriptions. Most graphs showing group data should show error bars so that the reader can see the amount of variability within the data (28,48). As with statistical analysis programs, there are several computer programs available to help with graphic presentations, such as KaleidaGraph *(www.synergy.com)*, GraphPad *(www.graphpad.com)*, GB Stat *(www.gbstat.com)*, and Microsoft Excel. One of the most common errors in presenting data in a paper is to have graphics that are misleading, confusing, or not readily interpretable.

As stated earlier, the discussion section is where the author can express his or her opinions on the outcomes of the study. It is often helpful to begin the discussion section with a bullet recap of the major results. This helps both the writer and the reader to focus on the important aspects of the data. The discussion allows the author a place to express opinions about the meaning of the data and interpret it for the reader. Of course, the reader does not have to agree with the writer's interpretations.

The reference section should list the sources consulted by the author. All references that are cited in the text or that contributed to the ideas in the article should be cited. It is a serious ethical problem to use the material of others and not give attribution to them. Plagiarism is poorly looked on. It is a good idea to be inclusive rather than exclusive in referencing others' work.

The beginning and even the seasoned author can get help in writing articles by consulting the instructions for authors given in most medical journals. The only osteopathic journal fully indexed in the Index Medicus library is the *Journal of the American Osteopathic Association* (JAOA). It publishes instructions to authors in each issue, and these can be viewed on the internet at the AOA web site, *www.aoa-net.org*. Another invaluable source of information on writing style is the *Publication Manual of the American Psychological Association* (49). This invaluable book gives not only style guidelines but also information on presenting graphics, writing theses, plagiarism, and much more.

When considering a journal for publication of an article, first choice should be given to journals indexed in the Index Medicus or similar worldwide listings. The target audience should be identified and the chosen journal should target that audience. The journal should be peer-reviewed to insure quality of the articles published.

If the study is not sufficient for stand-alone publication, the author should consider presenting the data at a medical or scientific meeting from which abstracts are published. This provides a public reference of the work. The AOA research conference held each year in conjunction with the AOA convention is such a venue. The abstracts of the scientific presentations are published in the JAOA and indexed in the world literature.

SPECIAL CONSIDERATIONS IN OSTEOPATHIC CLINICAL RESEARCH

In the sections on research design, several ideas were introduced that require discussion in terms of osteopathic research questions.

The areas that are of special interest to the design of osteopathic studies are:

The "gold standard" for medical research
The question being asked
Blinding
Control groups
Patient populations
Pilot studies and statistical power
Inclusion/exclusion criteria
Dependent variables

The "Gold Standard" for Clinical Research

The randomized, double-blind, placebo-controlled study (RDBPC) has evolved as the "gold standard" for clinical research studies. This design was developed in the 1940s and 1950s as the appropriate design to test the effects of drug treatments. The major elements of this particular design are:

Randomization of subjects into the treatment groups (or arms)
Blinding of subjects, drug givers, and data collectors as to treatment given
Provision to the control subjects of a "placebo" or inactive substance that is indistinguishable from the active drug

This design was developed to answer a very specific question in drug therapy. For practical purposes, the question or experimental hypothesis to be answered is, "What is the effect of this drug on the natural course of a disease process in the human unaware of what drug is given?"

The random assignment of subjects to the experimental or control group hopefully assures that the experimental and control groups (or more groups if, for example, a group given neither drug nor placebo is used) have the same characteristics to begin the study. The blinding of the patient to what is being received (active drug or inactive substance) will hopefully assure that the patients in the experimental group do not feel better simply because they are getting an active drug. In other words, the psychological aspects of the treatment should be equal for the two groups. Blinding the drug giver and caregivers as to which group the patient is in hopefully insures that the treated patients do not get subtle cues that they are being given an active substance; blinding the data gatherers assures that bias is not introduced by knowing the patients receiving the active drug. Thus, for the question being asked, this design is a good one. Unfortunately, studies of manipulative treatment are not always amenable to this design, and may often ask different questions. Thus, we must examine briefly what affects the interpretation of clinical trials.

Validity and Bias

The validity of a study is simply how strongly we can believe that the results are a reflection of what is actually the case. Did the manipulative technique really cause the observed change or was some other mechanism at work? Will the technique work with other patients, or was the result limited to the patients being studied? Many factors can influence how results can be interpreted, and these factors are called biases.

The definition of bias in a research study is basically anything that could interfere with the correct interpretation of the results of the study. If the study asks about the effect of a technique on low back pain, then measuring the pain differently in experimental and control groups would constitute a bias that would invalidate the results. There are many forms of bias that affect the validity of a study.

External Validity

Simply put, an external bias is something that interferes with the generalization of the results of a study from the patients in the study to other patients (32). If an experimenter wanted to have an externally valid study of the effects of a manipulative technique on asthma in the general population, the study group would be chosen not from a hospitalized population but from the whole group of people with asthma. If the asthma study patients were all hospitalized, the effects of a manipulative technique might well be different than if the technique were performed on patients with a less severe form of the disease. The study would not be externally valid because it would not be generalizable to the whole population of asthma sufferers. Of course, if the intent of the study were to study the effects of manipulative interventions on asthma in hospitalized patients, it would be externally valid. Thus, it is very important to frame the hypothesis with knowledge of whom the subjects will be and to whom the data will be generalized. Many things can affect external validity, including:

Lack of proper control procedures
Improper selection of patients
Simple length of time the patient is in the study (symptoms may change over time even without treatment)

Biases that threaten the external validity of a study are often fairly easily seen and recognized. For the example above, the bias of using only hospitalized patients as subjects obviously limits the results to that population of patients. Other problems of generalizability are not so obvious. For this reason, the investigator must keep records of the patients and be able to define at least the demographics of the patients so that the reader will be able to judge which population the results are most likely to be applicable to.

Internal Validity

Much more serious are the threats to internal validity. These biases are often very subtle and can make statements about the actual meaning of results difficult if not impossible. A nonblinded observer who takes data in a study and who knows whether or not the subject was treated is an obvious source of bias that will almost surely make interpretation of between-group differences impossible. Other sources of biases threatening internal validity include (32):

Inappropriate control groups
Measures that do not accurately determine the response being studied
Objectivity in the measures being used
Small numbers of patients in the groups
Initial differences between experimental and control groups

Random fluctuations in the course of a disease process
Regression of symptoms to the mean
Many others

Thus, the investigator must pay close attention to issues affecting the internal validity of the study design and would be well advised to consult an experienced clinical trials designer on the issue.

DESIGN OF OSTEOPATHIC CLINICAL TRIALS

Blinding

As noted above, the design of clinical trials of osteopathic manipulation is more complex and may ask different questions than drug trials. Obviously, the person providing the treatment cannot be blinded to whether manipulation is given or not. In some cases, the patient can be blinded to treatment condition, as in the Irvine study. None of the patients included in the study had any experience with manipulative treatment, and results showed that there was no difference between the groups as to their recognition of whether manipulation had been given or not. Blinding was done for the data gatherers, so the study can be considered a blinded trial with the exception of the treating physician. Although patient blinding is possible in cases of technique studies like the Irvine study, it is not as likely in studies of full treatment effects. In addition, it is difficult to find large numbers of patients in most osteopathic practices that are completely naïve to manipulation. Thus, the question of patient blinding is one that must be examined for each study and dealt with as the study and situation allow. The consequences of not blinding the patients to treatment are considered under the section on control groups, below. In any event, it is imperative to have the data collectors blinded as to group assignment.

Population Selection

In most cases, studies of manipulative treatment will use patients from the investigators' practices. The study design should include recording the demographics of the patients so that there will be a basis to generalize from the study population to other patients. It is obvious that the patients coming to an osteopathic practice are not a random sample of the general population, but a highly self-selected group that may be motivated to seek osteopathic care. Thus, caution must be taken when generalizing results of manipulative trials to the general population, and this bias must be taken into account.

Control Groups

One of the most contentious issues in osteopathic research design is the issue of appropriate control groups. The idea of the control group stems from the necessity of having some way to compare the active treatment with some baseline. As mentioned above, historical controls are sometimes used, but are far from ideal. Historical controls may differ widely from the contemporary study group in many aspects, so give only an impression of effects. Historical controls are used only as a last resort.

The "gold standard" control is the placebo control. Defined above, the placebo control is designed to mask from the patient the knowledge of whether the active drug or the inactive substance is being given. Such a control is meant to take the psychological effects of the patient's knowledge on the interaction between drug and disease natural history out of the therapeutic picture. It has been widely assumed that the simple knowledge of treatment had about a 30% effect on the patients response to the treatment (the "placebo effect") (50). Thus, according to the commonly held view, the simple psychological effect of knowing that a treatment was being given could alleviate symptoms by a large amount. Thus, the placebo control is designed to keep the placebo effect from entering into the difference a drug would make in the course of a disease.

Significant questions are being raised about the placebo as an effective control condition (51–54). For example, is the "placebo effect" really as robust as has been assumed? Is factoring out the psychological effect giving a true picture of the actual effect of a drug or treatment on the course of a disease, or is the placebo control consistently causing an underestimation of the total effect of drug plus knowledge? It is now well known that an individual's psychological status has real and measurable effects on their physiologic processes (see Willard, Chapter 8). Is the placebo the best control for treatment studies? The placebo's sister control group, the sham control, is often used in studies of manipulative treatments and techniques. With a sham control, some type of "hands-on" experience is given to the patient so that the physiologic and psychological effects of placing the hands on the patient are equal in the treatment and control groups. The Irvine study is a good example of a sham treatment control. Because the question being asked was regarding the effectiveness of the thrust alone, a sham was appropriate.

However, what if the question being asked is of the effect of the osteopathic treatment as a total treatment effect? Is it then not appropriate to test the total treatment, including the effect of hands-on and patient knowledge, against giving the patient no treatment? The question being asked determines the control group. If the question is to test the totality of the treatment effect against no treatment, and treatment includes the effect of putting hands on the patient, then the appropriate control is a patient receiving only rest during the treatment time. It may also be appropriate to use the musculoskeletal examination as the "sham" in such cases. Here, both groups would receive the structural examination, but the control group would then rest while the manipulative treatment was given to experimental group. Blinding of the subjects to treatment group in many cases is simply impossible, thus leaving the concept of a "placebo" group as a moot point.

Another control often used in manipulation studies is the "community standard" control in which, for example, low back pain is treated manipulatively in the experimental group, but by drugs, physical therapy, and counseling in the control group. This type of active control group is asking yet another question: Is the effect of manipulation equal to or better than standard care? The recent Andersson study (38) on manipulative treatment for low back pain is a good example of this type of control group. Because of the ethical considerations of giving no care to a patient in a "do nothing" control group, the active or community standard of care control may be the only way some conditions can be examined.

Thus, the osteopathic researcher must carefully determine the actual intent of the experimental question prior to determining the appropriate control group. The myth of the "gold standard" must not be forced onto research designs for manipulation. If the question of the study is whether the manipulative treatment is better than nothing, a rest or nothing control is appropriate. If the question is whether the manipulation is better than community standard care, the appropriate control is the active community standard treatment. If the question is whether the manipulation is better than simply placing hands on the patient, probably the best control is the examination-only control.

Thus, careful consideration of what is being asked will determine the appropriate control group, not a preconceived notion of what a control should be.

Study Size and Power

Studies on the effects of manipulative treatment are in their infancy. It is difficult for an individual investigator to procure sufficient subjects for a large study. In fact, it is now becoming increasingly evident that many studies have not been sufficiently large for their results to be reliable. The term for the probability that a study contains sufficient subjects for an effect to be accurately found if, in fact, there is an effect of the independent variable, is called "power." The measure of the power of a study is called power analysis (55). The probability that the statistical analysis of a clinical trial will show a significant *p* value is remarkably large if the number of subjects in the study is small. In a study with few subjects, one subject's large change in findings may result in a significant effect, although the effect is not general. In this case, a "type I" error will result; the experimental hypothesis that there is a treatment effect will be accepted although no such effect is present. Thus, power analysis gives an estimate of the number of subjects required in a study to be reasonably sure that if there is an effect it will be found. Power calculations can be made with relatively simple formulas found in standard books (55) or on the internet (*http://ebook.stat.ucla.edu/calculator/powercalc/*, for example).

Pilot Versus Full Studies

Thus, the Andersson study, although well done with about 178 patients, is most likely still lacking sufficient patient numbers to fulfill power requirements (38). Studies not meeting standard power requirements must be termed "pilot studies," and their results should be viewed with caution. Pilot studies are very useful in giving indications of what effects may be valuable to further study and in providing data on the amount of variability inherent in outcome measures; therefore, they are very valuable. Studies that meet the required numbers of subjects indicated by power calculations are considered full-scale studies and, other things equal, are more reliable than studies with fewer subjects.

Drop-Outs

The problem of drop-outs can be acute in any clinical study. In studies of manipulation, the investigator must account for patients not finishing the study. This is important because of the potential for causing imbalances between the experimental and control groups. For example, if all the patients with more severe disease dropped out of the experimental group but stayed in the control group, the results would be inaccurate or biased toward a larger effect in the experimental group. The usual practice is to try to determine the cause of the patient's failure to finish the study and to carefully examine the drop-outs for commonalities that could affect study results.

Inclusion/Exclusion Criteria

The issue of inclusion/exclusion criteria is also difficult in many studies of manipulative treatment. The inclusion criteria are those things that make the patient eligible for the study, such as low back pain. However, the inclusion criteria must be well specified and measurable prior to the study. In the example of low back pain, the type, duration, and other factors should be carefully delineated. An area that needs special attention in inclusion criteria is that of a well-defined diagnosis. Often, studies of manipulation do not have well-defined structural diagnoses that can be justified and defended to the greater medical community, which results in poor acceptance of the study.

Exclusion criteria are those factors that exclude a patient from a study. These can be age, pregnancy, drug use, and so forth. Exclusion criteria must also be clearly specified in the study design. It had been standard practice to exclude women from many drug studies because of the danger of pregnancy. This practice resulted in a lack of information on the effects of drugs on females (poor external validity), and the effects were often different than the effects on males. It is now unacceptable to simply exclude females; if a study does so, explicit reasons must be given.

Dependent Variables

Selecting Appropriate Measures

The best measures to determine if a manipulative procedure had an effect are often difficult to decide. These measures are known as the dependent variables because their values are supposedly dependent on the experimental treatment. In studies of the efficacy of a manipulative technique or a manipulative treatment on the outcome of a specific disease process, the measures are presumably some aspect of the disease process or of the natural course of the symptoms. In assessing the contributions of manipulative treatment to resolution of somatic dysfunction or to the maintenance of health, the task of defining sensitive dependent variables becomes more difficult. Some dependent measures include:

Measures of immune system function
Studies of the activities of daily living
Episodes of loss of health (for long-term studies)
Other measures of body function, including reports of feelings of well-being and comfort

One of the problems in many studies of manipulative treatment is the use of purely subjective, dependent variables in the study. Typically in these cases, an examiner performs a musculoskeletal examination of a patient and records the somatic dysfunction found. The treating physician typically repeats the examination and treats the findings for experimental subjects and simply does nothing for control subjects. The blinded examiner then performs a second examination and reports differences between the two examinations. The problems inherent in this design are mainly a lack of any knowledge of the reliability of the examiner. How much do the findings vary between examinations (repeat reliability) and how do the examinations of the two examiners correlate (interexaminer reliability)? These are significant issues that must be acknowledged in such a study.

The answer to such issues is to use dependent variables that are not dependent on the subjective examination of either a blinded examiner or the treating physican. Such measures can be instrumented measures, such as Doppler blood flow, respiratory volumes, and so on.

Whatever the dependent variable or variables, the measures of manipulative treatment results should include an evaluation of whether the treating physician determined that the treatment given actually did what it was designed to do. Sometimes the manipulation fails to accomplish the desired immediate outcome in restoring range of motion or proper muscle relaxation. These facts must be recorded and used in analysis of the outcome of the treatment so that unsuccessful treatments can be looked at separately from those judged to achieve the desired end points. This will help reduce the variability of the data.

Another problem in choosing dependent variables is the temptation to simply measure everything available and hope to find a few that change. This may be a good strategy for a preliminary exploration of a treatment technique, but holds many pitfalls. In fact, this is sometimes called "oh heck" research design: Oh heck, let's do this and see what happens!

Given enough measures, the probability that one or a few will show significant changes is very high. In fact, if 20 dependent measures are chosen for measurement, expect that one will show a significant outcome by chance (when no effect actually exists). Thus, special statistical tests must be used when several measures are studied to guard against chance significant results. It is best to design a study with a few dependent variables that have either been shown to be affected by the independent variable, or to have good reason for suspecting that they may be so affected.

Characteristics of Well-Designed and Pitfalls of Poorly Designed Osteopathic Research

Good osteopathic research will have the characteristics of any well-designed clinical study. These characteristics include:

A complete and well-documented literature search
A well-defined working hypothesis
Research design is logical and fits the hypothesis
Complete and well-documented methodology
Statistical methods and data processing procedures defined in advance
Power calculations completed
Well-defined inclusion and exclusion criteria
Both objective and subjective dependent variables
Adequate statistic and logistic support
IRB approval obtained

These characteristics of a well-designed osteopathic trial should lead to reliable and believable data.

On the other hand, some of the pitfalls, especially for novice investigators, include the converse of the above, but also some perhaps less-obvious points when planning and conducting research:

Planning is incomplete and not well documented
Protocols are not rigorously followed
Record keeping is not complete
Time for study completion is underestimated
Patients cannot be recruited in sufficient numbers
Study is too complex
Too many dependent variables

Many of these areas have been covered earlier in the chapter. However some deserve brief mention here. As a study is carried out, it is very important for the investigator to make sure the protocols are followed at every step. If a mistake is made, it must be noted and any problem corrected. Mistakes will be made in any protocol; difficulties arise if the mistakes are not acknowledged.

Many investigators underestimate the time needed to complete a study. At times, patients cannot be recruited readily or replacement patients must be sought. These things can add significantly to the time required for study completion. A careful investigator plans extra time into the study design. It is good to offer a bonus to key personnel for subject recruitment and for help with the protocol.

As stated in the hypothesis section, a simple study is often the best one. A study with too many hypotheses to be tested or too many dependent variables or measures can become uncontrollable and even impossible to analyze. It is often better to perform several small, well-designed studies that together paint a picture, than one large, complex study that is not interpretable.

CONCLUSION

Clinical research in osteopathic medicine is at the cutting edge of research design technology. The uncertainties surrounding controls, dependent variable measures, and interpretation of results makes it a difficult and challenging field. Well-designed studies that make a small contribution to understanding the mechanisms and efficacy of manipulative treatment, such as are now coming out in the osteopathic literature, will eventually paint a compelling and fascinating picture of this treatment modality. The profession must take full advantage of the fourth osteopathic period of research to strengthen its foundation in the coming years.

REFERENCES

1. Smith WA. Skiagraphy and the circulation. *J Osteopath.* 1899;5(8):365–384.
2. Northup GW, ed. *Osteopathic Research: Growth and Development.* Chicago, IL: American Osteopathic Association; 1987.
3. Burns L. *The Nerve Centers,* vol II. Cincinnati, OH: Monfort and Company; 1911.
4. Burns L. *Basic Principles,* vol I. Los Angeles, CA: The Occident Printery; 1907.

5. Burns L. *The Physiology of Consciousness,* vol III. Cincinnati, OH: Monfort and Company; 1911.
6. Burns L. *Cells of the Blood,* vol IV. A. T. Still Research Institute; 1931.
7. Burns L, ed. *Pathogenesis of Visceral Disease Following Vertebral Lesions.* Chicago, IL: American Osteopathic Association; 1948.
8. Kelso AF, Townsend AA. The status and future of osteopathic research. In: Northup GW, ed. *Osteopathic Research: Growth and Development.* Chicago, IL: American Osteopathic Association; 1987:93–117.
9. Denslow JS. *The Early Years of Research at the Kirksville College of Osteopathic Medicine.* Kirksville, MO: Kirksville College of Osteopathic Medicine Press; 1982.
10. Denslow JS, Korr IM, Krems AD. Quantitative studies of chronic facilitation in human motoneuron pools. *Am J Physiol.* 1947;105(2):229–238.
11. Korr IM. The neural basis of the osteopathic lesion. *J Am Osteopath Assoc.* 1947:191–198.
12. Korr IM. The emerging concept of the osteopathic lesion. *J Am Osteopath Assoc.* 1948;Nov:1–8.
13. Beckwith CG. Thoracic vertebral mechanics. *J Am Osteopath Assoc.* 1944;43:436–439.
14. Still AT. *Autobiography of A. T. Still.* Kirksville, MO: A. T. Still; 1897.
15. Still AT. *Osteopathy Research and Practice.* Kirksville, MO: The Pioneer Press; 1910.
16. Northup GW. *Osteopathic Medicine: An American Reformation.* Chicago, IL: American Osteopathic Association; 1966.
17. Patterson MM, Howell JN, eds. *The Central Connection: Somatovisceral Viscerosomatic Interaction.* Indianapolis, IN: American Academy of Osteopathy; 1992.
18. Enserink M. Helsinki's new clinical rules: Fewer placebos, more disclosure. *Science.* 2000;290(20 October):418–419.
19. Emanuel EJ, Wendler D, Grady C. What makes clinical research ethical? *JAMA.* 2000;283(20):2701–2711.
20. Taylor TE. Increased Supervision of Clinical Research at Home and Abroad. *J Am Osteopath Assoc.* 2001;101(12):696–698.
21. Patterson MM, Steinmetz JE. Long-lasting alterations of spinal reflexes: A potential basis for somatic dysfunction. *J Am Osteopath Assoc.* 1986;2:38–42.
22. Willard FW, Patterson MM, eds. *Nociception and the Neuroendocrine-Immune Connection.* Indianapolis, IN: American Academy of Osteopathy; 1994.
23. Van Buskirk RL. Nociceptive reflexes and the somatic dysfunction: A model. *J Am Osteopath Assoc.* 1990;90(9):792–794.
24. Denslow JS, Korr IM, Krems AD. Quantitative studies of chronic facilitation in human motoneuron pools. *Am J Physiol.* 1947:229–238.
25. Patterson, MM. Mechanisms of classical conditioning and fixation in spinal mammals. *Adv Psychobiol.* 1976;3:381–436.
26. Patterson MM, Grau JW, eds. *Spinal Cord Plasticity.* Boston, MA: Kluwer Academic Publishers; 2001.
27. Shekelle PG, Adams AH, Chassin MR, et al. Spinal manipulation for low-back pain. *Ann Intern Med.* 1992;117(7):590–598.
28. Dawson B, Trapp RG. *Basic and Clinical Biostatistics,* 3rd ed. New York, NY: Lang Medical Books/McGraw-Hill; 2001.
29. Johnson SM, Bordinat D. Professional identity: key to the future of the osteopathic medical profession in the United States. *J Am Osteopath Assoc.* 1998;98(6):325–331.
30. Johnson SM, Kurtz ME. Diminished use of osteopathic manipulative treatment and its impact on the uniqueness of the osteopathic profession. *Acad Med.* 2001;76(8):821–828.
31. Johnson SM, Kurtz ME, Kurtz JC. Variables influencing the use of

osteopathic manipulative treatment in family. *J Am Osteopath Assoc.* 1997;97(2):80–87.
32. Trochim WMK. *The Research Methods Knowledge Base,* 2nd ed. Cincinnati, OH: Atomic Dog Publishing; 2001.
33. Greenberg RS. *Medical Epidemiology,* 2nd ed. New York, NY: Appleton & Lange; 1966.
34. Buerger AA. A controlled trial of rotational manipulation in low back pain. *Man Med.* 1980;2:17–26.
35. Hoehler F, Tobis J, Buerger AA. Spinal manipulation for low back pain. *JAMA.* 1981;245(18):1835–1838.
36. Wells MR, Giantinoto S, D'Agate D, et al. Standard osteopathic manipulative treatment acutely improves gait performance in patients with Parkinson's disease. *J Am Osteopath Assoc.* 1999;99(2):92–98.
37. Korr IM. Osteopathic medicine: the profession's role in society. *J Am Osteopath Assoc.* 1990;90(9):824–832.
38. Andersson GBJ, Lucente T, Davis A, et al. A comparison of osteopathic spinal manipulation with standard care for patients with low back pain. *N Engl J Med.* 1999;341(19):1426–1431.
39. Jones LH. *Jones Strain-Counterstrain.* Boise, ID: Jones Strain-Counterstrain; 1995. (Available from the American Academy of Osteopathy, Indianapolis, IN.)
40. Willard FH, Swartzlander B. Basic Research and Osteopathic Medicine. In: Ward RC, ed. *Foundations for Osteopathic Medicine.* Baltimore, MD: Williams & Wilkins; 1997;1107–1114.
41. Hoehler FK, Tobis JK, Buerger AA. Spinal manipulation for low back pain. *JAMA.* 1981;245(18):1835–1838.
42. Hulley SB, Cummings SR. *Designing Clinical Research: An Epidemiologic Approach.* Baltimore, MD: Williams & Wilkins; 1988.
43. Kaprow MG, Sandhouse M. Refractory torticollis after a fall. *J Am Osteopath Assoc.* 2000;100(3):148–150.
44. Pocock SJ. *Clinical Trials: A Practical Approach.* New York, NY: John Wiley and Sons; 1983.
45. Keating JC, Seville J, Meeder WC, et al. Intrasubject experimental designs in osteopathic medicine: Applications in clinical practice. *J Am Osteopath Assoc.* 1985;85:192–203.
46. Frymann VM, Carney RE, Springall P. Effect of osteopathic medical management on neurologic development in children. *J Am Osteopath Assoc.* 1992;92(6):729–744.
47. Daniel WW. *Biostatistics: A Foundation for Analysis in the Health Sciences.* New York, NY: John Wiley and Sons; 1999.
48. Byrne DW. *Publishing Your Medical Research Paper: What They Don't Teach You in Medical School,* 2nd ed. Baltimore, MD: Williams & Wilkins; 1998.
49. *Publication Manual of the American Psychological Association,* 5th ed. Washington, DC: American Psychological Association; 2001.
50. Beecher HK. The powerful placebo. *JAMA.* 1955;159(17):1602–1606.
51. Hrobjartsson A, Gotzsche PC. Is the placebo powerless? An analysis of clinical trials comparing placebo with no treatment. *N Engl J Med.* 2001;344(21):1594–1602.
52. Kiene H. A critique of the double-blind clinical trial. *Altern Ther Health Med.* 1996;2(1):74–80.
53. Al-Khatib SM, Kaliff RM, Hasselblad V, et al. Placebo controls in short-term clinical trials of hypertension. *Science.* 2001;292(15 June):2013–2015.
54. Kienle GS, Kiene H. Placebo effect and placebo concept: A critical methodological and conceptual analysis of reports on the magnitude of the placebo effect. *Altern Ther Health Med.* 1996;2(6):39–54.
55. Murphy KR, Myors B. *Statistical Power Analysis.* Mahwah, NJ: Lawrence Erlbaum Associates; 1998.

THE RESEARCH STATUS OF SOMATIC DYSFUNCTION

DEBORAH M. HEATH
NORMAN GEVITZ

KEY CONCEPTS

- History and definition of somatic dysfunction
- Interexaminer agreement of palpatory findings
- Instrumentation and identification of somatic dysfunction
- Clinical correlations of somatic dysfunction
- Current challenges of clinical research

HISTORY

One of the many challenges facing osteopathic clinical research is to simulate the clinical encounter as closely as possible. Another is to capture the distinctiveness of the operating osteopathic principles while studying the influences of the practical application of these principles (1). Although individual osteopathic clinicians have claimed positive clinical results, systematic and controlled research has been progressing slowly. Historically, scientific inquiry at osteopathic colleges and hospitals has not had a high priority in a profession where the major emphasis has been placed on the laudable service goal of producing primary care physicians (2). Consequently, osteopathic researchers have often struggled to find the resources and the time to conduct scientific studies on the distinctive diagnostic and therapeutic aspects of osteopathic principles and practices. External sources of funding have been difficult to secure. Through its Bureau of Research, the American Osteopathic Association has annually devoted a small pool of funds to support mostly pilot studies. It has, however, committed several hundreds of thousands of dollars to underwrite Andersson and associates' (3) large outcome study comparing the management of back pain by MDs and DOs, which was recently published in the *New England Journal of Medicine.*

A distinctive aspect of osteopathic practice is the identification of the presence of "somatic dysfunction" and its relevance to health. The particular role of somatic dysfunction, once referred to as "the osteopathic lesion," in health and illness has its roots in studies initially conducted at the A. T. Still Research Institute in Chicago by John Deason early in the century, later by Louisa Burns on the Pacific Coast, and then by J. Stedman Denslow and Irwin Korr and their associates at Kirksville in the 1940s and beyond (4). Although basic science research on the phenomenon that became known as somatic dysfunction made considerable strides in decades past, clinical research has been difficult to conduct due to several methodological and resource-based factors. Ideally, an instrument that could objectively identify somatic dysfunction and its relationship to physiologic and pathologic processes would expedite the understanding of palpatory findings and simplify some of the unique challenges in osteopathic clinical research. To date, objective measurement of somatic dysfunction remains elusive.

The term somatic dysfunction is of relatively recent origin. As early as 1863, the English anatomist and surgeon, John Hilton, identified what he called "sore spots" along the spinal column, which he associated with pathology at segmentally related viscera (5). Andrew Taylor Still used several descriptive terms to denote the meaning of his palpatory findings (6). The term "osteopathic or bony lesion" gained currency with the work of Louisa Burns (7); however, the term "osteopathic lesion" gradually declined as a physiologic understanding of the phenomenon gained favor over the conception of an anatomic displacement. Denslow and Korr's work led to the concept of the "facilitated segment," which helped explain certain patterns of spinal findings that were not necessarily segmentally related to pathology elsewhere (8). In recent decades, the Educational Council on Osteopathic Principles (ECOP), using consensus-based discussions, fleshed out the concept of somatic dysfunction.

Somatic dysfunction is currently described as an "impaired or altered function of related components of the somatic (body framework) system: skeletal, arthrodial, and myofascial structures, and related vascular, lymphatic, and neural elements ... The positional and motion aspects of the somatic dysfunction may be described using at least one of three parameters: a) the position of the element as determined by palpation and referenced to its adjacent structure, b) the directions in which motion is freer, and c) the directions in which motion is restricted" (9).

The early 1980s marked a transition for several forms of osteopathic clinical research. Increased attention was devoted to understanding the distinctive diagnostic procedures osteopathic physicians employed to identify somatic dysfunction. For example, Dinnar, Beal and associates (10) videotaped 15 actual doctor-patient encounters and categorized five classes of musculoskeletal diagnostic procedures. Three classes of diagnostic tests (i.e., general impression, regional motion testing, and position of landmarks) were not considered unique to osteopathic diagnosis. However, in two classes of procedures, involving vertebral segment location and motion characteristics, the authors concluded that these constituted distinctly osteopathic procedures. They noted that tests in these two latter classes required high levels of sensory skill, precise anatomic knowledge, and were subject to considerable individuality in their application by different physicians. Knowing more about these distinctive osteopathic diagnostic procedures was fundamental in steering the direction and amplifying the quality of osteopathic clinical research. By incorporating these unique diagnostic procedures into osteopathic clinical research, it was believed that the somatic component of health and disease could be more precisely identified, and its role in health and disease could be elucidated. The nature of the somatic component and how it is exhibited in health and disease continues to be a crucial question for the osteopathic profession.

This chapter on somatic dysfunction will focus on clinically oriented research that has been published in the *Journal of the American Osteopathic Association* (JAOA) since 1980. Research studies involving certain forms of osteopathic diagnosis not focused on the spine will not be discussed here nor will research on general physiologic benefits of osteopathic manipulative treatment (OMT). Rather, we will consider three categories of somatic dysfunction–oriented clinical research over the last 2 decades. The first category is interexaminer agreement and somatic dysfunction. The second category is the use of instrumentation and somatic dysfunction. The third category is the clinical correlations of somatic dysfunction.

INTEREXAMINER AGREEMENT AND SOMATIC DYSFUNCTION

Throughout much of the osteopathic profession's history, clinicians have reported the presence of "lesions" or somatic dysfunction based on their own understandings. These findings were generally nonstandardized and lacked independent verification—either through other examiners or through instrumentation. Nevertheless, over the years, there have been studies where multiple examiners, blinded from each other's evaluation, have tried to determine whether there existed a high correlation of their palpatory findings. Beal reported on nine such studies completed from 1951 to 1985 that looked at patterns of somatic dysfunction throughout the spinal column (11). Beal graphed the distribution of somatic dysfunction findings of these researchers and concluded that the incidence of somatic dysfunction was not uniform throughout the spine. He noted there were peaks and valleys, with the peaks occurring at the transitional areas of the spine (i.e., the occipital area, the cervicothoracic area, the thoracolumbar area, and the lumbosacral area). Nevertheless, Beal noted great variation in reported findings between studies. He attributed these discrepancies to observer influence, differences in testing procedures and their interpretation, and different subject populations. He noted that osteopathic researchers did not share

a broadly accepted protocol of tests for the evaluation of spinal somatic dysfunction other than general categories of tissue texture, asymmetry of bony landmarks, and segmental joint motion.

Experience in doing structural examinations was also a critical variable. In 1980, Kappler reviewed the results of 837 examinations performed on the same patients by experienced osteopathic physicians and students in a hospital setting between 1969 and 1972 (12). He found that student examiners tended to record more findings and that the findings of experienced examiners were more localized in groups than specific areas. He concluded that the experienced examiner tends to discard "insignificant" findings prior to their possible entry onto the medical record.

McConnell, Beal, and associates (13) noted the problem of low interexaminer agreement in a study published in 1980. Six osteopathic physicians each examined upward of 15 of 21 volunteer patients with acute spinal complaints. They recorded their findings numerically on a scale of zero to three with respect to clinical significance. Interexaminer agreement on segmental location was low. Of 25 area-by-area comparisons, only four demonstrated significant agreement. The authors concluded that if high levels of interexaminer agreement were to be achieved, the examiners must first agree on the areas to be examined, the test procedures to be used, the method of quantifying the intensity of the findings, and the method of recording.

The effort to standardize diagnostic procedures among multiple examiners in research on spinal somatic dysfunction has been led by William Johnston and his associates. In their 1981 study of interexaminer agreement, Johnston and co-workers focused on passive gross motion characteristics along the vertebral columns of human subjects using a series of selected palpatory tests (14). Six gross motion tests were used on 161 subjects. Each of three examiners performed a test three times on the same subject and recorded three findings. Criteria were established for agreement among examiners and for subjects with inconsistent findings among examiners. Data from two tests revealed better than random agreement with a high confidence level for cervical rotation (less than 0.001). Subjects with inconsistent findings contributed greater than 25% of disagreement for each of the six tests.

In their next study, Johnston and associates (15) hypothesized that a high level of interexaminer agreement could be obtained on passive motion testing of selected subjects with "stable" (i.e., persistent) findings of regional motion asymmetry. They noted that because transient findings are more likely to change during the multiple examinations needed to test interexaminer agreement, subjects with major findings that were stable needed to be identified. The agreement of two examiners on the direction and the intensity of asymmetrical response to cervical rotation was used to identify 14 subjects with stable palpable findings from a total sample of 70 subjects. Data from examination of all 14 subjects by a second set of examiners revealed a high level of agreement on subjects with stable findings. Using a numerical scale to substitute for directions of findings, permutation testing revealed a confidence level of less than 0.01.

In a third study, Johnston and associates (16) selected procedures of palpatory examination and established criteria for finding segmental dysfunction in the thoracic spinal region. Five trained individuals examined 30 subjects for deep tissue tension about a bony segment. The intensity of findings was graded on a scale of zero (least) to three (most). For each of the five examiners, agreement levels exceeded 79% in distinguishing between two marked segments, one with relatively normal tension (less than one) and one with increased deep tissue tension (greater than two). Statistical analysis rejected the hypothesis that the distribution of agreements could have been reached by chance (chi square calculated 91.3 versus 3.84).

INSTRUMENTATION AND SOMATIC DYSFUNCTION

The validity of palpatory findings has been advanced through interexaminer studies. However, even if two or more examiners have a high degree of agreement as to the presence or absence of somatic dysfunction, it is highly desirable to have subjective findings documented through objective instrumentation. Indeed, while working with electromyography in the 1940s, Denslow and associates (17) wrote the first articles on what became known as somatic dysfunction for basic science research journals.

Beginning in 1985, Johnston, Vorro, and Hubbard (18) wrote the first of four papers on employing instrumentation in somatic dysfunction research. In the first study, 16 subjects were placed in groups according to their symmetry or asymmetry, as determined by a palpatory test for passive side-bending of the cervical region. Using kinematic analysis, the authors assessed both active and passive movement responses. Head orientation was measured at the end of range after six primary rotations. Two secondary deviations from each primary rotation were also observed. Data revealed a significant decrease in all six primary ranges in the combined asymmetric groups as compared with the symmetric group. A similar relationship was observed for secondary deviations. There was no significant difference in these motions between the right and left asymmetric subgroups. The authors concluded that the palpable clinical sign of asymmetry in response to passive cervical side-bending appears to be an early indicator of a measurable impairment of cervical function.

In the second publication of this series, Vorro and Johnston (19) reported myoelectric data collected simultaneously with their kinemetric study. Three specific muscle sites and three spinal sites on the paravertebral musculature were each monitored bilaterally. A profile analysis was used to examine relationships among subject groups, head motion, muscles, and side of recording for the time elapsed prior to the beginning of electrical activity. When all movements were considered and analyzed, a significant interaction between symmetry and side resulted ($p \leq 0.03$). This indicated that in regard to muscular activity at each of the six sites, symmetric subjects differed from asymmetric subjects when right- and left-side measures were considered. Asymmetric subjects were slower to initiate action, and the action was reduced in time and strength of contraction.

The third paper addressed additional kinematic data collected regarding three-dimensional orientations of the head accumulated throughout the paths of movement (not just at their end points, as in their previous reports) (20). The fourth paper evaluated 34 asymptomatic subjects categorized to symmetry group based on initial palpatory tests comparing regional motion responses of the head and neck to right and left side-bending (21).

Electromyographic techniques were used to study muscular activity, indicating contraction frequency for each muscle monitored during active and passive motions. Subjects diagnosed with regional motion asymmetry exhibited a significantly altered organization of electrically active and electrically silent muscles. This pattern of muscle contraction was compromised just as frequently in the passive as in the active phases of motion.

In addition to kinematic and electromyographic studies, a few osteopathic researchers have experimented with thermography as a means of correlating palpatory findings of somatic dysfunction with instrumental methods. Kelso, Grant, and Johnston (22) evaluated thermographic measurement of skin temperature of the back to determine the feasibility for its use on osteopathic examination and manipulative treatment. In 35 subjects, they found variation in skin temperature of 2° to 3° Celsius. Although they found no uniform pattern of variation, warm and cool areas could be identified. In another pilot study, Walko and Janouschek (23) employed thermography to provide information on how cervicothoracic pain responds to OMT. Of five women subjects receiving OMT, all demonstrated a decrease in skin temperature of the cervicothoracic region after treatment. To date, however, it would appear that thermographic findings do not offer sufficient specificity for research purposes on somatic dysfunction.

CLINICAL CORRELATIONS

The identification and location of somatic dysfunction, whether through interexaminer reliability studies or through the correlation of palpatory findings with instrumental measures, has particular meaning if somatic dysfunction can be associated with specific clinical entities for the purpose of diagnosis and treatment.

In 1980, Kelso, Larson, and Kappler (24) reported general findings of a study conducted a decade earlier on more than 6,000 hospital patients who received a structural examination. The authors concluded that there was an increased frequency of findings in somatic tissues segmentally related to diseased viscera. However, they also noted that it was evident from the results that the frequency of any one somatic finding in a region or segment did not predict the health status of a patient and that there was no specific segmental relationship that will signal probable presence of visceral disease.

In the 1970s, Johnston and associates (25) looked at the relationship between spinal findings through palpation and hypertension. They reported somatic findings on normotensive and hypertensive patients, providing evidence of a consistency in location of specific palpatory findings arranged in a pattern within the cervicothoracic region of some hypertensive patients.

In 1980, they reported a preliminary interexaminer reliability study of 132 subjects (26). Three trained examiners ascertained the presence or absence of three components of the somatic pattern that had been described. Twenty-seven agreements were possible based on three motion tests used to examine each of nine vertebral segment levels in the cervicothoracic region. There was a high frequency of agreement among the three examiners on the presence of pattern components in hypertensive subjects (77%), and low frequency of agreement on the presence of pattern components in normotensive patients (25%). Although the absolute level of interexaminer agreement in this study was only 40%, the difference between the value and the value predicted on the basis of a random distribution of agreements was highly significant.

In a third study, Johnston and associates (27) looked at 307 normotensive and hypertensive volunteers. In this study, they used agreement on findings of three independent trained examiners during three consecutive examinations of the spinal region C5 to T7 as the criteria for persistence of palpatory cues. Distribution of agreements on presence of stable findings was bimodal, with the values in the lower range of agreement fitting closely to the frequency predicted by a random model. Within this lower agreement range of 216 subjects with unstable findings, there were 48 hypertensive patients (22.2%). Within the group of 91 subjects with stable findings, there were 48 hypertensive patients (52.7%) The researchers concluded that a relationship exists between the hypertensive condition and a reproducible somatic component.

More recently, Johnston, Kelso, and associates (28) extended this general line of research. A standardized palpatory examination determined whether there were specific motion asymmetries centered at spinal segments C6, T2, and T6 in 253 normotensive and hypertensive subjects. The examiner was blinded as to whether a subject was hypertensive. Of 193 volunteers independently diagnosed as hypertensive, borderline, and graded, 113 (56%) were found by the researchers to have the C6T2T6 pattern. Of 61 normotensive patients, 24 (39%) were found with this pattern. Of these subjects, 184 (73%) agreed to return for follow-up examination 4 to 8 months later. Of the 132 returning hypertensive and normotensive patients with the C6T2T6 pattern on initial visit, this pattern persisted in 118 (89%) individuals. Johnston and Kelso (29) later completed a longitudinal study that demonstrated, among other findings, that the C6T2T6 pattern persisted from 3 to 10 years in 16 of 16 subjects with a grade two or greater hypertension.

Interestingly, several additional studies have focused on the role of somatic dysfunction in cardiovascular disease. Beal (30) looked for somatic dysfunction in 108 patients already diagnosed with a variety of cardiovascular problems, including coronary artery disease, ischemic heart disease, angina, myocardial infarction, hypertension, hypertensive cardiovascular disease, congestive heart failure, valvular disease, arrhythmia, and pericarditis. Of all the patients in his study, Beal found 94 (87%) had segmental dysfunction of two or more adjacent vertebrae from T1 to T5 on the left side. Somatic dysfunction at C2 on the left was also present in 69 (63%) patients. Beal recognized certain biases in his study. As patients were examined from the cardiac service, there was an expectation on the part of the examiner that a pattern of somatic dysfunction would be observed.

Cox and associates (31) studied a series of 97 consecutive patients who had cardiac catheterization. Within 1 week of angiography, patients underwent a musculoskeletal examination consisting of segmental evaluation of pain, range of motion, soft tissue texture, and "red reflex" by a blinded examiner. Univariate and multivariate analysis revealed a high correlation between coronary atherosclerosis and abnormalities of range of motion and soft tissue texture at T4.

In a study that was somewhat similar to that of Cox et al., Beal and Kleiber (32) looked for somatic dysfunction in 99 patients scheduled for cardiac catheterization on the day preceding angiography. Somatic dysfunction was found on the left side from T1-5 in 85 patients. In 70 patients, diagnosed somatic dysfunction correlated with evidence of coronary artery disease, although in 15 cases, somatic dysfunction was associated with the cardiologist's diagnosis of normal or subclinical disease. The authors considered the issues of "sensitivity" and "specificity" of their testing. The sensitivity of the test for left-sided somatic dysfunction in the T1-5 region as a predictor of the incidence of true positive results for the diagnosis of coronary artery disease in this study was 92%. However, the specificity of the test for left-sided somatic dysfunction in the same region as a predictor of the incidence of true negative results (i.e., patients who did not have coronary artery disease) was only 30%. Thus, the authors concluded that the palpatory test should not be used as a specific test for coronary artery disease.

A paper by Nicholas and associates (33), first published in the *British Medical Journal* and later reprinted in *JAOA,* looked at patterns of somatic dysfunction related to myocardial infarction (MI). Sixty-two patients were randomized for the purpose of being seen by DOs for palpation of segments T1-8. Twenty-five patients had clinically confirmed acute MI. Twenty-two patients without known cardiovascular disease served as controls, and 15 were excluded because of diagnosed cardiovascular disease other than MI. The control group was found to have a low incidence of palpable changes throughout the thoracic region uniformly distributed from T1-8. The MI group evidenced a significantly higher incidence of soft tissue changes confined almost entirely to the upper four thoracic levels. The authors concluded that their data suggest that myocardial infarction is accompanied by characteristic soft tissue changes that are readily detected by palpation.

In addition to cardiovascular studies, two other articles from the 1980s considered the relationship between somatic dysfunction and other organ systems. In reviewing historical literature, Beal and Morlock (34) determined that the majority of previously published palpatory findings of somatic dysfunction and pulmonary disease occurred within the spinal area of T2-7. To test these findings, the authors recruited 40 patients with diagnosed pulmonary disease. On examination, they found that all patients showed evidence of somatic dysfunction in the pulmonary reflex area of T2-7.

In a controlled clinical trial, Johnston, Kelso, and associates (35) examined three groups of patients to test the assumption that somatic manifestations of renal disease would be present in the spinal region of T9-12. One group had advanced renal disease; the two control groups consisted of normotensive and hypertensive patients without signs of renal disease. Recorded findings of both palpatory examination and thermography of the thoracic spinal region revealed a significantly higher frequency of segmental dysfunction and areas of elevated skin temperature in the region of T9-12 for the renal group.

More recently, as part of a broader study, Reeves and associates (36) found that the average gross number of somatic dysfunctions in 14 patients abstaining from caffeine increased from 3.57 at point of withdrawal to 7.78 on day four after withdrawal.

However, the specific locations of the somatic dysfunction were neither identified nor correlated.

The positive findings of some of these aforementioned clinical studies were subjected to serious methodological challenge by Tarr and associates (37). In this study, the researchers attempted to ascertain whether experienced DOs could diagnose disease states using palpatory findings as their source of diagnostic clues. Five examiners saw a total of 100 subjects. Two of the examiners were allowed to palpate the subject; the other three were not. None of the five examiners had any knowledge of the subject's medical history, and none were allowed to talk to the subjects. Nonpalpating examiners had only visual clues to aid in diagnosis while the palpating examiners had both visual and palpatory clues. Of the 100 subjects, 22 had documented gastrointestinal disease, 31 individuals were demonstrated to have asthma, and 47 control subjects had a negative history for either gastrointestinal pathology or asthma. The results showed that neither the palpating nor the nonpalpating physicians could correctly categorize the subjects as gastrointestinal patients, asthma patients, or controls. The authors noted that in some previous studies correlating palpatory findings with pathologic states, the researchers already knew their subjects were ill or even that they suffered from some specific condition. This knowledge could bias results. Tarr and associates concluded that reports of specific palpatory findings being associated with pathologic states required further studies on the accuracy of palpatory findings be conducted. The design of such studies, they maintained, should include an analysis of both total correct and incorrect observations. In addition, they argued that a well-designed investigation of the accuracy of palpatory diagnostic techniques required some control for nonpalpatory clues. The arguments of Tarr and associates with respect to the adequacy of prior clinical correlation studies, the results they obtained in their study, as well as the greater controls they recommended to be built in to this type of research, may have unintentionally contributed to a decline in conducting further clinical correlation projects. Some clinical researchers have instead turned their attention to conducting studies that look at various effects of osteopathic manipulation but do not directly tie the treatment given to the specific locations where spinal somatic dysfunction is located. Indeed, aside from the work of Johnston and Kelso on hypertension, it would be 10 years before another clinical correlation study by different authors would appear in the *JAOA*.

In 1997, Iwata, Rodos, and associates (38) obtained permission to perform a musculoskeletal structural examination on each of the subjects in a study of 60 hospitalized patients with psychotic and affective disorders. The results of this study indicated that psychotic and affective disorders each tend to affect a different portion of the musculoskeletal system. Psychotic patients exhibited increased musculoskeletal dysfunction in the lower extremities. Patients with affective disorders were found to exhibit increased cervical and thoracic dysfunction. The authors suggested that at the clinical level, the structural examination may be used to correlate psychiatric disorders with dysfunctional regions of the musculoskeletal system. Given Tarr and associates' aforementioned conclusions, it was perhaps not surprising that the author of a letter to the *JAOA* editor (39) critiquing this article observed that it suffered for not comparing psychiatric patients with appropriate control subjects.

CONCLUSION

Clinical research on somatic dysfunction is still in its formative stage. Despite a greater number of articles after 1980, inquiry into the nature of somatic dysfunction and its clinical significance remains modest. Nevertheless, research under osteopathic auspices has demonstrated that if appropriate training is provided, several examiners can achieve a high degree of agreement on the presence or absence of somatic dysfunction at specific spinal locations. Research has also demonstrated that some instrumentation, most notably electromyography, can provide objective instrument-based evidence confirming palpatory findings. Although several investigators have associated patterns of somatic dysfunction with specific pathologic states, methodological issues of researcher bias have been raised, and future studies will need to address these concerns. In addition, many of the studies reviewed here are notable for their small sample size. Importantly, none of the studies cited above test whether somatic dysfunction as specifically identified in subjects can be eliminated through the use of osteopathic manipulation, and that such treatments are correlated in any way with demonstrable physiologic changes elsewhere.

Osteopathic research on somatic dysfunction is currently at a crossroads. Many of the more productive contributors in the 1980s are now at or past the usual retirement age. In the last 10 years, research on somatic dysfunction has appeared to slow. There are currently few full-time faculty members in osteopathic colleges who devote a significant portion of their time to clinical research. A new generation of such researchers needs to be developed from today's students. Arguably, the osteopathic profession has a social and ethical obligation to support research on its distinctive diagnostic, prognostic, and therapeutic aspects. This research must take place to a considerable extent in and be supported by osteopathic colleges and hospitals. Expansion of resources to facilitate institutional research in the osteopathic profession is essential. The methodological difficulties and expense of conducting controlled clinical studies should not prevent increased investment in the ongoing obligation of determining the relative value of distinctive osteopathic approaches in maintaining or improving the health of patients and building on the body of osteopathic clinical research conducted during recent decades.

REFERENCES

1. Korr IM. Osteopathic research: The needed paradigm shift. *J Am Osteopath Assoc.* 1991;91:156–171.
2. Gevitz N. "Researched and demonstrated:" inquiry and infrastructure in osteopathic institutions. *J Am Osteopath Assoc.* 2001;101:174–179.
3. Andersson G, Lucente T, Davis A, et al. A comparison of osteopathic spinal manipulation with standard care for patients with low back pain. *N Engl J Med.* 1999;341:1426–1432.
4. Gevitz N. *The DO's: Osteopathic Medicine in America.* Baltimore, MD: Johns Hopkins University Press; 1982:53–55, 90–93.
5. Hilton J. *On Rest and Pain,* 2nd ed. New York, NY: W. Wood; 1879.
6. Still AT. *Osteopathy: Research and Practice.* Kirksville, MO: Published by the author; 1910.
7. Burns L. *Pathogenesis of Visceral Disease following Vertebral Lesions.* Chicago, IL: American Osteopathic Association; 1948.

8. Denslow JS, Korr IM. Quantitative studies of chronic facilitation in human motoneuron pools. *Am J Physiol.* 1947:150:229–238.

9. Glossary of Osteopathic Terminology. In: *Foundations for Osteopathic Medicine.* Baltimore, MD: Williams & Wilkins; 1997.

10. Dinnar U, Beal M, Goodridge J, et al. Classification of diagnostic tests used with osteopathic manipulation. *J Am Osteopath Assoc.*1980;79:451–455.

11. Beal M. Incidence of spinal palpatory findings: a review. *J Am Osteopath Assoc.* 1989;89:1027–1035.

12. Kappler R. A comparison of structural examination findings obtained by experienced physician examiners and student examiners on hospitalized patients. *J Am Osteopath Assoc.* 1980:79:468–471.

13. McConnell D, Beal M, Dinnar U, et al. Low agreement of findings in neuromusculoskeletal examinations by a group of osteopathic physicians using their own procedures. *J Am Osteopath Assoc.* 1980;79:441–450.

14. Johnston W, Elkins M, Marino R, et al. Passive gross motion testing: Part II. A study of interexaminer agreement. *J Am Osteopath Assoc.* 1982;81:304–308.

15. Johnston W, Beal M, Blum G, et al. Passive gross motion testing: Part III. Examiner agreement on selected subjects. *J Am Osteopath Assoc.* 1982;81:309–313.

16. Johnston W, Allan B, Hendra J, et al. Interexaminer study of palpation in detecting location of spinal segmental dysfunction. *J Am Osteopath Assoc.* 1983;82:839–845.

17. Denslow J. Pathophysiological evidence for the osteopathic lesion. In: Goldstein M, ed. *The Research Status of Spinal Manipulative Therapy.* Bethesda, MD: U. S. Dept. of Health, Education, and Welfare; 1975:227–234.

18. Johnston W, Vorro J, Hubbard R. Clinical/biomechanical correlates for cervical function: Part 1. A kinematic study. *J Am Osteopath Assoc.* 1985;85:429–437.

19. Vorro J, Johnston W. Clinical biomechanic correlates for cervical function: Part II. A myoelectric study. *J Am Osteopath Assoc.* 1987;87:353–367.

20. Vorro J, Johnston W, Hubbard R. Clinical biomechanic correlates for cervical function: Part III. Intermittent secondary movements. *J Am Osteopath Assoc.* 1991;91:145–155.

21. Vorro J, Johnston W. Clinical biomechanic correlates of cervical dysfunction: Part 4. Altered regional motor behavior. *J Am Osteopath Assoc.* 1998;98:317–323.

22. Kelso A, Grant R, Johnston W. Use of thermograms to support assessment of somatic dysfunction or effects of osteopathic manipulative treatment. *J Am Osteopath Assoc.* 1982;82:182–188.

23. Walko E, Janouschek C. Effects of osteopathic manipulative treatment in patients with cervicothoracic pain: Pilot study using thermography. *J Am Osteopath Assoc.* 1994;94:135–141.

24. Kelso A, Larson N, Kappler R. A clinical investigation of the osteopathic examination. *J Am Osteopath Assoc.* 1980;79:460–467.

25. Johnston W. Interexaminer reliability studies: spanning a gap in medical research. *J Am Osteopath Assoc.* 1982;81:819–829.

26. Johnston W, et al. Palpatory findings in the cervicothoracic region. Variations in normotensive and hypertensive subjects. A preliminary report. *J Am Osteopath Assoc.* 1980;79:300–308.

27. Johnston W, Hill J, Elkiss M, et al. Identification of stable somatic findings in hypertensive subjects by trained examiners using palpatory examination. *J Am Osteopath Assoc.* 1982;81:830–836.

28. Johnston W, Kelso A, Babcock H. Changes in presence of a segmental dysfunction pattern associated with hypertension: Part 1. A short-term longitudinal study. *J Am Osteopath Assoc.* 1995;95:243–255.

29. Johnston W, Kelso A. Changes in presence of a segmental dysfunction pattern associated with hypertension: Part 2. A long-term longitudinal study. *J Am Osteopath Assoc.* 1995;95:315–318.

30. Beal M. Palpatory testing for somatic dysfunction in patients with cardiovascular disease. *J Am Osteopath Assoc.* 1983;82:822–831.

31. Cox J, Gorbis S, Dick L, et al. Palpable musculoskeletal findings in coronary artery disease: Results of a double-blind study. *J Am Osteopath Assoc.*1983;82:832–836.

32. Beal M, Kleiber G. Somatic dysfunction as a predictor of coronary artery disease *J Am Osteopath Assoc.* 1985;85:302–307.

33. Nicholas A, DeBias D, Ehrenfeuchter W, et al. A somatic component to myocardial infarction. *J Am Osteopath Assoc.* 1987;87:123–129.

34. Beal M, Morlock J. Somatic dysfunction associated with pulmonary disease. *J Am Osteopath Assoc.* 1984;84:179–183.

35. Johnston W, Kelso A, Hollandsworth D, et al. Somatic manifestations in renal disease: A clinical research study. *J Am Osteopath Assoc.* 1987;87:22–35.

36. Reeves R, Struve F, Patrick G. Somatic dysfunction increase during caffeine withdrawal *J Am Osteopath Assoc.* 1997;97:454–456.

37. Tarr R, Feely R, Richardson D, et al. A controlled study of palpatory diagnostic procedures: Assessment of sensitivity and specificity. *J Am Osteopath Assoc.* 1987;87:296–301.

38. Iwata J, Rodos J, Glonek T, et al. Comparing psychotic and affective disorders by musculoskeletal structural examination. *J Am Osteopath Assoc.* 1997;97:715–720.

39. McPartland J. Clarifying inaccuracies made regarding neuropsychiatric disorders and musculoskeletal examinations. *J Am Osteopath Assoc.* 1998;98:477–478 (letter).

OUTCOMES RESEARCH AND DESIGN

RICHARD J. SNOW
JOHN C. LICCIARDONE
RUSSELL G. GAMBER

The various diagnostic and therapeutic interventions available to health care providers have grown exponentially over the last 3 decades. Although the efficacy (how well these interventions perform in a controlled setting) of many of these interventions is often demonstrated in randomized clinical trials, their effectiveness in larger populations is often unknown. For example, a surgical procedure that removes plaque from the carotid artery, carotid endarterectomy, had been used for 20 years before two large, randomized clinical trials, the North American Symptomatic Carotid Endarterectomy Trial (NASCET) (1) and the Asymptomatic Carotid Atherosclerosis Study (2) defined the procedure's efficacy in stroke reduction. These randomized clinical trials enrolled patients into surgical programs with low perioperative stroke and mortality rates. Thus, the actual results obtained in the general community may vary widely from those obtained in the controlled studies (3). This is one example of the importance of tracking outcomes in clinical practice. Understanding the principles of outcomes research, including its biostatistical and epidemiologic underpinnings, provides clinicians with the knowledge necessary to evaluate the strengths and weaknesses of various research designs and to better assess the therapeutic value of a given intervention. Also, as clinicians function under increased expectations of practicing evidence-based medicine, they will need to evaluate the biomedical literature and understand the rationale behind clinical practice guidelines.

EVALUATION OF OSTEOPATHIC HEALTH DELIVERY

A framework originally attributed to Donabedian (4) describes health care delivery systems in terms of structure, process, and outcomes. Structure can be defined as the physical plant, equipment, human resources, and governance of the health care delivery system. Process is best described as the interaction between the patient and the health care delivery system. Examples can range from the prescription of an antibiotic or diagnostic test to open-heart surgery. Outcomes, the results of such clinical interactions, are frequently used to make judgments about the quality of health care. Thus, it is important that osteopathic physicians become engaged as active participants in the evolution of outcomes measurement and management in health care (5).

Outcomes may be generally measured along four axes. First, clinical outcomes include such events as morbidity, disease complications, and mortality. Second, functional outcomes include measures of physical or mental functioning and may use generic instruments, such as the Medical Outcomes Study Short Form–36 (SF-36) or the health status survey (6), or may use condition-specific outcomes tools, such as the stroke impact scale (7), the Roland-Morris disability questionnaire, and the Oswestry disability index for low back pain (8–10), and the WOMAC osteoarthritis index for knee or hip osteoarthritis (11). Third, patients' perceived outcomes focus on patient satisfaction and use such tools as the patient satisfaction questionnaire (PSQ) (12) or the Press-Ganey instrument (13). Finally, financial outcomes are measured by costs, charges, or by surrogates, such as length of stay. The term "outcomes research" broadly encompasses the evaluation of health care delivery using the framework described above.

The plethora of medical procedures brought about by advances in biotechnology, combined with increased demands on health care delivery systems because of an aging population, will increase the need for information about the most efficient treatment protocols. Outcomes research will help supply this information. In the realm of osteopathic medicine, outcomes research will help meet increasing demands to quantify the effects that osteopathic treatment, particularly osteopathic manipulative treatment (OMT), has on health (14). The recent designation of the Texas College of Osteopathic Medicine as the home of the national Osteopathic Research Center represents a response to demands for research on the efficacy of OMT. The implications for osteopathic medicine are obvious as the profession continues to strive to demonstrate its unique contributions to health care delivery. Recently, as described below, the body of literature addressing the impact of osteopathic medicine on clinical outcomes has been growing. In part, the future of osteopathic medicine relies on continuing and expanding such efforts to empirically demonstrate the unique role that osteopathic physicians play in health care delivery.

Demands for improved and standardized health care are becoming more apparent to those involved in health care delivery. Administrators of hospitals and health care plans need information to understand the financial impact of evolving technologies for managing health care organizations. Physicians need to assimilate and understand the multitude of diagnostic and therapeutic options to determine the best ways to treat patients. The sensitivity (ability of a test to correctly identify patients with a disease) and specificity (ability of a test to correctly identify patients without a disease) of tests and the expected and observed outcomes of patients will become important aspects of communicating with and managing the health care of patients.

The need to develop methods to practice evidence-based medicine and to better understand the outcomes of patients was recently reinforced by the Institute of Medicine (15). Their report entitled *Crossing the Quality Chasm* cited deficiencies of current health care delivery in providing evidence-based medicine in a consistent manner. This latter approach has the potential to improve the health of patients under the care of osteopathic physicians.

This chapter will describe, in a general manner, the tools and methods available to conduct clinical outcomes research. It will touch on hypothesis testing, study design, and related methodological issues. The chapter provides an overview of the field, with the intent of encouraging those interested in becoming more avid consumers of outcomes research information, as well as those wishing to add to the body of knowledge regarding osteopathic medicine. Examples of outcomes research are provided to demonstrate various approaches to assessing the impact of osteopathic medicine.

HYPOTHESIS TESTING

The foundations of outcomes research are similar to and largely overlap those of clinical research. The basic tools include epidemiology and biostatistics, a field of statistics concentrating on the unique aspects of statistical testing in biomedical settings. Epidemiology has been defined as the study of the distribution of health-related events in specified populations and the application of such studies to control health problems (16). Initially, as a basic science for public health, epidemiology was used to describe diseases according to person, place, and time, and to identify the determinants of disease. Over time, however, epidemiologic methods were used for hypothesis generation and testing in the clinical arena. Biostatistics serves to complement epidemiology by providing the analytical framework for testing hypotheses.

A clinical outcomes study begins with the hypothesis. It is essential to develop rational and testable hypotheses by thoroughly reviewing prior research in the field of study. Classically, hypothesis development involves framing the fundamental question as a statement indicating that there is no difference in effect or outcomes between treatment and control groups. This so-called "null hypothesis" is then tested in a structured manner. As an example, the null hypothesis in a randomized clinical trial testing a new anticoagulant's effect on deep vein thrombosis would be stated as: "There is no difference between the rates of deep vein thrombosis in patients treated with the new anticoagulant and those treated by conventional methods." An example of the null hypothesis in an observational study examining the effectiveness of carotid endarterectomy in high- and low-volume hospitals would be stated as: "There is no difference in the clinical outcome of patients

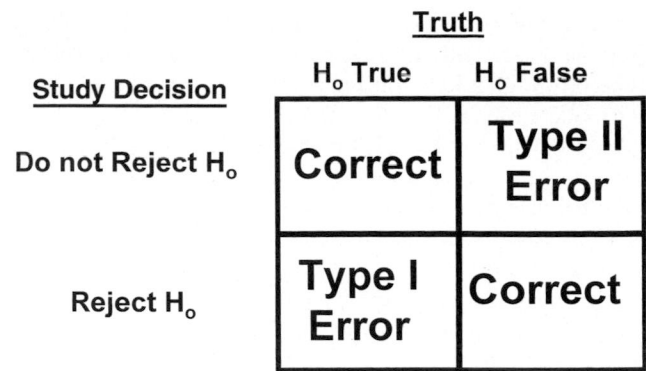

FIGURE 76.1. Schematic representation of the four possible, mutually exclusive, outcomes of hypothesis testing. H_0 denotes the null hypothesis.

receiving carotid endarterectomy in high-volume centers versus low-volume centers." Clinical outcomes may be measured by a variety of methods along the four axes previously described.

When testing the null hypothesis, two mutually exclusive types of errors may occur (Fig. 76.1). If, in the clinical trial of anticoagulation described above, it is erroneously concluded that there is a difference in the rates of deep vein thrombosis between the treatment and control groups, then a type I error is committed. The type I error, caused by rejecting the null hypothesis when it is in fact true, is considered the most important threat in hypothesis testing. Because this type of error results in the erroneous conclusion that a treatment improves patient care when, in fact, it is no better than placebo or conventional treatment, tolerance of a type I error is set at a low level. Scientific convention defines the acceptable risk of this event as α and sets its limit at one time out of twenty, or 0.05. The *p* value denotes the actual probability that a type I error was committed in a particular study.

The other type of hypothesis testing error that may occur in the anticoagulation trial example is to conclude that there is no difference in the rates of deep vein thrombosis between the treatment and control groups when a difference truly exists. This is known as a type II error and its acceptable risk is defined as β. Although scientific standards for an acceptable β are not as well established as for α, 0.20 is often used. Type II errors are attributed to insufficient numbers of research subjects for adequately performing hypothesis testing. The number of subjects in a study, or sample size, is a measure of the statistical power of a study. The relationship between risk, or probability, of a type II error and statistical power is given by the expression:

$$\text{(Probability of type II error)} = 1 - \text{(Power)}$$

Thus, all other things being equal, the probability of committing a type II error can be decreased by increasing the number of subjects in a study.

A common pitfall in interpreting the biomedical literature involves subgroup analyses, which consider only a subset of subjects in a study. Subgroup analyses that fail to demonstrate a significant difference in clinical outcomes between subgroups may be associated with high probabilities of type II errors because of limited numbers of subjects. Thus, such subgroup analyses must be adequately powered to address the research question or hypothesis at hand; otherwise type II errors will be likely. This concept has been summarized by the phrase, "the absence of proof is not the proof of absence."

An adequate sample size for randomized clinical trials, or subgroup analyses, may be computed by using four factors: the minimal difference between study groups that the investigator considers important enough to detect, the anticipated event rate in the control population, and the acceptable probabilities of committing type I and type II errors, α and β, respectively.

Type I and type II errors in clinical studies need to be understood when interpreting the biomedical literature. Because of the potential for these errors, several randomized clinical trials are needed to test the same hypothesis before statistical inferences can be comfortably applied in a clinical setting. For example, there were five randomized clinical trials examining the reduction of stroke risk afforded by the use of warfarin (an anticoagulant) in individuals with atrial fibrillation. The sixth study was stopped when evidence from the preceding studies was published, as it became unethical to withhold the drug from individuals based on the published information. By this account, it took five studies to define the use of warfarin in atrial fibrillation as the standard of care.

The exercise of computing the needed number of subjects for various hypothesis tests increases awareness of the cost of executing clinical studies. Testing a hypothesis that seeks to detect small differences between study groups, involving a low-frequency event or end point, can require several thousand subjects. The costs of subject recruiting, acquiring informed consent, collecting data, and tracking participants in such a large group can run into millions of dollars. Thus, it is important to estimate sample size to avoid embarking on a research project that cannot be realistically implemented within the available budget and scheduled time frame.

STUDY DESIGN

Experimental studies are best exemplified by randomized clinical trials. Such trials, with specific inclusion and exclusion criteria, enroll patients and randomly allocate them to treatment and control arms. The external generalizability of a randomized clinical trial is determined by how well the study subjects reflect the general population. This is determined, in part, by the selection of subjects through the applicable inclusion and exclusion criteria. In the previously cited NASCET randomized clinical trial, patients aged 80 years and greater were excluded. Because of this, the trial results cannot be adequately extrapolated to determine the effect of carotid endarterectomy on stroke risk reduction in individuals 80 years of age or older. A rationale for exclusion of older subjects is that the demonstration of a potentially beneficial surgery effect (carotid endarterectomy) over medical treatment requires the patient to be observed (i.e., to survive) long enough to offset the 2% risk of stroke or mortality associated with surgery.

The method of allocating subjects to the treatment or control arms in a randomized clinical trial involves random numbers or other statistical methods to ensure that no bias exists when patients are assigned to one arm or another (Fig. 76.2). This ex-

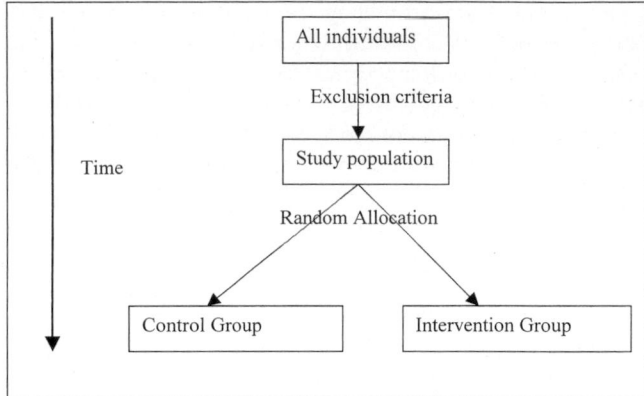

FIGURE 76.2. Selection of subjects for a randomized clinical trial.

perimental design provides the most valid approach to hypothesis testing. Theoretically, by randomizing the patients to either arm, the investigator removes any patient factors that might bias or confound the results of the study. As an example, if investigators testing the hypothesis that a new antacid reduces the incidence of ulcers sampled subjects in a way that resulted in higher numbers of subjects taking aspirin in the control group, they would likely find a lower rate of ulcers in the treatment group. The investigators may erroneously attribute the lower rate of ulcers to the antacid, when in reality it may be related to the confounding influence of greater aspirin use among controls compared with those in the treatment group. In this example, aspirin use is considered a confounder because it is associated with both the group assignment and the study outcome. A truly randomized study would eliminate the threat to validity posed by this confounder by apportioning comparable percentages of aspirin users to each arm of the study.

Inspection of the baseline characteristics of study groups in a randomized clinical trial is useful to assess the adequacy of the randomization process, particularly by checking for potential selection bias and by comparing the frequencies of potential confounders in each group. Similar characteristics in the treatment and control groups provide evidence that randomization has been properly executed. In such cases, randomized clinical trials provide the most accurate assessment of the effect of an intervention on patients who are included in the study. This represents high internal validity. When a comparison of treatment and control groups indicates a substantial imbalance in a baseline study variable or important confounder, potentially serious threats to validity are found. To maintain internal validity, more sophisticated multivariate statistical techniques may be needed to adjust for such confounder imbalances. Selection biases may be more subtle and difficult, if not impossible, to correct. They may seriously hamper the ability to extrapolate study results to other populations, resulting in poor external validity.

Experimental studies represent the most valid mechanism for hypothesis testing and are the standard of evidence required by the Food and Drug Administration when considering new drug approvals. Experimental studies generally are expensive because they require substantial resources to recruit, randomize, and follow patients over time. Because of these financial barriers, many interventions commonly used in health care delivery have not been tested by randomized clinical trials.

Other obstacles to conducting randomized clinical trials exist, including ethical issues. All scientific evidence linking tobacco use to lung cancer is based on nonrandomized studies. These are also known as pseudo-experimental, quasi-experimental, or observational studies. Because very early observational studies suggested there was a strong association between lung cancer and tobacco use, a randomized clinical trial testing the association became unethical because it would require randomizing individuals to a study arm exposing them to a cancer-causing agent.

Observational studies can test hypotheses without randomization of subjects to treatment and control groups. Although there are several different types of observational studies, two types are most commonly seen: case-control, or retrospective, studies (Fig. 76.3) and cohort, or prospective, studies (Fig. 76.4). Such studies often work well in situations when randomized clinical trials are not feasible or possible. The ability to detect statistical associations between naturally occurring events and outcomes cannot always be done using randomized clinical trials. An example of this involves exposure to electromagnetic fields and risk of leukemia. The association between the two has been hypothesized for the last several decades. Testing the hypothesis using a randomized clinical trial would be impractical for several reasons. First, the ethical issues regarding human research subjects are obvious when setting up an experiment that would be exposing individuals to a potential carcinogen. Second, because of the relative infrequency of the outcome (leukemia), the number of subjects in the treatment and control groups would have to be very large to ensure adequate statistical power and to maintain an acceptable risk of type II error. Finally, follow-up on a large number of subjects for 20 years or longer to determine if they develop leukemia would be very expensive. Under such circumstances, the hypothesis would be tested much more efficiently using a case-control study.

Despite concerns about potential biases and under- or overestimation of treatment effects in observational studies, there is little evidence for such problems in well-designed studies over the

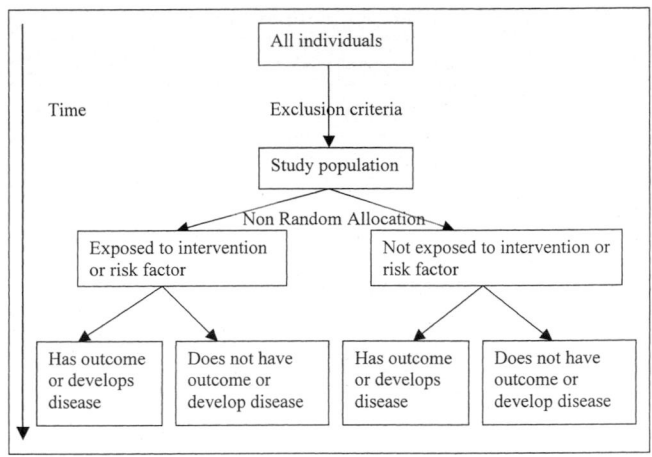

FIGURE 76.4. Design of a cohort, or prospective, study.

last two decades (17,18). Regardless of these concerns, observational studies provide an opportunity to test hypotheses that may otherwise not be testable using randomized clinical trials. Their use will continue to grow in clinical research and public health. It is incumbent on osteopathic physicians examining such studies and their results to understand the strengths and weaknesses of the study designs and the potential threats that such weaknesses and biases can pose to applying research findings in the clinical arena (Table 76.1).

In a case-control study, subjects are initially classified on the basis of whether they have (cases) or do not have (controls) the disease of interest. To avoid selection bias, controls should be representative of the same population that generated the cases. As an example, it is hypothesized that the use of aspirin is associated with an increased risk of developing ulcer disease. A case-control study would select subjects with diagnosed ulcer disease from a defined population and also identify a set of controls without ulcer disease from that same population. Sometimes controls may be matched to the cases on attributes that are related to disease occurrence, such as age, sex, caffeine use, tobacco use, nonsteroidal antiinflammatory use, and diet in this case. After selection of cases and controls, the past history and frequency of aspirin use is ascertained for subjects in each group. Statistical analysis of the amount and frequency of aspirin use in the cases and controls determines if any association between aspirin use and ulcer disease exists.

One advantage of the case-control study design is its ability to demonstrate an association using relatively small numbers of subjects. This advantage is most evident when examining diseases that occur infrequently. A good example of this is the above-mentioned relationship between electromagnetic forces and leukemia. Because leukemia is a rare disease, occurring in the range of one to five cases per 100,000 persons, it would be necessary to follow a large number of individuals exposed to electromagnetic forces to determine any relationship using a cohort, or prospective, study. The case-control study design dramatically decreases the number of subjects needed because of its retrospective nature. A case-control study starts with subjects known to have leukemia and identifies suitable controls. Thus, the total number of cases and controls numbers is in the hundreds compared to the hundreds of thousands using any other study design.

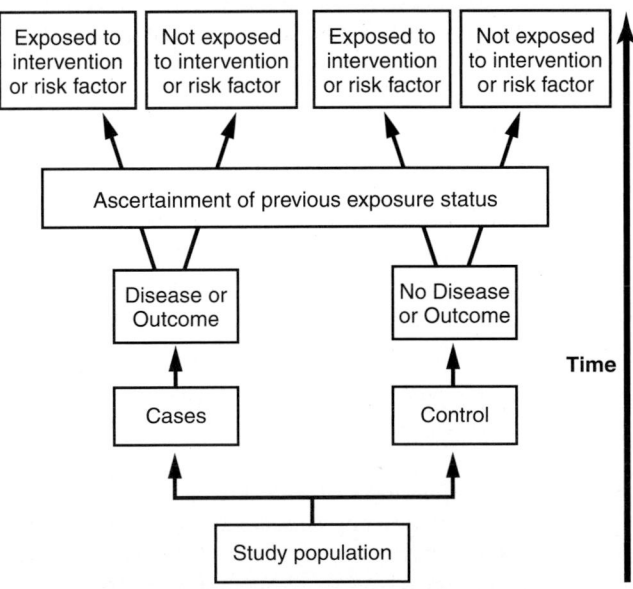

FIGURE 76.3. Design of a case-control, or retrospective, study.

TABLE 76.1. COMPARISON OF CASE-CONTROL AND COHORT STUDIES

Factor	Case-Control Studies (Retrospective)	Cohort Studies (Prospective)
Study group	Persons with disease	Exposed persons
Comparison group	Persons without the disease	Non-exposed persons
Outcome measures	Proportion of cases exposed and proportion of controls exposed	Incidence in exposed versus incidence in non-exposed
Measures of risk	Odds ratio	Absolute risk
	Attributable risk	Relative risk
		Attributable risk
Length of study	Relatively short	Generally long
Cost of study	Relatively inexpensive	Generally expensive
Population size needed	Relatively small	Relatively large
Potential bias	Assessment of exposure	Assessment of outcomes
Best when	Disease is rare	Exposure is rare
	Exposure is common among the diseased	Disease is frequent among exposed
Problems	Selection of appropriate controls often difficult	Selection of non-exposed comparison group often difficult
	Incomplete information on exposure	Loss to follow-up

Limitations of case-control studies result from potential biases that can be introduced when implementing the study. Recall bias, a problem introduced when asking subjects about exposures that may have occurred years before, can become a threat if there are long periods between exposure and manifestations of the disease. In the above example, there can be a long lag period between the exposure to electromagnetic forces and development of leukemia. Responses to questions about exposure to high-tension wires during childhood may be inaccurate. More importantly, subjects with leukemia, when compared with controls, may differentially recall (either inflate or deflate) their exposure to high-tension wires near their house as a child.

Other limitations of this type of study design include the potential bias introduced by improper selection of controls. A study that suggested an association between pancreatic cancer and coffee consumption was biased by the fact that potential controls were excluded if they had any previous gastrointestinal complaints. Because coffee is known to produce dyspepsia, eliminating subjects from the control group because of dyspepsia inappropriately reduced the number of coffee drinkers among the controls relative to the cases and made it appear that there was an association between coffee use and pancreatic cancer. The results were already published in a prestigious peer-reviewed journal before the bias was discovered and the association discounted (19,20).

The other type of observational study design is the cohort study, also known as a prospective study (Fig. 76.4). This type of study is commonly used in clinical research. Using a cohort study to test a hypothesis requires following subjects over a period of time to demonstrate an association between exposure to a risk factor or intervention and a specified outcome. The ongoing Framingham study is an excellent example of a cohort study. The Framingham study has provided the groundwork for many of the associations between risk factors and heart disease that are used for clinical decision making in primary and secondary prevention of heart disease. The Framingham study also identified the link between atrial fibrillation, a chaotic atrial rhythm, and stroke. By following subjects over a long period of time, investigators were able to identify a link between frequency of stroke and atrial fibrillation, even after adjusting for other factors that may be linked to stroke, including hypertension and age. The Framingham study was set up as a cohort study by measuring the baseline characteristics of a community of people and then following them over time for the occurrence of disease events. Analysis of the disease events includes a comparison of antecedent risk factors in those individuals experiencing the events and those not experiencing the events. The recruitment and follow-up of offspring of the early Framingham study subjects also affords a unique opportunity to study the effects of hereditary factors on heart disease.

Another example of a cohort study is the carotid endarterectomy outcome study mentioned previously (3). This study compared stroke morbidity and mortality rates in patients receiving carotid endarterectomy in high-volume versus low-volume centers. Patients entered the study when they received the surgery at either a high- or low-volume hospital. They were then tracked for 30 days to determine the occurrence of stroke or death, and statistical tests were used to compare the frequency of the end points in each of the two groups. Potential selection bias is an important factor to consider in interpreting the results of such studies. High-volume centers may serve as a referral site for complicated or high-risk cases, thereby attenuating the effects of technical expertise that may have been acquired by frequently performing carotid endarterectomy. Classification of patients' disease status may be used to control for this phenomenon when seeking to assess the surgical proficiency of high- and low-volume centers.

OUTCOMES RESEARCH IN THE REALM OF OSTEOPATHIC MEDICINE

Over the last 2 decades, there have been increasing efforts aimed at quantifying clinical outcomes associated with various aspects of osteopathic health care, particularly OMT. Perhaps most notably, there have been several randomized clinical trials to assess the efficacy of OMT in patients with low back pain. The first, a randomized clinical trial involving patients referred to a university-based back clinic in California from 1973 to 1979, found significant benefits with the first manipulative treatment when compared with a combined treatment involving soft-tissue massage and a sham manipulation technique (21). However, no significant benefits were attributed to manipulation at discharge, which, on average, occurred 30 days after the initial treatment. This trial has been criticized on the basis that it studied the effects of a particular manipulation technique rather than of OMT in general (22).

Another randomized clinical trial was performed at two medical offices of an Illinois-based health maintenance organization from 1992 to 1994 and involved patients with "subacute" low back pain lasting at least 3 weeks but less than 6 months (23). This trial compared OMT using a variety of techniques (each at the discretion of the treating provider) with standard care for low back pain. There were no significant differences in primary clinical outcomes between the OMT group and the standard-care group at 12 weeks. However, the OMT group used significantly less medication and physical therapy.

A recently completed randomized clinical trial examined the efficacy of OMT as a co-treatment in subjects with chronic low back pain of at least 3 months' duration (24). Subjects were randomized to either OMT, sham manipulation, or a no-intervention control group. OMT and sham manipulation subjects received interventions of comparable duration at the same intervals over 6 months. The main outcome measures included the SF-36 health status survey, the Roland-Morris disability questionnaire, a visual analog scale for back pain, and satisfaction with back care. Compared with no-intervention controls, OMT subjects reported less back pain and greater satisfaction with their back care throughout the trial, better physical functioning and mental health at 1 month, and fewer co-treatments at 6 months. Although there were no significant benefits associated with OMT when compared with sham manipulation, the trial was sufficiently powered to detect only moderate to large differences in treatment effects.

The most comprehensive evaluation of spinal manipulation for low back pain, including non-osteopathic approaches, was undertaken by the Agency for Healthcare Research and Quality, formerly known as the Agency for Health Care Policy and Research (25). A total of 112 articles were screened, and more extensive reviews of randomized clinical trials, meta-analyses, and cost analyses were conducted. The two highest-quality, randomized clinical trials that evaluated manipulation in patients with acute low back pain found significant improvements in pain and function in the manipulation groups compared with the control groups (26,27). Two meta-analyses, one based on 29 controlled trials (28) and another based on 23 randomized clinical trials (29), both attributed significant short-term benefits to manipulation for low back problems. The recommendation of the Agency for Healthcare Research and Quality concerning spinal manipulation is that manipulation can be helpful for patients with acute low back problems without radiculopathy when used within the first month of symptoms (25). The strength of evidence for this recommendation is graded as "B," indicating that moderate, research-based evidence was available from a relevant,

high-quality scientific study or multiple adequate scientific studies. A recent review of the continued validity of this clinical practice guideline found that only minor updating is needed, mostly involving the recommendations for back schools, lumbar corsets, and epidural steroid injections (30).

OMT has also been shown to be useful in ambulatory patients with other musculoskeletal conditions. A pilot study randomized female fibromyalgia patients to four groups that received various interventions in addition to their current medications (31). Those patients randomized to an OMT group were treated weekly with a combination of Jones strain/counterstrain techniques and other osteopathic modalities applied to troublesome tender points identified by the patient. Over 6 months, the patients receiving OMT reported significant benefits involving their perceived pain, attitudes toward treatment, activities of daily living, and perceived functional ability.

Another study randomized geriatric patients with chronic shoulder problems, such as tendonitis, bursitis, and osteoarthritis, to receive either OMT or sham manipulation in addition to their usual treatments (32). OMT included only the seven-step Spencer technique performed twice during each session. Sham manipulation consisted of the seven positions of the Spencer technique without administration of the actual corrective forces. Patients were initially treated biweekly and then monthly. Over the 14-week course of treatment, both groups experienced significantly increased range of motion and decreased pain compared to baseline; however, after treatment, the OMT group continued to demonstrate improved range of motion while the sham manipulation group experienced decreased mobility.

OMT has also been found to reduce hospital length of stay in several studies involving a variety of diseases. A small, randomized clinical trial compared patients who received a daily, standardized OMT protocol involving myofascial release, soft tissue, and strain-counterstrain techniques during their hospitalization for pancreatitis with those who received only conventional hospital care for pancreatitis (33). The OMT patients experienced a mean reduction of 3.5 days in their hospital stays. Another randomized clinical trial studied the efficacy of OMT in older patients hospitalized with acute pneumonia (34). In addition to conventional medical treatment for pneumonia, OMT patients received osteopathic manipulation and control patients received light touch sham treatments—each twice daily based on a standardized protocol to ensure comparable patient contact time. OMT patients experienced a shorter duration of antibiotic use and a mean reduction of 2.0 days in their hospital stays.

In the field of rehabilitation, two OMT studies in patients with knee or hip osteoarthritis who had recently undergone arthroplasty have yielded conflicting results. The first study, described as a "prospective, single-blinded, two-group, match-controlled outcome study," assessed the benefits of OMT as a complement to usual postsurgical care after knee or hip arthroplasty (35). OMT patients performed better than controls by negotiating stairs earlier and ambulating farther during their in-hospital rehabilitation. The study was limited, however, by lack of double blinding and sham treatments to control for anticipated therapeutic effect. A more recent study examined similar research questions using

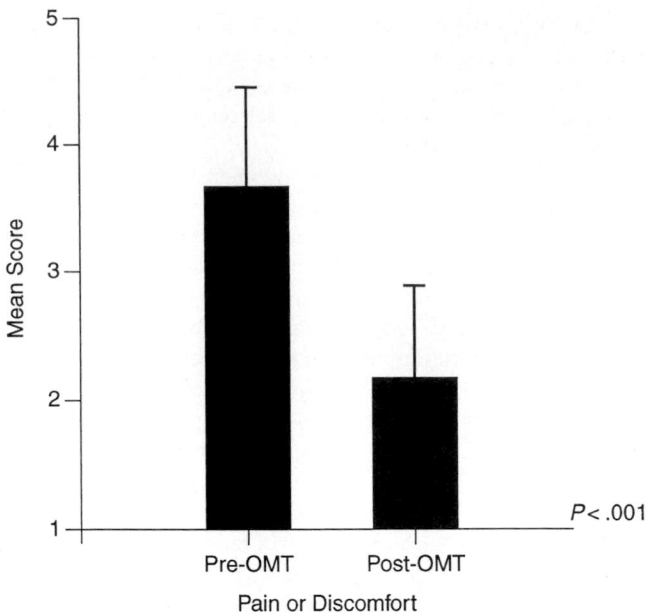

FIGURE 76.5. Comparison of reported pain or discomfort before and after receiving osteopathic manipulative treatment. A greater score indicates more pain or discomfort. The error bars represent one standard deviation.

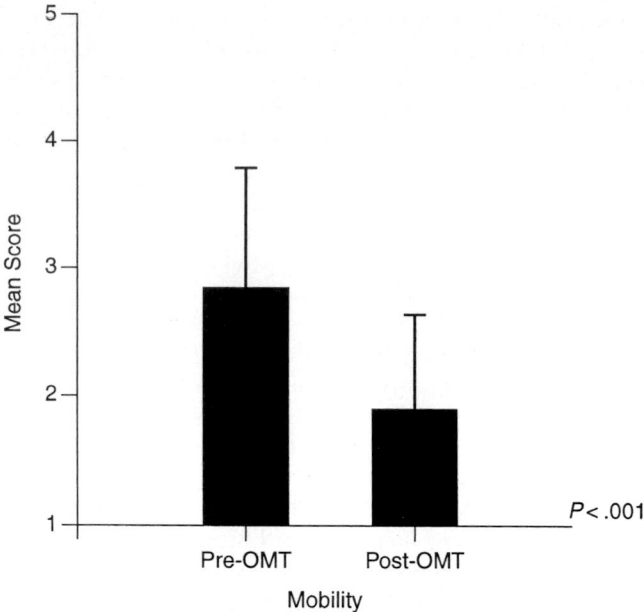

FIGURE 76.6. Comparison of reported mobility before and after receiving osteopathic manipulative treatment. A greater score indicates less mobility. The error bars represent one standard deviation.

a randomized clinical trial including double blinding and light touch sham treatments but failed to demonstrate any significant benefits associated with OMT in rehabilitation patients after knee or hip arthroplasty (36).

More recently, the clinical outcomes and satisfaction of patients attending a university-based specialty OMT clinic during 1998 were reported (37). Patients described OMT as being highly efficacious and reported significant reductions in pain and improvements in mobility associated with their OMT regimen (Figs. 76.5 and 76.6). A unique finding of this study is that women experienced significantly greater reductions in pain or discomfort than men. Patient satisfaction was generally high across all measured dimensions, with the sole exception of finances. More specifically, patients reported significant dissatisfaction with insurance coverage for OMT services.

Another study conducted within the same OMT clinic during 1997 examined quality of life, functional status, and patient satisfaction (38). This OMT clinic population was highly selected, often referred to the clinic after treatment failed elsewhere. Not surprisingly, clinic patients reported significantly poorer physical and mental functioning than patients in the general population on each of the eight SF-36 scales: physical functioning, role limitations because of physical problems, bodily pain, general health, vitality, social functioning, role limitations because of emotional problems, and mental health (Fig. 76.7). Perhaps the most interesting finding of the study was that patients referred to this OMT specialty clinic frequently reported poorer quality of life than national referents with hypertension, congestive heart failure, diabetes mellitus (type 2), recent myocardial infarction, or clinical depression. This highlights the difficulties that osteopathic physicians often face in treating patients with chronic musculoskeletal conditions. Despite such challenges, clinic

patients reported a high level of satisfaction with their health care.

The SF-36 health status survey was also used to ascertain the health of 2,700 patients attending six family medicine training clinics at a college of osteopathic medicine from 1996 through 1998 (39). As in the previously described study, clinic patients reported significantly poorer health status then the general population on all eight SF-36 scales. This has been attributed to the case mix of clinic patients, including a relatively high proportion of indigent and uninsured patients. Clinic patients were given the option of completing the SF-36 survey in their preferred language, either English or Spanish, and the results were then compared. English-language respondents reported significantly better health in the SF-36 scales measuring general health, social functioning, role limitations because of emotional problems, and mental health. Interestingly, however, Spanish-language respondents reported significantly greater vitality. Overall, patients reported high levels of satisfaction with their health care.

CONCLUSION

Osteopathic outcomes research is a fledgling enterprise. The basic tools afforded by biostatistics and epidemiology, as presented herein, are readily available to investigators seeking to add to our body of knowledge. The need to demonstrate the benefits of osteopathic medicine, as well as its distinctiveness, has never been greater. The future of osteopathic medicine may well hinge on its ability to satisfy this need by identifying, nurturing, and supporting a new breed of vibrant osteopathic clinical researchers.

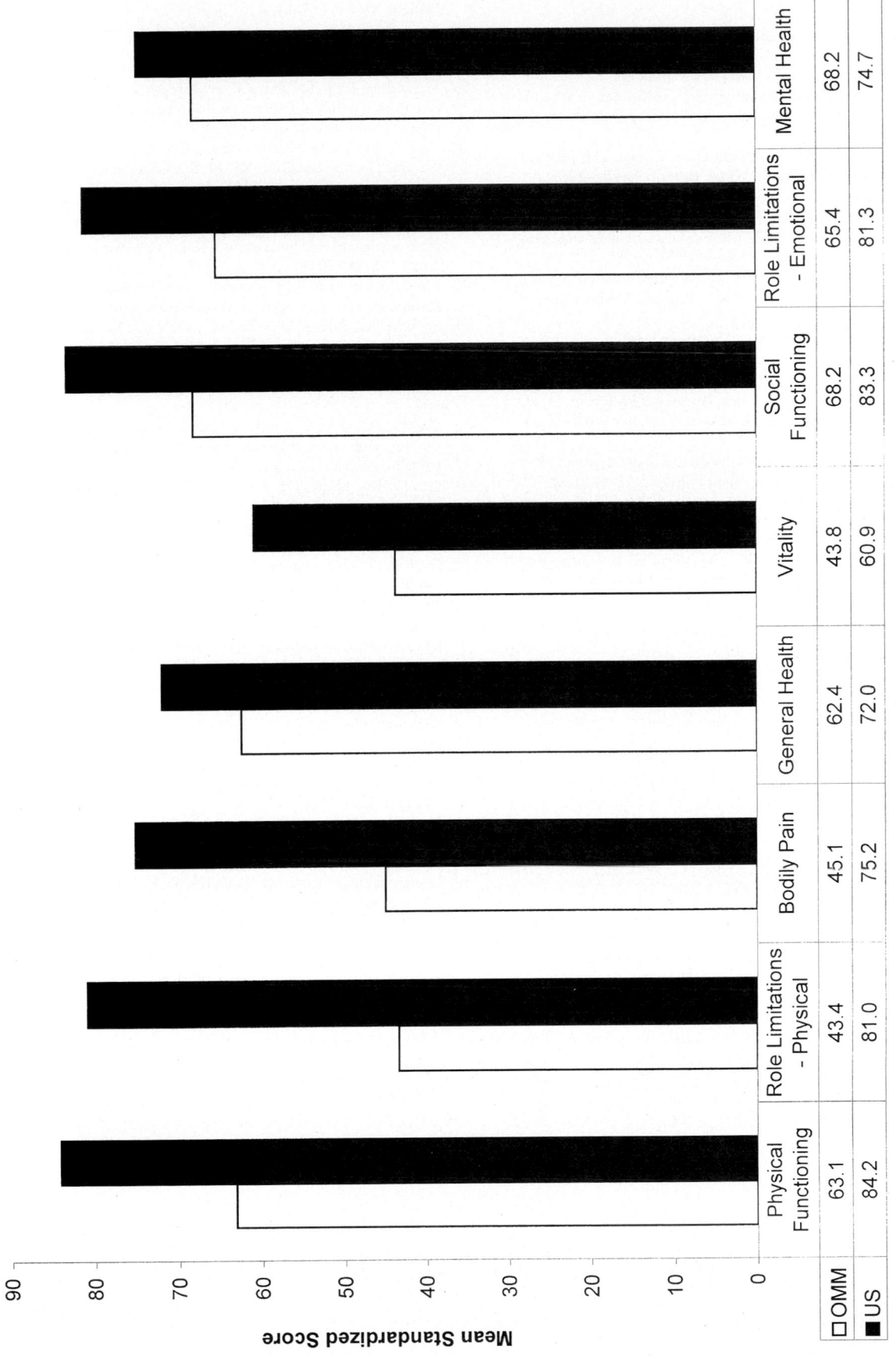

	Physical Functioning	Role Limitations - Physical	Bodily Pain	General Health	Vitality	Social Functioning	Role Limitations - Emotional	Mental Health
OMM	63.1	43.4	45.1	62.4	43.8	68.2	65.4	68.2
US	84.2	81.0	75.2	72.0	60.9	83.3	81.3	74.7

SF-36 Health Scale

FIGURE 76.7. Mean standardized scores according to SF-36 health scale for osteopathic manipulative medicine patients and the general United States population. Higher scores represent better health on each scale. Each of the eight comparisons is significant at the p less than 0.001 level. SF-36 denotes the Medical Outcomes Study Short Form–36.

REFERENCES

1. North American Symptomatic Carotid Endarterectomy Trial Collaborators. Beneficial effect of carotid endarterectomy in symptomatic patients with high-grade stenosis. *N Engl J Med.* 1991;325:445–453.
2. Executive Committee for the Asymptomatic Carotid Atherosclerosis Study. Endarterectomy for asymptomatic carotid artery stenosis. *JAMA.* 1995;273:1421–1428.
3. Cebul R, Snow R, Pine R, et al. Indications, outcomes, and provider volumes for carotid endarterectomy. *JAMA.* 1998;279:1282–1287.
4. Donabedian A. The role of outcomes in quality assessment and assurance. *Qual Rev Bull.* 1992;18:356–360.
5. Licciardone JC. The evolving role of outcomes measurement and management in healthcare. *J Am Osteopath Assoc.* 1997;97:290–292.
6. Ware JE, Snow KK, Kosinski M, et al. *SF-36 Health Survey: Manual and Interpretation Guide.* Boston, MA: New England Medical Center; 1993.
7. Duncan PW, Wallace D, Lai SM, et al. The stroke impact scale version 2.0. Evaluation of reliability, validity, and sensitivity to change. *Stroke.* 1999;30:2131–2140.
8. Roland M, Morris R. A study of the natural history of back pain: Part I. Development of a reliable and sensitive measure of disability in low-back pain. *Spine.* 1983;8:141–144.
9. Roland M, Fairbank J. The Roland-Morris disability questionnaire and the Oswestry disability questionnaire. *Spine.* 2000;25:3115–3124.
10. Stratford PW, Binkley J, Solomon P, et al. Assessing change over time in patients with low back pain. *Phys Ther.* 1994;74:528–533.
11. Bellamy N. WOMAC Osteoarthritis Index. User's Guide III, 1998.
12. Ware Jr JE, Snyder MK, Wright WR, et al. Defining and measuring patient satisfaction with medical care. *Evaluation and Program Planning.* 1983;6:247–263.
13. Press, Ganey Associates, Inc. Effective customer services practices. *Healthcare Executive.* 2001;16:64–65.
14. Goldstein M. A challenge to the profession: initiate evidence-based osteopathic medicine now [editorial]. *J Am Osteopath Assoc.* 1997;97:448, 451.
15. Committee on Quality of Health Care in America, Institute of Medicine. *Crossing the Quality Chasm: A New Health System for the 21st Century.* Washington, DC: National Academy of Sciences; 2001.
16. Last JM. *A Dictionary of Epidemiology,* 2nd ed. New York, NY: Oxford University Press; 1988.
17. Benson K, Hartz AJ. A comparison of observational studies and randomized, controlled trials. *N Engl J Med.* 2000;342:1878–1886.
18. Concato J, Shah N, Horwitz RI. Randomized, controlled trials, observational studies, and the hierarchy of research designs. *N Engl J Med.* 2000;342:1887–1892.
19. MacMahon B, Yen S, Trichopoulos D, et al. Coffee and cancer of the pancreas. *N Engl J Med.* 1981;304:630–633.
20. Hsieh C, MacMahon B, Yen S, et al. Coffee and pancreatic cancer (Chapter 2) [letter]. *N Engl J Med.* 1986;315:587–588.
21. Hoehler FK, Tobis JS, Buerger AA. Spinal manipulation for low back pain. *JAMA.* 1981;245:1835–1838.
22. Patterson MM. Osteopathic research: the future. In: Ward RC, ed. *Foundations for Osteopathic Medicine.* Baltimore, MD: Williams & Wilkins; 1997:1115–1124.
23. Andersson GB, Lucente T, Davis AM, et al. A comparison of osteopathic spinal manipulation with standard care for patients with low back pain. *N Engl J Med.* 1999;341:1426–1431.
24. Licciardone J, Stoll S, Fulda K, et al. A randomized, controlled trial of osteopathic manipulative treatment in patients with chronic low back pain. Unpublished manuscript, 2001.
25. Bigos S, Bowyer O, Braen G, et al. *Acute Low Back Problems in Adults. Clinical Practice Guideline No. 14.* Rockville, MD: Agency for Health Care Policy and Research, Public Health Service, U. S. Department of Health and Human Services; 1994.
26. Hadler NM, Curtis P, Gillings DB, et al. A benefit of spinal manipulation as adjunctive therapy for acute low-back pain: a stratified controlled trial. *Spine.* 1987;12:703–706.
27. McDonald RS, Bell CM. An open controlled assessment of osteopathic manipulation in nonspecific low-back pain. *Spine.* 1990;15:364–370.
28. Shekelle PG, Adams AH, Chassin MR, et al. Spinal manipulation for low-back pain. *Ann Intern Med.* 1992;117:590–598.
29. Anderson R, Meeker WC, Wirick BE, et al. A meta-analysis of clinical trials of spinal manipulation. *J Manipulative Physiol Ther.* 1992;15:181–194.
30. Shekelle PG, Ortiz E, Rhodes S, et al. Validity of the Agency for Healthcare Research and Quality clinical practice guidelines: how quickly do guidelines become outdated? *JAMA.* 2001;286:1461–1467.
31. Gamber RG, Shores JH, Russo DP, et al. Osteopathic manipulation in conjunction with medication relieves pain associated with fibromyalgia syndrome: results of a randomized clinical pilot project. *J Am Osteopath Assoc.* 2002 *(in press).*
32. Knebl J, Shores J, Gamber R, et al. Improving functional ability in the elderly by osteopathic manipulative treatment: a randomized, controlled trial. *J Am Osteopath Assoc.* 2002 *(in press).*
33. Radjieski JM, Lumley MA, Cantieri MS. Effect of osteopathic manipulative treatment on length of stay for pancreatitis: a randomized pilot study. *J Am Osteopath Assoc.* 1998;98:264–272.
34. Noll DR, Shores JH, Gamber RG, et al. Benefits of osteopathic manipulative treatment for hospitalized elderly patients with pneumonia. *J Am Osteopath Assoc.* 2000;100:776–782.
35. Jarski RW, Loniewski EG, Williams J, et al. The effectiveness of osteopathic manipulative treatment as complementary therapy following surgery: a prospective, match-controlled outcome study. *Altern Ther Health Med.* 2000;6:77–81.
36. Licciardone JC, Stoll ST, Herron KM, et al. A randomized controlled trial of osteopathic manipulative treatment following knee or hip arthroplasty. *J Am Osteopath Assoc.* 2002 *(in review).*
37. Licciardone JC, Gamber R, Cardarelli K. Patient satisfaction and clinical outcomes associated with osteopathic manipulative treatment. *J Am Osteopath Assoc.* 2002;102:13–20.
38. Licciardone JC, Gamber R, Russo D. Quality of life in referred patients presenting to a specialty clinic for osteopathic manipulative treatment. *J Am Osteopath Assoc.* 2002;102:151–155.
39. Licciardone JC, Brittain P, Coleridge S. Health status and satisfaction of patients attending osteopathic medical training clinics. *J Am Osteopath Assoc.* 2002 *(in press).*

BIOBEHAVIORAL INTERACTIONS WITH DISEASE AND HEALTH

BRIAN H. FORESMAN
GILBERT E. D'ALONZO, JR.
JOHN A. JEROME

KEY CONCEPTS

- Biobehavioral mechanisms alter health and disease through three basic pathways: physiologic responses that lead to disease, behaviors that increase or decrease health risk, and behaviors that alter surveillance activities or adherence with medical interventions.
- The major behavioral factors that have been studied and shown to have clear associations with health and disease include: diet, exercise, sleep, cigarette smoking, tobacco use, alcohol use, and prevention of excessive sun exposure.
- Placebos are also a biobehavioral mechanism that must be addressed in most forms of research. Results are affected by race, direct suggestion, patient belief in the treatment, trust in the physician, genetic variation, environmental effects, and nonspecific cause–effect relationships with placebos.
- Sleep and somatovisceral responses constitute major biobehavioral mechanisms that are common to all individuals, a rich area for research, and that suggest a strong role for biobehavioral approaches.
- As with other types of research, the biobehavioral research process begins with the acquisition of information and the development of a hypothesis about the mechanisms involved with the processes under consideration. Selection of the study design, subjects, methods to be used constitute the major components of the process and lead to a systematic analysis of the data.
- Biobehavioral measures and techniques may provide a more effective research paradigm and may render valuable insight into the impact of osteopathic principles and practice. Major topics in this area will likely focus on: behaviors leading to the development of somatic dysfunction, behaviors resulting from somatic dysfunction, quality of life (QOL), effects of pain, and relationships between locomotor function, somatic dysfunction, and subsequent behaviors.

Biobehavioral research involves the investigation of behaviors on the maintenance of health and the development of disease. The onset of disease is a complex phenomenon that incorporates the tissue pathology (musculoskeletal abnormalities), psychosocial and behavioral response to that physical insult, and the environmental factors that maintain or reinforce that disability (even after the initial cause has been resolved). A large portion of the variance in an individual response to any disease outcome is accounted for by the manner of behavior and emotional response to the stress of the illness (1). In fact, the majority of today's health woes—obesity, cancer, and anxiety disorders to heart disease, hypertension, and adult-onset diabetes—are actually relatively new "diseases of civilization" brought on by our behavioral choices and mind-body interactions. Although the concepts that the mind influences disease processes have long been a part of osteopathic medicine, research involving mechanisms of disease modification through a mind-body interaction have only recently become a part of mainstream medicine.

Our current understanding of biobehavioral interactions suggests that these processes are a complex interplay between genetic, physiologic, environmental, and behavioral factors that influence health and disease (2). Behavioral mechanisms can alter the nervous system, endocrine system, and the immune system, directly and indirectly, thereby influencing such medical illnesses as cancer and cardiovascular disease. Diet, exercise, drugs, alcohol, and tobacco use, along with a variety of other behaviors, modify disease progression and/or disease risk. Finally, behaviors directly related to seeking or avoiding medical care can have important consequences on prevention, early detection, and adherence with medical regimens. Thus, the implication is that biobehavioral factors may significantly affect health care and health maintenance through a variety of direct and indirect mechanisms (2), and these effects should be addressed in osteopathic research and clinical practice (3–5).

BIOBEHAVIORAL MECHANISMS IN HEALTH

Behavioral components of the mind-body interaction manifest in cognitive processes, emotions, and/or physical behaviors. The

**TABLE 77.1. ABBREVIATED LIST OF COGNITIVE PRO-
CESSES**

Language acquisition
Reading
Emotional appraisal
Memory
Attention
Mental models or representations
Learning and cognition
Problem solving
Ascribing meaning, abstraction
Action

study of cognitive processes (Table 77.1) primarily focuses on understanding the acquisition, retention, and processing of information. However, under most circumstances, thoughts, emotions, and cognitive processes must transmit information, be translated into motor actions, or have identifiable physiologic responses before a behavior can be identified. It is for these reasons that many consider mental phenomena to be a special form of physical phenomena (i.e., biobehavioral) and therefore inseparable from physiologic processes.

Biobehavioral factors exert their influence through three defined pathways (2,6) and at least one alternate pathway. In the first of these pathways, emotional reactions or behaviors are associated with or occur in parallel with physiologic alterations that contribute directly or indirectly to the pathophysiology of the disease (Fig. 77.1). An example is the stress response that is associated with increases in blood pressure and heart rate as part of global sympathetic arousal. Sympathetic alterations can, in turn, contribute directly to the development of cardiac disease and sudden death. Excessive stress, whether induced by external events or extreme exercise, can alter neural and hormonal responses, leading to enhanced vulnerability to infection and inappropriate response to disease (i.e., viral infections, wound healing, and cancer).

The second pathway for biobehavioral interactions involves behaviors associated with increasing or minimizing health risk (Fig. 77.1). These particular behaviors are referred to as health-enhancing or health-impairing behaviors. Examples of health-enhancing behaviors include diet and exercise (due to their ability to minimize the development cardiovascular disease and cancer).

Tobacco use and alcohol abuse are examples of health-impairing behaviors typically associated with adverse effects that frequently lead to emphysema, lung cancer, and cardiovascular disease. Other examples include drug use and high-risk sexual activity. Each of these activities conveys a risk or benefit to an alteration of the underlying physiology and/or exposure.

The third and final pathway (Fig. 77.1) involves behaviors that occur in response to the possibility that a disease may be, or is, present. For individuals without disease, the behaviors that lead to early detection include ongoing surveillance (i.e., retained breast examinations, sigmoidoscopy, etc.), recognition of symptoms, and the decision to seek medical care or follow-up care. Once a disease or a symptom is identified and a medical regimen is prescribed, adherence with the medical regimen (or lack thereof) is a behavior that can affect the outcome of the disease process. In addition, the sudden discontinuation of medications or their erratic administration may not only hinder the effectiveness of medical regimens; such behaviors may create secondary adverse consequences.

Prior investigations have not routinely included somatic or motor dysfunction as attributable to a biobehavioral pathway; however, there are many situations under which this theoretic framework would be applicable and might offer distinct advantages in understanding the relevant pathophysiologic relationships. The consideration of such pathways is in keeping with known responses of the somatic musculature and would represent a modification of pathway "A" (Fig. 77.1). In this instance, we would substitute musculoskeletal impairment for altered disease risk, and the pathway becomes more consistent with the concepts of viscerosomatic pathways. This theoretic framework is also consistent with the biologic and behavioral responses of individuals with acute and chronic pain (see Chapter 11).

Disease Development (Pathway "A")

The major biobehavioral influences on disease development that have been studied involve the effects of stress on health or illness (Chapter 15). Because of the scope of the data involving stress, physiologic response, and behavioral issues, our intent is to discuss the major mechanisms wherein stress responses affect select diseases.

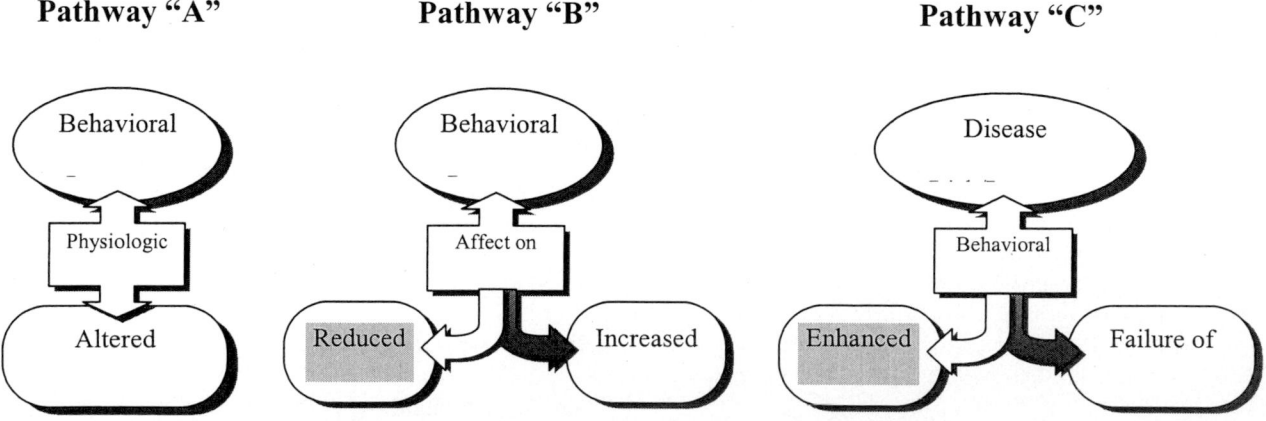

FIGURE 77.1. Common biobehavioral pathways in health and disease.

From an evolutionary standpoint, most neural events can be considered to develop and have been selected by evolutionary process associated with species survival (2). In this viewpoint, stress responses and other emotional patterns are hardwired into the central nervous system (CNS) and modified by learning and experience. Thus, content and environmental conditions give rise to particular responses that can modify the emotional or cognitive response. Essentially, our bodies "learn" about the external correlates of internal responses much like a baby learns that food and eating extinguish the uncomfortable response later learned as hunger. This process of "learning" can be significantly affected by the intensity and chronicity of the stress response under which the learning occurred. Less intense and intermittent stressors allow more complex and appropriate coping strategies to be learned; whereas more severe and prolonged stressors may cause a conditioned biobehavioral response that is less adaptable. In this sense, learning may be either adaptive or maladaptive and may affect predisposition to disease.

CARDIOVASCULAR DISEASE

Previous research has shown that stress, whether physical or emotional, perceived or real, often results in characteristic physiologic and behavior responses (Table 77.2). The physiologic and behavioral correlates may trigger acute, disease-related events and alter the pathophysiology of the disorders (7). Acute cardiovascular events, such as ischemic episodes, heart attacks, arterial occlusion, and arrhythmias, have been shown to occur with anxiety, bereavement, and anger (3,8,9). Similar effects are also seen with strong positive emotions associated with desirable events (e.g., weddings). Several mechanisms have been proposed to account for these responses, including alteration of sympathetic-parasympathetic balance, activation of platelets, alterations of intravascular flow dynamics, and changes of endothelial function (10,11).

Within these hardwired responses, heightened maladaptive processes may lead to secondary physiologic responses that may have additional adverse consequences. For example, when assessing cardiovascular responses, physiologic reactivity is measured by the magnitude and the duration of the particular response. Studies have shown that increased cardiac reactivity may be a direct index of the underlying predisposition toward developing cardiovascular disorders or may reflect the activity of mediators of cardiovascular risk (12). In several studies, exaggerated blood pressure responses identified individuals at risk for developing hypertension and atherosclerosis (13–15). Similarly, other behaviors may have adverse affects on serum lipid composition, silent ischemia oxidative damage (9,16) (such as that seen with smoking), personality styles (e.g., type A), and altered coping mechanisms (17). Through the use of biobehavioral approaches, cardiovascular researcher are now beginning to enhance our understanding of the complex relationships between the mind and the body in the development and progression of cardiovascular disease (6,9).

IMMUNE FUNCTION AND INFECTIOUS DISORDERS

Immunologic activity has also been shown to be altered by behavioral responses; however, the impact on disease development is less clear. Some of the difficulty in making assessments regarding immune function involves the variability of the stressors and the dynamic nature of the immune system (see Chapter 10). For instance, natural killer cells have a different response to acute and chronic stress exposures (18), and these responses are also subject to circadian variations. Changes in latent viral activity, lymphocyte proliferation, and natural killer cell activity have all been demonstrated in response to stress (19–21). These changes in immune function and cell numbers may also occur with physical stress, such as severe exercise (22). Several immunologic responses may also promote facilitating responses. The activation of inflammatory mediators, such as interleukin-6 and proinflammatory cytokines, may alter neural processes to enhance aspects of the CNS stress response (23). However, the role that stress-induced changes in immune function have on the development of subsequent disease has been debated and remains unclear.

Behaviors can have a more direct effect on the development of disease by altering bodily functions and behaviors associated with disease risk (24). Perhaps the most classic example involves human immunodeficiency virus (HIV) disease. The transmission of HIV typically occurs during sexual activity, intravenous drug use, or through other forms of direct contact with bodily fluids. An attenuation of these behaviors or the addition of protective measures can result in substantial decreases in the risk of acquiring

TABLE 77.2. SUMMARY OF MAJOR RESPONSES TO STRESS

Behavioral Response		Physiologic Response
Moderate/Short Duration	**Severe/Long Duration**	
Increased attention	Diminished attention	Increased heart rate
Increased alertness	Anxiety	Increased sympathetic activity (both neural and humoral)
Enhanced memory and problem-solving skills	Irritability	Increased blood pressure
	Reduced retention and recall	Increased catabolism
	Diminished problem solving	Altered immune function (dependent on the duration and intensity of the stressor)
	Insomnia	

HIV. Conversely, increases in risky behaviors or the occurrence of impulse behaviors, as can occur with individuals with certain types of mental health problems (25) or during drug and alcohol use (26,27), can change routine behaviors of the individual and increase the risk of acquiring HIV. In this setting, stress or drug use may initiate impulsive behaviors or may inhibit intentions to avoid the risky behaviors (28) leading to impaired judgment, a lack of attention to details, or in some instances, disregarding the potential consequences of their actions (29).

Evidence for a direct effect of behaviors on immune status leading to outcomes in HIV is limited (30). In a recent study of 100 HIV-positive individuals, somatic findings were associated with progression disease; however, there was no evidence to suggest that these effects were mediated by the immune system. Cole and colleagues (31) suggested that some specific behaviors may affect the progression of disease development when present. In their study, the investigators identified that concealment of sexual identity was positively related to cancer morbidity and the incidence of pneumonia. However, there was no clear link with alterations in immune function, which might be related to the behaviors themselves.

SLEEP AND CIRCADIAN BIOLOGY

Sleep and sleep wake activities also constitute a major biobehavioral mechanism. Sleep deprivation and sleep fragmentation result in excessive daytime sleepiness, chronic fatigue, and other symptoms. Many of the symptoms are indistinguishable from depression, and they may have some of the same adverse consequences on medical adherence as depression does (32). More recently, studies have suggested that alterations of sleep wake schedule may contribute to the development of disease. In one recent study, Bursztyn and colleagues (33) assessed daytime napping in an older patient cohort (n = 455). The findings suggested that an afternoon nap appeared to be an independent predictor of mortality with a risk odds ratio of 2.1. In a separate study using self-administered questionnaires on health status and lifestyle (34), the investigators identified that significantly longer and shorter sleep times, compared with 7 to 8 hours, were associated with increases in total mortality in men. In addition, female users of sleeping pills and those with self-reported poor sleep quality also shared an increased risk of mortality independent of sleep duration. Similar findings have been noted by others (35), and were noted to be unaffected by later arousal times. However, a recent review of the literature on shift work, an extreme form of late risers, suggested there is an overall increase in cardiovascular risk of 40%. These data suggest that disrupted sleep or significantly altered sleep schedules may have adverse effects on medical outcomes through biobehavioral mechanisms.

PAIN SYNDROMES

Specific diseases need not be the only focus of biobehavioral investigations. Major symptoms, and specifically chronic pain, may benefit from a biobehavioral approach to investigations (36–38). In a review from an NIH-sponsored workshop, the current status and major directions for biobehavioral pain research were out-

lined. Pain was identified as a subjective experience that could only be quantified through behavior (39), and there were many behavioral responses to chronic pain that impacted treatment and recovery. Consistent with the NIH initiative, investigators demonstrated that biobehavioral models offer significant insight into the mechanisms active in chronic pain (40,41). Several studies suggest that dysfunctional information processing occurs, accentuating the perception of pain and reinforcing the concept that learning plays a significant role in pain syndromes (40,42). Such mechanisms may also be actively involved in the disability associated with several disorders (e.g., low back pain, osteoarthritis, cardiac pain) (5,43), and may have a significant role in our understanding of the neurophysiology of somatic dysfunction (44).

Disease Risk (Pathway "B")

Several behaviors exert their primary effect by modifying disease risk or factors associated with disease risk. The major behavioral factors within this category that are also supported by substantial data include: diet, exercise, sleep, cigarette smoking, tobacco use, alcohol use, and the prevention of excessive sun exposure. In general, modifications of diet, exercise, sleep, and relaxation constitute factors associated with a protective influence over physiologic sources of risks. They also function in an indirect manner by minimizing the effects of stress and enhancing coping mechanisms. Smoking, excessive alcohol consumption, and drug abuse typically fall into the category of health-impairing behaviors that directly influence disease processes and have secondary effects on mood and other behaviors. Physical behaviors (e.g., exercise, aerobics, and other types of physical exertion) often exert a protective influence and therefore fall in the category of health-enhancing behaviors. The consequences of these physical behaviors may directly or indirectly affect pain syndromes, medical interventions, and the natural history of disease. For example, an individual attempting to undergo a weight control regimen without substantial lifestyle changes that include increases in activity may experience difficulty in achieving and maintaining weight loss (45,46).

In general, the preponderance of data demonstrating association between diet and disease outcomes is found in the cardiovascular literature. Weight gain, obesity, excessive salt consumption, and fat or cholesterol intake are major contributors in the development of coronary artery disease, hypertension, and stroke. Interventions directed at weight loss and weight maintenance have engendered some success when the interventions were maintained (47) and when the interventions target specific ethnic or socioeconomic groups (48). These interventions recognize that adherence and cultural affects were an important part of an effective regimen.

The role of dietary influence on cancer risk is more speculative than the data regarding cardiovascular disease. For example, there appears to be an association between fat/fiber content in the diet and the mammography profile associated with breast cancer (49) or recurrence of breast cancer among women with estrogen receptor–positive tumors (50). Whether patients can effectively alter their fat intake and weight has also been studied by investigators. Several studies have shown that diet can be effectively modified (51), secondarily leading to an increase in consumption of healthier food (52). These programs appear to be more effective when there is evidence to support the dietary changes and the individuals are aware of the evidence (53). However, the effect of dietary interventions on cancer-relevant outcomes has been questioned by some and may require further study, especially in patients with established malignancies.

Exercise appears to exert beneficial effects by reducing stress and increasing caloric consumption. The increasing caloric consumption is important in designing effective weight management programs. There are data to suggest that routine exercise programs reduce the relative risk of developing cancer (54) through either a reduction in sedentary activities or weight loss (55). Exercise also appears to be an effective coping strategy for stress (22). These effects may be related to alterations in mood and a reduction in perceived stress that occurs with routine exercise (56). The latter of these effects may relate more specifically to an attenuation of physiologic reactivity. Unfortunately, for many individuals, increasing stress reduces the amount of physical activity undertaken (57). Reduction of stress and an improvement in the physiologic adaptability have also been cited as possible mechanisms by which exercise could exert its effect in cancer.

Our knowledge of the effects of tobacco use dates back to the early 1960s. Since that time, extensive data have demonstrated the adverse health consequences of cigarette smoking and tobacco use. The habitual use of tobacco relates to physiologic responses to nicotine (e.g., sense of well-being, arousal, and appetite suppression) and the avoidance of or the relief from withdrawal (58). Smoking contributes to the development of atherosclerosis, coronary artery disease, hypertension, stroke, emphysema, bronchitis, and several malignancies through recognized physiologic mechanisms (59). Even secondhand smoke may carry some of the habituating and cardiovascular responses related to nicotine exposure (60). In this regard, prevention may be a more effective strategy for limiting cigarette smoking and its adverse health consequences (61). However, in individuals who smoke, stress appears to be a significant contributor to the amount and frequency of tobacco use (57), as well as to relapse after smoking cessation. Thus, the combination of stress and tobacco use is a self-reinforcing behavioral pattern that is complicated by nicotine addiction. Behavioral strategies designed to alter tobacco use must address these interactive behaviors to be effective (62). The biobehavioral components of successful addiction management are found in Table 77.3.

Understanding the issues relevant to the health consequences of sun exposure is illustrative of the complexity of some biobehavioral interactions. Ultraviolet (UV) radiation in sunlight has been linked to the development of basal-cell cancers, squamous-cell cancers, and melanomas (63–65). For basal-cell and squamous-cell cancers, the risk parallels cumulative lifetime UV exposure.

Routine use of avoidance measures or sunscreen can substantially decrease the risk of skin cancer. Unfortunately, despite increased awareness and knowledge of skin cancer, there has been little change in individual behavior. One reason is the belief that sun tanning makes an individual look healthier and that exposure to the sun is healthy (66). This persistence of beliefs and behaviors underlies several medical disorders and high-risk behaviors.

Disease-Related Biobehavioral Activities (Pathway "C")

The final general mechanism relating behavior with disease involves behaviors that occur when illness is present, suspected, or where there is risk of illness. Many factors influence individual behaviors under these conditions. When illnesses are suspected or where there is the potential for illness, the perception of illness (e.g., fear), and the potential impact (e.g., need for chemotherapy) may significantly alter the response of the individual. Socioeconomic factors, issues involved with physician support or confidence, the perception of risk, and emotional reaction of the individual all significantly affect surveillance efforts (67,68). Health beliefs, perceptions of risk, and generalized anxiety regarding disease or illness greatly contribute to avoidance on the part of the patient (67,69). Consistent with these concepts, Lerman and associates (69) reported heightened anxiety about developing breast cancer in association with intrusive thoughts and demonstrated some relationship with adherence (70). Similar findings were noted in women undergoing genetic counseling for breast cancer (71). However, the distress associated with disease risk does not have a consistent effect on surveillance activities (72). These findings have also been noted in screening for HIV. Studies have linked the associated anxiety with undergoing screening and failure to follow-up for test results. In general, stress, emotional responses, and past behavior are often the best predictors (73) of adherence.

A variety of behaviors related to the presence of illness may arise. Two major behavioral mechanisms affect outcomes in individuals with existing disease. The first of these mechanisms relates to adherence. Medical regimens are rarely effective when patients are nonadherent. However, nonadherence may arise from many sources, including inadequate understanding (74), forgetfulness, confusion, health beliefs, personal (naïve) theories of illness, and cost (75). There are few reliable predictors of adherence; however, high-quality communication, patient supervision, social support, and the recognition and management of underlying impairments, especially depression (32), all contribute to improving adherence (32,75).

TABLE 77.3. BIOBEHAVIORAL COMPONENTS OF ADDICTION-MANAGEMENT MODELS

1. A public declaration.
2. Attend to withdrawal syndrome.
3. Aerobic exercise.
4. Attacking learned behaviors.
5. A supportive group.
6. Diary of progress.
7. Track economic rewards.
8. Track interpersonal rewards.

PLACEBO AS A BIOBEHAVIORAL MECHANISM

Improvement of a condition during clinical trials or treatment can be attributable to one of three causes: natural history, specific effects of the intervention, and nonspecific effects of intervention. The latter of the three causes is typically termed a "placebo effect" (76). If this effect were to be represented in graphic form with the spectrum of intervention along the horizontal axis and clinical improvement along the vertical axis, the placebo effect would be represented by gradual improvement in the clinical condition.

Unwillingness to make the effort to explore an unfamiliar and seemingly out-of-the-mainstream topic

These challenges are severe but surmountable. The osteopathic profession is moving to provide the materials needed to acquaint its basic scientists with its background, theoretical basis, and research data. The Texas bibliographic project is soon to be available and should provide greater access to the literature of the profession. The AAO, as mentioned earlier, has provided its literature bibliography on CD-ROM. Such sources as this book and others now appearing provide the willing basic scientist with useful information.

The ready access to the profession's older research literature is poor. Ways must be found to make those sources more available, not only to basic scientists, but to clinician researchers and students as well. Many of the works of Burns and other early anatomists and physiologists investigating basic mechanisms of manipulation are available in only a few college libraries. This is a continuing challenge to the profession.

A basic scientist coming into an osteopathic school to teach is faced with the task of teaching in a profession about which he or she usually knows nothing. In this case, the only option is to teach a topic in the same way it was taught elsewhere. The osteopathic profession thinks of itself as a unique entity, implying that the teaching of its students should be somehow different from the experience of other medical students. How can that occur if the basic scientist does not know the basis of the profession? One way is to integrate osteopathic physicians into the teaching of the sciences. Of course, another is to inform the basic scientists of the profession. Clinicians and others knowledgeable of the profession can provide seminars and workshops on osteopathic medicine for their colleagues. Basic scientists can be encouraged to sit in on the osteopathic courses. Clinicians can take basic scientists as shadowers in their practices and discuss the unique aspects of osteopathic medicine with them. Administrators can provide expectations and rewards for basic scientists who show a willingness to avail themselves of opportunities to become knowledgeable about the profession. In general, the profession has not held sufficiently high expectations for its basic scientists nor has it provided good opportunities for them to become familiar with the theory and practice of osteopathic medicine.

A basic scientist coming into the profession with a budding or established research program faces real obstacles in retooling or realigning that program to the needs of osteopathic medicine. Funding may not be as readily available. The switch or realignment may take several years to accomplish. The comfort of a known research enterprise is lost. The schools can help this transition by providing funding for the transition, understanding that productivity may decrease for a time, and finding clinicians to supply information and experience to the investigator. In addition, the expectation should be clear that such a transition will be rewarded in tangible ways. Korr (4–11) has published several articles on the challenges posed by osteopathic theory and practice that can be given to entering faculty.

Although the school and profession can do much to help an investigator realign their research and intellectual efforts toward the questions of osteopathic medicine, there is also an onus on those coming into the profession to make an effort to gain this understanding. Honest intellectual effort would seem to demand of a person coming into a profession that knowledge of that profession be acquired. The investigator should have some intellectual curiosity and desire to find out about what it is he or she is getting into. Thus, an investigator may be expected to make efforts to seek out opportunities to become familiar with the backgrounds, theoretical underpinnings, and research basis of the profession. Too often, this does not happen, but should be encouraged. Osteopathic clinicians can be very helpful in this by offering manipulative treatment to their basic science colleagues. Osteopathic students can challenge their basic science professors to investigate the profession. In this way, a healthier interaction can be accomplished.

But what about osteopathic clinician researchers within the profession? They also need help in meeting the challenges of research. They often are not schooled in research methods and skills. They are pressured for time and are expected to provide patient care to generate income, not research studies. These individuals also need to be given the time, resources, and encouragement to pursue the difficult and often discouraging field of research. They need to have the backing of their administrators for time and resources to acquire research skills and protected time for intellectual pursuits. They need to become aware of the long-term nature of a research endeavor. They need collaborations with their basic science colleagues in designing and carrying out osteopathically oriented studies. In short, they have the same needs as do the basic scientists. The DO making a transition to research is venturing into unknown and uncertain territory, just as is the basic scientist trained in other institutions. Support and understanding are needed for both groups.

Academic Challenges: The Students

In planning for the long-term health of osteopathically oriented research, the role of the students must be considered. At present, in most osteopathic schools, little attention is given to providing the students with a background in prior research of the profession, let alone in the basics of research design and process relevant to the profession. One of the best ways to increase research power in the profession is to orient its students early in their training to the basic properties and needs for research. Only a small percentage will become researchers, but only a few are needed to make a large difference. If only one student per class aspired to become a full-time researcher in the profession and were provided sufficient support to pursue that goal, the profession would soon have an abundance of trained and functioning researchers in its institutions.

The schools can implement lectures on research background, methodology, and process for all students. For those showing more interest, mentors can be provided to work with the more motivated students to provide initial training, research opportunities, and support. These students can be integrated into ongoing investigations of osteopathic manipulation and technique. There have been some efforts to provide a model research curriculum to all the schools, and this should be encouraged. Too often, the schools are attracting students with research interests, only to destroy that interest by failing to provide opportunities and training.

In addition, opportunities can be made available for graduate training for students interested in well-recognized laboratories outside the profession. However, it is imperative that such opportunities incorporate aspects of research particularly pertinent to the profession, lest the student be discouraged from building the knowledge bridges to the important issues of the profession.

The profession is beginning to take steps to add a research basis to the curriculum. In late 2001, a workshop was held at the Osteopathic Clinical Trials Initiative Conference (OCCTIC) meetings for the purposed of outlining a research curriculum for the years of osteopathic medical training. The results of this meeting have been endorsed by the Educational Council on Osteopathic Principles (ECOP) and made available to the schools. Should the schools adopt these guidelines for research training, a real step forward in producing research-oriented students will have been taken. The recommended research curriculum consists of the following:

By the end of osteopathic medical school years one and two, the student should have the following capabilities:
1. History of osteopathic research
2. Knowledge of research vocabulary
3. Ability to do a literature search
4. Knowledge of basic statistics
5. Understanding of research problems that are uniquely osteopathic (OMT)
6. Awareness of support resources available consistent with level of competency expected

By the end of osteopathic medical school years three and four, the student should have the following capabilities:
1. Ability to review and summarize journal articles
2. Ability to formulate a research question/hypothesis
3. Awareness of support resources available consistent with level of competency expected

By the end of postgraduate years one through three, the student should have the following capabilities:
1. Understand the process of design and implementation of a research project
2. Ability to critique journal articles
3. Ability to write a manuscript suitable for publication or a grant application
4. Awareness of support resources available consistent with level of competency expected

Organizational Challenges: Other Osteopathic Institutions

As the profession moves into the fourth research period, it is increasingly evident that the challenges of providing a research basis for osteopathic theory and practice cannot be met by the COMs alone. The establishment of the new center for osteopathic research was not an isolated effort of one or more schools. It was an effort spanning several years and with its roots in the early days of the profession with the A. T. Still Research Institute. Several institutions of the profession came together to promote and fund the center's formation, including the AOA, AAO, AACOM, the American College of Osteopathic Family

Physicians, and the American Osteopathic Healthcare Association. These and other organizations within the profession have realized the necessity of promoting a research culture in the profession. These institutions, the profession's leaders, and the rank and file of the profession must continue to support (in concept and financially) the development of researchers who understand the osteopathic profession and can apply their skills and intellectual abilities to answering the vital questions posed by this unique philosophy and practice. Without continued support and encouragement from all, a research-friendly atmosphere will not flourish.

Collaborative Challenges: Building Research Networks

As the research efforts of the profession mature, clinical trials of the effects and efficacy of osteopathic techniques, osteopathic manipulative treatment, and osteopathic care will move from the pilot study format to full-blown clinical trials. These trials will be expensive and time consuming. A full clinical trial often requires hundreds of subjects (see Chapter 74) and many practitioners. The osteopathic profession is, despite its rapid growth, still a small profession. The conduct of full trials will require collaboration between multiple sites and practitioners. The basis for planning such studies has yet to be advanced in the profession. The center for osteopathic research, with its mandate to conduct studies on osteopathic manipulative themes, is an appropriate venue for such planning. However, there exist other avenues that can begin the process in preparation for these trials. One such avenue lies in the OPTI networks. These confederations of hospital training sites affiliated with osteopathic colleges provide ready-made resources for pilot studies of collaborative trials. Some OPTIs already have provision for research efforts and research training. The OPTI networks can be valuable testing grounds for collaborative efforts in the next few years. In addition, encouraging practitioners in their office practices to join research networks would lead to more viable clinical trials.

Recent developments in clinical research stimulated by the acquired immunodeficiency syndrome (AIDS) epidemic are also useful models for the osteopathic profession to follow. In the past, there has been little clinical research performed outside major research centers. In response to increasing pressure for clinical data on the AIDS epidemic, there has been an increasing use of smaller neighborhood clinics and solo practitioners to collect data on the disease (M. Goldstein, personal communication, 1992). It is becoming evident that there is an important role for the practicing physician in collecting data for clinical studies. Studies using this important resource for data collection must be designed to take advantage of the practice of medicine in the office setting so as not to disrupt the daily flow of the practice. However, it is here that the real practice of osteopathic medicine takes place. It is here that there is the best chance to ask such questions as:

What is the incidence of somatic dysfunction?
What is its natural course?
What is the effectiveness of manipulative treatment on it?

The questions of real life in osteopathic medicine can be approached at the office level. Such research must be encouraged.

That such research can be accomplished is seen in the recent report from the office of Frymann (12) on the effects of osteopathic care on neurologic development in children. Other office-based studies that include many practitioners would provide many important data on the basis for and efficacy of osteopathic care.

Collaborative Challenges: Isolation

The osteopathic profession began in the United States but quickly spread to other countries. Early in the 1900s, osteopathy was established in the United Kingdom; in 1916, an osteopathic school was established there. Currently, there are osteopathic movements in many countries of the world, some nascent, as in Russia, and some well developed, as in the United Kingdom. Although the practitioners of most of these schools are licensed to practice manipulation only, they are valuable resources for research collaboration. In addition, many countries have active allopathic groups who have traditions of manual medicine, and some have become well trained in osteopathic techniques and theory, as is the case in Germany. The International Federation of Manual Medicine, or FIMM, has an active research component. Canadian students of osteopathy, in fact, must complete an extensive research thesis, practically comparable to a U.S. doctoral thesis before becoming certified as diplomats in osteopathy.

The U.S. osteopathic movement has an opportunity to greatly enhance its research efforts by encouraging interactions with these movements. In fact, it may be that, taken together, these organized osteopathic schools outside the U.S. have more potential for research on efficacy and outcomes than does the U.S. profession. Clearly, there are aspects of osteopathic care that can only be studied in the U.S., because only here at present are osteopathic doctors fully licensed physicians; however, technique, reliability, and treatment studies can be collaboratively studied with many other sections of the world osteopathic community. These types of collaboration should not be wasted by isolationism.

CHALLENGES OF RESEARCH DESIGN

As pointed out in Chapter 74, the design of osteopathic clinical research faces unique challenges. The design of clinical research is actually in its infancy, beginning only about 50 to 60 years ago. Clinical research grew up around the testing of drug efficacy, and the gold standard design for such studies is the randomized, placebo-controlled, double-blind (RPCDB) study. The challenges facing the osteopathic and manipulative medicine communities are two:

Is the RPCDB methodology appropriate for studies of osteopathic manipulative treatment?
What research designs are appropriate for studies of osteopathic manipulative treatment?

These questions cannot be answered in a vacuum. The design of any study should flow from an understanding of the research question and the available research techniques. Parts of this challenge have been examined in the Foundations for Osteopathic Research, Chapter 74, but other aspects will be discussed here.

Shams and Placebos

One of the most interesting issues facing the design of research in osteopathic manipulative treatment or techniques is whether to use placebo or sham controls and, if so, what to use. The use of placebos is well known and documented in clinical research literature (as is the use of sham controls), but these are being called into question (13,14). The placebo treatment was initially developed for research on the effectiveness of drugs, and entails the delivery of a substance that is, from the standpoint of the patient and physician, indistinguishable from the drug being tested. Such a placebo is often in the form of a capsule that is the same color, size, and weight as the capsule containing the drug, but the placebo contains only inert substances. The patient is given either the drug-containing capsule or the inert-substance capsule, not knowing which is being given. The sham is a procedure given to the patient that has been shown or is thought to have no affect on the symptoms being treated. With both placebos and shams, the intent is to keep the patient from knowing whether he or she is receiving an active or inactive drug or procedure. This should keep the expectations of both the experimental and control groups equal and thus allow the effect of the active ingredient or procedure to be seen, independent of patient expectations.

In the case of drug tests or for testing specific manipulative techniques, placebo and sham controls are entirely appropriate. The intent of such studies is to ascertain the effect of the active ingredient alone. They look at the effect of either a certain molecule (or, more precisely, many millions of molecules) on the natural course of something like a bacterial invasion of the body, or of a particular procedure (such as a lateral recumbent roll) on the course of a particular symptom (15). The patient's expectations and conscious processes are not at issue. The use of placebo or sham procedures as control groups against which the drug or procedure groups can be compared gives the researcher a measure of the effectiveness of the drug or technique alone.

Thus, in the design of manipulative technique research, it seems entirely appropriate to use sham treatment control groups. Here, the rationale is to test the effectiveness of a certain specific technique that is administered in the same way to each patient for presumably the same symptom or symptoms. The treating physician has no leeway in how the maneuver is accomplished, and the patients are screened closely so that the symptoms are much the same from patient to patient.

However, at the heart of osteopathic philosophy is the premise that treatment should be aimed at normalization of function by removing the barriers to the body's ability to optimize its function. Once these barriers are removed, the body can regain its optimal function and return to or maintain health. To think that this is purely a physiologic function and has nothing to do with conscious processes or the mind (i.e., the patient's expectations, desires, beliefs, and will) is to return to a belief in mind/body dualism holding that the mind has nothing to do with physiologic function, and vice versa. It is to deny the most vital part of the whole equation of health and disease: the patients themselves. In addition, the treating physician is a part of the equation. Both the skill and the manner of the treating physician affect the results of the treatment, because both the patient's tactile and mental perceptions of the physician influence how the patient responds to the treatment.

In osteopathic treatment, the treatment is an interaction between patient and physician, each responding to the other throughout the treatment. The osteopathic physician relies on the very effect that is labeled placebo or expectation in drug testing to help with the alteration he or she is attempting to produce—that of normalized function. The patient's expectation is an important and vital factor in OMT; it must not be cast off as some spurious side effect. It is also a real and unusually safe therapeutic tool. There are few deleterious side effects to positive expectations.

In addition, the use of a sham treatment group in which the patient is exposed to a treatment that is considered ineffective presents another real problem for the evaluation of OMT (again, as contrasted to the evaluation of a particular technique). It is assumed that in the sham control group, the treatment of a body area distant from a particular somatic dysfunction does not influence the resolution of a diagnosed dysfunction being treated in the experimental group. Many available data show that the simple act of touching and moving an individual produces real changes in function and response. The act of manipulative treatment involves touching and moving the patient as an integral part of the process. To compare a manipulation group with some sham group that has also received touch and movement may well lead to an underestimation of the effects of manipulative treatment, unless it can be shown that the sham treatment had no effect on the total mind and body function of the patient.

Thus, initial attempts to evaluate the true effectiveness of manipulative treatment (as opposed to techniques) on either the progression of symptoms or on total body function requires the use of a control group that either receives some standard medical therapy not requiring manipulation or the use of a totally untreated control group that would simply undergo the natural course of the malfunction being studied. This could be done by simply requiring control subjects to come to the physician's office for diagnostic measurements. To try to factor out the mental process involved in manipulative treatment is to deny much of the actual treatment. It is akin to studying the effectiveness of a drug by giving only a partial dose.

To study the effects of osteopathic manipulation, one must study osteopathic manipulation as it is given, as an interaction between physician and patient, with all components intact and functioning. To factor out any particular component, such as the so-called hands-on effect, and call it an artifact is to underestimate the effect of manipulative treatment and deny that the natural power of cognitive and recuperative processes is a factor in the effects of OMT.

Once the overall effects of manipulative treatment have been established, studies can be designed to tease apart the various components of the treatment, including the effects of touching the patient, and so forth. However, to try to do such studies in the absence of demonstrated effects is both inefficient and impractical. The study of OMT must flow from the philosophy of osteopathy and not from some other philosophic orientation.

The investigator designing studies of OMT must determine what is really being asked of the study so that the appropriate contrast control can be used. Using the incorrect control may result in underestimation of the effect of manipulative treatment, although the same control may be the appropriate one for evaluation of a manipulative technique. The decision rests on whether the total response of the individual to the interaction between patient and physician is being evaluated or whether manipulative technique is being studied as a procedure. The challenge here is to actively defend the use of appropriate designs for osteopathic manipulative research, and not to be forced into inappropriate designs by preconceived notions of how research is done.

PRIORITY CHALLENGES: WHAT RESEARCH IS MOST IMPORTANT?

It is tempting to say that all research that can be done is important and no area should be singled out above others. However, some suggestions can be made as to areas that may be most valuable in determining the usefulness and value of osteopathic theory and practice.

Basic Research

Research on the mechanisms underlying osteopathic practice begins with either the theoretical underpinnings of the profession, or clinical observations of practitioners. As an example, Korr (16) followed both theory and clinical observation when beginning his line of research on transsynaptic delivery of proteins from nerve to muscle tissue. The nurturing of tissues by their nerve supply had long been a theme in osteopathic medicine, but almost ignored in other Western traditions. Clinical observations showed that muscles deprived of nerve supply would degenerate, but those only deprived of nerve activity would only atrophy. Certainly, Korr's research program was clearly driven by osteopathic clinical and theoretical considerations.

Clearly, some of the vital areas in the traditions and clinical experiences of the profession can lead to distinctive basic research programs. Examples of such areas include:

- The interactions between somatic and visceral structures are a vital issue that is receiving attention in laboratories now, but is very under-researched.
- How does the mechanoreceptor input from muscle affect sympathetic outflow?
- How does sympathetic activity affect somatic structure and function?
- How can virus and bacterial activity be influenced by sympathetic activity?
- What is the structure and function of the fasciae of the body?
- How do strains in the somatic structures affect visceral function over time?

Certainly one of the most basic questions in the area of osteopathic basic research is the prevalence and incidence of the entity known as somatic dysfunction. This is perhaps one of the most pressing and most difficult questions that remain unanswered in the profession. It actually crosses the bounds of basic and clinical areas.

The list of questions generated by osteopathic theory and clinical experience is almost endless. However, to tap these areas, the researcher must be able to see how they apply to the osteopathic experience.

Clinical Research

As long as the list of questions in the basic sciences is flowing from the osteopathic theory and practice, it is perhaps longer in the clinical arena. Various lists of the most important areas of clinical research have been generated, but consensus has not been reached. Areas that seem to be especially critical, although not prioritized, are included here.

Teaching Techniques in Osteopathic Manipulation

The area of research on educational techniques, although not clinical, would provide important information on how to pass on the techniques and skills of osteopathic medicine. Research into how to best teach palpation, recognition of tissues texture alterations, and so forth, is badly needed.

Inter- and Intraexaminer Reliability Studies

One of the basic unknowns in osteopathic medicine (and manual medicine in general) is how to assess and improve the reliability between the examination skills of practitioners, and indeed, how reliable the same individual is when examining the same patient twice. There are studies available on the reliability between examiners of the same patient (17), but the studies vary widely in quality and findings. In addition to being an important question in terms of how much value can be placed on palpatory findings, studies on the factors influencing the reliability within and between palpators would help inform the teaching of these skills. This is an area that probably should be a priority in the profession and on which several projects are being mounted.

Outcomes and Cost Effectiveness of Osteopathic Manipulative Treatment

Although seemingly obvious, simple outcome studies that look at what happens to patients, without the use of controls, is needed. One such study is under way at present in Maine (the Maine Osteopathic Outcomes Study, or MOOS), and more may be planned. However, with the amount of data collected by state, federal, and private entities, the numbers of epidemiologically related studies that are now possible are immense. Models for these types of studies must be generated more frequently in the profession.

Comparisons of Osteopathic Treatment Techniques with Other Forms of Manual Medicine

Many other forms of manual medicine exist. How do treatment techniques generated by the osteopathic profession compare with these? Is a manipulative treatment driven by osteopathic theory more effective than that given by other practitioners of manual medicine? Such questions are not only fascinating, but also vital to understanding the value of osteopathic medicine.

Comparing Different Modalities of Osteopathic Treatment with Each Other

There are several major treatment modalities used in the profession. How do they compare in outcomes when used on a common disease process? Is a high-velocity/low-amplitude thrust better than a muscle treatment for a sore neck? Comparing one modality with another would produce interesting insights into the potential mechanisms of the different modalities, as well as their efficacy in various conditions.

What Are the Effects of Manipulation on a Somatic Dysfunction?

Just as the questions of prevalence and incidence of somatic dysfunction are basic to the profession, so are the questions surrounding the actual influence of a manipulative treatment on a well-delineated somatic dysfunction. How do such parameters as chronicity and cause affect the outcome? Although it is assumed that an osteopathic treatment corrects somatic dysfunction, how long does the effect last in chronic cases, and how susceptible is the dysfunction to reoccurrence?

What Is the Effect of Manipulation on Diagnosed Disease Entities?

This question has been debated for years and is, in fact, a basic question for payment for services. Actually, the list of conditions to target for such research has received much attention. At a recent meeting, several conditions were targeted for special consideration:

Chronic low back pain
Headache (type unspecified)
Asthma
Otitis media

These conditions have a history of study in and outside the profession, and may be more amenable to tight research designs than many other conditions.

There is a wide range of studies either under way or in planning stages at osteopathic schools and other institutions. All should be encouraged, as each will add to the body of design knowledge about how to do research in osteopathic manipulative treatment. It is likely that a few conditions will have to be selected for full-scale studies due to cost and manpower limitations. Pilot studies will pave the way for selecting those conditions most likely to provide meaningful information on the large-scale effects of osteopathic treatment.

CHALLENGES OF THE BIGGER PICTURE: OSTEOPATHIC PHILOSOPHY AND LARGER RESEARCH QUESTIONS

Although these specific areas of research are important, the role of the osteopathic philosophy in shaping even larger questions, and directions of osteopathic research must be mentioned.

Basic to the philosophy and theory of osteopathy is the idea that the body is an integrated functional unit. This unit includes the physical, cognitive, and spiritual aspects of the individual. Indeed, there is a growing body of evidence suggesting positive effects of spiritual interventions, such as prayer, in the healing process (18–21). How these elements interact within the total individual and with the external environment determine the long-term health status of the person. From the beginning of osteopathic medicine, osteopathic practitioners have held that there was an entity that would adversely affect a person's health status. This entity, which could be palpated and specifically treated with manipulation, was first known as the osteopathic lesion and then, more recently, as somatic dysfunction. In the 1940s and 1950s, Denslow, Korr (22), and their colleagues postulated that a major component of the osteopathic lesion was the facilitated segment. The facilitated segment concept arose from the data gathered by these researchers, which showed that, in most individuals, there was no uniform excitability throughout the spinal cord. The areas of hyperexcitability were shown to react more strongly to afferent input, exposing innervated structures, both visceral and somatic, to increased activation. This break in body unity was postulated to lead to early breakdown and malfunction over time—in short, to disease. Clinical disease was, then, a consequence of earlier body dysfunction. Indeed, this was a data-based theory that truly embodied one of Still's basic insights; that clinical disease was a manifestation of body malfunction rather than a primary event.

DETERIORATION OF NORMAL FUNCTION AS A CENTRAL CONCEPT

That clinical disease is a result of earlier deterioration of normal function is central to osteopathic philosophy. It is perhaps best manifest in the treatment of somatic dysfunction, an entity not recognized by most medical practitioners as a clinical entity at all. Why treat it? Because it is the beginning of disease, the start of body breakdown. To treat the root of disease would seem to be more cost-effective than waiting until the final breakdown of clinical disease has occurred before beginning treatment.

OTHER ROLES FOR SOMATIC DYSFUNCTION

Given this view, osteopathic research should be aimed at elucidating the relationships between disturbances of body function and health status:

How does the presence of somatic dysfunction predict the health status of the individual?

What is the incidence of serious somatic dysfunction and its natural history?

What environmental and lifestyle attributes seem to contribute to the incidence of somatic dysfunction?

How does lifestyle contribute to the incidence of somatic dysfunction in old age?

Flowing from these questions are even larger questions that should be at the forefront of osteopathic thinking:

What is the contribution of early lifestyle or events that happen to the person and the health status of the individual in old age?

What regime of manipulative treatment in early life will contribute most to deterring the deterioration of health usually associated with old age?

More simply, why are some very old people vital and healthy and others completely overtaken by deterioration and disease?

What role does long-lasting somatic dysfunction play in the presence or absence of vitality in old age?

These questions are complex and not easily answered. The critical point is that at least some research of the profession should take as its starting point body unity and the concept that the start of disease is the deterioration of that functional unity, not a bacterial or viral invasion.

INTEGRATION AND SELF-REGULATION IN HEALTH

These questions suggest several important areas of research for the osteopathic profession. In the basic sciences, increasing attention must be paid to understanding the integration of body systems and what can cause the fine-tuned integration of body function to deteriorate. The capacity of the body to self-regulate (homeostasis) and the limits of that capacity in both the short-term and long-term must be better understood. Research aimed at elucidating the fine control and adaptation of body function would be especially useful. Integration of basic science data with data from studies of cognitive function gives a greater understanding of the role of the physician in the health maintenance process. A greater understanding of the effects of afferent input and cognitive function on the immune system, and how manipulative treatment can affect this system, would be useful.

HEALTH BENEFITS OF MANIPULATIVE TREATMENT

Within the clinical research areas, there must be studies of the efficacy of manipulative techniques and manipulative treatment. Measurements of the effects of manipulation on specific disease entities, such as those listed above, need to be carried out to demonstrate that manipulation can be used effectively in treating specific disease processes. To rely on such demonstration studies to show the most significant benefits of manipulation would, however, be unwise. The most beneficial and lasting effects of manipulation and, indeed, of osteopathic care should be searched for in the effects on total functional capacity of individuals and in their long-term health status. The current health care system is preoccupied with the treatment of disease, especially in the chronic degeneration of old age. It is by no means clear that the chronic diseases commonly associated with old age are inevitable. What are the enabling or protective roles of early and continued normal body function in the aging process? Osteopathy is ideally suited by its philosophy and clinical experience to look at the effects of early disruptions of body unity on the deterioration of old age. This is a golden opportunity for osteopathic research.

TOTAL NATURE OF SOMATIC DYSFUNCTION

Clinical research should continue to look at the effects of manipulation on specific disease processes. Such studies can be effectiveness studies, such as the use of manipulative treatment in low back and chronic pain syndromes. These studies could have fairly quick and valuable outcomes for the profession. Other less specific studies, such as the effects of manipulation on sympathetic tone, vasomotor reactivity, and muscle spasticity, contribute to an understanding of the more general effects of manipulation on body function. Studies of the effects of somatic dysfunction and its etiology, prevalence, and contributions to the long-term health of the individual form a solid base for a greater understanding of the fundamental dynamics of health and disease. Investigations of the effects of manipulation on somatic dysfunction and of osteopathic care on old age health status are probably the most important area of study to which the profession can aspire.

CONCLUSION

Northup (1) wisely noted that the future of the profession rested in the decisions and integrity of organized osteopathy. Organized osteopathy now must rise to the challenge of mounting and sustaining a research enterprise that will test the central tenets and beliefs of the profession. These studies must be done on the playing fields of the profession, not on those of other professions. The studies must test the profession's questions and assumptions and be interpreted by those knowledgeable in the theories and practices of osteopathic medicine, not by others. The risk of allowing others to do the studies or interpret the results from other points of view is simply unacceptable. The future of the profession now rests as much on its research endeavors as on its teaching and clinical endeavors. The three legs of the profession's stool are equal, and all are vital.

By closely following the basic philosophy of osteopathy and the insights from its years of clinical experience, the research efforts of the profession can truly add to the most beneficial aspects of health care to which osteopathy is fundamentally dedicated: the maintenance of health and optimal function of the total person throughout life.

REFERENCES

1. Northup GW. An adventure in excellence. *J Am Osteopath Assoc.* 2001;101(12):726–730.

2. Patterson MM, Howell JN, eds. *The Central Connection: Somatovisceral Viscerosomatic Interaction.* Indianapolis, IN: American Academy of Osteopathy; 1992.

3. Willard F, Patterson MM, eds. *Nociception and the Neuroendocrine-Immune Connection. Proceedings of the 1992 American Academy of Osteopathy International Symposium.* Indianapolis, IN: American Academy of Osteopathy; 1994.

4. Korr IM. Biological basis for the osteopathic concept. In: *1960 and 1963 Academy Yearbooks.* Indianapolis, IN: American Academy of Osteopathy; 1960:129 and 1963:114, respectively.

5. Korr IM. Some thoughts on an osteopathic curriculum. *J Am Osteopath Assoc.* 1975;74(8):685–688.

6. Korr IM. Biologic process in the context of human uniqueness and diversity. *Osteopath Ann.* 1978;6(1):10–13.

7. Korr IM. Osteopathic principles for basic scientists. *J Am Osteopath Assoc.* 1987;87(7):513–515.

8. Korr IM. Medical education: The resistance to change. *Advances.* 1987;4(2):5–10.

9. Korr IM. Osteopathic principles: A way of life. *The DO.* 1987;May:25–27.

10. Korr IM. An explication of osteopathic principles. In: Ward RC, ed. *Foundations for Osteopathic Medicine.* Baltimore, MD: Williams & Wilkins; 1997:7–12.

11. Korr IM. Pathways to excellence in clinical research. In: Beal MC, ed. *1994 Yearbook, Louisa Burns, DO Memorial.* Indianapolis, IN: American Academy of Osteopathy; 1994:60.

12. Frymann VM, Carney RE, Springall P. Effect of osteopathic medical management on neurologic development in children. *J Am Osteopath Assoc.* 1992;92(6):729–744.

13. Kienle GS, Kiene H. Placebo effect and placebo concept: A critical methodological and conceptual analysis of reports on the magnitude of the placebo effect. *Altern Ther Health Med.* 1996;2(6):39–54.

14. Kiene H. A critique of the double-blind clinical trial. *Altern Ther Health Med.* 1996;2(1):74–80.

15. Hoehler F, Tobis J, Buerger A. Spinal manipulation for low back pain. *JAMA.* 1981;245(18):1835–1838.

16. Korr IM, Wilkinson PN, Chornock FW. Axonal delivery of neuroplasmic components to muscle cells. *Science.* 1967;155(760):342–345.

17. Beal MC, Patriquin DA. Interexaminer agreement on palpatory diagnosis and patient self-assessment of disability: A pilot study. *J Am Osteopath Assoc.* 1995;95(2):97–100, 103–106.

18. Abbot NC, Harkness EF, Stevinson C, et al. Spiritual healing as a therapy for chronic pain: A randomized, clinical trial. *Pain.* 2001;91:79–89.

19. Dossey L. The return of prayer. *Altern Ther Health Med.* 1997;3(6):10–17.

20. Harris WS, Gowda M, Kolb JW, et al. A randomized, controlled trial of the effects of remote, intercessory prayer on outcomes in patients admitted to the coronary care unit. *Arch Intern Med.* 1999;159(Oct 25):2273–2278.

21. Thomson KS. The revival of experiments on prayer. *Am Scientist.* 1996;84:532–534.

22. Korr IM. The emerging concept of the osteopathic lesion. *J Am Osteopath Assoc.* 1948;47:1–8.

GLOSSARY OF OSTEOPATHIC TERMINOLOGY

Prepared by the Glossary Review Committee sponsored by the Educational Council on Osteopathic Principles (ECOP) of the American Association of Colleges of Osteopathic Medicine (AACOM).
—Revised April, 2002

The Glossary of Osteopathic Terminology is revised twice each year by the Educational Council on Osteopathic Principles (ECOP), Chairman, John C. Glover, DO. Forward any comments or suggestions to the Chairman of the Glossary Review Committee, William Thomas Crow, DO, Philadelphia College of Osteopathic Medicine, 4190 City Line Avenue, Philadelphia, PA 1913-1693. The Glossary first appeared in the *Journal of the American Osteopathic Association* (No. 80, pages 552–567) in April 1981. The 1995 version of the Glossary of Osteopathic Terminology was also published in the first edition of this textbook. The most current and revised version is printed annually in the *American Osteopathic Association Yearbook and Directory of Osteopathic Physicians.*

The February 2002 glossary review was performed by James Binkerd, DO; Jane Carreiro, DO; William Thomas Crow, DO; Robert Clark, DO; William H. Devine, DO; Dennis Dowling, DO, FAAO; John C. Glover, DO; Donald V. Hampton, DO; Robert Kappler, DO, FAAO; Michael Lockwood, DO; David Macon, DO; William Morris, DO; James Rechtien, DO; Mark Sandhouse, DO; Karen Steele, DO, FAAO; Edward G. Stiles, DO, FAAO; and Scott T. Stoll, DO, PhD.

The purpose of this osteopathic glossary is to present important and often used words, terms, and phrases of the osteopathic profession. It is not meant to replace a dictionary. The glossary offers the consensus of a large segment of the osteopathic profession and is to serve to standardize terminology. The ECOP Glossary Review Committee specifically seeks to include those definitions that are uniquely osteopathic in their origin or common usage, distinctive in the osteopathic usage of a common word, and/or important in describing osteopathic principles and philosophy and osteopathic manipulative treatment.

We also expect this glossary to be useful to the student of osteopathic medicine and to be helpful to authors and other professionals in understanding and making proper use of osteopathic vocabulary.

Dictionary definitions are included from:

Dorland's Medical Dictionary, 29th ed. Philadelphia, PA: WB Saunders; 2000.
Gray's Anatomy
Stedman's Medical Dictionary, 27th ed. Philadelphia, PA: Lippincott Williams & Wilkins; 2000.

A

abbreviations (for types of osteopathic manipulative techniques):

ART: articulatory treatment
BLT: balanced ligamentous tension treatment/ligamentous articular strain treatment
CR: osteopathy in the cranial field
CS: counterstrain treatment
D: direct treatment
DIR: direct treatment
FPR: facilitated positional release treatment
HVLA: high velocity/low amplitude treatment
I: indirect treatment
IND: indirect treatment
INR: integrated neuromusculoskeletal release treatment
LAS: ligamentous articular strain treatment/balanced ligamentous tension treatment
ME: muscle energy treatment
MFR: myofascial release technique
NMM-OMM: neuromusculoskeletal medicine
OCF: osteopathy in the cranial field/cranial treatment
OMT: osteopathic manipulative treatment
PINS: progressive inhibition of neuromuscular structures
ST: soft tissue treatment
VIS: visceral manipulative treatment

acceleration: Rate of increase in velocity. See also *deceleration.*
accessory joint motions: See *secondary joint motion.*
accessory movements: Movements used to potentiate, accentuate, or compensate for an impairment in a physiologic motion (e.g., the movements needed to move a paralyzed limb).
accommodation: A self-reversing and nonpersistent adaptation.
active motion: See *motion, active.*
acute somatic dysfunction: See *somatic dysfunction, acute.*
allopathy: 1. A therapeutic system in which a disease is treated by producing a second condition that is incompatible with or antagonistic to the first. (*Stedman's*) 2. A term used to refer those holding a Doctor of Medicine (MD) degree, a nonosteopathic medical degree.
anatomic barrier: See *barrier (motion barrier).*
angle:
    Ferguson a., see *angle, lumbosacral.*
    lumbolumbar lordotic a., an objective quantification of lumbar lordosis typically determined by measuring the angle between the superior surface of the second lumbar

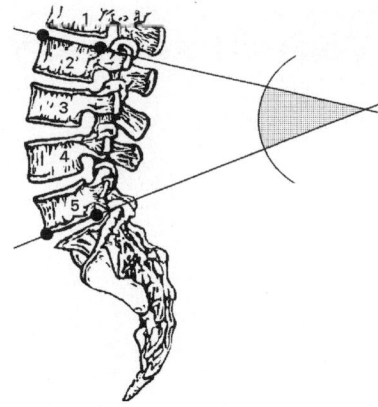

FIGURE 1. Lumbolumbar lordotic angle (L2-5).

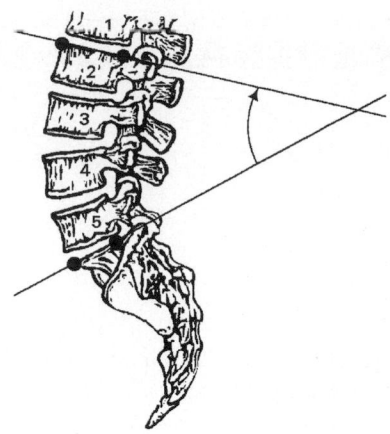

FIGURE 3. Lumbosacral lordotic angle.

vertebra and the inferior surface of the fifth lumbar vertebra; best measured from a standing lateral x-ray film (Fig. 1).

lumbosacral a., represents the angle of the lumbosacral junction as measured by the inclination of the superior surface of the first sacral vertebra to the horizontal (this is actually a sacral angle); usually measured from standing lateral x-ray films; also known as the Ferguson angle (Fig. 2).

lumbosacral lordotic a., an objective quantification of lumbar lordosis typically determined by measuring the angle between the superior surface of the second lumbar vertebra and the superior surface of the first sacral segment; best measured from a standing lateral x-ray film (Fig. 3).

anterior component: A positional descriptor used to identify the side of reference when rotation of a vertebra has occurred; in a condition of right rotation, the left side is the anterior component; usually refers to the less prominent transverse process; see also *posterior component.*

anterior compression test: See *ASIS (anterior superior iliac spine) compression test.*

anterior iliac rotation: See *ilium, somatic dysfunction of, anterior (forward) innominate (iliac) rotation.*

ART: See *TART.*

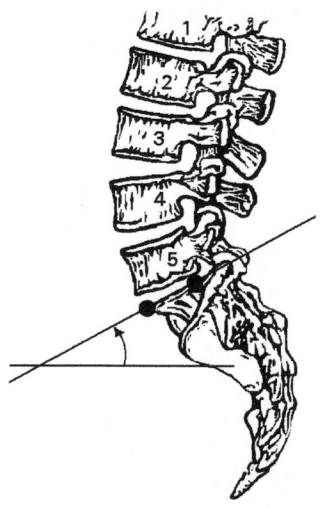

FIGURE 2. Lumbosacral angle (S1-horizon) (Ferguson angle).

articular pillar: 1. Refers to the columnar arrangement of the articular portions of the cervical vertebrae. 2. Those parts of the lateral arches of the cervical vertebrae that contain a superior and inferior articular facet.

articulation: 1. The place of union or junction between two or more bones of the skeleton. 2. The active or passive progress of moving a joint through its permitted anatomic range of motion. See also *osteopathic manipulative treatment, articulatory treatment (ART) system.*

articulatory pop: Sound made when cavitation occurs in a joint. See also *cavitation.*

articulatory technique: See also *technique; osteopathic manipulative treatment, articulatory treatment (ART) system.*

asymmetry: Absence of symmetry of position or motion; dissimilarity in corresponding parts or organs on opposite sides of the body that are normally alike; of particular use when describing position or motion alteration resulting from somatic dysfunction.

axis: 1. An imaginary line about which motion occurs. 2. The second cervical vertebra. 3. One component of an axis system.

axis of rib motion: An imaginary line through the costotransverse and the costovertebral articulations of the rib.

   anteroposterior rib axis, see *bucket handle rib motion.* See also Figs. 4 and 5.

   transverse rib axis, see *pump handle rib motion.* See also Figs. 6 and 7.

ASIS (anterior superior iliac spine) compression test: Test for determining the side of pelvic somatic dysfunction.

axis of sacral motion: See *sacral motion axis.*

axoplasmic flow: See *axoplasmic transport.*

axoplasmic transport: The antegrade movement of substances from the nerve cell along the axon toward the terminals, and the retrograde movement from the terminals toward the nerve cell.

B

backward bending: Opposite of forward bending. See *extension.*

backward bending test: 1. A test that discriminates between

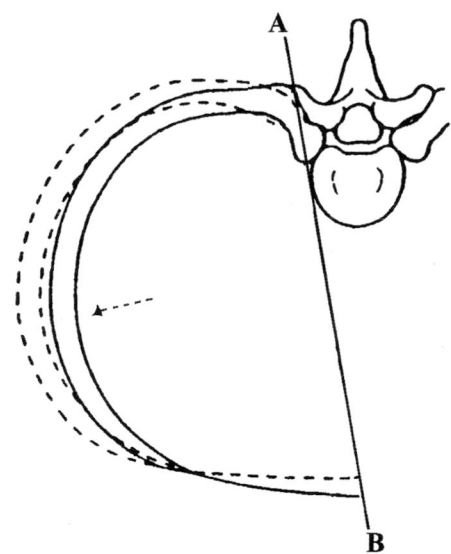

FIGURE 4. The functional anterior-posterior rib axis.

Anteroposterior Axes

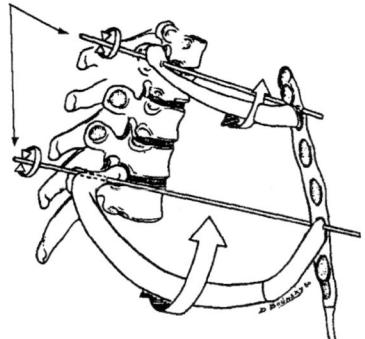

FIGURE 5. Bucket handle rib motion.

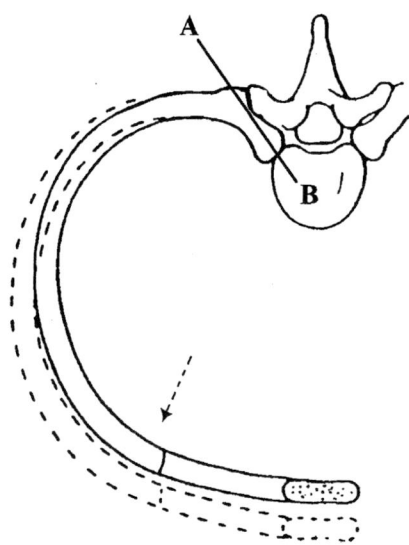

FIGURE 6. The functional transverse rib axis.

"Transverse Axes"

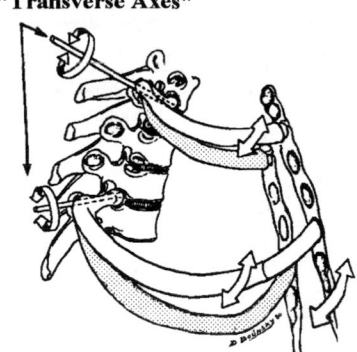

FIGURE 7. Pump handle rib motion.

forward and backward sacral torsion/rotation. 2. A test that discriminates between unilateral sacral flexion and unilateral sacral extension.

balanced ligamentous tension technique: See *osteopathic manipulative treatment, ligamentous articular strain.*

barrier (motion barrier): The limit to motion; in defining barriers, the palpatory end-feel characteristics are useful (Fig. 8).

anatomic b., the limit of motion imposed by anatomic structure; the limit of passive motion.

elastic b., the range between the physiologic and anatomic barrier of motion in which passive ligamentous stretching occurs before tissue disruption.

pathologic b., permanent restriction of joint motion associated with pathologic change of tissues (e.g., contracture, osteophytes).

physiologic b., the limit of active motion.

restrictive b., a functional limit within the anatomic range of motion, which abnormally diminishes the normal physiologic range.

batwing deformity: See *transitional vertebrae, sacralization.*

bind: Relative palpable resistance to motion of an articulation or tissue. Synonym: resistance; antonyms: ease, compliance, resilience.

biomechanics: Mechanical principles applied to the study of biologic functions; the application of mechanical laws to living structures; the study and knowledge of biologic function from an application of mechanical principles.

body unity: One of the basic tenets of the osteopathic philosophy; the human being is a dynamic unit of function; see also *osteopathic philosophy.*

bogginess: A tissue texture abnormality characterized principally by a palpable sense of sponginess in the tissue, interpreted as resulting from congestion due to increased fluid content.

bucket handle rib motion: Movement of the ribs during respiration such that, with inhalation, the lateral aspect of the rib moves cephalad, resulting in an increase of transverse diameter of the thorax. This type of rib motion is predominantly found in lower ribs (Figs. 4–6), increasing from the upper to the lower ribs. See also *axis of rib motion; pump handle rib motion.*

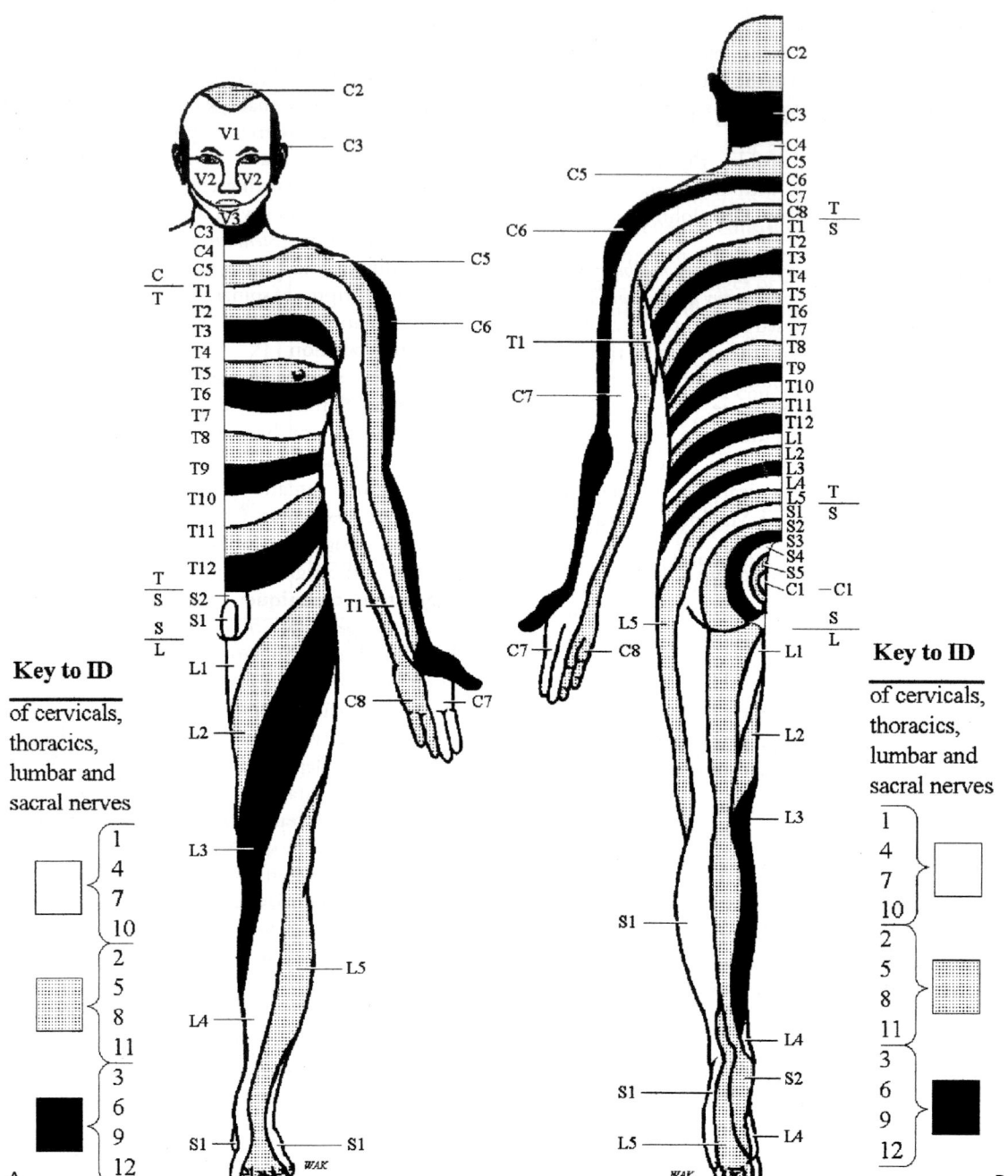

FIGURE 9. **A:** Dermatomal map (anterior). **B:** Dermatomal map (posterior). (Modified from Agur AMR. *Grant's Atlas of Anatomy*, 9th ed. Baltimore, MD: Williams & Wilkins; 1991:37.)

facilitated segment: See *facilitation*.

facilitation: 1. The maintenance of a pool of neurons (e.g., premotor neurons, motoneurons, or preganglionic sympathetic neurons in one or more segments of the spinal cord) in a state of partial or subthreshold excitation; in this state, less afferent stimulation is required to trigger the discharge of impulses. 2. A theory regarding the neurophysiologic mechanisms underlying the neuronal activity associated with somatic dysfunction. 3. Facilitation may be due to sustained increase in afferent input, aberrant patterns of afferent input, or changes within the affected neurons themselves or their chemical en-

vironment. Once established, facilitation can be sustained by normal central nervous system (CNS) activity.

fascial patterns: Systems for classifying and recording the preferred directions of fascial motion throughout the body. Major systems of fascial patterns include the observations of J. Gordon Zink, DO, FAAO, and W. Neidner, DO.

common compensatory pattern (CCP),   the specific finding of alternating fascial motion (Fig. 13A) preference at transitional regions of the body described by Zink.

uncommon compensatory pattern,   the finding of alternating fascial motion preference in the direction opposite that

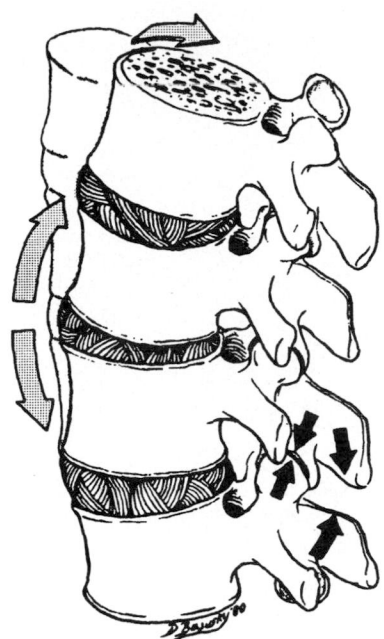

FIGURE 10. Extension.

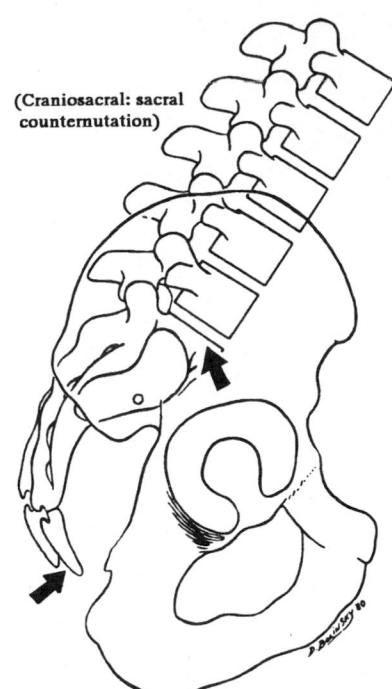

(Craniosacral: sacral counternutation)

FIGURE 12. Sacral extension.

of the common compensatory pattern described by Zink (Fig. 13B).

uncompensated fascial pattern, the finding of fascial preferences that do not demonstrate alternating patterns of findings at transitional regions. Because they occur following stress or trauma, they tend to be symptomatic.

fascial release technique: See *osteopathic manipulative treatment, fascial release treatment.*

FAAO: Fellow of American Academy of Osteopathy. An earned fellowship awarded by the American Academy of Osteopathy.

Ferguson angle: See *angle, lumbosacral.*

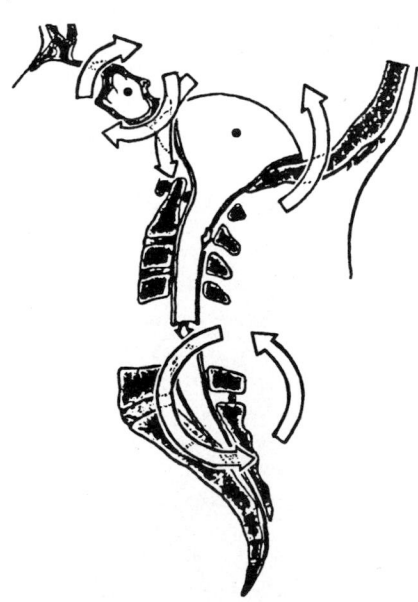

FIGURE 11. Craniosacral extension.

flexion: 1. Accepted universal term for forward motion in a sagittal plane of the spine about a transverse axis (Fig. 14); in a vertebral unit when the superior part moves forward; see *forward bending.* 2. In the extremities, an approximation of a curve or angle (biomechanics). 3. Approximation of the ends of a curve in a spinal region; see *flexion, regional.*

craniosacral f., motion occurring during the cranial rhythmic impulse, when the sphenobasilar symphysis ascends and the sacral base moves posteriorly (Fig. 15).

regional f., historically, the approximation of the ends of a curve in the sagittal plane of the spine; also called the Fryette regional flexion; see *flexion* (Fig. 14).

sacral f., anterior movement of sacral base in relation to the ilia. See also *extension, sacral* (Fig. 16).

flexion tests: Tests for iliosacral or sacroiliac somatic dysfunction.

seated, a screening test which determines the side of sacroiliac somatic dysfunction (motion of the sacrum on the ilium).

standing, a screening test which determines the side of iliosacral somatic dysfunction (motion of ilium on the sacrum).

forward bending: Reciprocal of backward bending. See *flexion.*

FRS: A descriptor of spinal somatic dysfunction used to denote a combination flexed (F), rotated (R), and side-bent (S) vertebral position.

FRS left, somatic dysfunction in which a vertebral unit is flexed, rotated, and side-bent left; usually preceded by a designation of the vertebral unit(s) involved (e.g., T5 FRS left or equivalent T5 FRLSL).

FRS right, somatic dysfunction in which a vertebral unit is flexed, rotated, and side-bent right; usually preceded by

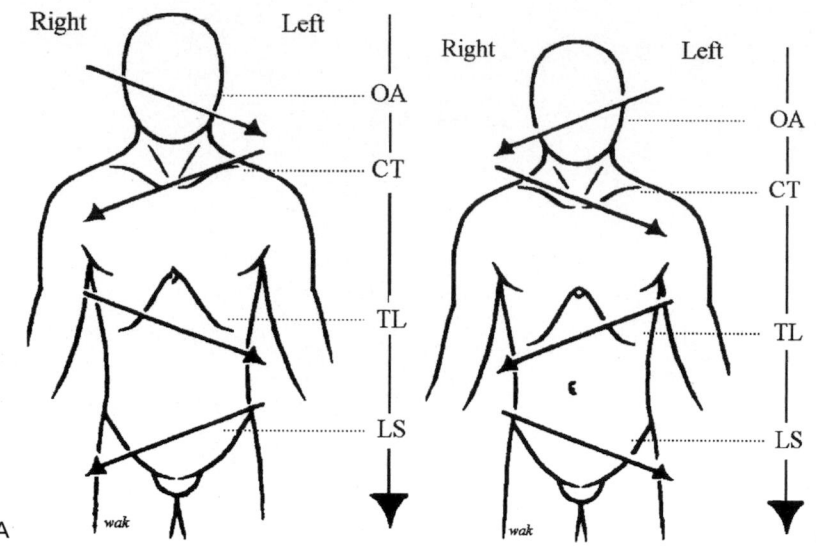

FIGURE 13. A: Common compensatory fascial pattern (Zink). **B:** Uncommon compensatory fascial pattern (Zink).

a designation of the vertebral unit(s) involved (e.g., C3-5 FRS right or equivalent C3-5 FRRSR).

Fryette principles: See *physiologic motion of the spine.*

FSR: A descriptor of spinal somatic dysfunction used to denote a combination flexed (F), side-bent (S), and rotated (R) vertebral position. Typically, the involved vertebral unit(s) are specified first and often a subscript is used to designate left (L) or right (R) in the formula. (e.g., T5-6 FSR$_{RL}$ is interpreted to mean that T5 on T6 and T6 on T7 are flexed, side-bent right, and rotated left).

functional technique: See *osteopathic manipulative treatment, functional method.*

G

Galbreath treatment: See *osteopathic manipulative treatment, mandibular drainage.*

gravitational line: Viewing the patient from the side, an imaginary line in a coronal plane which, in the theoretical ideal posture, starts slightly anterior to the lateral malleolus, passes across the lateral condyle of the knee, the greater trochanter, through the lateral head of the humerus at the tip of the shoulder to the external auditory meatus; if this were a plane through the body, it would intersect the middle of the third lumbar vertebra and the anterior one-third of the sacrum; it is used to evaluate the anteroposterior curves of the spine (Fig. 17). See also *mid-malleolar line.*

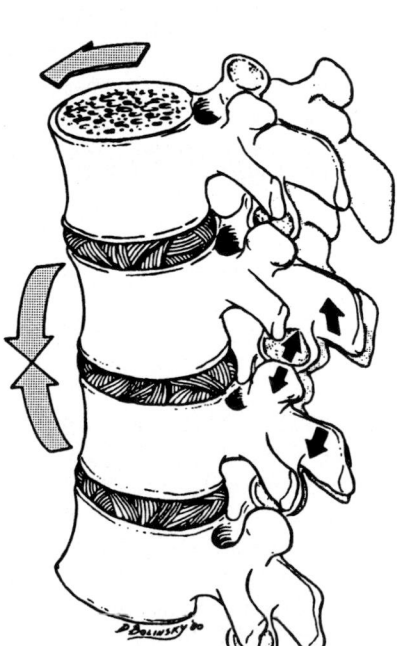

FIGURE 14. Flexion.

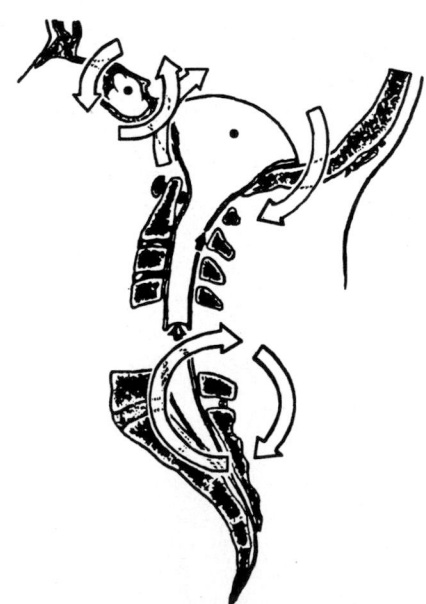

FIGURE 15. Craniosacral flexion.

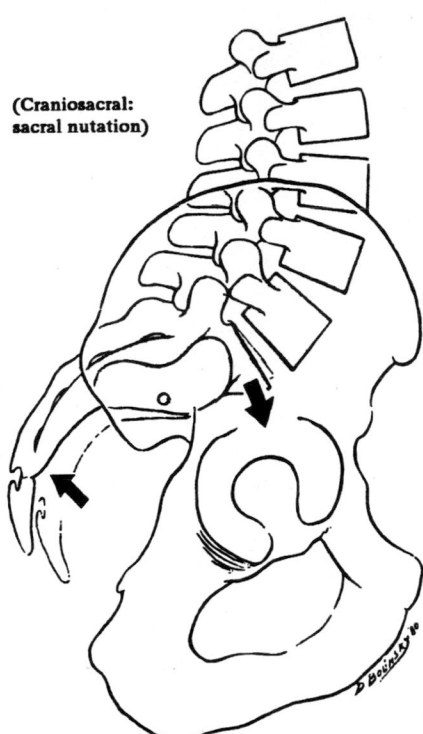

FIGURE 16. Sacral flexion.

(Craniosacral: sacral nutation)

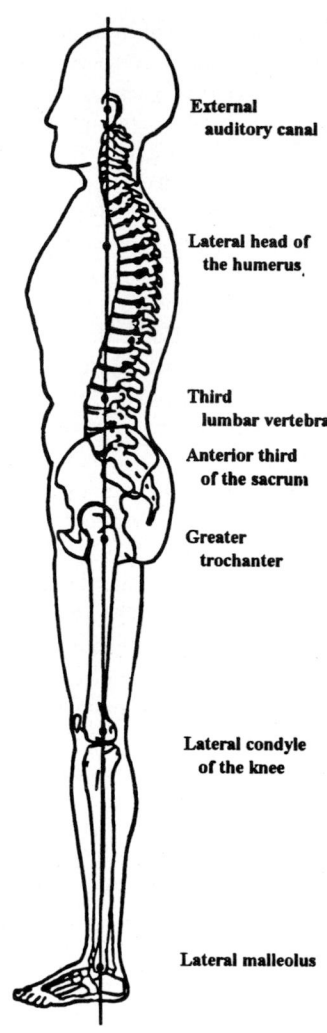

External auditory canal

Lateral head of the humerus

Third lumbar vertebra

Anterior third of the sacrum

Greater trochanter

Lateral condyle of the knee

Lateral malleolus

Gravitational Line

FIGURE 17. Gravitational line.

guiding: Gentle movement by the operator following the path of least resistance in the movement of a body part within its normal range.

H

habituation: Decreased response to repeated stimulation; hypothetically, a short-term (minutes or hours) decremental central nervous system (CNS) process; it interacts with the incremental CNS process of sensitization and yields a final behavioral outcome.

health: Adaptive and optimal attainment of physical, mental, emotional, spiritual, and environmental well-being.

hip bone: The os coxae; a large, irregular-shaped bone which consists of three parts: ilium, ischium, and pubis, which meet at the acetabulum, the cup-shaped cavity for the head of the femur at the hip (femoroacetabular) joint; the pelvis is made up of the right and left hip bones, the sacrum, and coccyx. Also called the innominate bone or pelvic bone; see *innominate, somatic dysfunctions of.*

homeostasis: 1. Maintenance of static or constant conditions in the internal environment. 2. The level of well-being of an individual maintained by internal physiologic harmony; it is the result of a relatively stable state or equilibrium among the interdependent body functions.

homeostatic mechanism: A system of control activated by negative feedback (*Dorland's*).

hypertonicity: A condition of excessive tone of the skeletal muscles; increased resistance of muscle to passive stretching.

I

ilia: See *inferior lateral angle (ILA) of the sacrum.*

ilial compression test: See *ASIS compression test.*

ilial rocking test: See *ASIS compression test.*

iliosacral motion: Motion of the ilia on an inferior transverse axis through the sacrum, as occurs in walking; considered to be primarily influenced by the attachments and movements of the pelvis, hips, and lower extremities.

ilium, somatic dysfunction of: See *innominate, somatic dysfunctions of.*

inferior ilium: See *innominate, somatic dysfunctions of.*

inferior lateral angle (ILA) of the sacrum: The point on the lateral surface of the sacrum where it curves medially to the body of the fifth sacral vertebrae (*Gray's*) (Fig. 25).

inferior pubis: See *pubic bone, somatic dysfunctions of.*

inhalation rib: A somatic dysfunction usually characterized by a rib being held in a position of inhalation such that motion toward inhalation is more free and motion toward exhalation is restricted. Synonyms: inhaled rib, anterior rib, inhalation strain, elevated rib, exhalation restriction.

inhibition reflex: 1. In osteopathic usage, a term that describes the application of steady pressure to soft tissues to effect relaxation and normalize reflex activity. 2. Effect on antagonist muscles due to reciprocal innervation when the agonist is stimulated. See also *law, Sherrington; osteopathic and manipulative treatment, inhibitory pressure technique.*

innominate bone: See *hip bone.*

innominate, somatic dysfunctions of:

anterior i. rotation, a somatic dysfunction in which the anterior superior iliac spine (ASIS) is anterior and inferior to the contralateral landmark and the innominate (os coxae) moves more freely in an anterior and inferior direction and is restricted from movement in a posterior and superior direction. The rotation occurs around the inferior transverse axis of the sacrum.

inferior i. shear, a somatic dysfunction in which the anterior superior iliac spine (ASIS) and posterior superior iliac spine (PSIS) are inferior to the contralateral landmarks, and the innominate (os coxae) moves more freely in an inferior direction and is restricted from movement in a superior direction.

inflared i., a somatic dysfunction of the innominate (os coxae) resulting in medial positioning of the anterior superior iliac spine (ASIS). The innominate moves more freely in a medial direction and is restricted from movement in a lateral direction.

outflared i., a somatic dysfunction of the innominate (os coxae) resulting in lateral positioning of the anterior superior iliac spine (ASIS). The innominate moves more freely in a lateral direction and is restricted from movement in a medial direction.

posterior i. rotation, a somatic dysfunction in which the anterior superior iliac spine (ASIS) is posterior and superior to the contralateral landmarks. The innominate (os coxae) moves more freely in a posterior and superior direction and is restricted from movement in an anterior and inferior direction. The rotation occurs around the inferior transverse axis of the sacrum.

superior i. shear, a somatic dysfunction in which the anterior superior iliac spine (ASIS) and posterior superior iliac spines (PSIS) are superior to the contralateral landmarks. The innominate (os coxae) moves more freely in a superior direction and is restricted from movement in an inferior direction.

intersegmental motion: Designates relative motion taking place between two adjacent vertebral segments or within a vertebral unit; described as the upper vertebral segment moving on the lower.

intrinsic corrective forces: Voluntary or involuntary forces from within the patient that assist in the manipulative treatment process. See also *extrinsic corrective forces.*

-ion: A suffix describing a process or movement (e.g., extension, flexion, rotation, restriction).

isokinetic exercise: Exercise using a constant speed of movement of the body part.

isolytic contraction: See *contraction, isolytic c.*

isometric contraction: See *contraction, isometric c.*

isotonic contraction: See *contraction, isotonic c.*

J

junctional region: See *transitional region.*

K

key lesion: the somatic dysfunction that maintains a total dysfunction pattern, including other secondary dysfunctions.

kinesthesia: The sense by which muscular motion, weight, position, etc. are perceived.

kinesthetic: Pertaining to kinesthesia.

kinetics: The body of knowledge that deals with the effects of forces that produce or modify body motion.

klapping: Striking the skin with cupped palms to produce vibrations with the intention of loosening material in the lumen of hollow tubes or sacs within the body, particularly the lungs.

kneading: A soft tissue technique which utilizes an intermittent force applied perpendicular to the long axis of the muscle.

kyphoscoliosis: A spinal curve pattern combining kyphosis and scoliosis; see also *kyphosis; scoliosis.*

kyphosis: 1. The exaggerated (pathologic) anteroposterior curve of the thoracic spine with concavity anteriorly. 2. Abnormally increased convexity in the curvature of the thoracic spine as viewed from the side (*Dorland's*).

kyphotic: Pertaining to or characterized by kyphosis.

L

lateral flexed: A term used to describe a position of a vertebral body; defined as the movement of a point on the anterosuperior aspect of the vertebral body about an anteroposterior axis in a coronal plane.

lateral flexion: Also called lateroflexion; see *side bending.*

lateral masses (of the atlas): The most bulky and solid parts of the atlas; they support the weight of the head.

law:

Fryette l., of motion; see *physiologic motion of the spine.*

Head l., when a painful stimulus is applied to a body part of low sensitivity (e.g., viscus) that is in close central connection with a point of higher sensitivity (e.g., soma), the pain is felt at the point of higher sensitivity rather than at the point where the stimulus was applied.

Sherrington l., 1. Every posterior spinal nerve root supplies a specific region of the skin, although fibers from adjacent spinal segments may invade such a region. 2. When a muscle receives a nerve impulse to contract, its antagonist receives, simultaneously, an impulse to relax. (These are only two of Sherrington's contributions to neurophysiology; they are the ones most relevant to osteopathic principles.)

Wolff l., every change in form and function of a bone, or in its function alone, is followed by certain definite changes in its internal architecture, and secondary alterations in its external conformations (*Stedman's*, 25th ed.) (e.g., bone is laid down along lines of stress).

lesion (osteopathic): See *osteopathic lesion.*

lesioned components: See *osteopathic lesion; somatic dysfunction.*

ligamentous:

l. articular strain, any somatic dysfunction resulting in abnormal ligamentous tension or strain; see *strain; ligamentous strain; osteopathic manipulative treatment, ligamentous articular strain.*

l. articular strain technique, see *osteopathic manipulative treatment, ligamentous articular strain.*

l. strain, motion and/or positional asymmetry associated with elastic deformation of connective tissue (fascia, ligament, membrane). See *strain; ligamentous articular strain.*

line of gravity: See *gravitational line.*

localization: 1. In manipulative technique, the precise positioning of the patient and vector application of forces required to produce a desired result. 2. The reference of a sense impression to a particular locality in the body.

lordosis: 1. The anterior convexity in the curvature of the lumbar and cervical spine as viewed from the side; the term is used to refer to abnormally increased curvature (hollow back, saddle back, sway back) and to the normal curvature (normal lordosis) (*Dorland's*). See also *kyphosis; scoliosis.* 2. Hollow back or saddle back; an abnormal extension deformity; anteroposterior curvature of the spine, generally lumbar with the convexity looking anteriorly (*Stedman's*).

lordotic: Pertaining to or characterized by lordosis.

lumbarization: See *transitional segment.*

lumbolumbar lordotic angle: See *angle, lumbolumbar lordotic.*

lumbosacral angle: See *angle, lumbosacral.*

lumbosacral lordotic angle: See *angle, lumbosacral lordotic.*

lumbosacral spring test: See *spring test.*

lymph pumps: See *osteopathic manipulative treatment, lymphatic pump.* See also *pedal pump* or *thoracic pump.*

M

mandibular drainage: Soft tissue manipulative technique using passively induced jaw motion to effect increased drainage of middle ear structures via the eustachian tube and lymphatics.

manipulation: Therapeutic application of manual force. See also *technique.*

manual medicine: Defined by the International Federation of Manual/Manipulative Medicine (FIMM).

massage: Therapeutic friction, stroking, and kneading of the body. See also *osteopathic manipulative treatment, soft tissue technique.*

mechanoreceptor: A receptor excited by mechanical pressures or distortions, such as those responding to touch and muscular contractions (*Dorland's*).

membranous articular strain: Any cranial somatic dysfunction resulting in abnormal dural membrane tensions.

membranous balance: The ideal physiologic state of harmonious equilibrium in the tension of the dura mater of the brain and spinal cord.

middle transverse axis: See *sacral, s. motion axis, middle transverse axis (postural).*

mid-heel line: A vertical line used as a reference in standing anteroposterior radiographs and postural evaluation, passing equidistant between the heels.

mid-malleolar line: A vertical line passing through the lateral malleolus, used as a point of reference in standing lateral radiographs and postural evaluation.

motion: 1. A change of position (rotation, and/or translation) with respect to a fixed system. 2. An act or process of a body changing position in terms of direction, course, and velocity.

active m., movement produced voluntarily by the patient.

inherent m., spontaneous motion of every cell, organ, system, and their component units within the body.

m. barrier, see *barrier (motion barrier).*

passive m., motion induced by the physician while the patient remains passive or relaxed.

physiologic m., changes in position of body structures within the normal range. See also *physiologic motion of the spine.*

translatory m., motion of a body part along an axis. See *translation.*

muscle energy technique: See *osteopathic manipulative treatment, muscle energy.*

myofascial release technique: See *osteopathic manipulative treatment, myofascial release.*

myofascial technique: See *osteopathic manipulative treatment, myofascial technique.*

myofascial trigger point: See *trigger point.*

myotome: 1. All muscles derived from one somite and innervated by one segmental spinal nerve. 2. That part of the somite that develops into skeletal muscle (*Stedman's*).

N

Neidner, W: See *fascial patterns.*

neurotrophicity: See *neurotrophy.*

neurotrophy: The nutrition and maintenance of tissues as regulated by direct innervation.

neutral: 1. The range of sagittal plane spinal positioning in which the first principle of physiologic motion of the spine applies (Fig. 18). See *physiologic motion of the spine.* 2. The point of balance of an articular surface from which all the motions physiologic to that articulation may take place.

NMM-OMM: Osteopathic neuromusculoskeletal medicine, certification granted by the American Osteopathic Association through the American Osteopathic Board of Neuromusculoskeletal Medicine. First granted in 1999.

nociceptor: A peripheral nerve organ or mechanism for the appreciation and transmission of painful or injurious stimuli (*Stedman's*).

nonneutral: The range of sagittal plane spinal positioning in which the second principle of physiologic motion of the spine applies. See *physiologic motion of the spine.*

normalization: The therapeutic use of anatomic and physiologic mechanisms to facilitate the body's response toward homeostasis and improved health.

NSR: A descriptor of spinal somatic dysfunction used to denote a combination neutral (N), side-bent (S), and rotated (R)

Spencer technique, a series of direct manipulative procedures to prevent or decrease soft tissue restrictions about the shoulder. See also *osteopathic manipulative treatment OMT, articulatory treatment (ART).*

splenic pump technique, rhythmic compression applied over the spleen for the purpose of enhancing the patient's immune response. See also *osteopathic manipulative treatment OMT, lymphatic pump.*

springing technique, a low velocity/moderate amplitude technique where the restrictive barrier is engaged repeatedly to produce an increased freedom of motion.

Still technique, 1. Characterized as a specific nonrepetitive articulatory method that is indirect then direct. A system of diagnosis and treatment attributed to A.T. Still. 2. A term coined by Richard Van Buskirk, DO, PhD.

thoracic pump, a technique developed by C. Earl Miller, DO, which consists of intermittent compression of the thoracic cage.

thrust treatment (HVLA), a direct technique which uses high velocity/low amplitude forces; also called mobilization with impulse treatment.

toggle technique, short lever technique using compression and shearing forces.

traction treatment, a procedure of high or low amplitude in which the parts are stretched or separated along a longitudinal axis with continuous or intermittent force.

v-spread, technique using forces transmitted across the diameter of the skull to accomplish sutural gapping.

ventral techniques, see *osteopathic manipulative treatment, visceral manipulation.*

visceral manipulation (VIS), a system of diagnosis and treatment directed to the viscera to improve physiologic function; typically the viscera are moved toward their fascial attachments to a point of fascial balance; also called ventral techniques.

osteopathic medicine: A complete system of medical care with a philosophy that combines the needs of the patient with the current practice of medicine, surgery, and obstetrics, that emphasizes the interrelationship between structure and function and that has an appreciation of the body's ability to heal itself.

osteopathic philosophy: A concept of health care supported by expanding scientific knowledge that embraces the concept of the unity of the living organism's structure (anatomy) and function (physiology). Osteopathic philosophy emphasizes the following principles: (a) The human being is a dynamic unit of function. (b) The body possesses self-regulatory mechanisms that are self-healing in nature. (c) Structure and function are interrelated at all levels. (d) Rational treatment is based on these principles.

osteopathic physician: a person with full, unlimited medical practice rights who has achieved the nationally recognized academic and professional standards within their country to practice diagnosis and treatment based upon the principles of osteopathic philosophy. Individual countries establish the national academic and professional standards for osteopathic physicians practicing within their countries.

osteopathic postural examination: The part of the osteopathic musculoskeletal examination that focuses on the static and dynamic responses of the body to gravity while in the erect position.

osteopathic structural examination: The examination of a patient by an osteopathic physician with emphasis on the neuromusculoskeletal system including palpatory diagnosis for somatic dysfunction and viscerosomatic change, in the context of total patient care. The examination is concerned with range of motion of all parts of the body, performed with the patient in multiple positions to provide static and dynamic evaluation.

osteopathy (osteopathic medicine): A system of medical care with a philosophy that combines the needs of the patient with current practice of medicine, surgery, and obstetrics, and emphasizes the interrelationships between structure and function, and an appreciation of the body's ability to heal itself. See *osteopathic philosophy.*

P

palpation: The application of the fingers to the surface of the skin or other tissues, using varying amounts of pressure, to selectively determine the condition of the parts beneath.

palpatory diagnosis: A term used by osteopathic physicians to denote the process of palpating the patient to evaluate the neuromusculoskeletal and visceral systems.

palpatory skills: Sensory skills used in performing palpatory diagnosis and osteopathic manipulative treatment.

passive motion: See *motion, passive m.*

patient cooperation: Voluntary movement by the patient (on instruction from the operator) to assist in the palpatory diagnosis and treatment process.

pedal pump: See *osteopathic manipulative treatment, pedal pump.*

pelvic bone: See *hip bone.*

pelvic declination (pelvic unleveling): Pelvic rotation about an anteroposterior axis.

pelvic index: An objective radiographic measurement representing the relative positions of the sacrum and innominates; normal values are age related and increase in subjects with sagittal plane postural decompensation.

pelvic rotation: Movement of the entire pelvis in a relatively horizontal plane about a vertical (longitudinal) axis.

pelvic side-shift: Deviation of the pelvis to the right or left of the central vertical axis as translation along the horizontal (z) axis, usually observed in the standing position.

pelvic tilt: Pelvic rotation about a transverse (horizontal) axis (forward or backward tilt) or about an anteroposterior axis (right or left side tilt).

percussion vibrator technique: See *osteopathic manipulative treatment, percussion vibrator technique.*

pétrissage: Deep kneading or squeezing action to express swelling.

physiologic barrier: See *barrier (motion barrier), physiologic b.*

physiologic motion: See *motion, physiologic.*

physiologic motion of the spine: Principles I and II of thoracic and lumbar spinal motion described by Harrison H. Fryette, DO, C.R. Nelson, DO (1948); see *rotation; r. of vertebra.* The

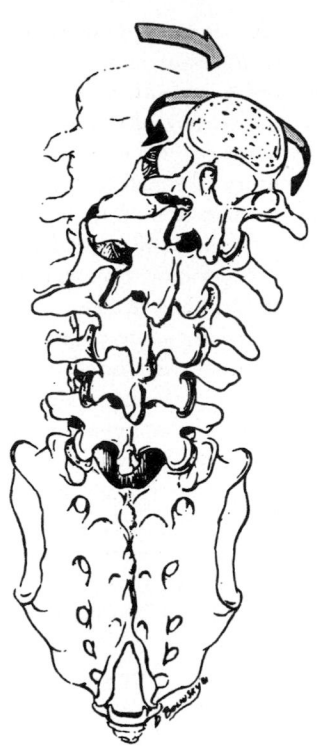

FIGURE 19. Physiologic motion of the spine (type I). Side-bending and rotation from neutral.

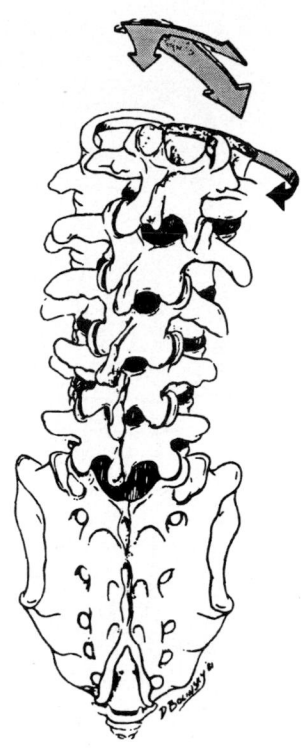

FIGURE 20. Physiologic motion of the spine (type II). Forward-bending and side-bending from a nonneutral position.

three major principles of physiologic motion are:

I: When the thoracic and lumbar spine is in a neutral position (Fig. 18) (easy normal), the coupled motions of side-bending and rotation for a group of vertebrae are such that side-bending and rotation occur in opposite directions (with rotation occurring toward the convexity) (Fig. 19); see *somatic dysfunction, type I.*

II: When the thoracic and lumbar spine is sufficiently forward or backward bent (nonneutral), the coupled motions of side-bending and rotation in a single vertebral unit occur in the same direction (Fig. 20). See *somatic dysfunction, type II.*

III: Initiating motion of a vertebral segment in any plane of motion will modify the movement of that segment in other planes of motion.

plagiocephaly: An asymmetric condition of the head.

plane: A flat surface determined by the position of three points in space; any of a number of imaginary surfaces passing through the body and dividing it into segments (Fig. 21).

    coronal p.,   frontal plane.

    frontal p.,   a plane passing longitudinally through the body from one side to the other, and dividing the body into anterior and posterior portions.

    sagittal p.,   a plane passing longitudinally through the body from front to back and dividing it into right and left portions; the median or midsagittal plane divides the body into approximately equal right and left portions.

    transverse p.,   a plane passing horizontally through the body perpendicular to the sagittal and frontal planes, dividing the body into upper and lower portions.

plastic deformation: A nonrecoverable deformation. See also *elastic deformation.*

plasticity: Ability to retain a shape attained by deformation. See also *elasticity; viscosity.*

posterior component: A positional descriptor used to identify the side of reference when rotation of a vertebral segment has occurred; in a condition of right rotation, the right side is the posterior component; usually refers to a prominent transverse process; see also *anterior component.*

postural balance: A condition of optimal distribution of body mass in relation to gravity.

postural decompensation: Distribution of body mass away from ideal when postural homeostatic mechanisms are overwhelmed; occurs in all cardinal planes but is classified by the major plane(s) affected (Fig. 21).

    coronal plane p. d.,   scoliotic changes.

    horizontal plane p. d.,   rotational changes.

    sagittal plane p. d.,   kyphotic and/or lordotic changes.

postural imbalance: A condition in which ideal body mass distribution is not achieved.

posture: Position of the body; the distribution of body mass in relation to gravity.

primary machinery of life: The neuromusculoskeletal system; a term used by I.M. Korr, Ph.D., to denote that body parts act together to transmit and modify force and motion through which man acts out his life. This integration is achieved via the central nervous system acting in response

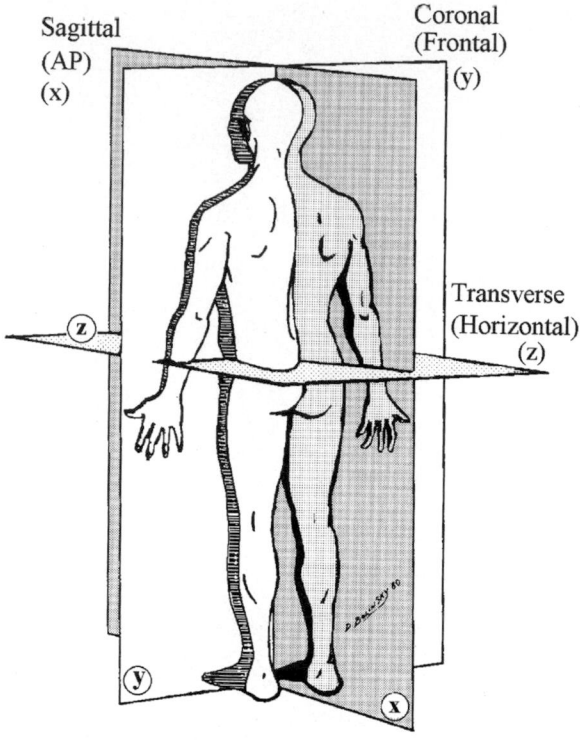

Sagittal
(AP)
(x)

Coronal
(Frontal)
(y)

Transverse
(Horizontal)
(z)

Planes of the body

FIGURE 21. Planes of the body.

to continued sensory input from the internal and external environment.

primary respiratory mechanism: A model proposed by William G. Sutherland, DO, to describe the interdependent functions among five body components as follows: a: The inherent motility of the brain and spinal cord. b: Fluctuation of the cerebrospinal fluid. c: Mobility of the intracranial and intraspinal membranes. d: Articular mobility of the cranial bones. e: The involuntary mobility of the sacrum between the ilia (pelvic bones). See also *osteopathic manipulative treatment, osteopathy in the cranial field.*

primary, refers to the internal tissue respiratory process.

respiratory, refers to the process of internal respiration (i.e., the exchange of respiratory gases between tissue cells and their internal environment, consisting of the fluids bathing the cells).

mechanism, refers to the interdependent movement of tissue and fluid with a specific purpose.

prime mover: A muscle primarily responsible for causing a specific joint action.

progressive inhibition of neuromuscular structures (PINS): See *osteopathic manipulation, progressive inhibition of neuromuscular structures.*

prolotherapy: See *sclerotherapy.*

pronation: In relation to the anatomic position, as applied to the hand, rotation of the forearm in such a way that the palmar surface turns backward (internal rotation) in relationship to the anatomic position. Applied to the foot, a combination of eversion and abduction movements taking place in the tarsal

and metatarsal joints, resulting in lowering of the medial margin of the foot. See also *supination.*

prone: Lying face downward (*Dorland's*).

proprioception: The sensing of motion and position of the body.

proprioceptor: Sensory terminals found in muscles, tendons, and joint capsules which give information concerning movements and position of the body (*Dorland's*).

psoas syndrome: A painful low back condition characterized by hypertonicity of psoas musculature. The syndrome consists of a constellation of typical related signs and symptoms:

typical associated somatic dysfunctions, as a long restrictor muscle, psoas hypertonicity is often associated with flexed dysfunctions of the upper lumbars, extended dysfunction of L5, and variable sacral and innominate dysfunctions. Tender points typically are found in the ipsilateral iliacus and contralateral piriformis muscles.

typical gait, Trendelenburg gait.

typical pain pattern, low back pain often accompanied by pain on the lateral aspect of the lower extremity extending no lower than the knee.

typical posture, flexion at the hip and side-bending of the lumbar spine to the side of the most hypertonic psoas muscle.

pubic bone, somatic dysfunctions of:

anterior pubic shear, a somatic dysfunction in which one pubic bone is displaced anteriorly with relation to its normal mate.

inferior pubic shear, a somatic dysfunction in which one pubic bone is displaced inferiorly with relation to its normal mate.

posterior pubic shear, a somatic dysfunction in which one pubic bone is displaced posteriorly with relation to its normal mate.

pubic abduction, see *pubic gapping.*

pubic adduction, see *pubic compression.*

pubic compression (p. adduction), a somatic dysfunction in which the pubic bones are forced toward each other at the pubic symphysis. This dysfunction is characterized by tenderness to palpation over the pubic symphysis, lack of apparent asymmetry, but associated with restricted motion of the pelvic ring.

pubic gapping (p. abduction), a somatic dysfunction in which the pubic bones are pulled away from each other at the pubic symphysis. This dysfunction is often seen in women following childbirth.

superior pubic shear, a somatic dysfunction in which one pubic bone is displaced superiorly with relation to its normal mate.

pubic symphysis: Somatic dysfunctions of. See *pubic bone, somatic dysfunctions of.*

pump handle rib motion: Movement of the ribs during respiration such that with inhalation the anterior aspect of the rib moves cephalad and causes an increase in the anteroposterior diameter of the thorax. This type of rib motion is found predominantly in the upper ribs (Fig. 7), decreasing from the upper to the lower ribs. See *axis of rib motion; bucket handle rib motion.*

R

reciprocal inhibition: The inhibition of antagonist muscles when the agonist is stimulated. See also *law, Sherrington*.

reciprocal tension membrane: The intracranial and spinal dural membrane including the falx cerebri, falx cerebelli, tentorium, and spinal dura.

reflex: An involuntary nervous system response to a sensory input. The sum total of any particular involuntary activity. See also *Chapman reflex*.

  cervicolumbar r., automatic contraction of the lumbar paravertebral muscles in response to contraction of postural muscles in the neck.

  conditioned r., one that does not occur naturally in the organism or system but that is developed by regular association of some physiologic function with an unrelated outside event; soon the physiologic function starts whenever the outside event occurs. See also *facilitation; somatic dysfunction*.

  oculocephalogyric r., (oculogyric reflex, cephalogyric reflex), automatic movement of the head which leads or accompanies movement of the eyes.

  red r., 1. The erythematous biochemical reaction (reactive hyperemia) of the skin in an area that has been stimulated mechanically by friction; the reflex is greater in degree and duration in an area of acute somatic dysfunction as compared to an area of chronic somatic dysfunction. It is a reflection of the segmentally related sympathicotonia commonly observed in the paraspinal area. 2. A red glow reflected from the fundus of the eye when a light is cast upon the retina.

  somato-somatic r., localized somatic stimuli producing patterns of reflex response in segmentally related somatic structures.

  somatovisceral r., localized somatic stimulation producing patterns of reflex response in segmentally related visceral structures.

  viscerosomatic r., localized visceral stimuli producing patterns of reflex response in segmentally related somatic structures.

  viscero-visceral r., localized visceral stimuli producing patterns of reflex response in segmentally related visceral structures.

regenerative injection therapy (RIT): See *sclerotherapy*.

region: An anatomic division of the body defined by either natural, functional, or arbitrary boundaries. 2. Body areas as defined in the *International Classification of Diseases, Ninth Revision, Clinical Modification (ICD-9-CM)* using the codes 739.0 to 739.9. See also *transitional region*.

resilience: Property of returning to the former shape or size after mechanical distortion. See also *elasticity; plasticity*.

respiratory axis of the sacrum: See *sacral motion, superior transverse axis (respiratory)*.

respiratory cooperation: A physician-directed inhalation and/or exhalation by the patient to assist the manipulative treatment process.

restriction: A resistance or impediment to movement; for joint restriction. See *barrier (motion barrier)*.

Anatomical vertical axis (y)

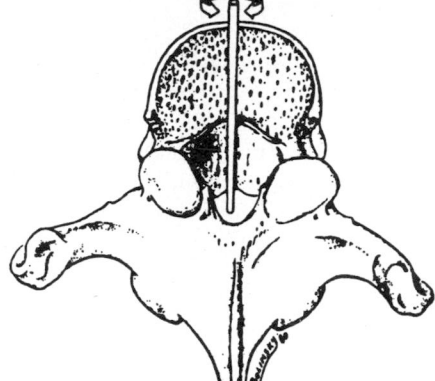

FIGURE 22. Rotation of the vertebra (thoracic).

retrolisthesis: Posterior displacement of one vertebra relative to the one immediately below.

rib dysfunction (rib lesion): A somatic dysfunction in which movement or position of one or several ribs is altered or disrupted; for example, an elevated rib is one held in a position of inhalation such that motion toward inhalation is freer, and motion toward exhalation is restricted. A depressed rib is one held in a position of exhalation such that motion toward exhalation is freer, and there is a restriction in inhalation. See also *inhalation rib; exhalation rib*.

rib motion: See *axis of rib motion; bucket handle rib motion; pump handle rib motion; caliper rib motion*.

ropiness: A tissue texture abnormality characterized by a cord-like feeling. See also *tissue texture abnormality*.

rotation: Motion about an axis.

  r. dysfunction of the sacrum, see *sacrum, somatic dysfunctions of*.

  r. of sacrum, movement of the sacrum about a vertical (y) axis (usually in relation to the innominate bones).

  r. of vertebra, movement about the anatomic vertical axis (y axis) of a vertebra; named by the motion of a midpoint on the anterior superior surface of the vertebral body (Fig. 22).

rule of threes: A method to locate the approximate position of the transverse process (TP) of a thoracic segment by using the location of the spinous process (SP) of that same vertebra. The relationship is as follows:

T1 to T3:	TP is at the same level as tip of the SP
T4 to T6:	TP is one half vertebral level above the tip of the SP
T7 to T9:	TP is one full vertebral level above the tip of the SP
T10:	TP is one full vertebral level above the tip of the SP
T11:	TP is one half vertebral level above the tip of the SP
T12:	TP is at the same level as the tip of the SP

S

Sacral:

s. base, 1. In osteopathic palpation, the uppermost posterior portion of the sacrum. 2. The most cephalad portion of the first sacral segment (*Gray's Anatomy*).

s. base declination (unleveling), with the patient in a standing or seated position, any deviation of the sacral base from the horizontal in a coronal plane; generally, the rotation of the sacrum about an anterior-posterior axis.

s. base unleveling, see *s. base declination*

sacralization, see *transitional vertebrae.*

s. motion axis, motion of the sacrum about any of its hypothetical axes (Fig. 23).

anterior-posterior (x) axis, axis formed at the line of intersection of a sagittal and transverse plane (Fig. 23).

inferior transverse axis (innominate), the hypothetical functional axis of ilial motion proposed by Fred Mitchell, Sr, DO, that passes from side to side on a line through the inferior auricular surface of the sacrum and ilia, and represents the axis for movement of the ilia on the sacrum (Fig. 24).

longitudinal axis, the hypothetical axis formed at the line of intersection of the midsagittal plane and a coronal plane, see *sacral, s. motion axis, vertical axis (y) axis (longitudinal)* (Fig. 23).

middle transverse axis (postural), the hypothetical functional axis of sacral nutation/counternutation in the standing position proposed by Fred Mitchell, Sr, DO, passing horizontally through the anterior aspect of the sacrum at the level of the second sacral segment (Fig. 24).

oblique axis (diagonal), a hypothetical functional axis proposed by Fred Mitchell, Sr, DO, that is from the superior area of a sacroiliac articulation to the contralateral inferior sacroiliac articulation; it is designated as right or left relevant to its superior point of origin (Fig. 23).

postural axis, see *sacral, s. motion axis, middle transverse axis (postural)* (Fig. 24).

respiratory axis, see *sacrum, s. motion axis, superior transverse axis (respiratory)* (Fig. 24).

superior transverse axis (respiratory), the hypothetical transverse axis about which the sacrum moves during the respiratory cycle proposed by Fred Mitchell, Sr, DO;

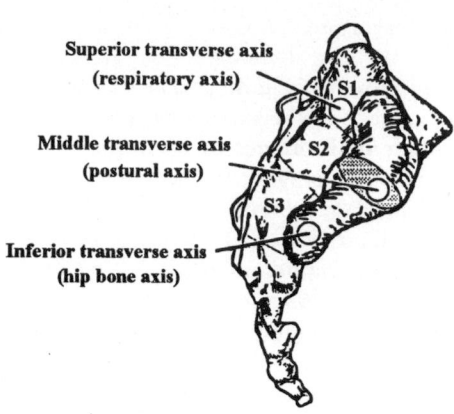

FIGURE 24. Sacral transverse axis.

it passes from side to side through the articular processes posterior to the point of attachment of the dura at the level of the second sacral segment; involuntary sacral motion occurring as a part of the craniosacral mechanism is believed to occur about this axis (Fig. 24).

transverse (z) axes, axes formed by intersection of the coronal and transverse planes about which nutation/counternutation occurs (Fig. 24).

vertical (y) axis (longitudinal), the axis formed by the intersection of the sagittal and coronal planes (Fig. 23).

s. somatic dysfunction, see *sacrum, somatic dysfunctions of.*

s. sulcus, a depression just medial to the posterior spine iliac spine (PSIS) as a result of the spatial relationship of the PSIS to the dorsal aspect of the sacrum (Fig. 25).

s. torsion, 1. A physiologic function occurring in the sacrum during ambulation and forward bending. 2. A sacral somatic dysfunction around an oblique axis in which a torque occurs between the sacrum and innominates. The L5 vertebra rotates in the opposite direction of the sacrum. 3. If the L5 does not rotate opposite to the sacrum, L5 is

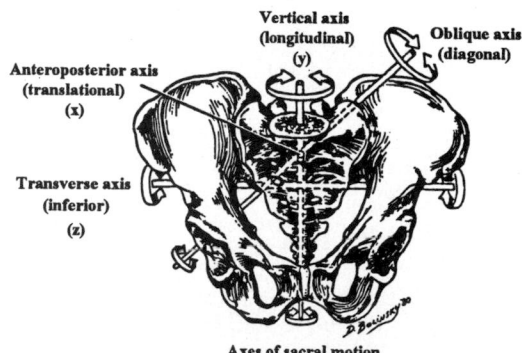

FIGURE 23. Axes of sacral motion.

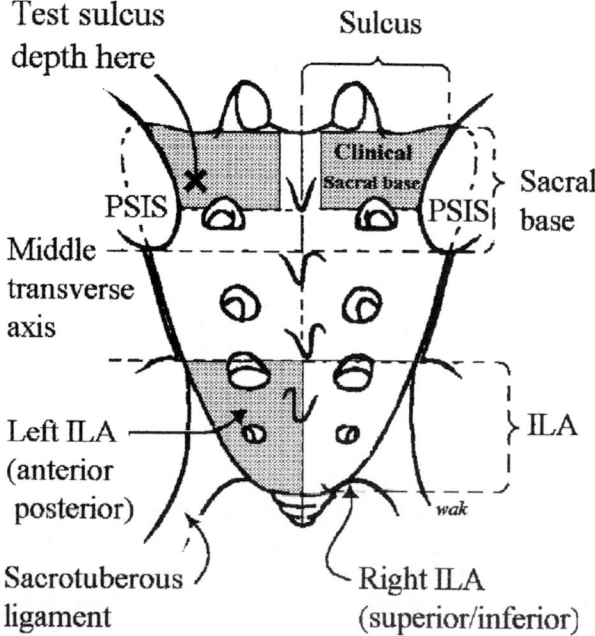

FIGURE 25. Sacral sulcus, anatomic base, clinical base, and inferior lateral angles (ILA) of the sacrum.

termed maladapted. 4. Other terms for this maladaption include: rotations about an oblique axis; anterior or posterior sacrum, and a torsion with a noncompensated L5 (Archaic use). See also *sacrum, somatic dysfunctions of.*

sacrum, somatic dysfunctions of, any of a group of somatic dysfunctions involving the sacrum. These may be the result of restriction of normal physiologic motion or trauma to the sacrum. See also *TART.*

anterior sacrum, a positional term based on the Chicago model referring to sacral somatic dysfunction in which the sacral base has rotated anterior and sidebent to the side opposite the rotation. The upper limb of the sacroiliac joint has restricted motion and is named for the side on which forward rotation has occurred. Tissue texture changes are found at the deep sulcus.

anterior translated sacrum, a sacral somatic dysfunction in which the entire sacrum has moved anteriorly (forward) between the ilia; anterior motion is freer, and there is a restriction to posterior motion (Fig. 26).

backward torsions, 1. A backward sacral torsion is a physiologic rotation of the sacrum around an oblique axis such that the side of the sacral base contralateral to the named axis rotates posteriorly. L5 rotates in the direction opposite to the rotation of the sacral base. 2. Referred to as nonneutral sacral somatic dysfunctions (Archaic use). Fred Mitchell, Sr, DO, described the backward torsion as being nonphysiologic in terms of the walking cycle.

bilateral sacral extension (sacral base posterior), 1. A sacral somatic dysfunction that involves rotation of the sacrum about a middle transverse axis such that the sacral base has moved posteriorly relative to the pelvic bones; backward movement of the sacral base is freer, forward movement is restricted, and both sulci are shallow. 2. The reverse of bilateral sacral flexion (Fig. 11).

bilateral sacral flexion (sacral base anterior), 1. A sacral somatic dysfunction that involves rotation of the sacrum about a middle transverse axis such that the sacral base has moved anteriorly between the pelvic bones; forward movement of the sacral base is freer, backward movement

is restricted, and both sacral sulci are deep. 2. The reverse of bilateral sacral extension (Fig. 15).

forward torsions, 1. A group of somatic dysfunctions described by Fred Mitchell, Sr, DO, based on the motion cycle of walking. Forward torsion is a physiologic rotation of the sacrum around an oblique axis such that the side of the sacral base contralateral to the named axis glides anteriorly and produces a deep sulcus. L5 rotates in the direction opposite to the rotation of the sacral base. 2. Referred to as neutral sacral somatic dysfunctions (Archaic use).

left on left (forward) sacral torsion, refers to left rotation torsion around a left oblique axis. See *sacrum, somatic dysfunctions of, sacral torsions.*

left on right (backward) sacral torsion, refers to left rotation around a right oblique axis. See *sacrum, somatic dysfunctions of, sacral torsions.*

posterior sacrum, a positional term based on the Chicago model referring to a sacral somatic dysfunction in which the sacral base has rotated posterior and sidebent to the side opposite to the rotation. The dysfunction is named for the side on which the posterior rotation occurs. The tissue texture changes are found at the lower pole on the side of rotation.

posterior translated sacrum, a sacral somatic dysfunction in which the entire sacrum has moved posteriorly (backward) between the ilia; posterior motion is freer, and there is a restriction to anterior motion (Fig. 27).

right on left (backward) torsion, Refers to right rotation about a left oblique axis. See *sacrum, somatic dysfunctions of, sacral torsions.*

right on right (forward) torsion, Refers to right rotation about a right oblique axis. See *sacrum, somatic dysfunctions of, sacral torsions.*

rotated dysfunction of the sacrum, a sacral somatic dysfunction in which the sacrum has rotated about an axis approximating the longitudinal (y) axis; motion is freer in the direction that rotation has occurred, and is restricted in the opposite direction.

sacral shear, a complex nonphysiologic translational

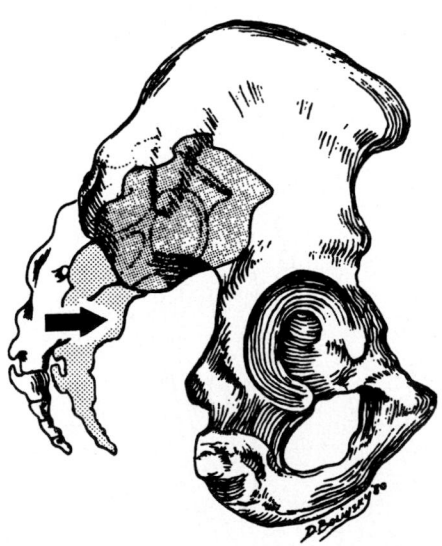

FIGURE 26. Anterior translated sacrum.

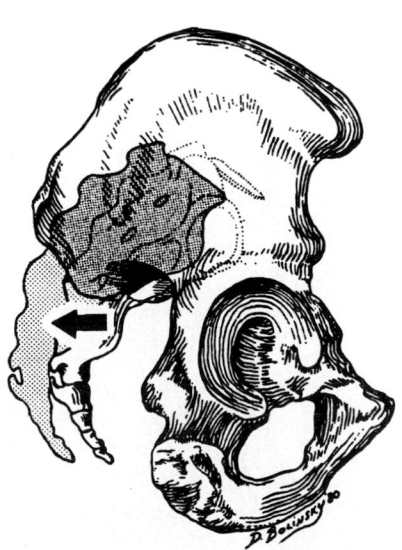

FIGURE 27. Posterior translated sacrum.

motion of the sacrum in its relationship to the innominates. (Sometimes described as a side-bending in one direction and rotation in the opposite direction. Alternatively described as a unilateral movement along the arc of the L-shaped curve of the sacroiliac joint.) See also *sacrum, unilateral sacral flexion; sacrum, unilateral sacral extension.*

sacral torsions, a group of physiologic motions and somatic dysfunctions of the sacrum around an oblique axis, in which a torque occurs between the sacrum and innominates. The L5 vertebra usually rotates in the direction opposite the sacrum. (If the L5 does not compensate, it is maladapted. Other terms for this maladaption include: rotations about an oblique axis; anterior or posterior sacrum, and a torsion with a noncompensated L5.) See *sacrum, somatic dysfunctions of.*

unilateral sacral extension, is a sacral somatic dysfunction described as a superior shear of one side of the sacrum resulting in a shallow (full) sacral sulcus and ipsilateral superior-anterior inferolateral angle of the sacrum. See *sacrum, sacral shear.*

unilateral sacral flexion, is a sacral somatic dysfunction described as an inferior shear of one side of the sacrum resulting in a deep sacral sulcus and ipsilateral inferior-posterior inferolateral angle of the sacrum. See *sacrum, sacral shear.*

scan: An intermediate detailed examination of specific body regions which have been identified by findings emerging from the initial examination.

scaphocephaly: Also called scaphoid head or hatchet head, it is a transverse compression of the cranium with a resultant midsagittal ridge.

sclerotherapy: 1. Treatment involving injection of a proliferant solution at the osseous-ligamentous junction. 2. Treatment involving injection of irritating substances into weakened connective tissue areas such as fasciae, varicose veins, hemorrhoids, esophageal varices, or weakened ligaments. The intended body's response to the irritant is fibrous proliferation with shortening/strengthening of the tissues injected.

sclerotome: 1. Sclerotomal area; the pattern (Fig. 28) of innervation of structures derived from embryonal mesenchyme (joint capsule, ligament, and bone). 2. The area of bone

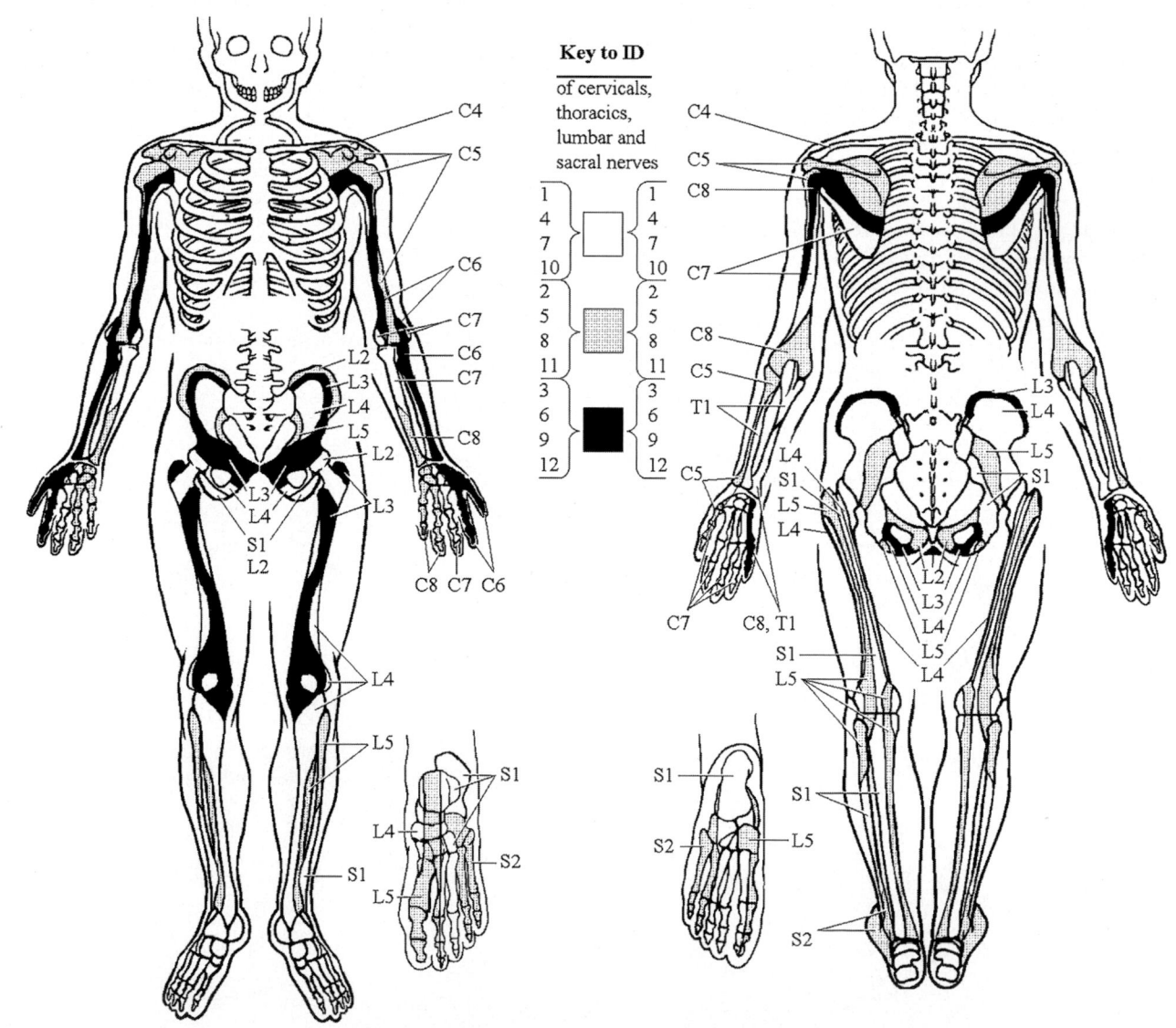

FIGURE 28. Anterior and posterior sclerotomal innervations.

innervated by a single spinal segment. 3. The group of mesenchymal cells emerging from the ventromedial part of a mesodermal somite and migrating toward the notochord. Sclerotomal cells from adjacent somites become merged in intersomatically located masses that are the primordia of the centra of the vertebrae.

(sclerotomal) pain, deep, dull achy pain associated with tissues derived from a common sclerotome (Fig. 28).

screen: The scan focuses on segmental areas for further definition or diagnosis.

scoliosis: 1. Pathologic or functional lateral curvature of the spine. 2. An appreciable lateral deviation in the normally straight vertical line of the spine (*Dorland's*) (Fig. 29).

screen: The initial general somatic examination to determine signs of somatic dysfunction in various regions of the body. See also *scan*.

secondary joint motion: Involuntary or passive motion of a joint. Also called accessory joint motion.

segment: A portion of a larger body or structure set off by natural or arbitrarily established boundaries, often equated with spinal segment. 1. To describe a single vertebra, such as a vertebral segment. 2. A portion of the spinal cord corresponding to the sites of origin of rootlets of individual spinal nerves.

segmental diagnosis: The final stage of the spinal somatic examination in which the nature of the somatic problem is detailed at a segmental level. See also *scan; screen*.

segmental motion: Movement within a vertebral unit described by displacement of a point at the anterior-superior aspect of the superior vertebral body.

sensitization: Hypothetically, a short-lived (minutes or hours) increase in central nervous system (CNS) response to repeated sensory stimulation that generally follows habituation (q.v.).

shear: An action or force causing or tending to cause two contiguous parts of an articulation to slide relative to each other

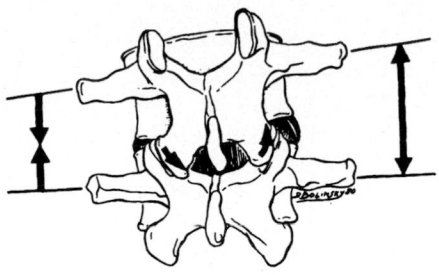

FIGURE 30. Side bent.

in a direction parallel to their plane of contact (e.g., pubic shear (q.v.); sacral shear, innominate shear).

Sherrington law: See *law, Sherrington*.

side bending: Movement in a coronal (frontal) plane about an anterior-posterior (x) axis. Also called lateral flexion, lateroflexion, or flexion right (or left).

side bent: The position of any one or several vertebral bodies after side bending has occurred (Fig. 30).

skin drag: Sense of resistance to light traction applied to the skin; related to the degree of moisture and degree of sympathetic nervous system activity.

soft tissue technique: See *osteopathic manipulative treatment, soft tissue technique*.

somatic dysfunction: Impaired or altered function of related components of the somatic (body framework) system: skeletal, arthrodial, and myofascial structures, and related vascular, lymphatic, and neural elements. Somatic dysfunction is treatable using osteopathic manipulative treatment. The positional and motion aspects of somatic dysfunction are best described using at least one of three parameters: (a) the position of a body part as determined by palpation and referenced to its adjacent defined structure; (b) the directions in which motion is freer; and (c) the directions in which motion is restricted. See also *STAR, TART*.

acute s. d., immediate or short-term impairment or altered function of related components of the somatic (body framework) system; characterized in early stages by vasodilation, edema, tenderness, pain, and tissue contraction; diagnosed by history and palpatory assessment of tenderness, asymmetry of motion and relative position, restriction of motion, and tissue texture change (TART). See also *TART*.

chronic s. d., impairment or altered function of related components of the somatic (body framework) system, characterized by tenderness, itching, fibrosis, paresthesias, tissue contraction; identified by TART (q.v.). See also *TART*.

primary s. d., 1. The somatic dysfunction that maintains a total pattern of dysfunction. See also *key lesion*. 2. The initial or first somatic dysfunction to appear temporally.

secondary s. d., somatic dysfunction (q.v.) arising either from mechanical or neurophysiologic response subsequent to or as a consequence of other etiologies.

type I s. d., 1. A group curve of thoracic and/or lumbar vertebrae in which the freedoms of motion are in neutral with side bending and rotation in opposite directions with maximum rotation at the apex (rotation occurs toward the convexity of the curve) based upon the principles

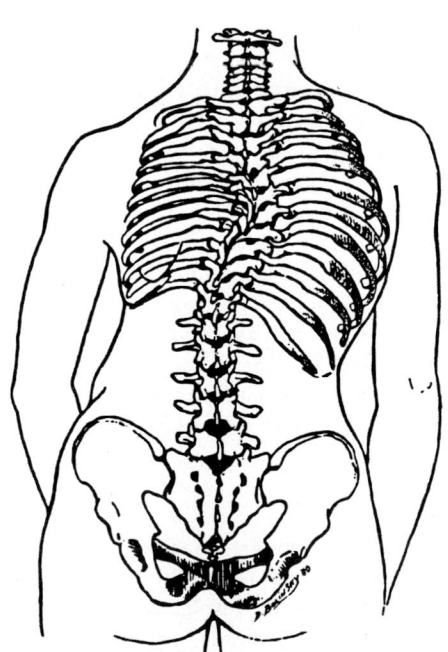

FIGURE 29. Scoliosis.

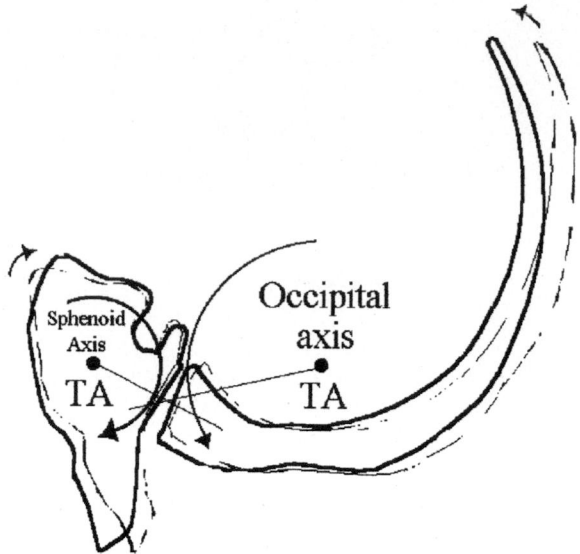

FIGURE 31. Extension (sphenobasilar synchondrosis).

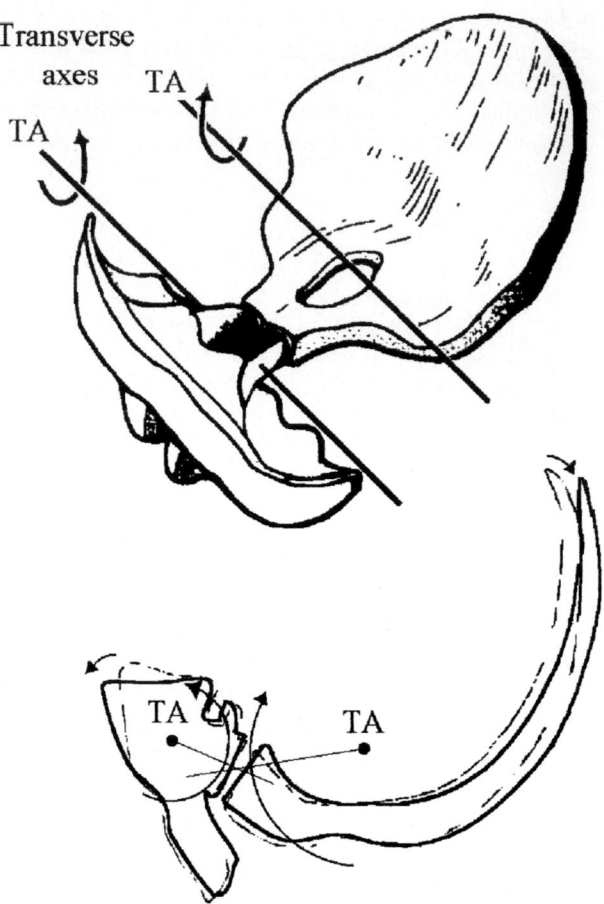

FIGURE 32. Flexion (sphenobasilar synchondrosis).

of Fryette (American usage). 2. Second degree dysfunction based upon the laws of Lovett (French usage).

type II s. d., thoracic or lumbar somatic dysfunction of a single vertebral unit in which the vertebra is significantly flexed or extended with side-bending and rotation in the same direction (rotation occurs into the concavity of the curve) based upon the principles of Fryette (American usage). 2. First-degree dysfunction based upon the laws of Lovett (French usage).

somatogenic: That which is produced by activity, reaction, and change originating in the musculoskeletal system.

somato-somatic reflex: See *reflex, somato-somatic reflex.*

somatovisceral reflex: See *reflex, somatovisceral reflex.*

spasm: (compare with hypertonicity) a sudden, violent, involuntary contraction of a muscle or group of muscles, attended by pain and interference with function, producing involuntary movement and distortion (*Dorland's*).

Spencer technique: See *osteopathic manipulative treatment, Spencer technique.*

sphenobasilar synchondrosis (symphysis), somatic dysfunctions of: any of a group of somatic dysfunctions involving primarily the interrelationship between the basilar portion of the sphenoid (basisphenoid) and the basilar portion of the occiput (basiocciput). The abbreviation, SBS, is often used in reporting the following somatic dysfunctions:

SBS compression, somatic dysfunction in which the basisphenoid and basiocciput are held forced together significantly limiting SBS motion.

SBS extension, sphenoid and occiput have rotated in opposite directions around parallel transverse axes; the basiocciput and basisphenoid are both inferior in SBS extension with a decrease in the dorsal convexity between these two bones (Fig. 31).

SBS flexion, sphenoid and occiput have rotated in opposite directions around parallel transverse axes; the basiocciput and basisphenoid are both superior in SBS extension with

an increase in the dorsal convexity between these two bones (Fig. 32).

lateral strain, sphenoid and occiput have rotated in the same direction around parallel vertical axes; lateral strains of the SBS are named for the position of the basisphenoid, right or left (Fig. 33).

side-bending/rotation, sphenoid and occiput have rotated in opposite directions around parallel vertical axes and rotate in the same direction around an anteroposterior axis; SBS side-bending/rotations are named for the convexity, right or left (Fig. 34).

torsion, sphenoid and occiput have rotated in opposite directions around an anteroposterior axis; SBS torsions are named for the high greater wing of the sphenoid, right or left (Fig. 35).

vertical strain, sphenoid and occiput have rotated in the same direction around parallel transverse axes; vertical strains of the SBS are named for the position of the basisphenoid, superior or inferior (Fig. 36).

spondylo-: Combining form denoting relationship to a vertebra, or to the spinal column (*Dorland's*).

spondylitis: Inflammation of vertebrae (*Dorland's*).

spondylolisthesis: Anterior displacement of one vertebra relative to one immediately below (usually L5 over the body of the sacrum or L4 over L5).

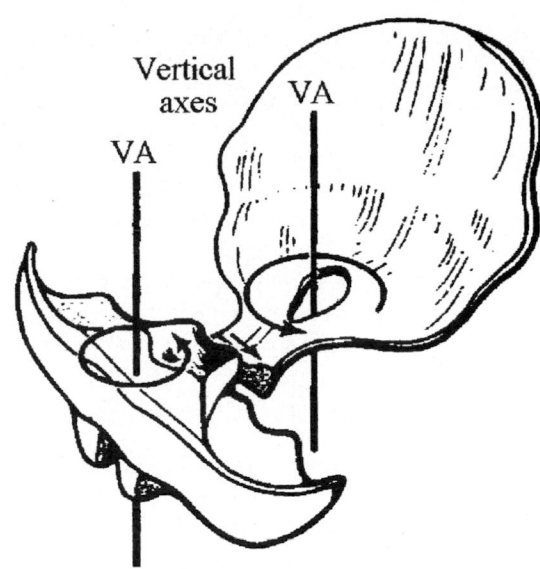

FIGURE 33. Right lateral strain (sphenobasilar synchondrosis).

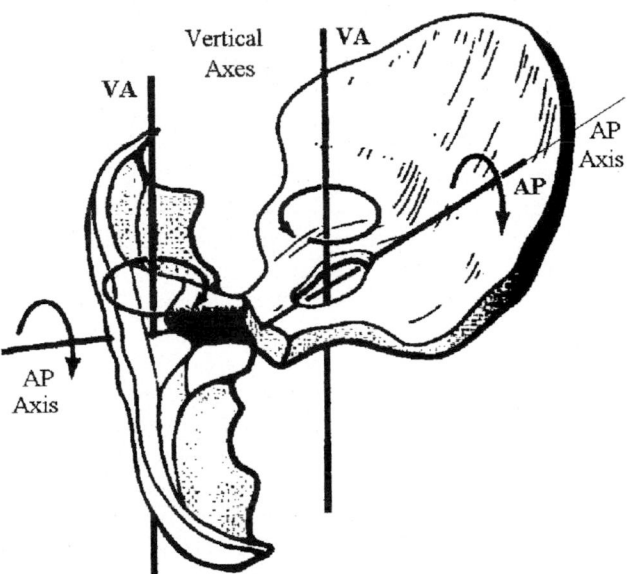

FIGURE 34. Left side-bending/rotation (sphenobasilar synchondrosis).

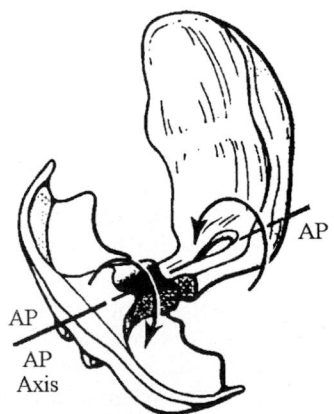

FIGURE 35. Right torsion (sphenobasilar synchondrosis).

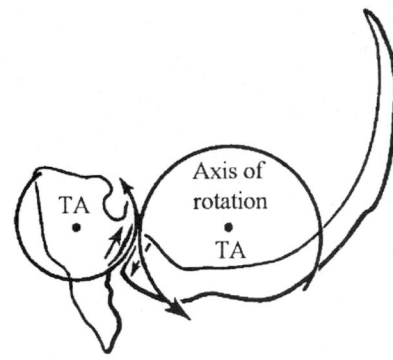

FIGURE 36. Superior vertical strain (sphenobasilar synchondrosis).

spondylolysis: Dissolution of a vertebra, aplasia of the vertebral arch, and separation at the pars interarticularis; platyspondylia; prespondylolisthesis.

spondylosis: 1. Ankylosis of adjacent vertebral bodies. 2. Degeneration of the intervertebral disc.

sprain: Stretching injuries of ligamentous tissue (compare with strain). First degree: microtrauma; second degree: partial tear; third degree: complete disruption.

springing technique: See *osteopathic manipulative treatment, springing technique.*

sphinx test: See *backward bending test.*

spring test: 1. A test used to differentiate between backward or forward sacral torsions/rotations. 2. A test used to differentiate bilateral sacral extension and bilateral sacral flexion. 3. A test used to differentiate unilateral sacral extension and unilateral sacral flexion.

STAR: A mnemonic for four diagnostic criteria of somatic dysfunction; *s*ensitivity changes, *t*issue texture abnormality, *a*symmetry, and alteration of the quality and quantity of *r*ange of motion.

static contraction: See *contraction, isometric c.*

Still, MD, DO: Andrew Taylor. Founder of osteopathy; 1828–1917; first announced the tenets of osteopathy on June 22, 1874, established the American School of Osteopathy in 1892 at Kirksville, MO.

still point: A term used by William G. Sutherland, DO, to identify and describe the brief cessation of rhythm attributed to the fluctuation of cerebrospinal fluid (a component of the primary respiratory mechanism which is observed by palpation during osteopathic manipulative treatment when a point of balanced membranous tension (or balanced ligamentous tension) is achieved.

strain: 1. Stretching injuries of muscle tissue. 2. Distortion with deformation of tissue. See also *ligamentous, l. strain.*

stretching: Separation of the origin and insertion of a muscle and/or attachments of fascia and ligaments.

stringiness: A palpable tissue texture abnormality characterized by fine or stringlike myofascial structures.

structural examination: See *osteopathic structural examination.*

subluxation: 1. A partial or incomplete dislocation. 2. A term describing an abnormal anatomic position of a joint that exceeds the normal physiologic limit but does not exceed the joint's anatomic limit.

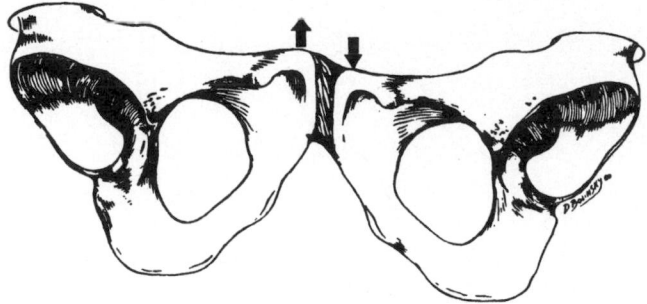

FIGURE 37. Symphyseal shear.

superior (upslipped) innominate: See *innominate, somatic dysfunctions of, superior innominate shear.*

superior pubic shear: See *pubic bone, somatic dysfunctions of.*

superior transverse axis: See *sacral, s. motion axis, superior transverse axis (respiratory);* and *transverse (z) axes.*

supination: 1. Beginning in anatomic position, applied to the hand, the act of turning the palm forward (anteriorly) or upward, performed by lateral external rotation of the forearm. 2. applied to the foot, it generally applies to movements (adduction and inversion) resulting in raising of the medial margin of the foot, hence of the longitudinal arch; a compound motion of plantar flexion, adduction and inversion; see also *pronation.*

supine: Lying with the face upward (*Dorland's*).

Sutherland fulcrum: A shifting suspension fulcrum of the reciprocal tension membrane located along the straight sinus at the junction of the falx cerebri and tentorium cerebelli.

symmetry: The similar arrangement in form and relationships of parts around a common axis, or on each side of a plane of the body (*Dorland's*).

symphyseal shear: The result of an action or force causing or tending to cause the two parts of the symphysis to slide relative to each other in a direction parallel to their plane of contact; it is usually found in an inferior/superior direction but is occasionally found to be in an anterior/posterior direction (Fig. 37).

T

tapotement: Striking the belly of a muscle with the hypothenar edge of the open hand in rapid succession in an attempt to increase its tone and arterial perfusion.

TART: A mnemonic for four diagnostic criteria of somatic dysfunction; *t*issue texture abnormality, *a*symmetry, *r*estriction of motion, and *t*enderness, any one of which must be present for the diagnosis.

technic: See *technique.*

technique: Methods, procedures, and details of a mechanical process or surgical operation. [. . . method, treatment, maneuver. . .] (*Dorland's*); see also *osteopathic manipulative treatment.*

tenderness: 1. Discomfort or pain elicited by the physician through palpation. 2. A state of unusual sensitivity to touch or pressure (*Dorland's*).

tender points: 1. System of points originally described by

Lawrence Jones, DO, FAAO, in strain/counterstrain diagnosis and treatment; see *osteopathic manipulative treatment, counterstrain.* 2. Small, hypersensitive points in the myofascial tissues of the body used as diagnostic criteria and treatment monitors.

terminal barrier: See *barrier (motion), physiologic b.*

thoracic aperture (superior): See *thoracic inlet.*

thoracic inlet: 1. The functional thoracic inlet consists of T1-4 vertebrae, ribs 1 and 2 plus their costicartilages, and the manubrium of the sternum; see *fascial patterns.* 2. The anatomic thoracic inlet consists of T1 vertebra, the first ribs and their costal cartilages, and the superior end of the manubrium (Moore).

thoracic pump: See *osteopathic manipulative treatment, thoracic pump.*

thrust: See *osteopathic manipulative treatment, thrust treatment (HVLA).*

tissue texture abnormality (TTA): A palpable change in tissues from skin to periarticular structures that represents any combination of the following signs: vasodilation, edema, flaccidity, hypertonicity, contracture, fibrosis; and the following symptoms: itching, pain, tenderness, paresthesias; types of TTAs include: bogginess (q.v.), thickening, stringiness (q.v.), ropiness (q.v.), firmness (hardening), increased/decreased temperature, and increased/decreased moisture.

tonus: The slight continuous contraction of muscle which, in skeletal muscles, aids in the maintenance of posture and in the return of blood to the heart (*Dorland's*).

 myogenic t., 1. Tonic contraction of muscle dependent on some property of the muscle itself or of its intrinsic nerve cells. 2. Contraction of a muscle caused by intrinsic properties of the muscle or by its intrinsic innervation (*Stedman's*).

torsion: 1. A motion or state where one end of a part is twisted about a longitudinal axis while the opposite end is held fast or turned in the opposite direction. 2. An unphysiologic motion pattern about an anteroposterior axis of the sphenobasilar symphysis/synchondrosis. 3. See also *sacrum, somatic dysfunctions of, sacral torsions.*

traction: A linear force acting to draw structures apart.

transitional region: Areas of the axial skeleton where structure changes significantly lead to functional change; transitional areas commonly include the following:

 occipitocervical (OA) region, typically the OA-atlantoaxial-C2 region is described.

 cervicothoracic (CT) region, typically C7-T1.

 lumbosacral (LS) region, typically L5-S1.

 thoracolumbar (TL) region, typically T10-L1.

transitional vertebrae: A congenital anomaly of a vertebra in which it develops characteristic(s) of the adjoining structure or region.

 lumbarization, a transitional segment in which the first sacral segment becomes like an additional lumbar vertebra articulating with the second sacral segment.

 sacralization. 1. Incomplete separation and differentiation of the fifth lumbar vertebra (L5) such that it takes on characteristics of a sacral vertebra. 2. When transverse processes of the fifth lumbar (L5) are atypically large, causing pseudoarthrosis with the sacrum and/or ilia(um); referred to as batwing deformity, if bilateral.

translation: Motion along an axis.

translatory motion: See *motion, translatory m.*

transverse axis of sacrum: See *sacral, s, motion axis, transverse (z) axes* (Fig. 24).

Travell trigger point: See *trigger point (myofascial trigger point).*

treatment, osteopathic manipulative techniques: See *osteopathic manipulative treatment.*

trigger point (myofascial trigger point): A small hypersensitive site that, when stimulated, consistently produces a reflex mechanism that gives rise to referred pain and/or other manifestations in a consistent reference zone which is consistent from person to person. These points were most extensively and systematically documented by Janet Travell, MD, and David Simons, MD.

trophic: Pertaining to nutrition, especially in the cellular environment (e.g., trophic function—a nutritional function).

trophicity: 1. A nutritional function or relation. 2. The natural tendency to replenish the body stores that have been depleted.

trophotropic: Concerned with or pertaining to the natural tendency for maintenance and/or restoration of nutritional stores.

-tropic: A word termination denoting turning toward, changing, or tendency to change.

tropism, facet: Unequal size and/or facing of the zygapophyseal joints of a vertebra; see also *facet asymmetry.*

type I somatic dysfunction: See *somatic dysfunction, type I.*

type II somatic dysfunction: See *somatic dysfunction, type II.*

U

uncommon compensatory pattern: See *fascial patterns.*

uncompensated fascial pattern: See *fascial patterns.*

V

velocity: The instantaneous rate of motion in a given direction.

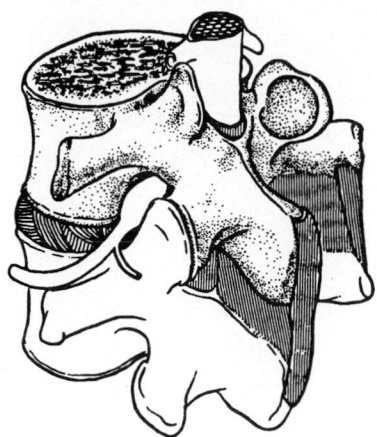

FIGURE 38. Vertebral unit.

ventral technique: See *osteopathic manipulative treatment, visceral manipulation.*

vertebral unit: Two adjacent vertebrae with their associated intervertebral disc, arthrodial, ligamentous, muscular, vascular, lymphatic, and neural elements (Fig. 38).

visceral dysfunction: Impaired or altered mobility or motility of the visceral system and related fascial, neurologic, vascular, skeletal, and lymphatic elements.

visceral manipulation: See *osteopathic manipulative treatment, visceral manipulation.*

viscerosomatic reflex: See *reflex, viscerosomatic r.*

viscosity: 1. A measurement of the rate of deformation of any material under load. 2. The capability possessed by a solid of yielding continually under stress; see also *elasticity; plasticity.*

W

weightbearing line of L3: See *gravitational line* (Fig. 17).

CRANIAL NERVES: ACTIONS AND USUAL SOMATIC DYSFUNCTIONS ACTIVATING SYMPTOMATOLOGY

Appendix II

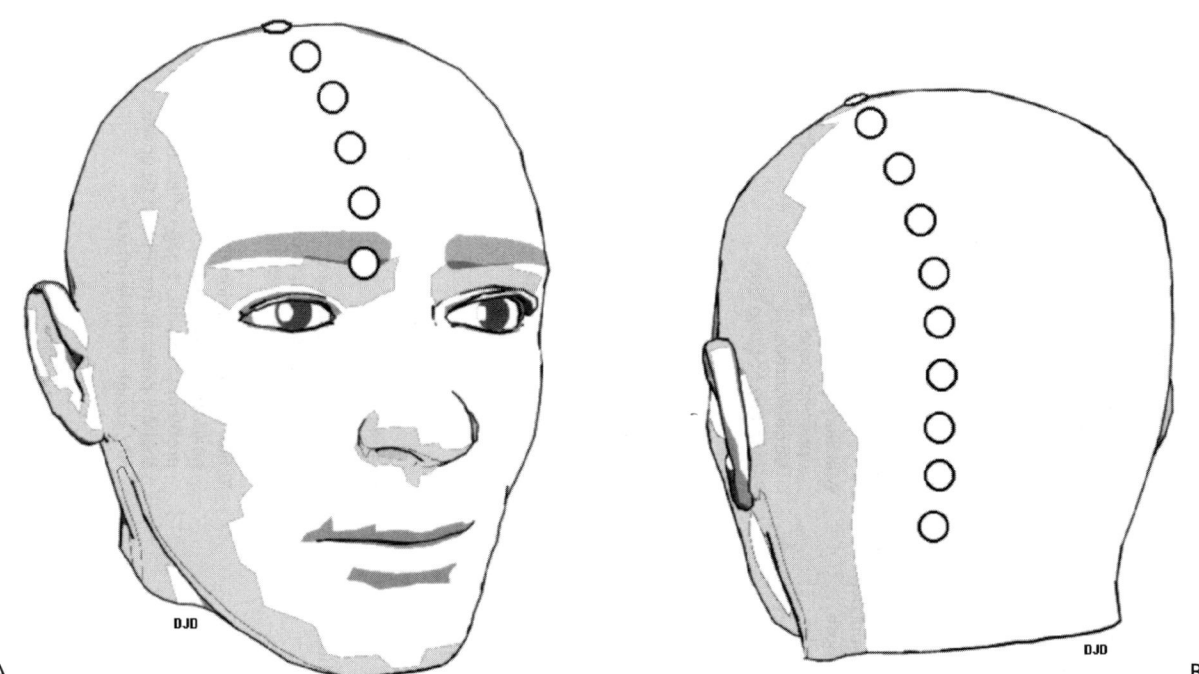

A

B

FIGURE Appendix II.1. Primary point: supraorbital notch; endpoint: suboccipital region; connection: frontalis-occipitalis muscles (**A**), trigeminal-greater occipital nerves (**B**).

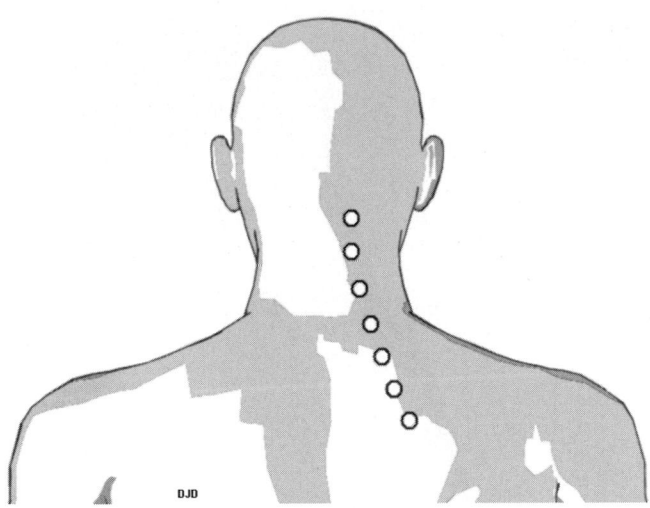

FIGURE Appendix II.2. Primary point: superior medical scapular border; endpoint: base of occiput; connection: levator scapula.

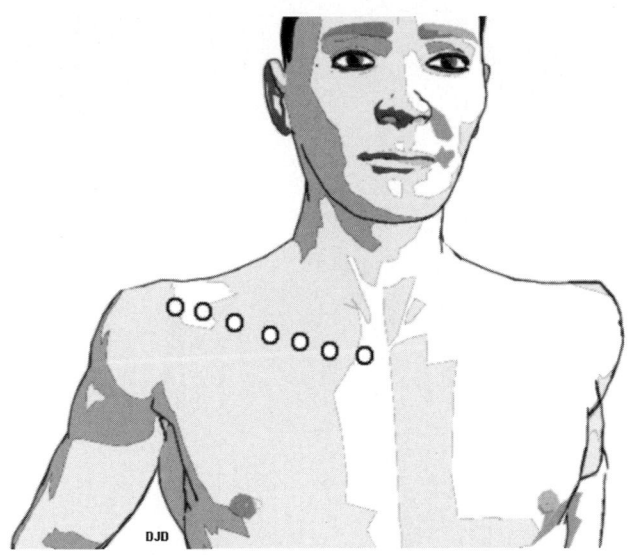

FIGURE Appendix II.4. Primary point: sternum at second rib; endpoint: coracoid process; connection: pectoralis minor.

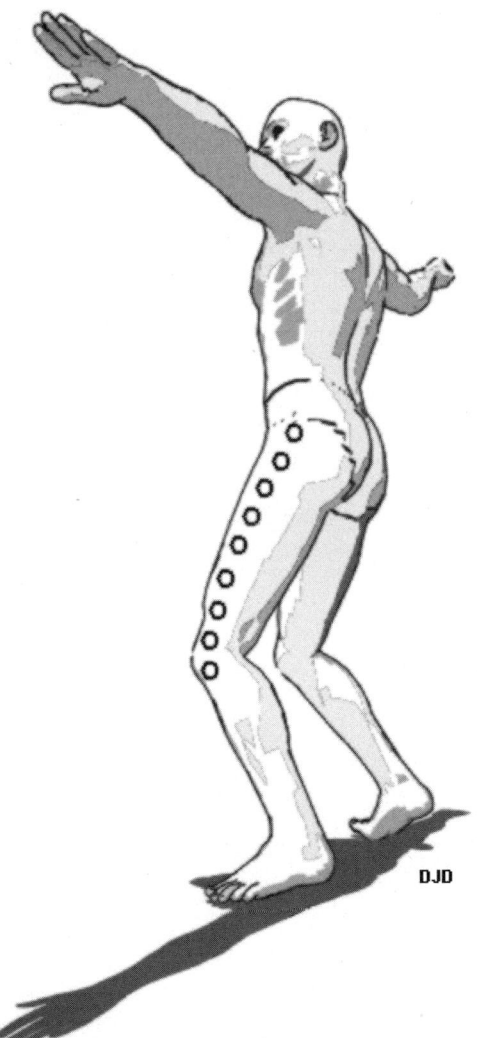

FIGURE Appendix II.3. Primary point: greater trochanter of femur; endpoint: fibular head; connection iliotibial band.

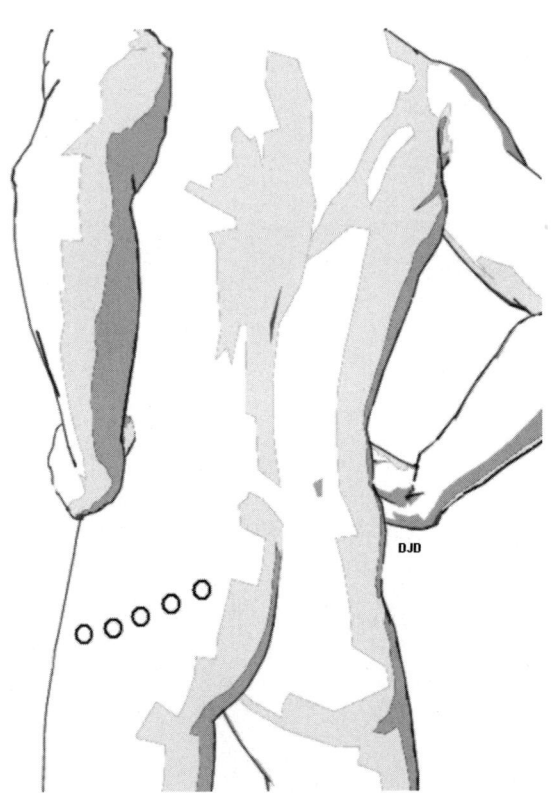

FIGURE Appendix II.5. Primary point: gluteal region; endpoint: greater trochanter; connection: piriformis muscle.

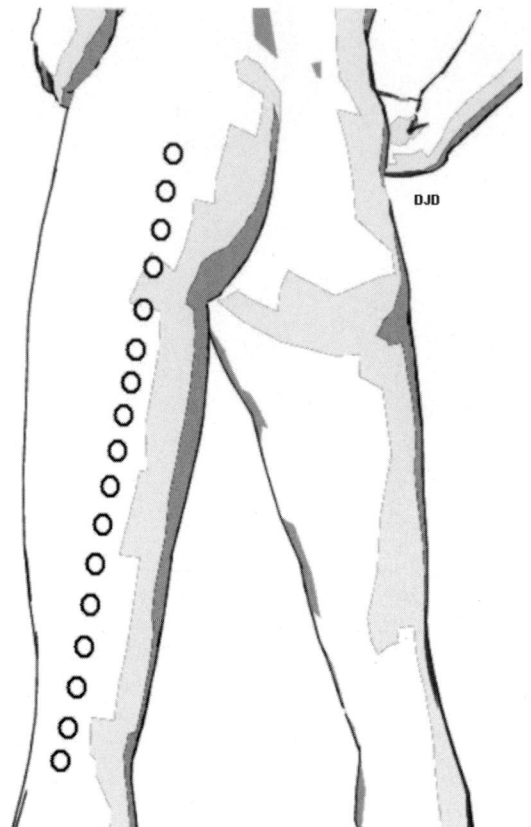

FIGURE Appendix II.6. Primary point: gluteal region; endpoint: popliteal region; connection: sciatic nerve.

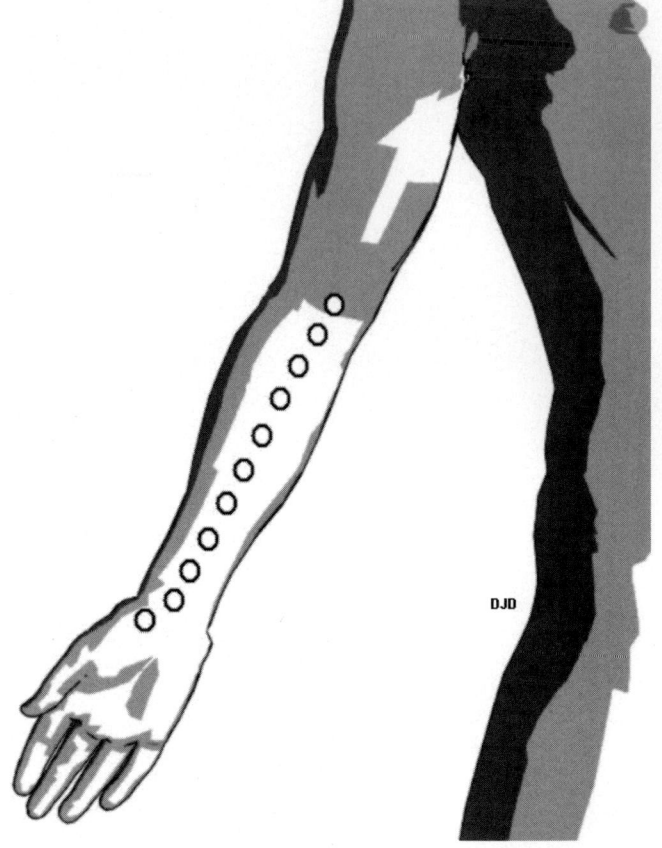

FIGURE Appendix II.8. Primary point: antecubital region; endpoint: wrist; connection: median nerve.

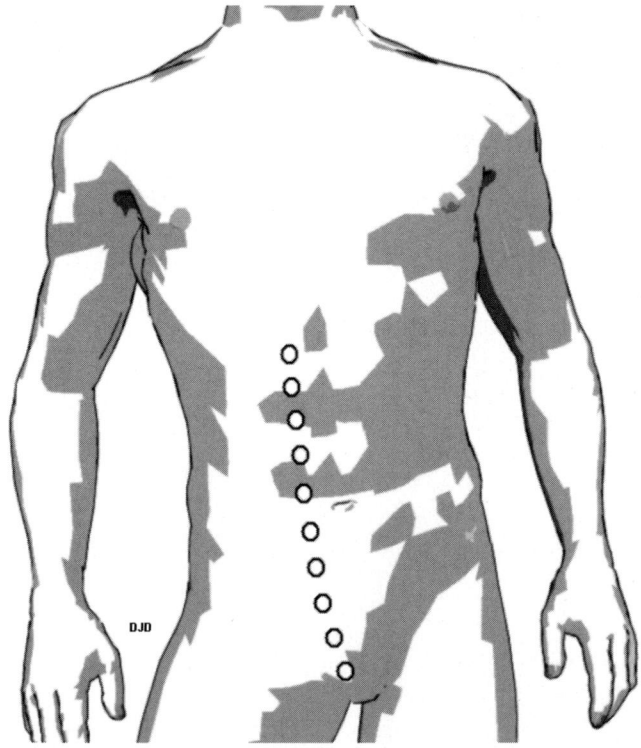

FIGURE Appendix II.7. Primary point: xiphoid process; endpoint: public ramus; connection: rectus abdominus.

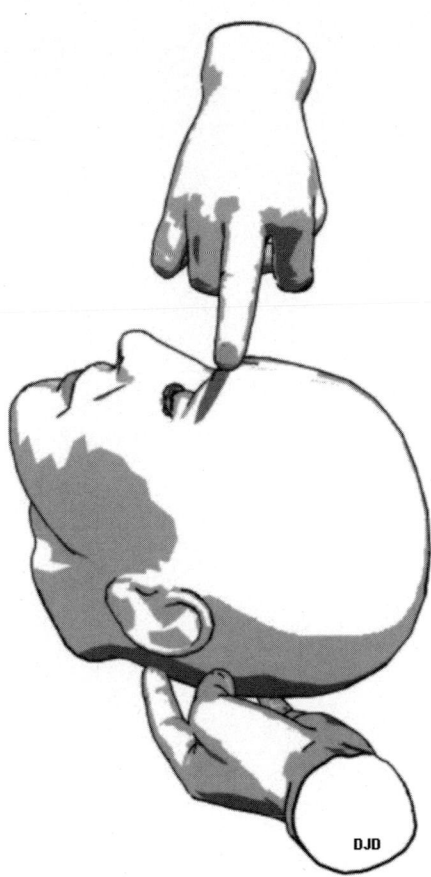

FIGURE Appendix II.9. Press both the primary point and the end point simultaneously using the pad region of a finger on each hand.

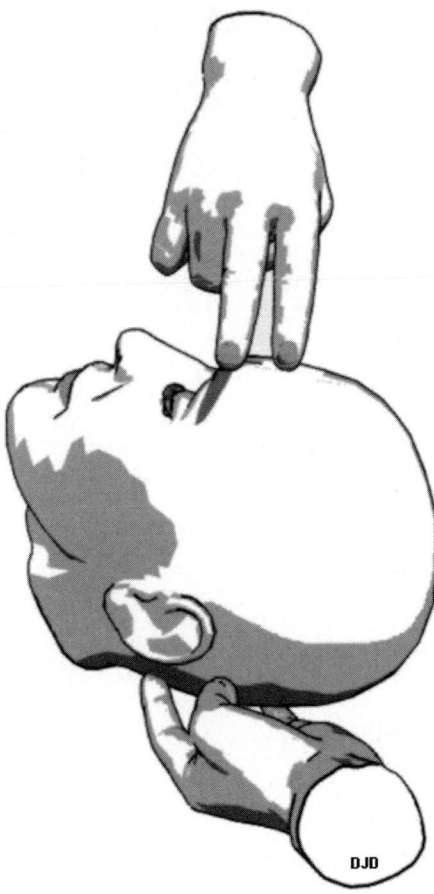

FIGURE Appendix II.10. One finger remains on the primary point. Use another finger of the same hand to locate a "secondary point." If the middle finger is on the primary point, then use the index finger to palpate the secondary point.

SUBJECT INDEX

Note: Page numbers in *italics* are figures; page numbers followed by t indicate tables.

Abdominal pain
emergency medicine, 395–397
surgery, 400–405
Abdominal region, 751–761
acutely ill patient, 1121–1123,
1131–1134, *1122,*
1131–1133
OMT, 1139–1140
definition, 752, *752*
diagnosis, 755–757
functional anatomy, 752–754
ligaments, muscles, and fascia,
752–753, 752t
nerves, 753, *755*
reflex of Morley, 753, *756*
skeleton, 752
vasculature and lymphatics, 752,
754–755
visceral pain, 753, *755*
viscerosomatic pain, 753, *755*
historical perspective, 751
key concepts, 751
lymphatic flow, 1069–1070, 1073–1075,
1070
osteopathic manipulation. *See* Visceral
manipulation.
topographic anatomy, 754, *756–758*
treatment, 757–758
osteopathic, 758–760
collateral ganglia inhibition,
759–760
falciform ligament release, 760
mesenteric releases, 760, *760*
paraspinal inhibition, 758–759
Abdominopelvic region, autonomic
innervation, 104–116, *106*
gastrointestinal tract, 105–111, *107–110,*
111t
hepatobiliary tree and pancreas, 111
kidney and urinary tract, 111–114, *112,*
114
reproductive tract, 114–116, *115*
Abducens nerve, 671–672
Abel, John J., 189
Academic institutions, 1220–1224
Acanthosis nigricans, in cancer, 466
Accessory nerve, 674
Acetabulum
angular structure, 80, *80*
hip dysplasia, 480–481
N-Acetyl aspartate, in pain transmission, 216
Acetylcholine, in cerebral vasculature, 99

Achilles tendon, 816
Acquired immunodeficiency syndrome
(AIDS)
hospital treatment, 428
osteopathic research, 1223
Acromion, 541, 690
Activities of daily living (ADL)
geriatric, 331–332
pelvic floor dysfunction, 416–417
physiologic mechanics, 571
Acupressure, 1028
Acupuncture, 474
Adaptation, and nociception, 138–139
Adenomyosis, 415
Adenosine triphosphate (ATP), in muscle
contraction, 75
Adrenal gland
See also Hypothalamic-pituitary-adrenal
axis.
hormone processing, 182
Adrenoceptors, in peripheral vasculature, 98
Adrenocorticotropin (ACTH), and
brainstem arousal system,
148–149, *149*
Adson test, 701
Adult attention deficit disorder, 252
Affective disorders, 1192
African sleeping sickness, 169
Age factors
See also Geriatrics.
bone properties, 70
cartilage wear, 71
ligaments and tendons, 73
pelvic floor dysfunction, 417
Agency for Healthcare Research and Quality,
1199
Airflow resistance, 502
Airway disease
in children, 319t
osteopathic manipulative therapy, 513
Alcohol use, 201–202
biobehavioral factors, 1206–1207
and fetal growth, 227
hospital treatment, 428
and stress, 239–240, 240t
Alendronate, 493
Allen test, 702
Allergic rhinitis, 376
Allodynia, primary afferent nociceptors, 140
Allostasis, 150–153
markers, 151t
Alternative medicine, in cancer, 474

Alzheimer's disease
and aging, 334
diagnosis, 251
Ambulatory patients, somatic dysfunction,
652–654, 650–652t
health forms, *655–658*
American Academy of Osteopathy,
international conferences,
1144
American Association for the Advancement
of Osteopathy, 25
American College of Osteopathic Surgeons
(ACOS), 400
American Medical Association (AMA), and
osteopathy, 22
American Osteopathic Association (AOA)
educational standards, 22
fellowship programs, 420–421
hospital examination form, 1115, *1116*
organization, 25–26
somatic dysfunction research, 1188
American Osteopathic Board of Emergency
Medicine, 383
American School of Osteopathy (ASO)
establishment of, 21–22
neurophysiology, 121
orthopedics, 478
vaccinations, 7
Amino acids, endocrine, 182, 184–185
Amphetamines, 549
Anabolic steroids, 548
Analgesia
adjuvants, 221–222
opioids
addiction, 221
side effects, 221
tolerance, 221
patient-controlled, 220
placebos, 221
transdermal patch, 220
Anatomy
abdomen, 752–754
ligaments, muscles, and fascia,
752–753, 752t, *753*
nerves, 753, *755*
skeletal, 752
vasculature and lymphatics, 753, *755*
abdominal pain, 400–401
autonomic nervous system. *See*
Autonomic nervous system.
brainstem reticular formation, 146
central nervous system, 435–436

Anatomy—*continued*
 cervical spine, 684–685
 key concepts, 37, 44
 limb anatomy, 58, *58*
  cartilage and bone, 47, *48*
  connective tissue, 46–47, *46*
  injury effects, 49
  microscopic, 46–49
  skeletal muscle, 49, *49*
 musculoskeletal function, 49–55
  fascia and neurovascular bundle,
    52–54, *53–54*
  joint play, 51–52
  muscle action, 54–55, *55*
  muscle-tendon complex, 52, *52*
  synovial and nonsynovial joints, 49–51,
    50–51
 myofascial continuity, 58–60, *59–61*
 neuromuscular system
  embryology, 44–46, *45, 46*
  segmental organization, 55–56, *55–57*
 pelvis and sacrum, 762–767, *763*
  female, 409–412, *410–411*
  muscles and connective tissue, 763–765
    primary, 763–764
    secondary, 764–765, *764*
  nerves, 767–777, *767*
  skeletal/ligaments, 762–763
  vascular/lymphatic, 765–766, *765*
 PINS method, 1030–1031
 rib cage, 718–720
  connective tissue and fascia, 720
  lymphatics, 720
  muscles, 719–720, *719*
  skeleton, 718–719, *719*
 rules of movement, 37–43
  connectedness with other sites, 41–42
  difference, 43
  drainage, 40
  functional anatomy, 38–39
  pain, 41
  proximity, 37–38
  supply, 39–40
 somatic dysfunction, 567–568,
    1153–1157
  facilitation, 1153–1154, *1154*
  mechanoreceptors, 1154–1155,
    1154t
  myofascia, 1156–1157
  spinal cord and nociception,
    1155–1156
 thorax, 705–712, *706*
  connective tissue and fascia, 710–711
  lymphatic system, 710, *711*
  muscles, 706–710, *707–710t*
  neural connections, 711–712, *712*
 upper extremities, 690–694, *691–693t,
    693*
Ancient writings, 8
Aneurysms, 681, 744
Angina pectoris, 355, *355*
Angioplasty, coronary, 356–357
Angiotensin, 98
Angles of lordosis, *1230*
Angular structure of hip, 80, *80*
Animal research, 1171

Ankle
 anatomy, 794–797
  pes planus and pes cavus, 796–797
  subtalar joint, 795–796, *797*
  tibiotalar joint, 795, *796*
 INR and MFR techniques, 961–962, *961*
 inversion sprain, 543–544, *543*
 muscle energy techniques, 905–906, *905*
Ankylosing spondylitis, 529
 back pain, 491
 in pregnancy, 452
Antecubital region, primary and endpoints,
    1260
Antibiotics, 175
Antibodies, and infections, 173
Antihistamines, for allergic rhinitis, 376
Anxiety
 diagnosis, 248–249
 management, 237–239, 238t
Aortic plexus, 104, *105*
Apley scratch test, 702
Apnea in children, 323
Aponeurosis
 definition, 908
 plantar, 799
 thoracolumbar, 733, *734*
Appendix, vermiform
 See also Lymphatic system.
 abdominal pain, 402
 Chapman reflexes, 1052
 functional technique, 982–983, *982*
Apprehension test, 702
Arches of foot, 798, *801*
Arteriovenous malformations, 681
Arteritis, temporal, 681
Arthritis
 See also Rheumatology.
 rheumatoid, HVLA complications, 1149
Arthrogryposis, 312
Arthroscopy, for knee osteoarthritis, 485
Articular processes
 acutely ill patient, 1135
 superior and interior, 729–730
Articulatory techniques, 834–851
 cervical
  extension, 837, *837*
  flexion, 837, *837*
  regional side-bending, 838, *838*
  rotation, 838
  segmental side-bending, 838
 cervicothoracic flexion, extension,
    side-bending, 838–839, *839*
 common questions, 834–835
 costal. *See also* rib cage
  anterior, 841, *841*
  lateral recumbent, 841–842, *842*
  posterior, 841, *842*
  posterior rib raising, 842–843, *842*
 design and use of, 834
 extremities, 848–851, *848–851*
 key concepts, 834
 lumbar
  extension, 844–845, *844, 845*
  flexion, 843–844, *843*
  rotation, 846, *846*
  side-bending, 845–846, *845, 846*

 pelvic
  rotation to innominate, 846–847, *847*
  sacroiliac joint gapping, 848, *847–848*
 regional treatment, 836–837
  contraindications, 837
  indications, 836
 sample clinical application, 835–836
 shoulder treatment, Spencer technique,
    836, 851
 thoracic
  extension, 839–840
  flexion, 839, *839*
  rotation, 840, *840*
  side-bending, 840–841
Ashmore, Edythe, 969–971
Asthma
 acutely ill patient, 1130–1131
 in children, 317–320
 osteopathic manipulative therapy,
    512–513
 somatic dysfunction research, 1192
 thoracic reflexes, 1125
Asylums, mental, 247
Asymptomatic Carotid Atherosclerosis
    Study, 1194
Atelectasis, 405–406, 513–514
 efficacy of OMT, 1147
Atlantal-axial joint
 balanced ligamentous tension, 930, *930*
 muscle energy techniques, 889–890, *890*
Atlas-axis, osteopathic manipulation, 1096,
    1096
ATP synthesis and function, 158–159
Atrioventricular (AV) node innervation, 101
Auditory nerve, 672–673
Auerbach's plexus, 103–104
Aura, migraine, 439, 679
Auscultation, lumbar, 740
Automobile accidents, 202, 660
 cranial dysfunction, 996
Autonomic nervous system, 33, 39, 90–119
 abdominal pain, 400–401
 brainstem reticular formation, 146
 catecholamine release, 148
 divisions of, 93–97, *94*
  parasympathetic ANS, 96–97, *96*
  primary afferent fibers, 97
  sympathetic ANS, 94–96, *95, 96*
 emergency medicine, 386, 387
 head and neck, 372–373, 374, *373*
 key concepts, 90
 myofascial trigger points, 1047–1048,
    1048
 organization, 91, *91*
 reflex arcs
  autonomic, 92–93, *92–93*
  somatic, 91–92, *92*
 regional distribution, 97–116
  abdominopelvic region, 104–116, *105*
   celiac ganglia, 106, *107–110*
   gastrointestinal tract, 105–111, *107*
   hepatobiliary tree and pancreas, 111
   kidney, 111–112, *112*
   reproductive tract, 114–116, *115*
    penis and clitoris, 116
    testis and ovary, 114–115

uterus, uterine tube, cervix, and
vagina, 115–116
ureter, 112–113
urinary bladder, 113–114, *114*
head and neck, 99–100
thorax, 100–104, *100–102*
aortic plexus, 104
cardiovascular plexus, 101–102
esophageal plexus, 103–104
respiratory plexus, 103
thoracic duct innervation, 104
trunk and limbs, 97–99
sweat glands and connective tissue,
98–99
vasculature, peripheral, 97–98
terminology, 90
Axon reflex, 164
Axoplasmic flow, 133–134

B lymphocytes, 1059
Babinski sign, 443
Back pain
See also Low back pain; Lumbar region.
in cancer, 465–466, 469
efficacy of OMT, 1145–1146
injured athletes, 539–544, *539*
iliopsoas spasm, 539–540, *540*
sacroiliac/sacral torsion dysfunction,
540, *540*
in pregnancy, 459
somatic dysfunction research, 1188
Balanced ligamentous tension (BLT)
techniques, 916–930
articular mechanisms, 916–917
diagnosis, 917–919
treatment principles, 918–919, *919*
key concepts, 916
reciprocal tension, 917
specific regions
atlantal-axial joint, 930, *930*
cervical spine, 927–930, *929–930*
clavicle, 926, *928*
hip capsule, 921–924, *922–923*
humerus/glenohumeral joint, 926–927,
928
innominates, 920–921, *921*
pelvis, 919–920, *920*
ribs, 924–926, *925*
sacroiliac joint, 927, *929*
scapulothoracic joint, 926, *927*
thorax, 924, *924*
Bankart lesion, 495, 541
Barlow test, 786
Baroreceptors, 128–129
Barriers
HVLA treatment, 855
joint motion, *1232*
Barr-Lieou syndrome, 667
Batson plexus, 469, 473
Bayes theorem, 278
Bedridden patients, somatic dysfunction,
649–659, 653–654t
Behavior modification, pain management,
223–224
Bell's palsy, 681–682
Bending, in biomechanics, 66

Bias, clinical research, 1183, 1197
Bickerstaff syndrome, 439
Bile ducts, osteopathic manipulation, 1086,
1086
Biobehavioral research, 1203–1214
cardiovascular disease, 1205, 1205t
disease development pathways,
1204–1205, *1204*
in health, 1203–1205
cognitive processes, 1204t
immune function and infections,
1205–1206
key concepts, 1203
opportunities, 1212
pain syndromes, 1206–1207, 1207t
placebos, 1207–1208
research process, 1208–1212
basic research, 1208
design and implementation, 1209t
group formation, 1210
instrumentation, 1210
intent to treat, 1210
maturation, 1210
measurement variance, 1210
multiple treatments, 1210
hypothesis, 1209, *1210*
quantitative measurement, 1210–1211
statistics, 1211–1212
sleep and circadian biology, 1206
Biofeedback
pain management, 223
stress management, 242
Biologic response modifiers, in cancer,
472–473
Biomaterials, in knee osteoarthritis,
484
Biomechanics, 63–89
articular cartilage, 70–71, *70*
behavior of materials, 66–68
elastic modulus, 66–67, *67*
fatigue, 68
isotropic or anisotropic, 66
strain vectors, 66, *66*
viscoelasticity, 67–68, *67*
bone, 68–70, *68–69*
cervical spine, 685
elbow, 81–82, *81*
entrapment neuropathies, 446
hip, 80–81, *80*
injured athletes, 538–539
key concepts, 63
knee, 78–80, *78*
ligaments and tendons, 71–73, *72*
locomotion, 86–87, *87*
motion and forces in three-dimensional
space, 64–66, *64–66*
musculoskeletal models, 75–78, *76–77*
myofascial trigger points, 1038–1039
postural decompensation, 605, *605–606*
in pregnancy, 456
rib cage, 720–721, *721*
shoulder, 82–83, *82*
skeletal muscle, 73–75, *73–74*
spine, 83–86, *83–85*
Bipolar disorders, 248
Birth canal, 458, *458*

Bisphophonates, 493
Bladder, osteopathic manipulation,
1090–1091, *1090*
Blinding, in research, 1180, 1184, 1217
Blood doping, 549
Blood flow
in cancers, 469
general mechanisms, 159–160, *160*
HVLA complications, 1149
local control of, 160–161
myocardial, 161–163, *162*
in pregnancy, 452, *453*
pulmonary, 503
in skin, 163–164, *163*
Blood pressure, and baroreceptors, 128–129
Blood vessels
abdominal, 753, *754–755*
brain, 996
cervical spine, 685
female pelvis, 411–412
of head and neck, 99, 662, *669*
hip, 806, 810, *815*
hip fractures, 482–483, *483*
innervation, 97–98
knee, 810
lower leg, 810, 813, *816*
lumbar, 735, *736*
pelvis and sacrum, 765–766, *765*
thoracic, 706
upper extremity, 691–692
Blood-brain barrier, 192
Bombesin, and lung cancer, 464
Bonding, infants, 228
Bone
abdominal, 752
biomechanics, 68–70, *68*
fractures, 69–70, *69*
remodeling, 70
cervical spine, 684
cranial, articular mobility of, 987,
989–990
lower extremity, 784–785, *785*
metastatic disease, 465–466, 468–469
microscopic anatomy, 47, *48–49*
pelvis and sacrum, 762–763
PINS method, 1030
in postural decompensation, 606–607
rib cage, 718–719, *719*
of skull, 660, *661–666*, 666t
Braces
in knee osteoarthritis, 485
postural, 589
for scoliosis, 622
for spondylolithesis, 630
Brachial plexus, 694
Bradykinins, in somatic dysfunction, 1154
Brain
autonomic innervation, 99–100
motility of, 986–988
tumors, 681
Brain natriuretic peptide (BNP), 360, 361
Brainstem
arousal system, 145–147
ascending pathways, 145–146
and neuroendocrine immune network,
147–152

Brainstem, arousal system—*continued*
    cytokines, 149
      hormonal release, 147–149, *149*
    reticular formation, 146
  and baroreceptors, 128–129
Breast cancer, biobehavioral factors, 1207
Breathing, work of. *See* Respiration.
Brief psychotic disorder, 249
Bronchi, osteopathic manipulation,
    1089–1090, *1089*
Bronchiolitis
  in children, 317–318
  osteopathic manipulative therapy, 513
Bronchitis
  osteopathic manipulative therapy, 512
  thoracic reflexes, 1125
Bucheim, Rudolph, 189
Bunions, 800–801
Burns, Louisa, 121, 1156, 1167
Bursitis, 814–816, *816*
  subacromial, 541

Cachectin, in cancer, 469–470
Caffeine
  performance enhancement, 549
  somatic dysfunction research, 1191–1192,
    1198
Calcitonin gene-related peptide (CGRP)
  in cardiovascular innervation, 102
  in cerebral vasculature, 99
  in respiratory plexus, 103
  in somatic dysfunction, 1154, 1155
Calcium, and ATP synthesis, 158–159
Calcium pyrophosphate deposition disease, 529
Capsulitis, adhesive, 703
Carbon dioxide, pulmonary, 504
Cardiology, 345–369
  angina pectoris, 355, *355*
  coronary artery disease, 350–355
    cases, 357–358
    diagnosis, 351–353, 352t
    pathophysiology and natural history,
      350, *350*
    therapy, 353–355, 354t
    vascular biology, 350–351
  heart failure, 358–363
    diagnosis, 360–361
    exercise, 361
    muscle hypothesis, 361–362, *362*
    osteopathy, 362–363
    treatment, 361
  key concepts, 345
  myocardial infarction, 355–357, *356*
  osteopathic overview, 345–349, *346, 348*,
    348t, 349t
  unstable angina, 355, 355t
Cardiopulmonary system, emergency
    medicine, 394–395
Cardiovascular disease
  allostasis, 151–152
  biobehavioral mechanisms, 1205, 1205t
  endocrine function, 184
  somatic dysfunction research, 1191
Cardiovascular plexus, 101–102
Carpal tunnel syndrome, 445–446
  myofascial trigger points, 1043

physiatry, 523
  in pregnancy, 454
  treatment, 702–703
Cartilage
  articular, 70–71, *70*
  in knee osteoarthritis, 484
  lower extremity, 792–793
  microscopic anatomy, 47, *48–49*
Casts, for spondylolithesis, 630
Catecholamines
  brainstem arousal system, 148
  hormone processing, 182, 184
Catheterization, cardiac, somatic
    dysfunction research, 1191
Cauda equina syndrome, 744
Cement line of bone, 68
Center of rotation, 78
Central nervous system
  allostasis, 152
  anatomy, 435–436
  autonomic components, 91
  in cancer, 467–468
  myofascial trigger points, 1038
Cephalgia, in emergency medicine, 389–391
Cerebellar degeneration, and lung cancer,
    464, 467
Cerebrospinal fluid, 674–675
  motility of, 987, 988
Cervical region
  articulatory techniques
    extension, 837, *837*
    flexion, 837, *837*
    rotation, 838
    side-bending
      regional, 838, *838*
      segmental, 838
    facilitated positional release (FPR),
      1018–1019, *1019*
    fascial-ligamentous release, 913, *913*
    functional technique, 976–977, *978*
    HVLA treatment, 857–859
      atlanto-axial joint, 857–858
      occipito-atlantal joint, 857, *857*
      rotational focus, 858–859, *859*
      side-bending focus, 858, *858*
    lymphatic flow, 1072–1073, *1072–1073*
    muscle energy techniques, 887–888, *888*
    soft tissue techniques
      forward bending, 820–821, *821*
      rotation, 820, *820*
      suboccipital inhibition, 820, *820*
      traction, 820
        contralateral, 821
        longitudinal, 821, *821*
Cervical spine, 86, 684–689
  anatomy
    blood supply, 685
    ligaments, 684
    lymphatic system, 685
    muscles, 684
    neural, 685
    skeletal, 684
  balanced ligamentous tension, 927–930,
    929–930
  biomechanics, 685
  clinical information, 688–689

key concepts, 684
  motion testing, 686–688, *687*
  osteopathic manipulation, 689,
    1094–1095, *1095*
  strain and counterstrain technique,
    1007–1009, *1008–1009*
Cervical sprain/strain, physiatry, 524
Cervicothoracic region, articulatory
    techniques, 838–839, *839*
Cervix
  autonomic innervation, 116
  osteopathic manipulation, 1091–1092,
    1092
Chapman reflexes, 1051–1055
  clinical use, 1052–1055
    specific reflexes, 1052–1053,
      1053–1054
    treatment, 1055
  emergency medicine, 386, 396
  history and philosophy, 1052
  key concepts, 1051
  palpation, 1051–1052, *1052*
  pelvic pain, 412
  point and pressure techniques, 1028
  in pregnancy, 454
  upper extremity, 704
Chemoreceptors, 139–140, 505
Chemotherapy, 174–175, *175*
Chest pain
  cardiovascular disease, 352
  emergency medicine, 392–394
Children, hospital treatment, 428–429
Cholecystitis
  abdominal pain, 403
  segmental facilitation, 1126
Cholesterol, hormone processing, 182
Chopart joint, 800
Chronic obstructive pulmonary disease
    (COPD)
  efficacy of OMT, 1147
  osteopathic manipulative therapy,
    512–513
Circadian rhythms, 1206
Circulatory system
  See also Respiration and circulation.
  connectors, 41–42
  in pregnancy, 452
Citric acid cycle, 158
Civil War medicine, 20
Claudication, 491
Clavicle
  acutely ill patient, 1120
  balanced ligamentous tension, 926, *928*
  muscle energy techniques, 906–907, *906*
  myofascial release technique, 88
Clinical problem solving, 257–279
  abdominal pain, 258–259
  Bayes theorem, 278
  caveats, 259–264
    decision analysis, 263–264
    diagnostic problems, 264–265
    hypothetico-deductive method,
      260–261
    problem-oriented perspective, 261–263
  coronary artery disease, 277–279
  data gathering, 258

examples, 257, 265–270, 272–276
key concepts, 257
manipulative treatment, 271
musculoskeletal system, 269
    pain, 270–271
patient as whole, 271
patterns, 258, 259
Clinical trials. *See* Research, osteopathic.
Clitoris, autonomic innervation, 116
Cocaine addiction, 250–251, 250–251t
Cognitive function
    geriatric, 332
    in health, 1204t
    pain transmission, 219
Cole, Wilbur V. 121
Colic, 322
Collagen
    in articular cartilage, 70–71
    in connective tissue, 46–47, *47*
    of fascia, 52
    in ligaments and tendons, 71–72
Colon
    Chapman reflexes, 1052–1053
    osteopathic manipulation, 1082–1083
        cecum and ascending colon, 1082,
            1082
        root of sigmoid, 1082–1083, *1083*
        sigmoid, 1083, *1083*
        transverse colon and flexures, 1082,
            1082
Common cold, 677–678
Compartment syndrome, 813–814
    bursae and bursitis, 814–816, *816*
Complementary medicine, in cancer, 474
Compliance
    biobehavioral factors, 1207
    pulmonary, 502
Complications of OMT, 1147–1150
    incidence, 1147–1149, 1148t
Compression
    in biomechanics, 65–66
        bone fracture, 69
    cervical spine, 688
    spinal, 742
    spinal disorders, 442–443
    vertebral body fractures, 727–728
Computed tomography (CT), 38
Computer resources
    graphics, 1182
    literature search, 1175–1177, 1176–1177t
    statistical analysis, 1181
Concussions, sports medicine, 543–548
Conferences, international, efficacy and
        complications of OMT,
        1143–1145
Confidentiality, 1170
Confusion, geriatric, 333–334, 333t
Connective tissue
    See also Ligaments; Tendons.
    as connectors, 42
    continuity. *See* Fascial-ligamentous release
        and myofascial release
        (indirect approach).
    of head, 660–661, *668*
    innervation of, 98–99
    microscopic anatomy, 46–47, *46–47*

pelvis and sacrum, 763–765
rib cage, 720
in somatic dysfunction, 1156–1158
thoracic, 710–711
Constipation
    Chapman reflexes, 1052
    in children, 321
Coronary artery bypass graft (CABG)
        surgery, 356–357
Coronary artery disease
    cases, 357–358
    diagnosis, 351–353, 352t
    efficacy of OMT, 1147
    pathophysiology and natural history, 350,
        350
    statistics, 277–279
    therapy, 353–355, 354t
    vascular biology, 350–351
Corticosteroids, for arthritis, 531
Corticotropin-releasing hormone, 186
    and brainstem arousal system, 148–149,
        149
Cost effectiveness studies, 1226
Costal region
    articulatory techniques
        anterior, 841, 841
        lateral recumbent, 841–842, *842*
        posterior, 841, *842*
        posterior rib raising, 842–843, *842*
    functional technique, 977–980, *979*
    INR and MFR techniques, 958–961
    muscle energy techniques, 890–894
    ribs, 890–894, *890–894*
Counseling, pain management, 223
Counterstrain. *See* Strain and counterstrain
        technique.
Cranial nerves, 667–674
    abducens (VI), 671–672
    accessory (XI), 670
    auditory (VIII), 672–673
    facial (VII), 672
    glossopharyngeal (IX), 673
    hypoglossal (XII), 674
    oculomotor (III), 669–670
    olfactory (I), 667–668
    optic (II), 668–669
    parasympathetic, 99
    and somatic dysfunction, 1255–1256t
    trigeminal (V), 670–671
    trochlear (IV), 670
    vagus (X), 673–674
Cranial region, 985–1001
    clinical problems, 994–997
        dentistry, 996–997
        neonatal, 994–996, *995*
        trauma, 996
        vascular supply, 996
    diagnosis, 993–994
        observation, 994
        palpation, 994
        patient history, 993
    fascial-ligamentous release, 914, *914*
    history of OMT, 19–29, 985–986
    INR and MFR techniques, 952–961
    key concepts, 985
    mechanics of physiologic motion,
        990–991, *991*

primary respiratory mechanism (PRM),
    986–987
    bone mobility, 987, 989–990, *989*
    brain and spinal cord motility,
        986–987, 988
    cerebrospinal fluid, 987, 988
    membrane mobility, 987, 988–989
    research results, 988–990
    sacral mobility, 987, 990
    strains, 992–993, *992*
    treatment, 997–999, *997–999*
Craniocervical spine, INR and MFR
        techniques, 952–955,
        955–958
Craniosacral region, complications of OMT,
    1150
Cranium
    development, 309–310
    myofascial continuity, 60
Creatine, performance enhancement, 548
Creep
    in biomechanics, 68
    ligaments and tendons, 72
Crossed extensor reflex, 883
Croup, 316–317
Curriculum, osteopathic schools, 22–23
Cushing syndrome, and lung cancer, 464,
    468
Cyriax, James, 477, 1028
Cytokines
    biobehavioral mechanisms, 1205
    and brainstem arousal system, 149

Data analysis, 1217–1218
Databases, computer, 1176
Delirium
    diagnosis, 251–252
    geriatric, 333, 333t
Dementia
    and cancer, 464, 467
    geriatric, 332, 332t, 333t
Demographics
    emergency medicine, 384–386, 385t
    geriatric, 327
Denslow, J.S.
    neurophysiology, 121, 129
    research in OMT, 1167–1168
Dentistry, cranial dysfunction, 996–997
Depression
    and arthritis, 527
    diagnosis, 248
    geriatric, 332, 332t
    management, 235–237, 236t
de Quervain tenosynovitis, in pregnancy, 459
Dermatomal bands, 56, *56*
Dermatomes, *1234*
    lumbar, 734–735
    thoracic, *772*
Descartes, pain theory, 212–213, *213*
Design of research
    between-subject, 1179–1180
        blinding, 1180, 1184
        independent and dependent variables,
            1179
        random assignment, 1179–1180
    biobehavioral mechanisms, 1211

Design of research—*continued*
case studies
prospective, 1178
retrospective, 1178
clinical research
control groups, 1184–1185
dependent variables, 1185–1186
drop-outs, 1185
inclusion/exclusion criteria, 1185
pilot vs. full studies, 1185
pitfalls, 1186
population selection, 1184
study size and power, 1185
experimental, 1179
hypothesis, 1177–1178
literature search, 1175–1177, 1176–1177t
observation, 1175
outcomes research, 1196–1198, 1198t, *1196–1197*
statistics, 1181–1182
within-subject and crossover, 1180–1181
data collection and analysis, 1180–1181
Development
hip dysplasia, 479–482, 480–481
hormonal control, 187
lymphatic system, 1056
musculoskeletal system, 308–314, 309t
Diabetes, and arthritis, 527
Diaphragm, abdominal
acutely ill patient, 1118–1121, 1129, 1131–1132, *1130, 1133*
OMT, 1139–1140
anatomy, 719–720, 724, *719*
functional testing, 740–741
innervation, 712
INR and MFR release, 949–951, *952–955*
and lymphatic system, 1060–1061, 1065–1067, *1066*
re-doming, 741
respiratory function, 501, 720
Diarrhea, in children, 321
Diathermy, 517
Diet
and asthma, 320
biobehavioral factors, 1206–1207
Dirty half-dozen, 746, *746*
Disability-Adjusted Life Years, 197
Disc, intervertebral, 83–84
anatomy, 729
sacroiliac dysfunction, 782
Diverticulitis, abdominal pain, 404
Doctor-patient relationship, 240–206, 205t
psychiatric, 247
Down syndrome, HVLA complications, 1149
Downing, C. Harrison, 970
Drainage systems, 40
Drop arm test, 701
DSM-IV (Diagnostic and Statistical Manual of Mental Disorders, Fourth Ed)
alcohol abuse, 201
classification, 248
depression, 235

Duodenum, osteopathic manipulation, 1080–1081, *1080–1081*
Dura mater, cranial, 51, 60
Dynorphin, in nociception, 132
Dysmenorrhea, 413, 413t

Ear, nose, and throat disease, 370–382
ears, 376–378, *377*, 377t
anatomy, 677, *677–678*
otitis media, 378–379
emergency medicine, 390–392
head and neck
autonomic nervous supply, 372–373, *373*
lymphatic system, 371–372, *372*
myofascia, 371, *371*
key concepts, 370
musculoskeletal system, 380–381, *381*
rhinitis, allergic, 376
sinuses, nose and paranasal, 373–375, *374*, 374t
sinusitis, 375–376, *376*
throat/pharynx, 379, *379*
tonsillitis/pharyngitis, 379–380, *380*
Eaton-Lambert syndrome, 468
Eclecticism, disease treatment, 21
Edema
and lymph flow, 1061
in pregnancy, 452, 455
somatic dysfunction, 137, 140
Edinger-Westphal nucleus, 99
Education, medical
AMA standards, 22
osteopathic colleges, 24
Educational Council on Osteopathic Principles, 1223
Educational Council on Osteopathic Principles (ECOP), 10–11
curriculum, 23
Efficacy and complications, 1143–1152
complications and contraindications, 1147–1150
choice of technique, 1149
counterstrain, 1150
craniosacral, 1150
HVLA, 1149
incidence, 1147–1149, 1148t
muscle energy, 1149
prevention of, 1150
guidelines, 1150–1151
international conferences, 1143–1144
key concepts, 1143
low back pain, 1145–1146
systemic disease, 1146–1147, *1146*
Effleurage
cancer patients, 473, 474
lymphatic flow, 1071–1072, *1071*
extremities, 1076–1077, *1076*
Egyptians, physical medicine, 517
Elastic modulus, 66–67, *67*
of ligaments and tendons, 72
Elbow
anatomy, 696–699, *697*
biomechanics, 81–82, *81*
force movements, 75–76, *76*
fractures in children, 312

HVLA treatment, 874–875, *875*
INR and MFR techniques, 964–966, *964–966*
somatic dysfunction, 699
Electrical stimulation
and posture, 589
for scoliosis, 622
Embryology, neuromusculoskeletal system, 44–46, *45–46*
Emergency medicine, 383–398
abdominal/pelvic pain, 395–397
autonomic nervous system, 387
cardiopulmonary system, 394–395
chest pain, 392–394
head and neck, 389–392
cephalgia, 389, 390, 391
eye and ear pain, 389–392
neck pain, 390–392
nosebleeds/upper respiratory infection, 390, 392
history of development, 383–384
key concepts, 383
lymphatic system, 387
osteopathic philosophy, 384–387, 385t, 387t
screening examination, 387–389
viscerosomatic activity, 387
Emotional stimuli, brainstem arousal system, 147
Emphysema, 502
Endarterectomy, carotid, 1194, 1198
Endocrine system, 34, 179–188
cardiovascular system, 184
key concepts, 179
nervous system, 184–185
regulation of, 185–188, *186*
processes regulated by hormones, 187–188
structure and function, 179–184, 180–181t
cellular processing, 181–182
hydrophilic hormones, 183
lipophilic hormones, 183–184
mechanism of action, 183
transport and metabolism, 182–183
terms and definitions, 179
Endometriosis, 414
Endomysium, 73
Endoplasmic reticulum, hormone processing, 181–182
Endothelin, in peripheral vasculature, 98
Endpoints. *See* Point and pressure techniques.
Energy metabolism, 187–188
Entrapment neuropathies, 444–447, 445t
Environment, and asthma, 320
Epidemiology
coronary artery disease, 350
definition, 1195
in emergency medicine, 389–390
heart failure, 358
mental disorders, 245
osteopathic research, 1173
Esophagus
autonomic innervation, 103–104
osteopathic manipulation, 1079–1081

Ethical factors, 1170, 1197
Eustachian tube, 677
Evolution, biobehavioral mechanisms, 1205
Exercise, 199–200
  and asthma, 320
  biobehavioral factors, 1206–1207
  Chinese tai chi, 483
  coronary artery disease, 354
  heart failure, 361, 362
  postural, 588–589
    decompensation, 612, *612*
  in pregnancy, 454
  prescription for, 284–287, *284–285*
  spinal dysfunction, 286–287
  spondylolithesis, 629
Extension, *1235*
Extracellular matrix
  of bone, 68
  ligaments and tendons, 71–72
Extremities
  See also Lower extremities.
  articulatory techniques
    stage 1: stretching tissues, pumping
      fluid, arm extended, 848
    stage 2: glenohumeral extension/flexion
      with flexed elbow, 848–849,
      849
    stage 3: glenohumeral flexion/extension
      with extended elbow, 849,
      849
    stage 4: circumduction and
      compression with elbow
      flexed/extended, 849–850,
      849–850
    stage 5: abduction and external rotation
      with flexed elbow, 850, *850*
    stage 6: adduction with internal
      rotation with arm behind
      back, 850–851, *850*
    stage 7: stretching tissues, pumping
      fluids with arm extended,
      851, *851*
  development, 311–313
  HVLA treatment
    lower, 875–879
      fibular head, 875–876, *876*
      Hiss plantar whip, 878–879, *879*
      malleolus, 877, *877*
      talotibial joint, 878, *878*
      talus in plantar flexion, 878, *878*
    upper, 874–875
      abducted elbow, 874–875, *875*
      posterior radial head, 874, *874*
      wrist, 875, *875*
  lymph flow, 1060, 1075–1077, *1076*
  muscle energy techniques, 900–907
    ankle, 905–906, *905*
    clavicle, 906–907, *906*
    hip, 901–904, *901–904*
    knee, 904–905, *904–905*
  strain and counterstrain technique,
    1014–1015, *1014–1015*
  upper, 690–704
    anatomy, 690–694
      blood supply, 691, 692
      brachial plexus, 694

lymphatic drainage, 692–693, *693*
muscles, 691, 692t
skeletal and arthrodial, 690–691,
  691t
sympathetics, 694
diagnosis, 694–696, 694t, 695t
  motion testing, 695–696
  motor strength, 695, 695t
elbow and forearm, 696–699, *697–699*
key concepts, 690
tennis elbow, 702
tests
  Adson test, 701
  Allen test, 702
  Apley scratch test, 702
  apprehension, 702
  bicipital tendonitis, 702
  drop arm, 701
  Phalen, 702
  Tinel sign, 702
  Yergason, 701
treatment, 702–704
  adhesive capsulitis, 703
  carpal tunnel syndrome, 702–703
  Chapman points, 704
  myofascial triggers, 703
  reflex sympathetic dystrophy, 703
  thoracic outlet syndrome, 704
wrist and hand, 699–701, *700*
Eyes
  anatomy, 675–677, *676*
  ciliary ganglion, 99
  emergency medicine, 390–392

FABERE acronym, 786–787
Face, myofascial continuity, 60, *61*
Facial nerve, 672
Facilitated positional release (FPR),
  1017–1025, 1027
  cervical region, 1018–1019, *1019*
  diagnosis and treatment, 1018
  effectiveness, 1017
  gluteal and hip regions, 1024
  history, 1018
  key concepts, 1017
  lumbar region, 1022–1024, *1022–1023*
  sacroiliac joint, 1024, *1024*
  thoracic region, 1019–1022, *1020*
    ribs, 1020–1022, *1021*
Facilitation
  emergency medicine, 386
  segmental, 436–437
    acutely ill patient, 1115–1120,
      1124–1126, 1135,
      1117–1119
  somatic dysfunction, 1153–1154
  spinal, 137
    See also Spinal cord facilitation.
    primary afferent nociceptors, 139, *139*
Falciform ligament (linea alba) release, 760
Falling, and aging, 335, 335t
Fallopian tubes
  autonomic innervation, 116
  osteopathic manipulation, 1091–1092
Family practice, 289–297
  community outreach, 296

disease management, 294
osteopathic diagnosis and treatment,
  290–293
person as whole, 293–294
pharmacotherapeutics, 294
preventive health, 295
psychosocial factors, 295–296
Fascia
  abdominal, 752–753
  acutely ill patient, 1135
  anatomy, 52–54, *52–54*
    continuity, 58–60, *59–61*
  definition, 908
  head and neck, 371, *371*
  innervation of, 98–99
  ligamentous laxity, 496–497
  lumbar region, 732–733
  PINS method, 1030
  rib cage, 720
  thoracic, 710–711
Fascial-ligamentous release (indirect
    approach), 908–915
  connective tissue continuity, 908–909
  key concepts, 908
  models, 909
  philosophy, 908
  supine treatment, 910–914
    cranium, 914, *914*
    diagnosis, 910
    lower body, 910–912, *911–912*
    observation and palpation, 910
    upper body, 912–914, *912–914*
  treatment issues, 909–910
Fatigue
  and arthritis, 527
  in biomechanics, 68
    bone fracture, 69
  in ligaments and tendons, 72
  and muscle contraction, 75
Federal government, commissions for DOs,
  26–27
Feedback, PINS method, 1029
Femoral head. *See* Hip.
Femur
  anatomy, 786–789, *788*
    ligaments, 787, *788*
    longitudinal axis, 786–787, *788*
    motion, 787–789
  hip dysplasia, 480–481
  primary and endpoints, *1259*
Fever, and inflammation, 171–172
Fibers, primary afferent, 97, 98
Fibrocartilage, 47, *48*
Fibroids, uterine, 415
Fibromyalgia, 530
  outcomes research, 1199
Fibrosis, lung, 502
Finger injuries in children, 312
Flare, 164
Flexion, *1236–1237*
  standing and seated, 773–774
Flexner Report, 22
Fluid balance, lymphatic system, 1059
Food and Drug Administration (FDA),
  clinical research, 1215
Food Pyramid, 198, *199*

Foot
    anatomy, 797–801, *797*
        arches, 798, *801*
        ligaments, 798, *800*
        plantar ligaments and fascia, 799, *802*
        sprains, 797–798, *798–799*
        transverse tarsal joint, 799–800
    fascial-ligamentous release, 912, *912*
    injuries in children, 312–313
    INR and MFR techniques, 961–962, *961*
    metatarsal and phalangeal findings,
            800–801
        hallus valgus, bunions, and hammer
                toes, 800–801
        somatic dysfunction, 801
    neuromuscular structures, 801, *803*
    radiculopathy, 801–804
        referred pain, 803–804, 805–806t
    tarsal somatic dysfunction, 800, *802–803*
Footware, spondylolithesis, 629
Foramen, intervertebral, 731, *731*
Force
    definition, 64
    in knee, 78–79
    three-dimensional, 64, *64*
Forearm
    anatomy, 696, *698*
    INR and MFR techniques, 964–966,
            964–966
    lymphatic fluctuation, 1141
    somatic dysfunction, 699
Foreign bodies
    emergency medicine, 390, 391
    in knee osteoarthritis, 484
Fourth ventricle, 674–675, *674–675*
Fractures
    bone, stress vectors, 69–70
    hip, geriatric, 482–483, *483*
    spinal disorders, 442
    vertebral, 493
Framingham study, 1198
Frankenhuser plexus, 115–116
Functional spinal unit, 488, *489*
Functional technique, 969–984, 1028
    appendicular regions, 982–983, *982*
    cervical region, 976–977, *978*
    costal region, 977–980, *979*
    historical perspectives, 969–973, *971–972*
    indirect method, 973–975, *973–974*
        concept, 974–975
        guidelines, 974
    innominate, 981–982, *982*
    key concepts, 969
    thoracic, lumbar, and sacral regions,
            975–976, *976–978*
    thoracic cage, 980–981, *981*
Funding for research, 1220–1221

Gait
    ankle rehabilitation, 543
    biomechanics, 86–87, *87*
    in knee osteoarthritis, 484
    in pregnancy, 456
    spinal disorders, 443
Galbreath mandibular drainage, 378, 380,
            380

Galen, 4
Gallbladder, 1085–1086, *1086*
Ganglia
    anatomy of, 91–93
    in esophageal plexus, 103–104
    in gastrointestinal tract, 105–106
        celiac, 106, *107*
        mesenteric, 107, *109, 110*
    of head and neck, 99–100
    of parasympathetic autonomic nervous
            system, 96–97, *96*
    paravertebral, acutely ill patient,
            1136–1137
    sympathetic nervous system, 95, *95*
Gas exchange, pulmonary, 503, *504*
Gastritis, segmental facilitation, 1126
Gastroesophageal reflux disease, in children,
            321
Gastrointestinal system
    See also Lymphatic system.
    acutely ill patient, 1126
    anatomic barrier, 171
    autonomic innervation, 105–111, 111t,
            107–110
        celiac ganglia, 106, *107*
        mesenteric ganglia, 107–111, *110*
    Chapman reflexes, 1053
    efficacy of OMT, 1146–1147, *1146*
    pediatric, 320–321
    somatic dysfunction research, 1192
Gene expression, in nociception, 132
Genetics, molecular, and cardiology, 348
Genitourinary system, Chapman reflexes, 1053
Geriatrics, 327–337
    clinical concerns, 333–336
        confusion, 333–334, 333t
        falling, 335, 335t
        hip fractures, 482–483, *483*
        iatrogenesis, 335–336
        urinary incontinence, 334–335
    functional assessment, 331–332
    historical aspects, 327
    key concepts, 327
    medical assessment, 330–331, 331t
    physiology, 329–330, 328–329t
    psychological assessment, 332, 332t
    social aspects, 333
    theories of aging, 327
Germ theory of disease, 167–168
Glenohumeral joint, fascial-ligamentous
            release, 913
Glossary of osteopathic terminology,
            1229–1253
Glossopharyngeal nerve, 672
Glucocorticoids, and brainstem arousal
            system, 148–149, *149*
Gluteal region
    osteopathic manipulation, 1110–1112,
            1111–1112
    primary and endpoints, *1259–1260*
Glycolytic fibers, in muscle contraction, 75
Glycosaminoglycans (GAGs), in somatic
            dysfunction, 1154,
            1156–1157
Golgi apparatus, hormone processing,
            181–182

Golgi tendon organ, 1032
Gout, 529
Gravitational line, *1237*
Gravity, and postural decompensation,
            603–607, *604*
    biomechanics, 605, *605–606*
    homeostasis, 604
    ligaments, 606, *607–608*
    muscle stress, 605–606, 606t
    skeletal stress, 606–607
Ground reaction force, gait
    in hip, 80–81, *80*
    in knee, 79
Ground substance, 47
Group curves
    See also Posture.
    manipulative treatment, 586–587,
            587–588
    mechanics and diagnosis, 581
    significance, 583
Growth, hormonal control, 187
Guidelines
    human subject research, 1171
    OMT, 1150–1151
    osteopathic principles, 11–12, 15–16, 11t
Gynecology, 409–419
    key concepts, 409
    pelvic pain
        anatomy, 409–412, 410–411t,
            410–411
        differential diagnosis, 413–417
            dysmenorrhea, 413, 413t
            endometriosis, 414
            ovarian pain, 414–415
            pelvic floor dysfunction, 416–417
            pelvic inflammatory disease,
                415–416
            premenstrual syndrome, 413–414,
                413t
            uterine pain, 415
        patient evaluation, 412, 4412t

Habituation, 130
Hahnemann, Samuel, 21
Hallus valgus, 800–801
Hammer toes, 800–801
Hamstrings, 774
    knee muscle forces, 78–79
Hand
    anatomy, 698, 699–700
    fascial-ligamentous release, 913–914, *914*
    osteopathic manipulation, 1112–1113,
            1114
    somatic dysfunction, 700–701
    washing of, 175–176
Haversian canal of bone, 68
Head and neck
    autonomic innervation of, 99–100
    autonomic nervous supply, 372–373, *373*
    diagnosis and treatment, 660–683
        anatomy
            blood vessels, 662, *669*
            connective tissue, 660–661, *668*
            cranial nerves, 667–674, *673*
            ear, 677, *677–678*
            eye, 675–677, *676*

fourth ventricle, 674–675, *674–675*
innervation, 663–667, *672*
lymphatic system, 662–663, *670*
muscles, 660, *667*
sinuses, 675
skeletal, 660, 666t, *661–666*
throat, 677
common cold, 677–678
headache, 678–683
cranial motion assessment, 683, *683*
key concepts, 660
emergency medicine, 389–392
cephalgia, 389–391
eyes and ears, 389–391
neck pain, 390–392
nosebleeds/upper respiratory infection, 390, 392
injuries in children, 323
lymphatic system, 371–372, *372*
myofascia, 371, *371*
primary and endpoints, *1258*
Headaches, 437–442, 678–683
classification, 427t
cluster, 439–441, 680
migraine, 438–439, 679–680, 440t
sports medicine, 543–548
tension-type, 441, 680
traction and inflammatory, 680–681
aneurysms, 681
arteriovenous malformations, 681
brain tumors, 681
cerebrovascular disease, 680–681
hydrocephalus, 681
large lobar hemorrhages, 681
temporal arteritis, 681
transient ischemic attacks, 681
treatment, 441–442
Health promotion and maintenance, 197–207
doctor-patient relationship, 204–206, 205t
family and work, 2023
key concepts, 197
nutrition, 198, 198t, *199*
obesity, 200
personal safety, 202
physical activity, 199–200
sexuality, 202–203
stress, 203–204
substance abuse
alcohol, 201–202
illegal drugs, 202
tobacco, 200–201
support systems, 204
Heart
acutely ill patient, 1125
blood flow, 161–163, *162*
innervation
See also Cardiovascular plexus.
parasympathetic, 126–127, *127*
sympathetic, 125–126, *125–127*
Heart failure
causes, 349t
diagnosis, 360–361
emergency medicine, 394
exercise, 361, 362

muscle hypothesis, 361–362, *362*
osteopathy, 362–363
pathophysiology and natural history, 358–360
treatment, 361
Heartburn, 104
Heilig formula, 616t
Hemorrhage, large lobar, 681
Hemorrhoids, in pregnancy, 452, 455
Hepatobiliary tree, autonomic innervation, 111
Herbal products, 474
Herniation, lumbar spine, 486, 489, 492
Hibernation, 162
High velocity low amplitude (HVLA) techniques, 473
See also Thrust (high velocity/low amplitude) techniques.
back pain, 1145
complications, 1148, 1149
somatic dysfunction, 1159
Hill-Sachs deformity, 542
Hip
anatomy, 786, *787*
muscles, 804
balanced ligamentous tension, 921–924, *921–923*
biomechanics, 80–81, *80*
developmental dysplasia, 479–482, *480–481*
facilitated positional release (FPR), 1024
muscle energy techniques, 901–904, *901–904*
osteopathic manipulation, 1109–1112, 1110t, *1111–1113*
fractures, geriatric, 482–483, *483*
Hip drop test, 741
Hippocrates, 4, 6, 8
physical medicine, 517
Hiss plantar whip, 878–879, *879*
Hoffman (H) reflex, 1159
Home safety, 202, 203t
Homeopathy, 21
Homeostasis
allostasis, 150, 153
emergency medicine, 386
endocrine function, 18–185
postural decompensation, 604
Hormones
See also Endocrine system.
and brainstem arousal system, *147–149*
in cancer, 467
in pregnancy, 453
Horner syndrome, 664
Hospice care, 472
Hospitalization
acutely ill patient, 1115–1142
key concepts, 1115
structural examination, 1115, *1116*
abdomen, 1121–1123, *1122*
lymphatic system, 1123, 1124t
segmental facilitation, 1115–1120, *1117–1119*
thorax, 1120–1121
treatment, 1134–1135

abdomen/pelvis, 1131–1134, *1131–1133*
inflammation, 1123–1124
neuroendocrine immune system, 1126–1127
segmental facilitation, 1124–1126
specific techniques, 1135–1141
abdomen, 1139–1140
lymph mobilization, 1140–1141
paravertebral ganglia, 1136–1137
thoracic region, 1137–1139
thorax, 1127–1131, *1128–1130*
in elderly, 335–336
and osteopathic manipulative therapy, 512–513
outcomes research, 1199
patient treatment, 426–429
Hospitals, osteopathic, 27
Hot packs, 222
Hulett, C.M.T., 8
Hulett, G.D., 9
Human Genomic Project, 348
Human growth hormone, performance enhancement, 548
Human immunodeficiency virus (HIV) infection, 166
biobehavioral mechanisms, 1205–1206
Humerus/glenohumeral joint, balanced ligamentous tension, 926–927, *928*
Hyaline cartilage
anatomy, 47
in synovial joints, 70
of synovial joints, 49
Hyaluronic acid, in articular cartilage, 70–71
Hydrocephalus, 681
Hygiene, 175–176
Hyperactivity, in children, 323–325
Hyperalgesia, primary afferent nociceptors, 140
Hypercalcemia, in cancers, 464, 465, 468
Hypercapnia, pulmonary, 504
Hyperemia, 160–161
Hypermobility, 747
Hypertension
efficacy of OMT, 1147
headaches, 680–681
and heart failure, 359–361
pharmacology, 192–193
pulmonary, 503–504
Hyperviscosity syndrome, in multiple myeloma, 465
Hypoglossal nerve, 674
Hypotension, in pregnancy, 455
Hypothalamic-pituitary-adrenal axis, 186
and glucocorticoid release, 148–149, *149*
Hypothalamus, in acutely ill patient, 1126–1127
Hypothesis testing, 1195–1196, *1195*
biobehavioral research, 1208–1209
Hysteresis, 1158, *1158*

Iatrogenesis, and aging, 335–336
ICE (ice, compression, and elevation), 494
IDET (Intra Discal Electrothermal Therapy), 492

Ileus, 406–407
    acutely ill patient, 1126
    efficacy of OMT, 1147
Iliac crest, 773
Iliac spine, motion testing, 774–775, 776, *776*
Iliolumbar ligament syndrome, 746–747
Iliopsoas spasm, 549–540, *540*
Ilium
    HVLA treatment, 872–874, *872–874*
    osteopathic manipulation, 1103–1105, 1104t, *1104–1105*
Image analysis, 37–38
Immune system
    acutely ill patient, 1126–1127
    allostasis, 152
    biobehavioral mechanisms, 1205–1206
    cancer patients, 472–473
    and infections, 172–173
    lymphatic system, 1059–1060
Immunoglobulin A, in multiple myeloma, 465
Impingement syndromes, 541–542, *542*
Inclusion/exclusion criteria, 1185, 1217
Incontinence, pelvic floor dysfunction, 416–417
Individualization, pain management, 220
Inertia, 64
Infants
    See also Pediatrics.
    birth history, 307–310
    cranial dysfunction, 993–994, 994–996
    developmental dysplasia of hip, 479–482, *480–481*
    hospital treatment, 428–429
    respiratory distress syndrome, 513
    respiratory dysfunction, 314–315
Infectious diseases, 165–178
    antimicrobial therapy, 174–175, *175*
    back pain, 491
    biobehavioral mechanisms, 1205–1206
    germ theory, 167–168
    global significance, 165–167
    hygiene, 175–176
    immunity, 170–173, *171*
    inflammation, 171–172
    key concepts, 165
    knee osteoarthritis, 485
    nutrition, 173–174
    pelvic pain, 416
    respiratory, 511–512
    smallpox, 176
    vaccines, 176–177
    virulence and pathogenicity, 168–170, *168–170*
Inflammation
    acutely ill patient, 1123–1124
    biobehavioral mechanisms, 1205
    infections, 171–172
    nociception, 130
    somatic dysfunction, 137
Influenza outbreaks, 165, 1174
Informed consent, 1170, 1217
Innervation
    acutely ill patient, 1125–1126

autonomic. *See* Autonomic nervous system.
    of cervical spine, 685
    female pelvis, 410–411
    of head
        parasympathetic, 663, *672*
        sympathetic, 663–667, *672*
    pulmonary structures, 506
    in somatic dysfunction, 1155–1156
    thoracic, 706, 711–712, *712*
    upper extremity, 694
Innominate dysfunction
    See also Pelvis and sacrum.
    balanced ligamentous tension, 920–921, *921*
    functional technique, 981–982, *982*
    muscle energy techniques, 894–897, *895–897*
    osteopathic manipulation, 1103–1105, 1104t, *1104–1106*
Insomnia management, 242–243, 242t
Institutional Review Board, 1170–1171, 1217
Instrumentation
    biobehavioral research, 1210
    somatic dysfunction research, 1190
Intensive care unit, 428
Interleukin-6, biobehavioral mechanisms, 1205
Intermuscular septa, 53
Internal medicine, 298–304
    key concepts, 298
    osteopathic, 298–299
    patient management, 299–302
    pneumonia, 303, 303t
    visceral and systemic disorders, 302–303
International Federation of Manual/Musculoskeletal Medicine (FIMM), 1144, 1224
Ionic binding, in articular cartilage, 70–71
Iron deficiency, 174
Irritable bowel syndrome, Chapman reflexes, 1052
Irritation, PINS method, 1032
Irvine study, 1173–1174
Ischemic heart disease. *See* Heart failure.
Isolation patients, 428

Jenner, 7
Joint reaction force, 76
    hip, 81
    in knee, 79
    shoulder, 83
Joints
    See also specific joints.
    anatomy
        joint play, 51–52
        synovial and nonsynovial, 49–51, *50–51*
    ankle, 795–796, *796*
    in cancer, 466
    dysfunction, upper extremity screen, 639–640, *639*
    lower extremity, 784–785
    movement types, 77–78, *77*

in musculoskeletal biomechanics, 75–76, *76*
    patellofemoral, 541
    in pregnancy, 451
    replacement, for knee osteoarthritis, 485
    rib cage, 718
    of shoulder, 82, *82*
    in somatic dysfunction, 1156–1158
    thoracic, 705–706
    upper extremity, 690
Jones, Lawrence H, 971, 1002
Journal of the American Osteopathic Association (JAOA), 1175, 1182
    future research, 1219
    somatic dysfunction research, 1189
Jungmann pelvic index, 611

Kegel exercises, 417
Kennedy, John F., 1034
Kidneys
    autonomic innervation, 111–112, *112*
    osteopathic manipulation, 1086–1087, *1087*
Kinematic analysis, somatic dysfunction research, 1190
Knee
    anatomy, 789–794, *789–791*
        ligaments and cartilage, 792–793, *792–794*
        Q-angle and patella, 791–792, *791*
    athlete injuries, 541, *541*
    biomechanics, 78–80, *78*
        intraarticular movements, 79
        joint structure, 79
        movement efficiency, 79–80
        muscle forces, 78–79
        range of motion, 78
        reaction stress forces, 79
    injuries in children, 312–313
    lymphatic fluctuation, 1141
    motion, 793–794, *795*
    muscle energy techniques, 904–905, *904–905*
    osteoarthritis, 483–485, *484*
    osteopathic manipulation, 1113–1114, *1114*
Knee jerk reflex, 122
Knee joint, 50
Koch's postulates, 167–168
Korr, Irvin M., 8–9
    osteopathic principles, 12–17
    neurophysiology, 121, 129
    research in OMT, 1168
Kyphoplasty, 493
Kyphosis, in pregnancy, 451

Labor and delivery, 457–459, *457–458*
Lamina, lumbar region, 730, *730*
Langley, J.N., 189
Lasegue sign, 443
Learning disorders, 323–325
Leg. *See* Lower extremities.
Legg-Calve-Perthes disease, 312
Leiomyomas, uterine, 415
Length, and muscle contraction, 74

Leptomeningeal carcinomatosis, 466
Levator ani studies syndrome, 417
Lhermitte sign, 443
Licensure, 24–25
Life expectancy, 165, 197
Life phases and health, 227–232
 adolescence, 229–230
 adulthood, 230
 ages one to five, 228–229
 development, 227
 elderly, 230–231
 infancy, 228
 prenatal period, 227
 school-age child, 229
Lifting, lumbar spine, 86
Ligaments
 See also Balanced ligamentous tension
  (BLT) techniques.
 abdominal, 752–753, 792–793
 biomechanics, 71–73, *72*
 of cervical spine, 684
 laxity, 496–498
 lower extremity, 784–785
 lumbar region, 731–732, 731–732t
 pelvis and sacrum, 762–763
 PINS method, 1030
 in postural decompensation, 606,
  607–608
 of shoulder, 495
 of synovial joints, 50
Lightening, in pregnancy, 452
Limbs
 anatomy, 58, *58*
 embryology, 46, *46*
Lippincott, Howard A., 970–971
Literature sources, 1175–1177, 1222,
  1176–1177t
 glossary, 1229
Littlejohn, J. Martin, 8–9
Liver
 See also Lymphatic system.
 fascial-ligamentous release, 911
 lymphatic pumps, 1070–1071, *1071*
 osteopathic manipulation, 1083–1085,
  1084–1085
Load bearing
 in biomechanics, 66
  bone fracture, 69
  muscle moments, 76
 in knee, 79
 and muscle contraction, 74
 by spine, 85–86, *85*
Locomotion biomechanics, 86–87, *87*
Locus coeruleus, and brainstem arousal
  system, 148–149, *149*
Lordosis
 angles, *1230*
 in pregnancy, 451
 radiography, 611
Lordotic curve, normal, 727
Low back pain
 orthopedics, 485–494
  causes, 486t
  differential diagnosis, 490–491, *492*
  history and physical examination,
   486–488

management, 491–494, *493*
  pathophysiology, 488–490, *489–490*
 physiatry, 522–523
 in pregnancy, 450–452, 456
Lower extremities, 784–818
 See also Extremities.
 anatomy, 784–785, *785*
 ankle, 794–797, *796*
 fascial-ligamentous release, 911–912,
  912
 femur, 786–789, *788*
 foot, 797–801, *797–803*
 hip, 786, *787*
 INR and MFR techniques, *958–961*
 key concepts, 784
 knee, 789–794, *789–79*
  Q angle and patella, 791–792, *791*
 ligamentous sprains, 785–786
 muscles, 804–806, *805–806t*, 807–809t
 nerves, 804, 806, *811, 814*
 neuromuscular structure and function,
  801, *803*
 radiculopathy, 801–804
  referred pain, 803–804, 805–806t
 soft tissue techniques
  arch springing, 832, *832*
  fascia lata, 830–831, *830–831*
  piriformis, 831–832, *832*
  plantar fascia, 832, *832*
 vascular and lymphatic systems, 806–813,
  815
Lubricin, 71
Lumbar region, 727–750
 anatomy, 727–737
  anterior element, 727–728
   intervertebral disc, 729
   vertebral body, 727–728, *728*
  foramen, intervertebral, 731, *731*
  ligaments, 731–732, 731t
  muscles and fascia, 732–733, 732–732t
  posterior elements, 729–731
   articular processes, 729–730
   lamina, 730, *730*
   pedicles, 729, *729*
   spinal canal, 730–731
   spinous processes, 730
   transverse processes, 729
  spinal cord and lumbar nerves,
   733–735
   dermatomes, myotomes, and
    sclerotomes, 734–735, *736*
   lumbar plexus, 734, 736t
   spinal cord, 733–734, *735*
  vasculature and lymphatics, 735–737,
   736–737
 articulatory techniques
  extension, 844–845, *844*
  flexion, 843–844, *843*
  rotation, 846, *846*
  side-bending, 845–846, *845, 846*
 examination, 739–743, *739*
  auscultation, 740
  palpation and motion testing, 740,
   740–741
  specific tests, 740–743
   diaphragm, 740–741

hip drop test, 741, *742*
   lumbar rotation, 742–743
   paraspinal palpation, 743
   psoas test variation, 743
   spinal compression, 742
   spinal spring test, 742
   tender points and trigger points,
    743
   Thomas test, 743, *743*
   thoracolumbar rotation, 741–742
 exercise prescription, 286–287
 facilitated positional release (FPR),
  1022–1024, *1022–1023*
 fascial-ligamentous release, 910–911, *911*
 functional technique, 975–976, *976–978*
 INR and MFR techniques, 936–951,
  937–955
 key concepts, 727
 motion, 737–739
  normal motion, 737–738, *737*
  somatic dysfunction, 738–739
  vertebral unit, 737
 muscle energy techniques, 885–886, *885*
 osteopathic manipulation, 1102–1103,
  1103
 soft tissue techniques
  bilateral thumb pressure, 827
  lateral recumbent, 827, *828*
  prone pressure with counterleverage,
   826, *826*
  prone scissors technique, 826–827, *826*
  prone traction, 827, *827*
  seated, 828, *828*
  supine, 827
  supine fixation, 825
   with counterleverage, 825–826
 strain and counterstrain technique,
  1012–1013, *1012–1013*
 treatment, 743–750
  abdominal aneurysm, 794
  cauda equina syndrome, 744
  dirty half-dozen, 746, *746*
  hypermobility, 747
  iliolumbar ligament syndrome,
   746–747, *747*
  meralgia parestheticaa, 747
  psoas syndrome, 747–748, *748*
  radiculopathy, 748–750, *749*
Lumbar spine, 86
Lumbosacral arch, acutely ill patient, 1132
Lumbosacral pain, exercise prescription,
  286–287
Lungs
 See also Pulmonology; Respiration.
 acutely ill patient, 1125–1126
 carcinoma, 464–465
 osteopathic manipulation, 1089, *1089*
Lymph. *See* Lymphatic system.
Lymphatic pumps
 cancer patients, 473, 474
 thoracic drainage, 507–508
Lymphatic system, 1056–1077
 abdominal, 753, *754–755*
 acutely ill patient, 1123–1124, 1129,
  1124t
 OMT, 1140–1141

Lymphatic system—*continued*
  anatomy, 1057–1059
    channels, 1058–1059, *1058*
    lymph, 1059
    organized tissues, 1057
  cervical spine, 685
  emergency treatment, 386, 387
  embryologic development, 1056
  head and neck, 371–372, 374, , 662–663,
      372, 670–671
  key concepts, 1056
  lumbar, 736–737, *737*
  manipulative techniques, 1062–1077
    flow improvement, 1068–1077
      abdominal and pedal pumps,
          1069–1070, *1070*
      abdominal techniques, 1073–1075,
          1074–1075
      cervical soft tissue, 1072–1073,
          1073–1074
      direct pressure, 1071–1072,
          1071–1072
      extremities, 1075–1077, *1076–1077*
      liver and spleen pumps, 1070–1071,
          1070–1071
      pump techniques, 1068–1069,
          1068–1069
      thoracic soft tissue, 1073
    impediment removal, 1063–1068
      diaphragm, 1065–1067, *1066–1067*
      extrinsic pump, 1065
      open thoracic inlet fascia,
          1063–1064, *1063–1064*
      sympathetic activity, 1064–1065,
          1065
    myofascial trigger points, 1045,
        1045–1047
  pathophysiology, 1061
  pelvis and sacrum, 765–766
  physiology, 1059–1061
    fluid balance, 1059–1060
    mechanisms of flow, 1060–1061
  protocol for osteopathic examination, 426
  rib cage, 720
  thoracic, 710, *711*
  treatment, 1061–1062
  upper extremity, 692–693

Magnetic healing, 21
Magnetic resonance imaging (MRI), 38
Major histocompatibility complex (MHC),
    and infections, 172–173
Malaria, 166, 168
Mandibular nerve, 670–671
Mathematical models, load resistance, 76
Maxillary nerve, 670
McConnell, Carl P., 970
Mechanoreceptors, 1154–1155, 1154t
  In kidney, 112
Medial malleoli levelness, 774
Mediastinum, 1090, *1090*
Medications
  adverse reactions, in aging, 335–336
  for arthritis, 531
  for asthma, 320
  in osteopathy, 7

for spondylolithesis, 630
MEDLINE, 1175
Meissner corpuscles, 138
Meissner's ganglia, 103
Membranes, intracranial and intraspinal,
    987–989
Menopause, 417
Menstruation, pelvic pain, 413
Meralgia paresthetica, 747
Merkel discs, 138
Mesenteric release, 760, *760*
Mesenteries
  lumbar, 733, *734*
  lymphatic flow, 1074, *1075*
Meta-analysis research, 1172
Methotrexate, for rheumatoid arthritis, 531
N-Methyl-D-aspartate (NMDA)
  in nociception, 132
  pain transmission, 216
  in somatic dysfunction, 1155
Michigan State University, international
    conferences, 1144
Microbial diseases. *See* Infectious diseases.
Microbiology, 34
Migraine, 438–439, 679–680, 440t
  sports medicine, 543–548
Models, theoretical, 1172
Moment arm, 65
Mood disorders, 209–210
Morning sickness, 454
Motion
  cervical spine, 686–688, *689*
  in cranial region. *See* Cranial region.
  injured athletes, 538
  of knee, 793–794, *795*
  lumbar, 737–739, *737*
  palpatory skills, 561–562
  pelvis and sacrum, 767–768
    axis of motion, 768
    walk cycle, 768–769
  segmental testing, 646–649
    cervical, 646
    lumbar, 647–648
    patient position, 647t
    pelvic, 648–649
    rib, 647
    thoracic, 716–717
  shoulder, 695–696
    spinal segments, 83, *83*
    thoracic, 715–716
    three-dimensional, 64, *64*
    upper extremity, 695–696
    vertebral and costal cage, 712–713
Motor neurons
  definition, 73
  in heart innervation, 126
  structure, 122–123
Muscle energy techniques, 881–907
  complications, 1149
  contraindications, 884
  diagnosis, 882
  efficiency factors, 884
  history, 881–882
  key concepts, 881
  physiologic principles
    crossed extensor reflex, 883

joint mobilization, 882–883
    oculocephalogyric reflex, 883
    post-isometric relaxation, 882
    reciprocal inhibition, 883
    respiratory assistance, 883
  sequential steps, 883–884
  somatic dysfunction, 1159
  technical principles, 881
  techniques
    costal somatic dysfunction, 890–894,
        890–894
    extremities, 900–907, *901–906*
    innominate dysfunction, 894–897,
        895–896
    sacrum, 897–900, *897–900*
    spinal segmental somatic dysfunction,
        885–890, *885–890*
Muscle hypothesis, 361–362, *362*
Muscles
  See also specific muscles.
  abdominal, 752–753
  acutely ill patient, 1120–1121,
      1133–1134
  in cancer, 466
  of cervical spine, 684
  contraction, 54–55
    biomechanics, 73–75, *74*
    hip, 80–81, *80*
    in knee, 79
  of head, 660, *667*
  hip, 804, 805–806t
  lumbar region, 732–733, 732t, 733t
  myofascial continuity, 53, 58–60
  pelvis and sacrum, 763–765
  PINS method, 1030
  in postural decompensation, 605–606,
      606t
  rib cage, 719–720, *719*
  of shoulder, 495
  thigh and leg, 804–806, 807–809t
  thoracic, 706–710, 707–710t
  upper extremity, 691
  of urinary bladder, 113–114
Muscle-tendon complex, 52, *52*
Musculoskeletal system
  biomechanics, 75–78
    center of rotation, 78
    force moments, 75–76, *76*
    joint structure, 77
    joint surfaces, 77–78, *77*
    load resistance, 76
    mechanical advantage, 77
    range of motion, 77
    segment movement, 75
    tendon actions, 76, *76*
  in cancer, 465–467
    back pain, 465–466
    joints, 466
    muscle and skin, 466–467
    occult symptoms, 467
  core of diagnosis and treatment, 14–16,
      11
  development, 308–314, 309t
    costal cage, 310
    cranium, 309–310
    lower extremity, 312–313

upper extremity, 311–312
vertebral spine, 310–311
ear, nose, and throat, 380–381
embryology, 44–46, *45–46*
in emergency medicine, 388
functions, 49–55
  fascia and neurovascular bundle,
    52–54, *52–54*
  joint play, 51–52
  muscle action, 54–55, *55*
  muscle-tendon complex, 52, *52*
  synovial and nonsynovial joints, 49–51,
    50–51
geriatric, 329–330
limb anatomy, 58, *58*
microscopic anatomy, 46–49
  cartilage and bone, 47, *48–49*
  connective tissue, 46–47, *46, 47*
  injury effects, 49
  skeletal muscle, 49, *49*
myofascial continuity, 58–60, *59–61*
in pregnancy, 450–452
protocol for osteopathic examination,
    422–426, *424–427*
somatic dysfunction, 633–659
  in ambulatory or bedridden patients,
    649–659
    ambulatory, 650–652t
    bedridden patient, 654
    outpatient or hospitalized, 652–654,
      653–654t
  key concepts, 633
  outpatient forms, *655–658*
  specific tests, 635, 636t, *637*
    anterior screen of horizontal planes,
      639, *639*
    joint dysfunction, 639–640, *639*
    patient position, 646–649, 647t,
      650–652t
    posterior screen of horizontal planes,
      638, *638*
    standing spinal flexion, 640, *640–641*
      active screening, 640–641,
        640–641
      passive screening, 641–646,
        642–647
  TART mnemonic, 633–634
  and vascular systems, segmental
    organization, 55–56, *55–57*
Musculotendoinous unit, 74
Myasthenia gravis, 468
Myeloma, multiple, 465
  back pain, 491
Myocardial infarction, 355, *356*
  efficacy of OMT, 1146–1147, *1146*
  emergency medicine, 386
  somatic dysfunction research, 1191
Myofascia
  See also Fascia.
  in somatic dysfunction, 1156–1158
  trigger points. *See* Trigger points,
    myofascial.
Myotomes, lumbar, 734–735

Naffziger sign, 443
National Institute of Aging, 327

National Institute of Communicative
    Diseases and Stroke, 1143
National Institutes of Health, 1168
National Library of Medicine, 1175
Nausea, in pregnancy, 454
Neck
  autonomic innervation of, 99–100
  exercise prescription, 286–287
Neidner technique, 324t
Nerve blocks, 222–223
  ethyl chloride, 223
  hot packs, 222
  ice, 223
  transcutaneous nerve stimulation, 222
  vibration, 223
Nerve growth factor (NGF), 133
Nerves
  See also Autonomic nervous system;
        central nervous system;
        peripheral nervous system.
  abdominal, 753, *755*
  in children, 321–325, 323t
    apnea, 323
    closed head injury, 323
    colic, 322
    learning disorders/hyperactivity,
      323–325
  cranial. *See* Cranial nerves.
  endocrine function, 184–185
  lower extremities, 804, 806, *811, 814*
  origin of, 39
  pelvis and sacrum, 766–767, *767*
  spinal cord and lumbar, 733–735, *735–736*
Neuralgia, cranial, 681–683
  Bell palsy, 681–682
  temporomandibular joint dysfunction,
    682–683, *682*
  trigeminal neuralgia, 681
Neuroendocrine-immune network, and
      brainstem arousal system,
      147–152
Neurologic deficits, sports medicine,
      543–548
Neurology, 435–449
  anatomy, 435–436
  chronic pain syndrome, 447
  entrapment neuropathies, 444–447, 445t
    carpal tunnel syndrome, 445–446
    thoracic outlet syndrome, 446–447
  headaches, 437–442, 437t
    cluster, 430–441
    migraine, 438–439, 440t
    tension-type, 441
    treatment, 441–442
  key concepts, 435
  osteopathic lesion, 436–437
  spinal disorders, 442–444
Neuromusculoskeletal medicine, 420–434
  AIDS, 428
  case study, 431–433
  children, 428–429
  drug and alcohol detoxification, 428
  hospital chart, 429, *430*
  hospital-based, 421
  hospitalization, 426–429
    treatment protocol, 428

intensive care unit, 428
isolation patients, 428
key concepts, 420
OMM specialty, 421, 422t, 423t
osteopathic consultation, 429–431
patient examination, 422–426
  history taking, 422
  physical examination, 422–426,
    424–427
postoperative or trauma patients, 429
psychiatric patients, 429
rehabilitation, 428
Neuromusculoskeletal system
  inhibition of. *See* Progressive inhibition of
      neuromuscular structures
      (PINS).
  lower extremity, 801, *802*
  and myofascia, integrated release,
      931–968
    clinical assessment, 935
    definition, 931–932
    exercise role, 936
    key concepts, 931
    mechanics and forces, 932–934
      asymmetry sensing, 933–934
      force effects, 932–933, *933*
      palpation to develop haptic skills,
        933
    posttreatment discomfort, 936
    specific areas
      carpal and palmar tunnel, 966–967,
        966–967
      craniocervical spine, 952–955,
        955–958
      foot and ankle, 961–962, *961*
      forearm, elbow, and wrist, 964–966,
        964–966
      lower limb, 956–961, *958–961*
      lumbosacral spine and pelvis,
        936–951, *937–955*
      upper limb and shoulder, 962–964,
        962–963
    three-dimensional patterns, 935
    treatment goals, 935–936
    treatment skills, 934–935
      pain at loose sites, 934–935
      tight-loose concept, 934
Neuropathic pain, 215–216
Neuropeptide Y
  in cerebral vasculature, 99
  in ureter, 112
Neuropeptides
  See also specific neuropeptides.
  in somatic dysfunction, 1156
Neurophysiology, 33, 120–136
  heart innervation
    parasympathetic, 126–127, *127*
    sympathetic, 125–126, *125–126*
  integrative function, 129–130
  key concepts, 120
  nociceptive stimuli, 130–133
  nonimpulse-based integration, 133–134
  in osteopathy, 121
  reflexes, 121–123
    excitability, 130
    interactions, 123–125, *124–125*

Neurophysiology, reflexes—*continued*
    somato-somatic, 123
    structure, 122–123, *122*
    viscero-visceral, 123
    somatic afferents and baroreceptor
            control, 128–129, *128, 129*
    visceral function control, 127–128, *127,
            128*
Neurotransmitters, lymphatic system,
        1057
Neurovascular accidents, HVLA
            complications, 1149
Neurovascular bundle, 52–54, *52–54*
Newton, definition, 65
Nitric oxide
    in myocardial blood flow, 162–163
    in peripheral vasculature, 98
Nociception, 137–156
    abdominal pain, 400–401
    acutely ill patient, 1135
    headaches, 441
    neuroendocrine immune network,
            147–152, *150*
        allostasis, 150–153
        allostatic load, 151–153, 151t
        arousal system, 147–149, *149*
        cytokine network, 149
    pain management, 216
    pulmonary, 505
    in respiratory plexus, 103
    and somatic dysfunction, 137–140, 1154,
            138, 1154
        fiber systems, 138–139
        pathophysiology, 137–138
        peripheral sensitization, 139–140, *139*
    spinal facilitation, 140–145
        brainstem arousal system, 145–147
            ascending pathways, 145–146
            reticular formation, 146
        central sensitization, 144
        dorsal horn, 140–144, *141–144*
        PANS model, 145
        spinal cord output, 145, 1155–1156
Nodes, lymphatic, 1057
Nonsteroidal antiinflammatory drugs
            (NSAIDS)
    for arthritis, 531
    orthopedic conditions, 496
North American Symptomatic Carotid
            Endarterectomy Trial
            (NASCET), 1194
Nose. *See* Ear, nose, and throat disease.
Nosebleeds, 390–392
Null hypothesis, 1195, 1217
Nurses' Health study, 356
Nutrition
    cancer patients, 472
    geriatric, 330
    health promotion, 198, 198t, *199*
    and infections, 173–174
    lymphatic system, 1060
    performance enhancement, 549

Obesity, 200
Obstetrics, 450–461
    body fluids and circulation, 452, *453*

    first trimester, 453–454, *454*
    hormonal changes, 453
    key concepts, 450
    labor and delivery, 457–459, *457–458*
    postpartum, 459
    second trimester, 454, *455–457*
    somatic dysfunction, 450–453, *451*
        low back pain, 450–452
    third trimester, 455–457
Obturator foramen, 1091, *1091*
Occipital-atlas, 1095–1096, *1096*
Occipito-atlantal joint, muscle energy
            techniques, 888–889,
            888–889
Oculocephalogyric reflex, 883
Oculomotor nerve, 669–670
Olfactory nerve, 667–668
Oncology, 462–476
    biologic response modifiers, 472–473
    central nervous system, 467–468
        cerebral malignancy, 467
        indirect paraneoplastic, 467–468
    complementary and alternative medicine,
            474
    ethics of presentation to patient, 470–471
    key concepts, 462
    lung carcinoma, 464–465
    musculoskeletal system, 465–467
        in adults, 467
        back pain, 465–466
        in children, 467
        joints, 466
        muscle and skin, 466–467
    osteopathic manipulative therapy,
            473–474
        contraindications, 473, 473t
        indications, 474, 474t
    peripheral nervous system, 468–469
        neuropathies, 469
        peripheral manifestations, 468
        spinal cord compression, 468–469
    plasma cell neoplasm, 465
    renal cell cancer, 464
    supportive care, 471–472
    touching as communication, 463
    viscerosomatic response, 469–470
        tumor necrosis factor, 469–470
    whole patient, 463
Onuf's nucleus, 116
Ophthalmic nerve, 670
Opioids. *See* Analgesia.
Optic nerve, 668–669
Orthopedics, 477–499
    developmental dysplasia of hip, 479–482,
            480–481
    hip fracture, geriatric, 482–483, *483*
    key concepts, 477
    ligamentous laxity, 496–498
    low back pain, 485–494, 486t
        differential diagnosis, 490–491, *492*
        history and physical examination,
            486–488, *487*
        management, 491–494
        pathophysiology, 488–490, *489*
    osteoarthritis of knee, 483–485, *484*
    patient examination, 479

    principle of, *478*
    shoulder instability, 494–496, *495*
Orthotics
    postural, 589, 613–614, *613*
    for spondylolithesis, 630
Ortolani sign, 479, 786
Osmotic pressure, and lymph flow,
            1060–1061
Osteoarthritis, 529–530
    knee, 483–485, *484*
    Osteons of bone, 68–69, *68*
Osteopathic manipulative therapy
            (OMT)
    See also specific techniques.
    of abdomen, 758–760
        collateral ganglia inhibition, 759–760
        falciform ligament (linea alba) release,
            760
        mesenteric release, 760, *760*
        paraspinal inhibition, 758–759
    atelectasis, 405–406
    in cancer
        contraindications, 473, 473t
        indications, 474, 474t
    complications, 1147–1150
    coronary artery disease, 357
    ear, nose, and throat disease, 371,
            380–381, *381*
    efficacy, 1143–1147
    in emergency medicine, 393–397
    group curves, 586–587, *587–588*
    headaches, 439, 441–442
    ileus, 407
    ligamentous laxity, 496–498
    lung disease, 508–514
    neuromusculoskeletal medicine. *See*
            Neuromusculoskeletal
            medicine.
    otitis media, 378–379
    in physiatry, 519–520
    postural homeostasis, 613
    in pregnancy, 459
    rehabilitation, 545
    for rheumatoid arthritis, 532
    for scoliosis, 622
    sinusitis, 375
    somatic dysfunction, 569
    spinal disorders, 442–444
    spondylolithesis, 629
Osteopathy
    cardiology, 345–349
    definition of, 9–10
    diagnosis and treatment, 574–579
        dose guidelines, 577–578
        key concepts, 574
        SOAP method, 578
        somatic dysfunction, 574–577
        TART acronym, 574
    Educational Council, 10–11
    emergency medicine. *See* Emergency
            medicine.
    examination and diagnosis, 566–573
        key concepts, 566
        somatic dysfunction, 567–568
            anatomy, 567–568
            OMT, 569

physiologic mechanics, 571
structure, 568–569
spinal motion, 569–572, *570*
active and passive testing, 571
germ theory of disease, 167
history of, 19–29
education and growth, 21–24
conflict with AMA, 22
curriculum, 22–23
research, 23–24
schools, 21–22
federal government recognition, 26–27
hospitals, 27
key concepts, 19
organizations, 25–26
specialties, 26–27
state licensure, 24–25
internal medicine, 298–304
organization, 25–26
pain management, 223–224
pediatrics. *See* Pediatrics.
and pharmacology, 190–193
philosophy of, 4–6, 32, 5t
allostatic response, 153–154
historic development, 8–11, 19–29
holistic aspects, 6
patient care, 6–8
medications and vaccinations, 7
practice guidelines, 11–12, 11t
primary care. *See* Family practice.
principles, 12–17
musculoskeletal system, 14–16
person as a whole, 13–14
personal health care systems, 15
psychiatry. *See* Psychiatry, osteopathic.
Osteotomy, for knee osteoarthritis, 485
Otitis media, 315–316, 378–379
emergency medicine, 389–390
Outcomes research, 1194–1202
cost effectiveness, 1226
hypothesis testing, 1195–1196, *1195*
osteopathic medicine, 1194–1195,
1198–1200, *1200–1201*
osteopathic research, 1173
study design, 1196–1198, 1198t,
1196–1197
Ovary
autonomic innervation, 114–115
cysts, 414–415
osteopathic manipulation, 1091–1092
Oxidative fibers, in muscle contraction, 75
Oxidative phosphorylation, 158–159
Oxygen, pulmonary, 504

Pacinian corpuscles, 138
Pain
abdominal, 753, *755*
acutely ill patient, 1118–1119
biobehavioral factors, 1206–1207
in cancer, 471
chronic, 447
physical medicine, 521
definition, 214–215
discogenic, 1023–1024, *1023*
and embryologic development, 401
growth, in children, 313

history of theories, 212–214, *213*
information flow, 217–219
cognitive/emotional appraisals, 219
perception of pain, 217, 219, *218*
key concepts, 212
in kidney, 112
management, 219–220, 220t
analgesics, 220–222
addiction, 220–221
adjuvants, 221–222
placebos, 221
side effects, 221
tolerance, 221
coping strategies, 224
individualization, 220
medications, 220
nerve blocks, 222–223
osteopathic, 223–224
behavior modification, 223–224
biofeedback, 223
cardiovascular fitness, 223
counseling, 223
gait training, 223
proprioceptive neuromuscular
facilitation, 223
stretching and strengthening, 223
support groups, 224
neuropathic, 215–216
nociception, 130, 216
pelvic. *See* Gynecology.
psychology of, 214
referred, 386
lower extremities, 803–804, 805–806t
myofascial trigger points, 1038–1039
thoracic, 712
reflex interactions, 123–124
rule of, 41
spinal, exercise prescription, 286–287
spinothalamic pathways, 216–217
Palpation
See also Touch.
abdomen, 757
acutely ill patient, 1117–1123
cervical spine, 686
Chapman reflexes, 1051–1052, *1052*
cranial dysfunction, 994
injured athletes, 537–538
lumbar, 740
paraspinal, 743
pelvic and sacrum, 770–771
postural diagnosis, 608–609, *608*
primary and endpoints, *1261*
skills and exercises, 557–565
dominant eye, 558–559, *559*
dominant hand, 558
forearm, 560–561
with hands and fingers, 558
inanimate objects, 558
key concepts, 557
layer palpation, 559–560
motion perception, 561–562
sensitivity, 561
somatic dysfunction, 562–565, 562t
cervical region, 563, *563*
lumbar region, 564, *564*
research, 1191

sacroiliac region, 564–565, *564–565*
thoracic region, 563–564, *564*
spondylolithesis, 628, *628*
thoracic region, 715
upper extremity, 694
Pancoast syndrome, 464
Pancreas
autonomic innervation, 111
osteopathic manipulation, 1087–1088,
1088
Pancreatitis, segmental facilitation, 1126
Parasympathetic nervous system, 96–97, *96*
abdominal pain, 401
head, 663, *672*
heart innervation, 126–127, *127*
protocol for osteopathic examination, 426
Parathyroid hormone-related peptide, in
renal cell cancer, 464, 468
Pasteur, 6
Patch, transdermal, 220
Patella. *See* Knee.
Patellofemoral joint. *See* Knee.
Patient education
ear, nose, and throat disease, 371
spondylolithesis, 629
Patient satisfaction
back pain OMT, 1145
osteopathic health delivery, 1194
outcomes research, 1200
See also Orthopedics
Patterning
fascial, 583–585
musculoligamentous, 585, 587t, *586*
spinal, 583, *584*
Pavlik harness, 480, *480*
Pedal lymphatic pumps, 1069–1070, *1070*
Pediatrics, 305–326
gastrointestinal system, 320–321
constipation, 321
diarrhea, 321
gastroesophageal reflux disease, 321
history and examination, 307–308
key concepts, 305
musculoskeletal development, 308–314,
309t
costal cage, 310
cranium, 309–310
juvenile rheumatoid arthritis, 313–314
lower extremity, 312–313
upper extremity, 311–312
vertebral spine, 310–311
neurologic dysfunction, 321–325, 323t
apnea, 323
closed head injury, 323
colic, 322
learning disorders/hyperactivity,
323–325
Neidner technique, 324t
respiratory dysfunction, 314–320
asthma, 318–320, 319t
bronchiolitis, 317–318
croup, 316–317
newborn, 314–315
otitis media, 315–316
pharyngitis, 316
Pedicles, 729, *729*
Pelvic floor dysfunction, 416–417

Pelvic inflammatory disease, 415–416
Pelvis
  See also Gynecology.
  acutely ill patient, 1126, 1131–1134,
    1133
  anatomic landmarks, 772
  articulatory techniques
    rotation to innominate, 846–847,
      847
    sacroiliac joint gapping, 848, *848*
  balanced ligamentous tension, 919–920,
    920
  emergency medicine, 395–397
  fascial-ligamentous release, 910, *911*
  HVLA treatment, 871–874
    extremities
      lower, 875–879, *876–879*
      upper, 874–875, *874–875*
    ilium, 872–874, *872–874*
    sacrum, 871–872, *871–872*
  INR and MFR techniques, 936–951,
    937–955
  lymphatic system, 1067–1068, *1067*
  osteopathic manipulation. *See* Visceral
    manipulation.
  in pregnancy, 451
  and sacrum, 762–783
    anatomy, 762–767
      muscles and connective tissue,
        763–765
        primary, 763–764
        secondary, 764–765, *764*
      nerves, 766–767, *767*
      skeletal/ligaments, 762–763, *763*
      vascular/lymphatic, 765–766,
        765
    history and physical examination,
      769–772, 770t
      neurology, 771–772
      palpation, 770–771
    key concepts, 762
    motion and dysfunction, 767–768
      axes of motion, 768
      normal walk cycle, 768–769
      sacral motion, 768
    motion testing, 772–777
      anatomic landmarks, 772
      special tests
        backward bending, 776
        fascial restriction, 777
        hamstring, 774
        iliac crest, 773
        iliac spine, 774, 775
          compression, 776–777, *776*
        medial malleoli, 774
        oblique axis, 775–776
        pubic symphysis, 774
        sacral base, 775
        sacral inferolateral angles, 775
        sacrum, 774–775
          posterior, 776
        seated flexion, 773–774
        spring, lumbosacral, 776
        standing flexion, 773–774
        transverse axis, 775
        Trendelenburg test, 772–773

pelvic diagnoses
  iliosacral somatic dysfunction,
    777–778
  sacroiliac dysfunction, 778–782,
    779t
    anterior sacrum, 779
    causes of, 782
    posterior sacrum, 779–782
      torsion, 780–781, 780t
  strain and counterstrain technique,
    1013–1014, *1013–1014*
Penis, autonomic innervation, 116
Peptides, endocrine, 181–182, 184
Percutaneous reflex of Morley, 401
Performance enhancement, 548–549
Perimysium, 73
Periodontal disease, 166
Peripheral nervous system
  autonomic components, 91
  in cancer, 468–469
  myofascial trigger points, 1038
  primary afferent nociceptors (PANs),
    138–139
Person as whole, Chapman reflexes, 1052
Personality disorders, 252–253
Personalized treatment, 7–8, 13–14
Pes planus, 796
Petrissage, lymphatic flow, 1074–1075, *1075*
  extremities, 1076–1077, *1076–1077*
Phalen test, 702
Pharmacology, 34, 189–193
  history of, 189–190
  hypertension, 192–193
  key concepts, 189
  osteopathic principles, 190–192
Pharyngitis, 316, 379–380
Phosphocreatine, as ATP source, 158
Physiatry. *See* Physical medicine and
    rehabilitation.
Physical medicine and rehabilitation,
    516–525
  carpal tunnel syndrome, 523
  cervical sprain/strain, 524
  history of, 517–518
  key concepts, 516
  low back pain, 522–523
  manipulation, 519–520
    research, 520–522
  patient evaluation, 518–519
  return to work issues, 522
  sports medicine, 524–525
  training, 516
Physical training, of ligaments and tendons,
    72
Piriformis muscle
  osteopathic manipulation, 1112, *1113*
  primary and endpoints, *1259*
  strain and counterstrain, 1014, *1014*
Pituitary gland, segmental facilitation, 1127
Pituitary hormones. *See* Hypothalamic-
    pituitary-adrenal
    axis.
Placebos
  biobehavioral factors, 1207–1208
  osteopathic research, 1224–1225
  pain management, 221

Plagiocephaly, 309
Planes of body, *1244*
Plasma cell neoplasm, 465
Plasticity, in biomechanics, 67
Pneumonia
  emergency medicine, 394
  osteopathic manipulative therapy, 303,
    511–512, 303t
  thoracic reflexes, 1125
Point and pressure techniques
  See also Progressive inhibition of
      neuromuscular structures
      (PINS).
  antecubital region, *1260*
  femur and gluteal region, *1259–1260*
  head, *1258*
  palpation, *1261*
  shoulder and sternum, *1259*
  xiphoid process, *1260*
Position of patient, visceral manipulation,
    1092, *1092*
Posture
  coronal, horizontal, and sagittal planes,
    603–632
    diagnosis, 607–612
      observation and palpation, 608–609,
        608–609
      radiography, 609–612, *610–611*
    gravitational strain, 603–607, *604*
      biomechanics, 605, *605*
      homeostasis, 604
      ligament stress, 606, *607–608*
      muscle stress, 605–606, 606t
      skeletal-arthrodial stress, 606–607
    key concepts, 603
    sagittal plane disorders, 622
    scoliosis, 618–622
      diagnosis, 618–620, *619–620*
      radiography, 620–622
      symptoms and screening, 620
      treatment, 622, *621*
        braces, 622, *623*
        electrical stimulation, 622
        OMT, 622
        surgery, 622, *624*
    short leg syndrome, 614–618, *614*
      diagnosis, 614–615, *616*
      lift therapy, 615–618, *617, 616t*
      pelvic rotation, 618, *618*
    spondylolisthesis, 625–630
      causes, 625
      classification, 625, 626t
      diagnosis, 625s–628, *628*
      treatment, 628–630
    treatment, 612–614
      exercise, 612, *612*
      OMT, 613
      orthotics, braces, 613–614, *613*
  group curves, 581
    mechanics and diagnosis, 581
  key concepts, 580
  myofascial trigger points, 1045, *1045*
  patterning, 583–585
    fascial, 583–585
    musculoligamentous, 585, *586*, 587t
    spinal, 583, *584*

posture
  bracing, 589
  compensated, 581
  decompensation, 581–583
  education and exercise, 588–589
  optimal, 580
  orthotics, 589
  radiography, 591–602
    equipment, 591–592, *592–593*
    key concepts, 591
    measurement exercises, 599–601
    procedure, 592–595, *594,* 594t
      anteroposterior postural, 593–594, *595*
      general considerations, 594–595
      lateral postural, 594, *595*
      results, 595–598, *596*
        anteroposterior pelvis, 596–597
        anteroposterior thoracic, 596
        lateral postural of pelvis, 597–598, *599–600*
        lumbar postural, 596, *597*
  treatment, 585–588, *587–588*
    electrical stimulation, 589
    prolotherapy, 589
    surgery, 589
Pregnancy
  See also Obstetrics.
  spondylolithesis, 629
  uterine innervation, 116
Premenstrual syndrome, 413–413, 413t
Pressure, 64
Primary afferent nociceptors (PANs), 138–139
  peripheral sensitization of, 139–140, *139*
Primary care
  See also Family practice.
  osteopathic, 26–27
Primary points. *See* Point and pressure techniques.
Primary respiratory mechanism. *See* Cranial region.
Probability, 1195
Procaine, myofascial trigger points, 1041–1042
Progressive inhibition of neuromuscular structures (PINS), 1026–1033
  contraindications and side effects, 1032
  inhibition, 1026–1027
  key concepts, 1026
  mechanism of action, 1032
  point and pressure techniques, 1027–1028
  procedure, 1029–1032, 1030t
Prolotherapy, 497–498
  postural, 589
Proprioception, large fiber system, 138
Prostacyclin, in peripheral vasculature, 98
Prostaglandins, in somatic dysfunction, 1154
Proteins, endocrine, 181–182
Proteoglycans
  in articular cartilage, 70–71
  in ligaments and tendons, 72
Psoas muscle, 743, 1110, *1111*
  sacroiliac dysfunction, 782

Psoas syndrome, 747–748, *748*
Psychiatry, osteopathic, 245–254
  adult attention deficit disorder, 252
  Alzheimer's disease, 251
  asylums, 247
  bipolar disorders, 248
  brief psychotic disorder, 249
  cocaine addiction, 250–251, 250t
  delirium, 251–252
  depression and anxiety disorders, 248–249
  doctor/patient relationships, 247
  epidemiology, 245–246
  hospital treatment, 429
  key concepts, 245
  mental health and illness, 246–247
  nomenclature, 247
  personality disorders, 252–253
  schizophrenia, 249
  somatoform disorders, 249
  substance abuse, 250
Psychoneurobiology, 472
Psychoneuroimmunology, 208–211
  key concepts, 208
  mood disorders, 209–210
  research, 208–209
  stress effects, 210
  treatment recommendations, 210
Psychosocial factors in family practice, 295–296
Psychotic disorders, somatic dysfunction research, 1192
Pubic ramus, 1106–1107, *1107–1108*
Pubic symphysis
  INR and MFR release, 945–946, *945–946*
  motion testing, 774
  muscle energy techniques, 896–897, *896*
Pubovesicular ligaments, 1091, *1091*
Pulmonology, 500–515
  See also Lymphatic system.
  acutely ill patient, 1127–1131
  efficacy of OMT, 1147
  key concepts, 500
  lung disease
    chronic obstructive pulmonary disease, 512–513
    infections, 511–512
    postoperative complications, 513–514
    prevention and treatment, 511
    respiratory distress syndrome, 513
  osteopathic approach, 506–509, *506*
    manipulative treatment, 508–509
    thoracic lymphatic drainage, 507–508
    viscerosomatic reflex, 507, *508*
  pulmonary function, 509–510
  respiratory function, 501–506
    gas exchange, 504
    pulmonary circulation, 503–504, *504*
    ventilation, 501–503, *502*
    ventilatory control, 505–506
  somatic dysfunction research, 1191
  thoracic pump, 510–511
Pulses, upper extremity, 694
Pumps, lymphatic, 1065, 1068–1077
  abdominal and pedal, 1069–1070, *1070*
  liver and spleen, 1070–1071, *1071*

pectoral traction, 1068, *1068*
  thoracic, 1068–1069, *1069*

Q-angle, 791–792, *791*
Quadriceps tendon, knee muscle forces, 78–79
Quality of life, outcomes research, 1200
Questionnaires
  osteopathic health delivery, 1194
  sleep behavior, 1206

Radiculopathy
  lower extremity, 801–804
  lumbar region, 748–750, *749*
  spinal, 442–443
Radiography
  postural. *See* Posture.
  postural diagnosis, 607–608, 609–612, *610–611*
  spondylolithesis, 611, 626–628
Randomization in research, 1196–1197, 1208, 1217, 1224
Range of motion
  See also Balanced ligamentous tension (BLT) techniques.
  arthritis, 528
  elbow, 81, *81*
  hip, 80
  knee, 78
  lower extremity, 788, 791
  muscle movement, 77
  myofascial trigger points, 1043
  shoulder, 82
  somatic dysfunction, 575
  spine, 84, 85, *84*
Rapid eye motion (REM), and cluster headache, 439
Receptors
  in pharmacology, 192
  pulmonary, 505
Reciprocal inhibition, 883, 917
Recruitment, 73
Reflex of Morley, 753, *756*
Reflex sympathetic dystrophy, 703
Reflexes
  See also specific reflexes.
  acutely ill patient, 1125–1126
  arcs
    autonomic, 92–93, *92, 93*
    somatic, 91–92, *92*
  excitability, 130
  facilitation, 130
  fatigue, 130
  interactions of, 123–125, *124, 125*
  in pregnancy, 453–454
  sensitization, 130–132
  in somatic dysfunction, 1156
  somato-somatic, 123
  structure, 122–123, *122*
  upper extremity, 694–695
  viscerosomatic and somatovisceral, 406
  viscero-visceral, 123
Reflexology, 1028
Rehabilitation
  See also Physical medicine and rehabilitation.

Somatic dysfunction, osteopathic
    manipulation—*continued*
  hand, 1112–1113, *1114*
  hip muscles, 1109–1112, 1110t,
      1111–1113
  ilium or innominate, 1103–1105,
      1104t, *1104–1106*
  knee, 1113–1114, *1114*
  lumbar spine, 1102–1103, *1102–1103*
  occipital-atlas, 1095–1096, *1096*
  pubic ramus, 1106–1107, *1106–1107*
  ribs, 1096–1097, 1099–1102,
      1097–1098, 1100–1102
  sacrum, 1107–1109, 1108t,
      1108–1109
  thoracic spine, 1098–1099, *1099*
palpatory skills, 562–565, *563–565,* 562t
pathophysiology, 137–138, 140, *138*
pre- and postoperative, 406–407
in pregnancy, 450–453, *451*
primary afferent nociceptors, 139, *139*
research studies, 1188–1193
  clinical correlations, 1190–1192
  history, 1188–1189
  instrumentation, 1190
  interexaminer agreement, 1189–1190
spinal disorders, 442–444
spinal facilitation, 137
Somatoform disorders, 249
Somatosympathetic reflexes, 127
Somatovisceral reflexes
  myofascial trigger points, 1048–1049,
      1048
  sinusitis, 375
Spencer, Herbert, 8
Sphenobasilar synchondrosis, 991,
    1250–1251
Sphincters
  of Oddi, 1086, *1086*
  upper esophageal, 103
Spinal canal, 730–731
Spinal cord
  compression, in cancer, 468–469
  facilitation, 137, 140–145
    brainstem arousal system, 145–147
      ascending pathways, 145–146
      reticular formation, 146
    central sensitization, 144
    PANs in dorsal horn, 140–144,
        141–144
    spinal cord output, 145
  innervation, 733–734, *734*
  motility of, 986–988
  Rexed layers, 124, *124*
Spinal nerves, segmental organization,
    55–56
Spine
  biomechanics, 83–86
    atlas and axis, 86
    cervical spine, 86
    intervertebral discs, 83–84
    loading, 85–86, *85*
    lumbar spine, 86
    motion segment, 83, *83*
    range of motion, 84, 85, *84*
    soft tissues, 83

  translation and rotation, 86
  vertebrae movements, 84–85, *85*
development, 310–311
dysfunction, 442–444
exercise prescription, 286–287
motion
  examination and diagnosis, 569–572,
      570
    active and passive testing, 571
    hip flop test, 645
    seated flexion test, 645
    standing flexion tests
      active screening, 640–641, *640–641*
      passive screening, 641–646
        cervical rotation, 641
        costal cage motion, 644, *645–646*
        hip drop test, 642, *642*
        pelvic side-shift, 642–643, *643*
        rib angle tenderness, 644, *644*
        rib elevation, 643, *643*
        straight-leg raising, 644–645
        thoracolumbar side bending, 642
        trunk side-bending (acromion
            drop test), 641
  muscle energy techniques, 885–890
    atlanto-axial dysfunction, 889–890,
        890
    cervical, 887–888, *888*
    lumbar dysfunction, 885–886, *885*
    occipito-atlantal joint, 888–889,
        888–889
    thoracic dysfunction, 886–887,
        886–887
  neutral position, *1240*
  physiologic motion, *1243*
Spinothalamic pathways, pain management,
    216–217
Spleen
  See also Lymphatic system.
  lymphatic pumps, 1070–1071, *1071*
  osteopathic manipulation, 1087, *1087*
Spondyarthropathies, 529
Spondylolisthesis
  causes, 625
  classification, 625, 626t
  diagnosis, 625–628
    neurologic, 628
    palpatory, 628, *628*
    radiography, 626–628
  treatment, 628–630
    exercise, 629
    manipulation, 629–630
    medication, 630
    orthotics, braces, and casts, 630
    patient education, 629
Spondylolysis, 490
Sports drinks, 549
  Sports medicine, 477, 534–550
  in children, 312–313
  concussions, headaches, and neurologic
      deficits, 546–548, 547t
  history of, 535
  injured athlete, 536–544
    ankle sprain, 543–544, *543*
    back pain and spondylolysis, 539–544,
        539

    iliopsoas spasm, 539–540, *540*
    sacroiliac/sacral torsion dysfunction,
        540, *540*
  functional biomechanical examination,
      538–539
  history, 536–537
  knee pain, 541, *541*
  motion testing, 538
  palpatory examination, 537–538
  physical examination, 537
  rotator cuff tendon/impingement
      syndrome, 541–542, *542*
  somatic dysfunction, 539
  standing screening examination, 537
key concepts, 534
performance enhancement, 548–549
physical medicine, 521, 524–525
practitioners, 535
pre-participation physical, 535–536
rehabilitation, 544–546
  compensations, 545
  functional approach, 544–545
  muscle function, 545
  osteopathic manipulative therapy,
      545
  pronation and supination, 545
return-to-play, 548
sideline and event medical management,
    549
somatic component, 542, *543*
training, 535
Sprains
  of ankle, 543–544, *543*
  ligamentous, 785–786
  of shoulder, 494
Sprays, vapocoolant, 1041
Spring test
  lumbosacral, 776
  spinal, 742
Spurling sign, 443
Statistics
  coronary artery disease, 277–279
  in research, 1181–1182, 1210–1211,
      1217–1218
Sternclavicular joint, 50
Sternum
  acutely ill patient, 1120, 1139
  anatomy, 718–719
  compression, 724–726, *724–725*
  primary and endpoints, *1259*
Steroids, endocrine, 182, 184
Stiffness
  biomechanical, 67
  ligaments and tendons, 72
Still, Andrew Taylor, 3–12
  abdominal OMT, 751
  biography, 19–21
  education, 21–24
  integration of body units, 120
  mental disorders, 245–246
  osteopathic philosophy, 4–6
    historic development, 8–11
    patient care, 6–8
    practice guidelines, 11–12, 11t
  research in OMT, 1167
  surgical training, 399–400

Stomach, osteopathic manipulation, 1079–1080, *1080*

Strains
  in biomechanics, 66, *66*
  and counterstrain techniques, 1002–1016
    complications, 1150
    history, 1002–1003
    instructions to patient, 1006–1007
    key concepts, 1002
    physiology, 1003–1004
    somatic dysfunction, 1158–1159
    treatment, 1004–1006
      cervical spine, 1007–1009, *1008–1009*
      lower extremity, 1015, *1015*
      lumbar spine, 1012–1013, *1012–1013*
      patient position, 1005–1006
      pelvis, 1013–1014, *1013–1014*
      ribs, 1011–1012, *1011–1012*
      tender point, 1004–1005
      thoracic spine, 1009–1011, *1009–1011*
      upper extremity, 1014–1015, *1014–1015*
  cranial, 992–993, *992*

Stress
  alcohol use, 239–240, 240t
  anxiety, 237–239, 238t
  biobehavioral mechanisms, 1204–1205
  biomechanics, 65–66
  and bone fracture, 69–70, *69*
  depression, 235–237, 236t
  health promotion, 203–204
  injuries in children, 313
  key concepts, 233
  in knee, 79
  in ligaments and tendons, 72
  management, 240–243
    biofeedback, 242
    cognitive function, 241–242
    desensitization, 241
    insomnia, 242–243, 242t
    learning and relaxation, 241
    risk perception, 241
    social and spiritual support, 240
  psychoneuroimmunology, 210
  theories, 234–235

Stretch receptors, pulmonary, 505
Stretching and cooling, myofascial trigger points, 1041, *1042*
Subluxation, iliosacral, 778
Substance abuse
  alcohol, 201–202
  biobehavioral mechanisms, 1204, 1206
  diagnosis, 250
  hospital treatment, 428
  illegal drugs, 202
  performance enhancement, 548–549
  tobacco, 200–201

Substance P
  in cardiovascular innervation, 102
  in cerebral vasculature, 99
  in nociception, 131
  pain transmission, 216
  in peripheral vasculature, 98

in respiratory plexus, 103
in somatic dysfunction, 1155
Summation, 73
Sun exposure, 1206–1207
Support groups
  pain management, 224
  stress management, 240
Support personnel, for research, 1221
Surgery, 399–408
  abdominal pain, 400–405
  key concepts, 399
  orthopedic. *See* Orthopedics.
  postoperative complications, 405–406, 405t
    atelectasis, 405–406
  pre- and postoperative somatic dysfunction, 406–407
    ileus, 406–407
  pulmonary complications, 513–514
  for scoliosis, 622
  viscerosomatic and somatovisceral reflexes, 406
Surveillance, biobehavioral mechanisms, 1204, 1207
Sutherland, William G., 985–986, *985*
Sweat gland innervation, 98–99
Sydenham, medical practices, 4
Sympathetic nervous system, 94–96, *95–96*
  abdominal pain, 401
  head, 663–667, *672*
  heart innervation, 125–126, *125–127*
  protocol for osteopathic examination, 425–426
  thoracic, 712
Symphysis pubis, 459
Syndrome of inappropriate antidiuretic hormone (SIADH), and lung cancer, 464, 468
Synovial joints
  anatomy, 49–51, *50–51*
  hyaline cartilage, 70
Systemic disease, efficacy of OMT, 1146–1147, *1146*

T lymphocytes, 1059
TART (tenderness, asymmetry, restriction of motion, tissue texture changes), 574, 633–634, 972
  abdominal, 753
  myofascial trigger points, 1034
  somatic dysfunction, 1153
Temperature
  and muscle contraction, 74–75
  somatic dysfunction, 1153
Temporal bone dysfunction, newborn, 314–315
Temporomandibular joint, 50, 682–683, *682*
Tender points. *See* Strain and counterstrain technique.
Tendon tap reflex, 122–123
Tendonitis, bicipital, 702
Tendonosis, 496
Tendons
  anatomy, 52, *52*
  biomechanics, 71–73, *72*

definition, 908
knee muscle forces, 78–79
transfer of muscle moments, 76, *76*
Tennis elbow, 702
  myofascial trigger points, 1043
Tensegrity, 497
Tension in biomechanics, 65–66
  ligaments and tendons, 71–72
Terminology
  functional technique, 969–970
  glossary, 1229–1253
Testis, autonomic innervation, 114–115
Tetanus toxin transport by nerve terminals, 133
Tetany, 73
Theater cocktail syndrome, 747
Theatre sign, 541
Thomas test, 743, *743*
Thoracic duct
  innervation, 104
  lymphatic system, 1058, 1141
Thoracic lymphatic pump, 510–511
  atelectasis, 406
Thoracic outlet syndrome, 446–447
  treatment, 704
Thoracolumbar region
  HVLA treatment, 868–871, *871–870*
  INR and MFR release, 936–938, *937*
Thorax
  acutely ill patient, 1120–1121, 1127–1131, *1128–1130*
    OMT, 1137–1139
  anatomy and physiology, 705–712
    connective tissue and fascia, 710–711
    divisions, 705–706, *706*
    lymphatic system, 710, *711*
    muscles, 706–710, *707–710t*
    neural connections, 711–712, *712*
    variations and dysfunction, 712–713
      clinical characteristics, 713
      spinal motion, 713
      vertebral and costal cage motion, 712–713
  articulatory techniques
    extension, 839–840
    flexion, 839, *839*
    rotation, 840, *840*
    side-bending, 840–841
  autonomic innervation, 100–104, *100–102*
    aortic plexus, 104
    cardiovascular plexus, 101–102
    esophageal plexus, 103–104
    respiratory plexus, 103
    thoracic duct innervation, 104
  balanced ligamentous tension, 924, *924*
  diagnosis, 716–717
  facilitated positional release (FPR), 1019–1022, *1020*
  fascial-ligamentous release, 912–913, *912–913*
  functional technique, 975–976, *976–978*
  history and physical examination, 713–715
    palpation, 715

Thorax—*continued*
  HVLA treatment, 859–864
    multiple planes, 860–864, *860–864*
    single plane, 859–860, *859*
  key concepts, 705
  lymphatic system, 1063–1064, *1063*
  motion testing, 715–716
  muscle energy techniques, 886–887,
    886–887
  osteopathic manipulation, 1088–1090,
    1088–1090
  osteopathic manipulation, 1098–1099,
    1099
  soft tissue techniques
    lateral recumbent, 823, *823*
    midthoracic extension, 825, *825*
    prone pressure, 822, *822*
    prone pressure with counterpressure,
      822–823
    prone thumb pressure, 822
    seated, over/under, 824, *824*
    side leverage, 824, *824*
    supine extension, 824–825, *825*
  strain and counterstrain technique,
    1009–1011, *1009–1011*
Throat, 677
  See also Ear, nose, and throat disease.
Thrust (high velocity/low amplitude)
    techniques, 852–880
  classification and mechanisms, 854–855,
    854
  clinical application, 855–857
    barrier engagement, 855
    dose of thrust technique, 856
    end-feel at restrictive barrier, 855
    final corrective force velocity and
      amplitude, 856
    force accumulation at restriction, 855
    guidelines for safety, 857
    indications, 855
    precautions and contraindications, 856
    technique improvements, 856
  historic perspective, 852
  key concepts, 852
  motion loss and somatic dysfunction,
    852–854, *853*
    quality of motion, 853–854
  regional treatment, 857–879
    cervicals, 857–859, *857–859*
    extremities
      lower, 875–879, *876–879*
      upper, 874–875, *874–875*
    pelvis, 871–874, *871–874*
    ribs, 864–868, *864–868*
    thoracic, 859–864, *859–864*
    thoracolumbar region, 868–871,
      868–870
  unstable hypermobile joint, 854
Thymus. *See* Lymphatic system.
Thyroid gland, 182
Tibiofemoral joint. *See* Knee.
Time commitments for research, 1221
Tinel sign, 702
Tinnitus, 389–390
Tissue texture changes, 574
  acutely ill patient, 1117

Chapman reflexes, 1053
facilitated positional release (FPR),
  1018
  lumbar, 743
Tobacco, 200–201
  biobehavioral mechanisms, 1204
  and fetal growth, 227
  and lung cancer, 464–465
  and sinusitis, 376
Tolerance, pain management, 221
Tonsillitis, 379–380
Tonsils. *See* Lymphatic system.
Torque, 65
Torsions
  bone fracture, 69
  pelvic and sacral, 780–781, 780t, 781t
  stress, 65
Torticollis, 310, 688
Touch
  arthritis, 527–528
  discriminative, 138, 140
Trachea, lymphatic flow, 1073, *1073*
Transcutaneous nerve stimulation (TNS),
  222
Transient ischemic attacks, 681
Transport of hormones, 182–1813
Transverse processes, 729
Trauma
  cranial, 993, 996
  emergency medicine, 389–390
  hospital treatment, 429
  sacroiliac dysfunction, 782
  spinal disorders, 442–444
  tender points, 1003
Travell, Janet, 1034, 1045–1048
Trendelenburg test, 772–773
Trigeminal nerve, 670–671
Trigger points, 1028
  In emergency medicine, 388
  lower extremity, 804
  myofascial, 703, 1034–1050
    diagnosis, 1039–1040, 1041t
    incidence, 1037–1038
    key concepts, 1034
    point systems, 1034–1039,
      1035–1037
    referred pain, 1038–1039, *1039*
    treatment, 1040–1042
      cooling with stretching, 1041, *1042*
      injection, 1041–1042, *1043*
      osteopathic, 1042–1049
      posture, 1045, *1045*
      regional trigger points, 1042–1044,
        1043t, *1044*
      Travell points, 1047–1048, *1048*
      venous and lymphatic drainage,
        1045–1047, *1046–1047*
      viscerosomatic and somatovisceral
        reflexes, 1048–1049,
        1048–1049
  strain and counterstrain technique, 1002
Trochlear nerve, 670
Tuberculosis, 165–166
Tumor necrosis factor
  in cancer, 469–470
Twitch, 73

Typhoid Mary, 168
Tyrosine hydroxylase, in ureter, 112

Ulcers, segmental facilitation, 1126
Ulnomeniscotriquetral joint, 50
Upper extremity
  See also Extremities.
  fascial-ligamentous release, 913–914, *913*
  soft tissue techniques
    interosseous membrane of forearm, 830
    pectoral traction, 829, *829*
    posterior axillary folds, 829–830, *829*
    rhomboids, 830, *830*
Ureter
  autonomic innervation, 112–113
  osteopathic manipulation, 1087, *1087*
  segmental facilitation, 1126
Urinary bladder
  autonomic innervation, 113–114, *114*
  incontinence, and aging, 334–335
Uterus
  autonomic innervation, 115–116
  osteopathic manipulation, 1091–1092
  pelvic pain, 415

Vaccinations, 176–177
  in osteopathy, 7
Vagina, autonomic innervation, 116
Vagus nerve
  acutely ill patient, 1125
  anatomy, 97, 99, 673–674
  cardiovascular innervation, 102
  in esophageal plexus, 103–104
  in heart innervation, 126–127
Validity in clinical research, 1183
Varicosities, in pregnancy, 452
Vasoactive intestinal polypeptide
  in cerebral vasculature, 99
  in respiratory plexus, 103
Vasodilators, 163–164
Vectors, force and motion, 64–66
Ventilation, 501–503, *502*
  control of, 505–506
Vertebrae
  rotation, *1245*
  in spinal movement, 84–85, *85*
  thoracic, 706
Vertebral body anatomy, 727–728
Vertebral unit, 737, *1253*
Vertigo, 389–390
Virulence, and pathogenicity, 168–170
Viscera
  dysfunction
    brainstem arousal system, 147
    emergency medicine, 387, 388
    protocol for osteopathic examination,
      426
  innervation of, 127–128, *127–128*
  manipulation, 1078–1093
    abdomen, 1079–1088
    cervix, uterus, fallopian tubes, ovaries,
      1091–1092, *1092*
    colon, 1082–1083, *1082–1083*
    esophagus, stomach, and duodenum,
      1079–1081, *1080*
    gallbladder, 1085–1086, *1086*

kidneys, 1086–1087, *1087*
liver, 1083–1085, *1084–1085*
pancreas, 1087–1088, *1088*
small intestine, 1081–1082, *1081–1082*
spleen, 1087, *1087*
ureter, 1087, *1087*
diagnosis, 1079
history, 1078
key concepts, 1078
pelvis, 1090–1091
bladder, 1090–1091, *1090*
obturator foramen, 1091, *1091*
pubovesicular ligaments, 1091, *1091*
theory, 1078–1079
thorax, 1088–1090, *1088–1090*
treatment, 1079
treatment positions, 1092, *1092*
Viscerosomatic reflex
acutely ill patient, 1117, *1117*
lumbar region, 744
and lung disease, 507, *508*

myofascial trigger points, 1048–1049, *1048*
in pregnancy, 453–454
Viscoelasticity
of articular cartilage, 70–71
in biomechanics, 67–68, *67*
in ligaments and tendons, 72
and muscle contraction, 75
Vision, geriatric, 329, 330
Vitamin A deficiency, 173
Vitamin E deficiency, 174

Walk cycle, 768–769
Walking, knee movements, 79
Wallace, Alfred Russel, 8
"Warming up", and muscle contraction, 75
Water cure, 21
Wear damage, articular cartilage, 71
Wheal, 164
Whiplash injury, 496, 524, 688
Whole patient
with cancer, 463, 470–471
family practice, 293–294

Whooping cough, OMT, 512
Wind-up phenomenon, 128–129, 130, *128*
Wolff's law, 70, 568, 712
Workmen's compensation, 1146
Wrist
anatomy, 697, 699–700
fascial-ligamentous release, 913–914, *914*
fractures in children, 312
HVLA treatment, 875, *875*
INR and MFR techniques, 964–966, *964–966*
somatic dysfunction, 700
Wristberg's ganglion, 101
Writing and publication of research, 1182

Xiphoid process, primary and endpoints, *1260*

Yergason test, 701

Zinc deficiency, 174